TRAUMA NURSING

From Resuscitation Through Rehabilitation

VIRGINIA D. CARDONA, RN, MS

Associate Director for Professional Development
Maryland Institute for Emergency Medical Services Systems
Baltimore, Maryland

PATRICIA D. HURN, PhD, RN

Assistant Professor, Department of Anesthesiology and Critical Care Medicine
Assistant Professor of Nursing
The Johns Hopkins University and Medical Institutions
Baltimore, Maryland

PAULA J. BASTNAGEL MASON, RN, MS, CNA

President, Health Care Management Systems Inc.
Annapolis, Maryland
Faculty Associate, Trauma Critical Care
Graduate Program, School of Nursing
University of Maryland
Baltimore, Maryland

ANN M. SCANLON, RN, MS, CS

Director, Psychiatric Nursing
University of Maryland Medical System
Baltimore, Maryland

SUSAN W. VEISE-BERRY, RN, MS

Nurse Consultant
Former Clinical Nurse Specialist
Trauma Resuscitation Unit
Maryland Institute for Emergency Medical Services Systems
Baltimore, Maryland

TRAUMA NURSING

From Resuscitation Through Rehabilitation

SECOND EDITION

W.B. SAUNDERS COMPANY
A Division of Harcourt Brace & Company
PHILADELPHIA, LONDON, TORONTO, MONTREAL, SYDNEY, TOKYO

W.B. SAUNDERS COMPANY
A Division of
Harcourt Brace & Company

The Curtis Center
Independence Square West
Philadelphia, Pennsylvania 19106

Library of Congress Cataloging-in-Publication Data

Trauma nursing: from resuscitation through rehabilitation/[edited by] Virginia D. Cardona . . . [et al.].—2nd ed.

p. cm.

Includes bibliographical references and index.

ISBN 0–7216–4333–7

1. Wounds and injuries—Nursing. I. Cardona, Virginia D.
[DNLM: 1. Emergencies—nursing.
2. Wounds and Injuries—nursing. WY 154 T777]

RD93.95.T73 1994 617.1′026′024613—dc20

DNLM/DLC 92–49094

TRAUMA NURSING:
From Resuscitation Through Rehabilitation ISBN 0–7216–4333–7

Printed in the United States of America.

Last digit is the print number: 9 8 7 6 5 4 3 2

This book is dedicated to our colleagues in trauma care
and to those who believed in us and supported us
through these endeavors.

VDC, PDH, PBM, AMS, SWV-B

Contributors

MARY BEACHLEY, RN, MS, CEN

State Trauma Nurse Coordinator, EMS Nursing and Specialty Care, Maryland Institute for Emergency Medical Services Systems, Baltimore, Maryland

Evolution of the Trauma Cycle

JUDITH K. BOBB, RN, MSN

Research Associate, Department of Pathology, University of Maryland School of Medicine; Research Associate, University of Maryland Medical System, Department of Veterans Affairs Medical Center, Ft. Howard Veterans Administration Medical Center, Baltimore, Maryland

Trauma in the Elderly

T. CATHERINE BOWER, RN, BSN, CPDN

Nursing Representative and Coordinator, Acute Pain Service, University of Maryland Medical Systems; Senior Partner, Maryland Institute for Emergency Medical Services Systems, Baltimore, Maryland

Maxillofacial and Soft Tissue Injuries

VIRGINIA D. CARDONA, RN, MS

Faculty Associate, University of Maryland Graduate Nursing Program (Trauma/Critical Care); Associate Director for Professional Development, Maryland Institute for Emergency Medical Services Systems, Baltimore, Maryland

Nursing Practice Through the Cycles of Trauma

HOWARD R. CHAMPION, FRCS(EDIN), FACS

Professor of Surgery and Chief, Division of Surgery for Trauma, Uniformed Services University of the Health Sciences, Bethesda, Maryland; Senior Attending Surgeon and Chief, Trauma Service; Director, Surgical Critical Care and Emergency Services, Washington Hospital Center, Washington, DC

Economic Issues in Trauma Care

WARREN T. CHAVE, ESQ.

Baltimore, Maryland

Legal Concerns in Trauma Care

CHRISTINE COTTINGHAM, RN, CCRN

Staff Nurse–Full Partner, Multiple Trauma ICU; Co-Director, Acute Hemofiltration Service, Maryland Institute for Emergency Medical Services Systems, Baltimore, Maryland

Genitourinary Injuries and Renal Management

MARGARETA K. CUCCIA, RN
Donor Advocate, Johns Hopkins Hospital, Baltimore, Maryland
The Organ Donor

JOCELYN A. FARRAR, RN, MS, CCRN
Education Specialist, Maryland Institute for Emergency Medical Services Systems, Baltimore, Maryland
Genitourinary Injuries and Renal Management

PAMELA PHILLIPS GAUL, RN
Staff, Bay Area Home Health Care (STAPA); Formerly Organ Procurement Coordinator, Transplant Resource Center of Maryland, Baltimore, Maryland
The Organ Donor

ROBBI L. HARTSOCK, RN, MSN, CCRN
Faculty Associate, University of Maryland Graduate Nursing Program (Trauma/Critical Care); Clinical Nurse Specialist, Maryland Institute for Emergency Medical Services Systems, Baltimore, Maryland
Thoracic Injuries

ERKAN HASSAN, PHARM D
Assistant Professor of Pharmacy, University of Maryland School of Pharmacy; Critical Care Consultant, University of Maryland Medical Systems, Baltimore, Maryland
The Trauma Patient with a History of Substance Abuse

KAREN KLENDER HEIST, RN, MS
Director of Subacute Operations, Meridian Healthcare, Towson, Maryland
The Demand for Trauma Rehabilitation

NANCY J. HOYT, MA, CIC
Clinical Infection Control Consultant, Severna Park, Maryland; Formerly Infection Control Officer, Maryland Institute for Emergency Medical Services Systems, Baltimore, Maryland
Infection and Infection Control

PATRICIA D. HURN, PhD, RN
Assistant Professor of Anesthesiology and Critical Care Medicine, School of Medicine; Assistant Professor of Nursing, School of Medicine and Nursing, The Johns Hopkins University and Medical Institutions, Baltimore, Maryland
Thoracic Injuries

CONNIE JOY, RN, MSN
Director of Nursing, Alfred I. duPont Institute of the Nemours Foundation, Wilmington, Delaware
Administrative Issues in Trauma Care

JAMES W. KARESH, MD, FACS
Assistant Professor, University of Maryland School of Medicine; Assistant Professor, Johns Hopkins University School of Medicine and Nursing; The Krieger Eye Institute, Sinai Hospital of Baltimore, The University of Maryland, The Johns Hopkins Medical Institutions, Baltimore, Maryland
Ocular Injuries

MARGUERITE T. LITTLETON KEARNEY, DNSc, RN
Associate Professor, Department of Acute and Long-Term Care, University of Maryland School of Nursing; Visiting Assistant Professor, Department of Anesthesia and Critical Care, Johns Hopkins University School of Medicine, Baltimore, Maryland
Pathophysiology of Traumatic Shock and Multiple Organ System Failure

PAULA M. KELLY, RN, BA
Clinical Nurse-Senior Partner, Trauma Resuscitation Unit, Maryland Institute for Emergency Medical Services Systems, Baltimore, Maryland
Musculoskeletal Injuries

BARBARA J. KEYES, RN, BS, MAS
Nurse Manager, University of Maryland Medical Systems, Baltimore, Maryland
Ocular Injuries

KAREN M. KLEEMAN, PhD, RN, CS
Associate Professor, Department of Acute and Long-Term Care, University of Maryland School of Nursing, Baltimore, Maryland
Family Systems Adaptation

JORIE D. KLEIN, RN
Clinical Instructor, Department of Surgery, University of Texas Southwestern Medical Center; Trauma Program Director, Trauma Department, Parkland Memorial Hospital, Dallas, Texas
Mechanism of Injury

MARCIA S. MABEE, MPH, PhD
Senior Vice President, Timothy Bell and Company; Executive Director, Coalition for Health Funding, and Executive Director, The Coalition for American Trauma Care, Reston, Virginia
Economic Issues in Trauma Care

JANET A. MARVIN, MN, RN
Director of Nursing, Shriners Burns Institute, Galveston, Texas
Thermal Injuries

PAULA J. BASTNAGEL MASON, RN, MS, CNA
Faculty Associate, Trauma/Critical Care, University of Maryland School of Nursing; President, Healthcare Management Systems Inc., Annapolis, Maryland
Abdominal Injuries

PATRICIA E. McCABE, RN
Clinical Practice Coordinator for Managed Care, University of Maryland Medical Center, Baltimore, Maryland
The Trauma Patient with a History of Substance Abuse

JOAN M. PRYOR McCANN, RN, MN, MA
Assistant Professor of Nursing, Otterbein College, Westerville, Ohio
Ethics in Trauma Nursing

PAUL McCLELLAND, MD
Chairman, Department of Psychiatry, Greater Baltimore Medical Center, Baltimore, Maryland
The Trauma Patient with a Preexisting Psychiatric Disorder

KAREN A. McQUILLAN, RN, MS, CCRN
Faculty Associate, University of Maryland Graduate Nursing Program (Trauma/Critical Care); Clinical Nurse Specialist, Maryland Institute for Emergency Medical Services Systems, Baltimore, Maryland
Initial Management of Traumatic Shock

PAMELA H. MITCHELL, PhD, ARNP, CNRN, FAAN

Professor, Department of Physiological Nursing, University of Washington; Neuroscience Nurse Specialist, University of Washington Medical Center, Seattle, Washington

Central Nervous System I: Closed Head Injuries

PATRICIA MOLONEY-HARMON, RN, MS, CCRN

Clinical Nurse Specialist, Women's and Children's Services, Sinai Hospital of Baltimore, Baltimore, Maryland

Pediatric Trauma

MARY MURPHY-RUTTER, RN, MS

Full Partner, Oncology ICU, University of Maryland Cancer Center; Formerly Primary Nurse, Maryland Institute for Emergency Medical Services Systems, Baltimore, Maryland

Genitourinary Injuries and Renal Management

ANN M. SCANLON, RN, MS, CS

Faculty Associate, University of Maryland Graduate Nursing Program (Psychiatric Nursing); Director, Psychiatric Nursing, University of Maryland Medical System, Baltimore, Maryland

Psychosocial Responses of the Human Spirit: The Journey of Trauma

ELLEN K. SHAIR, MA

Analyst/Writer, Trauma/Surgical Critical Care and Emergency Services, Washington Hospital Center, Washington, DC

Economic Issues in Trauma Care

LYNN GERBER SMITH, RN, MS

Instructor of Nursing, Division of Allied Health, Anne Arundel Community College; Full Partner, Trauma Resuscitation Unit, Maryland Institute for Emergency Medical Services Systems, Baltimore, Maryland

The Pregnant Trauma Patient

GENA STIVER STANEK, RN, MS, CCRN

Faculty Associate, University of Maryland Graduate Nursing Program (Trauma/Critical Care); Clinical Nurse Specialist, Neurotrauma, Maryland Institute for Emergency Medical Services Systems, Baltimore, Maryland

Metabolic and Nutritional Management of the Trauma Patient

JULIE MULL STRANGE, RN

Maryland Organ Procurement Center, Inc., Baltimore, Maryland

Musculoskeletal Injuries

THOMAS C. VARY, PhD

Associate Professor, Department of Cellular and Molecular Physiology, Pennsylvania State University; Milton S. Hershey College of Medicine, Hershey, Pennsylvania

Pathophysiology of Traumatic Shock and Multiple Organ System Failure

SUSAN W. VEISE-BERRY, RN, MS

Nurse Consultant; Former Clinical Nurse Specialist, Trauma Resuscitation Unit, Maryland Institute for Emergency Medical Services Systems, Baltimore, Maryland

Evolution of the Trauma Cycle

KATHRYN T. VON RUEDEN, RN, MS, CCRN, FCCM

Acute Multitrauma Clinical Nurse Specialist, Maryland Institute for Emergency Medical Services Systems, Baltimore, Maryland

Nursing Practice Through the Cycles of Trauma

CONSTANCE A. WALLECK, RN, MS, FCCM

Adjunct Clinical Assistant Professor, SUNY Health Science Center College of Nursing; Director of Critical Care and Emergency Nursing, University Hospital, SUNY Health Science Center, Syracuse, New York

Central Nervous System II: Spinal Cord Injury

NEIL WARRES, MD

Clinical Assistant Professor of Psychiatry, University of Maryland Medical School; Director of Psychiatry, Maryland Institute for Emergency Medical Services Systems; Director of Psychiatry, Montebello Rehabilitation Hospital, Baltimore, Maryland

The Trauma Patient with a Preexisting Psychiatric Disorder

JOHN A. WEIGELT, MS, FACS

Professor and Vice Chairman, Department of Surgery, University of Minnesota; Chairman, Department of Surgery, St Paul-Ramsey Medical Center, St. Paul, Minnesota

Mechanism of Injury

JoANNE D. WHITNEY, PhD, RN

Assistant Professor, Department of Physiological Nursing, University of Washington, Seattle, Washington

Wound Healing

MARGARET WIDNER-KOLBERG, MA, RN

Pediatric Quality Assurance Specialist, Emergency Trauma Service, Children's National Medical Center, Washington, DC

Pediatric Trauma

JOYCE S. WILLENS, RN, MSN

Instructor, Villanova University College of Nursing, Villanova, Pennsylvania; Doctoral Candidate, University of Maryland School of Nursing, Baltimore, Maryland

Pain Management in the Trauma Patient

Reviewers

H. NEAL REYNOLDS, MD
Critical Care Attending, Assistant Professor of Medicine, University of Maryland; Director of Biomedical Engineering, Maryland Institute for Emergency Medical Services Systems, Baltimore, Maryland

PAUL MANSON, MD
Chief, Plastic Surgery, Maryland Institute for Emergency Medical Services Systems, Baltimore, Maryland

MARGUERITE T. LITTLETON KEARNEY, DNSc, RN
Associate Professor, University of Maryland School of Nursing, Baltimore, Maryland

ART KURZ, BS, CPTC
Transplant Coordinator, Transplant Resource Center of Maryland, Inc., Baltimore, Maryland

JANET A. MARVIN, MN, RS
Director of Nursing, Shriners Burns Institute, Galveston, Texas

KAREN A. McQUILLAN, MS, RN, CCRN
Clinical Specialist, Neurotrauma Center, Maryland Institute for Emergency Medical Services Systems, Baltimore, Maryland

DAVID A. NAGEY, PhD, MD, PE, FACOG
Director, Division of Maternal-Fetal Medicine; Associate Professor, Departments of Obstetrics and Gynecology and Epidemiology and Preventive Medicine, University of Maryland School of Medicine, Baltimore, Maryland

JOYCE E. MASLYK, BSN, RN
Associate Director for Administrative Nursing, Maryland Institute for Emergency Medical Services Systems, Baltimore, Maryland

KATHLEEN M. DRISCOLL, RN, MS, JD
Associate Professor, University of Cincinnati, Cincinnati, Ohio

MARTHA ELLIOTT, MSW, MPH, MA
Director of Social Work, Mt. Washington Pediatric Hospital, Baltimore, Maryland

Foreword

The first edition of this text was critically acclaimed for initiating a framework for trauma nursing care that clearly delineates the art and science required of the dedicated trauma nurse. The cycles of trauma is the framework that makes this text unique, by focusing attention on the journey of trauma for the patient and the nurse. This framework has also encouraged an in-depth pathophysiological approach to the injured in which state-of-the-art science is reviewed for practice. This combination of sophisticated science and the caring aspects of nursing truly make *Trauma Nursing: From Resuscitation Through Rehabilitation* irresistible for the trauma nurse involved in clinical practice, administration, education, or research.

Trauma remains a major controversial topic for even the casual observer of the 1990's health care scene. In the public media more than ever before, trauma as a result of urban violence, drunk driving, and high speed injury is portrayed as an ongoing health care problem without simple solutions. The injury problem in this country cries out for the same dedication and unified support as the war waged on cancer and heart disease. We know that trauma care systems save lives and should be a national public health priority. Consumer demand for quality trauma services will only increase with tighter control of the federal health care dollar. What does this mean for trauma nursing? Trauma nurses serving on collaborative trauma teams in traditional and advanced roles will be more in demand and expected to demonstrate efficiency and effectiveness in terms of patient outcome. The cycles of trauma requires that nurses acquire special expertise in the resuscitative, operative, critical, intermediate, or rehabilitative phase of care. Moreover, it requires that the nurse be sufficiently familiar with the patient's progression through all phases to help the individual and family meet positive, measurable outcomes. This text assists nurses in meeting the challenges of trauma care in the 1990s by providing comprehensive coverage of the key issues, trends, and controversies in trauma care today.

While this text is authored by health care providers from many disciplines and various regions of the country, it truly showcases the talent and expertise of trauma nursing at the R A Cowley Shock Trauma Center. This 138-bed center, devoted exclusively to providing excellent practice, teaching, and research in trauma, continues to receive world-wide praise and imitation for innovations in multidisciplinary trauma care. It is not uncommon for nurses throughout the country and abroad to be attracted enough to the clinical learning environment at the Shock Trauma Center to move to Baltimore for work and graduate study. It is this text, widely cited in the literature and quoted at national meetings, that has successfully demonstrated the importance of bringing together necessary state-of-the-art practices in trauma nursing care.

The second edition continues to carry the strength, beauty, and utility of the first while expanding upon known concepts, introducing new issues, and projecting future trends in trauma nursing. *Trauma Nursing* is admired and used. The text's great strength lies in its depth and breadth, which make it unlike other trauma books. Well-researched chapters with scientific rationale and suggestions for future nursing research are included. Updated appendices serve as readily available sources of reference for the nurse functioning in the trauma arena. This text highlights the journey of the trauma patient and nurse through the cycles of care—this is the beauty and substance of the text and the place where the art of nursing shines. Thorough yet succinct guidelines on how to make this journey successful are provided. The nurse committed to the provision of optimal trauma patient care knows that promoting quality of life and not just survival for the trauma patient enriches both their lives. Finally, the usefulness of this text is demonstrated by its extensive use by clinicians, educators, and managers, who have relied on the first edition as a sound and authoritative source for clinical problem-solving, professional presentation content referencing, and trauma care standards and policies review. My own trauma/critical care graduate students use the text extensively for trauma theory, practice, and research referencing.

I have special gratitude for the achievement of these editors, all of whom I worked with when they were dedicated clinical nurse specialists at the Shock Trauma Center throughout the turbulent decade of the 1980s. They had the insight to know that trauma nurses needed a sophisticated research-based reference text that could be utilized by nurses in a wide variety of practice settings—whether it be in clinical practice, education, research, or administration. The high practice standards held by these editors are reflected throughout this revised and updated second edition, which will most assuredly continue to be referred to as "the classic" on trauma nursing.

Expectations are high for the trauma nurses of the 1990s. This trauma text helps nurses to meet this challenge with optimism. A positive approach to our role as trauma nurses is best exemplified by a statement on nursing from a scholar and leader in nursing. A decade ago, Donna Diers, then professor and Dean of the School of Nursing at Yale University, described the uniqueness of our profession: "Nursing puts us in touch with being human. Without even asking, nurses are invited into the inner spaces of other people's existence—for where there is suffering, loneliness, the tolerable pain of cure or the solitary pain of permanent change, there is a need for the kind of human service we call nursing."* In trauma care, nurses are continually confronted with patients who experience great physiologic instability and suffering, with patients who must learn to cope with permanent disability, and with those who must integrate the pain of loss into a meaningful existence. There is a need for ever more skilled, competent, and caring trauma nurses. There is a need for this remarkable second edition on trauma nursing.

DORRIE K. FONTAINE, DNSC, RN, CCRN
Associate Professor and Coordinator
Trauma/Critical Care Nursing
School of Nursing
University of Maryland
Baltimore, Maryland

*Diers, D: Nursing reclaims its role. Nurs Outlook 30:459–463, 1982.

Acknowledgments

The editors wish to thank the following authors whose contributions to the first edition made this textbook such a successful endeavor:

Mary E. Mancini
Benny Hopper
Carolyn Milligan
Peggy Trimble
Roy L. Mason
Anne F. McCormack
Steven Linberg
Charles E. Wiles, III
Lisa Robinson
Patricia C. Epifanio
Barbara E. Schott
Susan M. Luff
Gerri Spielman McGinnis
Sandra L. Deli
Linda S. Cook
Melva Kravitz
Paul McClelland
Elizabeth Scanlan

Preface

When *Trauma Nursing: From Resuscitation Through Rehabilitation* was introduced five years ago, it proposed a unique framework. Since then comments and reviews from our trauma nurse colleagues have validated our cyclical concept of care. Prevention will always remain the key. But once trauma is experienced, the care furnished at any point in the cycle alters the patient's adaptation physically, psychologically, and emotionally. Health care practitioners at each stage must comprehend the process for the individual and family from the moment they enter the trauma system. Without this knowledge, the patient will seldom receive the best care at each juncture. With the cycle principle thus reaffirmed, we have continued with it in the second edition, enhancing the content with more recent developments.

The cycle framework has been adopted at many sites throughout the United States. This broad acceptance is reflected by the geographical distribution of contributors for this edition. The careful reader will recognize many different authors and coauthors, who have added their expertise and provided a new vitality to the writing. We also welcome back the strong voices of many of the first edition authors, who have shown renewed commitment to participating in another state-of-the-art edition.

Part One, "General Concepts in Trauma Nursing," reviews the broad health care system issues that affect all trauma facilities. Any site dedicated to the care of trauma patients must deal with philosophical, economic, ethical, and legal issues. How an institution handles these issues often affects the nursing care offered to the trauma patient.

The second part, "Clinical Management Concepts," develops those aspects of care that cross all patient groups. The topics of mechanism of injury, pathophysiology and management of shock, psychological response to traumatic injury, the family's adaptation, management of wound healing, nutrition, and pain, and the patient's needs in rehabilitation are presented in detail, with a clear focus on the ever-changing nursing obligations at each phase of the cycle.

Part Three, "Single System Injuries," supplies the state-of-the-art care for each body system. This section stands alone as a quick, thorough reference for the practitioner. The chapters have been updated to include the latest research guiding medical and nursing interventions today. Each chapter projects a future research direction.

Part Four, "Unique Patient Populations," addresses the needs of those patient groups whose care must be altered because of the complicated demands they place on the system. Here the reader will find information to guide practice and promote system adaptations to meet the extraordinary demands of these special populations.

Finally, the appendices have been revised and updated to include new procedures, worksheets, evaluation scales, and more.

The dynamic field of trauma nursing demanded a prompt second edition. The vanguard research frequently highlighted in these pages illustrates that trauma patient care has, in many instances, changed dramatically in just five years. Issues such as sepsis, multiple organ failure, treatment of pain, demand for early mobilization of the patient, respiratory care technologies, management of traumatic wounds, advances in infection control, ethical decision-making, and many other concerns have continued their rapid development. They are covered here. Accordingly, we are confident *Trauma Nursing: From Resuscitation Through Rehabilitation, Second Edition* will satisfy your professional resource requirements in the practice of contemporary trauma nursing.

VIRGINIA D. CARDONA
PATRICIA D. HURN
PAULA J. BASTNAGEL MASON
ANN M. SCANLON
SUSAN W. VEISE-BERRY

CONTENTS

PART I

General Concepts in Trauma Nursing

1

EVOLUTION OF THE TRAUMA CYCLE

SUSAN VEISE-BERRY and MARY BEACHLEY

For everything there is a season, and a time for every matter under heaven:
a time to be born, and a time to die;
a time to plant, and a time to pluck up what is planted;
a time to kill, and a time to heal;
a time to break down, and a time to build up;
a time to weep, and a time to laugh;
a time to mourn, and a time to dance;
a time to cast away stones, and a time to gather stones together;
a time to embrace, and a time to refrain from embracing;
a time to seek, and a time to lose;
a time to keep, and a time to cast away;
a time to rend, and a time to sew;
a time to keep silence, and a time to speak;
a time to love, and a time to hate;
a time for war, and a time for peace.

Ecclesiastes 3:1–9 (RSV)

INTRODUCTION

Trauma occurs in epidemic proportions in our society today; however, this is not a new phenomenon. Traumatic injury has been recognized as a part of the human experience since early civilization. Anthropological studies of the bony remains of Neanderthal man have shown that this group of people sustained a great deal of trauma during their lifetime.[1] Disfigured skeletal structures and long-term bony calcification are evidence that the trauma that this group of people experienced was a result of their relatively dangerous lifestyle. Reportedly, many injuries were sustained secondary to constant exposure to the raw elements of nature, including frequent encounters with wild animals.

Although the concept of traumatic injury as a recognized societal affliction has remained unchanged since the time of Neanderthal man, the incidence, magnitude, cause, and mechanism of traumatic injury *has* changed. Human interaction with the environment at given points throughout our lifespan and the effect of a variety of forces—industrialization, societal influences (including belief systems), and educational orientation and level—have influenced the way in which trauma occurs in our society today. No matter what the reasons for traumatic injury, however, its occurrence has reached mammoth proportions.

TRAUMA SYSTEMS DEVELOPMENT

Trauma nursing is one of the major challenges in emergency, critical care, and rehabilitation practices today. To recognize and develop a keen appreciation for trauma nursing as a specialty field, one must not only examine state-of-the-art practices but also review historically the events that led to the creation of a systems approach to care and to the development of the clinical knowledge base that has formed the foundation for this distinct area of clinical nursing practice.

The term *trauma* is used to describe a variety of injuries, and the concept of trauma embodies several associated terms—*shock, injury, accident, accidental injury, fatality,* and *casualty.* These terms are sometimes used synonymously and, in this book, may be used interchangeably, although use of the term *accidental* is avoided, when possible, because it implies that an event is unexpected or unavoidable. The belief that most unintentional events are predictable and therefore preventable is widely accepted. Over the years, a deeper understanding of the underlying causes of traumatic injury has led to this belief.

Magnitude of the Problem

Trauma is the most common cause of death in the United States in individuals less than 44 years of age. It is the fourth leading cause of death in individuals of all age groups, exceeded only by deaths occurring from cardiovascular disease, cancer, or cerebrovascular disease.[2] It is estimated that close to 60 million injuries occur annually in this country. In 1990, of the total number of injuries that occurred, 93,500 resulted in death.[2] This was only 2 per cent below the fatality rate of the previous year, still representing an exorbitant figure. Although ranked fourth as the cause of death for all age groups, trauma is the leading killer of one of our nation's most valued resources—young people. Children and youths between 15 and 24 years of age have a greater chance of dying from unintentional injury than from any other cause. More than three of four individuals in this age group are male.[2]

Motor vehicle crashes, falls, ingestion, drowning, and burns represent the primary causes of unintentional injury.[2] Motor vehicle crashes caused 46,300 deaths in 1990 (18.6 per 100,000 population), a 2 per cent decrease from 1989.

In 1990, fatalities resulting from falls totaled 12,400 (5.0 per 100,000 population).[2] Seventy-five per cent of these deaths involved individuals 65 years or older; over one half of the falls occurred in the home.

In 1990, deaths occurring from ingestion of drugs, medicines, mushrooms, and shellfish as well as commonly recognized poisons totaled 5700 (2.3 per 100,000).[2] Deaths occurring from accidental ingestion or inhalation of objects or food that resulted in airway obstruction totaled 3200 (1.3 per 100,000) in 1990.

Drownings from boating accidents, swimming, playing in water, or falling in water accounted for 5200 deaths in 1990. This figure represents a 2.1 per 100,000 population death rate, a 4 per cent increase from the previous year.[2]

Deaths from fires, burns, and injuries in conflagrations totaled 4300 in 1990 (1.7 per 100,000 death rate), representing a 9 per cent decrease from the 1989 figures. The most frequent victims are children 0 to 4 years of age and the elderly (65 years and older).[2]

The trends in accidental death rates between 1912 and 1990 have shown a gradual improvement. Since 1912, accidental deaths decreased 55 per cent from 82 to 37 per 100,000. The decline in non–motor vehicle death rate from 79 to 19 (per 100,000) represented a 75 per cent reduction. This, however, was offset in part by the sixfold increase in the motor vehicle death rate from 3 to 19 per 100,000, which occurred during the same period—a trend that should cause every American to be concerned.

In addition to the human loss resulting from trauma, the economic cost to our nation also must be considered. The National Safety Council defines a disabling injury as one that results in death or in some degree of permanent impairment or that renders the injured person unable to perform effectively regular duties or activities for a full day beyond the day of the injury. Cost estimates therefore include wage losses, medical expenses, insurance administration costs, property damages in motor vehicle accidents, fire losses, and indirect work loss from accidents.* The cost for unintentional injuries, including those in which deaths or disabling injuries occurred together with motor vehicle accidents and fires in which no injury took place, was estimated as $173.8 billion in 1990.[2]

Despite an alarmingly high incidence of unintentional injury over the years, the significance of this problem has not always been recognized by the public sector. The first sign that this issue had reached the level of national politics appeared in 1960 when John F. Kennedy during his presidential campaign issued a statement acknowledging that "traffic accidents constitute one of the greatest, perhaps the greatest, of the nation's public problems."[3] Since that time, attention has been directed toward raising public awareness about this sizable problem, while concurrent efforts have been made to identify fundamental elements that would render the nation's health care delivery system more responsive to the needs of those who have sustained traumatic injury.

The Military Experience

Many of the advances in the care of the critically injured prior to the 1960s were made by the military. The injuries sustained by military personnel as well as civilians during times of war were the primary focus of studies of traumatic injury and shock, which became the initial source of information regarding traumatic injuries.

The concepts guiding medical personnel in their attempts to care for the wounded during the Civil War (1861 to 1865) and the Spanish–American War (April 1898 to August 1898) were vague, at best. Prior to World War I, a variety of theories regarding traumatic injury and its treatment had been advanced, but there was a tremendous need to generate hard data to describe what became known as the "shock state" following injury.

In 1916, during World War I, the United States National Research Council of the National Academy of Sciences formed a Committee on Physiology, whose Subcommittee

*Indirect loss from work accidents is the money value of time lost by noninjured workers and includes time spent filling out accident reports or giving first aid to injured workers and time lost owing to production slowdowns.

on Traumatic Shock began to produce objective data regarding the physiology of circulation and its relationship to the various models that had been defined for the study of shock.[4] This was the first coordinated prospective work project organized for the purpose of obtaining a better understanding of the body's responses to severe trauma. The information from these studies was discussed at formal meetings and conferences, which resulted in more widespread dissemination of knowledge about shock resulting from traumatic injury. Although by the mid-nineteenth century the term *shock* began to be applied to the clinical state of individuals who had sustained severe trauma, the nature of clinical shock remained a mystery.[4]

It has only been since World War II that the nature of shock has been better understood and that the treatment regimen has become more clearly defined. During World War II, the care of trauma patients significantly improved. This was due largely to the prompt application of information obtained by the Medical Board for the Study of the Treatment of the Severely Wounded. This 22-member board was appointed on September 3, 1943, by the Theater Commander, Lt. General Jacob B. Devers, and was made up of medical officers, nurses, technicians, and support personnel who worked as a research team.[4] This team responded to any medical request from the field and compiled casualty data over an 8-month period in Italy. The data from observations of 186 military casualties comprised the first volume of the historical series by the Medical Department of the United States Army. It was entitled *Surgery in World War II: The Physiologic Effects of Wounds.*[5] The information obtained by the board was disseminated not only in the field hospitals that were treating and studying the wounded but also throughout the front-line and base hospitals. The study results were impressive and led to a change in policy regarding the treatment of wound shock. Resuscitation practices improved as hemodynamic alterations became better understood and knowledge about posttraumatic renal failure, an often fatal complication of severe shock, emerged.

A similar but more extensive program was established during the Korean War (1950 to 1953) and later during the Vietnam War (1957 to 1975). The research efforts put forth during World War II by the Medical Board for the Study of the Treatment of the Severely Wounded continued and were strengthened by a newly established Surgical Research Team. The study results of this team were of laboratory research quality and sophistication. This was made possible in part by the support services that had been made available from stateside organizations and institutions in the form of high-tech equipment sent to the combat zone. The emergence of the research team represented a significant achievement of the military medical efforts during the 20th century and contributed to the further refinement of the care delivered to trauma patients during the Korean War. Through these efforts, progress was made in the clarification of the hemodynamic disturbances that occur with different forms of traumatic injury, and much knowledge was gained about organ function and the metabolic disturbances in shock and acute circulatory failure.

The pressing demands of war surgery coupled with the advances in medical care that occurred during the previous century contributed in part to the high level of performance that was realized during the Vietnam War. Improvements in field resuscitation, increased efficiency of transportation, and aggressive treatment of war casualties proved to be major factors contributing to livesaving endeavors. The death rates of war casualties reaching designated facilities decreased from 8 per cent in World War I, to 4.5 per cent in World War II, to 2.5 per cent during the Korean War, to less than 2 per cent in the Vietnam War.[6]

The Military Influence

Based on what had been learned by the military during war regarding the significant impact of time on saving lives, coupled with scientific knowledge regarding the human physiological response to injury, it became apparent that changes and adjustments within our health care delivery system were necessary.

Many have questioned with dismay why the information learned about the care of the injured during our nation's military experiences was so delayed in being applied to injuries occurring in civilian life. This is indeed baffling, since changes in patient care delivery that occurred during the Civil War and which were refined and improved on during each subsequent military conflict, were known to be responsible for the favorable trends in casualty survival. The need for an effective civilian system to care for the severely injured was just as prevalent as the need for one in the military arena. Yet this civilian need was not generally recognized or, if recognized, not accepted. As had been demonstrated consistently during wartime, rapid evacuation of the seriously injured from the battlefield to advanced treatment stations (Mobile Army Surgical Hospital [MASH] units), which were equipped with necessary supplies and staffed with highly skilled personnel, saved lives. The principles on which this system was designed have since been found to be easily transferable—although long overdue—and as effective in civilian life.

The modern era of a civilian systems approach that focused on more efficient emergency health care for the accidentally injured began in 1966 with the publication of a document by the National Academy of Sciences, National Research Council. This document, "Accidental Death and Disability—The Neglected Disease of Modern Society," was a far-sighted approach to the development of an effective emergency medical services system throughout our nation. It was the product of a 3-year study conducted by a committee on trauma, shock, and anesthesia in conjunction with special task forces from the Division of Medical Sciences, National Academy of Sciences, National Research Council. The results were compiled after representatives from health care organizations reviewed the status of initial emergency care provided to individuals following accidental injury. The study groups reviewed a broad spectrum of factors, including ambulance services, voice communication systems, hospital emergency departments, and intensive care units, while incorporating research results in shock, trauma, and resuscitation. Based on identified deficiencies, the general areas of consideration recommended by the committee and outlined in the published document[7] included the following:

- Accident prevention
- Emergency first aid and medical care
    - Ambulance services

  - Communications
  - Emergency departments
  - Interrelationships between the emergency department and the intensive care unit
- Development of trauma registries
- Hospital trauma committees
- Convalescence, disability, and rehabilitation
- Medicolegal problems
- Autopsy of the victim
- Care of casualties under conditions of natural disaster
- Research in trauma

The national effort for establishing an improved emergency health care system and much of the basic framework on which the nation's emergency medical services (EMS) system has subsequently been built were presented in this document. This classic white paper represented the first major governmental report acknowledging that significant numbers of people were killed or disabled as a result of unintentional injuries in the civilian population, which was costing the nation billions of dollars each year. Contributing significantly to the high mortality and morbidity rates were the inefficiencies in the nation's emergency health care delivery system. Unskilled health care personnel working with inadequate transportation and communication system policies and guidelines were taking the injured to facilities that were not sufficiently prepared to treat them. It became apparent that the problems of initial care and management of accidentally injured persons were similar in kind, although different in magnitude and scope, to those encountered by the military during war. The time was right for the application of new knowledge and skills in caring for the injured.

Early Pioneering Efforts

During the late 1960s and early 1970s, the need for a systems approach to the care of the seriously injured patient became apparent. The initial efforts to design and develop emergency medical clinical delivery systems were based on the care requirements of specific types of injury (e.g., trauma, burns, spinal cord injuries).[8] The conceptual design of a systems approach required that effective medical and surgical treatment regimens be applied in situations other than the traditional in-hospital setting. This necessitated the reorganization of preexisting health care structures, the implementation of new technologies, and the development of educational programs so that clinical treatment modalities proven effective in the hospital environment could be applied and tested in the prehospital and interhospital phases. Physician-supervised educational programs and extrahospital emergency care programs began to emerge, with emergency medical technicians–ambulance (EMT-A) and advanced life support emergency medical technicians–paramedic (EMT-P) assuming key roles.[8]

In several parts of the country hospitals were categorized regionally, and those with demonstrated expertise were designated as trauma, burn, or spinal cord injury centers. In Illinois, for example, the regionalization of emergency care for multiple and critical injuries was initiated and developed statewide in 1971. As the Illinois trauma program began to develop and mature, a program of patient transfer and burn center care also was initiated for the four burn units and major burn center (Cook County Hospital) in Chicago, which utilized a patient distribution program and central bed registry.[9]

In 1972, in collaboration with the Illinois trauma program, representatives from the Midwest Regional Spinal Cord Injury Care Systems at Northwestern Memorial Hospital and Rehabilitation Institute of Chicago (McGaw Medical Center, Northwestern University) formulated a macroregional catchment program for acute spinal cord injuries.[10] In 1973, the shock-trauma program of the University of Maryland, supported by the Maryland state government, was expanded statewide and became the Maryland Institute for Emergency Medicine (MIEM).[11]

These pioneering efforts were significant because they represented working models for further regional trauma/EMS systems development. The apparent successes resulting from these system designs became the catalysts for a more intense national effort to plan and to implement improved trauma/EMS systems.

Federal Support of Trauma/EMS Systems

Federal support of emergency medical services started during the early 1970s when congressional hearings were held to promote the development of a comprehensive EMS law. In 1973, the Emergency Medical Services Systems (EMSS) Act was passed, which contained guidelines and specific technical measures that would support a nationally coordinated and comprehensive system of emergency health care accessible to all citizens. The identification of fundamental elements of the EMS system deemed necessary for the comprehensive care of the critically ill and injured was accomplished with this mandate. Included in the EMSS Act were 15 requirements that would assist EMS system project planners and health care professionals in establishing comprehensive, area-wide, and regional EMS programs.[12] These components consisted of the following:

1. Provision of manpower
2. Training of personnel
3. Communications
4. Transportation
5. Facilities
6. Critical care units
7. Use of public safety agencies
8. Consumer participation
9. Accessibility to care
10. Transfer of patients
11. Standard medical record keeping
12. Consumer information and education
13. Independent review and evaluation
14. Disaster linkage
15. Mutual aid agreements

The 1973 EMSS Act, with its subsequent changes in 1976, is considered one of the most important factors influencing the development of EMS systems throughout this country. This act focused on improving the nation's emergency death and disability statistics by mandating that the emergency medical care programs that were federally funded by the Department of Health and Human Services (DHHS) must plan and implement a systems approach on a regional basis for emergency response and immediate care provisions. Although many emergency medical conditions had been identified, the seven critical target patient care areas for regional EMS systems planning were major trauma, burns, spinal cord injuries, poisonings, acute cardiac conditions, high-risk infants and mothers, and behavioral emergencies. In-depth knowledge of the incidence, epidemiology, and clinical aspects associated with these categories is considered essential for appreciating a systems approach to regional planning and delivery of care. Much of this information, specifically that related to multiple trauma, spinal cord injuries, and burns, will be explored in greater detail in this book in the respective chapters.

The federal government withdrew from its lead role in EMS development in 1981 with the passage of the Reconciliation Act, which integrated the EMS program into the Health Prevention Block Grants and gave responsibility back to the states for direction and development of EMS. The General Accounting Office (GAO) report of 1986[13] disclosed the effect of this transition of EMS system programs from federal to state leadership under the block grant program, concluding that a major sector of the United States (more than 50 per cent) lacked the universal phone access number 911, advanced life-support ambulance services were lacking or limited in rural areas, and many areas had not developed trauma care systems at all. Senators Alan Cranston and Edward M. Kennedy first introduced legislation to address the recommendations of the 1986 GAO report in the 100th Congress in January of 1987.

This legislation was finally signed into law as Public Law 101-590 by President Bush on November 16, 1990. This legislation, entitled the Trauma Care Systems Planning and Development Act of 1990, is significant because it provides federal assistance for the development of emergency/trauma care systems throughout the United States. This act amended the Public Health Services Act by adding a new title, Title XII. The major provisions of this act include[14]

1. *A council on trauma care systems.* The purpose of the council is to report needs to the trauma care system and how states are responding to such needs. This council has 12 public members, including two nurse positions (one critical care position and one emergency medical training position).

2. *A clearinghouse on trauma care and EMS.* This is to be established by contract to serve as a collection, compilation, and dissemination point for information relating to all aspects of emergency medical services and trauma care.

3. *Programs for improving trauma care in rural areas.* Grants will be authorized to be made to public and private nonprofit entities for research and demonstration projects for the purpose of improving the availability and quality of emergency medical/trauma care in rural areas.

4. *Formula grants with respect to modification of state plans.* Most of the appropriated funds (80 per cent) will be allotted by formula for each state and territory. Beginning in the second fiscal year that states receive funds, they must make a matching nonfederal contribution (in cash or in kind) in specified ratios.

5. *State plans and modifications.* Each state must submit to the Secretary of Health and Human Services the trauma care component of the state's EMS plan. The funds allotted for each state may be used only to make such modifications to the state plan as are necessary to ensure access to the highest quality of trauma care.

6. *Trauma care standards and a model trauma care plan.* Each state must adopt standards for designating trauma centers and for triage, transfer, and transportation policies. In addition, the Secretary must develop in the first year of this act a model trauma care plan that may be adopted for guidance by the states.

7. *Data and reporting requirements.* Each state must report annually to the Secretary the number of severely injured patients, the cause of injury and contributing factors, the nature and severity of the injury, monitoring data sufficient to evaluate the diagnoses, treatment, and outcomes of such trauma patients in each trauma center, and expenditures.

8. *Technical assistance and supplies and services in lieu of grant funds.* The Secretary shall provide technical assistance with respect to planning, development, and operation of any program carried out with the allotted funds, at no charge to the state.

9. *Waiver.* Under certain limited conditions, the Secretary may allow a state to use a percentage of allotted funds to reimburse designated trauma centers for uncompensated care.

Trauma/EMS System Development

As EMS systems have developed, the design seems to represent a composite of individual and unique systems of care for the particular patient group (e.g., multiple trauma, spinal cord injury, burns). Although it is necessary for these systems to utilize common EMS components, such as transportation, communications, and specially skilled prehospital health team members, the care, resources, and facilities must be specifically designed for each patient group. EMS system components must be adapted to address and accommodate specific clinical needs if accurate and effective planning is to occur. For example, unlike EMS systems planning for cardiac emergencies or for poisonings, the key EMS components for the trauma patient population are facilities categorization and trauma center designation (Table 1–1). For these patients, the establishment of triage and transfer protocols is critical so that immediate interventions are consistent and decisions regarding transfer to a designated trauma facility for definitive care are facilitated. Thus it is of utmost importance that regional trauma/EMS systems plan and develop clinically sound trauma care programs on a geographical basis. Because of the complex requirements, the care of the trauma patient has provided an excellent model from which to design a basic health care delivery system. This has since been expanded to include other types of emergency medical conditions.[15]

The clinical significance of the systems approach in developing a regional trauma/EMS system was clearly identified by the Division of Emergency Medical Services of the Department of Health and Human Services and reflected in their program guidelines. In congressional testimony, this agency described the unique clinical requirements of the multiple trauma patient, the need for a regionalized system of care, and the key EMS system components crucial to a successful and efficient trauma care program (i.e., facilities,

TABLE 1–1. KEY COMPONENTS OF A CLINICAL EMS SYSTEM

Trauma
Facilities categorization
Trauma center designation
Transfer agreements and triage protocols
Cardiac emergency
Patient access (911)
Citizen cardiopulmonary resuscitation (CPR)
Advanced cardiac life support (ACLS) paramedic response
Poisonings
Information specialists
Toxicologic information and treatment protocols
Telephone-directed home care and physician consultation

From Boyd DR, Edlich RF, Micik S: Systems Approach to Emergency Medical Care. Norwalk, Appleton-Century-Crofts, 1983.

critical care units, and transfer of patients). Although it was felt that a trauma/EMS system must adequately respond to all declared emergency calls within its designated geographical region, which included nonemergency cases (80 per cent), truly emergent cases (15 per cent), and critical cases (5 per cent),[8] emphasis was placed on the need to identify effectively the critical patient whose chance of survival so desperately depended on a competent trauma care delivery system. It was toward increasing the chance of survival for these critical patients that conceptual systems planning and initial program development were directed.

In 1987, the American College of Emergency Physicians' Trauma Committee published "Guidelines for Trauma Care Systems."[16] The ACEP guidelines state that "trauma care represents a continuum that is best provided by an integrated system extending from prevention through rehabilitation and requiring close cooperation among specialists in each phase of care."

Facilities Categorization

In the 1976 report, "Optimal Resources for Care of the Seriously Injured,"[17] the Task Force of the Committee on Trauma of the American College of Surgeons called for hospitals to commit personnel and facility resources to caring for seriously injured patients. The original proposal presented in the 1966 landmark document "Accidental Death and Disability: The Neglected Disease of Modern Society" suggested that the categorization of facilities should be based on the individual institution's capacity to handle a broad spectrum of emergency conditions.[7] This plan—the implementation of a variety of categorization schemes—proved to be unsuccessful, and a more detailed set of guidelines was provided by the Task Force of the Committee on Trauma of the American College of Surgeons in 1979. This revised document, "Hospital Resources for Optimal Care of the Injured Patient," replaced the 1976 report.[18] Emphasis was placed on special problems of geography, population density, availability of community and regional resources and personnel, and the pervasive demands of cost-effectiveness, with the most significant element being commitment—personal as well as institutional. Institutional commitment was defined as the immediate availability of capable personnel and accessibility to sophisticated equipment, laboratory and radiological facilities, operating rooms, and intensive care units. The personal commitment of hospital trustees, administrators, physicians, nurses, and other health care professionals also was imperative, since the responsibility for providing optimal hospital resources for the care of the seriously injured patient rests with these individuals.

Trauma Center Designation

In the 1979 report,[18] optimal standards for categorization of trauma care facilities were expanded and refined. Three distinct levels of trauma care services were identified, with functional responsibilities, capabilities, and comparable nomenclature outlined for the three levels. These were intended to serve as a guide for assessing an institution's potential for trauma center designation. The most recent revision appears in Appendix 1–1.

In the latest document by the American College of Surgeons' Committee on Trauma, "Resources for Optimal Care of the Injured Patient,"[19] a distinction is made between patient components and societal components of the system, and the sequence of events necessary to develop a trauma care system is presented. A level I trauma care facility is likely to be a teaching hospital of over 500 beds and is usually located in a large metropolitan area. This institution must make a firm but costly commitment in personnel and equipment.[18] Highly sophisticated equipment that is expensive to purchase and to maintain, the availability of skilled and experienced clinicians, and the need for the continuous educational preparation of all professional health care providers suggest that at least 1000 seriously injured admissions per year are needed to offset the enormous cost to the institution and to ensure that clinical skills are maintained at a high level. Extensive clinical experience enhances the management of multiple, complicated injuries. The 24-hour availability of staff specialists and skilled clinicians is essential to a level I trauma care facility (see Chapter 3 for further discussion of trauma costs).

A level II trauma care facility is most likely a tertiary institution that can handle a substantial volume of seriously injured trauma patients in a geographical area that lacks a teaching hospital necessary for level I trauma center designation. The most significant differences between a level I and level II institution are the formal trauma training programs and the research focus.

A level III facility is most often a community hospital located in an area that lacks level I or level II hospital facilities. It must make a strong commitment to the optimal care of the trauma patient, and clear and concise transfer protocols are essential.

Many other hospitals, both large and small, that have emergency department capabilities but have made no official commitment to an organized approach to the care of the seriously injured patient must upgrade their trauma care. This type of institution is an implied fourth level of trauma care and requires strict treatment protocols and transfer agreements with higher-level facilities.

Each institution should constantly monitor its capabilities

as a trauma care facility and continue to strive to upgrade its resources. Ideally, the severity of the injury should be equally matched with appropriate facility resources and personnel expertise. Health care professionals working within a hospital who have an interest in trauma care, who are educated and skilled in managing the special problems of trauma patients, and who assume a well-defined role on a trauma team organized especially to provide optimal care will produce more favorable patient outcomes than those who view trauma care as another general service.

Although there is a distinct difference between the categorization of hospital emergency and critical care capabilities and the more formal process of selecting and designating certain facilities for specialty clinical services, the categorization of all hospitals within a particular trauma/EMS region is beneficial in two respects. First, categorization allows for assessment of the hospital's general emergency department capabilities in caring for seriously injured patients and of its overall critical care capabilities for specific patient groups. This is considered an integral part of the planning activity helpful in documenting the existing resources and in identifying deficits that may ultimately lead to appropriate improvements in trauma/EMS systems. This information is considered when decisions are made concerning the official designation of specialty care centers. Second, once designated, these specialty referral centers are held accountable for maintaining their capabilities.

Transfer Agreements and Triage Protocols

The relationship of a regional trauma/EMS system to the overall EMS system is an important consideration when planning a comprehensive systems approach to trauma care. EMS and trauma/EMS systems involve a complex series of events which must be coordinated effectively to provide a consistent mechanism for efficient health care delivery. Clinical research has provided a deeper understanding of the natural course of traumatic disease and has proved that time is of the essence in treating these diseases. A standard mortality curve clearly shows that if a medical emergency is measured against time, death will eventually result if effective emergency care is not initiated promptly. The time constraints that exist for the seriously injured patient have served as the impetus for creating more effective mortality and morbidity controls.

Experience has shown that the outcome of traumatic injury is more favorable if resuscitation and stabilization efforts are initiated early and sustained. Although the time of patient death varies depending on the magnitude and variety of the traumatic pathology, a prompt trauma/EMS system response, the provision of initial basic field care, the use of a sophisticated communications system, and the rapid and safe transport of the patient will save valuable time, and eventual death may be prevented. Each phase of EMS activity has a critical effect on mortality. Every single act can save time. Rescue squads and first responders are prepared to perform basic life-support skills in the field. In many parts of the country, more sophisticated and advanced measures are being taken by EMT–paramedics in caring for critically injured patients both during extrication efforts and during transport within the EMS system.[20]

The EMS process begins when notification is received by EMS system operators that an accident has occurred; an ambulance team is dispatched to the scene. The patient's condition is assessed, and resuscitation and stabilization efforts are initiated in the field. The interventions and skill levels of the ambulance team members and field personnel are dictated by their level of educational preparation and certification. A sophisticated communications system allows the field personnel to contact authorized personnel at an appropriate trauma center for instructions concerning triage and treatment and provides the receiving hospital with an estimated time of patient arrival. Measures are then taken to transfer the patient to the most appropriate facility. This decision must be guided not only by the patient's condition and injury type but also by the geographical dynamics of that area. Thus each regional trauma/EMS system must be organized in such a way as to accommodate the unique needs of the area. Because there are distinct differences between urban and rural areas, three sociogeographical regional trauma/EMS models have been proposed for incorporation into the planning of trauma/EMS systems throughout the country.[8] When developing these sociogeographical models (the urban–suburban model, the rural–metropolitan model, and the wilderness–metropolitan model), population density, trauma care resources, and geography were considered.[8] Although some absolute examples of these models exist within regional trauma/EMS systems, most systems have more than one type model as seen in Maryland, Oregon, Pennsylvania, Virginia, and San Diego County, California. Generally, attempts are made to centralize designated trauma or specialty care facilities within regional trauma/EMS systems to facilitate timely and efficient primary triage or secondary transfer of patients, if necessary. Protocols for field identification, triage, resuscitation, and transportation to designated trauma centers have been adopted and have become operational in many communities. These protocols not only facilitate consistency within the trauma/EMS system but also ensure that injured patients are taken to hospitals capable of continuing and expanding life-support measures initiated in the field. A sophisticated systems approach to triage, communication, and transport is of little avail if clinical expertise of the highest quality does not await the injured patient's arrival.

The trauma facility notified of a pending admission has the responsibility of alerting the in-house trauma team, whose members will report to the designated resuscitation area to prepare for the patient's arrival. Staff specialists and expert clinicians, equipment, supplies, and ancillary support systems must be immediately available if the complex problems of the seriously injured patient are to be managed in a timely fashion. Effective resuscitation and stabilization efforts are based on the implementation of a predetermined series of activities performed simultaneously by appropriate trauma team members. Once the patient is stabilized, priorities are established for definitive care. Dependent on the type, magnitude, and severity of the patient's injuries, subsequent treatment may include surgical intervention, intensive care management, or long-term rehabilitation.

In summary, the trauma/EMS system by design must provide immediate and appropriate care at the scene of an incident, safe and efficient transportation to the trauma center, definitive surgical interventions, critical care management, and rehabilitation services. This broad scope of capabilities may be available within the respective geographical region. If not, the trauma/EMS system must respond by transferring patients out of that region to a distant trauma care facility where the specific needs of patients can be met. It has become apparent that all EMS systems throughout the country need a stratified, or graded, echelon system of trauma/EMS care so that flexibility within the emergency health care system is guaranteed. In order to support an effective trauma care system, integration of and cooperation among all hospitals treating injured persons in a region are crucial. An inclusive systems approach can minimize geographical and geopolitical constraints, allowing for efficient and effective use of resources to provide optimal trauma care to all injured persons served by the region.[21]

THE EVOLUTION OF TRAUMA NURSING

Historical Background

Nurses have long been challenged by the complexity of the health care needs of seriously injured patients and their families. Because wars have been responsible for producing traumatic injuries in epidemic proportions, nurses have gained experience in caring for the wounded. Although no clear records exist, perhaps the first organized nursing effort focusing on battlefield injuries was pioneered during the Crimean War (1854) when Florence Nightingale, Lady Superintendent-in-Chief of female nursing in the English General Military Hospitals, led a group of women in caring for war casualties.[22] For approximately 2 years, this group of nurses provided makeshift hospital facilities, bathed and dressed wounds, and painstakingly sought proper sanitation, hygiene, and control of infection. In October of 1861, Miss Nightingale was asked by the United States Secretary of War for advice on setting up military hospitals for the Union Army, and her suggestions were widely adopted throughout the course of the Civil War (1861–1865).[23] Clara Barton, the first woman clerk of the U.S. Patent Office, served as a nurse caring for wounded men on the battlefield after the outbreak of the Civil War in 1861 and later during the Franco-Prussian War (1869). In 1881, after her return to the United States, Miss Barton organized the American Red Cross, a volunteer society that was modeled after the International Red Cross (established in 1863 by Jean Henri Dunant).

In subsequent wars, nurses have cared for the wounded on and off the battlefield, seeking new ways to manage the devastating injuries resulting from the ever-increasing power of weaponry. Under the most adverse circumstances, combat nurses worked to help salvage mutilated extremities, tried to replace massive losses of blood, and attempted to administer appropriate medications, when available, to those with severe clinical complications. All actions were taken to prolong life; if initial efforts proved to be successful, death due to infection following a complicated clinical course was always a possibility.

Enormous problems existed for the nurses who cared for the wounded. They found that the scars of battle extended far beyond those from burns or bayonet or bullet wounds. The psychological implications for nursing care were just as pervasive as the physical demands: The mind and spirit were scarred as well. While caring for the wounded, nurses came to understand that the long-term effects and difficulties their patients faced as a result of war were far greater than the bullets, bombs, or missiles.

The knowledge gained from the experiences of the front-line nurses has provided valuable information in helping to understand trauma in civilian life. Moving from the war zone to the home front awakens us to the realities of our modern life-style. Influenced by the evolution of wounding forces unique to different historical periods, the occurrence of death and disability in our nation is astounding, and the effects are far-reaching.[24, 25]

Changes Within the Hospital Setting

During the 1970s, because of improved access to emergency medical services, the expanded educational preparation of emergency medical technicians, the development of sophisticated communication systems (including telemetry), and the use of more efficient means of transportation (including air evacuation), more viable patients were being brought to hospital facilities. During this same 10- to 15-year period of improved prehospital care, however, commensurate changes were not necessarily being made in the hospital. Reports indicated that basic errors in assessment and treatment of seriously injured patients were occurring with alarming regularity.[26–29] These errors, coupled with inadequate preplanning on the part of the hospital and poor mobilization and organization of hospital resources, often resulted in unnecessary death. The task of overcoming these unfavorable statistics presented a tremendous challenge to nurses, physicians, other health care professionals, and hospital officials.

Evolution of the Trauma Resuscitation Team

Categorization of hospital facilities had been one strategy demanded by the federal government in an attempt to ensure that patients were taken to institutions capable of caring for their injuries. Unfortunately, in most parts of the country this trend was occurring very slowly, if at all. However, a few facilities throughout the country began to make tremendous advances in caring for seriously injured trauma patients. These institutions, because they cared for a large number of injured patients, developed a staff of physicians and nurses proficient in caring for complex injuries. Statistical trends began to indicate that mortality and morbidity were substantially lower in these designated hospitals, which had more qualified and experienced personnel and more extensive facilities.[30] The success of the nurses and physicians was dependent on a number of factors, including the implementation of an interdisciplinary team approach to care, which facilitated the coordination of resuscitation efforts, evaluation, and definitive management plans. The success of the trauma team depended not only on the knowledge base and skill level of each physician and nurse but also on the consistency and repetition of their practices as a team. Proven in both military and civilian settings, a dedicated trauma team approach is the most effective and efficient means to care for the critically injured trauma patient. The predetermined delegation of specialized role responsibilities to each nurse and physician team member fosters the efficient organization of talents, which decreases the time between the patient's arrival and the onset of definitive care. Thus the hospital trauma team's efforts to save lives support the activities during the prehospital phase of care.

The development of rapid and more efficient transport systems was instrumental in reducing the precious time interval between the onset of injury and the patient's arrival at the hospital. This time factor underlies many of the principles upon which the initial care of the trauma patient was based. A firmer understanding of the volume requirements for circulatory resuscitation on the part of nurse and physician team members also had a significant impact on the team's approach to care. Success during the resuscitation phase of care increased the number of patients who then needed to be monitored closely and managed in an environment that provided continuity of intense nursing supervision and care. The extent of the patient's injuries, compounded by the potential for postresuscitation complications (e.g., respiratory insufficiency, renal failure, sepsis, coagulopathy), represented a new phase that required critical care medical and nursing management.

Trauma Critical Care Nursing

The critical care phase of nursing has provided unique challenges for nurses as new concepts of physiology and biochemistry have been applied. Concurrently, new evaluation techniques and management therapies have been introduced, which contributed to the advances made in the care of the seriously injured trauma patient. With the advent of miraculous technological advances affecting physiological monitoring and improvements in diagnostic procedures and medical treatments, trauma nursing faced a new frontier. One of the natural outcomes of this rapidly expanding technology was the nurse's increasing responsibility for complex decisions.

The introduction of innovative diagnostic tools contributed to greater efficiency in the clinical evaluation process. The computed tomographic (CT) scanner allowed precise diagnosis of intracranial injuries and provided more exact diagnoses for vertebral, acetabular, mediastinal, and some abdominal injuries. Simultaneously, advances in angiography provided a mechanism for precise diagnosis of vessel injuries in the chest, pelvis, and extremities. The strengths of peritoneal lavage as a diagnostic tool were recognized, sparing many trauma patients unnecessary operative procedures.

With the introduction and increasing clinical use of the blood gas instrument in the late 1960s, pulmonary problems occurring during the posttraumatic period were recognized early.[31] Volume-cycled ventilators with versatile control systems became available, and positive end-expiratory pressure (PEEP) was introduced as a therapeutic measure as soon as signs of impending pulmonary failure were recognized.

The nutritional needs of the critically injured patient also became a focal point of attention. Clinical research suggested that patients with multiple systems organ failure who allegedly died of complications actually died of protein malnutrition.[31] The therapeutic concept of intravenous hyperalimentation was introduced in 1968, and the nutritional support or nonsupport of the critically injured patient became an area of controversy.

Wound management theories were introduced in the 1970s. Basic characteristics of wound infection were not clearly identified prior to that time. New information focusing on the deterioration of the host's defense and of retained necrotic tissue and bacterial growth was, in part, responsible for changes in wound management techniques.[31]

During the 1970s, although not accepted on a widespread basis for years, new techniques for caring for musculoskeletal injuries were introduced by a new generation of surgeons. Principles of operative fracture management expanded to include the care of soft tissue as well. The potential for cardiopulmonary metabolic failures associated with fracture management began to receive more attention. The conservative treatment of fractures by traction or plaster devices, which for many years had been the general practice, began to receive much criticism as the undesirable consequences of immobility began to be recognized. This type of treatment regimen restricted movement; the patient was forced to be in a supine position while the bone injury was healing. This immobility was detrimental to heart and lung function, created a continuing source of pain, and led to a state in which large hematomas, crushed muscle and tissue, and devitalized fat were left in place to be reabsorbed by phagocytosis and endogenous body processes, thus placing tremendous demands on the patient's metabolic system.[31] These concerns led to the introduction of new treatment modalities.

Because of the complicated care required by the critically injured patient, many trauma specialty fields within medicine began to emerge. These specialty services included traumatology, neurosurgery, orthopedic surgery, thoracic surgery, plastic surgery, oral surgery, and critical care and infectious disease medicine. With this trend came the potential for these specialists to care for the patient by focusing on the area of their expertise in partial or complete isolation of the patient's other health care problems. The unfavorable consequences of this fragmented approach to care became obvious. Nurses, because they provided bedside care on a 24-hour basis, were in a position to facilitate the coordination of multidisciplinary patient care activities. They appropriately began to take measures to incorporate a comprehensive and total approach in planning care for the critical trauma patient. The role of the trauma nurse expanded as problem-solving and decision-making responsibilities increased, leading to a new era in collegial relationships.

Trauma Rehabilitation Nursing

During previous decades, as advances in the care of the seriously injured patient were made and incorporated into the resuscitation and critical care cycles, more lives were saved, and another phase of trauma care was recognized. As trauma patients emerged from intensive care settings, it became apparent that the focus of their medical and nursing care would need to take a new direction. The rehabilitation needs of trauma patients were identified, since a more stable condition allowed them more independence and, thus, more involvement in their own care. Attention also needed to be placed on assisting patients as they prepared for reintegration into their homes, jobs, and social groups. The nursing care during this intermediate or rehabilitation phase required the acquisition of new knowledge and skills in areas such as patient–family teaching, cognitive retraining, occupational and physical therapy, and discharge planning.

Despite the evolution of effective rehabilitation methods and procedures for improving the clinical care of the trauma patient, the widespread utilization of such practices has been more the exception than the rule. Failure to incorporate such advances into the care plan for trauma patients results in preventable yet significant societal health care costs. The socioeconomic impact of this unfortunate trend is believed to be so great that for every dollar spent on rehabilitation services, it is estimated that in this country between $6 and $35 could be saved by state and federal agencies.[32, 33] More widespread application of the knowledge and skills associated with advanced rehabilitation practices may result in substantial economic savings and a more productive and improved quality of life for the trauma patient population.

In order to minimize social and economic disability in the trauma patient, it is essential that the rehabilitation components of care begin immediately. Appropriate interventions in managing the critically injured patient from injury through return to home enhance clinical outcomes (reduced disability and mortality), promote personal autonomy, and, since an independent noninstitutional life-style is fostered, may result in shortened inpatient stays. Rehabilitation within this framework represents a process whereby the patient and family collaborate with nurses, physicians, and other specialists to identify mutual goals and plans to assist the trauma patient in achieving an optimal level of recovery. By striving to overcome limitations in functional cognition, communication, self-care, mobility, hygiene, vocation, family role, and coping abilities, a multidisciplinary rehabilitation system can provide all trauma patients with the opportunity to achieve maximum physical, social, psychological, and vocational recovery.

Trauma Nursing—The Focus of Care

Along with the changes in incidence, magnitude, and severity of injuries, the complexity of the therapeutic needs of the trauma patient population, and thus the demands on the entire health care system, the specialty field of trauma nursing has carved its niche. Influenced by a rapidly expanding body of knowledge focusing on how the human system responds to traumatic injury and which factors may make a difference in improving care, trauma nursing has expanded beyond the traditional practice mode. The effects of stress and adaptability on the course of illness, factors traditionally recognized by nurses, have become more readily valued as critical variables in the trauma patient's recovery. This is supportive of the holistic approach to the patient's care—attention on the whole individual, which is easily contrasted with a fragmented approach that focuses on specific pieces of information without acknowledging that these pieces are woven in an intricate fashion into the human fabric. Holistic care of the trauma patient requires continuity in the delivery of expert nursing care. Several significant factors must be considered if this continuity is to be accomplished.

The Human Response to Traumatic Injury

The impact of trauma on the individual can be viewed from various angles, including physiological, psychological, emotional, and socioeconomic perspectives. The biological makeup provides the human species with miraculous capabilities for maintaining itself in a relative state of homeostasis. As insults such as infectious agents, foreign bodies, and/or traumatic injuries are imposed on the human system, various physiological components are activated in an attempt to counteract the insult and its effects. The human system has the function of maintaining a sense of equilibrium or balance; the function or process often referred to as the "natural healing power" of the human species. This healing energy exists within all of us in some form to varying degrees. The biological response of the individual to insult such as traumatic injury is in part dependent on the human organism's natural ability to adjust or adapt physiologically. How and to what degree the individual is able to adapt can be determined by observing behavioral responses as well as monitoring certain physiological parameters. These findings can often be translated by nurses and used as measurable therapeutic tools to predict outcomes.

The human organism cannot, however, be viewed simply from a biological perspective. To do so would defy the laws of nature. No organism can be understood completely by studying only one aspect of it without acknowledging the effects of others on the composition of the entire system. This is not to say that scientific studies cannot be organized so that separate bodies of knowledge are identified and developed according to established processes. However, the scientific exploration of one human parameter in isolation, without considering the effects on the total human configuration, results in fragmented, useless information.

In keeping with this theme, the individual human response to traumatic injury also must be examined from the psychological, emotional, and socioeconomic perspectives. In order to provide efficient and effective nursing care that encompasses all realms of human response, the trauma nurse must employ a systematic means of observing and assessing the patient. Part of the challenge for trauma nurses is to identify negative adaptation responses, behaviors, and attitudes and to help the patient adapt more positively.

Trauma patients face other hazards in addition to the physiological effects of injury. They also must face the effects of traumatic insult on their thought patterns and attitudes. These conditions also may be worsened by deprived sensory systems, a situation that frequently occurs in an intensive care setting or from a prolonged hospital stay. In making compensatory adjustments, the mind may create illusions, hallucinations, and visions. When the patient is unable to cope with or to adapt independently to increasing tension, the trauma nurse must apply energies to provide emotional and psychological support as well as physical support until the patient regains enough energy to resume independent functioning. This requires that the nurse formulate a plan of action based on open communication, especially important in the emotional atmosphere of an acute care environment. Thus, at the first available opportunity, the nurse should encourage the trauma patient to communicate fears, frustrations, and anxieties about the traumatic incident, the injuries sustained, the medical and nursing management regimen, and the future course of events.

Following comprehensive assessment, the nurse must choose appropriate nursing actions to enhance the forces of adaptation by redirecting the dynamic processes in a positive direction. The nurse can assist the patient in developing a new future based on assessment of the past and appraisal of realistic goals or limitations in the present. Ideally, the trauma nurse's support and understanding will help the patient to accept the limitations caused by the traumatic injury.

In developing a comprehensive plan of care, the trauma nurse also must be alert to socioeconomic dynamics. Trauma has an impact on the social groups of which the patient is a member. In addition to the family system, these groups include work and church groups as well as clubs and other social affiliations, all of which have an impact on the individual trauma patient. In order to enable the trauma nurse to assist the injured patient effectively in adapting, the reactions and expectations of family members and friends must be considered. Generally, the way in which injury and disability are viewed depends on a variety of factors, including the type of injury, previous personal experience with illness or injury, norms and values of the individual and particular social groups, and the perceived expectations for social reintegration. Understanding the social dynamics unique to each patient's situation will assist the nurse in identifying appropriate resources within the hospital and community that will help in planning for the patient's discharge.

The impact that an injured family member has on the entire family structure must not be overlooked. Considered an important and essential component in the nursing care plan, the family must receive attention and support from the trauma nurse. It is important and essential that the trauma nurse establish a firm base of knowledge and develop skills in interacting with the patient's family members. The nature and severity of the impact of trauma on the members of the family will vary as a function of (1) the type of traumatic injury, (2) the phase or point at which the family is observed, (3) the family structure, (4) the identity of the injured person (e.g., mother, daughter, grandfather), (5) the point at which the traumatic injury occurs during the course of the individual's life, and (6) the point at which it occurs in the life of the family. The family's response to a sudden and traumatic injury that represents a crisis event is dynamic and interactive. To understand the family system and its individual members, the nurse should assess the crisis response in all family members or other significant relationships.

Family function may be affected in different ways by the sudden traumatic injury of a family member. As the impact of the traumatic injury on the patient is considered from the biological, psychological, emotional, and socio-economic perspectives, so may the impact on the family structure.

The biological functions of a family unit include the nurturing and physical care of a family member: the feeding, cleaning, and tending to the injury or illness. This may include identifying, preventing, and attempting to cure health threats and determining when advice or assistance from others outside the family unit is necessary. Trauma nurses should identify themselves as supportive resources to family members so that open lines of communication are established, thus fostering the sharing of valuable information between the patient's family and the trauma health care team.

The development and maintenance of the patient's self-image and self-esteem are among the psychological functions of the family system. This is accomplished through emotional communication patterns, which involve the expression of fear, anger, anxiety, frustration, joy, excitement, and contentment. The conditions under which these emotional expressions are permitted, not permitted, or controlled also must be identified by the family.

Included among the family's social functions are the tasks of defining group membership and group boundaries and establishing norms for the relationships that exist within the group as well as outside the group. The family is also considered within the context of the formal or informal societal structure and is viewed as a wage-earning, product-consuming, help-giving, tax-paying unit within our socioeconomic system.

Each of the functions described represents an important component for assessing how well the family unit is fulfilling biological, psychological, emotional, and social functions.[34] The trauma nurse must be alert to the patterns of family system functions and incorporate the unique characteristics of patient–family life-styles into the comprehensive plan of care.

Nurses' Role in Prevention

An examination of the impact that trauma has on the community raises issues that must be addressed. In most communities, unintentional injuries are taken for granted. Perhaps a major problem relates to the knowledge, or lack of it, that communities have about injury and the effects not only on the individual and family but also on the community as a whole. The cost of trauma to the community must be seen in health care costs as well as in the monetary expenditure resulting from reduced worker hours. As responsible members of the health care community, nurses should take responsibility for disseminating information about the nation's trauma problem. Health care professionals and consumers need to be alert to the causes of unintentional injuries and how they can be prevented.

As with many health care problems today, the cause of injury cannot be reduced to a single factor but must be viewed within the context of a broad spectrum of related factors. Sudden illness such as cerebral vascular accident or myocardial infarction and chronic illnessess account for only a small percentage of unintentional injuries. The predominant factor is human error. In 1990, 78 per cent of the total number of injuries (fatal and nonfatal) involving a motor vehicle were due to improper driving practices. A much smaller percentage was due to vehicle defects or poor road conditions. Exceeding the posted speed limit or driving at an unsafe speed was the most common error reported in rural injury of all severities and in fatal urbal motor vehicle injuries. Right-of-way violations predominated in the occurrence of urban motor vehicle injuries.[2] Alcohol is a factor in approximately 50 per cent of fatal motor vehicle mishaps,[2] and illegal drugs as well as many legally prescribed medications can cause a slowing of reaction time, thus contributing to the occurrence of injury.

The home can be a dangerous place as well. In 1990, mishaps that occurred in and around the home resulted in 21,500 deaths and 3,200,000 disabling injuries. With an injury total of this magnitude, it is estimated that 1 in 78 Americans was disabled one or more days by injuries received in home mishaps; 90,000 of these injuries resulted in some degree of permanent impairment. Disabling injuries are more numerous for home mishaps than for any other class of injury occurrence.[2] Falls, poisonings, fires, criminal violence (including child abuse, domestic violence, and injuries from bullets and bombs), and sporting injuries, although representing a smaller proportion of the total number of deaths or cases requiring hospitalization each year, should alert the public to the importance of prevention.

Just as many trauma injuries are both predictable and preventable, many impairments are treatable and the resulting disabilities are preventable. The development of effective trauma prevention programs can provide countless opportunities for addressing the trauma problem as it currently exists in our society. Likewise, the ample availability of rehabilitation programs can create a proliferation of opportunities for thousands of trauma patients. Yet despite these common truths, a passive societal posture seems to prevail that has been described as a "pervasive fatalistic attitude that equates impairment with disability and concludes that accidents just happen and nothing can be done to prevent them."[35]

Consumer involvement is imperative in gaining legislative support for issues pertaining to health, safety, and the prevention of unintentional injury. Unfortunately, the beneficial economic impact of trauma prevention has not been adequately and effectively translated into compelling public policy. The following situation serves as a case in point. A general feeling of optimism prevailed after Tennessee enacted a child restraint law, making it the 50th state to do so. Optimism continued as a similar trend with regard to general safety belt use laws seemed to emerge. Yet the reversal of safety belt laws in Massachusetts, Nebraska, and, more recently, Oregon, occurred despite supportive evidence that shows that the savings in health care costs afforded by routine safety belt use are substantial.[35]

Trauma nurses have spoken out and should continue to do so as they assume a leadership role in influencing issues of injury prevention and control, refusing to accept the grim statistics regarding trauma in our society. A considerable number of currently active prevention programs have been initiated and maintained by trauma nurses throughout the country—courageous testimony to the energy, interest, and accountability exemplified by nurses on behalf of the public. Although a complete title list of such programs is not available and a program-specific description and an in-depth discussion are beyond the scope of this chapter, it is important to note that trauma nurse-activists are addressing issues regarding alcohol and drug abuse and their implications for every injury mechanism and etiology; highway safety issues, including safety belt use, child restraint, and helmet laws[36, 37]; and domestic violence issues, including child abuse, firearms, and environmental influences, to name a few. Most important, trauma nurses continue to voice the strong belief that in matters pertaining to trauma care, those who have assumed an intricate role in meeting the complex needs of the trauma patient population should play a key role in shaping policy.

TRAUMA NURSING TODAY

When considering the evolution of the trauma nursing specialty, one must understand several significant developments and historical events of the past three decades. A review of pertinent factual information in congressional testimony, technical reports, and the literature has served to establish a historical perspective for the development of trauma/emergency medical services systems[3, 5, 7, 12, 15, 17, 18] (Table 1–2). The proliferation of designated trauma care facilities and the increasing regularity of formal meetings and conferences joining major organizations and professionals together are measures of the progress in recognizing trauma patients as a unique population requiring specialty services. These professional gatherings are indicative of the need for increased coordination, and clearly defined responsibilities are needed if each group—nurses, physicians, paramedics, and other allied health care professionals—is to deliver effective and efficient care.

In the past 30 years, achievements and advances in this direction have been monumental and drastically surpass all efforts made during the preceding century. The technological advances, the unquestioned recognition of need, and the impetus from many concerned individuals and professional groups have made this possible. These factors have resulted

TABLE 1–2. MILESTONES OF TRAUMA NURSING

1961	First shock trauma nurses. Elizabeth Scanlan, RN, and Jane Tarrant, RN, pioneered the nurse's role in the first two-bed shock/trauma research center with R Adams Cowley, MD, at University of Maryland Hospital, Baltimore, Maryland.
1963	National Research Center awarded a first-of-a-kind grant to the University of Maryland in Baltimore to establish a center for the study of trauma.
1966	Cook County Hospital in Chicago opened a trauma unit with Robert Freeark, MD, as medical director and Norma Shoemaker, RN, nursing supervisor.
1966	"Accidental Death and Disability: The Neglected Disease of Modern Society" (the white paper on trauma) published, citing needs of trauma population. This led to federal funding of trauma centers.
1971	David Boyd, MD, hired Theresa Romano, RN, to direct the education and training of nurses working in the designated trauma centers in Illinois.
1971	First trauma nurse coordinators hired for level I trauma centers in Illinois.
1973	Federal contracts awarded to Texas Women's University, University of Cincinnati, and University of Washington to begin graduate nursing programs in burns. These programs were the model for the first graduate trauma nursing programs.
1975	Maryland State EMS System established trauma nurse coordinator position for training, designation, and evaluation.
1982	ATLS for Nurses (pilot program) taught in conjunction with physician course. Nursing track was developed by MIEMSS Field Nursing, Baltimore.
1983	Trauma Nurse Network organized to provide communication link for trauma nurses.
1986	TNCC Course, Emergency Nurses Association
1987	First national census forum on Development of Trauma Nurse Coordinator Role, Washington, DC.
1989	Society of Trauma Nurses formed.

Adapted from J.B. Lippincott: Developing Trauma Care Systems: The Trauma Nurse Coordinator. JONA 18(7,8):34–42, 1980.

in support from local, state, and national government for regional planning and implementation of efficient trauma care services. It is essential that nurses become involved in this regional trauma EMS planning, implementation, and evaluation locally, nationally, and internationally.

Many of the goals of the white paper "Accidental Death and Disability—The Neglected Disease of Modern Society"[7] have been attained or at least begun. An increasing number of institutions specialize in the care of the severely injured patient. The development and designation of such institutions may be viewed as a natural evolution due to the dramatically increasing magnitude of the trauma problem and the demands of the trauma patient population on the entire health care system.

Likewise, the demanding clinical needs of the critically injured trauma patients, coupled with trauma nursing's crossing of established boundaries within the traditional nursing educational structure, have led to the natural evolution of trauma nursing as a specialty field within the larger emergency health care system. As with all systems that change over time, trauma nursing continues to develop toward a higher level of organization. As trauma patient care requirements have become more complex, nurses have emerged as coordinators capable of integrating the actions of other health care professionals. This process has allowed for the integration of the total care regimen, including all trauma specialty fields, which potentiates the process of unified action. Several expanded roles have been established as a means for meeting the special care needs and complexities of the trauma patient population and their families, among them being the trauma nurse coordinator, the trauma nurse practitioner, and the trauma nurse manager.[38, 39] This book presents a working body of knowledge based on principles from traditional nursing models and from the theoretical frameworks of medicine, psychology, physical science, education, and behavioral and social sciences. Perhaps it is this broad spectrum of required knowledge that has attracted a pioneering breed of nurses to accept the challenge of contributing the integral components of a multidimensional and holistic focus in caring for the trauma patient. The nature of severe injuries resulting in multisystem disruptions requires the trauma nurse to comprehend extensive scientific data, to synthesize care in life-threatening emergencies, and to lead, assist, and support the patient and family on the long journey toward recovery. Daily, this group of caregivers is bombarded with uncharted pathophysiological phenomena and unceasing psychological and emotional crises. For the nurse to function efficiently in this situation, high levels of energy and stamina are required. To do this, each nurse must take responsibility for periodically examining his or her stress levels while constantly being alert to the stress levels of others. This fosters an atmosphere of caring, not only for the patients and families, but also for one another.

THE TRAUMA CYCLE—CONCEPTUAL DEVELOPMENT

In closely examining the cycle of events that occur throughout the many phases of trauma care—from the time of injury; through the resuscitation, critical, intermediate, and rehabilitation phases of care; to the return to home and community—a wealth of information can be derived and added to the existing body of knowledge and skills of trauma nursing. This process of continued growth and development will determine the future direction of trauma nursing practice.

Although a traumatic injury occurs within a very short time frame, it has long-term effects. Trauma can therefore be viewed as a disease process with far-reaching consequences.

Many of the changes that occur during and after a traumatic incident are a direct result of the individual's ability to adapt to the injured state. For this reason, this book is organized with the subject content presented in the context of time and space. In other words, we believe that it is beneficial to look at the individual's traumatic incident and subsequent care as it occurs in a cyclic pattern. What happens to an individual when an unintentional injury occurs will be described in blocks of time, or cycles. This method takes into account what circumstances existed prior to the injury, which may or may not have precipitated the incident; what occurs at the exact time of the incident, with consideration of the biomechanics of the injury as well as the circumstances that may have contributed to its nature and extent; and what changes occur following a traumatic injury. This exploration of events will begin with time representing the resuscitation phase and will continue through the operative, critical care, and intermediate and rehabilitation phases to the time at which the individual is integrated into the community. At any time during this cyclic pattern, valuable information can be learned that will assist the skilled nurse in assessing and planning, implementing, and evaluating a special plan of care for the trauma patient and his or her family.

Reflected throughout the book is the view that the care of the trauma patient is not performed on a linear continuum with a beginning and an end but instead throughout a cyclic process. The trauma cycle represents a series of changes that leads back to its starting point: The patient enters the emergency health care system from the community and at some point reenters the community. As the individual returns to the community, the cycle is completed, yet the potential always exists for the cycle to be repeated—there is no end point. Accordingly, prevention is a concept that must receive prime consideration when caring for patients throughout the process. Based on the strong belief that prevention is better than cure, much emphasis will be placed not only on the prevention of traumatic injury but also on the prevention of complications, disability, and maladaptive adjustments on the part of the patient and family once a traumatic injury has occurred. The trauma sequel represents a complete cycle of phenomena and operations—changes that lead toward the restoration of a state of well-being. Helping the patient and family return to a healthy state is the goal of the trauma nurse—and the target of all interventions.

REFERENCES

1. Trinkaus E, Zimmerman MR: Trauma among the Shanidar Neanderthals. Am J Phys Anthropol 57:61–76, 1982.
2. Accident Facts. Chicago, National Safety Council, 1991.

3. Report of the Secretary's Advisory Committee on Traffic Safety. US Department of Health, Education and Welfare. Washington, DC, US Government Printing Office, February 29, 1968.
4. Simeone FA: Studies of trauma and shock in man: William S. Stone's role in the military effort (1983 William S. Stone Lecture). J Trauma 24:181–187, 1984.
5. The Board for the Study of the Severely Wounded (Medical Department, United States Army). In Beecher HR (ed): Surgery in World War II: The Physiologic Effects of Wounds. Washington, DC, US Government Printing Office, 1952.
6. Heaton LD: Army medical service activities in Vietnam. Milit Med 131:646, 1966.
7. National Academy of Sciences, National Research Council: Accidental Death and Disability: The Neglected Disease of Modern Society. Washington, DC, US Government Printing Office, 1966.
8. Boyd D, Edlich RF, Micik SH: Systems Approach to Emergency Medical Care. Norwalk, Appleton-Century-Crofts, 1983.
9. Ogilivie RB: Special message on health care. Springfield, State of Illinois Printing Office, April 1, 1971.
10. Meyer P, Rosen HB, Hall W: Fracture dislocations of the cervical spine: Transportation assessment, and immediate management. Am Acad Orthop Surg 25:171–183, 1976.
11. Cowley RA: Trauma center—A new concept for the delivery of critical care. J Med Soc NJ 74:979–986, 1977.
12. United States Congress: Emergency Medical Services Systems Act (Public Law 93–154). Ninety-third Congress, SB2 410. Washington, DC, US Government Printing Office, November 16, 1973.
13. United States General Accounting Office: States Assume Leadership Role in Providing Emergency Medical Services (GAO/HRD-86-132). Washington, DC, US Government Printing Office, 1986.
14. Public Law 101–590, November 16, 1990 104 Stat. 2915, Trauma Care Systems Planning and Development Act of 1990. Washington, DC, US Government Printing Office, 1990.
15. Emergency Medical Services Systems Program Guidelines. DHHS Publication No. (HSA) 75-2013. Washington, DC, Division of Emergency Medical Services, Health Services Administration, Bureau of Medical Services Administration, February, 1975.
16. American College of Emergency Physicians' Trauma Committee: Guidelines for trauma care systems. Ann Emerg Med 16(4):459–463, 1987.
17. Committee on Trauma of the American College of Surgeons: Optimal hospital resources for care of the severely injured. Bull Am Coll Surg 61:15–22, 1976.
18. Committee on Trauma of the American College of Surgeons: Hospital resources for optimal care of the injured patient. Bull Am Coll Surg 64:43–48, 1979.
19. American College of Surgeons' Committee on Trauma: Resources for the Optimal Care of the Injured Patient. Chicago, American College of Surgeons, 1990, pp 5–8.
20. Caroline N: Emergency Care in the Streets. Boston, Little, Brown, 1982.
21. Trauma Care Systems Panel Position Paper in the Third National Injury Control Conference: Injury Control. Washington, DC, US Department of Health and Human Services, Public Health Services, Centers for Disease Control, April 1992, pp 377–426.
22. Nightingale F: Notes on Nursing: What It is and What It is Not. New York, Dover Publications, 1969.
23. Huxley EJ: Florence Nightingale. New York, Putman, 1975.
24. Mays ET: Clinical Evaluation of the Critically Ill. Springfield, Charles C Thomas, 1975.
25. Oakes AR: Trauma: Twentieth-century epidemic. Heart Lung 8:918–922, 1979.
26. Von Wagoner FH: Died in hospital: A three year study of deaths following trauma. J Trauma 1:401–408, 1961.
27. Gertner HR, Baker SP, Rutherford RB, et al: Evaluation of the management of vehicular fatalities secondary to abdominal injury. J Trauma 12:425–431, 1972.
28. Foley FW, Harris LS, Pilcher DB: Abdominal injuries in automobile accidents: Review of care of fatally injured patients. J Trauma 17:611–615, 1977.
29. Houtchens BA: Major trauma in the rural mountains west. J Am Coll Emerg Phys 6:343–350, 1977.
30. Frey CF, Huelke DF, Gikas PW: Resuscitation and survival in motor vehicle accidents. J Trauma 9:292–310, 1969.
31. Allgöwer M, Border JR: Advances in the care of the multiple trauma patient: Introduction. World J Surg 7:1–3, 1983.
32. Committee on Trauma Research Commission on Life Sciences, National Research Council and the Institute of Medicine: Injury in America: A Continuing Public Health Problem. Washington, DC, National Academy Press, 1985.
33. Hammerman SR, Maikowski S: The economics of disability from an international perspective. Annu Rev Rehabil 3:178–202, 1983.
34. Tuck, D, Kerns R: Health, Illness and Families: A Life Span Prospective. New York, Wiley, 1985.
35. Maull K: Dispelling fatalism in a cause-and-effect world (1989 E.A.S.T. Presidential Address). J Trauma 29:752–756, 1989.
36. Straight Talk on Prevention (S.T.O.P.) Program. Maryland EMS Newsletter 17(10):1–2, 1991.
37. Dearing-Stuck B: Trauma prevention. In Cardona G (ed): Trauma Nursing. Oradell, NJ, Medical Economics Press, 1985.
38. Beachley M, Snow S, Trimble P: Developing trauma care systems: The trauma nurse coordinator. JONA 18(7,8):34–42, 1988.
39. Spisso J, et al: Improved quality of care and reduction of housestaff workload using trauma nurse practitioners. J Trauma 30(6):660–663, 1990.

2

ADMINISTRATIVE ISSUES IN TRAUMA CARE

CONNIE JOY

INTRODUCTION

The successful management of any area of health care requires skill, talent, and creative leadership. The scope of responsibilities is as complex and challenging as any clinical situation and as important to patient outcome. Knowledge of current health care issues, such as changes in reimbursement practices, legal and political implications of such changes, and personnel management, is essential in administration. Health care is no longer viewed as being equally available to all people. It is a business, requiring managers to provide a business-like approach in their decisions with cost containment as a goal. Almost every activity needs to be questioned in order to evaluate its outcome and justify its expense. Innovative approaches to management are greatly valued, and nursing leaders have frequently been at the forefront of ensuring quality patient care while responding thoughtfully to institutional fiscal concerns.

SEASONALITY OF TRAUMA INJURIES

Health care is in transition, and trauma care is no exception. The clear direction of trauma care has been toward the development of trauma care systems using a rational approach based on the concept of centralization, or tertiary care.[1] Administration of trauma nursing requires vision, planning, and implementation of methods that support trauma system access, prehospital triage, treatment and transport, emergency department resuscitation, operative intervention, postanesthesia recovery, intensive care, and rehabilitation services. This process is complicated by the requirement that all services be available at all times and the knowledge that their need and use cannot always be easily anticipated. Costs related to trauma services are high because injury occurs episodically and these services are frequently over- or under-utilized at different times. Standby costs are most notable in the operating room and postanesthesia recovery area, specifically when multiple trauma patients are being managed simultaneously. Whenever the total number of trauma patients is higher than average, costs in the intensive care unit also climb as a result of the need for additional personnel. Because of the seasonality of trauma, costs related to care are also high during time periods that are less busy. Successful management of trauma means that personnel are paid to be available, waiting for trauma to happen. Recognition of this concept and the willingness to commit money to a perceived under-utilization of resources are essential concepts in trauma nursing care administration.

The focus of nursing administration within a trauma service is on the allocation of resources to care for the severely injured individual, the family, and the care providers. It is important that nursing administrations support adequate availability of systems that help nurses to provide this care and to gain self-support when care-related stress occurs. Today's trauma nurses are a highly specialized, expensive, and scarce resource. As this country's largest group of health care professionals, registered nurses are essential to the success or failure of current health care systems, including trauma. Present models of nursing address patient care needs and the use of technology in a supportive role, extending the productivity of nurses and increasing the quality and quantity of their work. Designing methods of nursing care delivery includes customizing systems for each facility based on its patient population. The nursing administrative and management issues addressed in this chapter are not necessarily limited to areas or organizations that care just for trauma patients but are important aspects of management in most health care settings.

ORGANIZATIONAL ISSUES

Organizational Culture

A culture constitutes the organizational boundaries inside of which individuals and groups function. These boundaries represent fiscal, behavioral, intellectual, and philosophical constraints while providing at the same time guidelines for success within the environment. An understanding of both the organizational culture and how to successfully interact with it is essential to all managers, regardless of level or department.

The culture of an institution that provides care to trauma patients typically is very different from that of other health care organizations. Frequently, there is a greater tendency to manage with anticipation and preparation rather than with reactions after a problem or need is recognized. Strategic planning is essential for trauma services as well as for other major health care programs. Forward thinking is apparent through the active sharing of information about anticipated changes and the provision of opportunities for involvement of personnel from all disciplines and levels in planning. Management is often aggressive, with attention being paid to streamlining services and making them readily available while limiting redundancy. Trauma patients require the services of almost every department within a hospital, which can create a natural common bond among these departments, as well as improve the working relationships among personnel. Trauma patients also can add extreme stress to both individuals and systems, which emphasizes the need to recognize and address issues effectively as they arise.[2]

Imaging Trauma Programs

In some communities, a hospital with a successful trauma program is viewed as having an important role within the community, sometimes resulting in a positive "halo" effect for the hospital. This halo effect, or the presumption that a trauma center has better services overall than other non-trauma-center hospitals, has both advantages and disadvantages. The largest advantage is the potential for increased market share for health care programs in the trauma hospital. The major disadvantages are the political struggles that a trauma hospital may need to endure because of other community hospitals' dislike of prehospital bypass and the potential loss of health care dollars. The exceptions to this are large urban hospitals or hospitals in areas of the country where there is a large uninsured population. In these areas, the opposite is true. Trauma programs that provide care for patients with low or no reimbursement potential lose tremendous amounts of money, sometimes placing the overall mission of the hospital at risk. Within the past 5 years, many hospitals with outstanding trauma programs have chosen to remove themselves from regional trauma systems. This is due largely to the inability to maintain services because of the amount of revenue lost from trauma patients unable to pay for services rendered. Therefore, inherent within the organizational culture of any hospital caring for large numbers of trauma patients is the need to understand the implications that trauma care has on the institution and community.

Hospital Accreditation

The Joint Commission on Accreditation of Healthcare Organizations (JCAHO) was established in 1951. Through a voluntary accreditation process, organizations can receive recognition for the standard of services they provide while receiving guidance for evaluating and improving the quality of those services. JCAHO standards for accreditation are updated and published on a regular basis and include guidelines for all essential departments within differing types of health care organizations. Accreditation occurs through a site-survey review process that compares existing services with JCAHO standards and rates them on the basis of scoring guidelines.

In 1986, JCAHO began to publicize a new evaluation methodology that was under development and scheduled to become part of the accreditation process in the early 1990s.

This process was entitled *Agenda for Change*.[3] Included was an innovative patient-centered performance evaluation that focuses on measures of health care quality as derived from clinical and organizational indicators. Emphasis was placed on principles of organizational and management effectiveness within health care organizations and their relationship with the clinical outcome of patients. Total organizational commitment to continuously improve the quality of patient care was the central concern of these principles. Evidence of this commitment is demonstrated through a system of on-going monitoring and evaluation of clinical and organizational performance that provides both managerial and clinical leadership information on patient care decisions and outcomes while also promoting fiscally responsible organizational change that will improve the quality of patient care.[4] The *Agenda for Change* called for an evaluation by the JCAHO in 11 areas:

1. Organizational mission
2. Organizational culture
3. Organizational change
4. Role of governing board and managerial and clinical leadership
5. Leadership qualifications, evaluation, and development
6. Independent practitioners' qualifications, evaluation, and development
7. Human resources
8. Support resources
9. Evaluation and improvement of patient care
10. Organizational integration and coordination
11. Continuity and comprehensiveness of care

Clinical Indicators

A major component of the JCAHO's *Agenda for Change* involves creation of a data-based performance-monitoring mechanism for accredited health care organizations. Through this process, it is anticipated that hospitals will routinely collect a limited set of important clinical and organizational process and outcome data, send them to the JCAHO, and receive back aggregate comparative data. Several expert task forces were established by the JCAHO to identify clinical indicators believed to be useful for monitoring systems for the care of differing patient populations, including trauma patients.[5] These indicators are intended to help hospitals and clinicians to improve patient outcomes by revealing problem areas, hospital systems, or other components of care delivery that warrant further evaluation. They are not intended to be used as direct measures of quality, but rather as a filter upon which to base more extensive review. These indicators are also not intended as a basis for accreditation by the JCAHO, although future accreditation of a hospital may be influenced by how effectively such indicators are used in their internal quality improvement programs.

The JCAHO standards for nursing services also were revised recently, and the revisions became effective in 1992. The new nursing standards place emphasis on the need for nursing to have a prominent place in organizational decision making and to have clearly defined and implemented standards of care. Quality assessment of patient services rendered is a critical component, involving appropriate response and follow-up when concerns are recognized.

Trauma Accreditation

Trauma accreditation or designation is an option for hospitals wishing to demonstrate consistent compliance with recognized standards of care for trauma patients. Throughout the country, a number of states have developed regionalized systems that identify a method for achieving the status of a "trauma hospital." All standards used are based on the work of the Committee on Trauma of the American College of Surgeons, which initially published their standards in 1976. The standards are significant and not easily implemented or maintained. However, it has been demonstrated that hospitals meeting or exceeding these standards have a positive impact on the outcome of severely injured patients.[6–9]

It is important that managers at all levels have an understanding of both the JCAHO standards and the trauma standards so that the implications for their own departments are clear.

Marketing Health Care Services

In the last decade, hospitals have recognized the need to become more consumer-oriented. After examination of their internal operations, many health care organizations have discovered that their services were frequently driven by the needs of departments rather than by the needs of patients. Restructuring services in order to be more patient-driven involves creating a dynamic system that allows personnel to respond to the needs of patients rather than the routine of the hospital.

Recognizing the need for a consumer-driven response to health care, marketing strategies promoting hospital services have become commonplace, especially in areas of the country where health care is competitive. Striving for, achieving, and monitoring patient satisfaction, as well as third-party payor satisfaction, have emerged as important issues for hospitals. Although the average patient is not technically competent to judge the appropriateness of the interventions and procedures he underwent, he will inevitably judge the adequacy, skill, and acceptability with which the care was delivered. These perceptions are based on the patient's own expectations, rather than on a professional's definition of appropriate care. Marketing initiatives to field providers as well as to the community at large are instrumental, because they can reflect on patient volumes as well as awareness of services.

Physicians also play a significant role in supplying hospitals with patients and defining care requirements as well as resources needed. It is important that hospital managers understand physician preferences related to hospital services. Studies have identified the specific hospitals attributes which rank as most important to physicians and act as a determinants for patient admission. In every study reviewed, including studies that addressed cross sections of all medical specialties, the top-ranking attribute that attracted physicians to specific hospitals was excellence in nursing care. Physicians send their patients to systems that are perceived as being at a higher level based on the education and excellence of nursing personnel.[10] Traditionally, where emphasis was placed on technology and ancillary services, it is becoming apparent that closer attention must be paid to the quality of services being delivered by all providers.

As demonstrated through research, nurses are a crucial

link in the patient–physician–hospital relationship. The quality of nursing services, as well as the physician–nurse relationship, will influence the hospital's strategy in competing for doctors and patients.

NURSING MANAGEMENT ISSUES

Leadership Responsibilities

Nurse managers are in a position to respond to pressures from hospital administration and from society to motivate nurses to economize, innovate, and maintain or improve the quality of nursing services. At the same time, nurses expect their managers to energize and lead them, solve problems, and represent their interests to hospital administration. One of the most essential attributes for a nurse manager to possess is the knowledge and ability to influence systems.[11, 12]

It is important to demonstrate nursing management expertise in a visible way. Displaying knowledge of current strategies for improving patient care services while diminishing costs will enhance the perception of nursing management expertise greatly. The use of effort to gain influence should not be underestimated. Obvious effort expended toward a project or goal that is highly valued within an organization will focus positive attention on the manager and department and enhance the manager's ability to influence. Persuasion is related most often to communication, involving style, timing, and articulation as components. Persuasion as a part of negotiation relies on the manager's expertise with and knowledge about the issue being discussed, as well as the manager's ability to present her argument in an influential manner.

Credibility is important in any management role. Trauma nursing's credibility comes primarily from skill and knowledge related to clinical patient care and services utilized to support this process. This does not imply that all nurse managers must be clinical experts. Managerial credibility is gained through an astute understanding of nursing resource requirements in terms of the patient population serviced and how best to gain and keep them. One of the most important concepts in nursing management is that all activities relate to patient care, either directly or indirectly. Managing budgets, personnel issues, and business plans for new services are all indirect patient care activities. Meetings and work sessions with other department managers are frequently time-consuming, but they are a vital dimension in the coordination of services.

Nursing Governance

The organizational structures of hospital nursing departments vary widely, but several trends are emerging. The impetus behind these trends is twofold: (1) authority over practice within a nurse's range of competence is important to job satisfaction, and (2) health care today is changing at such a rapid pace that the only way to accomplish outcomes is for clinical decisions to be made at the point of encounter. The implication of both these factors is that the trauma nurse must be educated, experienced, highly clinically capable, confident with decision making, and empowered to make decisions. The trauma nurse works in an environment that promotes professional independence as well as excellence in trauma nursing practice. It is the role of nursing leaders to create this environment and support nurses in attaining these outcomes.

Trauma nurses are an integral part of the health care team, and they desire both to participate and to be autonomous, in clinical as well as organizational issues. Professional motivation includes having a strong need for accomplishment and a desire to grow both within an organization and within a profession.[13] An organizational climate and structure that does not offer opportunities for staff decision making places the professional nurse in a position in which she suffers role confusion, conflict, and job dissatisfaction. Hierarchical bureaucracy and nonparticipative supervision are often cited as reasons for nurse turnover or departure from the nursing profession. *Shared governance* describes the management model that promotes autonomous operation at the unit level and systematic, participative representation by staff nurses in department-wide governance issues. Governance models may range from administrative decision making with staff nurse input to fully developed departmental governance structures that have a central coordinating council consisting of staff nurses.[14] Within this type of governance structure, emphasis is on placing decision making in the hands of the individuals who then implement the plans. Clinicians are consulted for clinical decisions, managers for administrative decisions, and educators for education or staff development decisions. Essential to the functioning of shared-governance models is open communication and an environment of trust. This involves recognition of the contributions of others and commitment to developing modes of timely, effective decision making.

Governance is also a key element in determining the system used for nursing care delivery and has been identified as being related to positive patient outcomes.[15] The association between enhanced patient outcomes and shared governance in nursing care can be seen clearly in the trauma setting. An organization that promotes the success of the care provider creates an environment with adequate resources, ample opportunities to develop healthy interpersonal relationships, and the freedom to engage in consensus decision making. Trauma care demands extensive resources and creative applications of nursing theory and practice. Trauma nursing frequently calls for thinking and working in unstructured situations, and nursing self-governance provides the framework and the tools to support this process.

Shared governance is a method of placing organizational decision making, responsibility, and accountability with the staff nurse. When implemented successfully, such an approach brings positive recognition to nursing and assists in meeting the expectations of professional nurses. There is little doubt that shared governance has a strong future within trauma nursing systems.[16]

Nursing Organizational Structure

The current trend in most health care organizations is to create a much more streamlined administrative and management structure. Greater emphasis is placed on leaders who are specialists in budget and financial planning, strategic and operational planning, education, research, and personnel management, specifically mentoring and guiding. This is a distinct difference from models that demand directing and controlling behaviors from their managers. There is also a greater need for leaders to support clinicians by facilitating the forces in the health care environment. This facilitation allows staff to achieve better departmental, organizational, and patient outcomes because they can better concentrate on issues that most directly affect patient care.[17]

One significant change in nursing organizational structure involves expansion of the nurse manager role to one similar to that for all other department heads. This expansion provides organizational influence and parity with other department heads, such as pharmacy, materials management, and radiology. As staff nurses become increasingly responsible, accountable, and clinically proficient, the need for direct supervision diminishes. The scope of managerial responsibility then increases to encompass a much broader area of responsibility.[18] The current trend focuses on increasing the span of control of the nurse managers so that they are responsible for multiple clinical areas.

Nursing Care Delivery Systems

One of the biggest changes in nursing within this decade has been and will continue to be the system for the delivery of nursing care—who will deliver it (type of care provider) and in what manner. A 1982 study identified 41 institutions as "magnet hospitals" because they had been particularly successful in attracting and retaining nursing staff. They also were identified by professional nurses as good places to work and places where they were able to provide excellent nursing care.[19] Two follow-up studies have been done since 1982 to determine if representative magnet hospitals were continuing to experience similar success.[20, 21]

Nursing Satisfaction and Retention

The question of what provides people with satisfaction has been addressed in many publications. In his classic work, Herzberg investigated engineers and accountants and found that job satisfaction was improved by fulfillment of human needs or motivators. These include achievement, recognition, responsibility, advancement, and contribution related to the work itself.[22] Job dissatisfaction may result from salary, working conditions, interpersonal relationships, and company policies. Work-related stress, regardless of its cause, is the single greatest reason for dissatisfaction.

Several studies have attempted to determine specific issues that lead to nursing satisfaction and job retention. The following have been identified as significant organizational retention factors:[23]

Staffing and Scheduling

Fewer weekend and holiday shifts for senior nurses
Day shift with minimal or no rotation for senior staff
12-hour weekend shifts

Salary and Benefits

More pay steps for senior nurses
More vacation for senior nurses
Weekend salary bonuses
Payback for unused sick hours
Increased shift differential

Educational Opportunities

Paid educational days
Free continuing education opportunities within the organization, including workshops
Increased tuition reimbursement
Advanced training in specialty areas

Each area described provides an opportunity for successful and creative management. Managers must be willing and able to move from an authority–obedience style of supervision to one of involvement, participation, and commitment. Systems should be established that encourage greater opportunity for employees to express their innate motivation to contribute. In many organizations, a select few individuals act as gatekeepers of both information and control. Managers need to recognize their role as being one of facilitating, mentoring, coaching, and rewarding. Designing methods of sharing managerial prerogatives will result in both increased job satisfaction and performance excellence.

Advanced Clinical Practitioners

Unit-based clinical nurse specialists, responsible for the definition and development of patient care standards as well as staff education, are increasingly integrated into and viewed as vital components in achieving good patient outcomes and quality nursing care. Advanced nursing practitioners within trauma nursing systems frequently include nurse practitioners, nurse anesthetists, and clinical nurse specialists. Post-basic education in an aspect of advanced nursing practice and/or national certification in a nursing specialty is required by the majority of state licensure boards.[24] There is variation in the scope of practice from state to state, most frequently related to medication prescriptive authority and level or amount of physician involvement in the practices of advanced nurses. Although adequate research has not been completed, there is strong evidence that increasing trauma patient access to advanced-practice nurses, on both an inpatient and an outpatient basis, may serve to decrease the length of hospitalization and improve long-term patient outcomes.

Primary Nursing

In 1982, the dominant system of nursing care delivery in the magnet hospitals was primary nursing. Philosophically, *primary nursing* was defined as a commitment to registered nurse accountability and responsibility for individualized, planned patient care from time of admission to discharge and, in some cases, after discharge. This system became operational with the help of an increasingly all-registered-nurse staff and was highly valued.

In the years since, primary nursing has become more difficult to operationalize. Decreased length of hospital stay related to reimbursement restrictions has forced hospitals and trauma systems to efficiently move patients through their systems and back into the community. Creativity, diversity, and experimentation in care delivery systems have been notable, and many novel delivery systems have emerged that support flexibility based on patient care requirements. Two specific trends seem to be emerging: (1) a change in staffing mix and (2) an increase in differentiated practice at the registered nurse level.

Staffing Mix

The change in staffing mix is related to an attempt to increase the percentage of registered nurses assuming responsibility for providing patient care while ensuring that there are adequate nonprofessional assistants to perform the nonnursing and environmental tasks. It is currently estimated that a nurse spends 31 per cent of her time in direct patient care.[25] This translates into an average of 25 to 30 minutes per shift with each patient, or a total of 2 ½ hours in care for all patients, based on an average daily assignment of medical/surgical adults. The majority of time is spent in indirect clinical activities, which include documentation, preparation of therapies, shift-change activities, professional interaction, and other miscellaneous tasks performed on behalf of a specific patient or group of patients. In addition to these activities, there is unit-related work, which consists of activities that contribute to the general maintenance of the nursing unit, such as attending meetings, classifying patients, attending unit rounds, preparing reports, and supervising other staff and students. All of these activities are essential components of the professional role.

Differentiated Professional Nurse Practice

Many hospitals and trauma centers are attempting to discriminate competencies through the use of clinical "ladders." A *clinical ladder* is a system that promotes nurses on the basis of their ability to meet specific performance criteria. Nurses differentiated through clinical ladders function at levels that expand both their responsibility and their accountability based on role expectations and clinical expertise. Movement through a clinical ladder is most frequently voluntary, allowing individual nurses to self-determine their own level of differentiation.

Another approach to differentiated practice involves case management. Several case-management systems have been described and operationalized, the most prevalent being the New England–Tufts and Carondelet models.[26] These systems focus on accountability and responsibility of the individual nurse for the planning and evaluation of nursing services to a trauma patient and family throughout the cycle of recovery. This service extends into the home environment. The case associate is responsible for complete nursing care during episodic hospitalizations based on the case manager's plan for nursing care. The case-management system has several similarities with a primary nursing system of care delivery, with two distinct differences. Within the case management system, it is recognized that not all trauma patients require the services of case management. Less complex patients who have rapid and uncomplicated recoveries without anticipation of relapse or prolonged illness typically do not require a case manager. In a primary nurse system, all patients are usually assigned to a primary nurse. Additionally, the case manager concentrates on planning, coordinating, and evaluating patient care and performing specific direct nursing care activities on a selected basis. The primary nurse usually performs the entire spectrum of nursing practice for the trauma patient.

Proposals for Change in Delivery Systems

Several elements have emerged that indicate a need to restructure the delivery of trauma care within the hospital setting. These elements include the shortage of registered nurses, the prospective payment system, consumer expectations, and federal, state, and independent regulatory agencies that have placed increased emphasis on standardization of practice, as well as continuous monitoring of the quality of care.[27] Any system that is used as a method of nursing care delivery to trauma patients must be created within a patient-centered environment. There needs to be a commitment to excellence in trauma nursing practice, with emphasis on quality of care outcomes. It is also necessary to contribute to the fiscal health of the organization through cost containment and a high level of productivity. The ideal system of trauma care delivery will be one through which both patients and staff can be empowered.

Two essential components of any system of nursing care delivery are work distribution and accountability for the appropriate standard of care. Important elements include patient assignment or individual nurse workload, initial patient assessment, planning of care, continuous patient reassessment, coordinating and providing necessary interventions, patient education, communication of patient information, and documentation. Within each of these elements is a defined standard of practice based on institutional policies and procedures. Models of nursing care delivery—such as team, primary, and case management—each address these elements differently by identifying the scope of practice and work responsibilities differently.

Proposals for improving the delivery of nursing care in hospitals include the following suggestions, regardless of the model of nursing care delivery system used:

- Develop roles for assistive nursing personnel or nurse extenders—persons who are available and equipped to assist with selected direct care clinical activities as well as certain indirect responsibilities.
- Restructure the roles of support services and health care disciplines to make their work more patient-centered rather than departmentally segmented.
- Implement labor-saving technologies, such as computer systems that are departmentally integrated, allowing improved information flow.
- Restructure the role of the registered nurse to increase her authority, accountability, and autonomy.

Support Personnel

Anticipating change should lead to retrospective learning from previous experience. In the past, widespread use of nursing assistants has decreased the time spent by registered nurses in direct patient care, with the exception of selected tasks, such as medication administration. The resulting increase of nonprofessional direct care may have affected quality, as well as patient outcome. Emphasis on length of hospital stay was one impetus for increasing the percentages of professional care providers. Assistive personnel should be used to augment, not replace, the practice of the professional nurse. Structuring of the nonprofessional's activities can occur by standardization of educational requirements and defined authorization through state practice acts to perform specific functions delegated and supervised by a licensed nurse. Maximizing individual performance also occurs by assigning the nonprofessional to a nurse rather than to a patient. Permanent, dedicated working relationships between a professional nurse and a nurse extender can help to avoid potential patient care problems and allow the registered nurse to redirect her own patient care to more complex issues that require professional judgment.[28] Providing adequate nurse extenders may ease the pressure on dwindling nursing resources while reducing the cost and maintaining the quality of patient care.

Support Services and Health Care Disciplines

Better use of support services can improve delivery of nursing services. Increasing the availability and response of a variety of workers can positively affect the time that nurses have to deliver nursing care.[29] Services such as secretarial, dietary, housekeeping, transport, equipment and supplies management, respiratory therapy, pharmacy, social service, and other nonnursing activities have important responsibilities within any health care setting. However, nursing is frequently called on to supplement or assume responsibility for these services in the absence of other personnel. This may be particularly true on off-shifts, weekends, and holidays, when nursing is frequently the department with the greatest representation within the hospital. Within any organization, objective evaluation of the costs related to nurses supplying these services rather than a less expensive worker may be helpful in obtaining the justification necessary to establish personnel availability.

Patient Satisfaction

With health care focusing increasingly on consumer satisfaction, patient perception of care has important implications. Judgments made by patients concerning their hospital experiences are often perceived to be areas in which nursing has responsibility. Attention to individual concerns is as important as patient expectations. A non-nurse unit representative can be responsible for answering patient call lights and providing amenities of care. Such an individual also can be effective in communicating relevant patient issues to the nurse. This type of worker can improve patient satisfaction while also allowing the nurse to provide more uninterrupted patient care.

Nurses spend approximately 48 minutes, or 10 per cent of their shift, in the direct preparation of therapies.[25] This includes preparing, dispensing, changing, labeling, and recording intravenous therapy solutions and other prescribed medications. Additional time is spent on completing pharmacy request slips or entering pharmacy orders into the computer, telephoning and transporting medications to and from the pharmacy, checking emergency carts, counting narcotics, and verifying physician orders. This is particularly true in the trauma setting because of the increased use of antibiotics, narcotics, total parenteral nutrition, and blood products. Many of these duties currently performed by nurses could be assumed by pharmacists, pharmacy technicians, or other unlicensed personnel. While many hospitals have instituted unit dose-distribution systems as well as intravenous admixture programs, very few offer clinical services. A pharmacist or pharmacy technician, ideally satellited on the unit, could assist in the preparation of medications. Delivery, receipt, and timely administration of drugs would be enhanced because of decreased turnaround time and the integration of drug-distribution and clinical services. Cost-effectiveness is also demonstrated through reduced floor stock and increased drug-handling efficiency resulting in less wastage. Similarly, nurses frequently provide patient services that could be provided by respiratory therapists or less expensive technicians. Expansion of the role of these workers to include all therapies that may be performed within their scope of practice would release nurses to concentrate on appropriate nursing activities.

Clinical Information Systems

Effective and efficient delivery of nursing care depends on labor-saving technologies. Computerization is probably one of the most critically important technologies at this time. Health care, particularly in hospitals, has lagged significantly behind other industries in the installation of automated information systems. The primary reason for this relates to cost. Traditionally, priorities in hospital capital expenditures have centered on patient care equipment. Today, trauma systems and hospitals are beginning to recognize the need for sophisticated computer systems that address three different needs: a hospital information system, the departmental support system, and a clinical information system. Integration of all three is necessary if an automated system is to be used to full capacity.

Hospital Information Systems

Hospital information systems are designed to deal with the problem of moving data rapidly through a complex organization. This is important in the trauma setting because of the unpredictability of patient admission and the constant need for updated, current patient care data. Transactions such as admission, discharge, transfer, charging, and billing have priority. Departmental support systems, such as laboratory or pharmacy information systems, function primarily to enhance the efficiency of the department in both accomplishing some of the work and in recording and communicating it.

Clinical information systems serve to provide nurses, physicians, and other patient care workers with a means to convey and obtain patient information. Integration of all three systems and the ability to control and use information result in an important quality assurance benefit. Nursing's involvement in the selection of the information system and nursing's use of the system are critical to its ultimate effectiveness.

It has been estimated that 1 ½ hours per nursing service employee per 8-hour shift could be saved by using appropriate information technology.[30] Almost a third of a nurse's day is spent communicating patient information, some of which is clerical in purpose and some requiring professional judgment. The crucial contribution of information by nursing, matched with nursing's need for information, emphasized the requirement that nursing be involved in system choice.

Support for this involvement is reflected in the 1992 *Accreditation Manual for Hospitals*, in which the JCAHO specifies that nurses must "be involved in evaluating, selecting, and integrating healthcare technology and information management systems that support patient care needs and the efficient utilization of nursing resources." Defining the needs of nursing as they relates to information systems and staying involved throughout the entire selection process will be critical.

Cost Savings

With today's emphasis on cost-containment strategies, more hospitals are recognizing that computer systems can do more than save money through automation of information. They can generate money if the computer system improves the operation of the hospital. If the use of an automated system can effectively reduce operating expenses, the dollars saved can be spent in other areas of need. The installation of bedside computer terminals is based on this premise.

Point-of-Service Technology

Point-of-service technology is not a new concept. Bank tellers, ticket reservationists, and stock analysts do not share a central terminal. Neither do registration clerks in busy hospital admissions or emergency departments. Since nursing care delivery occurs primarily at the patient's bedside, automated systems that allow rapid, effective entry and retrieval of information can maximize the amount of time a nurse has to deliver care.

Trauma care in particular is enhanced through the use of clinical information systems. As patients progress through the cycles of care, plans can be communicated effectively.

Fiscal Management

Budgeting Nursing Personnel for Trauma Care

More than half of all hospital employees are nursing personnel, so nursing salaries are a significant part of any hospital budget.[31] Hospital and nursing administrators are dedicated to ensuring that the budgetary systems used to determine the cost of nursing personnel are as accurate and as objective as possible. The ability to project future cost trends is also important because budgets are most typically completed on an annual basis with minimal opportunity to influence it midyear.

Budget planning includes several factors, most of which fall in the category of either personnel, which is concerned with individual workers, or nonlabor, which relates to supplies and capital equipment. In the anticipation of preparing a budget demonstrating personnel costs, several issues that relate to trauma nursing specifically need to be considered. These include (1) the forecasted workload, which is the number of patient days anticipated for the unit, (2) the number of budgeted patient care hours that nursing has for trauma patient care on a daily basis, (3) planned productive and nonproductive time for individual workers, (4) the productivity goal for both the specific patient care area that is preparing the budget and the entire nursing department, and (5) the seasonality of trauma. Summer, weekends, and nights are times of greatest resource consumption and are cultural indicators to be addressed in budget planning.

The forecasted workload, or budgeted patient days, is most frequently determined by the hospital finance department through review of retrospective budget data, with addition of anticipated changes within the hospital that may affect workload. Nurse managers of trauma service are influential in decisions about workload because they recognize changes that need to be considered when determining workload. Increases or reductions in medical services can directly affect patient days, as can the installation of a new process, such as a clinical or management information system. New services of any type, even those intended to streamline a function, will slow work to some degree and require time for a learning curve to occur.

Patient Classification Systems

Budgeted patient care hours are determined in many ways, the most frequent of which is a patient classification system. Classification systems are not intended to relate to the medical diagnosis or condition of the patient. They are indicative of the time requirements for providing nursing care based on patient needs. In the case of trauma patients, this includes both instructional and emotional support needs.

The process of developing classification criteria for trauma patients involves definition of each criterion and testing of each criterion for validity. Training of staff in the use of the classification system is critical to successful implementation, as is consistent on-going evaluation of its use. Time related to the performance and management of the classification system itself should be built into the personnel budget.

Budgeting Supplies and Equipment for a Trauma Service

Budgeting supplies for an entire fiscal year requires an understanding of how to project patient supply use trends, census trends, and inflation. Trauma patients will require the use of supplies at differing rates depending on their reason for and length of hospitalization. Overall, trauma patients use supplies at a high rate as a result of the surgical nature of trauma and need for wound intervention. Success in ensuring that needed supplies are always available while also managing unit costs is directly related to a system that allows for two things to occur easily: ready availability of adequate supplies on the unit and a patient charging system that is performed with great ease at the time that the supplies are used. Budgeting for supplies and equipment needs to address these issues.

Historical trending of either the total numbers of supplies used per year or actual charges for supplies is necessary. To do so, use either figure for at least 4 to 5 years and the actual patient days for each year, and take an average of both. Divide the average number of supplies based on the budgeted patient days for the new fiscal year. A specific rate of inflation can then be added, which is typically calculated by the hospital fiscal management based on anticipated contractual increases. It is important at this time to anticipate any changes that may influence the need for supplies in the next year. Newly implemented services and the opening or closing of other patient units may cause significant fluctuations in census or type of patient. In addition, unusual expenses that may occur on a one time only basis during the year but may be costly also need to be anticipated and added into budget projections. This method is far from exact, but it serves to build an annual projection through use of accurate historical information.

Capital Equipment Expenditures

Budgeting for capital equipment expenditures typically requires significant justification because of the costs involved. Prioritization of capital expenses occurs on the basis of several factors. Equipment that will contribute to the revenue of the hospital will most likely receive high priority in the budget process. Ideally, the costs of the equipment and the anticipated annual operating costs will be either less than or at a minimum balanced against the revenue. Equipment necessary for patient safety and quality care is also given high priority in budgeting, even though there is no revenue anticipated directly from its use. The largest percentage of nursing capital equipment budgeted will fall into the latter category.

QUALITY ASSURANCE: TOTAL QUALITY MANAGEMENT

The concept of total quality management has emerged as the current and most comprehensive approach to ensuring excellence in patient care. It is accomplished through the establishment of standards and measurement of compliance with those standards. The primary focus is moving from quality assurance to continuous quality improvement and creating management systems that can address quality improvement in all areas of operation.

One current leader in the area of quality management is William Edward Deming, who is well known for having influenced the executives of Japan's leading industries, and is credited with having a role in the transformation and success of the Japanese economy.[32] One interesting aspect of Deming's management theory is his belief that there are direct relationships between quality, costs, productivity, and profit and that as quality increases, so does productivity. With increased productivity, costs decrease. This savings in costs can then be passed on to the consumer, who is receives a higher-quality product at a lower cost. The satisfied consumer returning to the company allows it to capture more market share, thrive in business, and provide more and better products. It is a win–win scenario for all involved. Deming's theory has applications within health care.

In any health care organization, there are three areas of major responsibility essential to survival: (1) patient results or outcome, (2) organizational performance, and (3) profit potential.[33] Individual employee behavior (performance) has an impact on both patient outcome and patient satisfaction, but frequently the organizational systems have more direct influence, either in a positive or a negative manner. Both patient outcome and consumer satisfaction (including the third-party payor) determine organizational profit and market share. Standards for all areas of hospital operation are used to provide guidelines for and define a desired level of performance and patient outcome. It is these standards that form the basis of a total quality management program with emphasis on continuous quality improvement.

Transition from Quality Assurance to Continuous Quality Improvement

The JCAHO has made some important modifications to its standards in order to foster continuous improvements in quality. Revisions in the 1992 *Accreditation Manual for Hospitals* include

- Emphasis on the role of leadership in improving quality.
- Expanding the scope of assessment and improvement activities beyond the clinical areas into the interrelated areas of governance, managerial support, and clinical process that all affect patient outcomes.
- Use of multiple sources of feedback (in addition to ongoing quality monitoring) to trigger evaluation and improvement of care and services.
- Organization of assessment and improvement activities around the flow of patient care and services, with particular attention to how the consumer and supplier relationships between departments and within departments can be improved.
- Focusing first on the processes of care and service rather than on the performance of individuals.
- Emphasis on continuous improvement rather than on problem solving.
- Maintaining improvement over time.

In 1982, JCAHO described the "10-Step Process for Monitoring and Evaluation," which 10 years later has been revised in order to place increased emphasis on continuous quality improvement (CQI).

Trauma Care Indicators

Areas within trauma nursing to examine for the development of indicators include direct patient care functions that are performed frequently or affect large numbers of patients. Examples of high-priority functions include patient admission, patient discharge, and patient teaching. Other high-priority indicators may be related to specific patient populations that are frequently managed in a specific area, such as an orthopedic unit. The concentration of orthopedic patients on a single unit allows for direct clinical evaluation of orthopedic nursing care through identification of indicators that relate to key factors of care.

Another area to examine for trauma care indicators involves functions that focus on a significant aspect of care and expose individual patients to a greater chance of adverse occurrences if the functions are not carried out correctly. These functions are sometimes referred to as *intrinsically risky*, even when they are performed perfectly, because certain attributes of the functions make them hazardous. Transfusion of blood is one example. There are many points along the continuum of blood handling and administration where a deficiency in the process may result in substantial patient harm or even death. Other trauma care indicators can be related to complex and/or new procedures. An example would be the introduction within the past 5 years of totally implanted devices that are used for long-term venous access. As a newly implemented nursing procedure, monitoring aspects of access and care of these devices could be considered a high-risk indicator because the functions required have been performed only a relatively few times.

The recent emphasis on continuous quality improvement empowers nursing to take a more active role in reviewing the services provided. It encourages nursing to communicate effectively among departments in terms of patient care requirements. It also encourages nurses to become leaders in systems innovation, constantly improving processes that relate to planning, production, and service.

Trauma Program Quality Management

Within a hospital-wide trauma program, nursing is only one aspect of care that requires quality management. A trauma quality management program needs integration of all services used by trauma patients in order to have a clear understanding of the total care provided to trauma patients.

The same process described for nursing quality improvement is also useful within a trauma quality improvement program, with emphasis on the need to evaluate trauma care on the basis of a systems approach. Areas of evaluation for trauma patients might include

- System access
- Prehospital triage
- Prehospital treatment
- Prehospital transport
- Emergency department resuscitation
- Operative intervention/postanesthesia recovery
- Intensive care
- General surgical care
- Rehabilitation

Almost all seriously injured patients move through each one of these cycles, so the care within each area should be evaluated. In addition, many hospital departments are often involved in providing a service to these patients, such as radiology, respiratory therapy, and social services. The service each department provides should be evaluated within the overall scope of care that a trauma patient receives. Trauma programs should define performance standards in all areas of trauma care, allowing for their monitoring as indicators. Each indicator should then be trending in an on-going manner, with problems identified and resolved. Historical trending of trauma program issues and problems is the best method of demonstrating programmatic growth corresponding with positive patient outcomes.

The review of trauma patients against indicators is frequently based on the trauma patient meeting specific criteria, which are sometimes called *quality screens* or *filters*. However, it is important that all trauma patients be reviewed through at least one mechanism in order to identify areas of needed improvement. One component of a trauma quality improvement program should be the patient-specific trending of risk incidents, as well as overall risk incident trending of the trauma patient population.

EDUCATION

Continuing Education

Most trauma center hospitals have specific requirements regarding the continued staff development of trauma nurses. Many require nurses to have a form of trauma certification, frequently obtained through successful completion of a trauma course designed to provide basic and advanced information on trauma nursing. Nurses frequently attend and participate in "Advanced Trauma Life Support," a course designed especially for nurses. Advanced courses in trauma care should be provided for veteran nursing staff on a regular basis. The following content information should be included in on-going trauma continuing education, as well as in a generic trauma course for the beginning trauma nurse:

1. Methods of trauma prevention and their current use
2. Principles of the mechanisms of traumatic injury and their application to clinical patient management
3. Description of the prehospital care system
4. Methods to anticipate and prepare for a patient's arrival
5. The components of the primary and secondary surveys
6. Demonstration of skills needed for performance of the primary and secondary surveys
7. Priorities of patient management based on assessment surveys
8. Methods of providing definitive care
9. Methods and goals of rehabilitation
10. Descriptions of the care of patients with specific injuries, including burns, smoke inhalation, drowning, poisoning
11. Differences in management of pediatric trauma patients
12. Common complications of traumatic injuries and their clinical management
13. Organ transplantation in relation to trauma
14. Current moral, legal, ethical, and political issues in trauma care

SUMMARY

Since trauma nursing administration is an interpersonal process, it relies greatly on managers to influence, motivate, catalyze, and facilitate activities that lead to the fulfillment of the organization's mission. The challenge of trauma care provides an unparalleled opportunity for innovative managers to effect systems changes. Although the challenges presented to the trauma nurse manager are constantly changing and evolving, it is the astute individual who uses this opportunity to design innovative systems that support quality outcomes.

REFERENCES

1. Cales RH, Heilig RW: Trauma Care Systems. Rockville, MD, Aspen, 1986.
2. Curtin L: Creating a culture of competence. Nurs Management 21(9):7–8, 1990.
3. JCAH Perspectives. A publication of the Joint Commission of Accreditation of Hospitals, March 1989.
4. Agenda for Change. A publication of the Joint Commission of Accreditation of Hospitals, March 1989.
5. Agenda for Change. A publication of the Joint Commission of Accreditation of Hospitals, September 1989.
6. Cales RH: Trauma mortality in Orange County: The effect of implementation of a regional trauma system. Ann Emerg Med 13:1–10, 1984.

7. Boyd DR, Crowley RA: Comprehensive regional trauma/emergency medical services (EMS) delivery systems: The United States experience. World J Surg 7:149–57, 1983.
8. McKoy C, Bell MJ: Preventable traumatic deaths in children. J Pediatr Surg 18:505–509, 1983.
9. Ramenofsky ML, Luterman A, Quindlen E, et al: Maximum survival in pediatric trauma: The ideal system. J Trauma 24:818–820, 1984.
10. Muller A, Bledsoe P: Physician's ranking of hospital attributes: A comparison by use group. Health Care Management Rev 14(3):77–84, 1989.
11. Daft RL: Organization Theory and Design, 3d ed. St. Paul, MN, Citadel Press, 1989.
12. Professional Research Consultants: Hospitals 63(9):8–11, 1989.
13. McConnell CR: Managing the Health Care Professional. Rockville, MD, Aspen, 1984.
14. O'Grady T, Finnegan S: Shared Governance for Nursing: A Creative Approach to Professional Accountability. Rockville, MD, Aspen, 1984.
15. Jenkins, JE: Professional governance: The missing link. Nurs Management 22(8):26–30, 1991.
16. Rungl KK, Dotson L: Self-scheduling for professional nurses. Nurs Management 20(2):42–44, 1989.
17. Smith HL, Mitry NW: Nursing leadership: A buffering perspective. Nurs Adm Q Spring 8(2):12–18, 1984.
18. Peters T: Thriving on Chaos. New York, Harper & Row, 1989.
19. McClure M, Poulin M, Sovie M, Wandelt M: Magnet Hospitals: Attraction and Retention of Professional Nurses. Kansas City, American Nurses Association, 1982.
20. Kramer M, Schmalenberg C: Magnet hospitals: Institutions of excellence, parts 1 and 2. JONA 18(1):13–24 and 19(2):11–19, 1988.
21. Kramer M: The magnet hospitals: Excellence revisited. JONA 20(3):30–35, 1989.
22. Herzberg F: Dual-factor theory of job satisfaction. Personnel Psych Winter, 1967.
23. Adams BA, Rentfro AR: Strengthening hospital nursing: An approach to restructuring care delivery. JONA 21(6):12–19, 1991.
24. Advance Practice Survey Results. National Council of State Boards of Nursing Report, 12(2), 1991.
25. Hendrickson G, Doddato T, Kovner C: How do nurses use their time? JONA 20(3):31–37, 1990.
26. Ethridge P, Lamb G: Professional nurse case management improves quality, access, and costs. Nurs Management 20(3):30–35, 1989.
27. Robinson NC: A patient-centered framework for restructuring care. JONA 21(9):29–32, 1991.
28. Manthey, M: Practice partnerships: The newest concept in care delivery. JONA 19(2):33–35, 1989.
29. Manthey M: Practice partnership (a nurse extender system). Nurs Management 19(3):58–59, 1988.
30. Mowry N, Korpman R: Evaluating automated information systems. Nurs Econ 5:7–12, 1987.
31. Villemaire M, Lane-McGraw C: Nursing personnel budgets: A step-by-step guide. Nurs Management 17(1):28–32, 1986.
32. Aguayo R: Mr. Deming. New York, Simon & Schuster, 1991.
33. Hoesing H, Kirk, R: Common sense quality management. JONA 20(10):10–15, 1990.

3

ECONOMIC ISSUES IN TRAUMA CARE

HOWARD R. CHAMPION, MARCIA S. MABEE, and ELLEN K. SHAIR

Editor's Note: This chapter addresses the magnitude of the problem of the cost of care for trauma patients in this country. The loss of trauma services resulting from cost cutbacks has had and will continue to have a devastating effect on our nation's greatest resource, its youth. The issues of cost are multidimensional. We thought it would be of value to include a comprehensive review of these issues so that trauma nurses would be cognizant of changes in reimbursement that have occurred to date and of the forces that drive the high cost of trauma care. In addition, we hope that the reader will come to understand the efforts required to support policies intended to continue and expand access to much-needed, highly specialized trauma services.

Injury, with its high personal, social, and economic costs, has been named the most serious public health problem in the United States.[1] Injury is the major cause of death among children and adults under age 45, and it is the fourth leading cause of all deaths in the nation.[1] Because of its disproportionate prevalence among the young, injury is the main cause of years of lost work life; at least 4 million productive work years are lost each year. The 1989 report entitled *Cost of Injury in the United States*[2] estimated that the total lifetime cost to the nation for both intentional and unintentional injury was $180 billion in 1988.[3] This is far greater than the cost of any other single disease, including cancer.

Trauma accounts for 12 per cent of hospital bed occupancy, almost 7 per cent of the nation's total health expenditures, and 14 per cent of the U.S. gross national product.[3–5, 5a] Each year, one in three Americans is injured; more than 160,000 die and 340,000 are permanently disabled.[1, 6–8] It is estimated that at least 25,000 of these deaths (16 per cent) could be prevented if regional systems of trauma care were in place nationwide.

The National Academy of Sciences focused attention on the nation's injury problem with its 1966 and 1985 studies.[1, 9] In the 1970s, the American College of Surgeons (ACS) published guidelines for establishing three levels of trauma center care. Through the years, these guidelines have expanded to provide a blueprint for implementing regional systems of trauma care.[10] As a result of these developments, specialized trauma care units in the United States currently number 457.[11] This, coupled with organized emergency medical services (EMS) systems providing more effective prehospital treatment and triage, has been instrumental in saving countless lives.[12, 13]

Trauma care providers, however, are on the front lines of the nation's on-going health care crisis and face an uncertain future. The scenario that threatens trauma care is a complicated one. First, the number of people who cannot afford insurance coverage has risen astronomically, especially among young adults. A recent Census Bureau study showed, for example, that fully one-half of those between the ages of 18 and 21 lacked health insurance for at least 1 month between 1987 and 1989.[14] The combination of poverty and youth has become predictive of a higher rate of injury. (For example, it is well documented that unfavorable socioeconomic conditions create a climate that fosters violence.[15, 16]) Further, the per-unit cost of in-hospital trauma care is approximately three times the cost of other types of hospital care.[12, 17] Therefore, the highest costs are incurred by those who can least afford to pay them: typically the young and uninsured. Another complicating factor is the inadequate rate of reimbursement for trauma services by government medical assistance programs like Medicaid and Medicare. These and other factors are proving lethal to the nation's trauma centers. In a 1991 General Accounting Office (GAO) study,[18] the closure of more than 60 U.S. trauma centers was attributed to the problem of uncompensated care, i.e., the gap between costs and payments. A 1992 telephone survey conducted through the Eastern Association for the Surgery of Trauma (EAST) revealed that uncompensated care was responsible for the closure of a total of 92 trauma centers between 1985 and 1991.[11]

In this chapter we will further describe the components of regional trauma systems, weigh the benefits and costs, detail the forces that threaten to weaken or destroy these systems, offer solutions on the federal and state/local level, provide some conclusions about the cost-effectiveness of trauma care, and speculate briefly on the potential impacts of impending health care reform on trauma systems.

REGIONAL TRAUMA SYSTEMS

Severe trauma is a time-sensitive disease; without prompt intervention, trauma victims often die or suffer permanent disability between 1 and 4 hours after injury. More specifically, the first 60 minutes after a severe injury, known as the "golden hour," is the focus of most trauma center efforts because it is during this period that the most lives are saved and permanent disability has the best chance of being prevented or minimized. Other characteristics of severe trauma are that it frequently occurs at night and on weekends; effective response often requires maximum use of hospital resources during times when most hospitals would prefer to reduce staffing levels. Further, of all those injured, only a relatively small proportion sustain injuries severe enough to require the advanced technology and expertise available at a trauma center. Improved patient outcomes are directly proportional to patient volume and the resultant expertise gained by health care providers.[19] For these reasons, trauma care should be restrictive, confined to a few committed institutions, focused, and, above all, prompt.

The Korean War and the Vietnam conflict taught the U.S. medical community valuable lessons about responding to traumatic injury, introducing, in particular, the use of helicopters and triage techniques for prehospital care and the use of mobile army surgical hospitals (MASH units) as movable trauma centers. These concepts have been expanded to three-tiered regional systems that consist of (1) prehospital care, the first opportunity to save the 50 per cent of trauma patients who die before reaching a hospital, (2) trauma centers, which are organized by the level of care they are capable of providing, and (3) rehabilitation, the final stage in the spectrum of trauma care. Therefore, regional systems of trauma care are organized to meet the needs of the severely injured individual from the moment of injury until discharge. The three phases of this holistic approach are described below.

Prehospital Care

The elements of prehospital care are

- Triage—appropriate identification of the nature and extent of injury
- Treatment—application of advanced trauma life support (ATLS) techniques by prehospital personnel
- Transport—prompt transfer to a qualified trauma center via ambulance or helicopter

Trauma Center

Trauma center care includes resuscitation and other surgical or nonsurgical emergency treatment as necessary. Trauma centers operate in designated hospitals and are stratified according to criteria developed by the ACS.[20] Level I trauma centers provide 24-hour immediate care by in-house trauma surgeons and physicians. Hospitals with level I trauma centers are active in trauma research, teaching, and trauma system development. Criteria for level II trauma centers vary throughout the country; however, these centers must have physical facilities similar to level I centers, a trauma team coordinator in-house around the clock, and on-call surgeons no more than 20 to 30 minutes away. Level III trauma centers are set up to provide ATLS services to patients in rural areas. Because they do not have sophisticated facilities or trauma teams, one responsibility of level III trauma center physicians and surgeons is patient triage, when required, to the nearest level I or II trauma center.

Rehabilitation

The rehabilitation process begins in the acute phase and continues after hospital discharge, either in the outpatient/home setting or rehabilitation center. Rehabilitation gives certain trauma patients the greatest chance to regain productive functioning.

BENEFITS AND COSTS OF TRAUMA SYSTEMS

Studies have demonstrated that organized regional systems of trauma care can significantly improve survival and reduce the level of disability that otherwise results from severe injury.[21–24] For example, after only 1 year of operation, implementation of regional trauma systems in several major metropolitan areas reduced the preventable death rate by half. Between 20,000 and 25,000 Americans die each year because of inadequate technology or unskilled personnel at the nearest hospital.[25] Most of these unnecessary deaths would be prevented if regional trauma systems that ensure prompt access to a qualified trauma center were in place across the nation, thus reducing the 20 to 30 per cent preventable mortality rate to 2 to 3 per cent.[21]

On a local level, following implementation of a trauma system in Orange County, California, preventable deaths declined from 34 to 15 per cent, with most of the latter resulting when treatment was not rendered in a trauma center.[21] In San Diego County, California, trauma deaths fell 55 per cent in the first year of trauma system implementation, and the preventable death rate dropped from 13.6 to 2.7 per cent.[23, 26] In Washington, D.C., trauma deaths declined 50 per cent over a 5-year period at one trauma center after implementation of that city's trauma system.[22] The most recent validation of the role of trauma centers in saving lives is a 1992 study by Rutledge and colleagues[24] in which multivariate population-based analysis revealed that the presence of a trauma center was a main cause of declining trauma death rates, by county, in North Carolina.

Outcome studies of the severely injured who are treated in qualified, designated trauma centers have shown dramatically improved outcomes.[27] At least 80 per cent of these individuals return to full-time productivity within 4 years of their injury, with most resuming full-time activities within 1 year of injury.[28–30]

Providing this highly skilled, often technologically intensive, 24-hour care, however, is very expensive. The approximated 1991 cost (estimated at 65 per cent of charges) of the average non-trauma acute care admission was $3,428, while the equivalent trauma admission ranged from $6,640 to $14,942, with an average of almost $9,902.[12] In some parts of the country, however, trauma care costs can average three to four times the national figure.[31] The higher expense of trauma care is due to the expensive resources, both in terms of equipment and specially trained personnel, that must be maintained in constant readiness. Helicopters and state-of-the-art diagnostic and treatment modalities are costly to acquire and maintain. Further, intensive care and extended hospital stays add to costs (e.g., 57 per cent of major trauma patients require intensive care unit care, vs. 19 per cent of nontrauma patients).[11] Finally, the rehabilitative care component ranges from 6 to 30 per cent of costs, depending on severity of injury.[31] In the United States, the total cost of initial hospitalization or injury can be estimated at $22.4 billion in 1991 dollars.[29] Severe injury accounts for almost half this amount.

The situation will only worsen. As reported almost daily in the media, the nation's health care costs continue to spiral. By the end of 1993, U.S. health care spending will approach $940 billion (up from $738 billion in 1991 and $839 billion in 1992), accounting for a highr percentage (over 14 per cent) of the gross national product than in any other country.[5a, 32, 33] Significant annual increases (estimated at 12 to 15 per cent) are projected to result in health care expenditures exceeding $1 trillion in 1994, with increasing monopolization of the GNP.[33a] Unchecked, health care spending (which accounted for 6 per cent of the GNP in 1960), is expected to account for 17 per cent of the GNP by the year 2000 and 44 per cent by the year 2030.[34, 34a] Further, health care increases outpace inflation, for example, a compounded rate of 9.1 per cent for medical care for the first quarter of 1991 compared with a 6.1 per cent increase in the consumer price index in 1990.[34b] At this rate, costs could more than double by the year 2000, greatly enlarging the already gaping holes in what the Conference on Metropolitan Hospital Associations (CMHA) calls "a Swiss-cheese style safety net that no longer protects the disadvantaged and dispossessed in our society."[35]

THE CRISIS IN TRAUMA CENTER REIMBURSEMENT

Who pays these enormous costs? In short, an alarming number of people have no insurance and cannot or do not pay any, or even part, of their medical bills, which results in hospitals and trauma centers absorbing the costs. Further, government programs do not provide medical coverage for all who are injured and do not pay for all the medical expenses of those who are covered. These factors pose a real threat to the viability of trauma centers, which operate at huge deficits that continue to grow year after year.

Uncompensated Care

A recent Census Bureau study of 1987–1990 data revealed that 50 million people, one out of every five, did not have health insurance for at least 1 month at any given point in 1987, with an average monthly total of 32 million, or 13 per cent of the population, uninsured.[14] The situation is often worse in urban areas, where almost 45 per cent of the trauma patients admitted to most urban trauma centers are uninsured.[18] And these figures are increasing at an alarming rate. The number of uninsured individuals under age 65 grew from 28.4 million in 1979 to almost 37 million in 1986 to more than 40 million in 1990.[14]

The American Hospital Association reports that between 1980 and 1986 the amount of uncompensated care (charity care plus bad debt, minus state and local tax appropriations) that hospitals provided more than doubled, outpacing health care inflation by 40 per cent. Nationally, estimates indicate that the uninsured account for 68 per cent of these costs. Uncompensated care costs, which hospitals had to absorb, increased from $3 billion in 1980 to $7.2 billion in 1986, representing 5 percent of total hospital costs.[35] By 1988, the amount of uncompensated care provided by U.S. hospitals had risen to $8.3 billion. A conservative estimate places $1 to $2 billion (12–24 per cent) of this figure for acute trauma care (initial hospitalization and professional fees only).[12, 36] On the local level, bad debt alone accounted for a total loss of approximately $16 million in fiscal year 1988 for the five Washington, D.C., hospitals that provide level I trauma service.[12]

Inadequate Reimbursement

The other major contributor to this difficult scenario is the problem of inadequate reimbursement for trauma services by public medical assistance programs such as Medicaid and Medicare. Medicaid, or title XIX of the Social Security Act, was signed into law in 1965 to provide joint federal and state assistance with medical costs for the economically disadvantaged. Also in 1965, under title XVIII of the Social Security Amendments, the Medicare program was created to provide similar assistance for those over the age of 65. Currently, Medicaid pays for 11 per cent of the nation's health care costs.[37]

Restrictive Medicaid Coverage

Problems with Medicaid are many and greatly affect the delivery of trauma care. The first is that although the program was set up to protect the poor from devastating medical bills, very few uninsured trauma patients—who tend to be young, male, and able-bodied workers or students prior to injury—actually qualify for Medicaid coverage. Permanent disability from injury is almost always the prerequisite for qualification for Medicaid for a young male. Consequently, a patient with a gunshot wound to the abdomen requiring a 3-month stay in a surgical intensive care unit but who sustains no permanent disability would not be eligible for Medicaid coverage. Only 8 per cent of Washington Hospital Center trauma patients, for example, were covered by Medicaid in 1989 (14 per cent received D.C. Medical Assistance and 42 per cent lacked insurance of any kind).[12] Medicaid, which originally covered over 60 per cent of those in need, covered only 45 per cent in 1986 and undoubtedly covers a far lower proportion today.[38] And there are wide variations in coverage throughout the country because each state can link Medicaid eligibility to any income level it chooses. Medicaid coverage for trauma care may depend on whether a state has a medically needy program and, if so, what levels and criteria for "neediness" are operating and what levels of reimbursement and limits on coverage apply.[12]

Services that are covered by Medicaid are not reimbursed at a level that adequately covers costs, and Medicaid payments do not keep pace with inflation. Nationwide, annual losses attributed by trauma centers to inadequate Medicaid reimbursement ranged from $58,000 to $3.3 million, and more than a dozen states recently have challenged this low level of reimbursement in the courts.[18] In fiscal year 1989, D.C. Medicaid reimbursed the Washington Hospital Center (WHC) at a rate of only 18 per cent of charges (29 per cent of costs) for care of trauma patients.[12] When added to the losses incurred by bad debt, Washington, D.C., trauma patients alone cost hospitals more than $10 million in 1990[12] (Fig. 3–1). Losses of this type often force trauma centers to close, restrict patient access (e.g., at Houston's Hermann Hospital, which had to set a limit on the number of trauma patients it will admit), or remove resources in favor of more lucrative medical services in order to stay afloat.

A complicating factor is reimbursement for rehabilitation services. Because of the high financial losses associated with trauma care, trauma centers have a financial incentive to release their patients as soon as possible to rehabilitation facilities.[39] Medicaid, however, not only frequently fails to pay for entry of the uninsured trauma patient into the trauma system but also, like private insurers, often restricts coverage for rehabilitation to acute inpatient care only. The accepted approach to rehabilitative care generally calls for several weeks of inpatient care and then outpatient visits, home care services, and, simultaneously, use of durable medical equipment.[12] Failure to pay for some or all of these critical services (depending on the state) often halts the restoration of an otherwise disabled individual, who imposes huge costs on the health care system, to a functioning, contributing member of society.

Medicare Prospective Payment System

By the 1980s, federal reimbursement for health services was becoming a far bigger budget item than anticipated. In 1983, in an effort to contain hospital costs, which rose over 300 per cent between 1960 and 1972, the Health Care Financing Administration (HCFA) introduced a system of prospective payment for hospital services based on the concept of diagnosis-related groups (DRGs).[4, 40] DRGs collapse all of an individual patient's various diagnoses into the single most severe or complex diagnosis and assign a predetermined average length of stay (LOS) and associated fixed amount for reimbursement. The DRG system is used by the Medicare program, by at least 14 states under the Medicaid program, and in a few states (e.g., New Jersey) by all payors. Cost-containment efforts have recently been expanded to include physician services for surgery, including trauma care, under the resource-based relative value scale (RBRVS).

Use of DRGs has substantially reduced payments and subsequently dried up the profit margins that had helped cover the growing costs of uncompensated care. A 1988 study by the Prospective Payment Assessment Review Commission

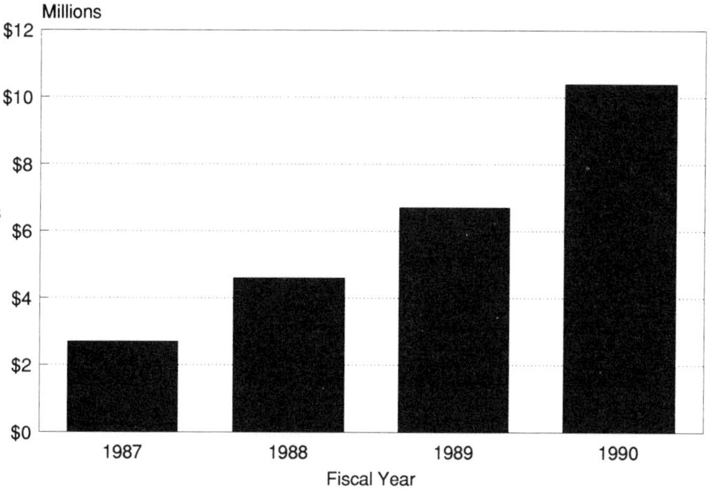

Figure 3–1. Washington Hospital Center D.C. trauma care losses in costs. Includes self-pay/contractual losses.

revealed that hospitals' Medicare revenue margins (Medicare payments less costs) declined from 14 per cent in 1984–1985 to 2 per cent in 1987 to zero in 1988.[40a]

DRGs are extraordinarily poor descriptors of injury, burying the complex list of diagnoses that generally accompanies multisystem trauma with other diseases and procedures. Because DRGs do not take into account the severity of injury and the necessarily higher costs of trauma care, trauma centers and other institutions that accept trauma patients are not adequately reimbursed for the services they perform.[40] Studies have shown that the DRG system covers anywhere from 0 to 50 per cent of the actual hospital costs of acute trauma care.[40–43] DRGs do not account for the cost involved in treating trauma patients, who often have multiple injuries and complications, nor do they adequately account for the comorbid factors and complications that are typical of geriatric trauma patients. As a trauma patient's bill increases, so does the trauma center's losses. For a bill of $10,000, for example, an estimated 150 per cent of the designated DRG would need to be collected just to break even.[4] The situation subsequently worsens every year because DRGs fail to keep pace with inflation. And, while at present comparatively few (8–11 per cent) severe trauma patients are elderly and covered by Medicare, they consume a disproportionate share (25 per cent) of trauma care resources. Further, the aging trend in the U.S. population is expected to result in this group's accounting for 39 per cent of trauma admissions by the year 2050.[36] Before implementing large-scale healthcare reform, the Clinton administration has proposed many short-term cost-containment measures.[43a] Together, Medicare and Medicaid are expected to be cut by more than $62 billion over a five-year period.[43b] For Medicare, 25 "short-term savings proposals" are listed; at least two have ominous overtones for trauma care. In one, radiology, anesthesia, and pathology services would be included in the already insufficient hospital DRG payment instead of being billed separately by physicians. Adoption of this measure would place an additional financial burden on hospitals, providing further disincentive to offer costly trauma care services, which depend heavily on the auxiliary services above. In the second, financial disincentives for primary surgeons to use surgical assistants (which increase with the skill level of the assistant) have direct implications for quality of care.

Resource-Based Relative Value Scale

In an attempt to reform Medicare's physician reimbursement policy, a resource-based relative value scale (RBRVS) was implemented by HCFA in 1992. Under RBRVS, physician reimbursement for services is determined by physician resources expended (including time and intensity of effort) and expenses (including malpractice insurance). Planned to be fully effective by 1996, RBRVS poses two major threats to trauma care reimbursement.[44] First, the global surgical fee lumps together pre-and postoperative care, an approach that severely undervalues the effort expended on trauma patients with multisystem injuries who need the services of specialists from many different disciplines. Further, proposed codes severely undervalued the work of critical care physicians, although recent code revisions have partially corrected this undervaluing. HCFA's final response to these and other problems with RBRVS will have a significant effect on trauma care reimbursement.

Effects on Provision of Trauma Care

These factors have reduced hospitals' operating margins and dramatically weakened their ability to cover uncompensated costs generated by inadequate reimbursement and mounting bad debt. In fact, many designated trauma centers are losing anywhere between $1 million and $10 million annually. Total losses for trauma care reported by 28 institutions in their most recent year of operation were $65.5 million.[18] An internal study of trauma patients treated at the Washington Hospital Center in 1989 found that 42 per cent of the patients who resided in Washington D.C., were uninsured and also were ineligible for Medicaid. Consequently, the hospital was reimbursed for only 16 per cent of costs.[12] In another example, Detroit Receiving Hospital, which operates primarily as a trauma center, had $30 million in unpaid bills for 1989 alone.[45] In Texas, uncompensated care of more than 30,000 trauma patients in 1989 alone resulted in losses of $157.5 million (25 per cent of total costs), with each trauma hospital losing between $0.8 and $8.3 million.[46] Chicago's six trauma centers (down from 10 in 1986) sustained losses totaling $12 million in 1991, mainly due to the high costs of caring for victims of drug violence whose volume has increased 29 per cent between 1990 and 1991 and who have much more severe injuries (i.e., multiple gunshot wounds) than ever before.[11] Cases such as that of a drug-related gunshot wound victim whose trauma care and subsequent 5-month hospitalization cost $190,000 are common, as is the shockingly poor amount recovered for payment; in this case, Medicaid covered only $5000, 3 per cent of the total charges.[45]

In the past, hospitals were able to shift much of their uncompensated care costs to privately insured patients, in effect subsidizing their uninsured patients by charging higher prices to their insured patients.[12] These inflated prices were, in turn, passed on to the insured patients' employers in the form of higher premiums. This forced many large employers to change to managed care plans, reduce or eliminate benefits, or withdraw entirely from the commercial insurance scene and set up their own insurance carriers. The escalating proportion of self-insuring employers, along with the rapidly growing number of managed care plans, has forced hospitals to be more competitive in their pricing to attract patients. As a consequence, hospitals have been forced into the classic strategy of supply versus demand; i.e., they often must discount their rates in an effort to increase patient volume and therefore have less income to cover the rising costs of uncompensated care.

These financial problems are exacerbated by worsening social ills such as drug and alcohol abuse, poverty, gang violence, homelessness, and mental illness, which have a tremendous impact on the medical community, especially in urban areas.[35] Some urban trauma centers, affected by increased violence (both in incidence and severity) stemming from drug-related activity, have seen their losses double in the past 2 years. "Not only is the number of [drug-related] gunshot victims increasing," stated the director of Chicago's Cook County Hospital Trauma Unit, "but their wounds are becoming more difficult and expensive to treat—thanks to the replacement of 'Saturday night specials' with higher-power, semiautomatic and automatic assault weapons."[11]

Mounting costs have forced many hospital administrators to close down their trauma services in order to protect the financial viability of their institutions and to preserve other vital community services. A study of trauma center closures found the top three reasons to be (1) the high costs of providing uncompensated care to uninsured or underinsured patients, (2) high operating costs, and (3) inadequate reimbursement by medical assistance programs.[47] The 1991 GAO study[18] concurred with these findings in that closure was primarily due to financial losses from trauma care provided to the uninsured and underinsured (i.e., patients covered by public programs). The GAO study also pointed out that the provision of trauma care could be considered an institutional burden for a hospital in that it disrupts nontrauma care and uses high-demand resources such as specialty beds, operating room time, and blood bank and laboratory services.

Closing trauma centers, however, in addition to placing the population served at increased risk, has the domino effect of placing additional economic pressure on the centers that remain open, making more of them likely to buckle under the same strains. With each day that passes, hospital administrators, to protect the financial viability of their institutions and their overall mission to their communities, consider withdrawing resources from the injured patient in favor of patients who can pay.[12] Although certain patient populations other than trauma patients are poor payors (e.g., neonates and AIDS patients), they have strong, specialized constituencies to work for preservation and even expansion of services. Conversely, trauma care, which provides a safety net for all segments of the population, is disproportionately burdened by those who have no constituency (i.e., the young, the poor, and the uninsured) and is, therefore, particularly vulnerable to "medical apartheid"—or rationing of services by ability to pay.

In the past 7 years, 92 designated trauma centers have withdrawn from regional trauma systems or have shut down operations altogether due to financial losses. The number of trauma centers in Los Angeles County, California, for example, dropped from 23 in 1984 to 16 in 1989 to 10 in 1990.[4, 35] In Dade County, Florida, the number dropped from 8 to 1.[4] As a consequence, the preventable death toll will undoubtedly rise, as will the number of seriously injured individuals who will become permanently disabled at great societal cost.

RECOMMENDATIONS

Many solutions have been proposed to avert a collapse of trauma care systems. These solutions range from modest changes to the current system to far-reaching programs that would completely restructure the nation's health care delivery system. The remainder of this chapter will focus on proposed solutions to address the economic challenges facing trauma care providers.

Federal Initiatives

In its quest to simultaneously provide affordable health care to all Americans and control runaway costs, the Clinton administration has focused on the dual-pronged concept of managed competition combined with budget caps. As described by Starr and Zelman among others, managed competition would be effected by "health alliances" that would act as purchasing managers by providing consumers with information on cost and quality of care and negotiating discounts with health care plans.[47a] Both the proposed short-term fixes and systemic reform under a managed competition model are likely to have drastic, unfavorable consequences for trauma care. First, cuts in Medicaid and Medicare will worsen the already untenable reimbursement situation. Second, managed competition incorporates many elements of health maintenance organization (HMO) plans, that have, in their short history, exhibited practices that hinder trauma care delivery. These include roadblocks to immediate care such as plan exclusions/conditions and patient disposition according to cost rather than medical considerations (i.e., cost-driven interhospital transfers). The time-sensitive nature of trauma (as well as ethical and legal considerations) precludes consideration of any but essential medical factors in the patient care decision.

Conspicuous by its absence in the current dialogue on health care reform is any mention of trauma care. Whatever model is chosen, however, must ensure access to care for the severely injured by supporting, not destroying, the nation's weakening trauma systems and by acting to preserve trauma centers. As outlined by Champion and Mabee,[12] the federal government has many potential avenues for action on these fronts.

Institute a System of Universal Access

Trauma care would be well served by a federal program to ensure universal access to the nation's health care system. Elements of this approach, introduced by the U.S. Bipartisan Commission on Comprehensive Reform (the Pepper Commission), include guaranteed health coverage to all workers and their dependents, guaranteed coverage for nonworkers through federal subsidies, and establishment of cost-containment and budgetary initiatives at the federal level.[48]

Develop a Trauma Financing Pool

To reduce the staggering $1 to $2 billion annual loss from uncompensated care, the federal government could create a federal/state/private sector financing pool to reimburse those ACS-accredited trauma centers for documented uncompensated care losses in the areas of acute hospitalization, physician services, and rehabilitation care. The financing pool should aim to accumulate at least $1 billion in assets annually, with a 50:50 federal/state match.

Federal matching funds could be raised, in part, by taxing the use of goods that have been proven to contribute to a disproportionate amount of health care costs: alcohol, tobacco, firearms and firearm-related products (e.g., bullets), and motor vehicles.

Alcohol is a factor in at least half of the approximately 42,500 fatal motor vehicle accidents that occur each year and in countless motor vehicle accidents that result in temporary as well as permanent disability, at an estimated annual cost of $46 billion.[48a] And it often is not the drinker who is injured; in the 22,084 alcohol-related traffic deaths that occurred in 1990, 8500 victims (35 per cent) had not been drinking prior to the accident.[49] The level of blood alcohol has been shown to be directly proportional to severity of injury and patient outcome.[52, 53] The use of alcohol also has been listed as a contributing factor in stabbings (75 per cent), drownings/boating accidents (68 per cent), homicides (64 per cent), burns (61 per cent), domestic violence (56 per cent), fatal falls (50 per cent), rapes (50 per cent), and suicides (30 per cent).[51, 54–57] Alcohol-related medical care costs for injury have been shown to be three times as high as those in which alcohol is not a factor, and problem drinkers seek medical attention for injuries at a rate 1.6 times higher than do nondrinkers.[58]

A 1981 study[59] indicates that the high costs (including collectively financed health insurance, pensions, motor vehicle accidents, disability insurance and group life insurance, as well as court costs) imposed by alcohol consumers classified as "heavy drinkers" could be recovered by raising federal and state taxes on alcohol. A 1989 economic analysis[60] reveals that alcohol consumption costs the public 48 cents per ounce, while the average federal and state excise and sales tax on alcohol totals only 23 cents per ounce.[61] Because alcohol is such a major contributor to violence and accidents, particularly motor vehicle accidents, a strong case can be made for raising federal alcohol taxes and allocating a certain percentage for trauma care.[12] Raising the federal excise tax on beer and wine to the level of that for distilled spirits and then correcting for inflation could produce an estimated $20.6 billion in revenues, with the additional benefit that consumption would likely drop in response to a price increase, subsequently averting 8400 to 11,000 (19–25 per cent) alcohol-related traffic deaths each year.[59, 62]

Increasing the tax on tobacco products also should be considered because one-fourth of the U.S. population are smokers and smoking is thought to be the nation's leading cause of preventable death.[63, 64] At least 434,000 people per year (more than 1000 per day) die from smoking-related illness (cancer, chronic obstructive pulmonary disease, and heart disease) or injury (including burns).[64, 65] The annual health care and other costs of smoking are approximately $52 million, and smokers pay approximately 7 cents per pack more in medical costs than do nonsmokers.[66, 67]

The federal–state match could be augmented by contributions from the private sector to provide the base for supporting trauma systems. Increased federal regulation of the insurance industry could encourage this private-sector participation. States, in turn, could fund their portion by imposing value-added taxes on firearms and motor vehicle licensing and registration, by increasing the fines for traffic violations, and by adding sales tax to firearms-related products such as ammunition.

Expand Medicaid Eligibility for the Severely Injured

To eliminate the inequitable variations in state eligibility requirements for Medicaid that deny medical coverage for such a large number of people, the federal government should set a national standard income requirement for eligibility.[68] In addition, a transitional partial-subsidy program should be established between Medicaid and expensive private insurance to cover the large numbers of people whose incomes place them just over the Medicaid eligibility cutoff.[68] And for the otherwise uninsured trauma patient specifically, a Medicaid "catastrophic" plan is needed, which would provide reimbursement at a rate of 80 per cent of acute care and rehabilitative services.[12]

Because the highest costs are incurred by patients who sustain the most severe injuries, Medicaid coverage should be expanded to cover all severely injured trauma patients who are treated in ACS-accredited trauma centers. The definition of *severe injury* has been refined and well documented in the literature. Injuries are classified by ICD-9-CM (*International Classification of Diseases*, 9th revision, *Clinical Modification*) codes for purposes of standardization. The codes that represent trauma-related injuries generally fall in the 800 to 959 range (excluding certain ranges) and include, for example, blunt and penetrating injuries, poisonings, and burns.[69] Injury severity can be quantified by the Injury Severity Score (ISS), a summary measure of anatomic injury based on an ascending severity scale of 1 to 75, and/or the revised trauma score (RTS), a physiologic measure of injury severity that assigns numerical values (on a descending severity scale of 0 to 8) to the patient's respiratory rate, systolic blood pressure, and Glasgow coma scale score.[70, 71]

That losses mount as severity of injury increases is documented in a 1988 study of the 103,644 trauma patients discharged from Florida's 226 hospitals. In this study, the average hospital charge for patients with an ISS in the 1 to 8 range (nonserious) was $5332; the average hospital charge for those with an ISS of 9+ (more severe) was $24,725, almost five times higher.[72] And reimbursement is inversely proportional to injury severity. In the preceding study, the reimbursement rate dropped more than 10 per cent between the ISS 1 to 8 and ISS 15 + patient groups. If Medicaid were to cover trauma and rehabilitation services for the severely injured, trauma centers would gain better footing in their precarious financial situation.

Revise Prospective Payment for Trauma Care

Adapting the DRG system to account for severity of injury or implementation of diagnostically based trauma-related groupings (TRGs) that utilize recognized trauma-specific guidelines will help close the gap between costs and reimbursement.[12] Current initiatives in this area include categorization systems that more truly calculate the resource needs for trauma care, such as that adopted by the state of Florida for level I trauma patients.[73]

Earmark Trauma Care in Proposals Addressing the Uninsured

Trauma care in the United States is clearly in crisis, manifesting perhaps the most visible symptom of the ills that affect the country's health care system as a whole. Consequently, health care policy initiatives need to be developed that are responsive to the unique demands of trauma care. Proposals that seek to provide health care benefits for the uninsured should include appropriate trauma care and accompanying rehabilitative care as part of any benefit package. A specific, coordinated trauma services benefit should be included in all proposals to finance health care for the uninsured, whether they address expansion of the Medicaid program, mandates for employers, insurance risk pools, or other such proposals. The trauma care portion of the benefit package should provide for comprehensive trauma care services, including rehabilitative care, with coverage for acute care limited to that provided in a designated trauma center and limited to instances of severe injury (ISS 9+) or life-threatening injury (ISS 15+). This type of benefit would ensure access to regional trauma care systems for severely injured individuals by providing for 1 year of coordinated trauma care (acute, rehabilitative, and follow-up) at an ACS-accredited trauma center. To be eligible for reimbursement under the benefit, trauma center hospitals would need to be active participants in regional systems of trauma care. Patients, in turn, would need to be severely injured according to accepted triage guidelines to qualify for coverage (trauma score of ≤ 12 or an ISS of ≥ 10). Uninsured patients who are permanently disabled would, after the 1-year period, apply for disability benefits under Medicaid or Medicare if they meet the eligibility requirements.

Further Develop Regional Systems of Trauma Care

More efficient use of expensive health care resources may produce direct cost savings. For example, consolidating trauma care resources in a few hospitals within a given metropolitan area can reduce duplication of services, lower marginal costs, boost occupancy rates, and improve the quality of patient care by concentrating the skills of trauma care professionals.[20] This would have the additional benefit of more equitably allocating trauma care resources across the country, since the 457 trauma centers currently in operation only serve 25 per cent of the population.[12] Comprehensive guidelines for patient triage are necessary to make this work, however. The goal is to triage the less seriously injured to the nearest hospital or other health care facility and to route the severely injured to a level I or II trauma center (or a level III center in rural areas). Concentrating the most severely injured patients in a few strategically located trauma center hospitals allows for the most cost-effective use of highly trained personnel, sophisticated technology, and other expensive resources.[12]

The efficiency and effectiveness of regionalizing trauma care is reflected in data collected by the Health Services Cost Review Commission in the state of Maryland, one of only two states reported to have fairly complete state-wide trauma systems in place. Of all Maryland trauma discharges, two-thirds of those with less severe injuries (ISS 1–8) were routed to a non-trauma center hospital, and 84 per cent of severely injured patients (ISS 20–75) were treated in a designated trauma center.

Structuring regional systems of trauma care must be done carefully so as to avoid the pitfalls of inequitable concentrations of resources. As evidenced by the high numbers of trauma center closures, a disproportionate concentration of severely injured patients who are uninsured or underinsured often proves fatal to trauma centers. Closure of even one trauma center sets in motion a domino effect, whereby the remaining trauma centers in a geographic area face increased financial pressure and begin to teeter precariously on the brink of financial disaster. An appropriate geographical distribution of trauma centers can equitably distribute the indigent care burden, minimize transport time, and maximize the public's access to life-saving care.[12]

Implementing regional systems of trauma care across the nation (as in Germany) would significantly lower the annual financial drain on the nation's trauma care resources.[12] It has been well documented that the provision of comprehensive trauma care significantly reduces overall costs. This appears to be particularly true of indirect costs—those associated with loss of productivity and social welfare services.

To assess the actual financial impact of regional trauma systems, however, a demonstration project should be implemented that would provide 100 per cent reimbursement for ACS-accredited trauma centers that provide services on a managed-care basis and as part of regional systems of trauma care. A cost comparison subsequently could be done among metropolitan areas of similar size to assess the cost-effectiveness of this type of reimbursement scheme. Direct and indirect cost factors would be compared, including acute care, rehabilitative care, long-term care, return to productivity, and utilization of social welfare services.[12]

State and Local Initiatives

Several states have made progress in financing trauma care. Initiatives range from increasing motor vehicle registration fees and taxing motor vehicle citations to setting up subsidy or grant programs for trauma care and trauma research.[73]

Impose Surcharges and Taxes

The state of Maryland, for example, added a one-time fee of $10 to automobile registrations; the $35 million collected was used to set up a state helicopter system. Colorado added $1 to vehicle registrations as well, with the funds to be used exclusively for EMS. The Florida legislature has received a recommendation that the state create a funding pool to reimburse trauma centers by adding a surcharge to automobile registrations and driver's license fees and increasing automobile personal injury protection coverage.[72] Dade County, Florida, uses revenues from a recently added sales tax to support the county's trauma and emergency services. In Texas, a grant program has been set up for EMS and hospitals, to be funded by increasing motor vehicle registration and driver's license fees and by taxing automobile liability insurance.[73] California has added a $2 fee for every $10 charged for moving violations, with the proceeds going to an EMS fund for all levels of trauma care.[73] Pennsylvania passed an EMS act that levies an additional $10 fine for moving violations; most of the revenues collected go to support the commonwealth's EMS system, and the remainder goes to patients in need of extensive rehabilitative services.[73] And Kansas City voters approved a property tax increase that raised $25 million to subsidize uncompensated care costs at the city's Truman Medical Center.[73]

Provide Subsidies and Grants

Washington state provides the city of Seattle with some medical care funding ($16 million in 1989) because Seattle provides a disproportionate amount of the state's indigent care.[73] Florida collects 1.5 per cent of the gross revenues of its hospitals and redistributes the money according to a funding formula based on severity of injury and ability to pay.[73] Minnesota keeps people from falling through the

Medicaid/Medicare net by providing funding for patients who are not eligible for these programs. In addition, Milwaukee county has implemented a medical assistance program for its uninsured residents that combines state subsidy funding and a financing (or "spend-down") plan.[73] The Washington, D.C., Department of Transportation funds the area's trauma registry.[73] The state of Maryland funded the creation of, and continues to subsidize, its state university's shock/trauma center. In addition, Maryland obtained a waiver from HCFA from the cap on Medicaid reimbursement for trauma patients, which provides almost $15 million in funding for Medicaid trauma patients.[12]

TRAUMA CARE IS COST-EFFECTIVE

These funding initiatives are being developed because trauma care increasingly is being viewed at the grassroots level as a top health care priority. The high costs associated with trauma care, however, lead many to ask whether it is cost-effective to allocate what seems like such a disproportionate amount of money for such a relatively small percentage of the population. There often is the view that those without health insurance are also without jobs and therefore would be unable to "pay back" the expense of their trauma care.

Contrary to popular assumption, however, most uninsured Americans (83.5 per cent) are considered the working poor: Almost 90 per cent of the uninsured either work for one of the 44 per cent of the nation's companies that do not have health benefits for their employees or are self employed.[68, 74] Therefore, saving and rehabilitating the typical trauma patient, aside from having obvious humanitarian benefits, most often restores to society a productive member of the workforce who can "pay back" his or her "debt" through taxes.

The average trauma patient is a 20-year-old male injured in a car crash. According to human capital theory, society has invested heavily in this individual through its provision of public education and health services (e.g., immunizations and water and sewage treatment services). At age 20, however, the typical trauma patient is most likely a student or new employee who has not yet provided society with a return on its investment. According to several studies of trauma patient outcomes, the typical trauma patient in 1988 incurred approximately $45,000 in acute medical and 1 year of rehabilitative care costs.[28, 29, 31] If this individual receives prompt, expert trauma care, he has a greater than 80 per cent chance of regaining full productivity and has, therefore, 40 years of work life ahead of him. At an average yearly salary of $20,000 and at a 22.2 per cent tax rate (federal, state, and local), this young man would have paid approximately $4444 in taxes in 1988. Combined with a payroll withholding tax of $3004 (7.51 per cent for 1988), the total tax contribution the average rehabilitated trauma patient (and his employer) would make is $7448. If he works for 40 years, his lifetime tax contribution would total $206,416 (assuming a 6 per cent discount rate to equate future earnings with 1988 dollars). Although much of these funds cover his use of other public services, he would, in effect, pay society back for the cost of his trauma care in taxes alone within 7 years. Also, over his 40-year work history, this individual contributes a total of $554,918 to the gross national product in salary—12 times greater than the original $45,000 invested to save his life and restore him to full productivity.[12]

Multiplied by the 25,000 individuals annually who would be saved if regional systems of trauma care were in place across the nation, the total lifetime savings to the nation in tax contributions alone would be $5.16 billion each year.[12] Minus the $45,000 in trauma care expenditures per patient, net savings in lifetime tax contributions would total $4 billion per year. Within a 10-year period, organized systems of trauma care easily could generate lifetime tax savings of $50 billion, with a net savings of $41 billion. These numbers certainly are too conservative; as early as 1982, approximately 125,000 annual trauma-related deaths and 8 million injuries occurred, which cost over $60 billion.[4]

Alternatively, if this patient dies, the lifetime costs to the nation would total over $438,000.[2]

This is clearly an oversimplification of the cost benefit ratio of providing quality trauma care. First, it does not account for the other, nonmonetary contributions this person may make as a member of the community and contributor to his family.[12] Additionally, it does not figure in the expenses of operating regional EMS and trauma centers; for example, the San Diego County EMS system costs the county $3 million per year, or $3 for each county resident.[12] Nor does it account for the goods and services this individual consumes during the course of his lifetime. This simplified look at the cost-effectiveness of trauma care also does not account for the cost to society of the 15 per cent of trauma patients who, despite expert trauma care, do not regain full-time productivity, even 4 or more years after their injury occurred.[30] Although many people with permanent disabilities work part time or can live independently, some require on-going care that ranges from minimal to "maintenance" care (i.e., for quadriplegics or those in long-term coma or persistent vegetative state). The costs of providing lifetime care for the small proportion of those in the latter category are indeed great, but these costs do not outweigh the social and economic benefits of returning 80 to 85 per cent of injured patients to full-time productivity.

The high costs of trauma care must, however, be balanced against the considerable benefits of saving lives and restoring injured people to productivity. A 1992 multistate analysis of data on patients hospitalized for traumatic injuries showed dramatically reduced medical care costs and faster recovery times in states with regionalized systems of trauma care (unpublished data). In areas without trauma centers, many more seriously injured people die or become permanently disabled than do those in areas with the appropriate trauma resources. In dollars, as mentioned above, the death of the typical trauma patient costs the nation more than $438,000 in lost tax revenues.[2] Without trauma care, the rate of posttrauma disability, both in incidence and severity, would increase, and rehabilitation costs would soar. Implemented nationwide, however, organized systems of trauma care have the potential to save approximately $14 billion, or almost 8 per cent of the national costs of injury, while providing the seriously injured person with the best opportunity for survival and continued productivity (unpublished data[30]).

To adequately and equitably serve the population, the United States should have 350 to 400 strategically located level I or II trauma centers, each served by a regional system of trauma care. Although the nation currently has 457 trauma centers designated by state or local government, many are overly concentrated in large urban centers and only a few are part of regional systems. As a result, these 457 centers serve only a fraction of the population.[12]

The crisis that faces trauma centers is a crisis that affects us all. If the nation's health care system is teetering on the brink of collapse, emergency patients, particularly trauma patients, will be the first to fall. For trauma patients, even minor delays in treatment can mean the difference between life and death and return to productive functioning or permanent disability. The most acutely ill patients, those who have been severely injured, increasingly have no place to go for treatment. Trauma centers, uniquely organized to provide lifesaving services and prevent disability, are closing across the nation, and in their wake, the lives of the injured, many of them children and young adults who could have been saved and fully restored, are lost.[12]

Tragic outcomes, such as the unnecessary death of a 7-year-old girl in Houston, which had only two area hospitals that offered trauma care, will become commonplace. When Hermann Hospital shut its doors to trauma patients because its uncompensated care costs had skyrocketed to $1 million per month, Ben Taub General Hospital became inundated with emergency patients. When the girl was hit by a car, the prehospital personnel on the scene, acutely aware of the severe overcrowding at Ben Taub, took her to a nearby community hospital. Although her condition initially did not appear to be serious, the absence of an on-staff neurosurgeon, coupled with unsuccessful attempts to locate any available surgeon, made it impossible to confirm the extent of her injuries. Her condition subsequently worsened, and she was rushed to Ben Taub. The 4-hour delay in appropriate trauma care cost the child her life.[75] Similar incidents occur all too often throughout the country.

The crisis in trauma care reimbursement is resulting, daily, in unnecessary death and disability that is robbing the nation of its youth and future. Recognizing the widespread effects of diminishing trauma care, policymakers need to develop health care policy initiatives that will ensure access to trauma centers for the insured and uninsured alike. The human consequences of ignoring this crisis will be devastating.

REFERENCES

1. National Academy of Sciences: Injury in America: A Continuing Public Health Problem. Washington, National Academy Press, 1985.
2. Rice DP, MacKenzie EJ: Cost of Injury in the United States: A Report to Congress. San Francisco, Institute for Health & Aging, University of California and Injury Prevention Center, The Johns Hopkins University, 1989.
3. White JH: A grand design for quality. Health Progress June:18–24, 1990.
4. Shapiro MJ, Keegan M, Copeland J: The misconception of trauma reimbursement. Arch Surg 124:1237–1240, 1989.
5. Pories SE, Gamelli RL, Vacek P, et al: Predicting hospital charges for trauma care. Arch Surg 123:579–582, 1988.

5a. National Health Lawyers Association: Spotlight on healthcare reform: Commerce projects $940 billion health tab. Health Lawyers News Report 21(2):3–4, 1993.

6. Baker SP, O'Neill B, Karpt RS: The Injury Fact Book. Lexington, MA, Lexington/Heath and Co, 1984.
7. American College of Surgeons: Fact Sheet on Trauma. Chicago, ACS, 1988.
8. Thal ER, Rochon RB: Inner-city trauma centers: Financial burdens or community saviors? Surg Clin North Am 71(2):209–219, 1991.
9. National Academy of Sciences: Accidental Death and Disability: The Neglected Disease of Modern Society. Washington, National Academy Press, 1966.
10. Champion HR: Legislative issues in trauma: The need for a federal presence. Probl Gen Surg 7(2):192–202, 1990.
11. Skolnick AA: Congress acts to resuscitate nation's financially ailing trauma care systems. JAMA 267(22):2994–2996, 1992.
12. Champion HR, Mabee MS: An American Crisis in Trauma Care Reimbursement: An Issues Analysis Monograph. Washington, Champion & Mabee, 1990.
13. Curreri WP: Editorial: Academic consequences of a trauma system failure. J Trauma 30(7):834, 1990.
14. Bureau of the Census: Health Insurance Coverage: 1987–1990. Selected Data from the Survey of Income and Program Participation. Washington, US Department of Commerce, Economics and Statistics Administration, Bureau of the Census, Current Population Reports/ Household Economic Studies, Series P-70, No. 29, 1992.
15. Mercy JA, Davidson LS, Goodman RA, Rosenberg ML: Alcohol and Intentional Violence: Implications for Research and Public Policy. Background paper for the National Institute on Alcohol Abuse and Alcoholism, Conference on Research Issues in the Prevention of Alcohol-Related Injuries, Berkeley, CA, 1986.
16. Willin KR: Economic sources of homicides: Reestimating the effects of poverty and inequality. Am Sociol Rev 49:283–289, 1984.
17. Health Care Cost Containment Board: A Study of Trauma Costs in Florida. Tallahassee, Health Care Cost Containment Board, in cooperation with the Center for Human Services Policy and Administration of Florida State University and the Department of Health and Rehabilitative Services, Office of Emergency Medical Services, 1989.
18. General Accounting Office: Trauma Care: Lifesaving System Threatened by Unreimbursed Costs and Other Factors. Report to the Chairman, Subcommittee on Health for Family and the Uninsured, Committee on Finance, U.S. Senate. Washington, U.S. General Accounting Office (GAO/HRD-91-57), 1991.
19. Luft HS, Buner JP, Enthoven AC: Should operations be regionalized? The empirical relation between surgical volume and mortality. N Engl J Med 301:1364, 1979.
20. American College of Surgeons: Resources for Optimal Care of the Injured Patient. Chicago, ACS, 1990.
21. Cales RH: Trauma mortality in Orange County: The effect of implementation of a regional trauma system. Ann Emerg Med 13:1–10, 1984.
22. National Highway Traffic Safety Administration: The NHTSA Emergency Medical Services Program and its Relationship to Highway Safety. Washington, U.S. Department of Transportation, National Highway Traffic Safety Administration, Technical Report DOT HS 806 832, 1985.
23. San Diego County Division of Emergency Medical Services: First Year Trauma System Assessment. County of San Diego, August 1984–July 1985.
24. Rutledge R, Messick J, Baker CC, et al: Multivariate population-based analysis of the association of county trauma centers with per capita county trauma death rates. J Trauma 33(1):29–38, 1992.
25. Cales RH, Trunkey DD: Preventable deaths: A review of trauma care systems development. JAMA 254:1059, 1985.
26. Shackford SR, Hollingworth-Fridlund P, Cooper GF, et al: The effect of regionalization upon the quality of trauma care as assessed by concurrent audit before and after institution of a trauma system: A preliminary report. J Trauma 26:812, 1986.
27. Champion HR, Sacco WJ, Copes WS: Improvement in outcome from trauma center care. Arch Surg 127(3):333–338, 1992.
28. MacKenzie EJ, Shapiro S, Smith RT, et al: Factors influencing return to work following hospitalization for traumatic injury. Am J Public Health 77(3):329–334, 1987.

29. MacKenzie EJ, Siegel JH, Shapiro S, et al: Functional recovery and medical costs of trauma: An analysis by type and severity of injury. J Trauma 28(3):281–297, 1988.
30. Rhodes M, Aronson J, Moerkirk G, et al: Quality of life after the trauma center. J Trauma 28(7):931–938, 1988.
31. MacKenzie E, Shapiro S, Siegel JH: The economic impact of traumatic injuries. JAMA 260(22), 1988.
32. Rich S: Tracing medical costs to social problems. The Washington Post, August 28, 1991, p A21.
33. Mahrenholz DM: Are health care costs really the costs of caring for health? Nurs Connect 5(1):27–30, 1992.
33a. Schwartz RM: Clinton emphasizes curb on "spiraling healthcare costs." Group Practice Managed Healthcare News 9(2):5,24–25, 1993.
34. Public Agenda Foundation: The Health Care Crisis: Containing Costs, Expanding Coverage. New York, McGraw-Hill, 1992.
34a. Dobson A, Clarke RL: Shifting—no solution to problem of increasing costs. Healthcare Financial Management 46(7):25–32, 1992.
34b. Wasik JF: The crisis in health insurance. Consumers Digest 30(4):49–58, 1991.
35. Conference of Metropolitan Hospital Associations: The Health of 1990 Urban America. Minneapolis/St. Paul, Urban Health Issues Group, 1990.
36. MacKenzie E, et al: Acute Hospital Costs of Trauma in the United States: Implications for Regionalized Systems of Care. Chicago, American Association for the Surgery of Trauma, Annual Meeting, October 1989.
37. Healthcare delivery: Marginalizing Medicaid. Health Progress, November 9, 1990.
38. Curtis R: The role of state governments in assuring access to care. Inquiry 23(fall):277–285, 1986.
39. Batavia AI: The Payment of Medical Rehabilitation Services: Current Mechanisms and Potential Models. Chicago, American Hospital Association, 1988.
40. Jacobs LM, Schwartz RJ: The impact of prospective reimbursement on trauma centers. Arch Surg 121(4):479–483, 1986.
40a. Prospective Payment Assessment Commission: Report and Recommendations to the Secretary, U.S. Department of Health and Human Services, April 1, 1987. Washington, ProPAC.
41. Schwab WC, Young G, Civil I, et al: DRG reimbursement for trauma: The demise of the trauma center (the use of ISS grouping as an early predictor of total hospital cost). J Trauma 28(7):939–946, 1988.
42. Bennett BR, Jacobs LM, Schwartz RJ: Incidence, costs and DRG-based reimbursement for traumatic brain injured patients: A 3-year experience. J Trauma 29(5): 556–565, 1989.
43. Demaria EJ, Merriam MA, Casanova LA, et al: Do DRG payments adequately reimburse the costs of trauma care in geriatric patients? J Trauma 28(8):1244–1249, 1988.
43a. Clinton WJ: Report to Congress, "A Vision of Change for America." Washington, U.S. Bureau of National Affairs. Released February 18, 1993.
43b. Priest D, Rich S: Proposed Medicare, Medicaid cuts total $62.6 billion over five years. The Washington Post, February 18, 1993, p A14.
44. Champion HR: EAST Presidential Address: Reflections on and directions for trauma care. J Trauma 33(2):270–278, 1992.
45. Price D: Field hospitals of the drug wars. The Detroit News and Free Press, September 16, 1990, pp 1A–14A.
46. The Texas Trauma Data Study: Executive summary. West Palm Beach, FL: Udell Research Associates, under contract to the Texas Department of Health, Emergency Medical Services Division, 1990.
47. Dailey JT, Teter H, Provenzano G: Trauma Center Closures: A National Assessment. Baltimore, The Charles McC. Mathias, Jr., National Study Center for Trauma and Emergency Medical Systems at the Maryland Institute for EMS Systems, 1991.
47a. Starr P, Zelman WA: A ridge to compromise: Competition under a budget. Health Affairs 12(Supplement):7–23, 1993.
48. Feder J, Rowland D: Government. JAMA 268(3):362–364, 1992.
48a. National Highway Traffic Safety Administration: Economic Cost of Motor Vehicle Crashes to Society. Washington, U.S. Department of Transportation, 1992.
49. US Department of Transportation: Drunk Driving Facts. Washington, National Highway Traffic Safety Administration, 1986.
50. Cigarette smoking among adults—United States, 1990. MMWR 41:354–355, 361–362, 1992.
51. Marwick C: Counteracting alcohol's "glamour image." JAMA 267(17):2289, 1992.
52. House EG, Waller PF, Stewart JR: Blood alcohol level and injury in traffic crashes. In American Association of Automotive Medicine, 26th Annual Proceedings. Des Plaines, IL: AAAM, 1982, pp 349–373.
53. Waller PF, Stewart JR, Hansen AR, et al: The potentiating effects of alcohol on driver injury. JAMA 256:1461, 1986.
54. Zuska JZ: Wounds without cause. Bull Am Coll Surg October 66(10):5–10, 1981.
55. Maull KI: Alcohol abuse: Its implications in trauma care. South Med J 75:794, 1982.
56. Niven RG: Alcoholism—A problem in perspective. JAMA 252:1912, 1984.
57. Pories SE, Gamelli RL, Vacek P, et al: Intoxication and injury. J Trauma 32(1):60–64, 1992.
58. Blose JO, Holder HD: Injury-related medical care utilization in a problem drinking population. Am J Public Health 81(12):1571–1575, 1991.
59. Cook PJ: The effect of liquor taxes on drinking, cirrhosis and auto accidents. In Moore MH, Gerstein DR (eds): Alcohol and Public Policy: Beyond the Shadow of Prohibition. Washington, National Academy Press, 1981.
60. Manning WG, Keeler EB, Newhouse JP, et al: The taxes of sin: Do smokers and drinkers pay their way? JAMA 261(11):1604–1609, 1989.
61. Distilled Spirits Council of the United States: Public Revenues from Alcohol Beverages. Washington, DSCUS, 1985.
62. Saffer H, Grossman M: Beer taxes, the legal drinking age, and youth motor-vehicle fatalities. J Legal Studies 16:351–374, 1987.
63. April through June 1991 table reporting alcohol involvement in fatal motor-vehicle crashes. MMWR 41:434, 1992.
64. Manley M, Epps RP, Husten C, et al: Clinical interventions in tobacco control: A National Cancer Institute training program for physicians. JAMA 266(22):3172–3173, 1991.
65. Schultz JM: Smoking-attributable mortality and years of potential life lost—United States, 1988. MMWR 40:62–71, 1991.
66. US Department of Health and Human Services: Smoking and Health: A National Status Report, 2d ed. Rockville, MD: USDHHS, CDC 87-8396, 1990.
67. Guerra LG, Verghese A: Health costs. Book review of Manning WG, Keeler EB, Newhouse JP, et al: The Costs of Poor Health Habits. JAMA 267(18):2534, 1992.
68. Wilensky GR: Viable strategies for dealing with the uninsured. Health Affairs Spring:33–46, 1987.
69. Commission on Professional Hospital Activities: International Classification of Diseases, 9th Revision, Clinical Modification. Ann Arbor, Edwards Brothers, 1977.
70. Baker SP, O'Neill B, Haddon W, et al: The Injury Severity Score: A method for describing patients with multiple injuries and evaluating emergency care. J Trauma, 14:187–196, 1974.
71. Champion HR, Sacco WJ, Copes WS, et al: A revision of the trauma score. J Trauma 20:623, 1989.
72. Florida Department of Health and Rehabilitative Services: A Proposal for State-Sponsored Trauma Centers: Draft Report. Tallahassee, Emergency Medical Service, Center for Human Services Policy, Administration of Florida State University, Committee on State-Sponsored Trauma Centers, 1990.
73. Charhut M, Lippitt E, Oberman D: Survey Results of Trauma Care Systems in 21 U.S. Cities. Submitted to Health Commissioner Richard M. Krieg, City of Chicago, October 13, 1989.
74. Schroepfer L: Who are the uninsured? Special Report on Health May-July:20, 1991.
75. Belkin L: Houston accident care: Options are cut. New York Times, National Section, Sunday, October 22, 1989, p 22.

4

LEGAL CONCERNS IN TRAUMA NURSING

WARREN CHAVE

INTRODUCTION

Trauma nursing is undergoing rapid change, as is evident by the nursing as well as medical and scientific content of this book. Prior to the 1950s, any nursing book that dealt with the law could do so in the context of ethical or administrative considerations. Up to that time, the law for nurses was subordinate to the law for physicians, as was the nurse's role in patient care.

The legal notion of independent judgment by nurses was established in the late 1950s and early 1960s.[1, 2] Today the nurse in a trauma setting performs highly skilled functions in the care of patients, including the coordination and delivery of services to the patient, the monitoring of complex physiological data, the diagnosis of psychological and physical states, and the operation of sophisticated life-saving equipment. The performance of such functions mandates the regular exercise of independent judgment without the supervision of a physician.[3]

This increased sophistication and the added authority bring additional responsibility. This, in turn, requires that the nurse have greater knowledge of medical, scientific, and especially legal issues. Trauma nursing takes place against the backdrop of a legal system growing increasingly complex and vigilant of professionals.

The purpose of this chapter is to provide trauma nurses with a survey of the primary legal issues that affect their professional lives. Its main themes are the patient's right to control over his or her body and life and the nurse's obligation to act reasonably and prudently according to current standards of nursing care. This chapter will not substitute for the advice of an attorney in particular cases, but it will provide nurses with a working knowledge of those subject areas in which they or their patients have specific rights or responsibilities.

SOURCES OF LAW

United States law is divisible into three main areas: common law, statutory law, and administrative law. These divisions correspond to the three branches of government at the federal and state level: judicial, legislative, and executive.

Common law results from the decisions of the courts. The judiciary is given the responsibility of seeking the facts in particular cases and controversies and of applying the law to reach a decision. *Statutory law* derives from acts passed by legislatures. The legislatures (Congress at the federal level and legislative bodies at the state level) are empowered to pass laws dealing with subjects for which the respective constitutions have granted them authority. *Administrative law* stems from the rule-making process and results in regulations promulgated by the executive branch. The President of the United States and the governors of individual states preside over the operation of executive or regulatory agencies that have been given specific authority to make rules by acts of the legislatures. All three branches of federal and state government are restricted by the "higher" law of the Constitution of the United States. Actions that are contrary to its provisions cannot be incorporated into common, statutory, or administrative law. State governments are also restricted by any additional provisions contained in the constitutions of the individual states.

Each of these three sources of law influences the legal issues discussed in this chapter. These issues are undergoing change as the law evolves. The methods by which the law is created and the manner in which it changes will be discussed in the following section.

Common Law

Common law is the term used to describe the body of principles that arise from court decisions. More generally, it is known as case law and consists of the accumulation of judicial opinions prepared by judges at the trial and appellate levels from lawsuits initiated by parties (litigants) to a controversy. The common law traces its roots to cases dating back to the 11th century in England. The underlying principle of the common law is *stare decisis*, that the law will provide continuity by deciding cases consistent with the precedents set by earlier cases. This only means that two controversies between litigants that are the same factually and that raise the same legal issues will be decided the same way. This continuity is dependent on there being no changes in statutory law and no changes in public policy. Since both evolve as society changes, the common law also evolves. The reliance on precedent in judicial decrees generally guarantees controlled change in the common law upon which the public can rely.

Over the years, judges have recognized the existence of a number of rights that are necessary for the orderly operation of society. Many of these have been embodied in the law of torts. For nursing, the common law is most relevant to torts such as malpractice and assault and battery (unauthorized and unprivileged contact between two people) and to the judicially recognized right to privacy.

Torts are civil as opposed to criminal "wrongs" committed by one person on another which can be "righted" through an action brought before a judge and jury. For example, hundreds of years ago, courts established both the individual's right to be free of the negligent acts of another which cause harm and the remedy to this harm, monetary damages to compensate the injured party. Where civil law speaks to the relations between people, criminal law speaks to actions prohibited by society as a whole. Legal actions under civil law are between private parties, whereas actions under criminal law are brought by the government against individuals (or corporations).

Statutory Law

Statutes are the acts of Congress and state legislatures that regulate the lives of the people. Unlike the common law, statutory law does not change through time and evolution but rather by the deliberate acts of the legislatures to create, amend, or repeal statutes. Statutory law deals with such diverse topics as taxation, interstate commerce, and, pertinent to nursing, regulation of the professions.

Trauma nursing is affected by state laws that define the minimum standards required of a licensed nurse. These laws, called *Nurse Practice Acts*,[4, 5] exist to protect citizens from "unskilled and incompetent persons who would practice or offer to practice nursing."[6] They regulate nursing by defining the types of acts that licensed practical nurses (LPNs) and registered nurses (RNs) can perform and by providing a mechanism to exclude from the profession those who are incompetent.[6]

Trauma nursing is also affected by statutes dealing with brain death and by laws requiring that nurses report incidents of child or spousal abuse or of abuse of the elderly. Other legislative acts prescribe the manner in which criminal evidence must be handled in order for it to be admissible in a criminal action. These statutes have been the subject of many judicial proceedings over the past 30 years so that the law relative to the handling of criminal evidence is grounded in common law as well as statutory law.

Administrative Law

Administrative law is created when a regulatory agency is empowered by the legislature through a statute to make rules to control the actions of a class of individuals. The rules and regulations must be consistent with the intent of the legislature.

Administrative law is a relatively modern and uniquely American form of law. Rules and regulations can be and are changed by the executive agencies that administer them as the circumstances underlying them change. The administrative procedures statutes of the state and federal governments control the process for developing and changing regulations. This means that regulatory agencies are empowered to make rules and to change them only after the class of individuals affected has had the opportunity to comment on the changes. The purpose of these requirements is to ensure that regulations reflect the reality of, for example, nursing practice and that they not be unreasonable. Furthermore, the rules cannot be made in an arbitrary or capricious manner. Regulations change not exclusively as a result of societal evolution and not exclusively by the act of a legislative body. Rather they are the result of statutory changes as well as changes in the work of the people regulated.

Trauma nursing is affected by administrative law through the state boards of nursing. They exist as a result of the legislature empowering the boards to regulate nursing through Nurse Practice Acts.[7] These boards establish and enforce the rules which define requirements for licensure, but they also are empowered to further define allowable nursing acts and the education requirements for nurses. State boards of nursing decide cases involving violations of the professional standards of care embodied in these regulations or set forth in the enabling legislation. Nurses can be disciplined by the board of nursing if they violate the standards established for practice. These standards do vary slightly from state to state, and the reader is encouraged to investigate the particulars of the state where licensed. Some of the bases for disciplinary action common to all states include fraud in obtaining or in using a nursing license, conviction of a felony or other crime involving moral turpitude (acts involving abusive behavior, dishonesty, or immodesty), knowingly failing to file a required record or report or knowingly filing a false record or report, and drug or alcohol addiction or other physical or mental condition rendering the individual nurse incapable of acting as a nurse. The grounds for disciplinary action also may include refusing to provide, withholding of, denial of, or discrimination in providing nursing services to patients who have tested HIV positive.[8] Suspension or revocation of one's license is likely to occur for a serious violation of the standards of practice or for repeated violations.

Law affects the lives of all professionals. The types of laws and the manner in which they come into being have been explained. What remains is to relate these concepts to the specific aspects of trauma nursing practice.

LEGAL ISSUES OF TRAUMA NURSING

The issues of law that affect trauma nursing derive from the three sources of law and the actions of the corresponding branches of government. Issues that affect all nursing equally are contained in other sources, and the reader is referred to them for a detailed discussion.[9–13] The general legal concepts discussed in the following sections contain both the pertinent elements of the law and their relevance to nursing actions. Many of these concepts are interwoven with ethical considerations discussed in Chapter 5.

Consent to Treatment

The nature of trauma practice requires that nurses touch patients and administer therapeutic care. The law, on the other hand, has as a basic principle the right of the individual to determine who shall touch him or her and in what manner[14] and that the competent individual can refuse to be treated.[15] Violation of this right of the individual is a violation of the common law.[16]

> Every human being of adult years and sound mind has a right to determine what shall be done with his own body; and a [professional who provides treatment] without his patient's consent commits an assault for which he is liable in damages.[17]

In this right, the law is quite rigid, and failure to obtain consent for a treatment will subject the professional to a lawsuit.

Three elements must be present if consent is to be valid: (1) capacity, (2) information, and (3) voluntariness. *Capacity* refers to the right of the patient to give consent. Minors and incompetent adults lack the capacity to give consent. *Information* refers to the sufficiency of the patient's understanding of what is being consented to. If the descriptions of treatments given on consent forms or made verbally fail to state clearly what is to be done in such a way that the patient can understand, then consent is not valid. *Voluntariness* refers to lack of coercion. Consent obtained by trick or by threat is not valid.

The requirement to obtain consent applies to all treatments done to a patient. Specific consent for invasive procedures must be obtained by the person performing the procedure, generally the physician. Nurses frequently are involved in obtaining consent for such procedures on behalf of the physician. While the nurse is not directly responsible for the performance of these procedures and the particulars of such consent are not required of nurses, it is prudent to be aware of them. For nursing practice separate from physician practice, the reasonable act for the nurse is to inform the patient of any touching to be performed and the reason for the touching and to obtain the patient's consent.

Violations of the common law for obtaining valid consent require that the patient show that the treatment caused some harm and that the treatment would not have been permitted if the possibility of this harm were known. This is true even if there is no lack of care in administering the treatment. It is no defense that the patient would have permitted the treatment if consent had been obtained.[18] It is therefore *critical* to obtain consent to stay within the law.[15] Note that harm does not necessarily equate to injury, and nonconsensual contact, even if beneficial to the health of the patient, is not permitted under the law.[14]

Informed Consent

Over the years, the concept of consent has been refined so that it is now referred to generally as *informed consent.* The adjective *informed* is not superfluous in this concept. It exists because the courts mandate that consent can only be given if the patient is knowledgeable about the effects of the treatment[18] and has made an affirmative decision to receive the treatment.[14]

Hospitals and trauma centers all require patients to sign a consent to treatment form upon admission. This form should be looked on by nurses as constituting consent by the patient to be taken care of in the facility and not as consent to all procedures, treatments, and therapies. Each time the patient is to be touched, the action involved should be explained, and either verbal or written agreement or some action demonstrating willingness to participate in the treatment[14] should be received from the patient. Consent forms that specifically list the procedures to be performed and the risks or consequences are gaining increasing favor under the law. Mandatory use of these forms, where possible, is likely to be universally legislated in the future.[14] Note, however, that a signed consent form that is obtained from a patient who does not understand its contents is not valid consent.

The general rule of consent is that the patient should be told everything that is to be done each time something is to be done to or for the patient and that the patient should agree to the treatment or procedure. The patient should be informed of the nature of the treatment, its benefits and risks, and any reasonable alternatives. Furthermore, the explanation should be couched in terms *understandable* to patients, because courts are tending to favor what the "reasonable patient would expect to know to make an informed decision regarding consent for treatment"[15] as opposed to the prior practice of relying on what a "reasonable practitioner" would tell the patient.

Of course, not all patients are capable of giving consent. The law has permitted exceptions to the requirement of informed consent.

Emergency Doctrine

The first such exception is one that has great application in trauma care. When a patient is unconscious or otherwise unable to give consent, treatment can proceed under the emergency doctrine, which implies consent. This implication frees the nurse from liability for violation of the common law. *Implied consent* means that the patient would have consented to the treatment required to maintain health had that patient been able because the alternative would have been death or serious disability. The law assumes that the patient would act reasonably, and the maintenance of bodily integrity is a reasonable act.[19] Note, however, that the emergency doctrine's implication of consent terminates as soon as the patient's disabling condition (e.g., unconsciousness) abates.

Competency to Give Consent

A second exception to the informed consent rule is that of competency. Consent is legally valid only if it is given by someone who is recognized as being of "adult years and sound mind."[17] What this means is that someone not of legal age or who is judged to be in some way incompetent cannot give the consent that would constitute a valid defense to a lawsuit for battery. A parent or legal guardian must give consent for the treatment of a minor. Even under circumstances where an emergency exists, the parent should be contacted or some notation that the parent is unavailable should be made on the chart.[19] A listing of the steps taken to find the parent will be critical in the event that a lawsuit is filed.

There are further considerations to this exception to the informed consent rule. A minor is generally considered to be any one under the age of 18. In some states, an individual under the age of 18 who is married, has a child,[20] or is otherwise emancipated from the parents is considered an adult for purposes of giving consent to medical treatment. In addition, some states permit a minor to consent to emergency medical treatment without a parent's consent.[21] The reader is referred to hospital policy and state law for additional information on this subject (the state's board of nursing, a local professional nursing association, or a law school library may all have specific details).

A second consideration, and one that bears some watching in the future, is that of consent by the state as legal guardian. The majority of the states protect parents from criminal liability for denying life-saving medical care to their children on religious grounds. While uncommon, the state may consent to the treatment of a minor after the parents have refused consent. The reason is that some states, in order to protect the child's rights, will consent to the life-saving treatment when the parents will not. This is most likely to occur when the parents' religious beliefs preclude use of blood transfusions or other medical techniques. This type of consent is not common and is given only under extreme circumstances, since the states are loathe to interfere in the parent–child relationship. The consent given, however, is effective in the same way as described previously.

Some patients, although not minors, may not be competent to give consent. The concept of being of sound mind is the second half of the competency equation. Any person who is not competent because of some mental disability (e.g., lack of mental capacity or senility), chronic alcoholism, drug addiction, or physical disability or disease[22] that renders the individual incapable of making reasoned judgments should be under the control of a guardian. In cases where there is no guardian, one may have to be appointed by the courts. Consent for these individuals is obtained in the same manner as for minors, with the guardian substituted for the parent. Consent is implied by law for such patients where emergency medical treatment is required.[23] If there is no guardian and no durable power of attorney relative to medical care (a document by which a person grants a designated other person the authority to make health care decisions in the event of the person's incapacity to make decisions), state law may provide that the consent of a spouse, adult child, adult sibling, adult grandchild, or a grandparent[24] be substituted.[25]

Issues of consent must be considered before each treatment or procedure is commenced whether in the resuscitation, operative, critical care, or intermediate/rehabilitative cycles. It is important that the nurse be knowledgeable about consents obtained by or for physicians, since the primary nurse is the consistent coordinator for patient care.

Refusal of Treatment

One of the reasons that consent should be obtained separately for each treatment or procedure is that the patient has the right to control all touching of the body not only through consent but also through refusal of treatment. The nurse needs to be aware of the consent obtained by the physician so that a patient's subsequent refusal of treatment can be identified. The withdrawal of consent or any other refusal of treatment must be properly documented in the chart and, because it is often against medical advice, should be witnessed by several people.[19] Hospital policy will likely identify the individuals who should witness such refusal and will likely require that the patient sign a form. Readers are encouraged to investigate the policies at their institutions. Any treatment or procedure done after a patient refuses treatment is a violation of that patient's legal rights and may become the subject of a successful lawsuit even if the treatment has beneficial results.

Assault and Battery: Failed Consent

Assault and *battery* are common law torts that protect the individual from the threat of contact and from unpermitted contact, respectively. They are intentional torts as distinguished from negligent torts. The legal elements of battery are that the person committing the action intends to cause a harmful or offensive contact and that the act is unpermitted and unprivileged. Assault is similar except that actual contact is not required; only the immediate apprehension of a harmful or offensive contact is needed. The good intentions of the nurse do not justify action constituting assault or battery.[26] The nurse may have the patient's best interests in mind, but if the contact is not consensual, a lawsuit may follow.[15]

In a nursing context, failure to obtain informed consent followed by the performance of a procedure is battery. Continued treatment after the patient's refusal of treatment is also battery. While this may seem bizarre in the face of successful treatment or the saving of the patient's life, a patient's deeply held belief may make the contact sufficiently offensive to take it to court.

Patient Confidentiality and the Right to Privacy

Nurses, by ethical code and through the policies of hospitals, are required to keep the identity and condition of their patients confidential. In law, this concept of confidentiality is expressed as the common law right to privacy. It has been called the "right to be let alone" and was first introduced in American law in 1890.[27] While there is no clearly recognized right to privacy under the federal constitution, many of the states have explicitly enacted a privacy clause in their state constitutions or by statute.

An action for invasion of privacy can be brought for monetary damages. Such action is divided into four major themes: (1) appropriation of the individual's name or picture without consent, (2) intrusion into the person's seclusion (as in a hospital bed), (3) public disclosure of private facts, and (4) placing the individual in a false light in the public eye.[28] The first three are particularly relevant to the trauma nurse.

Hospital and university policies require that consent be obtained from a patient prior to photographing injuries for use in a professional journal. Appropriation of the patient's picture or name is outside the law. The second theme, intrusion into the patient's seclusion, involves the unauthorized entry of a person such as a member of the press into an area where the patient has an expectation of privacy. This doctrine forms the legal basis for visiting policies. The third forms the legal basis for hospital policies that restrict employees from discussing patients with the press or public.[29] The confidentiality of diagnoses, treatments, test results, and procedures takes on added significance for patients with AIDS, because it is almost certain that they will require hospitalization at some time during the course of their illness.[30]

The right to privacy applies to the whole continuum of trauma care. During resuscitation or critical care, information about the patient may be increasingly sought by distant relatives, friends, and business associates. Nurses must be particularly careful to avoid divulging information from a patient's medical record or committing unwarranted intrusions into the patient's personal affairs. Pressure from the press and public may be most intense at the beginning of an accident involving a prominent person; however, the right to privacy remains throughout the patient's stay. While it is a regular practice of researchers to use a series of photographs of the progress of a patient's treatment in scholarly works, consent must first be obtained.

As with most of the legal rights and responsibilities detailed so far, there are exceptions to the stringency of the privacy right. Society has determined that the individual's right to privacy is secondary to the prevention and prosecution of spousal, child, and elderly abuse. Nurses, therefore, are empowered by statute to report incidents of abuse without fear of liability in a civil action for invasion of privacy. Mandatory reporting requirements relative to abuse and other prohibited acts are described below.

Mandatory Reporting

Mandatory reporting requirements in the law exist to identify actions that society abhors. The general rule stated earlier is that the facts of a patient's injuries and treatments are confidential and protected by the right to privacy. That right is superseded by mandatory reporting requirements because public policy dictates that these reportable actions are illegal.

Reporting laws require that hospitals, doctors, and nurses notify the appropriate state agency when an incident occurs. They also protect the individual reporting the incident from liability for an inaccurate report unless the false report was made with knowledge of its falsity.[19] There is a flip side to this protection from liability. If a nurse or doctor fails to report an incident and a further injury occurs from the same proscribed action, that individual may be held liable for the failure to report it.[31]

The trauma or emergency nurse must see if the trauma was the result of an act proscribed by law. Examples include child and spousal abuse. Many states have reporting requirements when such abuse is identified. When injuries resulting from abuse are discovered, the trauma nurse must take two actions: (1) notify the physician in charge of the patient's case and any other person identified by hospital policy and (2) make sure the report is filed with the appropriate agency. Failure to follow these two steps in the reporting of an abuse may subject the nurse to liability even though all internal policies have been followed.

Additional examples of incidents with mandatory reporting requirements are abuse in nursing facilities, attempted suicide, and injuries resulting from violence, illegal abortions, animal bites, and motor vehicle accidents. The reader is encouraged to obtain a complete list of reportable incidents from appropriate risk-management personnel.

Negligence/Malpractice

The main theme of the common law that pervades the legal issues discussed thus far is that of reasonableness. Patients expect that their injuries and conditions will be explained to them in a manner that they can reasonably be expected to understand. A patient incapable of giving consent because of injuries will consent to the course of life-saving treatment because it is reasonable to do so or so the law presumes. The patient has the right to have reasonable expectations of privacy protected by the nurse.

The issue of law discussed in this section also focuses principally on this notion of reasonableness. Suits for malpractice, or professional negligence, are actions brought by patients against nurses because the nurse is seen by the patient as not having exercised reasonable care in the treatment of the patient's injuries.

The law of negligence, simply stated, is the breach of a duty owed by the nurse to the patient that results in injury to the patient. Four elements are identified in the law: (1) a duty of care, (2) breach of this duty, (3) a causal connection between the flawed conduct and injury, and (4) the injury or damage suffered by the patient.[32] The crux of the action for negligence is that the nurse did not use reasonable care and an injury resulted.

When applied to professionals, *negligence* is referred to as *malpractice*. The law measures the professional's duty of care differently than the duty of care owed by nonprofessionals. This one distinction separates ordinary negligence from malpractice. It is mentioned here because, while it is generally accepted that nurses exercise independent professional judgment and should be treated as professionals, not all states allow nurses to be sued for malpractice. Such states hold nurses to the standard of negligence only.[33]

In daily life, individuals must act with reasonable caution so as not to cause harm to others. Drivers are expected to exercise reasonable care. Failure to do so (such as when a car runs a red light, strikes a pedestrian, and breaks his leg) is a failure to use reasonable care. It is negligence because (1) the driver had a duty to drive carefully, (2) the driver breached that duty by running the red light, (3) the pedestrian was struck by the car, and (4) the pedestrian suffered a broken leg.

Establishing the Nurse's Liability

The nurse has the duty to provide competent care to patients. If that care is provided in a less than competent manner and the patient is injured as a result, malpractice occurs. The critical definition is of the duty of care and its measurement by the law. The causal connection between the nurse's conduct and the injury must then be established and damages assessed.

Duty of care in negligence is defined as what the reasonably prudent person would do in the same or similar circumstances. This is a fiction recognized by the law because there is no person or group of people identifiable as the "reasonably prudent person." It is not what the average person does, but rather what the law thinks the average person should have done. Due care requires that people not engage in conduct that involves unreasonable danger to others. Critical to the understanding of this duty is that it is conduct which is being evaluated and not state of mind.[32]

In states that do not have malpractice standards for nurses, the duty of nursing care is based on what the reasonably prudent person (not nurse) would do.[33] The specialized training and knowledge of the nurse are not considered when the standard of care is measured in negligence suits in these states.

Malpractice differs from negligence for precisely this reason. The knowledge and training of the nursing profession define the standard for malpractice. This means that nursing as a profession establishes certain minimum qualifications of education through, for example, the licensure requirements of the boards of nursing. All nurses must meet such professional standards to be considered "reasonably prudent nurses." An action that falls below these minimum qualifications and causes injury is malpractice. In addition, specially qualified nurses (e.g., CCRNs) must maintain educational and practice requirements set down by the boards and, in addition, may be held to a standard for all such specialty qualified nurses on a national basis.[34] These requirements form the basis for the duty of care required of such a certified nurse over and above the qualifications of all nurses.

A description of emergency nursing, which shares many common traits with trauma nursing, helps to illustrate these qualifications.

> Emergency nursing practice is the nursing care of individuals of all ages with perceived physical and/or emotional alterations which are undiagnosed and may require prompt intervention. Emergency nursing care is unscheduled and most commonly occurs in a specific care setting, i.e., an emergency department, a mobile unit, or a suicide prevention center. Thus, the nursing care is episodic, primary, and acute in nature.
>
> The scope of emergency nursing practice encompasses nursing activities which are directed toward health problems of various levels of complexity. A rapidly changing physiological and/or psychological status, which may be life-threatening, requires assessment of the severity of the health problem, definitive intervention, on-going reassessment, and supportive care to significant others. The level of physiological and/or psychological complexity may require life-support measures, appropriate health education, and referral. The scope of emergency nursing practice not only encompasses nursing activities which are directed toward health problems presented by the individuals, but also encompasses knowledge of and the observance of legal aspects, such as reporting an incident to reporting governmental agencies, i.e., police or public health departments, when a situation calls for such action. Emergency nursing practice is affected by the brevity of patient interaction with the nurse, the stressful climate created by lack of control over the number of individuals seeking emergency care, and the limited time frame in which to evaluate the effectiveness of intervention.[35]

In emergency settings, nurses have assumed an increasingly independent, professional role. With this change comes the added burden of legal responsibility for their actions. One particular legal problem that may confront the nurse in the field occurs when an accident victim is treated on the scene with physician support provided only through radio communication. If the doctor orders treatment that will be harmful to the patient, the nurse can be held responsible (and the trauma center vicariously) if the orders are followed and the nurse knew or should have known that the harm would occur.[36] This is a dilemma for the nurse at the scene. If the prescribed treatment fails, the doctor will be subject to a malpractice action. However, the increased knowledge and ability of currently practicing nurses exposes them to liability if the doctor's orders result in an injury.

Particularly important is the responsibility of the trauma nurse to document the operative events accurately and thoroughly. The rush to prepare the patient for surgery often requires deviations from standard protocols. Compromises in required nursing routines open the professionals to liability if uncorrected later in the patient's course of recovery.

A trauma operation often lasts 12 hours or more, resulting in nursing shift changes and rotation of other staff. Ideally, all sponges, needles, and instruments are accounted for after an operation. In lengthy surgeries with multiple concurrent procedures, the tracking of these accoutrements of surgery may be faulty. Where there is a discrepancy, it should be documented in the nurse's notes. A radiograph should be ordered at a later time to determine if the discrepancy is a counting error or if the missing sponge or instrument is still in the patient's body. Later recovery of such an intruder in the patient will mitigate, if not eliminate, the liability of the hospital and of the surgical team.

Another area of exposure to liability for the nurse involves cautery burns from the patient's being inadequately grounded. Even in the face of an emergent surgical procedure, the law may not be understanding of injuries caused by improper procedure. The best course of action for the operative nurse remains to ensure that the ground is in place to lessen the exposure to malpractice liability.

Particularly critical in the immediate aftermath of an operation is the responsibility to record and document procedures and their future implications to the course of care of the patient. Exposure to infection, for example, is important to the later cycles, and failure to record these exposures may adversely affect the patient's recovery. These complications expose the operative nurse to liability for malpractice if not properly documented. The length and complexity of trauma surgery compounded by difficulty in achieving proper patient positioning can result in the development of peripheral nerve damage and ischemic tissue injury related to pressure. Proper care mandates that the patient's body be padded at weight-bearing points; however, the later development of skin breakdown may still occur. The nurse's responsibility in this event is to document complications so that nurses in the postoperative care cycle can initiate treatment.

Standards of reasonable nursing care are required of nurses at all stages of the patient's treatment. This is particularly true in managing the discharge process. A patient being prepared for discharge must be thoroughly educated in, for example, wound care and the use of pharmaceuticals. Reasonable care mandates that the patient be given oral and written instructions explaining how to perform the daily tasks that will ensure recovery.[19] Where appropriate, the patient must have demonstrated the ability to perform these tasks. In all cases, the patient's understanding of the instructions must be clearly demonstrated to the nurse. The patient's support system, whether it is family, home health care providers, or a rehabilitation facility, must be prepared to care for the patient.

Elements of a Malpractice Suit

In a patient's suit for malpractice, what constitutes due care is established through the testimony of expert witnesses. An expert is qualified in court through educational credentials and experience and is then permitted to state an opinion about what is or is not proper care. No one other than a duly qualified expert is permitted to give opinions about what is the duty of care in a court of law. This expert will, in all likelihood, be a nurse who will give testimony about what constitutes proper care for nursing. Physician experts also may be called to differentiate between the duties of physicians and nurses' practice, especially where a nurse is claimed to have exceeded the limits of nursing practice.

As with duty of care, the proximate cause of the injury is established in court by the expert witness.[37] The patient's experts can be expected to state that the injury was a result of the nurse's failure to follow proper practice protocols. The nurse's experts will, of course, state that the injury occurred in a different way. While this creates a "battle of the experts," this process has been deemed necessary by the judiciary because the knowledge of professional practice is not within the common knowledge of jurors as laypersons.

Expert witnesses are needed in proving the nexus, or connection, between the care and the injury because the patient as plaintiff has the burden of proof to show that malpractice occurred. There is an exception to the rule that only experts can prove the causal nexus between action and injury which is rarely applied but bears noting. Some injuries are considered to be of a type that most likely do not happen in the absence of malpractice. This narrow class of injuries shifts the burden of proof to the defendant without the need for expert testimony for the patient. The legal concept is *res ipsa loquitur*, which translated literally is "it speaks for itself." The nurse as defendant, in these cases, must prove that the injury did not occur from the treatment.[37]

Once the first three elements of malpractice are established, damages must be proved in order for the nurse to be liable to the patient. Damages are characterized as either compensatory or punitive. *Compensatory* damages are the monies necessary to make the patient "whole." They include the medical expenses associated with the injury, past and future; lost earnings and earning potential; pain and suffering; and loss of consortium (inability to function as a spouse). The injury is viewed as a continuum beginning at the time of injury and extending until cured. If the elapsed time between these points is short, damages are assessed for only that brief time. If, however, the resulting injury is permanent, damages are estimated for the whole of the patient's estimated lifespan. Damages awarded to pay for pain and suffering are usually the largest part of the award, although some state legislatures have acted recently to place a cap on the amount of awards for pain and suffering. They are to pay for what the patient must endure as a result of the nurse's breach of the professional duty of care.

Punitive damages are monies awarded in excess of compensatory damages to punish the nurse's conduct. Since there is this element of punishment, punitive damages are rarely awarded and then only in cases involving "gross negligence," where the nurse acted maliciously or in reckless disregard of the patient's life.

Respondeat Superior and Vicarious Liability

The law of malpractice does not view the nurse's actions in isolation. A trauma nurse is generally an employee of a hospital or trauma center. The employer–employee relationship is established when the employer has the ability to control and direct the performance and duties of the employee. The nurse's actions, by this definition, are considered to be those of an employee if they are within the scope of employment.

If all the conditions of an employer–employee relationship are satisfied, then the negligence of the nurse will be imputed to the hospital as well. This is the doctrine of *respondeat superior. Respondeat superior* applies only to employees, not independent contractors. Courts recognize that a hospital employs nurses to work for it rather than merely providing a place where nurses can act of their own volition. This means that the trauma center is liable for the negligence of its nurses who are operating within the scope of their employment.

The only complication in the application of *respondeat superior* occurs when, for example, the nurse is assisting a surgeon who is not a "house officer." A surgeon employed and paid by the trauma center is an employee of that center in the same way the nurse is. *Respondeat superior* applies equally to both as they share a "master," the trauma center. The difficulty arises when the surgeon is not an employee of the hospital but is reimbursed by fees charged directly to the patient. In those states which apply this distinction to a lawsuit, the doctrine of the "borrowed servant" applies. This rule states that the negligence of the nurse is imputed to the surgeon even though the surgeon does not employ the nurse. Furthermore, the liability of the surgeon for the nurse's negligence accrues only if the negligence occurred when the surgeon exercised control over the nurse's actions. The accepted rule in states that apply the "borrowed servant" doctrine is to hold the hospital liable for the nurse's negligence and to hold the surgeon jointly liable. Vicarious liability does not extend to the nurse supervisor for the malpractice of subordinates because a true employer–employee relationship does not exist. The supervisor is an employee of the trauma center, as is the staff nurse. Nurse supervisors can be held liable, however, if acts of commission or omission in supervising cause a patient's injury.

While the discussion of vicarious liability and *respondeat superior* has centered on the nurse's malpractice, these concepts apply equally to the other torts previously discussed. They, like malpractice, occur during the course of the nurse's duties and are therefore imputed to the employer.

Good Samaritan Rule

As with many of the legal issues discussed in this chapter, there is an exception to the law of malpractice where a negligent nurse may not be held liable. The trauma nurse who becomes involved in the care of the victim of an accident or of a violent crime during off-duty hours is not liable for negligent acts. When an off-duty nurse happens on an accident, there is an ethical and moral, if not legal, duty to stop and render assistance. In order to encourage professionals to help accident victims, the legislatures of all states have passed statutes that grant nurses immunity for liability for negligent acts. These statutes, named after the biblical Good Samaritan, state that health care professionals who stop and aid accident victims without compensation for that help will not be liable for their acts even if negligent.[38, 39]

There is also, however, an exception to the Good Samaritan rule. The law will not exempt the nurse from acts that constitute gross negligence, acts that manifest a reckless disregard for the life of the patient.[40] The rule is that if the care was rendered in good faith that an emergency existed, then the nurse will be free from liability.[19] The nurse who is a member of an emergency team sent to the scene of an accident is not covered by the Good Samaritan rule. The professional duty of care is required of this type of nurse.

The Nurse as Expert Witness

Expert witnesses are used to establish standards of nursing care and to give opinions about the care provided by a nurse being sued for malpractice. While it is not within the scope of this chapter to provide detail for the nurse acting as an expert witness, a few suggestions can be made. The nurse should be currently practicing in the field in which testimony is required. A nurse with a master's degree or a doctorate is preferred over one with a bachelor's degree. Affiliation with a school of nursing and a record of publication is also highly desired.[41] The expert witness is qualified by counsel before the court based on education, publications, and experience.

The role of the expert witness is to educate the jury as laypersons about nursing practice, to give opinions about what constitutes good nursing practice, and to state whether the nurse's actions were negligent (for the plaintiff) or not (for the defendant).[42] The expert witness is the only type of witness permitted in American courts to state opinions about standards of care and about the cause of an injury and to answer hypothetical questions.

The Nurse as Factual Witness

Nurses are also called to testify as factual witnesses. A factual witness is asked to describe what happened or what was done. Nurses may testify about the handling of evidence such as blood specimens, tissue samples, or bullets removed from a patient. They may be asked to state what nursing procedures were performed and what actions physicians took. They may be asked what patients said or did as it relates to giving consent.

Trauma nurses also may be called on to repeat what a dying patient said. While it is generally true that a witness cannot testify about what someone else said about a third party (the rule against hearsay) because it is better to have that person testify, the law makes an exception when the statement is a dying declaration.

Unlike expert witnesses, however, factual witnesses may not express an opinion about the standard of care in court, nor can they answer hypothetical questions.

Law of Death and the Dying Patient

Brain Death

Brain death, simply stated, is the irreversible cessation of brain activity as determined in accordance with reasonable medical standards. The essence of brain death statutes is that the traditional definition of death—cessation of respiration and heart action—still holds but that death may occur even if the body is kept alive by mechanical means in the absence of brain activity.

Trauma nurses have a need to understand brain death for two reasons. First, the families of patients who have suffered extensive head injuries must be counseled about the death of their loved ones. Second, trauma patients are often organ donors, since they are frequently young and healthy prior to trauma. Many organs remain viable for transplantation. Knowledge of the law of brain death is important in both these situations.

There is no single law that defines when death occurs in the United States, although 27 states and the District of

TABLE 4–1. STATES THAT HAVE ADOPTED THE UNIFORM DETERMINATION OF DEATH ACT

Arkansas	Nevada
California	New Hampshire
Colorado	North Dakota
Delaware	Ohio
Georgia	Oklahoma
Idaho	Oregon
Indiana	Pennsylvania
Kansas	Rhode Island
Maine	South Carolina
Maryland	South Dakota
Minnesota	Vermont
Mississippi	West Virginia
Missouri	Wyoming
Montana	

Adapted from West's Ann. Cal. Health and Safety Code, Sec. 7180. St. Paul, Minn., West Publishing Co., 1992.

Columbia had adopted the Uniform Determination of Death Act by the end of 1990–1992 (Table 4–1). This statute states that an individual is dead when, based on accepted standards of medical practice, either irreversible cessation of circulatory and respiratory function or irreversible cessation of all function of the entire brain including the brainstem occurs.

Clinical criteria for establishing brain death have been developed. These criteria are only examples of the medical criteria employed. There is, at present, no single list that encompasses all tests applied to satisfy the standard of reasonable medical practice. The reasonable and prudent approach above incorporates tests performed by two separate neurologists or neurosurgeons at least 12 hours apart:[43]

1. Isoelectric EEG indicating no brain wave activity
2. Drug screens to eliminate drugs as the cause of a reversible comatose state
3. Body temperature no greater than 35°C
4. No response to stimuli, even noxious ones
5. No pupillary response to light
6. No eye movement in response to head turning
7. No corneal reflexes
8. Confirmatory arterial blood gas studies

The drug screen is important because patients with no brain activity measured by an EEG have been known to recover following a drug overdose.[43]

The brain death statutes are all couched in terms of the cessation of brain activity as determined by reasonable medical standards. The language of the laws permits changes in the determination of death as medical techniques improve. Trauma nurses need to stay informed of these changes so that they can fulfill their role in family support as well as remain alert to appropriate opportunities for organ procurement. A discussion of the law can do no more than state that medical techniques underlie the standards for the determination of death. Nurses must independently keep abreast of changes in the state where they practice.

Anatomical Gift Act

A corollary to the brain death statutes is the organ donation laws now in existence in many states. These laws include the Uniform Anatomical Gift Act (Table 4–2), which specifies how an organ donation, an anatomical gift, can be made by a patient. The law includes a requirement of written authorization from the patient. Notice that a patient is an organ donor may be included on a driver's license so long as an affirmative statement of intent to donate was obtained when the license was issued. The act also usually states that the physician or surgeon who pronounces death is prohibited from removing or transplanting the donated organs.[44] The reader is referred to Chapter 32 for further discussion of this topic.

Living Wills

Legal issues in caring for a dying patient center on two key concepts: living wills and withdrawing or withholding treatment, including cardiopulmonary resuscitation. The issues raised here recently gained added importance to trauma nurses through the federal Patient Self-Determination Act. Under this law, health care providers are now required to provide information to patients about living wills and other similar proxy documents.

Increasingly, states are accepting directives made by patients long before they are ill or injured. By 1992, 33 states and the District of Columbia had adopted laws that state that competent adults have the right to control decisions about their medical care (Table 4–3). These laws specifically state that the decision to withhold or withdraw treatment for a terminal patient resides with that patient. These wills outline patients' wishes in the event that they become comatose or otherwise mentally incapacitated and dependent on extraordinary means of life support. These directives are called *living wills* (Fig. 4–1). Their purpose is to state the patient's desire that extraordinary care be withheld or discontinued in the event that it would be fruitless and to relieve the emotional burden on the families of these patients.[45, 46]

The underlying concept for these wills is that adults of

TABLE 4–2. STATES THAT HAVE ADOPTED THE UNIFORM ANATOMICAL GIFT ACT

Alabama	Montana
Alaska	Nevada
Arizona	New Hampshire
Arkansas	New Jersey
California	New Mexico
Colorado	New York
Connecticut	North Carolina
District of Columbia	North Dakota
Florida	Oklahoma
Georgia	Oregon
Hawaii	Pennsylvania
Idaho	Rhode Island
Illinois	South Carolina
Indiana	South Dakota
Iowa	Tennessee
Kansas	Texas
Kentucky	Utah
Louisiana	Vermont
Maine	Virginia
Maryland	Washington
Michigan	Wisconsin
Minnesota	Wyoming
Missouri	

Adapted from West's Ann. Cal. Health and Safety Code, Sec. 7150. St. Paul, Minn., West Publishing Co., 1992.

sound mind have the right to determine what treatments they will consent to and which they will refuse. The wishes of the patient are of paramount importance. It is no surprise, then, that a method of prospectively stating the individual's will about use of life support has been created.

The use of living wills has not reached all the states.[43] However, they are sufficiently pervasive that trauma nurses should be familiar enough with them to be able to identify a living will if it is presented to them.

Withholding or Withdrawing Treatment

Many courts have grappled with the problem of withholding or withdrawing treatment from a dying patient. There is, at present, no set of legal doctrines that apply to all clinical situations or to all states. The basis of common law decisions permitting the patient to die has been the same as for giving informed consent. The patient may consent to have treatment withheld or withdrawn.[47]

In 1990 in the *Cruzan* case, the Supreme Court of the United States held that a state's policy which favors continuation of life support supersedes the opinions of a patient's close family members where there is no clear and convincing evidence of the patient's wishes to withhold or withdraw treatment. The Court held that the states may indicate the kind of evidence required to establish a patient's wishes.

In this case, the family of Nancy Cruzan stated that they believed that she would not want treatments to continue after they had become futile. The state of Missouri refused to recognize these opinions as Nancy Cruzan's wishes and, instead, required that life support be continued. Missouri's public policy is to continue life support unless a written directive from the patient states otherwise.

Cruzan does not say that all states must follow Missouri's policy of continuing life support, only that the states *may* do so. It also does not state that written directives are required to discontinue life support for a patient, but it does state that individual states such as Missouri may so require while others may apply different evidentiary standards.

Cruzan may cause the unfortunate consequence of "jurisdiction shopping." Because the Court recognized that individual states may act as the final arbiter in maintaining or withdrawing treatment, there will be large differences in these policies. As a result, family members seeking to have treatment withdrawn from a patient may seek to move the patient from a state that requires maintaining treatment to one that leaves the decision to the family. Isolated cases of family members seeking to move patients to states with more liberal rules for withholding or withdrawing treatment have occurred since the *Cruzan* decision.

While the right of the individual to terminate extraordinary (or life-sustaining) care is well established, what constitutes such care is less clear. In the case of Karen Ann Quinlan, the court distinguished between what constituted ordinary and extraordinary care. A respirator, in this case, represented extraordinary care for a comatose patient in a persistent vegetative state with no hope of recovery. The guardians were permitted to have the respirator withdrawn.[48]

The distinction between ordinary and extraordinary care is dependent on the individual situation and the judgment of those involved. A widely quoted definition, however, was formulated by Gerald Kelly, a Roman Catholic ethicist. It states

> Ordinary means all medicines, treatments and operations which offer a reasonable hope of benefit and which can be obtained and used without excessive cost or other inconvenience. Extraordinary means are all machines, treatments and operations which cannot be obtained or used without excessive expense, pain or other inconvenience, or if used would not offer a reasonable hope of benefit.[9]

A *life-sustaining procedure* has been defined as any "medical procedure, treatment, or intervention which uses mechanical or other artificial means to sustain, restore, or supplant a spontaneous vital function or is otherwise of such a nature as to afford a patient no reasonable expectation of recovery from a terminal condition and which, when applied to a patient in a terminal condition, would serve to secure only a precarious and burdensome prolongation of life."[49]

Withholding or withdrawal of extraordinary treatment does not eliminate all duties owed to the patient. Ordinary supportive care must be continued. There are still differences of opinion regarding supportive care, especially special mechanisms for feeding, although many living wills specifically state that nutrition is to be discontinued.

Do Not Resuscitate Orders

Living wills express the individual's wish that extraordinary means not be used to prolong the life of the body when such action will be fruitless. This wish is a form of a *do not resuscitate* (DNR) order from the patient. Since living wills are not yet universally used, a DNR order usually originates from the attending physician in consultation with the patient or family members. Ensuring that the order is based on a correct legal foundation is imperative so that there are no adverse ramifications.

DNR orders must be written on an order sheet, and an accompanying note should appear in the progress notes with the rationale for the order. A written order documents the fact that a decision has been made and by whom. It ensures that the decision is clearly communicated to all nurses so that cardiopulmonary resuscitation (CPR) is not initiated inappropriately. It also acts to assure nurses that they can withhold CPR without fear that they have neglected the patient.[9]

DNR orders take on different character depending on the physician who enters the order. The order may simply state that CPR not be initiated should the patient suffer cardiac arrest. This is a recognition that death is imminent and that CPR will not save the life, only temporarily prolong it. An alternative order is one that continues life support such as feeding and ventilatory support but that orders no additional initiation of therapeutic treatments. The distinction between an order that terminates existing treatments and one that does not initiate new therapies is often based on the practitioner's ethical framework and has no legal significance. The importance at law centers on the existence of a DNR order rather than the order's clinical characteristics.[43] All hospitals must have policies for dealing with DNR orders, and such policies are the best source of information for the trauma nurse.

The principal issue in the use of DNR orders is what would be the wishes of the patient. Living wills eliminate this concern, since the patient has clearly stated what should be done. In all other cases, consent must be obtained from someone who is substituting judgment for that patient. The

TABLE 4–3. STATES THAT HAVE ADOPTED LAWS GUARANTEEING THE PATIENT'S RIGHT TO CONTROL DECISIONS ABOUT WITHHOLDING OR WITHDRAWING TREATMENT

Alabama	Mississippi
Arizona	Nevada
California	New Hampshire
Colorado	New Mexico
Connecticut	New York
Delaware	North Carolina
District of Columbia	Oregon
Florida	South Carolina
Georgia	Tennessee
Hawaii	Texas
Idaho	Utah
Illinois	Vermont
Indiana	Virginia
Kansas	Washington
Louisiana	West Virginia
Maryland	Wisconsin
Minnesota	Wyoming

Adapted from West's Ann. Cal. Health and Safety Code, Sec. 7185. St. Paul, Minn., West Publishing Co., 1992.

next of kin (spouse or children, for example) and the patient's legal guardian (parents or court-appointed guardian) are prime examples. Hospital policies as a reflection of state law also may permit the physician in charge of the patient's case, an administrator, or the hospital attorney to act as this substitute.[43]

The nurse who receives a DNR order from a physician must be conversant with the current law in the state in which she practices. It is an order which, if permitted in the particular jurisdiction, should be renewed by the physician every day.[43]

DECLARATION

On this (date) day of (month, year), I (person's name), being of sound mind, willfully and voluntarily direct that my dying shall not be artificially prolonged under the circumstances set forth in this declaration:

If at any time I should have an incurable injury, disease, or illness certified to be a terminal condition by two (2) physicians who have personally examined me, one (1) of whom shall be my attending physician, and the physicians have determined that my death is imminent and will occur whether or not life-sustaining procedures are utilized and where the application of such procedures would serve only to artificially prolong the dying process, I direct that such procedures be withheld or withdrawn, and that I be permitted to die naturally with only the administration of medication, the administration of food and water, and the performance of any medical procedure that is necessary to provide comfort care or alleviate pain. In the absence of my ability to give directions regarding the use of such life-sustaining procedures, it is my intention that this declaration shall be honored by my family and physician(s) as the final expression of my right to control my medical care and treatment.

I am legally competent to make this declaration, and I understand its full import.

(Signature)

(Witnesses' signatures)

Figure 4–1. Sample Living Will. (Adapted from Annotated Code of Maryland, Sec. 5-602c.)

Physical Evidence and Chain of Custody

Chain of custody of physical evidence is particularly applicable in cases in which the injury resulted from a violent crime such as a shooting or rape, although it also has application in civil matters. *Chain of custody* consists of two parts: a documentation component and a handling component. The first mandates meticulous recording of all evidence discovered (or samples taken), where it came from, when and to whom it was given. Receipts should be maintained as each piece of physical evidence or sample is given by the nurse to, for example, a laboratory technician. These receipts should list what was given, who gave it, to whom it was given, and the date and time of the transfer of possession.

The handling component speaks to the need for purity in a sample and the need to keep physical evidence in its original condition.[19] Potential contaminants should be kept away from tissue samples. A gun should not be handled except as absolutely necessary so that fingerprints are retained.

Protection of Patient's Property

When a patient is first brought into a trauma center, the trauma nurse is engaged in many activities that may involve resuscitation and preparation for surgery. The protection of a patient's property can easily be forgotten. While this may seem to be a relatively mundane concern during resuscitation, surgery, or critical care, property loss and damage frequently result in monetary claims against the hospital.[19] The law underlying the responsibility to protect the patient's personal possessions is that of a bailment.

The patient entrusts the trauma center through the trauma nurse to hold property and clothing until reclaimed at a later time. Property should be marked and stored so that it can be returned to the patient upon request or discharge or upon death to the family. The patient is the only person authorized to determine its disposition. Proper documentation is therefore necessary.[19]

DISCUSSION

If given the obligation of advising nurses with a single phrase, an attorney would most likely say "act reasonably." While this phrase is fundamentally true, it only provides the nurse with a general framework for guarding patient rights and for protection from professional liability. Handling the day-to-day legal dilemmas inherent in the practice of trauma nursing requires both this framework of reasonableness and specific knowledge of common points of law as applied to the patient-oriented situation in question.

Acting reasonably means that patients should be consulted at all possible times so that they are aware of the nature and rationale of nursing interventions. This will promote the patients' cooperation in recovery, which is critical to the nurse's protection against subsequent legal actions.

Acting reasonably means knowing and following standing orders and protocols for the assessment and care of the patient at the time of arrival at the emergency room. These protocols ensure that medically appropriate assessment and triage are performed even in the absence of a physician. Clearly, standing orders do not take the place of nursing judgment and are not to be blindly followed when additional injury to the patient may result. Objective self-assessment is also inherent in reasonable practice. Tasks and procedures for which the nurse is inadequately trained should not be done without seeking help from a more senior nursing colleague, supervisor, or physician.

There is no complete protection from malpractice litigation, and recent trends suggest that nurses suffer expanded susceptibility to lawsuits. However, liability can be limited through a number of actions. Since nurses are often in a position in which they possess exclusive patient information, the importance of proper documentation and communication of this information takes on great significance. It must be stressed that the entire medical record plays a crucial role as evidence in determining the standard of care provided by the nurse. It also can be used by the nurse during a lawsuit to help recall the details of the actions taken in the patient's care long after they are over. Documentation must be accurate and complete, describing the patient's changing condition, nursing diagnoses, plans and actions, and reports to physicians and other professionals. Effective verbal and written communication provides continuity among nurses and between nurse and physician.

Incident reporting is a specific type of documentation that is reasonable in the eyes of the law. A well-written incident report states facts rather than conclusions without supporting observations. Hospital policies detail the steps to follow in reporting an incident such as a patient fall or the injection of the wrong drug or an incorrect dosage. The policies should include how an incident report is prepared and who is responsible for its disposition. Incident reports are important to the hospital as indicators of areas of potential liability. As employees, nurses are required to report incidents promptly and thoroughly. The reports can mitigate the nurse's liability to the patient. They also can limit the nurse's potential liability to the hospital if the nurse is sued by the hospital to recover judgments against it based on the nurse's negligent actions.

Maintaining current and adequate levels of malpractice insurance is another prudent and protective action. Hospitals may provide malpractice insurance for their nurses. Nurses should be aware of the extent of this coverage, as well as any exclusionary clauses present in the insurance agreements that leave them open to personal liability for adverse judgments. Nurses must be aware of the relevant time periods the policies cover. There are two types of malpractice insurance. The first covers claims made during the period of coverage. The second covers claims resulting from occurrences during the period of coverage even if the claim is made after the policy's expiration date.

Being aware of new medical and scientific issues through continuing education is also important. Nursing supervisors and administrators must be responsive to the need of nurses to remain current on hospital policies and changes in state law that affect their practice.

These reasonable acts, coupled with adherence to the standards of quality nursing care, will generally keep trauma nurses free from legal liability for their actions. While such acts may not always keep the nurse out of court, they will significantly reduce the chance of an adverse judgment in a lawsuit.

The legal issues of this chapter identify areas of exposure of the trauma nurse to liability. They also speak of responsibilities that nurses have to society, to the hospital where they are employed, and to themselves. In the future, trauma nurses' actions will be subject to increasing scrutiny. There may be changes so that emergency and critical care nurses are granted a different license to practice based on higher educational and experience requirements. Higher standards of professional conduct will, in turn, be expected. Trauma nurses as expert witnesses will become more commonplace as their professionalism is more widely recognized by the law. By offering the court the benefit of years of special training, skill, and education, trauma nurses may perform a valuable service in advocating for the nursing specialty and potentially bringing about changes in the law that reflect the realities and expertise of trauma nursing practice.

CONCLUSION

Central to American jurisprudence and the legal issues presented in this chapter is the right to control one's own life and to expect others to act in a reasonable fashion. Trauma patients, despite their incapacitation, are accorded these rights by the laws of the United States and of the individual states. Trauma nurses must operate within this framework to be legally effective.

The law need not be viewed as the nurse's adversary. A rapport can easily be established in which nurses maintain respect for the rights of patients while exercising their judgment about types of treatment and quality of care. Knowledge of the law and legal responsibilities can enhance the nurse's relationship with patients.

REFERENCES

1. *Goff v. Doctors General Hospital*, 333 P. 2d 29 (Cal. App. 1958).
2. *Darling v. Charleston Community Hospital*, 33 Ill. 2d 326, 211 N.E. 2d 253 (1965), *cert. denied*, 383 U.S. 946 (1966).
3. Louisell DH, Williams H: Medical Malpractice. New York, Matthew Bender, 1985, p 16A-2.
4. Annotated Code of Maryland, Health Occupations, sec 8–101ff.
5. West's Annotated California Business and Professions Code, sec 2725.
6. Hayt E: Law of Hospital and Nurse. New York, Hospital Textbook Company, 1958, pp 20–21.
7. Annotated Code of Maryland, Health Occupations, sec 8–201.
8. Annotated Code of Maryland, Health Occupations, sec 8–316(a).
9. Rhodes AM, Miller RD: Nursing and the Law, 4th ed. Rockville, Md, Aspen Systems, 1984.
10. Rocereto LR, Maleski CM: The Legal Dimensions of Nursing Practice. New York, Springer, 1982.
11. Calloway SD: Nursing and the Law, 2nd ed. Eau Claire, Wisc, Professional Education Systems, 1987.
12. Guido GW: Legal Issues in Nursing. Norwalk, Conn, Appleton & Lange, 1988.

13. Northrop CE, Kelly ME: Legal Issues in Nursing. St. Louis, CV Mosby, 1987.
14. Guido GW: Legal Issues in Nursing. Norwalk, Conn, Appleton & Lange, 1988, pp 71–79.
15. Rocereto LR, Maleski CM: The Legal Dimensions of Nursing Practice. New York, Springer, 1982, pp 1–2.
16. *Nancy Beth Cruzan v. Missouri*, 497 U.S. 261, 269 (1990).
17. *Schloendorf v. Society of New York Hospital*, 211 N.Y. 125, 105 N.E. 92 (1914).
18. Strickler MM: The Rights of Patients. In Strickler MM, Ballard FL Jr (eds): Representing Health Care Facilities. New York, Practicing Law Institute, 1981, pp 1–17.
19. Cahill JA: Legal aspects of emergency medical care. In Cosgriff JH Jr, Anderson DL (eds): The Practice of Emergency Care, 2nd ed. Philadelphia, JB Lippincott, 1984, pp 17–28.
20. Annotated Code of Maryland, Health—General, sec 20–102(a).
21. Annotated Code of Maryland, Health—General, sec 20–102(b).
22. Annotated Code of Maryland, Health—General, sec 20–107.
23. Annotated Code of Maryland, Health—General, sec 20–107(c).
24. Annotated Code of Maryland, Health—General, sec 20–107(d).
25. *Anonymous v. State*, 17 App. Div. 2d 495, 236 N.Y.S. 2d 88 (1963).
26. Prosser WL: Handbook of the Law of Torts, 4th ed. St. Paul, Minn, West Publishing, 1971, pp 34–41.
27. Warren S, Brandeis L: The right to privacy. Harvard Law Rev 4:193, 1890.
28. Prosser WL: Handbook of the Law of Torts, 4th ed. St. Paul, Minn, West Publishing, 1971, pp 802–818.
29. American Hospital Association: A Patient's Bill of Rights. Management and Advisory Series. American Hospital Association, Chicago, Illinois, 1990.
30. Wold JL: AIDS testing: An ethical question. J Neurosci Nurs 22:258, 1990.
31. *Landeros v. Flood*, 551 P. 2d 389 (Cal. Sup. Ct. 1976).
32. Prosser WL: Handbook of the Law of Torts, 4th ed. St. Paul, Minn, West Publishing, 1971, pp 139–180.
33. Morris WO: The negligent nurse: The physician and the hospital. Baylor Law Rev 33:109, 1981.
34. Rocereto LR, Maleski CM: The Legal Dimensions of Nursing Practice. New York, Springer, 1982, p 99.
35. American Nurses' Association: Standards of Emergency Nursing Practice. Kansas City, ANA, 1975.
36. Connors JP: Nursing errors. In Mackauf SH (chairman): Hospital Liability. New York, Law Journal Seminars Press, 1985, pp 33–66.
37. King J Jr: The Law of Medical Malpractice. St. Paul, Minn, West Publishing, 1977, p 82.
38. Annotated Code of Maryland, Courts and Judicial Proceedings, sec 5–309.
39. West's Annotated California Business and Professions Code, sec 2727.5.
40. Black's Law Dictionary, 4th rev ed. St. Paul, Minn, West Publishing, 1968, p 1185.
41. Quigley FM: Expert testimony. Focus Crit Care 18:164, 1991.
42. Quigley FM: Responsibilities of the consultant and expert witness. Focus Crit Care 18:238, 1991.
43. Rheingold PD: Codes and death. In Mackauf SH (chairman): Hospital Liability. New York, Law Journal Seminars Press, 1985, pp 113–132.
44. West's Annotated California Health and Safety Code, sec 7182.
45. Annotated Code of Maryland, Health—General, sec 5–602.
46. West's Annotated California Health and Safety Code, sec 7188.
47. *Nancy Beth Cruzan v. Missouri*, 497 U.S. 261, 277 (1990).
48. *In re Quinlan*, 70 N.J. 10, 355 A. 2d 647, *cert. denied sub. nom. Garger v. New Jersey*, 429 U.S. 922 (1976).
49. Annotated Code of Maryland, Health—General, sec 5–601(3).

5

ETHICS IN TRAUMA NURSING

JOAN M. PRYOR-McCANN

Mr. Jones, 84 years old, is rushed to City Hospital's trauma unit from the site of an automobile accident. He was a passenger in an automobile that hit a guard rail at 60 mi/h. The driver of the car, a neighbor of Mr. Jones, died at the scene, but Mr. Jones survived, sustaining mild head trauma and multiple fractures, including a compound fracture of his right leg. The on-call physician, Dr. Brown, tells Nurse Smith that Mr. Jones will "probably never survive these injuries," and he questions the judiciousness of providing aggressive treatment. However, because of "legal concerns," Dr. Brown writes orders that include preparing Mr. Jones for the operating room and initiating a full code if his heart stops. Mr. Jones is stuporous and is unable to provide any information to the health care team, but from documents found in his wallet it is determined that his wife is deceased and he lives alone. He has no known relatives. While his vital signs are stable, Nurse Smith thinks that Mr. Jones "looks bad" and continues to monitor him very closely. She has her own misgivings about what is appropriate treatment for Mr. Jones. As she prepares him for surgery to repair his leg fracture, he suffers a cardiac arrest. Should Nurse Smith initiate a code procedure on Mr. Jones?

This question is similar to many of the ethical questions that confront nurses in their everyday practice. Trauma nurses, however, especially those in emergency settings, face a unique set of problems that make the resolution of ethical issues more difficult than in other nursing settings. For example, patients admitted to trauma units often have not chosen to be admitted there. Usually, these persons have incurred a medical emergency requiring immediate health care intervention and admission. A trauma-induced hospital visit differs markedly from an elective surgery hospital admission or even an admission in which the patient walks into the emergency unit under his own power. If a voluntarily admitted patient arrests, the nurse can reasonably infer that the patient himself sought and wanted care, but in the event of an arrest in an involuntarily admitted trauma patient, this inference cannot be made.

Not only is it unknown whether the trauma patient wants care, but often the trauma nurse cannot ascertain what the patient's wishes are regarding particular treatment options. For example, the trauma patient's decision-making ability is commonly incapacitated by an altered level of consciousness or is impaired by severe pain, anxiety, anger, or drugs. Sometimes such alterations are amenable to reversal with short-term treatment, when direction for care can then be obtained from the patient. More often than not, however, crucial life-or-death decisions must be made immediately, before these conditions can be reversed, in which case temporary alterations in decision-making ability are as problematic as any long-term ones. Community health nurses or hospital floor nurses are generally familiar with the patient's wishes and those of his family, but the trauma nurse is not, and gaining speedy access to such information is often difficult or impossible.

At the same time, the experienced trauma nurse is all too familiar with the practical implications of her ethical decisions. For example, she is keenly aware that if she places a 75-year-old chronic obstructive pulmonary disease (COPD) patient on a ventilator, that person may never be able to be weaned from the machine. She also knows that many people survive initial trauma but are unable to obtain or afford quality rehabilitative care. These considerations weigh on Nurse Smith's mind as she tries to resolve the question of whether or not she should initiate a code on Mr. Jones.

The trauma setting is very fast-paced when compared with other health care settings. Trauma settings require quick decision making and allow very little time for information gathering, deliberation, or weighing of alternatives. This, of course, is part of the reason why emergency care guidelines for particular health care interventions are necessary in this setting. Yet, while trauma nurses usually have clearly delineated procedures to follow in health care emergencies, there are no similar guidelines to assist them in making crucial ethical decisions. Frequently, treatment decisions involve both issues. The decision whether or not to code Mr. Jones, for example, is an ethical as well as a health care decision.

This chapter attempts to provide the trauma nurse with some guidance for making ethical decisions. Knowledge of nursing's code of ethics, as well as knowledge of moral principles and theories, will help the trauma nurse resolve troublesome ethical issues that arise in this setting. It is vitally important that the trauma nurse become familiar with these aspects of ethics so that she can make sound ethical decisions in her practice.

THE DIFFERENCE BETWEEN ETHICS AND LAW

Consider the case of Mr. Jones described earlier. The question is whether or not Nurse Smith should initiate a code procedure on Mr. Jones. Some nurses (those not acquainted with ethics) think the answer is obvious and quickly reply that Nurse Smith should follow Dr. Brown's orders. These nurses believe that when their legal obligation is clear, their ethical obligation is clear, and that is what they must do. Some nurses claim even more, i.e., that their legal obligation always coincides with or determines their ethical obligation. In other words, these nurses hold that when a nurse knows that the doctor's orders call for a code to be initiated, this fact alone ends any deliberation about whether or not it is ethical to code the particular patient in question. Although this may sometimes be true, it is certainly not always true. There are several crucial distinctions that need to be made between ethical and legal decisions.

First of all, ethics and law are not the same thing. The former deals with moral behavior and the latter with legal behavior. Admittedly, ethical choices are often reduced by pressures of the moment to worries about legal risk, but compliance with the law does not guarantee ethical behavior, nor is it an excuse for ignoring the ethical aspects of a decision.[9] For example, slavery was once legal in parts of the United States, but even at that time many persons questioned its morality, and most of us would agree today that slavery is ethically unacceptable. Similarly, abortion is now a legal alternative for pregnant women, but many persons question the morality of abortion. Laws themselves are not necessarily ethically sound. In fact, laws themselves are properly the subject of ethical appraisal and evaluation. Therefore, the assumption that if Nurse Smith does her legal duty and follows the doctor's orders she will also be performing her ethical duty is incorrect.

Another difference between law and ethics is evident in the fact that existing laws do not always give direction for particular ethical problems. The law often lags behind current ethical questions. For example, it took years for legislatures to enact statutes accepting brain death criteria as part of the legal definition of biological death, yet nurses were faced with ethical decisions about the care of such patients long before these laws were enacted. The status of living wills is another legal issue that remains unresolved in many states, but ethical questions about the care of people who express their wishes in living wills must be addressed now. Ethics, then, is broader and more inclusive than law, and the nurse is not always able to gain direction for current ethical difficulties by consulting the law.

On the other hand, law is not irrelevant to ethics. Difficult ethical decisions can often be clarified by referring to the reasoning employed by courts and legal scholars on the issue in question or related issues. This is true because legal reasoning reflects our society's perceptions on a subject and because the law has its roots in public acceptance and its adherence to fair and reasonable procedures for decisions on issues. Some ethicists also claim that knowledge of one's legal obligations, although not decisive for answering ethical questions, is necessary for discerning one's ethical obligation.[2] Such obligations are often taken to be limited by the risks of legal liability or financial loss that an agent might incur secondary to a particular choice. For example, in the case of Mr. Jones, Nurse Smith should consider the legal risk she would be taking if she does not act consistently with her legal obligation to follow the doctor's orders. This is certainly not the only data she should consider, but it is relevant to whether or not she should code Mr. Jones, and most nurses would consider it very important indeed.

Curiously, nurses often consider physicians who make treatment decisions based on considerations of legal risk as morally pernicious. Consider Dr. Brown in the case of Mr. Jones. Dr. Brown admittedly ordered a code on Mr. Jones because he feared legal liability if he did otherwise. Many nurses would assess Dr. Brown as unprincipled or immoral. Interestingly, nurses usually do not apply the same negative assessment standard to themselves. What if Nurse Smith conducts a code on Mr. Jones merely because the doctor ordered it and despite her own ethical concerns about such an intervention? Is she also without principles or perhaps immoral? One could argue that the nurse and the doctor are in somewhat different positions, and, of course, to some extent this is true. For example, the doctor writes the orders, and the nurse is legally bound to follow them. However, in assessing the nurse's or the doctor's moral culpability for ordering or initiating a code out of sole regard for her or his own legal risks, it is apparent that they seem to be on an equal footing. If the assessment of the physician is valid, then, logically speaking, a similar assessment of the nurse is required. The truth of the matter is that it is unclear whether Dr. Brown and Nurse Smith are acting immorally merely because they are concerned with legal risks. Legal risks are relevant data to consider when making moral decisions, and more analysis of this case is needed before a judgment of moral culpability can be made. The process of analyzing ethical decisions will be discussed later in this chapter, but there is an important lesson to be gained from this case as it now stands. Nurses must be more careful and more consistent in their assessments of the ethical implications of both their own actions and those of other health care workers.

In order to approach such assessments properly, nurses need more knowledge. Clearly, compliance with the law is not enough to guarantee morally correct decisions, so many nurses look for guidance to the ethical code proposed by the their professional association. The next section will discuss this document.

THE *CODE FOR NURSES*

In 1950, the American Nurses' Association adopted a code of ethics to guide professional nursing practice.[32] This document codifies nursing's traditional involvement with the obligations that health care workers owe to those under their care.[34] After several revisions, the code is now known as the *Code for Nurses with Interpretive Statements* (1976, 1985).[1] (Hereafter it is referred to as the *Code for Nurses,* or simply the *Code.*) The *Code* serves as a public declaration of the standards and values by which all professional nurses are expected to practice. The *Code* has what is called "performative force" because of its influence on nursing licensure, institutional accreditation, and curricula, as well as its use in court cases as the document representing accepted professional values standards.[3]

Professional codes of ethics are always mixtures of creed and commandments (beliefs and rules). The belief aspects of the *Code for Nurses* can be found in the preamble, and the rule aspects are delineated in the 11 statements and the interpretations that follow. While the ethical codes of some health professions have been criticized as overly paternalistic and limited, nursing's code has garnered much praise for its comprehensiveness and the emphasis it places on the autonomy of the patient.[26] Every professional nurse should familiarize herself with the *Code for Nurses* because its ideals are those deemed by the profession as essential for ethical nursing practice.

The *Code for Nurses* also serves to inform the public that nurses acknowledge their unique position of care and assures the public of the standards and values by which all nurses are expected to function.[3] Duties such as veracity (truth-telling) and advocacy are mentioned explicitly in the code. The preamble speaks to nurses' regard for the moral principles of beneficence (doing good), autonomy (patient self-determination), and justice (fairness).[23]

However, as impressive and important as the *Code* is, it cannot provide a specific answer to all the ethical questions that arise in nursing practice. Like other professional codes, the *Code for Nurses* provides general guidelines that must then be applied in specific situations. Making this shift from the general to the specific is especially difficult in trauma settings, where treatment decisions often have to be made quite rapidly, where patients may be either upset or unresponsive, and where adequate information about the patient and the patient's life situation is lacking.

For example, Section 1.1 of the *Code for Nurses* states

> Clients have the moral right to determine what will be done with their own person. . . . to accept, refuse or terminate treatment . . .

How should the trauma nurse respond to a very anxious and despondent battered woman who insists: "Don't you dare treat me; I just want to die." Does this patient's statement constitute a refusal of treatment? Should the trauma nurse abide by this woman's expressed wishes? Can a trauma nurse always get permission to render necessary life-saving treatment? If the patient ends up in the trauma unit after a suicide attempt, does the suicide victim have the right to refuse emergency life-saving treatment? Clearly the *Code for Nurses* does not address these complex questions in which the nurse's obligations and duties conflict and a resolution is not immediately apparent.

The same section of the *Code* states

> . . . truth-telling and the process of reaching informed choice underlies the exercise of self-determination, which is basic to respect for persons.

Should the trauma nurse tell the truth to a mother whose baby has just died in the next room, knowing that the mother has said that she wants to die if her baby dies? This is a classic case of a conflict of duty. The nurse has both the duty of veracity (to tell the truth) and the duty of beneficence (to do good for her patient). The *Code for Nurses* expects nurses to maximize these duties, but in the preceding case it seems that both cannot be maximized. The interpretive statements do say that the nurse should always tell the truth to the patient unless telling the truth will do more harm than good. The difficulty for the nurse in the preceding case is determining whether this particular situation qualifies as one of the latter exceptions. One can see that the *Code for Nurses* does not completely answer this difficult and crucial question.

Trauma nurses also must make decisions about triaging patients and distributing scarce resources. The *Code for Nurses* simply does not provide much direction for these essential activities. In fact, Section I of the *Code* directs nurses to "provide services . . . unrestricted by considerations of social or economic status, personal attributes, or the nature of the health problems." Taken at face value, this requirement possibly undermines the very practice of nursing itself. Currently, it is unquestionably understood that prognosis and illness are valid considerations for triage decisions, but obviously little guidance is provided by the *Code for Nurses* about how this process should be carried out.

Admittedly, no professional ethical code could capture all the myriad of ethical questions that arise within the scope of that profession's practice. The limits in the *Code for Nurses* just discussed point out that strict adherence to the *Code* is not enough to guarantee ethical behavior on the part of professional nurses. More important, however, is the fact that practicing nurses need to evaluate the *Code for Nurses.* Just as laws should be evaluated in light of ethical principles, so too should the *Code for Nurses* be ethically critiqued by practicing nurses. Is the current accepted *Code for Nurses* the very best code of ethics for a nurse to practice by? Can a nurse always act ethically if she adheres to the beliefs and rules included in the *Code?* What general standards or principles can be used to evaluate the *Code for Nurses?* In order to gain expertise to answer these questions, one needs to explore both moral principles and ethical theories.

ETHICS

What is ethics? *Ethics* can be defined as the philosophical study of moral conduct, whereas *morals* or *morality* is understood philosophically as dealing with what is right and what is wrong in a practical sense.[12] In this chapter, as in common usage, the terms *ethics* or *morals* will be used interchangeably. Thus I will sometimes refer to theories about what is right or wrong as *moral theories* or as *ethical theories*. Likewise, I will discuss the *morality of an action* by looking at the *ethical justification* for the action. Ethics involves a systematic appraisal of moral situations using moral principles and ethical theories to justify resolution of the question: What, all things considered, ought to be done in this situation?[24]

Ethics is a human enterprise that requires one to look at one's own obligations and provide justification for one's own actions. Nursing ethics requires nurses to look at their professional obligations and explore how these obligations coincide with or are justified by general ethical principles and theories.

As already noted, trauma nurses deal with a myriad of ethical issues in their everyday practice, and some of these issues are clear and easily answered by referring to the *Code for Nurses*. However, many more ethical issues are ambiguous and difficult to answer. An ethical dilemma occurs either when there is no obvious answer to the issue at hand or the available alternative actions are each somewhat morally justifiable or are all morally undesirable. Many ethical dilemmas routinely confront nurses who practice in the technologically complex and economically stressed modern health care system. The ethical code for the nursing profession cannot and should not be expected to resolve all these cases. Each case has numerous facets and considerations to take into account. Despite the complexity and uniqueness of each individual case, however, there are some commonalities upon which the nurse can and should base her ethical decisions. These are the general moral principles that provide the foundation of ethical nursing practice.

MORAL PRINCIPLES

Ethicists discuss four basic moral principles that affect nursing practice.[22] The first is the principle of *beneficence*, which requires that the nurse "ought to do good for and prevent or avoid doing harm to" her patient. This latter obligation, i.e., that of avoiding harm, is called *nonmaleficence*, and in general ethics it is usually considered more binding than the duty to do good. However, given the nurse's specialized education and training, coupled with the reasonable expectation by the public that nurses can resolve or ameliorate many health care problems, professional nurses do have a responsibility of beneficence as well as one of nonmaleficence to their patients. Sometimes a nurse cannot avoid causing some harm to a patient in order to properly perform her professional responsibilities. For example, nurses give injections or deliver other types of painful treatments such as debriding burn wounds or changing nasogastric tubes. These treatments are considered ethically acceptable only if the harm is minimized as much as possible and the benefit to be gained is worth the pain. One great difficulty with the principle of beneficence involves determining just what constitutes good or worthwhile gain for a particular patient. For example, is it beneficent to withhold food and water from a patient who has no likely chance of recovering from a terrible head injury and remains comatose? Withholding food clearly does constitute some harm, but does the good of allowing nature to take its course and letting the patient die outweigh the harm of not feeding him? Some nurses and ethicists reason that it does, whereas others claim that it does not. How should this issue be resolved? Perhaps investigating other moral principles will provide some guidance.

Autonomy is another moral principle that has gained prominence in health care settings as patient rights and informed consent issues have arisen.[14] It has a long history in general ethics, most notably in Immanuel Kant's writings. *Autonomy* refers to the freedom to rule oneself. It includes the right of informed consent, the right to accept or refuse treatment, and the right to confidentiality. The principle of beneficence often conflicts with the moral principle of autonomy. For example, when a patient chooses not to have a recommended treatment needed to save his life, the nurse must decide whether she should override the patient's decision in order to do the beneficent thing and administer the treatment or abide by the patient's refusal. In other words, which principle should have the most weight for the trauma nurse in such a situation, the principle of autonomy or the principle of beneficence? Most ethicists today agree that autonomy has more weight in moral decision making than beneficence, but despite this, nurses often take a paternalistic stance vis-à-vis their patients.

Benjamin and Curtis[6] point out how difficult it is to justify any paternalistic actions with adults. They list three criteria that must be met in order to decide ethically to take and carry out any paternalistic action.

1. *The autonomy condition:* where the patient is under the circumstances irretrievably ignorant of relevant information, or his capacity for rational reflection is significantly impaired.
2. *The harm condition:* where the patient is likely to be significantly harmed unless interfered with.
3. *The ratification condition:* where it is reasonable to assume that if the patient would regain at a later time, greater knowledge or recovery of his capacity for rational reflection, he would ratify the decision to interfere by consenting to it.[6]

These are strong criteria, and they require much justification to warrant any overriding of a patient's autonomy. Often trauma nurses restrain patients against their wishes for safety reasons or out of legal or medical concerns. In cases in which the patient is awake and alert enough to make decisions and refuses to be restrained, if the nurse continues with the restraining, she is clearly choosing to override the patient's own autonomous wishes. The more difficult case is one in which the patient is refusing, but the nurse has reason to think that his capacity to decide is impaired. The criteria listed above require more than this to justify overriding the patient's wishes, such as knowing that the harm is significant and that there is reason to assume that the patient would authorize the restraining if he could reason better. If these conditions are met, then the restraining is justified. Use of placebos also can be contrary to a patient's autonomy rights, and yet health care workers continue to try to justify the use of placebos solely on the basis of beneficence.

Most ethicists agree that the autonomy rights of a patient override the professional's beneficence obligations in usual cases.[11, 17, 30, 31] Therefore, in the preceding case in which the patient is in a coma and the question is whether or not to continue nutrients and water, many think the issue is resolved if a living will made by the patient requests withdrawal, because this is akin to the patient exercising his autonomy, and such autonomy should be respected. Unfortunately, many people do not have a living will, or the document itself may be unclear on this issue. In such cases, the nurse is in a difficult position in trying to determine what action beneficence requires, since the patient's autonomous wishes are unclear.

Several recent cases have explored the horizons of patient autonomy and beneficence obligations of health care workers in new ways. One case involved an 87-year-old woman from Minnesota, a victim of a stroke, who was comatose and on a ventilator for almost a year. She and her husband had lifelong moral compunctions against removing life support. The husband was an attorney and had substantial means to support his wife's care. However, the hospital and doctors took the husband to court to force him to remove her life support. Their claim was at least partially based on the tenet that continuing life support was cruel and inhumane treatment. In other words, they thought that their beneficent obligation to the woman was to remove her from life support. The court, however, held that the husband's and patient's wishes were to be honored (*Columbus Dispatch,* July 6, 1991).

Thus the court considered the principle of autonomy as primary in this case. What is important, for our purposes, is whether it is just or wise for any health care worker to claim to have the right to exercise beneficent obligations when to do so requires overriding a patient's autonomy.

Another more recent case involved a 3-year-old girl who was in an automobile accident and sustained severe head trauma resulting in a coma for 8 months. The child was not brain dead, but the hospital and doctors were convinced that she would only live "as a vegetable" connected to life support for the rest of her days. The parents were divided about what to do. The mother had mixed feelings about keeping her daughter on the ventilator, while the father still hoped that God would "wake her up." The parents were taken to court by the hospital and physicians in an attempt to remove the girl from life support. The health care workers asserted that the parents were guilty of child abuse. Again, the court upheld the principle of autonomy over the principle of beneficence and ruled that the ventilator was to remain on unless and until the parents agreed to remove it (*Columbus Dispatch,* Oct. 21, 1991).

Since this case involves a child, the issues are even more complex. However, it is important to note the point that health care workers, seeing themselves as advocates for the patient's beneficent outcomes, have in some cases expanded this obligation to the extent of deciding to let a patient die based on the health care workers' terms rather than those of the patient or family. I believe that this is an erroneous and dangerous application of the principle of beneficence and that the principle of autonomy deserves more weight than the health care workers in these cases are giving it.

The third ethical principle is that of *justice,* which requires that nurses treat all their patients fairly. This does not necessarily mean that each and every patient is treated exactly alike, but rather that equals are to be treated equally and that those who are unequal should be treated differently according to their differences.[5, 19] This means that patients with similar health care problems deserve the same care and those who have different needs should be attended to according to those needs. It also means that the nurse should take into consideration a patient's cultural and religious preferences. However, when one looks at the way the general principle of justice functions in mainstream ethics, a possible problem does arise for the nurse.

General ethics requires everyone to be fair to everyone. When justice is limited in scope to a particular nurse's patients, her duty to those patients may conflict with her general ethical duty to everyone at large. This issue rears its head vociferously when scarcity of resources comes into play. Consider a case in which a trauma nurse is to receive a large number of patients from a disaster site. Does she owe a duty to the patients she already has or to the ones she might get or both?[27] What if the two seem to conflict? This difficult issue will occur more and more as health care resources become increasingly scarce. Can the trauma nurse justify using current resources on patients who have a lower chance of recovery rather than saving those resources for potential patients who will have a better chance to recover? What if the latter patients never arrive? The answers to these questions remain unclear, especially when one acknowledges the special obligations nurses are taken to have to patients already in their care.[28] Furthermore, if the public decides that nurses have obligations of justice to persons not included in the nurses' current patient load, this decision would be bound to have profound implications for the principle of fairness in future health care decisions. It is unclear whether the nurse could ethically function under such a requirement because of the traditional nursing commitment of special duties owed to current patients. These issues are only part of the conundrum of gray areas currently under consideration in the arena of public and professional ethics.

The last moral principle, *fidelity,* may shed some light on the appropriate actions of a nurse in promise-making situations. Fidelity involves being faithful to one's promises. What are the promises a nurse implicitly makes to a patient in her care? Minimally, the nurse promises that she will do no harm to that person and, hopefully, that she will do as much good for the patient as she can. Note that this promise is made implicitly to patients already under the nurse's care. However, this principle does not provide very clear directions for what obligations (if any) the nurse owes to any potential or future patients. What is clear is that if a nurse makes an individual promise to a patient, then she has an obligation to follow through on it. The proper content of any promise a nurse should make to a patient, however, is still a gray area. Should the nurse remain faithful to a promise not to code a patient even if a physician has ordered such a procedure? What if the nurse needs her job to feed her five children and has reason to believe that if she resists the order she could be fired? Considerations about the nurse's own risks in making certain choices seem relevant to the moral weight of her promise, but to what extent should they prevail? Should the trauma nurse withhold pain medication from a patient because of lower vital sign readings, despite the explicit promise to try to relieve his pain? These complex questions are not entirely resolvable using only moral principles as guidelines. Perhaps a review of ethical theories will help to clarify the nurse's obligations in these complex cases.

MORAL THEORIES

Moral or ethical theories are more general than rules and principles and provide the most basic foundation for ethical decision making, especially when rules or principles conflict. Theories set priorities on which rules or principles override others in specific instances.[4] There are two major types of moral theories: teleological and deontological. The term *teleological* is derived from the Greek word *telos,* meaning "goal" or "end." Teleological moral theories are consequentialist theories because they hold that the rightness or wrongness of an act is determined solely by the consequences the act produces or is foreseen to produce. All consequentialist theories are alike in that they require that a moral agent's actions maximize the good; however, they differ in what they consider the good to be. Such theories view no particular act as morally wrong in and of itself; only the consequences determine the morality of any action. Thus a particular act can be right in one situation and wrong in another situation as long as the consequences of the act differ in terms of the amount of good they result in.[24]

The term *deontology* is rooted in the Greek word *deon,* meaning "duty." Deontological theories deny what consequentialist theories affirm. Deontological theories claim that the morality of an act is determined by more than the consequences of that action. The moral status of an act is a result of other relevant factors such as the nature of the act itself. Using this type of theory to evaluate the morality of actions involves looking at established rules and principles that govern human conduct such as the Ten Commandments, the *Code for Nurses,* or other procedures for determining formal duties.[12]

Although there are many differ kinds of consequentialist or deontological theories, the most familiar ones are utilitarian consequentialism and Kantian deontology. These two kinds of theories serve to illustrate the reasoning often offered in discussions of ethical questions facing trauma nurses.

Utilitarianism

Classical utilitarianism has its roots in the early 19th century works of Jeremy Bentham and John Stuart Mill. Despite the variations in their particular theories, both held that actions are to be judged by the amount of happiness or unhappiness that results from the action and that no one person's happiness or unhappiness counts any more importantly than another's. Each person's welfare is equally weighted in the utilitarian calculus.

The power of utilitarianism lies in two important points. First, promoting the "most good overall" has strong intuitive appeal. It certainly seems like a laudable thing to do and may be the very best that one can hope to accomplish in the complex cases that face trauma nurses. Second, utilitarianism offers an objective way (in theory) to determine the answer to any and every ethical dilemma. One merely assesses the consequences of the various alternatives and chooses the one that leads to the greatest happiness. In effect, utilitarianism does away with every ethical dilemma, and all cases have a decisive, determinative best way to proceed.

Despite the obvious advantages of utilitarianism, there remain some grave difficulties for nurses who accept this as their sole theory of morality. Beneficence, autonomy, justice, and fidelity are accepted principles that apply to nursing practice. These principles cannot be accommodated in their appropriate weight for proper ethical decision making of nurses in a utilitarian framework. This is so because utilitarianism gives no particular moral status to any principle beyond the absolute moral status it accords to maximizing overall good.[23]

Here is an example showing the type of difficulty that a nurse might face if she accepts utilitarianism as the appropriate ethical theory to guide her actions. Suppose a wealthy, famous patient was admitted to the trauma unit from the scene of an accident, and imagine that all the currently available nursing resources were lavished on this patient, while other needy patients went unattended. Such an action would clearly seem to be unethical and violates the basic principle of fairness. However, if this patient then went on to give a huge donation to the trauma center, which resulted in equipment being available for a greater number of patients than those left unserved originally, the actions of the nursing staff would be judged as right using utilitarian standards, because a greater good resulted from the lavishing of resources on this one patient than would have occurred if the nurses had not done that act. Surely this is an unacceptable outcome of moral decision making. Nurses do believe that unfair treatment of patients is morally wrong, just as the *Code for Nurses* claims. Thus utilitarianism falls short of capturing some of the basic moral principles that nurses incorporate into their professional practice in this case. It does not have the theoretical flexibility to allow for the special duties that nurses believe they owe to their patients.

However, utilitarianism does have some insights to offer nurses when considering ethical questions. It does seem that consequences should have some bearing on ethical decisions. Although it is apparent that nurses cannot consider consequences as the only relevant moral factor, it remains to be determined just how much weight consequences should be given by the nurse. An exploration of deontology will shed some light on this difficult question.

Deontology

An 18th century philosopher named Immanuel Kant[18] believed that morality consisted of following absolute rules no matter what the consequences. His primary test of whether a rule should be followed was to apply the categorical imperative of universality to the considered action. Whether or not the action was moral did not depend on the desire of the agent or the consequences of the action, but rather on whether one's duty was to perform the action as determined by his moral test, better known as the *categorical imperative.* Kant explored several applications of his categorical imperative in assessing the morality of lying, stealing, and suicide. These have been studied intensely and nearly uniformly rejected by later ethicists. For example, Kant concluded that stealing and suicide are always wrong and one must always tell the truth in all circumstances. However, the appeal of Kantian ethics remains for persons who believe that acting on principle rather than because of good results is an important ethical insight. Kant places a high value on autonomy and respect and can accommodate the special duties nurses are thought to owe their patients. Most contemporary deontologists think Kant went too far in concluding that morality requires absolute rules that do not take into account any consequences of actions. His theory is also limited in that it cannot adjudicate cases in which more than one duty applies but no alternative action can maximize both. Conflict-of-duty situations are common in nursing practice, but Kant's ethics offers no way to resolve them. There are several ethicists who have tried to remain faithful to the spirit of Kantian ethics but have tried to accommodate these commonsensical well-established aspects of morality.

W. D. Ross[12] proposes a theory that provides some guidance in this regard. He claims that duties originate from the social relationships one finds oneself in and eventually these duties are coalesced by humans into general duties. Ross claims that general duties have *prima facie* status and are only overridable in very particular circumstances. Furthermore, any overriding of a *prima facie* principle requires its own justification. He lists fidelity, reparation, gratitude, justice, beneficence, and nonmaleficence as *prima facie* duties owed to others. Ross does not prioritize these duties but says that some apply more stringently than others and all can be overridden at times. Presumably, circumstances and possible consequences play a role in defining the proper kind of justification for overriding a general principle. Thus this theory manages to support some of the special duties of a nurse while allowing for mitigating circumstances such as the consequences of the act being considered. Unfortunately, Ross's theory gives little direction about the way that justification is to proceed. He offers no rules or procedures to use in weighing the stringency of application of a particular principle in a specific moral situation nor ways to justify one principle being applicable over another. Thus, although Ross allows for more flexibility regarding rules and consequences than Kant, his theory is incomplete in that it provides little guidance for deciding difficult cases.

W. K. Frankena,[13] another modern deontologist, posits a theory in which the principles of beneficence and justice are considered to be the most basic of all moral principles. Thus, for Frankena, in cases in which there is a conflict between one of these primary principles and autonomy or fidelity, the right moral action will be the one that maximizes the basic principle. In a nursing situation in which justice and autonomy conflict, justice prevails. Or if beneficence and fidelity conflict, beneficence triumphs. However, a major problem persists, for how is a case of conflict between beneficence and justice to be decided? Some of the cases discussed previously involving scarcity of resources and duties owed to very ill patients with questionable prognoses have this exact issue at their heart. If two patients have equal need to go to the intensive care unit (ICU) but there is only one ICU bed available, how does one decide which patient to send? Frankena's theory does not provide specific guidance for these difficult yet pressing cases.

As can be seen, both the utilitarian and deontological theories have their own unique contributions to moral reasoning as well as their own sets of difficulties. In fact, no moral theory is without some problems. All moral theories fall short of some commonsensical and well-accepted portion of ethical judgment. This does not necessarily mean that any one of the moral theories is itself in error, since it could also be the case that more than one moral theory is needed to deal with new and complex issues in health care settings. It also should be noted, however, that each theory provides the nurse with some very important ethical insights and therefore can provide assistance to the nurse when she deals with difficult ethical problems.

THE ETHICS OF CARING

Some nursing ethicists and theorists such as Gadow,[15] Benner, Bishop,[7] Watson, and others[3] have described the ethic of nursing as the "ethic of caring." Although definitions vary, *caring* is most often associated with the principle of beneficence. Some say caring is the same thing as beneficence. Others believe that the nurse's obligation to care for her patients is merely supported by the principle of beneficence, whereas some describe caring as a way of acting that fulfills the obligations required by the principle of beneficence. As discussed earlier, beneficence is not without its problems. Paternalism has often clouded the moral ideal of "doing good," and the ethic of caring is vulnerable to this difficulty. Perhaps this is why *advocacy* is often linked by nursing scholars to the ethic of caring, but Winslow[33] and Trandel-Korenchuk[29] point out several complex difficulties inherent in the concept of advocacy. Much of the difficulty lies in the need to clarify exactly what advocacy requires. For example, is advocacy *doing* for a patient, *assisting* a patient, *defending* a patient, or some combination of these actions? Other problems involve clarifying *what* is to be advocated; that is, should the nurse advocate the patient's actual wishes or rather what is in the best interest of the patient? Furthermore, who is to define what constitutes the "best interest" of the patient? Should it be the patient himself, or his family, or the most expert health care professional, or someone else? How do the rules change with patients of different ages, competencies, or levels of consciousness?

Gadow[15] describes a model of "existential advocacy" that is claimed to avoid paternalism while maintaining the nurse as an involved, caring participant in the patient's decision-making process, but aspects of her model remain controversial.[33] For example, Gadow states that as an advocate, the nurse should answer a patient directly if he asks her opinion about treatment options. Yet many question whether the nurse can ever recommend a course of action for the patient without interfering with the patient's autonomy by inadvertently manipulating or coercing him. Others question Gadow's claim that nurses gain ethical knowledge about where the boundary between benefit and harm lies for the patient based on the nurse's special role as the touching, ministering caregiver.[15]

Bandman and Bandman[3] point out that the caring ethic has its roots in both the history of philosophy and the contemporary work of Carol Gilligan.[16] Bishop and Scudder[7] hold that nursing's caring ethic belongs primarily to its own history and practice. Whatever the basis for the approach, the caring ethic clearly offers important insights to nurses as they seek to practice ethically. For example, the caring ethic describes the orientation a nurse should have vis-à-vis a patient; therefore, it provides a basis for explaining the special duties that a nurse owes to her patient, such as beneficence and advocacy. When described in this way, the ethic of caring can be classified as a theory of virtue ethics that deals with the moral excellence of a person's character. The caring ethic describes the moral character requirements of a nurse; i.e., she must be caring toward her patients. However, difficulties arise when one attempts (as Gadow[15] and Gilligan[16] do) to use the ethic of caring as a theory of moral obligation, i.e., a theory that determines what actions are morally permissible, impermissible, or required. One difficulty is that the ethic of caring seems to be based on feelings, values, and intuition in such a way that the charge of pernicious relativism and subjectivism is hard to defend. It may be that the theory itself is simply less fully developed than the traditional theories of ethics discussed earlier.[3] Perhaps as nurses explore and clarify the ethic of caring it will become a more helpful tool to use when assessing the proper ethical action in particular situations. For now, however, I believe that the traditional theories of moral obligation offer more definitive help to practicing trauma nurses for resolving ethical issues.

The question remaining is how the nurse is to decide among the various moral principles and theories when trying to make actual ethical choices in her practice. Today's nurse requires a framework for decision making that is not arbitrary and considers all the relevant moral factors. The process of reflective equilibrium provides a structure for trauma nurses to use in ethical decision making.

ETHICAL DECISION-MAKING APPROACHES

A Harvard philosopher named John Rawls[28] has proposed a theory of justice that uses a process that he calls "wide reflective equilibrium." Callahan,[8] Curtin,[10] and others have endorsed an adaptation of Rawls' approach to justice as a guide for nurses in their ethical decision making. The reflective equilibrium process helps nurses to clarify their own moral framework by comparing and contrasting three important ethical data bases: their own beliefs, values, and considered moral judgments; moral principles; and ethical theories. It is the preferred decision-making process to use in making ethically supportable choices. However, it has its limits. I will explore the advantages and disadvantages of the reflective equilibrium process by applying it to the case of Mr. Jones presented at the beginning of this chapter.

When beginning the reflective equilibrium process, the nurse should clarify the pertinent facts of the case, the ethical question it presents, and the possible alternative actions that are available. In the case of Mr. Jones, Nurse Smith needs to know the patient's medical status, including his prognosis, and she needs to formulate the ethical dilemma of the case, i.e., whether to code or not to code Mr. Jones. Finally, Nurse Smith should list the alternative actions available to her, such as calling a code, not calling a code, calling Dr. Brown, beginning some code measures and not others, and so on. Then, while considering each alternative in turn, Nurse Smith should clarify her own moral judgments about the alternative by exploring her background beliefs and considered moral judgments and then cross-reference these with known and accepted moral principles and theories. The deliberation by Nurse Smith might proceed something like this:

Considering the first alternative, i.e., calling a code, Nurse Smith initially identifies her values and beliefs about the morality of calling the code. Given Nurse Smith's concerns about calling a code, it is likely that she has a moral compunction against taking this action. However, this is not enough to assure her that her judgment is ethically sound. Nurse Smith must then examine her moral judgment for validity by comparing it with accepted moral beliefs, principles, and theories. Nurse Smith would find that while some people question the rightness of coding an 84-year-old person even if their prognosis is fairly good, not all do.

In reflecting on the principle of beneficence, Nurse Smith should consider her obligation not to harm Mr. Jones and her responsibility to do good for him. She therefore needs to clarify whether or not death is a good in this situation and whether the harm incurred in conducting a code is warranted. If she feels that death is more desirable than coding Mr. Jones, she then needs to test this judgment by looking at the moral theories of utilitarianism and deontology.

Utilitarianism would confirm Nurse Smith's tentative conclusion that coding Mr. Jones is wrong if the good of not coding him outweighs the bad of coding him. Things to consider are the consequences for Mr. Jones, the outcomes for society in terms of resource use, and the possible legal, financial, and other outcomes for the nurse, the doctor, and the hospital. Note that in utilitarianism the possible legal difficulties for the health care team count in this assessment just as much as the actual outcome for Mr. Jones. Presumably, this moral theory, given the harmful consequences that may occur for the nurse, would lead to the conclusion that the coding of Mr. Jones is a correct moral action.

In addition, Frankena's deontological theory as well as Ross's could support coding of Mr. Jones given the status of the principle of beneficence in their systems and the fact that no one knows the patient's autonomous wishes. At this point in the analysis, the coding of Mr. Jones would be considered an ethically supportable action. Nurse Smith should then begin the same inquiry concerning the next alternative and each other one in turn.

Obviously this type of analysis is very thorough and as such gives much credence to the decisions made. It is the preferable approach when the nurse has the time for prolonged deliberation; however, this process is very time consuming, and it is not very feasible in situations that require quick decision making. Kenneth Iserson[21] has suggested another approach to ethical decision making when a rapid appraisal is needed, such as in the situation of Nurse Smith.

He claims that one should begin by asking oneself if the ethical problem at hand is similar in type to any other ethical problem for which one has already worked out a rule about how to proceed. If so, he suggests that the individual follow that rule, not because it is necessarily correct, but rather because it is more likely than not to be an ethically acceptable action, given that the individual has used it before and discussed it with others. I would add that the rule should be an ethically comfortable stance for the nurse and that the nurse should already have clarified the facts, the moral question, and the alternative actions available in the situation. If the rule is ethically unacceptable for the nurse, or if she has no rule for this type of situation, then she must consider whether any option exists that would buy time for further deliberation without excessive risk to the patient. If there is such an option, the nurse should take it. If there is no available option, then the nurse should perform three quick moral assessment tests on the alternative action under consideration:

1. *Impartiality test:* in which the nurse asks if she would be willing to have this action performed if she were in the patient's place.
2. *Universalizability test:* in which the nurse asks if she would be willing to have this action performed in all relevantly similar circumstances.
3. *Interpersonal justifiability test:* in which the nurse asks if she is able to provide good reasons to justify her actions to others.[21]

The first test is not infallible, but it is a good way to correct one obvious source of moral error, that of partiality or self-interested bias. The second test is also designed to eliminate a moral decision difficulty, shortsightedness. It enables the nurse to evaluate the action by considering whether it should be followed as a general practice in all similar circumstances. This is important because, although one may approve of the action in the particular situation, it may not be an acceptable practice to follow in similar circumstances. Moral rules are supposed to apply generally, and it is this that the nurse is assessing with this test. The final test requires that the nurse has reasons for proceeding in the way she decides and further that others would approve of her reasons. This ensures that the nurse has considered her decision thoughtfully and that her reasons are sound and nonidiosyncratic.

Nurse Smith may have had a rule to follow in the situation in which Mr. Jones suffers a cardiac arrest. More than likely, she would have previously opted to code other patients in Mr. Jones' situation. If so, she should call the code. However, if she is uncomfortable with this previously used rule, or if the situation with Mr. Jones is new, she should consider whether or not there is an option to gain time without excessive risk to the patient. It again seems that this point warrants Nurse Smith coding Mr. Jones, since delaying the code would result in the death of the patient.

However, if Nurse Smith decides to hesitate beginning the code because she considers Mr. Jones' death as a good, she should then quickly proceed to consider Iserson's three tests. She may find that she would not want to be coded herself in Mr. Jones' situation, but she might have more difficulty accepting not coding an 84-year-old patient as a matter of practice. Admittedly, this test is somewhat problematic because it is unclear exactly what factors are relevant to consider. For example, should the general comparison include Mr. Jones' injuries, the fact that his wishes are unknown, or the fact that his prognosis is poor? Even if all these factors are considered relevant, it would still be difficult to agree to a general practice of not coding such patients. In addition, it is not clear that Nurse Smith's reasons would be acceptable to many people, since many ethicists and nurses alike question the acceptability of using age as a criterion for limiting health care interventions. Therefore, it seems clear that on this assessment Nurse Smith should proceed to code Mr. Jones. Iserson's decision-making process takes less time for consideration and allows for much more rapid responses on the part of nurses. However, after the initial crisis is over, the nurse should reassess her ethical decision using the reflective equilibrium process. All ethical stands should be reviewed periodically for relevance and credence. Sometimes this process results in rule adjustments, while at other times it merely confirms the nurse's preexisting stance. Whichever way it goes, the review process will help to clarify and reinforce sound ethical decision making on the part of the nurse.

Ethical dilemmas in trauma nursing practice are ubiquitous and recalcitrant. However, the trauma nurse can be prepared to deal with these problems if she is knowledgeable about nursing's code of ethics, general moral principles, ethical theories, and ethical decision-making processes. Armed with these guideposts, the trauma nurse has at her fingertips the tools she needs to make sound ethical decisions in her nursing practice.

REFERENCES

1. American Nurses Association: Code for Nurses with Interpretive Statements, Kansas City, MO, ANA, 1976, 1985.
2. Buchanan AE: What is ethics? In Iserson KV et al (eds): Ethics in Emergency Medicine. Baltimore, Williams & Wilkins, 1986.
3. Bandman E, Bandman B: Nursing Ethics Through the Life Span. Norwalk, CT, Appleton & Lange, 1990.
4. Bandman EL, Bandman B: Ethical aspects of nursing. In Flynn JB, Heffron PB (eds): Nursing from Concept to Practice, 2nd ed. Norwalk, CT: Appleton & Lange, 1988.
5. Beauchamp TL, Walters L (eds): Contemporary Issues in Bioethics, 3rd ed. Belmont, CA, Wadsworth, 1989.
6. Benjamin M, Curtis J: Ethics in Nursing, 2nd ed. New York, Oxford University Press, 1986.
7. Bishop AH, Scudder JR: The Practical, Moral, and Personal Sense of Nursing. Albany, State University of New York Press, 1990.
8. Callahan JC (ed): Ethical Issues in Professional Life, New York, Oxford University Press, 1988.
9. Capron AM: Legal setting of emergency medicine. In Iserson KV et al (eds): Ethics in Emergency Medicine. Baltimore, Williams & Wilkins, 1986.
10. Curtin LL: Nursing ethics: Theories and pragmatics. Nurs Forum 17:4–11, 1978.
11. Davis AJ, Aroskar MA: Ethical Dilemmas and Nursing Practice, 2nd ed. New York, Appleton-Century-Crofts, 1983.
12. Feldman F: Introductory Ethics. Englewood Cliffs, NJ, Prentice-Hall, 1978.
13. Frankena WK: Ethics, 2nd ed. Englewood Cliffs, NJ, Prentice-Hall, 1973.
14. Fry ST: Ethical principles in nursing education and practice: A

missing link in the unification issue. Nurs Health Care 3(9):363–368, 1982.
15. Gadow S: Ethical dimensions. In Beare PG, Myers JL (eds): Principles and Practice of Adult Health Nursing. St. Louis, CV Mosby, 1990.
16. Gilligan C: In a Different Voice. Cambridge, MA, Harvard University Press, 1982.
17. Jameton A: Nursing Practice: The Ethical Issues. Englewood Cliffs, NJ, Prentice-Hall, 1984.
18. Kant I: Fundamental Principles of the Metaphysics of Morals. New York, Liberal Arts, 1949.
19. Beauchamp T, Childress JF: Principles of Biomedical Ethics. New York, Oxford, 1983.
20. Mitchell C: Integrity in interprofessional relationships. In Agich GJ (ed): Responsibility in Health Care. Dordrecht, Holland, Reidel Publishing Company, 1982, pp 163–184.
21. Iserson KV: An approach to ethical problems in emergency medicine. In Iserson KV et al (eds): Ethics in Emergency Medicine. Baltimore, Williams & Wilkins, 1986.
22. Mitchell C, Achtenberg B: Study Guide for Code Gray Film. Boston, Fanlight Productions, 1984.
23. Pryor-McCann J: Ethical issues in critical care nursing. Crit Care Nurs Clin North Am 2(1):1–13, 1990.
24. Rachels J: The Elements of Moral Philosophy. New York, Random House, 1986.
25. Rawls J: A Theory of Justice. Cambridge, MA, Harvard University Press, 1971.
26. Reich WT (ed): Encyclopedia of Bioethics, vol 4. New York, Free Press, 1978.
27. Reverly S: An historical perspective. In Study Guide for Code Gray Film. Boston, Fanlight Productions, 1984, pp 20–21.
28. Smith SJ, Davis AJ: Ethical dilemmas: Conflicts among rights, duties and obligations. Am J Nurs 80(8):1463–1466, 1980.
29. Trandel-Korenchuk DK: Nursing advocacy of patients' rights: Myth or reality. Nurse Pract March: 53–59, 1989.
30. Thompson JE, Thompson HO: Bioethical Decision-Making of Nurses. New York, Appleton-Century-Crofts, 1985.
31. Veatch RM: A Theory of Medical Ethics. New York, Basic Books, 1981.
32. Veins DC: A history of nursing's code of ethics. Nurs Outlook 37(1):45–49, 1989.
33. Winslow GR: From Loyalty to Advocacy: A New Metaphor for Nursing. The Hasting Center Report, June, 1984.
34. Yeaworth RC: The ANA Code: A comparative perspective. J Nurs Scholarship 17(3):94–98, 1985.

6

NURSING PRACTICE THROUGH THE CYCLES OF TRAUMA

VIRGINIA D. CARDONA and
KATHRYN T. VON RUEDEN

INTRODUCTION

The field of traumatology has come to be recognized as a specialized branch of health care. Concurrently, because of the uniqueness and complexity of patients with multiple injuries, trauma nursing also has evolved in its own right as a specialized field of nursing.

One of the most challenging aspects of caring for trauma patients is the development of a plan of care that addresses every component of the patient's needs in a logical, organized fashion to ensure continuity and coordination of all health disciplines. Formulation of such a plan of care requires incorporation of the five components of the nursing process: assessment, diagnosis, planning, implementation, and evaluation. In addition, the nursing care plan is necessarily intertwined with and reflects the plans of other health team members as the overall plan of care is developed and implemented throughout the cycles of trauma care.

Coordination of patient care in this fashion requires a multifaceted professional. Trauma nurses must have an understanding of the significance of the impact of the traumatic injury on the patient, the patient's family, and society. They must be adept at sophisticated monitoring and at caring for the intense physiological needs as well as psychological and social demands of the patient. They also must be able to assist the family to cope with the stress and emotional devastation that often accompany sudden traumatic events. Patient and family recovery is heavily dependent on the skills of the nurse as caregiver, communicator, collaborator, and coordinator throughout the cycles of trauma.

TRAUMA NURSING PRACTICE

Dorothy Johnson in 1961 defined nursing practice in terms of three major components: nursing care, delegated medical care, and health care. The nursing process is incorporated in each of these components and provides a framework for bringing the three components together. In describing the overall purpose of *nursing care,* she stated, "The achievement and maintenance of a stable state is nursing's distinctive contribution to patient welfare and the specific purpose of nursing care. The change of any magnitude toward recovery from illness or toward more desirable health practice depends upon the periodic achievement and maintenance, perhaps only for a short time, of this stable state."[1]

Delegated medical care refers to the care given by the nurse, which contributes to the development and implementation of medical care plans. *Health care* refers to the service that has as its purpose the promotion and maintenance of desirable health practices.

When developing a plan of care for the multiply injured patient, all three of these components are relevant. During the initial phase of care immediately after the injury and during the stabilization phase, it is vital that the focus include both nursing care and delegated medical care components. As patients enter the rehabilitative phase, the health care component takes on more significance as they learn ways in which to live with residual impairments from their injury and as they become reintegrated into society.

Health care also implies the education of the public related to trauma prevention. Trauma nurses have a crucial role in the educational process by providing information not only to adults and high-school students but also to small children.

Through all the cycles of trauma care, specialized expertise is required to provide quality care and to achieve optimal outcomes for this complex patient population. Credentialing of trauma nurses is a way to ensure accountability in practice by ensuring competence in performance. Competency-based orientation and periodic required cognitive and psychomotor certifications are a means to this end. In addition, annual competency verification serves to update staff on new or revised procedures as well as complex or high-risk procedures.[2]

Profile of the Trauma Patient

Several unique characteristics of the multiply injured trauma patient contribute to the complexity of the plan of care:

- Traumatic injuries are sudden. Unlike the patient who is hospitalized for elective surgery, the trauma patient and his family have no warning. The injury is an unexpected, severe interruption of normal life. There is no time to plan or prepare; one must simply cope with the injury once it occurs.
- Drug and alcohol abuse often play an important role in traumatic injury. The multiply injured patient whose history includes substance abuse is typically more difficult to initially assess and later to manage effectively. Often, the family's feelings of guilt over the inability to convince the patient to receive help for a drug or alcohol abuse problem may affect their ability to cope effectively with their family member's injury.
- Because of the severity and complexity of traumatic injury, most of these patients require long-term rehabilitative care. Systemic sequelae and physical handicaps also may result. Learning to cope adequately, both physically and psychologically, is a process that needs to begin early after hospitalization.
- Psychological sequelae are extremely common in multiply injured patients. Many experience a posttraumatic stress syndrome and grieving process after the injury, and depending on the individual's existing support systems and coping mechanisms, adaptation to severe injuries may be difficult.
- Trauma is a disease of the young adult. The average age of the multiply injured patient is 16 to 44.[3] These patients' inexperience with life crises, their developmental stage, and their level of maturity create special needs that must be considered when planning effective interventions.
- The number of elderly trauma patients is increasing,[3] and it will continue to do so with the "graying of America." This population has unique needs, which include alterations in the typical approaches to resuscitation, intensive care, and rehabilitative practices. More emphasis is required on modifying nursing and medical management of trauma patients who are over the age of 55 or 60.[4]
- Many traumatically injured patients who do not survive are potential subjects of a medical examiner's investigation because their injuries are a result of violence or accidents. Legal implications are therefore already inherent even before a plan of care can be developed. Once the plan of care has been developed, it is usually subjected to greater scrutiny by staff, hospital administrators, criminal investigators, attorneys, and patients' families than the care plan of a patient admitted for elective surgery.
- Traumatic injuries are often subtle. Many injuries are obvious, and they often mask other injuries that may be even more life-threatening. Nursing assessment takes on even greater significance when the occurrence of subtle injuries is considered, since the diagnosis may be delayed.
- Due to the complexity and/or severity of the injuries, the multiply injured patient has a tremendous potential for developing complications during the hospitalization phase. The nurse is largely responsible for prevention and early detection of such complications as well as minimizing the consequences.
- Initial injuries or the treatments necessary as a result of injuries create additional problems that greatly influence care planning for multiply injured patients. Many are immobilized due to hemodynamic instability, severe respiratory dysfunction, or as a result of orthopedic or neurological injuries. Communication is often difficult if an endotracheal tube or a tracheostomy tube is necessary for ventilatory support. Infection is prevalent in many of these patients because of the nature of their injuries, multiple invasive procedures, and exposure to numerous health care team members who provide care for them.
- Due to the existence of multiple injuries affecting several body systems, implementation of standard and accepted methods of treatment for each injury is often difficult or contraindicated. The existence of a severe head injury, for example, may prohibit routine repositioning and chest

physiotherapy treatments ordinarily required by a patient with thoracic injuries. Alternative methods of treatment that do not compromise the patient's existing injuries must be explored.

- The treatment of traumatically injured patients often imposes serious economic burdens on their families. The cost of critical care and rehabilitative care can be staggering.

These characteristics and the necessarily complex treatment modes make planning care for the multiply injured patient a difficult and challenging task.

Implementation of a philosophy of care that focuses on a well-communicated and organized approach to the delivery of available health services and medical expertise is essential. This approach includes the following:[5]

1. Immediate identification of the injured patient and provision for transport to the trauma care center.
2. Triage of all hospitalized patients in a single location by an experienced team of surgeons.
3. Resuscitation and comprehensive initial evaluation in a single, fully staffed and equipped area of the trauma unit.
4. Utilization of the team approach to the individual patient, with a senior surgeon functioning as the team coordinator.
5. Establishment of an integral intensive care area dedicated to the needs of the critically injured patient.
6. Ensurance of special education of nurses and other health care professionals to staff the unit.
7. Consolidation of all related hospital resources for the injured patient in a central location.
8. Arrangement for necessary supporting laboratory resources nearby.
9. Establishment of a priority system in the hospital's radiology department and blood bank, in which trauma patients are given high priority at any time of the day or night.

CRUCIAL CONSIDERATIONS WHEN PLANNING CARE

Collaborative Practice

When initiating the plan of care for the multiply injured patient, collaborative practice is crucial. This concept has become a common theme in recent medical and nursing literature. It describes the ideal working relationship between the physician, nurse, and other disciplines, resulting in higher-quality care. The purpose of collaborative practice is to integrate care regimens into a comprehensive approach to patient needs. It is a relationship in which professionals define specific roles and jointly determine a relationship that is most beneficial to the patient.

Collaborative practice may significantly affect morbidity and mortality of the critically ill.[6,7] Critical care units in large educational institutions do not always have the lowest mortality rates nor the most effective care. Highly coordinated systems for patient management that result in quality patient care are often lacking. Excluding other variables, investigators have concluded that the *process* of care is essential to reduce morbidity and mortality. Inherent in the process is the positive interaction and collaboration of physicians and nurses in achieving optimal results and the adherence to established protocols and procedures to guide their care.[6] Collaborative practice, when utilized in treating the multiply injured patient, includes all members of the health care team, from paramedics in the field to the physical therapist during rehabilitative care, who work together toward the common goal of providing the best possible care. Without collaborative practice, this common goal and optimal patient outcomes cannot be realized.

Hope for the survival of the multiple trauma patient rests with the collaborative efforts of the trauma nurses, physicians, technicians, and therapists who constitute the trauma team. Nurses and physicians labor together to resuscitate, stabilize, diagnose, and treat the severely injured patient. Because patients with multiple injuries require prompt attention and rapid stabilization, the trauma nurse *must* assume a collaborative role with surgeons,[8] critical care physicians, and other trauma team members.

Optimal care of trauma patients, which implies minimal errors and complications and maximal efficency and continuity, is provided by a team that accurately and consistently communicates, beginning with initial field providers and subsequently with the nurse and physician who follow the patient from admission throughout the resuscitative and operative phases. Communication and collaboration must continue throughout the cycles of trauma care.

Collaborative practice exists when there is mutual respect and understanding of the unique contributions that each professional brings to the care of the patient. It develops as a result of careful planning by physicians and nurses in identifying guidelines that may increase life expectancy and reduce complications. The benefits of collaboration[8] include the following:

1. Systematic, high-quality care
2. Increased nurse-to-physician accountability
3. Increased nurse-to-physician communication
4. Organized collection of patient data
5. Improved care of individual patients and their families

In a collaborative environment, care becomes directed and focused. Optimal patient care is achieved because a skilled clinical nurse follows the patient through resuscitation, diagnosis, and stabilization prior to surgery. With one nurse accountable to the physician team, communication improves and physician–nurse conflict is minimal. Postoperatively, a primary nurse or case manager coordinates a plan of care that addresses all the patient's needs, involving and integrating all members of the health care team.

The multiple trauma patient must be viewed as a "system" with several subsystems, whose internal environment has been interrupted by the stressor of a traumatic injury and will continue to be subjected to repeated stressors from the external environment during the journey through the cycles of care. When planning care, the nurse and others must anticipate the system-wide impact from change in any one part and appreciate the simultaneous nature of change in an open system. Successful management through the phases, and often patient survival, is therefore dependent on coordination and collaboration within the health care team.

Patient Advocacy

The role of the professional nurse as client advocate has evolved along with the development of practice based on nursing theory. Founded on the assumption of nursing science that humans are always capable of growing and developing, the nursing profession has focused the advocate role on its "supporting" aspect, the behavior of "maintaining or recommending a cause" (the cause being health and an individual's right to receive adequate health care).[9]

Many situations during the cycles of trauma care necessitate that the nurse assume the patient advocate role. The patient may be comatose, paralyzed, sedated, or in pain. These conditions alter his ability to participate actively in decision making. Such conditions also may contribute to a communication deficit, increasing the potential for care to become disjointed among the many involved services and personnel. Through the advocacy role, the trauma nurse participates with the patient and his family and professional colleagues in the advancement of processes that ultimately promote health. The advocate role consists of four basic behaviors: mutuality, facilitation, protection, and coordination.[9]

Mutuality implies that the nurse and patient are equally able and responsible for the outcomes of the nursing process. Thus, as the plan of care is developed and implemented, both the trauma patient, when able, and the trauma nurse must participate.

As a facilitator, the advocate must assume that every patient has strengths and must aid him to realize and use those strengths to achieve the highest level of functioning. Assisting the patient to identify and use supportive coping mechanisms that will aid in the adjustment to injury is one example of *facilitation.* The patient devastated by traumatic injury may feel powerless to make decisions—the nurse must facilitate and encourage the patient to do so.

Patient *protection* is a component of advocacy that the trauma nurse faces daily. Patient protection broadly encompasses a variety of activities as simple as enforcing infection-control policies or protecting a restless, brain-injured patient from harming himself to participation in complex ethical decisions. Prevention of premature discharge for the sake of bed space and the duty to protect the patient from possible iatrogenic complications throughout hospitalization are typical examples of the protector role.[9] The nurse should be involved in ethical discussions between physicians and families related to therapeutic decisions for hopelessly ill or incapacitated trauma victims. The nurse, based on her knowledge of the patient and/or family desires, needs to decide what actions are appropriate in terms of protecting the patient from either forced or withheld treatments. The Task Force on Ethics of the Society of Critical Care Medicine has developed useful, widely accepted guidelines and a framework for decision making related to foregoing life-sustaining treatment. Incorporation of such a framework into the ethical decision-making process provides a structure on which the health care team can base such difficult decisions.[10]

The *coordination* component of the advocate role occurs on a continuing basis as the patient progresses through the cycles of care. Since the nurse is often the one professional who focuses on the patient's whole response to the situation, she must use coordination techniques to ensure that the patient has access to all the health care delivery system and to enlist the resources appropriately.

Curtain[11] emphasizes that if one believes in the autonomy of the individual and respects the rights of that individual to make choices and decisions, one assumes certain obligations. Trauma nurses as patient advocates are morally obligated to carry out professional duties in relation to the rights of the severely injured. Chenevert[12] identifies three rights that are tempered with responsibility—rights that are integral to the care of trauma patients:

1. When there is a right to speak, there is the responsibility to listen.
2. When there is the right to have problems, there is the responsibility to find solutions.
3. Where there is the right to cry, there is a responsibility to dry tears.

DEVELOPING AN INTEGRATED PLAN OF CARE

It is generally recognized that a specialized plan of care is a necessity for the multitrauma patient, but actualizing such a plan requires several components. Regardless of the health care facility (a designated trauma center or a community or large university hospital), these mechanisms addressing solely the trauma patient's needs *must* exist, for these patients form a unique population that requires highly specialized care.

Mechanisms to Assist in Planning Quality Care

This highly specialized trauma care requires several mechanisms for guidance and direction. Policies and protocols specifically addressing care of these patients must be developed based on current modes of therapy, must be followed, and must be consistently updated as new therapies, equipment, and research dictate. It is imperative that the established protocols, policies, standards, and procedures be reviewed on a consistent basis and changed to reflect and incorporate new modes of therapy and current research findings. State-of-the-art trauma care changes rapidly, and so must the policies, protocols, and standards that guide and direct that care. The policies, protocols, and procedures should be consistent with the guidelines set forth by organizations such as the American Association of Critical Care Nurses, the Society of Critical Care Medicine, and the American College of Surgeons. From these elements, trauma nursing standards are developed; they are based on, and facilitate the implementation of, these policies and protocols. These standards should reflect the highest levels of care for which each caregiver strives, yet they must be realistic, based on the resources available to implement them. These standards also form the basis for nursing care evaluation. In addition, nursing procedures must be written to implement the policies, protocols, and nursing standards. It is important to note that if the standardized guidelines and procedures promulgated by the preceding organizations are used they must be reviewed and, if necessary, revised specifically for the trauma patient; for example, a procedure outlining the proper use of the hypothermia blanket, a standard procedure in most hospitals, will vary and must include special precautions in relation to aspects of the trauma patient's care, e.g., its use in spinal cord–injured patients whose thermoregulation mechanisms may be significantly impaired. Because the trauma patient requires so many highly specialized procedures, a procedure manual should be readily available as a resource in the patient care area.

System of Care Delivery

Because trauma patients require highly specialized care, a system of nursing care delivery capable of providing such care must be established. One system that best facilitates the coordination of specialized care is that of primary nursing, where the nurse in each cycle serves as the patient's case manager. Primary nursing facilitates goal-directed coordination of the many teams of professional and paraprofessional personnel that are necessary to provide the highest possible quality of care. Other systems of care delivery may be equally effective, as long as they ensure nursing accountability for the goal-directed care and for communication and coordination of the health care team.

One member of the health team must be in charge of coordinating this care, and the primary nurse who sees and cares for the patient on a consistent basis is the only one who can adequately carry out this overwhelming responsibility. The nurse must recognize and assume this responsibility and be able to hold herself and all others involved in the care accountable. The nurse sees the patient for 8 or 12 consecutive hours compared with other health care team members, who intervene in the care sporadically. Thus she can ensure that treatment plans and interventions from the various disciplines are congruent with the overall plan of care. If at all possible, only registered professional nurses should provide care for trauma patients, especially the multiply injured. The registered nurses' level of assessment skills, professional practice, accountability, and educational preparation are all necessary to provide the highly technical and complicated care that the trauma patient demands.

Some institutions have chosen to implement a case-management system to ensure collaboration and continuity of trauma patient care. This approach may be especially effective in hospitals that do not receive more than two or three trauma admissions per day. Typically, the trauma case manager is a master's-prepared clinical nurse specialist with expertise in the care of trauma patients. The case manager is responsible for the day-to-day review and coordination of multidisciplinary services, efficient use of resources, patient disposition through the system, and arrangement of follow-up care. The trauma case-manager role may be particularly valuable in hospitals, large or small, where a strong primary nursing system is not in place, the trauma patient population is small, and trauma care is not a major area of expertise of the nursing staff and other disciplines.[13, 14]

A philosophy of trauma nursing must exist that encompasses beliefs about the trauma patient's care from prevention through reintegration into the community. This philosophy must be adopted by every nurse caring for these patients as care is planned and delivered.

In addition to a philosophy of trauma nursing, nurses caring for these patients also must possess a strong pathophysiological knowledge base. This base is needed to assess the patient and to plan and direct care throughout the cycles. Especially for the resuscitation and critical care cycles, it is advantageous for the trauma nurse to have a strong background in emergency and critical care nursing before she takes on the responsibility of caring for patients whose injuries may involve many body systems and whose psychological responses are often complex.

THE PLAN OF CARE

The written plan of care is a vital component of the trauma patient's care. The Joint Commission on Accreditation of Healthcare Organizations requires a documented plan of care that addresses physiological, psychological, and environmental factors.[15] The care plan for the trauma patient must not be written only with the idea of satisfying this requirement but rather must be looked on as the link between injury and readaptation—the base from which all care is delivered. This plan should be familiar to and utilized by *all* members of the health care team. It should be reviewed at the beginning of each shift by the nurse caring for the patient and by each health team member prior to delivering care to the patient. The plan must be succinct and reflect changes in care immediately as they become necessary. The plan also should be evaluated and revised at regular intervals, dictated by patient acuity and specific goals or outcomes.

Problems in Actualizing the Written Care Plan

The complex nature of the multitrauma patient often necessitates an involved plan of care. It is often difficult to develop such a plan for many reasons. First and foremost, time may be a constraint. The ideal situation exists if nursing administration has the financial ability to provide nurses with paid time for writing the care plan aside from their actual patient care time. But with the increased emphasis on decreasing health care costs, this is typically not possible. The primary nurse must provide time during patient care hours to write the plan and make the needed changes. Documenting a complex plan is often difficult when the patient in the critical care area is unstable or if the nurse in the rehabilitation unit is caring for several patients. It is important not to lose sight of the value of the written plan when time constraints are inevitable.

Educating the nursing staff on how to develop and write an effective plan of care is essential. Workshops given at specified periods each year are one way, but again, staffing constraints often prevent their feasibility. One alternative might be a library of videotapes on subjects such as developing a plan of care, nursing diagnosis, writing patient and family goals, and selected leadership concepts that might be applicable to their role. Whatever the method, it is important that this education take place so that all nurses caring for these patients operate from the same baseline and can produce quality plans of care.

It is also necessary to ensure that the plan of care is followed, evaluated, and revised even when the primary nurse is off duty or on vacation. A consistent "relief nurse" should assume all the primary nursing responsibilities in the absence of the primary nurse. Continuity of care is absolutely essential with trauma patients; the plan of care must continue even in the primary nurse's absence.

Standardized Care Plans and Critical Pathways

In the past decade, standardized or master care plans have been developed in many specialty units to save time and ensure quality care for trauma patients. Plans such as these are extremely beneficial when planning care for the trauma patient and may be utilized throughout the cycles (see Appendix 6–1 for a sample). Many trauma patients exhibit the same unhealthful responses in relation to specific injuries. Care plans addressing these unhealthful responses, once developed, have several advantages. They conserve valuable nursing time, ensure that patients with a specific nursing diagnosis receive the highest standard of care, and promote continuity of care.

The reluctance of some nurses to use these standardized plans usually stems from the concern that patient individuality would be lost. However, built-in flexibility (spaces provided between several nursing interventions for adding specific patient and family needs) can avoid this hazard.

Critical pathways are a more recently developed means of planning patient care. *Critical pathways* prescribe day-to-day multidisciplinary activities such as interventions, consultations, diagnostic testing, and patient and family education for trauma patients with common physiological alterations or those with similar injuries. Developed and agreed on by a multidisciplinary group, critical pathways very concretely direct the efforts of all services (see Appendixes 6–2 and 6–3 for examples of critical pathways). The critical pathways presented are examples of those implemented in various populations within the United States. Due to the often complex and unpredictable nature of the trauma patient's path of recovery, it is difficult to predict which of the proposed models best serves the trauma population.

Regardless of the type of plan of care chosen by an institution, standardized care plans or critical pathways, it must have the following characteristics:

- Must be based on physiological priorities
- Must provide an organized, logical approach to trauma patient care
- Must identify specific goals or outcomes and interventions
- Must be usable by multidisciplines
- Must be usable over time, throughout the cycles of trauma care

Jointly made approaches to therapy, documented via nursing care plans or critical pathways, increase the efficiency of resource utilization and care delivery and ensure that energies are directed toward common patient goals and outcomes.[16]

CYCLE I: FIELD STABILIZATION AND RESUSCITATION

The ultimate goal in the prehospital phase is to stabilize and then to transport the multiply injured patient to the appropriate level trauma center via the safest and most rapid transport mode. Accomplishment of this goal requires collaboration which begins at the scene of an accident. An effective emergency medical services (EMS) system provides a means for specially trained paramedics to communicate with trauma physicians at the receiving hospital and a centralized communications center to assist in planning the appropriate mode of transport for that patient. Conditions at the scene also may require calls for additional personnel, such as firefighters to help with extrication or additional police officers to assist with care or to direct traffic to prevent further injuries. In addition to the indispensable role of the paramedic, the role of the nurse and physician in the field is gaining increased recognition as the concepts of "go teams" (medical and nursing personnel who go from the hospital to the scene of an accident) and flight trauma nurses (who care for the patient while en route to the trauma center) are becoming more popular.

Assessment and Diagnosis

The Advanced Trauma Life Support guidelines for initial assessment provide a standardized approach.[17] When communicating assessment findings to the receiving hospital, it is imperative that a common language and standardized approach be utilized, e.g., a specific trauma injury scoring system or the Glasgow Coma Scale.

In the field or at the site of an accident, the priorities are *always* the ABCs: airway, breathing, and circulation. Establishing an airway at the scene is often difficult. The individual may be trapped inside a vehicle with a steering wheel crushed against his chest or may have been thrown out of the vehicle, resulting in serious head and facial injuries with severe bleeding causing airway obstruction. *In almost every case, field personnel should suspect the trauma patient of having a cervical spine injury until proved otherwise, and an airway should be established with this possibility in mind.*

Immediately following attention to the ABCs, emergency medical personnel should note the patient's neurological status. The baseline neurological status (level of consciousness and pupillary size and reaction) of the trauma patient is of such a critical nature that it must be included as part of the primary assessment.[18] Once the primary survey has been completed, a secondary survey is performed to establish the presence of further injuries.

External evidence of trauma should alert the caregiver to the possibility of internal injury. These signs may be easily overlooked in the presence of obvious hemorrhage or other significant wounds. Abrasions, contusions, and pain on movement can be observed at the accident scene and may lead to early recognition of occult injuries. Back and neck pain suggest spine injury. Abrasion and contusion of the chest and abdomen may herald occult internal injuries and concomitant head injury. Deformity and pain suggest extremity injury. All patients should be managed as though they have sustained serious injuries until a thorough examination can be made at an appropriate medical facility. If the patient is unresponsive, it should be assumed that spine, thoracic, and abdominal injuries are present until proved otherwise. In this phase, the mechanism of injury should always be considered when assessing for signs of obvious or occult injury. It is essential that field personnel provide as much information as possible about how the accident occurred and relate specific assessment findings to the receiving facility (see Chap. 7).

Developing and Implementing the Plan

Assessment, diagnosis, and initiation of planned interventions are nearly simultaneous activities. As quickly as alterations in the ABCs are identified, treatment is instituted. Several first aid principles are followed at the scene of accident or injury:

1. Remove the patient from a hazard only when the risk (e.g., fire) outweighs the danger of moving the patient.
2. Establish the airway, usually by elevating the jaw. An esophageal obturator airway (EOA) or endotracheal intubation may be utilized to secure the airway if personnel are certified to do so.
3. Initiate cardiopulmonary resuscitation (CPR) as indicated; a mechanical resuscitator may need to be utilized.
4. Control obvious hemorrhage, usually with direct pressure. Use a tourniquet *only* as a last resort.
5. Splint spine and extremity injuries.
6. Apply pneumatic antishock garment (PASG) if indicated.
7. Establish intravenous access.
8. Move and transport as soon as possible.

A primary objective of care at the accident scene is to prevent further injury. Care in extracting and transporting patients to avoid further damage in spinal injuries cannot be overemphasized. Attention to limb position and simple handling and splinting may decrease the possibility of neurovascular damage and/or fat emboli. Further contamination of open wounds should be avoided, which may decrease the occurrence of overwhelming infection at a later stage.

In the prehospital phase, trained paramedic or nursing personnel should be able to identify specific injuries when they are obvious, but more important, they must assess the overall stability of the patient. Once the patient's condition is determined, effective triage in this phase of care is vital to ensure that the patient is sent to the most appropriate treatment facility based on the injuries present. Specific guidelines for making these decisions must be in place and rigorously adhered to. Triage of the patient from the scene of the accident is defined in the protocols of each state's emergency medical services system. As EMS systems become more sophisticated, specialty centers that treat specific injuries may exist. Hand trauma centers, eye trauma centers, spinal cord injury centers, and/or pediatric trauma centers are only a few examples.

Once the appropriate level of trauma center is identified, decisions about which method of immobilization and which mode of transport will be utilized are the next priority. Transportation and communication are essential in coordinating any multiply injured patient's entrance into the emergency/critical care system and in facilitating the patient's progression through that system. The patient's survival depends on health care professionals to describe his condition accurately. The reports must provide data and information that are succinct, specific, accurate, and easily understood. Transporting the patient from the site of trauma into the hospital or through various departments of the emergency facility requires selection of the method best suited to avoid or reduce complications.

The communication system utilized during this prehospital phase must be clear, accurate, rapid, and cost-effective. Depending on the EMS system, biomedical telemetry systems, radio transmitters, or standard telephones may be utilized to accomplish effective communication. Once the patient arrives at the treatment facility, a more detailed account of the accident history, assessment findings, and treatment administered at the scene must be given to the hospital admitting team.

Documentation is crucial in the field management plan of care. Records should include information on patient status, vital signs, Glasgow Coma Scale, accident data (including mechanism of injury), therapy received, past and present medical history, and whether or not other parties were involved. Accident data should include time of injury, geographical location, and patient body position. These written records should be examined closely by the receiving trauma team. Any obvious treatment methods, such as the application of a tourniquet to a limb or pain medication administered, must be communicated not only verbally but also by easily visible means, such as writing those details on adhesive tape placed across the forehead of the patient.

Evaluation

During the prehospital phase, ongoing evaluation of the treatment and transport plans is imperative. Continuous assessment of the patient's condition is vital to detect any signs of deterioration that may call for a change in plans. If the patient's condition worsens, transport to a nearby hospital for stabilization with subsequent transfer to an appropriate level trauma center may be required. If delays in the planned transport mode occur, alternate transport might be necessary to save time and, thus, the patient's life. Changes in the patient's condition also must be relayed to the receiving facility to allow alternate orders for treatment to be issued. In situations in which field personnel are without a physician and are unable to make triage or treatment decisions, the existence of a means for consultation with a trauma physician is essential. Many facilities that treat trauma patients have established "trauma hot lines" that allow field personnel to communicate directly with a trauma physician before vital decisions are made.

After the patient has reached the trauma facility, follow-up evaluation by the health care team will determine whether appropriate triage, treatment, and transport of the patient took place. Information gained from individual cases over a period of time will enable effective planning and care to take place for future trauma victims.

As was emphasized earlier, an effective plan of care for the traumatized victim must begin at the scene of the accident. Assessment, treatment, and communication during this phase will all impact later stages of the patient's care. R. Adams Cowley found that multiple trauma patients who received definitive care within 60 minutes of their injuries (the "golden hour") had the best chance for recovery. The

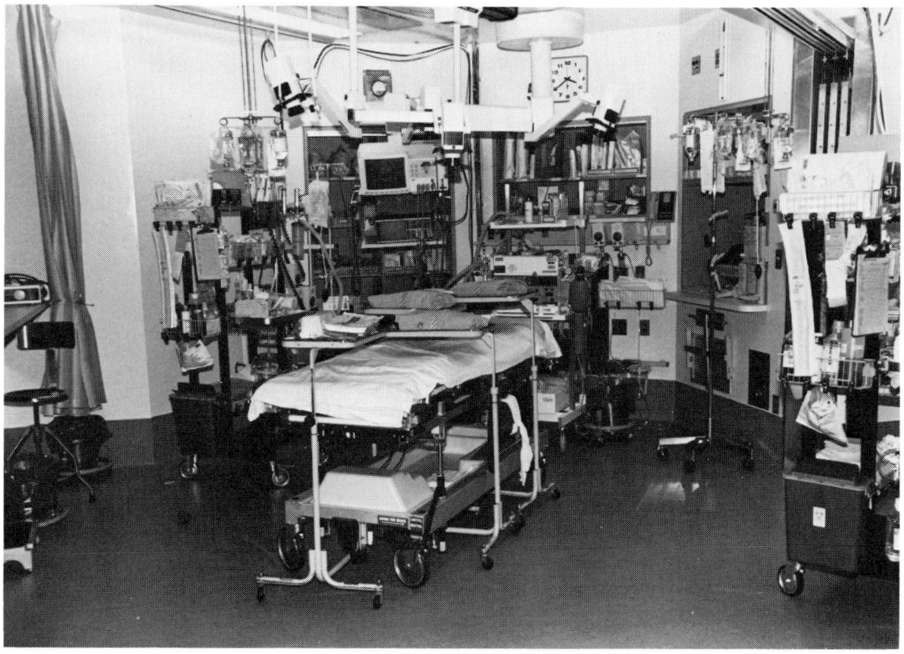

Figure 6–1. Trauma receiving bay prepared with equipment and supplies and ready for an admission. (Reprinted with permission from Maryland Institute for Emergency Medical Services Systems, Baltimore, Md, 1992.)

overall mortality rate of 15 to 20 per cent doubled for every hour lost in receiving that care.[19]

CYCLE II: IN-HOUSE RESUSCITATION AND OPERATIVE PHASE

Since the patient often arrives at the receiving facility from the scene of the accident with little of the "golden hour" remaining, immediate life-saving measures are required. A coordinated, collaborative, unified approach is the cornerstone of trauma patient care in the resuscitation unit. Philosophically, all trauma patients are in critical condition until diagnosed otherwise. Advance preparation for immediate access to equipment, supplies, and personnel that the patient might need for survival is essential.[20] Therefore, upon arrival in the emergency room, there should be an orderly transition from field to hospital personnel. Notifying the appropriate hospital personnel of the patient's condition prior to arrival allows for mobilization of the trauma team.

Preparation and Initial Contact

The resuscitation nurse plays a vital role even before the patient arrives. Routine, basic equipment for treating all injury priorities established by the American College of Surgeons Committee on Trauma Resuscitation[17] should be located in the area where the trauma patient will be admitted and should be readily accessible. In some institutions, proximity of the patients in the resuscitation area to the operating room is prohibitive, and therefore, the trauma admitting area must be able to support major surgical procedures. The design of some small resuscitation areas or emergency rooms makes this a challenge, but it must be recognized that every second lost because of disorganization decreases the patient's chance of survival. Figure 6–1 shows an admitting bay at the Maryland Institute for Emergency Medical Systems Services (MIEMSS) Shock Trauma Center; it demonstrates how a small area can be fully equipped in an organized manner (see Appendix 6–4 for an equipment list).

The trauma resuscitation area should receive prior notice of a patient's arrival. This allows not only for routine equipment needed for every admission to be made ready but also for acquisition of any unusual equipment required for specific injuries.[20] Equipment for airway management is a first priority, and that for hemodynamic management, specifically fluid resuscitation, also must be readily available. Sterile trays must be on hand—some even opened and covered with a sterile barrier—to save valuable time[20] (Table 6–1).

Members of the trauma team must be notified and must be present when the patient arrives. In major trauma centers, this team usually consists of a trauma surgeon, an attending trauma surgeon, and two to three residents. Other hospitals may have designated surgeons who take trauma "call" and admit trauma patients. Whatever the plan, the team designated to admit the patient must be present, ready, and awaiting the arrival of the patient. Preparation also includes donning of appropriate protective attire (goggles/face shield,

TABLE 6–1. STERILE TRAYS THAT MUST BE READILY AVAILABLE DURING RESUSCITATION

1. Cutdown tray
2. Peritoneal lavage tray
3. Foley catheter tray
4. Line insertion sets
5. Thoracoabdominal tray
6. Arteriogram tray
7. Halo or Gardner-Wells tongs tray
8. Plastic surgery tray

mask, gloves, fluid-impermeable cover gown) prior to the patient's arrival.[21] Each member of the team must be aware of and perform the specific role assigned, with the ultimate goal of delivering rapid, organized team care.

Assessment

The resuscitation nurse plays a vital role in the quick assessment and stabilization of patients upon admission (see Appendix 6–5 for protocol). Following the call notifying an emergency room of an admission, trays should be opened, suction apparatus and overhead lights turned on, and IV lines primed with the appropriate fluids. Additional equipment is prepared based on specific information obtained from the field personnel. Trauma patients who arrive at the trauma facility by helicopter, should be met by the admitting nurse and anesthesia provider. The comprehensive plan of care for the hospital phase is initiated on the helipad by performing a rapid assessment to ensure that the ABCs of life support are in place. If the patient is conscious, the nurse also may obtain a brief initial history at this time.

While assessing the patient, communicating with him is a priority. The nurse meeting the patient at the helipad, ambulance, or in the emergency room establishes verbal communication and continues the exchange throughout this cycle of care. "While steps to protect the patient's life obviously take highest priority, the nurse needs to begin to address the patient's emotional and mental state as well. By orienting him to reality and providing support, you can do much to relieve his anxiety and assist him toward resolution of his crisis."[22] The trauma patient is often frightened and confused, which may be compounded by pain or hypoxia. Although the emphasis during this cycle is on assessment and stabilization of the patient's physical condition, full recovery demands that the patient's emotional state also be considered. Psychological support to calm the patient, prepare him for what is ahead, and establish trust is important during this stage.

Upon arrival in the resuscitation area, the nurse provides the trauma team with a succinct report of the assessment and clinical findings. The initial assessment and resuscitation activities are protocol-driven and should be "indelibly ingrained" in the minds of all team members[18] (see Table 6–2). Throughout the resuscitation and stabilization phase, the physician team leader and admitting nurse coordinate procedures not only to carry out the established protocols for treatment but also to individualize care when appropriate. Specialists may need to be consulted; sedation may need to be given so that a thorough medical examination may be obtained; and priorities of treatment need to be established.

Documentation is crucial during this phase of care. Records utilized should be short but must contain vital information that is crucial to the plan of care. Vital signs and hemodynamic stability must be monitored continuously to

TABLE 6–2. TRAUMA ADMISSION ASSESSMENT PROTOCOLS

First Priorities 1. Rapid evaluation for a. Labored respirations b. Noisy respirations c. Cyanosis d. Tachypnea e. Decreased chest wall motion f. Pallor g. Lack of spontaneous eye opening h. Agitation i. Lack of verbal response j. Extremity rigidity 2. Bilateral chest auscultation for absent breath sounds 3. Supplemental oxygen administration 4. Tracheal intubation and adequate ventilation for a. Overt respiratory distress b. Hypoventilation c. Shock d. Absence of verbal response e. Absence of purposeful extremity response to pain f. Uncontrollable agitation 5. Palpation of pulse to determine presence and quality 6. Establish cardiac monitoring 7. Determine blood pressure 8. Establish intravenous access and begin volume infusion 9. Control external hemorrhage with direct pressure 10. MAST deflation by section after volume infusion initiated 11. Assess ability to wiggle fingers or toes to command 12. Apply sternal compression to unconscious patients 13. Assess pupil response to light 14. Cervical spine stabilization 15. Obtain arterial blood gases (repeat if intubation is required) 16. Obtain blood for laboratory assessment 17. Obtain supine chest x-ray if respiratory or cardiovascular distress present and after intubation	**Second Priorities** 1. Obtain pertinent history 2. Conduct a brief external physical examination 3. Conduct a more complete neurological examination 4. Obtain lateral cervical spine x-ray (all blunt trauma and penetrating neck injuries) 5. Obtain thoracic and lumbar spine x-rays 7. Institute treatment for severe brain injury 8. Obtain an upright chest x-ray (if there is no spinal injury) 9. Obtain anteroposterior (AP) pelvic x-ray (all blunt trauma and selected penetrating trauma) 10. Insert urinary bladder catheter if no urethral damage suspected 11. Place an orogastric tube 12. Evaluate the abdomen by peritoneal lavage or ultrasound 13. Obtain a urine analysis 14. Insert an arterial line 15. Obtain a 12-lead EKG **Third Priorities** 1. Repeat a systematic physical examination 2. Further diagnostic evaluation based on previous findings 3. Emergency surgery and other life-saving interventions are performed based on previous evaluation 4. Consider nonurgent tracheal intubation 5. Insert pulmonary artery catheter in high-risk patients 6. Obtain an accurate core temperature 7. Administer prophylactic antibiotics if indicated 8. Consider specialty consultation 9. Obtain specialty consultation 10. Reduce and splint extremity fractures 11. Consider patients with minor brain injuries for admission and observation

From Dunham CM, Cowley RA: Shock Trauma/Critical Care Manual. Gaithersburg, Md, Aspen Systems, 1991.

detect subtle changes in the patient's condition. Particular attention must be paid to intake and output. Overloading the patient initially may appear inconsequential at this stage of care; however, it may predispose the patient to severe pulmonary dysfunction within a few hours. The nurse must be certain that accurate I&O records are kept so that problems such as volume overload are either avoided or acknowledged, in which case appropriate treatment may be initiated to avoid complications. Continuous monitoring following the collection of baseline data is done to detect changes in the patient's condition as early as possible. Recording vital signs and electrocardiographic changes as often as every 5 minutes may be necessary.

The team approach is the most important factor during both the assessment and treatment of the patient. Following established protocols, the trauma nurse and physician must approach the assessment of the patient in a systematic, organized fashion.

The assessment must be done quickly and efficiently. Priority-based trauma protocols provide the framework for detecting and treating life-threatening injuries. The first priorities focus on the traditional ABCs [airway, breathing, circulation, cortex (brain), and cord (spine)]. Second priorities identify less evident but still life-threatening respiratory, cardiovascular, or neurological dysfunctions. The purpose of the third priorities is to detect and evaluate more subtle pathology which may contribute to morbidity and mortality but which is not necessarily life-threatening. Subsequent treatment priorities are established on the basis of protocol-driven patient assessment.[18]

Developing and Implementing the Plan

Appropriate patient management consists of the rapid assessment and treatment of life-threatening pathology. Logical sequential treatment priorities must be established on the basis of overall patient assessment in any emergency involving a critical injury to the patient. Patient management must consist of a rapid initial evaluation, resuscitation of vital functions, more detailed secondary and tertiary assessments, and finally, the initiation of definitive care. Prevention of irreversible tissue hypoxia is the essence of trauma resuscitation. Treatment of life-threatening respiratory and cardiovascular instability, brain injury, and spinal cord injury before definitive diagnosis is often essential in the management of the multiply injured patient. The time taken to establish a firm diagnosis before life-saving measures are instituted may mean the difference between life and death for that patient.

History

The resuscitation nurse must obtain as accurate a data base as possible if the patient is alert. In addition to physical symptoms, initial information should include history of allergies, significant medical history, current medications, age, religion, and weight. A brief history can be rapidly accomplished by an "AMPLE" history: A, allergies; M, medications currently being taken; P, past illnesses; L, last meal; E, events preceding the injury.

These aspects of the patient's medical history are vital for the trauma physician and must be known prior to initiating treatment. It is often impossible to obtain such a history when families are not available and the patient is comatose. The belongings of the patient should be examined for evidence of medic alert cards, delineating allergies or medical problems, or prescription medications that might give a clue to underlying medical conditions. The Self-Determination Act (1990) requires that the hospital also seek information regarding any advanced directives that the patient may have made. This information may be useful to the trauma team in making ethical decisions regarding treatment in some cases.[23]

Diagnosis

The nurse must be aware of the actual or suspected medical diagnoses in the trauma patient to guide her plan of care. Nursing diagnoses also must be formulated, but at this stage of the patient's care these diagnoses may be more like medical diagnoses, while others are clearly nursing-oriented. Diagnoses, both medical and nursing, also may be based on a high index of suspicion if injuries or unhealthful responses to injuries are not obvious.

The concept of nursing diagnoses in emergency care areas is often not utilized because of the abbreviated stay and focus on life-saving procedures. However, with the complexity of the multiple trauma patient, nursing diagnoses can and should be developed during the admission/resuscitation process. One means of accomplishing this in a busy resuscitation area is through the use of standardized care plans or protocols.

Standardized protocols and plans of care for critical patients during initial resuscitation and stabilization facilitate a systematic approach to quality care (see Appendix 6–5). Since care in this phase focuses on rapid diagnosis and treatment, which often occur simultaneously, the standardized plans provide consistent and organized emergency nursing care for multiply injured patients in the same manner as physicians' standardized medical protocols provide well-planned and orderly emergency medical care. These care plans may be categorized according to specific injuries or integrated with corresponding medical protocols.

The format for these standardized patient care plans may include assessment findings according to the specified injury by system-based priorities, potential nursing diagnoses, goals or desired outcomes, and nursing interventions. The assessment provides specific information concerning signs and symptoms of injuries and includes mechanisms of injury. The nursing diagnoses describe potential health problems that patients with specific injuries are at risk of developing.

The nursing diagnoses in this phase of the patient's care are primarily physiological. According to Kim,[24] a *physiological nursing diagnosis* is defined as an inferential statement made by a professional nurse to describe physiological disturbances that impede optimal functioning; it directs the nurse to specific interventions, both independent and interdependent. Psychosocial nursing diagnoses and care plans are also relevant during this phase of the patient's care.

The trauma admitting nurse must establish a trauma data base that will help to guide patient care. The aim of the data base is to organize facts concerning the causes of injury, the nature of injury, and the degree of trauma sustained by the patient. This data base logs the patient's progress in response

TABLE 6–3. ADMISSION LABORATORY STUDIES

Blood type and crossmatch	Lactate
Complete blood count	Creatinine
Arterial blood gases	Blood urea nitrogen
Coagulation profile	Osmolality
Electrolytes	Toxicology screen
Urine analysis	

From Dunham CM, Cowley RA: Shock Trauma/Critical Care Manual. Gaithersburg, Md, Aspen Systems, 1991.

to resuscitative efforts and chronicles events in the care. The data collected provide a basis for both medical and nursing diagnoses.

Evaluation of prehospital status and care is essential to the data base. This provides an understanding of the mechanisms of injury, the initial physical findings, and other clues important to the management of the patient. Evaluation of a critical patient's status and the ultimate medical and nursing management are dependent on analysis of vital signs, fluid resuscitation, and other critical data entered in the trauma data base. Establishing and maintaining an accurate data base are key responsibilities of the admitting area trauma nurse. Accuracy of diagnosis, legitimacy of the medical and nursing plans of care, and patient outcomes are dependent on this function.

Diagnostic Studies

The multiply injured patient often requires several diagnostic studies before accurate medical diagnoses can be made. The nurse plays a vital role in preparing the patient and in coordinating these studies. Portable radiography equipment should be available in the admitting area, but often additional studies must be done in a main radiology department. Transporting the multiply injured patient in a safe and timely manner is the responsibility of the admitting nurse. During transport, patient care should be maintained at the same level as that provided in the resuscitation unit. This is a team effort, which often requires a trauma physician, nurse, and respiratory therapist to aid in the transport. A multipurpose cart, equipped with the materials required for resuscitating and maintaining patients after they have left the admitting area, should always accompany the patient.[20] Portable monitoring equipment (EKG and pressure monitors) should always be utilized during transport. Blood may also be transported safely with the use of an insulated container and commercially available stickers that monitor the temperature of the blood.

Appropriate laboratory tests are drawn (with typing and crossmatching for blood receiving first priority) (Table 6–3). Following these initial measures and a secondary survey, treatment of less serious injuries and more thorough radiographic studies are initiated (Table 6–4).

Following the initial stabilization procedures and the secondary assessment, nursing interventions are continued based on priorities of care. Continuous monitoring must be carried out, psychological support must be continued, and appropriate treatments must be administered.

Stabilization of Life-Threatening Conditions

The immediate objective in this phase of the trauma patient's care is the stabilization of life-threatening conditions. The concept of "treatment prior to diagnosis" is crucial during this phase and based on establishment of an airway, adequate ventilation, and perfusion. Control of hemorrhage and initiation of fluid resuscitation must be accomplished rapidly.

A chest tube may need to be inserted rapidly to relieve a tension pneumothorax or hemothorax. The amount of chest drainage must be monitored closely to assist in determining blood replacement needs and the need for surgical intervention. Type-specific blood may be given until crossmatching has been completed. In extreme emergencies, O negative blood may be administered until laboratory results are complete.

Nurses in a trauma admitting area or emergency room utilize the principles and techniques of advanced trauma life support. Although in most trauma centers nurses do not intubate or insert central venous lines, they must prepare equipment for and assist with these procedures in addition to understanding their priority in resuscitative care. They must be familiar with and adept at setting up and operating autotransfusion (see Chapter 18). After the patient is stabilized and emergency procedures are completed, a more thorough secondary survey can be done. An ultrasound and/or peritoneal lavage (see Chapter 19) may be performed to determine the need for exploratory abdominal surgery. Additional radiological studies can be obtained. Obvious or suspected fractures may be immobilized with the use of splints or backboards if they are not already in place. Relief of pain now becomes a consideration, but pain must be judiciously considered prior to the administration of any medication. Medication can make accurate neurological assessment difficult and may cause hypotension in a less than stable trauma patient. On the other hand, if a patient arrives in a combative or severe restless state that hinders airway control and thorough examination, anesthetic or paralyzing agents may need to be utilized. Nursing management during this phase is first directed by established protocols and then by priorities of care. The overall assessment of the patient by the physician and nurse will guide the plan of care as it evolves. Throughout this cycle, the nurse must continuously anticipate and assess changes in the patient's condition, prepare equipment, and assist the team with procedures aimed at stabilization.

Cardiac Arrest

Most patients who arrest during the resuscitation phase following traumatic injury do so secondary to profound intravascular volume depletion.[18] Thus closed chest massage in many cases is not sufficient to maintain an effective stroke

TABLE 6–4. ROUTINE RADIOGRAPHIC STUDIES FOR MULTIPLE TRAUMA

1. Lateral cervical spine
2. Upright AP chest radiograph (after cervical spine injury has been ruled out)
3. AP radiograph of the pelvis
4. Other radiographs as indicated

From Dunham CM, Cowley RA: Shock Trauma/Critical Care Manual. Gaithersburg, Md, Aspen Systems, 1991.

TABLE 6–5. CONDITIONS THAT WARRANT AN AGGRESSIVE APPROACH TO CARDIOPULMONARY RESUSCITATION

1. Young patient
2. Arrest less than 5 minutes in duration
3. Spontaneous movement of the extremities
4. Pupils reactive to light
5. Attempt at spontaneous respiration
6. Uncertainty regarding the effect of drugs, hypothermia, or timing of the arrest
7. History of an arrest greater than 5 minutes, but a situation in which a palpable pulse is obtainable with external cardiopulmonary resuscitation, i.e., effective stroke volume

From Dunham CM, Cowley RA: Shock Trauma/Critical Care Manual. Gaithersburg, Md, Aspen Systems, 1991.

volume. An arrest due to hypovolemia requires massive volume infusion with red blood cells and manual compression of the ventricles via open thoracotomy.

Table 6–5 lists the conditions in which an aggressive open thoracotomy approach regarding resuscitation would be indicated.[18] Table 6–6 lists the guidelines for the management of posttraumatic cardiac arrest.[18]

The nurse on the admitting team must ensure the accessibility of the necessary equipment for open or closed CPR and assist the trauma surgeon accordingly. Successful resuscitation requires a well-organized, collaborative effort on the part of the trauma team.

The potential for sudden cardiac arrest remains a priority into the critical care cycle and, although less likely to occur here, into the intermediate and/or rehabilitation cycles. In the critical care cycle, cardiac arrest may result from overwhelming sepsis, dysrhythmias secondary to myocardial damage, multiple organ failure, respiratory failure, tension pneumothorax, or pulmonary embolization. In the intermediate and/or rehabilitative cycles, a pulmonary embolus or complications from long-term care may precipitate an arrest.

Because cardiac arrest is often a sudden event that can occur in any cycle of care, standardized protocols that address resuscitation are imperative. Although arrest protocols will vary with each institution, they should address the following components: (1) physician coverage and the process for notification of the physician, (2) identification of team members, (3) specific role responsibilities for each team member (e.g., who is in charge, who is responsible for ventilating the patient), (4) coverage of the remaining patients in the area, (5) control of "traffic" in the area, and (6) restocking of emergency drugs and supplies.

Communication with the Family During the Resuscitation Cycle

The initial communication with the patient's family occurs during the resuscitation phase of care. Family members are generally in a state of crisis, having had no time to prepare for the suddenness of a traumatic injury to their loved one. The admitting nurse and trauma physician together provide information concerning the patient's injuries and condition. The initial patient and family history are obtained. The nurse thereafter serves as a liaison to the patient's family, keeping them updated on their family member's condition as often as time will allow. The initial approach with the family often sets the tone for the entire hospital stay of the patient (see Chapter 10).

Dearing and Dang[25] suggest the following guidelines for communicating with the family in crisis:

1. Be honest when giving information and answering questions about the patient's condition. Be realistic when offering hope.
2. Include all family members in the conversation.
3. Sit rather than stand when talking to the family. This establishes closeness and a more caring environment.
4. Provide information in short, succinct sentences rather than long explanations.
5. Let the family know that a crisis is time-limited and that the intense feelings they are experiencing will eventually decrease.
6. Convey support to the family during this difficult time.

Psychological Support

Psychological support for the patient is also a priority and should be carried out throughout this phase of care. Patients are in as much a state of crisis as their family members. Even though the total systems approach to trauma is utilized for treatment, it is essential to recognize that the total system being dealt with is a human being. The patient has had no time to anticipate the injury. Attempts to cope with this fact are often worsened by pain or hypoxia. The rapid sequence of unfamiliar activities, beginning with rescue, impairs the patient's ability to perceive events realistically.[5]

For full recovery, the patient's emotional state must be addressed from the very beginning. The nurse should introduce herself and provide the patient with a brief description of the surroundings and an explanation of procedures as they are performed. These explanations should be short and concise and may need to be repeated. Patients in the resuscitation phase feel very powerless. They have little control

TABLE 6–6. GUIDELINES FOR MANAGEMENT OF POSTTRAUMATIC CARDIAC ARREST

1. Immediate tracheal intubation and positive-pressure ventilation
2. Rapid venous access
3. Rapid volume infusion, preferably with red blood cells
4. Thoracotomy through the left fourth and fifth intercostal spaces
5. Manual ventricular compression
6. Compression of the thoracic aorta above the diaphragm
7. Opening of the pericardium to relieve possible tamponade
8. Control associated intrathoracic hemorrhage
9. Insert right pleural chest tube
10. Administer sodium bicarbonate, 1 mEq/kg IV; follow with arterial blood gas determination
11. Ventricular fibrillation: Apply 20 to 60 W/sec of current to the left ventricle; if the heart does not defibrillate, administer additional IV sodium bicarbonate, 50 to 100 mg lidocaine IV and 0.5 to 1.0 mg epinephrine IV
12. Asystole: Administer 0.5 to 1.0 mg (up to 5.0 mg) epinephrine and 0.5 to 2.0 mg atropine IV
13. Electromechanical dissociation: Administer epinephrine and/or atropine as above

From Dunham CM, Cowley RA: Shock Trauma/Critical Care Manual. Gaithersburg, Md, Aspen Systems, 1991.

and a significant amount of fear of the unknown. Keeping them informed aids in reducing these feelings.

Spiritual Considerations

The spiritual component is also vital to the multiply injured patient's plan of care. The nurse must consider the patient's religion as soon as that information is available, for it may have significant impact on the plan of care. If the patient is critically injured and death may be imminent, the need for a priest to administer the Sacrament of the Sick to a Catholic patient must be addressed. Often, it is the nurse who calls a priest, especially if the family has not yet arrived in the emergency area. If the patient is identified as a Jehovah's Witness, the treatment plan typically requires some modification, particularly during the resuscitation and critical care phases. Each trauma facility should have a clear policy covering the withholding or administration of blood for these patients.

Evaluation and Transition

During this phase of care, continuous assessment is required to reevaluate the appropriateness and effectiveness of medical and nursing interventions. As the patient's condition stabilizes or changes, the plan of care must be reevaluated and altered to accommodate the changing profile. The admitting team must always expect the unexpected, must continually determine and execute priorities of care, and must reevaluate periodically in a logical fashion. As the patient progresses to the next phase, care evolves from the plan already initiated by the field and admitting team members.

Determination of the patient's readiness to move into another phase or cycle is a collaborative decision. Clear communication with the nurses assuming responsibility for the patient is essential. Provision of pertinent information regarding injuries, treatments, psychosocial issues, and the plan of care is necessary to facilitate patient transition into the next cycle.

Operative Phase

Most traumatic injuries require surgical intervention. Once the patient has been resuscitated and it is determined that operative procedures are warranted, the work of the nurse in the trauma operating room begins. Many aspects of this role include the traditional responsibilities of any operating room (OR) nurse. In addition to these, however, the operative needs of the multiply injured patient make the nurse's role more complex and demanding. The primary nursing concept continues through this phase, since one OR nurse is assigned to the multiply injured patient.

Operating rooms in major trauma centers require fully staffed teams around the clock and the ready availability of at least one suite for direct admissions into the OR. In other facilities the operating room team must be prepared to react promptly when the trauma patient arrives. Trauma patients generally require repeated surgical procedures to treat their injuries successfully. Rooms must be available for these elective procedures without sacrificing ready availability of rooms for emergent trauma patients.

Assessment

The perioperative role of the OR nurse, which traditionally includes a preoperative assessment and interview of the patient, may be drastically altered during the resuscitation cycle for any of the following reasons:

1. The patient may be comatose or unable to communicate effectively if an endotracheal tube or a tracheostomy is in place.
2. The emergency care necessitated by the instability of the patient may render him inaccessible to the operative nurse until he arrives in the operating room.
3. The patient may have required induction of anesthesia immediately upon arrival to the emergency area to allow for the administration of resuscitation and diagnostic measures (e.g., a combative patient under the influence of alcohol or drugs).
4. If the patient is awake, the physiological and psychological impact of injury may be so overwhelming as to preclude any assimilation of information given.

In these situations the priorities for the trauma OR nurse in the perioperative phase include ascertaining the urgency of the need for surgical intervention, arranging for the availability of a room, preparing the necessary equipment for the procedures to be performed, and coordinating the participation of the various specialty surgical teams who will be operating on the patient. Any data collection needed would be obtained from the admitting trauma nurse or physician. The OR nurse must obtain a detailed summary of what occurred during resuscitation. As the patient progresses past the critical care phase, elective surgical procedures may be necessary to restore maximal function. In these cases, the OR nurse plays a vital role in establishing trust and in providing the appropriate patient education.

Diagnosis

From a medical standpoint, the trauma patient who arrives in the operating room is far different from the patient undergoing elective surgery. The latter has been diagnosed preoperatively, and surgical intervention has been prescribed to correct the disorder. The multiply injured trauma patient, on the other hand, often arrives in the operating room without a specific diagnosis. A peritoneal lavage may have identified the presence of a hemoperitoneum, but the specific organs injured will not be known until an exploratory laparotomy is performed. Nursing diagnoses continue to be an integral part of the plan of care even during the operative phase.

Developing and Implementing a Plan

As the multiply injured patient is transported into the operating room, the specialized plan of care continues. The nurse's role during the actual operative phase remains crucial. In collaboration with the surgical teams and anesthesiologist, continuous assessment of the patient's hemodynamic stability is a priority. Meticulous record keeping must continue. The circulating trauma nurse plays a major role as coordinator. Multiply injured patients often require procedures performed by several different specialty teams either simultaneously or sequentially. Equipment for all these procedures must be readily available and properly placed for easy access. Coordination between the teams is essential. The nurse must be able to set up equipment that might be needed to repair injuries that were totally unsuspected until surgical exploration identified them. The OR nurse and the services that will be performing the procedures generally determine the order of surgical procedures based on time and priority of surgical intervention. If conflict arises, the attending trauma surgeon makes the decision about which procedure has priority. A patient who has a hemoperitoneum, an open ankle fracture, a deep chin laceration, loose teeth, and multiple facial fractures might be treated in the following manner: One team of surgeons will perform the exploratory laparotomy, while the oral surgeon extracts teeth and applies arch bars. Upon completion of these procedures, the orthopedic surgeon may set the ankle, while the plastic surgeon closes the laceration of the chin.

Because of the necessity for multiple surgical procedures, the patient is often on the OR table for as many as 16 to 18 hours. The effects of prolonged positioning on the table and administration of anesthesia must be addressed. Pressure sores can occur even before the patient arrives in the critical care unit if vulnerable areas have not been protected. Decreased circulation from blood loss, hypothermia, and prolonged anesthesia all contribute to this problem.

It may be difficult to maintain accurate sponge counts, since emergent situations may not allow time for a preoperative count. Radiographic confirmation is often the only choice to ensure that a sponge has not inadvertently been left in the patient.

Blood and blood products must be readily available to the trauma operating rooms. Many trauma centers have established separate refrigerators in the OR area for the storage of blood and blood products. To prevent severe hypothermia, all blood and intravenous fluids should be warmed.

The role of the anesthesiologist or nurse anesthetist has additional implications when the trauma patient is under anesthesia than when elective surgery is performed. These patients must be accurately monitored, often for prolonged periods of time. Constant vigilance is an absolute requirement. Assessment of hemodynamic and pulmonary status, maintaining multiple intravenous lines, administering appropriate medications and/or fluids, and being prepared for sudden unexpected deterioration of the patient are responsibilities that make the trauma anesthesiologist unique.

Evaluation and Transition

Following surgery, the patient must be scrutinized and prepared for transport to the post-anesthesia care or critical care unit. Prior to transport, an accurate report to the receiving unit is required to allow the nurses in the next phase to prepare for the admission. The initial communication with the receiving unit should, however, occur soon after the patient's arrival in the OR. Periodic updates related to the patient's condition or disposition status assist other units to prepare for the patient's arrival. Often critical care units need to alter current patient assignments and obtain specific supplies and equipment to accommodate the needs of a postoperative trauma patient.

The multiply injured patient is often admitted directly to the critical care unit postoperatively. On arrival in the unit, a survey of vascular access sites, fluids and medications being infused, and drainage tubes by both the OR nurse or the anesthesia provider and the receiving trauma nurse in the critical care unit is necessary. An accurate report of the resuscitation efforts, surgical procedures performed, vital sign trends, fluid balance, estimated blood loss, and medications and anesthesia administered ensures continuity in the plan of care for the patient.

Frequently, severely injured patients later require multiple surgeries to treat injuries or complications that may have developed. Many of these occur while the patient is still requiring critical care and maximum technological support. The OR nurse has the responsibility, in conjunction with the critical care nurse and respiratory therapist, to transport the patient safely.

Communication with the Family

Another primary responsibility of the OR trauma nurse is family intervention. Every attempt should be made to keep them informed both prior to and during the surgical procedures. Prior to surgery, the information conveyed to them should include suspected injuries, the planned surgical procedures, estimated time the patient will be in surgery, and the potential for death if it is present. When operative procedures are prolonged, consistent communication with family members is imperative. Information given intraoperatively should include an update on the current status of the patient, what the family can expect postoperatively, the surgeon's name, necessary phone numbers to obtain information postoperatively, and the reiteration of the time estimate for completion of surgical procedures. Following the procedure, the trauma surgeon and OR nurse should explain which operative procedures were performed, the stability and prognosis of the patient, and the unit to which the patient will be admitted.

Comfortable waiting areas for families should be available as close to the operating room floor as possible. Beverages, a telephone, and pillows should be readily available. Often during this cycle the family members are at a loss for knowing what they can do to help. Sometimes the suggestion that they or their friends can donate blood to help replace that given to their loved one provides direction at a time of grief and uncertainty.

CYCLE III: CRITICAL CARE

The critical care aspect of the patient with multiple system injuries requires the skills of a variety of medical and related professional groups. These efforts must be coordinated in such a way as to provide optimal care and to minimize the physiological and psychological stress of the injury. In this phase of multidisciplinary care, it is essential that a primary physician and nurse coordinate the efforts of all members of the health care team. It is the primary nurse, however, who has the overall picture of the patient's plan of care. It is the nurse's responsibility to remain abreast of *all* aspects of the patient's progress and treatment and to keep each member of the health team informed of what others are doing. Trauma patients often have a wide variety of problems, both physical and psychological, and coordinating the efforts of all the health care providers is integral to their management.

Assessment

Just as the resuscitation area nurse must prepare for the emergency admission of a multitrauma patient, the critical care nurse also must assemble and have on hand the necessary equipment for the patient's arrival into the critical care unit (CCU). The resuscitation nurse, the anesthesia provider, or the post-anesthesia care unit nurse gives the CCU nurse a thorough report and identifies equipment that will be needed. Monitoring, suction, ventilatory, and emergency equipment must be available and checked thoroughly for proper functioning prior to the patient's arrival.

General

Admission to the critical care unit directly from the operating room is preferable. Utilization of a separate recovery room may interrupt the continuity of care, and the additional transportation often puts the critically ill patient at risk. If a separate recovery room is utilized, care should be taken to provide continuity in the plan of care and safe transport. Upon admission, the patient is immediately connected to monitoring equipment and placed on the ventilator. IV fluids or blood products being infused are noted, and the infusion site for each fluid should be identified immediately. If IV medication is needed, the nurse knows exactly which lines may be utilized safely. The position and patency of drains, condition of wound dressings, and the location and status of skeletal traction are established.

After establishing that vital physiological functions are intact, the CCU nurse continues the initial assessment. A total systems assessment and a careful examination of procedures performed in the admitting area and the operating room are necessary. The following information is minimally required: units of blood the patient received, estimated blood loss, hypotensive episodes prior to or during admission, fluid balance, type of anesthesia and medications administered, surgical procedures performed, and whether or not the family was notified and exactly which family members were told about the patient's injuries. This information should be recorded to provide a baseline for therapy and interventions during the critical care phase.

Physical

A total systems assessment should be conducted and recorded completely, system by system, in the nursing record at least once every 24 hours (see Appendix 6–6). A standardized assessment form decreases time needed for recording.

Frequent reassessment and documentation of changes are an ongoing responsibility. It is most often the nurse at the bedside who identifies the changes in the patient's condition which warrant notification of the medical team for corresponding changes in treatment.

Frequent evaluation of the multiply injured patient is vital during this phase for many reasons. The body responds to the stress of trauma with many physiological and emotional changes. The trauma patient may deteriorate as existing injuries worsen and the body fails to achieve system stability, and occasionally subtle injuries may be missed on admission. Possible life-threatening complications that often occur in this phase demand early detection for prevention or treatment to increase chances of survival, ongoing assessment data act as validating criteria for accurate nursing diagnoses and interventions, and the patient's tolerance of and response to prescribed medical and nursing therapies must be monitored.

Throughout the cycle of critical care, one of the major values of ongoing assessment is the early detection of actual or pending complications. For example, the patient with a severe pulmonary contusion may go on to develop adult respiratory distress syndrome (ARDS); early recognition of this condition allows for early therapeutic intervention. The primary objective in the assessment of major complications following traumatic injury is the anticipation by the nurse of complications that can occur with associated injuries. During assessment, the nurse must keep in mind the injuries that the patient has sustained and the complications commonly associated with them (see Appendix 6–7).

Laboratory Protocols

During the critical care cycle, serial laboratory studies play an important role in the overall assessment of the patient's status and are utilized with other data to alter a patient's treatment plan. Established protocols for obtaining these tests ensure that adequate monitoring takes place. Protocols should include the type of tests to be drawn, time intervals for obtaining them, the type of container to be utilized for each test, and where they are to be sent for analysis.

In this critical care cycle, blood samples for serial hematocrit and hemoglobins, coagulation profile, electrolytes, and arterial and venous blood gases should be drawn at least every 12 hours and more often if the patient's condition is unstable (Table 6–7). Although frequent laboratory studies provide necessary data for assessment, the amount of blood drawn from the patient must also be considered. The need for blood replacement should never be a result of too frequent, unnecessary blood sampling.

Bedside Diagnostic Studies

Multitrauma patients are often hemodynamically unstable or ventilator-dependent and therefore too unstable to be transported unnecessarily to areas outside the trauma unit for diagnostic studies. Interruption of traction devices also may be detrimental to a patient. In these cases, bedside studies may be necessary. These studies (e.g., evoked potentials, echocardiogram) are often time consuming and involve large pieces of equipment. The nurse caring for the patient should coordinate proper timing of the tests so they do not interfere with other needed treatments. While the test is being done, the monitoring of the patient must not be interrupted. Care should be scheduled so that necessary treatments may be completed just prior to or immediately following a test.

Psychosocial

The ongoing assessment of a trauma patient's psychological adjustment to injury is equally as important as ongoing physical assessment: It is a vital component of holistic care. A trauma patient often fluctuates dramatically as adjustment

TABLE 6–7. DIAGNOSTIC LABORATORY STUDIES PROTOCOL

TEST	UNSTABLE PATIENT 0700	UNSTABLE PATIENT 1900	STABLE PATIENT 0700
Arterial blood gas	X*	X*	X†
Venous blood gas	X*	X*	
Complete blood count	X	X	X
Electrolytes	X	X	X
Glucose	X	X	X
Blood urea nitrogen	X	X	X
Creatinine	X	X	X
Calcium	X		X
Ionized calcium	X		
Osmolarity	X		X
Coagulation profile	X	X	
Phosphorus	X		
Magnesium	X		
Total bilirubin	X		
Direct bilirubin	X		
AST/SGOT	X		
Alkaline phosphatase	X		
Amylase	X		
Albumin	X		
Cholesterol	X		
Triglycerides	X		
Lactate	X	X	

*Direct oxygen saturation (Co-oximetry).
†Mechanically ventilated patients.
Note: The frequency of blood testing is dictated by patient condition; the above are the minimum frequency for stable and unstable patients. Reprinted with permission from STAT Laboratory Manual, Maryland Institute for Emergency Medical Services Systems, Baltimore, Md, 1991.

to the injuries occurs. One moment the patient may demonstrate signs of adjustment to the injury; the next moment the patient may succumb to depression, not responding to or cooperating with treatment.

Trauma patients' psychological responses are often totally unpredictable. The 40-year-old patient with paraplegia secondary to a thoracic spine injury may adjust better than a 16-year-old boy whose severely fractured femur will keep him from fulfilling his life's dream of playing professional football. A continuous psychosocial assessment will enable the primary nurse to plan interventions that will help a trauma patient deal with the injuries more effectively. Knowledge of the patient's existent, or nonexistent, support systems, how the patient usually reacts to stressful situations, and previous coping mechanisms will enable the nurse to develop a more individualized plan of care.

Family

The critical care unit primary nurse, beginning on the first day of admission, must assess the family members for their knowledge of the patient's injuries and for their ability to interpret and accept what has been communicated to them.[26] Coping mechanisms and support systems that they use to deal with the crisis should also be identified and documented. All such family information, as well as the planned interventions to assist the family, should be carefully outlined in the nursing care plan. Families in crisis often latch on to a single piece of information, and unless it is clear to all those caring for the patient what the family has been told, family members may receive mixed messages. Upon initial contact with the family members, a spokesperson should be identified so that all communication relating to the patient's condition can be relayed to that one person to avoid the possibility of varied interpretations by several different family members. To prevent inaccurate or inconsistent information from being delivered to the family, all information should be given by the primary nurse or physician to the spokesperson. Early assessment and appropriate interventions such as providing information, active listening, facilitating flexibility in visiting, and family–caregiver conferences are key to effective management of families of trauma victims.[26] (Refer to Chapter 10 for a more complete discussion of family interactions with trauma care personnel.)

Diagnosis

Nursing diagnoses carry immense significance—and responsibility—during the multiply injured patient's critical care cycle. Most diagnoses will be physiological, as the patient strives to adapt to the stressors of severe injury. Some of these diagnoses will be easy to identify if the unhealthful responses are actually present, but the majority of the diagnoses during this phase are *potential,* with nursing interventions aimed at preventing their occurrence. The patient with a severe pulmonary contusion, for example, might have a nursing diagnosis of "potential for occluded airway related to tissue sloughing and copious bloody secretions." Interventions are thus aimed at preventing an occluded airway, e.g., use of a mucolytic agent and frequent suctioning.

At this stage, diagnoses are generated from frequent and thorough assessments and are based on the priority of patient needs. A patient with fractured ribs might have the diagnosis of "impaired gas exchange related to inability to cough adequately secondary to pain." Interventions to address this condition are of immediate priority. Multitrauma patients in this phase of care often exhibit similar unhealthful responses.

Psychological nursing diagnoses are often readily apparent during this cycle. One might see a diagnosis of "powerlessness related to inability to communicate effectively" in the spinal cord–injured patient who has a tracheostomy and is immobilized on a Stryker frame. Even though nursing diagnoses in this cycle primarily emphasize the body's physiological response to severe injury, the psychosocial component must not be overlooked.

Developing and Implementing the Plan

During the critical care cycle, the concept of collaborative practice, begun in the resuscitation cycle, becomes even more important. Many different medical services may be involved in the multiply injured patient's care: orthopedics, neurosurgery, plastic surgery, and critical care. Respiratory therapists, physical therapists, nutritionists, and others who have daily contact with the patient assume integral roles in the care plan. The primary nurse is the only one who has a global view of all the services involved, and her role as coordinator is of great significance. The trauma patient is totally dependent on the nurse at this stage of care. The patient looks to the nurse as the decision maker who controls his destiny.

It is beyond the scope of this chapter to address all nursing care concerns during the critical care phase. Much of it includes critical care practice. In caring for trauma patients, however, there are particular aspects of critical care nursing practice that have special relevance to this phase of care. Whereas medical protocols dictate actual treatment of the trauma patient, nursing protocols based on established standards of practice provide a basis for quality care. Individualized care planning then must follow, for each trauma patient is unique.

Multidisciplinary Approach to Patient Care

All aspects of the plan of care for the critically ill trauma patient involve multiple disciplines. Coordination of the efforts of these individuals, ensuring common patient goals, is uniquely the responsibility of the primary nurse. Daily multidisciplinary rounds facilitate sharing of information and objectives and development of the short- and long-term plans of care; the primary nurse, or designee, must be a part of these interactions and decisions. Planning caregiver conferences every 2 to 4 weeks, especially as the complexity of patient care increases, allows all disciplines to discuss their perspectives and agree on priorities and specific long-term goals. This plan should be documented by the primary nurse. Subsequent conferences focus on evaluation of progress and revising the plan. Caregiver conferences need to be attended by representatives from all disciplines and services involved in the patient's care.

Emergency Procedures

Polytrauma patients are often hemodynamically unstable immediately following injury or upon development of complications later in the critical care phase. The multitrauma patient also has the potential for developing sudden, potentially life-threatening complications that occur without warning. Critical care trauma nurses require the cognitive and psychomotor capabilities to deal with sudden, emergent situations. The need for emergency equipment is predictable, and making it accessible becomes automatic when planning care. The availability of up-to-date emergency equipment in good working condition is required at all times. Seconds count: Patients' lives may depend on the anticipation of critical events and the readiness of emergency equipment.

Bedside operative procedures are not unusual, and the critical care nurse should be prepared to facilitate these. Again, this nurse coordinates the efforts, obtaining necessary equipment, ensuring the presence of appropriate personnel (e.g., for provision of anesthesia and OR nurses), maintaining continued high-level care and monitoring, serving as the patient advocate, and communicating with the family.

Documentation

The physiological monitoring that occurs in the critical care unit generates a large amount of data that together with the clinical picture of the patient provides the basis on which to prescribe treatment. Identifying trends from these data is crucial to detecting subtle changes in the patient's condition and to altering therapy accordingly. To identify these trends in a timely and objective manner, documentation must be thorough and must allow for the visual examination of various categories of data in relation to other sets of data. For example, whether computers or a flow sheet is utilized, it is important to be able to look at *all* parameters (vital signs, intake and output values, medications, neurological status) simultaneously over a given time in the patient's course (see sample of flow sheet in Appendix 6–8).

Computers can be very useful for documenting physiological data. Automatic physiological monitoring capabilities, IV drug calculation programs, and recording of laboratory data can be helpful adjuncts to the development of a specialized and individualized plan of care. The computer allows data gathered by various disciplines involved in trauma patient care to be stored in one place and to be utilized by anyone at a given time.

Transporting Critical Care Patients

Effective diagnostic procedures and therapies for the multitrauma patient often depend on information obtained through special tests, such as computed tomography (CT) or nuclear medicine studies. Because the physical aspects of equipment for effectively performing these tests prohibit its transfer to the bedside, the nurse must move the patient to the equipment's location. Therefore, an already compromised, critically injured patient may have to undergo the additional stress of transport to other areas of the hospital. When the patient is multiply injured or unstable, the problems and the nurse's responsibilities increase in direct proportion to the number and severity of life-threatening injuries already present. To ensure patient safety before, during, and after the transfer, the trauma nurse must utilize advance planning to coordinate care requirements, personnel, backup equipment, and supplies.[27] The level of patient monitoring and care should not change during transport.

Once the risks have been weighed against the necessity of the test, the nurse assumes responsibility for the coordination of the transport. Patient needs during transport are many: (1) respiratory support, (2) medications (routine, emergency, and premedications for diagnostic tests) that must be given while out of the unit, (3) IV fluids, and (4) adequate monitoring.

During any transport, the nurse has the responsibility to protect and preserve all IV and monitoring lines and drains. The lines must remain patent—accidental dislodgment of lines or drains may be of significant risk to the patient.

The number and type of personnel accompanying the patient also must be decided. A transport policy should provide guidelines for these decisions. Backup equipment (e.g., extra oxygen tanks, batteries for portable monitoring equipment) also must accompany the patient. Because it is often necessary to transport blood with an unstable trauma patient, an insulated container with a temperature indicator to monitor the temperature range of the blood should be utilized. Any equipment specific to the individual patient also must be taken. The nurse must be aware of the nearest emergency equipment cart en route and at the destination.

Even after all plans have been made, a final checklist will ensure that all aspects have been covered and will often alert the nurse to facts that may affect the procedure for which the patient is being transported. For example, a patient with a pelvic Hoffmann device in place may need that device adjusted before transport to enable him to fit into the CT scanner or a patient who weighs more than 300 lb may not fit into the CT scanner. If such factors are overlooked, they may, at the last minute, cause cancellation of a test after the patient has already undergone the risk of transportation.

Special Considerations

Administration of IV Medications

Trauma patients with multisystem injuries are often unable to take medications orally or by the gastrointestinal route. They have an increased need for high doses of antibiotics to prevent infection, and these drugs are more effective if given intravenously. Agents that augment cardiac output are frequently administered to multiply injured patients: One patient may simultaneously receive many different cardiovascular medications at one time. Dosages are titrated frequently as the patient's hemodynamic status dictates.

In addition, most multitrauma patients typically receive total parenteral nutrition therapy and maintenance IV fluids on a continual basis. Thus one patient may have as many as eight or nine intravenous fluids/medications infusing simultaneously. This situation creates a situation risking medication errors, even when intravenous infusion pumps are utilized. Off-going and on-coming nurses must review all infusions together and ensure that infusion alarm limits are set to allow administration of only the volume that should be received.

Critical care nurses must often make independent judgments when administering IV medications. Their knowledge base must include an awareness of drug compatibilities and incompatibilities, specific actions of the drugs, and unique aspects for consideration when administering specific drugs. When patients receive multiple medications, changes in behavior or physical manifestations such as a skin rash must be examined closely. In emergency situations, which are common in the multiply injured patient, emergency drugs must be administered immediately to facilitate adequate resuscitation. An IV medication policy is essential not only to provide guidelines for the nurse but also to provide legal coverage for her actions.

Infection

Nosocomial infection is a serious problem for the multiply injured patient during this phase of care (see Chapter 11). Protocols that are aimed at preventing infection should be established and adhered to rigorously. Protocols addressing invasive catheter changes and dressing care, suctioning and endotracheal techniques, culture surveillance, tracheostomy changes, and isolation policies, for example, are a necessity. An established dress code for patient care procedures in the critical care area also should be followed. Employee compliance with recent OSHA regulations to protect health care workers from bodily fluid exposure needs to be standardized and consistently enforced.

Pain and Agitation Control

Traumatic injury often results in severe pain for the patient. Managing pain, anxiety, and agitation is a multifaceted challenge for the critical care nurse. Agitation and anxious behavior may be related to pain, hypoxia, sepsis, drug toxicity, and a multitude of other factors. The nurse must assess and differentiate the cause, also a challenge, particularly in the mechanically ventilated or brain-injured patient with impaired communication capabilities, prior to sedative or analgesia administration. Even a minimal dose of some medications may precipitate an acute hypotensive episode.

Patients with a history of alcohol or drug abuse prior to injury present a difficult problem. In these patients, determining the appropriate drug and dosage is a challenge. Combination analgesia and sedation or use of an alcohol infusion and methadone is often necessary.[28] The patient with a brain injury presents an additional problem for nurses and physicians. Evaluation of the neurological status of such a patient on a day-to-day basis restricts the use of analgesics and sedatives. These patients may become severely agitated and experience significant pain. Assessment of pain and caring for this population are indeed a challenge. The use of touch, soothing music, and other less conventional modes of therapy may be necessary alternatives.

The physiological effects of sedatives, narcotics, and other medications also must be considered. Large doses may reduce and prolong already slowed gastric motility and peristalsis and deter the early institution of enteral nutrition. In addition, high doses of morphine have been associated with the occurrence of acalculous cholecystitis in trauma patients.[29] Patients with severe thoracic or abdominal pain and oversedated patients often cannot cough effectively, thereby increasing their potential for developing atelectasis and pneumonia. Consulting the acute pain management service or an anesthesiologist is often most appropriate in the care of the trauma patient with poorly controlled pain and agitation. In nearly all situations, the management of pain needs to be a multidisciplinary effort to provide the most effective therapy. The nurse is in the optimal position to assess the patient, coordinate the services, and address the issue of the patient's pain.

The administration of pain medication should never be routine; it must be considered in relation to all facets of the patient's care (see Chapter 14).

Communication Issues

Communication from patient to health care team members, a crucial component for a therapeutic relationship, is often difficult in this critical care phase for several reasons: the presence of an artificial airway, paralytic agents, sedation, paralysis, unconsciousness, or sensory disturbances. Establishing a mode of communication that is effective for such a patient must be a priority in the care plan.

Wound Care

Although this subject is covered in depth elsewhere (see Chapter 12), its importance during this critical care cycle must be emphasized. Traumatic injury elicits a variety of wounds: penetrating, abrasive, avulsive, and/or lacerations. Many of them are contaminated wounds, depending on the source of traumatic injury, and many become infected after admission. Wound healing may be impaired by steroid therapy and nutritional deficiencies or immunocompromise related to the persistent inflammatory response associated with severe traumatic injuries. It is crucial to establish a protocol for individualized wound care, document it in the patient's care plan, and evaluate its effectiveness on a daily basis. Even the smallest laceration has the potential for becoming infected, thereby producing serious complications such as systemic sepsis or severe localized tissue and muscle damage. Careful attention must be paid to assessing all wounds and establishing consistent treatment measures immediately following the patient's admission to the critical care unit.

Pulmonary Complications

During this critical care cycle, pulmonary complications often occur related to a pulmonary injury, preexisting conditions such as fluid overload or multiple blood transfusions, and immobility. Aggressive pulmonary toilet must be a priority. Protocols for suctioning, tracheal lavage, tracheostomy care, and tracheostomy changes should exist for this phase of care. Chest physiotherapy should be a part of the pulmonary care regimen for all patients in whom it is not contraindicated. Frequent turning, repositioning, institution of kinetic therapy, and early mobilization are preventive measures to reduce the risk of nosocomial pneumonias. If respiratory therapists are included in the health care team, there should be a clear delineation of their responsibilities and those of the nurse to ensure the delivery of good pulmonary care (see Chapter 18 for details).

Rehabilitative Considerations

The belief that rehabilitation begins on admission has long been accepted, but it is particularly relevant when planning care for the trauma patient. At the time the patient enters the critical care cycle, rehabilitation needs must be addressed. Immobility has significant impact on all systems. Attention to reducing musculoskeletal alterations must begin in the critical care phase. Early splinting of extremities, when appropriate, active and passive range of motion, and frequent repositioning aid in prevention of serious contractures and other problems arising from immobilization. The application of pneumatic leg compression devices deters the development of deep vein thrombosis related to extremity injury and immobility.

The use of specialty beds and mattress overlays has become common practice in the care of the multiply injured patient. When prescribed appropriately, they enhance the patient's recovery process. Several types of beds are available to hospitals. Each one has unique features. Kinetic therapy beds have proven to be efficacious in reducing the incidence of nosocomial pneumonia[30] and other immobility-related complications. Air-fluidized beds relieve interface pressure and enhance healing of large wounds. Low-air-loss beds decrease interface pressure and pressure sore development. The placement of a patient on one of these beds should occur as a collaborative nursing and medical decision. It is helpful to develop specific criteria to use as guidelines in placing patients on these beds to prevent unnecessary or inappropriate use.

Planning for discharge needs to begin during the critical care cycle. Often the need for a rehabilitation facility or long-term ventilator unit is evident early in this cycle. Collaborative family and health care provider discussions and plans should take place to identify the desired facility and expedite transfer when the patient is sufficiently healed.

Visiting Considerations

Family visits are a vital part of the overall plan of care for the patient. Visiting by family members and significant others should be encouraged during the critical care cycle. Family members are often afraid that their loved one will appear grotesque or will have wounds exposed. The nurse can facilitate their first visit by describing how the patient looks, by providing a clear explanation of tubes and equipment, and by remaining with the family. Signs of visible trauma help the family accept reality. Family visits provide the nurse with an opportunity to assess their understanding and perception of their loved one's injuries and their acceptance of the information they have received from the nurse and physician. Families who are restricted from visiting a critically ill member often suffer from fear, anxiety, hopelessness, and helplessness. These may be displayed as hostility and anger toward the staff in an attempt to appear in control of the situation.[26]

High Technology

Trauma care has become a highly specialized health care field. With increasing recognition of the importance of specific physiological parameters in deciding on specific treatment modalities and development of intricate machinery to measure such parameters, the trauma nurse today faces additional responsibilities. She must have a thorough working knowledge of these devices and must be able to recognize and incorporate the value of the parameters they measure into the plan of care (Fig. 6–2).

The use of high technology in trauma care demands certain conditions. The nurses and other staff members who utilize the equipment to provide care must be properly educated before being expected to assume these responsibilities. A certified and experienced biomedical engineering staff must keep equipment in working condition and be available as a resource for staff when problems occur. A system of product control is useful. For example, it is advantageous to have all units utilize the same monitoring system or emergency equipment so that the entire staff can become familiar with and secure in its utilization. It also should be recognized that high technology is no longer limited to the critical care phases of care; more and more devices are being developed to assist in rehabilitation. Proper utilization is mandatory: Even seemingly simple devices such as the passive leg exerciser can be dangerous if not used properly.

The most important aspect to consider when using highly technical equipment, computer systems, and other devices is patient care. The patient must remain the main focus. Naisbitt's theory[31] of "high tech, high touch" is truly relevant to the trauma patient's care and should be incorporated in the plan of care. This theory is a formula to describe the way we have responded to technology. Whenever new technology is introduced into society, there must be a counterbalancing human response, i.e., high touch, or the technology is rejected.

In the health care field, high technology is inherent and ever-expanding. Consequently, the need for more high touch is increasing. For example, primary nursing, which Naisbitt believes is a very "high touch" mode of care, has slowly replaced team nursing.

Naisbitt acknowledges the fact that there is no way to keep

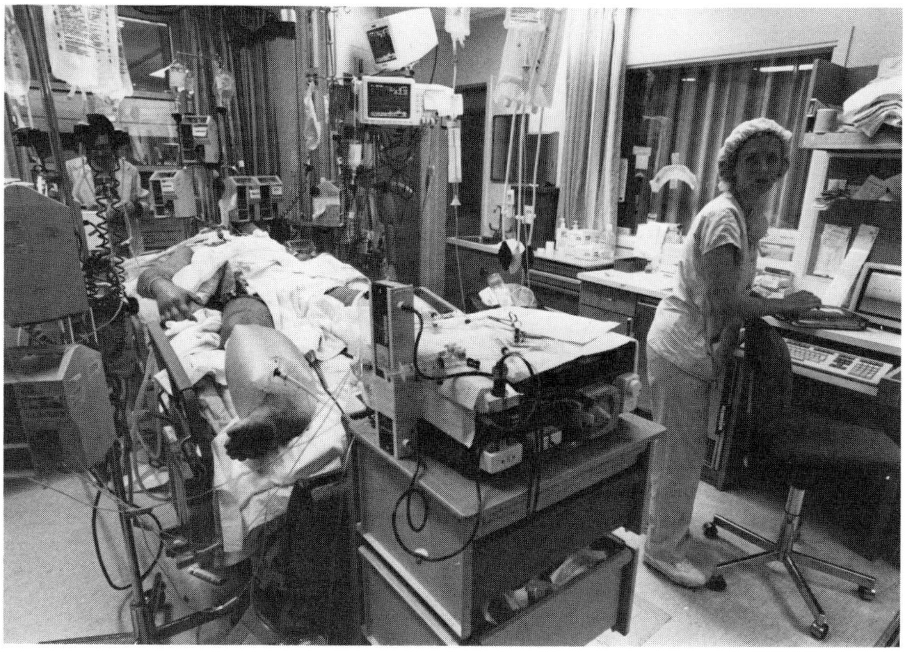

Figure 6–2. A critical care nurse with a severely injured trauma patient who has developed multisystem organ failure. The patient requires mechanical ventilation, multiple drug infusions, and continuous veno-veno hemofiltration with dialysis to maintain organ and system function. (Reprinted with permission from Maryland Institute for Emergency Medical Services Systems, Baltimore, Md, 1992.)

humans from devising new tools, but we must also take care not to see these tools as the sole solution. "When we fall into a trap of believing or hoping that technology will solve all of our problems, we are actually abdicating the high touch of personal responsibility. The more high technology around us, the more the need for human touch."[31] Nowhere in the medical field is this theory more relevant than in trauma care.

Computers have become commonplace in hospital care and are valuable adjuncts in providing trauma care. Once thought to be "dehumanizing," computers (if utilized correctly) can actually work *for* the practitioners in planning more effective care. Laboratory values are retrieved more quickly, drug calculation programs can reduce the possibility of medication error, and fluid intake and output programs will ensure accurate cumulative fluid totals, which are invaluable to the trauma patient's plan of care. Documentation of plans of care, progress toward goals, physician orders, and the like are easily accessible, and modifications can be made in the plan. As long as the patient remains the primary focus, computers are invaluable in providing higher-quality care.

Finally, as cost-cutting practices in hospital equipment budgets become more of a reality, there is a tendency to believe that practitioners can deliver the same care with less sophisticated and less expensive equipment. Caring for critically ill trauma patients often requires certain types of equipment and may necessitate a higher monetary investment to ensure quality care. Careful evaluation and balancing high quality with cost containment are an integral part of trauma nursing.

Research

Because of the complexity of traumatic injury, the multidisciplinary approach to trauma care is a rapidly evolving new specialized field, and efforts are continuously being made to encourage trauma practitioners to institute research directed toward this field. Characteristics of the population, multiple therapeutic interventions, and drugs and modes of therapy are continuously being studied to refine the process and improve the outcomes of trauma care. The multitrauma patient may suddenly become the host for a number of simultaneous medical and nursing research endeavors which can impact care and clinical operations. A trauma center must have an established committee for reviewing all proposed research studies and existing protocols to protect the patient (and family) yet facilitate both nursing and medical research projects.

There is much to be learned about the trauma patient's responses to injury and the effectiveness of specific treatments; therefore, research can and should be a vital component of the overall plan of care for each patient, as long as established protocols for performing research are followed. It is understood that every trauma patient has the right to a highly individualized plan of care, but some situations need special reflection and attention to ensure high-quality care.

Organ Donation

Traumatic injury, especially severe head injury, often creates the potential for organ donation (see Chapter 30). Traumatically injured individuals are frequently young, with healthy organs suitable for donation. The potential organ donor requires a specialized plan that involves physiological support, and the family requires intense psychological support. Once the patient has been identified as a potential donor, sets of specific guidelines as determined by the transplant coordination team must direct the care.

The Dying Patient

The terminal patient is not an uncommon situation in the field of trauma nursing. Overwhelming injuries or lethal complications often occur as a result of injury. Once it has been recognized and accepted that no more can be done for the patient, it is easy to label him as a "no CPR" patient who "can easily be combined with other patients in staff assignments because he is not busy." The truth is, however, that the dying patient is still in need of a highly "specialized" plan of care that involves the patient, the family, and various members of the health care team.

The definition of nursing by the International Council of Nurses addresses the nurse's role in the care of the dying:

> The unique function of the nurse is to assist the individual, sick or well, in the performance of those activities contributing to his health, his recovery, or to a peaceful death that he would perform unaided if he had the necessary strength, will or knowledge.[32]

The specialized component of this patient's plan of care is personalization. Each nurse has learned ways to personalize care for the dying patient in nursing practice. Although treatment may be withheld and only basic nursing care and comfort measures are appropriate, assignments should allow the nurse to spend time with the dying patient and the family. When trauma nurses tend to spend less time with such patients, it is often a mechanism that allows them to distance themselves from the reality that their hard work was to no avail. But one must step back and recognize that such a situation exists and make special efforts to personalize the plan of care and spend time with the patient. Often, this is the only comfort that family members have as the end draws near—the knowledge that someone is with their loved one at a time when they cannot be.

Occasionally, conflicting opinions among the medical staff, nurse, and family regarding the continuation of aggressive treatment will arise. In these situations, the primary nurse must assume the role of coordinator and patient advocate and work with all team members to finalize a plan of care that is implemented consistently. Specific documentation of such decisions must be present on the chart and care plan.

The dying patient, perhaps more than other trauma patients, has the right to an individualized plan of care that integrates "caring" as the most vital component. The transition from life to death is a voyage that requires the company and quiet reassurance of another. The potential exists, in those moments, for the exchange of many human gifts and values that otherwise may go unnoticed.

Evaluation and Transition

The evaluation component of the nursing process is ongoing during the critical care cycle, as it was during the resuscitation phase. During the initial postoperative period, emphasis is on stabilization of the patient as the body attempts to regain homeostasis following the stressor of traumatic injury. Just as assessment must be continuous and appropriate and interventions are initiated based on the assessment, the evaluation of the care plan must be continuous so that therapy may be altered accordingly. During this cycle, the plan of care may be altered initially, from shift to shift, and later, as the patient stabilizes, on a daily basis. The primary nurse and physician coordinate the health team to accomplish this.

As the patient achieves stability and therapies are found to be appropriate and effective, assessment again becomes a critical factor as the time approaches for the patient's transfer to a less critical care environment.

The transition from critical care to a less intensive care unit may be difficult for the patient and family who have for days or months depended on the critical care primary nurses and formed strong relationships and trust. Early planning for transfer will assist the patient and family to make the transition. Discussions related to patient readiness and characteristics of the new unit or rehabilitation facility help the patient and family to prepare. Ideally, this takes place as far in advance as possible and may serve as a motivator for the patient. Advance notification and communication with the receiving unit nurses, identifying the next primary nurse, reviewing the plan of care and personal details with her, and introducing the patient to the nurse will facilitate the transition and maintain continuity of patient care. The patient and family also need to be prepared for the necessity of a move to another unit related to other patient acuity changes or the need for the critical care unit to emergently accept new admissions.

CYCLE IV: INTERMEDIATE CARE

An integrated approach to care continues to be a vital concept in this stage, and many health team members need to be involved in planning and implementing patient care. One of the most effective means of planning is the patient-centered multidisciplinary care planning conference. Conferences should include all the disciplines impacting patient recovery. In addition to medicine and nursing, representatives from speech, occupational, and physical therapy should be involved. Needs assessments are presented, goals are set, and a specific plan to meet these goals, involving the whole team, is developed. Once the plan has been established, the patient again plays an important role in mutual goal setting. The plan should be flexible enough to allow the patient to take an active part in identifying long- and short-term goals and in outlining how these goals will be reached.

Tracking and documenting patient progress toward achievement of desired goals and outcomes are the responsibility of the primary nurse. Subsequent conferences should focus on evaluation of progress and identification of additional strategies to expedite the patient's recovery.

When feasible, advanced planning should take place in the intermediate care unit to reduce the stress of transfer for the previously critically ill patient and his family. Particularly in cases of long-term critical care unit patients, the preassigning of a primary nurse is useful to ease the transition. The nurse on the intermediate care unit can begin to establish a trusting relationship by visiting the patient and family prior to transfer from the critical care unit. These pretransfer visits also serve as early assessment opportunities and may elucidate special needs of the patient and/or the family.

Many trauma patients do not require critical care and are admitted directly to the intermediate care unit from the resuscitation unit or emergency department, or from the post-anesthesia care unit. These patients and their families have unique physical and psychological needs which should not be minimized because the patient is not injured severely enough to require critical care.

Assessment

Physical

The intermediate phase of care is still "critical" because physiological as well as psychological complications can occur. Ongoing assessment is vital. The nurse should perform and document a complete systems assessment once every shift, and any untoward changes noted must be reported to the physician quickly. During this cycle, the trauma patient often appears to be doing well. Subtle changes noted during the assessment have the potential of being overlooked or viewed as unimportant when, in fact, these changes may be signaling the onset of complications. Often, it may simply be a high index of suspicion that alerts the nurse to unmanifested changes in physiological status. It is important to recognize that complications following traumatic injury often occur on a delayed basis and may occur very unexpectedly in the postcritical phase. Laboratory protocols may change in this phase to allow less frequent blood sampling. Generally, patients in this phase need to have blood drawn once every 24 hours.

Patients who are admitted to the intermediate care unit from the resuscitation or post-anesthesia care unit, although not critically ill, still require very close observation, especially for the first 72 hours. Initially, undiagnosed injuries may become evident and require rapid interventions on the part of the nurse and physician team. Complications, most commonly infection and sepsis, also may develop within this time period. Astute assessment of vital signs, sensorium, physical signs and symptoms, laboratory values, and EKG changes allow for early identification of problems and interventions that may substantially reduce patient morbidity.

Psychological

The trauma patient may exhibit significant changes psychologically. During the critical phase, the predominant concern of the trauma patient is whether he will live or die. But once the patient recognizes that the immediate crisis is over and that he is going to live, other psychological problems may surface. For example, the patient may exhibit disproportionate sick-role behavior or have difficulty in expressing grief. Anger, blaming, and withdrawal are also signs of ineffective coping. This frequently occurs as the patient realizes that the incurred injuries will require a long period of rehabilitation for complete recovery. These are just a few examples of psychological problems that may surface during this cycle. Continuous assessment for symptoms that signal their actual or potential presence facilitates institution of appropriate preventive measures and interventions.

The families of these trauma patients experience similar shock and disbelief. The nurses must assess the family's ability to cope with the crisis of sudden injury, as discussed in Chapter 11.

Rehabilitative

It is also during this cycle that a more vigorous assessment of rehabilitation needs must occur. Assessing for potential complications that may prolong eventual rehabilitation is essential. The patient whose tibial fracture heals well with external fixation but who develops footdrop as a result of inconsistent passive range-of-motion exercises can expect a prolonged hospitalization course and the possible need for additional surgery to correct the problem. If it is evident that the patient will require extensive rehabilitation at a specialty center, the nurse and physician should assess the available rehabilitation centers to determine which one could provide the most appropriate care and discuss the options with the patient and family. Early identification of rehabilitation needs is essential to facilitate referral and timely placement in a rehabilitation facility.

Diagnosis

Unlike the potential nursing diagnoses that dominate the critical phase, diagnoses in this cycle are most often "actual." At this stage, diagnoses such as "prolonged denial of traumatic injury" or "depression" often surface. The patient psychologically attempts to adapt to the stressor of trauma that has so unexpectedly interrupted his life. At the same time, physiologically, the body is still striving to compensate and may regress periodically as complications occur. The following patient report serves as an example of how nursing diagnoses might change as the patient progresses from the critical to the intermediate care phase.

> *The patient, an 18-year-old female, had severe fractures of the right humerus and ulna, requiring external fixation and elevation of the extremity in a pronated, flexed position, and a fracture of the left humerus which was stabilized with a cast. The patient suffered severe nausea during the critical phase secondary to pain medication and stress. The diagnosis in the critical phase read "potential for alteration in nutrition related to severe nausea secondary to sedation and anxiety."*
>
> *After the patient was transferred to the intermediate care area, the nausea had subsided and her appetite had returned. However, because her right arm still required elevation in a fixed position and her left arm could not be bent, it was difficult for the patient to hold food on the fork long enough to bring it to her mouth. She became frustrated and discouraged when food would fall into the bed and she started to refuse her meals. The nursing diagnosis changed to "alteration in nutritional status related to inability to eat with conventional instruments."*

The interventions of using alternative ways to eat and serving foods with a manageable consistency were instituted. Although the end result of inadequate intake was the same, the cause was different as the patient progressed through the cycles. Accurate diagnosis of complications cannot be overemphasized during this phase. These are addressed in the section "Unique Considerations."

Developing and Implementing a Plan

Active Involvement

As the patient becomes more stabilized, the plan of care focuses on patient needs to maintain this stability and to prevent complications. The overall care plan is crucial at this stage even though the patient is more stable. Interventions become more consistent but continue to be outcome-driven. Outcomes are often more predictable during this phase and should be documented on a time line. In this cycle, the patient must begin to take a more active role in planning and participating in care. The overall goal is to move the trauma patient from a *dependent* role to a more *independent* one while striving toward regaining optimal function. Interventions directed toward aiding the patient and family to adapt to the injury are a priority.

Even an immobilized patient should be involved in making choices about his care. Initially, patient involvement may be limited to the opportunity to make simple choices, such as deciding when he would like to bathe. Or, for example, if there are three activities of daily living that he must relearn, which one is important enough to him to learn first? Allowing choices in care, collaboratively developing daily schedules, provides the patient with some control as well as encourages the patient to assume a more active role and strive toward independence.

Rehabilitation Needs

The familiar statement "rehabilitation begins upon admission" takes on greater relevancy when formulating the plan of care for the trauma patient, especially the multisystem-injured patient. During the operative and postoperative critical periods, rehabilitation is addressed appropriately, but the emphasis is clearly on immediate physiological needs. In the cycle of intermediate care, the rehabilitative focus begins to assume greater significance in the plan of care. The patient learns that he must take responsibility for some of his care and activities of daily living. Often, specific plans are required for the patient to relearn activities of daily living. This is especially true of patients with neurological dysfunction related to the injuries or to the long-term effects of paralytics used in the critical care phase. The overall long-term plan for rehabilitation needs is developed during this cycle of care (see Chapter 15).

Preparation for transfer to a rehabilitation facility requires collaborative planning and communication with the multidisciplinary team, the patient and family, and the receiving center. All must be aware of the time line or potential date of transfer to facilitate patient preparation and a timely, smooth transition.

Family Involvement

During this cycle, the family members begin to be less concerned about the physiological problems of the patient and start to focus more on what needs to be accomplished before discharge can occur. They begin to want to be involved with the patient's care. They no longer ask, "Will he live?" but now ask, "How long before he can go home?"

It is important at this stage to involve the family in patient teaching, especially if some procedures will need to be carried out after discharge. The family should be allowed to administer some care during their visits. This not only allows the nurse to evaluate how well the family member performs the care but also gives the family member a sense of self-satisfaction from actually assisting in the patient's care. In addition, this also may increase the patient's feelings of acceptance by family members, especially if disfiguring injuries are present.

The family-centered conference is an integral component of this stage of care. The family should be made aware of the goals that have been formulated and the plan of care that has been developed to meet these goals. The need for family members' involvement in this plan should be emphasized, and appropriate resources should be mobilized to assist them in this role. The family at this stage is often faced with finding and/or choosing an appropriate rehabilitative facility for the patient. The nurse, with the help of family service or social service counselors, should assist in providing the family with the information necessary to make this decision. The specific type of rehabilitation needed by the patient may require his being placed in a facility far from home. This can be a difficult decision for the family if they are not helped in understanding the importance of proper placement in successful rehabilitation. Financial counselors, visiting nurse associations, and self-help groups are resources commonly used.

Unique Considerations During the Intermediate Care Phase

Adjustment to Injury

Patients experience interrelated physical, cognitive, and personal responses to their traumatic injuries. The nurse needs to appreciate the extent of the impact of the cognitive and personal aspects on the patient's physical recovery. Understanding the full range of responses to trauma allows the nurse to "harness the patient's natural healing ability and promote optimal recovery."[33]

When these responses are identified as maladaptive, a specific and consistent care plan that mobilizes all resources must be developed. As the patient physically feels better, he may attempt to manipulate health care personnel, often resulting in a delayed progression toward discharge, especially if leaving the security of the hospital environment is threatening. Depression often occurs as the reality of the injury is recognized by the patient. This often leads to noncompliance with the therapeutic regimen or a delayed progression through the grief process.

Difficulties coping with alterations in body image often surface during this stage. It is important to recognize the behavior patterns that signal possible problems the patient may have in maintaining his body image following traumatic injury. If this is recognized early, a therapeutic approach to assist the patient in dealing with changes in body image may be planned and implemented. Family service counselors or a psychiatric liaison nurse may become valuable participants of the health care team when patients begin to elicit maladaptive responses to their injury. Assistance from self-help groups also may be utilized. A visit by a former trauma patient or an amputee if the patient has lost a limb may prove beneficial for the patient.

Immobilization

Even though most multitrauma patients are immobilized following injury, immobilization begins to assume greater significance during the intermediate phase of care. By the time the patient reaches this stage of care, he may already have been immobilized for a significant time, and complications of immobility may be apparent. Some of these include muscular and cardiac deconditioning; ventilation and perfusion abnormalities; orthostatic abnormalities; alterations in ingestion, digestion, and elimination; and development of deep vein thrombosis with embolization. The prevention and treatment of complications from immobility must remain a priority in the plan of care. Early and aggressive mobilization is beneficial and necessary to prevent sequelae from immobility. The more recent techniques of fracture management such as the use of intermedullary rods, plates, or screws, as well as the external fixator devices, allow earlier mobilization of patients with multiple fractures (see Chapter 20). However, even patients in traction may be mobilized, if creative methods for maintaining the traction are utilized. For example, hanging the traction rope and weights over a straight-backed chair may effectively maintain enough tibial traction so that the patient may sit up in a chair several times a day. The patient with turning restrictions who needs chest physiotherapy to prevent or treat atelectasis can still be treated if the nurse works with the physician to select the safest way to position the patient.

Infection

During the critical care cycle, the potential for the patient to acquire nosocomial infection is great. Septic episodes may occur and are always anticipated during the intermediate cycle of care. Whether or not the patient was in the critical care unit or is admitted from the resuscitation or post-anesthesia care units, the potential for infection and related sepsis exists. It is crucial that the care plan continue to emphasize the prevention of infection. The patient who is seemingly physiologically stable has the potential for suffering a serious setback if infection sets in and sepsis follows. Strict adherence to sterile technique and infection-control protocols must continue throughout this care cycle.

Pulmonary complications may persist or develop during this phase, particularly if the patient has limited mobility or injuries that impair ventilation and/or gas exchange. Nosocomial pneumonias are not uncommon during this cycle and significantly hinder recovery, impede the healing process, and may affect patient survival. A therapeutic modality that is most effective for the individual patient must be incorporated into the plan of care (see Chapter 18 for a summary of pulmonary therapeutics).

Nutrition

During the critical care cycle, the trauma patient is initially catabolic in response to the physiological stress of trauma and its sequential complications. Once physiological stability has been achieved, every effort should be made to return the body to an anabolic state. The primary nurse must work closely with the physician and dietitian to plan the most effective means of providing nutritional support for the patient. Hyperalimentation may continue to be utilized during this phase, but enteral feedings are usually given if oral feedings are contraindicated. Providing adequate nutrition with enteral feedings poses many challenges. It is often difficult to ensure the administration of the prescribed amount of feeding when therapies and trips to radiology and/or the physical therapy department are a routine part of the day. Feedings, especially if administered by a continuous infusion pump, need to be stopped prior to and during chest physiotherapy to prevent aspiration. All efforts should be made to provide the amount of feeding prescribed.

Patients often have problems with diarrhea or retention of feedings when hyperosmolar solutions are utilized. Systematic checking of residual feeding and auscultation of bowel sounds are mandatory to assess the patient's tolerance of the feeding. If diarrhea persists, antidiarrheal medication such as diphenoxylate hydrochloride (Lomotil) may be added to feedings. Placement of feeding tubes should be checked on a routine basis, including verification by radiographic film if pediatric-sized feeding tubes are being utilized. Preventing accidental dislodgment of the tube by the patient prevents the occurrence of aspiration. If feeding or needle catheter jejunostomies or gastrostomy tubes are utilized, feedings should be administered according to specific protocols and/or procedures. Serial weights are important to ascertain weight gain or loss.

Pain

The control of pain during this phase is a high priority, particularly for the patient with a severe isolated wound or for those with multiple injuries. Alternative methods of pain management may need to be trialed and evaluated to achieve the most effective pain control (see Chapter 14). Adequate pain control is essential for physical and psychological recovery and rehabilitation.

Evaluation

As in previous phases, nursing interventions need to be continuously evaluated for effectiveness. Overall evaluation is directed toward the patient's progressing toward discharge to home or a rehabilitation center. A discharge that occurs at the end of this cycle of care cannot be sudden. Goals that were set by the health care team must be met, and documentation of such should be present. Discharge should be a predicted and planned event so that when it does occur, the patient and family members look forward to it and feel comfortable when it arrives rather than feeling frightened or insecure.

CYCLE V: REHABILITATION

It is somewhat difficult to address rehabilitation as a cycle separate from the others because, as previously discussed, it begins on admission and continues throughout the patient's hospitalization. Once physiological stability is achieved, emphasis of care progresses to recovery and adaptation. The primary nursing objective in this cycle is to assist the patient in overcoming temporary disabilities or adapting to his environment within the confines of permanent disabilities resulting from the trauma. This involves dealing with his total needs, psychosocial as well as physical, regardless of whether the disabilities are temporary or permanent. The family is an integral part of the care in reorientation, teaching, and discharge planning and in helping to reintegrate the patient into the family system and the community. To accomplish this, nursing must be accountable for recruiting and mobilizing patient and family resources.

Assessment

The belief that "rehabilitation begins on admission" must be practiced when addressing rehabilitative needs of the multitrauma patient. Even during the resuscitation and operative cycles of care, when attention is primarily on hemodynamic and physiological stabilization, assessment for and prevention of potential problems that would prolong the period of rehabilitation must occur. For instance, early, proper immobilization of fractures during the resuscitation phase may prevent neurovascular damage that would ultimately prolong hospitalization. Improper positioning on the operating room table for the extensive multiple surgical procedures may cause a decubitus ulcer even before or immediately after the patient reaches the critical care area or intermediate care unit.

During the critical care cycle, assessment is crucial to recognizing conditions that may ultimately lead to prolonged rehabilitation. For example, a patient with bilateral tibia/fibula fractures that are treated with external fixation devices may need bilateral foot splints to prevent footdrop, which would complicate rehabilitative efforts.

Assessment continues to be imperative in the rehabilitation cycle even though the patient has stabilized. Assessment in this phase includes (1) determining the patient's psychological response to injury, (2) evaluating the patient's potential level of functioning, (3) ascertaining the availability of support mechanisms to assist the patient in injury adjustment and eventual reintegration into society, and (4) coordinating the various community resources and health disciplines that will facilitate a smooth rehabilitative process.

Assessment throughout the cycles also should focus on the patient's readiness to participate in care. Assessment of psychological responses to the injury must be continuous so that by the time the full rehabilitation cycle of care begins, the patient is ready to participate. Observation for signs of ineffective coping is key to appropriately planning interventions and expectations. When the patient cannot use direct strategies to cope with stress, he will often employ indirect strategies, such as defense mechanisms, which are unconscious maneuvers that deny, falsify, or distort reality.

The patient's and family's economic situation must be assessed. This begins on admission so that by the time the patient is ready for rehabilitation treatment, a plan can be developed that will pose the lowest possible economic burden on those involved. Insurance coverage and the patient's and/or family's economic status are vital components to consider when determining which rehabilitation center will be best for the patient. It not only must meet the patient's physical needs but also must be economically feasible.

Diagnosis

By the time the patient reaches the rehabilitation cycle, nursing diagnoses relating to the physical needs of the patient are fairly well formulated. They usually will address problems of immobilization, cognitive rehabilitation, and educational needs of the patient and family. The potential for infection and altered nutritional intake are still major considerations during this phase.

Nursing diagnoses addressing psychological and social needs may be somewhat difficult to formulate at this stage. In actuality, the patient who is noncompliant with therapy may be depressed, may be afraid to tackle returning to the community, may feel powerless about having any control over his situation, or may still be so angry about the injury that he cannot progress to the point of accepting therapy. It is vital that continuous assessment be performed utilizing all available resources to define an accurate nursing diagnosis so that appropriate interventions may be instituted. This procedure is often prolonged during this cycle: It may take weeks of data gathering before the nurse can isolate and label the patient's "real" unhealthful response. This "discovery" also depends on the collaborative effort of all health team members involved in the patient's care.

Developing and Implementing a Plan

If rehabilitative needs have been assessed as the patient moved through the initial and intermediate cycles of care, a well-developed plan should be in place (with the ultimate goal of returning the patient to the optimal level of functioning) by the time the patient moves into the rehabilitative cycle. During this cycle, the goal is for the patient to regain control—to become the decision maker with the support of the health care team. Problems that surface in this phase are unique and challenging. Life-support care in the resuscitation and critical care cycles can cause sleep deprivation due to sensory overload and hourly nursing functions. The care plan in this phase would allow for more normal cycles of activity, rest, and increased interaction with family and friends. Helping a paraplegic with a radically altered body image begin to cope with the reality of his injury can be difficult and at the same time gratifying. The goal during this cycle is to provide an atmosphere in which the patient can begin to work toward reentry into the community while at the same time to ensure that he remains medically stable. Each patient uniquely adapts to traumatic injury; thus planning care requires creativity and persistence.

When developing the rehabilitative plan, mutual goal setting is again a necessity. The patient must be, and perceive himself as, an integral part of this process. The plan should address physical, psychological, and teaching needs of both the patient and family. Family members may need assistance from social service counselors if they begin to feel they will be unable to cope with an injured family member's care or disability once he arrives home. During the rehabilitation cycle, it becomes even more important that the family be encouraged to participate as much as possible in the plan of care once it has been determined that they can effectively deal with the reality of the disabilities.

A consistent, planned approach is the essential component of the care plan during this phase. All members of the health team must be working toward the same defined goals and outcome-oriented time line, and each member should be aware of other members' roles as they strive to achieve these goals. The roles of physical therapists, speech therapists, and occupational therapists are vital to this care plan and must be included in its development and evaluation. Thorough discharge planning is crucial.

During the rehabilitation cycle, it is not uncommon to see a cycle of progression/regression on the part of the patient.

The patient may be fully cooperative and demonstrate consistent progress one day or for a period of several weeks, only suddenly to become uncooperative, depressed, and unwilling to comply with the care plan he helped develop. These periods of setback are not uncommon as the patient struggles to adopt to his injury and the changes it has imposed on his life.

Evaluation

Consistent weekly evaluation of the care plan is vital during the rehabilitation cycle. Assessment of interventions addressing physical and psychological needs of the patient may indicate a need to alter those interventions to meet the set goals effectively. As the patient's attitude toward and participation in the program designed for him fluctuates, so must the plan itself change in terms of anticipating possible regression. The primary nurse's role of coordinator of the health team takes on even more importance during the rehabilitation cycle as more and more health care team members and outside resources become actively involved in the care plan. The nurse must constantly be aware of the overall plan, be able to recognize and coordinate the process for altering the plan when the need arises, and be certain that all members of the health care team are kept up to date about changes that are proposed and implemented.

However, the rehabilitation cycle does not stop when the patient is discharged home or to a rehabilitation center. The process is not complete until the patient is successfully reintegrated into the community. This aspect of reintegration must be included in the overall specialized care plan primarily during the rehabilitation cycle. Reintegration is actually the final phase of this cycle, and all resources that are available to assist the patient toward this goal should be utilized.

Rehabilitation nursing is an integral part of acute nursing care and significantly impacts the patient's potential for maximal recovery. "Insight into the patient throughout the rehabilitation process may give him the ray of hope he needs to survive. Joint development of realistic and obtainable long-range goals often can be instrumental in allowing each patient to achieve optimal levels of independent function."[34]

Postdischarge Phase

Assessment of the trauma patient does not end at hospital discharge; rehabilitation also includes caring for the patient's physical and psychological status after leaving the hospital. This process must take into account the patient's family as well. Trauma patients, especially those requiring extended care, often develop significant support systems and "significant other" relationships while hospitalized. If these relationships are interrupted suddenly, the patients often face additional readjustment problems in their home. As demonstrated by war victims whose injuries have resulted in body image changes (such as amputation), trauma patients often display a facade of total acceptance of their injury while hospitalized, but after discharge they experience severe depression or loss of motivation when they reenter society. As long as their environment includes patients with similar injuries, they often do well psychologically. When they return home, however, they begin to feel they are "different" from the healthy, so-called normal people who surround them.

Postdischarge patient assessment can occur by several means: return clinic visits, home visits from a visiting nurse association or public health home referral, or home visits from trauma nurses who cared for the patient (if your facility provides for this). Assessment factors critical to the evaluation of the patient, such as coping mechanisms and response to family and friends, as well as general mood and affect, should be identified in a nursing discharge summary or a visiting nurse referral form.

PREVENTION

Throughout other chapters in this book, the authors have addressed the cycle of prevention in relation to their specific topic areas. It is an important cycle of a specialized plan of care. For the patient who is already injured, prevention of complications is a consistent goal through all cycles of care.

Nurses also play a vital role in the prevention of injury. Participation in community programs and events that educate the public about accident prevention is essential. Trauma nurses also can play an active role in lobbying for legislation that is aimed at preventing or reducing traumatic injury (e.g., seat belt, child safety seat, or helmet legislation). There is nothing more convincing to legislators than first-hand accounts of unnecessary devastating injury.

In addition to teaching prevention to the patient, families of trauma patients also should be educated. They generally will impart such information to other family members and friends, particularly if they recognize that injury to their loved one might have been prevented.

Traumatic injury will never be completely eradicated, but it can be drastically reduced with increased attention to prevention modalities. It is the responsibility of every member of the trauma team to address the cycle of prevention and become involved with its role in trauma care. It is no longer enough to know how to provide quality care to an injured patient—the trauma caregiver must also strive for its prevention.

SUMMARY

The multiply injured trauma patient is unique because of the nature of injuries, the suddenness of the traumatic event, and the multiplicity of health care professionals needed to organize and implement an effective plan of care, from the scene of the accident through reintegration into the community. The hope for survival of the trauma patient depends on the collaborative efforts of the trauma nurse, physicians, and therapists who make up the trauma team.

Three essential components are necessary to ensure high-quality care and the best possible outcomes for the multiply injured patient: collaborative practice; adherence to established protocols, procedures, and plan of care; and the often indefinable aspect labeled the "art" of nursing and medicine.

Primary nursing is a most effective model for delivering

quality care to the trauma patient through collaborative practice. The best care for the multiply injured, in terms of minimal errors, reduction of complications, and maximum continuity, is provided by a physician–nurse team that follows the patient from admission through the resuscitation and operative cycles and into the critical care cycle. A similar team coordinates care through the intermediate and rehabilitative cycles of care. The multidisciplinary approach to polytrauma ensures the ready availability of needed expertise. Inherent in this approach is the significant impact on the patient by numerous services, individuals, and environments. The strength of the multidisciplinary approach is the expertise that each group brings to the care of the patient. Essential are a primary physician and a primary nurse as key links to continuity and early coordinated care planning.

Florence Nightingale[35] saw the role of the nurse as having "charge of somebody's health," based on the knowledge of "how to put the body in such a state to be free of disease or to recover from disease." The primary nurse who coordinates the plan of care for the multiply injured patient exemplifies this historical definition. It is essential that one nurse coordinate the care to rid the patient of his disease—trauma.

Finally, in addition to the science of providing quality trauma care, the "art" of trauma care must be an essential component through all the cycles. For it is this art, the undefined humanistic element, that often determines whether a multiply injured patient lives or dies. It is often the trauma nurse who has a "sixth sense" that something is not "quite right" with the patient, even though physiological parameters may not suggest deterioration, who convinces the physician to investigate further and ultimately diagnose an early complication. The physician who perseveres until discovering a source for sepsis or who suspects subtle injuries practices the "art" of trauma care.

The multiply injured patient is truly complex and challenging. Through collaborative teamwork, quality care can be planned and delivered from resuscitation to reintegration into society.

REFERENCES

1. Johnson DE: The significance of nursing care. Am J Nurs 61:63–66, 1961.
2. Hesterly SC: Nurse credentialing in an acute care setting. J Nurs Qual Assur 5(3):18–26, 1991.
3. National Safety Council: Accident Facts. Washington, DC, National Safety Council, 1991.
4. Rauen C: Trauma and the elderly: The impact on critical care. AACN Clin Iss Crit Care Nurs 3(1):149–154, 1992.
5. Mann J, Oakes A: Critical Care Nursing of the Multi-injured Patient. Philadelphia, WB Saunders Co, 1980.
6. Knaus W, et al: An evaluation of outcome from intensive care in major medical centers. Ann Intern Med 104:410–418, 1986.
7. Baggs JG, et al: The association between interdisciplinary collaboration and patient outcomes in a medical intensive care unit. Heart Lung 21(1):18–24, 1992.
8. Adams H: Trauma nursing: A collaborative model. Top Emerg Med April:60–66, 1984.
9. Leddy S, Pepper JM: Conceptual Bases of Professional Nursing. Philadelphia, JB Lippincott, 1985.
10. Society of Critical Care Medicine, Task Force on Ethics: Consensus report on the ethics of foregoing life-sustaining treatments in the critically ill. Crit Care Med 18(12):1435–1439, 1990.
11. Curtain L: The nurse as advocate: A philosophical foundation for nursing. Adv Nurs Sci 1:1–10, 1979.
12. Chenevert M: STAT—Special Techniques in Assertiveness Training. 2nd ed. St. Louis, CV Mosby, 1983.
13. Holmquist P, et al: Trauma case manager development and implementation as a nursing role in a community trauma center. J Trauma 31(1):103–106, 1991.
14. Simmons FM: Developing the trauma nurse case manager role. Dimens Crit Care Nurs 11(3):164–170, 1992.
15. Joint Commission on Accreditation of Healthcare Organizations: Accreditation Manual for Hospitals. Oakbrook Terrace, Ill, JCAHO, 1992.
16. Zander K: Nursing case management: Strategic management of cost and quality outcomes. J Nurs Admin 18(5):23–30, 1988.
17. ATLS Course Manual. Chicago, American College of Surgeons, 1979.
18. Dunham CM, Cowley RA: Shock Trauma/Critical Care Manual. Gaithersburg, Md, Aspen Systems, 1991.
19. Cowley RA, Dunhamc M: Shock Trauma/Critical Care Manual. Baltimore, University Park Press, 1982.
20. Friend B, Harrell C: The trauma admitting area. In Cardona V (ed): Trauma Nursing. Montvale, NJ, Medical Economics, 1985, pp 1–13.
21. Occupational Safety and Health Administration, Department of Labor: 29CFR, Part 1910.1030. Occupational exposure to bloodborne pathogens: Final rule. Fed Reg 56(235):64175–64182, 1991.
22. Groves M: Initial communication with trauma patients. In Cardona V (ed): Trauma Nursing. Montvale, NJ, Medical Economics, 1985, pp 15–18.
23. U.S. Congress: Patient Self Determination Act. Washington, D.C., 1990.
24. Kim MJ: Physiologic nursing diagnosis: Its role and place in nursing taxonomy. In Kim MJ, McFarland G, McHane A (eds): Classification of Nursing Diagnosis: Proceedings of the Fifth National Conference. St. Louis, CV Mosby, 1984.
25. Dearing B, Dang D: The family in crisis. Life Support Nurs 3:15–25, 1980.
26. Hopkins AG: Trauma nurse's role with families in crisis. Crit Care Nurs (in press).
27. Keyes B: Safe and Effective In-House Transportation for Critically Ill Patients. Baltimore, Institute for Emergency Medical Services Systems, 1985.
28. Omert L: Agitation management. Trauma 1(3):365–372, 1990.
29. Fabian T, Hickerson W, Mangiante E: Posttraumatic and postoperative acute cholecystitis. Am Surg 52:188–192, 1985.
30. Choi S, Nelson L: Kinetic therapy in critically ill patients: Combined results based on meta-analysis. J Crit Care 7(1):57–62, 1992.
31. Naisbitt J: Megatrends: Ten New Directions Transforming Our Lives. New York, Warner Books, 1982, pp 39–53.
32. Potter P, Perry A: Fundamentals of Nursing. St. Louis, CV Mosby, 1985.
33. Fontaine DK: Physical, personal, and cognitive responses to trauma. Crit Care Nurs Clin North Am 1(1):11–22, 1989.
34. Summey L: Rehabilitation of trauma patients. In Cardona V (ed): Trauma Nursing. Montvale, NJ, Medical Economics, 1985, pp 221–231.
35. Nightingale F: Notes on Nursing: What It Is And What It Is Not. London, Harrison & Sons, 1860.

PART II

Clinical Management Concepts

7

MECHANISM OF INJURY

JOHN A. WEIGELT and JORIE D. KLEIN

Several definitions for trauma exist. In *Webster's Third New International Dictionary, trauma* is defined as "an injury or wound to a living body caused by the application of external violence." Injury is a public health problem of vast proportions. It is the leading cause of death for persons below the age of 44 years and the fourth leading cause for all ages. For ages 1 to 34, motor vehicle accidents (MVAs) are the most common cause of death. Approximately 150,000 Americans die annually from traumatic injuries, and an additional 400,000 people suffer permanent disability.[1] Trauma injuries produce 3.6 million hospital admissions each year, with an average of 7 days per hospital stay.[1a] More than 4 million potential years of productive life are lost annually due to trauma injuries, exceeding the loss produced from heart disease, cancer, and stroke combined. The annual cost to our nation from the injuries is estimated to be $118 billion. MVAs produce 50 per cent of the cost related to trauma injuries.

Injury results from acute exposure to energy such as kinetic (crash, fall, bullet), chemical, thermal, electrical, or ionizing radiation or from a lack of essential agents such as oxygen and heat (drowning and frostbite).[1b] The injury occurs owing to the body's inability to tolerate excessive exposure to the acute energy. Wounds vary depending on the injuring agent. For example, damage from a gunshot wound (GSW) is dependent on the missile's mass and velocity; degree of burn varies with temperature and duration of contact; injuries from deceleration depend on the victim's body mass, rate of deceleration, and area over which the energy is dissipated. Effects of an injury are also dependent on personal and environmental factors such as age, sex, nutrition, underlying disease processes, and geographical region (rural versus urban). These factors help define populations at risk for various types and severities of injuries.

RISK FACTORS

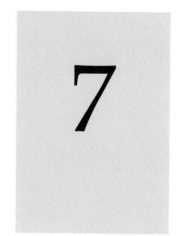

Risks of injury from different causes vary by age, sex, race and income, environment, alcohol abuse, geographical region, and temporal variation. Prevention measures can be focused on high-risk groups by identifying characteristics among different populations and subgroups for injury. Intentional and unintentional injuries provide one way to subdivide injury groups. Mechanism of injury for these two subdivisions is typically identical or similar, yet the events leading to the injury differ. For example, ingestion of a toxic substance can be intentional, as in a suicide attempt, or unintentional, as in an accidental ingestion. However, the mechanism of injury remains the same.

Age

Death rates from injuries are highest in patients 75 years of age or older.[2] This high death rate in the elderly may be secondary to associated medical conditions. The highest injury rate occurs in persons between the ages of 15 and 24 years[3] because of their exposure to high-risk activities. Poor judgment with the use of alcohol and drugs also contributes to the high injury rate. The lowest injury rate is for ages 5 to 14.[2] The highest homicide rate occurs among people between 20 and 29 years of age. Suicide rates for both sexes show little variation with age.

Sex

Injury rates are highest for 15- to 24-year-old males. The risk for males is 2.5 times that for females,[4] possibly because of male involvement in hazardous activities. The unintentional injury death rate for males peaks between the ages of 20 and 24 years and again in the elderly. Suicide has similar peaks. The rate of homicide peaks between 25 and 30 years. In females, the death rate peaks at 15 to 19 years for unintentional injury and at 20 to 24 years for homicide. Females in the late 40s have the highest suicide rate. Nonfatal injury rates for sexes do not differ significantly, suggesting that injuries to males are more severe than those to females.

Race and Income

Race and per capita socioeconomic level influence injury death rates. In a depressed economy, the suicide and homicide rates increase and MVAs decrease. Native Americans (Indians, Eskimos, Aleuts) have the highest death rate from unintentional injury, regardless of income. Blacks have the highest homicide rate. Whites and Native Americans have the highest suicide rate. Asian Americans (Chinese, Japanese, Koreans, Hawaiians, Filipinos, Guamanians) have the lowest death rates from unintentional injuries, homicide, and suicide. The unintentional injury rate is higher in low-income areas (71 per 100,000 population) in comparison with the wealthiest areas (34 per 100,000 population). An inverse relationship between income levels and death rates exists for blacks and whites: i.e., the higher the income, the lower the death rate.[2] For Asians, there is essentially no difference in death rates among all income groups.

Alcohol

Alcohol not only contributes to injury-producing events such as MVAs but also can increase the severity of injury, such as by preventing escape from a burning house.[4] Alcohol is a major factor in motor vehicle, home, industrial, and recreational accidents and in crime, suicide, and family abuse.[5] Automobile accident fatalities are alcohol-related 63 per cent of the time in persons between the ages of 21 and 34 years.[5a] Reyna and associates showed that for 16- to 30-year-olds, alcohol-related emergency department trauma visits were twice as common as for patients older than 30 years.[5] Alcoholism in the general population is believed to be approximately 5 to 10 per cent.[5] Many traumatic injuries may have alcohol as an underlying cause.

Geography

Geographical comparison of injury rates demonstrates the diversity in our population and exposure to hazards. This is reflected in the high unintentional injury rate in rural areas and high intentional injury rate in urban areas.[6] Rural unintentional injuries are commonly caused by MVAs and accidents involving lightning and chemical exposure. Urban unintentional injuries are most commonly seen as poisonings. Homicide is highest in the cities; suicides are highest in cities with populations of 250,000 to 1 million. Clearly, the physical environment is important in determining injury rate.

Temporal Variation

Deaths from injury occur most frequently on weekends, with a Saturday peak. Suicide rates show less variation: Monday is the peak time, with the fewest occurring Friday through Sunday. Unintentional injuries are most pronounced in July; major causes are summer activities, including swimming and motorcycle riding.

EFFECTS OF INJURY ON SOCIETY

A health problem can be examined by its cost to society, but this cost does not examine the grief, pain, and social disruption experienced by an individual and family. Death before 70 years of age is premature.[2] By considering the years of life lost prematurely due to health problems, it can be calculated that 4 million years of life are lost prematurely as a result of injury each year. Even when intentional injuries (homicide, suicide) are excluded, 3 million years of life are lost, which is greater than the loss from any other single disease.

Indicators used to compare health problems are cost to society, physician contacts, and hospital admissions. Injuries, one of the most expensive health problems, have direct and indirect costs amounting to 75 to 100 billion dollars a year.[7] The total cost to society for these injuries is not known. In 1975, MVAs cost society $15 billion, which is equivalent to $20 billion in 1980 dollars.[2] A recent noncomparative study by the National Highway Traffic Safety Administration estimated total societal cost of injuries from MVAs in 1980 at over $36 billion.[8] Only cancer costs society more. Unlike cancer, injury affects younger people, and a disabling injury will cost much more indirectly.

Injury ranks first as the reason for physician visits and contacts for treatment: In 1980, 99 million physician contacts were made as a result of injuries. Heart disease was second and respiratory disease third.[2] Over 25 per cent of all emergency department or hospital clinic visits are for treatment of injuries.[8] Injuries account for about 3.6 million hospital admissions yearly, which is 1 of every 10 short-term admissions. Injury admissions for all ages are greater than those for all other diseases except circulatory and digestive disorders. In 1979, injuries were the leading cause of admissions for people 45 years of age or younger.[8] The elderly have the highest hospitalization rate for injury, and a major cause is hip fracture. Other injuries accounting for hospitalization include head trauma in 15- to 24-year-olds, back and neck sprains in the 35- to 44-year-old group, and arm fractures in children between the ages of 5 and 14 years.

INITIAL ASSESSMENT AND HISTORY

In the initial evaluation of the trauma patient, a careful history of the events leading to the injury must be obtained. The practitioner must attend to urgent therapeutic needs along with the usual diagnostic evaluation.[9] Obtaining an accurate history—especially asking about the mechanism of injury—can reduce morbidity and mortality. Questions that are helpful in assessing potential injuries based on mechanism of injury for motor vehicle impacts (such as automobile, motorcycle, and pedestrian accidents) identify the circumstances of the impact. Prehospital personnel should quickly survey the scene, noting the appearance of the vehicle and the damages sustained to the passenger compartment.[9a] It is important to know the speed of the vehicle, the point of impact, and the type of impact (single-vehicle, high-speed, front-end, rear-end, or T-bone intersection collision). The evaluating team should identify if the patient was the driver or the passenger, whether safety devices (safety belt, child safety seat, airbag) were utilized, and where the victim was found at the scene. Death of an occupant in the vehicle should alert the team to potential energy forces within the collision. Patients from a vehicle in which an occupant has died and patients who are ejected from a vehicle have a higher morbidity and mortality and warrant a thorough evaluation for injury.

Frontal-impact collisions in which the vehicle has a bent steering wheel or column, knee imprints in the dashboard, and a broken windshield are associated with head injuries, hemopneumothoraces, injuries to the spleen or liver, and dislocation of the patella.[9a] Femur fractures with or without posterior fracture-dislocation of the ipsilateral hip must be considered. Deceleration injuries, such as aortic rupture, must be ruled out.

Side-impact collisions produce contralateral neck sprain, cervical fractures, head injuries, lacerations to the soft tissues, lateral rib fractures or flail chest, abdominal injuries, and pelvic and acetabular fractures.

Rear-impact collisions result in hyperextension neck injuries, and there may be rebound frontal-impact injuries. Ejection from the vehicle produces a multitude of injuries. Such victims may suffer penetrating impalement wounds, head injuries, cervical fractures, and road burns. The risk of injury is increased by 300 per cent when the occupant is ejected.

Motorcycle accidents comprise single or multiple impacts. The evaluating team must determine the type of collision (direct impact with stable object or impact with another vehicle), rate of speed, where the victim was found in relation to the cycle, and if protective devices were worn (helmet, gloves, boots). Head injuries, long-bone fractures, pelvic fractures, and soft tissue injuries are common. Pedestrians hit by vehicles may have many injuries. The prehospital team should identify (or estimate) how fast the vehicle was traveling, the type of vehicle, the point of impact, and whether the victim was thrown or dragged.

Penetrating trauma refers to any injury produced when a foreign object passes through the tissue. The energy is dissipated through the tissue, producing the injury. Penetrating trauma injuries are more predictable than those caused by blunt trauma. It is important to identify the type of weapon (caliber of gun, length of knife blade), stance of the assailant, distance from the assailant to victim, and potential number of wounds.

It is not always possible and sometimes it is impractical to obtain a detailed history, but information can be obtained from family members, paramedics, fire fighters, police officers, onlookers, or eyewitnesses. Priority is obviously given to managing life-threatening injuries, i.e., inadequate ventilation, hypoxia, and bleeding. After the patient is resuscitated and stabilized, the trauma practitioner should begin a detailed review of history, physical findings, and laboratory results to direct further investigations.

A quick examination must be performed during or immediately following resuscitation. This is easier to accomplish in patients with penetrating trauma than in those with blunt injury, since surface injury may or may not be present with blunt injury. It is important to systematically examine the *undressed patient* to avoid overlooking injuries. Failure to diagnose the patient's injuries correctly is associated with a high mortality rate.[10] An index of suspicion for associated injuries based on the mechanism of injury must be maintained, and a detailed physical examination must be performed to avoid missed injuries.

Some body areas do not lend themselves easily to physical examination, e.g., cranium, vertebral column, and bony thorax.[11] Injury may exist without classic signs, but the mechanism of injury may raise suspicion enough to warrant further diagnostic examinations. Examples include computed tomography for diagnosis of diffuse brain injury, angiography for blunt chest injury and possible aortic injury, and simple radiography for spinal column evaluation. All tests must be performed without placing the patient at risk of further injury. The patient is continually reexamined to identify changing physical findings.

Complete assessment of the trauma patient is aided by knowing the cause of injury. MVAs are the primary cause of injury, followed by falls.[10] Other causes of injury are pedestrian accidents, drownings, fires, explosions, poisoning, firearms, aspiration, machinery, and sports accidents. In some cases, the cause can be related to patterns of injury, which indicate expected types of injury. This information plus the events preceding the accident can provide clues to the practitioner regarding the patient's response, expected severity, and occult or missed injuries.

Waddell's triad occurs when a pedestrian is struck by a car.[10] Three injuries result when the victim is a child: (1) the bumper and hood impact the femur and/or chest, (2) the victim is thrown upon impact, and (3) the contralateral skull is injured by the force of impact. One of these injuries is often missed in the initial evaluation. Adult pedestrians receive a lateral impact from contact with the bumper and hood, injuring the lower and upper leg, since adults try to protect themselves by turning sideways (Fig. 7–1). Fractures to this area are recognized, but ligamental damage in the other knee is often overlooked.

Common areas where injuries are missed include the extremities (hand and foot), upper extremity (forearm and arm), and skin (scalp lacerations). Other injury patterns include sports injuries after sudden deceleration (diving, falling), excessive forces (twisting, hyperextension, hyperflexion), or changes in momentum (boxing).[10] Because of repeated blows to the head in boxing, cumulative brain damage may occur, with resultant neurological damage depending on the affected area. Spinal cord injuries can occur from gymnastics and football. Head injuries occur with football and horseback riding. Skiing can produce fractures, and knee injuries are common with skiing and football.

MECHANISM OF INJURY

The mechanics of injury are related to the type of injuring force and subsequent tissue response. A thorough understanding of these two facets of injury helps in determining the extent and nature of damage. Injury occurs when the force deforms tissues beyond their failure limits. This can result in anatomical and physiological damage. Anatomical damage, such as skeletal fractures, will usually heal, and function will return. Physiological damage, such as central nervous system injury, may be permanent despite the healing process. The mechanism of injury can help explain the type of injury, predict eventual outcome, and identify common injury combinations. All these improve trauma patient management.

Biomechanics

The principles of mechanics are used to investigate the mechanisms of physical and physiological responses to force. The injuring force can be penetrating or nonpenetrating. The resultant injury is dependent on the energy delivered and area of contact. Penetrating injury usually involves a concentration of injury to a small body area; nonpenetrating injury distributes energy over larger areas. Injury can occur by slow deformation of tissue, such as in a wringer injury[12]; however, the predominant feature is usually speed and violence, e.g., the impact of the head against a windshield or a bullet's penetration into an extremity.

The field of biomechanics involves a variety of disciplines, including engineering, physiology, medicine, biology, and anatomy. Knowledge of injury mechanisms allows the appropriate biomechanical measurements to be made to characterize injuries. No one approach to the field is available, and research is best conducted with representatives of as many of the disciplines as possible. Detailed reviews of various aspects of basic biomechanical research are available but are too encompassing for this report. Interested readers are referred to appropriate references.[13–21]

Injury Concepts

Among the factors that influence injury are velocity of collision, object shape, and tissue rigidity. Body tissue has inertial resistance as well as tensile, elastic, and compressive strength. *Tensile strength* equals the amount of tension a tissue can withstand and its ability to resist stretching forces. *Elasticity* is the ability of a tissue to resume its original shape and size after being stretched. *Compressive strength* refers to the tissue's ability to resist squeezing forces or inward pressure. Whenever the force exceeds maximum tissue strength, a fracture or tear occurs.[22]

Force is a physical factor that changes the motion of a body either at rest or already in motion. It is calculated[23] by the following equation:

$$\text{Force} = \text{mass} \times \text{acceleration}$$

The more slowly the force is applied, the more slowly energy is released, with less subsequent tissue deformation. If the same force is dissipated over a large surface area, the tissue disruption is further reduced. The forces most often applied are acceleration, deceleration, shearing, and compression. *Acceleration* is a change in the rate of velocity or speed of a moving body. As velocity increases, so does tissue damage. *Deceleration* is a decrease in the velocity of a moving object. *Shearing forces* occur across a plane, with structures slipping relative to each other. *Compressive resistance* is the ability of an object or structure to resist squeezing forces or inward pressure.[23]

Viscoelastic properties of tissue help absorb energy and protect vital organs from the effects of impact. If the energy transmitted to the tissue remains below the limit of injury, the energy will be absorbed without causing injury.[24] This phenomenon is used to protect against injury by using energy-absorbing structures and padding. These objects do not prevent deformation of tissues but can extend the duration of and reduce the force of impact below the limit of injury.

When the tissues are deformed beyond the recoverable limit, injury occurs. Tissue or structure deformation can be

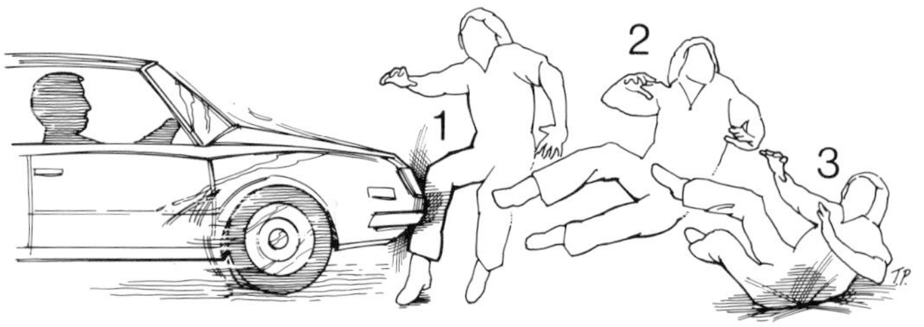

Figure 7–1. Waddell's triad in adult pedestrians. Impact *(1)* with the bumper or hood and lateral rotation *(2)* produces injury to the upper and/or lower leg *(3)*.

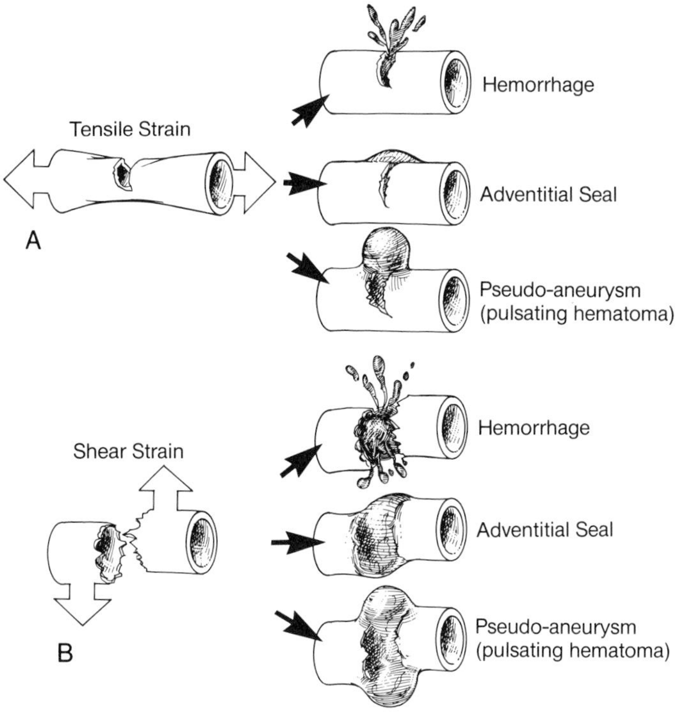

Figure 7–2. As the artery is stretched along its longitudinal axis, its length and amount of tissue strain increase *(A)*. An increase in length that exceeds tensile strength causes the artery to break. The injury can result in a complete tear or can produce lower degrees of damage if the strain is less. Shear strain occurs when the force is applied 90 degrees to the longitudinal axis *(B)*. Varying degrees of injury can occur with different levels of force. (Redrawn with permission from Committee on Trauma Research, National Research Council and the Institute of Medicine: Injury in America, Washington, National Academy Press, 1985, p 52.)

measured according to changes in shape, commonly defined as a change in length divided by the initial length.[24] Another term for this change is *strain*. Two major types of strain are tensile and shear. A third type is compressive, which is less common and responsible for crushing injuries. Tensile and shear strain in an artery is illustrated in Figure 7–2. Stretching of the artery along its longitudinal axis increases its length and tissue strain. If the strain or increase in length is too great, the tissue will break. An "all or none" phenomenon is not present, and the artery may completely or partially break. A similar result can be produced by a force applied at 90 degrees to the long axis of the artery. This shear strain occurs when the movement of tissue in opposite directions exceeds recoverable limits. Other examples of tensile strain injuries are femur and rib fractures. Shear strain injuries include hepatic vein laceration from differential movements of hepatic lobes and brain injury from movement of the brain within the skull. Compressive or deformation strain is a factor in contusion injury. This type of injury often leaves the surface of the tissue undamaged. An artery can be used again to illustrate this mechanism of injury (Fig. 7–3).

Another factor in strain injury is the rate of loading or strain rate.[24] A tissue response is dependent on both strain and rate of strain limits. Bony injuries can be used to demonstrate this principle. Compact bone will fail at lower strain values if applied at a rapid strain rate.[25] The same strain applied more slowly will not cause tissue failure. In general, the viscous tolerance of a tissue is proportional to the product of loading rate and amount of compression.[24] A tissue's tolerance to compression decreases as the rate of loading increases.

Our overall knowledge regarding injury mechanisms for specific organ systems is not great. Table 7–1 outlines current information. The following discussion will cover blunt forces, thermal injury, and penetrating trauma and various organ responses to these forces.

BLUNT INJURY

Injury with no communication to the outside environment is *blunt trauma*. Blunt trauma is caused by a combination of forces: deceleration, acceleration, shearing, crushing, and compression. Multiple injuries are common. Blunt trauma is often more life-threatening than penetrating trauma because the extent of injuries is less obvious, and diagnosis is difficult.

Laboratory, radiographical, and invasive studies along with physical examination aid in the diagnostic process. Knowledge of tissue properties can help decide what diagnostic studies are needed. Explosion injuries can occur in air-filled organs such as the bowel and lung. The forces are transmitted in all directions; if pressure is not released, tissues will break or burst. Solid organs sustain crush injury that may have little external evidence of injury. The automobile is respon-

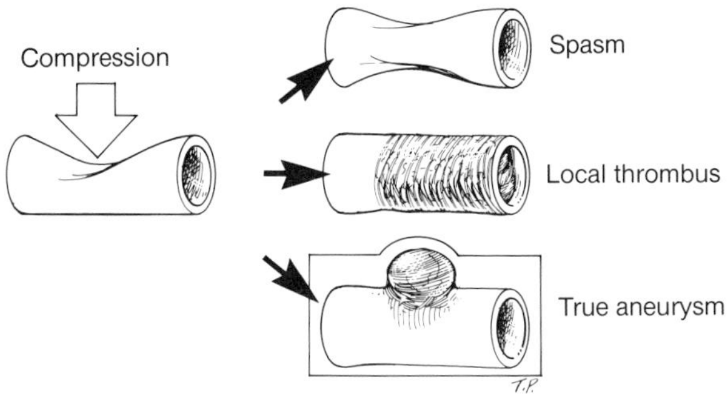

Figure 7–3. A crushing force can be applied over an artery, causing damage to the arterial wall. Little or no damage occurs to the overlying skin. The compression produces stretching and shear forces in the arterial wall, which cause injuries similar to those produced by a pure tensile or shear force. (Redrawn with permission from Committee on Trauma Research, National Research Council and the Institute of Medicine: Injury in America, Washington, National Academy Press, 1985, p 53.)

TABLE 7–1. SUMMARY OF KNOWN INFORMATION ABOUT MECHANISM OF INJURY FOR VARIOUS ORGAN SYSTEMS

HEAD
Information on skull fractures and brain contusions is available. Response and tolerance data on anatomical injuries are crude. Assessment technology for head injuries is available.

FACE
Fracture data on a few facial bones are available, but tolerance data are sparse. Assessment technology is limited.

NECK
A few injury mechanisms are known. Response and tolerance data are available for a few types of impact. Assessment technology is crude, although computed technology has been helpful.

THORACOLUMBAR SPINE
Vertical acceleration mechanisms are known, but combined accelerations have not been studied.

THORAX
Rib cage injuries are understood. Frontal impact mechanism of injury for heart and great vessels is available, but more precise information is needed. Other force mechanisms are poorly explained.

ABDOMEN
Isolated failure impact for liver is known. Many mechanisms are understood, but detailed information on differences between hollow and solid viscera is lacking.

EXTREMITIES
Long bone fracture mechanisms are understood as tensile strain failure. Tolerance data for adult femur are known.

SKIN AND MUSCLE
Lacerative and thermal injuries to skin are understood. Assessment technology exists for skin but not for muscle.

SENSORY ORGANS
Noise-induced threshold shift mechanisms are known.

REPRODUCTIVE ORGANS
Fetal injuries from frontal impacts are minimally understood.

Adapted from Grossblatt N (ed): Injury in America. Washington, National Academy Press, 1985.

sible for at least 50 per cent of these nonpenetrating injuries.[3] Blunt abdominal trauma is responsible for only 1 per cent of all trauma admissions but is associated with a 20 to 30 per cent mortality rate. Much of this mortality rate is attributed to associated head and chest injuries.

Common blunt forces include MVAs, falls, aggravated assaults, and contact sports. Direct impact causes greatest injury and occurs when there is direct contact between the body surface and injuring agent.[10] Indirect forces are transmitted internally, with dissipation of energy to the internal structure. The extent of injury from indirect forces depends on the transference of energy from an object to the body. Injury occurs as a result of energy released and the tendency for tissue to displace and move upon impact.

Acceleration–deceleration injuries are common with blunt forces. An example of the mechanism of injury associated with acceleration–deceleration forces is injury to the thoracic aorta. Rapid deceleration in MVAs can cause major vessels to undergo stretching and bowing.[26] Shearing is produced when stretching forces exceed the elasticity of vessels. Shearing damage is seen in the vessel walls, causing them to tear, dissect, rupture, or form an aneurysm.[24] This shearing damage occurs in the vessels as they decelerate at a different rate from the areas they perfuse. The aorta is fixed tightest to the chest wall at the isthmus just below the origin of the subclavian artery. The movement of the aorta above and below this fixation point produces a shearing force, causing the injury, which has a mortality of 80 per cent (Fig. 7–4).

Head Injuries

Head injury is a major health problem in the United States. Occurrence rates range from 200 to 610 per 100,000 population.[27] Mortality is a common outcome; survivors often

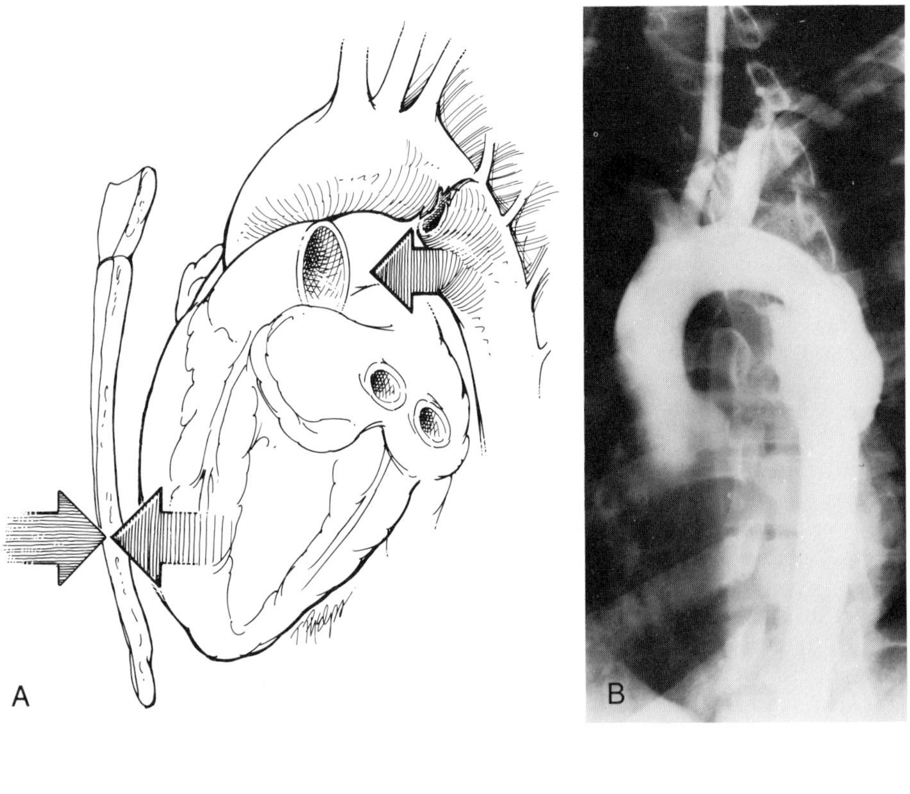

Figure 7–4. As the chest wall decelerates, the heart and aorta are still in motion. The aorta continues to move anteriorly after the chest wall has stopped, causing shear forces to be focused on the aorta at its point of attachment to the posterior chest wall. If the forces exceed tissue strength, an aortic laceration occurs. The aortogram reveals an aortic injury following a deceleration accident, with the dye column interrupted just beyond the aortic isthmus. Proper management dictates surgical repair as soon as possible.

TABLE 7–2. HEAD INJURY: RELATIONSHIP OF INJURING AGENT, FORCES APPLIED, PATHOPHYSIOLOGY, AND CLINICAL RESULTS

TYPE	IMPACT VELOCITY	FORCES* MOMENTUM	VELOCITY IMPARTED† (CHANGE)	SHEAR STRAIN‡	DAMAGE TO:					CLINICAL EFFECTS
					SCALP	BONE	VESSELS	BRAIN	STEM	
Stab	Low	Low	Small	Linear +	+ +	+	+	Local, mild	0	Specific, mild
Gunshot§	High	Low	Small	Linear +	+ +	+ +	Deep + + +	Specific, variable	0	Specific, variable
Crush	Very low	Very low	None	Linear +	+ + +	+ + + +	+	Diffuse, mild	0	General, mild
Blow, mild	Low	Low	Small	Linear + Rotary +	+	+	+	Local, mild	+	General, moderate
Blow, severe	Moderate	High	Large	Linear + + Rotary + + +	+ +	+ + +	+ +	Contrecoup	+ + +	General, moderate to severe
Fall, mild	Low	High	Large	Linear + + Rotary + + +	+	+	+ +	Contrecoup	+ +	General, moderate to severe
Fall, severe	Low	Very high	Very large	Linear + + + Rotary + + + +	+ + +	+ + +	Surface + + +	Diffuse, severe	+ + + +	General, severe

*Forces are either acceleration (as with an object striking the head) or deceleration (as with a head in motion striking an object).
†Velocity change is relative to velocity before impact.
‡Shear strain forces are for the brain relative to the skull.
§For gunshot wounds, the variability of injury is related to the kinetic energy of the missile.
Adapted from Walker AE, Ray CD, Laws ER, et al: Injuries of the head and spinal cord. In Zuidema GD, Rutherford RB, Ballinger WF (eds): The Management of Trauma. Philadelphia, WB Saunders Co, 1979, pp 181–253.

face debilitating sequelae. These results are especially sobering considering that the highest rate of injuries is in the 15- to 19-year-old age group. The three most common mechanisms of injury are motor vehicle crashes (114 per 100,000), falls (41 per 100,000), and aggravated assaults (23 per 100,000). The fatality rate is 5.2 per cent for MVAs, 6.2 per cent for falls, and 6.3 per cent for assaults.

Head injury is produced by the initial impact, but the momentum imparted to the head and brain dictates the eventual type and degree of injury.[28] This concept is detailed for a number of injury types in Table 7–2.

When a head is struck and its velocity is changed from rest to 1.7 m/sec (38 mph), a positive pressure is developed on the percussed side at the brain–skull interface.[29] This pressure is approximately 1 atm. Simultaneously, a negative atmospheric pressure develops at the opposite pole. This vacuum produces transient cavitation, which is a factor in contrecoup injuries. The other factor in contrecoup injuries is produced by the brain sliding within the cranial vault. The inside of the skull is not a smooth surface, and the brain substance is torn and damaged by rigid protuberances as it slides over them.

Acute subdural hematoma (ASDH) is the most important cause of death in head injury because of its high incidence (30 per cent), high mortality (60 per cent), and high severity of injury (Glasgow coma scale 3, 4, 5).[30] Three mechanisms of injury have been identified: (1) a direct laceration of cortical arteries and veins with penetrating injury, (2) large contusions with extensive "pulping" of brain tissue, and (3) the most common type, tearing of veins that bridge the subdural space as they travel from brain to dura. This last mechanism is more likely to occur following a fall or assault (72 per cent) than by motor vehicle accident (24 per cent).[30] In contrast, diffuse brain injury was found in 89 per cent of victims of MVAs and in only 10 per cent of victims of falls and assaults.

Injury biomechanics can be used to explain this difference. The parasagittal bridging veins have strong viscoelastic behavior, which makes their response to force dependent on the rate at which the vessel is strained. The ultimate strain to failure decreases with increasing strain rate. When acceleration or deceleration occurs very rapidly, the veins will fail. A person falling 25 ft and striking the head on concrete with a stopping distance of 0.1 cm has a deceleration force of 200 g with a duration of 3.5 msec. The equivalent deceleration would happen in a vehicle crashing into a rigid barrier at 40 mph. The dashboard deforms 10 cm and the duration is 35 msec. The longer deceleration time decreases the chance of ASDH but increases the chance of diffuse brain injury.[30]

Occipital skull fractures from backward falls have a high mortality.[31] This is related to direct injury to vital posterior fossa structures and to the countrecoup injury in the frontotemporal area. A third of 134 patients in one report suffered contrecoup injuries.[31] This high incidence of severe contrecoup injuries is related to the forces applied, the momentum generated, and the bony irregularities in the anterior skull.

Spinal Cord Injuries

The muscular and articular supports of the spinal cord are insufficient to tolerate violent forces. Areas where injury is most often seen are the junctional regions between the cervical, thoracic, lumbar, and sacral spine. Mechanisms of injury involved with spinal cord damage include axial loading, flexion, extension, rotation, lateral bending, and distraction[32] (Fig. 7–5).

Axial loading injury occurs when the force is applied upward and downward with no posterior or lateral bending of the neck.[26] A burst fracture of the vertebral body or disk extrusion results. This type of injury is common in MVAs when a person's head is thrown upward and strikes the roof of the car.

In a flexion injury, the force causes extreme movement of the spine beyond the normal range. The head is bent forward on the cervical spine. Flexion with rotation produces a more severe injury. A vertebral body is thrown forward, and the cord is compressed. The wedging force placed on an adjacent vertebra crushes it and drives fragments of bone into the

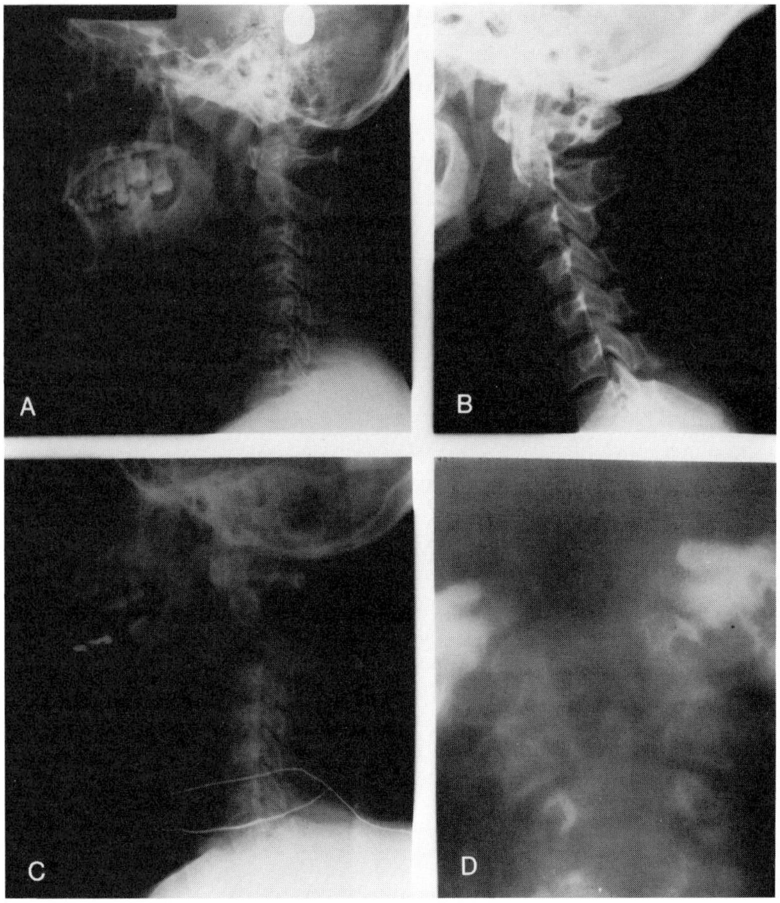

Figure 7–5. Flexion, extension, distraction, and axial loading injuries. *A*, Flexion injury with wedge compression of C5 with posterior retropulsion. *B*, Extension injury with teardrop extension avulsion of antero-inferior aspect of C2. *C*, Distraction injury with C2 disarticulated from C3 and a bilateral pedicular fracture of C2 with abnormal widening of spinous processes C1 and C2 (Hangman's fracture). *D*, Tomogram showing a Jefferson fracture caused by axial loading. There is lateral displacement of the lateral masses of C1 in relation to C2, which is more marked on the right side.

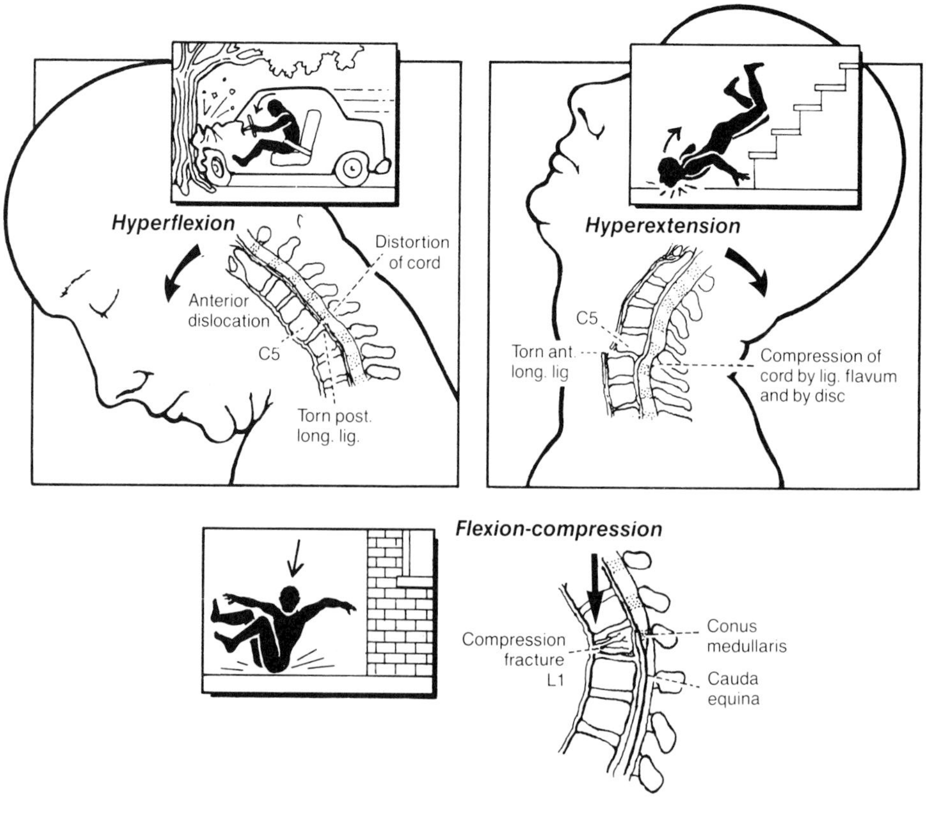

Figure 7–6. Mechanisms of injury for spinal column injuries. (Reprinted with permission from Black P: Common mechanisms of closed spinal injury. In Zuidema GD, Rutherford RB, Ballinger WF (eds): Management of Trauma. Philadelphia, WB Saunders Co, 1985, p 228.)

spinal canal. Flexion injury can occur with only a small amount of force. Posterior longitudinal or articular ligaments are torn, displacing the fracture forward into the lower vertebra (Fig. 7–6).

In hyperextension injuries, the cervical spinal cord is extended as the head is bent back sharply (see Fig. 7–6). Compression of the vertebral bodies is caused by a downward force. Fracture of the pedicles or lamina can be seen depending on the direction and intensity of the force.[26] Posterior dislocation of the upper vertebrae on the lower occurs, further complicating the injury. Acceleration forces can cause hyperextension of the neck, producing what is commonly known as "whiplash injury."[22] These injuries can squeeze the spinal cord, supplying the main stress in the center of the cord, resulting in the syndrome of acute central cervical cord injury. In this syndrome, there is greater motor impairment of the upper limbs as compared with the lower because the nerve fibers supplying the lower limbs are more peripherally situated and suffer less damage. Distraction injury to the cervical spine, a separation of the spinal column with resulting cord transection, is seen with hangings.[33]

Forces applied sufficiently to the anterior skull or face can displace the upper vertebrae backward, and the vertebral body above the distraction may separate.[22] This leaves the disk intact but strips the posterior longitudinal ligament from the vertebral body below. Spinal cord contusion against the lamina of the vertebra below can be seen.

Fractures

The biomechanics of fractures is an area in which knowledge is currently available.[24] Some basic definitions used to describe fracture biomechanics are helpful in understanding possible injuries. Force and strain have already been discussed and defined. *Stress* is defined as the internal resistance to deformation or the internal force generated from the application of a load:[25]

$$\text{Stress} = \frac{\text{load}}{\text{area on which the load acts}}$$

Stress cannot be measured directly. Stress is measured in force per unit area and expressed as pounds per square inch (psi) or kilograms per square centimeter (kg/cm^2). Other terms for force include pound force, kilogram force, and dynes.

Both extrinsic and intrinsic factors are important determinants of whether a bone will fracture when a stress is applied. Extrinsic factors include magnitude, duration, direction, and rate of force application. Intrinsic factors are properties of bone that determine its susceptibility to fracture. These include energy-absorbing capacity, modulus of elasticity (Young's modulus), fatigue, strength, and density.[34] Energy-absorbing capacity is related to the strain characteristics of the bone. The energy absorbed to produce femoral neck failure is 60 kg/cm^2. Stress-strain curves, or Young's modulus, measure elasticity. An imaginary curve is illustrated in Figure 7–7. Fatigue failure occurs when a material is subjected to repeated stresses that are below its breaking point, but the cumulative stress results in failure. Bone strength is directly related to its density. As bone density is

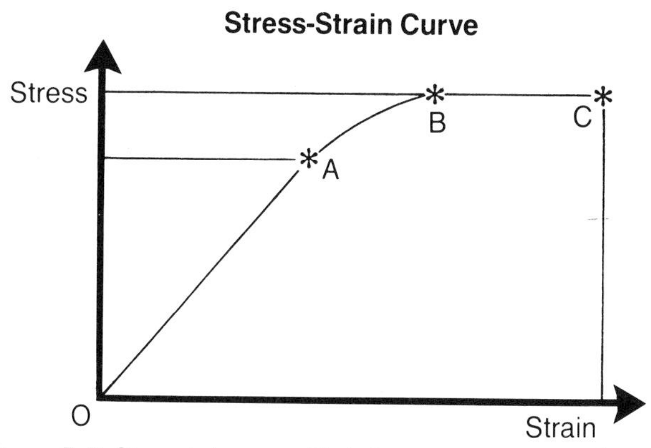

Figure 7–7. Stress-strain curve. Strain increases proportionately with stress to point A. From point A to point B, the strain is greater than the stress. Point A is called the *yield point*, or *limit of proportionality*, and point B represents the *ultimate tensile strength*.[25] Point C is the *break point*, or *breaking strain*, of the material. At C the material remains permanently deformed and does not recover its original shape.

reduced by osteoporosis, the stress required to fracture the bone decreases.

Fractures can be classified by their mechanism of injury (Fig. 7–8). Fractures caused by direct trauma are tapping, crush, low-velocity penetrating, and high-velocity penetrating.[25] Tapping injuries occur from kicks to the shin or blows with nightsticks to bony areas. Little energy is absorbed by soft tissue. Crush and high-velocity injuries produce multiple comminuted areas as well as soft-tissue damage. Indirect trauma also can produce fractures.[25] Traction injuries usually involve tendons pulling pieces of bone away at their attachments, such as external rotation injuries of the ankle. Angulation fractures are explained by tension and compression stress (Fig. 7–9). As a lever is angulated, the convex surface is under tension stress and the concave surface is under compression stress. The convex surface fails first, giving rise to a transverse fracture. Rotational fractures are rare because it is difficult to apply a true rotation force to a bone.[25] Compression fractures do occur and are explained by vector analysis. If a homogeneous cylinder is loaded axially until it fails, the fracture will appear at an angle of almost 45 degrees (Fig. 7–10). Since bones are not homogeneous, most axial loading produces T- or Y-shaped fractures at the lower end of the bone. Combinations of forces usually produce oblique or curved fracture lines.

Fractures in the thoracolumbar spine can present interesting clinical findings. Wedge or compression fractures are the most common spine fractures in this area. They result from acute flexion forces to the spine.[35] The injury can occur after a fall with feet landing first. An associated injury is an os calcis fracture. Burst fractures are produced when forces are applied perpendicularly to the spinal column. Spinous process fractures occur from direct force to the flexed spine or a violent muscle pull.

Pelvic fractures can be simple to manage or produce life-threatening hemorrhage. Injury to the lower genitourinary tract should always be a concern with any pelvic fracture. Open pelvic fractures have a mortality rate four times that of closed fractures.[36, 37] Traction fractures of the ischial tuberosity and anterior iliac spine represent stable simple

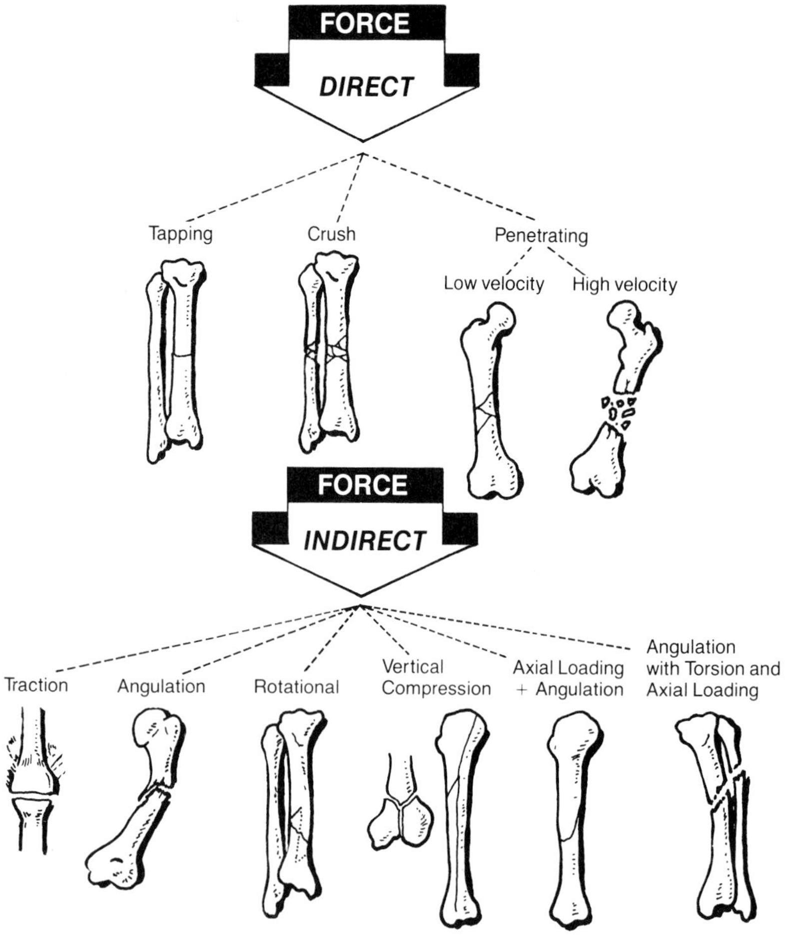

Figure 7–8. Types of fractures produced by various direct and indirect mechanisms of injury. (Reprinted with permission from Harkness JW: Principles of Fractures and Dislocations. In Rockwood CA, Green DP (eds): Fractures. Philadelphia, JB Lippincott Co, 1975, p 4.)

pelvic injuries. A shear fracture of the ilium is found in the motorcycle rider who is thrown forward and catches the iliac crest on the handlebars. Straddle fractures result from direct trauma to the perineum. Urethral injury should be sought in these patients, especially males. Patients with blood at the penile meatus, perineal or scrotal hematoma, or a nonpalpable prostate gland by rectal examination should not have a Foley catheter placed until a urethral injury is excluded by urethrogram. Malgaigne fractures are those with fracture lines through the sacroiliac joint and pubic rami on the same side (Fig. 7–11). This allows the two sides of the pelvis to float free; the resultant vascular disruption can produce massive bleeding.

Acetabular fractures happen when the hip is flexed and

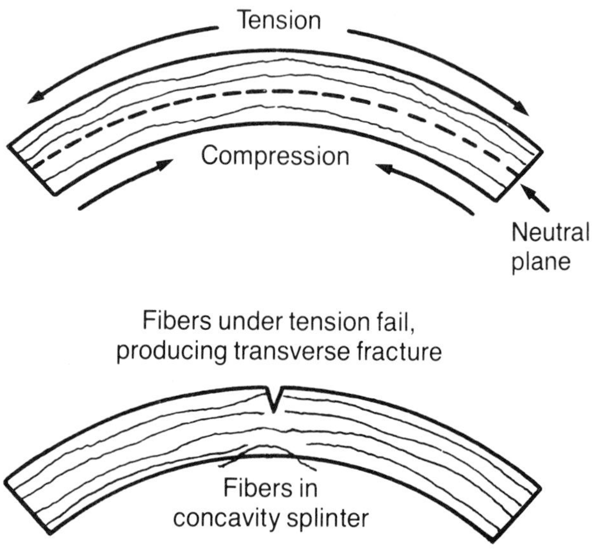

Figure 7–9. Forces sustained to produce an angulation fracture. (Reprinted with permission from Rockwood CA, Green DP (eds): Fractures in Adults. Philadelphia, JB Lippincott Co, 1984, p 13.)

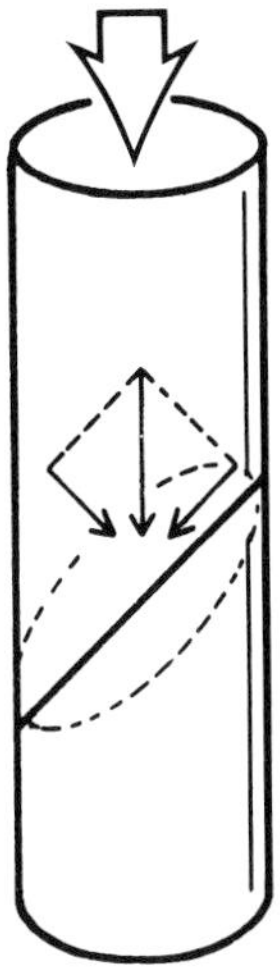

Figure 7–10. Vertical forces applied to a homogeneous cylinder will cause the structure to fail at an angle of 45 degrees to the long axis of the cylinder. The forces can be resolved into two forces, with the maximum shear force at 45 degrees to the long axis.

abducted during an MVA. The knee hits the dashboard during the forward body acceleration, and the femur is driven through the acetabulum. If the thigh is crossed at impact, a posterior dislocation of the hip is produced.[35, 38] The presence of these injuries should suggest the need for evaluation of the ipsilateral knee. An anterior dislocation of the hip is found when a posterior force is applied to an abducted, externally rotated thigh. The leg deformity in posterior and anterior hip dislocation is diagnostic (Fig. 7–12).

One of the most common and potentially most serious upper extremity fractures is a supracondylar humeral fracture in children.[25, 29] The anterior capsule and collateral ligaments are stronger than bone in children. Thus, as the elbow is locked in extension, the forces applied cause the weakest area, the supracondylar bone, to fracture. Even if the fracture is not displaced, the potential for swelling around the elbow is great and can produce arterial obstruction and vascular insufficiency of the forearm and hand. Volkmann's ischemic contracture can occur if the blood supply is occluded.

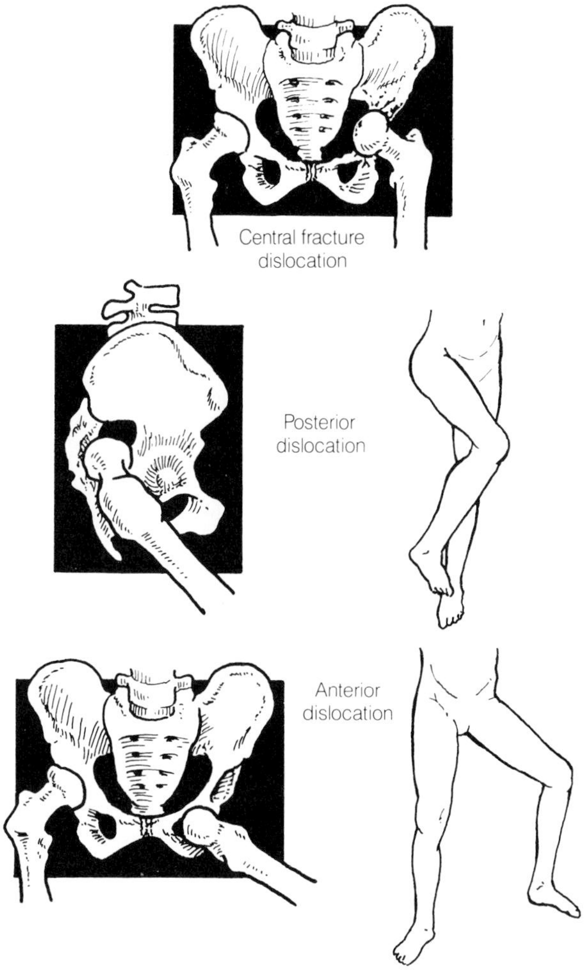

Figure 7–12. Three types of hip dislocation. (Reprinted with permission from Hughes JL: Initial Management of Fractures and Joint Injuries. In Zuidema GD, Ballinger RB, Rutherford RB (eds): Management of Trauma. Philadelphia, WB Saunders Co, 1985, p 621.)

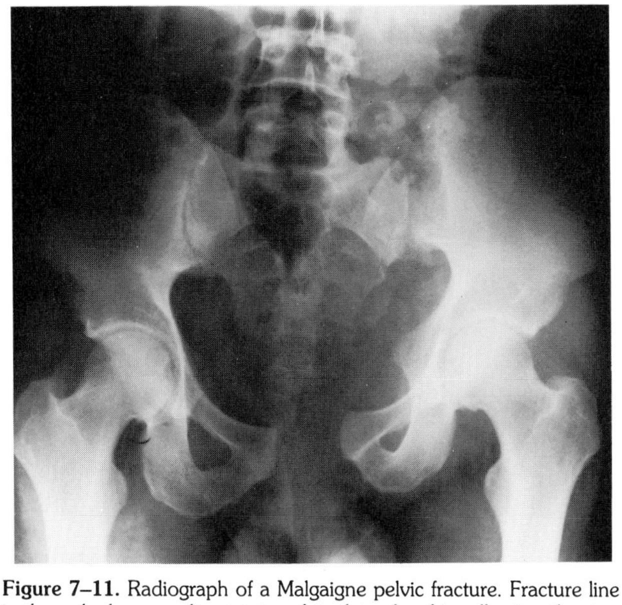

Figure 7–11. Radiograph of a Malgaigne pelvic fracture. Fracture line is through the sacroiliac joint and ipsilateral pubis, allowing the two sides of the pelvis to separate.

Abdominal Injuries

The automobile is responsible for at least 50 per cent of intra-abdominal injuries. The frequency of abdominal organ injury from blunt abdominal trauma is listed in Table 7–3. The National Crash Severity Study found that with Abbreviated Injury Scores of at least 3 and lateral impacts, the organs most likely to be injured were kidneys (43 per cent), spleen (33 per cent), and liver (24 per cent).[39] Animal experiments demonstrate that the risk of abdominal injury is a function of the impact velocity times the forced abdominal compression.[39] The mechanisms of blunt visceral injury include crushing, shearing, and bursting forces.[24, 32] In low-velocity, high-compression injuries, the mechanism is most likely due to organ motion and shearing forces. In high-velocity, low-compression injuries, the likely cause is bursting.

TABLE 7–3. ORGANS MOST COMMONLY INJURED FOLLOWING BLUNT ABDOMINAL TRAUMA

ORGAN	PER CENT
Spleen	26
Kidney	24
Liver	16
Intestine	16

Adapted from Anderson CB, Ballinger WF: Abdominal injuries. In Zuidema GD, Rutherford RB, Ballinger WF (eds): Management of Trauma. Philadelphia, WB Saunders Co, 1979, pp 429–482.

A crushing injury is represented by a midbody laceration of the pancreas. This can occur when the force is applied anterior to posterior, causing the pancreas to be crushed against the vertebral body. A shearing injury can result from acceleration–deceleration forces acting on the hepatic small bowel mesentery or renal vessels. In both cases, the momentum of the organ mass applies the force to the organ's vascular pedicle, causing injury. The apparent weight of the liver (actual weight, 1.8 kg) during a 36 km/hr impact would be 18 kg; a 72 km/hr impact, 72 kg; and a 108 km/hr impact, 162 kg.[29] It is easy to understand how vessels attaching this organ to its blood supply could be stretched and torn. Impact velocities for hepatic injuries have been studied.[40] Significant hepatic contusion occurs at velocities above 12 m/sec. At 20 m/sec, deep lacerations and transections are produced. A bursting injury can occur if the intestines are compressed in a closed loop formation, resulting in failure of the wall strength.

Causative Agents in Blunt Trauma

Motor Vehicle Accidents

Automobile accidents cause approximately 50,000 deaths annually.[1] Seventy-eight per cent involved automobiles, trucks, or motorcycles; 18 per cent involved pedestrians; 2 per cent involved bicyclists; and 2 per cent involved collisions with trains.[41] Some factors affecting the risk of occupant injury or death are amount of highway travel, road characteristics, speed, vehicle size, and restraint use.[6] Road characteristics, speed, vehicle size, and restraint use can affect the mechanism of injury.

Highway design can change the injury pattern. Crashes are reduced by separating opposing streams of traffic, eliminating intersections, removing obstacles from roadsides, using breakaway barriers, and surfacing roads with materials that decrease skidding. Successful examples of these changes include a death rate on interstate highways in 1979 of 1.6 per hundred million vehicle miles (mvm), while on rural, two-way roads it was 4.8 per hundred mvm.[24] Fatal accidents occur when roadside objects are struck within 40 ft of the road, emphasizing that road design should include a wide shoulder space free of obstacles.[6, 24] Speed becomes an important determinant of the likelihood and severity of injury once a crash occurs. The energy dissipated increases with the square of the change in velocity. Thus the forces on a properly restrained occupant in a forward crash at 70 mph might be roughly twice the forces at 50 mph (Fig. 7–13). It has been estimated that the 55 mph national speed limit when imposed had saved 5000 lives annually.[6] Vehicle size and design also change injury patterns. Small cars are involved in more crashes per mile and are associated with more deaths and injuries per crash than larger cars. The simple approach of making cars larger is not viable, since approximately 40 per cent of occupant deaths occur in single-vehicle crashes. Changing vehicle design, especially interior design, can improve the safety of the occupants. Incorporating design changes that are used in automobile racing also would increase the likelihood of escaping a vehicular accident without injury.[42]

Before a collision, the occupant is moving at the same speed as the vehicle. During the collision, the vehicle and occupant decelerate to a speed of zero, but not necessarily at the same rate. The deceleration forces are transmitted to the body according to the following relationship:[41]

$$\text{Gravity} = \text{mph}^2/30 \times \text{stopping distance (ft)}$$

Three collisions actually happen. The first is the car into another object. The second collision is the occupant's body with the interior of the car. A third collision may occur when internal tissues impact against rigid body surface structures. An example is the fracture of ribs by the steering wheel from the second collision and lung perforation by the ribs from the third collision (Fig. 7–14).

Unrestrained occupants are injured by contact with the steering wheel, instrument panel, or other car interior structures or by ejection. The most important cause of death is ejection from the vehicle, which was fatal in 27 per cent of cases.[43] Other causes of mortality are impact with front or rear doors (18 per cent), the steering assembly (16 per cent), and the instrument panel (13 per cent).[41]

Restraint systems allow occupants to decelerate with their vehicles rather than more abruptly when thrown against these unyielding structures inside or outside the vehicles.[44–46] Injuries are reduced by preventing ejection of the occupant

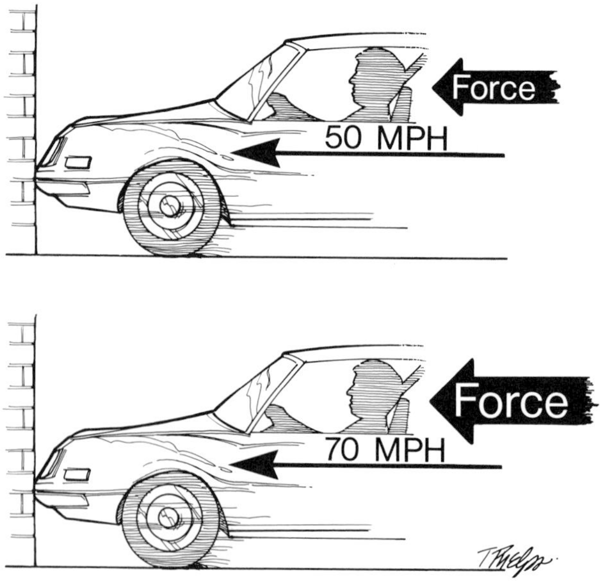

Figure 7–13. Force is increased approximately twofold when impact occurs at 70 mph in comparison to 50 mph.

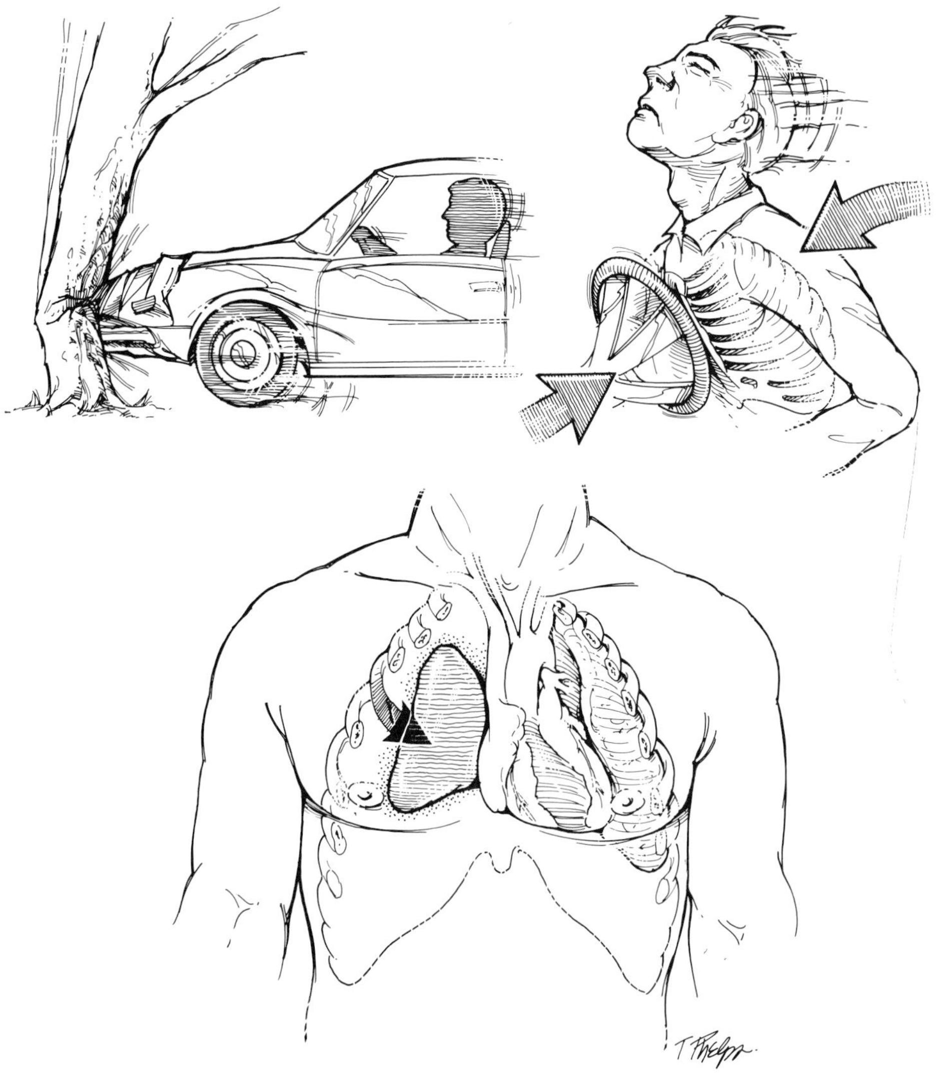

Figure 7–14. The three collisions of a head-on motor vehicle accident: The car impacts on an object, and the occupant's body impacts on some surface within the motor vehicle. The net result is collision between internal tissues and the rigid body surface structures.

during crashes, prolonging deceleration time, and reducing severity of impact by the occupant against the car interior.

Properly worn restraints decrease the number of fatalities and severity of injury. Major head injuries fell from 43 to 34 per cent in car passengers when laws were enacted requiring seat belt use.[6] A study by Volvo of Sweden showed no deaths under 60 mph when a harness-type restraint was worn.[47] Lap belts decrease the likelihood of ejection but not of impact with the vehicle interior. A three-point shoulder lap belt is the most effective restraint.[48] The harness belt reduces the impact of the second collision and thus reduces head and facial injuries, intra-abdominal solid viscus injuries, and long-bone fractures.[49] One study found that the use of seat belts would have prevented 40 per cent of deaths and lap belt/shoulder harnesses would have prevented another 13 per cent.[50] There is an increase in abdominal hollow viscus injury of patients using restraints.[51] This could be a result of a sudden increase in intraluminal pressure or shearing of relatively fixed ligaments and mesenteric attachments by the deceleration forces against the restraining device. These are the same forces that may cause an intra-abdominal aortic injury.[52] The increase in seat belt laws may produce new injuries related to their misuse. Seat belts can be misplaced intentionally or unintentionally. Examples of intentional misuse include placing small children in a harness designed for an adult. Defining injuries specific to malpositioning of seat belts is difficult. Recently, however, two blunt carotid injuries most likely related to a malpositioned seat belt were treated.

Collapsible steering columns and high-impact–resistant windshields help decrease injury from the second collision. The latest attempt to prevent these second collisions in MVAs is installation of the inflatable air bag activated on impact. This is a passive restraint mechanism.[53, 54]

Other motorized vehicles can present different mechanisms of injury. One type of transportation that is of growing concern is the three-wheeler all-terrain motorcycle.[55] A major problem with these vehicles is the perception of safety because of the wide tripod base. Injuries are produced by two mechanisms: A rider strikes an unseen wire or branch or the rider flips the motorcycle while turning or avoiding an obstacle. It is not uncommon for the vehicle to strike the rider after it flips. Few regulations concerning these motorcycles are in force, although strong recommendations from the manufacturers of these vehicles have resulted from consumer action.

Falls—Vertical Deceleration Injuries

Falls are the second leading cause of death due to trauma in the United States.[3] In falls, the relationship between physical forces of deceleration and biomechanical factors of the organism determines the type and severity of injury. Energy of a body in motion is expressed by kinetic energy (KE), which is a function of the body mass (m) and its velocity (v) and expressed as $KE = mV^2$. Mass, acceleration, and deceleration of the body in addition to the duration and area of application of the force are important when determining extent of injury in these accidents.[23, 56]

Duration of force application relates to whether the force is applied slowly or rapidly. The following formula describes the kinematics of vertical deceleration:

$$W = \frac{KE \times k}{TA}$$

Wounding (W) is directly related to the kinetic energy of the body modified inversely by the time of deceleration (T) and area through which the energy is dissipated (A).[23] The velocity at impact for a fall of 1 sec over a distance of 16 ft is 32.2 ft/sec or 21.9 mph. If duration is increased to 6 sec and distance to 580 ft, the velocity at impact is 193.2 ft/sec or 131.7 mph. The velocity at impact can be used as a measure of the kinetic energy of the body, which is related to the severity of tissue injury by the noted equation.

Tissue elasticity and viscosity must be considered as biomechanical factors of vertical deceleration. Elasticity is the tissue's ability to resist stretching and resume its previous shape. If the tissue remains distorted, it is said to be *plastic*. Viscosity is the tissue's resistance to change in shape when there are changes in motion. The body's ability to withstand deceleration forces is a combination of these two tissue properties.[23]

Tissue disruption at impact is caused by the motion of the tissues. The body's ability to withstand this force increases if there is uniform motion of all tissues. The injury can be minimized by increasing stopping distance or time of deceleration and enlarging the area of energy dissipation. These concepts are emphasized in a report of a female falling 50 ft and landing at a speed of 37 mph on her back and side, depressing the earth 4 in. There was no loss of consciousness or signs of injury.[44] The magnitude of injury increases as tissue cohesion is overcome. Forces transmitted at impact include compression, stretching, and shearing, which can occur singly or in combination.[23]

Skeletal injuries, especially of the lower extremities, are common with vertical deceleration. Wedge or compression fractures of vertebral bodies with fracture-dislocation of the spine are due to both flexion-compression and rotational injury forces. Torsion injury is also common and results from the force being transmitted to the feet and up the legs to the pelvis and supporting structures of bone, muscle, and cartilage[57] (Fig. 7–15).

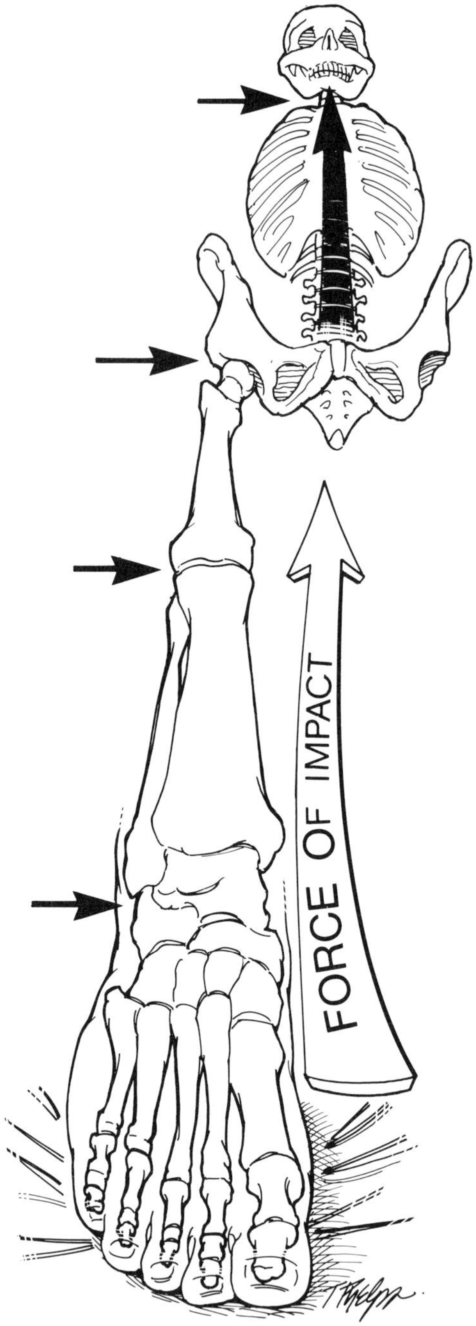

Figure 7–15 Forces resulting from a fall are transmitted up to the spine through the long leg bones and pelvis.

PENETRATING TRAUMA

Penetrating trauma refers to injury produced by foreign objects set into motion. Penetration of tissue occurs, and its severity is related to the structures damaged. The most commonly involved organs are intestines, liver, vascular structures, and spleen.[51] The mechanism of injury with penetrating trauma is the energy created and dissipated by the object into the surrounding areas.[58] Evaluation of injury is often difficult and dependent on the type and characteristic

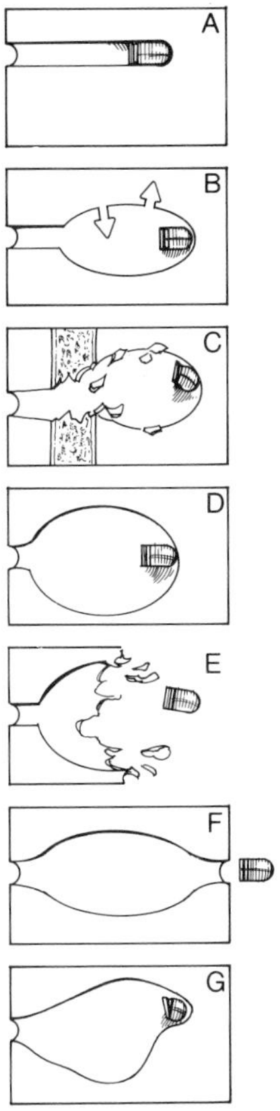

Figure 7–16. Patterns of injury in animal tissue secondary to variations in the ballistics of the missile and tissue characteristics. *A,* Low velocity, no cavitation, entrance and exit small. *B,* Higher velocity, formation of cavity, arrows show direction and magnitude of acceleration of tissue. *C,* Velocity as in *B,* but deformation of bullet and creation of secondary missiles upon penetrating bone. *D,* Very high velocity, large cavity, and small entrance. Exit may be small. *E,* Very high velocity, thin target, large and ragged exit. *F,* Velocity, caliber, and thickness of tissue such that cavitation occurs deep inside, and entrance and exit are small. *G,* Asymmetrical cavitation as bullet begins to deform and tumble. (Redrawn and adapted with permission from Swan KG, Swan RC (eds): Gunshot Wounds: Pathophysiology and Management. Littleton, MA, PSG Publishing, 1980, p 9.)

of injuring agent, energy dissipation, tissue characteristics, and distance from weapon to target (Fig. 7–16).

The extent of injury is proportional to the amount of kinetic energy (KE) that is lost by the missile:[59]

$$KE = \frac{\text{mass} \times (V1^2 - V2^2)}{2 \times g}$$

$V1$ is impact velocity, and $V2$ is exit or remaining velocity. It should be noted that doubling the mass only doubles the energy, whereas doubling the velocity quadruples the energy. Rotational energy is also a factor, since most missiles are shot from barrels that are rifled, causing the bullet to spin. Total kinetic energy can be estimated from adding velocity and rotational energy. Velocity at impact depends on three factors: muzzle velocity, distance of weapon from target, and influence of air friction on the missile (see Fig. 7–16).

Low-velocity weapons at a range less than 50 yards and high-velocity weapons at less than 100 yards have impact velocities that equal muzzle velocities. To penetrate skin, a missile must have an impact velocity of 150 ft/sec, and a velocity of 195 ft/sec is required to break bone. Increase in mass can affect total energy (magnum shells will usually increase energy by 20 to 60 per cent).[59]

The amount of kinetic energy lost by the missile is directly related to the tissue damage. The energy lost by the missile is transferred to the tissue. Factors that increase the amount of kinetic energy transferred effectively increase tissue destruction. As the missile penetrates, a tract is created, which temporarily displaces tissue forward and laterally. This tissue acceleration creates a temporary cavity as tissues are stretched and compressed, a process called *cavitation*. Cavitation is directly proportional to the amount of kinetic energy transmitted to the tissue.[42, 59] It commonly occurs with missiles traveling 1000 ft/sec or greater. The size of this cavity may be many times the diameter of the bullet. This phenomenon produces damage to structures outside the direct missile path and is commonly referred to as *blast effect*. The effect that cavitation has on wounding potential is illustrated in a wounding study that attempted to control the size of the temporary cavity.[60] The average tissue destruction was reduced by one third if the cavity size was limited by an external envelope.

The velocity of a missile determines the extent of cavitation and tissue deformation. Low-velocity missiles localize injury to a small radius from the center of the tract and have little disruptive effect. A low-velocity missile travels less than 1000 ft/sec or 305 m/sec.[42] Low-velocity bullets cause little cavitation and blast effect. They essentially only push the tissue aside. High-velocity missile injuries are more serious owing to the amount of energy lost and cavitation produced.

High-velocity missiles travel at greater than 3000 ft/sec or 914 m/sec.[42] Damage from high-velocity missiles is dependent on three factors: density and compressibility of tissue injured, missile velocity, and the primary missile's fragmentation.

High-velocity bullets compress and accelerate tissue away from the bullet, causing a cavity around the bullet and its entire tract. The cavity enlarges as the bullet transfers its kinetic energy to the tissue. A negative pressure is created behind the missile, producing contamination of the wound with foreign material. The diameter of the cavity might be 30 to 40 times the diameter of the bullet. This area is often devitalized and requires debridement. The cavity collapses and tissue recoils until all energy is dissipated. Tissue cohesiveness and elasticity resist expansion of the cavity. More cohesive and elastic tissues experience less damage. Dense tissue absorbs more kinetic energy, causing greater damage. This retarding factor can be related to tissue specific gravity. The higher the specific gravity, the more energy is imparted and the greater is the damage[59] (Table 7–4).

TABLE 7–4. SPECIFIC GRAVITY OF TISSUES

TISSUE	SPECIFIC GRAVITY
Rib	1.11
Skin	1.09
Muscle	1.04–1.02
Liver	1.02–1.01
Fat	0.8
Lung	0.5–0.4

In injuries from high-velocity missiles, the exit wound through narrow structures or tissue such as an extremity will be larger than the entrance wound because all energy is not dissipated at the exit point. Cavitation along with yawing and tumbling is still occurring. Through dense broad tissue, the exit wound is small because energy is dissipated and cavitation is complete.[61] If bullet fragmentation occurs, there may be no exit wound. The need for debridement can be extensive with high-velocity missile damage. Amputation and mortality rates are high.[42] High-velocity missile injuries to the head are destructive because the cranial vault is fixed and not able to yield to the expanding temporary cavity created by the missile.

After velocity, tissue yaw is the second most important factor in tissue destruction (Fig. 7–17). As a bullet's velocity increases, it becomes unstable in flight and may yaw or tumble.[61] *Yawing* is the deviation or deflection of the nose of the bullet from a straight path. The bullet strikes the body at an angle. With greater angles of yaw, the bullet is slowed, and more kinetic energy is lost to the tissue. *Tumbling* is the action of forward rotation around the center of mass, a somersault action of the missile that can create massive injury.[42, 59, 61] Yawing and tumbling increase the area of the missile as it hits the target. Impact increases these motions, which increases the amount of energy released by the bullet, producing more damage.

Various types of bullets are made to alter (in most cases, increase) the amount of energy transmitted. A bullet passing through tissue without deforming transfers little energy and causes less damage than the bullet that slows down or stops in the tissue. One way to increase the energy transferred is to allow the missile to alter shape upon impact. Bullets with hollow points mushroom upon impact and yield great amounts of kinetic energy. Soft-nosed and flat-nosed bullets have similar effects.[26, 59, 61]

Muzzle blast is another mechanism of injury for penetrating trauma. *Muzzle blast* refers to the cloud of hot gas and burning powder at the muzzle immediately after firing.[26] This is a factor when the gun is in contact with the skin or at close range (within 3 ft). The gas and powder enter the cavity and cause internal explosion by creating a burn.

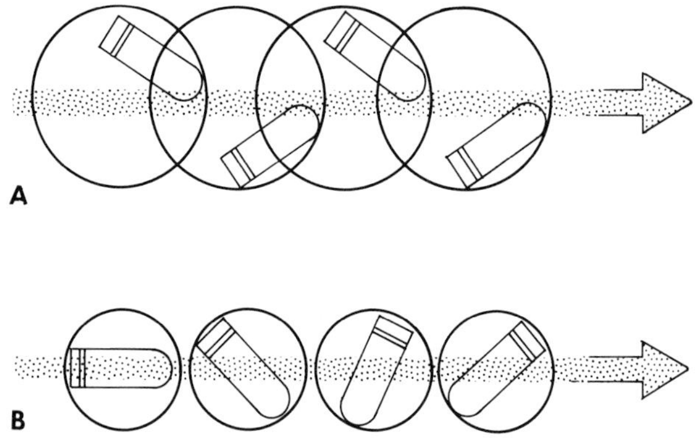

A

B

Figure 7–17. Effect of yaw on wounding potential. *A, Yawing* is the deviation of a bullet in its longitudinal axis from the straight line of flight. *B, Tumbling* is the action of forward rotation around the center of mass. (Redrawn with permission from Swan KG, Swan RC (eds): Gunshot Wounds: Pathophysiology and Management. Littleton, MA, PSG Publishing, 1980, p 11.)

Cavitation is from combustion of powder and the forceful expansion of gases. This is common with a shotgun wound but is not seen with handguns because the amount of gas released is less and the wound is too small for it to enter. As the gas is trapped between skin and bone, a stellate tear results from the ballooning of skin out from the bone.[22] This injury does not occur if subcutaneous tissue is present, because of tissue cohesiveness and elasticity.

Shotgun Injuries

Shotguns are short-range and low-velocity weapons with multiple lead pellets encased in a larger shell. Each pellet is considered a missile; there can be 9 to 200 small pellets, depending on the size of pellet and gauge of the gun.[22] The shell contains pellets, gunpowder, and a plastic or paper wad separating the pellets from the gunpowder. This wad of unsterile material increases the potential of infection in a shotgun wound.[62, 63] The wad is expelled with the pellets but loses momentum and drops about 6 ft from the barrel. The pellets leave the barrel closely together and separate as they move away from the barrel. The extent of injury depends on the distance of the target from the shotgun. At less than 6 ft, a tight, dense pattern is produced with extensive damage from the muzzle blast and mass of pellets. At 3 to 6 ft, the single entrance wound is 1.5 to 2 in in diameter with scalloping at the edges.[26] There is extensive contamination from shotgun wadding, clothing, skin, hair, burning, and powder entering the wound. At greater distances, a pellet does less damage because of the loss of velocity and energy. A brief description of the mechanism of shotgun injuries, including the weapon, ammunition, and ballistics, is important in understanding the clinical findings in patients sustaining wounds from these weapons.[64] Gauge designates the bore of the gun. Common gauges include 10, 12, 16, 20, 28, and .410. The shotgun shell is made up of the primer, powder, wad, and shot, in that order. Shotgun powder is fast burning and creates a low chamber pressure. Common shot sizes range from size 2 through 9 and have a respective pellet diameter of 0.15 to 0.08 in. Ninety #2 shot pellets equal 585 #9 shot pellets in weight. Larger shot sizes include buckshot and BBs. Buckshot sizes are designated as 4, 3, 2, 1, 0, and 00. Each 00 buckshot is 0.328 in in diameter. There are also single projectiles, called "slugs" or "pumpkin balls."

The shot pattern is of clinical importance. Most significant wounds occur between 0 and 15 yards. Wounding capacity is the function of mass and projectile velocity. Considering only ballistics, the shotgun is inferior to the single-projectile, high-velocity rifle such as the M–16. The average muzzle velocity of a shotgun is between 1100 and 1350 ft/sec. Rifle slugs have a muzzle velocity approaching 1850 ft/sec. The M–16, with a bullet weighing 55 gm has a muzzle velocity of 3200 ft/sec. The kinetic energy of the M–16 at the muzzle is 1248 foot-pounds (ft•lb). A #6 shotgun pellet, 0.11 in in diameter, has striking forces of 7.21 ft•lb per pellet at the muzzle and 3.88 ft•lb per pellet at 20 yards. A 12-gauge shotgun with 225 to 428 pellets in the load theoretically has 1694 ft•lb at the muzzle. Therefore, at point-blank or very close range, a shotgun injury has the potential for creating extensive tissue damage, similar to a high-velocity missile injury.

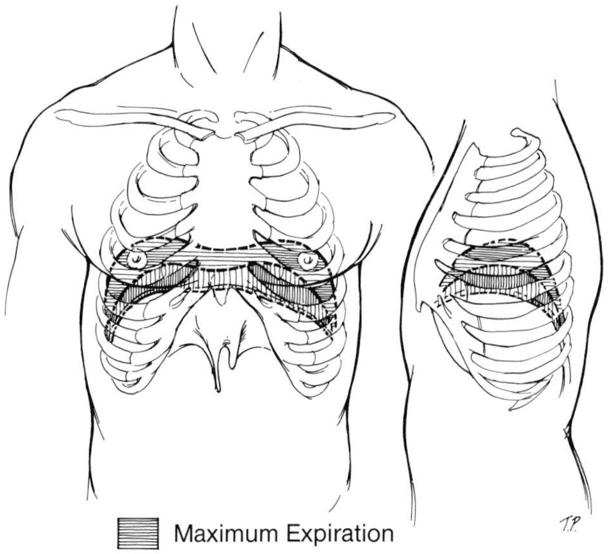

Figure 7–18. Diaphragmatic excursion during inspiration and expiration and its possible effect on penetrating injuries to the lower chest and upper abdomen.

The major factor affecting the nature of the shotgun wound is the range from the target at which the gun is discharged. If a 12-gauge shotgun loaded with #6 shot (275 pellets) were fired accurately at a distance of 40 yards into a 6-ft, 160-lb person, approximately 200 of the pellets would strike within a 30-in diameter. This would be between the midthigh to the shoulders, across the trunk, and extending about 9 in on either side. If the shot were absolutely evenly distributed, there would be about 2 in between each pellet. At a range of 10 yards, this wound would be only 7 in in diameter. These changes in pattern and clinical significance are used by Sherman and Parrish to classify shotgun wounds.[65] Type 1 are penetrating wounds at a range over 7 yards. Type 2 are perforating wounds at a range of 3 to 7 yards. Type 3 are massive pointblank wounds that are inflicted at a range of under 3 yards.

Low-Velocity Penetrating Wounds

Other types of penetrating wounds, such as stab wounds and impalements, are low-velocity wounds. These wounds are usually obvious, yet the patient must be undressed and inspected for entrance and exit wounds. If the offending agent remains in place, its trajectory can be traced and underlying trauma predicted. If removed, the gender of the assailant can be helpful in estimating the trajectory: males tend to stab with an upward thrust and females with a downward thrust.[10] This assessment should not be considered absolute, since intentional injuries often follow no pattern.

Stab wounds are low velocity and therefore low energy; the injuries produced depend on the location of penetration. Little damage occurs to tissue except in the locale of the injury. It must be remembered that multiple body cavities can be penetrated by a single wound. In particular, the thoracic and abdominal cavities can be injured by a wound whose entrance is located over one or the other cavity. Lower chest wounds, from the nipples to the costochondral margin, are frequently found to injure abdominal contents because the diaphragmatic excursion extends superiorly up to the nipple line or fifth intercostal space during exhalation (Fig. 7–18).

Impalement injuries usually result from a forceful collision between the object and patient during MVAs or falls or from falling objects. The spectacular nature of these injuries should not preclude proper management. The impaled object should be left in place until definite surgical therapy is available.[66–68] This recommendation dates back to 1862 in a treatise about arrow wounds and the ability of the arrow to tamponade vascular injuries.[67] Removal of these foreign bodies can remove the vascular control, causing exsanguinating hemorrhage. Another concern with these injuries is bacterial and foreign-body contamination. Care should be taken to remove all foreign material from these wounds, and occasionally extensive wound debridement is required.

SMOKE INHALATION AND PULMONARY BURNS

Inhalation injuries occur when the respiratory tract is exposed to the products of combustion. The type and severity of injury are determined by the type of gases inhaled, their concentration, and the duration of exposure. Thermal injury to the respiratory tree is uncommon because the heat-exchanging efficiency of the respiratory tract is so high that even superheated air is cooled before it gets below the larynx.[69] Steam inhalation can produce thermal injury of the lower respiratory tract because steam has 4000 times the heat capacity of air. The presence of these injuries should be suspected if certain circumstances are present: (1) fire in a closed space, (2) unconsciousness or inebriation associated with smoke exposure, (3) fires involving plastics, (4) presence of carbonaceous sputum, and (5) steam explosions.[69]

The most immediate concern in a patient exposed to a fire is carbon monoxide (CO) intoxication. This is the most frequent immediate cause of death. Carbon monoxide has an affinity for hemoglobin 210 times that of oxygen.[70] The signs and symptoms of CO intoxication are related to blood carboxyhemoglobin concentration (Table 7–5).

Inhalation of toxic constituents of smoke may damage alveolar epithelium and capillary endothelium. This results in increased permeability of the alveolar–capillary membrane, which can produce noncardiac pulmonary edema and

TABLE 7–5 SIGNS AND SYMPTOMS CAUSED BY VARIOUS CONCENTRATIONS OF CARBOXYHEMOGLOBIN

BLOOD SATURATION (% COHb)	SIGNS AND SYMPTOMS
0.3–10	None
10–20	Tightness across forehead; headache
20–30	Throbbing headache; abnormal fine manual dexterity
30–50	Severe headache; syncope; nausea and vomiting
60–70	Coma; convulsions; death

TABLE 7–6. COMMON TOXIC PRODUCTS OF COMBUSTION

SUBSTANCE	TOXIC PRODUCTS OF COMBUSTION
Polyvinyl chloride	Hydrogen chloride, phosgene, chloride
Wood, cotton, paper	Acrolein, acetaldehyde, acetic acid, formaldehyde, formic acid
Petroleum products	Acrolein, acetic acid, formic acid
Nitrocellulose	Oxides of nitrogen, acetic acid, formic acid
Polyurethane	Isocyanate, hydrogen cyanide
Polyfluorocarbons (Teflon)	Octafluoroisobutylene
Melamine resins	Ammonia, hydrogen cyanide

hypoxemia.[71] These toxic products also reduce bacterial clearance and mucociliary transport. Combustion of many common construction materials produces a large number of toxic by-products capable of this type of injury[70] (Table 7–6).

Motor vehicles provide some unique mechanisms of injury for burns. Carburetor priming resulted in 4 per cent of admissions to one burn center.[72] The burns most frequently involved the head, neck, and upper extremities. Gasoline is often used to prime an engine that has run out of gas. This practice is unnecessary and dangerous because it can produce an explosion and fire, which may happen when the gasoline comes in contact with hot metal, an electrical spark, or retrograde ignition from too much gasoline in the intake manifold. Burns sustained during an MVA are a second mechanism type and occur in two patterns: (1) the person is trapped in a burning vehicle, receiving facial and upper extremity burns with associated inhalation injury, or (2) the person is thrown from the vehicle and sustains less severe burns and no inhalation injury. Motorcycle accident victims are common in this second group. Associated injuries, including fractures, are common but do not correlate with mortality. The injury most commonly associated with mortality is inhalation injury (36 per cent).[73]

EXPLOSIVE BLASTS

Explosive blasts are a result of detonated explosives being converted to large volumes of gases.[74] The pressure created ruptures the casing, and resultant fragments become high-velocity projectiles. The blast shock wave created by the remaining energy has three components: positive phase, negative phase, and mass movement of air. The blast shock wave's velocity is as high as 3000 m/sec (10,000 ft/sec), which decreases to the speed of sound within a variable distance.[74] This is dependent on the composition and amount of explosive used. The positive-pressure phase is the maximum pressure reached by the blast wave and is greatest next to the immediate explosion. Pressure falls as the wave moves away from the explosion source. The negative-pressure phase follows immediately and lasts 10 times as long.[74] An equal volume of air is displaced along with the expanding gas and travels behind the blast wave. The mass movement of air can actually cause disruption of tissue, traumatic amputation, and evisceration.[74]

Blast injuries in water are more severe than in air because the blast wave travels farther and more rapidly in water owing to its greater density. Explosions in closed areas are more damaging than those in open spaces because of the toxic gases and smoke that are inhaled. Posttraumatic pulmonary insufficiency results and is reflected in blood gases with low Pa_{O_2} and increased Pa_{CO_2}.

Damage occurs most often at tissue–air interfaces. Damage in the lung is in the alveolar wall, with resultant hemorrhage and edema. The abdominal organs will show damage to the visceral wall and the trauma may cause perforation.[74] These types of injuries are rare if the explosion occurs in the open and the victim is not close to the detonation point. The ear is the most sensitive organ to explosions; eardrums will rupture at about 7 psi.[74] Burns also can be seen if a fireball effect is present. Penetrating injuries can occur if projectiles are released.

INJURY SCORING

An objective system to measure severity of injury is helpful in triaging patients, allocating and evaluating medical resources, assessing quality of medical care, conducting institutional auditing, and preparing comparative studies of morbidity and mortality.[75] A number of severity indices are available; however, each has its problems and limitations.[76–84] Three injury scales for trauma patients that have gained recent support are the Abbreviated Injury Scale (AIS), the Injury Severity Score (ISS), and the Trauma Score (TS).

The AIS was first published in 1971 as a single comprehensive scale for injuries secondary to MVAs. The most recent edition is AIS–85, which is now available.[83] The system divides the body into seven regions and uses a severity code for each injury. One is a minor injury, while six is a fatal injury. A deficiency with the system is that scores from different body systems cannot be added or averaged together to calculate an overall numerical indicator of severity.

This criticism is answered by the ISS.[79] Mortality increases with the AIS grade of most severe injury, and this increase is not linear, but quadratic. AIS scores from the second and third most severely injured body regions also tend to increase the risk of death and maintain the quadratic relationship. The AIS scores from the three most severely injured body regions are used to define a number score that relates to severity of injury. Since the association of the AIS score to mortality is quadratic, the ISS is defined as the sum of the squares of the highest AIS grade in each of the three most severely injured areas. A problem with the ISS is that it is a retrospective tool.

The need for a prospective physiological scoring mechanism produced the Trauma Score.[76] The components of the Revised Trauma Score (RTS) are listed in Table 7–7. The Glasgow coma scale is combined with simple physiological measurements to derive an RTS between 1 and 12. Lower scores are associated with higher mortality.[77] This severity index has considerable statistical support and can be combined with the ISS to yield the expected chance of patient

TABLE 7–7. REVISED TRAUMA SCORE

ASSESSMENT	METHOD	CODING
1. Respiratory rate	Count respiratory rate in 15 s and multiply by 4	10–29 = 4 >29 = 3 6–9 = 2 1–5 = 1 0 = 0
2. Systolic blood pressure	Measure systolic cuff pressure in either arm by auscultation or palpation	>89 = 4 76–89 = 3 50–75 = 2 1—49 = 1 0 = 0
3. Glasgow coma score		
EYE OPENING	**BEST VERBAL RESPONSE**	**BEST MOTOR RESPONSE**
Spontaneous = 4 To voice = 3 To pain = 2 None = 1	Oriented = 5 Confused = 4 Inappropriate words = 3 Incomprehensible sounds = 2 None = 1	Obeys command = 6 Localizes pain = 5 Withdraws to pain = 4 Flexion to pain = 3 Extension to pain = 2 None = 1
	Convert Glascow coma scale as follows: 13–15 = 4 9–12 = 3 6–8 = 2 4–5 = 1 <4 = 0	

To obtain the trauma score, add the final scores for respiratory rate, systolic blood pressure, and converted Glasgow coma score together.

Summary of survival probability in a trauma center:

TRAUMA SCORE	12	11	10	9	8	7	6	5	4	3	2	1	0
SURVIVAL	.995	.969	.879	.766	.667	.636	.630	.455	.333	.333	.286	.259	.037

survival (Fig. 7–19). The resulting TRISS method is based on regression equations, which consider patient age, severity of anatomical injury (ISS), and physiological status of the patient (TS). These comparisons are useful in identifying individual patients with statistically unexpected outcomes, whether good or bad. Survivors above the 50 per cent mortality line would be an unexpected favorable outcome, while deaths below the line would be an unfavorable outcome. TRISS also can be used to compare populations of trauma patients while controlling for severity mix.

PREVENTION

Injury prevention is a laudable goal but not an easy one. Injury-prevention programs that are successful require adequate and reliable data, an understanding of the mechanism of injury, and adequate planning.[85] The high-risk groups previously identified need to be the targets of such injury-prevention programs. Successful injury control must focus on these groups and use measures that minimize individual motivation and effort.[6] Adequate data yield numbers, types, and circumstances of injury which localize prevention needs. It is essential that the circumstances of injury are open to change. Protective measures require time for development and testing. Once an established protective device is found to be satisfactory, education and enforcement must be applied. The effects of these preventive measures are then monitored with appropriate revisions and improvements. Injury prevention needs to be a well-supported effort by established organizations in order to be effective and successful.

The health care professional needs to interface with multiple organizations and agencies in order to become involved in injury prevention programs. Several national organizations

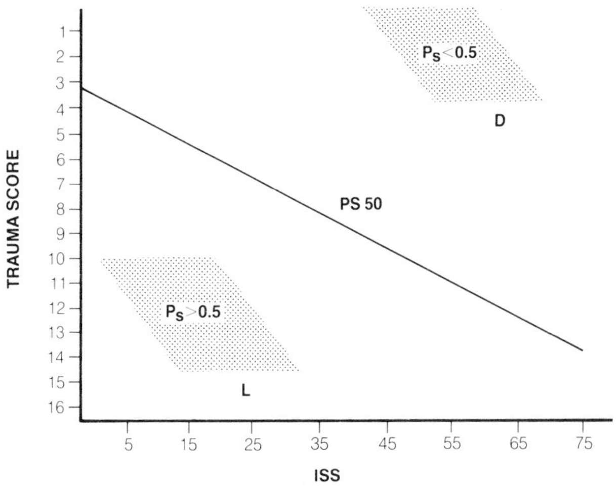

Figure 7–19. Trauma score plotted against the injury severity score. The probability of survival above the PS50 isobar is lower than 50 per cent, and the probability of survival below the isobar is higher than 50 per cent.

gather data on accidents and injuries, which can be useful in locating target areas and populations. These are the National Center for Health Statistics, National Ambulatory Medical Care Survey, National Medical Care Utilization and Expenditure Survey, and Vital Statistics programs. Two main national groups focus on the prevention of drunk driving and injuries: RID (Remove Intoxicated Drivers) and MADD (Mothers Against Drunk Driving). Both are citizen-oriented groups. RID focuses on public education and awareness about the present laws concerning drunk driving. It aids victims and their families as well as drunk drivers and their families. MADD is composed of citizens along with victims and survivors of drunk-driving accidents. They too are oriented toward public education and assistance along with active lobbying efforts for legislative reform. Staying Alive, a program directed at teenage drunk driving using educational material and a buddy system, has been developed by the Orange County, California, Trauma Society.

Automobile safety is an area where prevention measures have been focused. Seat belts have been shown to significantly decrease trauma from MVAs. About 60 per cent of people killed or injured in MVAs could have been spared serious injury if seat belts had been worn.[86] Mandatory safety seat use for children has been proposed and enacted in many states.[87] There is an active effort to develop passive automobile restraints. The mass media are used to educate the public about accident prevention, with some success in areas such as fire prevention and sports accidents. The Consumer Product Safety Commission has helped in these and other areas. Standards have been developed for product safety in sports equipment, stoves, fabrics, baby cribs, and child-proof containers. Safety standards attempt to ensure that products are safe when used as directed and that the consumer is protected even when foreseeable abuse occurs.[88]

Haddon and Baker have identified 10 logical approaches to reduce environmental hazards:[53]

1. Stop creating hazards.
2. Reduce the number of hazards.
3. Prevent the release of hazards that exist.
4. Modify the rate or spatial distribution of the hazard.
5. Separate by time and space the hazard from that which needs protection.
6. Separate by physical barriers.
7. Modify basic characteristics of the hazard.
8. Make the protected party more resistant to damage.
9. Respond quickly when damage is done.
10. Provide appropriate medical care for therapy and rehabilitation.

The last two are not preventive techniques but address the problem of adequate care. Baker and associates have identified how these strategies might be used in prevention of motor vehicle accidents, sports injuries, and handgun injuries[2] (Table 7–8).

When looking at injury prevention, three components need to be taken into account: (1) persuade high-risk groups to alter behavior for their self-protection, (2) require individuals to change behavior by law or regulations, and (3) provide

TABLE 7–8. STRATEGIES FOR REDUCING INJURIES AND DEATHS, AS APPLIED TO MOTOR VEHICLE, FOOTBALL, AND HANDGUN INJURIES

STRATEGY	INJURY TO MOTOR VEHICLE OCCUPANTS	INJURY TO FOOTBALL PLAYERS	INJURY RESULTING FROM HANDGUNS
Preventing marshalling of potentially injurious agents or reducing their amounts	Alternative travel modes; reductions in speed limits and speed capabilities of cars	Fewer games; shorter quarters; speed restrictions in tackling drills	Reduced production of handguns, bullets
Preventing inappropriate release of agent	Vehicle and road designs that simplify driver's task	Playing surfaces that reduce likelihood of falls	Locking up guns; eliminating incentive for shooting, e.g., no cash
Modifying release of agent	Use of seat belts to decelerate occupant with vehicle	Short cleats on shoes allowing foot to rotate rather than transmitting sudden force to knee	Single-shot guns requiring reloading between firings
Separating in time or space or with physical barriers	Restricting transport of hazardous materials to certain times and places; highway medians	Limited-contact practice drills; placing fixed structures farther from field; face masks	Bulletproof vests; bulletproof glass
Modifying surfaces, basic structures	Airbags to spread forces over wide area of body; removing projections in car	Changing outside of helmets to reduce injuries to other players	Soft, doughnut-shaped bullets for target shooting (require less initial velocity, unlikely to penetrate humans)
Increasing resistance to injury	Therapy for osteoporosis	Musculoskeletal conditioning	
Emergency response or medical care and rehabilitation	Systems that route patients to appropriately trained physicians	Personnel trained to recognize serious injuries; physicians on call	Occupational rehabilitation for paraplegics

Reprinted from Baker SP, Dietz PE: Examples of 10 basic strategies for reducing injuries and deaths. In Zuidema GD, Rutherford RB, Ballinger WF (eds): Management of Trauma. Philadelphia, WB Saunders Co, 1985, p 800.

automatic protection such as passive seat belts or sprinkler systems. Unfortunately, behavior change by law or regulation is apparently more effective than by persuasion and education. Automatic or passive protection is more effective than protection requiring active participation from the individual being protected.

Six recommendations for the prevention of injury have been developed and serve as goals:

1. Programs toward education, training, and information need to be evaluated experimentally.
2. Laws and regulation should be scientifically evaluated.
3. Research in the area of product design and modification should continue.
4. The barriers to injury control measures should be evaluated so that implementation is more effective.
5. Recreational, occupational, and home environments need to be assessed to identify the need for injury prevention.
6. Health care professionals and scientists need to be trained in injury control research in order to develop and apply new knowledge to the field of prevention.[89]

Successful community-based injury-prevention programs require several elements.[90] The first element is the selection of a leader. This individual is responsible for program coordination, including data and human resource management. The coordinator seeks out appropriate support from a lead agency that serves as a broker among other agencies and interested groups. In order to gain such support, the program must be clearly identified with an injury and population at risk. Its focus depends on the level of public awareness and publicity surrounding the injury, available funds, and the presence of motivated citizens.

The second element in program development is a systematic assessment of demographic, geographical, and economic data related to the injury. Important questions to be answered include (1) who in the community can influence and authorize public action, (2) who can focus the attention of the media on prevention of the injury, (3) who can raise funds, (4) who are the political, corporate, religious, and civic leaders most important to the community, and (5) what is the status of any preexisting or on-going injury-prevention legislation? The answers to these questions help to determine the direction of the program over its developmental course.

A third important factor is the development of clearly stated, measurable, and timely programmatic objectives. These objectives reflect the incidence rate, the community's knowledge of and response to the injury, public policy, and the physical environment. Lastly, a strategic plan as to how to decrease the incidence of injury within the target population is essential to any successful injury-prevention program. Most programs commonly integrate several approaches: legislative actions with enforcement by regulatory agencies, education centered on behavioral change, and promotion of engineering and technology specific to moderating or eliminating the injury. A review of previous injury-prevention programs helps to identify potential stumbling blocks to success.

With injury as our fourth leading cause of death and one of the most expensive health problems, a thorough understanding of the circumstances that result in injury is necessary for all health care personnel. Mechanism of injury helps to identify the type, extent, and pattern of injury and even relate to potential complications and outcome. Mechanism of injury affords the practitioner an opportunity to suspect certain injuries in addition to the obvious ones, thereby improving delivery of patient care. Prevention of injury is also aided by knowing the mechanism of injury. Active involvement of the trauma practitioner in organizations and programs aimed at injury prevention should be sought so their firsthand knowledge can be used to educate the public in injury prevention. This knowledge must be used if successful programs are to be developed that will impact on the currently dismal statistics of injury in the United States.

REFERENCES

1. National Safety Council: Accident Facts, 1987 Edition. Chicago, NSC, 1987.

1a. Haupt BJ, Graves E: Detailed Diagnostic Procedures for Patients Discharged from Short-Stay Hospitals: United States, 1979. DHHS Publication No. (PHS) 82–1274-1. Washington, U.S. Department of Health and Human Services, 1982.

1b. Waller JA: Injury Control: A Guide to the Causes and Prevention of Trauma. Lexington, Mass, Heath, 1985, pp 1–60.

2. Baker JP, O'Neill B, Karpf RS: The Injury Fact Book. Lexington, Mass, Heath, 1984.
3. Foege WH, Baker SP, Davis JH, et al: Epidemiology of injuries: The need for more adequate data. In Grossblatt N (ed): Injury in America. Washington, National Academy Press, 1985, pp 25–36.
4. Withers BF, Baker JP: Epidemiology and prevention of injuries. Emerg Med Clin North Am 2:701–715, 1984.
5. Reyna TM, Maj NC, Hollis HW, et al: Alcohol-related trauma. Ann Surg 201:194–197, 1985.

5a. Centers for Disease Control: Quarterly table reporting alcohol involvement in fatal motor vehicle crashes. MMWR 40:187–188, 1991.

6. Baker SP, Dietz PE: The epidemiology and prevention of injuries. In Zuidema DG, Rutherford RB, Ballinger WF (eds): The Management of Trauma. Philadelphia, WB Saunders Co, 1979, pp 794–821.
7. Foege WH, Baker SP, Davis JH, et al: Injury: Magnitude and characteristics of the problem. In Grossblatt N (ed): Injury in America. Washington, National Academy Press, 1985, pp 1–18.
8. Nahum AM, Melvin J: The Biomechanisms of Trauma. Norwalk, Conn, Appleton-Century-Crofts, 1985, pp 1–30.
9. Cowley RA, Dunham CM: Shock Trauma/Critical Care Manual. Baltimore, University Park Press, 1982.

9a. Weigelt JA, Klein JD: Mechanism of injury. In Mancini B, Klein JD (eds): Decision Making in Trauma Management. Philadelphia, BC Decker, 1991, pp 1–4.

10. Halpern JS: Patterns of trauma. J Emerg Nurs 8:170–175, 1982.
11. Zuidema GD, Cameron JL, Sabatier HS: Initial evaluation and resuscitation of the injured patient. In Zuidema GD, Rutherford RB, Ballinger WF (eds): The Management of Trauma. Philadelphia, WB Saunders Co, 1979, pp 1–27.
12. Golden T, Fisher JC, Edgerton MT: "Wringer arm" reevaluated: A survey of current surgical management of upper extremity compression injuries. Ann Surg 177:362–369, 1970.
13. Hess RL, Weber K, Melvin JW: Review of the literature and regulation relating to head impact tolerance and injury criteria. The University of Michigan Highway Safety Research Institute Report No. UM-HSRI-80-52-1. Springfield, Va, National Technical Information Service (PB81-123101), 1980.
14. King A: Survey of the state of the art of human biodynamics response. In Saczalski K, Singley GT, Pilkey WD, Huston RL (eds): Aircraft Crashworthiness. Charlottesville, University of Virginia Press, 1975, pp 83–120.
15. Kroell CK, Gadd CW, Schneider DC: Biomechanics in crash injury research. In Proceedings of the 19th International ISA Aerospace Instrumentation Symposium. Pittsburgh, Instrument Society of America, 1973, pp 199–219.

16. Smith GS, Coleman P: Unintentional injuries: Intervention strategies and their potential for reducing human losses. Presented at the "Closing the Gap" Health Policy Consultation, November 26–28, at the Carter Center of Emory University, Atlanta, Ga, 1984, p 129.
17. Snyder RG: Impact. In Parker JF, West VR (eds): Bioastronautics Data Book. NASA Publication No. SP-3006. Washington, National Aeronautics and Space Administration, 1973, pp 221–296.
18. Stapp JP: Whole body tolerance to impact. In Altman PL, Dittmer DS (eds): Environmental Biology. Bethesda, Md, Federation of American Societies for Experimental Biology, 1966, pp 228–230.
19. Staff JP: Voluntary human tolerance levels. In Gurdjian ES, Lange WA, Patrick LM, Thomas LM (eds): Impact Injury and Crash Protection. Springfield, Ill, Charles C Thomas, 1970, pp 308–351.
20. States JD: Case studies of racing accidents. In Proceedings of 8th Stapp Car Crash Conference, Society of Automotive Engineers. Warrendale, Pa, Society of Automotive Engineers, 1968, pp 251–258.
21. Von Gierke HE, Brinkley JW: Impact accelerations. In Calvin M, Gazenko OG (eds): Foundations of Space Biology and Medicine: Ecological and Physiological Bases of Space Biology and Medicine, vol II, book 1. Washington, National Aeronautics and Space Administration, 1975, pp 214–246.
22. Davis JE, Mason CB: Neurologic Critical Care. New York, Van Nostrand Reinhold, 1979, pp 101–110.
23. Maull KI, Whitley RE, Cardea JA: Vertical deceleration injuries. Surg Gynecol Obstet 153:233–236, 1981.
24. Foege WH, Baker SP, Davis JH, et al: Injury biomechanics research and the prevention of impact injury. In Grossblatt N (ed): Injury in America. Washington, National Academy Press, 1985, pp 48–64.
25. Rockwood CA, Green DP: Fractures. Philadelphia, JB Lippincott, 1975.
26. Kenner C, Guzzetta CE, Dossey B: Critical Care Nursing: Body—Mind—Spirit. Boston, Little, Brown, 1981, pp 627–642.
27. Jagger J, Levine JJ, Jane JA, Rimel RW: Epidemiologic features of head injury in a predominantly rural population. J Trauma 24:40–44, 1984.
28. Gikas PW: Mechanism of injury in automobile crashes. Clin Neurosurg 19:175–190, 1972.
29. Trunkey DD: Force in blunt trauma. In Trunkey DD, Lewis FR (eds): Current Therapy of Trauma—2. Burlington, Ontario, BC Decker, 1986, pp 102–104.
30. Gennarelli TA, Thibault LE: Biomechanics of acute subdural hematoma. J Trauma 22:680–686, 1982.
31. Young HA, Schmidek HH: Complications accompanying occipital skull fractures. J Trauma 22:914–920, 1982.
32. Walker AE, Ray CD, Laws ER, et al: Injuries of the head and spinal cord. In Zuidema GD, Rutherford RB, Ballinger WF (eds): The Management of Trauma. Philadelphia, WB Saunders Co, 1979, pp 181–253.
33. Bucholz RW: Unstable hangman's fractures. Clin Orthop 154:119–124, 1981.
34. Harkess JW: Principles of fractures and dislocations. In Rockwood CA, Green DP (eds): Fractures. Philadelphia, JB Lippincott, 1975, pp 1–90.
35. Hughes JL: Initial management of fractures and joint injuries: Thoracic and lumbar spine, pelvis and hip. In Zuidema GD, Rutherford RB, Ballinger WF (eds): The Management of Trauma. Philadelphia, WB Saunders Co, 1979, pp 610–625.
36. Mucha P: Recognizing and avoiding complications with pelvic fractures. Infect Surg, January:53–62, 1985.
37. Richardson JD, Harty J, Amin M, Flint LM: Open pelvic fractures. J Trauma 22:533–538, 1982.
38. Registad A: Traumatic dislocation of the hip. J Trauma 20:603–606, 1980.
39. Rouhana SW, Lau IV, Ridella SA: Influence of velocity and forced compression on the severity of abdominal injury in blunt, nonpenetrating lateral impct. J Trauma 25:490–500, 1985.
40. Lau VK, Viano DC: Influence of impact velocity on the severity of nonpenetrating hepatic injury. J Trauma 21:115–123, 1981.
41. Dolan WD, Gifford RW, Smith RJ, et al: Automobile-related injuries. JAMA 249:3216–3221, 1983.
42. Swan KG, Swan RC: Gunshot Wounds—Pathophysiology and Management. Littleton, Mass, PSG Publishing Co, 1980.
43. O'Day J, Scott R: Safety belt use: Ejection and entrapment. Health Educ Q 11:141–146, 1984.
44. DeHaven H: Mechanical analysis of survival in falls from heights of fifty to one hundred and fifty feet. War Med 2:586, 1942.
45. Newman RJ: A prospective evaluation of the protective effect of car seatbelts. J Trauma 26:561–564, 1986.
46. Wild BR, Kenwright J, Rastoji S: Effects of seat belts on injuries to front and rear seat passengers. Br Med J 290:1621–1623, 1985.
47. Denis R, Allard M, Atlas H, Farkouh E: Changing trends with abdominal injury in seatbelt wearers. J Trauma 231:1007–1008, 1983.
48. Williams JS, Kirkpatrick JR: The nature of seat belt injuries. J Trauma 11:207–218, 1971.
49. Woelfel GF, Moore EE, Cogbill TH, Van Way CW: Severe thoracic and abdominal injuries associated with lap-harness seatbelts. J Trauma 24:166–167, 1984.
50. Huelke DF, Gikas PW: Causes of deaths in automobile accidents. JAMA 203:1100–1107, 1968.
51. Anderson CB, Ballinger WF: Abdominal injuries. In Zuidema GD, Rutherford RB, Ballinger WF (eds): The Management of Trauma. Philadelphia, WB Saunders Co, 1979, pp 429–482.
52. Dajee H, Richardson IW, Iype MO: Seat belt aorta: Acute dissection and thrombosis of the abdominal aorta. Surgery 85:263–267, 1979.
53. Haddon W, Baker SP: Injury control. In Clark D, MacMahon B (eds): Preventive Medicine and Public Health. Boston, Little, Brown, 1981, pp 109–140.
54. Insurance Institute for Highway Safety: Background Manual on the Passive Restraint Issue. Washington, Insurance Institute for Highway Safety, Watergate 600, 1977.
55. Golladay ES, Slezak JW, Mollitt DL, Seibert RW: The three wheeler: A menace to the preadolescent child. J Trauma 25:232–233, 1985.
56. Lukas GM, Hutton JE, Lim RC, Mathewson C: Injuries sustained from high velocity impact with water: An experience from the Golden Gate bridge. J Trauma 21:612–618, 1981.
57. Champion HR, Sacco WJ, Hunt TK: Trauma severity scoring to predict mortality. World J Surg 7:4–11, 1983.
58. Graeber GM, Belville WD, Sepulveda RA: A safe model for creating blunt and penetrating ballistic injury. J Trauma 21:473–476, 1981.
59. Ordog GJ, Wasserberger J, Balasubramanium S: Wound ballistics: Theory and practice. Ann Emerg Med 13:1113–1122, 1984.
60. Janzon B, Seeman T: Muscle devitalization in high-energy missile wounds, and its dependence on energy transfer. J Trauma 25:138–144, 1985.
61. Fackler ML: Wound ballistics. In Trunkey DD, Lewis FR (eds): Current Therapy of Trauma—2. Burlington, Ontario, BC Decker, 1986, pp 94–101.
62. Deitch EA, Grimes WR: Experience with 112 shotgun wounds of the extremities. J Trauma 24:600–603, 1984.
63. Flint LM, Cryer HM, Howard DA, Richardson JD: Approaches to the management of shotgun injuries. J Trauma 24:415–419, 1984.
64. Hunt JL, Purdue GF: Shotgun injuries at Parkland Memorial Hospital. Presented at Current Topics in General Surgery Postgraduate Course, Maui, Hawaii, April 1986, pp 166–173.
65. Sherman R, Parrish A: Management of shotgun injuries: A review of 152 cases. J Trauma 3:76–86, 1963.
66. Bowsher WG, Smith WP: Severe facial injury by impalement. J Trauma 24:999–1000, 1984.
67. Horowitz MD, Dove DB, Eismont M, Green BA: Impalement injuries. J Trauma 25:914–916, 1985.
68. Ketterhagan JP, Wassermann DH: Impalement injuries: The preferred approach. J Trauma 23:258–259, 1983.
69. Crapo RO: Smoke-inhalation injuries. JAMA 246:1694–1696, 1981.
70. Fein A, Leff A, Hopewell PC: Pathophysiology and management of the complications resulting from fire and the inhaled

products of combustion: Review of the literature. Crit Care Med 8:94–98, 1980.
71. Herndon DN, Traber DL, Niehaus GD, et al: The pathophysiology of smoke inhalation injury in a sheep model. J Trauma 24:1044–1051, 1984.
72. Klabacha M, Nelson H, Parshley P, et al: Carburetor priming: A cause of gasoline burn. J Trauma 25:1096–1098, 1985.
73. Purdue GF, Hunt JL, Layton TR, et al: Burns in motor vehicle accidents. J Trauma 25:216–219, 1985.
74. Owen-Smith M: Bullet wounds: Explosive blast injuries. In Hughes S (ed): The Basis and Practice of Traumatology. Rockville, Md, Aspen Systems, 1983, pp 80–91.
75. Greenspan L, McLellan BA, Greig H: Abbreviated injury scale and injury severity score: A scoring chart. J Trauma 25:60–64, 1985.
76. Champion HR, Sacco WJ, Carnazzo AJ, et al: Trauma score. Crit Care Med 9:672–676, 1981.
77. Committee on Medical Aspects of Automotive Safety: Rating the severity of tissue damage: I. The abbreviated scale. JAMA 125:277–280, 1971.
78. Cullen DJ, Keene R, Waternaux C, Peterson H: Objective quantitative measurement of severity of illness in critically-ill patients. Crit Care Med 12:155–160, 1984.
79. Goris RJA: The injury severity score. World J Surg 7:12–18, 1983.
80. Knaus WA, Draper EA, Wagner DP, Zimmerman JE: APACHE II: A severity of disease classification system. Crit Care Med 13:818–829, 1985.
81. Ornato J, Mlinek EJ, Craren EJ, Nelson N: Ineffectiveness of the trauma score and the CRAMS scale for accurately triaging patients to trauma centers. Ann Emerg Med 14:1061–1064, 1985.
82. American Association for Automotive Medicine: The Abbreviated Injury Scale (AIS)—1985 Revision. Des Plaines, Ill, AAAM, 1985.
83. Abbreviated injury scale (AIS): 1985 Revision, Joint Committee on Injury Scaling. Arlington Heights, Ill, AAAM, 1985.
84. Goldberg JL, Goldberg J, Levy PS, et al: Measuring the severity of injury: The validity of the revised estimated survival probability index. J Trauma 24:420–427, 1984.
85. Jonah BA, Grant BA: Long-term effectiveness of selective traffic enforcement programs for increasing seat belt use. J Appl Psychol 70:257–261, 1985.
86. Cardona VD: Trauma Nursing. Montvale, NJ, Medical Economics, 1985, pp 233–244.
87. Decker MD, Dewey MJ, Hutcheson RH, Schaffner W: The use and efficacy of child restraint devices. JAMA 252:2571–2575, 1984.
88. Robertson LS: Highway injury. Texas Med 79:48–50, 1983.
89. Foege WH, Baker SP, Davis JH, et al: Prevention of injury. In Grossblatt N (ed): Injury in America. Washington, National Academy Press, 1985, pp 37–47.
90. The National Committee for Injury Prevention and Control: Injury Prevention: Meeting the Challenge. New York, Oxford University Press, 1989.

8

PATHOPHYSIOLOGY OF TRAUMATIC SHOCK AND MULTIPLE ORGAN SYSTEM FAILURE

THOMAS C. VARY and MARGUERITE T. LITTLETON KEARNEY

Shock, as clinically encountered, is the hemodynamic manifestation of cellular metabolic insufficiency, resulting from either inadequate cellular perfusion or a basic biochemical inability to utilize oxygen and other nutrients. Therefore, the basic clinical presentation can be either a cause or an effect of this hemodynamic disturbance. In *nonseptic shock*, the initial insult is generally a loss of cellular perfusion, which leads to cellular injury and, if allowed to persist, can result in an irreversible cellular structural and metabolic damage. In *septic shock*, the initial insult is believed to be at the cellular level, most likely resulting from an overwhelming inflammatory response initiated by bacterial invasion or activation of host-defense systems.

The etiologies of shock can be broadly placed into three categories: alteration in circulating volume, alteration in cardiac pump function, and alteration in peripheral vascular resistance. The most common cause of loss of circulating volume is hemorrhage. The response to hemorrhage will be covered in detail later. In addition to hemorrhage, there are a number of other conditions that result in inadequate intravascular volume leading to a shock state. In severe burns, loss of fluids and electrolytes through denuded areas results in enormous on-going losses of plasma volume. In addition to the decreased plasma volume, concentration of red blood cells increases the viscosity of the blood, which further alters cellular perfusion. Furthermore, conditions such as intestinal obstruction, which cause third-space sequestration of fluid without adequate volume replacement, can lead to decreased cardiac output with the development of shock as a consequence. High serum glucose levels can act as an osmotic agent, pulling fluids and electrolytes into the vascular compartment. This circulating volume is then lost via the urine. The result parallels that of dehydration via excessive sweating. Circulating volume is reduced, venous return decreases, cardiac output falls, and a shock state ensues.

While fluid loss represents a major process in the development of some shock states, in other conditions shock occurs without any decrease in the absolute plasma fluid volume through altered vascular tone. For example, in neurogenic shock, depression of the central nervous system results in a loss of vasomotor control, with pooling of blood in the systemic circulation. The decreased vascular tone causes a reduction in peripheral vascular resistance, which leads to inadequate venous return. The reduction of preload decreases end-diastolic fiber volume, which in turn reduces the cardiac output. Hence tissue perfusion is impaired. Neurogenic shock may be induced by deep general or spinal anesthesia or by brain damage, particularly in the basal regions near the vasomotor center. Spinal shock is seen when high cervical spinal cord injury occurs close to the sympathetic spinal ganglia outflow tracts (usually above T1), destroying the ability of the sympathetic nervous system to initiate reflex vasoconstriction. Consequently, the body is unable to vasoconstrict the peripheral vasculature. Altered peripheral vascular resistance is also responsible for anaphylatic shock. Anaphylactic shock occurs in some people following bee stings. In this situation, the body reacts to the foreign substance by activating the immune system against the antigen. The inflammatory responses to the antigen–antibody reactions directly damage the endothelial lining of the blood vessels, increasing vascular permeability. More important, the antigen–antibody reactions induce the release of histamine or histamine-like substances, which possess vasodilatory properties. Histamines increase vascular capacity through venodilation, reduce arterial pressure by dilating arterioles, and increase capillary permeability, promoting a rapid shift of fluids into the interstitial spaces. Both neurogenic and anaphylactic shock can be treated acutely by the rapid administration of norepinephrine or epinephrine, which vasoconstricts blood vessels, increases venous return, and increases myocardial contractility.

In shock states secondary to cardiac pump failure, the underlying pathogenesis of the disease is related primarily to the failure of the myocardium to adequately pump blood to the systemic circulation. This form of shock may be associated with heart failure, acute myocardial infarction, end-stage valvular disease, or severe pulmonary hypertension. Most often cardiogenic shock results from acute myocardial infarction. As perfusion to the heart muscle is reduced due to blockade of the major coronary arteries (commonly the left anterior descending), the myocardium loses the ability to adequately pump blood through the systemic vascular tree. Cardiac output falls drastically along with systemic tissue perfusion.

Trauma without acute hemorrhage may induce a shock state. Severe contusion or crushing damage to soft tissues often is sufficient to allow sequestration of blood and plasma in the interstitial spaces of the injured tissues. The resultant depletion of the effective circulating volume initiates a hypovolemia. The fall in cardiac output which accompanies the decrease in venous return may be succeeded by hypotension and shock. The hypotension may not become evident until the patient's position is changed for diagnostic procedures such as chest x-rays because the body may have compensated for the moderate volume loss. Furthermore, the pain associated with severe multiple trauma inhibits the vasomotor center in the brain, thereby dilating the peripheral vasculature and hindering the already compromised venous return.

COMPENSATORY CHANGES DUE TO HEMORRHAGE

Hemorrhage, regardless of its cause, results in a general pattern of bodily responses, or compensations, which is an attempt to stabilize a life-threatening situation. A small volume of blood (approximately 10 per cent of the total blood volume) can be removed without any significant effect on arterial blood pressure or cardiac output. Blood loss greater than 10 per cent initiates a powerful response designed to maintain blood flow to critical vital organs until restoration of the circulating fluid can occur either by volume replacement of blood and fluid during resuscitation or through a redistribution of fluid volumes in the body. As blood losses become greater than 10 to 15 per cent of the total blood volume, cardiac output diminishes due to decreased venous return. Venous return, a major contributor to the preload, determines the blood volume in the ventricles prior to contraction. A directly proportional relationship exists between preload and stroke volume. Consequently, a reduction in stroke volume leads to diminished cardiac output. The failure of cardiac output to be maintained leads to a fall in arterial pressure which is observed as hypotension. Hemorrhagic loss of more than 40 per cent of the total blood volume precipitates such a profound fall in the cardiac output that the body's ability to compensate is overwhelmed. Inaudible blood pressure, extreme tachycardia, and a nonresponsive patient are hallmarks of this stage of shock.

The shock episode can be divided into three major phases: compensatory stage, progressive stage, and irreversible stage. In the compensatory stage, tissue perfusion is altered, but cardiovascular deterioration is prevented by compensatory mechanisms. This stage of shock is reversible. During the progressive stage, the hypovolemia has progressed to a point of cardiovascular collapse, leading to a potentially vicious cycle that eventually leads to death if allowed to persist. In the irreversible stage, the organism becomes increasingly refractory to blood replacement. Eventually, all present forms of therapy are inadequate to save the individual, even though the person may still be alive at that point.

Circulatory Reflexes

The circulatory reflexes triggered by acute hemorrhage are designed to restore arterial pressure and blood volume toward normal and prevent the demise of the individual. An integrated response to blood losses greater than 10 per cent of the total blood volume is initiated by the baroreceptors, which respond to the fall in blood pressure, and by the atrial type B receptors, which respond to a fall in blood volume. Hypotension reduces the level of carotid and aortic baroreceptor afferent discharges, which normally inhibit the vasomotor center. In addition, the carotid artery chemoreceptors respond to decreases in the blood pH and a rise in P_{CO_2}. Activation of the carotid body chemoreceptors stimulates the vasomotor center (Figs. 8–1 and 8–2). The net effect of the response of the baroreceptors and carotid artery receptors is an increased sympathetic discharge by the medullary vasomotor center. The increased sympathetic discharge is carried over the sympathetic efferents to the heart, peripheral arterioles, and adrenals. At the level of the heart, increased sympathetic discharge has a positive inotropic effect that augments contractility. This ensures a more efficient ventricular emptying, manifested by an increased ejection fraction. The improved myocardial performance results from the direct release of catecholamines at the cardiac sympathetic nerve endings in the proximity of the myocardial β-receptors and by vasomotor center inhibition of vagal parasympathetic outflow. This change in the balance between the sympathetic and parasympathetic pathways increases atrial pacemaker activity and reduces atrioventricular conduction time, promoting an increased heart rate. Increased arteriolar constriction results in a redistribution of blood flow away from nonvital organs such as skin and skeletal muscle. If the cause of the hypovolemia is not corrected, eventually blood flow to the visceral organs will be diminished as well. Despite a reduced blood volume, venous constriction in response to the sympathetic output will tend to enhance venous return and prevent pooling of the blood in the venous circulation. Since the venous system has a capacitance of up to 60 per cent of the circulating volume, venoconstriction can markedly increase venous return, ensuring adequate blood volume for maintenance of myocardial preload. The neuronal homeostatic mechanisms function in a controlled and coordinated manner to restore arterial pressure, thereby preserving myocardial and cerebral blood flow, either by increasing venous return and cardiac output or by increasing peripheral vascular resistance. Hemodynamic compensation by stimulation of the sympathetic nervous system is extremely efficient if the shock state is not allowed to continue for a long period of time and blood and fluid losses do not persist.

Fluid Shifts

To compensate for the reduced circulating blood volume, there is a shift in fluids from extravascular to intravascular spaces. This occurs as a direct result of the decreased intracapillary hydrostatic pressure associated with the loss of blood volume. Normally, the balance between hydrostatic pressure tending to cause fluid to leave the capillary and the plasma oncotic pressure tending to cause fluid to be reabsorbed by the capillary favors a small net loss of fluid into the interstitial space. In a shock state, the reduction of blood pressure decreases the capillary hydrostatic pressure, decreasing filtration. The net effect is increased fluid volume in

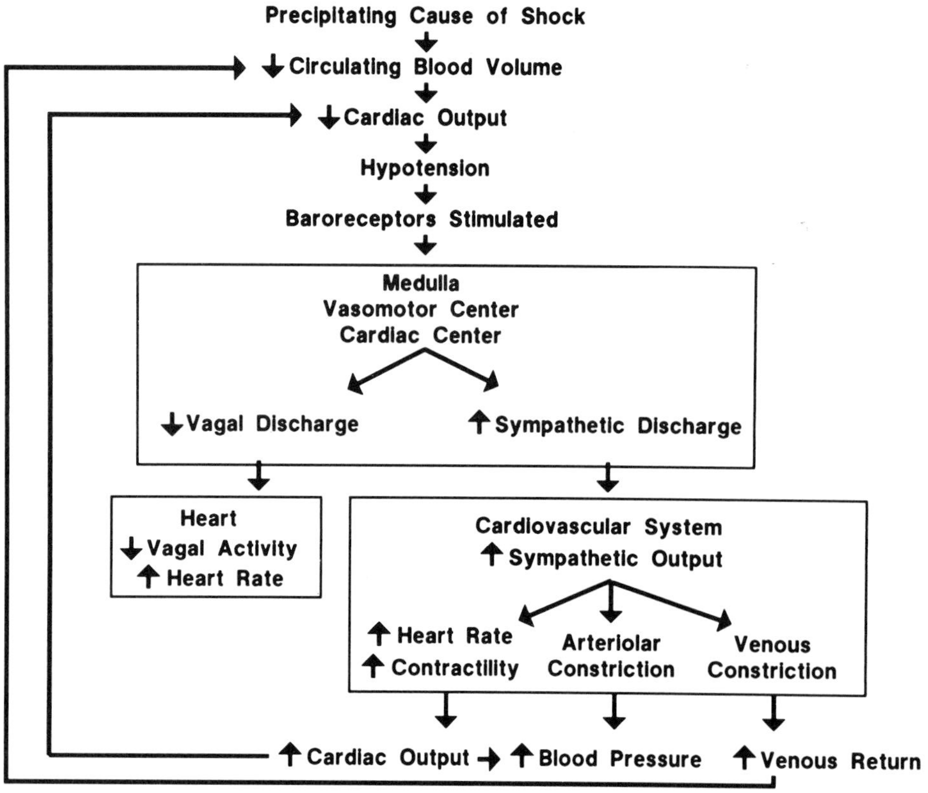

Figure 8–1. Compensatory mechanisms for the restoration of circulatory blood volume.

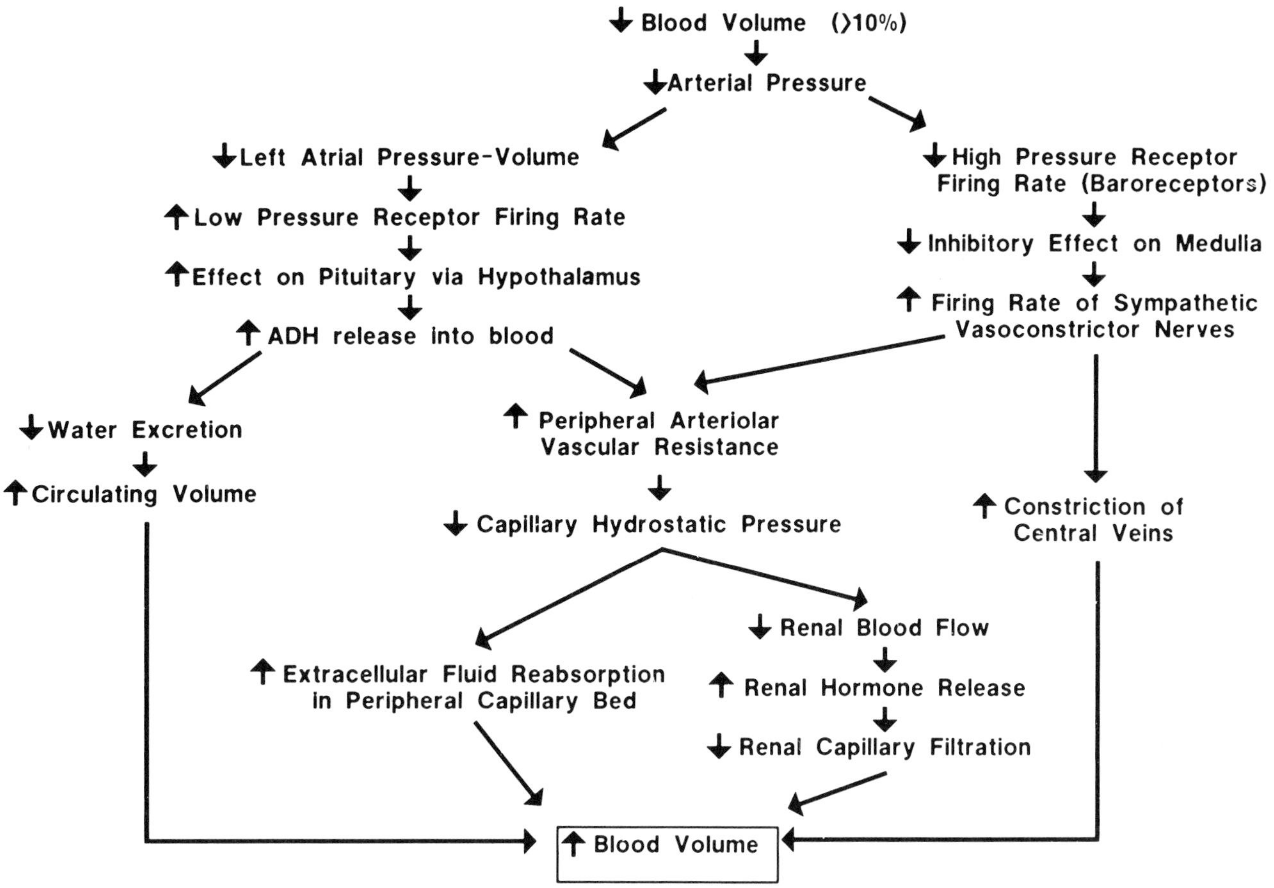

Figure 8–2. Compensatory mechanisms following loss of greater than 10 per cent of blood volume.

the capillary and enhanced vascular volume. The reduced venous pressure and arteriolar vasoconstriction are separate factors contributing to the reduced capillary pressure and outward fluid movement into the vascular compartment. This compensatory mechanism depends on the individual's hydration. Adequate hydration allows for better compensation.

Reduction in renal blood flow initiates efferent renal arteriolar vasoconstriction. Stimulation of the juxtaglomerular apparatus secondary to reduced renal blood flow ensues the subsequent release of renin. Renin is converted to angiotensin II by the endothelial cells of the lung. Angiotensin II, a potent vasoconstrictor, helps to increase arterial pressure and stimulates aldosterone secretion by the adrenal cortex. Aldosterone improves blood volume by decreasing water and salt excretion by the kidneys. The responses to hypovolemia can occur within seconds, as with the increased sympathetic discharge, or require days, as with the kidney-mediated changes in water and salt excretion. All the mechanisms result in an increased circulating blood volume from the low levels during hypovolemia back toward normal.

Limits of Compensation

The blood loss can be so severe that the compensatory mechanisms cannot restore the system to normal. If the hemorrhage is not arrested and/or volume replacement is insufficient, cardiovascular deterioration begins. When the arterial pressure falls low enough, coronary blood flow decreases below that required for adequate delivery of oxygen to the myocardium. The end result is deterioration of heart function. Decreased ventricular performance resulting from ischemia secondary to low perfusion pressures decreases cardiac output, further lowering arterial pressure. A positive-feedback cycle begins to develop, whereby the initial hypovolemia leads to dire consequences (Fig. 8–3). As cardiac output diminishes, cerebral blood flow is also reduced, as evidenced by a patient who becomes increasingly more obtunded. Eventually, blood flow to the vasomotor center of the medulla becomes so depressed that the vasomotor center becomes progressively less active and finally fails. Without adequate sympathetic activity, the peripheral vasculature is no longer able to maintain its vascular tone. Consequently, vasodilation and vascular collapse ensue. During this stage, the vascular beds behave more as passive distensible tubes and no longer exhibit active adjustment to circulatory changes. Arterial vasodilation can lead to reduced blood flow to capillary beds in critical organs, while venous dilation causes blood to pool in the veins, decreasing venous return and further reducing cardiac output. Eventually, this sluggish blood flow in the periphery leads to changes in the capillaries such that permeability gradually increases and large volumes of fluid move out of the vascular spaces, further lowering blood volume. Unless these situations are reversed rapidly, survival of the organism is doubtful. Irre-

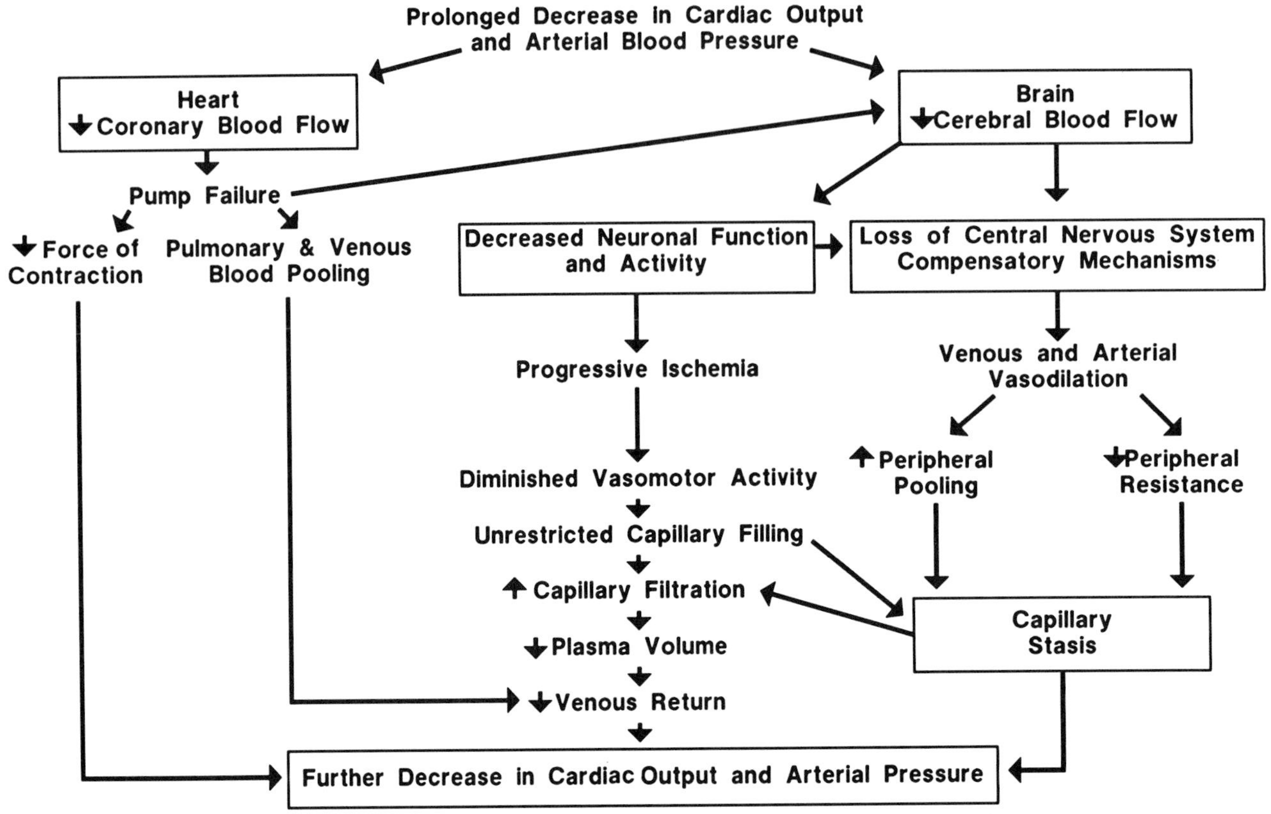

Figure 8–3. Negative effects of prolonged shock following loss of greater than 10 per cent of blood volume.

versible shock occurs when damage to the cells is sufficient to depress metabolic and structural functions. At this point, widespread cellular necrosis occurs in most tissues, leading to organ failure and death.

CELLULAR PATHOPHYSIOLOGY

Diminished blood flow reduces the delivery of oxygen. When oxygen delivery is insufficient to meet the demands of the cell for maintenance of normal function, a relative state of oxygen deficiency exists. This would be manifested by a fall in the oxygen consumption ($\dot{V}O_2$). Normally, not all the oxygen is extracted in a single pass through the organ bed. Therefore, a certain reserve exists, whereby when blood flow is reduced, the tissues can increase the per cent of oxygen extracted from the blood to maintain cellular oxidative metabolism. However, when the decrease in oxygen delivery is severe, cells of the body undergo a known series of changes.[1–7] The earliest stages show contraction of the inner mitochondrial compartment following the decrease in oxidative phosphorylation, followed by clumping of nuclear chromatin associated with the fall in intracellular pH (Fig. 8–4). The fall in oxidative phosphorylation results in a decrease in ATP, which is required for all cellular functioning. This sets the stage for the rest of the cellular response to injury. There is an early redistribution of cellular ions and water, evidenced by swelling of the cisternae of the endoplasmic reticulum. Blebs are seen on the cell surface, perhaps indicating ultrastructural damage. The mitochondria soon begin to shrink and become dense, indicating the degree of biochemical change that is occurring in these cellular energy factories. As the "point of no return" approaches, the mitochondria exhibit large-scale swelling, and many show tiny dense aggregates. Eventually, large flocculent densities appear in the mitochondria, and this event signals the death of that organelle. Nuclear chromatin soon dissolves, and the now swollen lysosomes are suspected of leaking hydrolases, which further destroy the cellular contents. Other changes occur, but it is clear that the original trigger is a loss of oxidative phosphorylation, with all other changes seen as a direct result of this primary event. A fall in oxygen consumption ($\dot{V}O_2$) is therefore an early and definite indicator of trouble, often identifying a potential clinical problem before it is clinically evident.

ENERGY METABOLISM

Normal Metabolism

Maintenance of normal cellular structure and function depends on the cell's ability to synthesize large amounts of energy. The energy requirements of different cells and organs vary depending on their functions. Continuous demands for energy are dictated by cellular and subcellular membrane ion pumps necessary to maintain the internal cellular environment; by the rate of protein synthesis, especially in cells with

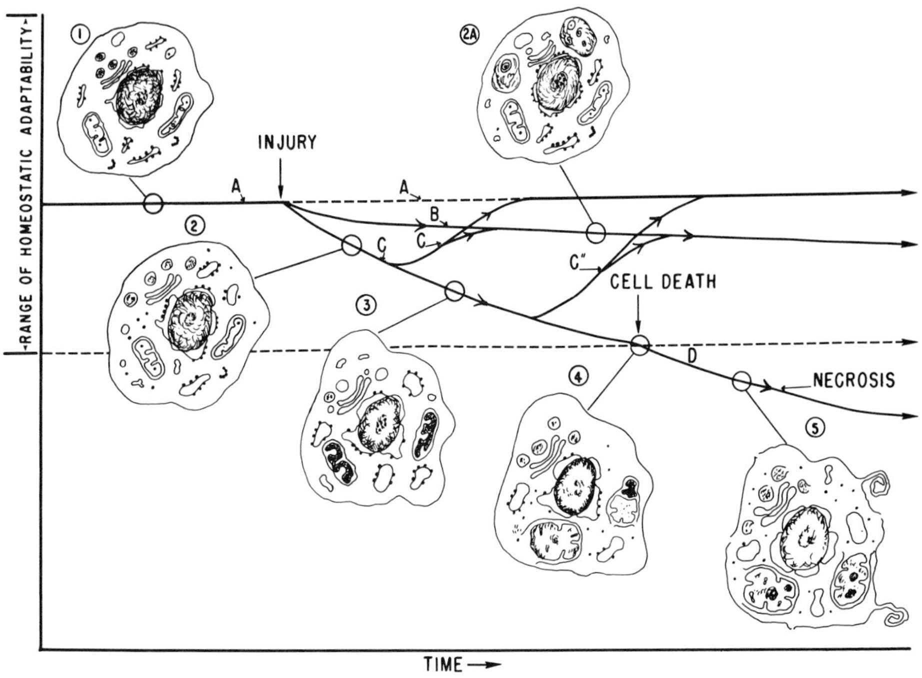

Figure 8–4. Diagram of the stages of cellular disorganization as a result of injury. The reversible field includes those stages from which the cell can recover to normal after removal of the insult. The irreversible field includes stages after cell death when removal of the insult no longer permits recovery. (From Trump BF, Valigorsky JM, Dees JH, et al: Cellular change in human disease. A new method of pathological analysis. Human Pathol 4:89, 1973.)

a high rate of protein turnover; and by mechanical work such as muscle contraction in cardiac and skeletal muscle (Fig. 8–5). The energy reserves of the cell are limited, and the demand for energy is generally derived from the continual catabolism of various fuels, particularly glucose and fatty acids. The energy derived from metabolism of these fuels is stored in the form of adenosine triphosphate (ATP). ATP is synthesized by the phosphorylation of adenosine diphosphate (ADP) via three processes: oxidative phosphorylation, utilizing the mitochondrial electron-transport chain; substrate phosphorylation; and conversion of creatine phosphate to creatine, with the synthesis of ATP and ADP catalyzed by the enzyme creatine phosphokinase. By far, oxidative phosphorylation is the most important pathway for ATP synthesis, accounting for as much as 95 per cent of the total ATP production over a wide range of ATP utilization rates.

Oxidative phosphorylation involves the utilization of energy derived from the transfer of electrons from NADH and FADH to molecular oxygen for the synthesis of ATP and ADP (Fig. 8–6). For each molecule of oxygen consumed, 6 moles of ATP are synthesized from ADP. In well-oxygenated tissues, the rate of oxidative phosphorylation and oxygen consumption is tightly coupled to the rate of ATP utilization. Mitochondrial ATP synthesis depends on a continuous supply of oxygen and substrates. Tissues cannot store oxygen; hence effective perfusion is necessary to provide sufficient delivery of oxygen for maintenance of adequate ATP production. Thus any condition that compromises oxygen delivery to the tissues would tend to alter the mitochondrial capability to synthesize ATP via oxidative phosphorylation.

Metabolic Changes in Impaired Oxygen Delivery

It is important to differentiate anoxia, hypoxia, and ischemia. Although all three conditions result in diminished oxygen delivery to the tissues, the causes and consequences of each condition with regard to energy metabolism are

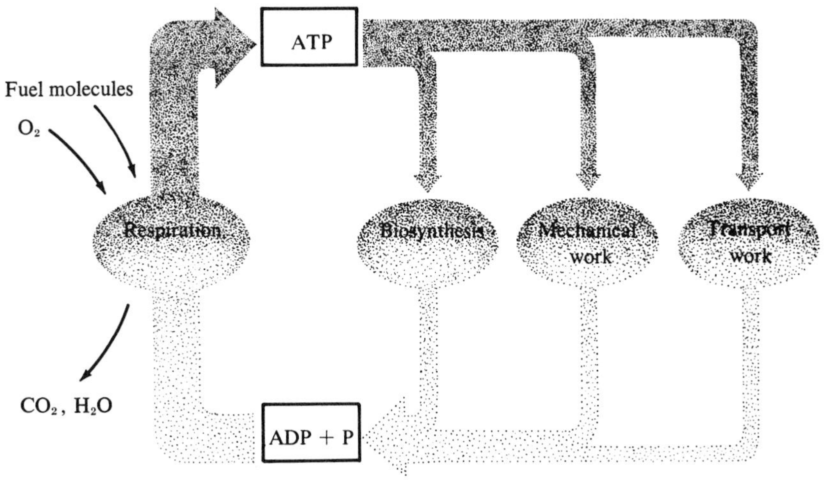

Figure 8–5. Relationship between energy production and energy utilization in maintenance of normal cell function. (From Lehninger AL: Bioenergetics, 2nd ed. Menlo Park, Calif., Benjamin, 1971, p 13.)

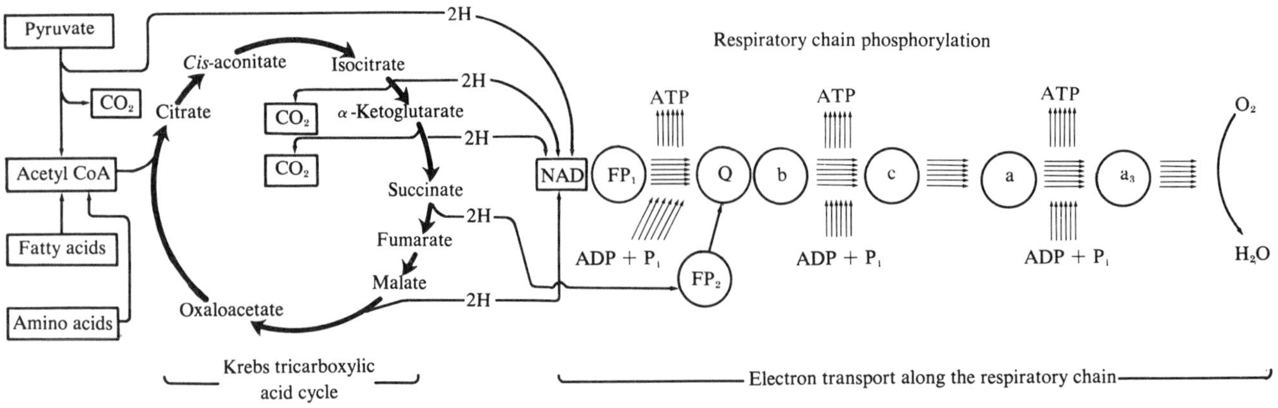

Figure 8–6. Flowsheet for oxidation of carbohydrates, fatty acids, and amino acids in mitochondria. (FP, FP_2) designate NADH and succinate dehydrogenases; (Q) coenzyme Q; (b, c, a, and a_3) designate cytochromes. (From Lehninger AL: Bioenergetics, 2nd ed. Menlo Park, Calif., Benjamin, 1971, p 74.)

different.[8] In the strict sense, *anoxia* is defined as an absence of oxygen, with blood flow either normal or increased. In *hypoxia*, the arterial oxygen content is decreased, but blood flow is normal. *Ischemia* is defined as a decreased blood flow resulting in diminished oxygen delivery. Ischemia differs from anoxia and hypoxia in that blood flow is curtailed. The consequence of this diminished blood flow, in addition to decreased oxygen delivery, is a decreased washout of the ischemic tissue leading to a buildup of potentially harmful metabolic products.[8, 9] An ischemic condition may exist when (1) blood flow falls below that required to meet the normal energy needs at rest or (2) blood flow fails to increase in response to an increased oxidative demand.

Normally, tissues do not extract all the available oxygen as blood passes through the organ. Cardiac muscle, for example, extracts 75 per cent of the available arterial oxygen. Therefore, with a small reduction in coronary flow, essentially all the available oxygen would be extracted from the arterial supply. At this point, oxygen delivery becomes rate-limiting for oxidative metabolism. Thus oxygen availability is the most important determinant of viable oxidative energy metabolism.

A reduction in oxygen delivery results in several characteristic changes. A decline in blood flow results in a greater extraction of arterial oxygen. When oxygen delivery becomes rate-limiting for oxidative metabolism, a linear relationship exists between oxygen consumption and flow, and oxygen delivery limits oxygen uptake (Fig. 8–7). The reduction in oxygen availability leaves intermediates in the electron-transport chain in a reduced state, and phosphorylation of ADP via oxidative phosphorylation ceases despite reduced ATP and increased ADP concentrations (Fig. 8–8). Creatine phosphate concentrations decline by 80 to 90 per cent within minutes, followed by a slower decline in ATP.[8–13]

This imbalance between energy production and energy utilization results in altered adenine nucleotide metabolism. Initially, high-energy phosphates stored as creatine phosphate are utilized to maintain cellular ATP concentrations near normal. However, the amount of high-energy phosphates the cell can store is limited, and creatine phosphate concentrations are depleted within 5 minutes of the onset of ischemia. Following the depletion of creatine phosphate, ATP concentrations begin to fall. The reduction in ATP concentrations is accompanied by a rise in ADP and AMP. As the duration of ischemia is increased, this alteration becomes more pronounced. In addition, there is a fall in the total sum on the adenine nucleotides (ATP + ADP + AMP). The concentration of adenine nucleotides may be of importance in maintaining cell viability, as well as in the ability of the cell to recover normal function following restoration of normal blood flow[8–13] (Fig. 8–9).

During ischemia, the breakdown of ATP for cellular metabolic needs leads to relatively high cellular concentra-

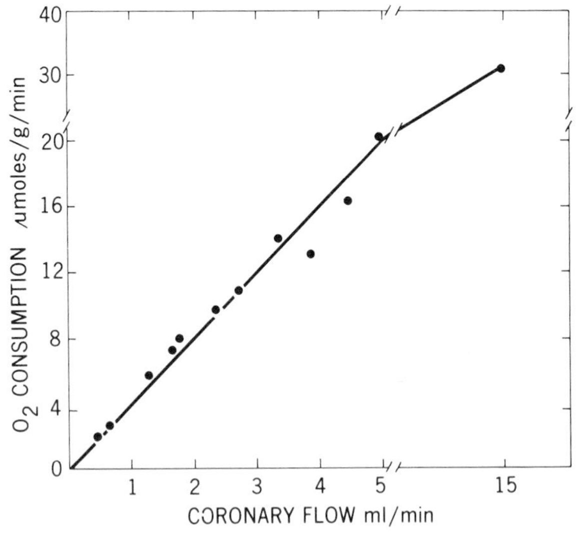

Figure 8–7. Effect of coronary flow on oxygen consumption in isolated rat hearts. Ischemia was induced in the whole heart by use of a one-way valve in the aortic outflow tract. This prevented retrograde aortic flow during diastole and reduced the perfusion pressure for the coronary arteries but did not alter preload or afterload on the ventricle. Coronary flow decreased initially from 15 to 5 ml/min. As a result, ventricular pressure development began to decrease after about 5 minutes, and coronary flow declined in proportion to the decrease in aortic systolic perfusion pressure. Oxygen consumption was calculated from the arterial–venous difference in P_{O_2} and the coronary flow rate. (From Neely JR, Vary TC, Liedtke AJ: Substrate delivery in ischemic myocardium. In Tillman H, Kubler W, Zebe H (eds): Microcirculation of the Heart. Berlin, Springer-Verlag, 1982, p 121.)

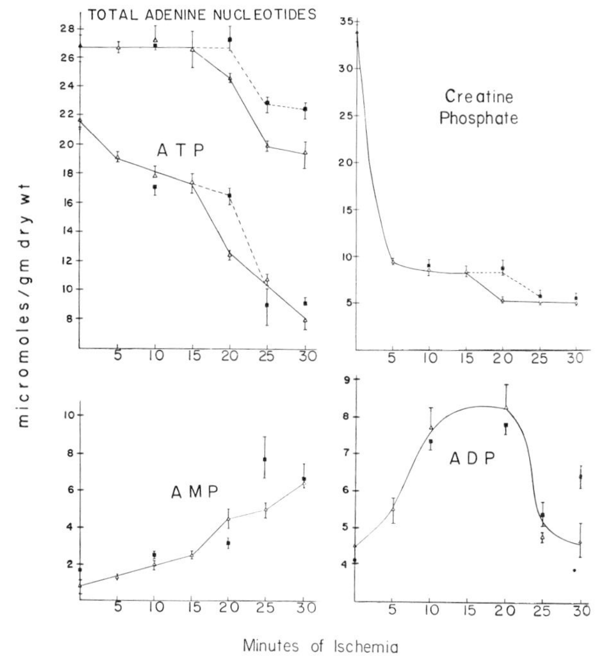

Figure 8–8. Effect of ischemia on tissue adenine nucleotide and creatine phosphate concentrations. Hearts were perfused with Krebs-Henseleit solution, supplemented with either glucose (△) or glucose plus acetate (■) for a 15-minute equilibration period. The hearts were then exposed to the appropriate period of severe global ischemia and rapidly frozen. (Reprinted by permission of the American Heart Association, Inc and Vary TC, Angelakos ET, Schaffer SW: Relationship between adenine nucleotide metabolism and irreversible tissue damage in isolated perfused rat heart. Circ Res 45:220, 1979.)

tions of hypoxanthine and xanthine. Reoxygenation of the ischemic area presents oxygen to the large pools of substrate and the enzyme xanthine oxidase, which is felt to be contained in the capillary endothelium, showering the capillary endothelium of the compromised tissues with superoxide free radicals and overwhelming the capacity of dismutation. Once the initial xanthine oxidase–mediated capillary injury has occurred, complement activation can attract leukocytes to the affected area, resulting in cellular death. This hypothesis has received considerable experimental validation in animal models of myocardial, intestinal, renal, skin, and lung tissue ischemia, with data also appearing on cerebral and hepatic ischemia.

When reduced oxygen supply limits oxidative energy production, ATP produced glycolytically via substrate phosphorylation is increased. In cardiac muscle, the maximal rate of glycolytically produced ATP represents only about 25 per cent of the normal energy requirements. In ischemia, there is a transient increase in glycolysis that results primarily from the breakdown of glycogen. However, if flow is reduced to a low enough level, the transient increase in glycolysis is succeeded by an inhibition of glycolysis to a rate about 10 per cent the rate observed in anoxia (Table 8–1). The mechanism responsible for this difference between ischemia and anoxia appears to be related to the buildup of metabolic products in ischemia. The inhibition of glycolysis in ischemia occurs at the level of the glyceraldehyde-3-phosphate dehydrogenase. Flux through the enzyme is restricted by the accumulation of metabolic products, particularly lactate, which are not removed from the ischemic tissue during poor perfusion.[8–13]

Although oxygen can become rate-limiting for energy production, a reduction in blood flow also decreases the delivery of carbon substrates for oxidative metabolism. A large percentage of the available oxygen is extracted but less than 5 per cent of the carbon substrates are extracted. Therefore, approximately 95 per cent of the available carbon substrates are not extracted, suggesting that there is a tremendous potential availability of carbon substrate, far above the tissue requirements. Hence the decreased supply of carbon substrates in ischemia would never be rate-limiting for their oxidation, except possibly if flow were reduced to zero.[11] A second factor preventing carbon substrates from becoming rate-limiting for energy production is that inhibition of glucose and fatty acid utilization develops secondary to the reduction in flow. In anoxia, the tissues are oxygen deficient, but flow is fast enough to remove metabolic products and prevent glycolytic inhibition. Under these condi-

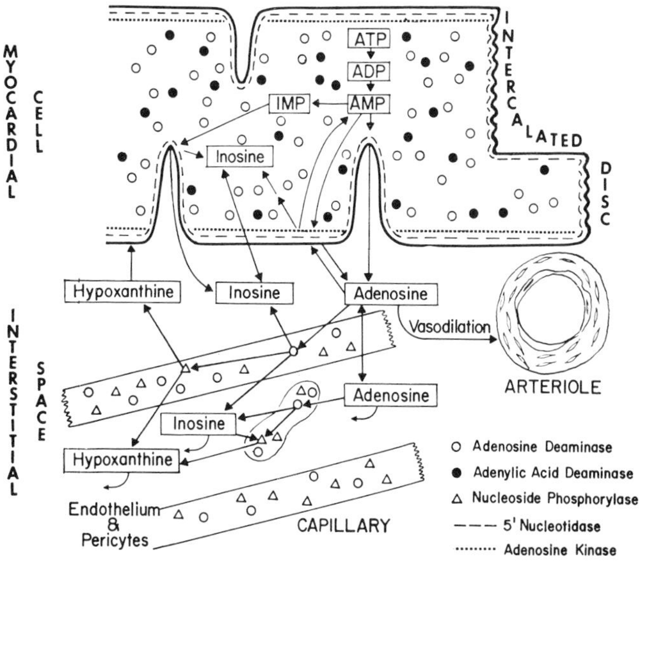

Figure 8–9. Diagram illustrating the formation, fate, and site of action of adenosine. The distribution of the different enzymes involved in the metabolism of adenosine is illustrated by the different symbols defined at the right of the diagram. (From Rubio R, Wiedmier T, Berne RM: Nucleoside phosphorylase: Localization and role in myocardial distribution of purines. Am J Physiol 222:554, 1972.)

TABLE 8–1. EFFECTS OF CORONARY FLOW ON GLUCOSE DELIVERY AND EXTRACTION BY HEART MUSCLE

CONDITION	CORONARY FLOW (ML/MIN/GM DRY WT)	GLUCOSE UTILIZATION (μM/GM DRY WT/MIN)	GLUCOSE DELIVERY (μM/GM DRY WT/MIN)	% EXTRACTION
Rat Heart				
Control	75	4.7 ± 0.7	825	0.6
Ischemic	30	9.6 ± 0.8	330	2.9
	10	7.0 ± 0.6	110	6.4
	3	2.0 ± 0.6	33	6.1
Pig Heart				
Control	8	3.0	42	7.2
Ischemic	3	0.4	16	2.7

Rat hearts were perfused with Krebs-Henseleit bicarbonate buffer containing 11 m*M* glucose and gassed with 95 per cent O_2 : 5 per cent CO_2. In situ pig hearts were made ischemic by cannulation of the left and right coronary arteries and coronary flow was controlled with an external pump. The heart was perfused with whole pig blood containing about 6 m*M* glucose and 0.4 m*M* fatty acid.

From Neely JR, Vary TC, Liedtke AJ: Substrate delivery in ischemic myocardium. In Tillmann H, Kubler W, Zebe H (eds): Microcirculation of the Heart. Berlin, Springer-Verlag, 1982, p 122.

tions, glycolysis is maximally stimulated. However, when flow is reduced (<3 ml/gm/min), glycolysis becomes inhibited. This suggests that glycolytic inhibition during ischemia is more dependent on flow than on oxygen availability. Oxidation of fatty acids is inhibited in proportion to decreased availability and is not flow-dependent other than to the extent that flow affects oxygen delivery (Table 8–2).

ROLE OF ATP IN CELL DAMAGE

Simple oxygen deficiency does not itself cause irreversible tissue damage. If the oxygen supply is restored within several minutes, both ATP synthesis and tissue function return to normal. However, if the reduction in oxygen supply is continued, the tissue becomes irreversibly damaged (Fig. 8–10). Many hypotheses have been put forward to account for this transition of viable to dead cells. Since ATP functions as the energy source, much attention has been focused on the role of ATP in reperfusion. Reperfusion and restoration of oxygen delivery to ischemic tissue result in the rapid resynthesis of creatine phosphate, but ATP concentrations remain depressed. The failure of ATP to be resynthesized can be due either to irreversible damage to the mitochondria such that oxidative phosphorylation cannot occur or to a loss of adenine nucleotides such that the mitochondria matrix concentration of adenine nucleotides limits oxidative metabolism. The depleted adenine nucleotide pool cannot be rapidly replenished by de novo synthesis. It is estimated that only 0.4 per cent of the total adenine nucleotide pool can be replaced per hour by de novo synthesis. While the rate of de novo synthesis of adenine nucleotides is slow, salvage of nucleosides (adenosine) occurs 10 times faster. Adenosine can be rephosphorylated to AMP by adenosine kinase. Increased adenine nucleotide concentrations have been demonstrated in hearts during reperfusion with buffer-containing adenosine following ischemia.

OXYGEN CONSUMPTION

Oxygen consumption ($\dot{V}O_2$) averages approximately 140 ml/m²/min (also calculated as 3.5 ml/kg/min or 250 ml/min in the 70-kg "textbook" man) not only in the normal, healthy individual but also in the afebrile, resting hospitalized patient.[14] This value remains constant, unless hypothermia or

TABLE 8–2. EFFECTS OF CORONARY FLOW ON FATTY ACID DELIVERY AND EXTRACTION

CONDITION	CORONARY FLOW (ML/MIN/GM DRY WT)	FA OXIDATION (μM/GM DRY WT/MIN)	FA DELIVERY (μM/GM DRY WT/MIN)	% EXTRACTION
Rat Heart				
Control	75	0.75 ± 0.1	75	1.0
Ischemic	25	0.55 ± 0.06	25	2.2
	5	0.18 ± 0.04	5	3.6
Pig Heart				
Control	8	0.22	4.2	5.3
Ischemic	3	0.07	1.6	4.5

Rat hearts were perfused with Krebs-Henseleit bicarbonate buffer containing 11 m*M* glucose and 1 m*M* palmitate bound to 3 per cent bovine serum albumin. Pig hearts were perfused with whole pig blood containing about 6 m*M* glucose and 0.4 m*M* fatty acid. Ischemia was induced as described in Table 8–1.

From Neely JR, Vary TC, Liedtke AJ: Substrate delivery in ischemic myocardium. In Tillmann H, Kubler W, Zebe H (eds): Microcirculation of the Heart. Berlin, Springer-Verlag, 1982, p 123.

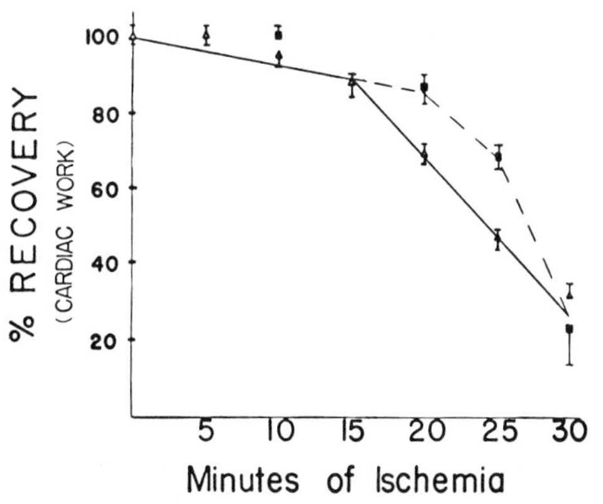

Figure 8–10. Plot of the per cent recovery versus duration of ischemia. Hearts were perfused with Krebs-Henseleit solution, supplemented with either 5 m*M* glucose (△) or 5 m*M* glucose plus 5 m*M* acetate (■) and insulin (2.5×10^{-3} U/ml) for a 15-minute equilibration period, followed by the appropriate period of severe global ischemia. Subsequently, the hearts were perfused under nonischemic conditions for 15 minutes. Coronary flow, coronary output, and aortic pressure were measured both before the induction of ischemia and following the 15-minute reperfusion period. The "per cent recovery" of cardiac work was calculated as the postischemia cardiac output × heart rate product divided by the preischemia cardiac output × heart rate product. Each point represents mean ± SEM of 9 to 12 hearts. (Reprinted by permission of the American Heart Association, Inc and Vary TC, Angelakos ET, Schaffer SW: Relationship between adenine nucleotide metabolism and irreversible tissue damage in isolated perfused rat heart. Circ Res 45:220, 1979.)

hyperthermia changes it (approximately 13 per cent for each degree-centigrade change in body temperature)[15] or sepsis occurs.[14] The normal stress response to trauma, surgery, or well-controlled sepsis is associated with an increase in oxygen consumption of 15 to 35 per cent.[16, 17] In the metabolically imbalanced state of septic multiple organ failure syndrome, however, cellular failures of oxidative metabolism may occur even at high body perfusion and oxygen delivery.[14] In the absence of such toxic metabolic failure, a mismatch between oxygen supply and tissue demand is caused by a reduced oxygen delivery, as in low body perfusion syndromes.[18, 19] Such a condition is encountered throughout the body during hypovolemic or cardiogenic shock or in a localized tissue bed during periods of inflow ischemia. The loss of perfusion volume and pressure peripherally causes the consequential reduction in oxygen delivery and $\dot{V}O_2$ (Fig. 8–11). The reduced oxygen delivery increases anaerobic metabolism, with a concomitant rise in serum lactate. Clinically, this is observed as a fall in the oxygen consumption index and a rise in serum lactate concentrations. In patients undergoing cardiac surgery, lactate concentrations rise when oxygen delivery falls below a critical value of 300 ml/min/m².[20]

The oxygen supply/demand relationship is difficult to measure in patients. However, it is possible to demonstrate this relationship by acutely increasing oxygen transport and evaluating a possible increase in consumption. Oxygen consumption should be measured directly to avoid the cardiac output measurement in calculation of oxygen consumption by the Fick method. Therefore, $\dot{V}O_2$ is potentially more useful for continuous monitoring than any one of the standard vital signs. However, it fails to accurately indicate oxygen supply. Neuhof and associates[21–23] and Siegel[14] demonstrated that the true condition of the unstable patient is often most accurately reflected by the $\dot{V}O_2$ and not quite so well by the heart rate and blood pressure. These latter measurements are modified as much or more by the compensatory response to injury than by the injury itself. Basing decisions on standard data can lead the clinician to a false sense of the ultimate outcome of the patient. The normal mechanisms of compensation may camouflage a slow but persistent intra-abdominal bleed, for instance, and the bedside cardiovascular assessment may not reveal the true nature of the problem until the patient decompensates, just prior to cardiovascular arrest. Cellular metabolic monitoring of $\dot{V}O_2$ may be of tremendous value in situations such as this.

OXYGEN DEFICIT AND REPAYMENT

The difference over time between the oxygen demand (equal to the "stable" $\dot{V}O_2$, assumed to equal demand for the given conditions) and the actual $\dot{V}O_2$ is referred to as the *oxygen deficit* (Figs. 8–12 and 8–13). The oxygen deficit is very closely tied to eventual survival in an experimental hemorrhagic model (Fig. 8–14), much more so than blood pressure, which has a strong positive correlation.[24, 25] Following the initiation of fluid resuscitation in hypovolemic survivors, there is a recovery of $\dot{V}O_2$ that exceeds the current "baseline" demands for oxygen for a period of time (Fig. 8–15). This "excessive" amount of oxygen consumed is referred to as the "repayment" of the oxygen debt and is quantitatively related to the preceding oxygen deficit. The actual mathematical relationship between the two is not known, although in another situation where oxygen demand temporarily exceeds consumption, severe exercise, the oxygen debt repaid is approximately twice the size of the calculated oxygen deficit.[26] In shock, this quantitative relationship is generally not found in animals and humans, which may be a direct result of a wide variety of factors, including the resuscitation therapy. Typically, fluid resuscitation using room-temperature fluids elicits a gradual fall in body temperature that lowers the "baseline" $\dot{V}O_2$ during this period. The true extent of the fall in baseline measurements compounds the efforts to clinically quantify the actual oxygen debt (Fig. 8–16) and estimate the extent of the metabolic injury resulting from the shock state.

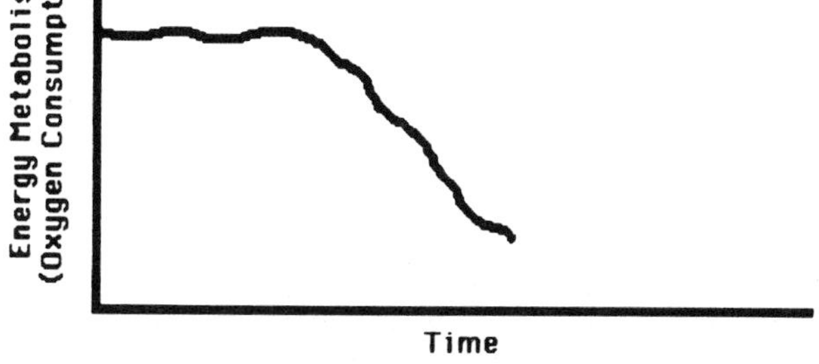

Figure 8–11. Oxygen consumption falls in hemorrhagic shock as the supply of oxygen to the body is reduced subsequent to the fall in circulating blood volume.

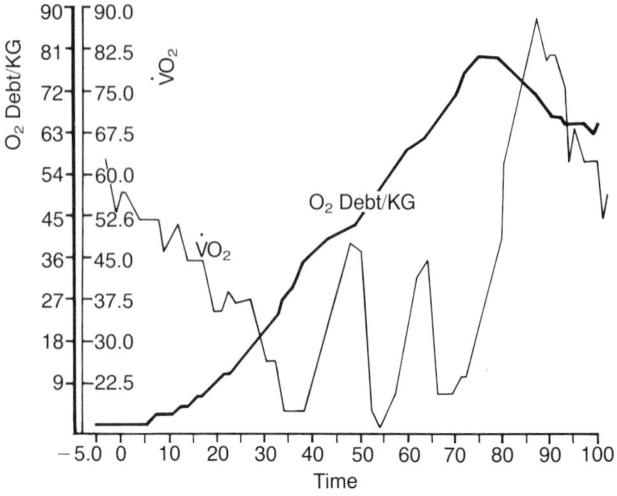

Figure 8–12. As the oxygen consumption falls, the oxygen debt gradually accumulates. With a recovery of oxygen (oxygen consumption above baseline demands), the oxygen debt is gradually repaid.

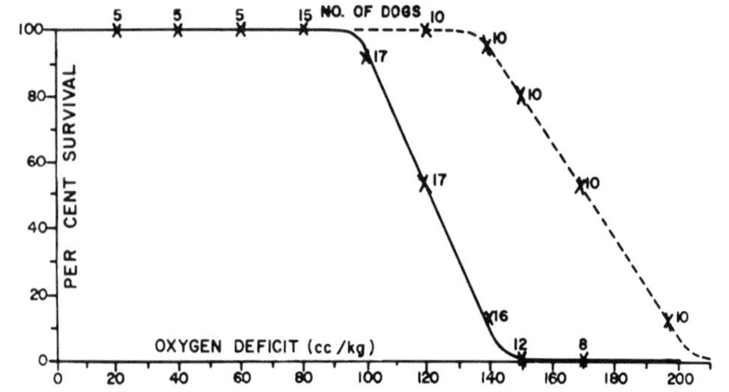

Figure 8–14. The total oxygen deficit has been shown to be an excellent quantitative predictor of survival following hemorrhagic shock in the dog model. The solid line shows the survival rate for control animals at various oxygen deficits; the dashed line shows the survival rate for digitalized animals. (From Crowell JW, Smith EE: Oxygen deficit and irreversible hemorrhagic shock. Am J Physiol 206:313, 1964.)

Cellular Pathology

While Crowell and Smith[25] demonstrated the relationship between survival and oxygen deficit, perhaps a finer relationship can be drawn between oxygen deficit and morphological and functional injury to cells. It appears that as ischemia worsens cellular perfusion, there is intracellular accumulation of lactic acid and hydrogen ions. Eventually, changes in cell membrane and function occur, followed by influx of sodium and potassium extrusion. This causes increased activity of sodium–potassium ATPase. As discussed earlier, there is a decreased production of ATP during ischemia. Consequently, the chemiosmotic balance of the intracellular environment is disrupted, leading to intracellular swelling. Mitochondria and cell organelles are disrupted, which ultimately results in cell death.

Some of these changes were demonstrated by the work of Trump's group.[1–7] In a canine hepatocyte taken by needle biopsy prior to shock, all cellular organelles appear normal (Fig. 8–17). At a moderate oxygen deficit of 60 ml/kg, autophagic vacuoles are present, indicating definite but reversible cellular injury (Fig. 8–18). At a much more severe oxygen deficit of 105 ml/kg, mitochondria are found to be swollen, and there is "blebbing" of the cytoplasmic vesicles (Fig. 8–19). Although the injury is significant, the shock is still thought to be reversible at this point, at least for the short term. This is in good agreement with the global short-term survival data from a study performed using dogs.[25] Whether this type of injury eventually leads to multiple organ failure after a few days is a very important, but as yet unanswered question.

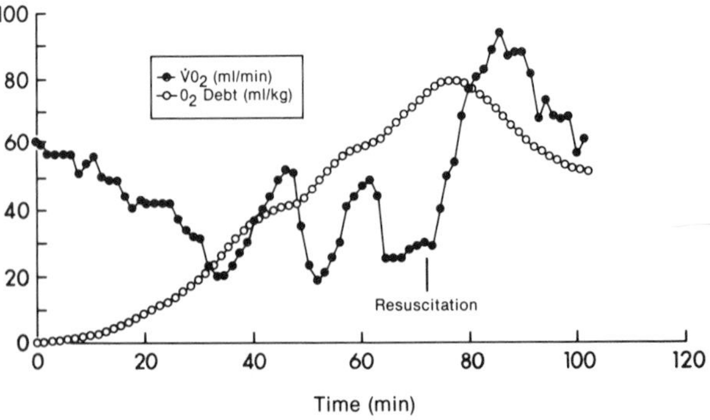

Figure 8–13. Actual data depicting the accumulating oxygen deficit that accompanies a fall in oxygen consumption as seen during experimental hemorrhagic shock in the dog. Note the spontaneous increases in $\dot{V}O_2$ as vasoconstriction and reperfusion occur with reduction in O_2 debt as volume resuscitation is instituted. (From Siegel JH, Linberg SE, Wiles CE: Therapy of low-flow shock states. In Siegel JH (ed): Trauma: Emergency Surgery and Critical Care. New York, Churchill Livingstone, 1987, p 206.)

Diagnosis

Using the $\dot{V}O_2$ data as a guide to resuscitation, a clinician can easily determine whether the patient is responding appropriately to therapy and use the data as a guide to volume replacement. Under actual resuscitation conditions, patients who arrive hypotensive, tachycardic, and tachypneic, with evidence of severe blood loss, have been found to fall into one of three groups.[27,28] The first group is composed of those patients who, in spite of their unstable cardiorespiratory status and apparent low blood pressure, are still not severely

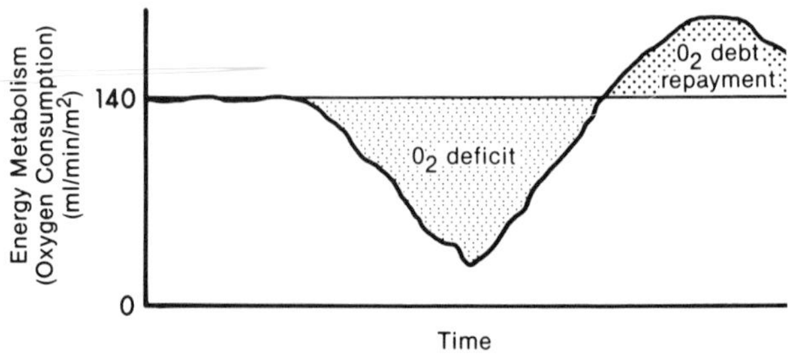

Figure 8–15. Graphic representation of the repayment of the oxygen debt when oxygen consumption following resuscitation exceeds the baseline requirements for oxygen. (From Siegel JH, Linberg SE, Wiles CE: Therapy of low-flow shock states. In Siegel JH (ed): Trauma: Emergency Surgery and Critical Care. New York, Churchill Livingstone, 1987, p 207.)

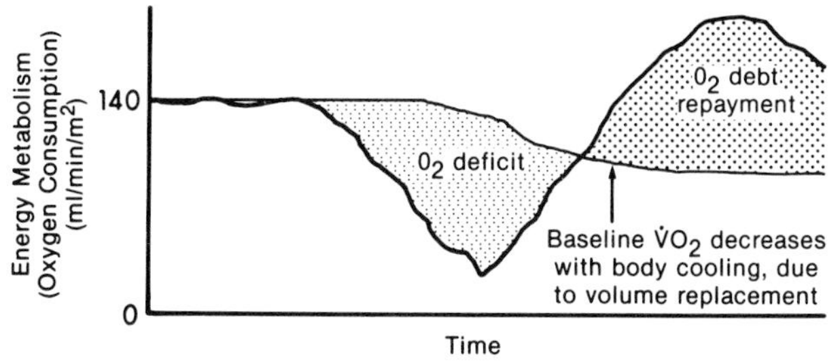

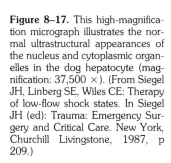

Figure 8–16. With hemorrhage and fluid volume resuscitation there is a significant hypothermia, with a fall in the baseline requirements for oxygen. Consequently, the increase in oxygen consumption required to exceed baseline needs is reduced, and repayment of the oxygen debt is achieved more quickly with an oxygen consumption that may not be that different from the preshock value. (From Siegel JH, Linberg SE, Wiles CE: Therapy of low-flow shock states. In Siegel JH (ed): Trauma: Emergency Surgery and Critical Care. New York, Churchill Livingstone, 1987, p 207.)

vasoconstricted, so organ perfusion persists, and they are metabolically stable. True circulatory shock may have developed only recently, and in that brief amount of time they have not experienced any significant loss of aerobic metabolic function. An actual example of this type of condition is presented in Figure 8–20, in which patient A presented with evidence of significant blood loss, hypotension, compensatory tachycardia, and decreased cognitive function. When resuscitated with volume, these patients should recover rapidly, as this depicted one actually did, except for any special considerations centered on their anatomical injuries.

A second grouping of patients who arrive in shock with an essentially identical clinical presentation are found to be severely depressed metabolically and are still accumulating an oxygen deficit at an alarming rate. The emergent needs of these patients are truly critical in that the oxygen deficit is accumulating so rapidly that the time between reversible and irreversible cellular injury is small. Patient B, whose data are depicted in Figure 8–21 along with those for two other patients, was admitted in hemorrhagic shock, with blood pressure undetectable by cuff, and accumulating an oxygen deficit at an initial rate of more than 1.5 ml/kg/min. At that rate, it would take less than 80 minutes to develop a lethal metabolic injury.[25, 29, 30] Those who regularly treat this type of patient know that the prehospital phase of accident extrication and transport may easily consume all or a large part of this total, leaving little time to treat the patient effectively, when time is truly critical. Patient A, who was not found to be accumulating an O_2 deficit when admitted, had an uneventful hospital course. Patient B, on the other hand, was not successfully resuscitated despite the heroic measures that were employed.

A third grouping of patients who arrive in shock initially appear essentially the same as the previous groups in clinical presentation but respond quickly to volume with an increase in $\dot{V}O_2$, as demonstrated by patient C. This patient arrived in a clinical condition similar to, and with a rate of oxygen deficit accumulation that was clinically indistinguishable from, the previously discussed patient B (Figs. 8–21 and 8–22). The unknown period during which the oxygen deficit was accumulating was apparently shorter; therefore, the size of the deficit was probably less than in patient B. Patient C also responded quickly to the intravenous fluid and blood component volume infusion, with an increase in $\dot{V}O_2$ to a level exceeding the expected baseline O_2 demands for a

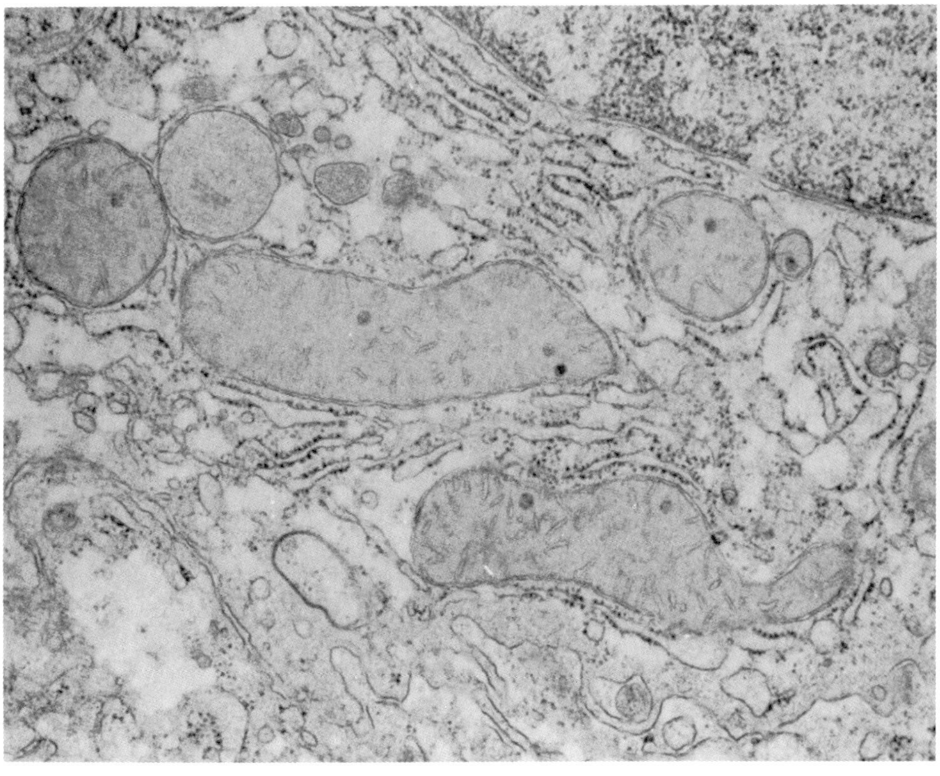

Figure 8–17. This high-magnification micrograph illustrates the normal ultrastructural appearances of the nucleus and cytoplasmic organelles in the dog hepatocyte (magnification: 37,500 ×). (From Siegel JH, Linberg SE, Wiles CE: Therapy of low-flow shock states. In Siegel JH (ed): Trauma: Emergency Surgery and Critical Care. New York, Churchill Livingstone, 1987, p 209.)

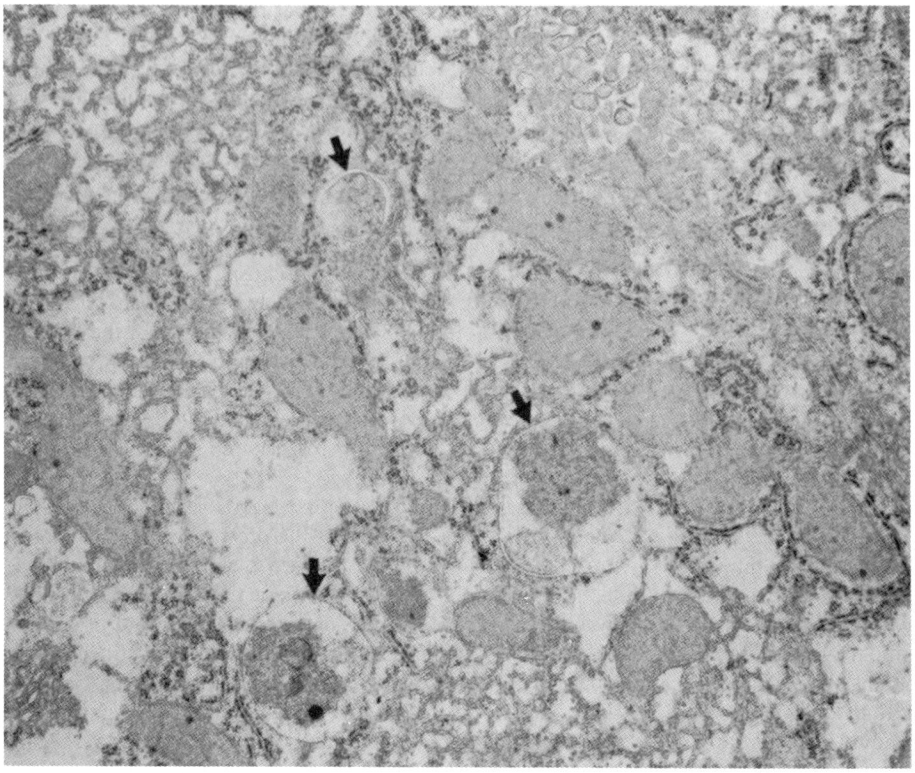

Figure 8–18. At the end of 1 hour of moderately severe hypovolemia (an O_2 deficit of 60 ml/kg after a 20-minute reinfusion), the only evidence of cell injury is an increase in the number of autophagic vacuoles (arrows). All other structures are normal (magnification: 25,000 ×). (From Siegel JH, Linberg SE, Wiles CE: Therapy of low-flow shock states. In Siegel JH (ed): Trauma: Emergency Surgery and Critical Care. New York, Churchill Livingstone, 1987, p 210.)

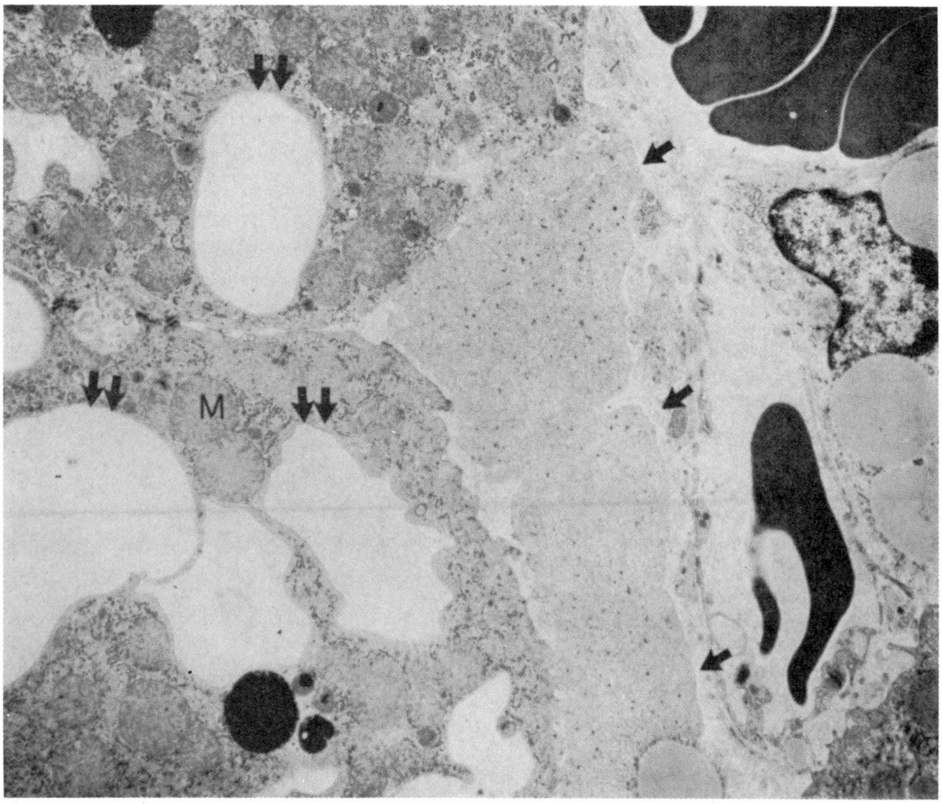

Figure 8–19. Effects of severe hypovolemia on hepatocyte ultrastructure. This animal was subjected to a 105 ml/kg oxygen deficit, and the micrograph illustrates the severe, although reversible, cellular injury. The mitochondria (M) are swollen, and there is blebbing of cytoplasmic vesicles into the space of Disse (single arrow). Several large toxic vacuoles are also seen in the hepatocytes (double arrow) (magnification: 15,000 ×). (From Siegel JH, Linberg SE, Wiles CE: Therapy of low-flow shock states. In Siegel JH (ed): Trauma: Emergency Surgery and Critical Care, New York, Churchill Livingstone, 1987, p 211.)

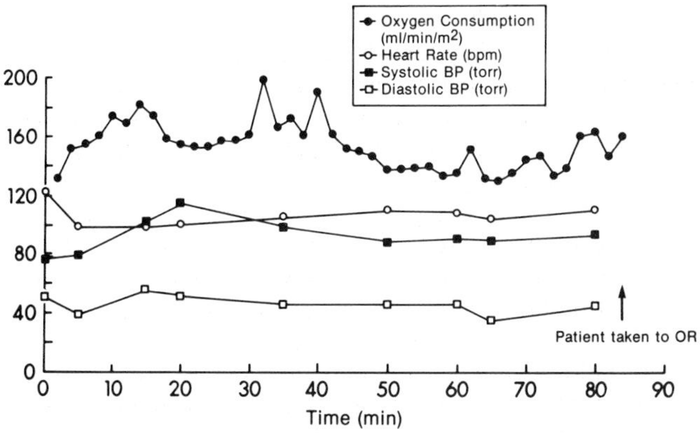

Figure 8–20. Hypotension following posttraumatic hypovolemia due to the lack of vasoconstriction about reduced blood volume. Data obtained during the resuscitation of patient A (see text). Although the patient was tachycardic and hypotensive upon admittance following traumatic injury, with obvious signs of significant blood loss, serial measurements of oxygen consumption indicated minimal detectable metabolic compromise. However, there was indication of a slight trend for an increase in oxygen consumption during the early resuscitation period as volume loss was replaced. (From Siegel JH, Linberg SE, Wiles CE: Therapy of low-flow shock states. In Siegel JH (ed): Trauma: Emergency Surgery and Critical Care. New York, Churchill Livingstone, 1987, p 214.)

normal individual, let alone an individual with a significantly reduced body temperature. It is worth mentioning that the improving metabolic status of patient C was evident long before the standard clinical data showed any sign of change.

Treatment

The immediate resuscitative efforts must be made with the fact in mind that the oxygen deficit accumulation must be halted and debt repayment begun as soon as possible. As mentioned, the size of the deficit is directly related to survival and most likely related also to the extent of multiple organ

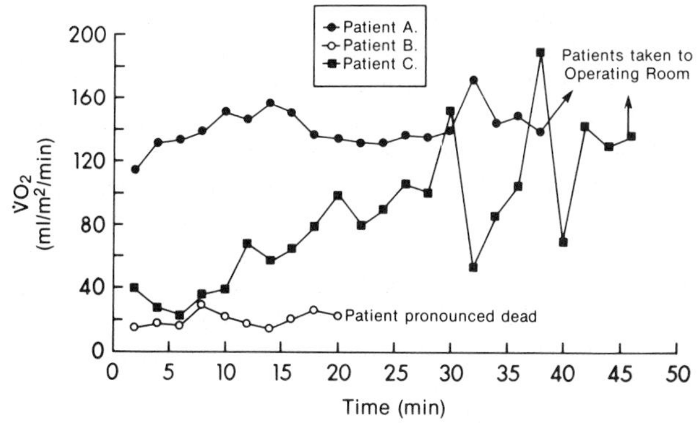

Figure 8–21. The data presented are from three patients and represent an example of each of three different classes of individuals who are seen in hemorrhagic shock: those who demonstrate no metabolic deficit (patient A), those who are metabolically unresponsive to therapy (patient B), and those who show severe metabolic depression on admission but quickly recover with appropriate volume resuscitation and related therapy (patient C). (From Siegel JH, Linberg SE, Wiles CE: Therapy of low-flow shock states. In Siegel JH (ed): Trauma: Emergency Surgery and Critical Care. New York, Churchill Livingstone, 1987, p 215.)

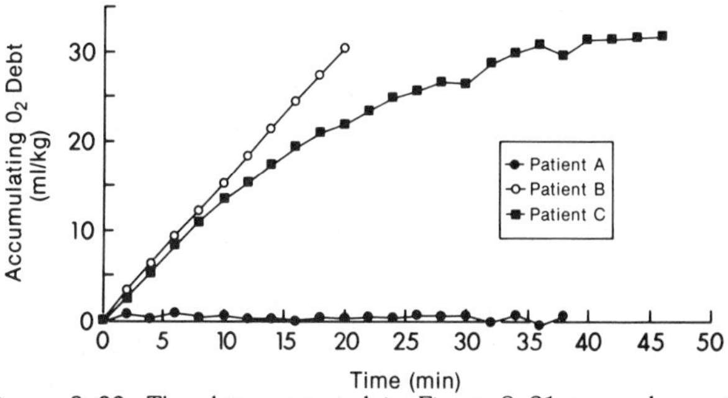

Figure 8–22. The data presented in Figure 8–21 are redrawn to demonstrate the varying rates of oxygen deficit accumulation (O_2 debt). Patient A was accumulating essentially no oxygen debt upon admission. Patients B and C were initially observed to be accumulating similar rates of oxygen debt. The difference between the two was that with volume resuscitation, the rate of accumulation for patient C leveled off to limit the total debt. (From Siegel JH, Linberg SE, Wiles CE: Therapy of low-flow shock states. In Siegel JH (ed): Trauma: Emergency Surgery and Critical Care. New York, Churchill Livingstone, 1987, p 215.)

failure that often follows a shock episode. It is not uncommon to find significant rates of deficit accumulation in patients upon arrival, which are rapidly developing into a lethal metabolic injury. The key to reversing this deadly trend is through the rapid correction of the oxygen supply/demand balance. This can be achieved by an increase in oxygen transport and/or a reduction in oxygen demand. One very large problem concerns the judicious use of volume in the resuscitation process. Oxygen transport is the product of arterial oxygen content and cardiac output. Arterial oxygen content depends on the hemoglobin concentration, the hemoglobin affinity, and the partial pressure of oxygen. Correction of any hypoxia is a step to restoration of oxygen transport. This can be achieved by the administration of oxygen. The hemoglobin should be maintained within a relatively narrow range (10 to 12.5 gm/dl) to avoid complications of increased viscosity or diluted oxygen-carrying capacity.[31] If the oxygen-carrying capacity is optimized, then the only other variable that can be manipulated to effectively increase oxygen delivery is cardiac output.

Fluid therapy represents the cornerstone of reversal of the hypovolemic event, by increasing total blood flow and correcting peripheral perfusion defects. There are experimental formulas that relate the reinfused volume to the hemorrhaged volume, although this value is rarely, if ever, known when a patient presents to the emergency or trauma service. Knowing the $\dot{V}O_2$ can aid the clinician in this situation, in that it can be used as a gauge of the effectiveness of the resuscitation.[30] While there is no magic number, efforts should be made to optimize $\dot{V}O_2$. If there is a rapid increase in $\dot{V}O_2$ with resuscitation, it indicates that the volume given is approaching the volume shed, and the question arises that if the source of bleeding is controlled, how much does the infusion rate need to be decreased in order to prevent fluid overload? Patients who show a slow response of $\dot{V}O_2$ to the resuscitation efforts must be treated much more aggressively. However, frequently the use of sophisticated methodology to determine the $\dot{V}O_2$ is unavailable, especially in smaller emergency departments. Therefore, other indices need to be correlated with the extent of oxygen debt. In one study designed to examine the effect of hypovolemia, a comparison was made of the ability to predict the oxygen debt from the cardiac output, mean blood pressure, shed blood volume, plasma base excess, and plasma lactate.[29, 30] The results of this study demonstrated that it is possible to predict the actual level of oxygen debt from the base deficit and lactate values during hypovolemia.

The question of the type of fluid to administer is one of the most troublesome problems in fluid resuscitation. Data that deserve mention on that issue are that $\dot{V}O_2$ recovers toward normal more quickly with colloid than with crystalloid.[22] Keep in mind that inadequate cellular perfusion exists and that the faster the $\dot{V}O_2$ recovers, the greater the chances are for a successful resuscitation.

In addition to fluid administration, positive inotropic agents may be beneficial by virtue of their ability to augment cardiac output. However, it should be remembered that significant increases in cardiac output require adequate ventricular filling. This can only be accomplished by use of fluids. For example, in a canine model of septic shock, fluid infusion was used to maintain cardiac filling pressures. The administration of dobutamine allowed a greater fluid administration than dopamine, resulting in a significantly higher oxygen transport and oxygen consumption.[138]

MULTIPLE ORGAN FAILURE SYNDROME

Clinical Description

Successful resuscitation with repayment of the oxygen debt may improve the patient's well-being in the hours immediately following the trauma episode. Adequate volume resuscitation is the cornerstone of all therapy. However, secondary complications resulting from the initial traumatic insult may ultimately be just as serious to the individual's survival as the hypovolemia in the immediate postinjury period. In fact, what has been described clinically is a sequential failure of the major organ systems of the body.[32] Often the patient survives the initial insult, be it hemorrhagic shock and/or severe multiple traumatic injuries, only to succumb to multiple organ failures (MOFs) later. Many patients with prolonged treatment in surgical intensive care units develop MOFs. Despite the most progressive medical management, mortality associated with MOFs remains high, approaching 100 per cent in some instances. Two clinical models which lead to MOFs have been proposed.[33, 34] In the "single hit" model, MOFs are initiated by the injury itself and subsequent resuscitation. The factors leading to the development of MOFs are related to the extent of injury, the time delay in resuscitation and admittance to a trauma center, and the quality of resuscitation. In the "two hit" model, there is an initial shock event which is adequately resuscitated, and the patient clinically appears to improve. Secondary to this initial shock event, a second insult such as infection or a second surgery precipitates the cascade of events leading to MOFs. Interestingly, there is little difference in the overall mortality rate between the two patterns of organ failure.[33, 34]

The clinical monitoring of the posttraumatic patient shows that the organ and system dysfunction is really the sum of many individual cellular failures. Thus there most likely exists at any given time a wide spectrum of metabolic and functional abnormalities within any given organ system. Organ dysfunction occurs only when enough cells of that particular organ system fail. The progressive deterioration at two or more organs over a brief period of time is defined as MOFs. In considering the failure of individual organs, the real potential problems arise because of the interdependence of all organ systems to the homeostatic mechanisms of the whole individual. For example, myocardial depression in cardiogenic shock also results in hypoperfusion of other organ systems, with the subsequent effects of decreased oxygen delivery to the previously healthy tissues.

Following trauma, respiratory distress is a common complication necessitating the need for ventilatory support. In addition, there may be renal, hepatic, gastrointestinal, cardiovascular, and/or metabolic failure. If each of these organ systems were to fail individually, chances of effective treatment may be high. The cardiovascular system can be supported with positive inotropic agents; the failed kidney can be supported with dialysis, whether acute or chronic; and the failed lung can be supported through advanced ventilatory assistance, including independent lung ventilation and jet ventilation as well as positive end-expiratory pressure techniques. Whenever two or more of these systems become involved, however, the survivability of the multiple organ failure syndrome decreases. A recent study placed the overall mortality rate for MOFs at 78 per cent.[35] Numerous reports have shown a relationship between the number of organ systems involved and the likelihood of death. One organ system failure is associated with a 40 per cent mortality. The mortality rate increases to 60 per cent with two dysfunctional organs and progresses to 100 per cent with four or more organ failures.[36] Particularly troublesome are the following combinations of organ failures (adapted from Baue[32]): (1) renal failure and respiratory failure (fluid overload affecting lung function that cannot be eliminated by the kidneys), (2) respiratory failure and metabolic failure (muscle strength is diminished to such an extent that spontaneous ventilation is no longer possible), (3) cardiac failure and respiratory failure (oxygen delivery is greatly impaired), and (4) sepsis, respiratory failure, and cardiovascular instability.

The classical MOF syndrome in surgical ICU patients is described by a pattern of injury, adult respiratory distress syndrome, and hypermetabolism followed by sequential organ failure.[37, 38] The onset of MOFs begins with a low-grade fever, tachycardia, and dyspnea, with appearance of infiltrates on the chest film, but normal liver and renal function tests (Fig. 8–23). Dyspnea progresses until endotracheal intubation and mechanical ventilatory assistance are required. The patient usually stabilizes hemodynamically with a cardiac index over 5 $l/min/m^2$ and a systemic vascular resistance of less than 600 dyn·cm. Metabolically, the $\dot{V}O_2$ is greater than 180 ml/m^2, hyperglycemia is prevalent in the absence of diabetes mellitus or pancreatitis, and hyperlactatemia and increased urea nitrogen excretion (>15 gm/day) are observed, consistent with a hypermetabolic state.

After 7 to 10 days, the bilirubin approaches 10 mg/dl and begins to rise progressively, heralding the onset of hepatic

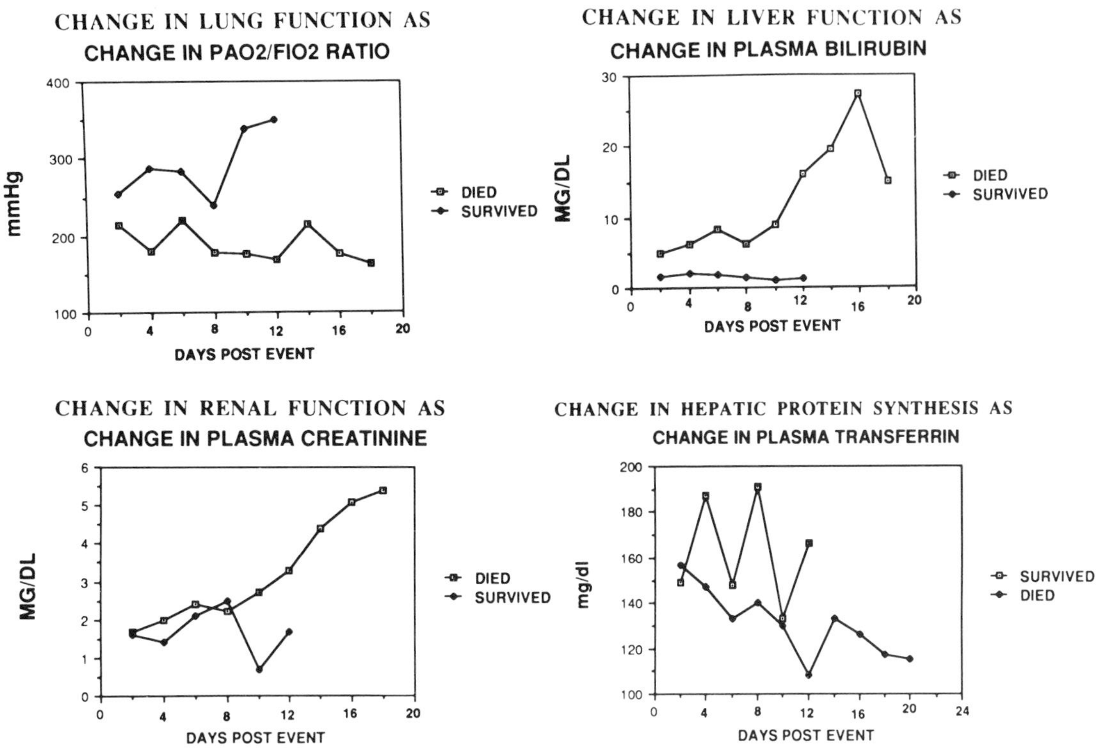

Figure 8–23. The characteristic changes of hypermetabolism and organ failure are presented in septic patients. Following the initial injury, the stable phase of hypermetabolism is entered. At day 7 to 10 after injury the progressive organ failure becomes apparent. (From Cerra FB, Alden PA, Negro F, Billiar T, et al: Sepsis and exogenous lipid metabolism. JPEN 12:645, 1988. © by American Society for Pharmacological and Experimental Therapy, 1986.)

dysfunction. Accompanying the rise in bilirubin, serum creatinine begins to rise. The hyperdynamic cardiovascular state and hypermetabolism become more pronounced. Bacteremia with enteric organisms is common, as is the culture of pathogens, usually gram-negative, from tracheal aspirate, urine, and wounds. Impaired wound healing leads to development of skin breakdown at pressure points. There is an increasing requirement for positive inotropic support in addition to fluids to maintain blood volume and cardiac preload as well as urinary output. Between 14 and 21 days, renal failure worsens, and dialysis may be required. By day 21, survivability is doubtful, and death often ensues within 21 to 28 days following the initial insult.

Multiple Etiological Factors

In a study of 553 patients requiring emergency surgery, it was shown clearly that uncontrolled bacterial infection (sepsis) was the primary cause of organ systems failure.[39] It has commonly been accepted that MOF is the expression of an occult septic focus (usually intra-abdominal). In operations for intra-abdominal sepsis, organ failure develops in 30 to 50 per cent of cases and carries a mortality rate of between 30 and 100 per cent, depending on the number of organ systems affected. In 1976, two-thirds of patients dying of MOFs demonstrated an intra-abdominal abscess as the bacterial focus.[40] However, as more patients with MOFs were subjected to exploratory laparotomies on the assumption of an intra-abdominal abscess, it became evident that MOFs could exist in the absence of any identifiable bacterial focus. In fact, one study showed that only 5 of 26 patients dying of MOFs possessed a major infection at autopsy, of which only one was intra-abdominal. It is now a common clinical observation that patients dying of MOFs and sepsis have enteric bacteremia for which no identifiable focus at autopsy is noted. The concept that has emerged over the past 5 years is that bacteria in the gut can lead to infection through translocation or surface spread following the disruption of the intestinal mucosa.[41]

Changes in the intestinal flora, coupled with an impairment of the normal barrier function of the gastrointestinal tract, allow the bowel to serve as a reservoir for pathogens so that the bacteria or their products (such as endotoxin) can enter the portal and systemic circulations and fuel the on-going septic process. Gut-derived bacteria or endotoxin contributes to the development of MOFs in the septic syndrome patient without evidence of infection. In a recent study, 2.5 nosocomial infections per ICU course were observed, and those patients developing MOFs had a higher incidence of infections caused by gram-positive and fungal organisms.[42] Even with appropriate antimicrobial therapy, the clinical course of organ failure continued. According to the translocation hypothesis, decontamination of the gut with selective suppression of lumina flora would be expected to reduce not only nosocomial infections but also mortality. Unfortunately, while a significant decline in infection rates was seen, there were no significant reductions in the incidence or mortality associated with MOFs.[42, 43] These studies point to alternative mechanisms to account for the development of the septic syndrome.

Activation of the body's host-defense mechanisms by the onset of sepsis precipitates a widespread inflammatory response that is apparently not organism-specific. Consequently, there is initiation of a complex series of biochemical cascades by inflammatory substances which set the stage for organ dysfunction.[44, 45] Recent data suggest that the complement system fragments are pivotal in the synthesis of cellular and humoral mediators associated with sepsis and MOFs. The severity of lesions in the lung, the intestine, the kidneys, and the liver of hemorrhagic, septic dogs correlated with high tissue levels of the complement split products C3a, C3b, and C5a. These data support the concept that complement provokes a sequence of events leading to eventual organ failure.

Stimulation of the complement system elicits the generation of complement split products, collectively known as anaphylatoxins. Three of the most notable are C3a, C3b, and C5a. Both C5a and C3b possess chemotactic properties for neutrophils, macrophages, and monocytes. They serve to attract these cells to areas of inflammation and enhance their adhesiveness and promote aggregation. All three cell types protect against bacterial invasion by virtue of their ability to engulf bacteria via phagocytosis. Nevertheless, large-scale infiltration and activation, such as that which occurs with sepsis and trauma, can be detrimental to tissues rather than protective. Activated neutrophils release oxygen free radicals (superoxide, peroxide, and the hydroxal radical) during phagocytosis. These toxic oxygen products normally serve a protective function by virtue of their bactericidal nature. However, if generated in sizable amounts, oxygen free radicals destroy membrane integrity, which could ultimately lead to widespread tissue injury and impairment of organ function.

Like other complement fragments, C3a exhibits chemotaxis. However, it also causes extensive mast cell degranulation, resulting in the liberation of histamine. Histamine loosens cell-to-cell junctions and permits the extravasation of fluid into the interstitial spaces. It is for this reason that C3a has been implicated in the genesis of permeability edema which may contribute to organ dysfunction.

Stimulation of the complement cascade has the indirect capability of triggering the activation of other enzyme cascades. These include fibrinolysis and coagulation systems, as well as the generation of prostaglandins and leukotrienes from granulocytes. These substances behave as mediators which modulate tissue injury during sepsis and MOFs. Nevertheless, the exact role of complement products has not been well elucidated at present.

Margination of neutrophils along vascular endothelium is likely to damage the cells composing the lining of blood vessels. This injury may be succeeded by exposure of plasma to the underlying collagen. Both are understood to effect activation of the coagulation cascade via Hageman factor (factor XII in the intrinsic pathway). In addition, activated neutrophils elaborate elastase, which may also cause Hageman factor formation. Conversion of biologically inactive precursors, initiated by Hageman factor, catalyzes the synthesis of the vasoactive kinins. The most commonly formed is bradykinin, a potent vasodilator, which also increases capillary permeability. Because of its rapid degradation, bradykinin cannot be measured directly; however, some data support that sepsis causes reduction in the levels of precursors. Presumably, changes in capillary permeability and vasodilation, exacerbated by such substances as bradykinin, have a role in local tissue injury and malperfusion, which may amplify organ dysfunction.

PHYSIOLOGICAL RESPONSES TO TRAUMA AND SEPSIS

Since sepsis is one of the primary initiators of MOFs, it is important to examine metabolic and hemodynamic differences between the clinical course of the septic episode and traumatic injury without sepsis. The evolution of the septic process can be contrasted with the clinical course of traumatized patients who do not become septic (Figs. 8–24 and

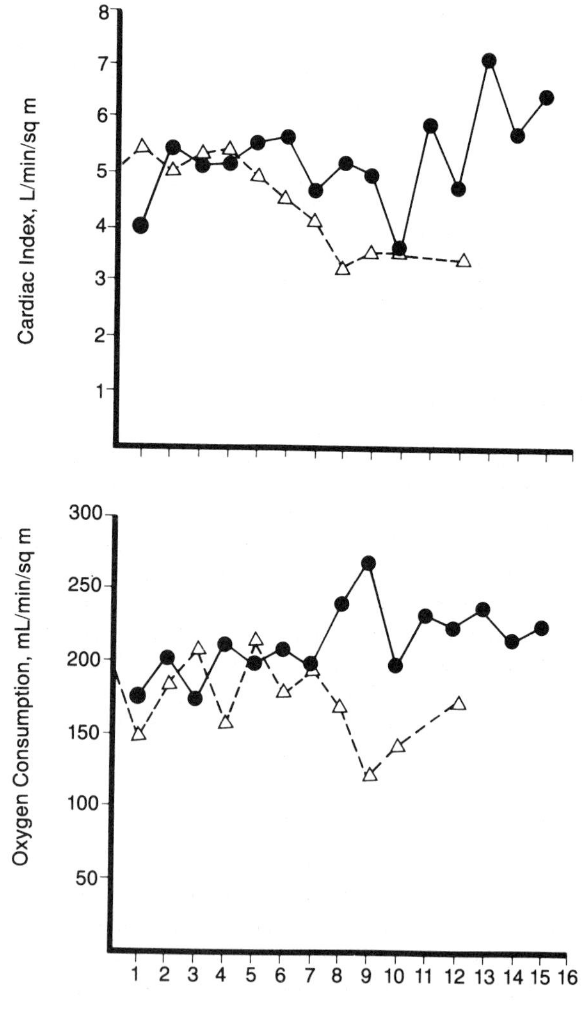

Figure 8–24. Cardiovascular and metabolic responses after trauma and sepsis in 10 septic and 16 nonseptic patients. Mean values over postinjury course for cardiac index (CI) (top) and oxygen consumption ($\dot{V}O_2$) (bottom) are shown for trauma patients who developed sepsis (ST) (closed circles) and compared with those who had nonseptic courses (NST) (open triangles). Note increase in cardiac index and $\dot{V}O_2$ in septic patients as sepsis becomes established between 5 and 7 days after injury. (From Sganga G, Siegel JH, Brown G, et al: Reprioritization of hepatic plasma protein release in trauma and sepsis. Arch Surg 120:190, 1985. Copyright 1985, American Medical Association.)

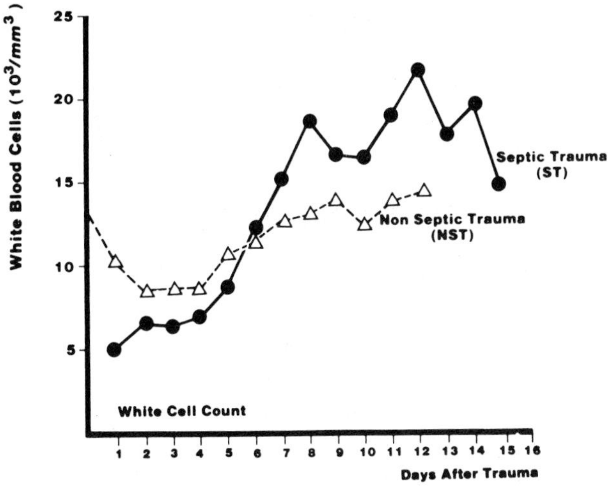

Figure 8–25. Nature of inflammatory response following trauma in 10 septic and 16 nonseptic patients. Comparison of the rise in white blood cell counts in patients with and without sepsis over a 16-day study period. (From Sganga G, Siegel JH, Brown G, et al: Reprioritization of hepatic plasma protein release in trauma and sepsis. Arch Surg 120:187, 1985. Copyright 1985, American Medical Association.)

8–25). Despite similar initial injury severity scores, age, and pattern of injury of 26 polytrauma patients, 10 patients developed fulminate sepsis, while 16 evidenced no signs of sepsis.[46] Initially, both groups had similar physiological responses. In fact, both had comparable increases in cardiac index during the first 5 days following resuscitation and/or surgery for their initial injury. However, after 5 days, the septic patients showed a gradual elevation in cardiac index over the previous 5 days, whereas in nonseptic trauma patients, the cardiac index returned toward normal levels. While oxygen consumption was raised for the first 7 days after trauma in the septic and the nonseptic groups, those patients who became septic continued to increase their oxygen consumption after the first 7 days. Furthermore, in the nonseptic trauma patients, the oxygen consumption dropped toward normal levels. Within the first 3 days following injury, the white cell count tended to be lower in those patients who developed sepsis. As the sepsis developed and became overt, a marked leukocytosis occurred (see Fig. 8–25). The posttraumatic nonseptic patients tended to have an increased white cell count but at an intermediate range, which fell during recovery. This latter course undoubtedly reflects the inflammatory processes associated with nonseptic traumatic injury.

Physiological Monitoring of Septic Patients

Since it has been possible to demonstrate that septic and nonseptic trauma patients show a differential response, the nature of the septic process can be followed through the identification of the pattern of physiological adaptations to sepsis. A method for quantitating the pattern of physiological abnormalities in patients with and without sepsis has been established; it relies on the principles of statistical pattern recognition[47, 48] (Fig. 8–26). Catheters are placed in the pulmonary artery for sampling of mixed venous blood gases and pH, as well as serving as a site for injection of dye or chilled saline for measurement of cardiac output. The pulmonary capillary wedge pressure also provides a good estimation of left ventricular preload. The dye or temperature is measured from an arterial cannula, from which arterial blood gases are drawn. Using either the dye dilution or thermal dilution technique, it is possible to obtain measurements of cardiac output, cardiac index, the pulmonary blood volume, and both mean cardiac ejection fraction and left ventricular end-diastolic volume. In addition, variables such as heart rate, mean arterial pressure, mean right atrial pressure, systolic ejection time, the arteriovenous oxygen difference, mixed venous oxygen tension, pH, and carbon dioxide can be measured. The analysis of these variables has

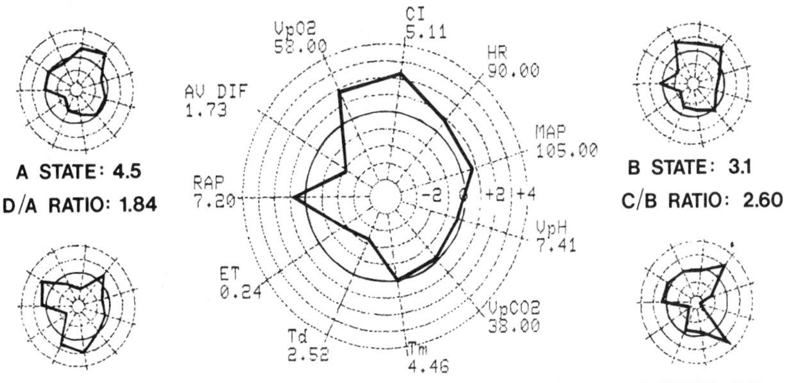

Figure 8–26. Circle diagrams of physiological state. At the corners are shown the prototype patterns for the A, B, C, and D states. In the *large circle* in the center is the physiological pattern manifested by a 56-year-old man with intra-abdominal sepsis and abscess. The perfect dark circle in the center equals 0 standard deviations from the reference control (R) state. Each dotted line represents 1 standard deviation from R, either increased or decreased. The rays of the circle diagram represent respectively cardiac index, heart rate, mean blood pressure, mixed venous pH (VpH), mixed venous CO_2 tension ($VpCO_2$), cardiac washout time (t_m), pulmonary mean transit time (t_d), cardiac ejection time, right atrial pressure (CVP), arteriovenous oxygen content difference (A–V Diff) and mixed venous oxygen tension (VpO_2). A state = compensated stress response (sepsis, postsurgery, posttrauma); B state = unbalanced septic; C state = decompensated septic; and D state = cardiogenic. (From Siegel JH, Cerra FB, Coleman B, et al: Physiological and metabolic correlations in human sepsis. Surgery 86:166, 1979.)

led to the understanding that the entire spectrum of clinical severity in patients with various forms of trauma, sepsis, or cardiogenic abnormalities could be viewed in terms of four basic patterns[47–49] (see Fig. 8–26). Once identified, specific treatment regimens can be instituted based on a particular pattern of physiological responses.

Patterns of Response

The normal response to stress observed in compensated sepsis and after trauma or major operative surgery is characterized by a sympathetic reaction in which heart rate, cardiac index, and contractility increase. This sympathetic adaptation occurs without any evidence of metabolic abnormalities and minimal respiratory dysfunction. The oxygen consumption index also increases. The failure to achieve this response in the presence of major stress is an abnormal response, indicative of complicating factors. The changing pattern of physiological variables is shown in Figure 8–27, which demonstrates the time course of the cardiac index, oxygen saturation, oxygen consumption, arterial P_{CO_2}, and total peripheral resistance from a 62-year-old woman with severe intra-abdominal sepsis. In contrast to hypovolemic shock, sepsis is characterized by an increased, rather than decreased, cardiac index. In this particular patient, the cardiac index tended to be greater than 4 l/min/m² throughout the course of study. Oxygen consumption was either normal, increased, or decreased when cardiac index was at its highest. Falling oxygen consumption was not due to an inadequate oxygen delivery, but rather to a failure of oxygen extraction. This can be seen by examining the time course of arterial and mixed venous oxygen saturations. At the time of lowest oxygen consumption, the mixed venous oxygen saturation and content rose so that the arteriovenous difference narrowed. There was also a tendency for hyperventilation in this spontaneously breathing patient such that the arterial P_{CO_2} also reached its lowest point. Throughout most of the clinical course, the peripheral pressure/flow relationships are also seen to be abnormal, with a marked reduction in total peripheral resistance at a time of increased cardiac output.[49–51]

Hyperdynamic State

Sepsis is characterized by an increased oxygen consumption, which must be met by an augmented oxygen delivery. Increased oxygen delivery is sustained by elevated cardiac output and minute ventilation. The primary induction of increased cardiac output consists of a combination of increased heart rate and a reduced afterload. The diminished afterload is a consequence of a fall in systemic vascular resistance.[52] This combination of an increased cardiac output with decreased vascular resistance characterizes a hyperdynamic cardiovascular state. Evidence suggests that this hyperdynamic state is necessary for survival in the compromised host in order to meet the energy demands of peripheral tissues trying to defend against the septic insult. A critical feature of the patient's ability to maintain the hyperdynamic cardiovascular response is the ability of the myocardium to sustain an increased cardiac output. Patients with hyperdynamic profiles typically have cardiac outputs greater than

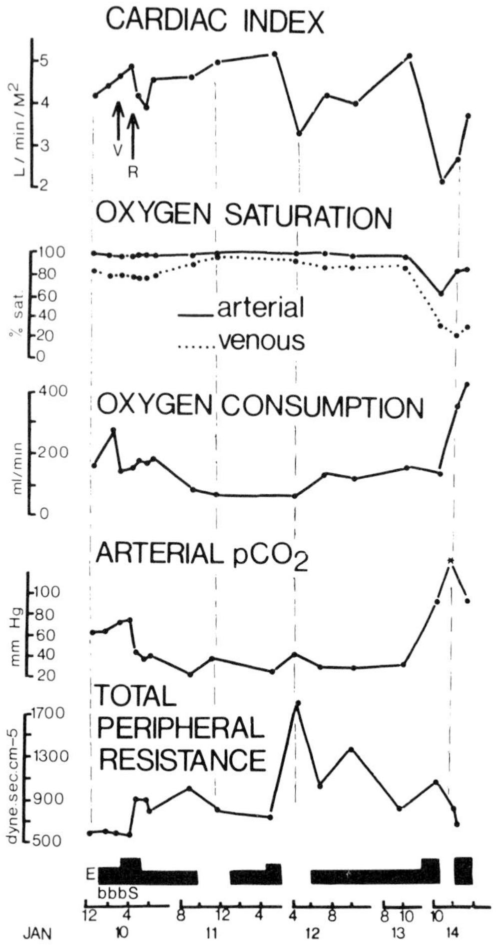

Figure 8–27. Clinical course of 62-year-old woman with subdiaphragmatic abscess in hyperdynamic septic shock. (From Siegel JH, Greenspan M, Del Guercio LRM: Abnormal vascular tone, defective oxygen transport and myocardial failure in human septic shock. Ann Surg 165:504, 1967.)

8 l/min, with a total peripheral resistance of less than 1100 dyn·sec·cm^{-5}. The difference is remarkable when these values are contrasted to those of normal nonseptic patients who demonstrate a cardiac output of 5 to 6 l/min at a total peripheral resistance in the range of 1200 to 1500 dyn·sec·cm^{-5}. Hyperdynamic septic patients can have cardiac work in the range of 10 to 17 kg/min, values similar to those obtained in healthy individuals exercising strenuously. While the myocardium has the potential to increase its cardiac work, in septic patients this increased level of cardiac work must be sustained for days or even weeks as the patient combats the septic episode.

It is not uncommon, therefore, that this large and continual demand on the heart leads to myocardial depression and high-output failure in sepsis.[49] Inadequate preload, preexisting cardiac disease, and acquired cardiac dysfunction all contribute to the failure to achieve the high-output state. Preexisting cardiac disease such as stenotic valvular lesions, cardiomyopathies, or scarring from previous myocardial infarction limits the ability of the heart to increase cardiac output. Acquired myocardial dysfunction arises from a primary reduction in contractility caused by sepsis or inadequate resuscitation following a hypovolemic episode. Under such a condition, the cardiac dysfunction arises from decreased ventricular compliance secondary to ischemic damage resulting from inadequate resuscitation. This cardiogenic failure is similar in its physiological response to other forms of myocardial failure such as myocardial infarction. The decreased myocardial function leads to a fall in cardiac index and a reduced ejection fraction. In the periphery, the arteriovenous difference widens as extraction of oxygen increases in an attempt to compensate for the reduced flow. Hypotension and acidosis may occur if the cardiac depression is severe enough to limit oxygen delivery to the tissues. Since, in the septic state, the increased cardiac output appears to support the peripheral tissues, a transition from a high-output to low-output state contributes to the mortality rate often associated with sepsis.

Therapeutic Implications

The importance of maintaining adequate myocardial function in the septic patient has vital therapeutic implications.[52] The positive inotropic agents commonly used to promote increased cardiac output during sepsis are dopamine, at nonvasoconstricting dosages (2 to 5 μg/kg/min), dobutamine in a similar low-dose inotropic concentration (3 to 5 μg/kg/min), or low-dose isoproterenol (0.25 to 1 μg/kg/min). At the lower level, isoproterenol has virtually no chronotropic toxicity, thus increasing myocardial contractility and augmenting cardiac output. Isoproterenol also has been used in conjunction with inotropic concentrations of dopamine and dobutamine, and the administration of two or three of these agents in low doses appears to have a synergistic effect with regard to positive inotropic action, but without excessive toxicity. Additional positive inotropic support in the hyperdynamic septic patient has been reported with digoxin. The positive inotropic effect of digoxin occurs at approximately 75 per cent of the normal digitalizing dose, provided serum potassium concentrations are maintained at approximately 4 mEq/l. Digoxin may be of particular usefulness in older patients, in whom some degree of preexisting myocardial disease may be present.

In general, it appears that the use of drugs possessing vasoconstrictor activity such as dopamine at doses greater than 8 to 10 μg/kg/min or of the α-agonist catecholamines norepinephrine and methoxamine would be counterproductive during hyperdynamic sepsis. Excessive systemic vasoconstriction caused by exogenous norepinephrine would restrict blood flow to critical organs and may potentiate any organ damage by superimposing the effects of relative ischemia on top of the organ's initial injury. Such agents may be of some limited usefulness during periods of frank hypotension, but infusion should be titrated down or eliminated as soon as possible.

The decreased vascular resistance necessitates an increased blood volume to maintain adequate preload. Therefore, judicious use of fluids may be warranted to maintain preload. The origin of the decreased vascular tone is unknown. The decrease in vascular resistance is independent of flow. Initially, it most likely stems from a local response to increased oxygen demand resulting in local vessel vasodilation. However, with increased duration of the septic episode, release of vasoactive substances may be induced by the bacterial or endotoxic challenge, which modulates vascular resistance.

Attempts to predict those ICU patients at risk to develop MOFs involve the use of different injury scoring systems. Injury severity scores, such as the APACHE II system, do not predict which patients will develop MOFs.[53] The indices of metabolic dysfunction are better able to predict those patients at risk. On the first day after injury, low PaO_2/FiO_2 is indicative of an impairment in oxygenation. A threefold increase in plasma lactate on day 2 indicates a glucose metabolism dyshomeostasis. Elevated serum bilirubin on day 6 after injury signifies an impairment of liver function, and increased serum creatinine on day 12 reflects renal failure. Therefore, monitoring of both the hemodynamic and metabolic components of injury assists in the ability to identify which patients are at risk.[37, 38, 42]

ROLE OF ENDOGENOUS MEDIATORS IN MULTIPLE ORGAN FAILURE

Central to the host's ability to combat a bacterial insult is the immune response. The immune system limits the spread of the pathogen, augments the flux of immune cells, and modulates the host's metabolism to enhance the environment necessary for the destruction of bacteria. These changes are mediated by the elaboration of factors secreted by cells of the immune system. Normally, this host response is limited to the local tissue when bacteria are present. However, a severe bacterial invasion results in an excessive release of the mediators. In its most severe form, the mediators elicit a shock state in which inadequate tissue perfusion may lead to organ damage.

The first line of defense in resisting bacterial invasion is the macrophages. In addition to the phagocytizing and bactericidal abilities of the macrophage, the macrophages release factors that activate other cells of the immune system and alter the host metabolism. These factors, termed *cytokines*, are rapidly released following an inflammatory insult. Initially, the overlapping stimulatory and inhibitory functions among the various cytokines regulate the host's response to injury, promoting control of the invading insult and tissue repair. However, prolonged or exaggerated elaboration of these cytokines can lead to adverse affects and organ failure.

Of the cytokines released by macrophages, tumor necrosis factor and interleukin 1 have received the most attention as mediators of the inflammatory response. Tumor necrosis factor is rapidly synthesized de novo following infectious or inflammatory stimulation of the macrophage and is released from the macrophage within 15 minutes of induction.[54–57] In rabbits, plasma tumor necrosis factor concentrations peak 90 to 120 minutes following administration of endotoxin. Thereafter, the plasma concentration falls as tumor necrosis factor is cleared from the circulatory system by internalization of membrane-bound TNF receptors on cells. The half-life of tumor necrosis factor is 6 to 7 minutes in the mouse but somewhat longer in humans. Infusion of tumor necrosis factor in animals elicits many of the clinical symptoms associated with MOFs, including hypotension, tachypnea, metabolite acidosis, hemoconcentration, and hyperglycemia that is superseded by hypoglycemia. At necropsy, severe thickening of the alveolar septum, ischemia of the gastrointestinal tract, renal and pancreatic hemorrhage, and antirenal tubular necrosis are observed. In addition, chronic exposure to low plasma concentrations of tumor necrosis factor induces the wasting diathesis observed in various disease states.

The rapid production and clearance of tumor necrosis factor must be reconciled with the observation that the shock phase can follow the administration of endotoxin by several hours. Hence the lethal effects of tumor necrosis factor occur temporally after the removal of tumor factor from the plasma compartment. Therefore, tumor necrosis factor must initiate a process that leads to tissue injury and shock. This is accomplished by the synthesis and release of other inflammatory mediators such as interleukins, leukotrienes, and platelet-activating factor.

Interleukin 1 is an additional macrophage-derived cytokine with potent biological effects. In myelohematopoietic tissues, interleukin 1 is required for optimal cellular activation and proliferation. Interleukin 1 is pyrogenic, accelerates the basal metabolic rate, increases oxygen consumption, and augments skeletal muscle catabolism and consequent release of amino acids.

The response of the host to the bacterial infection involves a complex interaction of humoral and cellular responses. The humoral response induces a primary sequence of relatively nonspecific immunological reactions. Acute-phase proteins such as C-reactive protein and opsonic fibronectin bind to antibody proteins on the cell walls of the offending organisms. This is followed by complement activation in which C5a enhances leukocyte or macrophage aggregation and opsonization of the bacterial or fungal organism and C3a by inducing leukocyte production of oxygen-derived free radicals in the form of superoxides which damage the microorganism's cell membrane. These events facilitate bacterial ingestion by defending white cells by promoting changes in the bacterial cell structure as well as the external environment which foster bacterial killing and lysis. Both interleukin 1 and 2 amplify host-defense responses by stimulation of lymphocyte propagation. Moreover, these immune responses effect blast transformation and proliferation of leukocytes and promote their migration and adherence to the invading organisms and to nonviable or damaged tissues. Consequently, the release of leukocyte proteases is increased, which completes the destruction of the bacteria and necrotic tissue, thereby facilitating their removal. Leukotrienes synthesized from white cells during this process also stimulate cellular immunity and alter the balance between suppressor, helper, and killer lymphocytes to deal with the secondary organism and tissue-specific aspects of this process.

Although cellular responses are aimed primarily at defense, sepsis seems to engender an overstimulation of some of these protective mechanisms. Subsequently, certain cells appear to make an abundance of a variety of substances which are postulated to intensify tissue malperfusion and/or injury. In a process termed "malignant inflammation," neutrophils, macrophages, lymphocytes, and perhaps platelets liberate vasoactive mediators which may amplify the pathogenesis of the septic process as well as organ failure.[44]

Once neutrophils become activated, they extrude proteases, including elastase, cathepsin G, and collagenase, that have the capability to degrade intracellular matrices if produced in surplus. Excessive free radical production associated with phagocytosis, combined with the release of these proteases, is thought to effect damage to surrounding tissues.[58] Neutrophils, macrophages, and monocytes all are known to synthesize metabolic products of arachidonic acid catabolism.[59, 60] These arachidonic acid derivatives, termed *eicosanoids*, include the leukotrienes, prostaglandins, and thromboxane, all of which have been implicated in modulating the physiological response to sepsis.

Collectively identified as *slow-reacting substance of anaphylaxis*, leukotrienes C4, D4, and E4 possess the ability to alter tissue permeability, produce bronchoconstriction, and trigger vasoconstriction in some vascular beds.[61] The exact role of LTC4, LTD4, and LTE4 in sepsis remains unknown; however, it is speculated that they participate in regional alterations in microvascular perfusion in addition to the exacerbation of tissue edema, particularly in the lung.[61, 62] Another leukotriene, LTB4, is a potent chemotactic agent for leukocytes. Like the stimulus for the other leukotrienes, inflammation and tissue ischemia can induce generation of LTB4. Once formed, it fosters neutrophil aggregation with release of granular constituents.[63] Consequently, more neutrophils are attracted to the area. The aggregation of substantial numbers of cells promotes increased free radical production and perpetuates eicosanoid synthesis. Additionally, leukocyte clumping in the microvasculature can effect mechanical obstruction to flow.

Thromboxane, known to be elevated in trauma and sepsis, is manufactured by white blood cells and platelets, as well as by other vascular and parenchymal tissues.[64, 65] An extremely potent vasoconstrictor, it has the additional ability to aggregate both platelets and neutrophils. Frequently, platelet abnormalities in septic shock are manifested by profound thrombocytopenia, probably as a result of complement system stimulation. However, once platelets aggregate, they release thromboxane, which also enhances leukocyte aggregation, thus creating a vicious cycle. Furthermore, aggregation of white cells and platelets by thromboxane may subsequently aggravate sluggish tissue blood flow. Vasoconstriction resulting from thromboxane synthesis may permit regions of malperfusion, intensifying tissue hypoxia.

One of the hallmarks of sepsis is vasodilation. Because the prostaglandin prostacyclin produces vessel dilation, it is a putative mediator of sepsis. Largely generated by vascular endothelium, elevated concentrations have been identified in patients with sepsis.[64] Since there appears to be widespread formation of this prostaglandin during sepsis, some evidence points toward possible modulation of the decrease in systemic vascular resistance by prostacyclin. Sustained vasodilation in certain organ beds may affect flow to the extent that sluggish movement of blood causes microvascular clot formation, which would further impede tissue oxygen delivery.

Although many prostaglandins are elevated in sepsis, much research has focused on prostacyclin and thromboxane. There is thought to be a physiological balance between the two due to their opposite biological properties. Sepsis, it is postulated, offsets this equilibrium, thereby potentiating tissue damage. In fact, elevated thromboxane concentrations correlate positively with the degree of organ dysfunction.[66]

Of the many pro-inflammatory substances manufactured

by white cells, tumor necrosis factor has stirred much recent interest. When studied in vivo, it engenders symptoms similar to those observed after endotoxin injection.[54–57, 67] This has led to the speculation that this factor is the primary mediator of gram-negative sepsis. Produced by macrophages, it elicits a dose-responsive hypotension, tachycardia, pyrexia, and hypermetabolism in both animals and human volunteers.[56, 57] Although the literature reflects much support of the contribution of tumor necrosis factor to the symptoms associated with sepsis, its exact contribution to the full pathology of the septic process is unclear.

Although the precise mechanisms involved in the failure of organ systems as a consequence of sepsis remains unknown, it is apparent that in those patients who die, the process of organ dysfunction appears metabolic in origin. In the process that culminates in the clinical syndrome of organ failure, instead of the metabolic response to injury abating, the hypermetabolism persists. Hypermetabolism represents a phase of altered metabolic regulation which becomes pathological as the organ failure phase begins. The metabolic dysfunction may be related to either altered hormonal environment, generation of host inflammatory or immunological mediators, and/or enhanced substrate fluxes overloading an already taxed organ system. Ultimately, it will probably be demonstrated that all three mechanisms are necessary for the manifestation of multiple organ failure in the critically ill patient. The sepsis-induced changes in metabolism produce fundamental abnormalities in the normal intraorgan dynamic relationships between muscle, liver, adipose tissue, and kidney. This metabolic dysfunction is associated with the development of profound anergy, lymphopenia, and inadequate wound healing, and if left uncorrected, death invariably follows. The metabolic adaptations in the posttraumatic or septic state are unique and are sometimes different from the physiological responses in fasting, exercise, starvation, diabetes, or other pathological conditions.

PHYSIOLOGICAL GLUCOSE CONSERVATION

In humans and animals there is a fine balance between *anabolism*, the building up of energy stores, and *catabolism*, the breakdown of these energy stores. Following a meal, anabolism predominates, with the sequestration of energy stores. These stores of energy include (1) glycogen, which is mainly amassed in liver and muscle, (2) triglycerides, which are derived from both ingested fatty acids and glucose and are deposited in adipose tissue, and (3) proteins, which can be considered amino acid reserves and are necessary for normal function of all tissues. Between meals and during some pathological conditions, these energy reserves are mobilized to provide fuels for normal function. Initially, when there is an increased demand for glucose in stress, glycogen is broken down to supply glucose for energy. For example, rats show a 99.5 per cent loss of liver glycogen and a 70.3 per cent loss of carcass glycogen after 48 hours of starvation.[68] However, the glucose released is not sufficient to sustain the energy needs of the whole body for more than a short time. Instead, the body adjusts to use alternative fuels for energy production. For example, in long-term starvation or diabetes mellitus, ketone bodies, derived from the incomplete oxidation of fatty acids in liver, are utilized as a primary energy source, thereby sparing glucose carbon, which would otherwise be oxidized.

The adaptive ability of the organism to use alternative fuels instead of glucose is of fundamental importance to the survival of the individual. This is because certain cells such as erythrocytes and cells of the renal medulla and central nervous system have an absolute requirement for glucose, amounting to approximately 180 gm/day. Less than one half of this demand can be supplied simply by the breakdown of glycogen to glucose in the liver (Fig. 8–28). However, the liver and, to a certain extent, the kidneys synthesize glucose from different carbon sources via the process of gluconeogenesis. Glucose is synthesized from glycerol, lactate, pyruvate, and certain amino acids. Glycerol is obtained from adipose tissue following the breakdown of triglycerides. Lactate and pyruvate are derived primarily from skeletal muscle tissue secondary to the breakdown of skeletal muscle glycogen. Amino acids are derived from protein degradation, particularly in skeletal muscle.

HORMONAL CONTROL OF SUBSTRATE FLOW

Many of the processes involved in glucose homeostasis are under hormonal control, which serves to regulate the flow of glucose carbon to ensure adequate blood glucose concentrations. These hormones, whose major effect involves the regulation of plasma glucose concentrations, can be broadly categorized into two groups: anabolic and catabolic hormones. At any time, the net effort of the hormones, whether to catabolize or store fuels, depends on the relative concentrations of each of the hormones to each other as well as their absolute concentration. The principal anabolic hormone

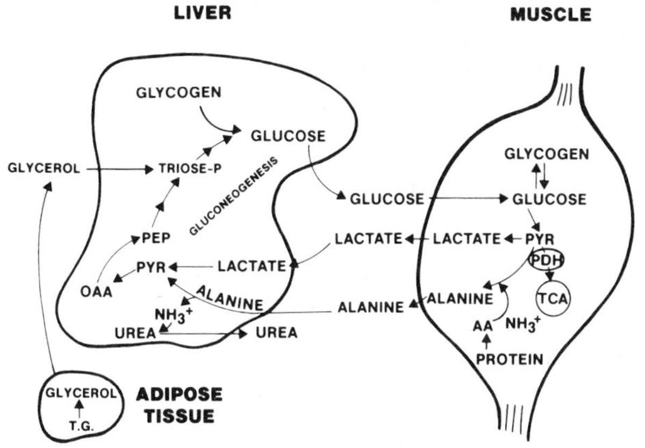

Figure 8–28. Role of liver, skeletal muscle, and adipose tissue in the regulation of plasma glucose concentrations. Pyr, pyruvate; PDH, pyruvate dehydrogenase complex; TCA, tricarboxylic acid cycle; AA, free amino acids; OAA, oxaloacetate; PEP, phosphoenolpyruvate; Triose-P, triosephosphate; TG, triglycerides. (From Siegel JH, Vary TC: Sepsis, abnormal metabolic control and multiple organ failure. In Siegel JH (ed): Trauma: Emergency Surgery and Critical Care. New York, Churchill Livingstone, 1987, p 452.)

is insulin. It is of major importance in fuel storage, promoting the deposition of glycogen, triglycerides, and proteins. At basal levels, insulin has an important anticatabolic role in restraining glycogenolysis, gluconeogenesis, and lipolysis. Growth hormone is also anabolic, but only with respect to protein metabolism, in which growth hormone stimulates amino acid transport and protein synthesis. The major catabolic hormones are glucagon, the adrenocortical hormones (cortisol), and catecholamines. None of these hormones individually totally opposes the action of insulin; instead, the hormones act together to counterbalance insulin action. Glucagon has its major effects on the liver, promoting gluconeogenesis, amino acid uptake, ureagenesis, and protein catabolism. Cortisol enhances net extrahepatic protein catabolism, thereby increasing the release of amino acids, and fosters hepatic utilization of the mobilized amino acids for gluconeogenesis.[69, 70] Catecholamines stimulate lipolysis and glycogenolysis in both hepatic and extrahepatic tissues and promote gluconeogenesis in liver.

Septic Catabolism

Physiological monitoring of the septic patient has demonstrated that the normal balance between anabolic and catabolic processes is altered in the direction of catabolic metabolism.[71, 72] This results in pathological alterations in glucose, fatty acid, and amino acid (protein) metabolism; often manifested clinically by mild hyperglycemia, a rise in serum triglycerides, and changes in plasma amino acid and acute-phase protein concentrations. The pattern of alterations in the plasma level of these fuels is superimposed over changes in the plasma concentration of hormones.[49, 52] Variations in carbohydrate metabolism following severe trauma and during sepsis include hyperglycemia, increased gluconeogenesis with an increased output of glucose from the liver, elevated blood lactate, and an insulin resistance. The metabolic alterations that occur in sepsis contribute to a cascade of secondary alterations which result from the initial traumatic or septic episode. Collectively, these variations lead to the observed plasma changes in hormones and substrates. The metabolic differences observed are most likely a result of changes in hormone concentrations and/or expression of inflammatory or immunological mediators.

Hormonal Changes in Sepsis

Typically, sepsis is characterized by a fall in the thyroid hormone T_3, whereas the other stress hormones (cortisol, epinephrine, and glucagon) are elevated. Glucagon concentrations rise to extraordinarily high levels. Although the rise in glucagon is accompanied by a rise in immunoassayable insulin, the insulin/glucagon ratio is reversed compared with its value in the postabsorptive state. This reversal of the insulin/glucagon ratio may be responsible in part for the accelerated rate of glucose production by the liver in sepsis. Both insulin and glucagon have immediate and delayed effects on hepatic glucose metabolism. The immediate effects of glucagon on hepatic glucose production are seen within seconds and are mediated by alterations in the concentration of cyclic adenine monophosphate (cAMP)[73] (Fig. 8–29).

Somewhat surprisingly, the action of cAMP appears to restrain the activity of phosphofructokinase and pyruvate kinase, which are both regulators of glycolysis in liver, rather than the gluconeogenic enzymes directly. Longer-term effects of glucagon on liver metabolism involve changes in the synthesis or degradation of enzymes in the metabolic pathway of glucose production and appear within hours.[74] In addition to stimulating the enzymes necessary for gluconeogenesis, glucagon also stimulates the breakdown of intracellular proteins. Although the precise mechanism of action of glucagon responsible for this is still unknown, glucagon does enhance the formation of autophagic vacuoles, which engulf and digest intracellular proteins via lysosomes. It is known that the stimulation of autophagic vacuole formation occurs secondary to a reduction in the amino acid glutamine levels in the liver and that glucagon reduces hepatic glutamine levels. By increasing the degradation of hepatic proteins, the action of glucagon on protein metabolism ensures that adequate substrate, in the form of amino acids, is available for gluconeogenesis.

Catecholamines also stimulate both glycogenolysis and gluconeogenesis. The levels of plasma catecholamines epinephrine and norepinephrine have been demonstrated to rise progressively with increasing severity of injury.[75, 76] Dopamine levels are also elevated, but this increase appears to be related to the rise in norepinephrine levels. Both epinephrine and norepinephrine rise to levels considered high enough to produce metabolic changes.[77] In this regard, plasma epineph-

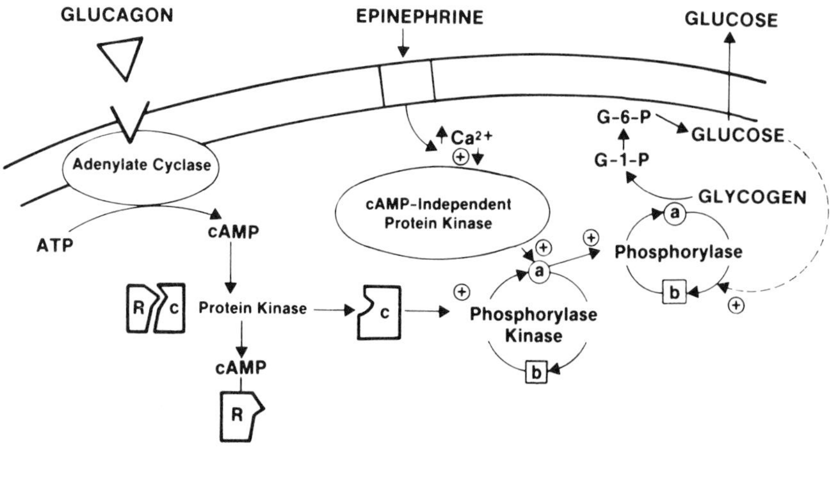

Figure 8–29. Hormonal regulation of glycogenolysis in liver by glucagon and epinephrine. Glucagon acts through a cAMP-dependent protein kinase, while epinephrine functions through a cAMP-independent protein kinase. Both protein kinases act to increase phosphorylase kinase, which in turn activates phosphorylase b. A (+) indicates sites of activation. G-6-P, glucose-6-phosphate; G-1-P, glucose-1-phosphate; cAMP, 5′-3′ cyclic adenosine monophosphate; R, regulatory subunit cAMP-dependent protein kinase; C, catalytic subunit cAMP-dependent protein kinase; Ca^{2+}, calcium stimulation of protein kinase. (From Siegel JH, Vary TC: Sepsis, abnormal metabolic control and multiple organ failure. In Siegel JH (ed): Trauma: Emergency Surgery and Critical Care. New York, Churchill Livingstone, 1987, p 453.)

rine concentrations are more important for stimulating hyperglycemia than is the severity of the injury itself. The stimulation of hepatic output of glucose by epinephrine involves the breakdown of glucagon with the release of glucose (see Fig. 8–29). However, changes in the hormonal milieu are not solely responsible for enhanced gluconeogenesis in sepsis. Unlike other pathological conditions such as starvation or diabetes, in sepsis, gluconeogenesis is not suppressed by the infusion of glucose.[78, 79] This lack of response to glucose has been proposed to occur as a result of enhanced and continual delivery of gluconeogenic precursors, namely lactate, alanine, glycine, serine, and glycerol, from peripheral tissues.

INSULIN RESISTANCE IN SEPSIS

The glucose space is increased in sepsis, as is the mass flow of glucose to peripheral organs. Abnormal glucose tolerance tests are commonly observed following traumatic injury, burn, shock, or sepsis despite normal or accentuated insulin secretion. Despite the responsiveness of the pancreatic β-cells to secrete insulin in response to a glucose load, glucose intolerance and hyperglycemia persist, suggesting that certain target organs in the injured or septic patient are relatively insensitive to the effects of circulating insulin. Since glucose consumption by central and peripheral nervous tissue, renal medulla, bone marrow, erythrocytes, and leukocytes is not insulin-sensitive, the primary sites of insulin resistance are in peripheral tissues, particularly skeletal muscle and adipose tissue, where insulin stimulates glucose uptake. Since only a small percentage (1%) of the glucose load is taken up by adipose tissue, the major effect of insulin appears to be in muscle tissue.

Resistance to the effects of circulating insulin exists in any situation in which a given dose of hormone produces a less than normal biological effect. In sepsis, this insulin resistance is manifested by either an abnormal glucose tolerance test or simply an elevated plasma glucose concentration for a given insulin concentration. This insulin resistance could occur by alterations at one of three levels: (1) prior to the interaction of insulin with the receptor, (2) at the receptor level, or (3) at steps distal to the insulin–receptor interaction, namely cellular metabolism. Causes of insulin resistance at the prereceptor level include factors that lower the effective plasma hormone concentration, such as increased degradation or anti-insulin antibodies. Present evidence suggests that the insulin concentration is the same or increased in sepsis; no anti-insulin antibodies have been detected. At the receptor level, alterations in receptor affinity or receptor number also would decrease the biological response for a given plasma insulin concentration. However, the sensitivity of the receptor to circulating insulin appears to be normal.[80] Hence it appears that insulin resistance in sepsis may be related to an intracellular defect in glucose metabolism.

Most physiological control of glucose utilization occurs at the level of glucose uptake (transport and phosphorylation), glycogenolysis (phosphorylase), glycolysis (phosphofructokinase), or oxidation (pyruvate dehydrogenase) (Fig. 8–30). In both septic patients[79, 81] and animal models,[82, 83] peripheral uptake of glucose is increased. However, the increased glucose uptake is not accompanied by a corresponding increase in glucose oxidation. The fractional oxidation of glucose as a per cent of total calories oxidized is reduced. Furthermore, increasing the insulin concentration accelerates glucose uptake but does not augment glucose oxidation. Instead, the glucose carbon is released from peripheral tissues into the venous blood as lactate, pyruvate, and alanine. Since the rates of pyruvate, lactate, and alanine production are normal or increased, it appears that glucose uptake and glycolysis are normal or accelerated in sepsis. Thus glucose carbon is conserved by the body, since oxidation would deplete the body stores of it. The lactate, pyruvate, and alanine released by skeletal muscle are returned to the liver and kidney, where glucose is synthesized from these three-carbon precursors by the process of gluconeogenesis. This interorgan relationship probably accounts for the increased rate of glucose carbon recycling observed in sepsis.

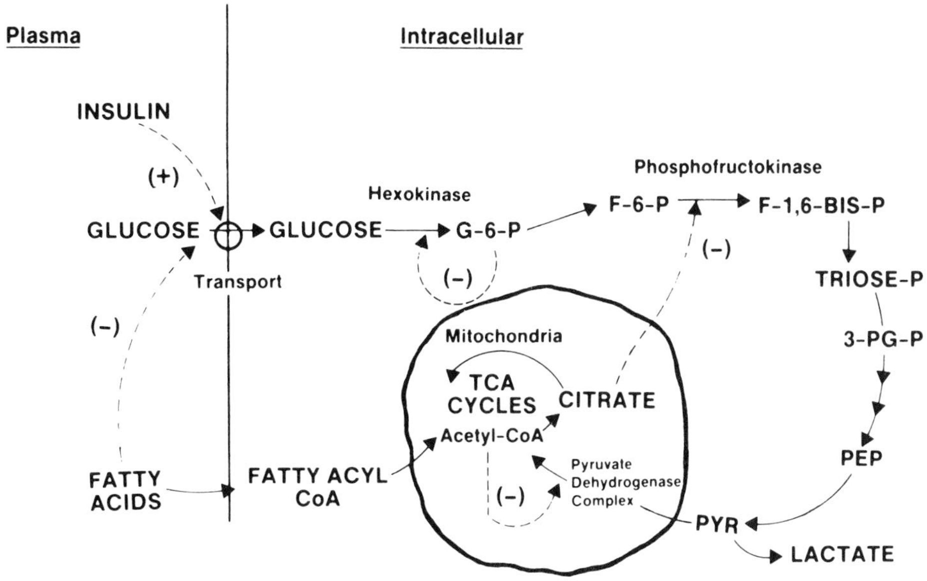

Figure 8–30. Diagram showing mechanisms by which increased FFA oxidation inhibits glucose utilization and oxidation. (+) Represents stimulation of glucose transport by insulin. (−) Represents inhibition of steps by the particular metabolite. G-6-P, glucose-6-phosphate; F-6-P, fructose-6-phosphate; F-1,6-BIS-P, fructose-1, 6-biphosphate; Triose-P, triosephosphate; 3-PG-P, 3-phosphoglycerate phosphate; PEP, phosphoenolypyruvate; PYR, pyruvate. (From Siegel JH, Vary TC: Sepsis, abnormal metabolic control and multiple organ failure. In Siegel JH (ed): Trauma: Emergency Surgery and Critical Care. New York, Churchill Livingstone, 1987, p 462.)

REGULATION OF GLUCOSE OXIDATION IN SEPSIS

Inhibition of Glucose Oxidation

Estimates of glucose recycling suggest that the rate of pyruvate formation from glucose is probably not rate-limiting for glucose oxidation. Impaired glucose oxidation in conjunction with normal or increased lactate, alanine, and/or pyruvate production suggests a specific inhibition of the pyruvate dehydrogenase reaction in sepsis. Thus entry of glucose carbon into the tricarboxylic acid cycle may be limiting for glucose oxidation in sepsis. The pyruvate dehydrogenase (PDH) complex catalyzes the oxidative decarboxylation of pyruvate and allows the entry of pyruvate into the tricarboxylic acid cycle as acetyl-CoA and has been identified as a key mechanism in the control of carbohydrate oxidation and the conservation of glucose carbon (Fig. 8–31). The PDH complex is regulated by end-product inhibition and by reversible phosphorylation.[84, 85] The phosphorylated form of the complex is inactive; the dephosphorylated form is active and allows flux through the complex. The oxidative decarboxylation of pyruvate to acetyl-CoA is of special importance to glucose homeostasis because it necessarily depletes the body of glucose carbon.

Inhibition (phosphorylation) of the PDH complex has been associated with impairment of glucose oxidation during starvation, in alloxan-induced diabetes, and by the oxidation of fatty acids and ketone bodies in liver, heart, and skeletal muscle. In these conditions, glucose oxidation is impaired, but lactate, pyruvate, and alanine production are undiminished.

Recent evidence in septic animal models suggests that a specific inhibition of the PDH complex exists in sepsis, and the degree of impairment is dependent on the severity of the septic episode[86, 87] (Fig. 8–32). Furthermore, while the cardiovascular response to sepsis appears to be independent of the bacterial organism, the metabolic response is dependent not only on the invading organism (aerobe versus anaerobe), but also on the concentration of the organism present. Hyperlactatemia was present only when an aerobe and anaerobe at sufficient concentrations were present.[88] Since decreased PDH activity is associated with a decreased pyruvate oxidation, the inhibition of the complex during sepsis may provide a biochemical explanation for the shift in skeletal muscle glucose metabolism in sepsis.

Intracellular Regulation

The effect of sepsis to lower the proportion of active PDH complex must arise from changes in the intracellular regulators of the interconversion of the PDH complex. In vivo the PDH kinase and phosphatase operate simultaneously, and the proportion of active PDH complex is dependent on the relative rates of these two reactions. The inhibition of the PDH complex may result from an accelerated phosphorylation of the enzyme by the PDH kinase secondary to a rise in the skeletal muscle acetyl-CoA/CoA concentration ratio (Fig. 8–33). In muscle tissue, elevated acetyl-CoA/CoA concentrations are indicative of accelerated fat oxidation. In a septic rat model, the acetyl-CoA/CoA ratio is increased in skeletal muscle, suggesting that the skeletal muscle may become more dependent on noncarbohydrate fuels.[87] The net effect of an increased dependence on noncarbohydrate fuels for energy production would be a decreased rate of glucose oxidation and a conservation of glucose carbon. These observations are supported by analysis of respiratory quotients,[89, 90] and indirect calorimetry data[91] in septic patients have demonstrated an increased dependence on fatty acid oxidation, supporting the concept of altered fuel utilization in sepsis.

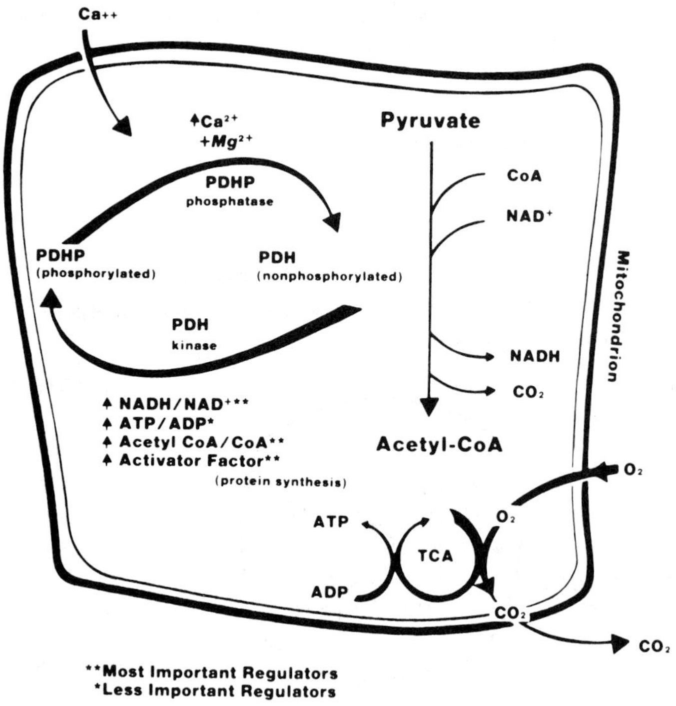

Figure 8–31. Interconversion cycle regulating the phosphorylation/dephosphorylation of pyruvate dehydrogenase complex (PDH) in mammalian cells. CoA, coenzyme A; PDH, pyruvate dehydrogenase complex; PDHP, phosphorylated pyruvate dehydrogenase complex; NAD^+ (H), nicotinamide adenine dinucleotide (reduced); ATP, adenosine 5′-triphosphate; ADP, adenosine 5′-diphosphate; TCA, tricarboxylic acid cycle. (From Siegel JH, Vary TC: Sepsis, abnormal metabolic control and multiple organ failure. In Siegel JH (ed): Trauma: Emergency Surgery and Critical Care. New York, Churchill Livingstone, 1987, p 456.)

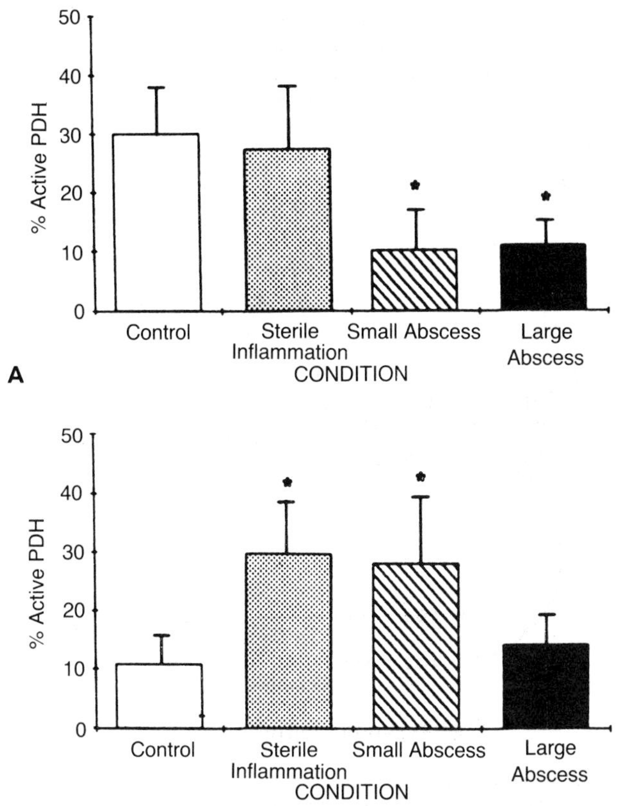

Figure 8–32. Effect of sepsis on activity of pyruvate dehydrogenase complex in skeletal muscle *(A)* and liver *(B)*. Skeletal muscle and liver samples were frozen in situ 5 days after intra-abdominal introduction of a rat fecal agar pellet. Four groups of animals were used: control (no pellet); sterile inflammation (no bacterial inoculation); small septic abscess (*Bacteroides fragilis* 10^8/ml + *Escherichia coli* 10^6/ml; 0.8 ml pellet); and large septic abscess (*B. fragilis* 10^8/ml + *E. coli* 10^2/ml; 1.5 ml pellet). Extracts of frozen tissue were assayed for active and total pyruvate dehydrogenase (PDH) activity in duplicate. Results are presented as a percentage of total PDH complex existing in active form. Values shown are means ± SE for 10 to 14 animals. **P* < 0.005 versus control, Scheffe's analysis for all contrasts. (From Vary TC, Siegel JH, Nakatani T, Sato T, Aoyama H: Effect of sepsis on activity of pyruvate dehydrogenase complex in skeletal muscle and liver. Am J Physiol 250:E636, 1986.)

There also is another longer-term mechanism which increases PDH kinase activity.[92] The effect of sepsis to decrease the proportion of active PDH complex persists into skeletal muscle mitochondria. This results from a 2.5-fold increase in the PDH kinase activity in mitochondria prepared from septic animals. Furthermore, the PDH kinase was less sensitive to the inhibitory effects of pyruvate or dichloroacetate in sepsis compared with control.[93] These results, taken together, suggest the mechanism must involve a rather stable change, since increased PDH kinase activity persists through isolation, incubation, and extraction of mitochondria.

Hyperlactatemia in Sepsis

Elevated plasma lactate concentrations are a characteristic feature of sepsis and have been correlated with increased mortality and morbidity.[94] Sepsis-induced hyperlactatemia can be easily explained when there exists tissue ischemia. However, in the hyperdynamic, hypermetabolic state of sepsis, oxygen consumption and oxygen delivery are increased with adequate tissue perfusion and maintenance of normal high-energy phosphate concentrations. Hence the hyperlactatemia is present under conditions where tissue oxygen delivery is elevated. The ratio of lactate to pyruvate is unchanged, suggesting that the increased plasma lactate does not result from inadequate oxygen delivery. Instead, sepsis-induced hyperlactatemia results from a metabolic dysfunction rather than a deficit in oxygen availability. Increased plasma lactate concentrations in sepsis are due to either an increased production or decreased utilization or both. Whole-body tracer studies in septic animal models and humans show a diversion of glucose carbon away from oxidation toward lactate and alanine formation.[80–84] The liver is the major organ responsible for lactate clearance by the body. Lactate taken up the liver is synthesized to glucose by the pathway of gluconeogenesis. While the rate of glucose production by the liver is increased in sepsis, the rate of lactate delivery may exceed the capacity for gluconeogenesis.

More important, there is accelerated lactate production in the periphery.[95] The sepsis-induced increases in plasma lactate probably result from a combination of metabolic abnormalities. There is an accelerated uptake of glucose in the absence of increased glycogen deposition. Therefore, pyruvate production is increased. While pyruvate production is increased, pyruvate oxidation is decreased owing to an inhibition of the PDH complex. Therefore, the pyruvate produced is channeled into lactate and alanine formation rather than oxidation.

Evidence for this mechanism is supported by studies in which the sepsis-induced inhibition of the PDH complex is partially reversed with dichloroacetate.[86, 96] Dichloroacetate activates the PDH complex, resulting in a stimulation of pyruvate oxidation. The increased pyruvate oxidation re-

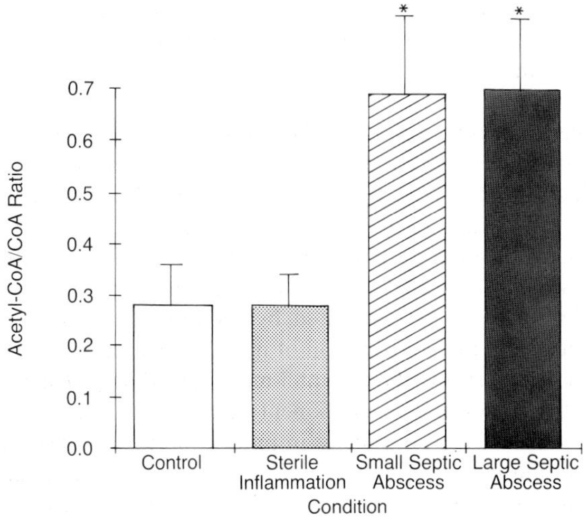

Figure 8–33. Effect of sepsis on skeletal muscle acetyl-CoA/CoA ratios. Skeletal muscle was frozen in situ 5 days after intra-abdominal introduction of a rat agar pellet, as described in Figure 8–32. Neutralized perchloric extracts of skeletal muscle were assayed for CoA and acetyl-CoA by reverse-phase, high-performance liquid chromatography. Values shown are means ± SE for 8 to 12 tissues in each group. **P* < 0.01 versus control. (From Vary TC, Siegel JH, Nakatani T, et al: Regulation of glucose metabolism by altered pyruvate dehydrogenase activity. JPEN 10:419, 1986. © by American Society for Pharmacological and Experimental Therapy, 1986.)

duces the availability of pyruvate for lactate formation, thereby reducing lactate production. Administration of dichloroacetate to septic animals activated the PDH complex and lowered both plasma and tissue lactate and alanine concentrations.[86, 96] Dichloroacetate also has been administered to a small number of patients with sepsis-induced lactic acidosis.[97, 98] In one of these patients, dichloroacetate administration was associated with a decreased blood lactate concentration and normalization of the blood pH. However, the other patients died, although there was some improvement in the plasma lactate concentrations. The latter patients belonged to a group in which the mortality was expected to be 90 to 100 per cent. Therefore, the role of dichloroacetate in the treatment of sepsis-induced hyperlactatemia needs to be examined in a randomized, prospective study during the clinical course where recovery is possible.

ALTERED SKELETAL MUSCLE PROTEIN METABOLISM

In addition to its role in locomotion, skeletal muscle, by virtue of its mass in relation to body weight, represents the major reservoir of amino acids (Fig. 8–34). Some of these amino acids are important substrates for gluconeogenesis in liver and kidney. Protein wasting is a general feature of trauma, septic, or burn patients as evidenced by profound weight losses which become obvious once the initial edema subsides.[81, 99, 100] The normal balance between synthesis and degradation is no longer maintained. The imbalance is first observed as tissue wasting and then as increased nitrogen excretion and increased amino acid concentrations in the blood. All the observed changes are the result of an imbalance in protein turnover, with the balance tipped in favor of catabolism. The clinical measurement of nitrogen excretion by the kidney can be used as an estimate of protein breakdown, since the nitrogen excreted is derived from amino acids released by proteolysis.

The increased net proteolysis results in the release of amino acids from structural protein stores, particularly in skeletal muscle (Fig. 8–35). The rate of release of amino acids across the lower extremities increases two- to fivefold in trauma or septic patients compared with healthy volunteers following an overnight fast. The protein economy of the whole body can be estimated by monitoring the nitrogen balance, and the contribution of muscle tissue can be monitored by measuring the rate of 3-methylhistidine production. 3-Methylhistidine is a component of actin–myosin proteins and is liberated from muscle in proportion to its concentration in muscle protein.[101] This catabolic phase is an intrinsic response to trauma and sepsis, with the amount of muscle loss exceeding that due simply to bed rest. In trauma patients, the catabolic phase abates within a few days of injury and is followed by the restoration of positive nitrogen balance and lean body mass. In contrast to trauma, the catabolic phase continues in sepsis, even when exogenous nutritional support is provided. Skeletal muscle makes a significant contribution to the rise in whole-body protein breakdown. The rate of muscle protein breakdown increases to a greater degree than that of the whole body, with the contribution of muscle proteolysis to whole-body protein degradation nearly doubling.

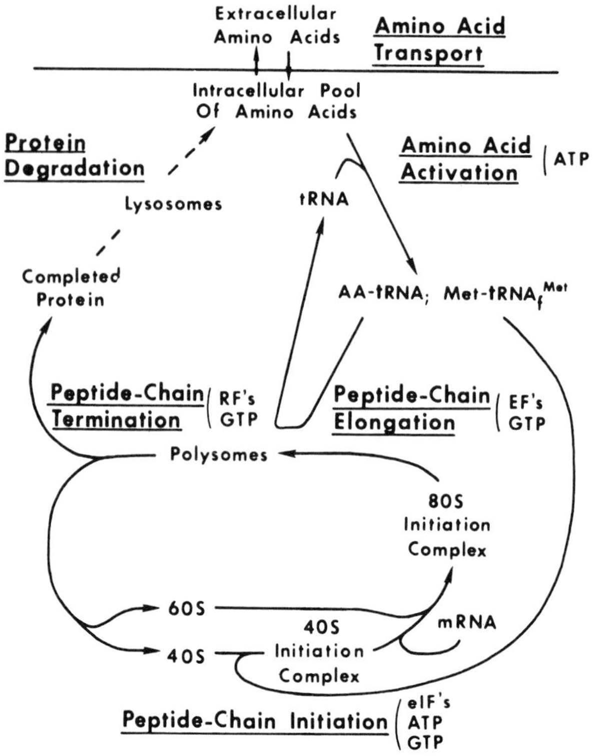

Figure 8–34. Pathway of skeletal muscle protein turnover. The figure schematically depicts the major steps involved in protein synthesis and in protein degradation. Abbreviations used are as follows: ATP, adenosine triphosphate; GTP, guanosine triphosphate; tRNA, transfer RNA; AA-tRNA, aminoacyl-transfer RNA; Met-tRNA$_f^{Met}$, the initiator methionyltransfer RNA; eIF's, eukaryotic initiation factors; mRNA, messenger RNA; EF's, elongation factors; RF's, releasing factors; 40S and 60S, the small and large ribosomal subunits, respectively. (From Jefferson LS: Role of insulin in the regulation of protein synthesis. Diabetes 29:488, 1980. Reproduced with permission from The American Diabetes Association, Inc.)

Mediators of Proteolysis

The stimulus for enhanced muscle catabolism during sepsis is unknown. A certain amount of muscle catabolism in the trauma patient can be attributed to direct injury to the muscle, with subsequent repair of the damaged tissues. However, enhanced catabolism also occurs in the septic patient with no overt signs of direct tissue trauma. Studies in burn patients have suggested that cortisol is a major determinant of the catabolic response.[81] Some of the effects of cortisol have been confirmed in healthy volunteers subjected to an artificial elevation of cortisol to levels seen in burn patients. However, in the postoperative state, and most probably sepsis, cortisol is of less importance, since the metabolic effects appear to be the net result of an integrated response to several hormones, with the possibility of additional factors.

Insulin conserves muscle protein by both stimulating protein synthesis and inhibiting protein degradation.[102, 103] However, in sepsis, the breakdown of muscle protein, as measured by 3-methylhistidine release, is increased despite increased

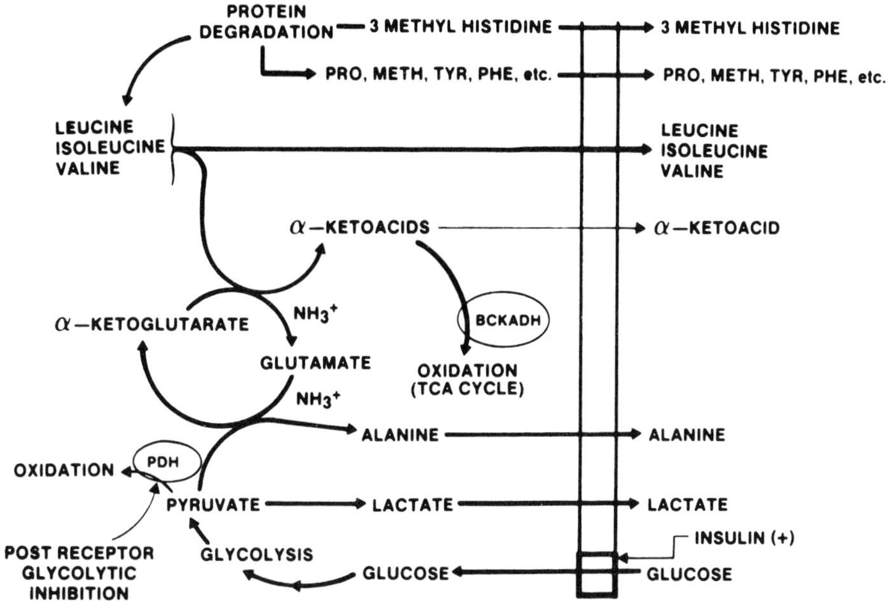

Figure 8–35. Effect of sepsis on skeletal muscle proteolysis, pathways of branched chain amino acid, and glucose metabolism. Septic protein degradation is accelerated with increased release of 3-methylhistidine. Proteolysis liberates branched chain amino acids (leucine, isoleucine, and valine), which are either released into blood or transaminated to α-ketoacid. The BCAA α-ketoacids are either released into blood or undergo oxidation via branched chain ketoacid dehydrogenase (BCKADH). In sepsis, glucose uptake at insulin-sensitive sites is either normal or increased. Glycolysis appears unaffected, but pyruvate oxidation is limited by postreceptor inhibition owing to decreased pyruvate dehydrogenase complex activity (PDH ↓). Glucose carbon (pyruvate) is either reduced to lactate or transaminated from BCAA liberated NH_3^+ via glutamate to form alanine. (Reprinted by permission of Siegel JH, Vary TC: Sepsis, abnormal metabolic control and multiple organ failure. In Siegel JH (ed): Trauma: Emergency and Critical Care. New York, Churchill Livingstone, 1987, p 440.)

insulin concentrations.[101] Furthermore, animal studies have shown both a decreased sensitivity and maximal response to the inhibitory effects of insulin on protein degradation in sepsis.[139] These observations also suggest that additional factors resulting from the septic episode accelerate muscle catabolism or that injury renders the muscle resistant to insulin action.

Increased muscle proteolysis induced by incubating muscle strips with serum from septic patients has led to the hypothesis that a serum factor expressed as a result of sepsis is responsible for the accelerated muscle catabolism.[104, 105] In particular, interleukin 1, which is secreted by macrophages activated by complement, has been proposed to mediate this effect on muscle proteolysis. Unfortunately, interleukin 1 has not been demonstrated in blood from septic patients. Instead, a small molecular weight protein, called *proteolysis-inducing factor*, has been isolated from blood obtained from trauma and septic patients.[105] Proteolysis-inducing factor stimulates protein degradation and release of free amino acids from muscle tissues incubated in vitro at rates three to five times above normal.

Protein Synthesis

The effects of trauma and sepsis on protein synthesis in skeletal muscle are not uniformly accepted, with rates of protein synthesis either unchanged, increased, or decreased. The maintenance or increased rates of protein synthesis during sepsis would seem uncharacteristic, since protein synthesis in muscle is sensitive to a wide range of insults. In muscle-wasting states where direct measurements have been made, skeletal muscle protein synthesis is depressed. It is not clear why some investigators have not observed a decreased rate of synthesis in sepsis, but part of the problem may lie in the use of incubated muscles. Incubated muscles which are not maintained at resting length show lower rates of synthesis.[106] Far more reliable are studies in vivo. In these studies, skeletal muscle protein synthesis is decreased following endotoxin administration,[107] acute exposure to *Streptococcus pneumoniae*,[108] or chronic intra-abdominal sepsis.[109] The reduction in protein synthesis during septic states was independent of prior food intake.[106]

Control of protein synthesis can occur at peptide chain initiation, elongation or termination by the number and distribution of ribosomes and by the amount and stability of translatable mRNA.[110] Synthesis of individual proteins is regulated in part by changes in the transcription of specific mRNAs in skeletal muscle. Once the mRNA is transcribed, it is translated, with the product being newly synthesized protein. Two general mechanisms modulate the translation of mRNA. There may be decreased capacity for translation. This means that there are fewer ribosomes than are necessary for protein synthesis to proceed. Since approximately 80 per cent of cellular RNA is ribosomal, changes in muscle RNA content presumably reflect changes in ribosomal RNA. Jepson and associates have proposed that a fall in tissue RNA is responsible, in part, for the decreased rate of protein synthesis in endotoxin-treated rats.[107] However, Young and associates reported that while the RNA falls over the short term (48 hr), over the longer term (5 days), RNA levels return to normal, and yet there is inhibition in protein synthesis.[111] Therefore, other mechanisms must be operating to account for discussed rates of protein synthesis in sepsis. In addition to the capacity for synthesis, there are decreases in the efficiency of translation. Efficiency of translation relates to how well available protein synthetic machinery is able to translate mRNA. The translational phase of protein synthesis involves peptide chain initiation, elongation, and termination. Each of these steps represents a complex sequence of reactions involving several enzymes, protein factors, and cofactors. A fall in translational efficiency also has been observed in the septic state, although the precise biochemical sites inhibited by the septic process are unknown.[112]

The signals responsible for the inhibition in protein synthesis are also unknown. In a recent study, injection of tumor necrosis factor caused a rapid and substantial decrease in muscle protein synthesis.[113] However, other investigators have failed to demonstrate any effect of either interleukin 1α or β or tumor necrosis factor on muscle protein synthesis.

Amino Acid Metabolism

The increased release of amino acids from skeletal muscle is intimately related to glucose homeostasis, since amino acids represent an important precursor for gluconeogenesis. When the molar percentage of amino acids in muscle protein is compared with the molar percentage of amino acids released, it is seen that the majority of amino acids are released in proportion to their concentration in muscle proteins. However, the exceptions to this are alanine and glutamine, which are released in excess of their concentration in muscle proteins. As described earlier, these amino acids serve as a major source of glucose carbon for gluconeogenesis in liver. In the postabsorptive state, plasma alanine can be derived from transamination of pyruvate with a nitrogen donor as well as from protein stores (see Fig. 8–35). The potential sources of nitrogen include the branched-chain amino acids (leucine, isoleucine, and valine), glutamine, and glutamate. In the postabsorptive human, about 40 per cent of the circulating plasma alanine could be derived from endogenous proteins, whereas 60 per cent is derived from de novo synthesis.[114] At least 20 per cent of the nitrogen required for the de novo alanine synthesis comes from leucine. Leucine (isoleucine and valine) nitrogen is incorporated into alanine through a series of reversible transamination reactions involving the nitrogen transfer from leucine to glutamate via the branched-chain aminotransferase and the subsequent transamination of glutamate with pyruvate, forming alanine. The rate of alanine synthesis will be determined by (1) the rate of leucine appearance and (2) the rate of pyruvate availability.

Branched-Chain Amino Acid Metabolism

Recent reports have suggested that administration of branched-chain amino acids is beneficial in septic patients and improves the survival of surgical patients with multiple organ failure.[114–118] Administration of branched-chain amino acids as part of the nutritional support for traumatized or septic persons results in decreased weight loss, reduced negative nitrogen balance, decreased protein catabolism, and increased protein synthesis. In surgical patients, nitrogen retention was greater in those patients receiving 45 per cent over those receiving 24 per cent as branched-chain amino acids in their total parenteral nutrition.[117, 118] One hypothesis for their efficacy is that they provide a fuel for skeletal muscle and liver energy metabolism at a time when glucose oxidative metabolism may be inhibited.

Branched-chain amino acids are one of the few amino acids oxidized in muscle tissues. In healthy animals and humans, there appears to be a differential pattern of branched-chain amino acid metabolism in muscle and liver.[119, 120] In muscle tissues, the aminotransferase activity is high, and the oxidative decarboxylation of the corresponding α-ketoacid is rate-limiting for leucine oxidation. Only about 50 per cent of the leucine undergoing transamination is oxidized. The corresponding α-ketoacids are released into the blood. The concentration of all three α-ketoacids of branched-chain amino acids in human plasma is approximately 0.04 to 0.1 m*M*. In contrast to muscle, the activity of the branched-chain dehydrogenase in hepatic tissue is higher than that of the transaminase, and α-ketoacids are readily oxidized.[120] The reason for the differential pattern may lie in the differential regulation of the branched-chain amino acid dehydrogenase in muscle and liver. The branched-chain α-ketoacid dehydrogenase is also regulated by a phosphorylation/dephosphorylation cycle, analogous to the PDH complex.[121–123] The branched-chain α-ketoacid dehydrogenase is inactivated in muscle tissue by ATP-dependent phosphorylation but is protected in some way from inactivation in liver. The liver appears to possess extra amounts of the catalytic subunit of the enzyme, called activator protein, which restores flux through the phosphorylated complex. Because of the presence of this activator protein, it is unlikely that the activity of the branched-chain dehydrogenase is rate-limiting for oxidation. This affords a mechanism whereby α-ketoacids released by extrahepatic tissues are taken up and utilized by the liver, with the possible formation of glucose and ketone bodies.

The absolute contribution of branched-chain amino acids to the overall energy metabolism (ATP generation) is still debatable. In the absence of any other exogenous substrate, leucine oxidation in cardiac muscle could account for only about 5 per cent of the total oxygen consumption, even at supraphysiological levels of leucine. Leucine could not provide sufficient energy to maintain normal cardiac function.[124] Hence it is doubtful that leucine represents a significant energy fuel.

CHANGES IN HEPATIC PROTEIN METABOLISM

While it is clear that net proteolysis occurs in skeletal muscle in sepsis, in liver, protein synthesis following trauma or infection is increased.[125] Liver is unique in that it synthesizes proteins for its own use, i.e., structural proteins essential for normal cell function, and proteins that are secreted into the blood, i.e., secretory proteins such as albumin. However, since most studies have simply measured whole-liver protein synthetic rates, it is not entirely clear whether there is a preferential synthesis of structural or secretory proteins in sepsis. In animal models when the synthesis rate has been measured, trauma or sepsis is associated with an increase in both secretory and structural proteins. The net effect is an increased liver weight. The increased rates of protein synthesis coincide with enhanced hepatic uptake (or clearance) of amino acids. Much of the evidence for a role of amino acids in regulating hepatic protein synthesis comes from isolated perfused liver studies.[126–128] Thus the increased hepatic protein synthesis has been suggested to be caused by or dependent on an increased supply of amino acids from the peripheral tissues.

Acute-Phase Protein Metabolism

Trauma and sepsis have been shown to increase the hepatic synthesis and secretion of a number of proteins referred to as *acute-phase proteins*. The acute-phase proteins include C-reactive protein, fibrinogen, ceruloplasmin, and α_1-antitrypsin. Many of these acute-phase proteins are linked to the host's ability to resist or control infection. These functions include complement activation and opsonization needed for bacterial killing (C-reactive protein), coagulation, surface structure and support lattice formations needed for leukocyte entrapment of foreign material (fibrinogen), superoxide scavenging (ceruloplasmin), and inactivation of excess proteases needed to prevent damage to viable cells (α_1-antitrypsin).

A differential pattern in the plasma acute-phase protein profile has been demonstrated in trauma and septic patients[46] (Figs. 8–36 and 8–37). The presence of sepsis, whether clinically evident or not, modifies the posttraumatic acute-phase protein response to favor the increase of some acute-phase proteins while affecting a decrease in the concentration of other proteins that may not be as critical for survival. In both nonseptic and septic patients, during the first 2 or 3 days after injury, there is a rise in C-reactive protein, fibrinogen, α_1-antitrypsin, and ceruloplasmin. After 3 days, the concentrations of C-reactive protein, fibrinogen, and ceruloplasmin all return toward normal values in nonseptic trauma patients, but α_1-antitrypsin concentrations remain elevated. In contrast, in trauma patients who develop clinical

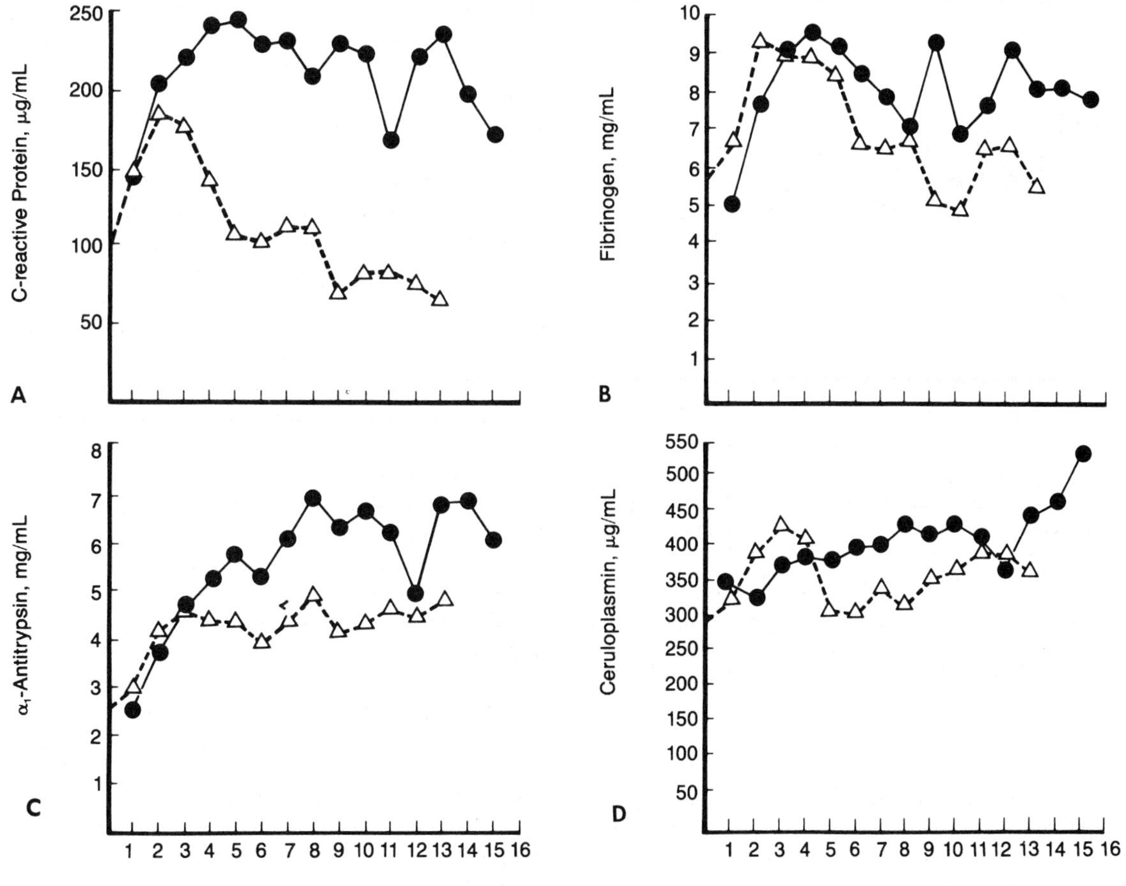

Figure 8–36. Plasma acute-phase protein concentrations after trauma in 16 patients (open triangles) and trauma complicated by sepsis in 10 patients (solid circles). Mean values for C-reactive protein *(A)*, fibrinogen *(B)*, α_1-antitrypsin *(C)*, and ceruloplasmin *(D)* in patients with sepsis developing after trauma are compared with nonseptic trauma patients. Note the early rise in both C-reactive protein and α_1-antitrypsin in those trauma patients who later became clinically septic between 5 and 7 days. (From Sganga G, Siegel JH, Brown G, et al: Reprioritization of hepatic plasma protein release in trauma and sepsis. Arch Surg 120:191, 1985. Copyright 1985, American Medical Association.)

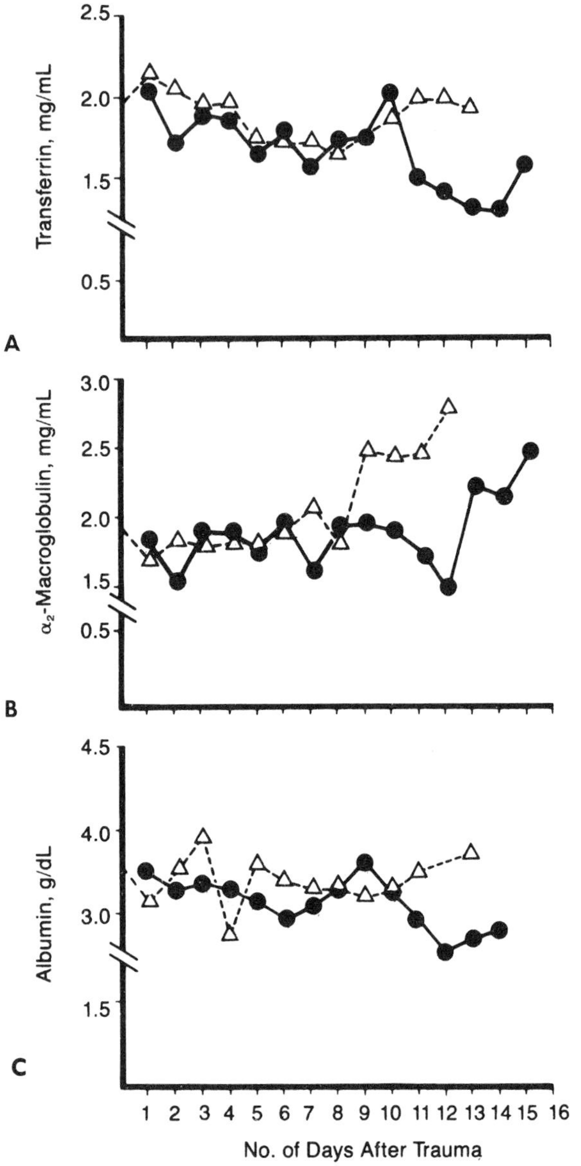

Figure 8–37. Plasma acute-phase protein concentrations after trauma in 16 patients (open triangles) and trauma complicated by sepsis in 10 patients (solid circles). Mean values for transferrin *(A)*, α_2-macroglobulin *(B)*, and albumin *(C)* in patients with sepsis developing after trauma are compared with nonseptic trauma patients. Most changes occur only after patients become clinically septic between 5 and 7 days. (Reprinted with permission from Sganga G, Siegel JH, Brown G, et al: Reprioritization of hepatic plasma protein release in trauma and sepsis. Arch Surg 120:192, 1985. Copyright 1985, American Medical Association.)

signs of sepsis, C-reactive protein, fibrinogen, α_1-antitrypsin, and ceruloplasmin all remained elevated. There is an early decrease in transferrin, but α_2-macroglobulin and albumin concentrations do not change in nonseptic trauma patients. The plasma concentrations of these latter proteins decrease as the septic episode progresses.

The mechanisms for these changes are unknown. In mouse liver, increased synthesis of acute-phase proteins is associated with increased mRNA for individual proteins, while decreased albumin synthesis in rats with an inflammatory insult is mediated by decreased mRNA concentrations.[139, 140] These findings suggest that a differential response in the synthesis of individual acute-phase proteins may occur through transcriptional control of mRNA synthesis.

DEPENDENCE ON FATTY ACID METABOLISM

The metabolic course of the traumatized or septic patient shows that fatty acids become the preferred fuel for oxidative metabolism. This conclusion is based on analysis of respiratory quotients[89, 90] and of indirect calorimetry studies.[91] The same dependence on fatty acid metabolism is observed under conditions of starvation and diabetes, in which the conservation of glucose carbon becomes pathological. In starvation and diabetes, fatty acid mobilization in adipose tissue is thought to occur as a result of a starvation- or diabetes-induced fall in plasma insulin concentrations. This enhanced mobilization of fatty acids from adipose tissue is coupled with an increased hepatic capacity to synthesize ketone bodies.[129] The mechanism responsible for the stimulation of ketone body production includes both increased substrate (fatty acids) delivery and an increased hepatic capacity to handle fatty acids. In addition to the effects in liver, fatty acid utilization in muscle tissue is also dependent upon delivery of fatty acid. As the level of fatty acids increases,[130] extraction and oxidation increase.[130]

The release of fatty acids from adipose tissue in sepsis is variable, with some reports of an increased release and other reports of a decreased release. Despite unaltered arterial fatty acid concentrations, fatty acids are continually released into the bloodstream and delivered to the liver. After removal from the plasma, fatty acids may undergo either oxidation for energy and ketone body production or esterification to triglycerides (Fig. 8–38). Increased hepatic triglycerides are a characteristic feature of sepsis, giving rise to the histological observations of increased lipid droplets in liver tissue at autopsy. Part of the increased triglycerides may be due to reesterification. This increased reesterification may be responsible in part for the increased secretion of triglycerides as very low lipoproteins (VLDL–TG).

Virtually all studies of fulminant sepsis have shown increased plasma triglycerides as the septic process worsens. Besides an increase in hepatic triglyceride synthesis, an impairment in the peripheral triglyceride disposal mechanisms may exist. The activity of lipoprotein lipase, the enzyme responsible for clearance of plasma triglycerides, is reduced in both adipose tissue and muscle from septic animals.[131, 132] Concomitant with the lowered lipoprotein lipase activity, plasma triglyceride concentrations are increased. Tumor necrosis factor is responsible for lowering lipoprotein lipase activity by reducing lipoprotein lipase synthesis in sepsis.

Reduced Ketone Bodies

The normal response of the liver to increased delivery of fatty acids is the synthesis of ketone bodies (3-L-hydroxybutyrate and acetoacetate). In addition, reversal of the insu-

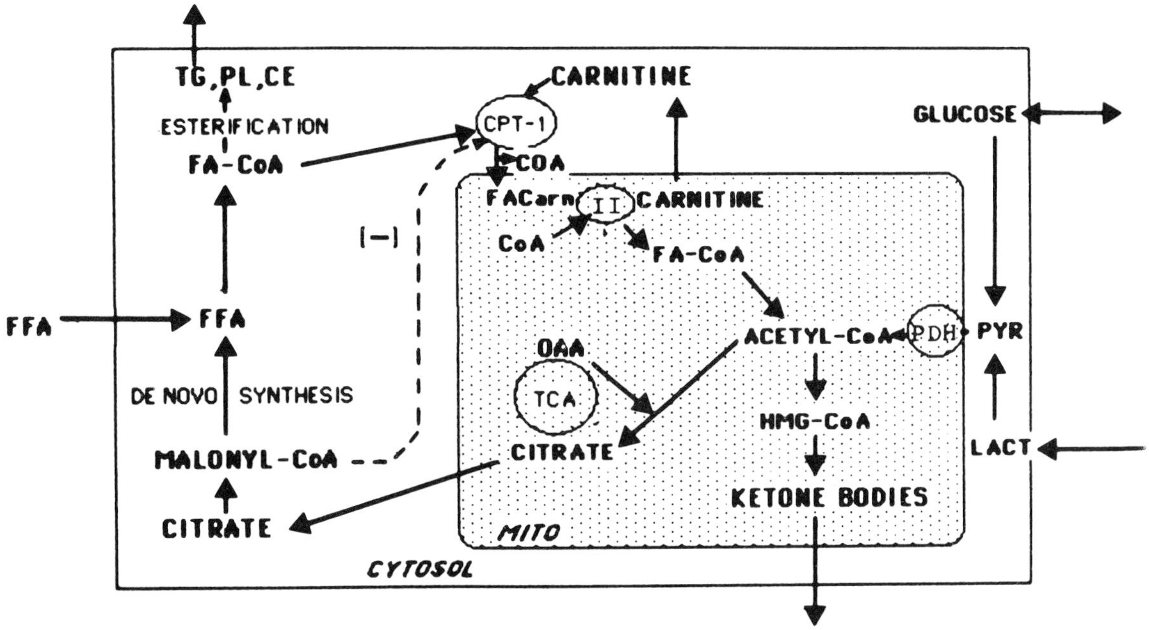

Figure 8–38. Relationships of hepatic fatty acid oxidation, ketogenesis, and fatty acid synthesis, (– –) Malonyl-CoA inhibition of carnitine:acyl-CoA transferase I. Carnitine:acyl-CoA transferases are bound to the inner mitochondrial membrane in vivo, but for clarity the reactions are shown away from membrane. FFA, long-chain fatty acids; FA-CoA, long-chain fatty acyl-CoA; FACarn, long-chain fatty acyl carnitine; CoA, coenzyme A; OAA, oxaloacetate; PYR, pyruvate; LACT, lactate; TCA, citric acid cycle; TG, triglycerides; PL, phospholipids; CPT-I, carnitine:acyl-CoA transferase I; II = Carnitine:acyl-CoA transferase II; PDH, pyruvate dehydrogenase complex; MITO, mitochondria. (From Vary TC, Siegel JH, Nakatani T, et al: A biochemical basis for depressed ketogenesis in sepsis. J Trauma 26:420, 1986. © by Williams & Wilkins, 1986.)

lin/glucagon ratio enhances the ketogenic capacity of the liver. In sepsis, there is a rise in the glucagon/insulin ratio, but the hepatic and plasma ketone body concentrations are lower than expected given the hormonal environment. Septic animals (Fig. 8–39) and patients undergoing a total fast will not demonstrate ketonemia. The lack of elevated plasma ketones does not indicate a lack of fatty acid oxidation, since these patients have respiratory quotients of 0.75, indicative of fatoxidation. Thus sepsis appears to induce changes in hepatic fatty acid metabolism, which prevents or reverses maximal rates of ketogenesis.[135] Part of this decreased ketogenic capacity may result from elevated malonyl-CoA concentrations in the liver. Malonyl-CoA is a competitive inhibitor of long-chain carnitine:acyl-CoA transferase, thereby preventing the mitochondrial uptake of fatty acid.[136]

The failure of hepatic tissue to enhance ketogenesis may be important to the clinical outcome of the septic episode, since survival is dependent on normal liver function. A decrease in the circulating ketone body concentrations would be expected to increase the dependence of peripheral tissues on alternative substrates for energy production when cellular metabolism is accelerated by sepsis. The failure to effect similar increases in plasma ketone bodies in nondiabetic septic patients may be an additional factor in the markedly increased rates of proteolysis in septic patients. Of considerable interest is the observation that enhanced muscle catabolism in response to injury is not observed if the blood concentration of ketone bodies is increased.[133, 134] However, it would be impractical to simply supply ketone bodies as nutritional support. To replace 5 per cent glucose, a patient would require 125 gm ketones per day. The amount of ketone bodies presents few problems, since ketone bodies are readily soluble in saline. The problem is that accompanying the ketone body infusion would be approximately 1200 mEq of a positive ion (Na^+). Such a salt load on kidneys is certainly not advised in healthy people and probably would be devastating to the septic patient who may have complicating renal dysfunction.

Lipogenesis in Sepsis

Ketogenesis may be inhibited during sepsis, but lipogenesis appears to be accelerated. In septic patients receiving only glucose in excess of 800 cal/m^2, the respiratory quotient rises above 1.0, indicative of net lipogenesis.[89] The capacity to synthesize lipids is increased, suggesting an increased flow of acetyl groups toward fatty acid synthesis and away from ketone body function. These observations support the concept of a reciprocal relationship between lipogenesis and ketogenesis, thus preventing both fatty acids and ketone bodies from being synthesized simultaneously, which would result in an energy-wasting futile cycle.

NUTRITIONAL SUPPORT

With this background in the metabolic alterations in sepsis, it may now be possible to better design nutritional support for the critically ill based on the knowledge of the sepsis-

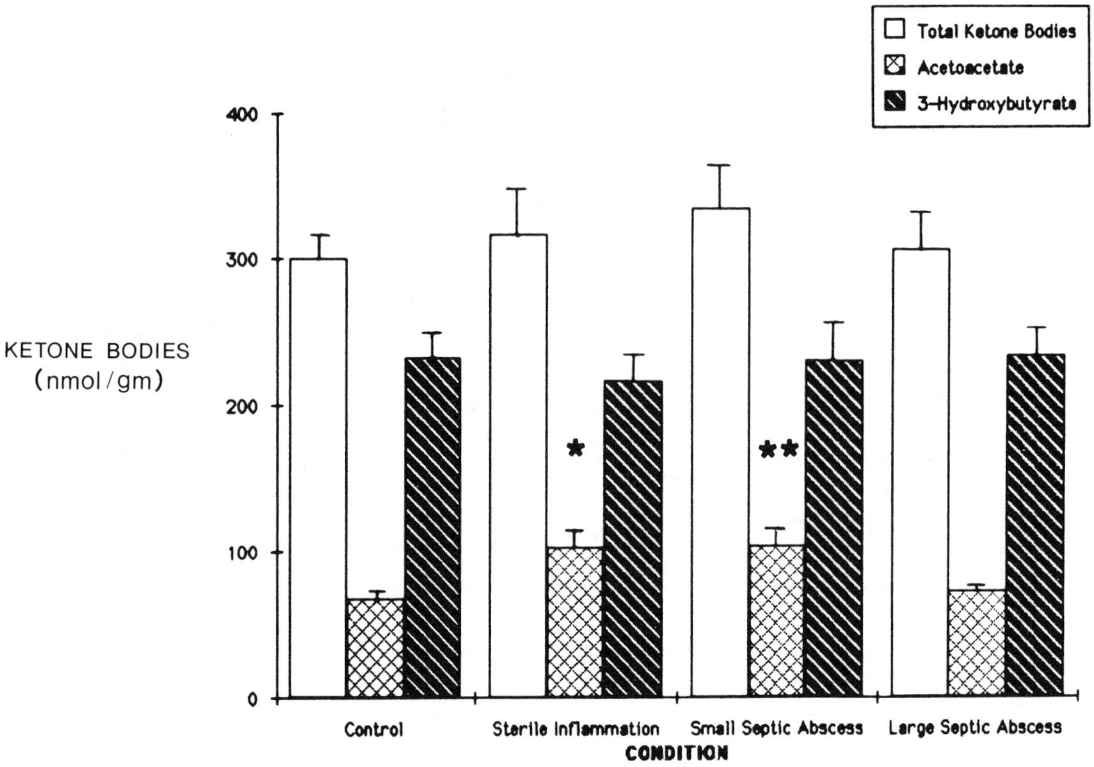

Figure 8–39. Effect of sterile inflammation and chronic sepsis on the hepatic ketone body levels. Livers from control, sterile inflammatory, and chronic septic abscess (small and large) animals were frozen in situ with clamps precooled to the temperature of liquid nitrogen 5 days following the intra-abdominal introduction of the rat fecal-agar pellet. Hepatic levels of total ketone bodies (sum of acetoacetate + β-hydroxybutyrate), acetoacetate, and 3-L-hydroxybutyrate were determined in neutralized perchloric acid extracts. Values are means ± SE for 6 to 13 livers in each group (*$P < 0.05$, **$P < 0.01$ compared with control). (Reprinted from Vary TC, Siegel JH, Nakatani T, et al: A biochemical basis for depressed ketogenesis in sepsis. J Trauma 26:422, 1986. © by Williams & Wilkins, 1986.)

induced alterations in substrate fluxes. The maintenance of adequate nutritional support is necessary to minimize skeletal muscle wasting, lessen postoperative weakness, and shorten convalescence. The objective nutritional support must be to provide adequate calories to account for energy expenditure and to attempt to arrest protein wasting of sepsis. These requirements can be satisfied with carbohydrate, fatty acids, and amino acids. Much debate exists, however, over the type and proportion of each fuel to be given. Evidence is given in previous sections regarding the metabolic consequences of different nutritional support therapies. In general, the kilocalories/nitrogen ratio reflects the quantities of nonprotein kilograms and nitrogen consumed in the diet of a normal healthy individual. This ratio is generally 159 to 200 nonprotein kilograms ingested per gram of nitrogen. Consequently, nutritional support should be geared to provide a ratio of 150:1 to promote positive nitrogen balance, weight gain, and protein synthesis. Pediatric patients may require a higher (250 to 300:1) ratio to achieve the same beneficial effects.

The total calories supplied to acutely ill patients varies between 1.2 and 1.5 times the predicted basal energy expenditure. The metabolic rate can be estimated by computing the patient's surface area from body weight and height and by measuring oxygen consumption. Burn patients require higher calorie intakes owing to their higher energy loss. The nonprotein calories are usually supplied as glucose or as a mixture of glucose and lipid. Glucose is used because of the absolute requirement of certain tissues or cells for glucose. In addition, glucose solutions are easy to prepare. As discussed in preceding sections in this chapter, the ability of certain tissues, particularly skeletal muscle, to oxidize glucose for energy in sepsis may be inhibited. Based upon these considerations, supplying all the nonprotein calories as glucose may not be the ideal nutritional support in sepsis. In addition, it was hypothesized that glucose infusions would improve nitrogen balance by virtue of decreasing gluconeogenesis from amino acids. Although this relationship between amino acid metabolism and glucose may be valid in nonseptic trauma patients, numerous reports have shown that glucose infusions fail to limit glucose output by the liver in septic patients. Hypertonic glucose infusions via peripheral veins may lead to complications such as thrombophlebitis, septicemia, water retention, and increased CO_2 output, which may limit weaning from the respirator. A combination of glucose and lipid is becoming more popular as a nutritional support therapy in sepsis. Based upon calculations from respiratory quotients in septic patients, it was suggested that up to 25 to 30 per cent of the calories should be as lipid. Lipid offers several advantages over glucose alone and is equally effective as nonprotein sources of calories in a concentrated form. Askanazi and associates recommend a minimum amount of glucose (50 to 150 gm, or about 2 gm/kg/day) with the remainder of calories supplied as lipid.[137] With this regimen, the central nervous system is supplied with adequate glucose, and acidosis and ketosis are prevented. Insulin concentrations remain low, gluconeogenesis is low, and fatty acid mobilization is enhanced.

SUMMARY

Severe multiple trauma that overwhelms the numerous compensatory mechanisms designed to stabilize a life-threatening situation results in a complex series of pathophysiological processes. Subsequent hemorrhagic shock and sepsis are cellular metabolic abnormalities reflected clinically in altered hemodynamic and metabolic status. The diagnosis and effective treatment of posttrauma shock states is guided by an understanding of these abnormalities and the ever present risk of sequential or multiple organ failure. Although many etiologies may cause MOFs in the patient with traumatic injuries, two of the most important are hypovolemia and sepsis. Of the two, the pathophysiology of hypovolemia is best understood and, as a consequence, more readily treated. Because of its more complex nature, sepsis makes treatment of the trauma patient difficult and increases mortality. Recently, many advances have been made in the understanding of the pathophysiology connected with the septic syndrome. However, there remains much yet to be elucidated. It is hoped that laboratory and clinical investigation will provide a fundamental understanding of the processes involved in sepsis and MOFs so that more effective treatment regimens can be generated.

ACKNOWLEDGMENTS: This work was supported in part by Grant GM 39277 from the National Institute of General Medical Services. TCV is the recipient of an NIH Career Development Award, KO4 GM 00570.

REFERENCES

1. Trump BF, Arstila AU: Cellular reaction to injury. In Hill RB Jr, LaVia MF (eds): Principles of Pathobiology, 2nd ed. New York, Oxford University Press, 1975, pp 9–96.
2. Trump BF, Ginn FL: The pathogenesis of subcellular reactions to lethal injury. In Bajusz E, Jasmin G (eds): Methods and Achievements in Experimental Pathology, vol 4. Basel, Karger, 1969, pp 1–29.
3. Trump BF, Laiho KU, Mergner WJ, Arstila AU: Studies on the subcellular pathophysiology of acute lethal cell injury. Beitr Pathol 152:243–271, 1974.
4. Trump BF, McDowell EM, Arstila AU: Cellular reaction to injury. In Hill RB, LaVia MF (eds): Principles of Pathobiology, 3rd ed. New York, Oxford University Press, 1980, pp 20–111.
5. Trump BF, Mergner WJ: Cell injury. In Zweifach BW, Grant L, McClusky RT (eds): The Inflammatory Process, 2nd ed, vol 1. New York, Academic Press, 1974, pp 115–125.
6. Trump BF, Berezesky IK, Laiho KU, et al: The role of calcium in cell injury: A review. Scan Electron Microsc 2:437–462, 1980.
7. Trump BF, Berezesky IK, Cowley RA: The cellular and subcellular characteristics of acute and chronic injury with emphasis on the role of calcium. In Cowley RA, Trump BF (eds): Pathophysiology of Shock, Anoxia, and Ischemia. Baltimore, Williams & Wilkins, 1982, pp 6–46.
8. Rovetto MJ, Whitmer JT, Neely JR: Comparison of the effects of anoxia and whole heart ischemia on carbohydrate utilization in isolated working rat heart. Circ Res 32:699–711, 1973.
9. Neely JR, Rovetto MJ, Whitmer JT, Morgan HE: Effects of ischemia on ventricular function and metabolism in isolated working rat heart. Am J Physiol 225:651–658, 1973.
10. Rovetto MJ, Lamberton WF, Neely JR: Mechanism of glycolytic inhibition in ischemic rat hearts. Circ Res 37:742–751, 1975.
11. Neely JR, Vary TC, Liedtke AJ: Substrate delivery in ischemic myocardium. In Tillsmanns H, Kubler W, Zebe H (eds): Microcirculation of the Heart. Berlin, Springer-Verlag, 1982.
12. Vary TC, Angelakos ET, Schaffer SW: Relationship between adenine nucleotide metabolism and irreversible tissue damage in isolated perfused rat heart. Circ Res 45:218–225, 1979.
13. Reibel DK, Rovetto MJ: Myocardial ATP synthesis and mechanical function following oxygen deficiency. Am J Physiol 234:H620–H624, 1978.
14. Siegel JH: Pattern and process in the evolution of and recovery from shock. In Siegel JH, Chodoff PD (eds): The Aged and High Risk Surgical Patient. New York, Grune & Stratton, 1976, pp 381–455.
15. DuBois EF: Basal Metabolism in Health and Disease, 3rd ed. Philadelphia, Lea & Febiger, 1936.
16. Cuthbertson DP: Post-shock metabolic response. Lancet 1:433–436, 1942.
17. Kinney JM, Long CL, Duke JH: Carbohydrate and nitrogen metabolism after injury. In Porter R, Knight J (eds): Energy Metabolism in Trauma. London, Churchill, 1970, pp 103–126.
18. Shoemaker WC, Lim L, Boyd DR: Sequential hemodynamic events after trauma to the unanesthetized patient. Surg Gynecol Obstet 132:1033–1038, 1971.
19. Shoemaker WC: Pathophysiologic basis of therapy for shock and trauma syndromes. Semin Drug Treat 3:211–229, 1973.
20. Komatsu T, Shibutani K, Okamoto K: Critical level of oxygen delivery of cardiopulmonary bypass. Crit Care Med 15:194–197, 1987.
21. Neuhof H, Hey D, Glaser E, et al: Monitoring of shock patients by direct and continuous measurement of oxygen uptake. In Current Topics in Critical Care, 3rd International Symposium, Rio de Janeiro 1974. Basel, Karger, 1976, pp 6–11.
22. Neuhof H, Wolf H: Oxygen uptake during hemodilution. Bibl Haematol 41:66–75, 1975.
23. Neuhof H, Wolf H: Method for continuously measured oxygen consumption and cardiac output for use in critically ill patients. Crit Care Med 6:155–161, 1978.
24. Crowell JW: Oxygen deficit as the common parameter in irreversible hemorrhagic shock. Fed Proc 20:116, 1961.
25. Crowell JW, Smith EE: Oxygen deficit and irreversible hemorrhagic shock. Am J Physiol 206:313–316, 1964.
26. Astrand PO, Rodahl K: Textbook of Work Physiology. New York, McGraw-Hill, 1970, pp 301–303.
27. Siegel JH, Linberg SE, Wiles CW: Therapy of low flow states. In Siegel JH (ed): Trauma: Emergency Surgery and Critical Care. New York, Churchill Livingstone, 1987.
28. Linberg SE, Dunham CM, Turney SZ: The response of oxygen consumption to volume resuscitation following hemorrhagic shock in man. Circ Shock (in press).
29. Linberg SE, Dunham CM, Mergner WJ, Marzella LL: The development of a clinically applicable hemorrhage shock model. Circ Shock 13:62, 1984.
30. Dunham CM, Siegel JH, Weireter L, Fabian M, Goodarzi S, Guadalupi P, Gettings L, Linberg SE, Vary TC: Oxygen debt and metabolic acidosis as qualitative predictors of mortality and the severity of ischemic insult in hemorrhagic shock. Crit Care Med 19:231–243, 1991.
31. Davidson I, Haglind E, Gelin L: Hemodilution and oxygen transport to tissue in shock. Acta Chir Scand 489(suppl):245–260, 1979.
32. Baue AE: Multiple, progressive or sequential systems failure: A syndrome of the 1970s. Arch Surg 110:779–781, 1975.
33. Faist E, Baue AE, Dittmer H, Hebecec G: Multiple organ failure in polytrauma patients. J Trauma 23:775–787, 1983.
34. Baue AE: Multiple organ failure: The setting, sequence, and domino effect. In Baue AE (ed): Multiple Organ Failure: Patient Care and Prevention. St. Louis, Mosby–Year Book, Inc., 1990, pp 421–428.

35. Fry DE: Diagnosis and epidemiology of multiple organ failure. In Deitch EA (ed): Multiple Organ Failure: Pathophysiology and Basic Concepts of Therapy. New York, Thieme, 1990, pp 13–25.
36. Kanus WA, Wagner DP: Multiple systems organ failure: Epidemiology and progress. Crit Care Clin 5:221–232, 1989.
37. Cerra FB: Hypermetabolism–organ failure syndrome: A metabolic response to injury. Crit Care Clin 5:289–301, 1989.
38. Cerra FB, Alden PA, Negro F, Billiar T, Sringen BA, Licari J, Johnson SB, Holman RT: Sepsis and exogenous lipid modulation. JPEN 12(suppl 1):63S–68S, 1988.
39. Fry DE, Pearlstein L, Fulton RL, et al: Multiple system organ failure: The role of uncontrolled infection. Arch Surg 115:136–140, 1980.
40. Meakins JL, Wicklund B, Forse RA, et al: The surgical intensive care unit: Current concepts in infection. Surg Clin North Am 60:117–132, 1980.
41. Dietch EA: Gut failure: Its role in the multiple organ failure syndrome. In Dietch EA (ed): Multiple Organ Failure: Pathophysiology and Basic Concepts of Therapy. New York, Thieme, 1990, pp 40–60.
42. Cerra FB, Abrams J, Negro F, et al: Multiple organ failure syndrome: Clinical epidemiology and effect of current therapy. In Vincent JL (ed): Update in Intensive Care and Emergency Medicine. Berlin, Springer-Verlag, 1990, pp 22–31.
43. Ramsey G, Ledingham I: Management of multiple organs: Control of the microbial environment. In Bihari DJ, Cerra FB (eds): New Horizons: Multiple Organ Failure Syndrome. Anaheim, California, Society of Critical Care Medicine, 1989, pp 327–337.
44. Pinsky MR, Matuschak GM: Multiple system organ failure: Failure of host defense homeostasis. Crit Care Clin 5:199–219, 1989.
45. Goris RJ, Bockhurst TP, Nuytinek JK, et al: MOF: Generalized autodestructive inflammation. Arch Surg 120:1109–1114, 1985.
46. Sganga G, Siegel JH, Brown G, et al: Reprioritization of hepatic plasma protein release in trauma and sepsis. Arch Surg 120:187–199, 1985.
47. Friedman HP, Goldwyn RM, Siegel JH: The use and interpretation of multivariable methods in the classification stages of serious disease processes in critically ill. In Elashoff R (ed): Perspectives in Biometrics. New York, Academic Press, 1975, pp 81–122.
48. Siegel JH, Cerra FB, Peters D, et al: The physiologic recovery trajectory as the organizing principle for the quantification of hormonometabolic adaptation to surgical stress and severe sepsis. Adv Shock Res 6:177–203, 1979.
49. Siegel JH, Cerra FB, Coleman B, et al: Physiological and metabolic correlations in human sepsis. Surgery 86:163–193, 1979.
50. Siegel JH, Greenspan M, DelGuerico LRM: Abnormal vascular tone, defective oxygen transport and myocardial failure in human septic shock. Ann Surg 165:504–517, 1967.
51. Siegel JH, Giovannini I, Coleman B, et al: Pathologic synergistic modulation of the cardiovascular, respiratory and metabolic response to injury by cirrhosis and/or sepsis. Arch Surg 117:225, 1982.
52. Siegel JH: Cardiorespiratory manifestations of metabolic failure in sepsis and the multiple organ failure syndrome. Surg Clin North Am 63:379–399, 1983.
53. Cerra FB, Abrams J, Negro F: Apache II score does not predict multiple organ failure or mortality in postoperative surgical patients. Arch Surg 125:519–522, 1990.
54. Tracey KJ, Beutler B, Lowry SF: Shock and tissue injury induced by recombinant human cachectin. Science 234:470–474, 1986.
55. Tracey KJ, Lowry SF, Fahey TJ, et al: Cachectin/tumor necrosis factor induces lethal shock and stress hormone responses in the dog. Surg Gynecol Obstet 164:415–422, 1987.
56. Evans DA, Jacobs DO, Revhaug A, et al: The effects of TNF and their selective inhibition by ibuprofen. Ann Surg 209:312–321, 1989.
57. Michie HR, Sprigss DR, Manogue KR, et al: Tumor necrosis factor and endotoxin induce similar metabolic responses in human beings. Surgery 104:280–286, 1988.
58. Brown KA, Sheagren JN: Recognition and emergent treatment of septic shock/multiple organ failure syndrome. Int Med 11:3–11, 1990.
59. Lewis RA, Austen KK: The biologically active leukotrienes: Biosynthesis, metabolism, receptors, functions and pharmacology. J Clin Invest 73:889–897, 1984.
60. Petrak RA, Balk RA, Bone RC: Prostaglandins, cyclo-oxygenase inhibitors and thromboxane synthetase inhibitors in the pathogenesis of multiple system organ failure. Crit Care Clin 2:303–314, 1989.
61. Sprague RS, Stephenson AH, Dahms TE, et al: Proposed role for leukotrienes in the pathophysiology of multiple system organ failure. Prostaglandins 2:315–330, 1989.
62. Knoller J, Schoenfeld W, Joka T, et al: Generation of leukotrienes in polytraumatic patients with adult respiratory distress syndrome. Prog Clin Biol 236:311–316, 1987.
63. Smith MJH, Ford-Hutchinson AW, Bray MA: Leukotriene B_4: A potential mediator of inflammation. J Pharm Pharmacol 32:517, 1980.
64. Halushka PV, Reines HD, Barrow SE: Elevated plasma 6-keto-prostaglandin$_{1alpha}$ in patients in septic shock. Crit Care Med 13:451–453, 1985.
65. Henderson WR: Eicosanoids and lung inflammation. Am Rev Respir Dis 135:1176–1185, 1987.
66. Oettinger W, Berger D, Beger HG: The clinical significance of prostaglandins and thromboxane as mediators of septic shock. Klin Wochenschr 65:61–68, 1987.
67. Schirmer WJ, Schirmer JM, Fry DE: Recombinant human TNF produces hemodynamic changes characteristic of sepsis and endotoxemia. Arch Surg 124:445–488, 1989.
68. Sugden MC, Sharples SC, Randle PJ: Carcass glycogen as a potential source of glucose during short-term starvation. Biochem J 160:817–819, 1976.
69. Goldberg AL: Protein turnover in skeletal muscle. J Biol Chem 244:3223–3229, 1969.
70. Millward DJ, Garlick PJ, Ananylugo DO, Waterlow JC: The relative importance of muscle protein synthesis and breakdown in the regulation of muscle mass. Biochem J 156:185–188, 1976.
71. Liddell MJ, Daniel AM, McClean LD, et al: Role of stress hormones in the catabolic metabolism of shock. Surg Gynecol Obstet 149:822, 1979.
72. Marchuk JB, Finley RJ, Groves AC, et al: Catabolic hormones and substrate pattern in septic patients. J Surg Res 233:117, 1977.
73. Exton JH, Park CR: The role of cyclic AMP in the control of liver metabolism. Adv Enzyme Reg 6:391, 1968.
74. Lardy HA, Foster DO, Young JW, et al: Hormonal control of enzymes participating in gluconeogenesis and lipogenesis. J Cell Comp Physiol 56:39–54, 1965.
75. Frayn KN, Little RA, Maycock PF, Stoner HB: The relationship of plasma catecholamines to acute metabolic and hormonal responses to injury in man. Circ Shock 16:229–240, 1985.
76. Davies CL, Newman CJ, Molyneaux SG, Grahme-Smith DG: The relationship between plasma catecholamines and severity of injury in man. J Trauma 24:99–105, 1984.
77. Clutter WE, Bier DF, Shah SD, Cryer PE: Epinephrine plasma metabolic rates and physiologic thresholds for metabolic and hemodynamic actions in man. J Clin Invest 66:94–101, 1980.
78. Long CL, Kinney JM, Geiger JW: Nonsuppressibility of gluconeogenesis by glucose in septic patients. Metabolism 25:193–201, 1976.
79. Shaw JHF, Klein FS, Wolfe RR: Assessment of alanine, urea, and glucose interrelationships in normal subjects and in patients with sepsis with stable isotope tracers. Surgery 97:557–567, 1985.
80. Black PR, Brooks DC, Bessey PQ, et al: Mechanism of insulin resistance following injury. Ann Surg 196:420–425, 1982.
81. Wilmore DW, Aulick LH, Mason AP, Pruitt BA: Influence of burn wound on local and systemic response to injury. Ann Surg 186:444–458, 1977.
82. Meszaros K, Lang CH, Bagby GJ, Spitzer JS: Contribution of different organs to increased glucose consumption after endotoxin administration. J Biol Chem 262:10965–10970, 1987.

83. Wolfe RR, Burke JF: Effect of burn trauma on glucose turnover, oxidation, and recycling in guinea pig. Am J Physiol 283:E880–E885, 1977.
84. Linn TC, Petit FH, Reed LJ: α-Ketoacid dehydrogenase complexes: X. Regulation of activity of pyruvate dehydrogenase complex from beef kidney mitochondria by phosphorylation dephosphorylation. Proc Natl Acad Sci USA 62:234–241, 1969.
85. Randle PJ, Fuller SK, Kerbey AL, et al: Molecular mechanisms regulating glucose oxidation in insulin deficient animals. Horm Cell Reg 8:139–150, 1984.
86. Vary TC, Siegel JH, Tall BD, Morris JG: Metabolic effects of partial reversal of pyruvate dehydrogenase activity by dichloroacetate in sepsis. Circ Shock 24:3–18, 1988.
87. Vary TC, Siegel JH, Nakatani T, et al: Effects of sepsis on activity of pyruvate dehydrogenase complex in skeletal muscle and liver. Am J Physiol 250:E634–E640, 1986.
88. Vary TC, Siegel JH, Tall BD, Morris JG: Role of anaerobic bacteria in intra-abdominal septic abscesses in mediating septic control of skeletal muscle glucose oxidation and lactic acidosis. J Trauma 29:1003–1014, 1989.
89. Nanni G, Siegel JH, Coleman B, et al: Increased lipid fuel dependence on critically ill septic patients. J Trauma 24:14–30, 1984.
90. Sganga G, Siegel JH, Coleman B, et al: The physiologic meaning of respiratory index in various types of critical illness. Circ Shock 17:179–193, 1985.
91. Stoner HB, Little RA, Frayn KN, et al: The effect of sepsis on the oxidation of carbohydrase and fat. Br J Surg 70:32–35, 1983.
92. Randle PJ, Kerbey AL, Espinal J: Mechanisms decreasing glucose oxidation in diabetes and starvation: Role of lipid fuels and hormones. Diabetes Metab Rev 4:623–638, 1988.
93. Vary TC: Increased pyruvate dehydrogenase kinase activity in response to sepsis. Am J Physiol 260(Endocrinol Metab 23):E669–E674, 1991.
94. Vary TC, Siegel JH, Rivkind A: Clinical and therapeutic significance of metabolic patterns of lactic acidosis. Perspect Crit Care 1:85–132, 1988.
95. Vary TC, Murphy JM: Role of extra-splanchnic organs in the metabolic response to sepsis: Effect of insulin. Circ Shock 29:41–57, 1989.
96. Vary TC, Placko R, Siegel JH: Pharmacologic modulation of increased release of gluconeogenic precursors from extrasplanchnic organs in sepsis. Circ Shock 29:59–76, 1989.
97. Stacpoole PW, Lorenz AC, Thomas RG, Harman EM: Dichloroacetate in the treatment of lactic acidosis. Ann Intern Med 108:58–63, 1988.
98. Stacpoole PW, Harman EM, Curry SH, et al: Treatment of lactic acidosis with dichloroacetate. N Engl J Med 309:390–396, 1983.
99. Beisel WR: Metabolic response to infection. Annu Rev Med 26:9–20, 1975.
100. Wilmore DW, Black PR, Muhlbacker F: Injured man: Trauma and sepsis. In Winters RW (ed): Nutritional Management of the Seriously Ill. New York, Academic Press, 1982.
101. Long CL, Birkhan RH, Geiger JW, et al: Urinary excretion of 3-methylhistidine: An assessment of muscle protein catabolism in adult normal subject and during malnutrition, sepsis and skeletal muscle trauma. Metabolism 30:765–776, 1981.
102. Jefferson LS: Role of insulin in the regulation of protein synthesis. Diabetes 29:487–490, 1980.
103. Morgan HE, Chua B, Beinlich CJ: Regulation of protein degradation in heart. In Wildenthal K (ed): Degradative Processes in Heart and Skeletal Muscle. Amsterdam, Elsevier–North Holland, 1980, pp 87–112.
104. Clowes GHA, George BC, Villee CA Jr, Saravis CA: Muscle proteolysis induced by a circulating peptide in septic and traumatized patients. N Engl J Med 308:545–552, 1983.
105. Loda M, Clowes GHA, Dinarello CA, et al: Induction of hepatic protein synthesis by a peptide in blood plasma of patients with sepsis and trauma. Surgery 96:204–213, 1984.
106. Sugden PH, Felber SJ: Regulation of protein turnover in skeletal and cardiac muscle. Biochem J 273:21–37, 1991.
107. Jepson MM, Pell J, Bates JM, et al: The effects of endotoxemia on protein metabolism in skeletal muscle and liver of fed and fasted rats. Biochem J 235:329–336, 1986.
108. Powanda MC, Wannemacher RW, Cockrell GL: Nitrogen metabolism and protein synthesis during pneumococcal sepsis in rats. Infect Immun 6:266–271, 1972.
109. Vary TC, Siegel JH, Tall BD, Morris JG, Smith JA: Inhibition of skeletal muscle protein synthesis in septic intra-abdominal abscess. J Trauma 28:981–988, 1988.
110. Kimball SR, Flaim KE, Peavy DE, Jefferson LS: Protein metabolism. In Rifkin H, Porte D (eds): Diabetes Mellitus Theory and Practice. New York, Elsevier–North Holland, 1990, pp 41–50.
111. Young VR, Chen SC, Newbeine PM: Effect of infection on skeletal muscle ribosomes in rat fed adequate or low protein. J Nutr 94:361–368, 1968.
112. Vary TC, Kimball SR: Translational regulation of protein synthesis in skeletal muscle of septic rats. Circ Shock 34:99, 1991.
113. Chartes Y, Grimble RF: Effect of recombinant human tumor necrosis factor α on protein synthesis in liver, skeletal muscle and skin of rat. Biochem J 258:493–497, 1989.
114. Haymond MW, Miles JM: Branched chain amino acids as a major source of alanine nitrogen in man. Diabetes 31:86–89, 1982.
115. Robert JJ, Bier DM, Zhao XH, et al: Glucose and insulin effects on de novo amino acid synthesis in young men. Metabolism 31:1210–1218, 1982.
116. Bower RH, Muggia-Sullan M, Vallgren S, et al: Branched chain amino acid–enriched solutions in septic patients. Ann Surg 203:13–20, 1986.
117. Cerra FB, Mazuki JE, Chute E, et al: Branched chain metabolic support. Ann Surg 199:286–291, 1984.
118. Freund HR, Ryan JA, Fischer JE: Amino acid derangements in patients with sepsis: Treatment with branched chain amino acid rich effusions. Ann Surg 188:423, 1978.
119. Livesey G, Lung P: Enzymatic determination of branched chain amino acid and 2-oxoacids in rat tissues. Biochem J 188:705–713, 1980.
120. Krebs HA, Lund P: Aspects of regulation of branched chain amino acids. Adv Enzyme Reg 15:375–394, 1977.
121. Lau KS, Fantania HR, Randle PJ: Inactivation of rat liver and kidney branched chain 2-oxoacid dehydrogenase complex by adenosine triphosphate. FEBS Lett 126:66–70, 1981.
122. Fantania HR, Lau KS, Randle PJ: Activation of phosphorylated branched chain 2-oxoacid dehydrogenase. FEBS Lett 147:35–39, 1981.
123. Fantania HR, Lau KS, Randle PJ: Inactivation of purified ox kidney branched chain 2-oxoacid dehydrogenase complex by phosphorylation. FEBS Lett 132:285–288, 1981.
124. Ichihara K, Neely JR, Siehl DL, Morgan HE: Utilization of leucine by working rat heart. Am J Physiol 239:E430–E436, 1980.
125. Wannemacher RW, Pekarek RS, Thompson WL, et al: A protein from polymorphonuclear leukocytes (LEM) which effects the rate of hepatic amino acid transport and synthesis of acute phase globulins. Endocrinology 96:651–661, 1975.
126. Flaim KE, Peavy DE, Everson WV, Jefferson LS: The role of amino acids in regulation of protein synthesis in perfused rat liver. J Biol Chem 257:2932–2938, 1982.
127. Flaim KE, Liao WS, Peavy DE, et al: The role of amino acids in regulation of protein synthesis in perfused rat liver. J Biol Chem 257:2939–2946, 1982.
128. Peavy DE, Taylor JM, Jefferson LS: Correlation of albumin production rate and albumin mRNA in normal, diabetic and insulin-diabetic rats. Proc Natl Acad Sci USA 75:5879–5883, 1978.
129. McGarry JD, Foster D: Regulation of hepatic fatty acid oxidation and ketone body production. Annu Rev Biochem 49:395–420, 1980.
130. Oram JF, Bennetch SL, Neely JR: Regulation of fatty acid utilization in isolated perfused rat hearts. J Biol Chem 248:5299–6309, 1973.
131. Pekela PH, Kawakami M, Angus CW, et al: Selective inhibition

of synthesis of enzymes for de novo fatty acid biosynthesis by an endotoxin-induced mediator from exudate cells. Proc Natl Acad Sci USA 80:2742–2747, 1983.

132. Scholl RA, Lang CH, Bagby GJ: Hypertriglyceridemia and its relation to tissue lipoprotein lipase activity in endotoxic escherichia coli bacteremia, and polymicrobial septic rats. J Surg Res 37:394–401, 1984.

133. Williamson DH: Regulation of ketone body metabolism and effects of injury. Acta Chir Scand 507(suppl):22–29, 1981.

134. Williamson DH, Farrell R, Kerr A, et al: Muscle protein catabolism after injury in man as measured by urinary excretion of 3-methylhistidine. Clin Sci Mol Med 52:527–533, 1977.

135. Wannemacher RW, Pace JG, Beall FA, et al: Role of liver in regulation of ketone body production during sepsis. J Clin Invest 64:1565, 1979.

136. Vary TC, Siegel JH, Nakatani T, et al: A biochemical basis for depressed ketogenesis in sepsis. J Trauma 26:419–425, 1986.

137. Askanazi J, Nordenstrom J, Rosenbaum SA, et al: Nutrition for the patient with respiratory failure: Glucose vs. fat. Anesthesiology 54:373, 1981.

138. Vincent JL, VanderLinden P, Domb M, et al: Relevance to fluid administration. Anesth Analg 66:565–571, 1987.

139. Hesselyren P-O, Warner BW, James JH, Takehara H, Fischer JE: Effect of insulin on amino acid uptake and protein turnover in skeletal muscle from septic rats. Arch Surg 122:228–223, 1987.

140. Liao WS, Jefferson LS, Taylor JM: Changes in plasma albumin concentration, synthesis rate and MRNA level during acute inflammation. Am J Physiol 251(Cell Physiol 20):C928–C934, 1986.

9

INITIAL MANAGEMENT OF TRAUMATIC SHOCK

KAREN A. McQUILLAN

Traumatic shock demands prompt and accurate assessment, competent planning, rapid and appropriate intervention, and continued evaluation by the trauma resuscitation team. Failure to recognize and correctly treat traumatic shock promptly will have a direct detrimental effect on early and delayed mortality and morbidity.[1, 2] Effective clinical judgment and swift, skilled responses must be demonstrated by the nurse to meet the challenge presented by the trauma patient in a shock state.

The clinical presentation, assessment, and initial management of the patient experiencing shock as a result of traumatic injury are the focus of this chapter. The essential components of diagnosis and current therapeutic modalities employed during resuscitation are outlined. Organizational aspects of trauma resuscitation are discussed to introduce the orderly interdisciplinary approach that is necessary for timely management of shock in the seriously injured patient. Measures evaluated to determine the effectiveness of initial resuscitation are also discussed.

As detailed in the preceding chapter, the complex pathophysiological process of shock occurs when altered hemodynamic function results in inadequate tissue perfusion and insufficient cell oxygenation.[3–8] In trauma, hemorrhage and tissue injury are the most common factors that alter hemodynamic function and produce a low-flow shock state.[2, 9] It is recognized that other etiologies of shock, such as sepsis, cardiac or neurological dysfunction, and fluid loss due to inflammatory processes or diuresis, may exist in the trauma patient. However, these causes of shock are discussed only briefly as adjuncts to the essential pathology in traumatic shock, that is, loss of circulating blood volume and subsequent insufficient oxygen transport to body cells.

The resuscitation from traumatic shock continues until designated physiological end points indicate cardiovascular and metabolic stability.[10] Achievement of these end points, evidenced by a normalization of the parameters the nurse monitors in the clinical setting, may not occur in the resuscitative cycle. Frequently, the assessment and treatment process begins in the field and emergency department and extends into the operating room and critical care areas. This chapter focuses primarily on the initial treatment of shock with the acknowledgment that full resuscitation may not be achieved until later in the patient's trauma course.

SHOCK ETIOLOGY IN THE TRAUMA PATIENT

It must be emphasized that the most common cause of shock in the injured patient is hypovolemia resulting from acute blood loss.[2, 11-13] Additional shock states and causative factors are discussed briefly, since the trauma patient may have more than one etiology of shock present simultaneously.[12, 14] The reader is referred to other chapters within this text for detailed discussions of pathophysiology relevant to specific injury or nonhypovolemic types of shock.

Acute Blood Loss

Acute blood loss may occur externally or internally in response to vascular injury. External hemorrhage resulting from lacerations, amputations, open fractures, or gunshot wounds is usually readily evident upon examination. However, a significant volume of blood may have been lost prior to the patient's hospital admission, and when possible, estimations of prehospital blood loss should be determined from field personnel.[1, 10]

Blood loss also may be concealed within body cavities such as the thorax, intraperitoneal space, and retroperitoneal space. For example, a hemothorax may represent a blood loss of 2 to 3 liters and the abdominal cavity may sequester as much as 6 liters of blood.[1, 9] Fracture sites also represent significant sites of hidden blood loss. Pelvic fractures are equated with up to 6 to 8 units of blood loss, while a femur fracture may result in 1 to 4 units of extravasated blood.[1, 15, 16] Body tissues also may sequester blood lost from fractures or vascular injuries. Such sites include the extremities, buttocks, perineum, neck, and shoulder girdle. Since the cranial vault is indistensible, it is not considered a likely site for concealing significant amounts of blood loss. Locating areas of overt and concealed hemorrhage by careful and comprehensive physical examination and diagnostic procedures is the first step in control of bleeding.

Fluid Losses in Injury

Fluid losses other than blood also occur as a result of tissue injury, establishing a second source of hypovolemia in the trauma patient. Soft tissue injury results in obligatory edema within the wounded area in amounts directly related to the magnitude of the injury.[11, 14] The edema occurs as a result of fluid translocation into the interstitial space at the injury site or where the tissues contain extravasated blood.[1, 11] The importance of edema as a causative factor in traumatic shock is frequently underestimated and must be viewed as an effective loss of circulating blood volume.[14, 16-18] Clearly, such volume loss has direct effects on systemic circulation. Extensive burn injury is a prime example in which very large amounts of extracellular fluid and plasma flood the burn wound and produce profound shock.[1, 19] Microcirculatory changes that occur in response to persistent hypovolemia and consequent cellular hypoperfusion create fluid shifts that further decrease effective circulating volume and compound the hypoperfusion state.[2, 7] Tissue response to injury can actually cause intravascular fluid losses in excess of the original blood volume loss.

Additional sources of fluid loss that should be considered include diuresis related to diabetes mellitus or diabetes insipidus. Increased insensible fluid losses also may occur during the operating room cycle or secondary to diaphoresis. Inflammatory processes occurring during the critical care phase of the patient's recovery also may cause diminished intravascular volume.

Hypovolemia and shock can be life-threatening and demand prompt and complete treatment. Fluid replacement is the fundamental treatment for fluid deficit and hypovolemic shock. Continued assessment and careful monitoring of fluid balance are important to detect unsuspected causes of fluid loss that may exacerbate the trauma patient's shock state or may cause its recrudescence.

Other Causes of Shock

Although some degree of hypovolemia exists in all multiple trauma patients, it is important to consider other causes of shock that may be present. Other etiological factors can serve to compound the hypovolemic shock state or in some rarer instances may serve as the primary cause of shock. Obtaining an accurate history, completing a thorough physical examination, monitoring the patient's reaction to initial treatments, and reviewing diagnostic studies permit determination of the shock sources,[11] thus allowing appropriate treatment modalities to be instituted.

Neurogenic Etiology. Neurogenic shock results from the loss of vasomotor tone and vasodilation in much of the peripheral vascular system. Direct injury to the medullary vasomotor center or interruption of sympathetic innervation secondary to cervical or high thoracic spinal cord injury causes such a loss of vascular control.[1, 19, 20] This directly inhibits compensatory vasoconstriction in response to intravascular fluid loss and thereby exacerbates the hypovolemic shock state. Appropriate treatment under these circumstances includes the use of vasoactive drugs as well as replacement of circulating volume.

Anaphylaxis. Anaphylactic shock, another form of vasogenic shock that occurs in response to an antibody–antigen reaction, is not commonly associated with trauma but may occur as an iatrogenic complication (i.e., transfusion reaction) during resuscitation.[19, 21] The antigen–antibody reaction stimulates release of vasoactive mediators resulting in a systemic vasodilation and increased capillary permeability.[19] Hypotension, laryngeal edema, bronchoconstriction, urticaria, dysrhythmias, and nausea are characteristic of the anaphylactic shock state.[20] Removal of the aggravating factor and use of agents such as epinephrine, antihistamines, bronchodilators, and steroids are indicated once anaphylaxis is recognized.[20, 22]

Septic Etiology. Shock associated with sepsis is uncommon immediately following a traumatic insult. However, septic shock may be suspected in the resuscitative cycle if preinjury infective foci exist or if transport has been considerably delayed. Trauma and its associated treatments offer multiple portals of entry for microorganisms. Sepsis associated with tissue damage is a major complication in the critical care cycle. This pathological state remains the principal cause of death in injured patients surviving the first 3 postinjury days.[4, 19]

The clinical presentation of septic shock is greatly dependent on the patient's volume status. In the normovolemic septic patient, a hyperdynamic cardiovascular state, evidenced by elevated cardiac output, low systemic vascular resistance, wide pulse pressure, tachycardia, and warm,

TABLE 9–1. CLINICAL MANIFESTATIONS OF TRAUMATIC SHOCK

PARAMETER (FOR A 70-kg MALE)	CLASS I EARLY	CLASS II MODERATE	CLASS III MAJOR OR PROGRESSIVE	CLASS IV SEVERE OR PROFOUND
Approximate blood volume loss (ml)	Up to 750	750–1500	1500–2000	2000 or more
Percent of blood volume	Up to 15%	15–30%	30–40%	40% or more
Neurological/ behavioral status	Slightly anxious	Mildly anxious, restless; muscle fatigue and weakness evident	Agitated, confused; progressive decrease in activity; progressive thirst evident	Confused, stuporous, lethargic, unconscious; dilated pupils may be evident
Heart rate	<100	>100 Mild tachycardia	>120 Tachycardia	140 or higher Irregular pulse, decreased pulse amplitude
Blood pressure	Normal	Normal	Decreased	Severe hypotension
Pulse pressure (mm Hg)	Normal or increased	Decreased	Decreased	Decreased
Respirations	14–20, normal	20–30, normal	30–40, hyperpnea	>35, shallow, irregular
Urine output (ml/ hr)	30 or more	20–30	5–15	Negligible
Capillary blanch test	Normal	Slight delay	Definite delay	No refilling observed
Skin	Pale pink, slightly cool	Slightly cold, pale	Cold and moist	Cold and cyanotic, mottled

Adapted from Committee on Trauma: Advanced Trauma Life Support Program: Instructor's Manual. Chicago, American College of Surgeons, 1989.

flushed extremities, may be demonstrated. Conversely, the hypovolemic patient appears hypodynamic, and the etiology of the septic shock state is difficult to distinguish.[11, 23] Underlying hypovolemia must be treated in these patients together with eradication of the septic foci. Antibiotics and inotropic and vasoactive pharmacological agents are usually indicated.[20, 23] In terminal septic shock, the patient is hypodynamic despite adequate fluid replacement.

Cardiogenic Etiology. Pump failure also may serve as a shock-inducing factor in the trauma patient. Cardiogenic shock may occur as a result of myocardial infarction or direct injury to the heart.[11, 12, 14, 19] Myocardial infarction may precede or even precipitate the events of the accident or injury. Cardiac lacerations, contusion, tamponade, and injury to cardiac valves, septa, or conductive tissue are examples of injuries that may cause compromised cardiac function and induce shock.[4, 14] The patient with preexisting heart disease, age-related cardiac reserve limitations, a history of excessive alcohol ingestion, or who requires myocardial depressants (e.g., anesthetics) has a high propensity for cardiac failure in the face of myocardial insult.[1, 5] These patients are also at greater risk for development of overt cardiac failure in response to rapid fluid infusion during trauma resuscitation.[5]

Other indirect injuries contribute on occasion to the development of cardiogenic shock states in the trauma patient. Tension pneumothorax reduces venous return and consequently impairs cardiac pump function. Less commonly cardiogenic shock may result from severe afterload elevation associated with pulmonary embolism or severe head injury. Eventually, myocardial function also may be compromised by myocardial depressant tissue factors released during progressive shock.[24, 25]

The classic symptoms of cardiogenic shock, such as pulmonary congestion, edema, neck vein distention, or hepatic congestion, may not be noted in trauma patients with coexisting acute hypovolemia. Recognition of the cardiogenic disorder is best achieved by noting a persistent low cardiac output in the face of large elevations in central venous or pulmonary capillary wedge pressures during volume resuscitation.[5, 19] Once myocardial failure is recognized, the underlying injury must be identified and treated rapidly. Appropriate treatment such as inotropic agents, vasoactive drugs, and, rarely, intra-aortic counterpulsation may be required to support myocardial function.

CLINICAL SIGNS USED IN DIAGNOSIS

The clinical manifestations of traumatic shock are the result of inadequate tissue perfusion and compensatory sympathetic nervous system and neuroendocrine activation.[2, 6, 9, 25] Clinical symptoms are dependent on both the relative or absolute volume of extracellular fluid lost and the rate of volume loss. Preexisting disease or coexistence of other etiological factors of shock also affects the clinical presentation of shock.[17, 18, 26] Physiological responses related to the amount of acute blood loss constitute the basis for defining four simplified categories or stages of shock symptomatology (Table 9–1).[9, 11]

Class I: Early Stage

Under conditions of mild blood loss (15 per cent of total blood volume), there are few clinical symptoms, and the patient may have essentially normal parameters. The effect of a small volume loss is minimized by well-known compensatory mechanisms, chiefly altered venous capacitance. Minimal pulse elevation and mild anxiety may occur in response to catecholamine release and sympathetic neural activation.[21, 26]

Class II: Moderate Stage

An acute blood loss of 15 to 30 per cent of the intravascular volume results in the appearance of multiple physiological responses. Cerebral stimulation caused by increased catecholamines or as a secondary response to hypoxia results in an increase in anxiety and restlessness.[20] Intense sympathetic discharge and catecholamine elevation raise the pulse rate and increase peripheral vascular resistance. Although at this stage there is rarely a significant effect on systolic blood pressure, peripheral vasoconstriction does create a rise in diastolic blood pressure and a subsequent decrease in pulse pressure. Unless an individual has impaired compensatory responses, it is not until at least 20 per cent of circulating blood volume is suddenly lost that a decline in systolic blood pressure occurs.[21] Orthostatic hypotension is frequently demonstrated with blood losses between 10 and 20 per cent.[27] Urine output is minimally diminished owing to compensatory vascular mechanisms and the activity of antidiuretic hormone and aldosterone.[6, 7, 9, 25] Sympathetic nervous system activation constricts cutaneous blood vessels and stimulates sweat glands, causing the skin to be cool, moist, and pale, especially at the extremities.[25, 28] Capillary filling is delayed due to peripheral vasoconstiction. Muscle fatigue and generalized weakness occurring during this stage correlate with a shift toward cellular anaerobic metabolism.[9]

Class III: Major or Progressive Stage

When effective circulating volume is rapidly depleted by 30 to 40 per cent, endogenous compensatory mechanisms are inadequate, and classic signs of inadequate tissue perfusion result.[7, 11, 16, 21] Cerebral hypoperfusion, hypoxia, and acid–base imbalance create progressive changes in level of consciousness.[25] Tachycardia persists. The class III stage represents the minimal amount of volume loss that consistently and significantly decreases systolic blood pressure.[11, 17] In the "average" patient, an acute 30 per cent blood volume loss results in a systolic blood pressure of 60 to 80 mm Hg.[29] Initially, tachypnea occurs in response to activation of the brainstem respiratory centers by sensory nociceptive impulses illicited from tissue injury, as well as receptor stimulation caused by reduced arterial pressure.[2, 20] Respiratory rate and depth also increase in response to hypoxemia.[25] As shock progresses, deep, rapid respirations are produced in response to progressive metabolic acidosis, presumably through stimulation of medullary respiratory centers.[9, 20] The decline in renal tissue perfusion is evidenced by reduced urine output. Poor cutaneous circulation persists, causing weak or absent peripheral pulses, a delay in capillary refill, and cold, clammy skin.

Class IV: Severe or Profound Stage

An acute loss of greater than 40 per cent of the circulating volume rapidly exhausts compensatory mechanisms, and symptoms of profound shock are readily evident.[7, 26, 30] Severe hypoperfusion further impairs organ function, eventually leading to failure of multiple organ systems.[25, 31] Inadequate cerebral blood flow causes progressive central nervous system depression, as evidenced by further deterioration in level of consciousness. Profound reduction in urine output occurs due to renal hypoperfusion. Insufficient myocardial oxygenation and acidosis may cause arrhythmias accompanied by persistent tachycardia. Stroke volume compromise leads to a significant reduction in blood pressure, usually within the range of 30 to 50 mm Hg in the "average" patient with a 40 per cent acute intravascular volume loss.[29] Diastolic pressure may be unobtainable as pulse pressure narrows.[11] Ischemia of the medullary vasomotor center eventually causes vasodilation and further decline of systemic blood pressure, often refractory to therapy.[7, 25] Eventual brainstem depression leads to shallow and irregular respirations. Reduction of oxyhemoglobin leads to cyanosis, and cutaneous perfusion is severely compromised. Patients showing all the signs of classic hypovolemic shock are in imminent danger of death; every effort must be made to immediately stabilize and resuscitate them.

Although these clinical descriptors are useful, it bears emphasis that no one clinical finding is a reliable diagnostic indicator of the extent and outcome of traumatic shock. One should keep in mind that many factors, including associated injuries, drugs, premorbid illnesses, and the presence of other forms of shock, will influence patient assessment findings, making the diagnosis of traumatic shock more difficult. As additional assessment parameters such as central venous pressures, laboratory values, radiographical findings, and other diagnostic study results become available during resuscitation, a clearer picture of the shock state is drawn. Each clinical manifestation must be viewed as part of this total picture that requires continuous monitoring to identify trends and responses to treatment. Undoubtedly, optimal shock management is based on rapid recognition of early, impending stages and prompt treatment before inadequate tissue perfusion becomes clinically apparent.[2, 25, 32]

ASSESSMENT AND TREATMENT OF TRAUMATIC SHOCK

Goals of Management

There are two essential rules of trauma management. First, the patient who has sustained traumatic injury is in shock until proven otherwise. Second, there is a finite period within which intervention must be instituted if death or disability is to be prevented. The longer tissue hypoperfusion and cellular anoxia are permitted to exist, the greater will be the detrimental influence on patient survival and incidence of shock-related complications.[2, 6]

The overall goal of therapy is to reestablish adequate tissue perfusion in order to restore oxygen delivery to metabolically active cells. Success in meeting this goal is dependent on restoring intravascular volume, providing adequate oxygenation, ensuring sufficient oxygen-carrying capacity of blood, and maintaining optimal cardiac filling and function. Therapy also must be aimed toward remedying the underlying pathological process in order to maximize the effectiveness of treatment efforts and prevent recurrence of the shock state.[10, 22]

Organization of the Resuscitation Team

An organized multidisciplinary team is essential to expedite efficient and effective care to the patient in traumatic shock. The composition of the trauma resuscitation team will vary from institution to institution depending on the organizational philosophy and availability of qualified personnel and resources.[9, 16] Generally, the team should consist of professional nurses, a trauma surgeon or trauma-trained emergency medicine physician, physician consultants from specialty groups, and various support services (Table 9–2).[9, 16, 33] A network of such health care personnel should be clearly designated in each hospital.

Each team member should have a clear role and predesignated responsibilities well known by all others on the team (see Table 9–2). These tasks are usually assigned by the team leader, usually the trauma surgeon, who is responsible for prioritizing and directing the initial resuscitation process.[10, 16] The nurse, an essential and integral component of the team, must work in concert with the team leader to coordinate team activities and to formulate an effective plan of care.

To facilitate the team concept, both direct and indirect caregivers alike must be considered valuable members. An atmosphere of collegial respect and open communication and a clear delineation of role responsibilities foster strong cooperative team practice.[33] Collaboration among team members conserves precious time during assessment, implementation, and evaluation of the plan of care. The multidisciplinary approach ensures comprehensive patient care and is continued throughout the cycles of trauma.

Trauma Protocol

Practitioners caring for a patient in traumatic shock are called on to make rapid and accurate diagnostic and treatment decisions, often under adverse conditions. This necessitates development and use of a systematic action plan.[6, 16, 34] Trauma protocol provides the necessary structural framework, which organizes and prioritizes the efforts of the trauma team. This framework serves as a blueprint to follow during high-intensity activities when time is critical. The use of protocol directs the trauma team in identifying the most lethal injuries first and prevents oversight of less serious injuries and delays in treatment.[4, 16, 29]

A fine balance is needed between definite protocols and rigid commandments. Unless protocols are evaluated in an on-going fashion, their use may lead to rigidity of thinking

TABLE 9–2. TRAUMA RESUSCITATION TEAM AND SUPPORT MEMBERS

PERSONNEL	RESPONSIBILITIES
Trauma surgeon	Serves as the leader in directing patient care
Trauma-trained emergency physician	Conducts initial physical examination Determines medical and surgical interventions according to priority Performs invasive procedures (may vary in individual emergency departments depending on the role responsibilities of the professional nurse) Determines necessary specialty consultations
Registered nurse 1	Serves as primary nurse in assessing, monitoring, and performing nursing interventions Intervenes with family or significant others at the appropriate time
Registered nurse 2	Serves as a support to registered nurse 1 May assist in establishing IV access, medication administration, documentation, obtaining lab work, preparing for procedures
Anesthesiologist, nurse anesthetist, or respiratory therapist (optional depending on the nature and severity of injuries)	Responsible for airway management, and ventilatory therapies (e.g., "ambuing" the intubated patient), O_2
Physician specialists	Consultation as required for specific injuries and medical problems (e.g., neurosurgery, plastic surgery, orthopedics)
Prehospital care personnel	Field resuscitation and transport Provide information regarding accident data base, initial findings, and preliminary interventions
Social workers/clergy	Provide support for the trauma patient's family Available for spiritual counseling
Emergency department orderly or technician (optional depending on organization of department)	Assists as directed by physician or nurse May assist in the performance of medical or surgical interventions Assists in patient transportation
Radiology technician	Obtain and develop diagnostic radiographs as needed
Laboratory personnel	Perform laboratory analyses on patient samples (i.e., blood, urine, etc.) and report results

Adapted from Balton DC, Harmon AR: The ABCs of trauma management. In Harmon AR (ed): Nursing Care of the Adult Trauma Patient. New York, John Wiley & Sons, Copyright © 1985.

and inflexibility of approach to unique situations. Annual reevaluation and modification of resuscitation protocol as new knowledge and techniques become available permit the team to operate within a structure but without inflexible doctrine.

Specific nursing management protocols are also essential in emergency trauma care settings. These guidelines should complement their medical counterparts to promote necessary interdisciplinary cooperation during resuscitation. Collaborative use of medical and nursing protocols can improve the trauma team's ability to provide optimal and efficient care for the critically injured patient.[33, 35]

General Plan for Resuscitation

The management plan for the patient in traumatic shock follows a sequence that prioritizes care with the clear objective of minimizing mortality and morbidity. The Advanced Trauma Life Support Protocol for initial assessment and management provides one such structure.[11] This plan is separated into four overlapping phases. The reader is referred to Chapter 6 for a comprehensive and more generalized discussion of the phasic management of the multiply injured patient.

First, a rapid primary survey is performed. The intent of this initial physical examination is to immediately identify injuries that pose an imminent threat to the patient's survival. The primary survey includes assessment of airway, breathing, circulation, and neurological disability. Rapid, thorough assessment and injury management are facilitated by undressing and exposing the patient as quickly as possible. Diagnosis and treatment proceed in rapid succession. Second, resuscitation begins with the management of identified life-threatening conditions as well as the shock state present. Once the primary survey is complete and resuscitation has been initiated, the third phase, a more timely in-depth secondary survey, is performed. This comprehensive head-to-toe patient evaluation is designed to detect less obvious injuries not necessarily apparent in the primary survey but which pose a latent threat to mortality and morbidity. For the patient in traumatic shock, the secondary survey presents an opportunity to identify a more occult source of hemorrhage and/or site of tissue injury causing blood/fluid volume loss. Definitive care constitutes the final phase of the management plan. During this phase, serious injuries are treated and definitive plans for the comprehensive care of the patient are made. A detailed description of assessment stragegies for each body area and definitive treatment for various injuries can be found in appropriate chapters elsewhere in this text.

The phases of shock management, although described as separate stages, must be viewed as an integrated entity. Lifesaving interventions are routinely initiated prior to completion of a comprehensive diagnostic assessment. Multiple tasks must be accomplished simultaneously to expedite diagnosis and implementation of resuscitative measures.[6] Any approach that provides a rational structure in which to organize the efforts of multiple care providers, some of whom may be new to the area of trauma care, can be used successfully to diagnose and manage the patient in shock. The following serves to describe one approach to team resuscitation.

The patient arrives immobilized on a long backboard with a cervical collar in place to prevent any potential or additional spinal cord damage. Usually, at least one intravenous line is already established and some type of crystalloid solution is infusing. On arrival in the resuscitation area, the simultaneous efforts of vital team members are essential. An anesthesiologist, nurse anesthetist, or respiratory therapist assumes control of the airway and ventilatory therapies. A patent airway is immediately ensured, and intubation with mechanical ventilatory support is initiated as needed.

The trauma team leader performs the primary survey. While this is being accomplished, one team member on either side of the patient establishes at least one large-bore intravenous catheter and obtains blood samples for laboratory analysis. The third team member, acting as a recorder, duplicates the primary survey and then begins the secondary survey immediately. A fourth member of the receiving team, usually the primary nurse, relays the known history. This individual then begins electrocardiographic monitoring and determines the blood pressure with a sphygmomanometer as soon as possible. The recording and assessing member of the team obtains initial arterial blood gas levels.

It is vitally important that the trauma team not neglect the established management priorities. Although a source of external hemorrhage may be readily apparent, it is futile to focus all efforts on controlling blood loss and stabilizing circulation if the patient has a lethal airway obstruction. Regardless if shock is present, airway, followed by breathing and then circulation, always takes management priority.

Primary Survey and Resuscitation

The primary survey, although most likely performed in the field by prehospital health care providers, is repeated on the patient's arrival in the emergency department. Airway, breathing, and circulation are continually reevaluated during resuscitation and throughout the phases of trauma care to ensure continued effectiveness of therapeutic interventions. Treatment initiated during resuscitation includes supplemental oxygen administration, establishment of vascular access, fluid replacement, cardiac rhythm monitoring, and, unless contraindicated, bladder and gastric catheter placement.[11]

Throughout shock resuscitation, survival of the physical being takes precedence, but consideration also must be given to the patient's psychological and spiritual welfare. Although the patient in shock may be confused or unresponsive, this does not imply that he or she is unaware of clinical procedures or the physical environment. It is likely that the patient feels helpless, anxious, and afraid. The nurse, as well as other team members, needs to remain cognizant of these feelings. Simple, brief explanations of procedures and emotional support should be given to the patient and family.

Accident Data Base. As in the management of any traumatic injury, a brief but thorough history is obtained from the field care providers. The data base includes all possible information about the mechanism of injury and events before, during, and after the incident and field resuscitation efforts. Changes in the patient's condition and initial responses to shock management are noted.

Ineffective Airway Clearance. Efforts to restore tissue oxygen delivery are first directed toward securing a patent airway. Severe traumatic shock, particularly when accompanied by head injury and/or concomitant substance abuse, may cause loss of consciousness and airway obstruction as jaw muscles relax and the tongue falls backward.[16] If the airway is not adequate, appropriate interventions are instituted immediately. This may be a simple maneuver such as a jaw thrust or may require endotracheal intubation or cricothyroidotomy. Removal of secretions and debris from the respiratory tract via suction is important to establish and maintain airway patency.[11, 18] Detailed discussion of the numerous causes of airway obstruction and immediate management is contained in Chapter 19.

Impaired Gas Exchange due to Ineffective Ventilation. Once the airway is secured, the next priority is ventilation. Respiratory rate and rhythm are quickly assessed. Hyperventilation is initially noted in major shock, followed by progressive deterioration of ventilatory efforts. Supplemental high-flow oxygen should be administered to improve oxygen availability for transport to hypoxic tissues. This may be all that is necessary in the spontaneously breathing patient who maintains adequate arterial blood gases. Any patient with compromised ventilation requires assistance in breathing to optimize oxygenation, and the patient in shock is clearly no exception. Injury-induced ventilatory insufficiency and/or the frequent need for surgical intervention in the patient in significant traumatic shock usually necessitates mechanical ventilatory support. Thoracic injuries that compromise ventilation and pose an imminent threat to survival need to be identified and treated at this time. Such conditions include tension pneumothorax, open pneumothorax, flail chest, and massive hemothorax.[11, 34]

Impaired Tissue Perfusion. Once it has been established that the airway is patent and that well-oxygenated gas is filling pulmonary alveoli, the priority becomes oxygen transport to body tissues. Assessment and stabilization of the circulation become the focus of shock management. The essential management components for a patient in shock or potential shock include a rapid evaluation for signs of internal and external hemorrhage and determination of the adequacy of the patient's circulatory system.

Common indicators of circulatory function evaluated in the primary survey include pulse rate and quality, skin color and temperature, capillary refill time, and mental status. Blood pressure measurements, which do not always accurately reflect blood flow or tissue perfusion, are generally obtained at a later point in the evaluation.[11, 14, 28] The pulse is readily assessed for rate, rhythm, and strength. The location at which the pulse is palpable can provide a general indication of the systolic blood pressure. However, the presence of palpable pulses does not ensure adequate tissue perfusion. A readily palpable radial pulse approximates a systolic pressure of 80 mm Hg, while the femoral and carotid pulses approximate pressures of 70 and 60 mm Hg, respectively.[36]

Pulse rate is thought to be relatively sensitive to shock, with tachycardia noted when as little as 15 per cent of total blood volume is depleted. Heart rate lacks specificity for hypovolemia and will rise in response to many factors. It cannot be relied on as a single assessment parameter for shock.[9, 29] Shock-induced tachycardia may not be noted in patients with artificial pacemakers, myocardial conduction abnormalities, age-related cardiac response limitations, or high spinal cord injuries. Individuals on medications such as digoxin and propranolol also may lack the tachycardic response to shock.

Assessment of the skin, including temperature, color, moisture, and capillary refill time, is a rapid and simple means of assessing peripheral perfusion. Although easy to assess, these parameters are difficult to quantify.[37] The injured patient who demonstrates cutaneous vasoconstriction, poor peripheral perfusion, and tachycardia of 120 beats/min should be assumed to be in shock unless proven otherwise.[11, 29] Although cutaneous hypoperfusion can be indicative of hypovolemic shock, it is important to remember that numerous other factors such as environmental temperature, various drugs, and neurohumoral alterations also can influence peripheral vascular diameter.[6, 16]

Level of consciousness is evaluated during the primary survey to assess neurological function. Increased anxiety may be the earliest sign of shock but also can be attributed to many other factors such as pain or fear. Symptoms of confusion and depression of consciousness are late signs indicating inadequate cerebral perfusion. These findings also may be attributed to other factors such as premorbid central nervous system dysfunction, metabolic disturbance, acute brain insult, or ingestion of drugs. A complete assessment should follow patient stabilization to make a differential diagnosis as to the exact cause(s) of altered neurological function.

Once it is recognized that inadequate tissue perfusion exists, the causative factor must be differentiated and the appropriate treatment begun promptly. The initial approach is to determine the adequacy of both intravascular volume and cardiac pump function to ensure volume circulation. During the primary survey and resuscitation, conditions that cause severe pump failure, including full cardiac arrest, are identified and treated. Simultaneously, measures to correct intravascular fluid volume deficits are initiated.

Cardiac Arrest Related to Profound Traumatic Shock

Cardiac arrest can occur for a number of reasons in the trauma patient and is discussed in detail in Chapter 6. Most commonly, cardiac arrest is a result of extreme intravascular volume loss or severe generalized hypoxia.[4] When greater than 50 per cent of the blood volume is rapidly lost, "exsanguination" cardiac arrest may result.[38] In milder forms of traumatic shock, ventricular fibrillation may occur owing to aggravation of underlying cardiac disease or heart injury (i.e., myocardial contusion). Infusion of cold fluids and/or use of cardiac stimulants during resuscitation also may trigger cardiac fibrillation.

Cardiac monitoring should be initiated as soon as possible to determine if shock- and/or injury-induced arrhythmias are present in the trauma patient. If there is no palpable carotid pulse, closed-chest cardiopulmonary resuscitation (CPR) per standard protocols should be instituted immediately regardless of the electrocardiograph (EKG) rhythm displayed.[9, 38] This directive is important, since trauma victims who rapidly exsanguinate and sustain a cardiac arrest may well have electromechanical dissociation.[38, 39]

The patient who has sustained a cardiac arrest secondary

to profound traumatic shock usually is severely hypovolemic and does not respond well to external cardiac massage.[16, 40–42] Therapeutic interventions to remedy traumatic shock and its underlying cause should never be delayed because of external cardiac massage.[41, 42] Blood volume must be rapidly restored and hemorrhage controlled to facilitate closed-chest resuscitation. Defibrillation is utilized as necessary, and CPR drugs such as cardiac stimulants, antiarrhythmics, and/or sodium bicarbonate should be administered as appropriate.[38]

Resuscitative thoracotomy in the trauma patient is a controversial topic. Immediate thoracotomy and internal cardiac massage are usually more hemodynamically effective for the patient with severe intravascular fluid depletion.[38, 41] This method of CPR also affords the physician the opportunity to relieve cardiac tamponade, repair myocardial injuries, control intrathoracic hemorrhage, and clamp the aorta to divert blood to vital organs.[1, 4, 9, 43]

Open-chest CPR has been shown to be most effective in improving survival of cardiac arrest patients who have sustained penetrating thoracic trauma.[16, 42, 44–47] Patients who have sustained blunt trauma, particularly those who present without signs of life or have had a prolonged cardiac arrest, do not respond favorably to resuscitative thoracotomy.[47–49] Patients not yet suffering cardiac arrest but in severe cardiovascular collapse, demonstrating progressive bradycardia and persistent hypotension refractory to inotropic support, fluid replacement, and pleural and pericardial decompression, also may benefit from internal cardiac massage.[10, 49]

Inadequate Cardiac Output Related to Myocardial Dysfunction

Severe myocardial dysfunction, short of cardiac arrest, may arise in the trauma patient, causing significant cardiac compromise. A number of contributing factors to cardiac pump insufficiency, such as blunt or penetrating cardiac injuries, ischemic damage secondary to profound shock, or less commonly myocardial infarction, have been described previously. During the primary survey and resuscitation, the patient is assessed for signs of failing cardiac pump function, and measures are instituted as needed to optimize myocardial performance.

Pericardial tamponade should be suspected in any patient with a history of thoracic trauma who remains unresponsive to resuscitative measures for traumatic shock.[11] In this case, the nurse should assist in promptly performing a needle pericardiocentesis. Decompression of the pericardium should result in vast improvements in cardiac pumping ability. Other myocardial injuries that may compromise pump function, such as infarction or contusion, may not be readily apparent during the primary survey because of lack of diagnostic data. Neck vein distention, although rarely noted in the face of hypovolemia, may be one indication that some degree of pump failure exists. Once hemodynamic monitoring has been instituted, a clearer picture can be obtained of the presence and degree of cardiac compromise.

Fluid Volume Deficit Related to Hemorrhage and Tissue Injury

In concert with efforts to ensure cardiac pump function, repletion of intravascular volume and restoration of oxygen-carrying capacity must be aggressively pursued. This is achieved by (1) control of external and internal hemorrhage and (2) administration of intravenous fluids and blood products. Each of the following therapeutic interventions described relates to one or both of these objectives.

Control of Hemorrhage

Exploration for sites of external and internal hemorrhage is a priority in resuscitation of the shock patient. The source of internal bleeding may not be readily apparent, and a variety of diagnostic measures are required. The assessment strategies and hemostatic interventions required for specific internal injuries that contribute to significant blood loss can be found in other appropriate chapters.

Obvious external hemorrhage is best managed by application of direct manual pressure over the bleeding site.[11, 14, 16, 22, 34] If practical, an extremity bleeding site may be elevated above the level of the patient's heart to augment hemorrhage control.[38] Application of pneumatic splints and traction can be instrumental in reducing blood loss from underlying fractures.[13, 16] As bleeding slows, a pressure dressing is applied to the wound to aid hemostasis. Rapid surgical intervention is necessary if these interventions fail to effectively control bleeding.[11]

Blind clamping and application of tourniquets are not recommended as measures for hemorrhage control, and their use should be avoided.[11, 16, 21, 34] Attempts to clamp blood vessels without adequate visibility can result in further vessel damage and inadvertent injury to nearby structures such as nerves.[13, 16] If transected vessels are visualized, carefully placed vascular clamps can be used to achieve temporary hemostasis until surgical repair is complete.[34] Tourniquets also obliterate circulation below the level of placement and result in further ischemia and potential loss of the affected limb. Their use is limited to emergencies when life-threatening hemorrhage is uncontrollable by any other means.[1, 16, 38] Under these circumstances, the tourniquet remains in place until shock therapy is under way and the physician is prepared to treat the bleeding site.

Emergency thoracotomy and temporary clamping of the thoracic aorta may be attempted to control massive, exsanginating hemorrhage from intra-abdominal and intrathoracic injuries in the patient suffering severe shock.[50, 51] This intervention also effectively redistributes the remaining circulating volume to vital organs, including the brain and the heart.[43, 50] The therapeutic merits of vascular occlusion remain very controversial. Occlusion of a major vessel such as the aorta can result in ischemic damage to the tissues and organs dependent on the vessel's perfusion. In addition, vascular unclamping is associated with multiple potential hemodynamic and metabolic derangements.[50]

Pneumatic Antishock Garment

The pneumatic antishock garment (PASG) is used in the treatment of traumatic shock for both hemorrhage control and blood pressure support (see Appendix 9–1). The PASG, also known as medical antishock trousers (MAST), is a trouser-like suit consisting of three independent inflatable compartments. The two inflatable leg chambers extend from the pubis to the ankle. The abdominal compartment extends from the upper abdomen to the pubis, surrounding the patient's lower torso. Each compartment is controlled independently by separate valve and footpump inflation systems.

Internal and external hemorrhage below the chest level may temporarily be controlled with the PASG because inflation of the device provides direct pressure to external bleeding sites and also to deeper blood vessels and tissue.[38, 52] The net effect is tamponade of soft tissue hemorrhage and reduction of hematoma expansion. The garment also serves to reduce bleeding when applied as a pneumatic splint for pelvic and lower extremity fractures.[11, 52–54]

The device is useful in rapidly raising blood pressure and in improving supradiaphragmatic tissue perfusion until adequate fluid volume has been restored.[1, 38, 52, 53, 55] Inflation of the suit translocates blood into the central circulation from the lower extremities and trunk. It was originally conjectured that the elevation of blood pressure occurred in response to this PASG autotransfusion effect.[55] However, more recent investigations indicate that only a limited amount of autotransfusion (approximately 150 to 300 ml blood volume) occurs during pneumatic compression.[53, 55–58] Current belief is that blood pressure elevation and improved upper body perfusion during PASG use are due to increased systemic vascular resistance.[53, 57–59]

Although still widely used as an adjunct in the management of traumatic shock, the therapeutic merits of the PASG have been questioned in the past few years. Analyses of one prospective, randomized trial evaluating prehospital use of the PASG concluded that use of this device may have no advantage and may even be detrimental in certain patient populations.[60–64] Field application of the PASG did not improve survival, reduce morbidity, or decrease hospital costs in hypotensive patients suffering primarily penetrating injury in an urban trauma center system with short transport times (30 minutes or less) and aggressive prehospital management.[60, 61] These same findings were true when only those hypotensive patients with penetrating abdominal injuries were analyzed.[63, 64] Patients with thoracic trauma, especially with myocardial or major thoracic vessel injury, had a much greater prehospital mortality rate when the PASG was applied in the field.[64] Because of findings such as these, PASG use has become controversial.

Indications for Use. Currently recommended indications for in-hospital use of the PASG include (1) splinting of pelvic and lower extremity fractures and control of associated hemorrhage and (2) tamponade of intra-abdominal or lower extremity hemorrhage.[4, 11] Hypotension associated with traumatic shock may be remedied by PASG placement until fluid resuscitation is sufficient.[53] Other causes of shock that may coexist with traumatic shock (i.e., neurogenic) also may gain therapeutic benefit from PASG application.[53, 59] These indications for PASG use are summarized in Table 9–3.[53, 55] Additional controlled clinical trials are necessary to better define the clinical indications and contraindications for PASG use.

Although the device may improve blood pressure and hemostasis, it must be emphasized that it is not a substitute for adequate blood volume replacement. Fluid administration should not be delayed because of PASG use.[11] The garment may assist in establishing intravenous access by enhancing upper torso and extremity venous filling and subsequent cannulation.[53]

Contraindications. The current absolute contraindications for the use of the PASG are pulmonary edema, left ventricular dysfunction, and known diaphragm rupture.[11, 53, 55] The increased peripheral vascular resistance associated with PASG use increases cardiac afterload and can be detrimental to an injured or diseased myocardium. Congestive heart failure and pulmonary congestion are therefore likely to be exacerbated.[11, 53] Inflation of the abdominal compartment may result in abdominal viscera herniation through the diaphragm if diaphragm rupture is present.[11, 65]

Several relative contraindications exist and are listed in Table 9–3. Due to the unknown effect on the fetus and potential decrease in placental perfusion pressure, compression of the maternal abdomen with the PASG must be

TABLE 9–3. USE OF THE PNEUMATIC ANTISHOCK GARMENT (PASG)

CURRENT INDICATIONS

Hypovolemic and traumatic shock
- Blood pressure less than 80 mm Hg systolic
- Blood pressure less than 100 mm Hg systolic accompanied by symptoms of shock

Stabilization of lower extremity or pelvic fractures
Control of hemorrhage within the confines of garment
Circulatory stabilization for patient transport
Maintenance of upper torso perfusion when intravenous fluids cannot be initiated
Circulatory support during volume replacement
Relative hypovolemia and hypotension
- Neurogenic shock
- Drug overdose
- Septic shock
- Anaphylaxis

CONTRAINDICATIONS

Absolute
Pulmonary edema
Left ventricle dysfunction
Known rupture of diaphragm

Relative
Pregnancy (abdominal compartment only)
Evisceration of abdominal contents
Impaled foreign body in lower torso
Compartment syndromes of lower extremity
Lumbar spine instability
Uncontrolled hemorrhage outside of garment

CONTROVERSIAL APPLICATIONS

Head injury with increased intracranial pressure
Intrathoracic injuries
- Tension pneumothorax
- Cardiac tamponade

COMPLICATIONS AND DISADVANTAGES

Hypotension after removal
Metabolic acidosis
Respiratory compromise
Decreased renal perfusion
Extension of diaphragmatic tear/herniation of abdominal viscera into thorax
Increased bleeding due to pressure elevation
Vomiting
Lower extremity tissue ischemia
Compartment syndrome
Skin breakdown
Pulmonary edema, congestive heart failure
Lumbar spine movement

Adapted from Frumpkin K: The pneumatic antishock garment (PASG). In Roberts JR, Hedges JR (eds): Clinical Procedures in Emergency Medicine. Philadelphia, WB Saunders Co, 1985.

approached cautiously.[55] Abdominal evisceration or the presence of an impaled object are also proposed as relative contraindications because of potential abdominal organ injury. The circumferential lower extremity pressure created by the PASG may exacerbate compartment syndrome, and its use should be avoided in a patient known to have this disorder.[53, 55] The abdominal compartment of the garment is used cautiously in a patient with possible lumbar spine trauma.[53] Inflation of the abdominal compartment may result in nerve injury in a patient with an unstable vertebral column fracture. Uncontrolled hemorrhage outside the pneumatic garment (i.e., intrathoracic) is a relative contraindication for PASG use, since an increase in blood pressure and perfusion may exacerbate blood loss.[11, 59, 64]

Controversial PASG Application. The use of the PASG remains controversial in conditions of head injury associated with increased intracranial pressure and certain intrathoracic injuries. Caution is clearly warranted when applying the device in the presence of these conditions.[53] It has been speculated that use of the PASG could result in increased intracranial pressure and a worsening of cerebral edema in the head-injured patient. However, improved blood pressure resulting from proper use of the device has been shown to positively affect cerebral perfusion pressure. This cerebrovascular benefit may outweigh the potential risk of intracranial hypertension.[55, 66]

The PASG may be hazardous in the presence of intrathoracic injuries, such as tension pneumothorax and cardiac tamponade, since it enhances the elevation in venous pressure associated with these pathologies.[55] If there is a decline in blood pressure following inflation of the device, the presence of tension pneumothorax or cardiac tamponade should be suspected. The garment inflation pressure should then be reduced.[53]

Technique. Frequently the patient is admitted to the emergency department with the PASG already in place. If the device has not already been applied, the nurse must determine the need for the PASG and rule out contraindications for its use. A procedure for application, maintenance, and removal of the PASG is found in Appendix 9–1.

Although time constraints in the initial survey may have postponed obtaining a blood pressure measurement for the patient, this parameter should be obtained as soon as possible during resuscitation. Blood pressure measurement varies as a priority initially since it can be estimated by the pulse, and the patient's baseline blood pressure for comparison is typically unknown. However, accurate determination and trending of blood pressure measurement are essential as a guide in using the PASG.

Once the PASG is in place, the patient's blood pressure and not the pressure of the inflation chamber directs the amount of inflation necessary to maintain an acceptable perfusion status.[11] The PASG can be maximally inflated to obtain an intrasuit pressure just above 100 mm Hg before pressure release valves are activated.[55, 67] Only the minimal intrasuit pressure necessary to maintain the systolic blood pressure at 90 to 100 mm Hg should be employed. In addition to monitoring blood pressure, one should closely observe the effect that garment inflation has on other indicators of the patient's status. Onset of respiratory distress and poor respiratory gas exchange during inflation of the abdominal section may signal the presence of diaphragm injury and visceral herniation.[11, 65] These findings require immediate abdominal compartment deflation, regardless of blood pressure readings.[11]

Once the PASG is inflated, the nurse continually monitors the patient's perfusion status and vital signs to determine if more or less pressure is necessary. The PASG should remain intact and inflated until the patient's circulatory status has stabilized.[9, 11] X-ray examination can be performed through the suit, and a 12-lead EKG can be done with the device in place.[9, 59] Urinary catheterization is somewhat difficult, especially in the female patient, but can be achieved through the perineal access space. The patient is transported to the operating room with the PASG still inflated if operative intervention is required to stop hemorrhage.[11, 53]

The PASG is usually left inflated if the patient requires transport to another institution.[11] Environmental factors that influence intrasuit pressures need to be considered during transfer. When air transport is used, the decrease in atmospheric pressure that occurs as the plane or helicopter ascends causes the air in the suit to expand. Consequently, intrasuit pressure is elevated. A similar expansion in intrasuit air and rise in suit pressure occurs when the patient is moved from a cold to a warm environment.[11, 52] Decreasing altitude and declining temperatures have opposite effects.

After the shock state has been controlled, vital signs stabilized, venous access established, and fluid volume replaced, the PASG can be *gradually* deflated. If the garment is deflated without adequate replacement of intravascular volume, severe shock and death of the patient may result.[11] Prior to beginning garment deflation, a pump should be made readily available in case reinflation is necessary.[13] The abdominal compartment is deflated first, followed by one leg compartment at a time. Again the patient's systolic blood pressure serves to direct the deflation process. When the patient's systolic blood pressure drops by 5 mm Hg, the deflation is halted, fluids are increased to regain an adequate blood pressure, and the deflation process is begun again.[11] Once deflated, the PASG may be left uninflated around the patient and removed at a later time.

Complications. There are several complications of PASG use that should be considered during the application and/or removal of the suit (see Table 9–3). A potentially lethal complication is severe hypotension resulting from inappropriate removal of the device prior to adequate fluid restoration.[53] Systemic metabolic acidosis may develop after suit deflation as metabolites accumulated in the underperfused lower extremities are washed into the central circulation.[53, 68] Arterial blood gas analysis and appropriate bicarbonate correction abate this complication.[53]

Abdominal compartment inflation elevates the diaphragm and restricts lung expansion.[53, 66] This may result in respiratory compromise which may require additional oxygen administration and ventilatory assistance.[38] Abdominal compression also may reduce renal blood flow and cause renal ischemia.[38, 53] Diaphragmatic ruptures or tears may increase in size as intra-abdominal pressure increases.[65] Abdominal compression also may stimulate vomiting, urination, or defecation.

Lower extremity PASG inflation compromises lower extremity circulation, which can result in tissue ischemia and compartment syndrome.[4, 60] Use of the PASG has been reported to cause lower extremity compartment syndrome which has resulted in cases of limb amputation,[61] rhabdomyolysis with renal failure,[69] and death.[70] This emphasizes the need to utilize minimal intrasuit pressure to maintain systolic blood pressure and to deflate the garment as soon as possible.[4, 71] Increase in lower extremity wound hemorrhage may occur with improved perfusion pressure and should not be allowed to go unnoticed beneath the PASG. Garment pressure over unprotected bony prominences or wrinkled clothing under the PASG may cause cutaneous breakdown.[53] Some serious but less frequently encountered complications of the PASG include pulmonary edema, congestive heart failure, and lumbar nerve injury, as described previously.

Fluid and Blood Component Therapy

Restoration of adequate circulating blood volume and oxygen-carrying capacity is essential for successful resuscitation of the patient in shock following traumatic injury. Volume replacement increases cardiac preload and output and consequently enhances tissue perfusion. Reestablishing tissue perfusion and oxygenation should resolve the shock state and prevent inherent complications.

Venous Access. The initial step in fluid resuscitation is to rapidly establish vascular access for controlled volume infusion. The severity of the patient's condition usually dictates the number and size of intravenous catheters inserted.[1] Generally, at least two large-bore (14- to 16-gauge) catheters are required.[4, 38, 67] Venous lines are preferably inserted percutaneously into the upper extremities. Lower extremities are generally not used for line placement due to interference of PASG placement, possible peripheral vascular disease, and potential for fluid extravasation in the presence of inferior vena cava injury.[28] A patient presenting with a penetrating neck or chest injury should preferably have at least one venous access established below the diaphragm into tributaries of the inferior vena cava to help ensure effective fluid resuscitation.[4, 28] Intravenous placement in an injured extremity or proximal to any suspected vascular injury should be avoided.[4, 16]

In some instances, peripheral cannulation is not possible due to vasoconstriction and venous collapse. Central venous access lines or venous cutdown then becomes essential. Subclavian, jugular, or femoral veins are employed for central cannulation. It is important to note that in the hypovolemic patient the subclavian approach carries significant risk of iatrogenic pneumothorax.[4] The saphenous and forearm veins are the sites of choice for venous cutdown.[4, 11, 16] Patient injuries, PASG placement, and physician experience will determine the exact location chosen for venous access.[4] Regardless of the site chosen, short, large-bore catheters should be used to provide maximal flow rates. For example, a 10-gauge catheter or No. 8 French introducer can be inserted by cutdown in order to administer quantities of blood or fluids in excess of 1000 ml/min.[72, 73]

Initially, crucial time constraints prohibit the insertion of central monitoring catheters. When time permits and fluid resuscitation is under way, a central venous pressure catheter is useful in evaluating patient response to fluid therapy and in the diagnosis of acute cardiac compromise. Similarly, a pulmonary artery catheter may be necessary in some patients for accurate and more detailed cardiopulmonary assessment.

Infusion Techniques. Rapid volume infusion is achieved by the use of short, large-diameter tubing and elevation of the infusing fluid as high as possible.[30, 38, 72, 74, 75] Only maximum drip administration sets are used to permit rapid fluid flow.[67, 76] Kinking of the intravascular catheter and tubing must be avoided to ensure that maximal flow rates are attained.[76] An inflatable pressure pack or blood pump can be inflated around the bag of intravenous solution to increase flow rate.[28, 75] This technique is somewhat time-consuming and poses the risk of fluid bag or tubing rupture, vascular injury, and infiltration.[38, 74]

Recently, several systems that enable large volumes of warmed fluids to be infused rapidly through a single large-bore venous catheter have been used successfully in resuscitation of traumatic shock.[77–79] Two examples of devices that have proven to be beneficial in initial management of the hypovolemic trauma patient are the R.I.S. (Rapid Infusion System, Haemonetics Corp., Braintree, Mass.)[77] and the modified Level I H-500 (Level One Technology, Marshfield, Mass.).[78] The R.I.S., composed of a roll-ahead pump, warmer, digital step motor, and multiple safety and infusion monitoring features, delivers normothermic fluids at rates up to 1500 ml/min. Crystalloids, colloids, or blood products, with the exception of platelets, can be used in the system. The less expensive and easy-to-use Level I H-500 delivers pressure-driven fluids that are warmed by a heat exchanger. Modification of this system by addition of compressor-driven pneumatic pumps enable infusion rates of up to 500 ml/min to be attained.[78]

Choice of Fluids. The resuscitation fluid best suited for the patient in shock remains controversial.[28, 80–82] A considerable number of experimental and clinical studies have compared crystalloid and colloid resuscitation solutions. These studies have yielded conflicting results about the effects and desirability of various fluids. The primary physiological difference between the two fluid types is that colloids possess oncotic capability not inherent in crystalloid solutions.[26, 81] Proponents of crystalloid therapy point out the benefits of cost-effectiveness, nonallergenic properties, and reduced viscosity which may improve microcirculation. Crystalloids also replete both the interstitial and intravascular spaces.[16, 21, 28, 67, 74, 80] Further arguments in favor of crystalloids include complications related to the use of colloid solutions, such as excessive fluid retention, pulmonary dysfunction, exacerbation of systemic or pulmonary edema, and reduction of renal filtration rate.[74, 83–85] Colloid proponents argue the greater effectiveness of colloid solution on a volume-for-volume basis in reversing signs of shock.[81, 86–89] The basis for this argument is that since crystalloids lack oncotic properties, such solutions readily move out of the intravascular space and increase the fluid required for effective resuscitation.[18, 26, 80, 81, 86] Large volume crystalloid infusions can dilute plasma proteins and red blood cells, which lowers hematocrit and reduces colloid oncotic pressure.[26, 28, 67, 74] Those supporting colloid use point out that its inherent oncotic properties act to minimize systemic and pulmonary edema,[87, 88] while reduction of colloid oncotic pressure caused by high-volume crystalloid infusion increases the likelihood of edema formation.[28, 80, 90] Contradicting this opinion, others report that despite a decrease in colloid oncotic pressure noted with crystalloid administration, there is not necessarily an increase in extravascular lung water.[82, 91]

Two points are agreed on by all. First, crystalloids are much cheaper than colloid solutions. Second, on a volume-for-volume basis, colloid solutions are more effective in restoring intravascular volume.[28, 83] The second point may be of significance in patients with central nervous system trauma, in whom increased intracranial pressure must be avoided.

One approach for choosing a fluid is to base the selection on the presence or absence of observable signs of shock. Isotonic electrolyte solutions, namely lactated Ringer's, normal saline, or Plasma-lyte A, are commonly the initial fluids used for resuscitation.[11, 14] Lactated Ringer's solution closely approximates the plasma electrolyte composition and is considered by many to be the resuscitation fluid of choice. Plasma-lyte A use is attractive due to inherent advantages which include that it is calcium-free and therefore compatible with blood, it has lower chloride levels so the risk of hyperchloremic metabolic acidosis is theoretically reduced, and it lacks lactate so exacerbation of lactic acidosis should not occur. Crystalloids are usually initiated in the field. If the patient has not shown signs of shock in the field or in the resuscitation area, crystalloid solutions are continued. Crystalloids alone may adequately replete the intravascular volume of patients only in early or moderate shock.[11, 16] Once hospitalized, the patient who demonstrates persistent symptoms of shock despite crystalloid infusion of 1500 ml or more will have colloid or possibly blood transfusion initiated.[4, 11, 28]

All the fluids discussed are capable of restoring circulating blood volume. The selection of the type of fluid used in resuscitation considers all the factors discussed and is weighted by each solution's advantages or disadvantages. Table 9–4 summarizes the parenteral fluids currently available, their uses, and factors that are important in fluid replacement.

In recent years, use of hypertonic saline (3 to 7.5 per cent) and hypertonic saline/dextran solutions for initial resuscitation from hemorrhage and traumatic shock has been investigated extensively in both animal shock models[92–103] and humans.[104–106] Multiple studies have reported that relatively small volumes of hypertonic saline (7.2 to 7.5 per cent) and hypertonic saline/dextran solutions can effectively improve hemodynamic parameters when administered during hemorrhage and traumatic shock.[92, 97, 101, 104, 105] Although the exact mechanisms remain controversial, the hemodynamic benefits provided by hypertonic saline solutions have been attributed to an increase in circulating volume due to recruitment of intracellular and interstitial fluid into the intravascular space, stimulation of a neurogenic reflex in the pulmonary circulation that causes venoconstriction, and increased myocardial contractility and precapillary vasodilation.[99, 100, 102, 107, 108] The addition of a hyperoncotic solution such as dextran enhances and prolongs the beneficial hemodynamic and microcirculatory effects associated with hypertonic saline administration.[97, 102, 103, 105]

Despite their apparent benefits, except for resuscitation from burns, hypertonic saline solutions are not typically the fluid of choice for management of hypovolemia in the trauma patient.[13, 82] Several studies have shown that although effective in improving cardiovascular status and animal survival in the state of controlled hemorrhage, hypertonic saline solutions may actually increase the rate of bleeding, further reduce arterial blood pressure, and increase mortality when administered during uncontrolled hemorrhagic shock.[94–96, 98] Administration of hypertonic saline also has other inherent potential complications, including development of hypernatremia, hyperosmolality, hypokalemia, and intracellular dehydration.[13, 97, 100, 101, 106] Further studies with human subjects are necessary to clarify the role of hypertonic saline as an alternative solution in resuscitation from traumatic shock.

Amount of Fluid Replacement. The amount and rate of fluid replacement required depend on the severity of intravascular volume depletion. Clinical observation of patient status guides fluid administration.[18] The best indices to determine the sufficiency of volume replacement are (1) amelioration of clinical signs of shock, (2) return of stable vital signs, including central venous pressure, and (3) urine output greater than 50 ml/hr.[1, 10, 11, 14, 16] When the shock state fails to show signs of resolution after 15 minutes of aggressive fluid replacement, then continued hemorrhage or a coexisting cause of shock should be suspected. The recurrence of signs of shock after initial correction similarly suggests continued blood loss, inadequate fluid delivery, or onset of complications.[29]

Clinical assessment and hemodynamic parameters are monitored to avoid fluid overload. Overhydration may precipitate posttraumatic cardiac or pulmonary complications. Special care should be taken to avoid excess fluid administration and consequent cerebral or spinal cord edema in patients with central nervous system injury.

Blood Component Therapy. Regardless of the initial solution chosen, it is important to remember that most trauma patients are in shock from hemorrhage. The logical replacement solution for blood is blood. Blood replacement is usually indicated for patients in major or severe shock in order to restore adequate oxygen-carrying capacity.

The decision to administer blood is based on the patient's response to initial fluid therapy.[11, 14, 28] Patients in severe shock with exsanguinating hemorrhage should receive universal, type O red blood cells (RBC) as soon as possible.[4, 14] Type O Rh-negative RBCs are preferred for women of childbearing age to decrease the risk of complications.[4, 11] Rh immune globulin should be administered to an Rh-negative female of childbearing age who has received Rh-positive blood transfusion.[4] Patients with less serious injuries may be stabilized with other resuscitation fluids until either type-specific blood or cross-matched blood becomes available. Type-specific blood can usually be obtained within 10 minutes and is appropriate for life-threatening shock states.[11, 67] Fully cross-matched blood is preferable but may require up to 1 hour to obtain. Transfusions are generally administered to maintain a hematocrit of at least 30 per cent.[12, 22, 29, 32, 37, 67] The optimal hematocrit, however, varies with the individual and is targeted for the level required to maximize oxygen transport and consumption.[32]

Consideration also should be given to the use of autologous blood, the safest source of red blood cells.[109, 110] Autotransfusion is particularly useful for replacement of blood lost from hemothorax or other intrathoracic injuries. A discussion of the indications, complications, and technical aspects of autotransfusion is found in Chapter 19.

The use of oxygen-carrying solutions as an alternative to blood transfusion is an on-going subject of experimental investigation.[111, 112] Fluorocarbon emulsions and stroma-free hemoglobin solutions have been described previously as effective oxygen-carrying fluids and promising blood substitutes.[26, 32, 38, 67, 112–114] The reader is referred to reviews of

TABLE 9–4. GUIDE TO PARENTERAL FLUIDS

TYPE	DESCRIPTION	COMPOSITION	USES/INDICATIONS	ADVANTAGES	DISADVANTAGES	SPECIAL CONSIDERATIONS
Blood and Blood Products						
Whole blood	500 ml unit of complete blood	Red blood cells Leukocytes Plasma Platelets Clotting factors	To replace blood volume and maintain adequate hemoglobin (Hgb)	Provides intravascular volume Increases the oxygen-carrying capacity of the blood	Possibility of limited supply Potential associated risks of hepatitis and HIV transmission and allergic reactions Delayed administration because of necessary typing and cross-matching Possibility of type and cross-match errors	Whole blood should be stored at 0–10° C, but warmed at least 20–30 minutes before administration (never infuse cold blood) (Use *fresh* whole blood whenever possible to avoid adverse metabolic changes related to stored blood (i.e., increased ammonia, potassium, and cellular debris)[22]
Red blood cells (packed, concentrate)			To increase the hematocrit	Concentrated form helps to prevent excess fluid administration in patients with cardiogenic shock (increases the oxygen-carrying capacity with less volume loading) Associated with fewer risks of metabolic complications when compared with stored whole blood (decreased amount of transfused antibodies, electrolytes, etc.) Provides economic use of blood as a resource; frees other blood components, such as platelets and clotting factors, to be concentrated and stored	Slow infusion rate because of increased viscosity Decreased content of plasma proteins and coagulation factors when compared with whole blood Inadequate (alone) for volume replacement and correction of hypovolemia Altered blood clotting with administration of more than 20 units; clotting factors need to be replenished as necessary High cost of frozen (thawed) red blood cells	Administer via Y-connector tubing with normal saline to increase infusion flow rate Washed red blood cells (resuspended in saline) can be given in shock to decrease red cell adhesiveness (washing decreases the cell's fibrinogen coating) Administration carries risk of blood-borne disease transmission and allergic reaction
Fresh	300 ml unit of whole blood minus 80% of plasma (hematocrit 70%)	Red blood cells 20% plasma Some leukocytes and platelets	To correct red blood cell deficiency and improve the oxygen-carrying capacity of the blood			
Frozen (also called leukocyte-poor)	200–250 ml unit with 85–90% of red blood cell mass contained in 1 unit of whole blood	Red blood cells No plasma Almost no leukocytes or platelets	Used in anemia and for modest blood loss (when hematocrit is below 25–30%)			
Human plasma (fresh, frozen, or dried)	200 ml unit of uncoagulated, unconcentrated plasma (separated from 1 unit of whole blood)	Plasma All plasma proteins, including albumin Clotting factors (no red cells, white cells, or platelets)	To restore plasma volume in hypovolemic shock without increasing the hematocrit To restore clotting factors (except platelets)	Effective for rapid volume replacement Contains clotting factors	Expensive Deficient of red blood cells	Human plasma carries the risk of viral hepatitis and HIV transmission and allergic reactions Administer fresh frozen plasma promptly after thawing to prevent deterioration of clotting factors V and VIII
Platelets	Platelet sediment from platelet-rich plasma, resuspended in 30–50 ml of plasma	Platelets Lymphocytes Some plasma	To control bleeding due to thrombocytopenia To maintain normal blood coagulability		Deficient of other coagulation factors	
Plasma protein fraction (e.g., Plasmanate, Plasma-Plex)	250 ml and 500 ml units of a 5% solution of human plasma proteins in normal saline	Albumin 44 gm/l α and β globulins 6 gm/l Sodium 130–160 mEq/l Potassium 2 mEq/l Osmolality 290 mOsm/l pH 6.7–7.3	To expand plasma volume in hypovolemic shock (while cross-matching is being completed) To increase the serum colloid osmotic pressure	Can be used interchangeably with 5% human serum albumin Osmotically equivalent to plasma Associated with low risk of hepatitis or HIV transmission	Expensive Deficient of clotting factors Associated with larger number of side effects, such as hypotension and hypersensitivity, than those reported with 5% albumin (due to presence of globulins) Hypotension induced by rapid intravenous administration (greater than 10 ml/min)	Plasma protein fraction is prepared from pooled plasma heated to 60° C for 10 hours; this procedure reduces the risk of transmission of HIV and viral hepatitis Rapid administration of large doses can alter blood coagulation This solution should be used cautiously in patients with congestive heart failure (due to added fluid and rapid plasma volume expansion) and in patients with renal failure (due to added proteins)
Albumin	Aqueous fraction of pooled plasma prepared from whole blood in buffered normal saline		To increase the plasma colloid osmotic pressure To rapidly expand the plasma volume	Rare allergic reactions (less than 0.011% in all albumin solutions combined) Rare transmission of hepatitis virus due to heating process (transmission only occurs secondary to accidents in its preparation)	Potential leakage from capillaries in shock states associated with increased capillary permeability Possible precipitation of congestive heart failure following rapid infusion in patients with circulatory overload and compromised cardiovascular function	Albumin does not contain preservatives; therefore, each opened bottle should be used at once The rate of administration of 5% albumin should not exceed 2–4 ml/min The rate of administration of 25% albumin should not exceed 1 ml/min 25% albumin is reserved for use in patients with pulmonary or peripheral edema and hypoproteinemia; administer with a diuretic to ensure diuresis
5%	250 and 500 ml units	Albumin 50 gm/l Sodium 130–160 mEq/l Potassium 1 mEq/l Osmolality 300 mOsm/l Colloid osmotic pressure 20 mm Hg pH 6.4–7.4				

Table continued on following page

TABLE 9–4. GUIDE TO PARENTERAL FLUIDS *Continued*

TYPE	DESCRIPTION	COMPOSITION	USES/INDICATIONS	ADVANTAGES	DISADVANTAGES	SPECIAL CONSIDERATIONS
BLOOD AND BLOOD PRODUCTS *Continued*						
25% (salt-poor)*	25 ml, 50 ml, and 100 ml units	Albumin 240 gm/l Globulins 10 gm/l Sodium 130–160 mEq/l Osmolality 1500 mOsm/l pH 6.4–7.4				
PHARMACEUTICAL PLASMA EXPANDERS						
Dextran	Biosynthesized Water soluble, large polysaccharide polymer of glucose		To rapidly expand plasma volume	All dextrans associated with low incidence of anaphylactic reactions (<0.01%) Less expensive than protein solutions LMWD associated with fewer allergic reactions than HMWD LMWD facilitates blood flow by decreasing red blood cell sludging and platelet aggregation HMWD leaks from the capillaries less readily than LMWD; can effectively increase plasma volume for up to 24 hours	LMWD 70% excreted unchanged in the urine, so the urine osmolality and specific gravity are altered Potential osmotic-nephrosis and renal tubular shutdown Possible bleeding from raw surfaces due to decreased platelet adhesiveness; side effects include decreased hemoglobin, hematocrit, fibrinogen, and clotting factors V, VIII, and IX HMWD 50% excreted unchanged in the urine, so the urine osmolality and specific gravity are altered Higher incidence of allergic reactions when compared with LMWD Increases blood viscosity and platelet adhesiveness	Avoid the use of dextran in patients with active hemorrhage, hemorrhagic shock, coagulation disorders, and thrombocytopenia Bleeding times can be prolonged when the correct dose of dextran 70 (1.2 gm/kg/day) or dextran 40 (2 gm/kg/day) are exceeded Administer dextran in dextrose solutions to patients with sodium restriction Dextran administration can interfere with typing and cross-matching of blood when the older (outdated) enzyme method is used
Low molecular weight dextran (LMWD; Dextran 40; Rheomacrodex; Gentran 40)	500 ml unit of solution that contains 10% dextran in either normal saline or 5% dextrose in water	Glucose polysaccharides with average molecular weight of 40,000				
High molecular weight dextran (HMWD; Dextran 70; Gentran 70–75; Macrodex)	500 ml unit of solution that contains 6% dextran in either normal saline or 5% dextrose in water	Glucose polysaccharides with average molecular weight of 70,000–75,000				
Hetastarch (Hespan; Volex)	500 ml unit of a 6% solution containing a synthetic polymer of hydroxyethyl starch in normal saline	Globular and branched-chain hydroxyethyl starch prepared from amylopectin Average molecular weight = 69,000–70,000 Sodium 154 mEq/l Chloride 154 mEq/l Osmolality 310 mOsm/l Colloid osmotic pressure 30–35 mm Hg	To expand plasma volume	Same volume expansion characteristics of albumin but with a longer duration of action (up to 36 hours) Associated with low risk of allergic and anaphylactic reactions (0.085%) Cost of hetastarch is about one half that of plasma protein fraction and albumin Nonantigenic No danger of transmission of hepatitis virus	Potential dilution of plasma proteins Potential dilution of clotting factors with resultant coagulation changes Potential circulatory overload in patients with severe congestive heart failure and compromised renal function Increased serum amylase level (>200 mg/100 ml), peaking within 1 hour of intravenous administration of hetastarch and persisting for 3 to 4 days (due to action of amylase in hetastarch degradation)	Do not use if the solution is cloudy or deep brown or if it contains crystals Monitor clotting studies and platelet counts, observing for prolonged prothrombin and partial thromboplastin times and thrombocytopenia The safety and compatibility of additives with hetastarch have not been established; the manufacturer recommends infusing hetastarch through a separate line, when possible, or piggybacking the second drug The maximum infusion rate in acute hemorrhagic shock is 20 ml/kg/hr Monitor serum albumin; if it falls below 2 gm/100 ml, consider substituting albumin for hetastarch
Mannitol (Osmitrol)	Solution of mannitol in water or normal saline	Mannitol (inert form of sugar mannose)	To raise intravascular volume To reduce interstitial and intracellular edema To promote osmotic diuresis	Reduces intracellular/interstitial swelling Increases urinary output	Potential circulatory overload in patients with congestive heart failure, pulmonary congestion, and renal dysfunction	
CRYSTALLOID SOLUTIONS						
Isotonic						
Normal saline	0.9% sodium chloride in water	Sodium 154 mEq/l Chloride 154 mEq/l Osmolality 308 mOsm/l	To raise plasma volume when red blood cell mass is adequate To replace body fluid	Considered by some to be the single most important salt for maintaining and replacing extracellular fluid Increases plasma volume without altering normal sodium concentration or serum osmolality	Potential fluid retention and circulatory overload due to sodium content Potential hyperchloremic metabolic acidosis due to high chloride content[14, 30, 81]	

TABLE 9–4. GUIDE TO PARENTERAL FLUIDS *Continued*

TYPE	DESCRIPTION	COMPOSITION	USES/INDICATIONS	ADVANTAGES	DISADVANTAGES	SPECIAL CONSIDERATIONS
CRYSTALLOID SOLUTIONS *Continued*						
Lactated Ringer's solution (Hartman's solution)	0.9% sodium chloride in water with added electrolytes and buffers	Sodium 130 mEq/l Potassium 4 mEq/l Calcium 2.7 mEq/l Chloride 109 mEq/l Lactate 27 mEq/l pH 6.5 Osmolality 273 mOsm/l	To replace body fluid To buffer acidosis	Lactate is converted to bicarbonate (in the liver), which buffers acidosis Lactate replaces bicarbonate, preventing precipitation of calcium bicarbonate and calcium carbonate Lactate is more stable than bicarbonate and more compatible with ions present in the solution	Increased lactic acidosis in shock due to lactate Fluid retention and circulatory overload due to sodium content	Lactate conversion requires aerobic metabolism; therefore, it should be used cautiously in shock and other hypoperfusion states Use cautiously in patients with liver failure since liver converts lactate[18, 81]
Plasma-lyte A	0.9% sodium chloride in water with added electrolytes, acetate, and glucagon	Sodium 140 mEq/l Potassium 5 mEq/l Magnesium 3 mEq/l Chloride 98 mEq/l Acetate 27 mEq/l Gluconate 23 mEq/l Osmolality 294 mOsm/l	To replace body fluids	Calcium-free, so can be administered with blood Lower chloride content decreases risk of hyperchloremic metabolic acidosis Lacks lactate, so will not exacerbate lactic acidosis Acetate acts to buffer acidosis	Fluid retention and circulatory overload due to sodium content	Give cautiously in patients with renal insufficiency due to potassium and magnesium load
Ringer's solution	0.9% sodium chloride in water with added potassium and calcium	Sodium 147 mEq/l Potassium 4 mEq/l Calcium 5 mEq/l Chloride 156 mEq/l	To replace body fluid To provide additional potassium and calcium	Does not contain lactate, so can be given to patients with hypoperfusion	Potential hyperchloremic metabolic acidosis due to high chloride concentration Potential fluid retention and circulatory overload due to sodium content	
Hypotonic						
½ normal saline	0.45% sodium chloride in water	Sodium 77 mEq/l Chloride 77 mEq/l	To raise total fluid volume		Potential interstitial and intracellular edema due to rapid movement of this fluid from the vascular space Dilution of plasma proteins and electrolytes	
5% dextrose in water (D_5W)	5% dextrose		To raise total fluid volume To provide calories for energy (200 calories/1000 ml)	Distributed evenly in every body compartment (acts like free water) Reverses dehydration Prevents hyperosmolar state Maintains adequate renal tubular flow (facilitates water excretion)	Dilution of plasma proteins and electrolytes due to rapid metabolism of glucose and resultant free water May cause or exacerbate interstitial and intracellular edema due to rapid movement of this solution from intravascular space	

*The term salt-poor designates the 25% albumin concentration and is a carryover from the days when acetyltryptophan replaced a 1.8% salt solution to increase the thermal stability of the product. The term salt-poor is erroneous because both concentrations of albumin contain sodium carbonate or sodium bicarbonate to adjust the pH and sodium caprylate and sodium acetyltryptophan as stabilizers.

Adapted from Rice V: Shock management. Part I: Fluid volume replacement. Crit Care Nurse 4:69–73, 1984.

these solutions and their potential use in shock resuscitation.[113, 115, 116]

MULTIPLE BLOOD TRANSFUSIONS. The patient who requires rapid, multiple transfusions to restore blood volume must be monitored for numerous potential complications. The problems associated with massive transfusion therapy are summarized in Table 9–5. In an effort to reduce hazardous effects, blood should be warmed during infusion and administered through a macropore intravenous filter.[11] Effective blood-warming measures include use of standard blood warmers or rapid infusion systems with blood-warming capabilities and administration of RBCs as an admixture with high-temperature saline solution.[11, 117] Calcium may be administered cautiously if the patient manifests symptoms of hypocalcemia. It is unlikely that supplemental calcium will be necessary within the first hour of treatment.[11]

Dilutional coagulopathy associated with massive blood transfusion is treated by administering fresh frozen plasma and/or platelets. The indications for these components include an abnormal coagulation profile and clinical evidence of coagulopathic or persistent bleeding.[4, 13, 28] Prophylactic administration of platelets or fresh frozen plasma is inappropriate and exposes the patient to unnecessary risk.[11, 14] Serum coagulation profile should be monitored frequently, with at

TABLE 9–5. PATHOPHYSIOLOGICAL CONSIDERATIONS IN THE MASSIVELY TRANSFUSED PATIENT

PROBLEM	RESULT
Citrate toxicity	Hypocalcemia
Coagulation abnormalities	Disseminated intravascular coagulation (DIC), hemorrhage
Altered hemoglobin function	Poor oxygen delivery to tissues
Acid–base alterations	Early acidosis followed by alkalosis
Hypothermia	Cardiac arrhythmias, platelet dysfunction below 32.2°C
Microembolization	Increased alveolar–arterial oxygen difference
Denatured proteins	DIC
Vasoactive amines	Hypotension
Potassium shifts	Initial elevation of serum potassium followed by hypokalemia
Impaired red cell deformability	Red blood cell sequestration and clearance
Inorganic phosphate and ammonia overload	Stresses liver function
Interdonor incompatibility	Potential hemolysis
Graft-versus-host syndrome	Fever, pulmonary infiltration, skin lesions
Hypoproteinemia	Decreased oncotic pressure, fluid extravasation[28]

Adapted from McMillen MA: The use of blood and blood products in surgical and critically ill patients. In Cerra FB (ed): Manual of Critical Care. St. Louis, CV Mosby, 1987.

least every 10 units of RBCs administered, to detect coagulopathy and the need for fresh frozen plasma, platelets, or other clotting factors.[4]

Generally, 1 to 2 units of fresh frozen plasma are administered for every 5 units of infused red blood cells to treat dilutional coagulopathy.[4, 10, 21, 81] When persistent coagulopathy is demonstrated, increased amounts of fresh frozen plasma are indicated. If fresh frozen plasma is unsuccessful in restoring adequate fibrinogen levels, cryoprecipitates are also given.[4] Platelet count evaluated in concert with the patient's clinical evidence of hemorrhage or coagulopathy is the determinant of whether or not platelets should be administered.[4] Platelet packs are usually given in the ratio of 6 to 10 units for each 8 to 10 units of infused red blood cells.[4, 10, 21]

PHARMACOLOGICAL THERAPY

There is little indication for the use of pharmacological agents in the initial treatment of traumatic shock. Administration of fluids and blood components to restore effective circulating blood volume is the primary therapy. Volume restoration is usually sufficient to remedy vascular instability, shock-induced cardiac dysfunction, and acidosis.[38, 118]

Once intravascular volume has been replaced and appropriate measures have been taken to repair mechanical sources of cardiovascular compromise, the patient's hemodynamic status is assessed to evaluate the need for pharmacological support. The patient with underlying cardiac disease, myocardial depression, or coexisting nonhypovolemic shock may require pharmacological support of cardiovascular function. Appropriate drug therapy requires knowledge of the underlying etiology of the shock state as well as an awareness of drug mechanism of action and pharmacology.

The majority of drugs used to support cardiovascular function in shock are amines that stimulate one or more sympathetic receptors or receptor subtypes. Since their actions mimic the sympathetic nervous system, they are commonly known as sympathomimetics. Table 9–6 lists several relevant receptor subtypes and their general effects on the vasculature.[119, 120] Knowledge of which receptors are stimulated by each drug at a given dosage guides their use clinically.

Pharmacological therapy is used to maximize myocardial contractility and regulate preload and afterload with the overall goal of optimizing cardiac output and oxygen transport. Drugs that may be employed during resuscitation include inotropes, vasopressors, and vasodilators for reduction of afterload. The pharmacology of these inotropic and vasopressor drugs is summarized in Table 9–7.[5, 22, 118, 119, 121, 124]

Not infrequently, multiple drugs are used to achieve a desired cardiovascular effect. For example, low-dose dopamine used for support of renal perfusion may be accompanied by dobutamine when inotropic support is needed. To avoid the complications of using any one inotrope at high dosages, it may be beneficial to use smaller doses of several agents simultaneously.

Inotropic Agents

Inotropic drugs are used to improve myocardial contractility in order to increase cardiac output and improve tissue perfusion. Dopamine, which stimulates α, β_1, and dopaminergic receptors in a dose-dependent fashion, is widely used in shock *following* intravascular volume repletion. At doses of 2 to 10 μg/kg/min, dopamine has predominantly inotropic and chronotropic activity by direct β_1 stimulation.[22, 122, 123] Its action also includes release of endogenous norepinephrine with subsequent β_1 activity.[122] Another sympathomimetic is dobutamine, which acts through β_1 receptor subtypes as an inotropic agent with minimal chronotropic effects.[37] Its lack of significant vasoconstrictive properties and mild β_2 vasodilator effect assist in reducing afterload and decreasing cardiac

TABLE 9–6. SUMMARY OF VASCULAR RECEPTOR SUBTYPES

RECEPTORS	SITE	ACTION
α	Peripheral blood vessels	Vasoconstriction of peripheral arterioles
β_1	Myocardium	Increased heart rate Increased contractility Enhanced conduction through atria and ventricles
β_2	Peripheral blood vessels	Vasodilation of peripheral arterioles
Dopaminergic	Blood vessels of the kidneys and mesentery	Vasodilation of renal and mesenteric vessels

work.[5, 22, 118, 121, 122] Of the agents currently available, dobutamine is the drug of choice for myocardial support.

Isoproterenol, a pure β-agonist, may be used at low doses in treating advanced cardiovascular insufficiency. Its β_1 effects produce improved myocardial contractility and elevated heart rate, while β_2 effects result in vasodilation.[5, 121] Undesirable effects such as arrhythmias, vasodilation-related hypotension, and increased myocardial oxygen consumption are dose dependent and may limit its usefulness.[118]

Other drugs improve myocardial contractile force by mechanisms other than sympathomimetic action. For example, amrinone lactate is both an inotropic agent and a vasodilator.[121] Although found to be effective in patients with low flow states due to congestive heart failure, its usefulness in the treatment of hypovolemic shock has not been well studied.[5, 22, 121] Digoxin may be effective in improving cardiac function in the patient with acute or preexisting heart failure.[5, 21, 124]

Two naturally occurring hormones, glucagon and insulin, have known inotropic properties but limited value in the treatment of shock.[5, 38, 125] Glucagon has not been shown to improve survival in hemorrhagic shock but may be used in critically ill patients with depleted myocardial norepinephrine or who have received β-blocking agents.[5, 125]

Vasopressors

Since the trauma patient frequently demonstrates considerable compensatory vasoconstriction, there is little role for these agents in traumatic shock management. Clearly, vasopressors are not to be used in place of fluid administration in the treatment of hypovolemic hypotension. However, vasopressors may be indicated in coexisting neurogenic, anaphylactic, or septic shock in addition to fluid volume replacement.[9, 38] These agents are used with caution, since the resulting vasoconstriction may produce renal ischemia or cardiac arrhythmias and may limit optimal fluid administration.[8, 38]

Most vasopressors act on α-adrenergic receptors to produce vasoconstriction of peripheral blood vessels. High-dose dopamine and epinephrine act as α-agonists.[22, 119, 121, 122] Norepinephrine has potent α effects that increase in a dose-dependent manner.[119, 122] Phenylephrine has pure α-agonist effects and also can be used to increase vasomotor tone.[22, 119]

Vasodilators

Several animal studies and clinical trials have suggested that vasodilators reduce catecholamine-induced vasoconstriction, which is believed to play a role in the development of irreversible shock.[118, 126] Such profound vasoconstriction can worsen shock by exacerbating inadequate perfusion.[2, 20] Careful use of vasodilators may improve blood flow to peripheral capillary beds, improve cardiac output by afterload reduction, optimize oxygen delivery, and subsequently decrease the shock state.[127] However, failure to ensure adequate circulating blood volume prior to administration of these drugs results in profound hypotension.[5, 38] For this reason, vasodilators are not indicated in the hypovolemic or hemorrhaging patient and have no role in the initial resuscitation of traumatic shock. After appropriate vascular volume expansion, vasodilator therapy may be attempted in the patient with refractory shock and high vascular resistance.[8, 38] Such drugs are described in Table 9–8 and include nitroprusside, nitroglycerin, and labetalol.[5, 22, 127–129] Therapeutic interventions to control pain and anxiety and to warm the hypothermic patient also should be initiated to reduce peripheral vasoconstriction and decrease afterload.[127, 130]

Acid–Base Management

The patient in shock usually develops metabolic acidosis as a result of inadequate tissue perfusion and oxygenation. Such acidosis is detrimental, since it depresses cardiac contractility and decreases the responses to other pharmacological therapies such as inotropic agents.[21] The majority of initial acid–base problems are remedied by ensuring adequate ventilation and restoring adequate tissue perfusion with fluid replacement. If such measures fail to restore the arterial pH to within the range of 7.2 to 7.3, then the judicious use of intravenous bicarbonate may be warranted.[14, 18, 21, 38]

The indiscriminate use of bicarbonate, particularly when used prior to pH determination, is not acceptable. Although administering bicarbonate may temporarily increase arterial pH, it is not without its own adverse effects and may mask signs of underlying tissue acidosis.[131–133] Metabolic alkalosis may result if bicarbonate is given in excess. Alkalosis shifts the oxyhemoglobin dissociation curve to the left, inhibiting oxygen release to tissue. Vigorous use of sodium bicarbonate potentially leads to sodium overload, elevated serum osmolarity, hypokalemia, and reduction in available ionized calcium as plasma pH is rapidly increased.[4] Finally, bicarbonate is incompatible with many of the sympathomimetic drugs, and care should be taken not to give the two simultaneously.

Steroids

The value of these drugs in human hypovolemic shock remains unproven.[5, 6, 21, 118] It has been suggested that steroid therapy may have beneficial effects in the treatment of lung injuries, posttraumatic respiratory distress syndrome, and cerebral ischemia.[38, 134] To date, such benefits have not clearly been demonstrated.

Opiate Antagonists

Endogenous opiate peptides, such as β-endorphins, have been shown to contribute to the cardiovascular dysfunction associated with many shock states.[118, 135, 136] Opiate receptor antagonists, such as naloxone and naltrexone, have been reported in animal studies to improve cardiovascular function and survival during hemorrhagic shock.[118, 122, 135–138] Similar therapeutic effects have been described in animal hemorrhagic shock models after administration of neuropeptides, such as thyroid-releasing hormone (TRH) and adrenocorticotropic hormone (ACTH), which are reported to act as endogenous physiological opiate antagonists.[122, 137, 139, 140–142] Preliminary clinical trials suggest that ACTH also can provide therapeutic benefit to humans suffering from hypovolemic shock.[143–145] The ability of opiate antagonists to promote cardiovascular performance can lengthen the time interval within which conventional interventions (i.e., fluid and blood infusions) remain effective.[135, 136, 140, 142] Although these drugs appear promising as an adjunctive therapy in the management of shock, controlled clinical trials are necessary to clearly define their role in treatment of traumatic shock.

TABLE 9–7. INOTROPIC AGENTS AND VASOPRESSORS

	DOBUTAMINE	DOPAMINE	ISOPROTERENOL	EPINEPHRINE
MECHANISM OF ACTION				
α	+	+ + + +[22, 119]	0[119]	+ + + +[119]
β_1	+ + + +	+ + + +	+ + + +	+ + + +
β_2	+ +	+ +	+ + + +	+ +
Dopaminergic	0	+ + + +	0	0
CLINICAL IMPLICATIONS				
Indications	Need for inotropic support[22] Myocardial infarction and congestive heart failure in absence of profound hypotension[119]	Low urine output[119] Hypotension with low or normal peripheral vascular resistance	Hypotension due to heart block Bronchoconstriction[119] Bradyarrhythmias unresponsive to atropine	Bronchoconstriction Loss of cardiac rhythm during cardiac arrest Anaphylactic shock Need for vasopressor support
Major actions	Increased cardiac contractility[22] Decreased systemic vascular resistance	Increased renal[22] perfusion (low doses)—0.5 to 3 μg/kg/min Increased cardiac contractility—2 to 10 μg/kg/min Vasoconstriction—over 10 μg/kg/min	Elevated heart rate Increased cardiac contractility Bronchodilation	Bronchodilation Peripheral constriction
Adverse effects	Arrhythmias[119] Tachycardia (elevated doses)	Tachycardia[119] Arrhythmias Infiltration, tissue sloughing Peripheral vasoconstriction	Arrhythmias Extreme tachycardia Increased myocardial oxygen consumption Tremors Headache	Arrhythmias[119] Tachycardia Hypertension Increased myocardial oxygen consumption Renal ischemia
ADMINISTRATION				
How supplied	250 mg/20 ml	200 mg/5 ml or 400 mg/5 ml	1 mg/5 ml	1:1000 1 mg/1 ml or 1:10,000 1 mg/10 ml
Mixed	Must be reconstituted and further diluted in at least 250 or 500 ml of normal saline (NS) or 5% dextrose in water (D_5W) Incompatible with alkaline solutions; do *not* mix with HCO_3	Must be diluted in at least 250 or 500 ml of NS or D_5W Incompatible with alkaline solutions; do *not* mix with HCO_3	Must be diluted in at least 250 or 500 ml of NS or D_5W	IV: must be diluted in at least 250 ml of NS or D_5W Unstable in alkaline solutions; do *not* mix with HCO_3
Route	IV	IV	IV	IV
Normal range of dosage	2.5–20 μg/kg/min[22] Titrate to desired effect	Initial: 2–5 μg/kg/min[119] Titrate to desired effect Up to 20–50 μg/kg/min or more Typical range: 2–20 μg/kg/min	Initial: 2–8 μg/min, then titrate to desired effect Range: 2–20 μg/min[121]	Bolus: 0.5–1 mg every 5 min[119] Infusion: 0.01–0.1 μg/kg/min[118] Titrate to desired effect

Data from Siegal et al.[5]; Rice[22]; Markowsky and Elenbass[118]; Hoffman and Lefkowitz[119]; Rice[121]; Hoffman and Bigger[124]

Other Pharmacological Agents Under Investigation

A number of pharmacological agents are the subject of intensive research and may prove therapeutic in the management of shock. Many of the drugs under investigation are antagonists toward specific mediators in the pathogenesis of shock, such as platelet-activating factor,[146–148] peptide leukotrienes,[149] and thromboxane.[150–152] Other notable groups of drugs include prostaglandins and prostaglandin antagonists,[122, 153] calcium-channel blockers,[138, 154] and oxygen-derived free radical scavengers.[155, 156] These agents have been found to have a range of beneficial effects and may act to preserve cell structure and organelle function in shock states. The interested reader is referred to one of several reviews of these investigational therapies.[118, 122, 157]

MONITORING AND EVALUATION

One fundamental component of shock management is continuous monitoring and evaluation of the patient's re-

USED IN THE TREATMENT OF SHOCK

NOREPINEPHRINE	PHENYLEPHRINE HYDROCHLORIDE	AMRINONE LACTATE	DIGOXIN
+ + + +[119]	+ + +[22, 119]	0[22, 124]	0
+ + + +	0	0	0
0	0	0	0
0	0	0	0
Profound hypotension with decreased vascular resistance	Hypotensive states[119]	Heart failure[124] Need for inotropic support	Heart failure (prevention and treatment) Selected atrial arrhythmias[124]
Increased cardiac contractility and peripheral vascular resistance	Vasoconstriction	Increased myocardial contractility Vasodilation	Increased myocardial contractility Slows atrioventricular conduction
Hypertension Arrhythmias Severe peripheral vasoconstriction Reduced renal blood flow Infiltration, tissue sloughing[119] Increased myocardial oxygen requirements	Infiltration and tissue sloughing Reflex bradycardia Headache Restlessness Reduced renal blood flow	Hypotension[124] Thrombocytopenia Hepatotoxicity	Arrhythmias Transient peripheral vasoconstriction Headache Confusion
4 mg/4 ml	10 mg/1 ml[119]	5 mg in 20 U ampule	0.1 mg/ml or 0.25 mg/ml
Must be diluted in at least 250 ml of D_5W or D_5NS; do *not* mix with NS alone	30 mg in 250 ml solution[22]	Dilute in NS or 1/2 NS for a 1–3 mg/ml concentration Do *not* mix with dextrose-containing solutions[121]	
IV Initial: 2–8 μg/min, then titrate to maintain desired blood pressure[121]	IV Dose range: 10–60 μg/min[22] Titrate to desired blood pressure	IV Bolus: 0.75–1.5 mg/kg over 2–3 min[22] Infusion: 5–20 μg/kg/min[22] Recommended maximal daily dose: 10 mg/kg[124]	IV 0.25 mg every 4–6 hours for a total of 0.75–1.0 mg[5, 124]

sponse to therapy. Careful reassessment of the patient's status determines if the shock state is resolving, as evidenced by improvements in tissue perfusion and oxygenation. Signs of failure to respond to therapy also may be observed and permit early recognition of potential complications. Repeated observation is crucial. Patients rarely deteriorate without giving notice to the careful observer. Meticulous attention to detail and thoughtful integration of available data can permit effective intervention before irreversible damage occurs.

Elementary Monitoring

Monitoring may be as simple as a trained finger on the carotid pulse or as complex as the latest technology permits. It begins on admission of the patient. The critical time factor in initial resuscitation requires the selection of a limited set of readily obtainable observations. Very sophisticated monitoring may need to be deferred initially in favor of more rapidly available techniques. Elementary monitoring in the

TABLE 9–8. PRIMARY VASODILATORS USED IN THE TREATMENT OF SHOCK

	SODIUM NITROPRUSSIDE	NITROGLYCERINE	LABETALOL
CLINICAL IMPLICATIONS			
Indications	Need to reduce preload and afterload[22] Hypertensive crisis Increased vascular resistance Refractory congestive heart failure	Acute ischemia syndromes Angina Congestive heart failure	Hypertension Increased vascular resistance May be preferred in brain-injured patients since it causes no increase in cerebral blood flow or intracranial pressure[127]
Major actions	Dilation of arterioles and veins[22] Preload and afterload effects	Venodilation at low dose: 10–100 μg/min Arteriodilation at high dose: 200–400 μg/min[127]	Selective α and nonselective β blocking effects Reduces vascular resistance
Adverse effects	Excessive vasodilation Hypotension Thiocyanate toxicity Cyanide poisoning	Hypotension[128] Tachycardia Dizziness Headache	Hypotension Bronchospasm Arrhythmias Congestive heart failure
ADMINISTRATION			
How supplied	50-mg ampule[129]	50-mg vial	5 mg/ml in 20-ml vial
Mixed	Dilute 50 mg in 2–5 ml of D_5W (no other diluent should be used), then add 250–1000 ml of fluid[129] Wrap in foil—light sensitive	50 mg in 500 ml of D_5W in a glass container[22]	2 vials in 150 ml D_5W or normal saline
Route	IV	Sublingual, topical, IV	IV, oral
Normal range of dosage	Infusion: 0.5–10 μg/kg/min Titrate to desired blood pressure[129]	Infusion: 5–500 μg/min[22] Titrate to achieve desired effect	IV bolus Initial: 5–20 mg, then increase by 10–20 mg every 15 minutes until a desired effect or 300 mg reached; 10–60 mg every 4–6 hours IV infusion Initial: 0.5 μg/kg/min, then increase 0.5 μg/kg/min every 15 minutes to obtain desired effect Typical rates: 200–800 μg/min Oral Inital: 100–200 mg twice a day Titrate upward to desired effect Typical dose: 200–400 mg twice a day

Data from Rice[22]; Simon and Reynolds[127]; Murad[128]; Gerber and Nies.[129]

resuscitation area consists of the physical examination findings described earlier in the primary survey, blood pressure measurement by auscultation, EKG monitoring, urine output via a Foley catheter, and laboratory data. These parameters continue to be serially monitored as shock resuscitation progresses.

A greater number of variables become accessible throughout resuscitation for monitoring and detection of significant trends. The comprehensive secondary survey provides additional diagnostic data. Physical assessment findings, patient history, hemodynamic variables, calculated cardiopulmonary values, and laboratory and radiological data form a more complete and detailed patient profile.

There is no one variable that is useful in monitoring the patient in shock. Noting trends, rather than static values, aids in early detection of a pathological process as it develops and in directing effective therapy. The following section presents an overview of parameters useful in monitoring the seriously injured patient in shock.

PATIENT HISTORY. The initial accident data base obtained from field personnel is expanded as much as possible into a complete patient history. The needed information can be gained from family members and friends. The data obtained should include allergies and currently used prescribed or illicit drugs, preexisting illnesses, and previous surgeries. The objective is to identify conditions that may aggravate the shock state or alter the patient's response to therapy. For example, a patient with a history of β-blocking drug therapy may not exhibit the tachycardia associated with early shock or may be predisposed to myocardial failure.

PHYSICAL ASSESSMENT. The same readily available parameters used to diagnose shock are used to evaluate the patient's response to shock management. As more sophisticated monitoring devices are incorporated, the importance of clinical observations such as level of consciousness, urine output, and skin quality should not be overlooked. In addition to basic circulatory parameters, other clinical findings are important in the eventual treatment plan. For example, flank

TABLE 9–9. DERIVED HEMODYNAMIC PARAMETERS

TERM	FORMULA	UNITS	NORMAL RANGE
Cardiac index	$CI = \frac{CO}{BSA}$	$l/min/m^2$	2.8–4.2
Stroke volume	$SV = \frac{CO}{HR}$	ml/beat	Varies with size
Stroke index	$SI = \frac{SV}{BSA}$	$ml/beat/m^2$	30–65
Mean arterial pressure	$MAP = DP + \frac{(SP - DP)}{3}$	mm Hg	70–105
Systemic vascular resistance	$SVR = \frac{MAP - CVP}{CO} \times 80$	$dyn\cdot sec\cdot cm^{-5}$	900–1400
Pulmonary vascular resistance	$PVR = \frac{MPAP - PAOP}{CO} \times 80$	$dyn\cdot sec\cdot cm^{-5}$	150–250
Left ventricular stroke work index	$LVSWI = SI(MAP - PAOP) \times 0.0136$	$gm \times m/m^2$	43–61
Right ventricular stroke work index	$RVSWI = SI(MPAP - CVP) \times 0.0136$	$gm \times m/m^2$	7–12
Coronary perfusion pressure	$CPP = DP - PAOP$	mm Hg	60–90

Hemodynamic parameters derived from intravascular pressure and flow measurements are used to select the optimal management for patients with inadequate cardiac output. CO, cardiac output; BSA, body surface area; HR, heart rate; DP, diastolic pressure; SP, systolic pressure; CVP, central venous pressure; MPAP, mean pulmonary artery pressure; PAOP, pulmonary artery occlusion pressure.

From Nelson LD: Monitoring and measurement in shock. In Barrett J, Nyhus LM (eds): Treatment of Shock—Principles and Practice. Philadelphia, Lea & Febiger, 1986.

ecchymosis or increasing leg girth may identify the source of intravascular fluid loss responsible for the shock state. The multiply injured patient with lower neck pain and lower extremity paralysis may demonstrate the presence of a spinal cord injury and the coexistence of neurogenic shock.

Cardiopulmonary Monitoring

Monitoring hemodynamic parameters via indwelling arterial, central venous, and pulmonary artery catheters provides more direct and precise measurement of vascular status and cardiac performance than the elementary techniques described. Continuous intra-arterial pressure monitoring is particularly useful in hypotensive states when blood pressure is difficult to accurately auscultate. During the administration of vasoactive drugs and when multiple arterial blood gas measurements are required, an arterial line is invaluable.

Central Venous Pressure. A single central venous pressure (CVP) measurement is not a reliable indicator of intravascular fluid volume in the shock patient.[6, 11, 29] Although intravascular volume is depleted, the CVP may appear normal in the patient with compensatory vasoconstriction.[11] CVP monitoring is best used in evaluating trends such as responses to fluid therapy. Hemodynamic instability accompanied by a CVP less than 5 mm Hg usually indicates that hypovolemic or vasogenic shock is present.[10, 14, 29] The hemodynamically unstable patient with an elevated CVP generally indicates cardiac compromise, possibly arising from pericardial tamponade, tension pneumothorax, or direct cardiac injury resulting in myocardial failure or exacerbation of preexisting cardiac disease.[10, 11, 14]

Pulmonary Artery Pressure Monitoring. Pulmonary artery (PA) catheter placement allows measurement of pulmonary artery pressures, pulmonary capillary wedge pressure, and cardiac output, which enables derived hemodynamic indices to be calculated (Table 9–9). These variables are useful in determining the need for fluid volume or drug therapy and for monitoring the patient's response to treatment. Persistent hypoperfusion after fluid resuscitation may require insertion of a PA catheter to evaluate the source of hemodynamic instability.[3, 10, 14] Certain patients, particularly those with underlying cardiac disease or with serious central nervous system injury, benefit greatly from the placement of a pulmonary artery catheter. Patients with potential organ failure, particularly pulmonary or renal failure, also benefit from PA monitoring.

Oxygen Transport and Consumption. To best assess tissue oxygenation, one should monitor not only the ability of the respiratory system to oxygenate the blood but also the adequacy of oxygen transport, delivery, and consumption.[8, 37, 130, 158, 159] Analysis of mixed venous oxygen tension ($P\bar{v}O_2$) and saturation ($S\bar{v}O_2$), sampled from the distal port of the PA catheter, provides additional information about these physiological parameters. Since mixed venous oxygen tension estimates tissue oxygenation, it serves as an index of circulatory sufficiency. $S\bar{v}O_2$ serves as an index of tissue oxygen extraction and allows insight into the balance between oxygen delivery and consumption. Serial measurements of $S\bar{v}O_2$ and $P\bar{v}O_2$ or continuous monitoring via fiberoptic PA catheter assists in monitoring the shock state and responses to the therapy.[160] Table 9–10 briefly outlines the implications of these parameters.[3, 21, 160, 161]

Derived cardiopulmonary indices such as those in Table 9–11 are also used to monitor oxygen transport and utiliza-

TABLE 9–10. MIXED VENOUS OXYGENATION PARAMETERS IN TRAUMATIC SHOCK

MIXED VENOUS PARAMETER	ABBREVIATION	NORMAL RANGE	IMPLICATIONS
Partial pressure of mixed venous oxygen	$P\bar{v}O_2$	35–40 mm Hg	Decreased in traumatic shock Decrease indicates tissues are extracting more O_2 to meet metabolic demand when circulation is insufficient Low values correlate with the severity of tissue hypoxia When less than 20 mm Hg, unable to maintain aerobic metabolism
Saturation of mixed venous oxygen	$S\bar{v}O_2$	60–80%	Decreased in traumatic shock Indicates increased O_2 extraction Source of low values may be: High $\dot{V}O_2$ Low O_2 delivery low cardiac output severe anemia arterial oxygen desaturation

$\bar{v}O_2$, mixed venous oxygen; $\dot{V}O_2$, oxygen consumption.

TABLE 9–11. CARDIORESPIRATORY FORMULAS DERIVED FROM ANALYSIS OF GASES

TERM	FORMULA	UNITS	NORMAL RANGE
Arterial O_2 content	$CaO_2 = (Hb \times 1.39 \times SaO_2) + (0.0031 \times PaO_2)$	ml O_2/dl	16–22
Mixed venous O_2 content	$C\bar{v}O_2 = (Hb \times 1.39 \times S\bar{v}O_2) + (0.0031 \times P\bar{v}O_2)$	ml O_2/dl	12–17
Pulmonary capillary O_2 content	$CcO_2 = (Hb \times 1.39) + (0.0031 \times P_AO_2)$	ml O_2/dl	varies with FiO_2
Alveolar O_2 tension	$P_AO_2 = (P_B - P_{H_2O})FiO_2 - \frac{PaCO_2}{RQ}$	mm Hg	varies with FiO_2
Arterial oxygen delivery	$DO_2 = CO \times CaO_2 \times 10$	ml/min	1000–1200
Arterial-venous O_2 content difference	$C(a - \bar{v})DO_2 = CaO_2 - C\bar{v}O_2$	ml O_2/dl	3–5
Oxygen extraction ratio	$OER = \frac{C(a - \bar{v})DO_2}{CaO_2}$	Percent	22–30
Respiratory quotient	$RQ = \frac{\dot{V}CO_2}{\dot{V}O_2}$	Fraction	0.7–1.0
CO_2 production	$\dot{V}CO_2 = V_E \times F_ECO_2$	ml/min	140–250
O_2 consumption (Fick)	$\dot{V}O_2 = C(a - \bar{v})DO_2 \times CO \times 10$	ml/min	180–280
O_2 consumption (measured)	$\dot{V}O_2 = V_E\left(\frac{FiO_2 - F_EO_2 - (FiO_2 \times F_ECO_2)}{1 - FiO_2}\right)$	ml/min	180–280
Intrapulmonary shunt (venous admixture)	$\dot{Q}s/\dot{Q}t = \frac{CcO_2 - CaO_2}{CcO_2 - C\bar{v}O_2} \times 100$	Percent	<10

Cardiorespiratory measurements derived from the analysis of blood and expired gases form the basis for understanding oxygen transport balance.

Hb	hemoglobin concentration	SaO_2	arterial O_2 saturation
PaO_2	arterial O_2 tension	$S\bar{v}O_2$	mixed venous O_2 saturation
$P\bar{v}O_2$	mixed venous O_2 tension	P_B	barometric pressure
P_{H_2O}	partial pressure of water vapor (47 mm Hg at 37°C)	V_E	expired minute ventilation
CO	cardiac output	F_ECO_2	mixed expired CO_2 fraction
F_EO_2	expired O_2 fraction	FiO_2	inspired O_2 fraction

Adapted from Nelson LD: Monitoring and measurement in shock. In Barrett J, Nyhus LM (eds): Treatment of Shock—Principles and Practice. Philadelphia, Lea & Febiger, 1986.

TABLE 9–12. COMMON LABORATORY DATA IN SHOCK

TEST	NORMAL	IN SHOCK	MECHANISM
BLOOD CHEMISTRIES			
Nutritional substances			
Glucose	70–100 mg/100 ml	↑ Early	Due to sympathetic stimulation
		↓ Late	Due to depletion of body glycogen stores and decreased liver function
Lactate	2 mEq/l 5–15 mg/100 ml	↑	Due to decreased tissue oxygenation and anaerobic metabolism
Total serum proteins			
Total	6.0–7.8 gm/100 ml	↓	Due to leakage from capillary and decreased synthesis in liver cells
Albumin	3.2–4.5 gm/100 ml	↓	
Globulin	2.3–3.5 gm/100 ml	N or ↓	Due to larger particle size, fewer leaks from capillary
Excretory substances			
Urea nitrogen	5.0–20.0 mg/100 ml	↑	Due to decreased renal excretion
Creatine	0.6–1.2 mg/100 ml	↑	Due to decreased renal excretion
Bilirubin			
Total	0.5–1.2 mg/100 ml	↑	
Direct (conjugated)	up to 0.2 mg/100 ml	↑	Due to liver cell damage
Indirect (unconjugated)	0.1–1.0 mg/100 ml	↑	
Functional substances			
Sodium	136–142 mEq/l	↑ Early	Due to increased aldosterone causing renal retention of sodium
		↑ or ↓ late	Due to altered renal function
Potassium	3.8–5.0 mEq/l	↓ Early	Due to increased aldosterone causing renal excretion of potassium
		↑ Late	Due to acidosis, cell necrosis, and decreased renal function
Chloride	95–103 mEq/l	↓ Early	Due to alkalotic state and bicarbonate excess
		↑ Late	Due to acidotic state and bicarbonate deficiency
Carbon dioxide (bicarbonate)	21–28 mEq/l	↑ Early	Due to alkalotic state
		↓ ↓ Late	Due to severe metabolic and respiratory acidosis
Serum enzymes			
Creatine phosphokinase (CPK)	5–35 μm/ml	↑	Due to necrosis of muscle cells and/or heart cells
Aspartate aminotransferase (AST)	15–40 U/ml	↑	Due to necrosis of heart cells and/or liver cells
Alanine aminotransferase (ALT)	15–35 U/ml	↑	Due to necrosis of liver cells
Lactic dehydrogenase (LDH)	150–450 Wroblewski units/ml	↑	Due to necrosis of liver and/or heart cells
Amylase	60–160 Somogyi units/100 ml	↑	Due to necrosis of pancreatic cells
Lipase	0–1.5 Cherry-Crandall U/ml	↑	Due to necrosis of pancreatic cells
HEMATOLOGY			
Hemoglobin	male 14.0–16.5 gm/100 ml female 12.6–14.2 gm/100 ml	↓	Due to hemorrhage and hemodilution; may be initially normal in mild blood loss
Hematocrit (packed cell volume = PCV)	male 42–52% female 37–47%	↑ or ↓	Due to fluid leakage from the capillary Due to loss of blood (Note: decrease lags behind blood loss)
Red blood cell count	male 4.6–6.2 million/ml female 4.5–5.4 million/ml	↓	Due to hemorrhage
White blood cell count	4500–11,000/ml	↑	Due to body's response to infection (if present)
Platelet count	150,000–400,000/ml	↓	Due to platelet aggregation and microemboli
Coagulation test			
Prothrombin time (PT)	12–14 sec	Prolonged	Due to hypercoagulable state (if present)
Partial thromboplastin time (PTT)	45–65 sec	Prolonged	Due to hypercoagulable state (if present)

Table continued on following page

TABLE 9–12. COMMON LABORATORY DATA IN SHOCK *Continued*

TEST	NORMAL	IN SHOCK	MECHANISM
ARTERIAL BLOOD GASES			
pH	7.38–7.42	↑ Early	Due to hyperventilation and carbon dioxide exhalation
		↓ Late	Due to carbon dioxide retention and lactic acid production
P_{CO_2}	35–45 mm Hg	↓ Early	Due to hyperventilation
		↑ Late	Due to hypoventilation
P_{O_2}	80–100 mm Hg	↓	Due to hypoventilation and hypoperfusion (ventilation/perfusion imbalances)
Bicarbonate	22–28 mEq/l	↓ Late	Due to severe acidotic state
URINE MEASUREMENTS			
Creatinine clearance	male 1.0–2.0 gm/24 hr female 0.8–1.8 gm/24 hr	↓	Due to impaired renal excretion
Osmolality	500–800 mOsm/l	↑ Early	Due to water retention, secondary to ADH
		↓ Late	Due to inability of the kidney to concentrate urine
Specific gravity	1.001–1.035	↑ Early	Same as above
		↓ Late	(Influenced by administration of dextran)
Sodium	80–180 mEq/24 hr	↓ Early	Due to sodium reabsorption secondary to aldosterone
		↓ or ↑ late	Due to abnormal renal function
Potassium	40–80 mEq/24 hr	↑ Early	Due to potassium excretion secondary to aldosterone
		↓ or ↑ late	Due to abnormal renal function

Adapted from Rice V: Shock, a clinical syndrome. Part III. Crit Care Nurse 1:1981. Normal values from Halstead JA: The Laboratory in Clinical Medicine. Philadelphia, WB Saunders Co, 1976.

tion in critically ill patients. One of the best indicators of adequate tissue perfusion and cellular metabolism is believed to be oxygen consumption ($\dot{V}O_2$).[5, 8, 32, 158, 162] As discussed in Chapter 8, a fall in $\dot{V}O_2$ is an early sign of low flow and inadequate tissue oxygenation. Therapeutic interventions for shock are aimed at optimizing the transport of oxygen to the tissues. Therefore, monitoring oxygen consumption and transport parameters is very useful for evaluating the shock state and patient responses to therapy.[8, 158, 162, 163]

Since shock is fundamentally related to cellular hypoxia, techniques for continuously monitoring arterial and tissue oxygenation have been advocated. Intra-arterial oxygen electrodes, ear and digital pulse oximetry, and transcutaneous and transconjunctival oxygen sensors have all been reported to be helpful in managing the shock patient. These devices are able to detect trends in oxygenation but require validation with direct arterial oxygen measurements.[164] Although the oximetric methods are noninvasive, each is dependent on tissue perfusion, which is known to be altered in the shock patient. The reader is directed to other sources for information about these techniques.[161, 164–166]

ADVANCED MONITORING TECHNIQUES. Monitoring techniques have continued to become sophisticated, enabling greater insight into the patient's condition and therapeutic responsiveness. Two such advanced monitoring techniques include multivariate physiological analysis and the computerized respiratory monitoring system. Multivariate physiological analysis, the computerized integration of multiple cardiopulmonary and metabolic parameters into an easily analyzed pattern, is used successfully in guiding shock resuscitation.[5, 163] This monitoring technique displays simultaneously multiple parameters that are compared against reference populations. The similarity of the patient to the reference state provides insight into the mechanism of shock and identifies possible alternatives for treatment.

A computerized respiratory monitoring system provides helpful information about the patient's metabolic and cardiorespiratory status and response to resuscitation therapy.[167] This monitoring system repeatedly samples inspiratory and expiratory gas composition, pressure, and volume and provides calculated clinical parameters. The nurse is able to observe trends in these parameters as early indicators of postresuscitation complications and treatment effectiveness. For example, oxygen consumption can be continually monitored as an index of the shock state and the patient's response to therapy.[5] Intrapulmonary shunt, airway resistance, lung compliance, and respiratory gas composition are useful parameters in evaluating the effect of fluid resuscitation on pulmonary function and oxygenation.

Laboratory Data

Laboratory tests that are usually evaluated in the shock patient are listed in Table 9–12 along with normal values and common alterations seen in the shock state. Blood samples for laboratory analysis should be obtained as soon as vascular access is established and periodically thereafter. Laboratory values must be analyzed in conjunction with clinical observations of the patient. For example, if the blood samples are evaluated soon after nonsevere hemorrhage, the hematocrit or hemoglobin value may be normal owing to vascular fluid shifts.[10, 11]

Lactate and calculated base deficit levels are two parameters that are particularly useful to monitor in the shock patient. Lactate levels have been found useful in indicating the severity and prognosis of circulatory shock.[14, 32] Level of blood lactate, considered one of the best markers of tissue oxygen balance, increases as tissue hypoxia worsens.[31] Base deficit has been identified as a reliable early indicator of the severity of hypovolemia. Therefore, base deficit may be a useful parameter to guide fluid therapy.[159]

In conclusion, monitoring and evaluation of patient responses to therapy are essential to the resuscitation of traumatic shock. Clinical evidence of hemodynamic stability and subsequent improved tissue perfusion becomes evident as desired physiological end points are attained. Inadequate or ineffective resuscitation is likely to progress to sequential system dysfunction and multiple organ failure.

SUMMARY

Traumatic shock undoubtedly presents an extraordinary challenge to the trauma care team. The general management goal, resolution of shock by restoring tissue perfusion and oxygenation, can be achieved only by prompt diagnosis and rapid, effective treatment. Knowledge of the causes of shock and their common clinical manifestations is important for early recognition of shock in the multiply injured patient. Collaborative practice and the use of protocol to guide resuscitation ensure effective and well-planned initial management.

Initiation of basic life support, control of hemorrhage, replacement of circulating blood volume, and support of myocardial performance are the priorities in shock management. Appropriate fluid therapy remains the key therapeutic modality. Accurate, continual monitoring is imperative in order to evaluate the patient's response to therapy and determine the need for pharmacological support. The nurse plays an integral role in all aspects of traumatic shock resuscitation.

REFERENCES

1. Trunkey DD, Sheldon GF, Collins JA: The treatment of shock. In Zuidema GD, Rutherford RB, Ballinger WF (eds): The Management of Trauma, 4th ed. Philadelphia, WB Saunders Co, 1985, pp 105–125.
2. Messmer KFW: Mechanisms of traumatic shock and their consequences. In Border JR, Allgower M, Hansen ST, Ruedi TP (eds): Blunt Multiple Trauma—Comprehensive Pathophysiology and Care. New York, Marcel Dekker, 1990, pp 39–49.
3. Nelson LD: Monitoring and measurement in shock. In Barrett J, Nyhus LN (eds): Treatment of Shock—Principles and Practices, 2nd ed. Philadelphia, Lea & Febiger, 1986, pp 35–55.
4. Cowley RA, Dunham CM: Shock Trauma Critical Care Manual. Rockville, Md, Aspen, 1991.
5. Siegel JH, Linberg SE, Wiles CE: Therapy of low-flow shock states. In Siegel JH (ed): Trauma: Emergency Surgery and Critical Care. New York, Churchill Livingstone, 1987, pp 201–283.
6. Skowronski GA: The pathophysiology of shock. Med J Aust 148:576–583, 1988.
7. Klein DG: Physiologic response to traumatic shock. AACN Clin Issues Crit Care Nurs 1:505–521, 1990.
8. Shoemaker WC: Relation of oxygen transport patterns to the pathophysiology and therapy of shock states. Intensive Care Med 13:230–243, 1987.
9. Bolton DC, Harmon AR: The ABCs of trauma management. In Harmon AR (ed): Nursing Care of the Adult Trauma Patient. New York, John Wiley & Sons, 1985, pp 1–26.
10. Dunham CM: Trauma protocols for resuscitation and evaluation. In Siegel JH (ed): Trauma: Emergency Surgery and Critical Care. New York, Churchill Livingstone, 1986, pp 803–842.
11. Committee on Trauma, American College of Surgeons: Advanced Trauma Life Support Program: Instructor's Manual. Chicago, American College of Surgeons, 1989.
12. Kreis DJ: Trauma and shock. In Kreis DJ, Gomez GA (eds): Trauma Management. Boston, Little, Brown, 1989, pp 29–46.
13. Lucas CE, Ledgerwood AM: Hemodynamic management of the injured. In Capan LM, Miller SM, Turndorf H (eds): Trauma, Anesthesia and Intensive Care. Philadelphia, JB Lippincott, 1991, pp. 83–113.
14. Carrico CJ, Rice CL: Shock. In Moore EE (ed): Early Care of the Injured Patient, 4th ed. Philadelphia, BC Decker, 1990, pp. 74–83.
15. McDonald K: Extremity injuries. In Harmon AR (ed): Nursing Care of the Adult Trauma Patient. New York, John Wiley & Sons, 1985, pp 221–249.
16. Maier RV: Evaluation and resuscitation. In Moore EE (ed): Early Care of the Injured Patient, 4th ed. Philadelphia, BC Decker, 1990, pp. 56–73.
17. Shires GT: Postoperative fluid management. In Shires GT (ed): Principles of Trauma Care, 3rd ed. New York, McGraw-Hill, 1985, pp 477–487.
18. Meyers KA, Hickey MK: Nursing management of hypovolemic shock. Crit Care Nurs Q 11:57–67, 1988.
19. Rice V: Shock, a clinical syndrome: An update, Part 1: An overview of shock. Crit Care Nurs 11:20–27, 1991.
20. De Angelis R: The cardiovascular system. In Alspach JG, Williams SM (eds): Core Curriculum for Critical Care Nursing, 4th ed. Philadelphia, WB Saunders Co, 1991, pp 132–314.
21. Kreis DJ, Baue AE: Clinical Management of Shock. Baltimore, University Park Press, 1984.
22. Rice V: Shock, a clinical syndrome: An update, Part 3: Therapeutic management. Crit Care Nurs 11:34–39, 1991.
23. Shires GT: Principles and management of hemorrhagic shock. In Shires GT (ed): Principles of Trauma Care. New York, McGraw-Hill, 1985, pp 3–42.
24. Mergner WJ, Marzella L: Heart in shock. In Barrett J, Nyhus LM (eds): Treatment of Shock—Principles and Practice, 2nd ed. Philadelphia, Lea & Febiger, 1986, pp 117–135.
25. Rice V: Shock, a clinical syndrome: An update, Part 2: The stages of shock. Crit Care Nurs 11:74–82, 1991.
26. Barrett J, Nyhus LM: Volume replacement in shock. In Barrett J, Nyhus LM (eds): Treatment of Shock—Principles and Practice, 2nd ed. Philadelphia, Lea & Febiger, 1986, pp 23–34.
27. Edmundowicz SA, Zuckerman GR: Gastrointestinal bleeding. In Dunagan WC, Ridner ML (eds): Manual of Medical Therapeutics, 26th ed. Boston, Little, Brown, 1989.
28. Giescke AH, Grande CM, Whitten CW: Fluid therapy and the resuscitation of traumatic shock. Crit Care Clin 6:61–72, 1990.
29. Lewis FR: Initial assessment and resuscitation. Emerg Med Clin North Am 2:733–748, 1984.
30. Sommers MS: Fluid resuscitation following multiple trauma. Crit Care Nurs 10:74–81, 1990.
31. Vincent JL, De Backer D: Initial management of circulatory shock as prevention of MSOF. Crit Care Clin 5:369–377, 1989.
32. Wilson RF: Future treatment of shock. In Cowley RA, Trump BF (eds): Pathophysiology of Shock, Anoxia and Ischemia. Baltimore, Williams & Wilkins, 1982, pp 500–506.
33. Strange JM: Shock Trauma Care Plans. Springhouse, Pa, Springhouse, 1987, pp 2–12.
34. Barrett J, Nyhus LM: Initial treatment of trauma. In Barrett J, Nyhus LM (eds): Treatment of Shock—Principles and Practice, 2nd ed. Philadelphia, Lea & Febiger, 1986, pp 163–169.

35. Kim MJ: Without collaboration, what's left? Am J Nurs 85:281–284, 1985.
36. McCormac M: Managing hemorrhagic shock. Am J Nurs 90:22–27, 1990.
37. Bryan-Brown CW: Blood flow to organs: Parameters for function and survival in critical illness. Crit Care Med 16:170–178, 1988.
38. Safar P: Resuscitation in hemorrhagic shock, coma and cardiac arrest. In Cowley RA, Trump BF (eds): Pathophysiology of Shock, Anoxia and Ischemia. Baltimore, Williams & Wilkins, 1982, pp 411–438.
39. Ornato JF: Special resuscitation situations, near drowning, traumatic injury, electric shock and hypothermia. Circulation 74:23–25, 1986.
40. Mattox KL, Feliciano DV: Role of external chest compression in truncal trauma. J Trauma 22:934–936, 1982.
41. Luna GK, Pavlin EG, Kirkman T, et al: Hemodynamic effects of external cardiac massage in trauma shock. J Trauma 29:1430–1433, 1989.
42. Pepe PE, Copass MK: Initial evaluation and resuscitation. In Moore EE (ed): Early Care of the Injured Patient, 4th ed. Philadelphia, BC Decker, 1990, pp. 37–55.
43. Markison RE, Trunkey DD: Establishment of care priorities. In Capan LM, Miller SM, Turndorf H (eds): Trauma, Anesthesia and Intensive Care. Philadelphia, JB Lippincott, 1991, pp. 29–42.
44. Tavares S, Hankins JR, Moulton AL, et al: Management of penetrating cardiac injuries: The role of emergency room thoracotomy. Ann Thorac Surg 38:183–187, 1984.
45. Vij D, Simoni E, Smith RF, et al: Resuscitative thoracotomy for patients with traumatic injury. Surgery 94:554, 1983.
46. Wahlstrom HE, Carroll BJ, Phillips EH: Emergency thoracotomy: Indications and techniques. Surg Rounds 9:23, 1986.
47. Feliciano DV, Bitondo CG, Cruse PA, et al: Liberal use of emergency center thoracotomy. Am J Surg 152:654–659, 1986.
48. Baxter BT, Moore EE, Moore JB, et al: Emergency department thoracotomy following injury: Critical determinants for patient salvage. World J Surg 12:671–675, 1988.
49. Cogbill TH, Moore EE, Millikan JS, et al: Rationale for selective application of emergency department thoracotomy in trauma. J Trauma 23:453–458, 1983.
50. Millikan S, Moore EE: Outcome of resuscitation thoracotomy and descending aortic occlusion performed in the operating room. J Trauma 24:387–392, 1984.
51. Wiencek RG, Wilson RF, DeMaeo P: Outcome of trauma patients who present to the operating room with hypotension. Am Surg 6:336–342, 1989.
52. Clark DE, Demers ML: Lower body positive pressure. Surg Gynecol Obstet 168:81–97, 1989.
53. Frumkin K: The pneumatic antishock garment (PASG). In Robert JR, Hedges JR (eds): Clinical Procedures in Emergency Medicine. Philadelphia, WB Saunders Co, 1985, pp 403–410.
54. Polando G, Huerta C, Shall J, et al: PASG use in pelvic fracture immobilization. J Emerg Med Serv 15:48–56, 1990.
55. Kemmer DL: Antishock trousers. Am Fam Physician 30:163–166, 1984.
56. Nieman JT, Rosborough JP, Criley JM: Continuous external counterpressure during closed chest resuscitation: A critical appraisal of the military antishock trouser garment and abdominal binder. Circulation 74:102–107, 1986.
57. Nieman JT, Stapczynski JS, Rosborough JP, et al: Hemodynamic effects of pneumatic external counterpressure in canine hemorrhagic shock. Ann Emerg Med 12:661–667, 1983.
58. Bivins HG, Knopp R, Tiernan C, et al: Blood volume displacement with inflation of antishock trousers. Ann Emerg Med 11:409–412, 1982.
59. Thal ER, Klein J: Military antishock trousers. In Mancini ME, Klein J (eds): Decision Making in Trauma Management: A Multidisciplinary Approach. Philadelphia, BC Decker, 1991, pp. 372–373.
60. Pepe PE, Bass RR, Mattox KL, et al: Clinical trials of the pneumatic antishock garment in the urban prehospital setting. Ann Emerg Med 15:1407–1410, 1986.
61. Mattox KL, Bickell WH, Pepe PE, et al: Prospective randomized evaluation of antishock MAST in posttraumatic hypotension. J Trauma 26:779–786, 1986.
62. Pepe PE, Bickell WH, Mattox KL: The effect of antishock garments on prehospital survival: The need for controlled clinical trials. J World Assn Emer Disaster Med 3:40–45, 1987.
63. Bickell W, Pepe PE, Bailey ML, et al: Randomized trial of pneumatic antishock garments in the prehospital management of penetrating abdominal injuries. Ann Emerg Med 16:653–658, 1987.
64. Mattox KL, Bickell W, Pepe PE, et al: Prospective MAST study in 911 patients. J Trauma 29:1104–1112, 1989.
65. Maull KI, Krahwinkel DJ, Rozycki GS, et al: Cardiopulmonary effects of the pneumatic antishock garment on swine with diaphragmatic hernia. Surg Gynecol Obstet 162:17–24, 1986.
66. Gardner SR, Maull KI, Swensson EE, et al: The effects of the pneumatic antishock garment on intracranial pressure in man: A prospective study of 12 patients with severe head injury. J Trauma 24:896–900, 1984.
67. Beckwith N, Carriere SR: Fluid resuscitation in trauma: An update. J Emerg Nurs 11:293–299, 1985.
68. Trunkey DD: Shock trauma. Can J Surg 27:479–484, 1984.
69. Taylor DC, Salvian AJ, Shackleton CR: Crush syndrome complicating pneumatic antishock garment (PASG) use. Injury 19:43–44, 1988.
70. Godbout B, Burchard KW, Slotman GJ, et al: Crush syndrome with death following pneumatic antishock garment application. J Trauma 24:1052–1056, 1984.
71. Kaplan BH, Soderstrom CA: Pneumatic antishock garments and the compartment syndrome. Am J Emerg Med 5:177–178, 1987.
72. Millikan KS, Cain TL, Hansbrough J: Rapid volume replacement for hypovolemic shock: A comparison of techniques and equipment. J Trauma 24:428–431, 1984.
73. Hansbrough JF, Cain TL, Millikan JS: Placement of 10-gauge catheter by cutdown for rapid fluid replacement. J Trauma 23:231–234, 1983.
74. Rice V. Shock management: 1. Fluid volume replacement. Crit Care Nurs 4:69–82, 1984.
75. Floccare DJ, Kelen GD, Altman RS, et al: Rapid infusion of additive red blood cells: Alternative techniques for massive hemorrhage. Ann Emerg Med 19:129–133, 1990.
76. Stevens S, Maull K: Rapid infusion catheters (abstract). Prehospital Disaster Med 4:183, 1989.
77. Dunham CM, Belzberg H, Lyles R, et al: The rapid infusion system: A superior method for the resuscitation of hypovolemic trauma patients. Resuscitation 21:207–227, 1991.
78. Buchman TG, Menker JB, Lipsett PA: Strategies for trauma resuscitation. Surg Gynecol Obstet 172:8–12, 1991.
79. Satiani B, Fried SJ, Zeeb P, et al: Normothermic rapid volume replacement in traumatic hypovolemia: A prospective analysis using a new device. Arch Surg 122:1044–1047, 1987.
80. Haupt MT: The use of crystalloidal and colloidal solutions for volume replacement in hypovolemic shock. Crit Rev Clin Lab Sci 27:1–26, 1989.
81. Kuhn MM: Colloids vs. crystalloids. Crit Care Nurs 11:37–51, 1991.
82. Moss GS, Gould SA: Plasma expanders—An update. Am Surg 155:425–434, 1988.
83. Ross AD, Angaran DM: Colloids versus crystalloids—A continuing controversy. Drug Intell Clin Pharmacol 18:202–212, 1984.
84. Lucas CE, Ledgerwood AM, Higgins RS, et al: Impaired pulmonary function after albumin resuscitation from shock. J Trauma 20:446–451, 1980.
85. Lucas CE: Resuscitation through the three phases of hemorrhagic shock after trauma. Can J Surg 33:451–456, 1990.
86. Haupt MT, Rackow EC: Colloid osmotic pressure and fluid resuscitation with hetastarch, albumin, and saline solutions. Crit Care Med 10:159–162, 1982.
87. Hauser CJ, Shoemaker WC, Turpin T, et al: Oxygen transport responses to colloids and crystalloids in critically ill surgical patients. Surg Gynecol Obstet 150:811–816, 1980.
88. Rackow EC, Falk JL, Fein IA, et al: Fluid resuscitation in

circulatory shock: A comparison of the cardiopulmonary effects of albumin, hetastarch, and saline solution in patients with hypovolemic and septic shock. Crit Care Med 11:839–849, 1983.
89. Hein LG, Albrecht M, Dworschak M, et al: Long-term observation following traumatic-hemorrhagic shock in the dog: A comparison of crystalloidal vs. colloidal fluids. Circ Shock 26:353–364, 1988.
90. Redl H, Krosl P, Schlag G, et al: Permeability studies in a hypovolemic traumatic shock model: Comparison of Ringer's lactate and albumin as volume replacement fluids. Resuscitation 17:77–90, 1989.
91. Shires GT, Peltzman AB, Albert SA, et al: Responses of extravascular lung water to intraoperative fluids. Ann Surg 197:515–519, 1983.
92. Chudnofsky CR, Dronen SC, Syverud SA, et al: Intravenous fluid therapy in the prehospital management of hemorrhagic shock: Improved outcome with hypertonic saline/6% Dextran 70 in a swine model. Am J Emerg Med 7:357–363, 1989.
93. Ducey JP, Mozingo DW, Lamiell JM, et al: A comparison of the cerebral and cardiovascular effects of complete resuscitation with isotonic and hypertonic saline, hetastarch, and whole blood following hemorrhage. J Trauma 29:1510–1518, 1989.
94. Gross D, Landau EH, Assalia A, et al: Is hypertonic saline resuscitation safe in "uncontrolled" hemorrhagic shock? J Trauma 28:751–756, 1988.
95. Gross D, Landau EH, Klin B, et al: Quantitative measurement of bleeding following hypertonic saline therapy in "uncontrolled" hemorrhagic shock. J Trauma 29:79–83, 1989.
96. Gross D, Landau EH, Klin B, et al: Treatment of uncontrolled hemorrhagic shock with hypertonic saline solution. Surg Gynecol Obstet 170:106–112, 1990.
97. Kreimeier U, Bruckner UB, Niemczyk S, et al: Hyperosmotic saline dextran for resuscitation from traumatic-hemorrhagic hypotension: Effect on regional blood flow. Circ Shock 32:83–99, 1990.
98. Landau EH, Gross D, Assalia A, et al: Treatment of uncontrolled hemorrhagic shock by hypertonic saline and external counterpressure. Ann Emerg Med 18:1039–1043, 1989.
99. Reinhart K, Rudolph T, Bredle DL, et al: O_2 uptake in bled dogs after resuscitation with hypertonic saline or hydroxyethylstarch. Am J Physiol 257:H238–H243, 1989.
100. Soliman MH, Ragab H, Waxman K: Survival after hypertonic saline resuscitation from hemorrhage. Am Surg 56:749–751, 1990.
101. Stanford GG, Patterson CR, Payne L, et al: Hypertonic saline resuscitation in a porcine model of severe hemorrhagic shock. Arch Surg 124:733–736, 1989.
102. Velasco IT, Rocha e Silva M, Oliveira MA, et al: Hypertonic and hyperoncotic resuscitation from severe hemorrhagic shock in dogs: A comparative study. Crit Care Med 17:261–264, 1989.
103. Wade CE, Hannon JP, Bossone CA, et al: Superiority of hypertonic saline/dextran over hypertonic saline during the first 30 minutes of resuscitation following hemorrhagic hypotension in conscious swine. Resuscitation 20:49–56, 1990.
104. Holcroft JW, Vassar MJ, Perry CA, et al: Perspectives on clinical trials for hypertonic saline/dextran solutions for the treatment of traumatic shock. Brazilian J Med Biol Res 22:291–293, 1989.
105. Maningas PA, Mattox KL, Pepe PE, et al: Hypertonic saline–dextran solutions for the prehospital management of traumatic hypotension. Am J Surg 157:528–533, 1989.
106. Vassar MJ, Perry CA, Holcroft JW: Analysis of potential risks associated with 7.5% sodium chloride resuscitation of traumatic shock. Arch Surg 125:1309–1315, 1990.
107. Rocha e Silva M, Velasco IT, Nogueira da Silva RI, et al: Hyperosmotic sodium salts reverse severe hemorrhagic shock: Other solutes do not. Am J Physiol 253:H751–H762, 1988.
108. Mazzoni MC, Borgstrom P, Arfors KE, et al: Dynamic fluid redistribution in hyperosmotic resuscitation of hypovolemic hemorrhage. Am J Physiol 255:H629–H637, 1988.
109. Moss GS, Gould SA, Rice CL: Crystalloids, colloids, and artificial blood substitutes in hypovolemia. In Siegel JH (ed): Trauma: Emergency Surgery and Critical Care. New York, Churchill Livingstone, 1987, pp 181–200.
110. Sympson GM: CATR: A new generation of autologous blood transfusion. Crit Care Nurs 11:60–64, 1991.
111. Elliott LA, Ledgerwood AM, Lucas CE, et al: Role of Fluosol-DA 20% in prehospital resuscitation. Crit Care Med 17:166–172, 1989.
112. DeVenuto F: Evaluation of human and bovine modified-hemoglobin solution as oxygen-carrying fluid for blood volume replacement. Biomater Artif Cells Artif Organs 16:77–83, 1988.
113. Maier RV, Carrico CJ: Developments in the resuscitation of critically ill surgical patients. Adv Surg 19:271–328, 1986.
114. Friedman HI, DeVenuto F, Schwartz BD, et al: In vivo evaluation of pyridoxalated-polymerized hemoglobin solution. Surg Gynecol Obstet 159:429–435, 1984.
115. Clark LC: Theoretical and practical considerations of florocarbon emulsions in the treatment of shock. In Cowley RA, Trump BF (eds): Pathophysiology of Shock, Anoxia and Ischemia. Baltimore, Williams & Wilkins, 1982, pp 507–522.
116. Bernstein DP: Transfusion therapy in trauma. In Capan LM, Miller SM, Turndorf H (eds): Trauma, Anesthesia and Intensive Care. Philadelphia, JB Lippincott, 1991, pp 167–205.
117. Wilson EB, Knauf MA, Donohoe K, et al: Red blood cell survival following admixture with heated saline: Evaluation of a new blood warming method for rapid transfusion. J Trauma 28:1274–1277, 1988.
118. Markowsky SJ, Elenbass RM: Pharmacologic treatment of shock. In Barrett J, Nyhus LM (eds): Treatment of Shock—Principles and Practice, 2nd ed. Philadelphia, Lea & Febiger, 1986, pp 195–210.
119. Hoffman BB, Lefkowitz RJ: Catecholamines and sympathomimetic drugs. In Gilman AG, Rall TW, Nies AS, et al (eds): Goodman and Gilman's The Pharmacological Basis of Therapeutics, 8th ed. New York, Pergamon Press, 1990.
120. Hancock BG, Eberhard NK: The pharmacologic management of shock. Crit Care Nurs Q 11:19–29, 1988.
121. Rice V: Shock management: 2. Pharmacologic intervention. Crit Care Nur 5:42–57, 1985.
122. Sharpe S, Chernow B: Newer pharmacologic approaches to shock. In Siegel J (ed): Trauma: Emergency Surgery and Critical Care. New York, Churchill Livingstone, 1987, pp 125–153.
123. American Regent Laboratories, Inc: Dopamine hydrochloride (package insert). New York, 1990.
124. Hoffman BF, Bigger JT: Digitalis and allied cardiac glycosides. In Gilman AG, Rall TW, Nies AS, et al (eds): Goodman and Gilman's The Pharmacological Basis of Therapeutics, 8th ed. New York, Pergamon Press, 1990.
125. Trachte GT: Endocrinology in shock. In Altura BM, Lefer AM, Schumer W (eds): Handbook of Shock and Trauma, vol 1: Basic Science. New York, Raven Press, 1983, pp 337–354.
126. Nickerson M: Sympathetic blockade in the therapy of shock. Am J Cardiol 12:619–623, 1963.
127. Simon R, Reynolds HN: Afterload reduction. Crit Care Rep 1:415–421, 1990.
128. Murad F: Drugs used for the treatment of angina: Organic nitrates, calcium-channel blockers and β-adrenergic antagonists. In Gilman AG, Rall TW, Nies AS, et al (eds): Goodman and Gilman's The Pharmacological Basis of Therapeutics, 8th ed. New York, Pergamon Press, 1990.
129. Gerber JG, Nies AS: Antihypertensive agents and the drug therapy of hypertension. In Gilman AG, Rall TW, Nies AS, et al (eds): Goodman and Gilman's The Pharmacological Basis of Therapeutics, 8th ed. New York, Pergamon Press, 1990.
130. Von Rueden KT: Cardiopulmonary assessment of the critically ill trauma patient. Crit Care Nurs Clin North Am 1:33–44, 1989.
131. Jaffe AS: Cardiovascular pharmacology I. Circulation 74:70–73, 1986.
132. Iberti TJ, Kelly KM, Gentili DR, et al: Effects of sodium

bicarbonate in canine hemorrhagic shock. Crit Care Med 16:779–782, 1988.
133. Makisalo HJ, Soini HO, Nordin AJ, et al: Effects of bicarbonate therapy on tissue oxygenation during resuscitation of hemorrhagic shock. Crit Care Med 17:1170–1174, 1989.
134. Svennevig JL, Bugge-Asperheim B, Geiran O, et al: High dose corticosteroids in thoracic trauma. Acta Chir Scand Suppl 526:110–119, 1985.
135. Reynolds DG, Gurll NJ, Holaday JW, et al: The therapeutic efficacy of opiate antagonists in hemorrhagic shock. Resuscitation 18:243–251, 1989.
136. Tuggle DW, Horton JW: Effect of naloxone on splanchnic perfusion in hemorrhagic shock. J Trauma 29:1341–1345, 1989.
137. Bernton EW: Naloxone and TRH in the treatment of shock and trauma: What future roles? Ann Emerg Med 14:729–735, 1985.
138. Chintala MS, Jandhyala BS: Comparative evaluation of the effects of felodipine, hydralazine, and naloxone on the survival rate in rats subjected to a "fixed volume" model of hemorrhagic shock. Circ Shock 32:219–229, 1990.
139. Gurll NJ, Holaday JW, Reynolds DG, et al: Thyrotropin-releasing hormone: Effects in monkeys and dogs subjected to experimental circulatory shock. Crit Care Med 15:574–581, 1987.
140. Guarini S, Tagliavini S, Bazzani C, et al: Early treatment with ACTH-(1-24) in a rat model of hemorrhagic shock prolongs survival and extends the time-limit for blood reinfusion to be effective. Crit Care Med 18:862–865, 1990.
141. Coppi G, Falcone A: The thyrotropin-releasing hormone analogue RGH 2202 reverses experimental haemorrhagic shock in rats. Eur J Pharmacol 182:185–188, 1990.
142. Bertolini A, Ferrari W, Guarini S: The adrenocorticotropic hormone (ACTH)–induced reversal of hemorrhagic shock. Resuscitation 18:253–267, 1989.
143. Noera C, Pensa P, Guelfi P, et al: ACTH-(1-24) and hemorrhagic shock: Preliminary clinical results. Resuscitation 18:145–147, 1989.
144. Bertolini A, Guarini S, Ferrari W, et al: ACTH-(1-24) restores blood pressure in acute hypovolaemia and haemorrhagic shock in humans. Eur J Clin Pharmacol 32:537–538, 1987.
145. Pinelli G, Chesi G, DiDonato C, et al: Preliminary data on the use of ACTH-(1-24) in human shock conditions. Resuscitation 18:149–150, 1989.
146. Stahl GL, Bitterman H, Terashita Z, et al: Salutary consequences of blockade of platelet activating factor in hemorrhagic shock. Eur J Pharmacol 149:233–240, 1988.
147. Stahl GL, Bitterman H, Lefer AM: Protective effects of a specific platelet activating factor (PAF) antagonist, WEB 2086, in traumatic shock. Thromb Res 53:327–338, 1989.
148. Karasawa A, Rochester JA, Lefer AM: Beneficial actions of BN 50739, a new PAF receptor antagonist, in murine traumatic shock. Methods Find Exp Clin Pharmacol 12:231–237, 1990.
149. Bitterman H, Smith BA, Lefer AM: Beneficial actions of antagonism of peptide leukotrienes in hemorrhagic shock. Circ Shock 24:159–168, 1988.
150. Karasawa A, Taylor PA, Lefer AM: Protective effects of KW-3635, a novel thromboxane A_2 antagonist, in murine traumatic shock. Eur J Pharmacol 182:1–8, 1990.
151. Aoki N, Johnson G, Siegfried MR, et al: Proctective effects of a combination thromboxane synthesis inhibitor-receptor antagonist, R-68070, during murine traumatic shock. Eicosanoids 2:169–174, 1989.
152. Levitt MA, Stahl G, Lefer AM: Efficacy of a combination thromboxane receptor antagonist and lipoxygenase inhibitor in traumatic shock. Resuscitation 16:211–220, 1988.
153. Bitterman H, Stahl GL, Terashita Z, et al: Mechanisms of action of PGE_1 in hemorrhagic shock in rats. Ann Emerg Med 17:457–462, 1988.
154. Carroll RG, Tams SG, Farmer PL, et al: Verapamil treatment of canine hemorrhagic shock. Ann Emerg Med 18:750–754, 1989.
155. Prasad K, Kalra J, Buchko G: Acute hemorrhage and oxygen free radicals. Angiology 39:1005–1013, 1988.
156. Aoki N, Lefer AM: Protective effects of a novel nonglucocorticoid 21-aminosteroid (U74006F) during traumatic shock in rats. J Cardiovasc Pharmacol 15:205–210, 1990.
157. Lefer A, Williams SK: Microcirculation in shock. In Barrett J, Nyhus LM (eds): Treatment of Shock—Principles and Practice. Philadelphia, Lea & Febiger, 1986, pp 3–21.
158. Shoemaker WC: Circulatory mechanisms of shock and their mediators. Crit Care Med 15:787–794, 1987.
159. Davis JW, Shackford SR, Mackersie RC, et al: Base deficit as a guide to volume resuscitation. J Trauma 28:1464–1467, 1988.
160. Jaquith SM: The oximetrix opticath. Crit Care Nurs 4:55–58, 1984.
161. Bernstein DP: Oxygen transport and utilization in trauma with special reference to hemorrhagic shock and rationale for transfusion. In Capan LM, Miller SM, Turndorf H (eds): Trauma, Anesthesia and Intensive Care. Philadelphia, JB Lippincott, 1991, pp 115–165.
162. Barone JE, Snyder AB: Treatment strategies in shock: Use of oxygen transport measurements. Heart Lung 20:81–85, 1991.
163. Maier RV, Carrico CJ: Developments in the resuscitation of critically ill surgical patients. Adv Surg 19:271–328, 1986.
164. Green GE, Hassell KT, Mahutte CK: Comparison of arterial blood gas with continuous intra-arterial and transcutaneous Po_2 in adult critically ill patients. Crit Care Med 15:491–494, 1987.
165. Von Reuden KT: Noninvasive assessment of gas exchange in the critically ill patient. AACN Clin Issues Crit Care Nurs 1:239–247, 1990.
166. Harris K: Noninvasive monitoring of gas exchange. Respir Care 32:544–557, 1987.
167. Turney SZ: Respiratory monitoring. In Applefeld JJ, Linberg SE (eds): Acute Respiratory Care. Boston, Blackwell Scientific, 1988.

10

PSYCHOSOCIAL RESPONSES OF THE HUMAN SPIRIT: THE JOURNEY OF TRAUMA

ANN M. SCANLON

> Miracles are to come. With you I leave a remembrance of miracles: they are by somebody who can love and who shall be continually reborn, a human being; somebody who said to those near him, when his fingers would not hold a brush, "tie it into my hand."[1]
>
> e. e. cummings

Today's health care system has made a national investment of monies, education, and research in attempting to address the life-threatening problems encountered by the traumatized person. Tremendous energy has been expended in developing highly complex and innovative systems of care for these patients from the moment they enter the system until they are discharged from the acute setting.

Although the emphasis continues to focus on the physiological stabilization of these patients, much more awareness regarding the effects of the environment on healing and recovery has emerged. Nursing literature reflects this attention and has begun to address the unique challenges that critical care environments present to nursing practitioners. Strategies that mediate the effects of the latest technologies pose opportunities for nurses to creatively care for patients in what can easily be viewed as a hostile environment.

Indeed, the experience of meeting and participating in another's life is no ordinary event: There is a certain intimacy that exists between patient and nurse, a presence that makes the other come alive and be real. In these unpredictable life situations, the capacity for openness allows both giving and receiving to occur. In these moments, nurse and patient cease to be strangers and become fellow travelers. By so journeying together, the devastating loneliness and fear of suffering encountered by the trauma patient is not experienced alone but in communion. The felt presence of the nurse often communicates a sense of aliveness, hope, and understanding to the patient, and this caring transforms and energizes the exchanges. These experiences lessen the aloneness and the patient's fears of being separate: These are the everyday miracles and mysteries that exist in critical care units. Qualitative nursing literature examines these dimensions of adaptation.

The nurse who elects to care for the traumatically injured patient has now available an extensive empirical and research data base that speaks to the many psychosocial dimensions of trauma.

The task at hand in this chapter is to comprehensively explore the major themes that traumatized patients must address to successfully adapt to the traumatic event and its sequelae. The journey that a person embarks on after severe injury is viewed from the patient's perspective. The questions to be answered are: What is the experience of the patient when the familiar patterns of life and relationships are radically disrupted? How does the traumatized person repair the fabric of his life and find hope and meaning once again? What is it that the nurse contributes in facilitating the patient's psychological movement through each phase of the trauma cycle? What is the art of trauma nursing?

ART AND SCIENCE OF TRAUMA NURSING

The trauma nurse, as artist, consciously uses skills, knowledge, and creative imagination that have been pragmatically acquired through experience with and observation of patients. The cognitive tool on which the art of trauma nursing hinges is perspective-taking: the ability and skill of the nursing practitioner to obtain knowledge about the subjective perceptions of the patient. The cognitive tool on which the science of psychological trauma nursing hinges is nursing judgment: the ability and skill of the nursing practitioner to recognize that prematurely intervening with a patient may teach the person something he needed to discover for himself and thus prevent him from experiencing, understanding, and assimilating events completely.

Many people will join the trauma patient in his journey back to health; among them and pivotal to the effort is the nurse. A part of both the art and the science of trauma nursing resides in the insight that the nurse brings to each interaction, be it verbal, physical, or nonverbal. It includes knowledge of the processes the patient undergoes and themes that he is addressing at specific moments in time. This knowledge allows the nurse to anticipate, support, and guide the patient as he moves toward recovery. Knowledge is but one piece. Empathy, courage, wisdom, and hope are the others. To adapt to these events, for meaning or purpose to be restored, all patients require the presence of another who will walk with them on this journey. It is most often the nurse who, critically weaving both knowledge and strength, walks the distance with the patient. A capacity for listening, caring, and communicating is essential. This demands that the nurse also have insight into herself and an acute awareness of her own values, strengths, and beliefs.

Part of the healing from a traumatic injury occurs because struggles and pains are shared and valued. Hope and concern for the future are embedded in these relationships. Most care providers have known patients with whom they have interacted on this empathic level and from whom they have grown themselves. The difference has been that the interchange occurred between two human beings and not only between patient and nurse.

INFORMATION PROCESSING: ESTABLISHMENT OF MEANING IN LIFE EXPERIENCES

Part of the difficulty in developing a comprehensive psychological model that reflects trauma patients' responses to catastrophic injury lies in the fact that each patient brings a unique personality and history to the traumatic event. Perception, life experiences, culture, education, and health all influence how the patient responds to a suddenly imposed, overwhelming situation. Bombarded by both physiologic and psychological stressors, the primary struggle for the patient is to make sense out of what is happening, to find meaning in what is meaningless.

To recognize what occurs for the trauma patient when meaningfulness and hope in life are absent, it is important to review how they are first established.

Throughout our lives there run threads of continuity that allow us to examine and interpret the many experiences we encounter. Our construction of life, simplistically, is based on the reliability of these connections and interpretations of experiences over time. These connections allow us the necessary security to find stability in life's experiences and to predict and learn from events and situations. Without the ability to predict and interpret new events in the light of past experience, life would be unmanageable[2] (Fig. 10–1).

Early in life, an infant begins to attach meaning to both people and objects. A person transfers this meaning from one situation or person to another. Although dissimilarities are also confronted, a person learns through generalization and gradually develops a repertoire of predictions based on past experience (Fig. 10–2). For learning to occur and for meaningfulness to be established, a person assimilates new knowledge into this predictable framework. Events and experiences that are unique and unfamiliar are placed in the context of what is known (Fig. 10–3).

A person's very survival rests largely on his ability to abstract what is familiar in the unique or unfamiliar event. Construction of reality is then based on the ability to interpret events because these interpretations have reliable connections with the past.[2] Growth is the continuing cataloging of experiences into this reliable repertoire.

Because not all new experiences fit into preexisting cognitive schemata, a person must sometimes either modify or form new ones that are capable of incorporating information

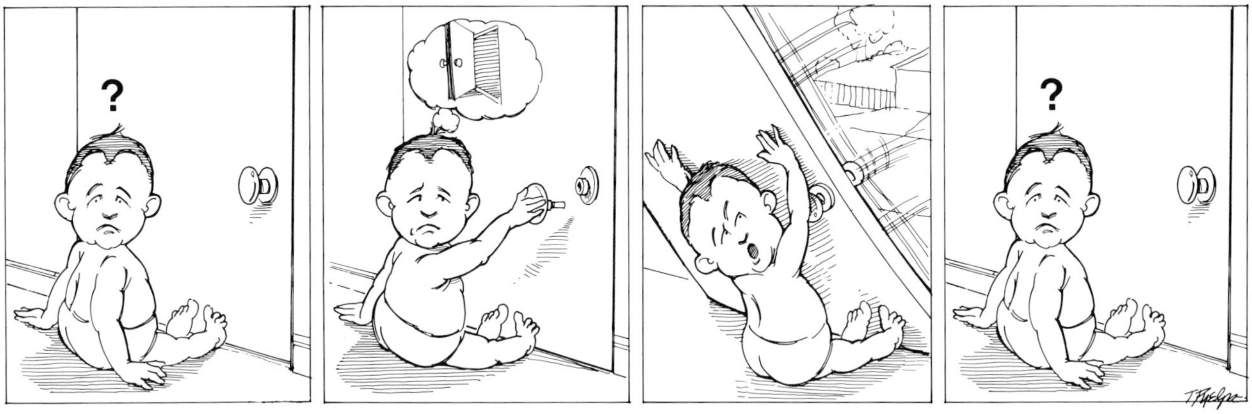

Figure 10–1.

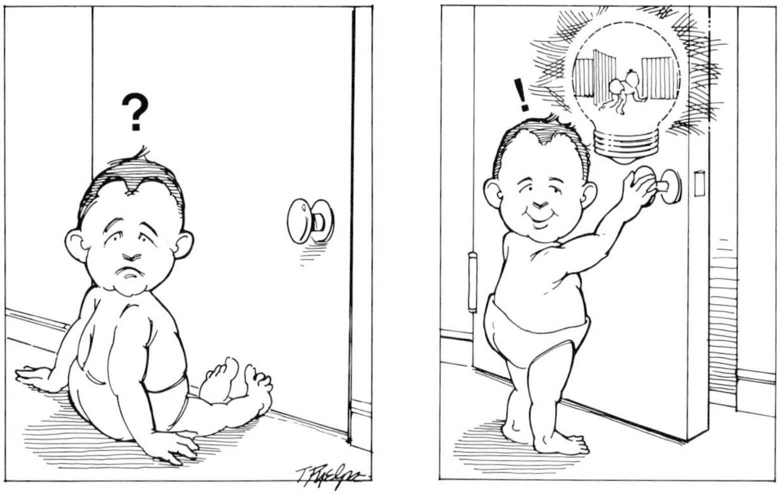

Figure 10–2.

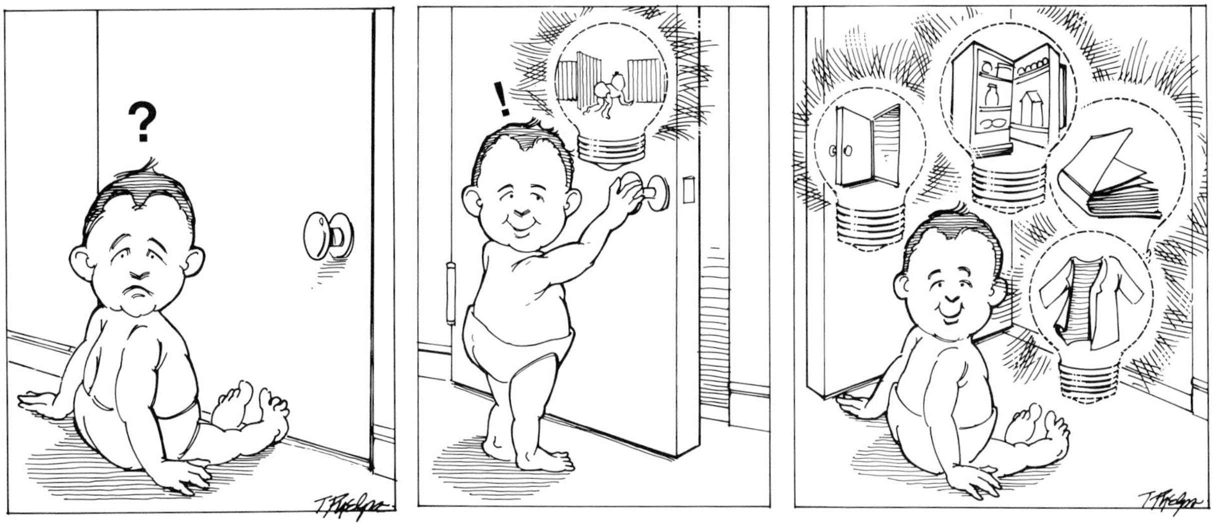

Figure 10–3.

or experiences that are incongruent with previous understandings. This process of accommodation results in the creation of new adaptive modes.

When a traumatic injury occurs, the predictability and continuity of life's experiences are dramatically interrupted. The fine strands of meaning that connected the past to the present and the future are broken, and with that break comes meaninglessness. A person is literally locked into the present: the predictability that was so intrinsic to his survival has been obliterated. To regain meaning, the trauma patient must reweave the strands of life experiences through assimilation and accommodation. When both these modes of processing the traumatic experiences are used, the person's scope of problem-solving is broadened and the potential exists for this life experience to be integrated and for meaning in life to be restored. Meaningfulness, which is simply the person's sense of continuity and connectedness of the self and life experience over time (past, present, future), is restored. Figure 10–4 summarizes the processes that lead to the reestablishment of meaningfulness.[3]

Coping Processes

The behaviors and processes the patient uses to tolerate, master, or control the numerous stressors that bombard him in the journey back to health are called *coping*. The stressors themselves are divergent, but whether they are perceived as stressful or not is largely determined by the meaning the patient imposes on them. Some events might be stressful to one patient but not to another. If an event is perceived as irrelevant or benign, the patient does not cope with it. If, however, the stressor is demanding, threatening, or harmful, the patient will attempt to master or tolerate it by coping. The nurse becomes instrumental in helping the patient to adapt by supporting and guiding the patient's choice of coping behaviors. Most healthy people are able to perceive stressors and cope without much assistance. In the case of the trauma patient, there is an acute and chronic summative crisis from the constant bombardment of multiple stressors. The energy demanded by the patient for continuous coping eventually exhausts him. Initially, professionals intervene in a timely manner through structuring and negotiating the environment for the patient. The nurse's judgment is critical in deciding where and how much constructive psychological energy the patient expends. Although each patient's perception of stressors is unique, certain commonalities in the trauma experience affect all patients to some degree. The simple provision of information by the nurse regarding the physical environment prevents the patient from having to expend psychic energy to process and construct information through trial and error.

Coping Behaviors

One of the most pervasive coping behaviors observed in trauma patients is grief work. This frequently is seen because loss is a significant theme in the trauma patient's experience.

The process of mourning (which is the response to loss) is painful, conflictual, work-centered, and ambivalent and can be done only by the self. Through mourning, a person is attempting to restore meaning and hope in life. The work of grief is to tie the past, present, and future together again, so that life becomes manageable and meaningful once more.[4–11]

Through empirical observation of trauma patients, it is well recognized that the actual traumatic event and its immediate sequelae are terrifying to those who experience it. Fear and helplessness are the predominant behavioral manifestations. Although some patients initially respond to the event by attempting to fight or flee the situation, most rapidly experience a profound emotional numbness. At this point, early on, after the injury, the work of grief is beginning. Unable to effectively process or interpret the event cognitively, the psychic compensating mechanism of numbness allows the patient time to distance himself from the

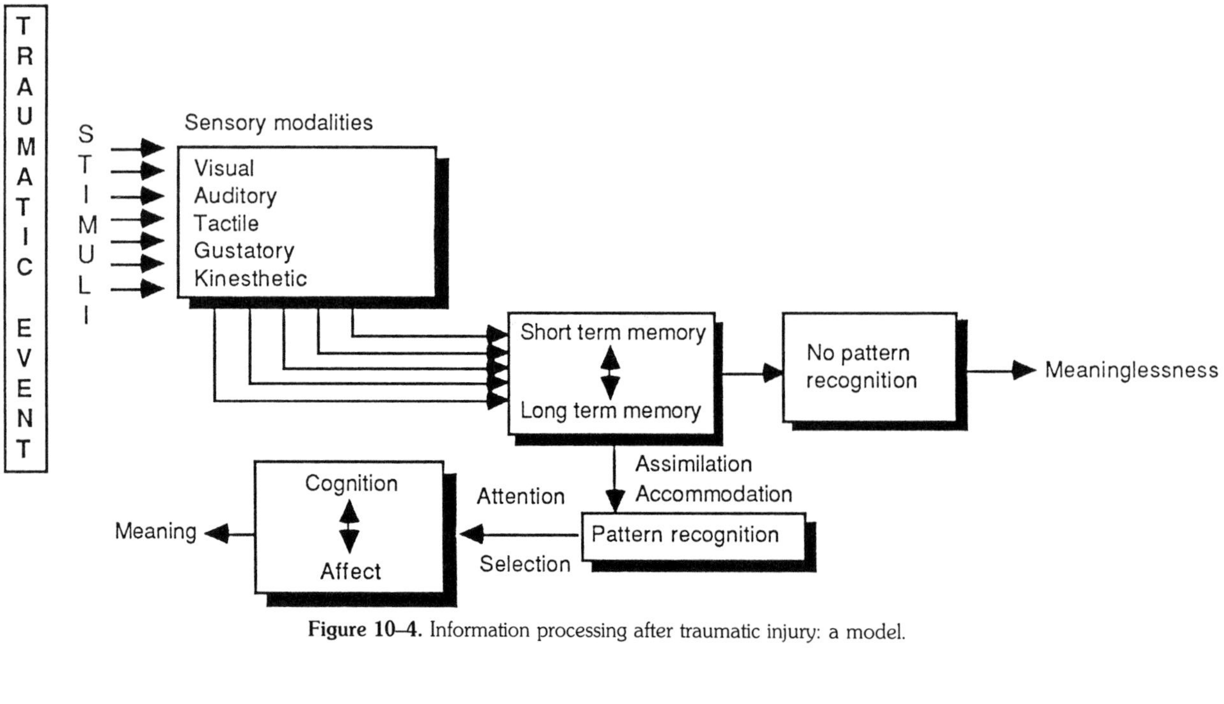

Figure 10–4. Information processing after traumatic injury: a model.

awareness that all his psychological systems have simultaneously become unbalanced and that he has lost control.[12] In effect, the patient psychologically disassociates himself from the event. Although the patient may provide accurate information and respond appropriately to helping professionals, the patient often is experiencing a sense of total disbelief that this event is happening to him.

As the sense of numbness dissipates, previous psychological defenses become activated and used by the patient in an attempt to make sense of what is happening and what has occurred. Initially, the trauma patient is unable to perceive any part of his life that the injury does not invade. He cannot distinguish between aspects of his life that have not been touched by the trauma: the loss is pervasive. The patient cannot focus on what is intact—only on what is gone. To him, all is lost. Locked into the present, he sees no future. All he experiences is pain and suffering that has no end. To look back at how he was generates pain: he no longer is the same—he is different. To look ahead is impossible: he cannot conceive of any future.

For the person to adapt healthily to the loss, the grief experienced must be worked through. It cannot simply be tolerated or endured. Understanding the loss takes time; it does not happen by the person's ceasing to care about what was lost or substituting something else for the loss. It occurs only when the person can abstract and redefine what was meaningful in the past, sees that meaning can still fit into the present, and can go on in the future, albeit in a different manner. He must discover that the meaning of the lost body part, value, or relationship can exist independently of the object in which it was originally invested.[13] Adaptation to the losses and changes encountered because of the traumatic event occurs when new meaning is imposed on the patient's experience of self. In effect, the patient experiences that although he no longer may be able to walk, his life is still worthwhile.

To support and guide the trauma patient's efforts at coping and moving toward reintegration of body and psyche and ultimate adaptation to his loss, it is necessary to explore the actual events with which the patient copes.

Although each patient's journey back to health is unique to him, some aspects of that trajectory are common to most patients. Because of the commonalities, it is appropriate to examine the stressors as they are embedded in a temporal framework, which can be divided into distinct cycles. These are the periods of resuscitation, critical care, intermediate care, rehabilitation, and community integration.

STRESSORS AND PATIENT/NURSE COPING RESPONSES DURING THE RESUSCITATION CYCLE

Fear of death and of mutilation are major stressors encountered by the trauma patient during the resuscitation cycle. The threat of annihilation arises from the patient's awareness of his loss of self-control and the actual visualization of his multilated, nonfunctioning body. Although the patient is not usually capable of careful cognitive processing because of extreme anxiety, on some level, he does appreciate the gravity of the situation. The astute clinician recognizes that the patient is in a state of psychological shock: the patient demonstrates a sense of numbness with tunneling of awareness, impaired memory, and disorientation. Behavior may be random with the loss of goal orientation. At this time, the specter of death looms large because of loss of self-control and body integrity and the perceived intensity of the caregivers' interventions. The patient is overwhelmed by the situation that forces him to give over control of his physical self to the ministrations of others in whom he must trust.

Many patients associate intense pain with thoughts of death. Perceptual coping styles, specifically the manner in which a person responds to anxiety, the context in which the pain occurs, and the cognitive processing of intrapsychic and extrapsychic inputs, contribute to the person's unique interpretation and expression of pain. Pain triggers automatic withdrawal reflexes that result in the patient's display of motivated avoidance and escape behaviors. Agitation, verbal and physical hostility, and emotional withdrawal reflect the patient's attempt to cope with and modulate the stressors assaulting the integrity of the body. As pain endures, despite the patient's attempts to flee from or control it, the ominous sense that something is terribly wrong persists. This perception, linked with the patient's rapidly deteriorating cognitive functioning, can result in the association of pain with impending death.

Coupled with the events that created the injury and the visualization of one's distorted body, the aforementioned stressors are present but seldom verbalized during resuscitation. It is usual for the trauma patient to express these fears later on when he is secure in the knowledge that he is not dying. Some patients do indirectly reflect this fear during resuscitation when they express their distress to nursing and medical personnel: "Help me, please . . . I don't want to die . . . Please, don't let me die . . . you're trying to kill me."

Data gleaned from trauma patients who retrospectively recall their experiences and feelings during the resuscitation cycle strongly indicate that these stressors exist. Because neither time nor circumstances allow a verbal assessment of these stressors, it is safe to assume that they potentially exist and therefore need to be addressed by the nurse. Fear swiftly moves toward increasing anxiety and, eventually, panic if information is not provided to the patient. Hence, before assessing the patient's sensorium, perception, cognition, or affect, it is critical for the nurse to support the patient in focusing his attention on her and on intervening. Eye contact is crucial when this mode is accessible. The nurse in fact may have to physically hold the patient's head with her hands, look him in the eyes, and give short succinct bits of information. "I'm Ann, I'm a nurse. You're in the hospital. You've been in a car accident. You've been hurt and the doctors and I are going to take care of you." Telling the patient what is going to be done before doing it allows the patient to anticipate and process what is happening to him. Because many people often are performing procedures on the patient simultaneously, the painful stimuli can be overwhelming. The nursing goal is to minimize the patient's anxiety level. This can be achieved to a degree by providing him with information regarding himself, his environment, what has happened and is happening, and who is with him. Out of what, to the patient, is perceived as a confusing, noisy environment, the reassurance of one calm person who consistently addresses his unspoken fears and organizes environmental information for him makes the situation somewhat safe.

Many patients also experience sensory input alterations at this juncture.[14–16] Visual, auditory, olfactory, and tactile receptors are all continuously bombarded with excessively familiar as well as meaningless stimuli. Auditory input consists mainly of unfamiliar sounds emanating from respirators, suction apparatus, and monitoring equipment. Recognizable sounds, such as voices of the staff and telephone rings, stress the patient.

Visual input generates fear. The patient may have only his damaged body to explore; the sight of tubes and machinery to which he is attached provides little help. If he is able to see other patients, his visual sense will be bombarded by the overwhelming mutilation of others around him. Privacy is minimal. Unpleasant smells emanate from various orifices. Tactile stimulation is constant, most of it being painful. Hence, much information contains excessively meaningless data. The result is sensory overload and the eventual impairment of the patient's thinking processes.

Patients admitted to the emergency department or trauma unit probably experience some, if not all, of these stressors. Some may appear to be inert and unresponsive. Others physically act out their terror; the nurse might observe crying, shouting, and agitated behavior. Other patients will lie still, revealing their inner turmoil only through a dazed, noncommunicative facial expression.

The extent and severity of injury vary in each trauma patient as well as the perception and intensity of the stressors encountered. The common thread that exists between the single-system–injured trauma patient and the multisystem-injured person is that stressors, potential or actual, are present for both. The intensity and degree to which the patient is affected depend largely on the person's perception and appraisal of the situation and the level of intactness of his biopsychological state. Hence, a person's response to traumatic injury is *not* directly related to the severity of the injury but to his unique perception and interpretation of the events and stressors as well as the coping strategies he is able to call forth. In effect, then, it is feasible that a minimally injured trauma patient may in fact experience and respond more intensely to stressors than a severely physiologically impaired person. The inverse also is possible: the more severely injured the patient is, the less able he may be to mediate the stressors himself. It becomes clear that the nurse's assessment and understanding of the patient's perception of stressors are what guide interventions, not simply the severity of injury.

Anxiety Related to Trauma State

The primary nursing diagnosis during the resuscitative phase is anxiety related to the disruption in the person's physiological and psychological integrity. Although closely related to fear and not affectively distinguishable, anxiety is not synonymous with fear. Fear is a response to specific environmental stimuli that appear to have a causal relation; anxiety is a vaguer and more diffuse affect for which there is no causative agent in the environment. Anxiety reflects the internal disequilibrium that occurs in a person in response to the impingement of multiple stressors. It is crucial to note that both fear and anxiety can and do usually exist in concert. Although the patient's behavioral responses to fear and anxiety are similar, different nursing interventions are based on the causative factor.

The physiological responses of a person to mild and moderate levels of anxiety are well documented in the nursing literature. A person's autonomic nervous system responds to fear and anxiety by increasing the heart and respiratory rates, which results in an increased state of arousal. This alerting effect has an adaptive and adjustment value in that the biophysical and behavioral systems maintain equilibrium, resulting in focused individual functioning. If stressors are not attenuated in a timely manner, anxiety increases and subsequent maladaption and disorganization occur, as reflected in the person's thought processes and behavior.

Patient Behavior

Excessive anxiety, from a psychological perspective, is reflected in impairment of a person's physical, cognitive, and affective abilities to process environmental information. When these intrapsychic mechanisms become useless in cataloging the external environment for the person, the confusion is reflected behaviorally. Characteristically, the nurse observes a disorganization in the patient's cognitive and affective processes:[17]

1. Attention span is shortened. The patient is not able to concentrate and focus thoughts, responds indiscriminately to stimuli in the environment, and is easily distracted. Eyes roam from one object to another. Verbalization reflects scattered thinking.
2. Perceptual abilities are narrowed. The patient is unable to process environmental stimuli, abstract essential information from the environment, and integrate multiple pieces of information. He also has a narrow focus of attention. Because of inability to process and interpret multiple stimuli, the patient may misperceive and misinterpret stimuli.
3. Memory function is impaired. The patient cannot retain and recall information over brief periods.
4. The patient is disoriented to person, place, time, and situation.
5. The patient is unable to problem solve. Behavior is not goal-directed.
6. Affective controls are lost: the patient is agitated, restless, hostile, and noncooperative.

Nursing Assessment

A comprehensive and usable tool for assessing the current psychological functioning of the trauma patient is the mental status examination (see Appendix 10–1). This tool allows the nurse to gather data systematically and objectively and focuses on the functioning of the person at the time the assessment is done. The tool's flexibility allows both general and specific observations to be made over time, so that a meaningful data base depicting trends and changes in cognition and affect can be accumulated. The four major areas of assessment are sensorium, perception, thought processes, and mood and affect. The extent and depth of the psychological assessment depend on the degree of intactness of the patient's sensorium. The ordering of the content of the tool moves from assessment of simple to complex functioning, so that the nurse is rapidly able to assess the patient's level of functioning. If the patient's sensorium should be markedly disorganized, the assessment process stops there.

The focus of the nursing assessment during the resuscitation cycle is evaluating the level of cognitive functioning of the patient. Through a rapid visual assessment of the patient, the nurse initially gathers subjective information. The patient's overall appearance is noted: clothing, hair, nails, body size, and age. In trauma patients, these parameters frequently are neither distinguishable nor meaningful. This brief assessment of appearance is aimed at gleaning some sense of the person's physical well-being before the traumatic event.

Any unusual, non–trauma-related behavior or psychomotor activity is noted, such as combativeness, retarded responses to following direction, stereotypical behavior, and echopraxia. The nurse can also make some judgment about the patient's attitude toward the personnel in the immediate environment: Is the patient cooperative, attentive, or guarded in his interactions? Is the patient's speech rapid, slow, or monotonous? Does the patient speak spontaneously, or does he only respond to questions when asked?

In assessing the patient's sensorium, the nurse is attempting to determine the patient's state of consciousness and any alterations or fluctuations in his alertness. During the resuscitation phase, the patient may be hyperalert: He responds unselectively to irrelevant stimuli in the environment and is quite distractable. This is assessed by the nurse who observes the patient's physical and verbal productions.

Assessing the patient's sensorium involves eliciting information from him regarding orientation to person, place, time, and situation; memory functioning (short, long, and immediate recall); general fund of knowledge; ability to concentrate; ability to think abstractly; and judgment abilities. On admission, initially, the nurse has provided information concerning the environment to the patient as well as information about his injury. In assessing the patient's orientation and memory functioning, the nurse asks questions about information that she knows the patient has been given:

Person: What is your name? What is my name?
Place: Where are you now, Mr. A? What is the name of this hospital?
Time: What is today's date, day of the week, month, season?
Situation: What happened? Why are you here?

In assessing memory functioning, the nurse asks specific questions, depending on the area of memory that is being tested:

Long-term memory: When is your birthdate? Are you married? When did you marry? What school did you attend when you were young?
Short-term memory: What did you do yesterday? What did you have for breakfast, lunch, or dinner?
Immediate retention and recall: Give patient six numbers; ask him to repeat them back to you.

Although the nurse can formally assess the patient's sensorium by asking these questions, this evaluation is best done by informal questioning as she is physically caring for the patient during resuscitation.

Goals and Interventions

The nursing goals during this cycle are aimed at supporting the patient in diminishing his anxiety level by providing him with information concerning his environment and making the environment understandable and as safe as possible for him.

By speaking calmly, empathetically, and slowly, by gently touching the patient, and by helping the patient focus his attention, the nurse begins a relationship with the patient that allows him to trust someone in a foreign and chaotic situation. In essence, the nurse conveys to the patient that although he may feel out of control, others are managing the crisis and he is safe and alive.

STRESSORS AND PATIENT/NURSE COPING RESPONSES DURING THE CRITICAL CARE CYCLE

Once the patient has survived the immediate postresuscitative cycle, he continues the complex and painful journey to recovery. At this time, the patient shifts from a major fear of death to increasing concerns about alterations of body functioning and significant losses. When it is established that life itself will not be suddenly lost, the patient gradually comes to terms with his altered body and with the pain that seems unceasing. At the same time, other struggles emerge; the patient must develop new ways of expressing self in relating to family, significant others, and, increasingly, the nurse.

Alteration of Body Image

Mutilation of the body, through both trauma and subsequent treatment, is stressful for the patient and the nurse. The patient recognizes that his once intact body now may have holes in it, tubes that emerge from his skin, and wires and pins that hold together his flesh and bone. He must address this change by coming to terms with the reality that these apparitions are now part of the self. To understand the dynamics of this process, it is necessary to review how body image is formed.

Body image develops through the child's use of his body and experiences that allow him to feel competent or incompetent. By way of social interaction, a mental image of the body and sense of personal identity is derived from the knowledge that one's body is intact in both form and function. Our conceptions of ourselves are a reflection of this mental image, which has been conceived through our active interactions with others in our environment. Hence, people are alert to the environment's responses to them.

The development of body image occurs in a sequential process. In infancy, by way of sensory modalities, a person experiences pain, mobility, and pleasure and learns the boundaries of himself that are distinguishable and separate from others in his environment.[18–20] As the toddler learns to control his body and its functions, he also learns that mastery of these functions brings a sense of competence and worth. If he does not master control of bodily functions, he experiences a sense of inadequacy. Through successful competition with peers, the child experiences and perceives himself as strong. If failure predominates, his perception of his body and self-image are weak. By the time a person reaches adulthood, his concept of body image is fairly solidified and he enjoys the total integration of body and mind. Greater emphasis is placed on the development of the inner self and less attention is paid to the physical self.[21] People whose conception of their body image is in transition (e.g., adolescents) or altered in some manner (e.g., anorexics) focus more attention and energy on the physical self and, hence, are more vulnerable to experiencing additional anxiety from the effects of any alterations in appearance.

Inevitably, in trauma, the physical body is altered in some manner, either temporarily or permanently. Whatever the actual physical alteration, there is a subsequent change in the person's perception of his body and, hence, in self-esteem. Loss of independent functioning and control of one's body coupled with a change in roles and functioning all must be addressed by the patient during the critical care cycle.

Both patient and nurse cope with the stress of altered body image. The nurse can withdraw from the sight when the shift is over. The nurse can isolate herself from the horror by saying, in effect, "This is not me." An alternative to withdrawal is valuing that which *is* the patient. The nurse can indicate her esteem and hope for the function of the patient's altered body in the future. The nurse can lay the groundwork for hope by talking about prostheses and compensation for loss of one part by the expanded functioning of another body part.

For the patient, "me" is pain, bandages, tubes, blood, wires, and gauze. "Me" must be reconstituted and tolerated—a complex adjustment because the patient must move beyond pain, through denial and the horror that he sees. Values and beliefs must be critically reviewed in order for the patient to accept the physical differences and loss, whether temporary or permanent, of self.

Loss

The theme of loss is pervasive in this phase of recovery. The patient faces loss of body integrity with all its attendant meanings: loss of control over his body, loss of control of the environment, and loss of control of his affective responses. Loss of function leads to loss of role(s) as well. The patient perceives himself as powerless. One means of coping with these numerous losses is to become dependent on the power of others and to regress to early phases of development when the psyche could tolerate such dependency.[22]

The patient's response to actual or perceived losses is to mourn or grieve for them. Grieving begins the moment the patient cognitively is aware that a change has occurred. The work of grief is displayed affectively by the patient throughout each of the cycles of trauma. The most frequently verbalized or displayed affects are denial, anger, guilt, bargaining, depression, and hope. Because the expression of grief is unique for each person, it is important that the trauma nurse be cognizant of the process and recognize each of the themes that the patient is expressing. Grief work is not a systematic process consisting of stages that occur sequentially. Rather, it is a complex array of affects and cognitions that the patient is sorting out and attempting to make sense of to integrate the changes in his life. The patient is struggling to hope and find meaning in his life. Mourning reflects the profound conflict that arises from the person's attempt to consolidate what was valuable in his past and preserve it from loss while simultaneously reconstructing a present and a future in which the loss is integrated.[23]

Assessment of Grief as a Response to Loss

The patient who is grieving reflects this process in both verbalization and behavior. It is important for the nurse to obtain from either the patient or some significant other information regarding the patient's previous coping patterns when he experienced a significant loss. Did he deny the loss initially? How did he reflect this denial? Did his motor and psyche activity diminish? Was he verbal or nonverbal? Did he cry frequently? Was he hostile or agitated? Did he stop functioning in other roles, such as work? Did he withdraw from the people and activities in his environment? Did his sleeping and eating patterns change? If so, how? Did he become dependent on others to direct his activities? Did he verbalize feelings of hopelessness? Did he become quiet, withdrawn, or apathetic? Was he preoccupied with the loss? What or who was significant in supporting him? What did they do or say that was helpful?[24]

As the patient's history of responding to previous losses is obtained, the nurse integrates this information into workable interventions with the patient.

Nursing Interventions

For the patient who uses denial, the nurse recognizes that the patient's behavior serves a purpose: he is indeed buying time and preparing himself intrapsychically to address the magnitude of the traumatic event. It is important that the nurse not strip away this defense. Reflecting verbalized content back to the patient confronts his thought processes in a nonthreatening manner. For example, if a patient in traction is inappropriately attempting to get out of bed to go to the bathroom, sincerely asking him a question such as "Do you think you would be able to walk with all that traction attached to your broken left leg?" helps the patient to focus on pieces of reality and allows the nurse to intervene with specific factual information. Simple explanations regarding the environment and procedures bring reality to the patient without forcing it on him.

Trauma patients often are hostile to and critical of staff. Anger exists because the patient has lost control and is dependent on others and because what has happened to him is perceived as unfair. Because the patient is virtually unable to change what has happened, by externalizing the anger to the environment, he at least maintains some sense of control by finding what is at fault externally. Frequently, this anger is reflected outwardly by complaining about unresponsiveness of staff to the patient's needs, by questioning of staff's ability to care for the patient adequately, and by constant demanding of attention from the staff. There are few, if any, answers to the question, "Why did this happen to me? It's so unfair." Blaming others initially relieves some of the patient's frustration. The astute nurse looks behind the angry verbalizations and recognizes the need they serve. The nurse must be nondefensive toward the patient, recognize and acknowledge with him that he is feeling angry, and help him focus on the reasons for the anger. It is also important that the nurse not be punitive in her actions or verbalizations.

Part of grief work is retreating from the environment by withdrawing invested energy from it. This internal retreat from external stimulation provides time for the patient to put the pieces together. Recognizing affects of sadness and depression and verbalizing them for the patient support him in acceptance of those feelings. The nurse supports this necessary introspection by minimizing environmental input and by spending quiet time with the patient. When the patient is depressed, small goals and choices that are achievable need to be set.[25]

As the loss begins to take on perspective for the patient, he comes to recognize abilities that he does retain. Hope becomes a bigger piece of the picture at this point, and the nurse now actively presents positive aspects of his life situation and acknowledges independent functioning and strengths. As the patient's self-image is beginning to integrate the changes that have occurred, renewed energy is applied to the task of healing. Often at this point, the patient shifts to more independent functioning; however, the patient moves back and forth in his utilization of coping behaviors throughout the phases of trauma as he mourns for his loss.

Affective coping behaviors such as denial, regression, anger, and depression do not alter the stressors, but they alter the perception of the patient experiencing them. At this juncture in the journey to recovery is the seed of a major conflict between nurse and patient. The patient may appear less anxious because he has often transformed the stressor, e.g., loss of control, by becoming markedly more dependent and tolerates this position by regressing to a level of development when it was appropriate; the nurse, on the other hand, perceives the situation without the aid of dependent and regressive eyes. The nurse often cannot tolerate the patient's level of dependency once there are physical signs that the patient's functioning can allow more autonomous behavior. In effect, nurse and patient may no longer be moving in the same direction. To cope with his anxiety, the patient has transformed the anxiety so that it is no longer experienced. The nurse becomes more anxious as a result of her need for the patient to continue progressing in their previously mutual direction and goals. This apparent dilemma can cause an alteration in the nurse-patient relationship as evidenced by increased conflict in their interactions. Acknowledgment of the tension by the nurse allows examination of causative factors, which in turn allows dialogue and resolution. Although there probably are alterations in the patient's other relationships, the interactions that the creative, skilled nurse has with the patient can pave the way for further healing and rehabilitation.

During the critical care cycle, the nurse is the dominating force that shapes the patient's experience. The nurse can tolerate the patient's dependency and regressive behavior and respond to it in such a way that hopelessness, helplessness, and powerlessness are not the patient's predominant experiences. Rather, the resourceful nurse continues to provide choices for the patient to act on. The patient's decisions in these matters of choice counteract the ever-present threat of powerlessness and helplessness. The nurse combats the patient's regressive tendencies by constantly presenting reality in terms of necessary treatments but leaves room for the patient to determine when and, as far as possible, how. The enterprising nurse constantly assesses the patient's functional level of responsibility, stepping in when the patient falters; when he is more active, the nurse withdraws, giving the patient freedom and legitimating his efforts to become more autonomous.

Critical care nurses need to be extremely flexible in order to respond to the patient's psychosocial needs during the critical care cycle. Because of pain and monotony and the constant danger of coping by regression, patients tend to be in flux. The nurse who intervenes as if the patient were constantly in the same position does either too much or too little for this person. Evaluation of the patient's status is easily accomplished by assessing his capacity to problem solve. This occurs when the nurse frames the day's schedule and seeks the patient's input about these events. The patient who is more regressed might simply wash his hands of the whole thing or say, "I don't care. Do what you want," or "You're going to do it anyway"; "Go away!" Each of these responses is a reasonably accurate reflection of the patient's willingness to act on his own behalf that day.

Impaired Verbal Communication

In the critical care phase, many patients are unable to verbalize their needs because they are intubated, have experienced facial trauma, or have tracheostomies. This compounds the problems of communication regarding the patient's psychological needs. It is important that the nurse support the patient in finding ways that he can make his needs, concerns, and feelings known. An environment that gives the patient permission, creative options, and time to communicate at his pace and in his own manner is crucial.

Nursing Assessment

A major component of the nursing assessment is to determine the ability of the patient to comprehend what is said to him. Because the patient's sensorium fluctuates in response to physiological shifts, pain, sedation, and environmental stimuli, a reliable assessment is best achieved when these factors are taken into account. Asking the patient to respond to simple commands that he is physically capable of performing, such as "Raise your left arm. Blink your eyes twice if you understand what I'm saying," aids in determining the patient's ability to comprehend information. Once the nurse assesses that the patient comprehends what is being said, creative modes for communicating must be devised.

Interventions

It is frustrating for the patient as well as the nurse when the patient has to repeat his communications because the nurse is not able to read his lips. It is important to acknowledge that frustration and to keep trying. Questions that require short answers should be asked so as not to tire the patient. Health professionals have a tendency to speak loudly to patients who are unable to talk, forgetting that the patient's comprehension and hearing are not altered. Speaking in a normal tone, facing the patient, modifying environmental stimuli, and being patient all facilitate communication. If a patient can write or use word and picture boards, these vehicles need to be incorporated into his care and made known to all those interacting with the patient. Mechanisms for contacting the nurse, such as call bells or buzzers, must also be determined, since the patient's sense of helplessness and his level of anxiety are compounded when he cannot call for help.

Impaired Thinking Processes

The trauma patient's thinking processes may be radically impaired secondary to physiological, psychosocial, and environmental factors. Hypoxia, kidney failure, electrolyte imbalances, and medications in concert with anxiety, sensory overload and deprivation, social isolation, sleep deprivation, and immobility all impact on the patient's cognitive functions, resulting in disorganized thinking and behavioral patterns.

Nursing Assessment

Using the mental status examination (Appendix 10–1), the nurse can find deficits in the patient's sensorium: the patient frequently is not oriented to place, time, and situation. Testing of memory functioning reveals that the patient's short-term memory and immediate recall abilities are impaired. The patient's thinking processes, as assessed through his spoken or written word, reflect unclear and loose association of ideas, indicative of scattered thinking processes. The flow of his speech may be slow and hesitant, slurred, or mumbled. Response time to questioning often is retarded. The content of his thought may indicate that he is misperceiving environmental stimuli, thus experiencing delusions. Repetitive themes often are present in his verbalizations. Illusions or hallucinations in any of the sensory modalities may be present. The patient's affect may also be inappropriate to his thought content. The patient's mood is labile: one minute he is crying, the next he is angry and hostile.

In assessing the patient whose thought processes are impaired, the nurse recognizes that the patient's attention span is minimal and that he is easily distracted by environmental stimuli. The patient's behavior is not goal-oriented: Because he misperceives stimuli, the patient may attempt to pull out tubes and tear off dressings. Eye contact is also poor, and the patient may not be responsive to touch.

Interventions

When a patient demonstrates that his thinking processes are impaired, the nursing goals are aimed at helping the patient differentiate reality from nonreality. Frequently providing the patient with information that supports orientation to place, time, and situation is paramount. Consistently modifying and interpreting the environment for the patient using his intact sensory modalities supports the patient in differentiating real from unreal. Respecting the patient's inappropriate thinking and asking for clarification in a calm, interested manner often allows the nurse to understand the patient's confusion. Because the patient is at risk for paranoid ideation, the nurse needs to explain all that she is doing.[26] Being cognizant of body posture and facial expressions is key: The patient's concerns are real, as is his fear, and must be taken seriously. Interpreting events realistically may not diminish the patient's concerns, but he relies on the nurse to support him in gaining clarity and control of his situation.

Social Isolation

While the nurse is constantly assessing the patient's level of interaction and modifying his regressive tendencies, the patient is acting out his dependency needs and other needs and wishes in his relationships with family, significant others, and friends. Because the latter are not usually cognizant of the patient's intrapsychic struggles, they may withdraw from him rather than be confronted with these seemingly unpleasant and meaningless outbursts. When this happens, the patient is socially isolated.

Although society places a high value on the independently functioning person, it is the unusual person who can exist without the acceptance and love of important others in his life. Whether imposed by the patient, the trauma, or the significant other(s), isolation from support and caring may occur at a time when support is sorely needed. Such a loss only adds to the already felt loss of self-esteem and worth.

Nursing Assessment and Interventions

Alterations in the usual methods of interacting with others compound the patient's isolation. Isolation is reflected in the patient's behavior by irritability, lack of activity, apathy, and anxiety. In essence, isolation can lead to impaired thinking processes. The trauma nurse is the bridge to social interaction. The nurse interfaces most often with the patient's significant others and must bring them, in tangible ways, into the narrow environment of the critical care unit. By encouraging the family to make tapes of their activities that can be played to the patient during the day, the patient is kept involved in family activities. Cards, pictures, and important objects from home can all be used to bring some familiarity into the hospital environment.

When the nurse is providing care to the patient, she can use that time to discuss what is happening in the world outside. Information about a patient's special hobbies or interests can be gleaned from both the patient and significant others. Talking about these interests provides the patient with some respite from his chronic concerns. It is also important to directly address the patient's feelings of loneliness and to seek his opinion as to what may be helpful. Introducing the patient to different staff members as they enter his room expands the scope of familiar faces with whom he can interact.

When family members visit the patient, they may initially feel uncomfortable in the intensive care unit. Explaining the environment and encouraging them to talk with, touch, or help the patient include them in his care. Simply giving family members some small task initiates a more comfortable feeling for them and involves them in this different relationship.

Although in this text we have chosen to artificially separate the patient's journey from that of the family, no such separation exists in reality. It is the task of the nurse to constantly bridge relationships during the critical care cycle so that each significant other is actively involved and connected. Social isolation is minimized to the degree that the nurse guides and involves the patient's interaction with significant others.

Extrapsychic Influences: Sensory-Perceptual Processes

Data from the immediate environment are received through functional sensory modalities. How reality is construed depends on the patient's ability to appropriately process the raw data: This occurs when end organs and cues are intact and appropriate. To determine meaningfulness, the patient has to have intact sensory receptors, stimuli of appropriate intensity, and information-processing capabilities that allow for interpretation of the information. Although the physical pathways involved in the perceptual processing of information are universal, the interpretation and assignment of meaning to events are uniquely individual. Imperative to an understanding of a person's interpretation and response to stressful environments is the understanding of the physiological activity and response to these.

As in the resuscitative cycle, sensory stimulation remains problematic. Orientation is promoted through continuous meaningful input from the environment. Perception of the environment rests on a person's ability to organize, synthesize, and categorize sensory information. Hence, the quantity, intensity, and familiarity of the stimuli are crucial. Whereas there was an overload of cues bombarding the patient on admission and during his resuscitation, throughout the critical care cycle the opposite tends to be the case as predictable stimuli occur with monotonous regularity. Overload is still a problem, however, in a crowded environment.

The literature describes a multiplicity of observable behavioral changes following deprivation of stimulation, but these changes are usually specific to healthy individuals participating in research studies. Similar responses are seen in patients in critical care units. Symptoms observed include disorientation; auditory, visual, and tactile hallucinations; delusions; impaired perception; impaired visual-motor coordination; increased sensitivity to pain; and impaired judgment and intellectual functioning.[27–30]

Neurobiological Nature of Stress

The primary biopsychosocial manifestations of the generalized stress response consists of redirecting behavior by way of the central nervous system and redirecting energy in the periphery. When homeostasis is threatened, the corticotropin-releasing hormone and locus ceruleus–norepinephrine systems act directly within the central nervous system to promote attention, arousal, and aggression. At the same time, they are inhibiting nonadaptive pathways that promote vegetative functions, such as feeding, sexual activity, activity cycle alterations, and mood variations.[31–37] Peripheral adaptation occurs through the redirection of blood flow to the central nervous system, which then mobilizes fuel for action. In the short run, this fight-or-flight response is beneficial. If sustained over time, however, the effects can be devastating (Fig. 10–5). This is particularly problematic during extended periods of emotional distress because resolution of issues seldom is achieved quickly or definitively. Table 10–1 reflects the acute behavioral and physiological changes that occur in response to stress.

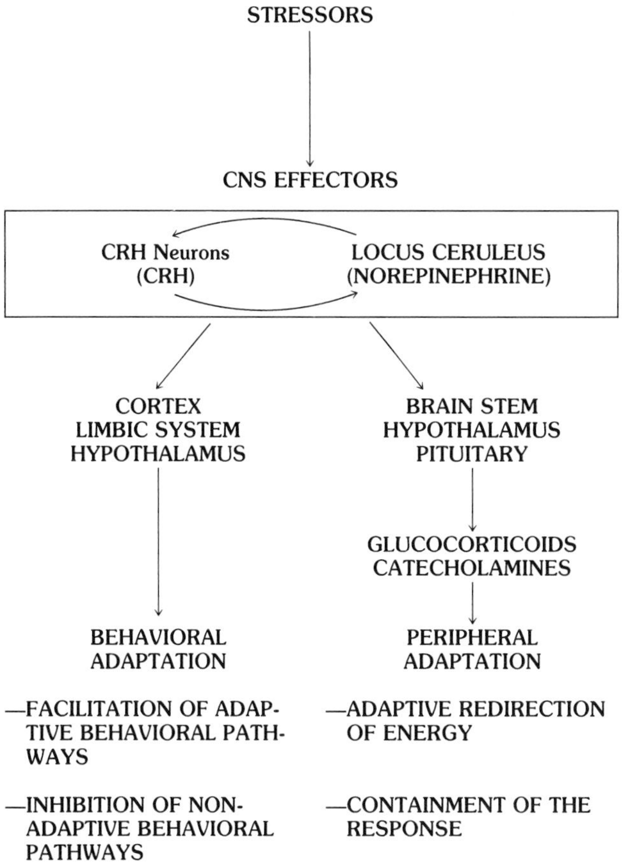

Figure 10–5. Schematic diagram of stress-mediated central effectors. Arrows show the function of central effectors in facilitating a characteristic behavioral and peripheral response to stress. CNS, central nervous system; CRH, corticotropin-releasing hormone. (Reprinted with permission from Gold PW, Goodwin FK, Chrousos GP: Clinical and biochemical manifestations of depression. Relation to the neurobiology of stress. N Engl J Med 319:413–420, 1988.)

Nursing Assessment

Injury to any or several of the sense organs, pain, isolation, and diminished mobility and environmental stimulation are some of the factors that result in alterations in the patient's sensory-perceptual processes. The nursing assessment includes evaluation of each of the patient's sensory modalities for their ability to provide environmental information. Immobility results in minimal input visually as well as kinesthetically: The patient is unable to receive feedback that allows him to orient his body and its parts in relation to the environment simply because movement is limited and the visual range from which to select input is narrow. Taste and smell are restricted if the critical care patient does not eat by mouth. Tactile stimulation is most often painful, and auditory input is restricted to the immediate, monotonous environment. After assessing the ability of sensory modalities to process information, the nurse can provide meaningful inputs into these modalities.

Interventions

Frequent orientation to the patient's surroundings, which includes equipment he can see or hear and people in the environment, is necessary. Using the patient's intact sensory modalities to explain the environment is critical. The patient can process facts more efficiently when he is able to touch, see, and hear an object rather than just perceive it through the provision of verbal information. Focusing attention on

TABLE 10–1. GENERAL ADAPTATIONAL RESPONSE TO STRESS

TYPE OF CHANGE	STRESS
Redirection of behavior by the central nervous system	Acute facilitation of adaptive neural pathways
	Arousal, alertness
	Increased vigilance, focused attention
	Aggressiveness when appropriate
	Acute inhibition of non-adaptive pathways
	Decreased eating
	Decreased libido and sexual behavior
	Appropriate caution or restraint
Redirection of energy in the periphery	Oxygen and nutrients to the stressed body site
	Increased blood pressure, heart and respiratory rates
	Increased gluconeogenesis
	Increased lipolysis
	Inhibition of programs for growth and reproduction
	Acute glucocorticoid-mediated counterregulatory responses
	Restraint of the corticotropin-releasing hormone system and the pituitary-adrenal axis
	Restraint of the norepinephrine–locus ceruleus system
	Restraint of the expected immunologic or inflammatory response

Adapted from Gold PW et al: Clinical and biochemical manifestations of depression. N Engl J Med 319:413–420, 1988.

and showing a patient part of his body when doing passive range-of-motion exercises helps the patient recognize his body in space. Involving the patient in the exercises also increases his attention span and concentration abilities. Because the patient tends to disassociate the injured part of his body from the rest of his self, the nurse supports the integration of the injured part by repersonalizing and identifying it as the patient's right leg or left arm. Patients who objectify body parts by referring to them as "that leg" or "that arm" psychologically have depersonalized a portion of their bodies and need the support of staff to integrate and own the injured part.

Time Orientation

Time orientation, which is influenced by light and dark, eating patterns, and sleeping patterns, no longer follows a consistent, cyclical pattern, and there is a loss of the usual references to time. Night may not be differentiated from day because the noise level may diminish only slightly; lights may remain on constantly, eating probably is contraindicated, and sleeping frequently is disrupted for nursing and medical procedures that often involve painful intrusions. Clocks, when present, provide no clue as to night or day. This beginning of time disruption in the alert patient often is exhibited by the gradual loss of a few hours, progressing to an inability to know the day, month, or season.

Nursing Assessment and Interventions

As with all the extrapsychic influences that can rapidly result in deterioration of the trauma patient's cognitive and affective functioning, it is crucial that the nurse anticipate the potential hazards the patient is exposed to by virtue of the environment. Preventive measures are by far the most significant in attenuating the impact on the patient's psyche. Recognizing that sensory overload and deprivation as well as time disruption are inherently present, the nurse minimizes the impact by structuring and making the environment meaningful.[38]

Assessment of time orientation is achieved by soliciting this information from the patient. At the beginning of each shift, the nurse provides the patient with this basic information and consistently reinforces it throughout the shift. Trauma patients frequently describe the passing of time as inexorably slow. Minutes seem like hours. Because environmental cues are not always informative, patients begin to pattern their recognition of time around people, treatments, and medications. These cues need constant reinforcement verbally from the nurse. Daytime can be further refined for the patient by referring to small blocks of time, e.g., early morning, breakfast, and late morning. Information that allows the patient to orient to season can be included in conversations: weather or sports results, for example. Physical cues, such as clocks and lights that are turned off at night, need to be present and used. Structured patterns of activities eventually become associated with time frames and also need verbal reinforcement.

Sleep Deprivation

Physiological systems function on a cyclical basis with activity cycles being followed by seemingly quiescent periods. The evidence of this rhythmic pattern is seen throughout nature: all life exhibits phases of activity counterbalanced by periods of inactivity. In humans, inactivity is exemplified most clearly in sleep cycles. During this period of rest, all physiological functions are maintained with a minimum expenditure of energy. The process of sleep occurs in stages, with gradual withdrawal from the environment and its stimuli. People usually get 5 to 8 hours of uninterrupted sleep. During this period, a person passes through the stages of sleep several times, with each cycle decreasing in length until he awakens.

Sleep Architecture

Normal sleep is divided into two phases: rapid eye movement (REM) and non-REM sleep. Non-REM sleep consists of four stages. Sleep begins at stage 1 and continues to stage 4. After a person has been asleep for about 70 to 90 minutes, the first period of REM occurs. Throughout the night, another three to five REM periods occur, usually in the latter part of the night. These REM periods increase in length as the night progresses.

Sleep and wake cycles normally follow the 24-hour cycle of light and dark. When continuous lighting exists, an endogenous oscillator drives this 24-hour rhythm with an intrinsic period of about 25 hours.[39, 40] In critically ill patients, after days of free-running, the sleep-wake cycle begins to lengthen and separates from the 25-hour intrinsic rhythm of temperature, adrenal, and REM sleep rhythms.[41] This desynchronization suggests the presence of related but independent oscillators.

Trauma patients experience abnormalities in sleep patterns and duration. These changes occur in both REM and non-REM sleep and appear to reflect a pathological state of arousal. This is reflected in non-REM abnormalities such as prolonged sleep latency, increased wakefulness, decreased arousal threshold, and early-morning awakening.[42, 43] Studies have shown that normal people who experience extended sleep and are in a state of sleep satiety[44] have REM abnormalities that are similar to those of depressed people: short REM latency and redistribution of REM sleep to the first half of the night.[45, 46] These studies suggest that trauma patients may be in a chronic state of sleep satiety or arousal and that the increased need for REM early in sleep may be in response to the trauma patient's attempts to compensate for his hyperaroused state. To restore normal patterns of REM sleep in these patients, antidepressants that diminish the overall locus ceruleus firing may reduce the frequency and intensity of REM sleep.[47, 48]

An important phase of sleep is when the person dreams; this particular phase, called REM, lasts for about 90 minutes and is followed by deeper levels of sleep. During REM sleep, the person may easily be aroused by environmental stimulation and, on awakening, remembers what he is dreaming about. At this point, disorientation is evident and the person is not aware of what is real and what is part of his dream as evidenced by hypnopompic hallucinations. In this type of hallucination, the person incorporates stimuli from the environment into his dream, hence often presenting bizarre thought content. Research has shown that people who are repeatedly awakened during the REM stage and not allowed to progress through an entire cycle of sleep exhibit varying degrees of inability to test reality and display signs of agitation and confusion. In the severely injured patient, procedures and excessive stimulation frequently prevent extended periods of sleep, with the result that sleep deprivation occurs in a matter of days. The importance of providing meaningful sleep time rests in the awareness of nursing staff in scheduling care. Sleeping medication, primarily barbiturates, blocks the REM stage of sleep and only contributes to sleep deprivation.[49]

Nursing Assessment and Interventions

In addition to excessive stimulation, medications, anxiety, fear, pain, and immobility all contribute to disruption of sleep patterns. Trauma patients who are experiencing sleep deprivation frequently are irritable and disoriented and display memory and thinking impairments. Many trauma patients doze for brief periods and claim that they are unable to fall asleep.

Assessment data that are critical to determining sleep disturbances must be collected from family and nursing staff. A reliable sleep history, before trauma, establishes the patient's baseline sleeping patterns and requirements. Information elicited from family or significant others should include usual bed and arising times, use of naps, use of adjuncts to sleep, bedtime rituals, problems in the past with falling asleep, and fears. A running data base of the actual time the patient sleeps in a 24-hour span can be collected and recorded by nursing staff. The nursing staff is also able to identify and address those factors that contribute to sleep disturbances.

The goal of the trauma nurse is to provide an environment that not only is conducive to sleeping but also allows the maximum quantity and quality of sleep.

Interventions focus on minimizing interruptions when the patient is attempting to rest. This requires the nurse to structure care and treatments so that the patient has blocks of uninterrupted sleep time. Decreasing environmental noise and lighting also facilitates sleep. Relaxation techniques such as back rubs, guided imagery, and music facilitate onset of sleep. Reassuring the frightened patient that the presence of the nurse remains while he is sleeping diminishes anxiety and his need for constant vigilance. Many trauma patients calmly drift off to sleep in the presence of someone they trust. Taking the time to sit and do charting quietly at the bedside provides the patient with a sense of security. Because patients need between 70 and 100 minutes of uninterrupted sleep to complete one full cycle of quality sleep, an ongoing chart that documents how well this is achieved is valuable. Quality sleep renews the patient both physically and psychologically and does much to enhance the healing process.

Loss of Emotional Control

Because traumatic injuries are accompanied by situations and procedures that cause pain and loss of normal emotional control of behavior, the patient, in an attempt to allay his anxiety, may react with loud crying, dependent behavior, use of obscenities, and questioning of the staff's ability to care for him. This may not be the person's normal repertoire of responses. The person feels extremely vulnerable to this lack of personal control, since it may lead to further isolation by staff as well as loss of self-esteem. If the response of the staff is one of ridicule of the behavior rather than insight into the emotional needs being expressed by the behavior, anxiety and fear are increased.

As the patient moves through the critical care cycle, the magnitude of the number and variety of losses he encounters and experiences is startling. This cycle has seen losses regarding his usual communication modalities, physical functioning, interpersonal relationships, environmental issues, alterations in roles, and invasion of boundaries of the self, to name but a few. The threat of powerlessness is profound. Patients respond with a variety of behavior ranging from hostility and dependence to withdrawal and lack of motivation and interest in their environment. The inability to make simple decisions or take an interest in what is happening to them reflects the deep sense of helplessness and hopelessness they are experiencing.

Throughout the patient's stay in the intensive care unit, the nurse constantly assesses and balances when and to what extent the patient can actively or passively make decisions and participate in his care. A sense of personal autonomy is enhanced every time the nurse solicits the patient's views, preferences, and opinions. As the nurse selects opportunities that allow and support the patient's decision making and control over his environment, personal control is enhanced. Small achievements are consistently pointed out and hope is renewed. The nurse's ability to diagnose, assess, and intervene in this phase of trauma sets the groundwork for psychological restoration.

STRESSORS AND NURSE/PATIENT COPING RESPONSES DURING THE INTERMEDIATE CYCLE

> Should you shield the canyons from the wind storms, you would never see the beauty of their carvings.
>
> Elisabeth Kübler-Ross[50]

At the juncture where the patient moves from critical to intermediate status, he is out of physical danger and ready to address the meaning of the sequelae resulting from the physical injuries that were incurred. At times, the patient's perception of his physical status is quite different from the nurse's. At the beginning of this cycle of the journey back to health, the patient may still perceive himself as seriously ill. The nurse knows that this is not the case, and much of the interaction between the two involves the nurse's fostering the belief that the patient is better and can act more in his own behalf. At this point, the patient usually is in a less constricted and more relaxed environment.

The patient, better physically, has more energy to focus on the meaning of his disability and the physical alterations of his body. He is no longer overwhelmed with the struggle to simply survive. Energy that was focused on that struggle is now freed up to grieve perceived losses and to act out needs and feelings that were promptly responded to when the patient was critically ill. When nursing actions are no longer prompt and responsive to the patient's immediate need, he may quickly feel unsafe and insecure. This fosters uncontrollable anxiety and sometimes rage. The intermediate cycle of care may be marked by interpersonal struggle and conflict because of these issues. Although the critical care cycle is undeniably dynamic, there usually exists a nonproblematic, nonconflictual relationship between patient and nurse in which the nurse advocates for and supports the patient. In the intermediate care phase, the patient begins to resume responsibility for his own care and activities of daily living. The process of reassumption is not without its struggles, both intrapsychically for the patient and interpersonally between nurse and patient. Once the patient realizes that he is indeed better, his struggle is to emerge from passive receptivity and become tolerant of the necessary delays between announcing his needs for assistance and the nurse's unavoidable delays in responding.

Continued Grief Work: Anger

Dominating the patient's psychosocial needs is the need to cope with his losses of body parts or functions by grieving. The grieving process, characterized by an initial denial of the loss, is more typically observed in patients during the critical care cycle of their recovery. Anger, minimally evidenced in the critical care cycle, is now expressed overtly in the intermediate care cycle because the patient has more available energy to feel and express anger. The anger may be projected, intellectualized, or disguised in some other ways. At times, it may be blatantly expressed. The patient may express hostility verbally and physically and project his hostility at the staff for their perceived inadequacies. He may also be excessively demanding or whining. This displacement of anger on the staff provides the patient with a sense of power in his helpless state: he has in fact placed the problem on the staff rather than acknowledging the problem that he is struggling to master. Guilt may be part of the clinical picture as well as a blaming process. One of the themes of this adjustment period is finding meaning in the loss by assigning blame to someone and then focusing anger on that person.

Nursing Assessment and Interventions

In both the resuscitation and the critical care cycles, the mental status examination's greatest utility is that it provides an objective tool in assessment of the patient's sensorium and perception. Although the tool measures the patient's functioning at the time of assessment, cumulative data are useful in recognizing trends and changes in the patient's cognitive functioning. Because the patient's sensorium usually stabilizes as he improves physiologically, the tool becomes valuable in the intermediate and rehabilitative cycles in assessing the trauma patient's thought processes, mood, and affect. Changes in affect related to thought content may now be accessible to discussion because the patient is able to verbalize his thinking with the nurse. Thought content usually focuses on concerns and fears about what effects the traumatic injury has on the patient's present and future life. Variation in mood can objectively be assessed by the nurse as it relates to specific thought content. Accurate assessment facilitates utilization of the most appropriate nursing interventions and highlights areas of concern where additional therapeutic support is indicated.

In this cycle, it is urgent that the nurse not get drawn into the patient's struggle with intrapsychic forces: the nurse must not defend or attack the patient. His behavior might be provocative, but the sensitive and skilled trauma nurse recognizes that this is a transient phase in which the patient is struggling with his own denial, anger, and feelings of helplessness and powerlessness. Responding to the patient's psychosocial needs appropriately requires that the nurse listen without defensiveness. She must hear, acknowledge that the patient has been heard, and introduce reality when the patient distorts it. The nurse must assess the cause of inappropriate behavior and modify that. The behavior itself is basically incidental to the larger issue of its underlying cause. The nurse identifies the behavior and labels it for the patient so that nurse and patient together can explore its meaning and underlying causes. For instance, if the patient is shouting and crying, the nurse might say, "You sound angry." The patient might then shout, "I am." The nurse responds, "Can we talk about what you are angry at?" This exchange fosters a further understanding of the patient's experience. If an environmental cause is established for the patient's anger, the nurse can try to modify that factor or she can seek the patient's assistance in modifying it so that the patient does not have to feel so angry. If the patient cannot identify a cause for his feeling, the nurse might infer that it reflects the struggle that the patient is undergoing in learning to control his needs and energy discharge.

Although anger was encountered in the critical care cycle, it is much more overtly and intensely expressed in the intermediate care cycle. Anger frequently may be seen in acting-out behaviors. These are actions in which the patient expresses his feelings without actually identifying them as such. Some examples of acting out are throwing food, trays, or other belongings and shouting for the nurse rather than using the call light. Acting out may be seen in depression when the patient is working through grief. In fact, any of these behaviors might be seen in any phase of grief work because it is a dynamic process that does not unfold in a systematic way. There are progressions and regressions; themes overlap and then come apart. The observation of grief work is inferred from the predominance of behaviors that are used over a period of time. When the patient is angry, energy is available for channeling. Sometimes the creative nurse can focus this energy into learning about the patient's needs and his self-care potential. At other times, the energy is too scattered for channeling.

Depression

On the heels of anger comes depression. The patient seems to withdraw; however, this is not an inert, passive stage. Unlike in the denial stage, when the patient would not deal with the loss, at this juncture, he is actively exploring the loss. Withdrawal seems to occur in the service of conservation of energy, which is then used to actively come to terms with the meaning of the loss and to integrate that loss into the present. Meaningfulness is attributed to events when causal relationships exist, when their predictability and regularity are a commonly occurring phenomenon, and when they are controlled and affected by the person's actions. Belief that one's actions do in fact affect change creates a personal sense of hopefulness that in turn motivates the person to respond.

After a traumatic injury, hope is lost. Depression signals the beginning of a trauma patient's search for confirmation of his existence. The patient still cannot envision a future, but he is no longer stuck in the past. There is a definite sense of struggle with what now is, and as the depression lightens, the struggle becomes one of what will be in the future.

Nursing Assessment and Intervention

Trauma patients who experience depression reflect changes in their mental status relating primarily to mood and affect. Physical appearance deteriorates; little attention is given to personal hygiene, so that a disheveled or unkempt appearance evolves. Posture often is stooped, and the facial expression suggests sadness. Interpersonal relationships deteriorate, especially with the nursing staff. The patient often is apathetic, unmotivated, and detached from events and people in his environment. Spontaneous interactions are minimal: the patient seldom initiates conversation. His appetite diminishes, and previous sleep patterns change, usually with the patient complaining of fatigue or sleeping excessively. Thought processes are slowed and content reflects negativity, primarily aimed at the self: self-criticism, negativity, and indecisiveness are verbalized. Motor activity diminishes, and vocal tone is monotonous. The patient often expresses lability in mood and may have crying spells. A complete mental status examination coupled with clinical observation reflects this profile.

The complex interaction that the trauma nurse now participates in challenges both her knowledge and her skill. To be responsive to the patient, the nurse must fight her natural inclination to withdraw. She must stay in meaningful contact with the patient by acknowledging the meaning of the patient's nonverbal behaviors and by a return to advocating the best possible environment for the patient. This may mean doing things for the patient that he was able to do for himself during the cycle of denial and anger. As the patient is withdrawing to conserve energy, so the nurse now has to expend more energy. During this cycle, as in other cycles, the nurse legitimates the patient's experience by interpreting and characterizing it for the patient as a normal albeit painful process, one through which the patient must work. As the depression lifts, the patient reinvolves self in his environment and the people in it. Once again, the nurse should set small, achievable goals so that the patient experiences mastery over his external environment. As the patient confirms his sense of competence, the nurse reaffirms his sense of worth.

Prolonged Depression

A percentage of trauma patients do experience prolonged despair and depression. The boundary between normal and pathological depression is difficult to draw initially, since the characteristics of both are similar in expression and content. Pathological depression is characterized by the severity and pervasiveness of the symptoms as well as by the person's loss of contact with his present reality.

Nursing Assessment and Interventions

In pathologically depressed people, the mental status examination reveals significant distortions in perception, thought processes, and mood and affect. Withdrawal from the environment is almost complete; the patient has little interest or energy in doing anything, including taking care of his basic needs. Significant weight loss, suicidal ideation, verbalized distorted perceptions of self, expressions of feelings of unreality, insomnia, and verbalizations that are incomprehensible to the listener are all symptoms of immediate concern. A psychiatric nursing consult should be initiated when the nurse's assessment of the patient's mental status reflects increasing severity of depressive symptoms. Antidepressants in conjunction with daily therapy are adjuncts to care. These alone, however, are not sufficient. In collaboration with the psychiatric clinical nurse specialist, psychiatrist, and patient, the nurse explores effective strategies and implements plans that support the patient in regaining his connectedness to himself and his environment. Continued belief in the patient's ability to successfully regain control of his feelings and environment is reflected in the nurse's consistent presence and interactions. This hopefulness, on some level, may be perceived by the depressed patient and ultimately experienced by him.[51]

Socialization

A marked difference between the critical care and the intermediate care cycles is the level of interaction and the diversity of people available for social exchange. These variables can be stressors, and they can also be experienced as supportive. The critically ill patient is aware first and foremost of himself. Next in frequency of perception is the presence of the nurse and intimate others. Once moved to intermediate care, the patient becomes aware of others like himself. There is both competition for care and cooperation such that patients themselves exchange care and services. It is also a time of networking and of comparing wounds and injuries. Patients use one another as confidants. They compare their own injuries with those of their peers. They soften their own harsh perceptions and expectations of others' perceptions of themselves through their positive interactions with one another. Mr. A.'s injuries typically are accepted without noticeable reactions by Mr. B. Mr. A. is then able to be more accepting of himself. In these microcosmic events, patients prepare themselves for the experiences they will have in the world beyond the hospital.

Environmental Expansion

In this cycle are further normative tendencies that evolve through the introduction of diversionary activities and return to more health status–related activities such as reading books, watching television, and listening to the radio. These diversionary activities also aid the patient in bringing back into his life factors that are not contaminated by the experience of the injury. This allows the patient some respite from the constant focusing on trauma, treatment, and recovery.

Activity Tolerance

Routines of care become comprehensible and more actively involve the participation of the patient. Normative routines such as eating, bathing, and participating in physical and occupational therapy have been introduced into the patient's day. All these activities tend to strengthen the patient's cognitive functioning, especially his problem-solving and decision-making abilities. Because the patient has been immobile and potentially nutritionally depleted, the nurse must systematically work with the patient to increase his ability to tolerate activity.

Nursing Assessment and Interventions

Trauma patients in the intermediate care cycle usually want to increase their physical activity rapidly because they see themselves progressing and want to return home. Careful assessment of the patient's tolerance of activity and structuring of mobility plans result in success and achievement of goals. The nurse assesses for physical, environmental, and treatment factors that can cause fatigue. Mobility plans are increased as patients demonstrate physical tolerance of them. Establishing small goals so that patients experience a sense of accomplishment and movement toward a larger goal is accomplished by nurse and patient together. Frequent rest periods are scheduled into the day's activities.

To prevent monotony, routines need to be varied. Patients need alternative choices that diminish the sense of boredom. Family and friends may need to have their time scheduled by the patient to avoid overstimulation when all arrive at once and monotony when none is present.

Encouraging patients to interact and help one another can be achieved through the provision of group learning situations. Patients with similar learning needs may be able to be brought together for instruction and support.

A nonstimulating environment can result in excessive sleeping and prolonged depression. The goal of nursing is to support the patient in recognizing activities and alternatives that are available and appropriate for him to engage in, given the constraints imposed by the injury. Once again, it is far simpler to prevent boredom and its sequelae by planning activities and structuring the environment so that diversion is possible.

Family Roles

Another characteristic of this cycle of recovery is the expanding role the family plays in the patient's physical care. Although the nurse was in constant attendance of both patient and family in the critical care cycle, her interactions with patient and family often were separate. Now there is a merging of patient and family interests and skills in the service of self-care for the patient. The nurse spends a larger proportion of time educating them as a unit. The family may lose track of the necessity of "making haste slowly," and the nurse must refocus both on setting short-term goals that are achievable for the patient, which inevitably will lead to meeting his long-term objectives. For instance, the patient and family are probably invested in an amputee's learning to walk again. Progressive daily and weekly goals aimed at facilitating the strengthening of musculature in concert with movement of the patient from the constricted environment of his cubicle to the wider environment of the corridor, albeit in a wheelchair, systematically prepare the patient for the long-anticipated day when self-mobility is achieved.

STRESSORS AND PATIENT/NURSE COPING RESPONSES IN THE REHABILITATION CYCLE

> Tho' much is taken, much abides; . . . that which we are, we are . . .[52]
>
> Alfred, Lord Tennyson

When the trauma patient has reached the rehabilitative cycle, he is well into his journey back to health. For the spinal cord–injured and the head-injured trauma patient, this cycle is longer. For the multisystem-injured person, this cycle may be shorter than that of critical and intermediate care. Almost all patients must address additional definable tasks to achieve adaptation to their losses. Included are a modification of values that facilitate incorporation of an altered body image, a resumption of prior roles and functions with appropriate modifications, a shift from dependence to expanded independent functioning, and a regaining of a future orientation. At this juncture, the patient usually does not deny the extent of disability or its long-term meaning. Psychological reintegration is very much a matter of incorporating the new identity into the boundaries of the old and learning to function as productively as possible, given the person's realistic capabilities. No longer is the impulse to return to the time before the trauma; rather, what was meaningful in the past must now be reinterpreted to fit into a new and different future. Continuity and predictability are restored.

Continuing the trend that emerged in the intermediate cycle, the patient uses the nurse and peer group increasingly to test reality by asking for feedback regarding his impact on them. Responses from significant people in the environment may be so subtly elicited and examined that the nurse may not be cognizant that her reactions and responses are being carefully evaluated by the patient.

Values Clarification

Perhaps the most significant shift that occurs in the psychosocial aspect of the patient's rehabilitation is the change of focus in the patient's value system. Although the patient's physical integrity abruptly changes after traumatic injury, it is only with time that the person can incorporate this alteration psychologically. Although physically different, the patient still holds the beliefs and values he had before his injury. Naturally, his reference point is that of a noninjured person. The patient brings to his current situation all the feelings and perceptions he had of injured people: they were less than whole, they were noncontributing members of society, they were burdens on those around them, they were unfortunate people. Now, *he* is one of those unfortunate people. To accurately realign these perceptions, the trauma patient must address the sense that he is an unfortunate person and extricate himself from his devalued position. To effect this change, he must rationally examine previously held beliefs and values, acknowledging the deficits and misperceptions that exist in his thinking. Devaluation occurs because the trauma patient's values are still those of a noninjured person. The first step on this voyage is to recognize that differences do exist: he is no longer a noninjured person. This is an incredibly difficult process because values and beliefs do not exist in isolation from each other. Alteration of one value has the potential to alter many others. The patient now must look to enlarging the scope of his values to identify other capabilities that the injury has not affected. He must place the lost values in a broader scope and in reference to his total value system. For example, in contending with the issue of physical appearance, the patient with a noticeable, disfiguring facial injury must first recognize that physically, his injury is unattractive. He may think that when others look at him, they see only the disfigurement and nothing else. This is perhaps an accurate reflection of his own values before his injury. What he must recognize now is that physical appearance, although certainly valuable, is but part of a bigger picture: that of his total personality presentation. His sense of devaluation will diminish as he is able to incorporate the importance of physical appearance into the larger scope that now includes the presentation of total personality. He must come to understand that people around him respond to his personality in positive or negative ways because the critical aspect of evaluation is personality, not physical appearance. Therefore, although physical appearance is a component of evaluation, it is not the primary factor for the valuing of a person.[53, 54]

The major shift that occurs in the person's value system pivots on the ability to change his frame of reference from a comparative belief system to one of an asset value system. Throughout life, most people hear, "Do the best you can, that's all that's expected." The reality is that people are taught to compare talents, abilities, and financial success with those around them. People learn to look at life comparing themselves with others: sometimes they have more than and sometimes less than those around them. When life is viewed from this framework, people indeed see themselves as less than acceptable in some ways and more than acceptable in others. The traumatized person, to adapt, must change this frame of reference. He must shift to an asset value system in which he is able to recognize and value his current assets, while mourning the loss of his former ones. This means that potentials and abilities, when present, are good; however, when they are absent, that is not bad. The trauma patient must focus on maximizing the assets he has. This does not mean that he minimizes what is no longer present; rather, he focuses on what is and what he can achieve. When capable of doing this, the trauma patient is free of the ghosts from his past. The trauma patient no longer focuses on the time before his accident. He values the present, what is. He no longer subscribes to the value system of a noninjured person. He accepts himself with both his differences and his assets.

New Body Image

Concurrent healing of the body and a successful shift in values and beliefs enable the trauma patient to gradually come to accept his new body image. His altered physical capacities foster tentative inquiry about new roles and functions. No longer does the patient say, "I can't," but instead he ponders, "How can I?" In the rehabilitative cycle, the patient tries out and modifies new body movements that will compensate for those that have been lost. New ways of thinking about solving problems emerge. The patient gives up his taken-for-granted "whole body" basis from which tasks used to be accomplished. Now, gradually, the patient comes to address new situations from the modified baseline of a disabled person. The double amputee who used to go to the cupboard to get a glass when thirsty now must think and grapple with the problem of *how* to get the glass off the shelf! In this cycle, frustration and intolerance give way to patience and acceptance of one's actual abilities. The trauma patient learns to *expect* the expenditure of time that is required to think through and execute a plan of action tailored to the deficits with which he lives. Related to this expanded capacity to problem solve is the trend to act autonomously. This potential, which emerged in the intermediate cycle, plays an ever increasing role in the patient's recovery as he assumes more and more responsibility while the nurse relinquishes her control.

Nursing Assessment and Interventions

Perhaps the greatest challenges for the trauma patient and nurse lie in the rehabilitative cycle because it is here that both the art and the science of trauma nursing must be precisely articulated. The focus of nursing interventions hinges on the accumulated assessment of the patient's physical and psychological strengths. Data regarding the patient's perceptions, thought processes, mood, and affect are reliably obtained from the mental status examination. The patient's decision-making ability is reflected in his adaptive responses. These responses indicate that the patient is attempting to incorporate and address the changes in his current life space. Assessment of his ability is ascertained through observation and listening to the types of questions the patient generates. Patients who actively participate in their own care, appropriately seek assistance when necessary, and ask questions regarding particular aspects of their injury are indicating that they are regaining control over their physical self. Adaptation is greatly affected by the degree of dialogue that exists between the patient and the nurse. When feelings of hopelessness, anger, despair, and frustration are met with tolerance, hope, acceptance, and appropriate challenges, the patient's self-esteem and sense of personal power are manifested in increasing self-confidence and independence. The delicate balance between success and frustration in achieving independent functioning relies significantly on the nurse's ability to appropriately challenge the patient's energies. Goals that are too difficult or too easy to achieve result in either failure or frustration. Self-esteem, which results from the patient's critical evaluation of his own competencies, is enhanced when he achieves success in doing things on his own that are perceived as both difficult and important. In the rehabilitative cycle, the nurse's primary goal is to support and guide the patient in his efforts to integrate, relearn, experiment, and address the challenges he encounters. The nurse listens for the directions the patient chooses to take, suggests modifications usually reflective of greater realism, and makes referral to people and agencies that are equipped to aid the patient in his endeavor. Reconciliation of the past with the constraints of the present facilitates the patient's looking to the future.

Future Vision

Notable are the shifts in temporal orientation throughout the trauma patient's journey back to health. The reader will recall that the critical care cycle was a time of numbness, denial, and terror that gave way to a grasping for the past and clinging to the memory of what was. In the intermediate cycle, the patient could be characterized as living in the here and now, dealing with surviving and beginning to try to improve the quality of life. In the rehabilitative phase, the patient returns to a more normative future orientation. A hallmark of the rehabilitative cycle is the linking together of past, present, and future. Meaning is conferred through these linkages. Loss has been confronted and placed in perspective. Although the future may not be defined, the patient looks to it with renewed confidence that he can overcome problems and lead a productive life again.

Community and Role Integration

Responsibility and accountability for the accidents that brought many trauma patients to the hospital must be addressed through litigation, worker's compensation, legal hearings, and incarceration. Although these considerations may be difficult for the nurse and patient to confront, the nurse must continue to support the patient in assuming the responsibilities that he must assume.

From the beginning of the trauma patient's journey back to health, he has been supported night and day by a caring staff and concerned family or significant others. Return to the community is marked by separation from the nurse and other care providers and a shift of total responsibility to the patient and family. Although the nurse has tried to educate patient and family about the patient's needs and treatment throughout the hospitalization, a rupture of this bond is still felt when the patient goes home.

The patient typically has dreamed about the day he could leave the confines of the hospital. Never in those fantasies does the patient deal with or even dream of the issues that are yet to ensue: the pain that will return; the social isolation that follows from moving into yet another confining room; the confusion that quickly emerges as family members scramble to hold onto or relinquish roles that they have taken on; the depression that ebbs and flows in response to the patient's frustrations when others view him as the poor, broken, handicapped victim—an image that the patient himself has struggled so hard to confront and change. There is no constant stream of well-wishers. Immobility makes the confines of the home close in when other family members leave to go to jobs all day. Pains return and it becomes obvious that they are chronic. The patient must now learn to cope with new and different concerns.

In the hospital, no sooner is the patient's bed cleaned and readied for a new trauma patient than the doors swing open once more, admitting the stretcher with another trauma patient. The nurse begins a new journey. The patient who has returned to the community and found it lonely may return to the hospital to help others, say hello, and perhaps visit the scene of his recent trauma to gain more perspective. When he returns, it is quickly noted that new faces occupy old beds. Staff are friendly and courteous, but they are also preoccupied with new concerns for new patients. A multitude of clues tell the former patient that he does not fit in anymore. The patient's journey is not complete until he makes a new place for himself outside the hospital, beyond the framework of illness and disability. The former patient must integrate the new meanings in his life and the new identity into the larger community beyond the hospital walls.

Nursing Assessment and Interventions

A major component of the discharge planning process must address the psychosocial issues that both patient and family will encounter on leaving the hospital. These issues have been well articulated by recovering trauma patients and are presented here so that trauma nurses can realistically present them to and therefore plan with the patient and family before discharge.

The trauma patient has usually adapted to the routines and patterns of hospital life. He frequently has found safety in its environment, established solid relationships with staff, and found ways to address his psychosocial needs. The process of returning into his own home, resuming peer relationships and role expectations, requires a new conceptualization and a shifting from patient to person. Assuming the nurse has worked with the family to adapt the home setting to meet the physiological and mobility requirements of the patient, she now must focus on the emotional experiences that both must address.

Structuring of daily activities, a process begun in the hospital, must continue at home to relieve monotony. The patient in the hospital was previously the focal point of family activities. At home, others will be vying for attention and time as well. Patients need to get to know spouses as well as rediscover children. Loneliness, fear, pain, and frustration are experienced once again. Significant others' lives have continued to go on while the patient was hospitalized; they continue to do so. Friends and family who visited in the hospital may not make the same effort once the patient is home. The recovering patient can feel deserted because the hospital's intense level of stimulation is different from that of the home. Whereas others perhaps reached out to him initially, he must now learn to initiate social contact with them. Whereas a disfiguring injury is acceptable within the environs of the hospital, people will now stare at the recovering patient in public places.

By exploring the reality of these issues, the trauma nurse cognitively presents the patient with a picture of what may be encountered and stimulates his thinking about ways to address these issues. When resources exist in a community, the trauma nurse facilitates their utilization through referral.

Self-help groups composed of recovering trauma patients and their families are valuable vehicles for support after discharge. These groups provide opportunities for trauma patients to share their experiences, to review and normalize their feelings, and to solve problems that are common to the majority. Members identify resources for one another and support one another in the recovering process. Foremost, the self-help group provides a social forum in which former trauma patients are able to explore and problem solve concerns they experience in common after hospitalization.[55]

SUMMARY

The journey of the trauma patient toward adaptation is a struggle that exposes him and those around him to a vulnerability to life's events. The recovering patient no longer believes that "this can't happen to me": it has indeed happened.

The metaphor of trauma as a journey symbolizes the passage of the patient from one place in life to another. Unlike a voyage or a trip, the route is relatively uncharted and the destination open-ended. The outcome of this journey depends on those nurses he meets along the way; they are the gifted ones who will consistently guide, encourage, and challenge him in rediscovering hope and meaning in life.

Because dyadic relationships are both interactive and dynamic, the exchange between the trauma nurse and the patient leaves its mark on both. The astute trauma clinician will recognize that although she brings knowledge, skill, and insight to these relationships, she often walks away with far more: a unique appreciation of and glimpse at the incredible abilities of human beings to adapt to unimaginable life events.

Research Directions

As noted in the beginning of this chapter, research in the area of the psychosocial responses to acute traumatic injury has not been prolific. Solid data bases do exist, however, for trauma patients who experience central nervous system trauma and thermal trauma (see references in these chapters). The focus of this literature is primarily on the long-term outcomes of these events on the psychosocial functioning of trauma patients.

The rehabilitation literature extensively examines physiological, psychosocial, and vocational adaptation after traumatic injury. These data bases are primarily limited to people who have participated in extended rehabilitation programs. For the patient who is discharged from the hospital setting to home, little is known as to how and to what degree this person recovers psychologically, since tracking systems are almost nonexistent. Posttraumatic stress disorder, a syndrome experienced by some trauma patients, is receiving greater attention in the literature as trauma patients themselves seek professional help after injury when they are unable to cope and function (see Chapter 29).

The research that exists focuses more on the outcomes to the trauma patient than the processes. Many studies are done retrospectively rather than concurrently, hence compounding reliability and validity issues. Greater contributions are being made by nurses to the research effort.

Trauma nurses are in a unique position in that they are significantly exposed to the actual course of events experienced by patients throughout all the phases of the trauma cycle. Their empirical data base is extensive. Awareness of the themes that present themselves in each of the phases lends the issues to systematic study. The focus of the research might center on validating specific nursing interventions that lead to effective outcomes for the patient from both a short- and a long-term perspective. The critical care environment is conducive to experimental, descriptive, and ethnographic research of this kind.

Because trauma patients simultaneously are physically and psychologically disrupted, current psychological models do not provide adequate structure for studying their responses. For a suitable model that encompasses and represents the traumatic experience, nursing input, by way of research, is critical. The clinician of today must develop data bases to direct the efforts of tomorrow's trauma nurse. Pivotal to this endeavor, the author also strongly affirms the need for the active presence of a nurse who is clinically knowledgeable in both trauma and the psychosocial nursing sciences. Utilization of a psychiatric trauma clinical nurse specialist facilitates optimal outcomes for the trauma patient as he moves through the phases of trauma as well as enhancement of the trauma nurse's understanding of the psychosocial dynamics the patient exhibits. This person can provide much-needed emotional support not only to the patient but also to the nursing staff as they care for these patients throughout the cycles of trauma.

REFERENCES

1. Cummings ee: Complete Poems, 1913–1962. New York, Harcourt Brace Jovanovich, 1972, pp 461–462.

2. Marris P: Loss and Change. New York, Pantheon Books, 1974, pp 2–12.
3. Norman DA: Memory and Attention: An Introduction to Human Information Processing. 2nd ed. New York, John Wiley & Sons, 1976, pp 23, 31.
4. Ramsay RW, Noorbergen R: Living with Loss: A Dramatic New Breakthrough in Grief Therapy. New York, William Morrow & Co, 1981.
5. Kübler-Ross E: On Death and Dying. New York, Macmillan, 1969.
6. Engle G: Is grief a disease? Psychosom Med 23:18, 1961.
7. Lindeman E: Symptomatology and management of acute grief. Am J Psychiatry 101:141–148, 1944.
8. Hofer MA: Relationships as regulators: A psychological perspective on bereavement. Psychosom Med 46:183–197, 1984.
9. Fromm E, et al: Self-hypnosis as a therapeutic aid in the mourning process. Am J Clin Hypn 25:3–14, 1982.
10. Bowlby J: Attachment and loss: Restrospect and prospect. Am J Orthopsychiatry 52:664–678, 1982.
11. Brice CW: Mourning throughout the life cycle. Am J Psychoanal 42:315–325, 1982.
12. Mattson EI: Psychological aspects of severe physical injury and its treatment. J Trauma 15:217–233, 1975.
13. Marris P: Loss and Change. New York, Pantheon Books, 1974, pp 90–91.
14. Zubeck JP, Pushkar D, Sansom W, Gowing J: Perceptual changes after prolonged sensory isolation (darkness and silence). Can J Psychol 15:83–100, 1961.
15. Freedman SJ, Grunebaum HV, Greenblatt M: Perceptual and cognitive changes in sensory deprivation. In Solomon P, et al (eds): Sensory Deprivation. Cambridge, Mass, Harvard University Press, 1961, p 58.
16. Leiderman PH, Mendelson JH, Wexler D, et al: Sensory deprivation: Clinical aspects. Arch Intern Med 101:389, 1958.
17. Lipowski ZJ: Delirium: Clouding of consciousness and confusion. J Nerv Ment Dis 145:227–255, 1967.
18. Piaget J: The Child's Conception of the World. New York, Harcourt, Brace & Co., 1929.
19. Weiner B, Peter N: A cognitive-developmental analysis of achievement and moral judgments. Dev Psychol 9:290–309, 1973.
20. Schilder P: The Image and Appearance of the Human Body. New York, International Universities Press, 1950.
21. Maslow AH: Psychological data and value theory. In Maslow AH (ed): New Knowledge in Human Values. New York, Harper & Row, 1959.
22. Hackett TP, Cassom NH, Wishne HA: The coronary care unit: An appraisal of its psychological hazards. N Engl J Med 279:365–370, 1968.
23. Marris P: Loss and Change. New York, Pantheon Books, 1974, pp 31–32.
24. Zesook S, et al: Measuring symptoms of grief and bereavement. Am J Psychiatry 139:1590–1593, 1982.
25. Reite M, et al: Attachment, loss and depression. J Child Psychol Psychiatry 22:141–169, 1981.
26. Schnaper N: The psychological implications of severe trauma: Emotional sequelae to unconsciousness. A preliminary study. J Trauma 15:94–98, 1975.
27. Nadelson T: The psychiatrist in the surgical intensive care unit. I. Postoperative delirium. Arch Surg 111:113–117, 1976.
28. Kleck HG: ICU syndrome: Onset, manifestations, treatment, stressors and prevention. Crit Care Q 6:21–28, 1984.
29. Snyder-Halpern R: The effect of critical care unit noise on patient sleep cycles. Crit Care Q 7:41–50, 1985.
30. Felton G: Human biologic rhythms. In Fitzpatrick JJ, Taunton RL (eds): Annual Review of Nursing Research. New York, Springer, pp 45–77.
31. Gold PW, et al: Clinical and biochemical manifestations of depression. N Engl J Med 319:413–420, 1988.
32. Calabrese JR, Kling MA, Gold PW: Alterations in immunocompetence during stress, bereavement and depression: Focus on neuroendocrine regulation. Am J Psychiatry 144: 1123–1134, 1987.
33. Ganong WF: The stress response: A dynamic overview. Hosp Pract 155–171, June 15, 1988.
34. Gold PW, et al: The clinical implications of corticotropin-releasing hormone. In Chrousos GP, Loriaux DL, Gold PW (eds): Mechanisms of Physical and Emotional Stress. New York, Plenum, 1988, pp 507–519.
35. Katon W: Panic disorder in the medical setting. Publ. No. 89-1629. Rockville, Md, US Department of Health and Human Services.
36. Stein M, Keller SE, Schleifer SJ: Stress and immunomodulation: The role of depression and neuroendocrine function. J Immunol 135:827–833, 1985.
37. Gurgius GN, Uhde TW: Anxiety disorders: A review of neurotransmitter systems and new directions in research. In Walker JR, Norton GR, Ross CA (eds): Panic Disorder and Agoraphobia: A Guide for the Practitioner. Pacific Grove, Calif, Brooks/Cole, 1990, pp 433–469.
38. Hackett TP, Cassom NH, Wishner HA: The coronary care unit: An appraisal of its psychological hazards. N Engl J Med 279: 365–370, 1968.
39. Aschoff J: Desynchronization and resynchronization of human circadian rhythms. Aerospace Med 40:844–849, 1969.
40. Wever RA: The Circadian System of Man: Results of Experiments Under Temporal Isolation. New York, Springer-Verlag, 1979.
41. Czeisler CA, et al: Timing of REM sleep is coupled to the circadian rhythm of body temperature in man. Sleep 7:126–136, 1980.
42. Coble P, Foster FG, Kupfer DJ: Electroencephalographic sleep diagnosis of primary depression. Arch Gen Psychiatry 33:1124–1127, 1976.
43. Gillin JC, Duncan W, Pettigrew KD, et al: Successful separation of depressed, normal and insomniac subjects by EEG sleep data. Arch Gen Psychiatry 36:85–90, 1979.
44. Aserinsky E: The maximal capacity for sleep: Rapid eye movement density as an index of sleep satiety. Biol Psychiatry 1:147–159, 1969.
45. Kupfer DJ, Foster FG: Interval between onset of sleep and rapid-eye movement sleep an indicator of depression. Lancet 2:684–686, 1972.
46. Foster FG, Kupfer DJ, Coble P, McPartland RJ: Rapid eye movement sleep density: An objective indicator in severe medical-depressive syndromes. Arch Gen Psychiatry 33:1119–1123, 1976.
47. Hartmann E, Cravens J: The effects of long term administration of psychotropic drugs on human sleep. III. The effects of amitriptyline. Psychopharmacology (Berlin) 33:185–202, 1973.
48. Kupfer DJ, Bowers MB Jr: REM sleep and central monoamine oxidase inhibition. Psychopharmacology (Berlin) 27:183–190, 1972.
49. Dement WC, Mitler MM: An overview of sleep research: Past, present and future. In Hamburt D, Brodie H (eds): American Handbook of Psychiatry. Vol. 6. New York, Basic Books, 1975.
50. Kübler-Ross E: On Children and Death. New York, Macmillan, 1983, p xix.
51. Zesook S, et al: Grief, unresolved grief and depression. Psychosomatics March:247–256, 1983.
52. Lord Tennyson, Alfred: Ulysses. The Oxford Dictionary of Quotations. 2nd ed. London, Oxford University Press, 1953, p 564.
53. Dembo T, Ladieu G, Wright BA: Adjustment to misfortune: A study in social and emotional relationships between injured and non-injured people. Final Report to the Office of the Surgeon General, 1948.
54. Ladieu G, Hanfmann E, Dembo T: Studies in adjustment to visible injuries: Evaluations of help by the injured. J Abnorm Social Psychol 42:169–192, 1947.
55. Scanlon-Schilpp A, Levesque J: Helping the patient cope with the sequelae of trauma through the self-help group approach. J Trauma 21:135–139, 1981.

11

FAMILY SYSTEMS ADAPTATION

KAREN M. KLEEMAN

Traumatic physical or cognitive disablement of a family member produces potentially severe crises for the families involved. The traumatic event and the subsequent changes are rapid and unanticipated, leaving most families openly vulnerable and ill-prepared for either the extent of the coping or the mobilization of necessary resources required almost instantaneously. Most families, having never faced any situation similar to the catastrophe of trauma in either degree of severity or complexity, have no clear knowledge of expected behaviors or responses. As one relative of a trauma victim described, "In one second, my entire world clouded over and I recognized no one in it—for the first time in my life, I didn't have any idea of what to do or what I could expect."

This chapter will focus on the impact of a traumatic event on the family as a whole and the potential role of the trauma nurse in both crisis and long-term intervention with these families. Bowen Family Systems Theory[1] will be utilized as an example within the cycle framework for the exploration of those characteristics in families which constitute a possible crisis-proneness as well as a tendency toward functional or dysfunctional coping with catastrophic events, such as traumatic injury. The utility of this particular approach to family intervention will be exemplified by specific application of assessment strategies and detailed interventions for use with trauma families. Special attention will be focused on delineation of the functional characteristics of the trauma care nurse that will best facilitate the families' potential mobilization of resources and enhance optimal coping.

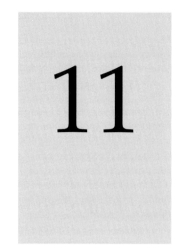

Family members function interdependently and reciprocally, with each member's behavior and experience affecting other members' behaviors and experience. Through the multiple generations of their own historical experiences, families come to have unique expectations of certain members and establish clear patterns of relationship function and process between family members. All families bring with them to a crisis event their own unique heritage in the form of values, communication patterns, coping mechanisms, and cultural traditions. When a sudden and traumatic injury occurs to one member, the entire family system reverberates in response to the crisis, with new and unfamiliar patterns of function often required. Some families incorporate this necessary change with seeming ease, whereas others are thrown into utter chaos and dysfunction.

All families experience stress during their developmental phases, but a traumatic injury or a critical injury calls on the family to absorb an extreme and sudden amount of anxiety attendant to the specific nature of the catastrophe, both immediate and long-term. To the extent that the family has a repertoire of coping skills already established and a wide relationship support system in place, the amount of stress able to be absorbed will increase. There may be an inherent fluidity in roles and assumption of alternative responsibilities, allowing flexibility and adaptation by individuals within the family.

However, in many cases, an already taxed family system is thrust into a crisis reaching proportions of stress and anxiety that cannot be functionally absorbed within the system. This can ultimately lead to family disequilibrium and subsequent breakdown in established family patterns. Families with unmanageable stress levels and little or no coping repertoire pose a special challenge for the nurse, since they seem to compose a significant proportion of the families in trauma/critical care settings.

It is essential that nurses focus on the family, since it is the family that provides critical support to the injured member. A family's ability to mobilize resources and adapt often prevents many emotional and medical consequences to the trauma. The family, serving as the social support network for the trauma victim, provides emotional support, advice and encouragement, essential companionship, and assistance in areas of tangible aid such as transportation, errands, and the like.

A number of factors influence a family's reaction to the catastrophe of a traumatic injury or a sudden critical illness (Table 11–1).

In most cases, the suddenness of the event prevents any anticipation or planning and requires almost immediate response from family members. This is a hallmark characteristic within trauma or sudden critical illness, and it is compounded by the fact that it is usually a novel experience for the family—in most cases, they have no direct experience in dealing with these situations. Until these situations strike, families are not inclined to seek advice or guidance from available literature or other resources on family coping. Although available literature abounds in the area of coping

TABLE 11–1. FACTORS INFLUENCING A FAMILY'S REACTION TO CRISIS OF SUDDEN ILLNESS OR TRAUMA

Having little or no time to prepare
Having little experience with this type of stressor, either for themselves or with others
Having little guidance available for what is expected
The loss of control; feelings of helplessness
The amount of time in the crisis state and its on-again, off-again nature
The degree of disruption/destruction to family roles, responsibilities, and routines
The perceived danger to and emotional impact on the family

Adapted from Figley CR: Catastrophes: An overview of family reactions. In Figley CR, McCubbin HI (eds): Stress and the Family, vol II: Coping with Catastrophe. New York, Brunner/Mazel, 1983, pp 3–20.

with normative family stresses, still very little has been written for the lay public dealing with catastrophic situational stresses and the potential impact on families. Having few resources for guidance or support, families are restricted by circumstance to a limited and select number of others who have had similar experiences and who can offer each other mutual support and guidance. But, for most, they remain few in both number and quality. Profound and overwhelming feelings of helplessness and powerlessness are often the result, with families who are unable to control the amount or nature of the stress experienced—they cannot order it or time it or remove it. All they can do is respond to the unwieldy and unpredictable nature of the course of the crisis.

Perhaps one of the most difficult factors influencing a family's reaction to this type of crisis is the indeterminant amount of time that it will last and the lability of its course. One set of events is no sooner adapted to than another set presents itself, most often in the form of physiological responses and/or psychological emergencies. There is rarely the feeling that the crisis is now past, but rather the sense that anything could still happen and, in fact, could be worse than the previous set of events. There is often very little recovery time as families mobilize repeatedly to adapt to crisis after crisis. Additionally, depending on which member of the family is injured, a family's entire life-style might be disrupted, with all major roles and responsibilities necessitating a shift.

Current trauma populations have become increasingly bimodal, with patients being under 25 years of age and over age 65. When patients are under 25, they usually tend to be male and, in many cases, just beginning the assumption of family roles and responsibilities. These cases are particularly catastrophic, since the family member involved in the trauma may be the pivotal resource for most major responsibilities in the younger, less established family.

Trauma patients over 65 years of age are an increasing challenge and reflect the drastically changing demographics of a "graying America." Families within this group are asked to respond to catastrophe at a time of decreasing coping capacity as well as less physiological capability for the stress response. Adult children of these trauma patients who often have young children of their own are called on to function as primary caregivers for their aged and now critically ill and potentially disabled parents.

Threat of physical harm or death involves the most intense reaction for an individual. News regarding these dangers for a family member may leave a profound emotional imprint, both acute and chronic, on the family as a whole.

It can be clearly identified that there is a very special nature to the crisis and stress experienced by victims and families of trauma or illnesses of a sudden, unexpected nature. It is both frightening and overwhelming in magnitude. Typical family responses to the crisis may include any or all of the following: anxiety, shock, and fright; denial, anger, hostility, distrust, remorse, and guilt; grief and depression; and/or hope. Families are called on to incorporate massive changes into previously predictable patterns and relationships on which they can no longer depend. Their responses may occur in no particular or orderly manner after the initial shock. Many families report the simultaneous competition of many of these emotions, leaving them feeling totally out of

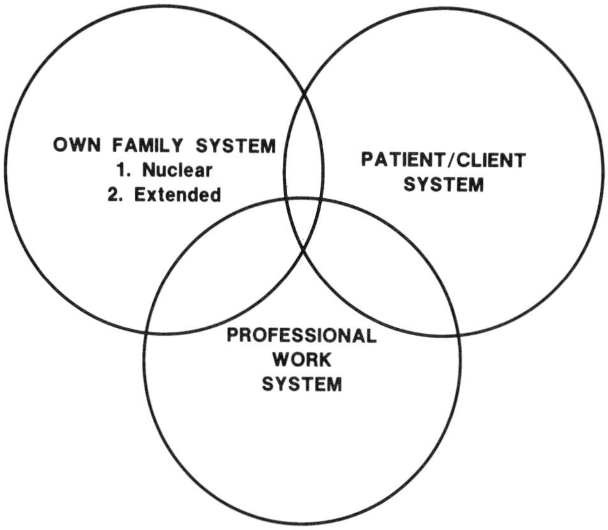

Figure 11–1. Interlocking emotional systems operational for nursing.

control and frightened by their emotional lability. There is frequently regression to denial and disbelief for periods of time after family members have essentially appeared to have handled this.[2] The trauma nurse is in an ideal position to intervene meaningfully with families. Whereas an entire team of highly skilled health professionals comes into the daily lives of the family, it is the nurse with whom there is established a close and special bond born out of the nature of the crisis, the clinical knowledge base, and the interpersonal skills exemplified by this particular member of the team. Assisting a family requires very sensitive judgments about when and where to intervene, just how much guidance and support to offer, and exposure to the best avenues of education, protection, and therapy. While most families may recover reasonably well regardless of the quality of the intervention, it is of special importance for the nurse to establish a firm body of skills to deal effectively with families in augmenting their response to stress, their adaptive methods of coping, and their progression from disorganization within the crisis state to crisis resolution and ultimate growth.

Nurses and helping professionals are simultaneously involved in three interlocking emotional systems: (1) their own family system, both nuclear (the family they live in now) and extended (the family in which they grew up), (2) their patient/client system, and (3) their professional work system (Fig. 11–1). Nurses have a unique opportunity to gain knowledge about the nature of and the effective functioning of these systems and how they interact with one another. The nurse's own family system experiences, both current and previous, will have an impact on functioning with particular clients and their family systems and will influence enactment of roles and responsibilities within the work place. To the extent that knowledge is gained as to how these three interlocking systems interconnect, the nurse can enhance objectivity in function and differentiation as a professional. The consequences of this awareness can be positive both personally and professionally in therapeutic endeavors.

Trauma nurses, by nature of their specialty area, are called on to assist families when they are at their most vulnerable state. High-level professional judgment is necessary to distinguish between overfunctioning for a family within the role of a health professional at this point and offering appropriate support, guidance, and structure for the family to function the most independently right from the impact phase of the injury. Too often sympathy for a family's situation overcomes empathy, and the nurse assumes function for the family that over time leads to dependence and underfunction. Sensitivity to a family's needs and wants is an essential component of effective nursing function; however, special skill is needed for the trauma nurse to be able to objectively incorporate a sensitivity to these needs that affords the family emotional support without jeopardizing their ultimate need to establish their own coping mechanisms and problem-solving skills.

Cleveland[3] has made a study of the impact on family adaptation with physical disablement of a family member. While her work focuses particularly on spinal cord injury, her research findings have applicability to how the crisis of trauma or critical, prolonged illness affects families as a whole (Table 11–2).

The time required by family members in terms of visitation to the hospital immediately effects task organizational changes within the family units. Tasks and responsibilities have to be reallocated, and this reallocation is on-going throughout the phases of the immediate injury to rehabilitation. Sibling and parental responsibilities are often altered dramatically. Changes in affection structure are seen initially as increases in feelings of intrafamily closeness; however, with time and the chronic, prolonged course of these illnesses, affection structural changes within families become more complex, and specific reciprocal relationships are more clearly established. "Responsibility for" and "dependence on" often determine to whom family members feel closest and with whom they align most consistently. Communication structure is drastically altered, with the focus on the crisis and family members often communicating with one another in protective, shielding ways. Fathers may think it is important to be strong and in control to help support mothers; siblings may communicate largely with one another about the crisis so as not to further upset parents. There are power shifts and struggles as family members are called on to make decisions and to incorporate new role responsibilities into their current functioning. Family unity is initially augmented by the crisis, but if it is prolonged or of a chronic nature, many families report a sharp decrease in feelings of closeness and often significant difficulties in holding the family together. There is mounting fear and anxiety about how the family will be called on to function in the future given the change in structural relationships. Significant changes in

TABLE 11–2. HOW CRISIS OF TRAUMA/CRITICAL ILLNESS AFFECTS A FAMILY

Changes in task organization
Changes in affection structure
Changes in communication process
Power shifts/struggles
Alterations in family unity
Alterations in specific interpersonal relationships

From Cleveland M: Family adaptation to traumatic spinal cord injury: Response to crisis. Fam Relations October: 558–565, 1980. Copyright 1980 by National Council on Family Relations, 1910 West County Rd B, Suite 147, St. Paul, MN 55113. Reprinted by permission.

TABLE 11–3. ASSESSMENT OF FAMILY CRISIS-PRONENESS AND/OR DYSFUNCTIONAL COPING

LEVEL OF CHRONIC ANXIETY	SAMPLE QUESTIONS*/OBSERVATIONS
How many intense relationship systems are there (either highly positive or highly negative)?	How do people in your family relate to one another generally? Are they very supportive? Are there a lot of conflicts? Who is most concerned over whom? Is your family loyal to one another? Who is most likely to be critical when they don't agree?
Who absorbs most of the anxiety?	Who in your family seems to be the most special? The most protected? Who seems to have the most problems? Who seems the most stressed?
How able is the family to distinguish *feelings* from *thinking*? Are they likely to do what feels better and impulsively react rather than measuring responsiveness for the future? Are they on the *defense* instead of the offense? "Out of control" instead of "in control"?	When there is a crisis in the family, what do you generally do first? How do you routinely react? How much do your "insides" rule what your behavior is in response to the problem? Is it important for you that problems/issues are settled immediately? What goes into that? Can you see problems coming before they hit, or are you often surprised and caught off guard?
How often do they tend to pull in others to blame or to help solve problems (i.e., police, school, alcohol, etc.)?	Who do you seek out when there is a crisis in your family? Who can you most depend on? Who would you try to keep the problem from? Where else might you go for help?
How many alternatives can they see to a problem, or do they see few choices and have fixed ways of responding?	What do you see as the possibilities here? What other kinds of approaches might help in resolving this problem? If that doesn't work, which might you think about trying next?
EMOTIONAL RELATIONSHIP STRUCTURES	**SAMPLE QUESTIONS†/OBSERVATIONS**
How much of a sense of "we" vs. a sense of "I" exists in the family? Does the "I" tend to get lost in the "we-ness"?	Do you sense that people in your family are respected for their own unique characteristics? How important is it in your family that people get along? How different can someone in your family be from everyone else without causing conflict?
What is the basic "caring index" of the family (emotional climate connoting affectional caring for one another)?	Describe how you feel about ________? How would you describe ________? (Note use of adjectives, tone of voice, vividness vs. ambiguity of description.) How do you show each other concern? caring?
How much *need* vs. *want* exists within significant relationship structures?	What is it that you know you really need from this relationship? What would it be "nice to have/get"? What can't you do without?
Is being different accepted or rejected?	How would your family react if you decided not to adopt their ideas about ________? How much leeway for disagreement would be given?
Are individuals' behaviors determined by other family members' desires?	What would it take for ________ to influence ________ to change his mind on that? to act differently? Who would be most likely to hold his ground no matter what the pressure from others?
Is sameness required to prove loyalty?	What are your family expectations for members' behaviors? How does ________ know you care for them? What is required of you by ________?
Who functions for whom? How often? In what capacities?	If things are going haywire, who can you always depend on? Who can you never depend on? If ________ is in trouble, who fills in? For how long? Who is most likely to pick up extra responsibilities in the family?
How sensitive are family members to one another?	How do you know when someone in your family doesn't agree with you? approve of your behavior? How influential is that in changing how you think or act? Can you criticize each other openly and honestly? How do people respond?
COMMUNICATION PROCESS	**SAMPLE QUESTIONS/OBSERVATIONS**
Is process flexible or rigid?	How are problems handled in your family? Is the process always the same or can it vary? What always happens? What never happens? What alternatives are tried? What if that doesn't work?
Is conflict resolution high or low? Can issues be confronted without threat to self or others?	How are issues resolved in your family? How do individuals respond to that? Who tends to feel the most threatened? The most in control? The most stressed? The most misunderstood?
How many issues are avoided or never discussed?	What do you discuss comfortably? Frequently? What is never discussed in your family?
Are there hierarchical boundaries between the generations? Are the appropriate generations "in charge"?	Who establishes the rules in your family? How are they enforced? By whom? For whom?
Is family affect impoverished? hysterical?	How would ________ react to a crisis with ________? How would they behave? How would you know something was wrong?
How much are members told what to do vs. deciding for self?	Who tells who what to do? How much of what you ultimately do is left up to you? How do members of your family give you advice and direction?
How much generalization is made to include all family members?	How are you like ________? How is ________ like ________? How are you different?
How much criticism exists (i.e., what is the "critical index")?	How much disagreement do you usually have with ________? How do you know there is disagreement?
Are there deceptions within the communication process?	(Observe for incongruities between family members' information.) ________ indicated that this often occurs; do you see it that way or do you see it differently?

*These are suggested questions that may be useful in eliciting the information under each of the four areas. They are not meant to be all-inclusive or exhaustive, and alternate phraseology may be appropriate depending on the individual case.

†Blanks are included where specific family members' names or relationships would be inserted by the nurse (i.e., Blanche, your mother, etc.).

TABLE 11–3. ASSESSMENT OF FAMILY CRISIS-PRONENESS AND/OR DYSFUNCTIONAL COPING *Continued*

MULTIGENERATIONAL HERITAGE AND PATTERNS	SAMPLE QUESTIONS‡/OBSERVATIONS
How much a part of the current generation is the previous generation?	How often do you see ________? How do you keep in touch with ________ ? How many times a week? month? year? What kinds of things do you let them know about you?
How available is the relationship network?	Do you sense that you can seek ________ out when you need to? How comfortable would that be? How much do you do it?
Are there open or closed boundaries between the generations?	With whom do you have the most open relationship? The most closed? With whom do you not communicate?
What myths, expectations have been handed down? Are there "secrets"?	What are the things in your family past that no one is supposed to know? How did you find out? What is expected of you by your grandparents? Are there certain beliefs/attitudes that have been handed down to you through the generations?
Are there patterns or repeated chronic physical, emotional, or social problems within the family?	From the genogram information, the nurse can observe multigenerational patterns of suicide, alcoholism, depression, heart trouble, and delinquency.

‡Questions here would refer to those family members who had preceded the present family generation—aunts, uncles, grandparents, great-grandparents, second cousins, and others.

interpersonal relationships occur among all family members, but with particular distinction between the injured or ill individual and other members of the family.

Explanations to the family by the nurse of these ranges of feelings and changes to increase their awareness of the usual "norms" within these situations can be invaluable to overall adaptation. By providing a baseline of what a family can expect to undergo during the course of response to the crisis, family functioning can be supported, and on-going self-evaluation by the family can be enhanced.

Richmond[4] identifies a major nursing function as assisting family members in giving support to the member who has sustained the injury. To do this, it is absolutely essential that family members clearly understand the adverse reactions that they will experience during this period and understand that such reactions are time-limited and that they will be assisted in the development of effective coping strategies.

PREVENTION CYCLE

Crisis-Proneness in Families

Some families exhibit certain characteristics and functional levels and abilities which constitute a predictable crisis-proneness in family members.[5] These same characteristics may herald a family's dysfunctional coping with the stress of traumatic injury or critical illness once it occurs. Four general functional areas are discussed in light of crisis-proneness and assessment of potential dysfunctional coping: (1) levels of chronic anxiety in the family, (2) family emotional relationship structure, (3) communication process, and (4) multigenerational heritage and patterns (Table 11–3).

Levels of Chronic Anxiety

Families prone to crisis and dysfunctional coping are usually shown to have very intense relationship systems: highly positive, highly negative and conflictual, or a combination of both. They are frequently characterized by a lesser ability to distinguish feeling process from intellectual process and are caught in a cycle of automatic emotional responses to each other over which they perceive they have no control.[1] Their behaviors are reactive and impulsive, with the goal of "feeling better" being paramount. Their emotional responses are frequently chaotic and repetitive, reflecting a controlled, rigid, and limited repertoire of skills with which to deal with one another. In these families, chronic anxiety tends to be absorbed by one family member, and that individual comes to be focused on in excess of either positive attention (i.e., "golden girl") or negative attitudes (i.e., "black sheep"). In this way, the level of chronic anxiety between two family members, such as spouses, is somewhat lessened by the focus and diversion of energy onto a third person in the system. This member who is focused on in this way is the one who comes to be the "most at risk" for development of physical, emotional, or social problems throughout life.[6]

Emotional Relationship Structure

Crisis-prone families and those likely to cope dysfunctionally tend to have a predominantly fixed and inflexible relationship structure, dominated by dependence and adaptiveness to one another. There is a strong sense of "we" and a loyalty to the family as a blended unit with autonomy of individuals often sacrificed to preserve harmony.[7] "Differentness" is not tolerated well, and members need approval from one another. Relationships tend to get fixed around one person underfunctioning in most of life's tasks and another reciprocally overfunctioning; there comes to be very little, if any, reciprocity within this pattern (i.e., one person always underfunctions and one always overfunctions). Members in this type of enmeshed, emotionally based family feel responsible for what another feels while they do not feel much responsibility for themselves. Rather than being sensitive to another, these individuals find that they allow their behaviors to often be determined by another's desires. There is a problem distinguishing "needs" from "wants," and even though family loyalty is rewarded, there may be an overall low caring index on the part of individuals for one another.

Communication Process

Crisis-prone families have few hierarchical boundaries and rules between the generations in communication and tend to be sensitive to praise or criticism for each other.[7] Communication sequences are predictable, rigid, and reactive with low levels of conflict resolution. Confrontation of issues tends to be avoided, and many conflictual issues either are never discussed or are fought about but never resolved. Communication is closed, with little taking in of new information, and is impoverished in affect. Generalizations are frequent, and blaming is heavily used to hold someone in the family, the school, the law, the society, or the institution at fault. Others are often told what to do rather than being encouraged to find their own solutions.

Multigenerational Heritage and Patterns

Crisis-prone families are often cut off from previous generations, being either geographically distant or, more frequently, emotionally disconnected. Boundaries around the family are closed, with little relationship network or few social supports available to help diffuse the family's chronic anxiety. There is a strong passing down of family "myths" and expectations for behavior and feelings on the part of individuals. Most often, there are multigenerational patterns of various physical, emotional, and/or social dysfunctions such as chronic physical illnesses, depression, violence, substance abuse, and repeated accidents.

While an assessment of these four functional areas may not prevent a future crisis or totally forestall dysfunctional family coping in light of a crisis, it can provide the nurse with a reasonably accurate predictor of what can be expected and what major areas for intervention will need to be targeted. In recent years, public education has played a crucial role in educating families regarding developmental family issues, parenting, adolescence, appropriate need for counseling, and the like. More and more families are aware, as a result, of their own strengths and weaknesses and their need for appropriate direction in seeking to improve function.

On the other hand, certain family characteristics are indications of potential ability to cope adaptively to the crisis of trauma or critical illness. They include low to moderate levels of anxiety, which allow the family to hear, understand, and repeat information; decreased reactivity to issues, which allows action rather than reaction and the adaption of a solution-oriented approach; high motivation and sense of personal identity distinct from collective identity with the patient; ultimate belief in one's ability to gain eventual control over one's life again; and evidence of role flexibility and high family caring and cohesion. These characteristics can be assessed by evaluating the family members' responses to the same types of sample questions provided in Table 11–3 for the assessment of crisis-proneness and dysfunctional coping. Additional useful questions may include the following:

- What will it take for you to be able to do what you have to do?
- What do you think is the most important next step for you?
- How do you see yourself as distinct from ________?
- How does ________'s condition influence you the most?
- How much control in what happens do you think you have?
- How can you go about assuming some of the responsibilities usually handled by ________?

If the nurse can accurately assess the presence or absence of these characteristics and plan interventions accordingly, many of the subsequent difficulties inherent within the prolonged course of treatment may well be avoided or sufficiently reduced in duration and scope.

RESUSCITATION/CRITICAL CARE CYCLE

Many sources are available in the literature to help direct the trauma nurse in the provision of immediate aid to families in the first few hours and days after the traumatic event.[8–13] These include a special focus on the family's perception of the traumatic event, identification of the problem, identification of coping abilities previously utilized in any similar situation, and identification of available social and situational supports for the family to tap. Crisis intervention models of this type are familiar, are effective, and have been widely adopted for use with families in crisis. However, the crisis of trauma is unique in that it often does not follow the time-limited range of a few minutes to 6 weeks' duration, as identified in the crisis literature. Hospitalizations of trauma victims may extend for months, with alternate periods of stabilization and physical emergency, often followed by extended rehabilitation. Recovery courses are unstable and often require that families adapt to long-term chronic levels of anxiety, uncertainty, unpredictability, and lack of overall resolution. The trauma nurse involved with the patient often has long-term involvement with families extending far beyond the 6-week crisis period. For this reason, a rather unique type of crisis assessment and intervention with these families is indicated. This not only involves taking into consideration the immediate needs for assistance and direction in repeated acute crisis episodes with resolution and restoration to at least the precrisis level of functioning but also requires an intervention framework that assists the family toward enhanced self-reliance and functional coping above that of the precrisis level. The skills needed by the nurse during this acute phase incorporate a mixture of crisis intervention and beginning family system assessment as family members are struggling with the uncertainty of whether their loved one will survive.

This phase involves particularly high anxiety levels for family members, which may be exhibited in a number of ways and which are capable of being maintained for prolonged periods. Individuals may be unable to sit still, may pace, have trouble processing verbal messages, shake, sigh deeply, or clench their fists, have difficulty breathing, not be able to complete a sentence, have flight-of-ideas, seem very labile in mood swings, and exhibit a host of other anxious behaviors. They feel overwhelmed, powerless, out of control, and frightened and have a sense of immobilization. Even the most stable individual in the face of sufficient anxiety may behave in a bizarre fashion. One very reserved middle-aged male executive, known for his usual calm demeanor in the face of business problems, was so anxious during the first 48 hours of his son's admission to the trauma center with multiple injuries from a hit-and-run accident that he would periodically seem to erupt from his chair in the waiting room and shout that he could not stand to hear one more announcement over the loudspeaker. His behavior frightened his family and himself because it was so out of character, yet all could be more calm about it and accepting when the nurse cast it within a normal range for the initial anxiety attendant to what he was experiencing.

Along with this high level of anxiety there may be accompanying shock, fright, disbelief, numbness, feeling of responsibility or blame, guilt, and distrust. It is important for the nurse to remember that a family's reaction to the present situation may be accentuated or blunted by previous experience with similar circumstances, and an initial question regarding whether the family has ever experienced anything of this nature/magnitude before may provide valuable initial direction. It is very important that families be afforded the opportunity to share all these initial responses, since they must be dealt with in order for them to move on with the crisis resolution.

Epperson[14] has identified a six-phase recovery process that families under severe and sudden stress undergo. How individuals within the same family respond remains unique and diverse, although there does seem to be an identifiable course that is common (Fig. 11–2).

During periods of high anxiety, family members often need repeated clarifications and restatements of information. This information should be brief, very explicit, and straightforward, or it may be more useful if it is actually written down for the family. To accurately ascertain that the family has actually heard what was being said, they should be asked to repeat what they understand at various points, as well as what they have been told and what that means to them. Even the most functional families may dysfunction for a time in the light of enough stress, and an initial period of confusion and the need for precise reinforcement and repetition of information are very normal. Often, the identification of one key family member with whom the health care team communicates regarding the patient's status is useful in limiting the confusion and defusing some of the anxiety.

Denial within the critical care phase serves a somewhat useful purpose for family members in that it may provide the time necessary to adapt and adjust to the actual reality of what has happened. Denial, as such, buys the family "psychological time." The nurse needs to "recognize" the purpose and function of denial while at the same time recognizing the family's need to deal with the reality of the present situation, still maintaining hope. Statements such as "Mrs. ________, your daughter has never been ill before and I know it must be very difficult for you to believe that she is in a coma from the auto accident" are often useful. In this way, the message is transmitted that the nurse is aware of the struggle between what is hoped for and what is the current reality.

If denial is prolonged and hampers the carrying out of necessary actions on the part of family members, additional interventions may have to be incorporated that are more directly nonsupportive of the denial and much more directive and confrontational. In the case of one 36-year-old mother of an 11-year-old daughter who was a drowning victim and had been in a coma with no physiological indication of functional improvement, the mother waited by the bedside every day for the child to wake up. She would say, "I just know that today Claudia's going to open her eyes and be OK." Her denial stemmed from the fact that the daughter's friend, who was with her and also had drowned and been initially unresponsive, had begun to respond and improve in 3 weeks after the initial accident. Also, on the news media that month was the story of a woman who had awoken after 11 years in a coma. Hence the mother's natural inclination toward denial and hope was buttressed by two cases evidencing improvement. However, given all medical indications, this was not predicted for Claudia, and her mother would make no perceptible move to investigate the possible institutional placements made available to her by the nurse and the rest of the team. A decision had to be made, and the mother had to be gently but firmly told that her daughter's case was different from the other little girl's. Clear distinctions were made in terms easily understandable as to the differences in initial signs and symptoms, sequencing of return of function, and the like. She was shown visual pictures of the extent of brain damage and told that all indications of what was known at this time indicated that this was the state in which Claudia would remain. Hope is an important ingredient and should not be totally removed, but to break through prolonged denial that may become pathological, a factual representation is essential along with the notion that miracles are always possible and, in this case, that is what would be necessary.

Families need to be able to verbalize their anger without the health care professional's personalizing it; they may be angry at the patient, at themselves, at the institutions giving care, at the physicians, at the nurses, at God, at society, and at life in general. Diffuse anger is often present and helps forestall the pain inherent in the grief that follows. Anger needs to be given expression and accepted as "OK" by the nurse, while at the same time direction is given in the form of questions that help families identify the actual legitimacy of the focus of their anger. When the "real thoughts behind the anger" can be pulled out by the family, they often realize that fear, guilt, and loss of control are driving the anger. They can then put that to rest and move on with the necessary grief work prior to reconciliation.

Epperson[14] refers to the remorse stage as the "if only . . ."

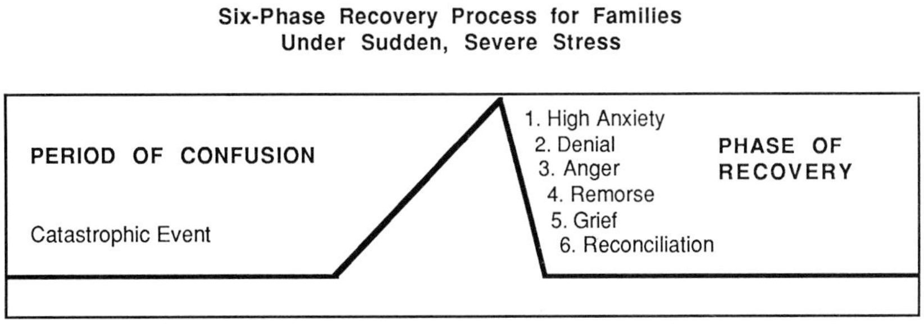

Figure 11–2. Six-phase recovery process for families under sudden, severe stress. (From Epperson MM: Families in sudden crisis: Process and intervention in a critical care center. Social Work Health Care 2:205–273, 1977.)

TABLE 11–4. INTERVENTIONS FOR INITIAL FAMILY RESPONSES TO CRISES

FAMILY RESPONSES	INTERVENTIONS
Anxiety, shock, fright	Giving information that is brief, concise, explicit, and concrete Repetition of information and frequent reinforcement—encourage families to record important facts in writing Ascertain comprehension by asking family to repeat back to you what information they have been given. Provide for and encourage or allow ventilation of feelings, even if they are extreme Maintain constant, nonanxious presence in the face of a highly anxious family Inform family as to the potential range of behaviors and feelings that are within the "norm" for crisis Maximize control within hospital environment, as possible
Denial	Identify what purpose denial is serving for family (e.g., Is it buying them "psychological time" for future coping and mobilization of resources?) Evaluate appropriateness of use of denial in terms of time; denial becomes inappropriate when it inhibits the family from taking necessary actions or when it is impinging on the course of treatment Do not actively support denial but neither dash hopes for the future (e.g., "It must be very difficult for you to believe your son is nonresponsive and in a trauma unit.") If denial is prolonged and dysfunctional, more direct and specific factual representation may be essential
Anger, hostility, distrust	Allow for ventilation of angry feelings, clarifying what thoughts, fears, and beliefs are behind the anger; let them know it's "OK" to be angry Don't personalize family's expression of these strong emotions Institute family control within the hospital environment when possible (e.g., arrange for set time(s) and set person(s) to give them information in reference to the patient and answer their questions Remain available to families during their venting of these emotions Ask families how they can take the energy in their anger and put it to positive use for themselves, for the patient, for the situation
Remorse and guilt	Do not try to "rationalize away" guilt for families Listen, support their expression of feeling and verbalizations (e.g., "I can understand how or why you might feel that way; however, . . .") Follow the "howevers" with careful, reality-oriented statements or questions (e.g., "None of us can truly control another's behavior"; "Kids make their own choices despite what parents think and want"; "How successful were you when you tried to control ____________'s behavior with that before?"; "So many things have happened for which there are no absolute answers.")
Grief and depression	Acknowledge family's grief and depression Encourage them to be precise about what it is they are grieving and depressed about; give grief and depression a context Allow the family appropriate time for grief Recognize that this is an essential step for future adaptation—do not try to rush the grief process Remain sensitive to your own unfinished business and hence, comfort/discomfort with family's grieving and depression
Hope	Clarify with families what their hopes are, individually, and with one another Clarify with families what their worst fears are in reference to the situation—Are the hopes/fears congruent? realistic? unrealistic? Support realistic hope Offer gentle factual information to reframe unrealistic hope (e.g., "With the information you have or the observations you have made, do you think that is still possible?") Assist families in reframing unrealistic hope in some other fashion (e.g., "What do you think others will have learned from ____________ if he doesn't make it?" "How do you think ____________ would like for you to remember him/her?")

From Kleeman KM: Families in crisis due to multiple trauma. *Crit Care Nurs Clin North Am 1(1):25, 1989.*

stage. Families struggle with sorrow and guilt over the part they played in the accident or injury or in not preventing the possibility of it. It is important not to rationalize this phase away as problem-solving questions are asked to help families reason out the thoughts, fears, and misperceptions they have. A mother's remorse and guilt over allowing her 19-year-old son to buy and ride the motorcycle on which he was struck by a truck should be listened to nonjudgmentally and without rationalization. Statements and questions such as "19-year-olds make their own choices." "No family is without conflict." "Have your efforts to control his use of his motorcycle worked before?" "Is it possible for even a mom to control a 19-year-old's behavior?" may be helpful in this phase. The more verbalization, the better, since this will defocus the issue and work toward problem solving. However, bear in mind that wide fluctuations in mood are normal within these early phases, and they may change very rapidly. Many family members share the fear that they are "going crazy" due to the lability of their emotional responses during the critical care phase, and it is crucial for the nurse to share the "norm" in ranges of feelings experienced by most families in similar situations.

Watching a family experience the necessary pain of the grief phase is especially difficult. Too often nurses intervene too rapidly to support, take care of, fix, or make better. Pain is a necessary component of grief work, and it must be allowed to run its course. To the extent that the nurse can be comfortable with staying connected to others' discomfort, the essential work for families within this phase will be augmented. This, in turn, allows the mobilization of resources and the realistic putting together of family life required for reconciliation. Table 11–4 summarizes the basic interventions for each of these initial family responses within the phases of recovery to crises.[2]

Throughout these phases, the art of nonjudgmental listening is essential. It is very easy to allow oneself to get pulled in by emotions to giving too much support, assuming too much responsibility for others' feelings, and/or siding and blaming. Nontherapeutic responses, questions, and statements made by the nurse such as "You shouldn't blame yourself." "How can you think you caused that to happen?" "Things will work out." "All things happen for a reason." "I would agree that ______ was wrong to do that!" do nothing to assist in long-term coping and may do much to alienate the nurse from the family she or he is endeavoring to support. It is not important to know the answers to many of the unanswerable questions that families pose but rather to ask the right questions so that families may begin to generate their own solutions, coping mechanisms, and resources. Questions such as "I hear what you say about ______; how do you see that as changeable?" "What goes into your thinking about that in that fashion?" "What would it take for you to feel less guilty? less hostile? less ______" are examples of the types of thought-producing stimuli that facilitate the family's own problem solving and ensure the transmission of a nonjudgmental attitude on the part of the nurse.

Several authors have conducted research on the perceived needs of family members of critically ill patients.[15–21] Hickey,[22] in a review of this literature since 1976, states that these reports present similar research methods, analyses, and findings. All are based on the earlier preliminary studies of Motter[15] and Hampe.[23] In eight research studies, family ratings of their 10 most important specific needs were found to be ranked in the following order:

- "To have questions answered honestly"
- "To know specific facts regarding what is wrong with the patient and the patient's progress"
- "To know the prognosis/outcome/chance for recovery"
- "To be called at home about changes in the patient's condition"
- "To receive information in understandable explanations"
- "To have hope"
- "To believe that hospital personnel care about the patient"
- "To know exactly what/why things are being done for the patient"
- "To have reassurance that the best possible care is being given to the patient"

In addition, the need "to see the patient frequently" was identified among the most important needs 50 per cent of the time.[22]

This list points to the identified need for relief of anxiety, operationalized by being informed of expected outcomes in understandable terms, receiving explanations of procedures and equipment, being called regarding changes in condition, trusting the care that is being given, and having questions answered honestly. Families need information consistently and frequently. Dracup[24, 25] advocates that the primary nurse assume this responsibility and suggests that 15 minutes per shift be set aside to talk with families, away from the bedside, to find out how they are doing, to give information, and to clarify explanations.

Families also need to maintain hope and identify this as a key factor in the maintenance of their coping ability. Table 11–4 offers possible interventions that the nurse can carry out to foster the maintenance of hope.

Families also need to be with or see the patient frequently. Although this is often difficult within the rigorous care schedules of a trauma unit or an ICU, family visiting within predetermined time limits is viewed as critical to the overall adaptation of family members to the crisis.[26] As the patient's condition worsens or the family perceives that there is an increase in severity, the family need to see the patient frequently increases, and yet this is often when nurses further restrict visiting.[27] Adequate preparation of the family by the nurse as to the care environment, the patient's appearance, surrounding equipment, and the like will facilitate family responses to strange and frighteningly unfamiliar sights and sounds. It is often the nurse's role modeling that is most instrumental in helping families cope with seeing a loved one. The nurse should indicate that it is OK to touch the patient ("It's OK to touch ______ and talk to him.") and should model how to do that, taking family members through the experience one by one. The nurse can tell family that it is OK to show emotion in front of the patient, to be demonstrative with affection toward him or her, and in other ways "give permission" for them to be as natural as possible while helping them to feel as unafraid as possible. No matter what the appearance of the patient, it is often the actual "seeing" that is instrumental in family coping, breakdown of denial, and commencement of necessary grief work.

Families need to feel that they are being helpful to the patient. This may be accomplished by actually providing some aspect of care, or by performing tasks for the patient outside the hospital setting, or even by providing valuable information to the nurse regarding the patient's previous, usual functioning. This is an area where the nurse can utilize creativity in getting family members involved in ways most meaningful for them.

Families also identify that they need support and allowance for ventilation of feelings. Families consistently identify their own personal needs as having low importance. While this is important for the nurse to be aware of, families also should be apprised that they are just as much a part of the plan of care as the patient and that attention to their own personal needs can ultimately benefit the patient. Family members need to maintain adequate rest and nutrition in order to mobilize the energy required during the hospitalization course, and pointing this out in terms of their overall, long-term contribution to the patient is frequently very beneficial.

In a crisis, habitual methods of problem solving do not work, and tension mounts. The most important question to be asked by the nurse regarding a crisis is, What do I need to know about this family to best help them do what needs to be done? The nurse is looking for those balancing factors which will best effect the family's return to equilibrium. Assessment of these factors involves three general areas[8] (Fig. 11–3).

1. REALISTIC PERCEPTION OF THE EVENT BY THE FAMILY

   Goal

   Clarification of the problem(s); situation(s).
   Focus of family on immediate situation(s).

   Useful Questions After Explanation

   What does this mean to you?
   How do you understand what was just explained?

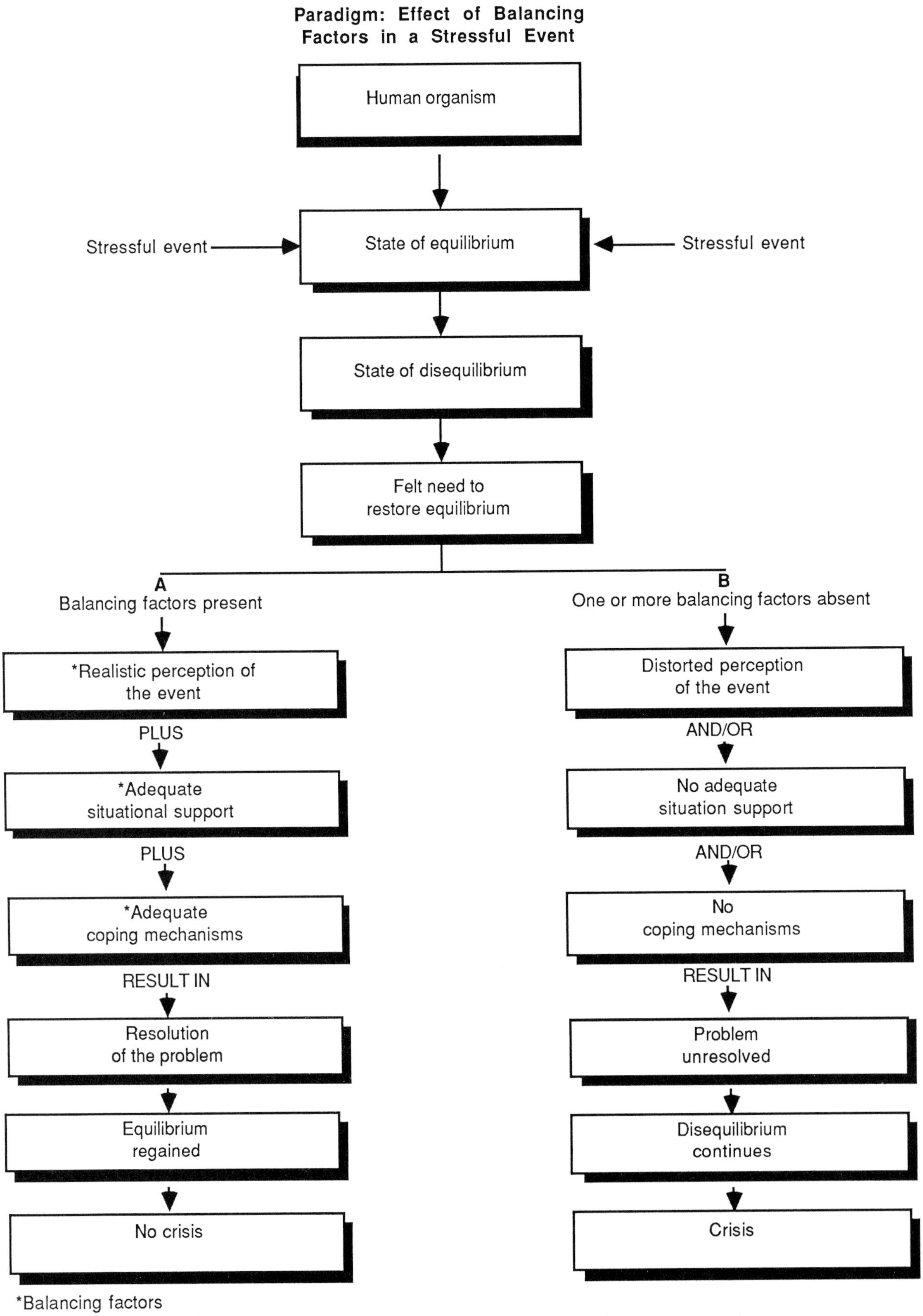

Figure 11–3. Paradigm: effect of balancing factors in a stressful event. (Reproduced by permission from Aquilera DC, Messick JM: Crisis Intervention: Theory and Methodology, 5th ed. St. Louis, CV Mosby, 1986, p 69.)

How does it affect you right now?
What does it mean for the future?

Intervention

Determination of whether family's perceptions are realistic or distorted. Support if realistic and redefine if distorted.

2. IDENTIFICATION OF ADEQUATE FAMILY COPING MECHANISMS

Goal

Clear delineation of methods either new or previously utilized to decrease anxiety and enhance coping.

Useful Questions

Have you ever experienced anything like this before?
How is this situation similar or different?
How have you coped with high anxiety situations in the past?
What did you try? What worked? What didn't?
What do you usually do when you feel like this?

Intervention

Establish specific and explicit procedure for coping with the varied emotions and responses to the current situation.

3. IDENTIFICATION OF FAMILY SITUATIONAL SUPPORTS

Goal

Delineation of family sources of emotional, physical, social, and spiritual support that may be tapped during the crisis.

Useful Questions

Are there people in your family or in your community upon whom you can depend or call on for help right now?
Who are they?
Can/should they be contacted?
Who can you most trust? Most use as a comfortable source of support?
With whom do you have the closest ties?

Intervention

Connect family with most accessible and most effective sources of support and encourage their consistent utilization.

It is difficult to separate assessment and intervention, particularly within initial crisis work; thus they are frequently undertaken jointly. This is depicted by the model for crisis intervention in trauma by Braulin, Rook, and Sills[9] in Figure 11–4. Overall, the nurse initially focuses on concurrent assessment and intervention regarding (1) how disrupted the family is and will be in the future because of the present situational crisis, (2) what available internal coping mechanisms the family can call on to utilize, and (3) who there is to work with and what other resources external to the immediate family members can be mobilized. Possible alternatives are explored; very specific directions are frequently necessary in this stage regarding what should be tried and what should be done by the family.

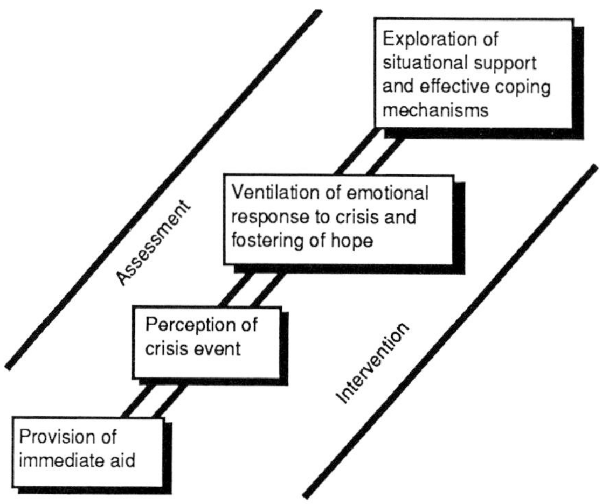

Figure 11–4. Model for crisis intervention in trauma. (From Braulin JLD, Rook J, Sillis GM: Families in crisis: The impact of trauma. Crit Care Q 5:38–46, 1982. Reprinted with permission of Aspen Publishers, Inc, ©1982.)

While the minimal goal of crisis intervention is resolution and restoration to at least the precrisis level of family functioning, the nurse should strive for the maximal goal of improvement of family functioning above precrisis level. This is possible through the acquisition of new knowledge, the acquisition of new skills, and the adoption of enhanced coping mechanisms. A noted family therapist, Virginia Satir, has said, "There is always hope as long as you can learn new things." A crisis, effectively managed, can strengthen the adaptive capacity of a family, promote growth and learning, and enhance problem-solving abilities. A potential growth curve in crisis is depicted in Figure 11–5 and depends on the timing of the intervention and the appropriateness of the intervention. In terms of the angle of recovery, the wider the angle (i.e., the longer the time), the longer the individual or family remains in crisis. Since contact with the nurse and other members of the health care team is immediate in most trauma critical care cases, there is great potential here for the instituting of rapid and effective crisis intervention.

Families are much more receptive in a crisis inasmuch as what they have used in the past to cope is not working. They are open for and often requesting assistance and direction. As such, they often listen better, have more motivation to try new behaviors, and may see the crisis as a "turning point" for the family's welfare. One such case involved the traumatic injury of a 31-year-old father of three who was hit head-on in his pickup truck by a drunk driver and sustained a severe closed-head injury and multiple internal injuries. With appropriate crisis intervention by the nurse and directions to utilize the identified support systems in the family, neighborhood, and community, the young mother and wife found that she had a wider circle of friends and supportive family than she ever would have expected. She remarked, "If it hadn't been that I was absolutely desperate and had to ask for help, I may never have known how much all these individuals cared for me and my family and what a wonderful blessing they are and will be in my future. I would never have dreamt of asking for help like I had to, and what I found out was that I didn't even need to ask and it was offered." The potential for growth is inherent in crisis. As Nietzsche has so aptly said, "that which does not kill me makes me stronger."

One very different situation necessitating special skill is that of sudden death of a family member. Sudden deaths give little warning and no time for resolution of relationship issues. There is no anticipatory mourning. Often, the family's contact with the health care setting and the nurse and/or health care team is short and highly emotional. In addition, it is often the nurse who is the one to first inform the family that a loved one has died. At the very least, most trauma nurses are in some way intimately linked to the sharing of this news with family. A calm, modulated voice on the part of the nurse coupled with eye contact, gentle supportive touch, and the careful choice of an appropriate setting for

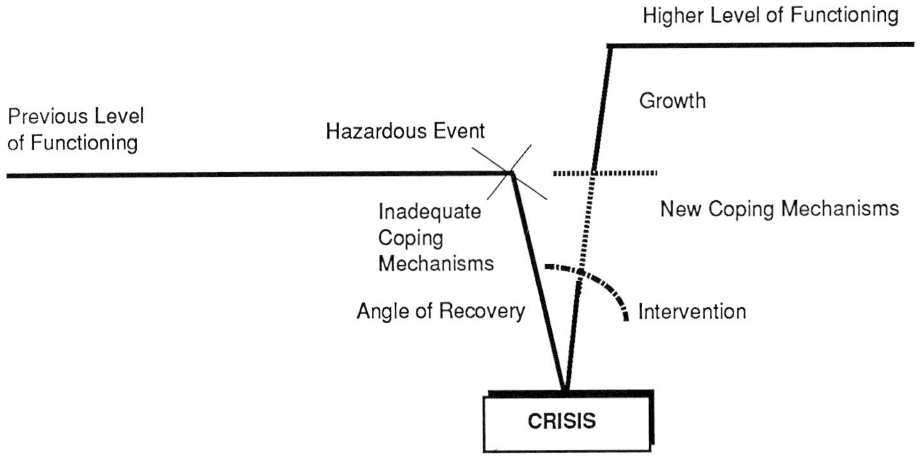

Figure 11–5. Potential growth curve of crisis. (Redrawn from Infante MS: Crisis Theory: A Framework for Nursing Practice. Englewood Cliffs, N.J., Prentice-Hall, 1982, p 19.)

informing the family that someone has died is essential. To the extent that the nurse has worked through her or his own feelings regarding the loss of a patient and death in general, the atmosphere provided will be much less anxious. It is crucial for trauma nurses to spend the time to explore their own attitudes about death because these ultimately affect the nurse's ability to be therapeutic with families dealing with death. Friedman[28] has said that by being a "nonanxious" presence in the face of anxiety in a family, the health care professional can provide the best catalyst for honest sharing of emotions and positive change. If the nurse has unfinished business and unresolved personal feelings regarding death, it is difficult to remain calm and nonanxious in transmitting that news to families.

Clear and open use of language is important here, with avoidance of terms or expressions that are indirect, such as "deceased," "passed away," or "passed on." These terms imply discomfort in speaking directly about death, and this will be relayed to the family. Using direct words such as "death" and "died" suggests to the family that the nurse is able to be open and relatively comfortable with such a discussion. Direct communication, such as "I'm sorry, but despite our efforts, ______ has died," should be used. If it is possible to ascertain (and if it is the case), it is often helpful for the nurse to state that the medical team did everything possible but met with no success, such as "Everything available to us was tried, but ______ did not respond." Families often fear that their loved one suffered or felt pain, and if the nurse is certain that due to the nature of the injury this was probably not true, it may be useful to share with the family that the patient was unconscious and not receptive to pain at this time.

When a family is first informed that their loved one has died, the impact is profound, and often nothing else is heard or comprehended as the family is thrown into chaos and disruption. It is often helpful to have the family sitting down in a private area. With sudden and unexpected death, the family system is thrown off balance, and the level of stress may seem intolerable. They react with shock. Death introduces multiple and immediate changes, and constructive grief work is dependent on permissiveness of feelings that is both accepting and supportive. With these cases, trauma nurses have as their main responsibility the provision of linkage to available support systems for the family. This may be in the form of attaching them to other members of the family and remaining with them until this can be arranged, attaching them to community support systems such as clergymen or neighbors and friends, or providing specific professional community resources for future utilization (i.e., names of therapists, local support groups, or others who are adept at supplementing the coping process). Social workers, psychologists, psychiatric nurses, psychiatrists, family life educators, therapists, and death professionals have varying expertise in assisting families in dealing with death. The trauma nurse can be instrumental in increasing family awareness of these resources and their availability.

Patients in whom trauma nurses have invested considerable caring and emotional energy over the course of their hospitalization may die suddenly of unexpected complications. In these cases, nurses must take special care to recognize and address their own feelings of loss and grief. Debriefing sessions with other staff members, including the entire team, are useful to resolve some of these issues.

It also may be appropriate for the nurse to contact the family at a later time. There are many things the family may not process at the time of the death and may now have questions regarding. The nurse can ask if they have any questions or concerns that they would like to share and can offer support and interest at the same time. It also may be necessary to present available resources to the family again for follow-up at this later time, when they are more able to hear.

In summary, special skills needed by the nurse within this phase include being able to distinguish between too much versus too little support or dependence on the part of family; avoiding taking sides or blaming; skillful posing of problem-solving, educative questions from which family may formulate their own answers; comfort in handling various emotions such as anger, guilt, and grief; awareness of the need to share "norms" of feelings and responses by families; and prediction for families of what they may expect to feel and how they may react based on these known "norms." In addition, the nurse's role in this phase should be one of emotional connectedness with the family while keeping emotional involvement to a minimum. Fogarty[29] has identified the need for the helping professional to exhibit "understanding detachment" in order to be most therapeutic for all family members. Family members should be encouraged to change, if necessary, for themselves, not for others in the family, with self-responsibility stressed. Emotional contact should be maintained with all significant members of the family, if possible. The focus is on questions, with guidance for the family to define and clarify their own direction and course. Content interpretations should be avoided while process in relationships is charted and clarified. Attention should be directed to extended family networks with the hope of decreasing emotional intensity around the present situation and sorting out more clearly the family's patterns and context of interactions.

The nurse can suggest possibilities for families that allow choice (i.e., "Other families have found this to be helpful; I don't know if it might work for you, but . . ."). Listening and observing are key ingredients of a therapeutic exchange, as are the skills of back-and-forth questioning—asking one family member if he or she would see a situation similarly or dissimilarly from another family member. Efforts should be made to get families talking and thinking about their feelings, as well as just expressing them. What can they do about these feelings? How did they come to be? The nurse should stay active but nonreactive in communication with the family, trying not to relieve anxiety too quickly. Some anxiety is necessary to increase function, and it can be supported without being totally removed.

A good clue to an overinvestment in a particular family situation is an exchange that leaves the nurse emotionally drained or feeling responsible. Keep in mind that families determine the degree of change they want, and the family does the "doing," not the nurse. It is important for the nurse to monitor self-levels of anxiety and reactivity and be aware of their origins to minimize their effect on the therapeutic outcome with the family. The issues reacted to most intensely in working with clinical families are probably similar to issues that engender the most reactivity on the part of the nurse within her own family.

One of the most useful and most efficient tools to collect factual information about the overall functioning patterns of a given family is the family history in the form of a genogram. This tool provides a pictorial, concrete, and easily understood structural framework in which to diagram general and specific family information (names, nicknames, family titles, ages, relationships, dates of births, deaths, marriages, separations, divorces and other significant family occurrences, illnesses, geographical locations, order of siblings in a given generation, education, occupation, adoptions, abortions, family "secrets," patterns of relationships either intensely close or conflictual, strengths and weaknesses of family members, how contact is maintained, and so on). More complex information can be elicited if prolonged work is to be done with the family (i.e., repetitive and highly intense family issues, relationship patterns and tone, operations of family triangles, and emotional climate); however, for the most part, during the critical care phase, a modified and shortened version of the genogram is the most functional, since it gives the family something factual upon which to focus and does not require a lot of analysis or thinking on their part. At the same time, even in its shortened version, the beginning genogram allows a variety of the facts about the family to be read at a glance, instead of a very wordy charting of the same information. It is a simple and concise yet thorough and organized tool, providing a "road map" of the on-going life in the family across three or more generations. In this way, a panoramic view is afforded that allows important issues and patterns in a family to be studied with relation to one another, one that includes a historical as well as a current picture of family functioning.

A genogram provides for the formation of questions along the four functional assessment areas of families previously outlined—levels of chronic anxiety, structure of emotional relationships, communication process, and multigenerational heritage and patterns. This, in turn, helps the nurse devise the most appropriate goals in intervention for a particular family, given their unique history, patterns, and relationship structure. Strengths and weaknesses in a family become obvious as relationships are tracked, allowing more accurate prediction of how family forces in the past and present can be used as a source of momentum for effecting change in the present. By following general areas of inquiry on a genogram, the nurse is acquiring crucial information about the family but is also educating families by directing their thinking toward an understanding of their family functioning within the context of what it has been in the past. Family members often see organization of family membership and relationship movement, which expands their view of "the problem" and enables them to free up somewhat from the guilt or blame they may be experiencing. Questions are based on the *who, what, when,* and *where* of a given multigenerational family, which facilitates problem definition and solution resources.

A simple genogram is provided in Figure 11–6 with a key to the use of various symbols commonly incorporated into a family diagram.

Many trauma units and critical care settings have incorporated routine and carefully planned meetings with families to reduce family stress, enhance coping, provide for emotional support of the family, share necessary information between the staff and the family, and help reduce any conflict or misunderstanding between the staff and the family. Each family meeting should use a team approach incorporating those health team members who deal with the patient and family most frequently. There should be specific goals, clear priorities, preestablished leadership, and provision for as much privacy as possible. Timing of the conferences is essential; they are held early in the course of hospitalization and at routine or critical junctures thereafter. Especially during the critical care phase, these family conferences can allay panic and prevent loss of control, as well as serve to introduce the family to the unit policies, procedures, and treatment team. Atkinson[30] outlines a series of preliminary questions that may serve to guide an initial family conference:

- Tell me about the circumstances of the accident/illness, as best you understand them.
- What do you know about the illness? What has _______ told you?
- How was the patient getting along with other family members?
- Has anyone else had this illness or other serious illnesses?
- How has your life changed with this illness?
- How are you spending your time?
- How are you sleeping and eating? How many hours of

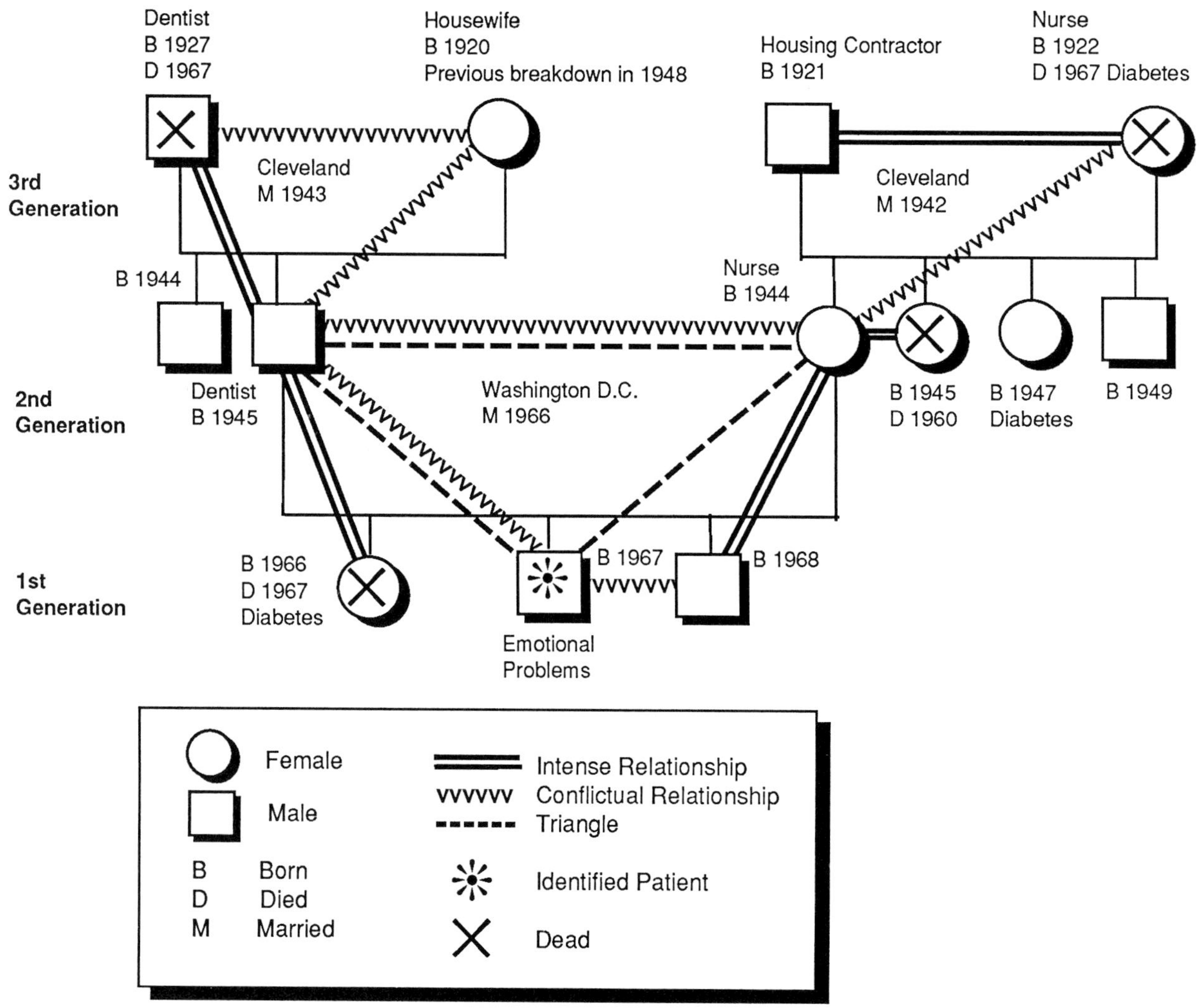

Figure 11–6. Family diagram. (From Miller JR, Janosik E: Family Focused Care. New York, McGraw-Hill, 1979, p 117.)

sleep did you get each day this week? What did you eat yesterday?

- Do you feel this was your fault (unfair, or a punishment)? (Only appropriate in those cases where guilt/blame are predictable responses by family.)
- What do you do when you get nervous and upset? What did you do when you first got the news?
- With whom can you share your feelings?

The actual family meeting, which routinely lasts 30 minutes to 1 hour, is only a small part of the entire process. Families are prepared prior to the conference and coached by the nurse with whom they have had the most contact and who is in the best position to help them identify issues of concern to them; in this way, they can formulate their questions ahead of time to optimize the use of time and the availability of resource people present. The designation by the family of a "family spokesperson" is a useful intervention. This person is the one who is designated to deal directly with the staff for information and is the one who is contacted by the staff both routinely and if there is any change in condition in the patient. It is important for the family to decide who this is to be, since it focuses them cognitively and provides the benefit of giving them a task they can problem solve through. Staff should meet ahead of time to formulate an agenda and identify priorities of needs and then determine who will follow up with the family around which particular issues. With appropriate rapport and empathic relaying of support, understanding, and interest, family conferences can be a very satisfying experience for staff and family.

Certain special management issues present themselves within the critical care phase. These include visiting rules and privileges, transfer of the patient from one care area to another, and use of other families as support for a family in need. Visiting within a trauma unit or critical care area poses procedural difficulties for staff, but it is widely recognized and established that family members need routine and frequent access to the patient. Contact does not have to be lengthy but should be scheduled, predictable, and vigorously allowed for. Within the uncertainties of this particular phase, one of the few things that families may count on is a visual verification of the status of their loved one. There is strong clinical evidence and substantial research to show that there are probably numerous beneficial psychophysiological responses on the part of the patient to the presence of family as well as staff offering encouragement and support.[31] It may be useful to time-limit visits and to restrict the number of family members at any one time. Families tend to respond more easily to this if it is clearly established early in the course of the critical care phase and well ahead of the actual initial visit. Within reason, attempts should be made for the provision of some alteration in the visiting schedule if relatives come from long distances or can come only infrequently to visit. Special care should be taken to alert family members to any changes, positive or negative, in the patient's status or appearance prior to visits. Family members should be encouraged to communicate freely with patients even though they often cannot respond; many patients, on recovery, report that communication by the bedside was very critical to their sense of orientation and well-being, even though they could make no response.

If small children are involved in the visiting issue, a number of special guidelines may be useful in deciding if it is appropriate for them to visit and how best to prepare them for a visit. Typically, in an effort to protect and shield children from anxiety and upset, decisions are made more on the basis of grown-ups' comfort levels than on the basis of what a child can cope with. When a parent or a sibling or any close member of a child's family is suddenly out of sight without warning, children are left to their own worst imaginings about what has actually happened. Even very young children, if adequately prepared for the differences in their loved one and appropriately supported throughout the visit, tend to respond positively to the opportunity to see where the person is, to see what is actually going on, and to be a part of the process. They should be encouraged to talk to the patient, to touch him or her, and to act as naturally as possible. They will tend to took to the family member accompanying them as their role model, and to the extent that this adult is calm, natural, and comfortable, the child or children visiting will tend to mirror that. All this is dependent on the functional level of other adults in the family system who will have to do the bulk of the preparation and support of the child before and after the visit. It is an exceedingly important role of the nurse to make provisions for children to visit and to be explicit with families about the positive benefits as well as the need for adequate preparation. It is equally important that children be afforded an opportunity to talk about their feelings and clarify their fears or misperceptions about the visit. Often the nurse can provide a well-appreciated backup to other adults in the system who may not be fully equipped to best deal with this. The research literature has shown that the adjustment of children over the years and even into adulthood to the loss or death of a parent is greatly augmented by their participation in the illness process throughout its course and an active participation in the funeral, if death does occur.

It remains the decision of the adult family members whether children visit or which other members of the family should be allowed to visit. In cases where it may seem more advisable not to have certain family members visit, innovative ways of communication and contact can be instituted. Tapes can be made by family members to be played at the bedside; telephone communication by family members can be arranged with the aid of the nurse for logistics; pictures, cards, and letters or written correspondence can all be utilized as effective means of communicating support and encouragement to a loved one when visiting is not possible or advisable.

Intense bonding usually occurs between family members and the nurse/health team on the first care area to which a patient is sent. This is due to the high emotional intensity and the extreme interdependence that operates in the first days of the critical care phase. As patients progress, they are often transferred to a different care unit with strange faces, different surroundings, divergent rules for visiting, and the like. This is an extremely difficult time for both the patient and the family who have grown secure in the familiarity and predictability of the previous unit. It is not uncommon for families to have greatly increased levels of anxiety and even anger over the transfer, largely owing to a lack of control and fear of the unknown, once again. Special care should be taken by the primary nurse of the first care area to formally introduce the patient/family to the nurse taking over on the next unit. Families should be told that an extensive report will be provided to the new team on the patient's course and that they are still available to the patient/family even though in a different capacity. Every effort should be made to inform families ahead of time of the transfer, allowing them to verbalize their feelings about the move and providing a viable explanation as to why the transfer is necessary. Adequate preparation ahead of a transfer can alleviate a magnitude of adjustment problems on the part of patients and families and is well worth planned time and effort.

Many times the only other people who share in the particular horror of a traumatic injury or sudden catastrophic illness for a family are the other families experiencing similar situations within the institution. Other families who have made it through the labile course of the first 72 hours, lived through a transfer, survived two or three emergency surgeries for their loved one, and are also struggling to hold life and limb together can prove to be invaluable resources to one another. There is little so powerful as the support gained from others who have actually lived through a similarly shared experience of this nature. It behooves the trauma nurse to link families together whom she identifies as having had experiences that could be shared to benefit others. This often provides one family with the support they need and another with a sense of usefulness in providing aid and something tangibly positive and productive as an outcome of their pain.

Regardless of technological advances and professional expertise, a certain percentage of families experience the eventual death of a loved one during this phase or well into later phases of the hospitalization. Survivors who accept the facts and consequences of the death, work through the various feelings associated with the deceased (guilt, anger, grief), and provide support and acceptance of other family members' reactions to the death will adapt most effectively.[32] Family should not be isolated from the family member who has died, and appropriate efforts should be made to allow the family time to say their goodbyes within the care area, even though this may cause procedural difficulties. The degree of disruption to the family system is affected most significantly by (1) the timing of the death in the life cycle (i.e., young child vs. grandparent), (2) the nature of the death (i.e., sudden, unexpected vs. anticipated), (3) the openness of the family system (i.e., can feelings be shared honestly or are they held in secret), and (4) the family position of the dying or dead family member (i.e., how emotionally significant the dead member is to the family).[33] The only factor in which the nurse can intervene is the openness of the family system. Open and factual terminology should be used and efforts made to open relationships within the family by discussing the death with various family members. The nurse should remain calm and nonreactive, checking empathically with various family members regarding their progress and any unresolved issues. Family rituals, customs, and styles should be respected. Ideally, for death to be resolved, the family will come to see the dead family member with both strengths and weaknesses and will be able to speak comfortably about him or her in time. There is probably no subject to which families react with more emotional intensity than death, and the effects on a family's emotional functioning can be widespread and prolonged. The composure and calm, empathetic understanding of a nurse with whom the family is acquainted are very useful in adequate coping with the process.

Thus, in the critical care phase, families are often in a state of chaos and are stressed, dependent, and dysfunctional initially. The nurse functions in a directive role, assessing appropriate time frames for various family emotional responses and sharing in family responsibility for decision making.

INTERMEDIATE CYCLE

Within the intermediate phase of a traumatic injury or critical illness, the focus for families shifts to the realization that "yes, the patient will live, within the limitations of the sustained injury and resultant changes." These changes are often of severe magnitude, and families are struck with the new realization that this will involve an entire lifetime of change, incorporation, and adaptation. One relative of a severely head-injured patient shared, "for weeks we prayed he'd live—now we know he'll live and my God, now what do we do?"

At the same time that families find they have a whole new set of difficulties to adjust to, their energy levels are more depleted. During the critical care cycle, energy for families runs high owing to the crisis situation, the anxiety, and the myriad other factors previously mentioned. By the time the family gets through the majority of the critical care cycle and enters the more lengthy intermediate phase, they are often experiencing very low energy levels, are often depressed more so than previously, and may act this out in a variety of ways. Visiting may decrease as family members recognize the need for some emotional refueling and distance. This does not connote less caring or commitment on the part of families; rather, the emotional system so hard at work for so long needs the distance to afford clearer thinking and some emotional "R and R" (rest and relaxation). However, most family members do not understand this mechanism if the nurse does not give the "OK" and explain the dynamics; instead, they feel guilty that they do not have the same motivation to keep up the previous pace.

On the other hand, visiting may increase at this point as the patient improves; family can be taught how to do physical care and be more heavily incorporated into the care regimen established for the patient. They are often very responsive to finally being able to *do* something for the patient, and feel more useful.

Depression is not uncommon for families in this cycle. A temporary emotional disengagement is often therapeutic for family members and, if assessed to be useful, should be advocated by the nurse—the key is that it is temporary and there are definite goals set for this time as to what will be accomplished emotionally. Again, provision for temporary emotional respites along the course of a prolonged traumatic illness and recovery may render family members much more able to sustain the prolonged coping that is necessary.

This is also a time for families when the effects of more chronic stress may be exhibited; other members of the family may exhibit physical, social, or emotional symptoms. If certain family members are prone to particular behaviors under stress, these may now surface, whereas during the critical care cycle the behaviors were held in check. A key responsibility of the nurse within this cycle is to educate the family about the long-term effects of chronic stress on the system, identify with them who may be the most vulnerable to exhibit the signs and symptoms of this system stress, and institute interventions to assist families in dealing with this. In one family of five adult siblings who were all very involved in the recovery course of their revered elderly father from a traumatic injury (he had fallen from a ladder while painting one of the children's homes), the nurse utilizing the genogram was able to identify which of the five siblings everyone worried about most and why. It turned out to be the youngest of the brothers, who had recently been diagnosed as severely hypertensive. Although his blood pressure was normal when checked at the trauma center, the nurse instituted a program whereby his brothers and sisters assisted him and each other in basic diaphragmatic breathing and stress-management strategies on a routine, preventive basis. This was seen as preventive and useful for all family members. It also provided them with a sense of purpose and usefulness during the interminable waiting periods associated with the resolution of their father's physical condition.

Various stress-management techniques may be taught, anxiety-reduction tape cassettes may be utilized, and sessions may be held with families to plan tasks and talk about the future, given their new perception of what that future involves with their injured family member. The more advanced process aspects of the genogram can be attended to, helping families identify specific patterns of relationships, emotional climate, strengths and weaknesses of family members, and mechanisms used by the family over the years to deal with interpersonal anxiety.

During this phase it may be apparent and become a source of conflict that the patient and the family are at different points in their grief work. In most cases, family members are ahead of the patient because all the patient's energy has gone into fighting for life while so acutely ill. When families may have moved through denial and resolved anger, patients may just be starting with those responses. The nurse can educate the family about the stages of grief and the fact that it is not uncommon for patients to fall behind the family in their progression through grief work. The nurse can encourage family members to be patient and tolerant, giving the patient the time necessary to progress. It is important that the nurse take an active role in supporting both the patient and the family with information as to what the differences in responses reflect and how to understand the divergence and work with it.

This is an active time in terms of education and teaching of the family by the nurse. In contrast to the empathic support and direct guidance given in the critical care cycle, the intermediate cycle necessitates a higher level intervention skill with restructuring of family patterns and renegotiation of tasks, and more advanced application of family systems theory. Families tend to be calmer during this period but less eager for intervention and more emotionally distant from the health care team as well as from the patient. Once again, this is a natural progression and should not be misinterpreted. There is nothing "magic" about the time that a family has had to cope with a situation. The course of coping for families on a trauma trajectory is often zigzag rather than linear, and allowances for shifts in family function should be made and accounted for on the basis of what the nurse understands regarding the need for some emotional distance and temporary emotional disengagement.

Ambiguity and nonresolution still remain for family members in this cycle as coping demands continue to vary from day to day; however, in this cycle most families who are functionally progressing have established a general system for the prolonged incorporation of the unexpected. Depending on the nurse's assessment of whether the family is functional or dysfunctional in coping at this point, consultants may be called in to deal with particular family issues of a more complex nature. Most trauma and critical care centers have highly skilled family service departments, psychiatric social workers, liaison psychiatric nurses, alcoholic counselors, and others to assist the nurse once a more complex need is identified. Also, families can be directed to professional and nonprofessional support groups for additional assistance.

Table 11–5 presents 12 characteristics useful in identifying a family system as basically functional. In contrast, dysfunctional progression may be heralded by the following behaviors:

- Prolonged denial
- Blaming—increased conflict
- Forgetting critical facts or necessary information
- Not hearing—decreased crisis or nonresolution of crisis
- Scapegoating—projecting all the problems onto one family member to relieve the overall anxiety in the system
- Unhealthy communication patterns:
  Secrets—keeping facts from the nurse or from other family members
  Deception—usually to protect a family member or an image; hiding information that is necessary to plan intervention course (social stigmas like drug abuse, alcohol addiction)
  Double messages—saying one thing and meaning another
  Evasiveness—vague answers or no answer; "yes" or "no" answers with no elaboration

TABLE 11–5. FOGARTY'S MODEL OF THE FUNCTIONAL FAMILY

Has the kind of balance that adapts to and welcomes change
Emotional problems are seen as existing in the family unit, with components in each person
Connectedness is maintained across generations with all members of family
Minimum of fusion; distance not used to solve problems
Each twosome can deal with problems occurring between them; triangling discouraged
Differences between people are not only tolerated but encouraged
Each can operate selectively using thinking and emotional systems with other members of family
Each knows what is gotten from self and what from others
Awareness of emptiness in each family member and there is no attempt to fill it up
The preservation of a positive emotional climate takes precedence over what "should" be done and what is "right"
Each member can say it is a pretty good family to live in, over time; if one or more members say there is a problem, there is a problem
Members of the family use each other for feedback and learning, not as the enemy

From Fogarty T: System concepts and the dimensions of self. In Guerin P (ed): Family Therapy: Theory and Practice. New York, Gardner Press, 1976, p 149.

The theory best suited for working with families, especially during the course of a prolonged traumatic or critical illness with the various cycles, is Bowen's Family Systems Theory.[1] This is a theory of human functioning based on relationship systems and patterns present in all families to some degree. How intense these patterns are is related to the level of anxiety within the system and to what degree individuals within the system can distinguish between feeling process and intellectual process. A very brief overview of the major concepts of this theory is presented to include only those aspects with the most relevance for trauma nurses in working with families in their settings.

Nuclear Family Emotional System. This refers to the emotional forces within a family that bind it together, that is, the emotional influence that occurs between any two people who are important to one another. When there is a high emotional meshing between two people, this is called *fusion*. When two people are fused, they have difficulty seeing themselves as distinct from the other, and what is experienced by one family member is perceived as experience for all. There is an "emotional oneness," with no clear boundary definition. This, in turn, causes anxiety due to potential loss of self, and family members may seek distance to reestablish self boundaries. So the counterbalancing forces of the need for togetherness (fusion) and for individuality (differentiation) are found in varying degrees within different families. These patterns are often the result of learning with one's original family (family of origin). If fusion is very high, four major mechanisms may be utilized to handle the attendant anxiety:

1. Conflict: open fighting, high disagreement.
2. Emotional distance: seeking space by involvement in other things (i.e., sports, work, excessive TV watching, extramarital affairs).
3. Physical, emotional, or social dysfunctions: one family member serves as the symptom-bearer and is adaptive and somewhat submissive to another family member who is more dominant. The adaptive person is less decisive and more dysfunctional. This may be exhibited by chronic physical problems, depressions, alcohol or drug abuse, and so on.
4. Projection to other family member: usually involves a child who is the targeted focus for the transmission of system

anxiety. May involve more than one child or other person in the system; typically, this person becomes symptomatic, thus expressing the anxiety for the family. Families often describe projected children as "different," "special," "the problem one," or "the perfect one." Projection may be highly positive or highly negative.

Most families use a combination of these four mechanisms at various times. The problem of a rigid, inflexible family system exists when only one mechanism is used exclusively.

Triangles. These are the basic emotional building blocks of the family in the face of tension. A triangle involves a three-person system that has definite patterns in relationships that are predictable and repetitive. Two members of the triangle are usually close, whereas one member is somewhat distant or closed out. The normal movement is toward closeness, except when anxiety runs high, at which point people seek the outside position. Families are composed of series of interlocking triangles and may even call in other persons from the outside to duplicate the same patterns (therapist, nurse, school authority, police). There is a constant emotional movement with triangles, and often families come to have fixed roles in how they relate within various triangles. It is essential for the nurse to identify how these triangles operate and what the automatic and repetitive emotional responses are for various family members. Families can be helped to identify those automatic responses ("triggers") and thus gain more control over relationship patterns and dynamics.

Differentiation. This refers to how family members distinguish between feeling and thinking as well as how one person sees himself or herself as distinct and autonomous from another. How well one person in a family can self-define in the face of the emotional climate depends on the degree of fusion present. Those individuals who are more feeling-dominated (tend to make decisions based on what "feels" right) tend to be less adaptable, less flexible, and more dependent on those around them. They are easily stressed and dysfunction more quickly than those who are more intellectual in function (tend to be more purposeful, principle-oriented, and goal-directed). The more highly differentiated are more adaptable, more flexible, and less ruled by emotions. They hold solid convictions/beliefs and do not give way on these in light of relationship conflict. Lower differentiated family members, on the other hand, acquire their beliefs from others and are influenced greatly by external pressures or relationship conflict.

Sibling Position. Toman[34] has identified roles based on sex (male or female) and age (eldest, middle, youngest, only) ranks that a person learns in his or her own family and tends to assume in future situations outside the original family. Sibling position implies certain behavioral tendencies, personality traits, social inclinations, and attitudes. While it is outside the purview of this chapter to highlight the various characteristics of the sibling positions identified by Toman, knowledge of one's sibling position can be very useful in understanding function and in gaining an overall picture of the entire family system.

Multigenerational Transmission Process (MGTP). This refers to successive generations dynamically linked to the preceding one and to subsequent generations through family relationships. Issues, problems, patterns, and beliefs are passed on from one generation to another, with relationship patterns remaining amazingly stable over generations. As relationship systems are traced across generations, current issues become clearer in the light of historical developments, and projections for the future of the family are feasible. Alcoholism, violence, depression, and many similar patterns may become very graphic when one explores the tradition of a family. The MGTP is the mechanism by which a family transmits relationship system patterns, tendencies, functioning, and habits from generation to generation. Families often find the tracking of these patterns exciting and freeing, in that it provides a context for understanding current problems/issues in light of the past. In many cases, the result is less blaming, less guilt, and enhanced awareness and understanding of behaviors.

Emotional Cutoff. This refers to high or extreme amounts of emotional disengagement between family members within intense relationship systems. There is little, if any, person-to-person relating, and interactions may cease totally through separation, withdrawal, cessation of all contact, or denial of attachment to or importance of that relationship. Emotional cutoffs always indicate unresolved emotional attachments, and the more intense this is within primary relationships, the more likely a person is to be symptomatic in present relationships. Viable emotional contact with previous generations is important to how one comes to define oneself and in how roles and patterns within future relationships are established.

These basic concepts of family systems theory can be assessed and utilized within the data base of a genogram for planning interventions with families. When the nurse is aware of some of these very basic patterns and tendencies, there is much more likelihood of instituting the type of intervention that a given family would be most likely to adopt. Without an accurate and adequate knowledge of the context of family relationships, both past and present, long-term intervention and change for families within this phase may turn out to be superficial and transitory. The overall goals of family interactions for this cycle and continuing into the rehabilitation cycle are outlined in Table 11–6. Discharge planning is often instituted during this phase and should be done based on adequate assessment of the family's coping (whether functional or dysfunctional). Appropriate referrals to specialized providers of services can be made, as well as direction to community groups and resources, and provision for the availability of system follow-up.

REHABILITATION CYCLE

A specific nursing management issue inherent in this cycle is chronicity and what that entails for a family. The entire family is involved in managing the chronic sequelae of a traumatic injury or critical illness, and this involves teamwork and collaborative effort on the part of family members. For some families, collaboration or teamwork has never existed even prior to the overlay of a chronic problem in one family member. Family interactions in these cases may be charac-

TABLE 11–6. GOALS OF FAMILY INTERACTION IN INTERMEDIATE AND REHABILITATION CYCLES

FAMILY INTERACTION GOALS	PROPOSED INTERVENTIONS
Translate the problem as a "family" problem	Collect a genogram Examine what the problem means to all individuals in the family; compare perceptions
View the treatment unit as a family one, rather than as an individual one	Track the process of family member involvement in the symptom What is the relationship of the symptom to each family member?
Assist family members in establishing a differentiated, autonomous function for self	Encourage "I positions" Encourage individual family members' speaking for themselves Engender novel approaches in problem solving for the family Support pursuit of individual goals
Expand relationship systems	Link family members to previous generations, or to other situational supports in the professional and nonprofessional community
Open "toxic" communication area	Encourage family members to discuss highly emotional issues so that anxiety around those issues can be defused; this is best achieved when the nurse can be matter-of-fact and nonanxious about the issue, thereby "detoxifying" it by her own nonreactivity to it

terized by resentment, criticism, manipulation, complaining, anger, and over- or underresponsibility. Families such as these pose a special challenge for the nurse in terms of coming to grips with how they will organize and plan their tasks, how they might utilize additional resources, and how they will effectively handle the inherent conflict in management of the chronically ill family member.

Corbin and Strauss[35] have identified a plan of intervention in these cases based on three basic nursing strategies: (1) assessing, (2) bringing someone into open awareness, and (3) assisting. The first step involves determining the actual cause of the conflict: Are there different goals? Do they have the necessary skills and resources? Have they renegotiated how tasks are accomplished? What do they see as their responsibilities? Second, identify what is seen as the problem, and have the family verify that, in fact, that is the nature of the problem. In this way, even though little may be amenable to change, a sensitivity to the source of the problem tends to lessen the conflict around it, and individuals can begin to do something about it. Last, the family can be assisted in talking out potential solutions and alternatives, negotiating reallocation of time and effort, developing new relationship patterns that are more functional, and identifying mechanisms for conflict resolution. Nurses can teach families the importance of open communication and the need for negotiation in the division of work and responsibility required by the nature of a chronic disability.

Within the rehabilitation phase, there is the ultimate potential of reentry of the patient back into the family unit. This may follow a prolonged hospital course and extended stays in rehabilitation centers. Families have adapted to "being without" this family member, and in many ways a family system may "shut down" to accommodate to this missing member. Others have taken over responsibilities once held by the injured family member and now may have a certain investment in keeping those new responsibilities. The very behavioral shifts that marked successful adaptation and coping in earlier stages may prove to be sources of conflict when there is a reentry into the system. Functional shifts, initially uncomfortable and fraught with anxiety for families, may have evolved into solid and comfortable modifications that family members do not want to renegotiate.

One 34-year-old wife and mother of three small children was left totally responsible for her husband's business and all the finances after he was accidentally run over by a tractor while clearing a field with his dad. She had never had anything to do with the business, had never handled finances for the family, and was completely immobilized and panicked by the prospects. However, with the able assistance of a few experienced friends, high motivation, and much encouragement, she slowly learned the business, often largely by trial and error. She found she could handle it, and it gave her a sense of self-esteem she previously had not known. When her husband came home from the rehabilitation center 6 months later, confined to a wheelchair and unable to assume an active role in his own business, he was faced with a wife who refused to give up the financial and behind-the-scenes, day-to-day functions in the business. She had grown to actually enjoy the responsibility and had successfully managed the affairs. She liked the way she ran things, but he wanted some modifications made. After much conflict and many sessions geared at renegotiation of tasks, compromises were made and a new set of operation principles was adopted, but consistent, periodic reevaluation was necessary. A system often readjusts to fill in for a missing person and can cause added conflict and anxiety when it is successfully accomplished.

This is a cycle in which family members need to educate one another regarding *who, what, when,* and *how* they have evolved during the course of the illness. Open communication is critical, since the family is now the context for management, rather than the nursing unit or the rehabilitation center. The realistic long-term outcomes and limitations in function are now known, and family members must channel their energy toward carrying out care regimens, monitoring symptoms and the illness course, and reorganizing their daily lives to incorporate a 24-hour a day reentry of a family member. They previously had to arrange visiting times or incorporate the patient into the home for weekends or holidays, but the full realization of 24-hour-a-day responsibility usually eludes families until they experience it in its fullest magnitude.

One of the primary concerns of families is the social isolation that is often felt with the added responsibilities of a chronically disabled family member. There tends to be less energy for socialization, guilt attendant to going out and "having fun" if it entails leaving the patient alone, and less formal or informal entertaining done from the home for any number of reasons. Social isolation can be a very real and very intense experience for families. Significant effort should be made in educating families in terms of the importance of friendship and relationship networks, the importance of time for self, and the monitoring of tendencies to overfunction (physically and emotionally) for the patient. Each family member has needs and rights, and it is critical to the overall effective functioning of the family that these needs be identified and efforts made to accommodate them.

Much attention has been paid to the growing number of family caregivers, whether spouses and adult children of impaired elderly or the burgeoning numbers of family members who must reincorporate moderately to severely disabled younger family members back into the home. The focus in much of the literature has been on the psychobiological stress-symptom experience[36] and has documented that generalized fatigue, mood swings, depression, sleep disruptions, gastrointestinal upsets, and headaches are among the most common symptoms experienced by caregivers. Caregivers need encouragement from health care providers to monitor their stress level, to take care of themselves, and to avail themselves of the numerous community support groups so that they can network with others in similar situations.

There is often high expectation on the part of the nurse and health care team for family function within this cycle. The expectation is often to discharge the patient to an "optimal home environment," since all the efforts have been toward optimizing functional abilities in the patient. What must be recognized is that now that the health care team's work is nearing an end, the family's real work is just beginning, and it extends for a lifetime. The nurse can do a great deal to prepare families for the differences in this phase by reinforcing that there will not be the same availability of a supportive network, the same checks for patient safety, and the same ready accessibility of resources found in the hospital. These links to community resources and referrals have to be made prior to discharge, and families must be educated as to their availability and usage.

There may be regression on the part of family, with resurgence of those initial emotional reactions of anger, ambivalence, guilt, remorse, and anxiety, as well as depression. At their most basic emotional level, the family may not really be ready for or may not want the patient back with the limits imposed by the injury. A workable reconciliation is necessary regarding the dynamics of "duty" versus "rights" versus "choice." Families may not like doing what they find themselves in a powerless position not to do. The most effective mechanisms available for ventilation of these feelings, for comfort in shared experiences, for validation and support, and for problem solving are the support groups and self-help groups readily available in most local communities. In many cases, sharing with a group of "like-kind" and the inherent understanding and compassion, as well as the practical advice afforded, meet certain families' needs more beneficially than normal psychotherapeutic intervention. The specifics of these self-help and support groups should be provided for families by the nurse, and they should be encouraged to participate. An opportunity for on-going communication with the nurse or a designated professional is essential here, and linkage to available supports is crucial for long-term adaptation to inherent chronicity of many of these cases.

RESEARCH INDICATIONS

There has been a growing focus on research in families of the critically ill, and nurses' awareness of the needs of families has increased significantly.[37] However, specific research foci should now be addressed so that there can be a fit between what has been well established in the area of needs and what interventions are best to facilitate coping. How and when are families best assessed for inherent strengths, and how are they best mobilized? How can the nurse determine if visitation will increase or decrease patient stress levels? What studies need to follow so varying results can be clarified?

Intervention studies are difficult at best, and yet these are precisely the types of studies that must be undertaken to document the best provision of care for families amid the growing technological world of the critically ill patient population.

SUMMARY

The trauma nurse is uniquely qualified to deal with the families of patients who have experienced a traumatic injury or a critical illness, throughout all cycles of the progressive course. A firm and sound knowledge base in family system structure, function, and process can serve to predict strengths as well as potential weaknesses in planning interventions with patients and families over time. The trauma nurse must be very aware of functional versus dysfunctional family adaptation and know when to appropriately utilize available support services, such as consultants, family services, social workers, alcohol counselors, financial counselors, and the like. Nurses in these settings are in ideal positions to further study the expectations and perceived needs of families as they experience the injury or illness of a loved one from initial entry to discharge.

Family systems theory applied to the various cycles provides a consistent and utilitarian framework from which to derive an accurate and thorough family data base. Family care plans can be individualized on the basis of genogram information, and more appropriate incorporation of family members into participatory care can be established from a firm theoretical base and assessment. New models of care delivery to families could well be on the horizon as more awareness is gained as to the critical nature of family dynamics on recovery trajectories. Trauma nurses with special focus on and preparation in family systems as well as with expertise in highly specialized nursing care may well herald the emergence of the image of the trauma nurse as an active, skilled, visible, and credible provider of family emotional support and guidance.

REFERENCES

1. Kerr ME, Bowen M: Family Evaluation: An Approach Based on Bowen Theory. New York, WW Norton, 1988.
2. Kleeman KM: Families in crisis due to multiple trauma. Crit Care Nurs Clin North Am 1:23–31, 1989.
3. Cleveland M: Adaptation to traumatic spinal cord injury: Response to crisis. Family Relations 29:558–565, 1980.
4. Richmond TS: Spinal cord injury: A family-centered approach to assessment and management. Trauma Q 4:58–72, 1988.
5. Hoff LA: Families in crisis. In Getty C, Humphreys W (eds): Understanding the Family: Stress and Change in American Family Life. New York, Appleton-Century Crofts, 1981, pp 418–434.

6. Kerr ME: Chronic anxiety and defining a self. Atlantic Monthly Sept:35–58, 1988.
7. Minuchin S: Structural Family Therapy. Cambridge: Harvard University Press, 1976.
8. Aquilera DC, Messick JM: Crisis Intervention: Theory and Methodology, 5th ed. St. Louis, CV Mosby, 1986.
9. Braulin JLD, Rook J, Sills GM: Families in crisis: The impact of trauma. Crit Care Q 5:38–46, 1982.
10. Infante MS: Crisis Theory: A Framework for Nursing Practice. Englewood Cliffs, NJ, Prentice-Hall, 1982.
11. Umana RE, Gross SJ, McConville MT: Crisis in the Family: Three Approaches. New York, Gardner Press, 1980.
12. Folkman S, Lazarus RS, Gruen RJ, et al: Appraisal, coping health status and psychological symptoms. J Pers Soc Psychol 50:572, 1986.
13. Lazarus RS, Folkman S: Stress, Appraisal and Coping. New York, Springer, 1984.
14. Epperson MM: Families in sudden crisis: Process and intervention in a critical care center. Social Work Health Care 2:265–273, 1977.
15. Molter NC: Needs of relatives of critically ill patients: A descriptive study. Heart Lung 8:332–339, 1979.
16. Rodgers CD: Needs of relatives of cardiac surgery patients living the critical care phase. Focus Crit Care 10:50–55, 1983.
17. Bouman CC: Identifying priority concerns of families of ill patients. Dimens Crit Care Nurs 13:313–319, 1984.
18. Daley L: The perceived immediate needs of families with relatives in the ICU. Heart Lung 13:231–237, 1984.
19. Mathis M: Personal needs of family members of critically ill patients with and without acute brain injury. J Neurosurg Nurs 16:36–44, 1984.
20. O'Neill-Norris L, Grove SK: Investigation of selected psychosocial needs of family members of critically ill patients. Heart Lung 15:194–199, 1986.
21. Leske J: Needs of relatives of critically ill patients: A follow-up. Heart Lung 15:189–193, 1986.
22. Hickey M: What are the needs of families of critically ill patients? A review of the literature since 1976. Heart Lung 19:401–415, 1990.
23. Hampe SO: Needs of the grieving spouse in the hospital setting. Nurs Res 245:113–120, 1975.
24. Dracup K, Breu C: Using nursing research findings to meet the needs of grieving spouses. Nurs Res 27:212–216, 1978.
25. Dracup K: Critical care nursing. Annu Rev Nurs Res 5:107–133, 1987.
26. Kirchhoff KT, Hansen CB, Evans, P, et al: Open visiting in the ICU: A debate. Dimens Crit Care Nurs 4:296–304, 1985.
27. Stillwell SB: Importance of visiting needs as perceived by family members of patients in the ICU. Heart Lung 13:238–242, 1984.
28. Friedman EH: Generation to Generation. New York, Guilford Press, 1985.
29. Fogarty T: Systems, concepts, and dimensions of self. In Guerin P (ed): Family Therapy: Theory and Practice. New York, Gardner Press, 1976, pp 144–153.
30. Atkinson JH, Stewart N, Gardner D: The family meeting in critical care settings. Trauma 20:43–46, 1980.
31. Simpson T, Shaver J: A comparison of hypertensive and non-hypertensive coronary care patients' cardiovascular responses to visitors. Heart Lung 20:213–220, 1991.
32. Figley CR: Catastrophes: An overview of family reactions. In Figley CR, McCubbin HI (eds): Stress and the Family, vol II: Coping with Catastrophe. New York, Brunner/Mazel, 1983, pp 3–20.
33. Herz F: The impact of death and serious illness on the family life cycle. In Carter E, McGoldrick (eds): The Family Life Cycle. New York, Gardner Press, 1980, pp 223–240.
34. Toman W: Family Constellations, 2nd ed. New York, Springer, 1982.
35. Corbin JM, Strauss AL: Collaboration: Couples working together to manage chronic illness. Image 16:109–116, 1984.
36. Baldwin BA, Kleeman KM, Stevens GL, Rasin J: Family caregiver stress: Clinical assessment and management. Int Psychogeriatr 1:185–194, 1989.
37. Riegel B: Families of the critically ill. In Riegel B, Ehrenreich D (eds): Psychological Aspects of Critical Care Nursing. Rockville, MD, Aspen, 1989, pp 31–46.

12

INFECTION AND INFECTION CONTROL

NANCY J. HOYT

OVERVIEW

Trauma and infectious diseases have been the leading cause of death, serious morbidity, and debilitating physical handicaps since the dawn of recorded history. Therefore, it is ironic that both trauma and infection control are viewed as newly defined subspecialties of modern health care delivery. Why is this true? It is only since World War II that technology has provided a means to treat these diseases and ameliorate the outcomes. For example, rapid-transport vehicles such as med-evac helicopters did not exist, so most trauma victims died either at the accident scene or during the transport to the hospital. Concomitantly, the evolution of sophisticated, invasive medical technology has made it possible to emergently resuscitate, sustain, and ultimately save the lives of critically injured trauma patients. Similarly, with the discovery of antibiotics and vaccines, many of the predominantly fatal and debilitating infectious diseases became treatable as well as preventable. Therefore, one would think that with all these new technological advances the development of infection in a trauma patient could be easily prevented or controlled. However, infection among severely traumatized patients surviving greater than 5 days is the predominant complication that will jeopardize the recovery and life of the patient. In fact, infection is ranked second only to severe head and high cervical spinal injury as the leading cause of death in this population.[1] It is a medical paradox that the many invasive therapies necessary to resuscitate and sustain these trauma victims become the precipitating agents of subsequent, often life-threatening infections.

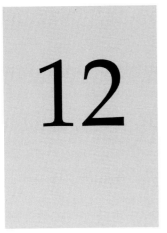

The purpose of this chapter is to give the reader an understanding of the relationships that exist among factors influencing the development of infection in severely traumatized patients. These factors include the nature of the underlying injuries, the multiplicity of invasive therapies and use of mechanical support devices, the loss of host defense mechanisms, the microorganisms of the body's resident flora and those of the hospital environment, antibiotic utilization, the clinical scenarios of resuscitation and patient care delivery, and the amount of attention paid to infection-control guidelines. It is only by understanding these relationships and the dynamic changes that occur during the patient's cycle from the initial injury through recovery that nursing care can directly affect the ultimate outcome.

HOST DEFENSE MECHANISMS

The compromise of the host defense mechanisms following trauma is the major determinant of subsequent infection. Therefore, the primary goal of nursing care throughout the trauma cycle is to promote and safeguard the patient's ability to resist infection. Careful evaluation of the patient's host defense compromise must be done continually with respect to the normal function of the mechanisms. It is absolutely crucial that nurses recognize and understand the relationship between the defense mechanisms and infection if they are to maximize the quality of their patient care.

The body's natural host defenses against infection consist of the external mechanisms of the anatomical barriers, the internal mechanisms of the humoral and cell-mediated immune responses, and the interactions that mediate between the external and internal defenses (i.e., the lytic enzymes such as lysozyme, secretory immunoglobulin A (IgA), and the phagocytes).[2] All these protective defense mechanisms can be impeded or in some cases completely obliterated as the consequence of injury, disease, invasive therapy, chemotherapy, nutrition, or age.

Multiply traumatized patients often compose a category in discussions of infection in immunosuppressed patients.[1, 3–5] While immunosuppression has been described more frequently in trauma patients sustaining thermal injury,[6–9] it has been demonstrated to occur in the multisystem trauma patient.[5, 9, 10] However, the suppression of the immune responses in these patients does not appear to be a sustained phenomenon.

It is important to realize that trauma patients are not immunosuppressed like cancer patients, who are compromised by direct immunosuppressive therapy, cytotoxic drugs, cellular immune dysfunction, or granulocytopenia.[11, 12] Trauma patients have functioning immune systems and can respond to invasion by exogenous antigens. Elevated white blood cell counts can occur even in patients receiving corticosteroid therapy following severe central nervous system injury. In addition, their infections are usually caused by virulent, pathogenic microorganisms and not the opportunistic, nonpathogenic organisms frequently associated with infection of immunocompromised patients. In addition, trauma is primarily an event of the young. The vast majority of clinical studies of the trauma population report the mean age between 29 and 31 years. Therefore, most trauma patients are not hospitalized with such underlying conditions as diabetes mellitus, chronic renal failure, cirrhosis, or cancer that jeopardize the defense mechanisms. Then, what are the primary mechanisms of host defense compromise in the trauma patient?

The major predisposing factor to infection in the trauma patient is the host defense failure caused by the nature of the injury as well as the invasive therapy necessary to treat and/or monitor the patient.[13–17] Local compromise in perfusion, hematoma formation, aggressive tissue handling, prolonged pressure on tissue, shock, necrosis, placement of foreign objects such as sutures, drains, and catheters, and the creation of dead space are all factors that lead to an increase in the probability of infection in a patient. It is primarily the break in the anatomical barriers coupled with the patient's exposure to the intensive care environment that produces the defense compromise (immunocompromise) in the trauma population.

External Defense Mechanisms

Skin

The skin acts as the major mechanical barrier, blocking invasion by pathogenic microorganisms. The skin's protective ability is enhanced by its normally acidic pH, which can inhibit the growth of some organisms.[18] Sebum, the oily secretion of the sebaceous glands, not only keeps the skin pliable and less susceptible to cracking, but its long-chain fatty acids also act as germicidal agents. Moreover, the biochemical characteristics are regulated by the resident microbes of the normal flora. The major inhabitants include both the coagulase-positive and -negative staphylococci, the streptococci, and diphtheroids.

Extensive tissue destruction from burns, degloving and avulsion injuries, traumatic amputations, and high-energy open fracture injuries totally obliterates the skin's protective barrier as well as the sensing mechanisms of the system. Massively burned patients also lose the skin's thermoregulatory mechanisms, thereby removing one assessment parameter (i.e., patient's temperature). The destruction of the skin prevents the delivery of cellular components of the immune system to the site of injury.

Compromise to the skin's perfusion from pressure on bony prominences, retraction by surgical instruments, or the presence of a hematoma or indwelling device can cause ischemia and subsequent necrosis, which can give the bacteria an enriched environment in which to thrive. Chemical irritation from degerming and defatting agents, adhesive tape, or excoriating exudates, as well as the mechanical irritations created from sheet burns or restraint friction abrasions, also contributes to loss of the skin's defense mechanisms.

Elderly patients have the added burden of the age-related changes that affect the skin's normal function. Their skin has less oil, blood flow, innervation, and subcutaneous fat. Therefore, elderly patients are more prone to skin breakdown and wound infection than younger patients. Similarly, obese patients, because of their increased amounts of subcutaneous fat, have a reduced ability to adequately perfuse the tissue. As a result, these patients have an increased risk for wound infection and skin breakdown.

Infection-control guidelines relative to the defense mechanisms of the skin are based on meticulous aseptic technique, gentle tissue handling, alleviation of pressure, selection of the least irritating but most effective antiseptic solutions, and diligent handwashing.

Respiratory Tract

The respiratory tract has a complex system of host defense mechanisms revolving around the cleansing and protective function of the mucociliated epithelium and the mechanical clearing actions of coughing, sneezing, and deep breathing. In addition, there are the interactions of secretory antibody IgA, the lytic action of lysozyme on the peptidoglycan of bacterial cell walls, and the engulfment mechanisms of the phagocytes.[19–21] All result in the normal lungs being sterile.

Although the respiratory defenses may be affected by chronic obstructive pulmonary disease, tobacco smoking, and immunosuppressive therapy, the primary loss of defenses in trauma patients occurs as soon as the patient is intubated. All the natural defense mechanisms are circumvented, and microorganisms from the environment can be afforded unobstructed entry into the lungs. The risk for the development of nosocomial infection also can be greatly increased if appropriate care of the respiratory equipment is not scrupulously maintained. Inadvertent contamination of the inspiratory circuits with an organism such as *Pseudomonas* could prove fatal to a trauma patient because the rapidly replicating bacteria could be continually aerosolized into the patient's lungs.

The patient can be further compromised if the clearing mechanisms of chest-wall function are impeded. In the critically injured patient, this occurs with flail chest injury, rib fractures, surgical incisions in the thorax or abdomen, placement of chest tubes, decreased level of consciousness, central nervous system dysfunction, or utilization of paralyzing agents such as pancuronium bromide. Furthermore, overall immobility of the patient from coma, traction and fixation devices, or spinal injury can facilitate retained secretions not only because the lung's clearing actions are compromised but also because it may be impossible to place the patient in a position optimal for drainage of the accumulated secretions. Damage from inhalation burn injuries secondary to heat, carbon monoxide, vaporization of toxic chemicals, and smoke can produce both temporary and permanent destruction of the lung's defense mechanisms. In addition, the restriction from unreleased circumferential thoracic eschars can impede breathing and contribute to hypoxemia. Elderly patients are prone to pneumonia secondary to the age-related changes that hinder their ability to cough and expectorate sputum. These factors are the result of decreases in the elasticity of the alveoli, the tonicity of their intercostal muscles and diaphragm, their vital capacity, and blood flow.

Aspiration can be a significant factor in the development of pneumonia, lung abscess, or empyema. This is a major concern in the unconscious, immobile, or intubated patient. The colonization of the normal respiratory flora can be shifted by coma, hypotension, leukocytosis, azotemia, intubation, or antibiotic therapy.

The placement of nasal, tracheal, and chest tubes can facilitate subsequent infection. Indwelling nasogastric and nasoendotracheal tubes can obstruct the drainage of the sinuses and result in nosocomial sinusitis. Similarly, these tubes can lead to obstruction of the eustachian tubes, and subsequent otitis media can develop. Hyperinflated cuffs on endotracheal tubes can cause ischemia of the trachea and lead to the presence of necrotic tissue that can become a medium for infection. Placement of chest tubes has been shown to be a highly significant factor in the development of nosocomial empyema.[13–15]

Nurses can facilitate the defense mechanisms of the respiratory tract by promoting pulmonary function, performing frequent pulmonary toilet on ventilator-dependent patients, frequently repositioning unconscious or immobile patients, and preventing the retention of pulmonary secretions by administering chest physiotherapy or frequently encouraging the patient to cough and deep breathe.

Gastrointestinal Tract

The heavily colonized gastrointestinal tract serves as a major reservoir for microorganisms that lead to nosocomial infection. The mouth, already abundant with resident flora, is continually exposed to the bacteria in the food that is consumed. The external defenses of the gastrointestinal tract include an intact mucosal epithelium, the acid barrier of the stomach, and peristalsis to continually evacuate the tract. The lytic enzymes in saliva, the interactions of IgA, lysozyme, and the function of the phagocytic cells work in concert to deplete bacteria that are ingested. The normal stomach, duodenum, and jejunum are essentially sterile, although low concentrations of swallowed mouth flora are occasionally present.[2]

Drug therapy can have a negative influence on the defense mechanisms of the gastrointestinal tract. Antacids and H_2-blocking agents affecting gastric acid secretions can elevate the normal pH of the stomach and eliminate the protective acid barrier.[22] Gastric motility can be hampered by skeletal muscle relaxants used as an adjunct to anesthesia.[23] Antibiotics shift the normal composition of the microbes colonizing gut flora. Often, and even despite the use of prophylactic antibiotics, peritonitis and deep-seated abscesses can develop when the integrity of the gastrointestinal mucosa has been broken. Other predisposing infection risks arise from hematoma formation, creation of dead spaces, abrasive tissue handling, compromised tissue perfusion, surgical misadventures, placement of drains, and the use of enteral feeding tubes (especially those which bypass the stomach).

Genitourinary Tract

The external defense mechanisms of the genitourinary tract include the interactions of a ciliated mucosa that blocks bacterial adherence and the flushing actions of a distensible bladder. The function of secretory IgA and the phagocytes affect the elimination of bacteria accessing the bladder. The bacteriostatic characteristic of urine is produced by both the low pH and the hyperosmolar composition. Therefore, urine is sterile because the environment of the bladder is not conducive to the growth of bacteria.[24]

By far the number one predisposing infection risk factor in the genitourinary tract is the use of an indwelling urinary catheter, which creates an easy portal of entry for the microorganisms colonizing the perineum. Infection risks are greater in females because they have a short urethra and the added reservoir of the organisms colonizing the vagina. In addition, a noninvasive drainage system, such as a condom catheter system for male patients, does not exist for females. Other clinical conditions that enhance the susceptibility to infection include obstructions in the urinary system, changes in the chemical composition of the urine, and renal failure. If the patient is hemodynamically unstable, hourly determinations of urinary output are necessary to determine the adequacy of circulatory volume. Therefore, frequent manipulations of the inlying drainage system can increase the risk of contamination of this "closed system" and ultimately enhance the probability of subsequent infection.

Central Nervous System

The central nervous system directs and controls the function of the body's other major organ systems. It allows the body to sense irritants of the external environment and internal metabolic imbalances and disturbances, regulates homeostasis, and allows the body to move and to communicate bodily needs. In other words, it provides the body with many mechanisms to defend itself against harm. However, if a patient sustains a severe central nervous system injury or is paralyzed or made unconscious secondary to drug therapy, many of these control mechanisms can be lost or impeded. Consequently, many of the body's normal functions must be mechanically supported, and the chances are that every one of the anatomical barriers against infection will be violated or circumvented.

The proper function of the central nervous system allows the body to move. As a result, circulation and perfusion are promoted, and the lung's clearing mechanisms of coughing and sneezing are facilitated. An immobile patient cannot turn or position himself, so the constant weight or pressure on one specific area can hinder perfusion, cause localized ischemia, and ultimately result in necrosis, producing a decubitus ulcer. Moreover, if a patient cannot move, the pulmonary secretions can be retained, so the patient is more prone to develop pneumonia.

Central nervous system dysfunction can prevent patients from sensing pain and communicating the problem. Such patients are unable to describe their symptoms. In these patients the diagnosis of infection can be difficult. For example, if a patient has sustained a cervical spinal cord injury, one of the consequences is gastrointestinal stress, which can lead to a ruptured viscus and/or an intra-abdominal abscess. However, the patient cannot sense abdominal pain or distention, so the early detection of this situation may be overlooked until a crisis develops. Physical examinations must include thorough evaluation of all body systems and a careful search for subtle changes in clinical parameters and trends.

Internal Defense Mechanisms

The internal defense mechanisms are the body's responses to tissue damage. Many complex cell-mediated and humoral immune responses that aid the patient's resistance against infection can be initiated by infection as well as injury. The loss, impedance, and dysfunction, as well as the stimulation, of some of these defenses are dependent on the characteristics and extent of the underlying trauma. The internal defense mechanisms primarily affected by trauma are the function of the spleen, the inflammatory response, and the fever response. Therefore, it is essential to understand the effects of these mechanisms as they relate to both the consequences of the trauma and the presence of infection in order to aid and ensure appropriate patient management.

Spleen

The immune responses mediated by the spleen include filtration, antibody synthesis, promotion of phagocytosis, and complement and T-cell amplification.[25] For many years it was thought that the nonsplenic portion of the reticuloendothelial system could compensate for mechanical loss of the spleen. However, with increasing research into the importance of the spleen's role in immunity, it is becoming evident that complete compensation for the spleen's loss does not occur.[26] Asplenic patients have been shown to have significantly decreased levels of the immunoglobulin M (IgM),[26, 27] to lack the ability to switch from IgM to IgG antibody production,[29] and to have diminished properdin activity (an alternative complement pathway factor).[30–33] The net effect of impaired antibody formation and of complement dysfunction is a reduction of the opsonic activity.[34] Opsonization facilitates the preliminary adherence of a bacterium to a phagocyte. This is especially important for the phagocytosis of encapsulated bacteria such as the pneumococci. Increased or decreased numbers of circulating blood cells, such as platelets and T-lymphocytes, have been reported at different times following splenectomy.

Because the spleen is a solid, highly vascularized organ, blunt abdominal trauma can produce splenic rupture and massive hemorrhage. In order to achieve prompt hemodynamic stability, in the past, emergent splenectomy was commonly performed. However, with the increasing awareness of the spleen's role in immunity and the reports of postsplenectomy sepsis, splenic salvage or splenorrhaphy is now becoming the treatment of choice.[35–37]

Although overwhelming postsplenectomy sepsis has been widely described in children, it is being increasingly reported in splenectomized adults.[25, 34, 37, 38] Overwhelming postsplenectomy sepsis is a fulminant, usually fatal infection. Onset of the disease has been reported to occur between 6 months and 25 years after splenectomy.[39] The initial characteristic events include the sudden onset of nausea, vomiting, and confusion leading to coma. Other pathological manifestations include disseminated intravascular coagulopathy (DIC), severe hypoglycemia, electrolyte imbalance, and refractory shock. Many of these events are irreversible, and death can occur within hours to 5 days of onset. The fatality rate has been reported as 50 to 75 per cent in most series. Although several different organisms have been cited as the causative organism, infection with *Streptococcus pneumoniae* (pneumococcus) is responsible for the most severe cases of this syndrome.[40] In fact, infection by this organism can be so overwhelming that the presence of diplococci can be seen on peripheral blood smears.[41] This is especially noteworthy because it is highly unlikely for bacteria to be seen on a peripheral blood smear of a bacteremic patient. Therapy must be aggressive, with early initiation of antibiotic therapy and vigorous hemodynamic support.

The incidence of postsplenectomy sepsis following trauma is relatively low, occurring in approximately 1.4 per cent of patients. However, since the associated mortality rate can be high, methods of preventing this syndrome should be sought. Patients undergoing splenectomy secondary to trauma should receive pneumococcal vaccine (Pneumovax 23), a polyvalent vaccine directed against 23 of the pneumococcal capsular antigens. One study has shown that the antibody response to a polyvalent pneumococcal vaccine among polytraumatized, splenectomized patients is similar to that in normal healthy controls.[42] Even though this study could not determine whether or not these patients were adequately protected from pneumococcal disease, it was recommended that vaccination be given within 72 hours of splenectomy. Revaccination in 5 years has been suggested, but further studies are needed to determine how long the response to vaccination will last. The prolonged prophylactic use of low-dose penicillin is no longer recommended[34, 36, 37] because (1) a wide variety of penicillin-resistant organisms, including penicillin-resistant strains of pneumococci, can cause later infection, (2) an antibiotic-resistant emergency can be promoted, (3) it is expensive therapy with questionable benefit, and (4) the patient cannot always be relied on to take the medication appropriately.

Even though infection rates in splenectomized patients have been reported to be 50 times greater than those in nonsplenectomized controls,[37] the overall impact of splenectomy and infection may never be known because infection following trauma is a multifactorial problem and the incidence of isolated splenic injury is extremely rare. Therefore, no clinical population exists that is large enough to significantly elucidate this question.

Throughout the trauma cycle, nurses can aid the prevention and/or outcome of postsplenectomy sepsis. They can ensure that vaccination has been given. This should always be verified prior to the patient's discharge. The most beneficial action may be to educate the patient about the infection risks as well as the signs and symptoms of disease. Nurses must carefully instruct the patient on the importance of immediate notification of a physician should any signs of postsplenectomy sepsis develop.

Inflammatory Response

Inflammation is a nonspecific response to tissue damage that can be caused by direct trauma or be induced by a variety of mechanical, chemical, and biological stimuli.[9] It is a complex pathological process consisting of cellular and histological reactions that occur in the affected blood vessels and adjacent tissues. The fundamental process includes the local reactions and resulting morphological changes, the destruction and removal of the injurious material, and the responses that lead to repair and healing.[43] The systemic response to inflammation is characterized by the hyperdynamic state and increased permeability of vascular endothelium.

When damage occurs, local blood flow, vasodilation, and capillary permeability are increased by multiple mediators to include histamine released from the mast cells. Edema is formed, and the increased volume of bound water results in a swelling of the inflamed area. The inflamed tissue induces leukocyte-promoting factor that attracts the circulating white cells and causes the reticuloendothelial system to release granulocytes, particularly neutrophils. Granulocytes and monocytes cross the walls of venules and capillaries via their ameboid movement and invade the affected area. This migration is called *diapedesis.* Inflammatory responses induced by infection can be brought under control by these phagocytic cells when they invade the inflamed tissue and engulf and kill the pathogenic organisms. This response is then amplified by the release and elaboration of several humoral mediators from the killed or injured cells. These substances include histamine, serotonin, leukotrienes, kinins, prostaglandins, and the early components of complement.[44] Other factors released from the inflamed tissue stimulate the liver to produce a number of proteins, including fibrinogen. The beneficial effect of the inflammatory response is derived from (1) the presence of leukocytosis, (2) the interaction of the plasma proteins (i.e., specific and nonspecific humoral agents), (3) the production of fibrinogen, which, when converted to fibrin, aids the localization of the infectious process by providing a matrix for phagocytosis, and (4) the increased blood and lymph flow that dilutes and flushes the toxic material.

Neutrophils (polymorphonuclear leukocytes) and macrophages (reticuloendothelial system cells) are the primary cells involved in phagocytosis. In the early stages of inflammation, the exudate is primarily alkaline, and polymorphonuclear leukocytes predominate. However, as the reactions persist, congestion of the capillaries leads to anoxia in the inflamed area. This induces anaerobic respiration. As glycolysis proceeds, lactic acid accumulates and causes a decrease in the pH of the exudate. If the inflammation is caused by bacteria, the lymphocytes can produce antibodies against the invading microorganisms. Macrophages then become the predominant cells of inflammatory exudate. Although the acidic pH and the antibodies of the exudate may inhibit many parasites, the major defense against infection is attributable to the actions of the phagocytic cells. All these cells interact to engulf the cell remnants and fibers altered by the tissue damage and the inflammatory response itself.

When the tissue damage is severe or the inflammation persists, large numbers of neutrophils migrate to the site. Many of these cells are killed by the inflammatory agent, and others die because of the acid pH of the exudate. Enzymes released from the stimulated, injured, or dead leukocytes can degrade the local connective tissue, causing further destruction, necrosis, and tissue liquefaction. This process is called *suppuration,* and the resulting inflammatory exudative fluid material is called *pus.* Pus consists of dead and dying leukocytes, the blood plasma, fibrin, and cellular debris (i.e., lipids, nucleic acids, etc.), as well as living and dead microorganisms if the inflammation was caused by infection. Resolution of the inflammatory response is impeded when extensive tissue damage and necrosis have occurred. Surgical débridement is then required.

Clinical manifestations of the inflammatory response include redness (rubor), heat (calor), swelling (tumor), pain (dolor), and loss or inhibited function (functio laesa). The redness and warmth result from the increased blood flow to the affected area. Swelling results from the congestion and exudation from the capillaries. Pain is caused by changes in osmotic pressure and pH of the exudate as well as the pressure and stretching of nerve endings. Loss of function may be secondary to injury or the destructive mechanisms of the inflammatory response.

Systemic pathological manifestations include peripheral leukocytosis, increased sedimentation rate, and fever. When tissue damage is overwhelmed by invasive infection and/or tissue necrosis, the inflammatory mechanisms cannot compensate for the insult, and septic shock ensues. In this condition, bacteria and/or the toxins of tissue necrosis invade the bloodstream, and septicemia develops. Septicemia produces a constellation of symptoms including fever, shaking chills, and confusion as well as signs and symptoms of shock (i.e., hypotension, tachycardia, tachypnea, and oliguria).

Although infection from a wide variety of bacteria, viruses, fungi, and rickettsiae can cause septic shock, the endotoxins from gram-negative enteric bacilli, gram-positive organisms such as *Staphylococcus aureus,* group A beta-hemolytic streptococci, and pneumococci and the histotoxic strains of anaerobic *Clostridium* most commonly induce septic shock in trauma patients.[17, 45] Exotoxins such as lecithinase (alpha-toxin), hemolysins, enterotoxins, coagulases, and hyaluronidases destroy cellular membranes, alter vascular permeability, and induce tissue necrosis. Bacterial toxins increase vascular permeability, which results in significant losses of plasma fluid into the interstitial spaces.[46–48] This is commonly referred to as "third-spacing." The net result is inadequate circulatory volume, circulatory collapse, and worsening of shock. It is the release of the exotoxins that is directly responsible for the progression of disease.[45, 48] Furthermore, when septic shock results from tissue necrosis, the progression of disease is rapid, and blood cultures are often negative.

The clinical presentation of septic shock is directly dependent on the patient's underlying volume status.[49] Septic shock in the normovolemic patient creates a hyperdynamic state with an elevated cardiac output, low systemic vascular resistance, wide pulse pressure, tachycardia, and warm, flushed extremities. On the other hand, the hypovolemic patient presents hypovolemic parameters with a decreased blood pressure, increased pulse rate, and cold, clammy skin. Since hypovolemic shock can be caused by factors other than sepsis in a trauma victim, determination of the precipitating cause can be difficult.[49]

No matter the etiology of hypovolemia in trauma patients, decreased perfusion of nonvital tissues produces deranged cellular metabolism.[45] Tissue anoxia results in anaerobic metabolism with increased production of lactate. This is the primary cause of metabolic acidosis in the shock state. The alteration in cellular metabolism, especially when coupled with the destructive effects of bacterial toxins, causes the lungs to compensate for the resultant hypoxia and acidosis. The patient's respirations become more rapid and shallow as the shock state progresses. This respiratory insufficiency can ultimately lead to acute respiratory failure. If hypovolemic shock is not corrected within 1 hour of injury or insult, the patient's survival is jeopardized.[50]

The inflammatory response results from a number of events and stimuli in the trauma population. Inflammation can occur directly from the injury. The more extensive the tissue destruction, the greater is the inflammatory response. Therefore, it is not uncommon to have very high white blood cell counts (i.e., 20,000 to 40,000 cells/mm^3) immediately following severe polytrauma. In addition to the trauma, inflammation can be induced by a variety of stimuli, including the presence of foreign objects such as bullets, stones, sutures, catheters, orthopedic hardware, and so on; exposure to toxic agents such as extremes of temperature, ionizing radiation, and chemicals; and the presence of biological agents such as microorganisms, bacterial toxins, antigen–antibody complexes, and devitalized and necrotic tissue.

It is important to determine the source of the inflammation so that appropriate therapy can be initiated. It may be virtually impossible to distinguish an inflammatory response that is induced by infection from one that is not. In such cases, the diagnosis of infection must be determined by the overall trend of the patient's clinical condition.[51, 52] Specific parameters facilitating this diagnosis are outlined later in this chapter.

The cellular immunological responses can be physically hampered by the inflammatory response, hematoma formation, edema, and the extent and characteristics of tissue destruction. The multifactorial effects of trauma on the complex interactions of the humoral and cell-mediated immune responses are often difficult to elucidate. Whether or not an overall depression of the immunological response occurs remains unclear.[53] Various defects of immunity following trauma have been identified. These include (1) responses and interactions of a variety of cellular populations, including neutrophils,[54–58] lymphocytes,[11, 29, 33, 59–61] monocytes, and macrophages,[33, 35, 60] (2) delayed hypersensitivity reactions,[62] (3) the function of the reticuloendothelial system,[26, 63] (4) opsonization,[25, 26, 31, 64] and (5) the activation of complement.[25, 30, 32, 64] Although there is some disagreement regarding the function of specific elements of these responses, it is generally agreed that the key determinants of immunological dysfunction emerge from the overall severity and characteristics of the trauma, the presence of shock, the obliteration of anatomical barriers, and the dilutional effects of massive fluid replacement.[53, 58]

As the patient progresses through the trauma cycle, the precipitating events of inflammation become less complex. Damaged tissues heal, function is restored, and fewer invasive interventions and mechanical support devices are required to maintain the patient. Therefore, increasing signs of inflammation developing during the later phase of recovery may be more easily attributed to infection than to some other cause.

Fever

Under normal conditions, body temperature is determined by the "set point" of the hypothalamic thermoregulatory system and a delicate balance between heat production and heat loss. Heat production is derived from the metabolism of food and body activity. Heat loss occurs via radiation, convection, and vaporization. It is accomplished by the peripheral blood flow in the skin, sweating, and heat loss with vapor from the lungs. The normal body temperature has a "set point" of 98.6°F (37.0°C), but variations of ±0.6°F can be observed. Therefore, the normal temperature range can vary from 98 to 99.2°F (36.6 to 37.5°C). Fever results from any disturbance in the hypothalamic thermoregulatory activity that leads to an increase of the thermal set point. Clinically, fever is defined as any temperature above 100.5°F (37.8°C) if taken orally or above 101.5°F (38.4°C) if taken rectally.

In normal healthy individuals, a fever is most frequently triggered by an infection from microorganisms, bacterial toxins, and/or antigens; an allergic reaction caused by the invasion of antigens; and/or the formation of antigen–antibody complexes.[65] These external agents, or *exogenous pyrogens,* stimulate the inflammatory response. The activation of the polymorphonuclear leukocytes, monocytes, and macrophages which mediate the inflammatory response releases an *endogenous pyrogen.*[66] When the fever pathway is triggered by antigenic stimulation, activation of the lymphocytes precedes activation of the phagocytic cells. In this case, the lymphocytes produce a "lymphokine" which then activates phagocytic cell populations. The exact mechanisms for the release of endogenous pyrogens are not known, but recent studies suggest the operation of more than one mechanism as well as the existence of more than one type of pyrogen.[67–70]

When endogenous pyrogen is released into the circulation, it travels to the thermosensitive neurons in the anterior hypothalamus. This, in turn, releases the inhibitory effect of these thermosensitive neurons on the "thermal-blind" neurons of the posterior hypothalamus, which leads to peripheral vasoconstriction.[71] Vasoconstriction is accompanied by a drop in body surface temperature. The thermal receptors in the skin activate somatic motor nerves which innervate the skeletal muscles. This leads to increased muscle contractions, expressed as shivering or shaking chills. A new thermal set point is established. The net results are increased body heat and a rise in body temperature (i.e., fever).

Fever is often described as one of the classical manifestations of infection. However, among trauma patients, the significance of the febrile response as well as the overall pattern of the temperature must be evaluated carefully. Many of the body's thermoregulatory mechanisms can be compromised by the nature of the underlying trauma. Patients sustaining massive burns, extensive soft-tissue injury, and severe spinal cord injury lose the skin's thermoregulatory functions. These patients can have a hypothermic set point, i.e., below 96°F (35.5°C). Therefore, a sudden increase of temperature to 99°F (37.2°C) may be indicative of fever in these patients. Elderly patients also can have a lower thermal set point, which is attributed to the deterioration of the skin's normal function. On the other hand, because of the chronic stimulation of the inflammatory response elicited by the implantation of a variety of mechanical devices as well as the damage and dysfunction of many organ systems, some patients may establish a higher than normal set point. These patients then appear to have a chronic fever. Patients sustaining severe brain injury resulting in compromise or injury of the hypothalamus can have highly irregular, widely variant temperature patterns. This condition is known as *central fever*.

Since fever is a manifestation of both infection and the noninfectious inflammatory responses, the diagnosis of infection can be difficult in trauma patients. These patients can have an intercurrent of multiple inflammatory responses occurring at the same time. Therefore, it is essential to continually evaluate the overall clinical condition against the trend of the temperature pattern. This is especially crucial during the early phases of the trauma cycle when the inflammatory responses are complex and acute. Nursing assessments can be enhanced by a clear understanding of the normal thermoregulatory mechanisms and the compromises induced by the characteristics of the underlying trauma. This is important throughout the trauma cycle.

THE MICROBIOLOGICAL RESERVOIR

As the trauma patient progresses through the cycle, the reservoirs of the microorganisms that can induce infection are continually changing. The contributory factors include the events of the initial trauma, the different locations of the patient in the health care delivery system, antibiotic utilization, and the underlying characteristics of the injuries and clinical condition.

There are both endogenous and exogenous sources of microorganisms.[72] The primary reservoir is the patient's own endogenous flora.[73] These are the organisms that abundantly colonize the skin, respiratory tract, gastrointestinal tract, and genitourinary tract. The predominant pathogen recovered from infections occurring in trauma patients has been shown to be coagulase-positive *Staphylococcus,*[13–17] which colonizes all four body systems. However, the organisms of the normal flora, the vast majority of which are nonpathogenic, act as pathogens when they are provided access into normally sterile body sites. These avenues are created by disruptions of the body's natural barriers. The overall composition of the normal flora as well as their usual patterns of antibiotic susceptibility can be altered by antibiotic therapy, changes in the patient's clinical condition, and exposure to the intensive care unit setting. The emergence of highly resistant strains creates complex dilemmas of therapy because more toxic antimicrobial agents must be employed should a serious infection develop. A summary of the normal flora is shown in Table 12–1.

The exogenous sources stem from the conditions at the accident scene and the hospital setting. Although relatively rare, organisms encountered from the accident scene can cause later serious, even fatal infection. These microorganisms become pathogenic when they are not debrided from

TABLE 12–1. THE MICROBIOLOGICAL RESERVOIR: THE NORMAL FLORA

SKIN	
Coagulase-positive staphylococci	*Bacillus* species
Coagulase-negative staphylococci	Diphtheroids
Aerobic and anaerobic streptococci	
RESPIRATORY TRACT	
Coagulase-positive staphylococci	*Acinetobacter* species
Aerobic and anaerobic streptococci	Lactobacilli
Neisseria species	*Actinomyces*
Bacteroides species	*Klebsiella* species
Fusobacterium species	*Pseudomonas* species
E. coli	
Hemophilus species	
Diphtheroids	
GASTROINTESTINAL TRACT	
Coagulase-positive staphylococci	Anaerobic staphylococci
Aerobic and anaerobic streptococci	Diphtheroids
Coagulase-negative staphylococci	*Bacteroides* species
Lactobacilli	*Fusobacterium* species
Clostridium species	*Klebsiella* species
Veillonella species	*Serratia* species
E. coli	*Pseudomonas* species
Enterobacter species	*Actinomyces* species
Proteus species	
Candida species	
GENITOURINARY TRACT	
Coagulase-positive staphylococci	Diphtheroids
Aerobic and anaerobic streptococci	*Hemophilus* species
Coagulase-negative staphylococci	*Fusobacterium* species
Lactobacilli	*Bacteroides* species
Neisseria species	*Candida* species
Clostridium species	
Actinomyces species	

open injuries, gain entry into tissues normally protected, or are aspirated into the lung.

On the other hand, the organisms encountered in the hospital setting are frequently the causative agents of infection.[74-76] Unwashed hands of the personnel, the use of contaminated equipment, and the sharing of supplies and equipment create a reservoir of potential pathogens and provide vehicles for cross-contamination among the patients. The primary objectives of infection control are to prevent these organisms from gaining access to sterile body sites, to eliminate the modes of transmission or cross-contamination, and to minimize any alteration of the patient's normal flora.

The presence of a microorganism in and of itself does not necessarily mean that an infection is evident. Nor does a positive culture necessarily mean that the patient is infected. A positive culture merely means that an organism is growing in the culture medium. Positive culture results must be evaluated from the perspective of the patient's clinical picture. In other words, there must be a specific host–parasite relationship in order for infection to occur.

Colonization occurs when the microorganisms exist in or on a body system and no detrimental effects result. In many instances, this can be a symbiotic relationship where both host and microorganism benefit. For example, the organisms colonizing the skin help to regulate the skin's pH and prevent pathogenic organisms from becoming established. Similarly, the gut flora provide the body with a natural source of vitamin K and add bulk to fecal material to promote peristalsis. Open wounds and the respiratory secretions of ventilator-dependent patients are often abundantly colonized with microorganisms, but their presence again does not necessarily mean that an infection has developed. Infection occurs when the organisms cause clinical injury or damage to the patient.

The relationship between the microorganisms and the patient and the development of infection is illustrated by the following formula:[72]

$$\text{Possibility of infection} = \frac{\text{no. of organisms} \times \text{virulence}}{\text{patient's resistance}}$$

The *number of organisms* means the dose or inoculum of microorganisms. The inoculum can stem from the patient's own endogenous flora, the hands of personnel, the environment of the hospital setting, and occasionally the accident scene. It can be reduced by the use of meticulous aseptic technique, adequate débridement of the wounds, proper cleaning and maintenance of equipment, strict compliance with infection-control guidelines, and handwashing.

The *virulence of the organism* means its ability to cause disease. For example, *Staphylococcus aureus,* which produces the enzyme coagulase, is more capable of inducing infection than *Staphylococcus epidermidis,* which does not produce coagulase. However, among critically ill patients, organisms such as coagulase-negative staphylococci and fungi that were thought to be nonpathogenic organisms are now emerging as the pathogens of serious and fatal infections.[77-81] Two factors contribute to this new trend of nosocomial pathogens: the increased use of invasive support devices and the availability of new potent antibiotics. Therefore, among the trauma population, it is important to remember that any microorganism, given the right opportunity, can cause serious and even fatal disease.

The major factor influencing the development of infection is the loss, dysfunction, circumvention, or impedance of the host defense mechanisms. It is crucial that nurses have a very clear understanding of these mechanisms and their relationship to infection risks so that the delivery of patient care can ultimately promote patient safety and minimize the outcome of infectious complications.

INFECTION RISK FACTORS

Contributory infection risks are constantly changing as the patient proceeds through the cycle of initial injury to recovery. These risks revolve around the the following factors: the clinical setting; the therapeutic interventions (e.g., antibiotics, surgery, invasive support devices, infusates, medications, and so forth); the amount of attention paid to infection-control guidelines; and most important, the nature and extent of the injuries and the compromise of the host defense mechanisms. Therefore, in order to facilitate the prevention of infection, one must not only identify these factors but also recognize the influences that each has on the other.

Clinical Setting

Time, organization, and the amount of attention paid to infection-control guidelines influence the environmental infection risks. Rapid institution of invasive therapy is crucial if patients are to survive. During these emergent conditions, there is literally no time to comply with accepted infection-control guidelines (i.e., meticulous skin preparation of operative and procedure sites, performance of scrupulous aseptic technique, gentle tissue handling, adherence to proper dress codes, or even handwashing). Sterile trays and fields can be easily contaminated as the attention of the staff focuses on the needs of the patient rather than the equipment in the environment. As more people become involved in the resuscitation, the less space there is for the staff to function, and the environment becomes more chaotic and cluttered. All these factors increase the probability of contamination. However, if the patient survives the crisis, the scenarios of this emergent situation are quickly forgotten. As soon as the patient is hemodynamically stable, the greatest infection threat is the failure to replace the resuscitation lines using stringent aseptic technique.

In nonemergent clinical settings, the lack of attention paid to infection-control measures by the hospital staff continues to be the primary cause of cross-contamination among the patients. The most important of these is the failure of the staff to frequently practice appropriate handwashing.[82] Handwashing involves only a few minutes of time, but the frequency with which handwashing should be performed—before and after each patient contact—can be time-consuming. In addition, traffic patterns of the hospital staff and the nurse/patient ratio can influence handwashing practices as well as overall compliance with infection-control guidelines.[83-87] The trauma team comprises many members: physicians, nurses, allied health professionals such as physical and respiratory therapists, and ancillary personnel. Therefore, it is not uncommon for one person to have multiple patient contacts during the course of his or her shift. Each time such personnel fail to wash their hands, the chances of cross-contamination increase. Similarly, handwashing prior to each and every patient contact or procedure may be difficult for the busy nurse responsible for the care of more than one patient. This is a particular hazard in the intensive care unit, where nurses must frequently manipulate vascular lines and other mechanical support devices. This equipment can be inoculated by the bacteria on their hands, and these bacteria can then gain direct access into the patient. Unfortunately, unless there is a constant reminder, as well as an awareness regarding the importance of handwashing, the practice of handwashing is too often forgotten. In addition, the hands of the patient, especially the fingernails, require care. This can be important for the confused or stuporous patient who may scratch off dressings or scratch suture lines. Other unconscious habits that can create infection hazards include spraying antibiotics into the environment, uncapping needles with one's teeth, touching sterile fields with bare hands, allowing fluid to reflux from drainage vessels back into the patient's body cavity, and dress code infractions.[87, 88]

The resuscitation and care of trauma patients often require a vast array and quantity of equipment and supplies. However, improper and inadequate cleaning of equipment, utilization of supplies and equipment beyond recommended sterility intervals, and sharing supplies and equipment among and between patients can promote infection hazards, create reservoirs of microorganisms, and facilitate infectious outbreaks and epidemic situations. Tape and scissors are common vehicles of cross-contamination. The misuse of tape when it is being applied to dressings can defeat the purpose of aseptic technique. Specifically, it is the practice of sticking strips of tape to such objects as bed rails, countertops, and IV poles prior to their application to the dressings that can result in problems. Tape is not sterile, but it is biologically clean. The surfaces of the equipment can be contaminated with bacteria that stick to the tape and thus inoculate the dressings. Scissors become a vehicle for cross-contamination when they are used to remove wound dressings. The grooves and notches of the scissor blades can become contaminated with wound drainage and exudates. This material is often teeming with bacteria, which can then be introduced into another patient's wounds at the next dressing change. Scissor blades should be washed and disinfected with alcohol after each dressing change. Disposable scissors may be best utilized for dressing changes on large open wounds.

Nurses can play a vital role in counteracting the environmental infection risks. The most important action is to increase their awareness and practice of infection-control guidelines. This must be emphasized in all phases of the trauma cycle.

Nature of the Injuries

It has been well documented that critically ill patients are predisposed to infection by the very nature of their underlying illness.[4, 12, 88–93] In the trauma population, those sustaining severe and multisystem injuries are at greatest risk.[3, 6, 13–17] Concomitantly, specific characteristics of each type of injury—open injuries, aspiration of fluids and objects into the lungs, extensive soft-tissue injuries and burns, crushing injuries, and blunt injuries—create specific infection risks. Open injuries, such as open bone fractures, traumatic amputations, degloving and avulsion injuries, and gunshot and stab wounds, annihilate many of the body's external barriers. In addition, these wounds can be heavily contaminated with microorganisms as well as a variety of foreign objects such as bullets, glass, leaves, and sticks. Shock, hypovolemia, hypoxia, localized ischemia, and hematoma formation can hinder inflammatory responses, cause tissue necrosis, and aid the creation of environments in which bacteria can thrive. The physiological aspects of the underlying injury, coupled with the consequences of invasive procedures and devices, break down the patient's resistance to infection.

The management of the consequences of trauma often requires complex chemotherapy, and drug therapy also can contribute to the patient's susceptibility to infection.[94] Antibiotics alter the composition of the normal flora, and their toxic side effects can cause the failure of many body organs.[95] Anesthetic agents, corticosteroids, antacids, and H_2-blocking agents are but a few of many medications that can alter the normal system functions and hinder both internal and external defense mechanisms.[11, 96, 97] Therefore, it is important that nurses understand and recognize the dual-edged nature of medication relative to infection risks.

Once the patient has undergone the resuscitative phase, an intercurrent of multiple pathological events can occur. This can confuse the overall clinical picture and hamper the diagnosis of infection. Examples of such events include coma, fever, hypotension, shock, atelectasis, respiratory distress syndrome, hyperglycemia, and renal failure. The severely injured patient may have one or many of these events occurring at the same time. Therefore, it is very important to clearly understand the characteristics and manifestations of these clinical conditions as well as their similarities and relationships to the diagnostic parameters delineating infection.

It is becoming increasingly apparent that effective infection-control practices for the trauma population must arise from the recognition of the patient's predisposing risks relative to the underlying nature of injuries as well as the consequences of therapy. As previously described, nurses must be ever alert throughout the trauma cycle to the continually changing status of the patient's host defense mechanisms relative to the consequences of injury and therapy.

Invasive Therapy

It is a paradox of modern medical care that the invasive interventions used to resuscitate and sustain the patient's life are equally responsible for the breakdown of the natural defenses and the subsequent development of infection.[4, 13–17, 72, 90, 91, 98–101] Trauma patients require the most extensive use of invasive therapy of any critically ill patient population. The vast majority of these patients must undergo at least one operative procedure, if not several. It is not uncommon for the patient to have several intravenous lines, an arterial line, a pulmonary arterial line, an endotracheal tube, a nasogastric tube, a urinary catheter, various types of surgical drainage devices, orthopedic hardware, cerebral pressure-sensing devices, and chest tubes. Each catheter, drain, device, and procedure creates a portal of entry for microorganisms. Once the microbes are established at a new site, the probability that infection will later develop is greatly increased. In addition, the immediate resuscitation may require massive fluid replacement with crystalloids as well as blood and blood products. All these fluids can become a reservoir of microorganisms should contamination occur.

The greatest infection risk occurs when the patient is in the intensive care unit because the patient has the maximum number of indwelling devices at the same time. The need to frequently handle and manipulate these devices, the failure to practice handwashing, and the failure to maintain the various catheter and drainage systems as *closed* systems can serve to inoculate the patient with the exogenous bacteria of the intensive care unit. This inoculation can be enhanced during linen changes or when the patient is being repositioned, moved in and out of bed, or transported to another area for diagnostic or operative procedures. All these situations require a number of people to have direct patient contact. Once again, the primary infection risk is the lack of attention paid by these personnel to the infection-control guidelines.

Concomitantly, these devices can be contaminated with substances that enhance bacterial colonization. The most common of these substances is dried blood, which can provide bacteria with essential nutrients. In addition, the tacky residue left by iodophor solutions can actually facilitate bacterial adherence as well as lead to the cracking and staining of some plastic or rubber materials.[102] Similarly, adhesive tape residue aids both bacterial adherence and nutrition. Respiratory secretions provide nutrients as well as their own source of intrinsic microorganisms. Therefore, nursing care includes keeping these devices clean and properly maintained. Dried blood can be easily removed with hydrogen peroxide, and lines used for frequent blood sampling should be thoroughly flushed. Alcohol rather than iodophor should be used to disinfect surfaces composed of inorganic material. Alcohol also can be used to remove iodophor residue. Tape should not be used on an IV line. If this is necessary, silk or paper tape rather than adhesive tape should be used.

As long as the patient is invaded with multiple devices, the possibility of autoinfection exists. *Autoinfection* occurs when organisms move from one body site and establish infection at another site. This can be a direct or secondary event. An example of direct autoinfection is the development of septic phlebitis at a catheter insertion site. If this infection is serious, a secondary bacteremia can develop. Then, if the bacteremia persists, this secondary event can cause infection at yet another site. The bacteremia can seed implanted devices such as orthopedic hardware and induce later bone infection, or it can directly infect another tissue such as the brain and induce a brain abscess.

Although, the infection risk associated with the use of invasive devices is greatest during the initial phases of resuscitation and in the intensive care unit setting, the risk remains as long as an invasive or implanted device is present. Therefore, it is absolutely essential that nurses search for methods to keep microorganisms in their normal habitats and to eliminate the modes of transmission of organisms and be ever attentive to infection-control guidelines.

Antibiotic Utilization

Although modern antibiotic therapy has dramatically reduced the morbidity and mortality of infectious disease, antibiotic utilization is a complex issue in patient care. Antibiotics are powerful drugs with dual-edged consequences. They can prevent and cure infection, but they also can alter the composition of the body's resident flora, promote superinfections, and induce the emergence of antibiotic-resistant flora. Therefore, antibiotic use must be judicious.

Antibiotic Selection

The factors guiding the selection of appropriate antibiotics for the treatment of infection[95] include

1. The *site* of infection. Certain organisms are associated with particular infections, and the effectiveness of the antibiotic varies for different tissues.
2. The *severity* of infection.
3. The *identity* of the organism.
4. The *antibiotic susceptibility* of the organism.
5. The *clinical condition* of the patient. More critically ill patients may have renal or liver failure, which could influence antibiotic selection, and sicker patients may require more aggressive and broad-spectrum therapy.
6. A basic knowledge of what organisms usually cause infection in a specific hospital unit.

When a patient develops a septic crisis, there is often no time to wait for culture results before initiating treatment. It takes approximately 72 hours to identify the organism and determine sensitivity patterns. Therefore, initial antibiotic selection can be aided by the use of a Gram stain, which can be performed in a matter of minutes. It is important to remember that this *does not* identify a specific organism—it qualitatively characterizes the nature of the specimen by demonstrating the presence and morphology of cells and organisms. Once the culture and sensitivity results are known, the antibiotics can be adjusted accordingly. The goal is to select a drug that maximizes effectiveness without inducing toxic side effects in the patient.

For severely traumatized patients, antibiotic utilization becomes more complex. Because of the nature of their injuries, the major compromise of their defense mechanisms, and their exposure to the intensive care unit, it is highly probable that the overall composition of their normal flora will change. It is not at all uncommon for these patients to be subjected to repeated courses of antibiotics. These drugs can be given both as prophylaxis for injury or surgery and as therapy for infection. Each time an antibiotic is used, the possibility of the emergence of resistant organisms increases. Thus, while the antibiotic is treating one infection, it may very well be inducing colonization at another site in the patient. This other site may then become the focus for a subsequent infection. Therefore, it is important to remember which antibiotics an individual patient has received so that the organism of an ensuing infection can be more readily determined.

Antibiotic Prophylaxis

Although the prophylactic use of antibiotics has been proven to be beneficial prior to some elective surgeries,[103] the benefits of prophylaxis for certain open injuries remains unclear.[104–108] Supporting the argument is the premise that administration of antibiotics following open injury is never prophylactic owing to the extensive presence of bacterial contamination. While it has been shown in animal models that there is a critical time period—within 3 to 4 hours of injury—when antibiotic administration appears to be effective in reducing the incidence of wound infection,[109] real-life situations may prevent early administration of prophylactic antibiotics. In addition, antibiotics are totally useless in the presence of devitalized tissue and indwelling contamination by foreign objects such as bullets.

Because of the complex dilemmas that antibiotic utilization presents, their prophylactic use must be considered carefully. Unfortunately, there is no one "wonder antibiotic" that can effectively eradicate all the microorganisms that can cause infection. No matter which antibiotic is selected, an advantage will always be given to another organism. For example, if a first-generation cephalosporin is given to minimize the subsequent infection from staphylococci, the composition of the patient's normal microbial flora can be shifted to favor *Pseudomonas*.

It is the prolonged administration of antibiotics that changes the flora and creates antibiotic-resistant organisms. Coupled with the use of invasive support devices that provide access to normally sterile body sites, it is easy to see how superinfection can be promoted. Therefore, the duration of prophylaxis should be kept short. Efficacy has been confirmed using a single preoperative dose and intervals equal to or less than 12 hours after the procedure. In addition, comparison studies of short courses (less than or equal to 24 hours) versus long courses (3 to 5 days) have had equivalent outcomes in certain injuries.[109–112]

Benefits versus risks must always be considered. Many prophylactic antibiotic uses once believed to be effective are now subject to controversy and debate. For example, it used to be standard practice to give prophylaxis to any patient sustaining a cerebrospinal fluid leak in order to minimize the possibility of meningitis. However, recent studies have shown that prophylactic antimicrobial therapy does not in fact prevent meningitis and may actually promote the development of gram-negative meningitis.[106, 113] Present recommendations for antibiotic prophylaxis in trauma patients include only those injuries producing open bone fractures, disruption of the intraoral mucosa, or penetrating injury of the colon. Courses of therapy should be short (i.e., 48 to 72 hours).[13–17, 114]

Antibiotic Resistance

Although some microorganisms can be naturally resistant to certain antibiotics, many, especially the gram-negative bacilli, can acquire drug resistance by extrachromosomal fragments of DNA known as *plasmids* or *R-factors*.[115, 116] Plasmids allow the organisms to synthesize enzymes that can inactivate the antibiotic, change the structure of the bacterial cell wall, or produce metabolic enzymes that make the cell resistant to inhibition by the antibiotic. The beta-lactamases, penicillinase, and cephalosporinase, which hydrolyze the peptide bond of the beta-lactam antibiotics, are good examples of enzymes that can inactivate an antibiotic. Expression of these enzymes is induced by exposure of the bacteria to the respective antibiotics.[115–120] Similarly, the emergence of aminoglycoside resistance also has been demonstrated to occur in patients exposed to repeated courses of aminoglycoside antibiotics.[121, 122] Expression of these enzymes gives the organisms a survival advantage.

The greatest impact of an antibiotic-resistance emergency occurs in the intensive care unit. Because of the many different procedures necessary to care for these patients, the opportunity for transmission of an antibiotic-resistant organism from one patient to another is always present. In addition, it has been demonstrated that the intensive care unit environment itself can promote this phenomenon.[123–127] This is caused by the aerosolization of antibiotics that spray off syringes or IV lines as nurses prepare to give the drugs.[127, 128] The environmental selection pressure can become so great that an outbreak of infection caused by these resistant organisms can develop. In fact, in one such outbreak, control of the epidemic could not be accomplished until there was a complete cessation of antibiotic use.[129] Therefore, it is important to monitor the antibiotic history of the patient as well as the overall antibiotic use of the unit and the antibiograms of the recovered pathogens.

Impact of Antibiotic Utilization

The medical management of the critically ill patients infected with resistant organisms can be a complex problem. A dilemma of therapy can be created, since the toxic side effects attributed to the use of the antibiotics may in some instances be as devastating as the infection itself. Sensitive monitoring procedures demonstrating the effectiveness of therapy are required. This may be accomplished via pharmacokinetic evaluation, synergy studies, or determination of minimum inhibitory concentrations or serum bactericidal levels of the antibiotics. Clinical parameters that may indicate the deleterious effects of therapy should be monitored daily. Moreover, because of the very complex characteristics of these patients, more than one infection process may be occurring simultaneously, and antibiotic selection must be constantly reevaluated. When antibiotics are started, the indication and length of therapy should be well defined. When the patient has received what is considered appropriate therapy, antibiotics should be discontinued.

If the patient is still febrile, new sites and new organisms should be looked for instead of continuing the antibiotics beyond the specific time period. This will ensure shorter courses of therapy that are much more site- and organism-directed and discourage continued long-term use of antibiotics, which could lead to increased colonization and subsequent infection with resistant and more opportunistic organisms.

The problem of antibiotic-resistance emergencies has promoted the search for new antimicrobial agents. During the middle to late 1980s, many new groups of antibiotics became available for use. These included the third-generation cephalosporins, the newer penicillins, and the quinolones.[130, 131] These newer antibiotics are more stable against attack by the bacterial enzymes, so the induction of resistance may be impeded. In addition, these drugs have an expanded spectrum of activity against a wide variety of microorganisms. The expanded spectrum may eliminate the need to give several antibiotics when treating infections caused by more than one organism. Many have longer half-lives and can be given less frequently. It should be remembered that newer antibiotics are very expensive drugs, so both these factors can reduce the cost of therapy. However, these advantages can be offset by an increased risk of superinfection, the toxic side effects, and a misuse in which a less expensive but therapeutically equivalent drug can adequately treat an infection. Therefore, the search for the "one wonder drug" will go on.

Because of the complexities of antibiotic therapy, the need to decrease the emergence of antibiotic-resistant microorganisms, and the demand for cost-containment measures for these very expensive drugs, overall antibiotic utilization must be continuously monitored.[132–134] In addition, mechanisms to enforce recommended prescription guidelines must be sought. In fact, the Joint Commission on Accreditation of Hospitals has required health care facilities to define prescribing guidelines and audit antibiotic utilization.[135] An example of guidelines for antibiotic utilization in the trauma patient is presented in Table 12–2.

As mentioned previously, the normal flora in the critically ill patient can be affected by the nature of the underlying injury as well as by compromise of the defense mechanisms. Therefore, it is difficult to clearly define the overall impact of antibiotic therapy. It is a constant challenge throughout the trauma cycle.

SURVEILLANCE AND IDENTIFICATION OF INFECTION

Evaluation of infection among the critically ill trauma population can be difficult and complex. The patients are usually unable to communicate or sense their symptoms as a result of a decreased level of consciousness, disorientation, sedation, endotracheal intubation, or central nervous system injury. Physical examination may be hampered by the placement of bandages; multiple indwelling devices; casts, traction, or fixation devices; the patient's immobility; and the use of isolation precautions. Diagnostic tests are frequently difficult to obtain because it is often cumbersome and risky to transport the patient to the proper department to obtain a particular evaluation. In addition, whether the patient is transported to the proper facility or portable studies are obtained, it may be impossible to place the patient in the optimal position for the study. Therefore, the results can be less definitive.

TABLE 12–2. GUIDELINES FOR ANTIMICROBIAL UTILIZATION

1. Restrict the prophylactic use of antibiotics to situations in which effectiveness has been demonstrated.
2. Use narrow-spectrum rather than broad-spectrum antibiotics.
3. Prescribe adequate dosages to ensure eradication of the organisms and minimal toxicity to the patient.
4. Use short therapeutic courses, i.e., 7 to 10 days, whenever possible.
5. Reserve third-generation cephalosporins, the new semisynthetic penicillins, and amikacin sulfate for use against resistant organisms.
6. Perform close monitoring of patients for adverse effects of antibiotics.
7. Conduct general audits of antibiotic utilization to evaluate the effectiveness of therapy as well as abuses in utilization.

Classical indicators of infection such as leukocytosis and fever may not be useful in the critically ill trauma patient. For example, fever may be the result of atelectasis, drug reactions, transfusion reactions, central nervous system dysfunction, hematoma formation, the presence of necrotic tissue, or inflammation alone. These patients can be hemodynamically unstable and in shock as a result of hemorrhage, cardiac and pulmonary dysfunction, or neurological dysfunction, not necessarily sepsis. It is these multiple aspects of the patient's underlying condition that must be differentiated from infection.

Since the evaluation of infection is complex in the critically ill trauma population, the most effective infection surveillance system is the infectious disease team, whose primary responsibility is to evaluate all high-risk patients.[114] However, whether the trauma center utilizes the infectious disease team approach or not, the key means for infection surveillance must stem from the prospective trend analysis of individual patients. Clinical parameters such as the pattern of the fever curve, white blood cell count, platelet count, creatinine level, use of corticosteroids and antibiotics, roentgenograms, Gram stain and culture results, and placement of indwelling devices should be documented and monitored daily by the team. Although time-consuming and cumbersome, this prospective surveillance facilitates trend analysis, the early diagnosis of infection, and the appropriateness of antibiotic therapy. It also establishes endemic infection rates, identifies infection hazards, monitors effectiveness of infection-control practice, and establishes baselines. Early diagnosis of infection may be enhanced by routine surveillance cultures of the sputum of patients on mechanical ventilators and of the urine of patients with indwelling urinary catheters, since colonization patterns, as well as the impact of antibiotic therapy, can be determined. Additionally, the use of a fever protocol may be beneficial. For example, with each temperature spike of 102.2°F (39°C) or change of 1.8°F (1°C), the following fever protocol could be automatically obtained: two sets of percutaneously drawn blood cultures, white blood cell count with differential, urine culture and urinalysis, sputum Gram stain and culture, and chest x-ray. Sites of wounds and indwelling catheters should be examined, suspect lines removed and cultured via semiquantitative technique, and any purulent drainage sent for culture and Gram stain. Sinus films should be obtained on patients with indwelling nasal tubes. If there is a suspicion of a central nervous system infection in patients sustaining head and spinal cord injury, the neurosurgeon should be consulted so that the safety of performing a lumbar puncture can be determined.

Although infection surveillance should be comprehensive and aggressive during the initial and intensive phases of the trauma cycle, it is a continuous process across the entire cycle. The infection risks are always in a dynamic state of change, and they must be constantly reevaluated as the status of the patient changes. As the patient recovers, the infection risks tend to decrease. However, eradication of many infections may be difficult during these later phases. These infections may be caused by the more resistant microorganisms or develop chronic patterns that are difficult to manage. Infection developing during any phase of the cycle always jeopardizes the final outcome—it prolongs the recovery and may even prevent saving the patient's life.

INFECTION RELATED TO DISRUPTION OF THE SKIN

Wound infection has been described extensively in literature and is the most frequently cited infectious complication following trauma.[3, 4, 136–144] However, it is important to realize that these infections comprise only 8 to 20 per cent of overall infections and that the majority of serious bacteremic illnesses in the severely traumatized patient are actually related to vascular and pulmonary infections.[13–17]

Any disruption or compromise of the skin's integrity can result in infection. These events include physical trauma, operative and invasive procedures, and inadequate tissue perfusion secondary to prolonged pressure, avascular necrosis, ischemia, hematoma, edema, or inflammation. At highest risk are massive open soft-tissue injuries such as traumatic amputations, degloving and avulsion injuries, burns, and high-energy open fractures. Stratification of the infection risks for operative wounds are defined by the class of surgery. These classes are outlined in Table 12–3 and are determined according to the degree of expected bacterial contamination relative to the surgical procedure.[145]

Management of the wound must overcome three basic factors if wound infection is to be prevented.[137] First, bacteria can contaminate any wound whether it results from trauma or an operative procedure. Second, the risk of infection increases proportionately with the extent of contamination.

TABLE 12–3. CLASSIFICATION OF SURGICAL PROCEDURES

Class I: Clean surgical procedures

Definition: Nontraumatic, uninfected operative wounds in which no inflammation is encountered, there is no break in technique, and neither the respiratory, alimentary, and/or genitourinary tracts nor the oropharyngeal cavities are entered.

Expected infection rate: 1 to 5 per cent

Class II: Clean-contaminated surgical procedures

Definition: Operations in which the respiratory, alimentary, and/or genitourinary tracts are entered under controlled conditions and without unusual contamination.

Expected infection rate: 8 to 11 per cent

Class III: Contaminated surgical procedures

Definition: Operations associated with open, fresh accidental wounds; major breaks in sterile technique or gross spillage from the gastrointestinal tract; or acute, nonpurulent inflammation is encountered.

Expected infection rate: 15 to 20 per cent

Class IV: Dirty and infected procedures

Definition: Operations involving old traumatic wounds with devitalized tissue and those which involve existing clinical infection.

Expected infection rate: >25 per cent

Third, devitalized tissue creates an environment supportive of bacterial growth. Therefore, the importance of meticulous aseptic and surgical technique cannot be overemphasized. It is well documented that sound surgical principles—gentle tissue handling, complete hemostasis, maintaining adequate blood supply, débridement of dead tissue, obliteration of dead space, avoidance of hematoma, and wound closure without tension—have significantly reduced the incidence of postoperative wound infections.[138–140, 146, 147] On the other hand, prolonged operative and anesthesia time, breaks in aseptic technique, and surgical misadventures significantly enhance the infection risks. In addition, practices determined not to reduce wound infection rates include preoperative shaving,[148] adhesive plastic drapes,[139] drains other than closed-suction systems,[139, 149, 150] ultraviolet lights,[151] and topical antibiotic and antiseptic irrigation solutions.[152–154]

Wound infections are divided into two broad categories—*superficial,* occurring above the fascial planes, and *deep-seated,* occurring below the fascial planes.[139, 140, 155] Therefore, wound infections can range from mild cases of cellulitis to deep-seated abscesses of the muscle, bone, and internal organ systems. The deep-seated infections are discussed elsewhere in this chapter.

Superficial Infections

Superficial infections range from mild conditions such as cellulitis to serious, fulminant conditions such as necrotizing fasciitis.[155] Clear definitions for some of these infections remain obscure because many underlying conditions present the same signs and symptoms. For example, pain, swelling, tenderness, redness, fever, and elevated white blood cell count are common signs and symptoms of the inflammatory response. Since inflammation can be induced by a variety of stimuli, it is virtually impossible to visually distinguish an inflammatory response induced by infection from one that is not. It is equally impossible to identify a causative organism by the color, odor, or consistency of drainage material. Therefore, the diagnosis of infection should stem from the evaluation of the overall trend of the patient's clinical condition, careful examination of the patient, the presence or absence of culture-positive material, and responses to therapy, such as wound débridement and antibiotic coverage. Cellulitis attributed to infection is characterized as an inflammatory reaction that dissipates as a response to antimicrobial therapy. Usually there is no purulent discharge. Suppurative wound infections are defined by inflammation, induration, and the presence of purulent, culture-positive material. Systemic manifestations such as fever, leukocytosis, and secondary bacteremia can occur. Surgical excision and débridement of the abscess and initiation of antibiotics are usually required. These infections are considered to be of nosocomial etiology when they are located along the margins of surgical incisions or around foreign bodies such as sutures, catheters, drains, or fixation devices. The most frequently isolated organism is *Staphylococcus aureus.* However, if these infections develop following prior antibiotic therapy or prolonged hospitalization, gram-negative bacilli such as *Escherichia coli, Pseudomonas aeruginosa,* or *Enterobacter* species or other gram-positive cocci such as coagulase-negative staphylococci may be recovered from the exudate.

The Gram stain, culture, and sensitivity testing of isolated organisms are key diagnostic tools for the evaluation of infection. It is important to always perform a Gram stain and culture of the purulent material. Usually, it takes approximately 72 hours before results of culture and sensitivity testing can be determined. However, the results of a Gram stain can be known in a matter of minutes. The Gram stain characterizes the nature of the pus. This includes the relative proportion of white blood cells and epithelial cells as well as the morphology and staining properties of any organisms (i.e., gram-positive cocci, gram-negative bacilli). The Gram stain cannot, however, identify specific microorganisms. It is the presence of a heavy concentration of polymorphonuclear leukocytes and the predominance of one or two organisms that are generally considered significant. Evaluation of the Gram stain enhances a "best guess" as to the possible identity of the organisms. This can facilitate appropriate antibiotic selection until the bacteria are identified by culture and antibiotic susceptibility is known. It is important to remember that two samples or swabs of material must be obtained from each suspicious site so that the laboratory can perform all the necessary tests. Intraoperative cultures should be sent for both aerobic and anaerobic evaluations.

The diagnosis of infection in large open wounds resulting from avulsion and degloving injuries, amputations, and fasciotomy following compartmental syndromes is often difficult. The diagnosis can be impeded by the underlying nature of the wound, especially when devitalized and necrotic tissues are present. All such wounds can be colonized with a wide variety of microorganisms. They also can visually appear to be clean even when they are actually infected. This can be a primary cause of subsequent skin-graft or muscle-flap failure. Therefore, the best determinant of whether tissues are viable for delayed closures or grafting procedures or incubating infection is the use of a quantitative tissue culture.[156–158] Bacterial colony counts are determined by the gram weight of the tissue biopsy. Culture results are considered to be significant when the colony count exceeds 100,000 organisms per gram of tissue.

Necrotizing Fasciitis

Necrotizing fasciitis is a rapidly progressive, potentially fatal infection of the skin and underlying fascia.[155, 159] It is a relatively rare phenomenon following trauma but can occur in any location on the skin. Patients with underlying vascular insufficiencies attributed to diabetes mellitus, obesity, and atherosclerosis are most susceptible. The causative organisms are group A streptococci, *Staphylococcus aureus,* and the anaerobic streptococci. Fournier's gangrene is a specific form of necrotizing fasciitis.[160, 161] Fournier's gangrene is most frequently cited as occurring in older men and seems to localize in the perineal and scrotal area. It is a synergistic infection among the staphylococci, the enteric gram-negative bacilli, and the anaerobic staphylococci and streptococci. These infections spread rapidly along the fascial planes and produce necrosis of the overlying skin but do not invade the underlying muscle. Necrotizing fasciitis is a serious infection because of the fulminant progression and propensity to spread to the lymphatics and bloodstream. Early recognition is crucial to ensure the patient's survival. Treatment involves emergent and aggressive excision of all involved skin and subcutaneous tissues and immediate institution of antibiotics.

Clostridial Infections

Fortunately, infections caused by *Clostridium* species are relatively rare. However, because they are rapidly progressive infections, when they occur, they are almost always fatal. Since clostridia are widely distributed in nature, wound contamination of open injuries is quite common. The pathogenic clostridia can be divided into three major groups according to the diseases they produce:[162] the histotoxic clostridia, *C. perfringens, C. novyi, C. septicum, C. histolyticum, C. bifermentans,* and *C. fallax,* which characteristically cause a variety of tissue infections—the most common being myonecrotic gas gangrene; *C. tetani,* the causative agent of tetanus; and *C. botulinum* type A, the causative agent of wound botulism. In all these infections, it is the production of potent exotoxins that is primarily responsible for the rapid progression of disease and the extent of damage to the involved tissues.

Gas Gangrene

Gas gangrene is a rapidly progressive, life-threatening toxemic infection of the skeletal muscle. It is most frequently associated with open bone fractures, but it can develop secondary to biliary and bowel surgery. Clostridial myonecrosis results when the wound is inoculated by clostridial spores. These spores can germinate and produce clinical disease in 72 hours. However, if vegetative forms of the organism are present, the onset of disease can occur within hours of inoculation. Lecithinase, or alpha-toxin, which has the ability to destroy cell membranes and alter capillary permeability is the exotoxin responsible for the progression of disease. Symptoms begin suddenly with severe local pain and tense swelling about the wound site. Accompanying systemic signs include tachycardia, hypotension, fever, agitation, and disorientation. Muscle necrosis is marked by distinct, advancing margins, and crepitance is usually evident. Serous hemorrhagic bullae can develop. A Gram stain of the exudate will show gram-positive rods and an absence of polymorphonuclear leukocytes. Early recognition is vitally important in order to save the involved limb, or even the life, of the patient.

Treatment necessitates immediate surgical exploration with excision of all necrotic tissue and emergent institution of large doses of penicillin. When the infection is related to open bone fracture and is limited to one or a few muscle groups, salvage of the limb may be possible. The majority of cases require open amputation. Patients developing infection of the abdominal wall have the poorest prognosis.[163]

Despite the lack of controlled clinical studies to verify the usefulness of hyperbaric oxygen therapy, patients may be transferred to a facility that can offer this type of care. The theoretical benefit is a promotion of wound healing after the initial surgery.[163, 165–170] Whether a consequence of injury or infection, the central area of wounds where the vasculature has been disrupted and the inflammatory reaction occurs is characteristically hypoxic. New vessel formation is suppressed by hypoxia.[171] However, hyperbaric oxygen has been shown to enhance the rate of wound healing in devascularized wounds by increasing the Po_2 in the damaged tissues.[172, 173] Therefore, hyperbaric oxygen therapy counteracts the effects of wound hypoxia. In addition, it may inhibit alpha-toxin production by the bacteria.[174] However, bactericidal effects of hyperbaric oxygen therapy have not been established. In fact, recent studies have shown that hyperbaric oxygen therapy of intensities and durations acceptable for human use may have little, if any, of the bacteriostatic effect reported with more vigorous in vitro oxygen-exposure protocols.[175]

The best treatment of gas gangrene is prevention by extensive initial débridement and open wound management.

Tetanus

The spores of *C. tetani* are ubiquitous. Simple puncture wounds from nails, splinters, thorns, or contaminated syringes and IV needles can provide conditions conducive for the development of tetanus. Open fractures, punctures by dirty metal objects, and injuries from farm cultivation equipment offer the same environment. However, tetanus is a preventable disease provided proper immunization has been given. Therefore, the key determinants of infection are the characterization of the wound and the patient's immunization history. Tetanus should be suspected in patients who have the appropriate risk factors and present with symptoms of neuromuscular dysfunction. This can be evident beginning with profound neuromuscular rigidity in the injured region followed by progressive central nervous system dysfunction: tremors and spasms of facial, pharyngeal, and laryngeal muscles (lockjaw); nuchal rigidity; and opisthotonos (hyperextension spasms of the paraspinous muscles). Seizures and autonomic nervous system involvement are common. Treatment involves sedation, paralytic agents, mechanical ventilation, high doses of penicillin, and large doses of tetanus immunoglobulin (TIG). Mortality has been reported at 50 per cent.[176, 177]

Wound Botulism

Wound botulism is an extremely rare, potentially fatal complication of open injury.[178, 179] It is caused by *C. botulinum* type A. Like all clostridial infections, it develops when the organisms or its spores are not adequately removed during initial débridement of a wound. The diagnosis is suggested in patients who complain of difficulty in swallowing or breathing several days following injury. Double vision and difficulty in speaking are also common complaints. The wound, however, may or may not appear infected. Death is generally attributed to respiratory failure. Treatment involves immediate respiratory support, administration of botulinum antitoxin, wound débridement, and administration of myoneural agents such as guanidine hydrochloride. The role of antibiotics remains unclear.

Since the ultimate salvage of limb and life is critically dependent on early recognition of the development of clostridial infection, it is essential that nurses have a basic understanding of these diseases. This is especially important for nurses who care for the patients during the first days to weeks of the injury.

Burn Wound Infections

A variety of infections can develop in burn patients. These infections are discussed in the sections of this chapter specific to each site. Therefore, only those infections related to burn wounds will be discussed here.

Burns have unique wound infection risks relative to the nature of the injury.[141, 180] The contributory factors include loss of the skin's mechanical barrier, an impeded ability to sense toxic stimuli, and the inability to control heat and water loss. Additional factors are related to the agent inducing the burn, the size and degree of the burn, and the injury of other organ systems. Patients with extensive third-degree burns are at greatest risk.

A full-thickness burn results in residual cutaneous tissue that is dead protein, called *eschar*. Therefore, eschar is always avascular and nonviable. Burns become contaminated and colonized with bacteria. This is true even in the early stages of injury. Infection develops when the colonization becomes dense and subsequently invades adjacent viable tissue.

A variety of microorganisms—bacteria, mycobacteria, yeast, fungi, and viruses—have been cited as the causative agents of burn infections. The pattern of infecting organisms tends to be cyclical. The first organisms are generally the invasive gram-positive cocci, i.e., coagulase-positive staphylococci and group A beta-hemolytic streptococci. Superinfection then follows with the gram-negative bacillary bacteria and then yeast. The emergence of multiply-antibiotic-resistant organisms is not uncommon, and the antibiotic selection pressures can evolve from both the topical antiseptic agents and the parenterally administered drugs.

The diagnosis of infection in burn patients is often difficult.[180] Purulence may be evident below the eschar, but wounds may appear clean even when they are infected. While the utility of quantitative tissue cultures remains controversial, this is the mainstay of diagnosis in many burn institutions. This is so because the types of organisms as well as the locations of organisms can vary within each burn. In addition, extensively burned patients lose their ability to regulate their temperature. Therefore, the assessment of infection must be made relative to the changes and trends in the patient's overall clinical condition and the pattern of the temperature curve. Systemic signs that may be indicative of infection include decreased level of consciousness, lethargy, or coma and the development of adynamic ileus. The consequences of infection can cause the conversion of a partial-thickness burn into a full-thickness burn. This may necessitate additional grafting procedures. However, if infection should incubate without recognition, overwhelming systemic infection, bacteremia, and death can result.

The management of the burn can influence the infection risks. The risk-to-benefit ratio must be carefully evaluated for each treatment modality. Adequate, atraumatic débridement of all nonviable tissue and early wound coverage are the single most important preventative measures.[180, 181] However, cadaver transplants and animal tissue grafts must be meticulously prepared so that additional contamination is not introduced into the wounds.[182] Care of the wounds mandates scrupulous aseptic technique.

A number of topical antiseptic agents have been recommended for burn care.[141, 180] Each agent has advantages and disadvantages. Silver nitrate has a limited effective range. Concentrations of 0.25% provide only bacteriostatic activity, whereas 1.0% concentrations can destroy epidermal buds, which can convert a second-degree burn into a third-degree burn. Therefore, the best concentration is 0.5%, which promotes epidermal growth while preventing bacterial growth. The outer layers of the dressing must remain dry, and this can retard the body's heat loss. The major disadvantage is the influence on electrolyte balances of the sodium, potassium, and chloride ions. Patients must be monitored carefully. Silver nitrate also may leave indelible stains.

Mafenide acetate at 10% concentration (Sulfamylon) can penetrate the eschar and retard growth of *Pseudomonas*. However, it can be painful to the patient. It is a powerful carbonic anhydrase inhibitor that hampers the renal tubular reabsorption of bicarbonate with resultant metabolic acidosis.

Silver sulfadizine at 1% concentration seems to combine the benefits of silver nitrate and mafenide acetate without producing metabolic complications.[183] However, this greasy cream must be completely removed at a minimum of every 24 hours.

Povodine-iodine solutions are not recommended because their prolonged use can be toxic to the wound and can cause necrosis of newly granulating tissue.[184, 185] Topical antibiotics such as aminoglycoside irrigants are not recommended because of a strong tendency to induce antibiotic-resistant organisms.[186, 187]

Hydrotherapy also can have dual-edged consequences. It is the single most effective means of removing topical antiseptic creams and superficially débriding wounds. In addition, adjustment of the pH of the whirlpool water may influence the kinds of organisms colonizing the wounds.[188] However, the infection risks associated with indwelling IV and urinary catheters can significantly increase if these devices are contaminated during hydrotherapy.[141] In addition, cross-contamination among the patients using the tubs can occur if the tubs are not adequately cleaned.

Protective isolation measures have been recommended, but the efficacy is questionable. The single most important measure is to avoid cross-contamination among the patients.[189] This is accomplished by frequent handwashing, not sharing supplies and equipment among patients, restricting traffic, and maintaining meticulous aseptic technique. Contact isolation precautions are necessary as discussed below.

Wound Care Through the Trauma Cycle

The primary objective of wound care throughout the trauma cycle is the prevention of infection. Nursing actions should minimize cross-contamination and promote wound healing. The most effective measures are meticulous aseptic technique and handwashing. Scissors and tape must always be handled properly. Contact isolation precautions are required for those patients with infections attributed to coagulase-positive staphylococci, group A beta-hemolytic streptococci, and aminoglycoside-resistant gram-negative bacillary organisms.[190]

Careful nursing assessment can detect the early development of infection. Early detection is especially crucial during the early phase of the trauma cycle, when rapidly progressive infections are most likely to develop. Deep-seated infections involving other organ systems tend to develop later. Therefore, nurses caring for patients during the recovery phases of the cycle must be ever alert to the underlying infection risks. Assessment in such situations involves a trend analysis. Increasing signs of inflammation, increased drainage or purulence, breakdown of the integrity of suture margins, and systemic signs of deterioration should be reported immediately. Nursing care must minimize patient immobility and stimulate tissue perfusion. Frequent turning and repositioning of the patient can prevent the development of decubitus ulcers. These lesions can become infected and dissect into the underlying muscle and bone. However, decubitus ulcers are entirely preventable with proper nursing care.

Nurses can promote wound healing as well as enhance the patient's resistance to infection by ensuring adequate nutrition. Burn patients have high caloric requirements. In addition, their diets should include foods that are rich in the nutrients that facilitate wound and bone healing. These nutrients include vitamin C, zinc, calcium, and phosphorus.

Throughout the trauma cycle, wound care must reflect the underlying nature of the patient's injuries. Guidelines for the care of wounds are found in Table 12–4. Further discussions on wound management and burns are found elsewhere in this book.

INFECTION RELATED TO ORTHOPEDIC INJURY

Certainly the primary goals of managing orthopedic injuries are to restore the patient to normal function, achieve union, avoid malunion, and prevent infection. However, despite many technological advances for the management of orthopedic injuries, infection remains a leading cause of postinjury morbidity (e.g., nonunion of long bones[191] and bone instability[192]), as well as a primary obstacle to an expedient recovery. Infection risk factors include the nature and extent of the underlying injury, management of the wound, use of fixation devices, and antibiotic therapy.

Nature of the Injury

The overall magnitude of the trauma is a key determinant of infection. Patients sustaining multisystem trauma coupled with orthopedic injury are at highest risk. Pulmonary compromise and hypovolemic shock must be emergently corrected if the patient is to survive. Therefore, the underlying hemodynamic instability of these patients can create a therapeutic dilemma for the orthopedic surgeon. Immediate fracture fixation and stabilization are certainly the primary

TABLE 12–4. INFECTION-CONTROL GUIDELINES FOR THE CARE OF WOUNDS

1. Wash hands before and after patient care.
2. Use aseptic technique for dressing changes of open wounds.
3. Change dressings that become saturated with drainage fluid, and notify the physician of changes in its character, i.e., amount, color, odor, viscosity. Document all changes.
4. Maintain the patency and function of wound drains.
5. Notify the physician of any signs of increasing inflammation, purulent drainage, or breakdown in the integrity of suture lines.
6. Perform wound cultures correctly. Obtain two samples or swabs from each culture site so that both Gram stain and culture can be performed.
7. Clean and disinfect scissor blades with alcohol after each use.

goals. To do so can lessen the degree of avascular necrosis at the fracture site and promote early mobilization of the patient in order to minimize and prevent the onset of pulmonary complications. However, fixation and stabilization may have to be delayed as indicated by the extent of the injuries and the priorities of resuscitation. Delay can contribute to the amount of local ischemia at the fracture site and increase the amount of soft tissue damage and bone loss. Not only does this promote the chance of infection, but it also can jeopardize the ultimate salvage of a limb as well as necessitate the later need for skin- and bone-graft procedures.

The primary index for fracture site infection is the severity of injury itself. Contributory factors include the amount of bone loss, comminution, displacement, and/or periosteal stripping; the extent of soft tissue injury; wound contamination; compromise to tissue perfusion; and vascular injury. The presence of foreign bodies, coupled with those conditions producing ischemia, hypovolemia, and avascular necrosis, creates an environment in which any bacterial inoculum can thrive.[138–140, 147] Long bone fractures, with their intrinsic problems of stabilization, tend to have greater infection risks than flat bone fractures. Traumatic amputations, open fractures with accompanying vascular injury resulting from high-energy events such as pedestrian road traffic accidents and gunshots, and fractures inducing compartmental syndromes have the greatest infection risks. All these injuries have extensive tissue damage and massive wound contamination. It should be clear that the nature of the injury determines both the contributory factors of infection and the requirements of fracture management. Paradoxically, the methods of fracture management also can augment infection risk.

Management of the Fracture

A primary objective in the management of fractures is the prevention of infection. Therefore, fracture management must minimize the consequences of bacterial contamination and the devitalization of tissues that occur secondary to the fracture itself.[137] Interventions generally accepted as preventative measures include early fixation and stabilization, adequate débridement, meticulous surgical technique, and antibiotic utilization.

As previously mentioned, the importance of meticulous surgical technique cannot be overemphasized. It is well documented that adherence to these principles has significantly reduced the incidence of postoperative wound infection.[138, 139, 147] However, extensive surgical dissection with loss of vital tissue attachments, failure to remove freed fracture fragments, and prolonged duration of operative time tend to induce later infectious complications.[193, 194]

Ideally, fixation of the fracture should occur as close to the initial time of injury as possible. A long bone fracture causes tearing of the periosteum as well as disruption of the longitudinally lying haversian system. Clot formation about the fracture site begins, but blood flow to the fracture and its surrounding tissue, the periosteum and bone marrow, ceases. The result is devitalized tissue and avascular necrosis. This creates an environment conducive to the growth of bacteria, which can be introduced by either trauma or surgical intervention. Therefore, early and adequate débridement of injury tends to reduce the infection risks.

Immobilization is an important adjunct to the healing of soft-tissue injury.[191, 192, 195, 196] Stabilization helps to restore the fracture to a near approximation of the bone's normal anatomical position. The stability realigns vital neurovascular structures, strengthens soft tissue planes, and promotes re-establishment of the microcirculation. Early revasculation of devitalized structures improves the local immune responses of the tissues and enhances resistance to infection. However, for some open fractures with accompanying soft tissue injury and a high level of contamination, the method of wound closure and stabilization is still controversial.[191, 192, 197, 198] Most agree that infection risk is reduced when open wounds are not closed primarily. Extensive redébridement as well as skin grafts and muscle flaps may be necessary to achieve adequate wound closure.

At the crux of the controversy surrounding open fracture management is the type of fixation—internal versus external. Some argue that the presence of a foreign body in an already heavily contaminated wound provides bacteria with a convenient surface on which to establish a habitat in an environment already conducive to their growth. Therefore, the risk of infection outweighs the benefits of closure. However, others feel that turning an open fracture into a closed fracture with extensive, repetitive débridements, delayed wound closure, and internal fixation provides the best environment for healing.[197] There is also clinical support for immediate internal fixation of open proximal long bone fractures, particularly to decrease pulmonary complications by early mobilization. These situations include open fractures in victims of multiple trauma, mutilated limbs, intra-articular fractures, open fractures with associated vascular injury, and open femur fractures in the elderly.[170] In these cases, the benefits of stabilization outweigh the risks of infection.

Fixation Devices

The use of external fixation devices can both facilitate and reduce infection risks.[192] The advantages include the relative ease and speed of application, achievement of reasonable anatomical reduction and stabilization, and the occurrence of minimal additional soft tissue trauma. The disadvantages include intricate and time-consuming application in large, complex open wounds, interference with soft tissue reconstructive surgery, and the development of pin tract infections.

Orthopedic appliances are foreign bodies that can provide surfaces for bacterial adherence, and this is but one infectious risk associated with their use. Their very presence can lead to local necrosis.[193] Technical placement also can be a contributory factor. The objective in placing orthopedic hardware is to minimize additional local tissue trauma. Technical factors that tend to promote infectious complications include the use of dull and worn drill bits, failure to control the direction of a cutting tool, and heat generated by drilling.[199] After insertion, any adverse stress and strain on the hardware or a loosening of the hardware can amplify the devitalization of the surrounding tissue and aid the development of infection.[193, 194, 196]

Antibiotic Use

Although the prophylactic use of antibiotics has been proven to be beneficial to the management of closed orthopedic injuries,[104] their utility in the management of open fractures remains controversial.[105, 106, 108, 109, 111, 197] Most antibiotic prophylaxis is directed against *Staphylococcus aureus*. First-generation cephalosporins such as cephalothin (Kelfin) or cefazolin (Ancef, Kefzol) or semisynthetic penicillins such as nafcillin are acceptable choices. Because of the previously described consequences of antibiotic therapy, the duration of prophylaxis should be kept short, and risk-to-benefit ratios must be evaluated individually for each patient.

Definition of Infections

The infections following orthopedic injury include wound infections, a wide variety of nosocomial infections, and deep-seated bone infections. Description of the wound infections and nosocomial infections are found elsewhere in this chapter. However, any of these infections that have an associated secondary bacteremia can subsequently induce a deep-seated bone infection. The bacteremia can cause hematogenous seeding of the fracture, the adjacent tissues, or an implanted fixation device. Therefore, patients developing bacteremic infections should be monitored carefully for any signs and symptoms of a later deep-seated infection.

Orthopedic Hardware–Associated Infections

Indwelling orthopedic hardware can precipitate both superficial and deep-seated infections. A common misnomer is to describe these as infections *of* the hardware itself (i.e., pin necrosis, infected compression plates, and so on). As mentioned previously, it is the implantation and presence of metal that contribute to factors predisposing the surrounding tissue to infection. Therefore, it is important to remember that the metal itself can become neither necrotic nor infected.

It has been reported that 4 to 30 per cent of patients in whom external fixation devices have been placed develop associated infections.[200–202] The associated infections include small areas of cellulitis and local abscess surrounding the pin insertion sites, muscle infections of the surrounding tract, and bone infections. A hallmark that a superficial infection has dissected into the deeper underlying tissues is the loosening of an implanted orthopedic bone pin. Pin/bone infection may necessitate pin removal for resolution of disease. It is a difficult decision because removal may decrease stability and further jeopardize the outcome.

Because of the local tissue responses to the presence of a pin, it is important to continually observe the pin–skin interface. Serous drainage is produced when tissues slide over the pin, and it may form a crust at the skin–pin interface. As long as this fluid can drain freely, infection risks are reduced. Consequently, crust formations must be gently removed. For newly placed pins, pin-site care may be necessary several times a day. Special care should be taken during cleansing so that additional trauma or cavitation about the pin–skin junction is not induced, since this can produce localized suppuration and necrosis. On the other hand, skin tension can impede the flow of fluid as well as promote inflammation, pain, necrosis, and infection. Increased frequency of cleansing and surgical débridement may be required to alleviate the tension. Therefore, the primary goals of pin-site care should be to promote the free drainage of fluid and minimize local tissue damage.

Whether or not one specific antiseptic solution is the best choice for pin cleansing remains unclear. Each solution has different advantages and disadvantages.[103] Iodophor solutions and alcohol are equally effective as intermediate-level antiseptics. The killing effects of iodophor occur as the solution dries. Once dry, a residue is left. On skin, this residue can hinder the reestablishment of bacteria. However, on inorganic surfaces such as metal, the residue becomes sticky and can enhance bacterial adherence. Both antiseptics require a previously cleaned surface to maximize effectiveness. It is probably best to use iodophors for skin and alcohol for metal. Hydrogen peroxide is a good débriding agent for the removal of blood and other body fluids. It can react strongly with iodophors. A combination of hydrogen peroxide and iodophor is a good agent for débriding necrotic or devitalized tissue; on healthy tissue, however, this combination can cause dermonecrosis. Therefore, on healthy tissue, hydrogen peroxide should be neutralized with saline before applying to an iodophor treatment area. The best agents for pin cleansing are probably a combination of solutions appropriately selected to meet the individualized needs of the patient.

As an adjunct to meticulous pin–skin cleansing, special attention must be paid to the fixator so that any unnecessary stress or strain can be reduced. Devices attached to traction apparatuses must be lubricated at the pin–traction junction. Similarly, when using a continuous passive motion (CPM) machine, the patient should be positioned so that no added pressure is applied to the pins.

Internal fixation devices (i.e., plates, nails, screws, pins, or prostheses) also can aid the development of infection. They cause a local tissue response as well as provide surfaces upon which bacteria can adhere and establish new habitats. Bacterial seeding can occur either at the time of insertion or by hematogenous spread from another site. Infection, then, can easily develop in the poorly vascularized crevices where the internal fixation devices adjoin the bone. Clinical manifestations can include pain, inflammation, fever, and leukocytosis. Resolution of infection cannot occur until the hardware is removed. These infections can range from low-grade infection around the hardware to deep-seated bone infections.

Infection-control guidelines for the care of external fixation devices are outlined in Table 12–5.

TABLE 12–5. INFECTION-CONTROL GUIDELINES FOR THE CARE OF EXTERNAL FIXATION DEVICES

1. Do not impede the flow of serous drainage fluid.
2. Do not use occlusive dressings or a thick coating of antimicrobial ointment at the skin–pin junction.
3. Notify the physician if skin tension develops at the skin–pin junction.
4. Gently remove any crust formation at the skin–pin junction.
5. Avoid inducing local tissue trauma or cavitation at the skin–pin junction.
6. Use a combination of antiseptic solutions determined by the needs of the patient.
7. Minimize any unnecessary stress and strain on the fixator, lubricate any pin–traction junctions, and carefully position patients on CPM machines.

Bone Infections

Osteomyelitis is described as an infection involving both the bone and its marrow. It can be caused by (1) hematogenous spread from another site of infection, (2) extension from a contiguous infection, or (3) direct introduction from trauma or a surgical procedure.[203] Osteomyelitis that develops as sequela to systemic diseases such as acute hematogenous osteomyelitis in children, hemodialysis, parenteral drug abuse, or prior infection at another site or osteomyelitis that develops from vascular insufficiencies such as diabetes mellitus or severe atherosclerosis, attacks previously normal bone. On the other hand, posttraumatic osteomyelitis or fracture infection is an infection that develops as a result of injury, impedance of the microcirculation, failure to débride necrotic tissue and/or evacuate hematomas, and the presence of indwelling fixation devices. This is the development of infection in bone that is devitalized and necrotic from the onset. Therefore, aggressive débridement with removal of bone sequestrum and appropriate antibiotic therapy often can prevent acute infections from becoming chronic problems.[196] Chronicity tends to be more commonly associated with nontraumatic osteomyelitis.[203]

Posttraumatic bone infections are not clearly defined in the medical literature. They can be caused by hematogenous seeding of implanted orthopedic hardware from a nosocomial bacteremia, dissection from an overlying superficial wound infection, or inadequate débridement and/or evacuation of a hematoma at the time of initial fixation. These infections can appear weeks, months, and even years following the initial injury. The clinical manifestations can include any combination of local pain, erythema, heat, tenderness, and draining sinuses over the involved site of bone infection. Elevated white blood cell count, rising sedimentation rates, and fever are not usually present. Treatment includes surgical débridement, removal of associated hardware, and appropriate parenteral antibiotic therapy for a minimum of 4 weeks.[204]

Prevention of infection in patients sustaining orthopedic injury is a challenge throughout the trauma cycle. Nursing interventions should be directed toward minimizing the compromise of the defenses attributed to the patient's immobility. Most important are actions that promote pulmonary function and maintain adequate perfusion of the skin. Meticulous care and evaluation of fixation devices and maintenance of proper alignment can reduce infection risks. During the later phase of the cycle, nurses should be ever alert to the development of bone infection.

CARDIOVASCULAR SYSTEM INFECTION

Bacteremia is defined as the presence of bacteria in the bloodstream.[205–208] It can be a transient phenomenon following the instrumentation of tissues abundant with microorganisms,[209] e.g., cystoscopic procedures on a patient with colonized urine, tracheal suctioning of a ventilator-dependent patient,[210] débridement of a local abscess, or simply brushing the teeth. Generally, this is a short-lived, self-limiting condition, and the organisms can be eradicated easily by the body's cellular immune responses. However, it is important to be aware of this phenomenon because blood cultures drawn immediately following such a procedure can be positive. The impact is that an accurate clinical diagnosis may be obscured by the positivity of these blood cultures, and inappropriate therapy subsequently may be begun by the physician.

On the other hand, bacteremia associated with sepsis or septicemia indicates a systemic reaction to the invasion of bacteria into the bloodstream. *Septicemia* is the name applied to a constellation of symptoms including fever, shaking chills, and confusion, as well as signs and symptoms of shock—hypotension, tachycardia, tachypnea, and oliguria. Septicemia often indicates clinically significant bacteremia but may occur as a consequence of tissue necrosis without bacteremia. The extreme form of septicemia is septic shock (discussed elsewhere in this chapter). Septic shock has been associated with many of the gram-negative bacillary organisms. It also may occur in association with gram-positive organisms (staphylococci and pneumococci) or fungi. Septic shock, like septicemia, may occur as a consequence of tissue necrosis without bacteremia.

It is important to remember that blood is a sterile body fluid and rarely is the origin of infection within the blood's tissue itself. Bacteremia originates from an underlying infection or reservoir at another site. It is important to determine both the origin of and the microorganism causing the infection so that appropriate antimicrobial and supportive therapy can be initiated. For example, if the bacteremia is secondary to an abscess or necrotic tissue, the abscess must be drained and the offensive tissue removed before the antibiotics can be effective in treating the infection. Since bacteremia can develop from a myriad of infections, sources, or organisms, one should be careful not to generalize the description of the systemic reactions to bacteremia with such terms as *gram-negative sepsis, septic shock,* or *sepsis*. It is more accurate to describe the disease as the primary infection with associated secondary bacteremia and/or episodes of shock; i.e., "The patient has a gram-negative bacillary pneumonia with secondary bacteremia and shock."

Primary Bacteremia

Primary or unexplained bacteremia is identified when the patient has a clinically significant bacteremia and no other site can be determined as the source. In other words, the organisms recovered from the blood cultures are not recovered from cultures taken from possible sites of infection, such as respiratory secretions, urine, wounds, intraoperative sites, cerebrospinal fluid, and so on. Most organisms responsible for primary bacteremia are very similar to those causing intravascular line–related infections. It is important to remember that the use of complex systems of IV fluid support and monitoring offers many opportunities for microorganisms to gain access to the bloodstream as well as sites for the organisms to colonize. It may be that some of these infections are related to contaminated fluids that have been infused into the patient prior to the discovery of the bacteremia. Similarly, it may be that the lines themselves have become colonized and are producing the source of the bacteremia. However, the line may have been removed prior to identification of the bacteremia, and it may be difficult to subsequently determine the line to be the source of the infection. Whatever the source, primary bacteremia points out the necessity for repeatedly obtaining blood cultures in the evaluation of such patients even when the site of infection is presumed to be known. In addition, these patients should have blood cultures repeated after appropriate treatment, as well as a continued search for the possible source.

In previous reports characterizing the infections among severely traumatized patients, approximately 40 per cent of serious bacteremic infections were related to the use of IV monitoring and fluid catheters.[13–17] The major infection risks for cardiovascular infection stem from the clinically urgent conditions under which the catheters were placed and the need to frequently manipulate the lines to obtain pressure readings or blood samples or to administer medications, fluids, blood, and blood products.[211–213] In these critically ill patients, vascular access may be difficult to maintain, and it can be compromised by the nature of the patient's injuries as well as the need for prolonged use of IV therapy. Infections related to invasion of the cardiovascular system include phlebitis, arterial abscesses, catheter-associated sepsis, endocarditis, and, as previously mentioned, unexplained bacteremias.

Phlebitis

Phlebitis, by definition, is an inflammation of a vein. It can develop from irritation produced by either mechanical trauma from the catheter or the chemical nature of the infusate and/or medications. Chemical phlebitis is generally not classified as an infection. Septic phlebitis may be defined as suppurative or septic nonsuppurative. Chemical and suppurative phlebitis may both present with signs of erythema, heat, tenderness, and/or a palpable cord. However, suppurative phlebitis is usually differentiated when purulent, culture-positive material can be expressed from the catheter insertion site. The causative organism is usually coagulase-positive staphylococci. When a systemic reaction (i.e., fever, elevated white blood cell count, and/or associated bacteremia) does not occur, heat and elevation of the afflicted body part may be adequate treatment. For those cases producing systemic involvement, parenteral antibiotics directed toward staphylococci are generally initiated. However, if there is no response within 24 hours, surgical excision of the vein may be necessary. Any local abscess should be drained.

Septic nonsuppurative thrombophlebitis should be suspected when a patient presents with a persistent gram-negative bacillary bacteremia with a member of the Klebsielleae tribe (*Enterobacter, Klebsiella,* and *Serratia* species) and no site of infection can be identified.[214] This diagnosis can be further supported when the patient is started on appropriate antimicrobial therapy and subsequent blood cultures continue to be positive. Excision of the infected vein is necessary. However, it may be very difficult to determine exactly which vein is involved, since there may be no evidence of purulence at an insertion site, nor will a palpable cord be detected. It is most likely to be the vein that was invaded at the time of the first positive blood culture or the vein through which the IV solutions are presently being administered. Unfortunately, several veins may be removed before such an infection is brought under control.

Arterial Abscesses

Arterial lines have been implicated as the source of serious infection.[215–217] *Arterial abscess* may result when a local stitch abscess at the catheter–skin interface dissects into the arterial wall or the tip of the indwelling catheter produces trauma to the arterial wall. Frequently, there is an associated secondary bacteremia as well as the presence of septic emboli distal to the insertion site. These emboli will be evident on the palm of the patient's hand if a radial or brachial artery is involved or on the sole of the patient's foot if a femoral artery is involved. Septic emboli appear as small hemorrhagic areas that may have necrotic centers. If emboli are observed, the line must be removed immediately and antibiotics begun. Careful observation for *pseudoaneurysm* must be initiated, and if one is found, the artery must be resected. Because of the possibility of stitch abscesses, arterial lines placed by radial cutdown have a higher probability of inducing subsequent infection than lines placed by percutaneous puncture. In one study, cannulation of the femoral artery was shown to result in fewer infectious complications than use of the radial artery.[218] Arterial abscesses and mycotic aneurysms also can be infectious complications of hemodialysis.[219, 220]

Catheter-Associated Sepsis

Catheter-associated sepsis may be defined as an infection or bacteremia developing secondary to either an IV catheter becoming colonized with microorganisms or contamination of the infusate. The patient may present with systemic signs and symptoms of infection, but once the offending line or fluid is removed, the patient's clinical status markedly improves. There may not be an actual infection of a specific tissue. If a catheter is suspected of being a source of infection, special care should be taken to properly culture the line. The line should be removed using strict aseptic technique, and a semiquantitative culture should be obtained by rolling the catheter across a blood agar plate.[221] A confluent growth of microorganisms is generally indicative of the catheter being the source of the infection. A culture of a line should not be taken by placing the catheter tip in a thioglycolate broth tube, since the presence of a single bacterium can produce a positive culture, and the clinical significance of this result may be obscure. Similarly, blood cultures should not be obtained by withdrawing blood through a line, since, once again, a single organism that may be colonizing the line can cause the culture result to be positive. Blood cultures drawn through a catheter have been considered to have a low sensitivity, a low positive predictive value for true infection, and a high false-positive rate.[222, 223] Therefore, in order to enhance the evaluation of catheter-related infection and the identification of the source of a bacteremia, two or more sets of blood cultures should be obtained via percutaneous puncture at the same time as semiquantitative catheter culture.[223, 224]

Infusate-Associated Sepsis

Hyperalimentation solutions are documented as being a source of catheter- and infusate-associated sepsis.[225–226] This may be due to the fact that these lines often must remain in place for a prolonged period of time, and therefore, the probability that the line will become colonized increases. Fungemia (candidemia) has often been associated with the use of hyperalimentation solutions.[227] However, since most of these solutions no longer contain casein hydrolysate, the viability of fungi in the fluid has been reduced. Rather, fungemia these days is most likely a consequence of broad-spectrum antibiotic therapy. Fat-emulsion solutions pose an infectious threat because they provide a rich medium for luxuriant microbial growth.[229]

Although relatively rare, septicemia associated with contaminated infusion fluids has been well documented. Outbreaks of *Enterobacter* bacteremia have been associated with contaminated dextrose solutions,[230] a *Pseudomonas cepacia* outbreak was attributed to normal serum albumin,[231] and *Salmonella* bacteremia has been related to contaminated platelet transfusions.[232] Surveillance of bacteremic illness can be instrumental in identifying infusion-related outbreaks in an intensive care unit. In addition, patients receiving massive blood transfusions should be followed for the acquisition of hepatitis and cytomegalovirus infection.

Endocarditis

Infective endocarditis (IE) is caused by the invasion of microorganisms into the endocardial surface of the heart.[233] Although infection may occur at any site on the endocardial surface, heart values are the most frequently affected. Historically, IE has been caused by a wide variety of microorganisms as well as many different predisposing illnesses, cardiac anomalies, and infections. Chronic parenteral drug abuse also can be a contributory factor. However, in severely traumatized patients and other critically ill patient populations, a new form of this disease is emerging as *nosocomial infective endocarditis* (NIE).[234–239] Development of NIE is directly related to the prolonged use of right-sided heart (Swan-Ganz) catheters, central venous catheters, hemodialysis shunts, intracardiac prostheses, vascular grafts, hyperalimentation lines, and intracardiac pacemaker wires. In addition, NIE may develop as a secondary complication of a serious bacteremic infection. Identification of NIE may be obscure. However, it should always be considered in patients demonstrating persistent bacteremia with the same organism and appropriate predisposing risk factors. Treatment requires prolonged parenteral antibiotic therapy (i.e., 4 to 6 weeks).

Intravascular Line Infection-Control Issues

Since critically injured and ill patients often require prolonged intravascular support and venous access may be difficult to maintain, infection-control guidelines must be stringent and carefully formulated.[13–17, 51, 53, 88, 100, 101, 224, 240, 241] It must be remembered that lines may have been placed during clinically urgent situations and that these lines are manipulated frequently to administer medications, blood and blood products, and nutritional support; obtain blood samples; and take pressure readings. Therefore, the situations and conditions unique to the intensive care unit patient must be considered when formulating guidelines. In addition, evaluation and application of infection-control guidelines for preventing and minimizing infection risks related to intravascular catheters as elucidated in the medical literature must be meticulously scrutinized. Comparisons of study results can be difficult, since all have been conducted with variable patient care conditions that can affect both outcomes and applications. These factors include underlying comorbidity conditions; catheter insertion techniques; frequency of catheter, dressings, tubing, and transducer changes; type of dressing (i.e., gauze versus transparent); culturing techniques; number of catheter lumens; type and/or use of topical antimicrobial ointment; use of the catheter; type of infusates; frequency of line manipulation; and use of designated IV personnel.

Some studies have suggested that it is safe to change delivery sets at intervals greater than 24 hours.[242–244] However, since these lines are manipulated so frequently, and since most people fail to wash their hands prior to each manipulation of the line, a guideline to change delivery sets at 48-hour intervals may not be applicable in the critically ill population. In fact, there have been at least nine epidemics in the past decade that have been linked to carriage of epidemic organisms on the hands of intensive care unit personnel manipulating the catheters and tubings.[217, 224, 245–251]

Antimicrobial ointments and antiseptic solutions should be used according to manufacturers' recommendations.[221] Ointments should be applied to catheter–skin interfaces as a thin coating. Povidone-iodine solutions should be allowed to air dry in order to maximize killing effects.

Special attention should be given to the type of material selected for line dressings. Many institutions use transparent dressings rather than the more traditional sterile gauze dressing. The rationale is that the transparent dressing allows continuous observation of the catheter insertion site. However, these dressings were initially designed to promote the healing of abrasions, burns, or skin-graft sites. Such dressings provide a protective barrier while still maintaining the dynamic characteristics of the skin. Application as a vascular line dressing was an afterthought. Therefore, such use of transparent dressings was initiated without the benefit of appropriate clinical trials. Recent reports in the medical literature indicate that transparent dressings have three to six times the bacterial colonization seen with gauze dressings and are significantly more expensive to use.[222] As previously mentioned, tape should always be handled appropriately. In addition, tape should never be applied directly to a catheter–skin interface.

Pressure-monitoring systems can become a bacterial reservoir when blood accumulates around stopcocks and access ports. The blood then becomes an ideal medium for organisms inoculated into the system from the hands of the personnel. Transducers as well as flush systems have been implicated as sources of infectious outbreaks in the intensive care setting.[199] Water and water–ice baths used for the preparation of syringes for thermodilution cardiac output studies and blood gas studies also can become infection hazards. Dextrose solutions are viable media for the Klebsielleae tribe and are frequently used as flushes for such systems.

Pressure transducers have been implicated as the source of bacteremia even when disposable domes have been utilized.[199] It is important to remember that these monitoring devices often interface directly with the blood. Therefore, the transducer should be sterilized after each use. A common misconception is that a disposable dome with its semipermeable membrane will not allow microorganisms that might contaminate the diaphragm access to the bloodstream. However, microscopic punctures can occur in these membranes, and if the transducer is contaminated, a bacteremia could be precipitated. In addition, the Centers for Disease Control (CDC) guidelines outlining the care of pressure transducers are contradictory.[223] Under CDC recommendations for proper sterilization techniques, any equipment that interfaces or invades the vascular system must be sterilized. However, the recommendations for the specific care of transducers states that either sterilization or high-level chemical disinfection is acceptable. The primary problem is packaging a piece of equipment that has a wet, disinfected end and a dry, contaminated end. In addition, the more frequent handling involved to achieve high-level chemical disinfection can damage the delicate sensing diaphragm of the transducer, rendering it unacceptable for patient use. Since reusable transducers are relatively expensive, breakage and maintenance costs should be considered when one is delineating infection-control guidelines. Therefore, the safest as well as the most cost-effective method for caring for transducers is sterilization or the use of disposable sterile transducers. Disposable sterile transducers reduce the risk of cross-contamination and can remain in use for a maximum of 96 hours, as opposed to the 48-hour maximal interval recommended for reusable transducers.[224]

Control Measures Through the Trauma Cycle

Minimizing the infection risks related to the use of IV devices is a challenge throughout the trauma cycle. Rapid insertion of IV lines is critical to a trauma patient's immediate survival; it is also a major precipitating factor for later infection. If the lines inserted under less than optimal conditions cannot be removed or changed within a few hours of the patient's admission to the intensive care unit, they should be débrided of all encrusted blood, redressed using meticulous aseptic technique, and reconnected to new sterile fluids and administration sets. Infection risks for the intensive care unit patient stem from the design of the administration and monitoring systems, the need for frequent manipulation, the number of lines utilized, and the continued need for IV support. Compromises of vascular access can result from the nature of the underlying injury as well as the prolonged use of the lines. Patients sustaining multiple extremity fractures or extensive burns, edematous patients, critically and chronically ill obese patients, and the elderly have the greatest disadvantage. Burn patients have an additional risk of catheter-associated infection when the lines must be placed through burned tissue.[225, 226] Vascular access proportionately decreases as the duration of therapy increases.

Infection-control guidelines for intravascular devices present many challenges for the future. Issues that still demand resolution include an assessment of the efficacy of using guidewires for the replacement of lines, identification of the safest and most cost-effective frequency of line changes, and determination of the myriad of infection risks that can be attributed to the complex systems of IV therapy (i.e., multi-medication drips, infusion pumps, etc.). Above all, nursing care for IV devices must be tailored to the individual needs of the patient throughout the trauma cycle.

Specific infection-control guidelines for the care of IV lines are outlined in Table 12–6.

CENTRAL NERVOUS SYSTEM INFECTION

Risk Factors

The major risk factor for development of a central nervous system (CNS) infection following CNS trauma is a violation of the dural membrane.[284–288] This disruption of the dura can result from direct penetrating injury such as gunshot wounds and stabbing injuries, cerebrospinal fluid (CSF) leaks, placement of intraventricular catheters, and extensive neurosurgical procedures. An additional risk is seen in patients who have sustained cranial fractures such as Le Fort II and III, and nasal and basilar skull fractures when a CSF leak has also occurred and is not evident.[289] As mentioned previously, prophylactic antibiotics following open CNS injuries are not recommended because they have been shown to be ineffective in preventing subsequent infection and tend to shift the patient's normal flora toward a predominance of gram-negative bacillary organisms.[106, 113, 286] Concomitantly, antibiotics are not effective on bullets, foreign objects, or devascularized and necrotic tissues. Therefore, the best preventive measures remain adequate débridement and meticulous surgical technique.

Infection risks are enhanced with the use of a variety of

TABLE 12–6. INFECTION-CONTROL GUIDELINES FOR THE CARE OF IV LINES

1. Use strict aseptic technique for insertion.
2. Use aseptic technique for dressing changes, which should be performed at 24-hour intervals. Inspect the catheter–skin interface and report any signs of inflammation or purulent drainage to the physician immediately.
3. Change fluid and flush solutions every 24 hours, and label with the date and time of change.
4. Change tubings every 24 hours, and label with the date and time of change.
5. Change site every 72 hours, whenever possible.
6. Change resuscitation lines using aseptic technique as soon as the patient is hemodynamically stable.
7. Remove lines immediately if they are suspected of being infected, and obtain a culture and Gram stain of any drainage from the insertion site.
8. Obtain a line culture using semiquantitative culture technique.
9. Document the site of each line with the length of time it remains indwelling.
10. Do not obtain blood cultures through IV lines but only by percutaneous puncture.
11. Begin hyperalimentation only through newly inserted lines, and use these solely for this purpose unless a clinical emergency arises.
12. Use disposable transducer domes, and sterilize the transducer itself after every use. If possible, utilize a disposable transducer.
13. Keep monitoring systems free of accumulated dried blood.
14. Minimize the utilization of stopcocks and access ports.

mechanical support devices. Special care should be taken not to place nasal tubes such as nasogastric and nasotracheal tubes in patients with known or suspected CSF leaks. Nasopharyngeal suctioning should not be performed. Both these procedures can significantly increase the risk of meningitis. Nurses also should remember that the vast majority of patients suffering CNS injuries are given high-dose antacids or H_2-blocking agents to help minimize gastrointestinal stress. These drugs raise the gastric pH so that the acidic barrier of the stomach is lost and an additional reservoir of microorganisms is created. Therefore, if a vented gastric tube such as a Salem sump is used, special attention must be given to preventing the reflux of the now microbiologically abundant gastric fluids onto neurosurgical drains or intracranial pressure-monitoring devices. The consequence could be the development of meningitis or ventriculitis.

The use of butterfly drains attached to vacutainer tubes as an adjunct for the repair of facial fractures can be a cryptic infection threat in those patients who have underlying CSF leaks. These tubes must be changed carefully so that no fluid is allowed to reflux into the drainage tract. Above all, nurses must ensure that only sterile vacutainer tubes are used.

Intracranial Pressure Monitoring Devices

Meningitis and ventriculitis can be associated with the use of intraventricular catheters.[286, 290, 291] The infection risks are related to the length of time these catheters remain indwelling, the ability of maintaining the monitoring and/or drainage system as a "closed system," and the need to vent CSF. Only drainage systems manufactured specifically for use as intraventricular monitoring and drainage devices should be used. These systems have special fused joints and stopcocks that minimize possible portals of entry for microorganisms. If these catheters are used, culture and Gram stain, complete cell count with differential, and glucose determinations should be obtained daily on a CSF sample withdrawn from the catheter. The results and trends of the cell count and glucose determination afford early detection of infection as well as aid in the evaluation of positive culture and Gram stain results. For example, if the glucose level is low or less than two-thirds the serum value and the cell count shows a predominance of polymorphonuclear leukocytes, the patient may have meningitis. Culture results take a minimum of 72 hours before identification and antibiotic susceptibility patterns can be determined. Therefore, antibiotic therapy should be initiated before culture results are complete and then, if needed, adjusted accordingly. Whenever possible, catheters should be inserted in the operating room and changed with a consistent protocol every 3 to 7 days. When the catheter is discontinued, it should be removed using aseptic technique, and a semiquantitative culture of the catheter tip should be obtained. The infectious hazards related to intracranial pressure monitoring devices can be reduced if subarachnoid bolts are used instead of the more invasive intraventricular catheter.[292] However, with the advent of fiberoptic intracranial pressure monitoring devices, infection rates are being further evaluated.

Cerebrospinal Fluid Shunts

Posttraumatic hydrocephalus can be a complication of head injury. Therefore, the management of hydrocephalus often necessitates the use of CSF shunts. These include ventriculoatrial, ventriculoperitoneal, lumbar-peritoneal, and ventriculopleural varieties.

Complications of infection developing secondary to the placement of these shunts can lead to impaired intellectual and neurological function and in some cases death.[293–298] These infections can include meningitis, brain abscess, wound infection, and peritonitis (for peritoneal shunts). The clinical manifestations of such an infection can be fever alone or any combination of the systemic signs of infection, such as peritoneal or meningeal inflammation, wound infection, induration along the shunt tract, or nonspecific symptoms of shunt malfunction. In addition, positive cultures of the CSF, blood, shunt apparatus, incisions, or peritoneal fluid may be seen. Treatment involves appropriate antimicrobial therapy and/or shunt removal, replacement, or revision.

Although *Staphylococcus aureus* and gram-negative bacillary organisms have been identified as the causative agents, most series report strains of coagulase-negative staphylococci as the predominant pathogen. This may be because this organism produces an excess of a mucoid substance that appears to promote adherence to smooth surfaces and may be protective against the lytic actions of lysozyme.[298] The major reservoir of this organism is the patient's skin. The predisposing infection risks are related to the technical placement, length of operative time, the time of placement relative to the initial injury, dissection from an overlying wound infection, and hematogenous seeding from a distant but bacteremic infection. The role of prophylactic antibiotics remains unclear.

Meningitis

Classical signs of meningitis may be obscure in patients sustaining severe head injury. It is difficult to determine a decreasing level of consciousness in an already unconscious patient. Nuchal rigidity may be absent secondary to loss of muscle tone or may not be evaluated in a patient with suspected neck trauma. Fever may be absent, demonstrate erratic patterns, or be the result of blood in the CSF. Leukocytosis can be influenced by the underlying injury or some of the medications the patient is receiving. If the patient has sustained a severe head injury, it may be impossible to perform a lumbar puncture because of the possibility of inducing brain herniation.

When a sample of the CSF can be obtained, diagnosis of meningitis is based on the presence of pleocytosis, hypoglycorrhachia, elevation of CSF protein not attributable to a noninfectious cause, and the isolation of an organism. Gram-negative meningitis is more likely to occur if the patient has received prior antibiotic therapy. When a sample of CSF is not obtainable, the diagnosis of infection is more difficult. In these patients, antibiotic therapy should be initiated when the patient shows signs of mental and clinical deterioration in conjunction with the suspicion of infection. An effective antibiotic regiment for the empirical treatment of meningitis when the causative organism is not known has been shown to be ticarcillin, amikacin sulfate, nafcillin, and chloramphenicol given in combination. This therapy provides coverage against both gram-positive cocci and gram-negative bacillary organisms.[299]

Brain abscess, epidural abscess, and osteomyelitis of the cranium or spine as well as infection of the CSF may develop from a dissecting wound infection. In addition, all these infections can result from inadequate débridement of the initial injury, failure to comply with the principles of meticulous surgical technique, or hematogenous seeding from a bacteremia. Eradication of infection may be difficult and requires prolonged antibiotic therapy (i.e., 6–8 weeks). Surgical intervention also may be necessary.

Infection-Control Measures Through the Trauma Cycle

The primary infection risks for CNS infection occur during the initial phase of the trauma cycle when the dura is broken. CSF infection is more likely to occur in the acute stages, whereas the deep-seated infections often develop much later. As a subgroup of the trauma population, patients sustaining CNS injury have the highest infection risks. This is because the dysfunction of the CNS necessitates the prolonged mechanical support of many organ systems. In addition, it is most important to remember that these patients lose their ability to communicate and sense the developing signs and symptoms of infection. Dysfunction of the CNS also compromises normal function of many organ systems as well as the defense mechanisms against infection. Therefore, the delineation of any infection in these patients requires refinement. Throughout the trauma cycle, nurses must be ever alert to the subtle changes in the patient's clinical condition that signal the presence of an incubating infection. This promotes earlier recognition of disease as well as the initiation of appropriate therapy. Infection-control guidelines for preventing CNS infection are found in Table 12–7. Infection problems of patients with CNS injury occurring in systems other than the CNS are detailed by specific sites elsewhere in this chapter, and further information on the management of patients with CNS injury is found elsewhere in this book.

TABLE 12–7. INFECTION-CONTROL GUIDELINES FOR PREVENTING CENTRAL NERVOUS SYSTEM INFECTION

1. Do not use prophylactic antibiotics in patients with CSF leaks.
2. Do not place nasal tubes or perform nasopharyngeal suctioning in patients with CSF leaks.
3. Use only sterile vacutainers on butterfly drains, and avoid reflux of fluid into drainage tract when changing the tube.
4. Use subarachnoid bolts instead of intraventricular catheters whenever possible.
5. Remove monitoring devices and drains as soon as possible.
6. Use strict aseptic technique for insertion of monitoring systems, and when possible, perform the placement procedure in an operating room.
7. Use strict aseptic technique to manipulate and calibrate monitoring systems.
8. Obtain daily CSF samples for culture, Gram stain, complete cell count, and glucose determination on patients with intraventricular catheters.
9. Whenever possible, change the catheter every 3 days, and obtain a semiquantitative culture of the catheter tip.
10. Use aseptic technique when manipulating any neurosurgical drain.
11. Prevent reflux from gastric tubes from cross-contaminating neurosurgical drains and intracranial pressure monitoring devices.
12. Continually assess the patient for signs and symptoms of incubating infection.

RESPIRATORY TRACT INFECTION

Nosocomial pulmonary infections are often a major complication of modern intensive care.[300–304] In fact, 10 to 40 per cent of nosocomial infections developing in trauma and other critically ill patient populations have been reported to occur in the respiratory tract.[1, 4, 5, 13–17, 53, 305] In addition, it has been estimated that 15 per cent of all hospital-associated deaths[300, 306] and 20 per cent of the infection-related mortality among trauma patients[17, 53] are attributed to lower respiratory tract infections. In the trauma patient, the infection risks are complex and are directly related to the degree of defense compromise induced by the injuries, preexisting underlying illnesses and clinical conditions, and the use of mechanical support devices.

Upper Respiratory Tract Infection

Sinusitis/Otitis

Upper respiratory tract infections are usually related to intubation, and most are of nosocomial etiology.[307–310] Nosocomial sinusitis usually presents as cryptic fever in patients with indwelling nasal tubes and a decreased level of consciousness.[307] The presence of a large-bore tube in the nose can cause inflammation and edema of the nasopharyngeal mucosa with blocked ventilation of the sinuses; this is the largest risk factor for the development of infection. Diagnosis is based on positive roentgenograms consistent with sinusitis and either purulent material aspirated from the sinuses or the presence of purulent nasal discharge. However, less than a third of patients described as having this disease have purulent nasal discharge. Most infections are polymicrobial, with a predominance of gram-negative bacilli. Similarly, otitis can develop secondary to indwelling nasal tubes or implanted myringotomy tubes. Purulent drainage may not be evident, and the diagnosis of infection in patients with appropriate risk factors may be overlooked. Careful examination and assessment of the patient are keys to the diagnosis. Failure to identify either sinusitis or otitis can result in the institution of inappropriate therapy if the source of the fever is attributed to other factors. Resolution of infection requires the removal of the tubes and appropriate antibiotics. Surgical drainage of an abscess or aspiration of the sinus also may be necessary.

Tracheitis

Tracheitis may be associated with endotracheal intubation. Prolonged hyperinflation of endotracheal cuffs causes localized tracheal ischemia, creating an environment which facilitates the growth of oral anaerobes. Purulent tracheitis that may have secondary cellulitis is generally attributed to anaerobes. Patients with tracheostomy tubes should be monitored for the development of purulent tracheitis. Discharges usually are copious, thin in viscosity, dirty brown in color, and very foul smelling. Most patients do well with appropriate antibiotic therapy, which is usually directed against the oral anaerobes.

Lower Respiratory Tract Infection

Pneumonia

Factors contributing to the development of pneumonia include coma or decreased level of consciousness, aspiration of oral secretions, major thoracic and/or abdominal injury or surgery, respiratory burns, immobilization, presence of pulmonary diseases such as COPD, and heavy tobacco smoking.[303–305, 311–313] Diagnosis of pneumonia in the critically ill patient is often difficult due to the influences of their underlying injury and the tendency to retain secretions. The diagnosis of pneumonia can easily be confused with other causes of infiltrates on chest x-ray, such as atelectasis, respiratory distress syndrome (ARDS), or lung contusions.[13–17, 53, 313–315] A useful definition for pneumonia in this population is an increasing temperature and white blood cell count trend, the production of copious sputum, the presence of polymorphonuclear leukocytes and a predominant organism on Gram stain, and a new infiltrate that does not clear with chest physiotherapy.[13–17, 53, 315] Prior isolation of pathogenic organisms is not necessary, since many patients in the intensive care unit will frequently be colonized with gram-negative pathogens early in their course.[316, 317] Patients on ventilators should be monitored with daily chest roentgenograms, and culture and Gram stain of sputum should be obtained frequently. By monitoring the Gram stains on a routine basis, the change in the nature of the sputum can easily be followed, and a diagnosis of pneumonia can be made with more certainty when a pulmonary infiltrate is found that does not clear with physiotherapy.

Patients with respiratory burns and burns of the head, neck, and thorax have added risks for pneumonia.[318] Respiratory burns cause direct alveolar damage, which can be the result of heat, smoke, or toxic chemical agents. This injury can produce additional compromise of pulmonary defense, lung dysfunction, and necrosis. Chemical pneumonitis is a frequent complication. Tracheostomy is generally avoided, since the added bacterial contamination of the wound is more easily introduced into the lungs. Pneumonias in burn patients are usually caused by the same organisms recovered from the wounds and can result from the hematogenous seeding from bacteremic wound infections. Otherwise, the infection risks are the same as in any other critically ill and ventilator-dependent patient.

A common complication among critically ill and injured patients is the physiological stress that can cause increased secretion of gastric acids with resultant upper GI ulceration and bleeding. Therefore, it is not uncommon to treat these patients with high-dose antacids or histamine (H_2) receptor antagonists such as cimetidine or ranitidine for stress ulcer prophylaxis. However, increasing gastric pH allows the stomach to become colonized with oral anaerobes and gram-negative bacillary organisms. The stomach, then, becomes a reservoir for organisms that can cause nosocomial pneumonia.[316, 317] Recent studies have suggested that the use of a gastric barrier agent such as sucralfate (Carafate), which preserves the natural gastric barrier against bacterial overgrowth, may counteract the effects of antacids and H_2-receptor blockers and ultimately reduce the incidence of nosocomial pneumonia.[319, 320] While these studies provide promising information and future direction for strategies to prevent and reduce the incidence of nosocomial pneumonia, the data remain inconclusive,[321] and the Food and Drug Administration (FDA) has noted that "administration of Carafate has not been demonstrated to result in lower rates of nosocomial pneumonia in hospitalized patients than do H_2 blockers."[322]

Another common problem for critically ill ventilator-dependent patients is the adverse consequences of tracheal suctioning for the removal of accumulated secretions. These complications can include arterial oxygen desaturation and periods of bradycardia and hypotension in unstable patients, as well as the opportunity to contaminate the airway.[323, 324] The complications often coincide with the need to disengage the patient from the ventilator while performing suctioning. Recently, new closed-circuit catheter systems have become available that eliminate the need to disconnect the patient from the ventilator for suctioning. One study has shown that the adverse consequences of suctioning can be markedly reduced.[325] In addition, infection risks in the intensive care unit may be reduced, since aerosolization of the patient's secretions will not occur. However, since these catheters are changed only when the ventilator circuits are changed, the catheters are repeatedly used during a 24- to 48-hour interval. It is a concern that the catheters may become a bacterial reservoir and increase the risk for subsequent pneumonia. Prospective, randomized clinical trials designed specifically to address the infection issues must be conducted to clearly define the risk-to-benefit ratio associated with the use of these catheters.

Nosocomial pneumonia is a serious disease. It is often complicated by bacteremia and has a high mortality rate. Pneumonia and aspiration can induce lung abscess and empyema. Therefore, all efforts to prevent it must be undertaken.

Preventative nursing actions center around frequent auscultation for changes in the quality of breath sounds, frequent pulmonary hygiene, turning and positioning of the patient, and routine chest physiotherapy.[326–328] Nurses and therapists performing tracheal suctioning should wear gloves on both hands to protect themselves against the acquisition of herpetic paronychia.[329]

Failure to maintain the care of respirators and respiratory support equipment can lead to infection risk, as well as outbreak situations.[330–337] This is a serious infection hazard, since a large bacterial inoculum can be introduced directly into the lungs. A fulminant, necrotizing pneumonia could develop, and death can result in a matter of hours.

Empyema

The second most frequently occurring lower respiratory infection among trauma patients is thoracic empyema.[13–17, 53, 305, 339, 340] Development of thoracic empyema has classically been described as a sequela of prior pneumonia, aspiration, or pleural effusion.[339–341] Nosocomial empyema has been shown to be significantly associated with prior chest tube insertion in the trauma population.[342, 343] Predisposing risk factors appear to be related to chest tube insertion for evacuation of blood following chest trauma or emergency intervention for internal cardiac massage and following barotrauma in patients requiring high levels of positive end-expiratory pressure or controlled mechanical ventilation.[344, 345] Infection may result from contamination during an emergency situation; the primary pathogen is usually coagulase-positive staphylococci. Empyema that follows barotrauma necessitating chest tube insertion generally develops relatively late in the patient's hospitalization, and therefore, patients may have a colonized lower respiratory tract. Organisms recovered from empyema via this mechanism are usually gram-negative bacilli and anaerobes. Empyema can develop as a secondary consequence of surgical misadventure during the placement of subclavian and jugular central venous catheters.[346–349] These accidents can cause pneumothorax, hemothorax, and/or hydrothorax, which contaminate the lungs and pleural space and often warrant the emergent insertion of chest tubes.

Diagnosis of nosocomial empyema is based on purulent drainage from the pleural space and increasing trends in the temperature and white blood cell count. Culture and Gram stain, complete cell count with differential, and pH and protein determinations of the drainage fluid can support the diagnosis.[341] Pleural fluid cultures obtained from drainage equipment must be properly taken. These cultures should not be obtained from the collection chambers, since this fluid may be contaminated and thus may not reflect the clinical picture. Samples should be drawn from a site on the latex tubing that is as close as possible to the thoracotomy tube. The tubing should be washed with an antiseptic soap and then disinfected with alcohol. Then, using a sterile 25-gauge needle, a small amount of pleural fluid can be aspirated. Specimens should be sent to the laboratory in the syringe, and the fluid should not be injected into blood culture bottles. Fluids injected into blood culture bottles cannot have Gram stain determination, and the use of this medium for fluids other than blood can result in inaccurate culture results. Treatment may require decortication and rib resection.[350] Appropriate parenteral antibiotics are given until the chest tube is converted to a treatment port.

Infection-control measures that may minimize the development of nosocomial empyema include strict aseptic insertion technique whenever possible and occlusive dressings that should be changed every 48 hours using aseptic technique. Nurses should be cautioned to gently milk and strip the latex tubings of the drainage system to prevent local trauma of the skin–tube interface and catapulting of organisms back into the pleural space.

Mediastinitis

A relatively rare thoracic infection in trauma patients is mediastinitis. The primary predisposing risks are esophageal perforation, penetrating thoracic injuries, and internal cardiac massage. Infection secondary to esophageal perforation is generally precipitated by the dissection of oral anaerobes into the mediastinum, whereas infection following open interventions is more likely to be from *Staphylococcus aureus*. Treatment requires appropriate antimicrobial therapy and may necessitate the placement of chest tubes and/or surgical intervention.

Infection-Control Measures Through the Trauma Cycle

Respiratory infections can develop in any phase of the trauma cycle subsequent to initial resuscitation. The greatest chance for pneumonia is when the patient is in the intensive care unit and is ventilator-dependent, unconscious, and/or immobilized. However, infection hazards are present throughout the cycle and may exist in the prehospital phase. Nursing actions must promote pulmonary function and prevent the retention of secretions. These actions can include chest physiotherapy, frequent repositioning and turning, encouraging cough and deep-breathing exercises in nonventilated patients, and providing frequent pulmonary toilet to ventilator-dependent patients. Infection-control guidelines are outlined in Table 12–8.

GASTROINTESTINAL TRACT INFECTION

The risks for the development of intra-abdominal infection following operative procedures have been well documented.[1, 3, 4, 72, 136–139, 142–146] The risk of developing an infection is influenced by the type and classification of surgery performed, the duration of the surgery, the skill of the surgeon, the manner in which the skin is prepared prior to incision, and the existence of trauma. Compromised tissue perfusion secondary to hypovolemia, shock, ischemia, and hypoxia can lead to devitalized tissue, which can ultimately provide a medium in which microorganisms can thrive. Other predisposing factors are hematoma formation, creation of dead spaces, abrasive tissue handling, surgical misadventures,

TABLE 12–8. INFECTION-CONTROL GUIDELINES FOR THE PREVENTION OF RESPIRATORY INFECTION

1. Frequent pulmonary toilet.
2. Frequent chest physiotherapy.
3. Frequent respiratory assessment.
4. Obtain routine sputum surveillance cultures on ventilator-dependent patients.
5. Change respirator circuits every 24 to 48 hours, and label tubes with date and time of change.
6. Change lavage fluid for tracheal suction tubing every 8 hours, and indicate time of change.
7. When replenishing nebulizers or humidifiers within 24-hour intervals, discard unused portion prior to filling unit with sterile water.
8. Do not allow bag-mask resuscitators (Ambu bags) to be shared among patients.
9. Do not allow condensate in tubings of patients on tracheal collars to reflux into the nebulizers.
10. Monitor the length of time nasal tubes remain indwelling, and where possible, switch to oral gastric or oral tracheal tubes.
11. Monitor cuff pressures frequently.
12. Milk and strip chest tubes gently.
13. Change chest tube dressings with aseptic technique every 48 hours.
14. Obtain culture and Gram stain of drainage fluid as clinically indicated.
15. Avoid placing anything in the nose if a CSF leak is suspected or evident.

placement of drains, peritoneal dialysis, CNS dysfunction, and the use of enteral feeding tubes, especially those which bypass the stomach. Often, despite the use of prophylactic antibiotic therapy, peritonitis and deep-seated abscesses can develop when the integrity of the GI mucosa has been broken.[13–17, 53, 351, 352] Mortality from these infections has been reported to approximate 30 per cent, and the prognosis worsens with increasing age, organ failure, bacteremia, and persistent abscess.[53, 352]

Infection risks for intra-abdominal abscess are enhanced by the nature of the patient's underlying illness, the type of trauma, and chemotherapy. Blunt and penetrating abdominal trauma often require emergent surgery. Penetrating trauma can disrupt the colonic mucosa, causing fecal contamination of the peritoneal cavity, and can sever the major deep vessels of the cardiovascular system. Blunt trauma causes rupture of the solid, highly perfused organs such as liver and spleen, which can produce massive hemorrhage. In order to control the hemorrhage, there simply is not time for meticulous skin preparation or gentle tissue handling. Performance of expedient stabilization techniques also increases the probability of surgical misadventure. In addition, trauma patients are prone to the development of infection as a result of noninvasive risks such as CNS injury, side effects of anesthetic agents and medications, and antibiotic utilization, which can alter normal GI function.[22, 23, 95, 97, 319, 320, 353] The most common sites for intra-abdominal abscess following trauma are within the subphrenic and subhepatic spaces.[53]

Contusion of the gallbladder secondary to trauma or a hepatobiliary procedure has been reported as one cause of acute acalculus cholecystitis.[354] The contusion impedes perfusion and creates a medium for bacterial growth. Concomitantly, a new reservoir of microorganisms is created when the upper intestinal tract, which is normally sterile, becomes colonized as a result of decreased gastric motility and elevated gastric pH. The gallbladder, then prone to necrosis, provides an environment conducive for microbial growth and proliferation as well as an access route for entry into the bloodstream. Therefore, the development of acute acalculous cholecystitis can be a serious, life-threatening disease. Creation of dead space as a result of tissue removal and the placement of drainage devices also increase the risk for the development of subsequent serious infection.

Intra-abdominal abscess, peritonitis, or local wound infection can be precipitated following diagnostic peritoneal lavage or the institution of peritoneal dialysis. Infection risks arise from poor aseptic technique and/or inadvertent bowel perforation during catheter insertion, inadequate drainage of the peritoneal cavity, leakage of the dialysate either through the incision or around the skin–catheter interface, and the contamination of the system from improperly warmed dialysate fluids or poor technique when emptying the drainage bag.

Diagnosis of intra-abdominal infection can be hindered by the patient's clinical condition. Examination may be difficult to perform due to the presence of drainage tubes and bandages or the patient's immobility. Many patients may not be able to communicate their symptoms owing to a decreased level of consciousness or the inability to sense pain or discomfort secondary to medication or CNS injury. Optimal diagnostic tests such as radioisotopic scans and x-rays may be unobtainable because the patient is too critically ill to be moved or the extent of the injury prevents the proper positioning of the patient for performance of the test.

Assessment of infection depends on repeated evaluation of bowel function, the integrity of suture lines, and the character of any drainage fluid as to amount, color, odor, and viscosity against the ongoing clinical trends of fever pattern and white blood cell count. Any purulent material from incisions or drainage tubes should be sent for Gram stain and culture. Persistent diarrhea must be evaluated, and culture and Gram stain of the fecal matter must be obtained.

Diarrhea occurs frequently in severely compromised patients. Usually it is due to the hyperosmolarity of the feeding solution given to the patient. However, infectious causes such as salmonellosis, shigellosis, pseudomembranous colitis, enterocolitis, and antibiotic-associated colitis must be considered. Persistent diarrhea, defined as three or more large, loose stools a day, in patients on or completing antibiotic therapy can be an indication of the presence of pseudomembranous colitis.[355, 356] Characteristically, the diarrhea is watery and large in volume, but evidence of blood and mucus may be absent. Fever, leukocytosis, and abdominal cramping are present in most cases. Antibiotic-related pseudomembranous colitis has been associated with almost every antimicrobial agent.[356–359] Diagnosis is based on onset of diarrhea during or following antibiotic therapy, presence of clostridial cytotoxin in stool specimens, and/or observation of pseudomembranes during endoscopic examination. Most patients do well with administration of oral vancomycin or metronidazole.[359] When patients are placed in close proximity to each other and the chance of cross-contamination is likely, enteric isolation precautions may be necessary for patients with diarrhea associated with GI infections.[190, 360, 361]

The presence of enteral feeding tubes can induce infection of the GI tract. Indwelling nasogastric tubes and gastrostomy tubes can result in staphylococcal enterocolitis.[362] The staphylococci invade the GI tract from the skin's reservoir via either the nares or the gastrostomy tube–skin interface and in some cases as a result of contamination of the feeding solution and apparatus. The presenting signs and symptoms include large volumes of watery green and mucous stools, abdominal cramping, and fever. Sheets of white cells and the presence of heavy quantities of gram-positive cocci can be seen on Gram stain of stool specimens. Needle jejunostomy tubes can produce localized ischemia, which can later lead to necrosis, intestinal perforation, peritonitis, and intra-abdominal abscess.

As a rule, sterile adminstration equipment is not necessary for enteral feeding. This is because ingested bacteria rarely survive the stomach's acid environment. However, special consideration must be given to trauma patients who have dysfunctional GI tracts or an increased gastric pH that is no longer protective.[353, 363, 364] The primary infection risk is related to residual solutions that accumulate within the administration sets. The feeding solution offers an enriched medium for bacterial growth.[365, 366] Therefore, any bacteria introduced into the system can rapidly replicate, and a large bacterial inoculum subsequently may be fed to the patient. This bioburden may then be too great for the patient to overcome. In fact, recent studies suggest that contaminated enteral nutrition represents a significant cause of bacteremic infection.[367–370] Infection risks for these patients can be reduced by thoroughly cleaning or changing the administration sets at a minimum of every 24 hours.[371–374]

Although many GI infections tend to manifest later in the trauma cycle, infection risks throughout the cycle are ever-present. Frequent assessment of GI function facilitates early diagnosis and treatment of disease. Therefore, any deviation from the patient's normal baseline may signal the presence of an incubating infection. Infection-control guidelines are shown in Table 12–9.

GENITOURINARY TRACT INFECTION

Catheter-associated urinary tract infection (UTI) is the most frequently cited nosocomial infection developed among hospitalized patient populations.[300, 303, 304, 375–378] Between 12 and 30 per cent of the infections developed among severely traumatized patients have been reported to be UTIs.[1, 4, 15, 13–17, 53] Underlying illness, advanced age, CNS injury, genitourinary injury, metabolic imbalances, and renal failure contribute to the infection risks.[377, 378] Females are prone to UTI secondary to the short urethra and the added microbial reservoir provided by the vagina and because an adequate noninvasive drainage system does not exist. Burn patients with indwelling catheters are at increased risk for UTI from the microorganisms colonizing the burns and the consequences of hydrotherapy.

In any case, the major influence is the indwelling catheter, which affords bacteria a direct portal of entry into the bladder.[377, 379] Bacteria may be inoculated into the system during catheter insertion, by traveling along the mucous coating that forms along the catheter as it remains indwelling,[380] from contamination of the drainage bag when urine is allowed to reflux into the bladder, and by frequent manipulations of the drainage system.[375, 379–382] The probability of developing bacteriuria and UTI increases proportionately as the duration of catheter indwelling time increases.[383, 384]

Because of the multiple aspects of a patient's disease and the high frequency for bacterial colonization of the urinary drainage system, the criteria for diagnosis of UTI[385] may require refinement. The urine is frequently colonized, and one must be cautious in ascribing the clinical signs of infection to the urinary tract solely because of a positive urine culture with greater than 100,000 colony-forming units per milliliter in the absence of white blood cells on microscopic urinalysis. This can be of particular importance in patients requiring prolonged bladder instrumentation, as in the care of spinal cord injury. Therefore, a useful definition for UTI in the catheterized patient is two or more consecutive positive urine cultures with greater than 100,000 colony-forming units per milliliter, pyuria of at least 10 white blood cells per high-power field of unspun fresh urine, and clinical signs of infection.[13–17, 53] Treatment of colonization rather than infection can encourage the emergence of antibiotic-resistant bacteria or mask the development of a more serious disease.

In patients sustaining spinal cord injury with concomitant neurogenic bladder, regimens for bladder training should be begun as soon as possible. There seems to be less of an associated risk for UTI from intermittent catherizations than with indwelling catheters. However, in male patients, epididymitis and/or prostate gland infection may be induced by repetitive instrumentations or intermittent catheterizations. Since these patients also have a high incidence of recurrent and chronic UTIs, they have an increased risk for the later development of pyelonephritis.

Although reports in the medical literature have cited UTI as the predominant type of nosocomial infection, UTIs have a comparatively low incidence of associated bacteremia. The vast majority of UTIs are caused by *E. coli* and other kinds of gram-negative bacillary bacteria. An indwelling catheter should never be changed during a fever spike or a septic crisis. If the patient has colonized or infected urine, the bacteria can gain access into the bloodstream as the catheter is being changed. The urethral mucosa also becomes more fragile with prolonged instrumentation. Therefore, the chance of inducing microscopic bleeding secondary to a traumatic insertion technique is increased. Catheter tips should never be sent for culture, since it is almost impossible to withdraw them without contamination from the urethral mucosa.[386] The appropriate tests to perform are urine culture and urinalysis of urine obtained by needle aspiration of the catheter system.

Infection-control practices and preventive efforts in the development of UTI have been widely examined in the medical literature.[387, 388] Certain measures have been found to be ineffective, such as routine irrigation of the bladder,[387] suppressive antibiotic therapy,[382, 389, 390] povidone-iodine solutions for meatal care,[391] and instillation of hydrogen peroxide into the drainage bag.[392] In the intensive care unit, the use of common urometers for measuring specific gravity and the sharing of collection vessels for emptying the drainage bags have been associated with outbreaks of gram-negative UTIs.[393, 394] Therefore, it is important not to share equipment among patients and to use clean, dry collection vessels when measuring urinary output.

TABLE 12–9. INFECTION-CONTROL GUIDELINES FOR THE GI TRACT

1. Use aseptic technique for wound and drain care.
2. Use sterile measuring devices when emptying drainage vessels.
3. Maintain the patency and function of all drainage tubes to ensure proper evacuation.
4. Document the characteristics of all drainage fluids as to amount, color, viscosity, and odor.
5. Document the appearance of surgical sites, and notify the physician of any leakage through the incision itself.
6. Obtain culture and Gram stain of any purulent material from wounds or drainage tubes.
7. Assess bowel sounds and function at the beginning of every shift.
8. Obtain culture and Gram stain of persistent diarrhea, and when indicated, test for clostridial cytotoxin.
9. Use strict aseptic technique for insertion of peritoneal and needle jejunostomy tubes.
10. Obtain culture, Gram stain, and complete cell counts daily on effluent dialysate.
11. Use a blood-warming apparatus for warming peritoneal solutions rather than water baths or placing bags under running hot water faucets.
12. Use closed systems for peritoneal dialysis and sterile containers for emptying drainage.
13. Inspect the catheter–skin interface of peritoneal catheters daily for signs of leakage or inflammation.
14. Change enteral feeding apparatus daily.

Bladder injury can promote UTI secondary to dysfunction of the bladder as well as the necessity for prolonged instrumentation. Indwelling suprapubic tubes can induce infection at the skin–tube junction. Patency of these tubes should always be maintained. Leakage from around the catheter as well as signs of inflammation or purulent drainage should be reported to the physician.

UTI can occur in any phase of the trauma cycle, even at the time of admission. Nosocomial UTI can develop within 3 days of admission. As the patient progresses through the trauma cycle, recurrent episodes of UTI can develop in patients requiring prolonged instrumentation. Concomitantly, the repeated courses of antibiotic therapy can increase the reservoir of antibiotic-resistant microorganisms. Because of the high risk for associated UTI, the use of indwelling catheters for the management of urinary incontinence should be considered carefully. Therefore, nurses should promote the use of noninvasive management (i.e., condom catheters in males and disposable diapers in females) whenever possible. A summary of infection-control guidelines is found in Table 12–10.

OCCUPATIONAL EXPOSURE TO BLOOD-BORNE DISEASES

As the acquired immune deficiency syndrome (AIDS) epidemic has emerged, occupational acquisition of an infectious disease while performing emergency medical services (EMS) has intensified.[395] This is true not only for prehospital and inhospital EMS providers, but for the entire health care community as well. In 1987, the CDC called for the institution of universal precautions for infection control to prevent the occupational acquisition of the blood-borne infections—hepatitis B virus (HBV) and human immunodeficiency virus (HIV).[396] These guidelines (1) suggested that all blood, bloody body fluids, and certain other body fluids be considered infectious, (2) required that appropriate protective attire (i.e., gloves, gowns, eyewear, and masks) be worn for tasks that could cause bloody fluid contamination of personnel performing the tasks, (3) defined the circumstances of exposures to blood and body fluids, and (4) outlined employee health guidelines for follow-up medical care for those personnel sustaining an exposure. However, the CDC has no powers of enforcement for their guidelines. Accordingly, in the fall of 1987, the U.S. Department of Labor through the Occupational Safety and Health Administration (OSHA) set out to codify the CDC guidelines into federal regulations.[397, 398] These were finalized in December of 1991 and became effective in March of 1992.[399] The OSHA regulations are much more explicit with regard to definitions of infectious blood and body fluids, requirements for education and training, mandating hepatitis B vaccine programs at the expense of the employer, guidelines for employee health programs, environmental controls, and documenting compliance with the regulations. OSHA is empowered to conduct unannounced inspections, either with or without prior complaint, and can levy heavy fines on employers who fail to comply.

TABLE 12–10. INFECTION-CONTROL GUIDELINES FOR THE CARE OF URINARY DRAINAGE SYSTEMS

1. Use strict aseptic, atraumatic insertion technique.
2. Maintain a closed drainage system.
3. Obtain urine cultures via needle aspiration and at routine frequency.
4. Obtain microscopic urinalysis with each urine culture.
5. Prevent urine reflux.
6. Do not irrigate the catheter unless it is obstructed, and then use aseptic technique.
7. Perform perineal care every shift.
8. Tape the catheter securely to the patient's abdomen in males or the inside of the thigh in females.
9. Do not change the catheter during a septic crisis.
10. Most important, remove the catheter as soon as possible.

Since 1987, much has been written about HIV and HBV concerning the modes of transmission of infection, the application of universal precautions, and the protection of health care workers from occupational infection. The purpose of this section is to address those issues which affect the application of OSHA regulations to emergency medical settings.

HIV and the Trauma Patient

Little has been written about HIV in the trauma patient. Most trauma patients admitted with HIV infection are in the asymptomatic carrier phase of the illness. The clinical presentation of AIDS can be masked by the underlying effects of the trauma; that is, both trauma and HIV infection can make the patient more susceptible to infection and cause CNS dysfunction.[400]

However, when one examines the demographic data concerning persons with HIV infection, some characteristics common to trauma patients can be seen.[401] For example, more than 90 per cent of all AIDS cases occur in people between 20 and 49 years. More than 93 per cent of these are male, with about 15 per cent of these IV drug abusers.[402] Similarly, trauma is the leading killer of Americans under the age of 38, most victims are male, and drug and alcohol abusers seem to have higher trauma rates. Of these patients, those sustaining gunshot wounds resulting from situations related to IV drug abuse or drug dealing are seen more frequently within large metropolitan areas and surrounding communities than in rural settings. Similarly, studies describing the seroprevalence rates of HIV antibody positivity among trauma patients reflect the demographic patterns of HIV infection within the community, with significantly greater numbers being concentrated within larger cities.[403–406] For example, the emergency department of a large metropolitan inner-city hospital reported a seropositivity rate of 18 per cent of IV drug abusers treated in the emergency room and 10.6 per cent of patients admitted for penetrating trauma.[405] On the other hand, a hospital approximately 2 miles away, whose trauma population was mostly referred from outside the same city limits, reported a seropositivity rate of 1.7 per cent of admissions.[406]

As of 1992, a reliable, cost-effective, and timely laboratory test for the presence of HIV does *not* exist. The only tests available are those which identify the presence of the HIV antibody. Therefore, identification of HIV-infected patients who may pose an occupational risk to emergency health care workers cannot be guaranteed. Two types of HIV antibody tests are widely utilized at present: ELISA (enzyme-linked immunosorbent assay) and Western blot electrophoresis. Both have intrinsic flaws.[407, 408] ELISA is a highly sensitive test for antibody response; however, it is not as specific because reactivity with similar antibodies can give false-positive results. Western blot electrophoresis is a highly specific test for HIV antibody proteins, which are identified on the basis of molecular weight. Adequate concentration of antibody proteins must be present before the results are considered positive. However, the Western blot is not a very sensitive test, and results can be inconclusive. Therefore, the most widely accepted criteria for HIV antibody positivity require that both tests be performed and both tests be reactive (i.e., positive). Another factor that may influence HIV antibody positivity is massive fluid replacement in trauma patients. In this situation, the antibodies may be diluted, and the patient's HIV antibody test could be falsely negative.[409] It is very important to realize that these tests identify antibodies to HIV, not the virus itself, so positivity is primarily a demonstration of past infection. Because these are antibody tests, newly infected individuals may test negative because their body has not had adequate time to mount an antibody response. These patients may have viral particles in their blood that can infect a health care worker who sustains a percutaneous or mucocutaneous exposure to that blood. Because this is true, knowledge of the patient's HIV antibody status could give the care provider a false sense of security, and thus infection-control precautions might be relaxed at a time when the patient's blood is most infectious. If, however, one of the blood-borne diseases or any communicable disease is diagnosed at the hospital, it is important to consider protection of prehospital EMS providers. Notification to prehospital care providers of exposure to infectious disease became federal law in August of 1990.[410] Notification mechanisms must ensure both accurate information and protection of the patient's and provider's legal rights.

It is important to note that informed consent is mandatory for HIV testing in most states and a requirement by OSHA for serotesting a patient in cases of occupational exposure.[399] This requirement exists because HIV antibody–positive persons have been severely discriminated against as a result of public awareness of their illness. Informed consent is particularly important for trauma patients because the circumstance for their admission is not HIV infection. For this reason, substitute consent of unconscious or cognitively impaired patients may not be legal unless formal legal guardianship has been established.[411]

Hepatitis B and Hepatitis B Vaccine

Unlike HIV, HBV can be easily and reliably detected in patients with a chronic carrier state or active state of infection. Serotesting for HBV is done by radioimmunoassay (RIA), which detects the presence of hepatitis B surface antigen (HBsAg), and positivity is an indication of existing HBV. However, HBsAg testing is not routinely performed by the majority of health care facilities. There are several reasons for this:

1. The prevalence of HBsAg carriers among the general U.S. population is approximately 0.5 to 2 per cent,[412] and the routine screening of all hospitalized patients may be prohibitively expensive for many hospitals.
2. Performance of an HBsAg test may be irrelevant to the underlying reason for the patient's admission to the hospital.
3. Many hospitals are not equipped to perform these tests on site.
4. Prophylactic treatment can be given for occupational misadventures such as needlestick injuries.
5. Employees can be vaccinated against HBV infection.

Therefore, it is estimated that approximately 90 per cent of HBsAg carriers who are hospitalized are undetected as carriers of the virus during admission.[413, 414]

In 1987, the CDC estimated that 500 to 600 health care workers whose jobs involved direct exposure to blood were hospitalized annually in the United States as a result of illness related to hepatitis B.[397] Of these, the CDC estimated that over 200 eventually die from the lethal sequelae of this disease (12 to 15 expiring from acute fulminant disease, 170 to 200 from cirrhosis, and 50 from hepatocellular carcinoma). In comparison with AIDS, 6 to 30 per cent of those not vaccinated or receiving prophylaxis who incur blood or body fluid misadventures involving patients with hepatitis B will develop disease,[413, 415] but fewer than 1 per cent of those incurring similar misadventures involving people with AIDS will become HIV antibody–positive.[416] There are rare reports of health care workers who have expired from documented or suspected occupational acquisition of HIV infection.

The occupational risk of HBV infection among health care workers is quite clear. Seroprevalence studies of HBsAg and hepatitis B antibody (anti-HB) among various groups of health care workers have been 5 to 30 per cent higher than those reported for the general public.[413, 417] Professional groups identified as having the highest rates of positivity include emergency medical personnel (18–30 per cent), surgeons (23–50 per cent), pathologists (27 per cent), blood bank personnel (25 per cent), laboratory workers (23–30 per cent), oral surgeons (21 per cent), intensive care nurses (15–28 per cent), and anesthesiologists (10–30 per cent).[413, 418–423] Contributory factors most associated with positivity have been identified as performance of invasive procedures, working in areas where splattering of blood and body fluids is likely, number of years practicing the profession, and age.[413, 418–421, 423] Transmission of HBV in health care settings can occur from personnel to patients. However, nosocomial transmission of HBV is comparatively rare.[424]

Despite these statistics and the CDC's recommendation[412, 414] that health care workers in high-risk settings be vaccinated with hepatitis B vaccine, vaccination programs have not met with much success.[425–428] Concern over safety and efficacy, lack of education regarding the vaccine, employees' unwillingness to share or assume the expense, and fear of needles have been identified as factors related to vaccine nonacceptance. However, the new OSHA regulations[399] mandate that employers make hepatitis B vaccine available at no charge to employees and require employers to document proof of vaccination refusal by employees not desiring to receive vaccination.

Active and long-lasting immunization can be achieved with either one of the hepatitis vaccines—plasma-derived (Hepatovax, MSD) and yeast-derived (Recombovax, MSD and Engerix, SKF). Both types of vaccines can elicit antibody response against determinants of HBsAg, the stimulator of HBV-neutralizing antibodies. For both vaccines, the binding of HBsAg and the vaccine-induced antibodies is equal to the antibody responses elicited by HBV infection.[429]

The plasma-derived variety consists of highly purified, formalin-inactive HBsAg particles from chronic carriers of HBsAg. This vaccine has been evaluated extensively for immunogenicity, safety, and efficacy.[412, 414, 429–431] Both local (soreness, pain, and tenderness) and systemic (headaches, fatigue, weakness, diarrhea, irritability) reactions have been transient and mild. In a large randomized, double-blind trial, vaccine was administered to one group of volunteers, and a second group received a normal saline placebo; there was no difference in occurrence of adverse complaints between the groups.[431]

Since advent of the AIDS epidemic, there has been concern about the possibility of transmitting HIV to vaccine recipients, since some chronic carriers of HBsAg may have participated in the high-risk behaviors that facilitate the acquisition of HIV infection. This is extraordinarily unlikely. The final vaccine is highly purified: only the noninfectious HBsAg protein is detected. HBV is inactivated in three steps: treatment with pepsin at pH 2, 8 *M* urea, and formalin. These steps inactivate HBV as well as all other known families of viruses (including slow viruses causing such diseases as Creutzfeld-Jakob disease and kuru) that infect humans.[429]

The yeast-derived vaccine is genetically engineered via recombinant DNA techniques using the yeast *Saccharomyces cerevisiae.* This technique involves cloning the HBV DNA into *E. coli* and isolating the portion of the DNA coding for HBsAg from restriction nuclease digestive enzymes. This DNA is then transformed into the yeast by a plasmid expression vector, which gives rise to the HBsAg-producing yeast strain. The HBsAg is released from the disrupted yeast and then purified by chromatographic procedures. The purified HBsAg is essentially free of contaminating yeast proteins and DNA, which, if present, would cause allergic reactions in some people.[432] The genetically engineered HBsAg is similar in appearance and chemical structure to that extracted from human plasma. Efficacy has been demonstrated in clinical trials, and adverse reactions (local and systemic) have been mild and transient.[432]

In general, plasma-derived HBV vaccine has induced seroconversion in similar proportions of vaccinees when vaccine has been administered by the intramuscular (IM) and intradermal (ID) routes.[433] Therefore, some organizations have attempted to decrease the cost of employee vaccination by administering one-tenth the recommended IM vaccine dose by the ID route.[434] However, immune responses to recombinant vaccine have not been equivalent after IM and ID vaccination.[435–437] In addition, inadequate immune response among public safety workers receiving ID vaccination against HBV has been reported.[434] Therefore, the Advisory Committee for Immunization Practices (ACIP) has recommended that vaccination programs should not use the ID route of administration.[438] It is important to note that HBV vaccine is not licensed by the FDA for ID administration except during a research protocol that includes informed consent from participants and postvaccination antibody testing to detect nonresponders, who would then be eligible for revaccination.

Occupational Protective Attire and Procedures

The need to guard against the acquisition of viral disease is very real. Because the performance of emergency medical services presents a high likelihood of occupational exposure to HBV and HIV, the application of OSHA guidelines must be carefully considered. Guidelines for the prevention of blood-borne diseases for the prehospital and in-hospital setting are outlined in Table 12–11.

Gloves

When the CDC recommended the implementation of universal precautions for the prevention of occupational acquisition of blood-borne diseases, glove utilization both inside and outside hospitals dramatically increased. Consequently, there was a national shortage of gloves, in particular sterile surgical and procedure gloves. While some of this shortage is attributed to increased demands, a major factor is inappropriate use of gloves. Gloves should be worn only when a task involves direct contact with blood or body fluids. They should be removed as soon as the task is completed, and handwashing should be performed. Wearing gloves should never be viewed as a substitute for handwashing. In addition, the failure to remove gloves promptly can facilitate cross-infection among hospitalized patients and increase nosocomial infection rates. Failure to remove gloves also can promote occupational acquisition of blood-borne infection because personnel can inoculate themselves with the blood

TABLE 12–11. INFECTION-CONTROL GUIDELINES FOR THE PREVENTION OF BLOOD-BORNE INFECTIONS IN THE HEALTH CARE ENVIRONMENT

1. Treat the blood and body fluids of all patients as if they were infectious.
2. Wear gloves when handling any blood or body fluid or performing invasive procedures. This would include IV insertions, percutaneous venous or arterial punctures, and manipulations of IV lines.
3. Wear masks and eye protection when the chance of blood or body fluids being splashed is probable.
4. Avoid needle stick injuries, and do not recap needles. All needles and sharps contaminated with blood must be disposed of in impervious, puncture-resistant (heavy plastic or metal) containers.
5. Before reporting to work, protect broken skin with Band-Aids or small dressings.
6. Wash hands after all patient care procedures.
7. Use respiratory assist devices when performing mouth-to-mouth resuscitation.
8. Change clothing or scrub attire contaminated with blood or body fluids as soon as patient care allows.
9. Report all percutaneous and mucocutaneous exposures to a patient's blood or body fluid, and provide appropriate follow-up care.
10. Prehospital providers should wear heavy-weight gloves, such as leather ones, during extrication procedures to prevent hand injury.
11. Use chemical disinfectants responsibly and according to manufacturers' guidelines for both equipment and disinfecting agent.
12. Establish vaccination programs for HBV.

or secretions on the outside of the gloves by unconscious habits such as wiping their eye, contaminating pens and placing them in their mouth, and so forth.

Some people think that only sterile medical-grade gloves can provide adequate protection. However, it is important to remember that glove strength, not sterility, and a proper fit of the gloves are the key factors for preventing occupational exposure. Sterile gloves should be worn only for procedures in which the patient needs protection from nosocomial infection. These include invasive and operative procedures. Sized nonsterile disposable gloves should be used for any other procedures or tasks in which finger dexterity is important to the task and that involve manipulation of blood samples, IV monitoring lines, or the performance of a variety of laboratory tasks. Midweight plastic or rubber gloves should be worn for cleaning procedures, and heavy gloves (e.g., leather) should be worn for prehospital extrication procedures or trash removal. Therefore, glove use must be task-specific, ensure the safety of both patients and personnel, and maximize availability.

Eye Protection

Selection of proper eye protection must facilitate safety as well as maintain vision. Visors or goggles are most appropriate for procedures that involve cutting or drilling bone, when using pulsatile-jet lavage irrigation systems, when controlling hemorrhage, and while performing vascular surgery or dental procedures. Plain glass or prescription eyeglasses may be suitable for areas of the hospital other than operative suites, emergency departments, invasive radiology suites, or labor and delivery suites.

Handling Sharp Medical Equipment

Although there is agreement that recapping needles is an unsafe practice, some procedures may require recapping a needle to remove it from a syringe of IV tubing. Examples include drawing a percutaneous arterial blood sample, exchanging needles when obtaining blood cultures, and connecting minidose intravenous medication. Therefore, all patient care procedures should be evaluated for safety; when appropriate, alternatives should be sought to minimize risks. In addition, technical proficiency should be monitored, and procedures identified as resulting in consistent needlestick injuries must be improved. The best mechanism to accomplish this is to document all needlestick misadventures. This allows monitoring of the acquisition of disease and the safety of patient care practices.

Handwashing

Handwashing is one the best methods of infection control in the health care environment. It facilitates protection of the patient from acquisition of nosocomial infection and of the provider from occupational acquisition of an infectious disease. Waterless hand cleaning products, especially in the prehospital setting, can be useful when there is no easy access to water sources and sinks. However, such products should not be considered a substitute for handwashing. If these products are used, the hands should be washed thoroughly as soon as patient care allows.

Failure to perform handwashing can be implicated in the acquisition of viral disease and may be an important factor in HBV transmission. While it is clear that HBV transmission occurs by direct percutaneous or mucocutaneous exposure in the workplace, a significant number of those infected disclaim any knowledge of previous misadventure.[439] Although the possibility that acquisition of infection could have resulted from an exposure in the community, the mode of transmission in most of these cases may be the unconscious habits of personnel and failure to comply with accepted practices of infection control. Health care professionals may easily contaminate their hands with a patient's blood or oral secretions when they fail to wear gloves while performing vascular punctures, inserting IV lines, intubating patients, and suctioning respiratory secretions. Blood and secretions can accumulate under their fingernails and around their cuticles.[440] If medical personnel then fail to adequately wash their hands, they can subsequently inoculate themselves with these body substances via unconscious habits such as using a pen and placing it in the mouth, biting fingernails and cuticles, picking up a syringe and pulling the needlecap with the teeth, scratching insect bites, rubbing abrasions, or eating and drinking in patient care areas.

Cleaning, Disinfection, and Sterilization

No other infection-control guidelines create more confusion than those outlining cleaning, disinfection, and sterilization recommendations. There is a misconception regarding basic terminology and the application of decontamination, disinfection, and sterilization techniques. It is not uncommon for these terms to be misused or inappropriately interchanged by supervisory personnel or those viewed as an authority on the subject. *Decontamination* is a process that removes disease-producing microorganisms and renders the object or the environment safe. It can be as simple as washing a surface with hot soapy water or rinsing an object under running water. *Disinfection* is a process that kills or destroys most disease-producing microorganisms except for the resistant bacterial endospores. The process can vary from low level (which kills vegetative bacteria, fungi, and lipid viruses) to high level (which kills vegetative bacteria, tubercle bacillus, some spores, and lipid and nonlipid viruses). *Sterilization* is a chemical or physical process that results in the total destruction of all microorganisms, including highly resistant bacterial spores.

Application of these procedures is determined by the specific use of the equipment or instrument.[441] Sterilization is required for *critical* items, defined as those which are inserted into or interface with the cardiovascular system, implanted into the body, or used for invasive surgical procedures. Disinfection is required for *semicritical* items, defined as those that touch or invade mucous membranes. High-level disinfection is recommended for respiratory equipment to ensure eradication of mycobacteria. All other items and surfaces are considered *noncritical* and require cleaning, decontamination, sanitizing, or low-level disinfection. To be effective, disinfection and sterilization procedures must be performed on precleaned surfaces.

Most disinfectants are inactivated in the presence of organic matter. Concentrations of disinfectants and sterilants must be exact and in accordance with label instructions. Spraying disinfectants on surfaces is ineffective and not recommended because neither appropriate concentrations of ingredients nor an even distribution of solution can be achieved.[442] Most disinfectants can be toxic to the personnel who use them. Anyone performing decontamination, disinfection, and sterilization procedures must wear appropriate protective attire. Toxicity of products can be assessed from a Materials Data Safety Sheet, which must be available from all disinfectant manufacturers. In addition, it is federal law[443] that all employees using disinfectants be educated about and protected against the hazards associated with the use of these chemicals.

No disinfectant is a panacea. Antimicrobial effects are variable, and a wide variety of chemical–inanimate object incompatibilities must be considered. Although there is variance among products, disinfectants and sterilants can corrode metal, leave ionic residues, stiffen and crack plastic, etch glass, stain plastic, short-circuit electronics, and dissolve adhesives and lens cement.[102] Therefore, selection of a sterilization or disinfection process must be in accordance with equipment manufacturers' recommendations. However, some manufacturers of hospital equipment may outline sterilization or disinfection procedures even though these practices may not be necessary.

All hospital-grade disinfectants, including glutaraldehydes, are solutions, and 97 to 99 per cent of ingredients may be unknown to the consumer. These are listed as "inert ingredients," but they are inert only with respect to their germicidal capabilities and not their ability to react with a variety of inanimate materials. For example, a 2% glutaraldehyde solution may contain a surfactant that, over time, can dissolve the lens cement of a fiberoptic endoscope. This ingredient is not listed on the label, and its presence may not be known unless a specific inquiry is made—an important question to ask, since not all glutaraldehyde solutions are manufactured with surfactants.

Many people assume that the Environmental Protection Agency (EPA) regulates the efficacy of disinfectants; however, this is not the case. Since 1979, the federal government has deregulated the chemical manufacturing industry with regard to disinfectants and antiseptics. The EPA no longer conducts efficacy testing of disinfectants,[444] and the FDA never completed its proposed guidelines for efficacy testing of antiseptics.[445]

Registration of a disinfectant requires the manufacturer to present data that support the labeling claims of its active ingredient; however, it does not require disclosure of the inert ingredients or the exact formulation of the solution.[446] Therefore, when evaluating the efficacy of a product, consumers must rely on the integrity of manufacturers and the laboratories they employ. Manufacturers may not have the technical data to support their claims. In a recent collaborative study of EPA-registered hospital disinfectants conducted among 18 laboratories routinely involved in efficacy testing of disinfectants, 20 per cent failed products for *Salmonella choleraesuis,* 37 per cent for *Staphylococcus aureus,* and 62 per cent for *Pseudomonas aeruginosa.*[447] In addition, four laboratories unknowingly tested their own product, and three of four failed their product with one or more of the test organisms. Ineffective disinfectants and antiseptics can have a major impact on the development of nosocomial infections, and selection of these products mandates meticulous scrutiny by the medical and nursing community. In 1988, Congress began to remedy this situation with House Bill 2355, the EPA Research Reauthorization Act[445]; however, the legislation was never finalized.

A major disinfectant dilemma of recent years has centered on the eradication of HIV and HBV in the environment. Early in the AIDS epidemic, most infection guidelines recommended the use of household bleach in 1:10 dilution for environmental cleaning. This recommendation was largely derived from those developed in the 1970s for HBV and the fact that bleach is inexpensive and widely available to the medical and general community. However, as our knowledge of HIV has advanced, no environmental mechanisms of HIV infection have been documented, and a variety of disinfectants have been proved to be effective against this virus.[448, 449] Subsequently, the CDC changed its recommendation to detergent disinfectants for environmental cleaning.[396] Therefore, standard recommendations for cleaning, disinfection, and sterilization are adequate measures to control this virus in health care settings.

HBV has often been considered as some sort of "super virus" because of its ability to survive under a variety of environmental conditions.[450] Because HBV is not easily adaptable to tissue-culture techniques in the laboratory, kinetic studies for its inactivation by physical and chemical agents were lacking, and many recommendations were predicated on the basis of empirical analysis of known biocidal activity of a particular treatment. In the mid-1970s, the CDC undertook intensive studies using radioimmunoassay (RIA) techniques for the detection of HBsAg and infectivity studies with chimpanzees to establish practical guidelines for environmental control of HBV in health care settings.[451] These studies demonstrated that undiluted serum from HBsAg carriers could be inactivated by a 1:10 dilution of household bleach in 30 minutes. Household bleach is 5.25% hypochlorite, and a 1:10 dilution gives 5000 ppm of active ingredients. However, even at much smaller concentrations (500–1000 ppm), bleach solutions still can be corrosive to metals.

During this series of studies, it also was demonstrated that HBsAg could be eliminated by the mechanical action of cloths soaked in water or moistened with hemolytic detergents used on smooth, hard surfaces such as asbestos floor tile; coarse-textured, nonabsorbent, rubber foam–backed upholstery material; or plastic instrument knobs. This was taken as reasonable proof of HBV eradication, since the ratio of HBV to HBsAg particles in serum is 1 to greater than 2000, and reduction of HBsAg below a detectable level implies an equally large reduction in the infective potential of the contamination. Therefore, detergent disinfectants were recommended for environmental cleaning even when the area was visibly contaminated with the blood or feces of a patient with hepatitis.[452] However, bleach solutions were still recommended for surfaces such as curled or grooved instrument knobs that could not be cleaned easily. Environmental disinfection with bleach solutions was recommended for hemodialysis units to reduce the nosocomial transmission of HBV. In this setting, it was theorized that critical and semicritical items used during dialysis could be contaminated by environmental HBV even if the person wore gloves.[453]

Since these studies, inactivation of HBV has been demonstrated by other intermediate- to high-level disinfectant chemicals.[454, 455] Most important, it has been shown that 70% isopropyl alcohol and 2% glutaraldehyde solutions can inactivate HBV in dried human plasma when exposed to these chemicals for 10 minutes at 20°C. From these chimpanzee infectivity models it was concluded that the resistance of HBV to disinfectant chemicals is not as extreme as once thought and that these disinfectants could be used on HBV contamination with a margin of safety.

Although HBV may survive in the environment, this does not mean that the modes of transmission are different. A mucocutaneous or percutaneous exposure to the virus is still necessary to cause disease. In addition, environmental survival does not mean that the virus is any less susceptible to chemical or physical inactivation. Therefore, the best means of protection is to wear gloves while performing cleaning, decontamination, and disinfection procedures and to meticulously clean the environment. Bleach must be used with caution because of its corrosive capabilities. Alternative methods of disinfection should be used when bleach is incompatible with the material being disinfected.

Prehospital Phase

Prehospital emergency medical service (EMS) providers deal with unique and complex infection-control issues. Nowhere within the trauma cycle is the application of infection-control guidelines a greater challenge. It is important for nurses working in emergency services, trauma, and infection control to understand the unique issues of infection control as it relates to EMS. It may well be the knowledge of such nurses that forms the basis for the infection-control guidelines and educational programs within a specific EMS system.

At the time of initial resuscitation of a patient, the presence of blood-borne viruses is generally unknown. Emergency care providers usually do not have knowledge of the patient's medical history or life-style. This information may never be obtained if the patient expires at the accident scene or shortly after admission or if the patient sustained an injury or complication of disease that results in permanent cognitive impairment. In most cases, these risks may never be subsequently determined by the receiving hospital, since knowledge of a "carrier state" of disease is not pertinent to the underlying condition necessitating admission. In addition, prehospital providers can be in situations where the blood of more than one patient contaminates the same environment, and it may be difficult or impossible to determine which blood came from which patient. To reiterate, any patient's blood or body fluids must be considered infectious. This means that appropriate protective attire must be worn. Any misadventures, such as needle sticks or cuts, causing percutaneous or mucocutaneous exposure should be treated at this time, and the provider should be reminded to report these exposures and receive follow-up care according to the individual EMS system's policy.

The unique nature of prehospital EMS care presents unusual situations that are associated with a high risk of infection. These can include crawling through blood-soaked environments strewn with sharp objects such as glass or twisted metal and performing complicated extrication procedures that could injure the provider. The physical environment can be unstable and adverse, and the EMS provider's life itself may be in jeopardy. There are no truly aseptic conditions in the field. EMS must often be performed under conditions of inclement weather, within very confined spaces, with limited supplies and equipment, and without adequate lighting or water sources. These situations help underscore the importance of wearing appropriate protective attire.

The most important factor in protecting EMS providers from acquiring a blood-borne infection is to carefully consider the different aspects of occupational infection control as previously described and adjust them according to the prehospital conditions. Guidelines for the prevention of blood-borne diseases for the prehospital and in-hospital setting are outlined in Table 12–11. The use of protective attire is essential for first responders to situations involving open injuries, such as gunshot and stab wounds, high-speed vehicular accidents, and child delivery. Therefore, if the chance of handling blood or body fluids is high (e.g., CPR, IV insertions, trauma, child delivery, surgical procedures), the provider should put on protective attire before beginning patient care. It is important to remember that time is a crucial factor in determining the patient's ultimate survival. Precious minutes can be lost if prehospital EMS providers arrive at the scene not wearing the appropriate protective attire and are unprepared for the resuscitation. For most situations, the possibility of the patient bleeding or requiring emergent medical care can be determined in advance.

Although there have been attempts to develop prehospital infection-control programs, many recommendations are impractical and unnecessary and can have a negative impact on the delivery of EMS.[456–458] Prehospital care providers must be protected from both biological and physical hazards. Heavy-duty hand protection such as leather gloves or gauntlets should be available for extrication procedures in order to prevent hand injury. Since water sources are unavailable, handwashing should be performed as soon as patient care allows once the providers have arrived at the hospital. Gowns are not recommended because they can be dangerous in rescue operations, be cumbersome, and are generally inadequate in the field. Turnout coats may offer a better alternative; however, blood should not be removed with bleach, since bleach can eliminate the fire-retardant properties of these coats.[459]

It is unnecessary to clean environmental splashes of blood with bleach solutions within EMS transport vehicles.[396] The most important point is to physically remove blood and organic matter. Bleach can corrode metal, damage equipment, and short-circuit electronics. Chemical disinfectants must be used with extreme caution.[102] Many germicidal solutions used within the hospital can have corrosive effects on the equipment or can leave strong ionic residues that can result in dysfunction of electrical equipment in transport vehicles. The use of disinfectants such as sprays or fogs has long been established as an ineffective means of infection control.[442] The vehicles should be kept clean. The practice of airing a vehicle for 1 to 2 hours following the transport of an infected patient is not necessary. This precaution is based on ritual and can manifest liability to the EMS system. Finally, the cleaning and disinfection of any equipment must be efficient, cost-effective, and in accordance with the disinfectant and equipment manufacturers' recommendations; they also must facilitate availability of the equipment in the field. A good example is the cleaning and decontamination of pneumatic antishock garments (PASGs). It is unnecessary, expensive, and impractical to utilize ethylene oxide. PASGs can withstand cleaning with a wide variety of chemical agents and temperatures.

Specific guidelines for cleaning and decontamination of PASGs are as follows:[460] The outer fabric of PASGs is made of nylon pack cloth with Scotchgard, and it will withstand cleaning with laundry detergents, hydrogen peroxide, 1:10 dilutions of chlorine bleach, and temperatures up to 200°F. PASGs can be washed in a standard washing machine using the "hot water" setting and one cup of bleach. Before placing them in the washing machine, be certain the air valves are closed. It is not necessary to remove the bladders. If a washing machine is not available, manual cleaning is acceptable, but all blood and organic matters must be removed. After washing, the fabric may be air dried or placed in a hot-air dryer. It is not advisable to use an ultrasonic washer, since soil and blood may only be loosened and not completely removed. If thorough cleaning cannot be performed when use of the trousers is initially discontinued, blood should be wiped off before it dries. Gloves should be worn throughout the cleaning procedure.

There is no nationwide standard system for the operation of EMS systems.[461] Therefore, systems vary from state to state and can include many different combinations of governmental, private, and volunteer personnel providing services to the various communities. Sources of revenue and resources are variable, as are mechanisms and requirements for provider and employee health programs. Educational and training programs are different. EMS providers often have no medical or nursing backgrounds, and their levels of basic education can range from incomplete secondary education to postdoctoral degrees. Education in infection is often too technical or incomplete, with access to knowledgeable infection-control practitioners with expertise in EMS limited. These factors must be kept in mind when developing infection-control guidelines for prehospital care.

The overall fear and anxiety generated by the AIDS epidemic are having a negative impact on the quality of emergency care.[461] The volunteers of the 27,000 volunteer fire companies in the United States are not bound to perform these duties, and the pool of personnel, both career and volunteer, is decreasing. In addition, many EMS systems have the option of providing care only to those they choose to treat, which can lead to patient discrimination and a decrease in the overall quality of EMS. Therefore, formulation of infection-control guidelines must be based on a clear understanding of a specific EMS system, i.e., how the system works, the kind of care provided, and the limitation of personnel, supplies, and financing. In addition, notification of prehospital care providers of the diagnosis of an infectious disease in persons transported by them is a federal law.[410]

INFECTION-CONTROL PROGRAM IN A TRAUMA UNIT

Infection control throughout the trauma cycle is a multifactorial problem. Trauma patients can have injuries that involve every organ system, the severity of injuries can be highly varied, and few patients seem to have exactly the same injuries. The infection risks as well as the reservoir of microorganisms are continually changing. Therefore, infection-control guidelines for patient care must be continually adjusted as the patient progresses through the trauma cycle. Infection-control guidelines must offer dual protection; that is, both the patients and staff must be protected from infection hazards. The overall infection-control program must be monitored constantly. The incidence and prevalence of the infections, the infection rates, the safety and efficacy of patient care practices, the colonization and antibiotic susceptibility patterns of the organisms, antibiotic utilization, and acquisition of infection among the staff must be prospectively and comprehensively evaluated on a daily, monthly, and yearly basis. All the members of the trauma team—physicians, nurses, allied health professionals, and ancillary personnel—must be adequately educated about infection-control principles and guidelines to ensure consistency of patient care and compliance with control measures. Therefore, the primary objectives of the infection-control program are (1) to identify the infection risks, (2) to determine the reservoirs of the microorganisms, (3) to provide a dual protection of both patients and staff, (4) to have comprehensive and prospective surveillance, (5) to determine the efficacy and cost-effectiveness of patient care practices, and (6) to provide adequate education to all staff.

Dress Codes

Recommendations for dress codes must address both the occupational protection of personnel and the protection of patients from nosocomial infection. Dress codes for preventing nosocomial infection have been a controversial issue in intensive care units and emergency departments.[462, 463] Although the use of scrub clothes and cover gowns is generally thought not to be effective for reducing nosocomial infection risks in these areas, there may still be benefits. The requirement for wearing scrub clothes can serve to regulate traffic of personnel and serve as a physical reminder to the personnel that they are caring for a special patient population. Additionally, some workers speculate that the wearing of scrub attire may help to protect the employees' health, especially the nursing staff, since they are frequently splattered with the patient's blood, secretions, excretions, and drainage fluids during the administration of care. On the other hand, some people believe that if nursing personnel wore white uniforms in the intensive care unit and emergency room, they would be more careful when they deliver care and this would reduce the incidences of nurses being contaminated with the patient's body fluids, secretions, and excretions.

The efficacy of wearing hats is not known. Although hair can be a reservoir for many microorganisms,[464, 465] the risk to the patient results when personnel unconsciously handle their hair and then fail to wash their hands prior to patient contact. The AORN standards require that all scalp and facial hair be covered when performing invasive procedures. This is a reasonable infection-control guideline. The efficacy of dress codes must be evaluated carefully in all phases of the trauma cycle.

One approach that may be beneficial in the prevention of nosocomial infection is the use of a procedural dress code. For example, insertion of a Swan-Ganz catheter should require sterile gowns, hats covering all hair, masks, and sterile gloves, whereas obtaining blood cultures would require sterile gloves only. In other words, each procedure would be assigned a specific dress code category.[93] For example:

Category I: Sterile gown, hat, mask, and sterile gloves
Category II: Clean scrub attire or cover gown, hat, mask, and sterile gloves
Category III: Hat, mask, and sterile gloves
Category IV: Sterile gloves only
Category V: Good handwashing

These guidelines may then require further refinement to comply with OSHA regulations.

New Product Evaluation

Another important aspect of infection control in a trauma center is new product evaluation. It is important to remember that new or innovative is not necessarily better and that the use of a new product in or on a patient requires special evaluation. The use and effectiveness of hospital devices have not been as carefully regulated as drugs and medications. Premarket evaluation of medical devices has only been required by the federal government since 1976.[466] Therefore, clinical trials demonstrating the utility and safety of a product may not be available, and the benefits to patient care may only be speculative. Second, apparent cost benefits may be obscure. For example, a change to a less expensive arterial catheter may appear to reduce cost. However, if the catheter cannot be inserted easily via percutaneous placement, a cutdown procedure may be necessary, and both cost and infection risk are substantially increased. Similarly, changes in procedure or policy should be examined carefully. Therefore, an on-going infection-surveillance baseline is mandatory for judicious decisions regarding changes in product and procedural policy.

Design of the Trauma Center

The design of a trauma center should provide an environment that minimizes infection hazards. The primary objective is to reduce mechanisms of cross-infection among the patients. An important factor is the separation of patients by either physical barriers or spatial arrangements. An effective design involves the use of individual patient cubicles. However, no matter how the patients are separated, each bed should have adequate space around it to contain all anticipated patient care equipment and still provide adequate access for health care workers.[467]

The organization of supplies and equipment should maximize efficiency. Patient care supplies must be adequate, but areas should not be overstocked. Supplies must be continually checked to ensure the sterility of the products (i.e., integrity of packaging, expiration dates, etc.). This can be a time-consuming process and may not be fully accomplished when the patient census is high and/or staffing is low. Therefore, overstocking can risk the use of nonsterile supplies and jeopardize patient safety. The arrangement must allow for rapid access during emergency situations as well as promote infection-control measures. Whenever possible, supplies and equipment should not be shared among patients. In addition, adequate space should be allocated for the proper cleaning and maintenance of equipment. Cross-contamination from dirty supplies to clean supplies must be avoided.

Because failure to comply with handwashing recommendations has been identified as the major cause of cross-contamination among patients,[75, 82] it is essential that sinks be readily available for this purpose. Government standards recommend that the ratio of beds to sinks be no more than 6:1 in a multibed unit.[467] Ideally, there should be a sink next to every patient bed, and these sinks should operate via foot pedal or knee mechanisms. Since sinks can become a reservoir for gram-negative organisms,[56, 345] special attention must be given to the proper maintenance of sinks, and aerators on faucets should be removed.

Flowers and flower water have been identified as a source of antibiotic-resistant microorganisms.[469, 470] Although there has never been an outbreak associated with the presence of flowers in a hospital setting, it is prudent to establish guidelines for the presence or handling of flowers in the intensive care unit[470] or to restrict cut flowers in the intensive care unit.

SUMMARY

Infection control throughout the trauma cycle is a challenging problem. Infection will always be a complication as long as the events of trauma produce the same kinds of devastating injuries and invasive therapy is necessary to resuscitate and support the patients. No matter the etiological factor, any infection can increase morbidity, prolong hospitalization, increase the cost of care, and jeopardize the final outcome. Therefore, every effort must be undertaken to prevent and minimize the infection risks.

Despite all the technological advances of medicine, the early lessons of Semmelweis and Lister[346] on the importance of handwashing, meticulous aseptic technique, and careful attention to and awareness of infection threats continue to be the most effective measures of preventing cross-contamination and infection in trauma patients. Valuable lessons of nosocomial infection control have been learned from trauma patients that can be applied to any critically ill population whose survival is dependent on mechanical and invasive support devices.

REFERENCES

1. Allgower M, Durig M, Wolff G: Infection and trauma. Surg Clin North Am 60:133–144, 1980.
2. Youmans GB: The Biological and Clinical Basis of Infectious Diseases. Philadelphia, WB Saunders Co., 1979, pp 9–18.
3. Fry DE: Infection in the trauma patient: The major deterrent to good recovery. Heart Lung 7:257–261, 1978.
4. Meakins JL, Wicklund B, Forse RA, et al: The surgical intensive care unit: Current concepts in infection. Surg Clin North Am 60:117–144, 1980.
5. Miller ES, Miller CL, Trunkey D: The immune consequences of trauma. Surg Clin North Am 62(1):162–181, 1982.
6. Michaels J, Moray V, Castermans A: A ten-year retrospective study of sepsis in severely burned patients treated with and

without silver sulfadiazinate. Scand J Plast Reconstr Surg 13(1):85–87, 1979.

7. Dobke M, Sztaba-Kania M: The occurrence of immune complexes in patients with thermal injuries. In Ninnemann JL (ed): Traumatic Injury, Infection, and Other Immunologic Sequelae. Baltimore, University Park Press, 1983, pp 153–161.
8. Bjornson AB, Altemeier WA, Bjornson HS, et al: Host defense against opportunist microorganisms following trauma: I. Studies to determine the association between changes in humoral components of host defenses and septicemia in burned patients. Ann Surg 188:93–101, 1978.
9. Howard RJ: Effect of burn injury, mechanical trauma, and operation on immune defenses. Surg Clin North Am 59:199–211, 1979.
10. Bauer AR, McNeil C, Trentelman E, et al: The depression of T lymphocytes after trauma. Am J Surg 136:674–680, 1978.
11. Craddock CG: Corticosteroid-induced lymphopenia, immunosuppression, and body defense. Ann Intern Med 88:564–566, 1978.
12. Eickhoff TC: Infections in immunosuppressed patients. Drug Ther November:19–29, 1972.
13. Caplan ES, Hoyt NJ, Cowley RA: Changing patterns of nosocomial infections in severely traumatized patients. Am Surg 39:204–210, 1979.
14. Caplan ES, Hoyt NJ: Infection surveillance and control in the severely traumatized patient. Am J Med 70:638–640, 1981.
15. Hoyt NJ, Caplan ES: Identification and prevention of infections in the critically ill trauma population. Crit Care Q 6:17–24, 1983.
16. Caplan ES, Hoyt NJ: Identification and treatment of infection in multiply traumatized patients. Am J Med 79(A):68–76, 1985.
17. Caplan ES, Joshi M, Hoyt NJ, et al: Changing patterns of infection and infection-related mortality in 10,308 multiply traumatized patients over a seven-year period. Presented before the American Association for the Surgery of Trauma, Honolulu, Hawaii, September 17, 1986.
18. Tramont EC: General or nonspecific host defense mechanisms. In Mandel GL, Douglas RG, Bennett JE (eds): Principles and Practice of Infectious Diseases, vol 1. New York, Wiley, 1979, pp 13–22.
19. Hand WL, Caney JR, Hughes CG: Antibacterial mechanisms of the lower respiratory tract: I. Immunoglobulin synthesis and secretion. J Clin Invest 53:354–362, 1974.
20. Reynolds HY, Thompson RE: Pulmonary host defenses: I. Analysis of protein and lipids in bronchial secretion and antibody responses after vaccination with *Pseudomonas aeruginosa.* J Immunol 111:358–368, 1973.
21. Reynolds HY, Thompson RE: Pulmonary host defenses: II. Interactions of respiratory antibodies with *Pseudomonas aeruginosa* and alveolar macrophages. J Immunol 111:369–380, 1973.
22. Donowitz LG, Page C, Mileur BL, et al: Alteration of normal gastric flora in critical care patients receiving antacid and cimetidine therapy. Infect Control 7:23–26, 1986.
23. Murray HS, Strottman MP, Cooke AR: Effects of several drugs on gastric potential difference in man. Br Med J 1:19–21, 1974.
24. Kaye D: Host defense mechanisms in the urinary tract. Urol Clin North Am 2:407–422, 1975.
25. Llende M, Santiago-Delphin EA, Lavergne J: Immunobiological consequences of splenectomy: A review. J Surg Res 40:85–94, 1986.
26. Lkhite VV: Immunologic impairment and susceptibility to infection after splenectomy. JAMA 236:1476–1477, 1976.
27. Schumacher MJ: Serum immunoglobulin and transferrin levels after childhood splenectomy. Arch Dis Child 45:114–117, 1979.
28. Claret I, Morales L, Montaner A: Immunologic studies in the postsplenectomy syndrome. J Pediatr Surg 10:59–64, 1975.
29. Sullivan JL, Ochs HD, Schiffman G, et al: Immune response after splenectomy. Lancet 1:178, 1978.
30. Najjar VA, Nishiokak K: "Tuftsin," a physiological phagocytosis stimulating peptide. Nature 228:672–673, 1970.
31. Carlisle HN, Saslow S: Properdin levels in splenectomized patients. Proc Soc Exp Biol Med 102:150–155, 1959.
32. Polhill RB, Johnson RB: Diminished alternative complement pathway after splenectomy. Pediatr Res 9:333–336, 1973.
33. Constantopoulos A, Najjar A, Wish JB: Defective phagocytosis due to tuftsin deficiency in splenectomized patients. Am J Dis Child 125:663–665, 1973.
34. Krivit W, Giebink GD, Leonard A: Overwhelming postsplenectomy infection. Surg Clin North Am 59(2):223–233, 1979.
35. Malangoni MA, Dawes LG, Droege EA, et al: Splenic phagocytic function after partial splenectomy and splenic autotransplantation. Arch Surg 120:275–278, 1975.
36. Scher KS, Scott-Conner C, Jones CW, et al: Methods of splenic preservation and their effect on clearance of pneumococcal bacteremia. Ann Surg 202:595–599, 1985.
37. Sherman R: Perspective in management of trauma to the spleen: 1979 presidential address, American Association for the Surgery of Trauma. J Trauma 20:1–13, 1980.
38. Chaikof EL, McCabe CJ: Fatal overwhelming postsplenectomy infection. Am J Surg 149:534–539, 1985.
39. Singer DB: Postsplenectomy sepsis. In Rosenberg HS, Bolande RP (eds): Perspectives in Pediatric Pathology, vol 1. Chicago, Year Book Medical Publishers, 1973, pp 285–311.
40. MMWR 30(33):410–412, 417–419, 1981.
41. Torres J, Bisno AL: Hyposplenism and pneumococcemia: Visualization of *Diplococcus pneumoniae* in peripheral blood smear. Am J Med 55:851–855, 1973.
42. Caplan ES, Boltansky H, Synder MJ, et al: Response of traumatized splenectomized patients to immediate vaccination with polyvalent pneumococcal vaccine. J Trauma 23:801–805, 1983.
43. Youmans GB: The Biological and Clinical Basis of Infectious Diseases. Philadelphia, WB Saunders Co, 1979, pp 97–112.
44. Mims C: The Pathogenesis of Infectious Disease. Orlando, FL, Academic Press, 1987, pp 55–62.
45. Schumer W: General treatment of septic shock. In Cowley RA, Trump BF (eds): Pathophysiology of Shock, Anoxia, and Ischemia. Baltimore, Williams & Wilkins, 1982, pp 479–482.
46. Emanuelsen SD: Shock. In Handbook of Critical Care Nursing. New York, Wiley, 1986, pp 417–431.
47. Muller-Eberhand HJ: The serum complement system. In Miescher PA, Muller-Eberhand HJ (eds): Textbook of Immunopathology. New York, Grune & Stratton, 1976, pp 45–73.
48. Schumer W: Septic shock. JAMA 242:1906, 1979.
49. McQuillen KA, Wiles CE: Initial management of traumatic shock. In Cardona V, Hurn PD, Mason P, et al (eds): Trauma Nursing: From Resuscitation to Rehabilitation. Philadelphia, WB Saunders Co, 1988, pp 160–193.
50. Attar S, Kirby WH, Masaitis C, et al: Coagulation changes in clinical shock: I. Effect of hemorraghic shock on clotting times in humans. Ann Surg 614:34, 1966.
51. Hoyt NJ: Preventing septic shock: Infection control in the intensive care unit. Crit Care Nurs Clin North Am 2(2):287–297, 1990.
52. Crowther CL, Hoyt NJ: Septic shock in the trauma patient. In Welton RH, Shane KA (eds): Case Studies in Trauma Nursing. Baltimore, Williams & Wilkins, 1990, pp 215–222.
53. Stillwell M, Caplan ES: The septic multiple-trauma patient. Crit Care Clin 4:345–373, 1988.
54. Fuenfer MM, Olson GE, Polk HC: Effects of various corticosteroids upon the phagocytic bactericidal activity of neutrophils. Surgery 78:27–33, 1975.
55. Heck E, Edgar M, Hunt J, et al: A comparison of leukocyte function and burn mortality. J Trauma 20:75, 1980.
56. Moderazo E, Albano S, Woronick C, et al: Polymorphonuclear leukocyte migration abnormalities and their significance in seriously traumatized patients. Ann Surg 198:736, 1983.
57. Palder S, O'Mahoney J, Rodrick M, et al: Alteration of polymorphonuclear leukocyte function in the trauma patient. J Trauma 23:655, 1983.
58. Polk H, Wellhausen S, Regan M, et al: A systematic study of host defense processes in badly injured patients. Ann Surg 104:282, 1986.

59. Bauer AR, McNeil C, Trentelman E, et al: The depression of T lymphocytes after trauma. Am J Surg 136:674–680, 1976.
60. Kane R, Munster A, Birmingham W, et al: Suppressor cell activity after major injury: Indirect and direct functional assays. J Trauma 22:770, 1982.
61. Salo M, Merikanto J, Eskela J, et al: Impaired lymphocyte transformation after accidental trauma. Acta Chir Scand 145:367, 1979.
62. Meakins J, Pietsch J, Rubenick O, et al: Delayed hypersensitivity: Indicator of acquired failure of host defenses in sepsis and trauma. Ann Surg 186:241, 1977.
63. Scovill W, Saba T, Kaplan J, et al: Disturbances in circulating opsonic activity in man after operative and blunt trauma. J Surg Res 22:709, 1979.
64. Alexander J, Stinnett J, Ogle C, et al: A comparison of immunologic profiles and their influence on bacteremia in surgical patients with high risk of infections. Surgery 86:94, 1979.
65. Dinarello CA, Wolff SM: Pathogenesis of fever in man. N Engl J Med 298:607–611, 1978.
66. Dinarello CA: Endogenous pyrogens. In Lipton JM (ed): Fever. New York, Raven Press, 1979, pp 1–10.
67. Bodel P: Studies on the mechanism of endogenous pyrogen production: II. Role of cell products in the regulation of pyrogen release from blood leukocytes. Infect Immun 10:451–457, 1974.
68. Bodel P, Atkins E: Release of endogenous pyrogen by human monocytes. N Engl J Med 276:1002–1008, 1967.
69. Bennett IL, Beeson PB: Studies on the pathogenesis of fever: II. Characteristics of fever-producing substance from polymorphonuclear leukocytes and from sterile exudates. J Exp Med 98:493–508, 1953.
70. Dinarello CA, Goldin NP, Wolff SM: Demonstration and characterization of two distinct human leukocyte pyrogens. J Exp Med 139:1369–1374, 1974.
71. Hellon RF: Monoamines, pyrogens, and cations: Their actions on central control of body temperature. Pharmacol Rev 26:289–321, 1975.
72. Altmeier WA, Culbertson WR: Surgical infections. In Moyer C, et al (eds): Surgery, Principles and Practice, 3rd ed. Philadelphia, JB Lippincott, 1965.
73. Mackowiak PA: The normal microbial flora. N Engl J Med 307:83–93, 1982.
74. Petras GY, Bognar SZ: Origin and spread of *Pseudomonas aeruginosa, Proteus,* and *Klebsiella* during twenty years in an infectious disease hospital. Acta Microbiol Acad Sci Hung 28:367–380, 1981.
75. Salzman TC, Clark JJ, Klenam L, et al: Hand contamination of personnel as a mechanism for cross-infection with antibiotic-resistant *Escherichia coli* and *Klebsiella-Aerobacter.* Antimicrob Agents Chemother 97:28–46, 1967.
76. Teres D, Schweers P, Bushnell LS, et al: Sources of *Pseudomonas aeruginosa* infections in a respiratory-surgical intensive therapy unit. Lancet 1:415–417, 1973.
77. Kallenbach I, Dusheiko J, Block CS, et al: Aspergillus pneumonia: A cluster of 4 cases in an intensive care unit. S Afr Med J 52:919–923, 1977.
78. Kirchhoff LV, Sheagren JN: Epidemiology and clinical significance of blood cultures positive for coagulase-negative staphylococcus. Infect Control 6:479–486, 1985.
79. Klein JJ, Watanakunakorn C: Hospital-acquired fungemia. Am J Med 76:51–58, 1979.
80. Walsh TJ, Bustamente C, Vlahov D, et al: Candidal suppurative peripheral thrombophlebitis: Recognition, prevention, and management. Infect Control 7:16–22, 1986.
81. Ponce de Leon S, Wenzel RP: Hospital-acquired bloodstream infections with *Staphylococcus epidermidis.* Am J Med 77:639–644, 1984.
82. Steere AC, Mallison GF: Handwashing practices for the prevention of nosocomial infections. Ann Intern Med 83:683–689, 1975.
83. Dascher FD: The transmission of infections in hospitals by staff carriers, methods of prevention and control (editorial review). Infect Control 6:97–99, 1985.
84. Haley RW, Bregman DA: The role of understaffing and overcrowding in recurrent outbreaks of staphylococcal infection in a neonatal special-care unit. J Infect Dis 145:875–885, 1982.
85. Russell B, Ehrenkranz NJ, Hyams PJ, et al: An outbreak of *Staphylococcus aureus* surgical wound infections associated with excess overtime employment of operating room personnel. J Infect Control 11:63–67, 1983.
86. McLane C, Chenelly S, Sylwestrak ML, et al: A nursing practice problem: Failure to observe aseptic technique. Am J Infect Control 11:178–182, 1983.
87. Caplan ES, Hoyt NJ: Infection control for adult and neonatal intensive care patients. In Gurevich I, et al (eds): Practical Aspects of Infection Control. New York, Praeger Publishers, 1984, pp 130–155.
88. Hoyt NJ: Infection control in trauma care. In Cardona V (ed): Trauma Nursing. Oradell, NJ, Medical Economics Books, 1985, pp 173–194.
89. Britt MR, Schleupner CJ, Matsumiya S: Severity of underlying disease as a predictor of nosocomial infection: Utility in the control of nosocomial infection. JAMA 239:1047–1051, 1978.
90. Hemming VG, Overall JC Jr, Britt MR, et al: Nosocomial infections in a newborn intensive care unit: Results of forty-one months of surveillance. N Eng J Med 294:1310–1318, 1976.
91. Cluff LE: Medical determinants of nosocomial infections. In Proceedings of the International Conference on Nosocomial Infections, August 3–6, 1970. Chicago, American Hospital Association, 1970, pp 164–168.
92. Schmipff SC: Infections in the compromised host. In Mandell GL, Douglas RG Jr, Bennett JE (eds): Principles and Practice of Infectious Diseases. New York, Wiley, 1979, pp 2257–2262.
93. Pietsch JB, Meakins JL: Predicting infections in surgical patients. Surg Clin North Am 59(2):185–198, 1979.
94. Murray HS, Strottman MP, Cooke AR: Effects of several drugs on gastric potential difference in man. Br Med J 1:19–21, 1974.
95. Moellering RC Jr: Principles of anti-infective therapy. In Mandell GL, Douglas RG Jr, Bennett JE (eds): Principles and Practice of Infectious Diseases. New York, Wiley, 1979, pp 201–217.
96. Fuenfer MM, Olson GE, Polk HC: Effect of various corticosteroids upon the phagocytic bactericidal activity of neutrophils. Surgery 78:27–33, 1975.
97. MacKercher PA, Ivey KJ, Baskin WN, et al: Protective effect of cimetidine on aspirin-induced gastric muscosal damage. Ann Intern Med 87:697–679, 1977.
98. Eickhoff TC. Nosocomial infections. J Epidemiol 101:93–97, 1975.
99. Gross PA, Neu HC, Aswapokee N, et al: Deaths from nosocomial infections: Experience in a community hospital. Am J Med 68:219–223, 1980.
100. Leviten DL, Shulman ST: Multiple nosocomial infections: A risk of modern intensive care. Clin Pediatr 19:205–209, 1980.
101. Maki DG: Risk factors for nosocomial infection in intensive care: "Devices vs. nature" and goals for the next decade. Arch Intern Med 149:30–33, 1989.
102. Block SS (ed): Disinfection, Sterilization and Preservation, 3rd ed. Philadelphia, Lea & Febiger, 1983, pp 183–196, 225–250, 469–504.
103. Boyd R, Burke J, Cloton T: A double blind clinical trial of prophylactic antibiotics in hip fractures. J Bone Joint Surg 58A:1251–1254, 1973.
104. Charnley J: Clean air in the operating room. Clev Clin Q 40:99–101, 1973.
105. Edlich RF, Smith QT, Edgerton MT: Resistance of the surgical wound to antimicrobial prophylaxis and its mechanism of development. Am J Surg 126:583–591, 1973.
106. Haines SJ: Systemic antibiotic prophylaxis in neurological surgery. Neurosurgery 6:355–356, 1980.
107. O'Riordan C, Adler J, Banks H, et al: Wound infections on an orthopedic service—A prospective study. Am J Epidemiol 95:442–445, 1972.
108. Patzakis MUJ, Harvey JP, Ivler D: The role of antibiotics in the management of open fractures. J Bone Joint Surg 56A:532–541, 1974.

109. Burke JF: The effective period of preventive antibiotic action in experimental incisions and dermal lesions. Surgery 50:161–168, 1961.
110. Caplan ES, Hoyt NJ, Burgess A, Brumback R: "Cefonicid vs. cefamandole" as prophylaxis against infections in polytrauma patients. Presented before the 14th International Congress on Chemotherapy, Kyoto, Japan, June 26, 1985.
111. Gustilio RB, Mendoza RM, Williams DN: Problems in the management of type III (severe) open fracture: A new classification of type III open fractures. J Trauma 24(8):742–746, 1984.
112. Oreskovich MR, Dellinger EP, Lennard ES, et al: Duration of preventive antibiotic administration for penetrating trauma. Arch Surg 117:200–205, 1982.
113. Caplan ES, Hoyt NJ: Nosocomial CNS infections. In Proceedings National Association for Practitioners in Infection Control, Atlanta, GA, June 1981.
114. Dunham CM, Cowley RA (eds): Infection Control. In Shock Trauma/Critical Care Manual: Initial Assessment and Management. Baltimore, University Park Press, 1982, pp 401–430.
115. Eickhoff TC: Antibiotics and nosocomial infections. In Bennet JV, Brachman PS (eds): Hospital Infections. Boston, Little, Brown, 1979, pp 195–222.
116. Neu HC: Antibiotic inactivating enzymes and bacterial resistance. In Lorian V (ed): Antibiotics in Laboratory Medicine. Baltimore, Williams & Wilkins, 1980.
117. Murray BE, Mollering RC Jr: Patterns and mechanisms of antibiotic resistance. Med Clin North Am 62:899–923, 1978.
118. Finland M: Emergence of antibiotic resistance in hospitals, 1935–1975. Rev Infect Dis 1:4–21, 1979.
119. Bulger RJE, Larson E, Sherris JC: Decreased incidences of resistance to antimicrobial agents among *Escherichia coli* and the *Klebsiella-Enterobacter*: Observations in a University hospital over a 10 year period. Ann Intern Med 72:65–69, 1970.
120. DeChamps C, Sauvant MP, Sirot D, et al: Prospective survey of colonization and infection caused by expanded-spectrum beta-lactamase–producing members of the family Enterobacteriaceae in an intensive care unit. J Clin Microbiol 27:2887–2890, 1989.
121. Weinstein RA, Nathan C, Gruensfelder R, et al: Endemic aminoglycoside resistance in gram-negative bacilli: Epidemiology and mechanisms. J Infect Dis 141:338–345, 1980.
122. Roberts NJ, Douglas RG: Gentamicin use and *Pseudomonas* and *Serratia* resistance: Effect of a surgical prophylaxis regimen. Antimicrob Agents Chemother 13:214–230, 1978.
123. Morse LJ, Williams HL, Grenn FP, et al: Septicemia due to *Klebsiella pneumoniae* originating from a hand cream dispenser. N Engl J Med 279:472–474, 1967.
124. Mouton RP, Glerum JH, Van Loenen AC: Relationship between antibiotic consumption and frequency of antibiotic resistance of four pathogens—A seven-year survey. J Antimicrob Chemother 2:9–16, 1976.
125. Crossley K, Landesman B, Zaske D: An outbreak of infections caused by strains of *Staphylococcus aureus* resistant to methicillin and aminoglycosides: II. Epidemiologic studies. J Infect Dis 139:280–287, 1979.
126. Jackson GG: Antibiotic policies, practices, and pressures. J Antimicrob Chemother 5:1–4, 1979.
127. Rorsova V, Urbaskova O, Vymola F: Bacterial multiresistance to antibiotics: Study of types of bacterial resistance to antibiotics in the environment and in clinical material of a resuscitation ward. J Hyg Epidemiol Microbiol Immunol 21:49–54, 1977.
128. Gould JC: Environmental penicillin and penicillin-resistant *Staphylococcus aureus*. Lancet 2:7019, 1958.
129. Price DJE, Sleigh JD: Control of infection due to *Klebsiella aerogenes* in a neurosurgical unit by withdrawal of all antibiotics. Lancet 2:1213–1215, 1970.
130. Marsh TD: Clinical pharmacology of antibiotics: The cephalosporin antibiotic agents. III. Third generation cephalosporins. Infect Control 6:78–83, 1985.
131. Interest rising in antibiotic quinolones. ASM News 51:614, 1985.
132. Kunin CM: Antibiotic accountability. N Engl J Med 301:380–381, 1979.
133. Nosocomial management of resistant gram negative bacilli (editorial). J Infect Dis 141:415–417, 1980.
134. Weinstein RA, Kabins SA: Strategies for prevention and control of multiple drug resistant nosocomial infections. Am J Med 70:449–454, 1981.
135. Joint Commission on Accreditation of Hospitals: Accreditation of Hospitals. Chicago, JCAH, 1992.
136. Brachman PS, Dan BB, Haley RW, et al: Nosocomial surgical infections: Incidence and cost. Surg Clin North Am 60:1–18, 1980.
137. Burke JF: Infection. In Hunt TK, Dunphy JE (eds): Fundamentals of Wound Management. New York, Appleton-Century-Crofts, 1979, pp 513–527.
138. Cruse PJE: Incidence of wound infection in the surgical services. Surg Clin North Am 55:1269–1280, 1975.
139. Cruse PJE, Foord R: The epidemiology of wound infections: A ten-year prospective study of 62,939 wounds. Surg Clin North Am 60(1):27–40, 1980.
140. Edwards LD: The epidemiology of 2056 remote site infections and 1966 surgical infections occurring in 1865 patients. Ann Surg 199:253–259, 1984.
141. MacMillan BG: Infections following burn injury. Surg Clin North Am 60:185–196, 1980.
142. Olson M, O'Conner M, Schwartz ML: Surgical wound infections: A five-year prospective study of 20,193 wounds at the Minneapolis VA Medical Center. Ann Surg 199:253–259, 1984.
143. Polk HC Jr: Overview of surgical infections. In Polk HC Jr, Stone HH (eds): Hospital Acquired Infections in Surgery. Baltimore, University Park Press, 1977, pp 1–18.
144. Polk HC: Prevention of surgical wound infection. Ann Intern Med 89(part 2):770, 1978.
145. Centers for Disease Control: Guidelines for Prevention of Surgical Wound Infections. Guidelines Activity, Hospital Infections Branch, Center for Infectious Diseases, Centers for Disease Control, Atlanta, GA, U.S. Department of Health and Human Services, 1982.
146. Altemeier WA: Surgical infections: Incisional wounds. In Bennett JV, Brachman PS (eds): Hospital Infections. Boston, Little, Brown, 1979, pp 287–306.
147. Altemeier WA, Culbertson WR, Hummel RP: Surgical considerations of endogenous infection: Sources, types, and methods of control. Surg Clin North Am 46:227–240, 1968.
148. Seropian Reynolds BM: Wound infections after preoperative dipilatory versus razor preparation. Am J Surg 121:251–254, 1971.
149. Alexander JW, Korelita J, Alexander NS: Prevention of wound infection: A case for closed suction drainage to remove fluids deficient in opsonic proteins. Am J Surg 132:59–66, 1976.
150. Nora PF, Vanecko RM, Branfield JJ: Prophylactic abdominal drains. Arch Surg 105:173–179, 1982.
151. Howard JM, Barker WF, Culbertson WR, et al: Postoperative wound infections: The influence of ultraviolet irradiation of the operating room and various other factors. Arch Surg 160(suppl):1–92, 1964.
152. Branemark PI, Ekholm R, Albrektsson B, et al: Tissue injury caused by wound disinfectants. J Bone Joint Surg 49A:48–62, 1967.
153. Joress SM: A study of disinfection of the skin: A comparison of povidone-iodine with other agents used for surgical scrubs. Ann Surg 152:296–304, 1962.
154. Galle PC, Homesley HD, Phyne AL: Reassessment of the surgical scrub. Surg Gynecol Obstet 147:215–218, 1978.
155. Swartz MN: Cellulitis and superficial infections. In Mandell GL, Douglas RG Jr, Bennett JE (eds): Principles and Practice of Infectious Diseases. New York, Wiley Medical, 1979, pp 797–817.
156. Woolfrey BF, Fox JM, Quall CO: An evaluation of burn wound quantitative microbiology: I. Quantitative eschar cultures. J Clin Pathol 75:532–537, 1981.
157. Baxter CR, Curreri PW, Marvin JA: The control of burn wound sepsis by the use of quantitative bacteriologic studies and subeschar lysis with antibiotics. Surg Clin North Am 53(6):1509–1519, 1973.

158. Pruitt BA Jr, Foley FD: The use of biopsies in burn patient care. Surgery 73:887–897, 1973.
159. Stone HH, Martin JD: Synergistic necrotizing cellulitis. Ann Surg 175:702–711, 1972.
160. Rudolph R, Soloway M, Depalma RG, et al: Fournier's syndrome: Synergistic gangrene of the scrotum. Am J Surg 129:591–596, 1975.
161. Campbell JC: Fournier's gangrene. Br J Urol 106–113, 1955.
162. Joklik WK, Willett HP, Amos DB (eds): Zinsser Microbiology, 17th ed. New York, Appleton-Century-Crofts, 1980, pp 832–863.
163. Caplan ES, Kluge RM: Gas gangrene: Review of 34 cases. Arch Intern Med 136:788–791, 1976.
164. Mohr JA, Griffiths W, Holm R, et al: Clostridial myonecrosis (gas gangrene) during cephalosporin prophylaxis. JAMA 239(9):847–850, 1978.
165. Duff JH, McLean PH, Mclean LD: Treatment of severe anaerobic infections. Arch Surg 101:314–317, 1970.
166. Lulu DJ, Riveria FJ: Gas gangrene. Am Surg 36:608–813, 1970.
167. Altemeier WA, Fullen WD: Prevention and treatment of gas gangrene. JAMA 217:806–813, 1971.
168. Demello FJ, Haglin JJ, Hitchcock CR: Comparative study of experimental *Clostridium perfringens* infections in dogs treated with antibiotics and hyperbaric oxygen. Surgery 73:936–941, 1973.
169. Schweigel JF, Shim SS: A comparison of the treatment of gas gangrene with and without hyperbaric oxygen. Surg Gynecol Obstet 136:969–970, 1973.
170. Roding D, Groenveld PHA, Boerema I: Ten years experience in the treatment of gas gangrene with hyperbaric oxygen. Surg Gynecol Obstet 134:579–585, 1972.
171. Hunt TK, Pai MP: The effects of varying ambient oxygen tensions on wound metabolism and collagen synthesis. Surg Gynecol Obstet 135:561–564, 1972.
172. Kivisaari J, Niinikoski J: Effects of hyperbaric oxygenation on the healing of open wounds. Acta Chir Scand 141:14–20, 1975.
173. Davis JC, Hunt TK (eds): Hyperbaric Oxygen Therapy. Bethesda, MD, Undersea Medical Society, Inc., 1977.
174. Holland JA, Hill GB, Wolfe WG, et al: Experimental and clinical experience with hyperbaric oxygen in the treatment of clostridial myonecrosis. Surgery 77:75–85, 1975.
175. Brown GL, Thomson PD, Mader JT, et al: Effects of hyperbaric oxygen upon *S. aureus, Ps. aeruginosa,* and *C. albicans.* Aviat Space Environ Med 50(7):717–720, 1979.
176. Rothstein RJ, Baker FJ II: Tetanus: Prevention and treatment. JAMA 240:675–678, 1978.
177. MMWR 34:405–414, 419–426, 1985.
178. Henson N, Tolo V: Wound botulism complicating an open fracture. J Bone Joint Surg 61A:312–316, 1979.
179. Merson MH, Dowell VR: Epidemiologic, clinical, and laboratory aspects of wound botulism. N Engl J Med. 289:1005–1010, 1973.
180. Mayhall CG: Infection in burn patients. In Wenzel RP (ed): Handbook of Hospital Acquired Infections. Boca Raton, FL, CRC Press, 1981, pp 317–339.
181. Marvin JA, Heck EL, Loebl EC, et al: Usefulness of blood cultures in confirming septic complications in burn patients: Evaluation of a new culture method. J Trauma 15:657–662, 1975.
182. Feller I, Tholen D, Cornell RG: Improvement in burn care, 1965–1979. JAMA 244:2074–2078, 1980.
183. Monafo WM, Tandon AN, Bradley RE, et al: Bacterial contamination of skin used as a biological dressing hazard. JAMA 235:1248–1249, 1976.
184. Moncrief JA, Lindberg RB, Switzer WE, et al: The use of a topical sulfonamide in the control of burn wound sepsis. J Trauma 6:407–419, 1966.
185. Bruber RP, Vistines V, Pardoe R: The effect of commonly used antiseptics on wound healing. Plast Reconstr Surg 55:472–476, 1975.
186. McCluskey B: A prospective trial of povidone-iodine solution in the prevention of wound sepsis. Aust NZ J Surg 46:254–256, 1976.
187. Schulman JA, Terry PM, Hough CE: Colonization with gentamicin-resistant *Pseudomonas aeruginosa,* pyocine type 5, in a burn unit. J Infect Dis 124(suppl):S18–S23, 1971.
188. Smith RF, Blasi D, Dayton SL, Chipps DD: Effects of sodium hypochlorite on the microbial flora and burns and normal skin. J Trauma 14:938–944, 1974.
189. Mayhall GC, Lamb VA, Gayle WE Jr, et al: *Enterobacter cloacae* septicemia in a burn center: Epidemiology and control of an outbreak. J Infect Dis 139:166–171, 1979.
190. U.S. Department of Health, Education and Welfare: Isolation techniques for use in hospitals. HEW Publication No. (CDC) 78-8314. Atlanta, GA, Centers for Disease Control, U.S. Public Health Service, 1985.
191. Clancy GJ, Hansen ST: Open fractures of the tibia. J Bone Joint Surg. 60A:118–122, 1978.
192. Chapman MW, Mahoney M: The role of early internal fixation in management of open fractures. Clin Orthop 138:120–131, 1979.
193. Turek SL (ed): Orthopaedics—Principles and Their Application. Philadelphia, JB Lippincott, 1977, pp 48–82.
194. Erhlich RF: Technical factors in wound management. In Hunt TK, Dunphy JE (eds): Fundamentals of Wound Management. New York, Appleton-Century-Crofts, 1979, pp 365–455.
195. Chapman MW, Hansen ST: Current concepts in the management of open fracture. In Rockwood CA, Green DP (eds): Fractures in Adults, 2nd ed, vol. 1. Philadelphia: JB Lippincott, 1984, pp 169–207.
196. Trafton PG: Infected fractures. In Complications of Fracture Management. New York, JB Lippincott, 1982, pp 51–78.
197. Gustilio RB, Anderson JT: Prevention of infection in the treatment of one thousand and twenty five open fractures of long bones. J Bone Joint Surg 58A:453–458, 1976.
198. Verrier ED, Bossart KJ, Heer WF: Reduction of infection rates in abdominal incisions by delayed wound closure techniques. Am J Surg 70:449–454, 1981.
199. Harkess JW, Ramsey WC, Admadi B: Definitive treatment of fractures and dislocations. In Rockwood CA, Green DP (eds): Fractures in Adults, 2nd ed, vol 1. Philadelphia, JB Lippincott, 1984, pp 1–139.
200. Anderson LD, Hutchins WC: Fractures of the tibia and fibula treated by casts and fixation devices. Clin Orthop 105:179–192, 1974.
201. Burney FL: Elastic external fixation of tibial fracture: Study of 1421 cases. In Brooker AF, Edwards CC (eds): External Fixation: The Current State of the Art. Baltimore, Williams & Wilkins, 1979, pp 55–73.
202. Edwards CC, Jaworski MF, Solana J, et al: Management of compound tibial fracture. Am Surg 45:190–202, 1979.
203. Hirschmann JV, Gilliland BC: Osteomyelitis and infectious arthritis. In Harrison's Principals of Internal Medicine, 9th ed. New York, McGraw-Hill, 1980, pp 1889–1891.
204. Dich V, Nelson J, Halalin K: Osteomyelitis in infants and children. Am J Dis Child 129:565–568, 1975.
205. Kreger BE, Craven DE, McCabe WR: Gram-negative bacteremia: IV. Reevaluation of clinical features and treatment in 621 patients. Am J Med 68:344–355, 1980.
206. Barza M: Finding and stopping bacteremia. Drug Ther April:83–97, 1975.
207. Spengler RF, Greenough WB: Hospital costs and mortality attributed to nosocomial bacteremias. JAMA 240:22, 1975.
208. McGowen JE, Parrott PL, Duty VP: Nosocomial bacteremia: Potential for prevention of procedure-related cases. JAMA 237:2727–2729, 1977.
209. LeFrock J, Ellis CA, Klainer AS, Weinstein L: Transient bacteremia associated with barium enema. Arch Intern Med 135:835–837, 1975.
210. Berry FA, Blankenbaker WL, Ball CG: A comparison of bacteremia occurring with nasotracheal and orotracheal intubation. Anesth Analg 52:873–876, 1973.
211. Applefeld JJ, Carother TE, Reno DJ, et al: Assessment of the sterility of long-term catheterization using the thermodilution Swan-Ganz catheter. Chest 74:377, 1978.
212. Cheesbrough JS, Finch RG, MacFarlane JT: The complications of intravenous cannulae incorporating a valved injection side port. J Hyg Camb 93:497–504, 1984.

213. Kopman EA, Sandza JG: Pulmonary-artery catheter after placement: Maintenance of sterility. Anesthesiology 48:373–374, 1978.
214. Zinner MJ, Zuidema GD, Lowery RD: Septic nonsuppurative thrombophlebitis. Arch Surg 111:122–125, 1976.
215. Band JD, Maki DG: Infections caused by arterial catheters used for hemodynamic monitoring. Am J Med 67:735–739, 1979.
216. Miyaska K, Edmond JF, Conn AW: Complications of radial artery lines in the paediatric patient. Can J Anaesth 23:9–13, 1976.
217. Weinstein RA: The design of pressure monitoring devices: Infection control considerations. Med Instrum 10:287–289, 1976.
218. Soderstrom CA, Wasserman DH, Dunham MC, et al: Superiority of the femoral artery for monitoring: A prospective study. Am J Surg 144:309–313, 1982.
219. Hopkins D: Unusual access infections in hemodialysis. Dialysis Transplant 8:7, 1979.
220. Tofte RW, Solliday J, Rotschafer J, Crossley KB: *Staphylococcus aureus* infection of dialysis shunt: Absence of synergy with vancomycin and rifampin. South Med J 74:612–617, 1981.
221. Maki DG, Weise CE, Sarafin HW: A semiquantitative method for identifying intravenous catheter-associated infection. N Engl J Med 296:1305, 1977.
222. Hudson-Civetta JA, Civetta JM, Martinez OV, et al: Risk and detection of pulmonary artery catheter-related infection in septic surgical patients. Crit Care Med 15:29–34, 1987.
223. Norwood S, Jenkins G: An evaluation of triple-lumen catheter infections using a guidewire exchange technique. J Trauma 30:706–712, 1990.
224. Mermel LA, Maki DG: Epidemic bloodstream infections from hemodynamic pressure monitoring: signs of the times. Infect Control Hosp Epidemiol 10:47–53, 1989.
225. Bjornson HS, Colley R, Bower RH, et al: Association between microorganism growth at the catheter insertion site and colonization of the catheter in patients receiving total parenteral nutrition. Surgery 92:720–726, 1982.
226. Dillon JD, Schaffner W, Van Way CW, et al: Septicemia and total parenteral nutrition: Distinguishing catheter-related from other septic episodes. JAMA 223:134, 1973.
227. Goldman DA, Martin WT, Worthington JW: Growth of bacteria and fungi in total parenteral nutrition solutions. Am J Surg 126:314–318, 1973.
228. Goldman DA, Maki DG: Infection control in total parenteral nutrition. JAMA 223:12, 1973.
229. Maki DG: Growth properties of microorganisms in lipid for infusion and implications for infection control (abstract). Am J Infect Control 8(3):89, 1980.
230. Maki DG, Martin WT: Nationwide epidemic of septicemia caused by contaminated infusion products: IV. Growth of microbial pathogens. J Infect Dis 131:276, 1975.
231. Steere AC, Tenney JH, Machel DC, et al: *Pseudomonas* spp. bacteremias caused by contaminated normal serum albumen. J Infect Dis 135:5, 1977.
232. Rhame FS, Root RK, MacLowry JD, et al: *Salmonella* septicemia for platelet transfusions. Ann Intern Med 78:633, 1973.
233. Scheld WM, Sande MA: Endocarditis and intravascular infections. In Mandell GL, Douglas RG Jr, Bennett JE (eds): Principles and Practice of Infectious Diseases. New York, Wiley Medical, 1979, pp 653–689.
234. Pelletier LL, Petersdorf RG: Infective endocarditis: 125 cases from the University of Washington hospitals, 1962–1973. Medicine 56:105, 1978.
235. Powell DC, Blivens BA, Bell RM, et al: Bacterial endocarditis in the critically surgical patient. Arch Surg 116:311–314, 1981.
236. Sasaki TM: The relationship of central venous and pulmonary artery catheter position to acute right-sided endocarditis. J Trauma 19:10, 1979.
237. Baskin TW, Rosenthal A, Pruitt BA Jr: Acute bacterial endocarditis: A silent source of sepsis in the burn patient. Ann Surg 184:618–621, 1976.
238. Hampers CL: Long Term Hemodialysis, 2nd ed. New York, Grune & Stratton, 1973.
239. Elliott CG, Zimmerman GA, Clemmer TP: Complications of pulmonary artery catheterization in the care of critically ill patients: A prospective study. Chest 76:647–652, 1979.
240. Maki DG, Goldman DA, Rhame FS: Infection control in intravenous therapy. Ann Intern Med 79:867, 1973.
241. Simmons BP: CDC guidelines for the prevention and control of nosocomial infections: Guideline for prevention of intravascular infections. Am J Infect Control 11(5):183, 1983.
242. Buxton AE, Highsmith AK, Garner JS, et al: Contamination of intravenous infusion fluid: Effects of changing administration sets. Ann Intern Med 90:764–768, 1979.
243. Band JD, Maki DG: Safety of changing intravenous delivery systems at intervals longer than 24 hours. Ann Intern Med 91:173, 1979.
244. Josephson A, Gornbert ME, Sierra MF, et al: The relationship between intravenous fluid contamination and the frequency of tubing replacement. Infect Control 6:367–370, 1985.
245. Donowitz LG, Marsik FJ, Hoyt JW, et al: *Serratia marcescens* bacteremia from contaminated pressure transducers. JAMA 16:1749–1752, 1979.
246. Cleary TJ, MacIntyre DS, Castro M: *Serratia marcescens* bacteremias in an intensive care unit: Contaminated heparinized saline solution as a reservoir. Am J Infect Control 9:107–111, 1981.
247. Solomon SL, Alexander J, Eley JW, et al: Nosocomial fungemia in neonates associated with intravascular pressure-monitoring devices. Ped Infect Dis 5:680–685, 1986.
248. Weems JJ, Chamberland ME, Ward J, et al: *Candida parapsilosis* fungemia associated with parenteral nutrition and contaminated pressure transducers. J Clin Microbiol 25:1029–1032, 1987.
249. Weinstein RA, Stamm WE, Kramer L, et al: Pressure monitoring devices. Overlooked source of nosocomial infection. JAMA 236:936–938, 1976.
250. Beck-Sague CM, Jarvis WR: Epidemic bloodstream infections associated with pressure transducers. Infect Control Hosp Epidemiol 10:54–59, 1989.
251. Peters G, Locci R, Pulverer G: Adherence and growth of coagulase-negative staphylococci on surfaces of intravenous catheters. J Infect Dis 146:479–482, 1982.
252. Martin MA, Pfaller MA, Wenzel RP: Coagulase-negative staphylococcal bacteremia. Ann Intern Med 110:9–16, 1989.
253. Beam TR: Vascular access catheters and infections. Infect Surg 5:156–161, 1989.
254. Cooper GL, Hopkins CC: Rapid diagnosis of intravascular catheter-associated infection by direct Gram staining of catheter segments. N Engl J Med 18:1142–1150, 1985.
255. Franceschi D, Gerding RL, Phillips G, et al: Risk factors associated with intravascular catheter infections in burned patients: A prospective randomized study. J Trauma 29:811–815, 1989.
256. Maki DG, Band JD: A comparative study of polyantibiotic and iodophor ointments in prevention of vascular catheter-related infection. Am J Med 70:739–744, 1981.
257. Prager RL, Silva J: Colonization of central venous catheters. South Med J 77:458–461, 1984.
258. Kamenski MV, Zamirowski T: Skin sterilization for percutaneous IV cannulation. In Proceedings World Congress on Antisepsis. New York, HP Publishing Co, 1978, pp 51–54.
259. Craven DW, Lichtenberg DH, Gonzalez M, et al: A prospective, randomized study comparing transparent polyurethane dressing (Op-Site) to a dry gauze dressing for peripheral intravenous sites. Infect Control 6:361–366, 1985.
260. Conly JM, Grieves K, Peters B: A prospective, randomized study comparing transparent and dry gauze dressings for central venous catheters. J Infect Dis 159:310–319, 1989.
261. Centers for Disease Control: Guideline for prevention of infection related to intravascular pressure-monitoring systems. Infect Control 3:61–72, 1982.
262. Luskin RL, Weinstein RA, Nathan C, et al: Extended use of disposable pressure transducers. JAMA 255(7):916–922, 1986.
263. Pemberton LB, Lyman B, Lander V, et al: Sepsis from triple- versus single-lumen catheters during total parenteral nutrition in surgical or critically ill patients. Arch Surg 121:591–594, 1986.

264. Apelgren KN: Triple-lumen catheters: Technological advance or setback? Am Surg 53:113–116, 1987.
265. McCarthy MC, Shives JK, Robinson RJ, et al: Prospective evaluation of single and triple-lumen catheters in total parenteral nutrition. JPEN 11:259–294, 1987.
266. Hilton E, Haslett TM, Bonenstein MT, et al: Central catheter infections: Single versus triple-lumen catheters. Am J Med 84:667–672, 1988.
267. Miller JJ, Venus B, Mathru M: Comparison of the sterility of long-term central catheterization using single lumen, triple lumen and pulmonary artery catheters. Crit Care Med 12:634–637, 1984.
268. Kelly CS, Ligas JR, Smith CA, et al: Sepsis due to triple lumen central venous catheters. Surg Gynecol Obstet 163:14–16, 1986.
269. Kaufman JL, Rodriguez JL, McFadden JA, et al: Clinical experience with the multiple lumen central venous catheter. JPEN 10:487–489, 1986.
270. Lee RB, Buckner M, Sharp KW: Do multi-lumen catheters increase central venous catheter sepsis compared to single-lumen catheters? J Trauma 28:1472–1475, 1988.
271. Pomp A, Varella L, Caldwell MD, et al: Catheter-related sepsis: Single-lumen catheters (SLC) versus triple-lumen catheters (TLC). JPEN 12:23S, 1988.
272. Blewett JH Jr, Kyger ER III, Patterson LT: Subclavian vein catheter replacement without venipuncture. Arch Surg 108:274, 1974.
273. Padberg FT Jr, Ruggiero J, Blackburn GL, et al: Central venous catheterization for parenteral nutrition. Ann Surg 193:264–270, 1981.
274. Eisenhauer ED, Derveloy RJ, Hastings PR: Prospective evaluation of central venous pressure (CVP) catheters in a large city-county hospital. Ann Surg 196:560–564, 1982.
275. Bozzetti F, Terno G, Bonfanti G, et al: Prevention and treatment of central venous catheter sepsis by exchange via a guidewire. A prospective controlled trial. Ann Surg 198:48–52, 1983.
276. Pettigrew RA, Lang SDR, Haydock DA, et al: Catheter-related sepsis in patients on intravenous nutrition: A prospective study of quantitative catheter cultures and guidewire changes for suspected sepsis. Br J Surg 72:52–55, 1985.
277. Sitzmann JV, Townsend TR, Siler MC, et al: Septic and technical complications of central venous catheterization: A prospective study of 200 consecutive patients. Ann Surg 202:766–770, 1985.
278. Armstrong CW, Mayhall G, Miller KB, et al: Prospective study of catheter replacement and other risk factors for infection of hyperalimentation catheters. J Infect Dis 154:808–816, 1986.
279. Krinsky AJ, Hoyt NJ, Joshi M, et al: Intravenous catheter usage and methods of catheter replacement in a major trauma center. Presented before the 27th Interscience Congress on Antimicrobial Agents and Chemotherapy, New York, New York, October 7, 1987.
280. Maki DG, Cobb L, Garman JK, et al: An attachable silver-impregnated cuff for prevention of infection with central venous catheters: A prospective randomized multicenter trial. Am J Med 85:307–312, 1988.
281. Trooskin SZ, Donetz AP, Harvey RA, et al: Prevention of catheter sepsis by antibiotic bonding. Surgery 97:547–551, 1987.
282. Parsa MH, Lau K, Jampayas I, et al: Intravenous catheter-related infection. Infect Surg 4:789–798, 1985.
283. Pruitt BA Jr, McManns WF, Kim SH, Treat RC: Diagnosis and treatment of cannula-related intravenous sepsis in burn patients. Ann Surg 191:546–554, 1980.
284. Berk SL, McCabe WR: Meningitis caused by gram-negative bacilli. Ann Intern Med 93:253–260, 1980.
285. MacGee EE, Cauthen JC, Brackett CE: Meningitis following acute traumatic cerebrospinal fistula. J Neurosurg 33:312–316, 1970.
286. Caplan ES, Hoyt NJ, Saul TS: Nosocomial CNS infections. In Proceedings of the National Association for Practitioners in Infection Control, Atlanta, GA, June 1981.
287. Caplan ES, Hoyt NJ: Meningitis due to *Acinetobacter calcoaceticus*. In Current Chemotherapy and Infectious Disease, vol 2. Washington, American Society for Microbiology, 1980, pp 1094–1096.
288. Buckwold FJ, Hand R, Hansebout RR: Hospital-acquired bacterial meningitis in neurosurgical patients. J Neurosurg 45:494–500, 1977.
289. Stillwell M, Hogue C, Hoyt NJ, et al: Post-traumatic meningococcal meningitis. J Trauma 31:1693–1695, 1991.
290. Smith RW, Alkane JF: Infections complicating the external ventriculostomy. J Neurosurg 44:567, 1976.
291. Mayhall CG, Archer NH, Lamb VA, et al: Ventriculostomy-related infection: A prospective epidemiologic study. N Engl J Med 310:553–559, 1984.
292. Winn HR, Dacey RG, Jane JA: Intracranial subarachnoid pressure recording: Experience with 650 patients. Surg Neurol 8:41–47, 1977.
293. Walters BC, Hoffman HJ, Hendrick EB, et al: Cerebrospinal fluid shunt infection: Influences on initial management and subsequent outcome. J Neurosurg 60:1014–1021, 1984.
294. Schoenbaum SC, Gardner P, Shilleto J: Infections of cerebrospinal fluid shunt: Epidemiology, clinical manifestations and therapy. J Infect Dis. 131:543–552, 1975.
295. Forrest DM, Cooper DG: Complications of ventricular-atrial shunts: A review of 455 cases. J Neurosurg 29:509–512, 1968.
296. Venes J: Control of shunt infections: Report of 150 consecutive cases. J Neurosurg 45:311–314, 1976.
297. Nelson J: Cerebrospinal fluid shunt infections. Pediatr Infect Dis May/June (3 suppl):530–532, 1984.
298. Holt RJ: The colonization of ventriculo-atrial shunts by coagulase-negative staphylococci. In Finland M, Marget W, Bartman K (eds): Bacterial Infections: Changes in Their Causative Agents, Trends, and Possible Bases. New York, Springer-Verlag, 1971, pp 81–87.
299. Caplan ES, Hoyt NJ: Empiric intravenous treatment of nosocomial gram negative meningitis. In Proceedings of 12th International Congress on Chemotherapy, Florence, Italy, July 1981.
300. Haley RW, Hooten TM, Culver DH, et al: Nosocomial infections in U.S. hospitals, 1975–1976: Estimated frequency by selected characteristics of patients. Am J Med 70:947–959, 1981.
301. Sanford JP, Pierce AK: Lower respiratory infections. In Bennett JV, Brachman PS (eds): Hospital Infection. Boston, Little, Brown, 1979, pp 225–286.
302. Stratton CW: Bacterial pneumonias—An overview with emphasis on pathogenesis, diagnosis and treatment. Heart Lung 15:226–244, 1986.
303. McLean APH, Boulanger MA: Epidemiology of infection in the surgical intensive care unit. In Meakins JL (ed): Surgical Infection in Critical Care Medicine. New York, Churchill Livingstone, 1985, pp 46–58.
304. Wenzel RP, Osterman CA, Hunting KJ: Hospital-acquired infections: II. Infection rates by site, service and common procedures in a university hospital. Am J Epidemiol 104(6):645–651, 1976.
305. Walker WE, Kapelanski DP, Weiland AL, et al: Patterns of infection and mortality in thoracic trauma. Ann Surg 210(6):752–757, 1985.
306. Gross PA, Neu HC, Aswapokee P, et al: Deaths from nosocomial infections: Experience in a university hospital and a community hospital. Am J Med 68:219–222, 1980.
307. Caplan ES, Hoyt NJ: Nosocomial sinusitis. JAMA 247(5):639, 1982.
308. Carter BL, Ankoff MS, Fisk JD: Computed tomographic detection of sinusitis responsible for intracranial and extracranial infections. Radiology 147:739–742, 1983.
309. Zwillich C, Pierson DJ: Nasal necrosis: A complication of nasotracheal intubation. Chest 64:376–378, 1973.
310. Pope TL, Stellin CB, Leitner YB: Maxillary sinusitis after nasotracheal intubation. South Med J 74:610–611, 1981.
311. Garibaldi RA, Britt MR, Coleman ML, et al: Risk factors for post operative pneumonia. Am J Med 70:677–700, 1981.
312. Lopez MM, Damoso D, Beltran MJ, et al: Epidemiology of respiratory infection in the intensive care unit. Antibiotics Chemother 21:99, 1976.

313. Bell RC, Coalson JJ, Smith JD, et al: Multiple organ failure and infection in adult respiratory distress syndrome. Ann Intern Med 99(3):293–297, 1983.
314. Meduri GU: Ventilator-associated pneumonia in patients with respiratory failure: A diagnostic approach. Chest 97:1208–1219, 1990.
315. Joshi M, Ciesla N, Caplan E: Diagnosis of pneumonia in critically ill patients. Chest 94:4S, 1988.
316. Johanson WG, Pierce AK, Sanford JP, et al: Changing pharyngeal bacterial flora of hospitalized patients: Emergence of gram negative bacilli. N Engl J Med 281:1137–1140, 1969.
317. Johanson WG, Pierce AK, Sanford JP, et al: Nosocomial respiratory infections with gram negative bacilli: The significance of colonization of the respiratory tract. Ann Intern Med 77:701–706, 1972.
318. Pruitt BA Jr, DeVincenti FC, Mason AD Jr, et al: The occurrence and significance of pneumonia and other pulmonary complications in burned patients: Comparison of conventional and topical treatments. J Trauma 10:519–531, 1970.
319. Dascher F, Kappstein I, Reuschenbach K, et al: Stress ulcer prophylaxis and ventilation pneumonia: Prevention by antibacterial cytoprotective agents? Infect Control Hosp Epidemiol 9:59–65, 1988.
320. Driks MR, Craven DE, Celli BA, et al: Nosocomial pneumonia in intubated patients randomized to sucralfate versus antacids and/or histamine type 2 blockers: The role of gastric colonization. N Engl J Med 217:1376–1382, 1987.
321. Karlstadt RG, Palmer RH: Risk factors for nosocomial pneumonia in intensive care. Arch Intern Med 150:919, 1990.
322. F-D-C Reports (The Pink Sheet). Chevy Chase, MD: F-D-C Reports, Inc, March 27, 1989, 51:13:9.
323. Craig KC, Benson MS, Pierson DJ: Prevention of arterial oxygen desaturation during closed-airway endotracheal suction: Effect of ventilatormode. Respir Care 29:1013–1018, 1984.
324. Demers RR: Complications of endotracheal suctioning procedures. Respir Care 27:453–457, 1982.
325. Ritz R, Scott LR, Coyle MB, et al: Contamination of multiple-use catheter in a closed-circuit system compared to contamination of a disposable single-use suction catheter. Respir Care 31:1086–1091, 1986.
326. Ciesla N, Klemic N, Imle PC: Chest physical therapy to the patient of multiple trauma. Phys Ther 61(2):202–205, 1981.
327. Mackenzie CF, Ciesla N, Imle PC, et al (eds): Chest Physiotherapy in Intensive Care. Baltimore, Williams & Wilkins, 1981.
328. Graham WGB, Bradley DA: Efficacy of chest physiotherapy and intermittent positive-pressure breathing in the resolution of pneumonia. N Engl J Med 299:624–627, 1978.
329. Rosato FE, Rosato EF, Plotkin SA: Herpetic paronychia: An occupational hazard of medical personnel. N Engl J Med 283:804, 1970.
330. Centers for Disease Control: Guideline for the prevention of nosocomial pneumonia. Guidelines Activity, Hospital Infections Branch, Center for Infectious Disease, U.S. Department of Health and Human Services, 1982.
331. Teres D: Management of respiratory infection in the intensive care unit. Int Anesth Clin 14:163, 1973.
332. Perea EJ, Criado A, Moreno N, et al: Mechanical ventilators as vehicles of infections. Acta Anaesthesiol Scand 19:180, 1975.
333. Pierce AK, Sanford JP, Thomas CD, et al: Long-term evaluation of decontamination of inhalation equipment and the occurrence of necrotizing pneumonia. N Engl J Med 282:528–531, 1970.
334. Reinarz JA, Pierce AK, Mays BB, et al: The potential role of inhalation equipment in nosocomial pulmonary infection. J Clin Invest 44:831, 1965.
335. Gervich DH, Grout CS: An outbreak of nosocomial *Acinetobacter* infection from humidifiers. Am J Infect Control 13:210–211, 1985.
336. Hoyt NJ, Caplan ES, Meidinski M, et al: Control of *Acinetobacter calcoaceticus* var. *anitratis* in a trauma unit. Presented at the National Association for Practitioners in Infection Control Meeting in Houston, Texas, 1979.
337. Craven DE, Connolly MG, Lichtenberg DA, et al: Contamination of mechanical ventilators with tubing changes every 24 or 48 hours. N Engl J Med 306:1505, 1982.
338. Hartstein AI, Rashad AL, Liebler JM, et al: Multiple intensive care unit outbreak of *Acinetobacter calcoaceticus* subspecies *anitratus* respiratory infection and colonization associated with contaminated, reusable ventilator circuits and resuscitation bags. Am J Med 85:624–631, 1988.
339. Weese WC, Shindler ER, Smith IM, et al: Empyema of the thorax then and now—A study of 122 cases over 4 decades. Arch Intern Med 131:516–520, 1973.
340. Emerson JD, Boruchow IB, Wheat MW: Pyogenic empyema. Am Surg April 43:205–209, 1972.
341. Light RW: Pleural effusion. Med Clin North Am 61:6, 1977.
342. Caplan ES, Hoyt NJ, Rodriguez A, et al: Empyema in the multiply traumatized patient. J Trauma 24:785–789, 1984.
343. Arom KV, Grover FL, Richardson JD, et al: Posttraumatic empyema. Ann Thorac Surg 23:254–258, 1977.
344. Kirby RR: Ventilatory support and barotrauma (editorial). Anesthesiology 50:181–182, 1978.
345. Cullen DJ, Calders DL: The incidence of ventilator-induced pulmonary barotrauma in critically ill patients. Anesthesiology 50:185–190, 1979.
346. Arnold S, Feathers RS, Gibbs E: Bilateral pneumothoraces and subcutaneous emphysema: A complication of internal jugular puncture. Br Med J 1:211–212, 1973.
347. Jacobsen WK, Smith DC, Briggs BA, et al: Aberrant catheter placement for total parenteral nutrition. Anesthesiology 50:152–154, 1979.
348. Oakes DD, Wilson RE: Malposition of subclavian line: Resultant pleural effusions, interstitial edema and chest wall abscess. JAMA 233:532–533, 1975.
349. Koch MJ: Bilateral IV hydrothorax (letter). N Engl J Med 286:218, 1972.
350. Coon JL, Shuck JM: Failure of tube thoracostomy for posttraumatic empyema: An indication for early decortication. J Trauma 15(7):588–594, 1975.
351. Dellinger EP, Oreskovich MR, Wertz MJ, et al: Risk of infection following laparotomy for penetrating abdominal trauma. Arch Surg 119:20–27, 1984.
352. Fry D, Garrison N, Heirtsh R, et al: Determinants of death in patients with intra-abdominal abscess. Surgery 88:517, 1980.
353. Drasar BS, Shiner M, McLeod GM: Studies on the intestinal flora: I. The bacterial flora of the gastrointestinal tract in healthy and achlorohydric persons. Gastroenterology 56:71, 1969.
354. DuPriest RW, Khaneja SC, Cowley RA: Acute cholecystitis complicating trauma. Ann Surg 189:84–89, 1979.
355. Bartlett JG, Chang TW, Gurwith M, et al: Antibiotic-associated pseudomembranous colitis due to toxin producing clostridia. N Engl J Med 298:531, 1978.
356. Bartlett JG, Moon N, Chang TW, et al: Role of *Clostridium difficile* in antibiotic-associated colitis. Gastroenterology 75:778–782, 1978.
357. Slagle GW, Boggs W: Drug-induced pseudomembranous enterocolitis: A new etiologic agent. Dis Colon Rectum 19:253–255, 1976.
358. Hutcheon DF, Milligan FD, Yardley JH, et al: Cephalosporin-associated pseudomembranous colitis. Dig Dis 23:321–326, 1978.
359. Tedesco F, Markham R, Gurwith M, et al: Oral vancomycin for antibiotic-associated pseudomembranous colitis. Lancet 1:226–228, 1978.
360. Kim KH, Fekety R, Batts DH, et al. Isolation of *Clostridium difficile* from the environment and contacts of patients with antibiotic-associated colitis. J Infect Dis 143:42–50, 1981.
361. Savage AM, Alford RM: Nosocomial spread of *Clostridium difficile*. Infect Control 4:31–33, 1983.
362. Gutman LT, Idriss ZH, Gelbach S, et al: Neonatal staphylococcal enterocolitis: Association with indwelling feeding catheter and *S. aureus* colonization. J Pediatr 88(5):836, 1976.
363. Gianella RA, Broitment SA, Zamcheck N: Influence of gastric acidity on bacterial and parasitic enteric infections: A perspective. Ann Intern Med 78:271, 1973.
364. Neale G, Gompertz D, Schonsby H, et al: The metabolic and

nutritional consequences of bacterial overgrowth in the small intestine. Am J Clin Nutr 25:1409, 1972.
365. White WT III, Acuff TE, Sykes TR, et al: Bacterial contamination of enteral nutrient solution: A preliminary report. JPEN 3:459, 1979.
366. Furtado D, Parrish A, Beyer P: Enteral nutrient solutions (ENS): In vitro growth supporting properties of ENS for bacteria. JPEN 4:594, 1980.
367. Levy J, Van Laethem Y, Verhaegen G, et al: Contaminated enteral nutrition solutions as a cause of nosocomial bloodstream infection: A study using plasmid fingerprinting. J Parenter Enter Nutr 14:288–234, 1989.
368. Baldwin BA, Zagoren AJ, Rose N: Bacterial contamination of continuously infused enteral alimentation with needle catheter jejunostomy: Clinical implications. JPEN 8:30–33, 1983.
369. Simmons BP, Gelfand MS, Haas M, et al: *Enterobacter sakazakii* infections in neonates associated with intrinsic contamination of a powdered infant formula. Infect Control Hosp Epidemiol 10:398–401, 1989.
370. Levy J: Enteral nutrition: An increasingly recognized cause of nosocomial bloodstream infection. Infect Control Hosp Epidemiol 10:395–397, 1989.
371. Schreiner RM: Nosocomial spread of *Clostridium difficile.* Infect Control 4:31–33, 1983.
372. Groschel DHM: Disposable enteral feeding bags should not be used. JAMA 248:2536, 1982.
373. Anderton A, Aidov KE: The effect of handling procedures on microbial contamination of enteral feeds. J Hosp Infect 11:364–372, 1988.
374. DeLeeuw I, Van Alsenoy L: Bacterial contamination of the feeding bag during catheter jejunostomy: Exogenous or endogenous origin? J Parenter Enter Nutr 8:591–592, 1984.
375. Kunin CM: Urinary tract infections. In Bennett JV, Brachman PS (eds): Hospital Infections. Boston, Little, Brown, 1979, pp 239–254.
376. Dixon RE (ed): Nosocomial Infections. New York, Yorke Medical Books, 1981.
377. Kunin CM: Detection, Prevention, and Management of Urinary Tract Infections, 2nd ed. Philadelphia, Lee & Febiger, 1974.
378. Turck M, Stamm WE: Nosocomial infection of the urinary tract. Am J Med 70:651, 1981.
379. Kunin CM, McCormick RC: Prevention of catheter-induced urinary tract infections by sterile closed drainage. N Engl J Med 274:1155–1162, 1966.
380. Kass EH, Schneiderman JL: Entry of bacteria into the urinary tracts of patients with inlying catheters. N Engl J Med 264:556, 1957.
381. Classen DC, Larsen RA, Burke JP, et al: Prevention of catheter-associated bacteriuria: Clinical trial of methods to block three known pathways. Am J Infect Control 19:136–142, 1991.
382. Platt R, Polk BF, Murdock B, et al: Prevention of catheter-associated urinary tract infection: A cost-benefit analysis. Infect Control Hosp Epidemiol 10:60–64, 1989.
383. Garibaldi RA, Burke JP, Dickman ML, et al: Factors predisposing to bacteriuria during indwelling urethral catheterization. N Engl J Med 291:215–218, 1974.
384. Garibaldi RA, Burke JP, Britt MR, et al: Meatal colonization and catheter-associated bacteriuria. N Engl J Med 303:315–318, 1980.
385. Macdonald RA, Levitin H, Mallory K, et al: Relationship between pyelonephritis and bacterial counts in the urine. N Engl J Med 256:915–922, 1957.
386. Gross PA, Messinger-Harkavy L, Barden GE, et al: Positive Foley catheter tip cultures—Fact or fancy? JAMA 228:72–73, 1974.
387. Stamm WE: Guidelines for the prevention of catheter-associated urinary tract infections. Ann Intern Med 82:386–390, 1975.
388. Centers for Disease Control: Guideline for the prevention of catheter-associated urinary tract infections. Guidelines Activity, Hospital Infections Branch, Center for Disease Control, Atlanta, GA, U.S. Department of Health and Human Services, 1982.
389. Warren JW, Platt R, Thomas RJ, et al: Antibiotic irrigation and catheter associated urinary tract infections. N Engl J Med 299:570, 1978.
390. Britt MR, Garibaldi RA, Miller WA: Antimicrobial prophylaxis for catheter associated bacteriuria. Antimicrob Agents Chemother 11:240, 1977.
391. Burke JP, Garibaldi RA, Britt MR, et al: Prevention of catheter-associated urinary tract infections. Efficacy of daily meatal regimens. Am J Med 70:655, 1981.
392. Thompson RL, Haley CE, Groschel DM, et al: Effect of installation of hydrogen peroxide into urinary drainage systems in the prevention of catheter-associated bacteriuria (abstract no 769). In Proceedings of the 22nd Interscience Conference on Antimicrobial Agents and Chemotherapy, ASM, Miami, FL, 1982.
393. Rutula WA, Kennedy VA, Loflin HB, et al: *Serratia marcescens* nosocomial infections of the urinary tract associated with urine measuring containers and urinometers. Am J Med 70:699, 1981.
394. Schaberg DR, Alford RH, Anderson R, et al: An outbreak of nosocomial infections due to multiply resistant *Serratia marcescens:* Evidence of intrahospital spread. J Infect Dis 134(2):181, 1976.
395. Hoyt NJ: Infection control and emergency medical services: Facts and myths. Md Med J 37:551–557, 1988.
396. Centers for Disease Control: Recommendations for prevention of HIV transmission in health care settings. MMWR Suppl 36:1S–16S, 1987.
397. Fed Reg 52(210), Friday, October 30, 1987, pp 41818–41823.
398. Fed Reg 52(228), Friday, November 27, 1987, proposed rules, pp 45438–45441.
399. Fed Reg 58(235), Friday, December 6, 1991, Occupational Exposure to Bloodborne Pathogens, pp 64174–64182.
400. Hoyt NJ, Crowther CL: The trauma patient with acquired immunodeficiency syndrome. In Welton RH, Shane KA (eds): Case Studies in Trauma Nursing. Baltimore, Williams & Wilkins, 1990, pp 260–265.
401. Meythaler JM, Cross LL: Traumatic spinal cord injury complicated by AIDS related complex. Arch Phys Med Rehabil 69:219, 1988.
402. Ward JW, Hardy AM, Drotman DP: AIDS in the United States. In Worman GP (ed): AIDS and Other Manifestations of HIV Infection. Park Ridge, NJ: Park Ridge Press, 1987, pp 18–35.
403. Aprahamian C, Olson D, Gottschall JL, et al: Potential risks of human immunodeficiency virus in critically injured patients. J Trauma 28:1081, 1988.
404. Kelen GD, Fritz S, Quiqish B, et al: Unrecognized human immunodeficiency virus infection in emergency department patients. N Engl J Med 318:16445–16450, 1988.
405. Baker JL, Kelen GC, Sivertson KT, et al: Unsuspected immunodeficiency virus in critically ill emergency patients. JAMA 257:2609–2611, 1987.
406. Soderstrom CA, Furth PA, Glasser D, et al: HIV infection rates in a center treating predominantly rural blunt trauma victims. J Trauma 29:1526–1530, 1989.
407. Weiss SH, Goedret JJ, Sarngadharan MG, et al: Screening test for HTLV-III (AIDS agent) antibodies: Specificity, sensitivity, and applications. JAMA 253:221–225, 1985.
408. Council on Scientific Affairs Report: Status report on the acquired immune deficiency syndrome: Human T-cell lymphotrophic virus type III testing. JAMA 254:1342–1345, 1985.
409. Lane TW, Ivey FD, Falk PS, et al: False-negative human immunodeficiency virus (HIV) testing in an organ donor (abstract). Am J Infect Control 15(2):87, 1987.
410. Ryan White: Comprehensive AIDS Resources Emergency Act of 1990. Public Law 101-381 (104 STAT 622).
411. 73 Opinions of the Attorney General at 34 (1988) [Opinion No. 88-046 (October 17, 1988)], Maryland.
412. Centers for Disease Control: Recommendations for protection against viral hepatitis. MMWR 31:317–324, 329–335, 1982.
413. Dienstag JL, Ryan DM: Occupational exposure to hepatitis B virus in hospital personnel: Infection or immunization? Am J Epidemiol 115:26–39, 1982.

414. Centers for Disease Control: The safety of hepatitis B virus vaccine. MMWR 31(10):134–137, 1983.
415. Seeff LB, Wright EC, Zimmerman HJ, et al: Type B hepatitis after needlestick exposure: Prevention with hepatitis B immune globulin. Ann Intern Med 88:285–293, 1978.
416. Vlahov D, Polk BF: Transmission of human immunodeficiency virus within health care setting. Occup Med 2:429–450, 1987.
417. Hoofnagle JH: Acute hepatitis. In Mandell GL, Douglas RG, Bennett JE (eds): Principles and Practice of Infectious Diseases. New York, Wiley, 1979, pp 1043–1059.
418. Janzen J, Tripatizis I, Wagner U, et al: Epidemiology of hepatitis B surface antigen (HBsAg) and antibody to HBsAg in hospital personnel. J Infect Dis 137:261–265, 1978.
419. Javanovich JF, Saravolatz LD: The risk of hepatitis B among select employee groups in an urban hospital. JAMA 250:1893–1894, 1983.
420. Denes AE, Smith JL, Maynard JE, et al: Hepatitis B infection in physicians: Results of a nationwide seroepidemiologic survey. JAMA 239:210–212, 1978.
421. Berry AJ, Isaacson IJ, Hunt D, et al: The prevalence of hepatitis B viral markers in anesthesia personnel. Anesthesiology 60:6–9, 1984.
422. Kunches LM, Craven DE, Werner BG, et al: Hepatitis B exposure in emergency medical personnel: Prevalence of serologic markers and need for immunization. Am J Med 75:269–272, 1983.
423. Hirchowitz BI, Dasher CA, Whitt FJ, et al: Hepatitis B antigen and antibody and test of liver function: A prospective study of 310 hospital laboratory workers. Am J Clin Pathol 73:63–68, 1980.
424. Redeker AG: Hepatitis B: Risk of infection from antigen-positive personnel and patients (commentary). JAMA 233:1061–1062, 1975.
425. Regenstein FG, Perrillo RP, Bodicky CJ, et al: Hepatitis B vaccine utilization by health care workers: A multi-analysis of factors relating to vaccine acceptance. Adv Ther 3:327–339, 1986.
426. Bodenheimer HC, Fulton JP, Kramer PD: Acceptance of hepatitis B vaccine among hospital workers. Am J Public Health 76:252–255, 1986.
427. Sienko D, Anda RF, McGee HB, et al: Hepatitis B vaccination programs for hospital workers: Results of a statewide survey. Am J Infect Control 16:193–197, 1983.
428. Christian MA: Influenza and hepatitis B vaccine acceptance: A survey of health care workers. Am J Infect Control 19:177–184, 1991.
429. Centers for Disease Control: Hepatitis B vaccine safety: Report of an interagency group. MMWR 31(34):465–467, 1982.
430. Gerety RJ: Hepatitis B. Curr Probl Pediatr May:309–339, 1987.
431. Szmuness W, Stevens CE, Harley EJ: Hepatitis B vaccine: Demonstration of efficacy in a controlled clinical trial in a high risk population in the United States. N Engl J Med 303:833–841, 1980.
432. Zajac BA, West DJ, McAleer WJ, et al: Overview of clinical studies with hepatitis B made by recombinant DNA. J Infect 13(suppl A):39–45, 1986.
433. Zuckerman AJ: Appraisal of intradermal immunisation against hepatitis B. Lancet 1:435–436, 1987.
434. Centers for Disease Control: Inadequate immune response among public safety workers receiving intradermal vaccination against hepatitis B—United States, 1990–1991. MMWR 40(33):569–571, 1991.
435. Gonzales ML, Usandizaga M, Alomar P, et al: Intradermal and intramuscular route for vaccination against hepatitis B. Vaccine 8:402–405, 1990.
436. Wistron J, Settergren B, Gustafsson A, Juto P, et al: Intradermal vs intramuscular route hepatitis B vaccinations (letter). JAMA 264:181–219, 1990.
437. Bryan JP, Sjogren M, Iqbal M, et al: Comparative trial of low-dose intradermal recombinant- and plasma-derived hepatitis B vaccines. J Infect Dis 162:789–793, 1990.
438. Centers for Disease Control: Protection against viral hepatitis: Recommendations of the Immunization Practices Advisory Committee (ACIP). MMWR 39(RR-3):5–22, 1990.
439. Grady DF: Hepatitis B immunity in hospital staff targeted for vaccination. JAMA 248:266–269, 1982.
440. Allen AL, Organ RJ: Occult blood accumulation under the fingernails: A mechanism for the spread of blood-borne infection. J Am Dental Assoc 105:455–459, 1982.
441. Garner JS, Favero MS: CDC guidelines for handwashing and environmental control, 1985. Infect Control 7:231–243, 1986.
442. Centers for Disease Control: Fogging an ineffective measure. National Nosocomial Infection Study Quarterly Report, Third Quarter, 1971, issued May 1972, 00-19-22.
443. 29 Code of Federal Regulations (CFR) Ch. XVII (7-1-85 Edition) 1910.1200, pp 878–889.
444. Administration Halts EPA Disinfectant Tests. Phoenix Sun, Sunday, March 6, 1983, pp A1–A21.
445. Myers T: Failing the test: Germicides or use dilution methodology. Am Soc Microbiol News 54:19–21, 1988.
446. Chemical Specialities Manufacturers Association v. United States Environmental Protection Agency, 484 F. Supp. 513, 1980.
447. Rutula WA, Cole EC: Ineffectiveness of hospital disinfectants against bacteria: A collaborative study. Infect Control 8:501–506, 1988.
448. Spire B, Barre-Sinoussi F, Montagnier L, et al: Inactivation of lymphadenopathy-associated virus by chemical disinfectants. Lancet 1:899–901, 1984.
449. Martin LS, McDougal JS, Loskoski SL: Disinfection and inactivation of the human T-lymphotrophic virus type III/lymphadenopathy-associated virus. J Infect Dis 52:400–403, 1985.
450. Bond WW, Peterson JJ, Favero MS: Viral hepatitis B: Aspects of environmental control series. U.S. Department of Health, Education and Welfare, September 1977, pp 2–19.
451. Bond WW, Petersen NJ, Favero M: Viral hepatitis B: Aspects of environmental control. Health Lab Sci 14:235–252, 1977.
452. Favero MS, Maynard JE, Leger RT, et al: Guidelines for the care of patients hospitalized with viral hepatitis. Ann Intern Med 91:872–876, 1979.
453. Maynard JE: Nosocomial viral hepatitis. Am J Med 70:439–444, 1981.
454. Bond WW, Favero MS, Petersen NJ, et al: Inactivation of hepatitis B virus by intermediate- to high-level disinfectant chemicals. J Clin Microbiol 18:535–538, 1983.
455. Kobayashi J, Tsuzuki M, Koshimizu K, et al: Susceptibility of hepatitis B virus to disinfectants or heat. J Clin Microbiol 20:214–215, 1984.
456. Thompson CJ, Gervin AS: Protect while you provide: Infection control guidelines for prehospital care providers. JEMS November: 44–46, 1987.
457. West KH: Infectious Disease Handbook for Emergency Care Personnel. Philadelphia, JB Lippincott, 1987.
458. West KH: On Guard (videotape). JEMS Publishers, 1988.
459. International Association of Fire Fighters: Hepatitis B Prevention Program (videotape). Philadelphia, PA.
460. Personal communication: Burton H Kaplan, M.D., inventor, pneumatic antishock trousers, and Dave Clark Company, Worcester, MA, manufacturer.
461. Background papers for the Multidisciplinary Curriculum Development Conference on HIV Infection: Report of the Emergency Medical Technicians Task Force on AIDS, September 1987. Washington, The Health Resources and Services Administration of the U.S. Public Health Services, U.S. Department of Health and Human Services, pp 5.1–5.10.
462. Hambraeus A, Ransjo U: Attempts to control clothes-borne infection in a burn unit: I. Experimental investigations of some clothes for barrier nursing. J Hyg Camb 79:193–203, 1977.
463. Forfar JP, MacCabe AF: Masking and gowning in nurseries for the newborn infant: Effect in staphylococcal carriage and infection. Br J Med 1:76, 1958.
464. Black DA, Bannerman CM, Black DA: Carriage of potentially pathogenic bacteria in the hair. Br J Surg 61:735–738, 1975.
465. Cozanitis DA, Makela P, Grant J: Microorganisms in the hair of staff and patients in an intensive care unit. Anaesthetist 26:578–580, 1977.
466. Medical Device Amendments of 1976 (90 Stat. 539).
467. Buxton AE: The intensive care unit. In Bennett JV, Brachman PS (eds): Hospital Infections. Boston, Little, Brown, 1979, pp 99–104.

468. U.S. Department of Health, Education and Welfare: Minimum requirements of construction and equipment for hospital and medical facilities. Health Resources Administration, USDHHS, 1978, DHHS publication No. 81-14500. Washington, U.S. Government Printing Office, 1981.
469. Ayliffe GS, Babb JR, Collins BJ, et al: *Pseudomonas aeruginosa* in hospital sinks. Lancet 1:578, 1974.
470. Taplin D, Mertz PM: Flower vases in hospitals as reservoirs for pathogens. Lancet 2:1279–1280, 1973.
471. Kates SG, McGinley KJ, Larson EL, et al: Indigenous multiresistant bacteria from flowers in hospital and nonhospital environments. Am J Infect Control 19:156–161, 1991.
472. Lister, J: An address on the effect of the antiseptic treatment upon the general salubrity of surgical hospitals. Br Med J 2:769, 1875.

13

WOUND HEALING

JOANNE D. WHITNEY

The concept of healing is central to the care of patients experiencing trauma. Trauma, by definition, implies injury to tissues, including the possible involvement of supporting structures. The extent of wounding varies from minor abrasions, contusions, lacerations, and surgical wounds sustained during treatment to extensive avulsion where tissue separates from underlying structures as a consequence of injury. Following accidental injury, tissue integrity is reestablished through integrated physiological processes and careful therapeutic management. Traumatic wounds differ from wounds that occur as a consequence of surgery, and this has implications for both the healing process and treatment. Major differences associated with trauma include the fact that injuries are often multiple in nature, trauma elicits extensive stress with catecholamine release, there is often concomitant shock, and body reserves are depleted in response to the extent of injury and from shock.[1] These differences and the likelihood of bacterial contamination at the time of injury present the potential for impairment of wound healing. Therefore, care is directed toward the avoidance of complications such as wound infection and delayed healing in addition to maximizing postinjury function of the affected body part.

All wounds, regardless of their origin, heal through the interaction of a complex set of physiological and biochemical responses. This chapter addresses the physical properties of the skin, the physiology of wound healing, and factors that affect healing in order to provide a basis for understanding treatment modalities. Selected aspects of care and wound assessment and management throughout the trauma cycles also will be discussed. Specific information about the use of wound dressings will be addressed in a separate section focusing on choices based on wound characteristics. The latter section diverges from the framework of the trauma cycles because the nature of the wound could be similar regardless of the trauma phase; e.g., primary closure wounds can occur in the resuscitation, critical care, and intermediate care phases.

ANATOMY OF SKIN

The skin or cutis has a surface area of 1.5 to 2.0 m^2 and accounts for 16 per cent of the total body weight, making it the largest organ of the body. It is one of the fastest growing tissues of the body, evidenced by complete replacement every 4 to 6 weeks. Normal skin is critical to survival through its

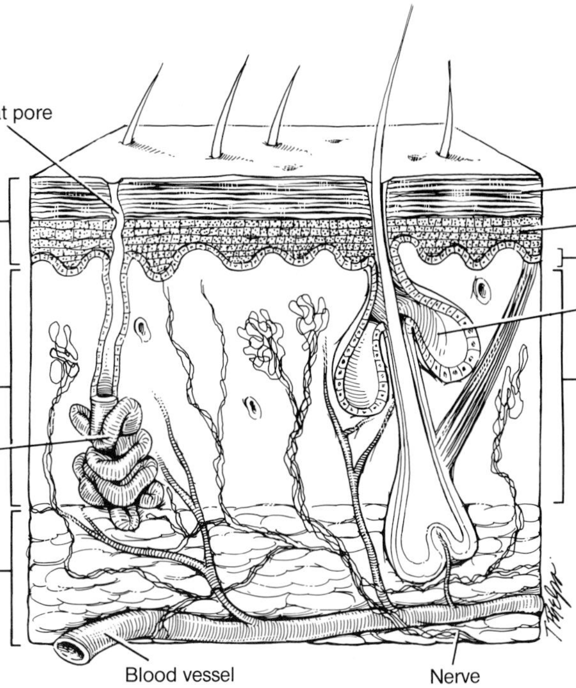

Figure 13–1. Anatomy of the skin.

provision of thermal regulation, prevention of dehydration, and function as a barrier to external insults such as chemicals and microorganisms. The integumentary system is composed of the skin and its appendages: hair, nails, and sweat and sebaceous glands.

The skin is divided anatomically into two major layers: the epidermis and the dermis. The *epidermis* is the external, protective layer, and the *dermis,* composed largely of collagen and elastic fibers, provides strength, elasticity, and protection against mechanical shearing forces. The epidermis, or cuticle, is the outermost layer of the skin and is further divided into the *stratum corneum* (cornified layer), *stratum lucidum* (clear layer), *stratum granulosum* (granular layer), *stratum spinosum* (prickle-cell layer), and *stratum basale* (basal layer) which borders the basement membrane zone.[2] The stratum corneum makes up the most superficial skin layer and is composed of nonviable, desiccated cells that are continually shed; below this horny layer are the living cells in the basal, spinous, and granular layers. The columnar basal cells undergo continual mitosis and are the source of new cells that eventually reach the stratum corneum. The epidermis provides the exit for hair follicles and glands. The thickness of the epidermis varies with body surface location, the eyelids having thinner layers with thicker layers found in the soles of the feet and palms of the hands.

The dermis, or corium, lies between the epidermis and the subcutaneous tissue. The dermis is a connective tissue composed of fibrous proteins (collagen and elastin) in a gel of ground substance (glycosaminoglycans).[2] The junction between epidermis and dermis is undulated with upward-projecting dermal papillae and downward-projecting rete ridges. The dermis nourishes the epidermis through its rich supply of vascular and lymphatic structures. There is a superficial layer, the papillary dermis, composed of interlacing fine collagen fibers, blood vessels, nerve endings, and thermoreceptors and a deeper reticular layer of thicker bundles of collagen which provide the skin with structural support (Fig. 13–1). Sensory receptors within the papillary dermis respond to pain, cold, heat, touch, and pressure. Dermal appendages, hair follicles, and sweat glands are within the reticular dermis and extend upward through the epidermis. These serve as an important source of epidermal regeneration during wound healing.[3]

The subcutaneous tissue, or panniculus, lies between the lower border of the dermis and the deeper fascia and muscle tissues. Though not generally considered part of the true skin, it is closely associated with the dermis and is an important tissue to consider in terms of wound healing. The subcutaneous tissue functions to absorb shock, insulate, store nutrients, and shape the body contour. It is composed of many cells: adipocytes, fibroblasts, histiocytes, plasma cells, lymphocytes, and mast cells. Fat lobules of the panniculus are surrounded by strands of collagen that contain nerves and vascular and lymphatic networks that travel from the fascia to supply the dermis. There are few vascular connections between fat lobules and neighboring structures, which leaves the subcutaneous tissue vulnerable to decreases in vascular supply.[4] This, in turn, has implications for wound healing. Complications of impaired healing such as infection often have their origin in subcutaneous tissue.

The integumentary system functions as a barrier and buffer zone against environmental insults and provides an essential means of communication, particularly for the visually impaired. Tactile stimulation is vital for normal growth and development and for normal psychophysiological function. Accidental injury may result in damage to any or all layers of the integument. A superficial abrasion involves the epidermal layer of the skin. Full-thickness injuries involve the epidermal and dermal skin layers and also may affect subcutaneous tissue, muscle, and bone.

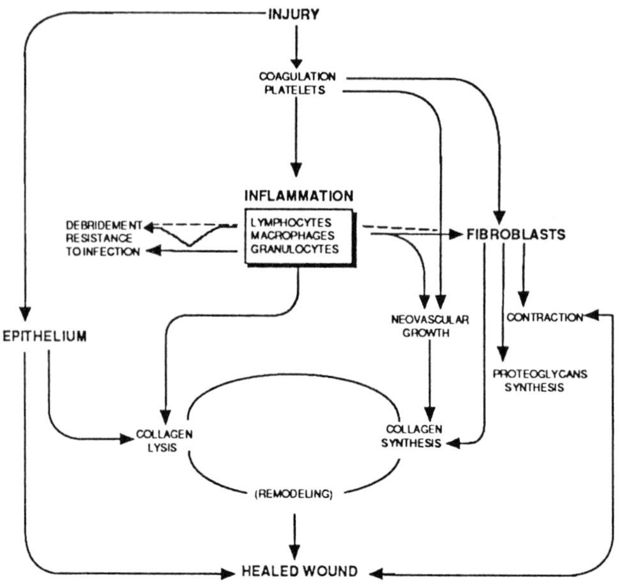

Figure 13–2. Flow diagram of normal repair. (From Hunt TK: Disorders of wound healing. World J Surg 4(3):272–277, 1980.)

WOUND HEALING PHYSIOLOGY

When the skin or internal organs are disrupted by trauma or surgery, a series of interdependent physiological events occur that result in tissue repair (Fig. 13–2). These occur within the three major phases of healing—inflammation, proliferation, and remodeling. The tissue response has seven major components: (1) hemostasis, (2) inflammation, (3) fibroblast proliferation, (4) matrix deposition, (5) angiogenesis, (6) or epithelialization, and (7) contraction.[5] Through these responses, the process of healing is initiated, directed, and finally completed with the formation of scar tissue.

Wound healing occurs through *primary* or *secondary intention* or, alternately, by *delayed primary closure,* also called *third-intention healing.* In primary-intention healing, wound edges are reapproximated using suture material or staples, and healing occurs through the formation of new blood vessels, scar tissue, and epidermal repair. In second-intention healing, wounds are left open, and healing occurs through formation of granulation tissue, contraction, and reepithelialization. In wounds in which initial bacteria counts are high, the technique of delayed primary closure is often used. The wound is left open temporarily until bacterial load is decreased, at which point wound edges are reapproximated or the area is closed by skin graft.

Tissue repair is a complex process with multiple vascular, cellular, and biochemical responses. A number of cells are important to the healing process. Polymorphonuclear leukocytes, macrophages, fibroblasts, endothelial cells, and epithelial cells function interdependently to restore tissue integrity. The actual time frame for healing varies depending on several factors, such as wound type (e.g., primary- or secondary-intention healing) and host factors (e.g., nutritional status, general physical condition). Generally, in acute wounds inflammatory events occur in the first days after injury. Collagen synthesis begins within days of injury and peaks at 7 to 9 days. Collagen remodeling begins about 3 weeks after injury and may continue for 6 months or a year. The first days and weeks following injury are critical periods in the healing process when multiple cellular events occur.

Hemostasis and Inflammation

Inflammation is a critical component of healing. Altered vascularity, coagulation, and inflammation occur immediately after wounding, beginning the process of normal repair. The initial response to injury is vasoconstriction, which produces hypoxia, tissue acidosis, and lactate accumulation. When blood is exposed to collagen, Hageman factor is activated and initiates platelet degranulation and the coagulation cascade (Fig. 13–3). Platelets are activated, and platelet factors that enhance fibroblast and monocyte migration and proliferation are released. The platelet factors include serotonin and thromboxane A_2 (which cause vasoconstriction), adenosine diphosphate, platelet-derived growth factor (PDGF), platelet-derived angiogenic factor (PDAF), platelet-derived epidermal growth factor (PDEGF), transforming growth factors alpha and beta (TGF-α, TGF-β), and platelet factor 4 (PF-4).[5, 6] PDGF is mitogenic and chemotactic for fibro-

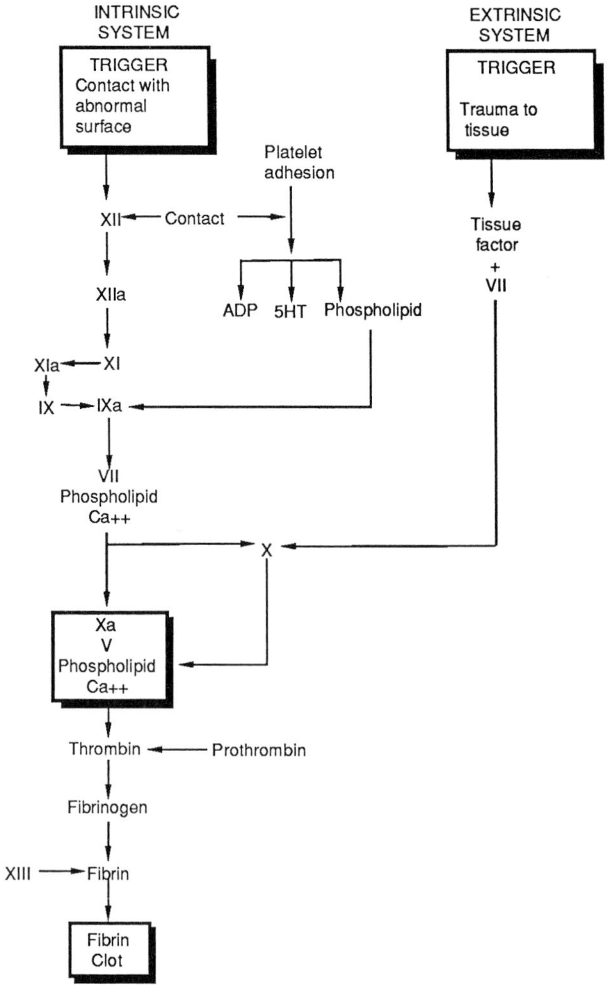

Figure 13–3. The clotting cascade.

blasts,[7] PDAF is chemotactic for capillary endothelial cells,[8] PDEGF is a mitogenic chemoattractant for epidermal cells, and TGF-β attracts monocytes and stimulates the production of collagen by fibroblasts.[9, 10] Platelet factor 4 is a chemoattractant for neutrophils.[11] The interaction of wound healing events and growth factors is diagramed in Figure 13–4.

Hageman factor also activates the plasma proteins of the complement system and the vasodilator peptides of the kinin cascade. Activation of the complement cascade produces biologically active molecules that opsonize and lyse bacteria, cause histamine release from mast cells, and act as chemotactic factors that attract inflammatory cells, i.e., polymorphonuclear leukocytes (PMNs) and monocytes, to the area of injury.[12] PMNs help protect the wound from infection initiated by foreign organisms. Monocytes ingest material and become tissue macrophages that phagocytose debris and destroy bacteria. Macrophages are required for healing and play a role in collagen synthesis through stimulation of fibroblasts.[13, 14] Histamine and the kinins act to relax vascular smooth muscle, producing vasodilation and increased blood flow to the area of injury. In addition, kinins attract inflammatory cells and cause capillary permeability to increase.[15] Once vasodilation and increased capillary permeability occur, intravascular elements, protein, enzymes, and cells leak into the wound area. In summary, the early physiologic responses to injury accomplish hemostasis through clot formation, increase blood flow to the wound, and begin to clear the wound of cellular debris and provide substrates to the tissues.

Fibroblast Proliferation and Synthesis of Connective Tissue

The proliferative phase of healing is characterized by the activity of fibroblasts. Soon after injury, undifferentiated mesenchymal cells in the area of injury are stimulated by growth factors and begin to differentiate into migratory fibroblasts.[16] The migrating fibroblasts use strands of fibrin and fibronectin as a scaffold for migration across the wound. The major function of fibroblasts in wound healing is to synthesize the basic monomer of the collagen fiber. In addition, fibroblasts also synthesize proteoglycans and elastin.[17] Fibroblasts are stimulated to produce collagen. Data from experiments of cultured fibroblasts suggest that an area of hypoxia and high lactate concentration or a high ascorbic acid concentration may activate some of the collagen-synthesizing enzymes of the fibroblasts.[16]

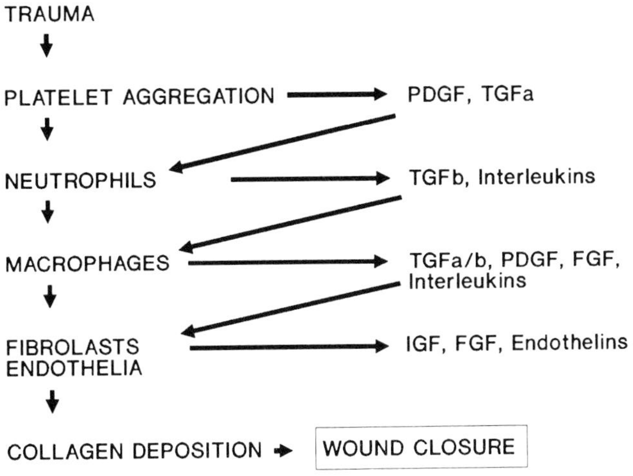

Figure 13–4. Sequence of cellular events following injury. (From Herndon DN, Hayward PG, Rutan RL, Barrow RE: Growth hormones and factors in surgical patients. Adv Surg 25:65–97, 1992.)

Collagen provides strength and support to new tissues through its deposition and cross-linking in the injured area. There are several types of collagen with different tissue distributions. Type I is the predominant collagen in skin, tendon, and bone. Type II collagen is distributed primarily in cartilage, type III in fetal skin and the cardiovascular system, and type IV in basement membranes.[18] Fibroblasts synthesize the basic structural unit of collagen, procollagen. Collagen formation (Fig. 13–5) depends on the enzymes lysyl and prolyl hydroxylase and the presence of molecular oxygen. As collagen is formed on ribosomes, transfer RNA (tRNA) brings specific amino acids to the chain; there is no tRNA for the amino acids hydroxyproline or hydroxylysine. Proline and lysine residues are incorporated into the growing collagen chains and are converted to hydroxyproline and hydroxylysine through enzymatic attachment of an oxygen atom by the hydroxylases.[18] Alpha-ketoglutarate, ascorbate, and iron are other cofactors required for collagen synthesis. The precursor chain of collagen is subsequently glycosylated and assembled into procollagen. Procollagen molecules are secreted into the extracellular wound space, where they become tropocollagen through enzymatic cleavage of peptidases. Tropocollagen has three polypeptide chains of the same size; chain composition varies depending on the collagen type.[18] The tropocollagen then forms larger collagen fibers. The fibers band together by cross-linking and overlapping. Collagen is both synthesized and degraded in a continual process of turnover.[19] The strength of older collagen in the wound decreases with lysis as the strength of new collagen increases with synthesis.[16] Collagen fibrils also become compressed as water and mucopolysaccharides are lost from the wound, promoting intermolecular cross-links that strengthen the collagen polymer.[17]

Over several weeks the collagen is remodeled, and the fibers that remain are those oriented parallel to lines of tension. By the third week after injury the wound has its greatest mass, and net collagen loss begins. The processes of collagen synthesis, lysis, and fiber cross-linking result in collagen with greater organization and a stronger, tighter matrix.

Angiogenesis

New capillary formation closely follows the entry of fibroblasts into the wound. New capillaries result from endothelial budding of existing capillaries in tissues surrounding the wound and are supported by the collagen produced by fibroblasts. Tissue hypoxia, such as that occurring in the central space of a wound where tissue oxygen levels are close to 0 mm Hg, appears to act as one stimulus for angiogenesis. New capillary buds and loops have been shown to advance toward tumor implants in rabbit corneas.[20] Hypoxic wound gradients stimulate macrophages to produce plasminogen activator, mitogenesis factor(s), and angiogenesis factor(s), which in turn stimulate angiogenesis.[21] The investigators proposed a mechanism by which these factors stimulate

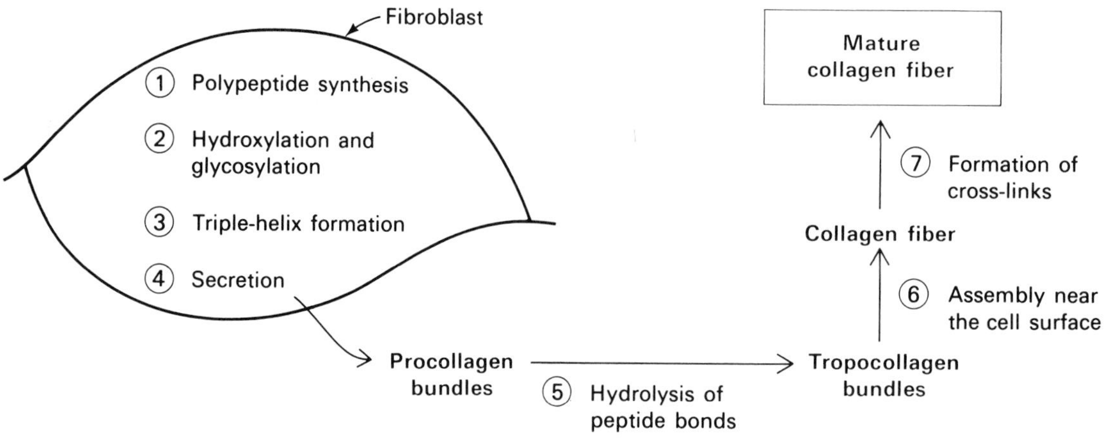

Figure 13–5. Steps in the formation of mature collagen fibers. (From Stryer L: Biochemistry, 2nd ed. New York, Freeman, 1981.)

proliferation of surrounding connective tissue; when the wound heals to the extent that oxygen tension in the wound space increases, secretion of the macrophage angiogenesis factor is suppressed.[21] In addition, platelets release angiogenic factor that stimulates endothelial cells either directly or through other cells such as macrophages.[22] As endothelial cells grow toward the hypoxic wound edge, capillary buds join with other similar buds, forming new capillary loops and reestablishing blood flow.[16] The new vasculature provides a continued supply of nutrients for wound healing and formation of the granulation bed consisting of fibroblasts, collagen, new vessels, and macrophages.

Epithelialization

The migration of epithelial cells across a wound provides protection against entry of bacteria into the wound and wound fluid loss. Within 24 to 48 hours of wounding, epithelial marginal basal cells enlarge, flatten, undergo mitosis, and migrate over the defect.[23] When the layer is complete, the cells again divide, forming another layer of epithelium. Hair follicles also serve as a source of epithelial cells, forming islands of epithelial tissue in wounds. The cells migrate a distance of one cell diameter an hour.[24] Desiccation of wounds and eschar on the wound surface act as a deterrent to movement of epithelial cells. In wounds allowed to heal in a moist, protected environment, epithelial cells migrate on top of the wound. This is in contrast to wounds that epithelialize by cell migration under eschar that forms when a wound is allowed to become dry. The rate of epithelialization in surgically formed epidermal wounds that were kept moist was twice as fast as in wounds exposed to air, showing that moist healing is a faster and more economical process than healing in a dry wound bed.[25]

Contraction

Wound contraction occurs in open wounds that are closing through the deposition of granulation tissue. It is the active process by which the area of a full-thickness wound is decreased by movement of the whole thickness of surrounding skin.[23] In this process, new tissue is not formed; the area of the wound is closed by inward movement of existing tissue at the wound edge. The mechanism by which contraction occurs is not well understood but is attributed to the activity of fibroblasts and is a process that is independent of changes in collagen.[23] Myofibroblasts, cells with microfibril and microtubule components, present within the granulation tissue are thought to be the cells responsible for contraction.[26] Myofibroblasts have been identified in granulating skin wounds of rabbits and have been shown to respond similarly to smooth muscle in response to pharmacological stimulants and relaxants.[26, 27] It also has been proposed that contraction results from the combined effects of vascular supply, fibroblasts, and the connective-tissue matrix within the healing wound.[28]

Remodeling

As healing progresses, edema decreases, and the numbers of fibroblasts and blood vessels recede.[16] The local metabolic needs of the tissue decrease and no longer require the support of a dense cellular and vascular network. The tissue enters into the final repair process, remodeling. This begins around 3 weeks after injury and continues over many months. As described earlier, the scar tissue loses mass and gradually gains strength as collagen remodels into an organized and tighter matrix. As the scar tissue matures, it also generally changes color and form. The early red, edematous, firm scar softens, lightens to pink, and becomes smaller. The scar tissue is strengthened through remodeling; however, skin and fascia only achieve approximately 80 per cent of their original strength. This degree of strength is achieved somewhere between 3 and 6 months after injury in wounds closed primarily.

DETERMINANTS OF THE HEALING PROCESS

Physiologically, wound healing begins at the moment of injury and proceeds through cellular recruitment and interaction until tissue continuity is reestablished. Several factors

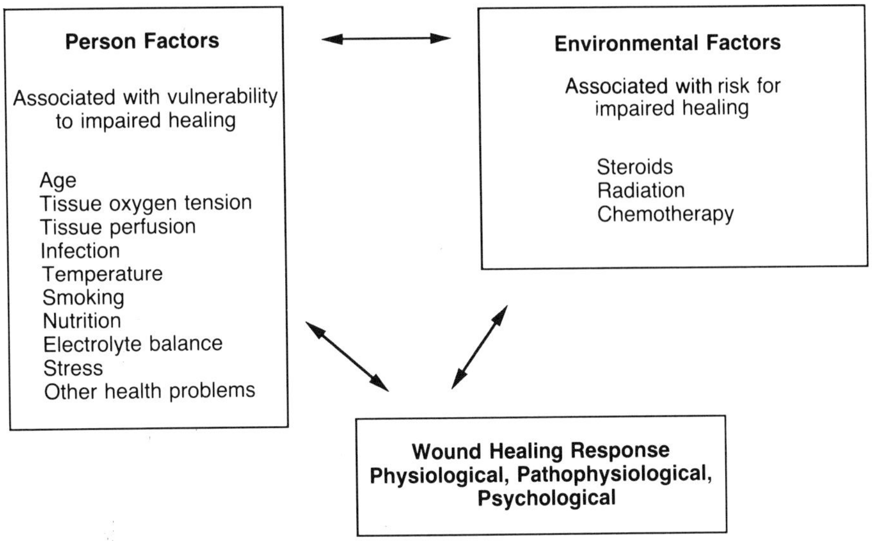

Figure 13–6. Human response model of factors that influence wound healing.

influence the healing process. These can be organized conceptually into a human response model that includes factors inherent in the person that increase vulnerability for impaired healing and environmental factors that present a risk for impairment of healing[29] (Fig. 13–6). Some of the factors may be modifiable, while others are not; all are worthy of consideration in order to provide appropriate therapy and an environment that supports healing.

Person Factors

Age

Advancing age influences healing. In general, it takes longer for healing to occur as a person ages. Though not a controlled study, observations of wounds made during World War I showed an increase in time required for contraction and closure with each decade between the ages 20 and 40.[30] Delay in other healing processes such as epithelialization and decreases in wound breaking strength have been reported in subsequent studies. Factors associated with aging, such as lowered immunological resistance, circulatory changes, and poor nutritional status, may contribute to these healing changes. Studies of cell migration, DNA synthesis, cell division, biosynthetic activity, and enzyme activity in both human and animal models suggest a delay in these processes with increased age.[31]

Tissue Oxygen Tension and Perfusion

Oxygen is essential to meet the energy needs of biologic activity; it is the ultimate acceptor of electrons in the electron-transport chain where ATP is produced. More specifically, in wounds, oxygen and perfusion play critical roles in the healing process and are related to a number of host factors that influence healing. Clinicians have long known that ischemic and hypoxic tissues do not heal. An adequate supply of oxygen to the wounded area is needed for synthesis and accumulation of collagen, and an increased oxygen supply enhances angiogenesis and epithelialization.[32–34] Increasing the supply of ambient oxygen to 35 to 45 per cent significantly increased hydroxyproline content (a measure of collagen content) of healing wounds in experimental animals.[32] Similarly, the rate of epithelialization in open wounds increased in a hyperoxic environment and decreased under conditions of hypoxia.[33] Through the use of a wound chamber method where observation of healing is possible, angiogenesis was noted to be faster for animals breathing 45 per cent oxygen versus those breathing 12 per cent oxygen.[34] These and other studies have enhanced our understanding of the importance of oxygen to several healing processes and provide evidence that increasing the supply of oxygen produces favorable healing results.

A complex physiological system determines tissue oxygen levels and is depicted in Figure 13–7. In terms of wound healing, blood supply is of particular concern and is discussed in greater detail. In addition, the relationship of oxygen to control of bacteria in the wound space is given special attention, as are selected variables that have been studied to advance understanding of their influence on oxygen supply

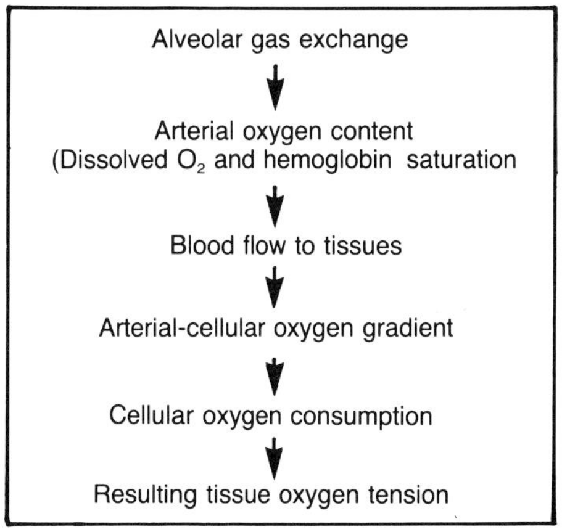

Figure 13–7. Determinants of tissue oxygen tension. (From Whitney JD: The influence of tissue oxygen and perfusion on wound healing. In Stotts NA (ed): Wound Healing: AACN Clinical Issues in Critical Care. Philadelphia, JB Lippincott, 1990.)

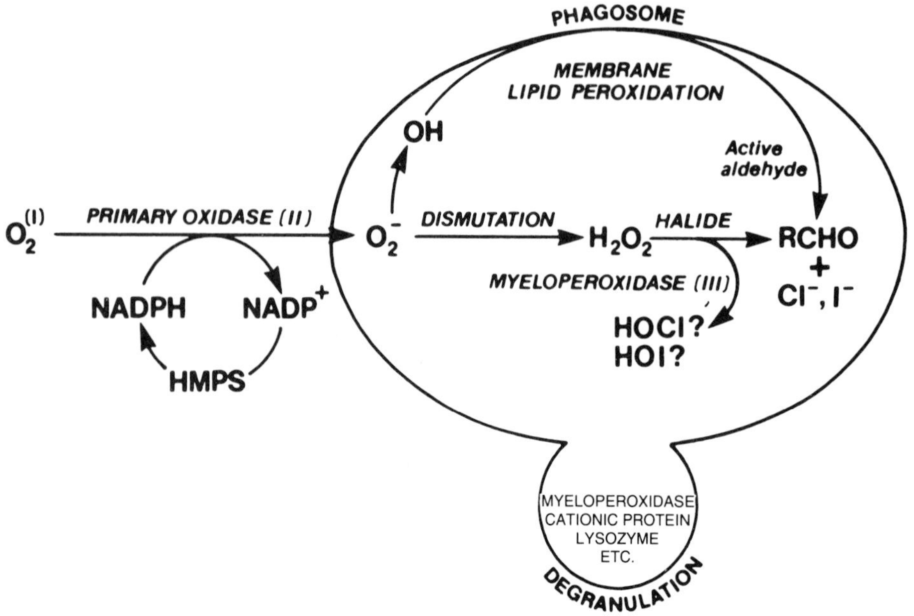

Figure 13–8. Schema of oxidative killing mechanisms. (Reprinted by permission of the publisher from Rabkin JM, Hunt TK: Infection and oxygen. In Davis JC, Hunt TK (eds): Problem Wounds and the Role of Oxygen. New York, Elsevier, 1988. Copyright 1988 by Elsevier Science Publishing Co., Inc.)

and healing. Many of these are frequently encountered in clinical practice.

Perfusion. Oxygen delivery, along with supply of neutrophils, monocytes, other cells, and nutrients, is closely linked to perfusion. Measurement of tissue oxygen tension has provided information about blood flow to peripheral tissues. Decreases in tissue oxygen reflect decreases in blood flow, provided pulmonary status is normal. This has become apparent through studies in human and animal systems where tissue oxygen has been measured during blood volume changes. In these studies there has been a clear response of decreased oxygen tension in the tissue with a slow recovery to baseline once volume is replaced despite the observation that both blood pressure and cardiac output return to normal levels.[35] The sacrifice of blood flow to connective tissues when vascular volume is depleted even marginally has been demonstrated in surgical populations. Low subcutaneous tissue oxygen tensions in the range of 25 to 40 mm Hg (normal is approximately 70 mm Hg) have been recorded in the presence of adequate urine output and normal parameters for other clinical indicators of peripheral perfusion.[36, 37] In these studies, tissue oxygen levels increased markedly when patients were given supplemental intravenous fluids, demonstrating the need for support of vascular volume to ensure adequate perfusion of peripheral tissue beds. This has implications for trauma patients, who are likely to experience hypovolemia and sepsis; blood volume needs to be maintained, sometimes above normal, in order to preserve wound perfusion and tissue oxygenation.[38]

In certain cases where tissue oxygen needs cannot be met through standard treatment modalities, hyperbaric treatment may be considered. Hyperbaric delivery of oxygen increases oxygen levels in soft tissues that are infected (e.g., necrotizing fasciitis) or slow to heal because of damage to the circulation.[39] It should be remembered that although these tissues are often hypoperfused, at least some degree of blood supply must be present in order to effectively deliver oxygen to the wound site. The cellular use of oxygen is the same as in any wound; it is used by leukocytes, fibroblasts, endothelial cells, and other cells in their reparative roles of bacterial control, collagen synthesis, and angiogenesis.

Infection. Traumatic wounds are often contaminated with the bacteria from the environment where the wound occurred. Wounds that contain greater than 10^5 organisms per gram of tissue are at risk for subsequent infection. Fewer bacteria may result in wound infection in cases where local defense is compromised by necrotic tissue, dead space, or foreign bodies. Oxygen is used in the aerobic pathway of leukocytes for the killing of bacteria that have been introduced or migrated to the wound site (Fig. 13–8). Oxygen is converted into free radicals that form a system of bactericidal agents. As leukocytes phagocytose bacteria, a primary oxidase in the cell membrane is activated that catalyzes an oxidation reaction with subsequent killing of the bacteria. In the process, the cells increase their respirations and oxygen consumption in what has been termed the *respiratory burst.*[40] Recent experimental evidence has shown that sufficient tissue oxygen levels are needed to resist infection. A local tissue Po_2 of 30 mm Hg or greater is needed for phagocytes to kill bacteria effectively.[41] Furthermore, the clearance of bacteria in infected wounds is significantly higher under conditions of relative hyperoxia (45 per cent supplemental oxygen) compared with anoxic or normoxic states.[42] Providing supplemental oxygen also has been shown to significantly decrease the size of infected lesions both by itself and in combination with antibiotics, which led investigators to coin the phrase "oxygen as an antibiotic."[43] Recent study of general surgery patients indicates that there is a level of tissue oxygen below which risk of wound infection increases.[44] The investigators reported that patients with subcutaneous oxygen tensions below 72 mm Hg had significantly higher rates of infection in relation to their predicted rate of wound infection based on Centers for Disease Control criteria.

Anemia, Temperature, and Smoking. Several factors

can restrict tissue oxygen supply. Anemia and smoking are two host elements that influence tissue oxygen and potentially healing. Because oxygen is transported primarily by hemoglobin, there is concern that oxygen supply will be limited due to anemia. However, a number of studies to date indicate that anemia is not as serious a threat to healing as once thought. Anemia in the presence of normal vascular volume and cardiac function does not impair wound healing until the hematocrit reaches a very low level (15–17 per cent).[45] At that point, transfusion is beneficial in terms of maintaining tissue oxygen supply. This was confirmed in a study of surgical patients that emphasized that provided perfusion is maintained, anemia does not interfere with wound healing because wounds consume relatively little oxygen.[46]

Hypothermia may indirectly influence healing through the thermoregulatory responses it elicits with subsequent vasoconstriction and lowered tissue oxygen.[47] During and after extensive surgery, body temperature may drop below 36°C, invoking cutaneous vasoconstriction and shivering mediated through the sympathetic nervous system. Energy and oxygen consumption rise above resting levels, further increasing the need for adequate oxygen supply to tissues. In addition, leukocyte activity is also adversely affected by decreases in body temperature. In contrast, local hyperthermia, as well as maintaining a normothermic state, may be beneficial in terms of supporting tissue oxygen tension and wound healing, although these have not been well studied. Application of a local heat source has been shown to improve tissue oxygen levels. Oxygen tension in the subcutaneous tissue of a small sample of hospitalized patients showed a mean increase of 39.5 mm Hg in response to application of a heat pack.[48] The duration of the increase in tissue oxygenation and its influence on healing outcomes were not evaluated. The use of local heat as a wound therapy, including the type of wound where its use is appropriate, remains an area for further study.

Smoking has several detrimental effects, including decreased amounts of functional hemoglobin and, more important, peripheral vasoconstriction. A recent study has documented that smoking lowers subcutaneous oxygen tension acutely, with oxygen levels remaining depressed for 30 to 50 minutes.[49] Lowered tissue oxygen can in part explain clinical observations and other research evidence that indicates that smokers are vulnerable to a variety of healing problems.

Nutritional Status

Nutritional assessment and maintenance of the trauma patient are discussed in detail in Chapter 14; however, several areas are notable for their effect on healing. A sufficient amount of glucose is important in local wound metabolism because it provides fuel for a number of cells, including leukocytes. Multiple trauma frequently leads to depleted protein status and lowered serum proteins; fewer amino acids are available for fibroplasia, collagen synthesis, and the formation of antibodies and leukocytes. If the patient has sustained a recent weight loss of greater than 10 per cent of lean body mass, there is an increased chance for wound complications.[50] Vitamins and trace minerals are important for several biochemical processes. Collagen formation requires vitamin C, iron, and zinc as cofactors. Vitamin C is necessary for hydroxylation reactions involving proline and lysine during collagen synthesis. Collagen that is synthesized in conditions of vitamin C depletion is insufficiently hydroxylated and lacks strength because normal collagen fibers cannot be formed.[18] Iron and zinc are also involved in hydroxylation reactions. In addition, iron plays a critical role in oxygen transport. Zinc is necessary for certain enzyme systems pertinent to healing, e.g., superoxide dismutase, which is involved in the dismutation of superoxide radicals in activated neutrophils.[51] The contributions of specific nutrients to wound healing are listed in Table 13–1. A review of the numerous processes related to healing that are linked to nutrition emphasizes the profound impact that nutrient depletion and elevation of the basal metabolic rate have on healing.

Electrolyte Balance

Normal serum electrolytes are essential for cell function. Potassium is necessary for maintaining protein anabolism for wound repair and may be lowered through loss of body fluids and in response to adrenocortical hormone release in trauma. Release of aldosterone can result in potassium loss and sodium retention, which, in turn, alter cellular responses. Phagocytosis is inhibited by serum sodium levels in excess of 300 mmol/l and by elevated serum glucose levels. Serum pH has direct effects on cell motility. Acidosis decreases phagocytosis, thereby diminishing an essential component of the inflammatory response.

Stress

Stress has the potential to impair healing in two ways: through physical and/or psychological stressors. Physical stress to the edges of a wound can lead to partial or complete separation. The stress may be the result of strain, movement, or weight bearing on an injured extremity. Vomiting and abdominal distention also can disrupt chest or abdominal wounds. For this reason, adequate gastric decompression and drainage of bladder or wound cavities are important to avoid unnecessary stress to healing suture lines. Psychological stress increases metabolic rate, oxygen consumption, and glucocorticoid levels. Natural and synthetic glucocorticoids alter the healing process. Cortisol, a major hormone released during stress, affects collagen metabolism and has been shown to decrease wound tensile strength in experimental models.[52] Minimizing stressors may indirectly influence wound healing by reducing the stress response. Only recently have reports from studies directed at stress reduction and wound healing in humans become available. In addition, investigators are beginning to examine cellular and physiological effects of factors such as noise that can contribute to stress. These studies provide the beginnings of a scientific basis indicating that stress reduction may be a useful strategy to positively affect wound healing and related biological events.[53, 54]

Preexisting Health Conditions

Primary vascular disease, immunological disorders, or diseases where depression of immune function is common such as cancer, diabetes, and uremia contribute to vulnerability to impaired healing. Diabetes is associated with small vessel disease that can limit blood supply to the wound area, and hyperglycemia retards neutrophil function so that infection

TABLE 13–1. NUTRIENTS AFFECTING WOUND HEALING

NUTRIENT	SPECIFIC COMPONENT	CONTRIBUTION TO WOUND HEALING
Proteins	Amino acids	Needed for neovascularization, lymphocyte formation, fibroblast proliferation, collagen synthesis, and wound remodeling Required for certain cell-mediated responses, including phagocytosis and intracellular killing of bacteria
	Albumin	Prevents wound edema secondary to low serum oncotic pressure
Carbohydrates	Glucose	Needed for energy requirement of leukocytes and fibroblasts to function in inhibiting activities of wound infection
Fats	Essential unsaturated fatty acids a. Linoleic b. Linolenic c. Arachidonic	Serve as building blocks for prostaglandins that regulate cellular metabolism, inflammation, and circulation Are constituents of triglycerides and fatty acids contained in cellular and subcellular membranes
Vitamins	Ascorbic acid	Hydroxylates proline and lysine in collagen synthesis Enhances capillary formation and decreases capillary fragility Is a necessary component of complement that functions in immune reactions and increases defenses to infection
	B complex	Serve as cofactors of enzyme systems
	Pyridoxine, pantothenic and folic acid	Required for antibody formation and white blood cell function
	A	Enhances epithelialization of cell membranes Enhances rate of collagen synthesis and cross-linking of newly formed collagen Antagonizes the inhibitory effects of glucocorticoids on cell membranes
	D	Necessary for absorption, transport, and metabolism of calcium Indirectly affects phosphorus metabolism
	E	No special role known; may be important if there is a fatty acid deficiency
	K	Needed for synthesis of prothrombin and clotting factors VII, IX, and X Required for synthesis of calcium-binding protein
Minerals	Zinc	Stabilizes cell membranes Needed for cell mitosis and cell proliferation in wound repair
	Iron	Needed for hydroxylation of proline and lysine in collagen synthesis Enhances bactericidal activity of leukocytes Secondarily, deficiency may cause decrease in oxygen transport to wound
	Copper	Is an integral part of the enzyme lysyloxidase, which catalyzes formation of stable collagen cross-links

From Schumann D: Preoperative measures to promote wound healing. Nurs Clin North Am 14:683–697, 1979.

becomes a greater risk. Control of serum glucose levels to below 200 mg/dl in the first 72 hours after injury will decrease wound-healing complications.[55] Uremia adversely affects healing through a reduction in granulation tissue formation and collagen polymerization; hypovolemia with tissue hypoxia has been suggested as a possible explanation for decreased healing in these patients.[50] Chronic use of alcohol studied in a murine model was associated with impairment of collagen accumulation.[56] The potential mechanism for this effect is not known. The acute effects of high blood alcohol levels often present in trauma victims may impair healing through metabolic disturbances associated with alcohol.[1]

Environmental Factors

Glucocorticoid Steroids

Glucocorticoids, cortisone in particular, have an inhibitory effect on inflammation, collagen formation, angiogenesis, and contraction. Early work provided information about the temporal relationship between administration of cortisone and healing.[57] The tensile strength of wounds was significantly lowered when cortisone was given either within 3 days of wounding or throughout the healing period after wounding. If cortisone treatment was started 2 days after wounding, tensile strength was not affected. Administration of vitamin A has been shown to counteract the detrimental effects of cortisone on wound strength.[58] However, it should be noted that vitamin A does not reverse the effects of steroids on wound contraction. The known inhibitory effects of steroids on healing underscore the importance of assessing the patient's medication history so that appropriate counteractive systemic therapy can be provided. In addition, because of the immunosuppression associated with steroid therapy, careful monitoring for infection is critical.

Radiation and Chemotherapy

Wounds that occur in tissue that has previously received radiation are likely to have impaired healing. Radiation alters the normal cellularity and vasculature of tissue, which, in turn, renders the tissue incapable of mounting a normal response to injury. The epidermis is thinned, the numbers and quality of blood vessels are decreased, and the dermis is fibrotic with many irregular fibroblasts.[59] Potentially, chemotherapeutic agents impair healing because they interrupt the natural cell cycle. In addition, these agents induce thrombocytopenia and leukopenia, reducing the inflammatory response to injury. Experimental models have suggested that in the presence of specific chemotherapeutic agents, healing is impaired; however, there is less evidence available to support these findings in clinical populations.[59] Based on existing knowledge, patients who have recently received either radiation or chemotherapy should be considered candidates for potential healing problems.

PRINCIPLES OF WOUND ASSESSMENT THROUGHOUT THE TRAUMA CYCLES

Traumatic wounds result from the impact of an energy source applied against the skin and underlying structures. The initial assessment is focused on the treatment of life-threatening conditions and, of necessity, precedes the exterior wound assessment and subsequent treatment. Once the patient's condition is stabilized, wound assessment is done concurrently with the physical examination and the patient's history. Assessment information throughout all the cycles provides the basis for development of the wound-management plan. During this process, the patient is assessed thoroughly and is included as an active participant to the greatest extent possible. Patient involvement is generally limited only by physical condition. Many injuries that involve the skin are not life-threatening, but they may have considerable psychological impact depending on a number of factors. For this reason, information about the patient's perception of the injury, its impact on daily living, and available support systems is included in the assessment.

Wound History

The wound history includes the details of the accident, including the time and the mechanism of injury (see also Chapter 7). The age of the wound and the environment in which it occurred must be identified. The "golden period" or "period of grace" is the amount of time before the inoculum introduced into the wound reaches critical proportions in terms of numbers of bacteria increasing the likelihood of infection. Study of wounds in an emergency department indicates that a delay in treatment of 3 hours or greater is associated with an increase in bacteria to levels above 10^5 per gram of tissue.[60] This places patients for whom treatment is delayed by several hours at considerable risk for the development of infection.

The environment of the wound includes both the location on the body and the source of the injury. The distribution of microorganisms on the body varies; in general, moister body areas harbor greater numbers than drier areas.[61] Table 13–2 identifies the typical concentration of skin microflora. Information about the physical environment in which the wound occurs helps to predict the existence of foreign bodies in the wound space, e.g., clothing fragments, and types of soil and dirt, which may vary depending on the source.[62] Similarly, an injury caused by a clean knife from the kitchen has different implications than one caused by mechanical equipment on a farm or a motorcycle accident on a city street. The organic components of soil and inorganic clay fragments have been associated with the development of wound infections due presumably to their inhibitory effect on host defense systems.[62] Organic fractions are heavily concentrated in swamps, bogs, and marshes, while clay fractions are largely located in the subsoil.[58] Thus there is an increased risk of contamination and wound infection if injury occurs in swamps or excavation areas. Injuries that occur in farm areas have the potential for contamination with *Clostridium tetani;* the bacteria's natural habitat is the intestinal tract of domesticated animals, and it is consequently found in their excretions.

The patient's history also includes an assessment of concomitant disease, which may influence the course of healing, as discussed earlier. History of medication use, allergies, previous healing impairment, and tetanus immunization status (Fig. 13–9) is also pertinent to the wound treatment regimen.

Physical Examination

Examination begins in order to detect sensory, motor, and vascular complications that may have resulted from the injury in addition to the physical wound. This is followed by assessment of the wound status, location, configuration, and viability of tissue, after which initial wound treatments are implemented.

Neurovascular Assessment

A comprehensive neurovascular assessment is performed and documented prior to initiating wound treatment in order to document the existence of complications related to the injury itself as opposed to treatment-induced complications. The components of the assessment are movement, sensation, color, temperature, presence of pulses, and edema. Comparison of the affected wounded area with its contralateral anatomical site is useful to determine disruption in neurovascular function.

Sensory-Motor Function. The patient is tested for both sensory and motor integrity within the affected area. Both gross and fine motor functions are tested, including the flexion and extension of each joint and full range of motion of each extremity. Sensation distal to the wound can be tested grossly by discrimination between sharp and dull sensations. Systematic evaluation is based on knowledge of the major nerves serving the extremities.

TABLE 13–2. COMPOSITION AND CONCENTRATION OF SKIN MICROFLORA

SKIN REGION	TOTAL BACTERIAL CONCENTRATIONS	AEROBE/ANAEROBE RATIO
Moister areas (axillae, perineum)	10^4 to 10^6	10:1
Drier areas (trunk, upper arms, and legs)	10^1 to 10^3	5 to 10:1
Exposed areas (head, face, and feet)*	10^4 to 10^6	5 to 10:1

*Anaerobes may outnumber aerobes in the skin of the cheeks, upper back, and presternum.
From Edlich RF, Rodeheaver GT, Morgan RF, et al: Principles of emergency wound management. Ann Emerg Med 17:1284–1302, 1988.

General principles

I. The attending physician must determine for each patient with a wound, individually, what is required for adequate prophylaxis against tetanus.

II. Regardless of the active immunization status of the patient, meticulous surgical care, including removal of all devitalized tissue and foreign bodies, should be provided immediately for all wounds. Such care is essential as part of the prophylaxis against tetanus.

III. Passive immunization with Tetanus Immune Globulin—Human (called human T.A.T.) must be considered individually for each patient. The characteristics of the wound, conditions under which it was incurred, its treatment, its age, and the previous active immunization status of the patient must be considered. It is not indicated, however, if the patient has ever received two or more injections of toxoid.[4]

IV. To every wounded patient, give a written record of the immunization provided, instructing him to carry the record at all times, and if indicated, to complete active immunization. For precise tetanus prophylaxis, an accurate and immediately available history regarding previous active immunization against tetanus is required.

V. Immunization in *adults* requires at least three injections of toxoid. A routine booster of adsorbed toxoid is indicated every ten years thereafter.[1] In *children* under seven, immunization requires four injections of diphtheria and tetanus toxoids combined with pertussis vaccine. A fifth dose may be administered at four to six years of age. Thereafter, a routine booster of tetanus and diphtheria toxoid is indicated at ten-year intervals.[2]

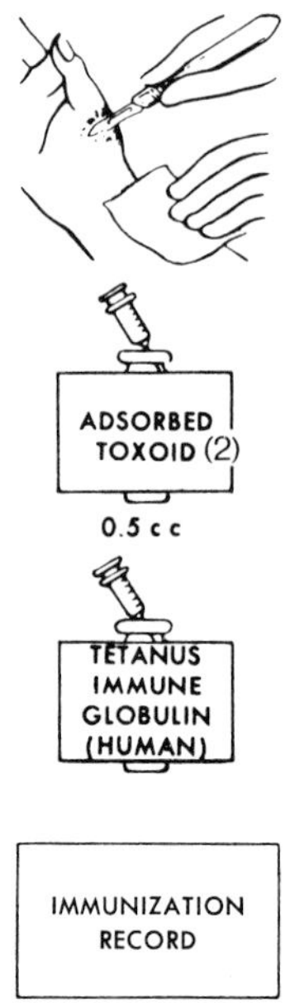

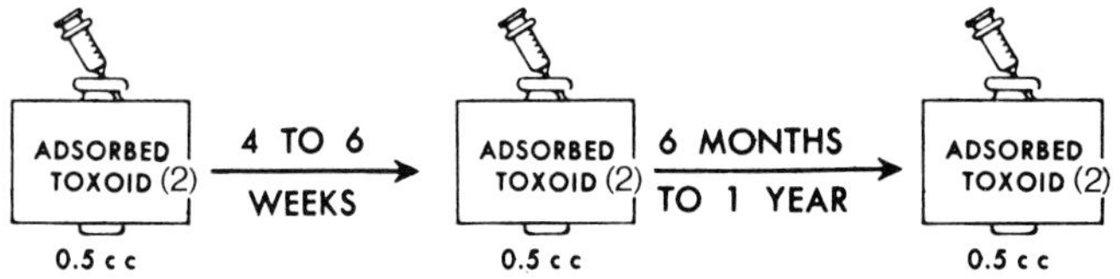

Figure 13–9. A guide against tetanus in wound management. (From Zuidema GD, Rutherford RB, Ballinger WR: Management of Trauma. Philadelphia, WB Saunders Co., 1985.)

The radial nerve innervates the extrinsic extensor muscles and the radial three-quarters of the dorsum of the hand and thumb. The ulnar nerve supplies several lower arm flexors and the majority of the intrinsic muscles of the hand. The skin on both surfaces of the little finger and ulnar side of the ring finger is innervated by the ulnar nerve. The median nerve supplies the remaining flexors and intrinsic hand muscles, the skin on the radial three-quarters of volar surface, and the distal dorsum of the hand and fingers. This nerve is frequently referred to as the "eye of the hand" because it innervates most of the palm.

The integrity of three lower extremity nerves is tested by similar examination techniques. The femoral nerve innervates muscles and skin of the anterior region of the thigh and the lateral aspect of the calf and foot. The tibial nerve supplies the hamstring muscles, muscle and skin of the back of the leg, and plantar aspect of the foot. Lastly, the peroneal nerve supplies anterior lower leg muscles and the dorsal skin of the foot and toes. Figures 13–10 and 13–11 summarize a sensory-motor screening examination for wounds that occur in the upper or lower extremities.

Color. Skin color is best assessed in a bright light, comparing the site of injury with a similar, uninjured area. Assessment of color hues is particularly important for individuals with darkly pigmented skin. The best areas of the body in which to observe color hues are the sclerae, conjunctivae, buccal mucosa, tongue, lips, nailbeds, palms of the hands, and soles of the feet. Heavily calloused areas exhibit an opaque, yellowish hue. Areas of ecchymosis appear as dark tones in the skin. Such areas are more easily identified in lighter-skinned patients. Erythema may be distinguished from ecchymosis by blanching the area. Areas of erythema will blanch, whereas areas of ecchymosis will not. Pallor may be very difficult to assess objectively. The body areas to evaluate for pallor are the nailbeds, earlobes, and lips. Pallor in a very dark-skinned patient will produce a gray cast, whereas in a moderately dark-skinned patient the skin will appear yellowish brown. The color hue findings are evaluated in light of the patient's respiratory status and sensorium.

Perfusion. The critical components of wound repair during the resuscitation phase, hemostasis and the initiation of the inflammatory process, are dependent on perfusion. Therefore, clinical monitoring of circulation is essential.

Specific measures for patients with wounds

I. Previously immunized individuals

A. When the attending physician has determined that the patient has been previously fully immunized and the last dose of toxoid was given *within ten years:*

1. For nontetanus-prone wounds, no booster dose of toxoid is indicated;
2. For tetanus-prone wounds and if more than five years has elapsed since the last dose, give 0.5 cc adsorbed toxoid. If excessive prior toxoid injections have been given, this booster may be omitted.

B. When the patient has had two or more prior injections of toxoid and received the last dose *more than ten years previously,* give 0.5 cc adsorbed toxoid for both tetanus-prone and nontetanus-prone wounds. Passive immunization is not considered necessary.

II. Individuals NOT adequately immunized

A. When the patient has received only one or no prior injection of toxoid, or the immunization history is unknown:

1. For nontetanus-prone wounds:
   a. Give 0.5 cc adsorbed toxoid,[1]

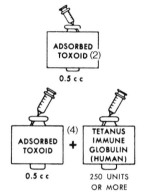

2. For tetanus-prone wounds:
   a. Give 0.5 cc adsorbed toxoid,[1]
   b. Give 250 units (or more) of human T.A.T.,[3]
   c. Consider providing antibiotics, although the effectiveness of antibiotics for prophylaxis of tetanus remains unproved.

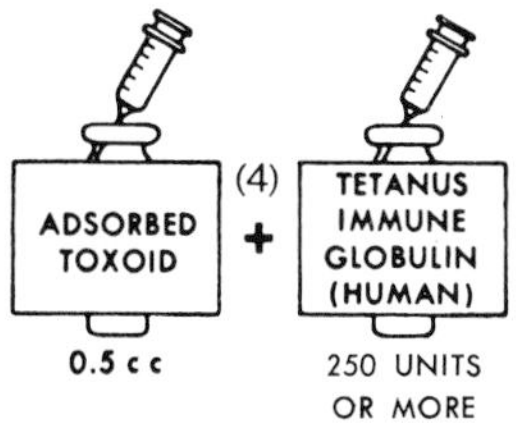

Footnotes

(1) The Public Health Service Advisory Committee on Immunization Practices in 1977 recommended DTP (diphtheria and tetanus toxoids combined with pertussis vaccine) for basic immunization in infants and children from two months through the sixth year of age, and Td (combined tetanus and diphtheria toxoids: adult type) for basic immunization of those over six years of age. For the latter group, Td toxoid was recommended for routine or wound boosters; but if there is any reason to suspect hypersensitivity to the diphtheria component, tetanus toxoid (T) should be substituted for Td.
(Morbidity and Mortality Weekly Report, Vol. 26, No. 49, p 402, Dec 9, 1977, Center for Disease Control.)

(2) Report of the Committee on Infectious Diseases, ed 18. Evanston, IL. American Academy of Pediatrics, 1977, p 2-11, 278-285.

(3) Use different syringes, needles, and sites of injection.

(4) Equine Tetanus Antitoxin: *Do not* administer equine T.A.T. except when human T.A.T. is not available, and only if the possibility of tetanus outweighs the danger of reaction to horse serum.

This guide from the Committee on Trauma of the American College of Surgeons is the work of an ad hoc subcommittee on prophylaxis against tetanus: Roger T. Sherman, MD, FACS, Tampa, Florida, Chairman; Wesley Furste, MD, FACS, Columbus, Ohio; and Richard Faust, MD, FACS, New Orleans, Louisiana.

Posters and reprints may be obtained from the Committee on Trauma, American College of Surgeons, 55 East Erie Street, Chicago, Illinois 60611.

Figure 13–9 *Continued*

Distal and proximal pulses are assessed during the neurovascular examination to confirm the presence or absence of circulation to the affected area. Strong distal pulses provide a gross estimate of vascular supply to distal areas. Pulses are palpated bilaterally and documented using a 0 to 3+ scale characterizing the pulse as absent (0), weak or thready (1+), normal (2+), full or bounding (3+). Use of a Doppler ultrasound blood flow detector provides an auditory pulse when palpation is not possible.

A systematic clinical examination estimates the adequacy of peripheral perfusion using the following indicators:[63]

1. Capillary return in the skin between and above the eyes is less than 1.5 seconds.
2. Eye turgor is equivalent to that of the examiner.
3. Mucous membranes are moist, and the patient is not thirsty (differentiate thirst versus dry mouth).
4. The skin feels normally moist (perspiration may indicate hypovolemia).
5. Skin temperature over the patella is equal or close to that of the thighs and calves, with capillary return of less than 5 seconds.
6. Postural hypotension is minimal. Compensation should

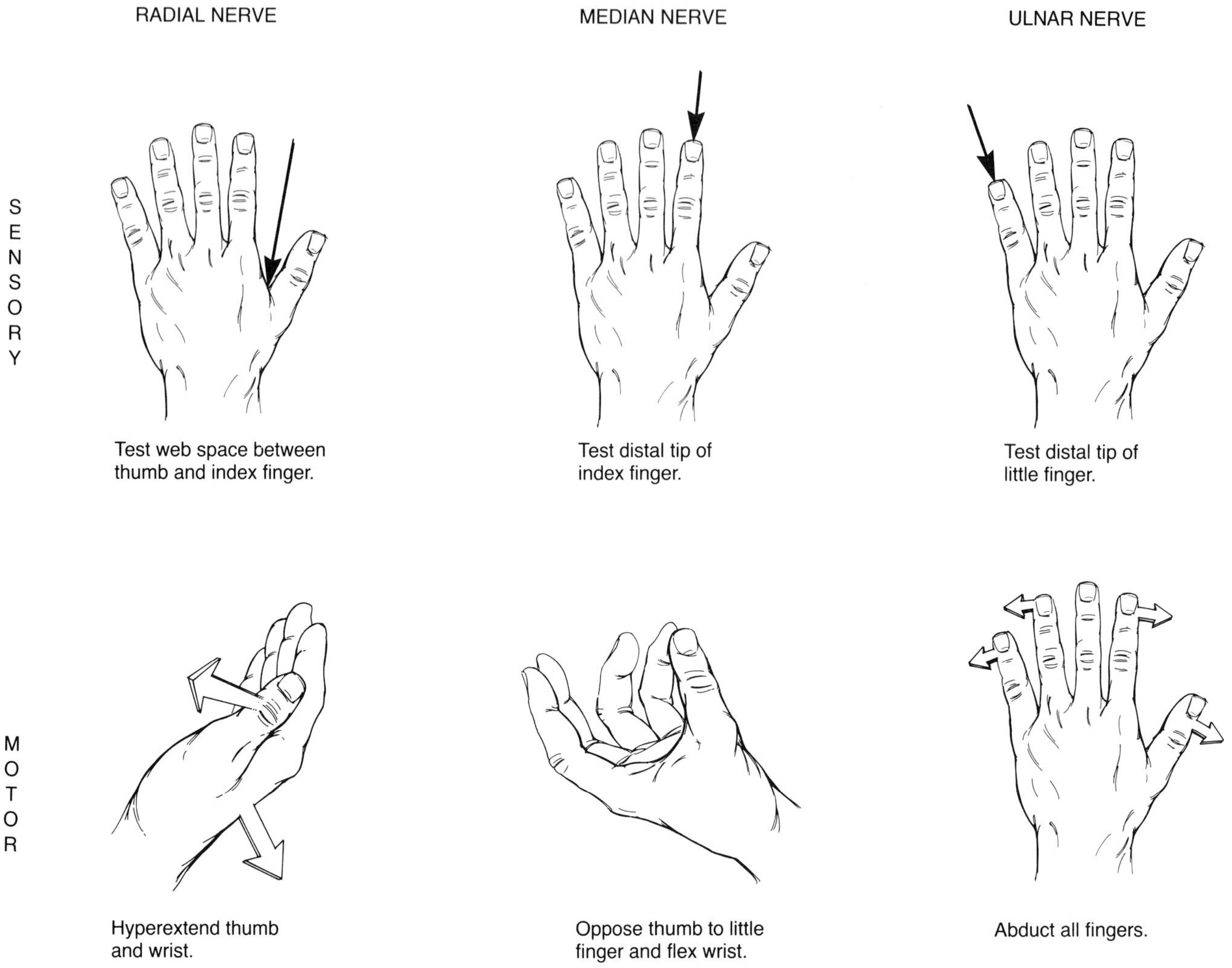

Figure 13–10. Upper extremity sensory-motor assessment.

be complete within seconds unless the patient is heavily narcotized.

Relative tissue oxygen levels can be quantified clinically using noninvasive techniques such as transcutaneous oximetry. The system uses a miniaturized polarographic electrode heated to 43 to 45°C that measures skin surface Po_2 and indirectly Pao_2. Heating the electrode enhances blood flow, and under normal cardiovascular conditions, Pao_2 and $Ptco_2$ are highly correlated. When perfusion is limited, $Ptco_2$ falls, reflecting the decrease in blood flow and subsequent limit to the supply of oxygen to the periphery.[64] A transcutaneous index ($Ptco_2/Pao_2$) will fall from 1 and approach zero as blood is preferentially shifted away from the skin to vital organs during volume loss or shock. Transcutaneous monitoring is a useful clinical tool in the sense that it provides information about changes in blood flow. However, in relation to tissue oxygen, it should be remembered that it does not measure true tissue oxygen levels because heat alters the vascular dynamics of normal tissue. Transcutaneous monitoring is not sensitive to tissue oxygen or blood flow decreases that occur with small volume deficits, e.g., 400 to 500 cc.[65]

Temperature of the wounded area is assessed by palpation using the dorsum of the hand and compared bilaterally. Temperature is significant to perfusion in the sense that cold elicits catecholamine release, which, in turn, decreases blood flow to connective tissues. A significant reduction in tissue oxygen, and presumably blood flow, has been demonstrated in subcutaneous tissue in response to epinephrine infusion.[66] Blood flow to anatomical areas varies and is reflected in differences in skin temperature of up to 4.8°C from head to foot.[67]

Wound Assessment in the Resuscitation Phase

Initially, wound location and configuration are assessed. The location is considered in terms of the distribution of microflora on the skin and also the proximity of the wound to sources of contamination, its vascular supply, weight bearing, and static and dynamic stress on the tissue. The natural static and dynamic skin tensions that occur following wound closure influence the final appearance of the scar. A prediction of the final wound appearance can be made by noting the extent that the wound edges are retracted.[61] Wound edges that are retracted greater than 5 mm are exposed to stronger static skin tensions and heal with wider scars than do wounds where the edges are separated less

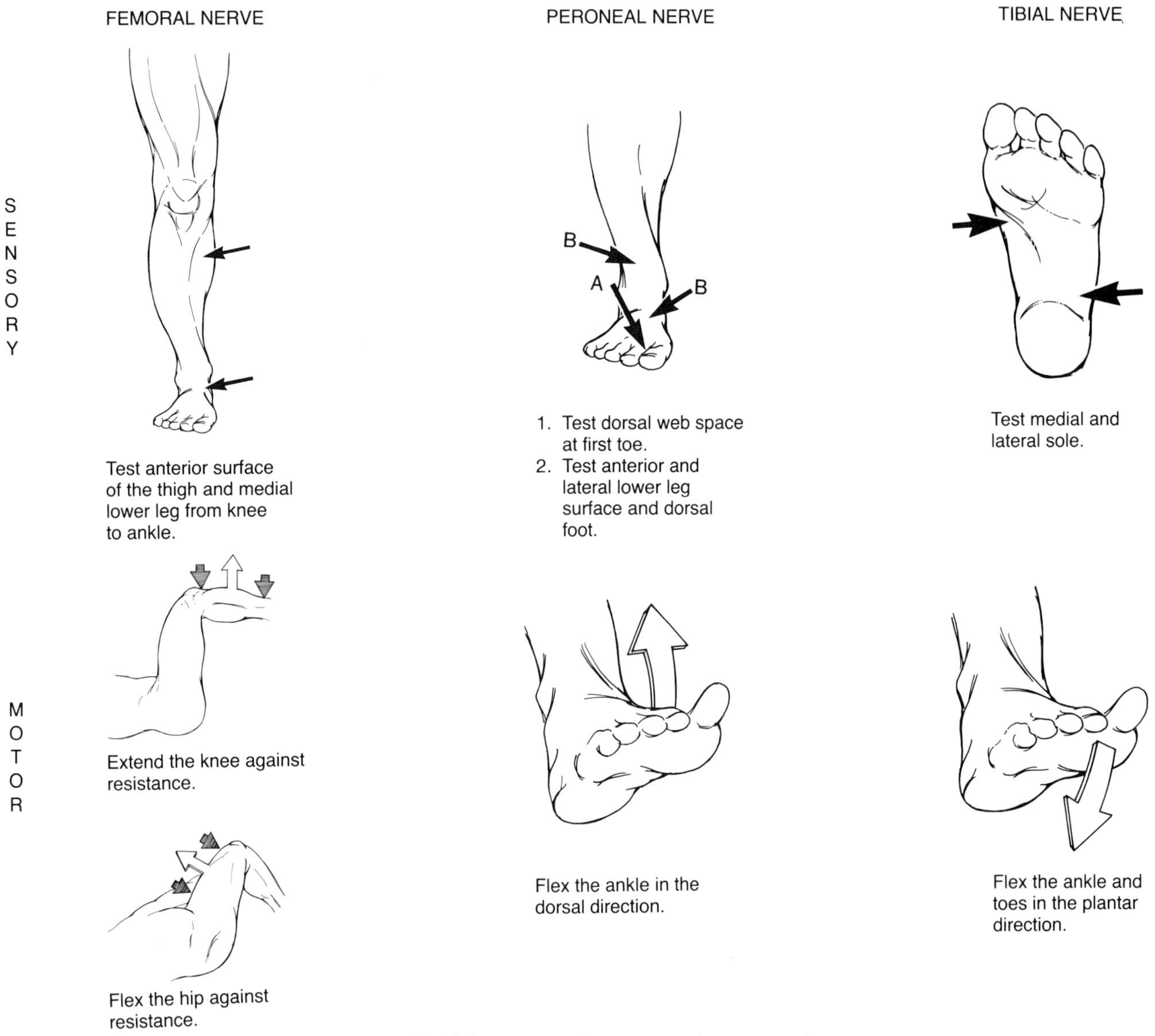
FEMORAL NERVE
PERONEAL NERVE
TIBIAL NERVE
SENSORY
B
A
B
Test anterior surface of the thigh and medial lower leg from knee to ankle.
1. Test dorsal web space at first toe.
2. Test anterior and lateral lower leg surface and dorsal foot.
Test medial and lateral sole.
MOTOR
Extend the knee against resistance.
Flex the hip against resistance.
Flex the ankle in the dorsal direction.
Flex the ankle and toes in the plantar direction.

Figure 13–11. Lower extremity sensory-motor assessment.

than 5 mm. Static tension is also influenced by wound configuration. It is sometimes not fully appreciated that jagged edged wounds, if carefully reapproximated, yield narrower scars than straight wounds because the magnitude of static tension is less per unit of wound length.[61]

The extent of injury and tissue loss is considered as well as the presence of nonviable tissue. There are many categories of soft-tissue injuries. These are summarized in Table 13–3 along with information relevant to assessment and treatment of the specific injury. Table 13–4 summarizes treatment in the event of potential exposure to rabies.

Wound Assessment in the Critical Care Phase

Healing processes that coincide with the critical care phase include fibroplasia and matrix deposition, angiogenesis, and epithelialization. Wounds that have been cleanly incised and closed will generally heal without problems; inflammation is minimal, and the distance required for new vessels to reestablish capillary networks is small.[63] There is also relatively little need for matrix deposition and epithelial repair. These wounds present the host with less of a metabolic burden than open wounds; however, in a compromised host, healing may be problematic. Assessment of primary-closure wounds includes observation initially for normal responses of inflammation, erythema, warmth, and induration along the suture line. Inflammation usually abates by the 3rd to 5th day after injury, and by the 7th to 9th day a palpable healing ridge of collagen is present.[68] The wound edges should be approximated. Impaired healing is indicated by the absence of an inflammatory response, absence of a healing ridge by the 9th day, and continued drainage along the incision, which indicates the lack of an epithelial seal.

Assessment of open wounds is vital in order to evaluate the progress of healing and make decisions regarding therapy. Unfortunately, no standardized clinical wound assessment instruments are currently available for open wounds, al-

TABLE 13–3. SUMMARY TABLE OF TRAUMATIC WOUNDS

TYPE	DESCRIPTION	MECHANISM OF INJURY	ASSESSMENT	THERAPEUTICS	COMPLICATIONS
Abrasion	A scraping or rubbing away of a layer or layers of the skin caused by friction with a hard object or surface. Abrasions vary in depth but are never deeper than the dermis. Also known as a "brush burn."	Caused often by motorcycle accidents or in any accident in which the patient is dragged across a rough surface.	Assess for size, depth, location, and degree of contamination. An abrasion covering a large amount of the body surface should raise concern for lost body fluids. Depth and number of exposed nerve endings affect the amount of pain experienced. Location affects limitation of movement, especially if the abrasion occurs over a joint. Dirt and debris are commonly embedded.	Local infiltration or topical application of anesthetic. Parenteral sedation for extensive abrasions. Meticulous cleansing by scrubbing with a saline- or surfactant cleanser–soaked sponge or surgical brush and copious irrigation. Do *not* use detergents, as they produce additional pain. A needle, no. 11 surgical blade, or forceps may be required to remove embedded particles. Coat with antibiotic ointment and leave open or cover with a nonadherent or occlusive dressing. Healing time varies with depth, location, and degree of contamination.	Direct sunlight may cause changes in skin pigmentation. "Traumatic tattooing," or the retention of foreign debris such as gunpowder, asphalt, and sand in the wound after healing, is characterized by a blue hue and a rough appearance.
Avulsion	A tearing away of tissue resulting in full thickness loss. Wound edges cannot be approximated. Degloving injuries, which result from shearing types of force, are one type of avulsion.	Caused when an extremity is cut by a meat slicer or saw or when an individual is thrown through the window in a motor vehicle accident.	Assess for amount of lost tissue, location, loss of function, and damage to underlying structures. The amount of tissue lost determines the course of treatment (e.g., grafting vs. revision and use of a flap). A large avulsion may result in fluid loss. Disability and disfigurement particularly occur when the avulsion involves the hand or face.	Thorough cleansing as described above. Control bleeding by direct pressure. Thorough irrigation with saline and early debridement of damaged tissue. Split-thickness grafting for closure when required. Complex avulsions may require use of a free flap placed with microvascular surgical techniques.	Disfigurement and loss of function of the affected limb may result in changes in patient's body image and may affect vocation and/or avocations.
Amputation	An avulsion in which the affected limb is completely separated from the body.	Caused when a finger or extremity is caught in a piece of equipment and is sheared off. Guillotine type of injury is caused when a finger or extremity is cleanly cut off by a power saw or similar tool.	As with an avulsion, assess for amount of lost tissue, location, loss of function, and damage to underlying structures. In addition, the separated part must be assessed for its viability following transport.	Thorough cleansing as described above. Wrap amputated part in dry, sterile dressing and place in a sterile plastic bag or container. Place wrapped part in an insulated cooler with ice. *Do not freeze* the amputated part. Properly managed, the part may be maintained for 6 to 12 hours before replantation.	Infection and hypertropic scarring are the most frequent complications of amputations. Loss of viability or inability to replant amputation part is related to mechanism of injury and warm-ischemic time. Amount of muscle contained in amputated part is sensitive to ischemia and may have adverse effect on its viability.
Laceration/ incision	An open wound resulting from tearing or cutting of the skin. It is termed superficial if it involves only the dermis and epidermis and deep when it extends into the underlying tissues or structures.	Caused by the rupturing of the skin when struck by a blunt force, producing a torn, jagged wound.	Assess for damage to underlying structures and degree of contamination. Perform neurovascular checks to determine any sensory or motor deficits. Assess age of injury for degree of contamination and desiccation.	Thorough cleansing and irrigation, with hemostasis by pressure and elevation. Necrotic wound edges should be excised, and edges approximated and closed with suture or skin tape. Use antibiotic ointment and nonadherent or occlusive dressing. Dressing should provide some pressure to reduce swelling and hematoma formation. Splints or casts are used when immobilization is required.	Sutures too tight cause unsightly cross-hatching; too loose sutures cause wide scars. Improper approximation of the wound edges causes raised scars or tunnels that permit infection and hematoma formation. A loose dressing permits the wound to bleed and gaping to occur; a tight dressing causes wound ischemia.

TABLE 13–3. SUMMARY TABLE OF TRAUMATIC WOUNDS *Continued*

TYPE	DESCRIPTION	MECHANISM OF INJURY	ASSESSMENT	THERAPEUTICS	COMPLICATIONS
Contusion/ hematoma	An injury that does not involve the breaking of the skin. It is characterized by swelling, pain, and discoloration. The rupture of small blood vessels causes extravasation of blood into the tissues, forming a hematoma.	Caused by the blow from a blunt instrument.	Test for sensation and movement. Assess vascular involvement by measuring changes in the surface area of the bruise. Check for any underlying fractures.	Elevate the injured part and apply cold packs. Administer mild analgesics as required. May require up to 2 to 3 weeks for the hematoma to be reabsorbed.	Development of compartment syndrome where blood collects and increases pressure, compromising the circulation and function of the affected area.
Puncture wound	A wound in which there is a small external opening in the skin but deep penetration of the underlying tissue.	Caused by the penetration of the skin by a sharp or pointed object. A high-pressure spray gun or similar equipment produces numerous punctures.	Assess for depth of penetration, degree of contamination, and any retained or injected foreign material. Appearance of surface injury may be benign. Assess for underlying tissue damage.	Soak the wound and examine the tract of the penetrating object. Remove any foreign bodies and irrigate the wound. Packing may also be required.	Complications most frequently involve infection related to retained foreign material.
Crush injury	A composite injury involving two or more tissue types and graded severity of injury.	Accident involving high energy exchange such as a fall of significant distance or a motor vehicle accident in which a part of the body is run over and crushed.	Assess for size and anatomical location of crushed area. Check neurological status and test for loss of function. Assess for tissue and blood loss and effect on underlying structures. Invasive or noninvasive transcutaneous monitoring for increased compartment pressure (pressure exceeds diastolic arterial pressure).	Apply a pressure dressing, elevate, and cool. Treat open portions as described above. Surgical intervention may be required for serial debridement, fasciotomy, and fracture stabilization. Measure urine myoglobin when extensive muscle damage is present.	Complications include those of abrasions, avulsions, amputations, lacerations and contusions. High risk of compartment syndrome. Amputation of crushed extremity may result.
Mammalian bites	An animal or human bite causing puncture and a crushing wound by the teeth and jaws of the mammal and resulting in a grossly contaminated injury.	Caused by animal or human teeth and pressure from jaw force (which may be as much as 400 psi in dog bites).[73]	Determine the source of the bite and potential for infection. Assess wound's age, depth and size, and damage to underlying tissue.	Scrub and irrigate with povidone-iodine solution and apply cold pack. Bites over 12 hours old should not have primary closure. Hand bites should be covered with a large bulky dressing. Plastic surgery may be required for facial bites. Antibiotic treatment is required in human and some animal bites. Tetanus and rabies prophylaxis may be needed.	Infection from microorganisms in the saliva. Human bites produce both gram-negative and gram-positive infections.

though some are in the process of being developed and tested.[69] Despite the lack of rigorously tested assessment tools, and until such instruments become available, there are some practical assessment approaches described in recent literature to guide wound observations.[69] The location, size, and depth of open wounds need to be documented. This can be accomplished with wound tracings or by measuring the wound diameter, length, and depth. One method, developed by Kundin and called the "wound gauge," consists of cardboard rulers that can be used to measure wound volume.[70] Regardless of the technique selected, the patient should be in the same position each time measurements are made to control for the influence of body position on wound shape and dimensions. The wound is also assessed for tracts and pockets, and the location and depth of these are noted. It is important to remember that when wounds are debrided, they will likely increase in size, and this need not be interpreted as a delay in healing but a necessity for healing to proceed.

An assessment approach proposed in recent years addresses critical aspects of the wound, including the character of tissue in the base and sides and new epithelium on the edges as well as the presence of exudate.[71] The characteristics of tissue and exudate, including color, moisture, and distribution, are documented. Healthy granulation tissue is deep pink to bright red in color and moist with minimal amounts of exudate present. Exudate, when present, varies in consistency, color, and odor; these characteristics should be documented as well as its distribution. Differences in exudate moisture and amount may dictate different management regimens, e.g., dressings that are more absorbent, the need for irrigation, and so forth. Exudate or tissue that is very dark or black is necrotic and must be removed for healing to progress. Growth of new epithelium is assessed on the wound edges. Its color and extent are important to note. Normally, it is a light pink or pearl color. It should eventually be observable around the entire edge extending across the wound as healing progresses. New epithelium also may be present, forming small pink islands around hair follicles.

A thorough wound assessment with documentation of the character of tissue, exudate, and epithelium is made daily and ideally with each dressing change. Exceptions to daily assessment are made when the type of dressing dictates a less frequent changing schedule, which is the case with some of the biosynthetic dressings. There are no research-based clinical standards for frequency of measuring wound size. It probably is not necessary to monitor as frequently as tissue assessment. In the acute care setting, a frequency of twice weekly is reasonable, provided assessment indicates that healing is progressing.

Wound Assessment in the Intermediate and Rehabilitation Phases

The extent to which a wound has healed in the presence of trauma is at best imprecise and depends on a number of factors. These include the balance between metabolic demand and nutritional supply, cardiovascular and respiratory status, as well as the existence of pertinent host and environmental factors reviewed previously. As the patient enters the intermediate and rehabilitation phases, the process of wound healing should be well established. The biological processes of collagen synthesis, angiogenesis, and epithelial regeneration will likely continue through the intermediate phase, while remodeling and contraction will be the predominant processes in the rehabilitation phase. Primarily closed wounds should at this point have an epithelial seal and be gaining strength. Tensile strength of human wounds cannot be observed nor measured. However, the wound can be assessed for complete closure and the absence of inflammation and infection. If the wound is healing by secondary intention, the assessment strategy used in the critical care phase remains appropriate. Generally, the wound should decrease in both size and volume as granulation tissue accrues and contractile forces operate to close the wound.

WOUND MANAGEMENT THROUGHOUT THE TRAUMA CYCLES

Systemic Support

Perfusion and Oxygenation

In the resuscitation and critical care phases of recovery, adequate perfusion and supply of oxygen and nutrients to the wound area are crucial for optimal healing and in particular for the avoidance of infection. Systematic clinical assessment of perfusion and in some cases oxygen tension and blood flow, as described under assessment, remain appropriate evaluation strategies. Support of vascular volume is essential to ensure that needed nutrients reach the reparative cells. Clinical studies have documented that low tissue oxygen tensions are most common in the first 24 to 48 hours after surgery or injury and point to the necessity of maintaining tissue perfusion in the critical care period.[36] In the presence of adequate perfusion, the use of supplemental oxygen is a rational therapeutic choice to sustain tissue oxygenation in patients who are at high risk for infection.[72] Treatment of hypothermia is important to consider, particularly if the patient has experienced surgery. Restoring normothermia will help prevent cutaneous vasoconstriction and may be important for resistance to infection by maintaining perfusion to injured tissues.[47] Although many clinical therapies for promoting tissue perfusion, oxygen supply, and healing have not been tested experimentally, their use as part of an individualized plan of care should be considered. These include an aggressive pulmonary hygiene plan, position changes, and ambulation, if possible.[73]

As healing progresses in the intermediate and rehabilitation phases of recovery, perfusion and tissue oxygen supply remain important and should continue to be supported. The emphasis and extent of treatment depend on assessment of wound status. In primarily closed wounds that are healing

TABLE 13–4. RABIES POSTEXPOSURE PROPHYLAXIS GUIDE

ANIMAL SPECIES	CONDITION OF ANIMAL AT TIME OF ATTACK	TREATMENT OF EXPOSED PERSON
Household pets: dogs and cats	Healthy and available for 10 days of observation	None unless animal develops rabies. At first sign of rabies in animal, treat patient with RIG* and HDCV.† Symptomatic animal should be killed and tested as soon as possible.
	Rabid or suspect unknown (escaped)	RIG and HDCV Consult public health officials. If treatment is indicated, give RIG and HDCV.
Wild animals: skunks, bats, foxes, coyotes, raccoons, bobcats, other carnivores	Regard as rabid unless proved negative by laboratory tests. If available, animal should be killed and tested as soon as possible.	
Other animals: livestock, rodents, lagomorphs (e.g., rabbits, hares)	Consider individually. Local and state public health officials should be consulted on the need for prophylaxis. Bites by the following almost never call for antirabies prophylaxis: squirrels, hamsters, guinea pigs, gerbils, chipmunks, rats, mice, other rodents, rabbits, and hares.	

*RIG (human rabies immunoglobulin)
†HDVC (rabies human diploid cell vaccine)
Adapted from Morbidity and Mortality Weekly Report, Centers for Disease Control, USPHS, Atlanta, June 13, 1980.

without complications, interventions focused on optimal pulmonary status and adequate oral intake to avoid dehydration are likely to be sufficient. Wounds healing by secondary intention present greater metabolic demands. Regular clinical assessment of peripheral perfusion with careful attention to volume status and in some cases supplemental oxygen may be necessary to sustain healing.

Nutrition

Nutritional status should be assessed in the resuscitation phase and a plan for support developed. In the critical care phase, it is important to provide energy for phagocytosis and the beginning reparative processes such as angiogenesis, collagen synthesis, and matrix deposition. Recall that vitamin C, iron, and zinc all contribute to the production of collagen. It is also critical to the support of wound healing that provision of nutrients be implemented quickly in the course of treatment and not be delayed.[74] The reader is referred to Chapter 14 for detailed information on nutritional therapy during this phase.

Depending on the status of the wound, nutritional demands for healing will vary in subsequent trauma cycles. Open wounds that continue to synthesize new tissue will naturally have greater energy requirements than wounds that are reapproximated. For wounds that are progressing, if the nutritional needs of the whole patient are met, it is likely that nutrition for the purposes of wound healing is adequate.[63]

Infection Control and Antibiotics

The use of antibiotics can affect the outcome of healing, but successful therapy depends largely on when they are administered. Prophylactic antibiotics are considered when the risk of infection is high or when the results of an infection would be life-threatening. Wound infection must be treated regardless of when it occurs. However, heavy bacterial load is most commonly associated with the resuscitation phase, and infection is most likely to occur in the early trauma phases. Tissue where repair is well established with development of a healthy granulation bed or the presence of an epithelial seal is highly resistant to infection. Ideally, this situation exists by the time the patient enters the intermediate and rehabilitation phases of recovery. Antibiotics are most effective when they are given prior to injury (e.g., preoperatively) or, in the case of trauma, as soon after injury as possible and when they are matched to the sensitivities of the infecting organism. When there is delay in treatment, it is thought that fibrin coats the bacteria, forming a barrier and preventing contact with the antibiotic.[62] Furthermore, due to the damage of the vasculature in the wound area, delivery of the drug becomes problematic. Delivery of antibiotics with resuscitation fluid that supports perfusion and débridement of necrotic tissue will enhance the effects of the antibiotics.[63] The reader is referred to Chapter 12 for an extensive discussion of antibiotic therapy.

Progressive Physical Activity

The effects of activity on wound healing are not well documented. In the early phases of recovery from trauma, some immobilization and physical support of the actual wound area to avoid stress on newly injured tissues are important. At the same time, activity that the patient can tolerate, of low intensity (e.g., turning), is likely to be beneficial through indirect cardiopulmonary effects. For example, the use of kinetic therapy (continuous rotation) compared with steep lateral positioning was found to restore arterial oxygen tension to supine values in a small study of patients in a surgical intensive care unit.[75] Lateral positioning of some patients in this study decreased markedly but was corrected by the kinetic therapy. This suggests that physical activity could potentially improve oxygenation in peripheral tissues through improvement of the ventilation to perfusion, provided that cardiac output and peripheral flow are adequate. Preliminary studies on the effects of activity on peripheral perfusion indicate that position and intensity of activity may be important determinants of tissue oxygenation and blood flow.[76] Studies are currently underway to evaluate peripheral oxygen tension and wound healing in response to activity in patients following surgery.

In the intermediate and rehabilitation phases, a progressive plan for physical activity may enhance healing. Motion and mild stress applied to wounds have been associated with increased wound strength, although the mechanism is not clear.[77] This, again, is an area in need of further study, since specific knowledge of activity effects during the later phases of healing is not available. Until such scientifically based information is available, known benefits related to activity in terms of maintaining strength and reducing cardiovascular deconditioning substantiate its importance for patient recovery.

Wound Closure and Débridement

Wound Closure

Decisions about wound closure depend on the type of wound and amount of tissue loss. In wounds in which tissue loss and contamination are minimal, primary closure is the likely method of choice. Factors that influence the decision as to the type of closure material include wound location, configuration, tension that will be applied to the wound, and desired cosmetic result. Sutures are used most commonly for primary closure. Suture that loses its tensile strength within 60 days is classified as *absorbable,* while *nonabsorbable* suture maintains its tensile strength beyond 60 days. Techniques of suture closure for skin include percutaneous (passing through epidermal and dermal layers) and dermal (epidermis is not penetrated). Small wounds that are not exposed to significant tension or stress can be closed using adhesive strips. Tape closure is useful for linear wounds in areas where static and dynamic tensions are low.[61] Where tissue loss is extensive, grafts or flaps will be required. In some cases, the wound heals by secondary intention through the processes of granulation tissue formation, contraction, and epithelial migration. However, the final scar is generally larger and the resulting deformity greater.[78] The timing for wound closure is dependent to a large extent on the degree of contamination.[61] Wounds inoculated with feces, saliva, or organic or clay soil fractions and where treatment is delayed 6 hours or more from the time of injury are often left open to heal by secondary intention or delayed primary closure. The benefits of delayed wound closure for contaminated wounds are well recognized; wound infection and dehiscence can often be avoided. The use of delayed primary closure enhances the development of a healthy granulation bed that resists infection and is prepared for subsequent grafting or closure, usually within a few days of the original injury.[79]

Débridement

Débridement is a traditional, accepted approach for the removal of necrotic tissue and debris from the wound. Devitalized tissue promotes bacterial growth and diminishes leukocyte function. Its presence serves only to make the wound increasingly hypoxic. Therefore, its removal via sharp débridement is of great importance in order to prepare a healthy wound bed regardless of whether the wound is closed primarily, left open for delayed primary closure, or left open to heal by secondary intention (Fig. 13–12).

Wound Débridement Using Mechanical Force. Irrigation utilizes mechanical force to remove debris and bacteria from the surface of wounds. Contaminants and particles are removed when irrigation pressure exceeds adhesive forces.[80] High-pressure irrigation, defined as 8 lb/in^2 or more, will more effectively remove particulate matter and bacteria than low-pressure irrigation.[81] Low-pressure syringe irrigation, e.g., with an asepto syringe, removes large particles but not smaller contaminants, bacteria in particular. An effective high-pressure system can be created using a 19-gauge plastic needle, a 35-cc syringe, and sterile normal saline. Concern has been raised about potential damage to tissues from high-pressure irrigation systems. There is evidence that high-pressure irrigation damages wound tissue, decreasing resistance to subsequent experimentally induced infection in the wound.[82] For this reason, it should be reserved for use in wounds that are highly contaminated or those which have occurred under conditions where pathogen inoculation is quite probable.

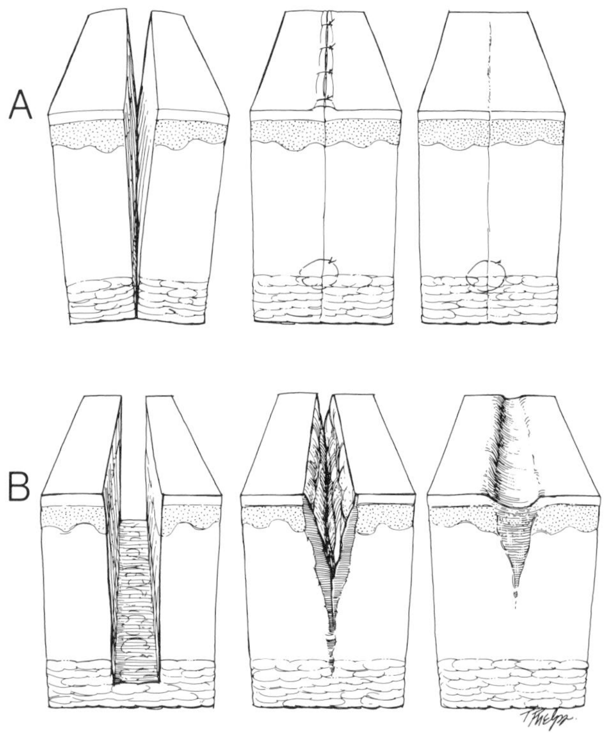

Figure 13–12. Wound healing status. Healing by primary *(A)* and secondary *(B)* intention.

Contaminated wounds also may be cleansed with a saline-soaked sponge. The direct contact and mechanical force applied remove particulate matter and bacteria. While this method effectively removes debris from the wound initially, the concomitant tissue injury impairs the ability of the wound to resist infection from remaining bacteria and/or new contaminants.[61] Several solutions that are commonly used for wound cleansing (povidone-iodine 1 per cent, sodium hypochlorite 0.5 per cent, hydrogen peroxide 3 per cent) are associated with toxic effects to leukocytes and fibroblasts and have retarded epithelial repair in experimental wound models.[83] In recent years, surfactant wound cleansers have been developed that appear to be less damaging to tissue and are useful for the removal of wound contaminants. Surfactant cleansers are nonionic solutions that contain block copolymers that consist of hydrophilic polyoxyethylene groups and a hydrophobic core of polyoxypropylene. In extensive clinical and animal studies, one such agent has been shown to be nontoxic to white blood cells and other cellular components of blood.[84] In addition, when it was applied to a sponge and used to scrub contaminated wounds, subsequent infection was prevented. Data concerning the cytotoxic effects of various antiseptic solutions suggest that they be used with caution and that preferably normal saline or a surfactant cleanser be used for removal of bacteria and particulate matter from wounds.

Dressings: Principles and Techniques

Once the wound has been cleansed, débrided if necessary, and assessed, appropriate dressing materials must be chosen. The dressing of choice during any phase of wound healing depends to a large extent on the characteristics of the wound, including whether it is closed primarily or left open. A myriad of wound covering products are available, and it is probably best to make choices based on some simple but important principles. In general, wound treatments are selected in order to support granulation tissue formation and epithelial repair while keeping contamination and dehydration to a minimum. In addition, dressings provide support to the wound and stabilize reapproximated wound edges. Figure 13–13 illustrates the basic characteristics and design of commonly available dressings. The reader is referred to Table 13–5 for suggestions on matching the dressing to the type of wound. Information on the application and use of specific products should be sought from manufacturer guidelines.

Primary-Closure Wounds

A primarily closed wound is most often covered with a dry gauze dressing that is layered if drainage is expected. Petrolatum-coated gauze or a nonadherent dressing may be used as the first layer to avoid adherence to the wound and the disruption of new epithelium when the dressing is removed. The next layer is absorbent to collect exudate, provide light pressure and support, and immobilize the local tissues. The top layer provides external support and protection. Coverings over primary-closure wounds are usually

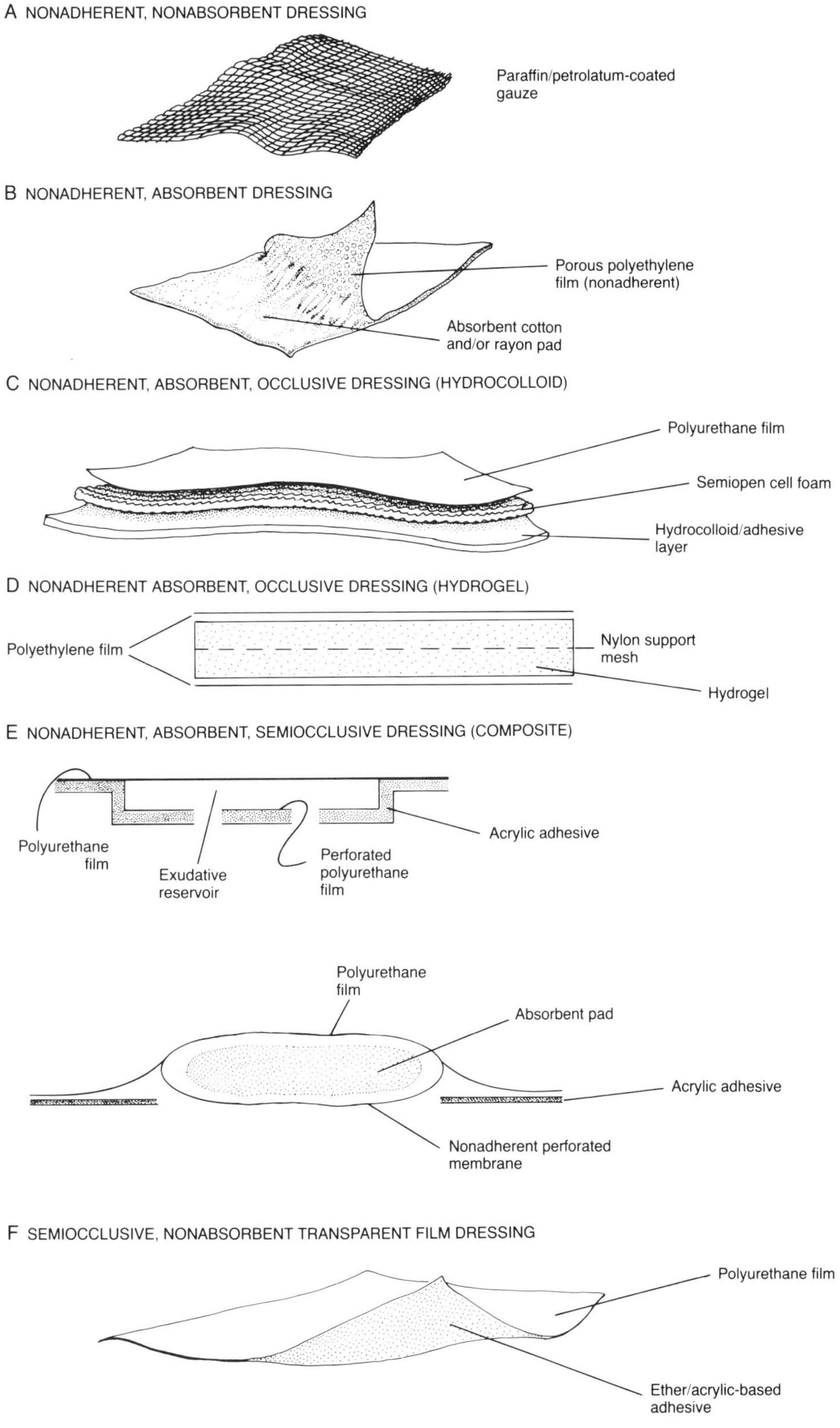

Figure 13–13. Dressing construction and design. (From Wiseman DM, Rovee DT, Alvarez OM. Wound dressings: Design and use. In Cohen IK, Diegelmann RF, Lindblad WJ (eds): Wound Healing: Biochemical and Clinical Aspects. Philadelphia, WB Saunders Co, 1992.)

TABLE 13–5. WHICH DRESSING FOR WHICH WOUND?

		TYPES OF DRESSINGS*						
WOUND DRAINAGE	**TYPES OF WOUNDS**	**ADHERENT, ABSORBENT**	**NONADHERENT NONABSORBENT†**	**NONADHERENT ABSORBENT**	**HYDRO-COLLOIDS**	**OCCLUSIVE ABSORBENT COMPOSITES**	**HYDROGELS§**	**OCCLUSIVE NON-ABSORBENT**
Heavy (>5 ml/day)	Penetrating abdominal trauma Draining incisions Large excisions Stage 3–4 leg ulcer	Use with nonadherent primary dressing	Use with absorbent secondary dressing					
Moderate (3–5 ml/day)	Stage 3–4 ulcer‡ (above knee—pressure sore) Stage 2 ulcer (leg) Excisions—deep PT¶ Dermabrasion (large) Drainage incisions	Use with nonadherent primary dressing	Use with absorbent secondary dressing					
Light (1–2 ml/day)	Excisions—(curettage/shallow PT) Dermabrasion (small) Stage 2 ulcer‡ (above knee—pressure sore) Burns (outpatient) Dry incisions							
None	Partial thickness Stage 1 ulcer Minor burns Minor excisions Minor abrasions Minor incisions							
Protection	Areas liable to develop pressure sores Cannulation sites							

*Shading indicates that the particular dressing is recommended for the corresponding wound.
†Maintain moisture to prevent adherence.
‡Ulcers on lower extremities tend to exude more heavily than similar wounds in sacral or trochanter areas.
§Tape is required to fix hydrogel dressings in place.
¶PT = partial thickness.
From Wiseman DM, Rovee DT, Alvarez UM: Wound dressings: Design and use. In Cohen IK, Diegelmann RF, Lindblad WJ (eds): Wound Healing: Biochemical and Clinical Aspects. Philadelphia, WB Saunders Co, 1992, p 575.

needed for 2 to 3 days until the wound surface is sealed with epithelial cells.

Partial-Thickness Wounds

Wounds that are open will require different dressings depending on their characteristics. Partial-thickness wounds, such as dermabrasions, that mainly require epithelialization in order to heal and are not heavily exudative can be covered with a product designed to provide a moist environment that supports cell migration. It has been understood for many years that maintaining a moist environment in epithelial wounds increases the speed of repair.[25] Semiocclusive/occlusive nonadherent transparent polyurethane film dressings were developed to provide this type of healing environment and also allow observation of the wound. Polyurethane film dressings trap fluid next to the wound and do not adhere to the wound surface. They also do not absorb fluid.

Other semiocclusive/occlusive dressings include hydrocolloid dressings and hydrogel dressings. Hydrocolloid dressings are composed of an inner hydroactive layer of gelatin, pectin, and carboxymethylcellulose with a water- and vapor-impermeable outer layer. Hydrogel dressings are composed of a water and polyethylene oxide gel between layers of polyethylene film. Hydrogel dressings are generally water- and gas-permeable. Both hydrocolloid and hydrogel dressings absorb moderate amounts of fluid and do not adhere to the wound. Both also can be used to cover partial-thickness wounds.

Bacterial growth under semiocclusive/occlusive dressings has been a concern. In experimental studies, hydrocolloid dressings have not supported the growth of normal skin flora, and *Staphylococcus aureus* and other bacteria have been shown to decrease as wound healing progresses.[85, 86] Hydrogel dressings have been found to support the growth of *S. aureus, Escherichia coli,* or *Pseudomonas aeruginosa* in wounds that were covered and then inoculated with these bacteria, suggesting that frequent dressing changes would be prudent.[87] A recent review of the literature on occlusive dressings indicates there have been no published reports of infection when these dressings are placed on "clean" wounds.[88] The wound fluid trapped beneath these dressings contains antibacterial elements, complement, immunoglobulins, lysozymes, and leukocytes, which help to control proliferation of bacteria.[89] However, the dressings should be used with caution in the presence of gram-negative bacteria, which thrive in moist environments, and in patients who are immunosuppressed. Care also should be taken to avoid the entry of microorganisms from outside the wound.

An additional apparent benefit of semiocclusive/occlusive dressings is the relief of pain associated with the wound, particularly for dermabrasions and skin-graft donor sites. The mechanism of this effect is not clear. Potential explanations that have been proposed include a reduction in the formation of certain prostaglandins that are known to cause pain, decreased inflammation, and protection of nerve endings.[90] In addition to pain relief, there are advantages in terms of the final cosmetic result when semiocclusive dressings are used. Patients whose facial wounds were dressed with polyurethane film dressings as opposed to gauze and ointment after micrographic surgery for squamous or basal cell carcinomas had significantly less deformity and smaller, smoother scars.[91] The relevance of these benefits should not be minimized. Increasing patient comfort is a significant contribution to care, and improved scar appearance and quality are particularly important for wounds that occur in highly visible areas.

Full-Thickness Wounds Healing by Secondary Intention or Delayed Closure

Full-thickness wounds may require more extensive dressings that offer greater absorption in addition to maintaining wound moisture. In wounds that are not necrotic or heavily exudative but have some depth, a simple wet-to-damp saline, fine-mesh gauze dressing will provide a moist environment for the wound bed and margins. If removal of exudate is needed, then coarse gauze is recommended, since fluids will move from the wound into the interstices of the gauze layers and then can be removed when the dressing is changed.[92] Wet-to-damp or wet-to-wet dressings are removed before they dry, thus protecting fragile new capillaries from damage that occurs when dressings are allowed to dry and adhere to the wound bed.

Hydrocolloid or hydrogel dressings can be applied to full-thickness wounds. In wounds with exudate, they are absorbent to the extent that there is gel available. These dressings, as discussed earlier, provide a moist healing environment, conform to the wound, and are associated with enhancement of healing and increased comfort.

Open wounds that produce large amounts of exudate can be dressed traditionally with gauze packing and multiple superficial layers to absorb fluid. Frequent changes of these dressings will manage excess drainage and remove contaminants for highly exudative wounds. Absorbent bead dressings are also available. These are hydrophilic dextran polymer porous beads that absorb wound fluid. They are placed into the wound cavity and covered with a transparent dressing. The beads absorb small molecules in the wound fluid, and larger molecules, including bacteria, become trapped in the spaces between the beads. Fluid and bacteria are moved away from the surface of the wound, reducing mediators of inflammation and infection and improving the granulation bed.[93]

A number of new dressings categorized as biological and biosynthetic membranes have been developed in recent years. In addition, epidermal grafts produced in cell culture are also now available in some medical facilities. All these can be considered as *skin substitutes*. This type of dressing is used to cover large areas of tissue loss to prevent invasive infection and loss of fluid and heat through evaporation.[50] *Biological dressings* consist of previously living tissues, while *biosynthetic dressings* consist of synthetic materials (nylon/silicone) combined with collagen. Biosynthetic dressings have prolonged shelf life and are more readily available than biological dressings. The dressing does not have adhesive materials and adheres to the wound surface by entrapment of fibrin.[94] Grafts of epidermal cells harvested from the patient can be grown in tissue culture over several weeks and then placed on the open wound area. The advantage of this type of permanent wound coverage is that creation of large donor sites in a person who is already injured is not necessary. The use of these newer dressings is not at present extensive, and many are still undergoing clinical trials to determine their impact on healing.

Alterations in Healing

Keloids and Excessive Scarring

Hypertrophic scarring and keloids are two alterations in healing that may become evident in the rehabilitation phase of trauma. They are significant because of their cosmetic and symptomatic consequences for the patient. *Hypertrophic scars* are an overgrowth of collagenous scar tissue within the wound margins that may spontaneously regress. A *keloid* is distinguished as a fibrous growth resulting from abnormal connective-tissue response that extends beyond the wound margins and rarely regresses. The pathophysiology of keloids is not completely understood. It is thought that excessive deposition of collagen may be the result of decreased collagenase activity with diminished degradation of newly synthesized collagen compared with normal wound healing.[95] Keloids are often seen among family members and are more prevalent in dark-skinned populations. Keloids tend to form in areas where skin tension is high, e.g., the upper back, shoulders, anterior chest, and upper arms; in other areas, the person may have normal-appearing scars indicating the contribution of local factors.[95]

Treatment for keloids and hypertrophic scars includes surgical scar revision, intralesional injection of corticosteroids, radiation, oral antihistamines, and various pressure devices. Surgical intervention is considered carefully, because it may worsen the keloid. If surgery is done, care is taken to avoid tissue trauma, dead space, foreign bodies, and wound tension, and adjuvant therapy such as steroid injections, pressure, or radiation is often included. Surgical scar revision is delayed for at least 6 months after injury to allow for maturational development of the scar.

Intralesional injection requires frequent treatments and careful monitoring. This type of therapy may be used alone or in combination with surgery or other therapies. Monthly or weekly injections are directed into the keloid, and infiltration into normal tissues is avoided. Steroids are responsible for some local complications, e.g., atrophy, depigmentation, necrosis, ulceration, and telangiectasia, seen within the scar and surrounding tissue.[95]

Radiation therapy may have a positive effect on the defect but is not selective for abnormal cells. Possible complications of the therapy, including carcinogenic effects, quite often outweigh the benefits.

The goal of gradient-pressure therapy is to maintain the capillary hydrostatic pressure above 22 mm Hg for a prolonged period, which will flatten and soften the scar.[96] The therapy is most effective if initiated early. A custom-made garment is fitted to supply the pressure and is worn for several months. The patient is fitted for more than one garment to allow for laundering without interrupting the therapy. The patient receiving this type of therapy needs to understand the importance of skin care and treatment should skin breakdown occur.

Scar Contracture

Scar contracture is the result of contractile processes in healed scars that result in a fixed, rigid scar that causes functional or cosmetic deformity.[97] Thick tendinous fibers tend to pull points of flexion together, limiting movement and causing considerable disability. The most common sites involve areas of flexion, such as fingers, arms, legs, and neck. Treatment modalities include physical therapy, splinting, and surgical release with full-thickness grafting. Range-of-motion exercises affect the remodeling of collagen as it is deposited within the wound. Splinting procedures impede contraction mechanically, and full-thickness skin grafts effectively inhibit contractile-related contracture.[96]

Pressure Ulcers

Although pressure ulcers are not the direct result of trauma, they are associated with acute illness and critical care patients; the elderly and patients who are immobile are among those at risk of developing a pressure ulcer. Pressure ulcers occur in areas where pressure, shearing force, friction, and moisture have damaged the epidermis, dermis, and underlying tissue layers. They often occur over a bony prominence. The smaller the area over which the pressure is distributed, the greater is the potential for the development of an ulcer. Shearing forces caused by sliding adjacent surfaces produce friction and tissue damage. Excess skin moisture from perspiration and incontinence increases the risk of decubitus ulcer fivefold.[98] Patients who remain immobile or have other factors present placing them at risk of pressure ulcer development need to be assessed continually throughout all the trauma cycles.

Recently, guidelines for pressure ulcer prevention were issued by the Agency for Health Care Policy and Research (AHCPR) that stress the need for assessment of pressure ulcer risk at admission. Two scales used to rate risk factors are recommended by the AHCPR, the Braden and Norton scales.[99–101] Elderly patients and those whose movements are restricted because of traction, casts, or the presence of life-support equipment are at risk and must be assessed. Shea's classification system is a useful classification system for skin condition that is used in addition to evaluating risk factors. It includes the following categories:

Stage 1: Acute inflammatory response. The epidermis is red, and an abrasion type of wound is present.
Stage 2: Persistent inflammation with dermal involvement. Blistering and erosion are apparent.
Stage 3: Full-thickness skin defect. The ulcer extends into the subcutaneous tissue.
Stage 4: Extension into deep fascia, with muscle and bone involvement.

Assessment is accompanied by preventive measures to relieve pressure and shearing forces while providing meticulous skin care, nutritional support, and patient education. The AHCPR recommends that skin be kept dry, warm, well moisturized, and protected with lubricants or protective coverings. Regular skin cleansing with a mild cleanser and the use of barrier sprays and creams to repel moisture when needed are suggested. Massage over bony prominences is contraindicated. To relieve pressure, patients require repositioning every 2 hours at a minimum if on bed rest. Static support surfaces filled with foam, water, gel, or air can be used as well as dynamic systems such as alternating-pressure mattresses, air-fluidized systems, air support systems, and water beds. Smaller supports such as foam cushions, wedges, or pillows can keep knees, elbows, ankles, and heels from receiving too much pressure. To avoid shearing and friction during positioning, patients should be lifted with linens or a lifting device.

The principles of assessment for open wounds apply to pressure ulcers. Location, size, and tissue and exudate characteristics are evaluated on a regular basis. A plan of treatment is established based on assessment of the wound status and the risk factors that are specific to the patient. In addition to choosing an appropriate dressing, a plan of care that addresses positioning and pressure relief is essential.

SUMMARY

Knowledge development in the area of wound healing has advanced rapidly in recent years. An increased understanding of this complex process and the effects of various therapies on its progression has altered some traditional beliefs about wound care and healing and has provided an empirical basis for treatment. There is still much to learn. Available data emphasize the need for early assessment of wound and patient status. Steps taken to provide systemic support in the early trauma cycles contribute significantly to the healing process and can prevent a number of complications, including infection. Many therapies for wound healing have yet to be studied to discern their mechanism of action and to define the limits of their use clinically to promote and ideally improve healing. Continued research will extend the science of wound healing and provide rational direction for optimal assessment and treatment strategies.

REFERENCES

1. Goodson WH: Traumatic injury. In Cohen IK, Diegelmann RF, Lindblad WJ (eds): Wound Healing, Biochemical and Clinical Aspects. Philadelphia, WB Saunders Co, 1992, p 316.
2. Parker F: Structure and function of the skin. In Orkin M, Maibach HI, Dahl MV (eds): Dermatology. Norwalk, Appleton & Lange, 1991, p 1.
3. Mast BA: The skin. In Cohen IK, Diegelmann RF, Lindblad WJ (eds): Wound Healing, Biochemical and Clinical Aspects. Philadelphia, WB Saunders Co, 1992, p 344.
4. Moragas JM: Disorders of the subcutaneous tissue. In Orkin M, Maibach HI, Dahl MV (eds): Dermatology. Norwalk, Appleton & Lange, 1991, p 325.
5. Hunt TK: Basic principles of wound healing. J Trauma 30(suppl 12):S122–S128, 1990.
6. Knighton DR, Fiegel VD, Doucette MM, et al: The use of topically applied platelet growth factors in chronic nonhealing wounds: A review. Wounds 1:71–78, 1989.
7. Seppa H, Grotendorst GR, Seppa S, et al: Platelet-derived

growth factor is chemotactic for fibroblasts. J Cell Biol 92:584, 1982.
8. Knighton DR, Hunt TK, Thakral KK, Goodson WH: Role of platelets and fibrin in the healing sequence: An in vivo study of angiogenesis and collagen synthesis. Ann Surg 196:379–384, 1982.
9. Oka Y, Orth DN: Human plasma epidermal growth factor/beta-urogastrone is associated with blood platelets. J Clin Invest 72:249–259, 1983.
10. Sporn MB, Roberts AB, Wakefield LM, de Cormbrugghe B: Some recent advances in the chemistry and biology of transforming growth factor-beta. J Cell Biol 105:1039–1045, 1987.
11. Deuel TF, Senior KM, Chang D, et al: Platelet factor 4 is chemotactic for neutrophils and monocytes. Proc Natl Acad Sci USA 78:4584–4587, 1981.
12. Leibovich SJ: Mesenchymal cell proliferation in wound repair: The role of macrophages. In Hunt TK, Heppenstall RB, Pines E, Rovee D (eds): Soft and Hard Tissue Repair. New York, Praeger, 1984.
13. Leibovich SJ, Ross R: A macrophage dependent factor that stimulates proliferation of fibroblasts in vitro. Am J Pathol 84:501, 1976.
14. Olsen CE: Macrophage factors effecting wound healing. In Hunt TK, Heppenstall RB, Pines E, Rovee D (eds): Soft and Hard Tissue Repair. New York, Praeger, 1984.
15. Malmsten CL: Some aspects of prostaglandins, thromboxanes and leukotrienes in inflammation. In Venge P (ed): The Inflammatory Process: An Introduction to the Study of Cellular and Humoral Mechanisms. Stockholm, Almquist & Wiksell, 1981, p 73.
16. Hunt TK, Goodson WH: Wound healing. In Way LW (ed): Current Surgical Diagnosis and Treatment. Norwalk, Appleton & Lange, 1988, p 86.
17. Pollack SV: Wound healing: A review. J Dermatol Surg Oncol 5:389–393, 1979.
18. Stryer L: Biochemistry, 2nd ed. New York, Freeman, 1981.
19. Enquist IF, Adamson RJ: Collagen synthesis and lysis in healing wounds. Minn Med 48:1695–1698, 1965.
20. Folkman J: Tumor angiogenesis. Adv Can Res 19:331–358, 1974.
21. Knighton DR, Oredsson S, Banda M, et al: Hypoxia stimulates production of angiogenesis factor, plasminogen activator and growth factor by rabbit bone marrow macrophages. Fed Proc 41:270, 1982.
22. Michaeli D, Hunt TK, Knighton DR: The role of platelets in wound healing: Demonstration of angiogenic activity. In Hunt TK, Heppenstall RB, Pines E, Rovee D (eds): Soft and Hard Tissue Repair. New York, Praeger, 1984, p 380.
23. Peacock EE: Wound Repair, 3rd ed. Philadelphia, WB Saunders Co, 1984.
24. Winter GD: Some factors affecting skin and wound healing. In Kenedi RM, Cowden JM (eds): Bedsore Biomechanics. Baltimore, University Park Press, 1976, p 47.
25. Winter GD: Formation of the scab and the rate of epithelialization of superficial wounds in the skin of the young domestic pig. Nature 193:293–294, 1962.
26. Majno G, Gabbiani G, Hirshcel BJ, et al: Contraction of granulation tissue in vitro: Similarity to smooth muscle. Science 173:548–550, 1971.
27. Rudolph R, Woodward M, Hurn I: Ultrastructure of active versus passive contracture of wounds. Surg Gynecol Obstet 151:396–400, 1980.
28. Ehrlich HP: The role of connective tissue matrix in hypertrophic scar contracture. In Hunt TK, Heppenstall RB, Pines E, Rovee D (eds): Soft and Hard Tissue Repair. New York, Praeger, 1984, p 533.
29. Shaver JF: A biopsychosocial view of human health. Nurs Outlook 33:186–191, 1985.
30. Carrell A, DuNouy P: Cicatrization of wounds. J Exp Biol 34:339–348, 1921.
31. Eaglstein WH: Wound healing and aging. Dermatol Clin 4:481–483, 1986.
32. Hunt TK, Pai MP: The effect of varying ambient oxygen tensions on wound metabolism and collagen synthesis. Surg Gynecol Obstet 135:561–567, 1972.
33. Pai MP, Hunt TK: Effect of varying oxygen tensions on healing of open wounds. Surg Gynecol Obstet 135:756–758, 1972.
34. Knighton DR, Silver IA, Hunt TK: Regulation of wound-healing angiogenesis: Effect of oxygen gradients and inspired oxygen concentration. Surgery 90:262–269, 1981.
35. Gottrup F, Firmin R, Rabkin J, et al: Directly measured tissue oxygen tension and arterial oxygen tension assess tissue perfusion. Crit Care Med 15:1030–1036, 1987.
36. Chang N, Goodson WH, Gottrup F, Hunt TK: Direct measurement of wound and tissue oxygen tension in postoperative patients. Ann Surg 197:470–478, 1983.
37. Jonsson K, Jensen JA, Goodson WH, et al: Assessment of perfusion in postoperative patients using tissue oxygen measurements. Br J Surg 74:263–267, 1987.
38. Heppenstall RB, Littooy FN, Fuchs R, et al: Gas tensions in healing tissues of traumatized patients. Surgery 75:874–880, 1974.
39. Davis JC, Buckley CJ, Barr P: Compromised soft tissue wounds: Correction of wound hypoxia. In Hunt TK, Davis JC (eds): Problem Wounds: the Role of Oxygen. New York, Elsevier, 1988, pp 143–152.
40. Babior BM: Oxygen-dependent microbial killing by phagocytes. N Engl J Med 298:659–668, 1978.
41. Hohn DC, MacKay RD, Hunt TK: The effect of oxygen tension on the microbicidal function of leukocytes in wounds and in vitro. Surg Forum 27:18–20, 1976.
42. Hunt TK, Linsey M, Grislis G, et al: The effect of differing ambient oxygen tensions on wound infection. Ann Surg 181:35–39, 1975.
43. Knighton DR, Halliday BJ, Hunt TK: Oxygen as an antibiotic: A comparison of inspired oxygen concentration and antibiotic administration on in vivo bacterial clearance. Arch Surg 121:191–195, 1986.
44. Hopf HW, Hunt TK, Goodson WH, et al: Infection risk is proportional to wound oxygenation. In Proceedings of the Wound Healing Society Second Annual Scientific Meeting. Richmond, VA, 1992, p 31.
45. Hunt TK, Goodson WH: Uncomplicated anemia does not influence wound healing. In Tuma RF, White JV, Messmer K (eds): The Role of Hemodilution in Optimal Patient Care. Munich, W Zuckschwerdt, 1989.
46. Jonsson K, Jensen JA, Goodson WH, et al: Tissue oxygenation, anemia, and perfusion in relation to wound healing in surgical patients. Ann Surg 214:605–613, 1991.
47. West JM: Wound healing in the surgical patient: Influence of the perioperative stress response on perfusion. In Stotts NA (ed): Wound Care: AACN Clinical Issues in Critical Care Nursing, vol 1, no 3. Philadelphia, JB Lippincott, 1990.
48. Rabkin JM, Hunt TK: Local heat increases blood flow and oxygen tension in wounds. Arch Surg 122:221–225, 1987.
49. Jensen JA, Goodson WH, Hopf HW, Hunt TK: Cigarette smoking decreases tissue oxygen. Arch Surg 126:1131–1134, 1991.
50. Orgill D, Demling RH: Current concepts and approaches to wound healing. Crit Care Med 16:899–908, 1988.
51. Prasad AS: Clinical manifestations of zinc deficiency. Annu Rev Nutr 5:341–363, 1985.
52. Oxlund H, Fogdestam I, Viidik A: The influence of cortisol on wound healing of the skin and distant connective tissue response. Surg Gynecol Obstet 148:876–880, 1979.
53. Holden-Lund C: Effects of relaxation with guided imagery on surgical stress and wound healing. Res Nurs Health 11:235–244, 1988.
54. McCarthy DO, Ouimet ME, Daun JM: The effects of noise stress on leukocyte function in rats. Res Nurs Health 15:131–137, 1992.
55. Goodson WH, Hunt TK: Studies of wound healing in experimental diabetes mellitus. J Surg Res 22:221–227, 1977.
56. Benveniste K, Thut P: The effect of chronic alcoholism on wound healing. Proc Soc Exp Biol Med 166:568–575, 1981.
57. Sandberg N: Time relationship between administration of cortisone and wound healing in rats. Acta Chir Scand 127:446–455, 1964.
58. Ehrlich HP, Hunt TK: Effects of cortisone and vitamin A on wound healing. Ann Surg 167:324–328, 1968.

59. Lawrence WT: Clinical management of nonhealing wounds. In Cohen IK, Diegelmann RF, Lindblad WJ (eds): Wound Healing: Biochemical and Clinical Aspects. Philadelphia, WB Saunders Co, 1992, p 541.
60. Robson MC, Duke WF, Krizek TJ: Rapid bacterial screening in the treatment of civilian wounds. J Surg Res 16:299–306, 1974.
61. Edlich RF, Rodeheaver GT, Morgan RF, et al: Principles of emergency wound management. Ann Emerg Med 17:1284–1302, 1988.
62. Rodeheaver G, Pettry D, Turnbull V, et al: Identification of the wound infection-potentiating factors in soil. Am J Surg 128:8–14, 1974.
63. Hunt TK: Physiology of wound healing. In Clowes GHA (ed): Trauma, Sepsis and Shock: The Physiological Basis of Therapy. New York, Marcel Dekker, 1988, p 443.
64. Tremper KK, Shoemaker WC: Transcutaneous oxygen monitoring of critically ill adults, with and without low flow shock. Crit Care Med 9:706–709, 1981.
65. Podolsky S, Baraff LJ, Geehr E: Transcutaneous oximetry measurements during acute blood loss. Ann Emerg Med 11:523–525, 1982.
66. Jensen JA, Jonsson K, Goodson WH, et al: Epinephrine lowers subcutaneous wound oxygen tension. Curr Surg 42:572–574, 1985.
67. Robson MC: Disturbances of wound healing. Ann Emerg Med 17:1274–1278, 1988.
68. Stotts NA: Impaired wound healing. In Carrieri VK, Lindsey AM, West CM (eds): Pathophysiological Phenomena in Nursing Human Responses to Illness. Philadelphia, WB Saunders Co, 1986, pp 343–366.
69. Cooper DM: Human wound assessment: Status report and implications for clinicians. In Stotts NA, Clochesy JM (eds): Wound Care: AACN Clinical Issues in Critical Care Nursing, vol 1, no 3. Philadelphia, JB Lippincott, 1990, pp 553–563.
70. Kundin JI: Designing and developing a new measuring instrument. Periop Nurs Q 1:40–45, 1985.
71. Stotts NA, Cooper DM: Development of an instrument to measure wound healing (abstract). Presented at the Twelfth Annual Nursing Research Conference, Tucson, University of Arizona, 1984.
72. LaVan FB, Hunt TK: Oxygen and wound healing. Clin Plast Surg 17:463–472, 1990.
73. Whitney JD: The influence of tissue oxygen and perfusion on wound healing. In Stotts NA, Clochesy JM (eds): Wound Care: AACN Clinical Issues in Critical Care Nursing, vol 1, no 3. Philadelphia, JB Lippincott, 1990, pp 578–584.
74. Stotts NA, Washington DF: Nutrition: A critical component of wound healing. In Stotts NA, Clochesy JM (eds): Wound Healing: AACN Clinical Issues in Critical Care Nursing, vol 1, no 3. Philadelphia, JB Lippincott, 1990, pp 585–592.
75. Nelson LD, Anderson HB: Physiologic effects of steep positioning in the surgical intensive care unit. Arch Surg 124:352–355, 1989.
76. Whitney JD: An experimental study of the effects of activity and inactivity on subcutaneous oxygen tension, subcutaneous perfusion and plasma volume. Dissertation, University of California, San Francisco, 1991.
77. Stephens FO, Hunt TK, Dunphy JE: Study of traditional methods of care on the tensile strength of skin wounds in rats. Am J Surg 122:78–80, 1971.
78. Dimick AR: Delayed wound closure: Indications and techniques. Ann Emerg Med 17:1303–1304, 1988.
79. Gottrup F, Fogdestam I, Hunt TK: Delayed primary closure: An experimental and clinical review. J Clin Surg 1:113–124, 1982.
80. Stevenson TR, Thacker JG, Rodeheaver GT, et al: Cleansing the traumatic wound by high pressure irrigation. J Am Coll Emerg Physicians 5:17–21, 1976.
81. Brown LL, Shelton HT, Bornside GH, Cohn, I: Evaluation of wound irrigation by pulsatile jet and conventional methods. Ann Surg 187:170–173, 1978.
82. Wheeler CB, Rodeheaver GT, Thacker JG, et al: Side effects of high pressure irrigation. Surg Gynecol Obstet 243:775–778, 1976.
83. Lineweaver W, Howard R, Soucy D, et al: Topical antimicrobial toxicity. Arch Surg 120:267–270, 1985.
84. Rodeheaver GT, Kurtz L, Kircher BJ, Edlich RF: Pluronic F-68: A promising new skin wound cleanser. Ann Emerg Med 9:572–576, 1980.
85. Lawrence JC, Lilly HA: Bacteriological properties of a new hydrocolloid dressing on intact skin of normal volunteers. In Ryan TJ (ed): An Environment for Healing: The Role of Occlusion. London, Royal Society of Medicine, 1985, pp 51–53.
86. Eriksson, G: Comparative study of hydrocolloid dressing and double layer bandage in treatment of venous stasis ulceration. In Ryan TJ (ed): An Environment for Healing: The Role of Occlusion. London, Royal Society of Medicine, 1985, pp 111–113.
87. Leaper DJ, Brennan SS, Simpson RA, Foster ME: Experimental infection and hydrogel dressings. J Hosp Infect 5(suppl A):69–73, 1984.
88. Hebda PA, Lee CI: Occlusive dressings for surgical and other acute wounds. Wounds 4:84–87, 1992.
89. May SR: Physiology, immunology and clinical efficacy of an adherent polyurethane wound dressing: Op site. In Wise DL (ed): Burn Wound Coverings, vol 2. Boca Raton, FL, CRC Press, 1984, pp 54–78.
90. Silver IA: Oxygen and tissue repair. In Ryan TJ (ed): An Environment for Healing: The Role of Occlusion. London, Royal Society of Medicine, 1985, pp 15–21.
91. Hien NT, Prawer SE, Katz HI: Facilitated wound healing using transparent film dressing following Mohs micrographic surgery. Arch Dermatol 124:903–906, 1988.
92. Noe JM, Kalish S: The mechanism of capillarity in surgical dressings. Surg Gynecol Obstet 143:454–456, 1976.
93. Jacobsson S, Jonsson L, Rank F, Rothman U: Studies on healing of Debrisan-treated wounds. Scand J Plast Reconstr Surg 10:97–101, 1976.
94. Wheeland RG: The newer surgical dressings and wound healing. Dermatol Clin 5:393–407, 1987.
95. Murray JC, Pinnell SR: Keloids and excessive dermal scarring. In Cohen IK, Diegelmann RF, Lindblad WJ (eds): Wound Healing, Biochemical and Clinical Aspects. Philadelphia, WB Saunders Co, 1992, pp 500–509.
96. Riley WB: Wound healing. Am Fam Pract 24:107–113, 1981.
97. Rudolph R, Vande Berg J, Ehrlich HP: Wound contraction and scar contracture. In Cohen IK, Diegelmann RF, Lindblad WJ (eds): Wound Healing, Biochemical and Clinical Aspects. Philadelphia, WB Saunders Co, 1992, pp 96–114.
98. Reuler JB: The pressure sore: Pathophysiology and principles of management. Ann Emerg Med 94:661–666, 1981.
99. AHCPR announces pressure ulcer prevention guidelines. Wounds 4:A18–A27, 1992.
100. Bergstrom N, Braden BJ, Laguzza A, Holman V: The Braden scale for predicting pressure sore risk. Nurs Res 36:205–210, 1987.
101. Norton D, Mclaren R, Exton-Smith AN: An Investigation of Geriatric Nursing Problems in Hospitals. London, National Corporation for the Care of Older People, 1962.

14

METABOLIC AND NUTRITIONAL MANAGEMENT OF THE TRAUMA PATIENT

GENA STIVER STANEK

OVERVIEW OF METABOLISM AND NUTRITION IN TRAUMA

In the healthy person, a balance exists between anabolism and catabolism. Normal dietary intake replenishes the stores of carbohydrate and fat for oxidation and provides the proteins necessary for maintenance of enzyme function, muscle mass, and visceral proteins.[1] Once a person is traumatically injured, the delicate balance between these processes is seriously disrupted. Critically ill trauma patients are characterized by metabolic alterations that favor catabolism (i.e., metabolic breakdown).

In trauma, glycogen stores are rapidly depleted, and the body must use endogenous substrates (protein and fat, respectively) to provide for the constant high-magnitude energy needs to maintain physiological functions. Increased demands coupled with the inability to ingest food set the stage for serious nutritional deficiencies. Although most patients contain enough reserve to support the metabolic and healing process for extended periods of time, severe trauma and sepsis may be associated with an (energy crisis).[1] The increased metabolic demands associated with traumatic injuries, wound healing, and complications such as sepsis can produce long-term high calorie and protein demands. Despite the fact that a large number of patients admitted to trauma centers are young, previously healthy people, the sequelae of trauma lead to malnutrition. In fact, protein depletion appears to be accelerated in the athletic and/or muscular young trauma victim.[2] In addition, trauma is not limited to the young; therefore, a certain percentage of people are older and/or have preexisting nutritional deficits. This portion of the trauma population needs early identification and intervention. One example is the elderly patient with a hip fracture.[3] Although the extent of protein catabolism is decreased in malnourished patients, it cannot be considered beneficial, since morbidity and mortality are particularly severe in this population.[4]

Protein depletion is common in the patient with a combination of severe catabolic stress and low nutrient intake. Trauma patients and those with major burns frequently exhibit this syndrome.[5] Protein malnutrition has been shown to result in decreased resistance to infection and poor wound healing. Malnutrition is widespread among patients who are hospitalized longer than 2 weeks, and in most cases, malnutrition is avoidable.[6] Trauma and burns have been noted to have a phenomenal impact on a patient's nutritional status. A well-planned, multidisciplinary nutritional assessment is needed for initial and ongoing evaluation of these critically ill patients.

Nutritional assessment is an art rather than a science. Available nutritional assessment strategies remain useful if analyzed in combination and critiqued in relation to individual patients. For example, specific anthropometric measures such as midarm muscle circumference is not valid in a patient with edema. Similarly, serial weight measurements reveal little information regarding nutritional status in a critically ill trauma patient whose casts, Hoffman apparatus, and unstable hemodynamic status invalidate accurate interpretation. Standard nutritional assessment as initially proposed, composed of biochemical and anthropometric measurements, must be abandoned as an end in itself, although it remains useful as one piece in a large mass of information necessary to reach a sound clinical evaluation.[7] Several new nutritional assessment strategies are being studied; however, similar problems exist with their validity. Further research needs to be done on this specific population, in areas of assessment as well as optimal replacement composition and modalities.

When oral intake is prohibited, both enteral and parenteral nutrients provide substrates that support faster convalescence and may be life-saving. The exact number of calories and the benefit of specific solutions (i.e., branched-chain amino acids, glutamine, and lipid composition) remain somewhat controversial and, therefore, in need of further research. Although total parenteral nutrition (TPN) has been vital in nutrient replacement, it is not a panacea. It is interesting that attempts to rehabilitate protein-calorie malnourished patients are usually associated with little recovery of gastrointestinal tract function if TPN is used.[7] Research suggests that the gastrointestinal (GI) tract is not only an absorptive organ but also an important metabolic organ. Studies by Windmueller[8] demonstrate that the GI tract plays an important role in amino acid metabolism. During TPN, there is a marked reduction in the mass of the large and small intestine.[9, 10] The cause of these changes remains unclear. It appears that utilizing the gut to some degree during TPN may be beneficial to retain intestinal mass as well as function.

Numerous studies have been published describing more specific complications related to TPN use. Significant differences in the number of circulating neutrophils, neutrophil function, and plasma complement levels in parenterally and enterally fed patients have been documented.[11] Bacterial translocation or migration of gut organisms through intact epithelial into mesenteric lymph nodes and into the bloodstream is a widely accepted concept. This links GI tract function or disuse to severe complications. Studies have shown significant differences in major infections and septic complications in TPN groups when compared with enterally fed groups.[12]

Specific nutrient formulations are being studied as they relate to improved GT tract function and nitrogen retention. For example, glutamine supplementation is thought to decrease bacterial translocation. Glutamine deficiencies are associated with prolonged TPN feedings. Similarly, branched-chain amino acid solutions have been studied relative to nitrogen retention in different critically ill populations.

As one can see, nutritional assessment and management are in a state of evolution. This chapter addresses the state-of-the-art metabolic and technical management of the trauma patient. Familiarity with this information enhances the nurse's understanding and ability to be actively involved in a truly multidisciplinary aspect of the trauma patient's care. Nutritional assessment techniques inappropriate in one phase of recovery may be acceptable in another. Similarly, feeding modalities change as the patient begins to recover. Therefore, this chapter addresses phase-specific patient alterations, nutritional assessments, goals, and feeding modalities.

METABOLISM

Normal Metabolism/Substrates in Humans

Metabolism is the cyclical assimilation and production of energy from exogenous and endogenous sources based on cellular need, and the energy is transported by way of various pathways mediated through enzymes and hormones for the purpose of sustaining life.[13] In healthy people, there is a balance between anabolism and catabolism. Anabolism is considered the process of food assimilation, or constructive metabolism. In contrast, catabolism involves a series of changes by which living matter is broken down into less complex and stabler substances within a cell or organism. Although oxygen, trace elements, vitamins, and minerals are nutrients that play an integral role in metabolism, only the macronutrients—carbohydrates, fats, and proteins—are discussed. These macronutrients serve specific functions and have specific normal metabolic pathways.

Carbohydrates

Carbohydrates, fats, and proteins are the three forms of energy stored in the human body. Carbohydrates are the preferred energy source for the brain and formed blood elements. Glucose becomes the final compound for transport of almost all carbohydrates to tissue cells. The major purpose of carbohydrates is to supply direct as well as potential energy to spare the use of protein and fat. Burning of these substrates for energy rather than carbohydrates may lead to functional losses and ketosis and can lead to potentially life-threatening problems.

When adequate amounts of carbohydrates are available, the remaining amounts are stored in the form of glycogen. Although all cells can store glycogen, the liver and muscle cells store large amounts. This stored glucose is an important reservoir for maintaining constant blood glucose levels. The process of forming glycogen is called glycogenesis. Conversely, when glycogen stores are metabolized, this process is called glycogenolysis (Fig. 14–1). The two principal hormones secreted by the pancreas to control glucose metabolism are insulin and glucagon.

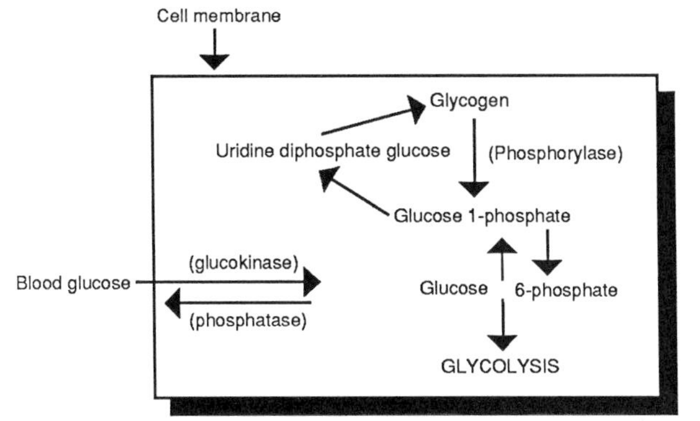

Figure 14–1. The chemical reactions of glycogenesis and glycogenolysis maintenance of blood glucose. (From Crocker KS, Gerber F, Shearer J: Metabolism of carbohydrates, proteins and fat. Nurs Clin North Am 18:4, 1983.)

Insulin affects the rate of glucose transport into the cells. When a person eats a meal, blood glucose levels rise and cause an increased insulin production from the beta cells of the pancreas. The presence of insulin aids in facilitated transport of glucose into the cell, allowing for more rapid transport. As glucose enters the cell, blood levels of glucose return to normal. In the opposite manner, low levels of glucose stimulate glucagon production and secretion from the alpha cells of the pancreas, thus converting glycogen stores into glucose. Therefore, the low blood glucose levels return to normal (see Fig. 14–1). Average glycogen stores amount to about 1200 kilocalories (Kcal).

Production of Energy

As stated earlier, the major function of glucose is to ensure adequate energy in the form of adenosine triphosphate (ATP). To form ATP, glucose undergoes four phases of metabolic reactions. ATP is necessary for muscle contraction, secretion, membrane transport, and synthesis of new substances. It is therefore found in the cytoplasm and nucleoplasm of all cells in the body (Fig. 14–2). The two high-energy phosphate bonds in a mole of ATP yield about 8000 Kcal of energy per bond. When one phosphate bond is lost, ATP becomes adenosine diphosphate (ADP). Similarly, the loss of a second phosphate bond yields adenosine monophosphate (AMP). These conversions occur and energy is released while food is gradually being oxidized to reform ATP from AMP and ADP (Fig. 14–3).

The first phase of glucose metabolism is called glycolysis. Glycolysis is the splitting of glucose to form two molecules

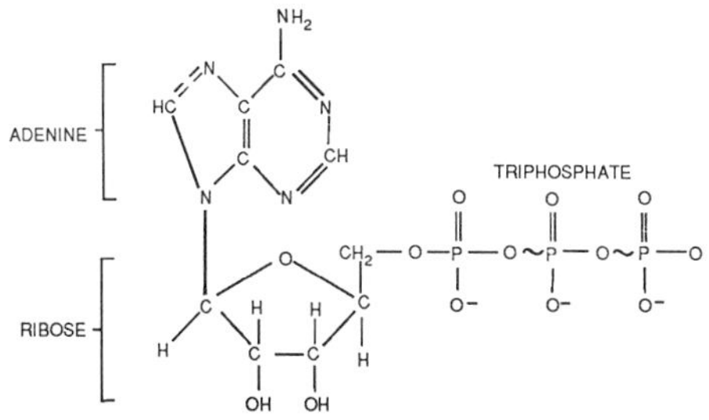

Figure 14–2. Adenosine triphosphate (ATP).

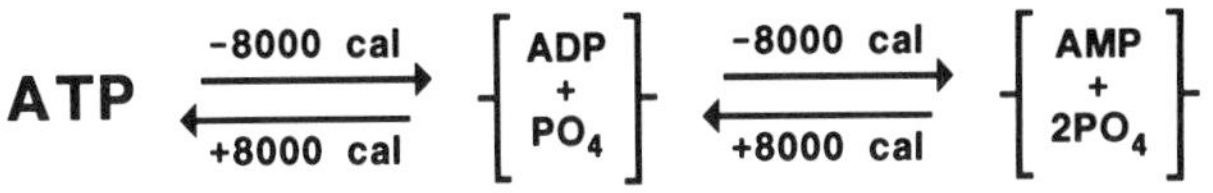

Figure 14–3. ATP conversion process. (From Guyton A: Textbook of Medical Physiology. 7th ed. Philadelphia, WB Saunders Co, 1985.)

of pyruvic acid. For each mole of glucose oxidized, there is a net gain of two ATP moles. This requires 10 successive steps (Fig. 14–4) in which ATP is needed to fuel the chemical conversions. The four hydrogens that are also released are utilized in the final phase of glucose metabolism.

During the second phase, pyruvic acid is converted to acetyl-coenzyme A, which allows entrance to the citric acid cycle (CAC), also known as Krebs' cycle or tricarboxylic acid cycle (TAC). Acetyl-coenzyme A is a key compound for the interconversions among fat and protein. No ATP is formed; however, four hydrogen ions are produced that later result in net ATP gain. The net reaction is as follows:

$$2\ (\text{pyruvic acid}) + 2\ (\text{coenzyme A}) \rightarrow 2\ (\text{acetyl CoA}) + 2\ CO_2 + 4H$$

In the third phase of the CAC, the net reaction is as follows:

$$2\ \text{acetyl CoA} + 6\ H_2O + 2\ ADP \rightarrow 4\ CO_2 + 16H + 2\ CoA + 2\ ATP$$

Figure 14–5 shows the chemical reactions that begin and end

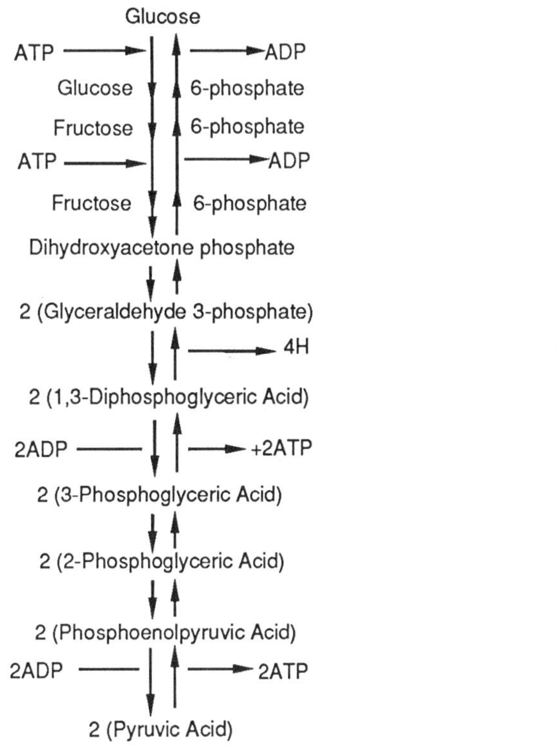

Net reaction:

$$\text{Glucose} + 2ADP + 2PO_4^{---} \rightarrow 2\ \text{Pyruvic Acid} + 2ATP + 4H^+$$

Figure 14–4. Glycolysis.

with oxaloacetic acid. There is a net gain of 16 hydrogen ions, 4 carbon dioxide as well as 2 ATP.

During the final phase, or electron transport chain, the bulk of ATP is formed. Before this phase, 24 hydrogen ions are produced. These hydrogen ions are converted to H_2O by oxidative phosphorylation. During this sequence, 34 ATP are produced. The end products are carbon dioxide and water. In summation, the phases of glucose metabolism yield a net gain of 38 ATP molecules for each molecule of glucose degraded into carbon dioxide and water. This represents an overall efficiency rate of 44 per cent (304,000 Kcal stored in the form of ATP, while 686,000 calories are released during complete oxidation). The remaining 56 per cent of the energy is lost in the form of heat.

Under anaerobic conditions, this process is extremely wasteful of glucose. This is because only 16,000 Kcal of energy is used to form ATP for each molecule of glucose utilized, representing only a little more than 2 per cent of the total energy in the glucose molecule.[14] Despite this inefficiency, glycolysis can still produce 2 ATP, since the conversion of glucose to pyruvic acid does not require oxygen. In addition, under anaerobic conditions, pyruvic acid and hydrogen ions build up. If not channeled into another pathway, they would halt the small amount of ATP formed in this glycolytic process. These two end products react with each other and form lactic acid, which diffuses easily out of the cells into extracellular fluids. This process only allows for several minutes of continued function.

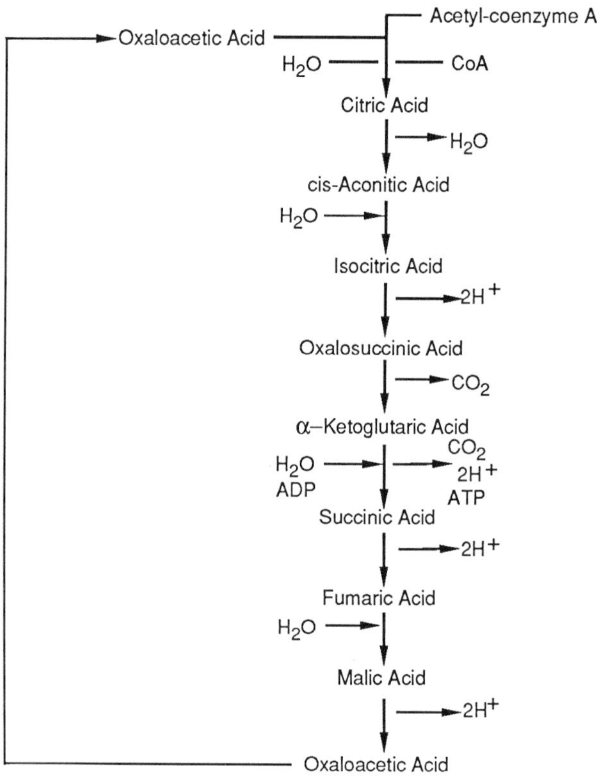

Net Reaction per molecule of glucose:

2 Acetyl CoA + $6H_2O$ + 2ADP - - -> $4CO_2$ + $16H^+$ + 2CoA + 2ATP

Figure 14–5. Citric acid cycle.

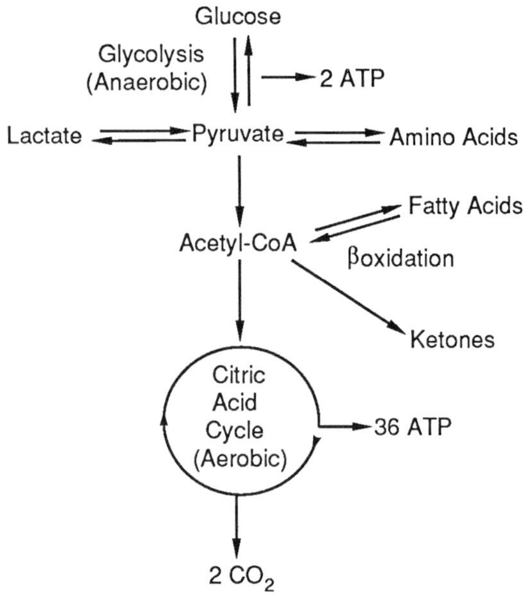

Figure 14–6. Formation of carbohydrates from proteins and fats. (From Wolfe BM, Chock E: Energy sources, stores and hormonal control. Surg Clin North Am 61:510, 1981.)

Formation of Carbohydrates from Proteins and Fats

Gluconeogenesis is the formation of glucose from protein amino acids and fat. When carbohydrate stores are low, a moderate quantity of glucose can be formed from certain amino acids and the glycerol portion of fat. It is the diminished carbohydrates in the cells as well as a decreased blood glucose that are the basic stimuli for gluconeogenesis. In addition, several hormones secreted by the endocrine glands are especially important in modulating this response. Figure 14–6 shows how amino acids and fatty acids enter glucose metabolic pathways to be utilized by the body for energy. Regulation of these pathways are discussed later in this chapter.

Proteins

Proteins are not stored, as are carbohydrates and particularly fat. Proteins can provide a source of calories in an emergency, as depicted in gluconeogenesis. Proteins are mainly used for tissue synthesis. In addition, they serve such functions as a transport system, instigating chemical reactions and maintaining osmotic pressure and blood neutrality, muscle and organ structure, antibodies, enzymes, and hormones. Protein has specific functions, and low supply may have devastating effects on any of the valuable functions previously described. Amino acids are the building blocks of protein.

Proteins are constantly undergoing turnover. In a steady state, the total body protein pool remains relatively constant. Synthesis of protein from endogenous and exogenous amino acids is equal to degradation and external losses. This normal turnover varies from active turnover occurring in the GI tract, liver, and kidneys (about 3 days) to a relatively long turnover in skeletal muscle (about 18 days). Some proteins are relatively inert, such as those that make up bone, cartilage, and tendons (Fig. 14–7).

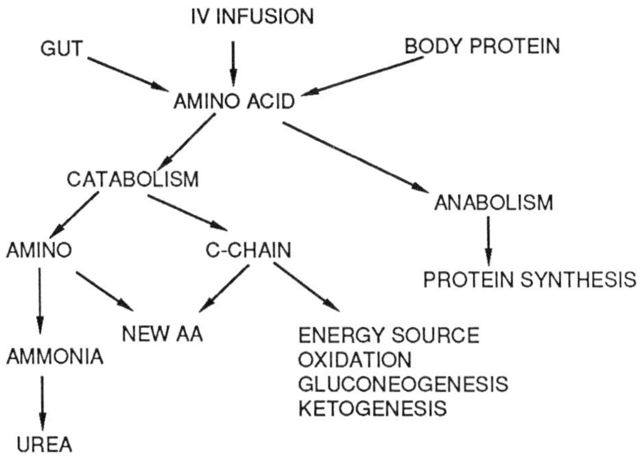

Figure 14–7. Amino acid flux. (From Wolfe BM, Chock M: Energy sources, stores and hormonal control. Surg Clin North Am 61:512, 1981.)

There are essentially two protein compartments. Somatic proteins are the skeletal and accessory muscle proteins, and visceral proteins are all the internal organ proteins—especially the plasma proteins, including retinal-binding protein, prealbumin, albumin, transferrin, and the immune competency proteins. These proteins are discussed later in this chapter. Figure 14–7 shows the amino acid flux that occurs with and without exogenous protein substrate in humans.

Multiple hormones regulate protein metabolism. When insulin levels fall to zero, so does protein synthesis. Although not completely understood, insulin does increase amino acid transport into cells, which could be a stimulus to protein synthesis. The glucocorticoids decrease the quantity of amino acids in most tissue while increasing plasma levels. In contrast, growth hormone increases protein synthesis. Testosterone increases protein deposits in tissue throughout the body. Thyroxine has an indirect effect on protein metabolism by increasing the rates of both normal anabolic and catabolic protein reactions.

Fats and Lipids

A number of compounds in food as well as in the body are classified as lipids. These include (1) neutral fat (known as triglycerides), (2) phospholipids, (3) cholesterol, and (4) a few others of less importance.[14] Fat serves as a major energy reservoir. It is the triglycerides that are utilized by the body to provide energy to fuel different metabolic processes, which are discussed here. The triglyceride molecule has three long-chain fatty acid molecules bound to one molecule of glycerol. It is the glycerol portion that enters the third phase of glucose metabolism. Once fat has been stored in the fat cells, it is transported to various tissues in the form of free fatty acid (FFA).

Insulin plays the primary role in fat synthesis and storage. Insulin rises owing to high blood levels of glucose. For example, after a meal, the lipoprotein lipase is activated, which increases the rate of fat storage. In addition, insulin promotes glucose entry into fat cells, where, in small quantities, it is converted into triglycerides. Further, insulin provides glycerol, a product of breakdown of glucose, which is an important part of the triglyceride molecule. If this does not occur, no fat could be stored. Fat is stored for the most part in adipose tissue or the liver, with a small amount circulating in the plasma.

The rate of turnover of FFA in the plasma is rapid (every 2 to 3 minutes). Any condition that causes an increase in the need for fat for energy increases the concentration of FFA in the blood. For example, conditions such as stress and starvation increase the blood levels of FFA. When FFA leaves the fat cell for the purpose of providing energy, it combines with the plasma protein albumin to allow for circulatory transport. During times of high energy needs, more than the average amount of FFA can be carried by albumin. The exchange of fat from the adipose tissue and the blood is modulated by the hormone-sensitive lipases. Some lipases favor deposition, whereas others cause splitting of the stored triglyceride. The triglyceride in fat cells is renewed every 2 to 3 weeks.

Excessive protein and carbohydrate intake promotes the synthesis and deposition of fat, whereas low intake with decreased insulin stimulates fat mobilization. In addition, the following hormones have fat-mobilizing capabilities: glucocorticoids, corticotropin, growth hormone, thyroid hormone, epinephrine, and norepinephrine.

In summary, balances normally exist among substrate utilization. Carbohydrates in appropriate amounts are primarily utilized to form ATP, whose high-energy phosphate bonds fuel essentially all metabolic processes. In time of excess, carbohydrates can be stored in the form of glycogen for rapid energy needs. Because glycogen stores are limited, additional carbohydrates are stored as fat and provide a large reservoir of calories. In contrast, proteins have specific tasks, such as building muscle tissue, creating antibodies, and synthesizing hormones and enzymes and therefore are not utilized for energy except in extreme situations. In addition to providing the body with padding and insulation, fat serves as a vast store of energy in times of need. Multiple enzymes and hormones regulate the storage, utilization, and synthesis of these substrates.

Starvation Metabolism

Alterations in metabolism occur during periods of starvation and stress. Death would ensue rapidly if the body did not have the capacity to adapt to changes. A decrease or absence of nutrient intake alters how the body utilizes or conserves carbohydrates, fats, and proteins. There are different mechanisms that work, depending on the length of time the body is deprived of food. Starvation is the lack of food intake from several days to the time of death.

Normal postabsorptive states are characterized by food intake and general allocation of substrates as follows: (1) protein compartments, (2) ATP demand, and (3) excess calories to adipose stores. Figure 14–8 shows this rather dynamic state. In contrast, early starvation that lasts from several hours to several days is shown in Figure 14–9. Low nutrient intake causes blood glucose levels to decrease with a concomitant fall in circulating insulin. The hormone glucagon is secreted by the alpha cells in the pancreas in response to low insulin levels. Therefore, it is the glycogen stores that are utilized initially to increase blood glucose. These stores are depleted in about 24 hours.

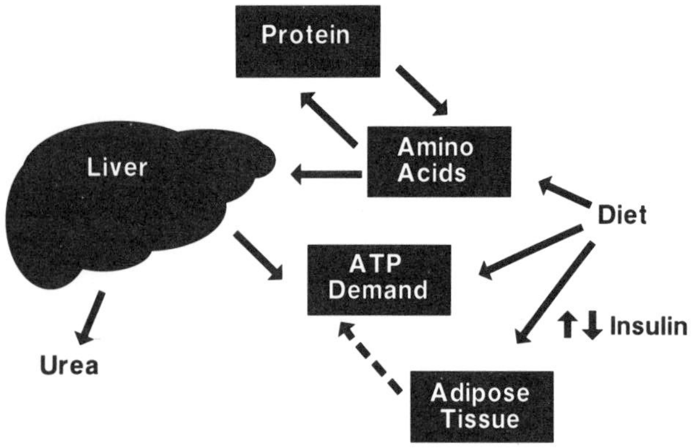

Figure 14–8. Postabsorptive state. (From Crocker KS, Gerber F, Shearer J: Metabolism of carbohydrates, protein and fat. Nurs Clin North Am 18:12, 1983.)

Once glycogen stores are depleted, protein and fat stores are oxidized for the purpose of supplying continued glucose demands (glyconeogenesis). The low levels of glucose and insulin allow the hormone-sensitive triglyceride lipase (an enzyme) to mobilize fatty acids from lipid reserves (Fig. 14–9). The overriding goal in starvation is to preserve tissue mass; initially, protein is metabolized for the first few days for energy provision. Again, low insulin levels stimulate amino acid release from skeletal muscle, some of which is converted by the liver to new glucose. This results in increased urinary nitrogen excretion, a by-product of protein metabolism. In addition, during the first several days, catecholamine excretion is increased, which accelerates release of FFA and amino acids. Other hormones, such as corticotropin, thyroid-stimulating hormone, and growth hormone, are altered but are of minor importance in the overall adaptation.[2] See Table 14–1 for a summary of brief and early starvation.

The brain and central nervous system utilize about 80 per cent of the glucose produced hepatically. Similarly, other tissues that primarily utilize glucose are red cells, white cells, bone marrow, and renal medulla. These tissues convert glucose to lactate and pyruvate, which enter the blood and travel to the liver, where they are reconverted to new glucose.

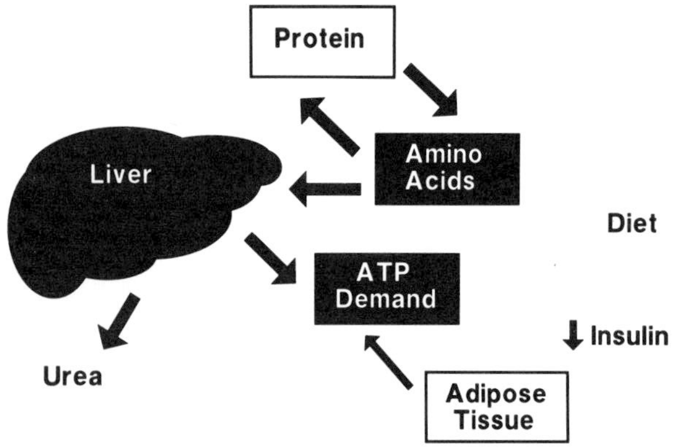

Figure 14–9. Acute fast. (From Crocker KS, Gerber F, Shearer J: Metabolism of carbohydrates, protein and fat. Nurs Clin North Am 18:12, 1983.)

TABLE 14–1. BRIEF/EARLY STARVATION

Insulin levels	Decrease
Blood glucose levels	Decrease
Gluconeogenesis (fat and protein)	Decrease
Urine urea nitrogen	Increase
Free fatty acid levels	Increase
Blood glucagon levels	Increase
Body temperature	No change
Catecholamines	Slight increase
Muscle mass	Slight decrease
Weight	Slight decrease

This is called the Cori cycle (Fig. 14–10). This cycle must begin with a molecule of hepatic glucose, which travels to peripheral tissues and is converted to lactate (energy-producing). Lactate is then recycled to the liver to be reconverted to new glucose (energy-requiring). This hepatic gluconeogenesis derives its energy from the oxidation of fat in the liver. Fats, therefore, assist in providing energy for gluconeogenesis so that glycolytic tissue has glucose. The remainder of the body utilizes fatty acids released directly into the circulation or partially oxidized in the liver to ketone bodies. Gluconeogenesis from protein is spared by limiting complete oxidation of glucose to CO_2 and water. Similarly, tissues that utilize glucose (skeletal muscle) shift to fat oxidation, and the glucose that enters is converted to lactate and sent to the liver. Therefore, the need for glucose is minimized, and protein is spared (Fig. 14–11).

As starvation continues, the brain and other glucose-dependent tissues begin to utilize more ketone bodies to meet energy demands. Metabolic acidosis occurs, which is usually mild and of little consequence unless the patient is stressed; then, buffer capacity is limited.[2] In addition, a gradual decrease in overall body temperature and metabolic rate occurs. The Cori cycle continues to be an important adaptive process. Fat stores eventually are depleted, and proteins are used to meet energy demands. Alanine and glutamine are the major glucogenic amino acids released from skeletal muscle. Alanine leaves the muscle by way of the blood, where it travels to the liver to form new glucose. Urea and pyruvate are the end products of this glucose–alanine shuttle system, and the kidneys excrete the urea while the liver uses the pyruvate. Ammonia is the end product of glutamine metabolism, and it is used by the kidneys and the gut to synthesize alanine. The kidneys therefore become a source of glucose as they recycle the end products of protein metabolism.

TABLE 14–2. PROLONGED STARVATION

Insulin levels	Decrease
Blood glucose levels	Decrease
Gluconeogenesis (protein)	Decrease
Gluconeogenesis (fat)	Increase
Weight loss	Decrease
Muscle mass loss	Decrease
Urine urea nitrogen	Decrease
Basal metabolic rate	Decrease
Body temperature	Decrease
Urine ammonia levels	Increase
Free fatty acid levels	Increase

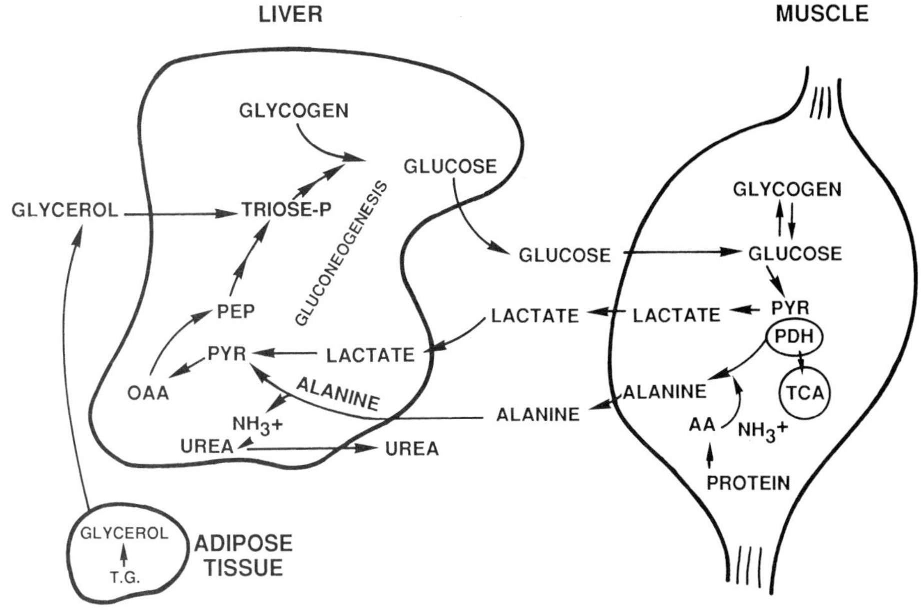

Figure 14–10. Interorgan glucose homeostasis. (From Siegel JH, Vary TC: Sepsis, abnormal metabolic control and multiple organ failure syndrome. In Siegel JH [ed]: Trauma: Emergency and Critical Care. New York, Churchill Livingstone, 1987, p. 452.)

The overall consequences of long-term starvation are loss of fat stores, muscle wasting, and peripheral edema due to hypoalbuminemia. The gluconeogenesis of body serum proteins are reflected by decreased osmotic gradients, slowed enzymatic activity, decreased immune competence, and the inability of the body to respond efficiently to stressful situations such as infection or injury. Table 14–2 summarizes the effects of prolonged starvation. As prolonged starvation continues, fat stores are depleted, protein compartments (both visceral and somatic) become severely depleted, and there is rapid weight loss. Without intervention, death ensues, usually from overwhelming infection. Table 14–3 provides a summary of premorbid starvation.

In summary, in fasting states, glycogen stores are depleted rapidly, and the body relies on gluconeogenesis from both protein and fat. The body tissues that once depended on glucose eventually adapt to ketone bodies from oxidation of fat stores to supply energy needs. The liver serves as the transformer, synthesizing glucose from its precursors and using fatty acid oxidation to ketones as its main energy source. Protein compartments are spared until fat stores are depleted. Proteins are task specific, thus depletion of this body store leads to severe consequences. Poor immune functioning altered osmotic gradients eventually lead to death if not corrected. This starvation continuum can take months to become fatal. Unlike starvation, in which the body has adaptive mechanisms that allow it to adjust to the absence of food, the metabolic response to stress such as trauma, burns, or sepsis evokes a hypermetabolic response.

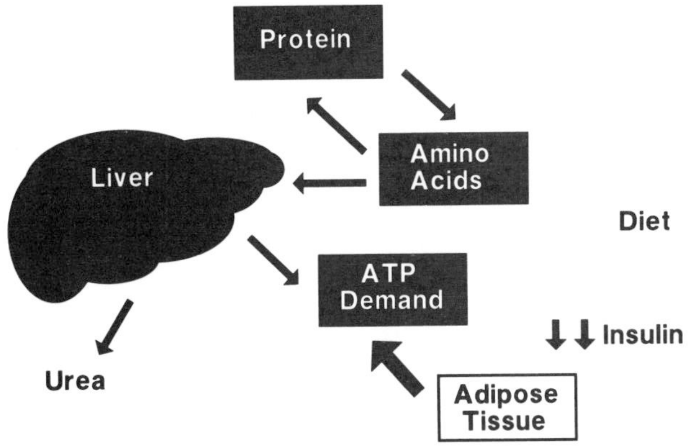

Figure 14–11. Prolonged starvation. (From Crocker KS, Gerber F, Shearer J: Metabolism of carbohydrates, proteins and fat. Nurs Clin North Am 18:12, 1983.)

Metabolic Alterations in Injury

Critically ill trauma patients are characterized by metabolic alterations that favor catabolism. Increased demands coupled with the inability to ingest food set the stage for serious nutritional deficiencies. Metabolic alterations occur immediately after injury because of increased neurohormonal activity. In a starvation state, the body gradually adapts by lowering the metabolic rate and increasing utilization of fatty acids for energy while sparing protein. In contrast, the physiological milieu of anti-insulin hormones results in severe proteolysis, gluconeogenesis, lipolysis, ketogenesis, and glycogenolysis[15] (Fig. 14–12). These catabolic processes are occurring in a population that needs energy for anabolic processes due to massive tissue injury.

TABLE 14–3. PREMORBID/LATE STARVATION

Insulin levels	Decrease
Blood glucose levels	Decrease
Gluconeogenesis (protein)	Increase
Gluconeogenesis (fat)	Decrease
Weight loss	Increase
Muscle mass loss	Decrease
Urine urea nitrogen	Decrease
Basal metabolic rate	Decrease
Temperature	Decrease
Visceral protein loss	Increase

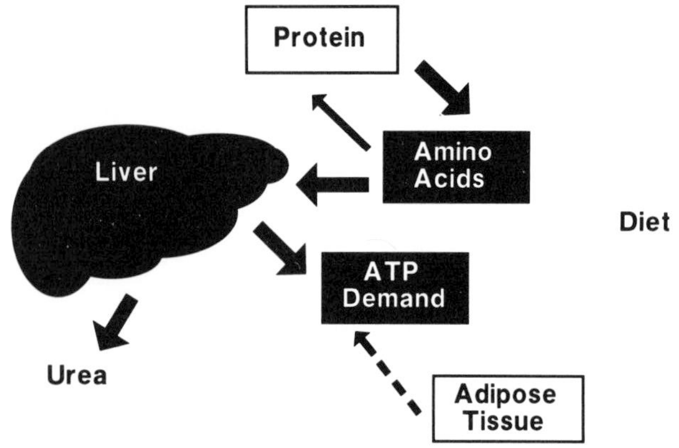

Figure 14–12. Stress/hypermetabolism. (From Crocker KS, Gerber F, Shearer J: Metabolism of carbohydrates, proteins and fat. Nurs Clin North Am 18:12, 1983.)

Various factors may elicit the metabolic response to injury. The exact stimuli and mediators for this response remain obscure.[16] It is hypothesized that immediate sympathetic discharge results from direct stimulation to the central nervous system. Hypoxia, anoxia, decreased blood volume, pain, and anxiety are all factors that result in an immediate sympathetic discharge.[2] Once resuscitation occurs and these initial insults are managed effectively, other factors play an important role in the degree and/or duration of the metabolic response. The cross-sectional mass of injured tissue, loss of normal barriers to infection, and starvation contribute to the hypermetabolic stress response to injury. Further, the metabolic response to injury is influenced by age, sex, and previous state of health and nutrition as well as the extent of primary injury and related complications. In addition, blood-borne chemical mediators are liberated directly from the site of injury by white blood cells as a result of the offending organisms (Fig. 14–13). Endogenous pyrogen, more recently known as interleukin-1 (IL-1), and a leukocyte endogenous mediator (LEM) may be elaborated by phagocytosis (see Fig. 14–13), both of which produce a fever.[2] These mediators have specific effects on the liver metabolism of trace elements and amino acids. They stimulate the synthesis of acute-phase globulins that participate in the host defense mechanisms. Therefore, these factors produce the changes in the metabolism of specific substrates.

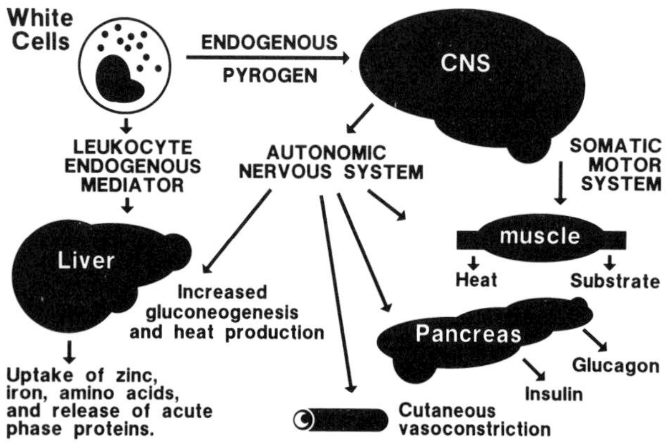

Figure 14–13. Intermediary metabolism/response to injury. (From Wilmore DW: The Metabolic Management of the Critically Ill. New York, Plenum Medical Book Co, 1977, p 147.)

In addition, tumor necrosis factor/cachectic (TNF) and interferon have been reviewed.[17] IL-1 and TNF seem to work by triggering metabolic responses in some organs and working synergistically in others during stress. TNF is thought to be responsible for protein breakdown in muscle as well as the transfer of amino acids to the liver (i.e., alanine) and GI tract (i.e., glutamine). Similarly, IL-1 is responsible for stimulating the increased secretion of glucagon and insulin and hence increased glucose production. As the ability to study these monokinines has developed through recombinant DNA techniques, future studies are expected to explain the complex sequence of events during stress and injury.

Endogenous carbohydrates, proteins, and fats must be utilized to provide for the high-magnitude energy needs. As in starvation, glycogen stores are the first to be depleted. There is an increase in autonomic nervous system discharge resulting in increased catecholamines (epinephrine and norepinephrine), cortisol, and glucogen. The hypothalamus secretes corticotropin-releasing hormone, which stimulates the anterior pituitary gland to secrete corticotropin, which stimulates the adrenal cortex to secrete cortisol. The sympathetic nervous system stimulates the adrenal medulla to secrete epinephrine and norepinephrine. These substances are responsible for the increased rate of glucose turnover, oxidation, and increased metabolic rate. As a result, there is an increase in blood glucose. This hyperglycemia is resistant to control by insulin probably because of the high hormone levels. Therefore, the insulin level is normal or slightly elevated relative to the existing hyperglycemia. Once glycogen stores are depleted, glucose is obtained at the expense of body protein stores.

Both the rate of protein synthesis and the rate of breakdown are increased. Breakdown rates are higher than synthesis. As stated previously, acute-phase proteins that assist in immune functioning are being produced. Similarly, the liver produces other acute-phase proteins that are manifested by progressive wound healing despite little to no protein intake. The priorities of protein utilization in stress appear to be utilizing skeletal muscle protein first so visceral proteins can continue their important organ and immune functioning. A reprioritization of protein synthesis occurs as acute-phase reactants (e.g., C-reactive protein, ceruloplasmin, α_1-acid glycoprotein) increase and other proteins (e.g., albumin and transferrin) decrease by redistribution and decreased synthesis.[18] In acute injury, there is a larger number of proteins catabolized than is necessary for protein synthesis, with the additional breakdown being used for glucose synthesis.[19]

The branched-chain amino acids (valine, leucine, and isoleucine) are oxidized and shuttled by way of the glucose–alanine cycle to the liver to supply continued energy needs (Fig. 14–14). Increased lactate levels are due not only to the glucose–alanine cycle but also to incomplete breakdown of glucose under anaerobic conditions. This increased protein breakdown is measured by way of nitrogen excretion and closely parallels the severity of injury. The peak metabolic response closely parallels peak nitrogen excretion, which occurs between 5 and 10 days (Fig. 14–15). Breakdown is influenced by previous nutritional status and age. A young, healthy, muscular patient has a much greater degree of

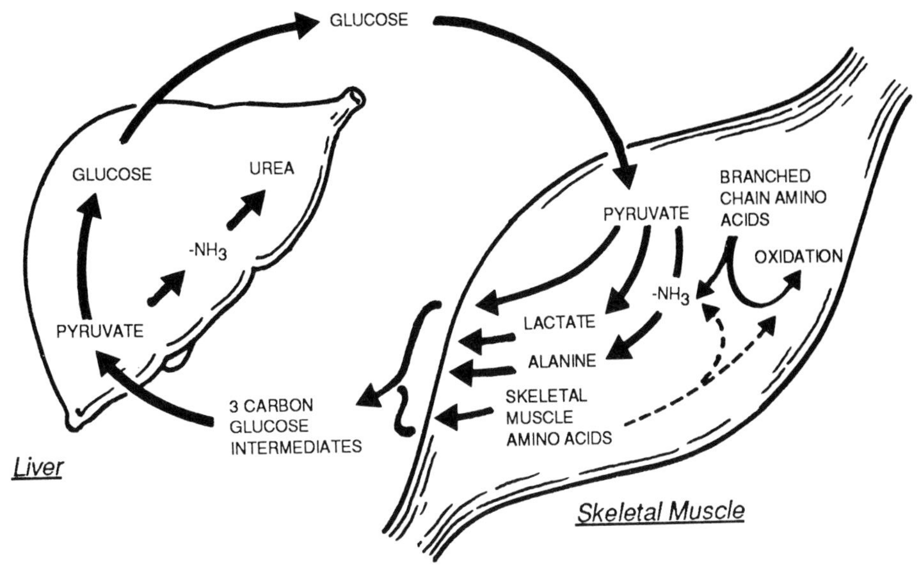

Figure 14–14. Process of skeletal muscle breakdown in injury. (From Wilmore DW: The Metabolic Management of the Critically Ill. New York, Plenum Medical Book Co, 1977, p 155.)

protein wasting. In contrast, an older, malnourished person has a lower rate of muscle catabolism.

Glutamine is produced by peripheral tissue, where it is then carried to the splanchnic circulation and metabolized by the GI tract into alanine and then by the liver into glucose. Although glutamine and alanine account for about 10 to 15 per cent of the amino acids in skeletal muscle, these amino acids account for up to 70 per cent of those released during sepsis.[20]

The catecholamines and the glucocorticoids act permissively, allowing an overwhelming gluconeogenesis from skeletal muscle. Insulin that is not abnormally low should be able to inhibit gluconeogenesis; in injury, this ability is dampened. Although this response can be slightly modified by exogenous substrate administration, this catabolic process cannot be significantly altered.[21] Research is studying administration of branched-chain amino acid solutions as an attempt to alter this destructive process.

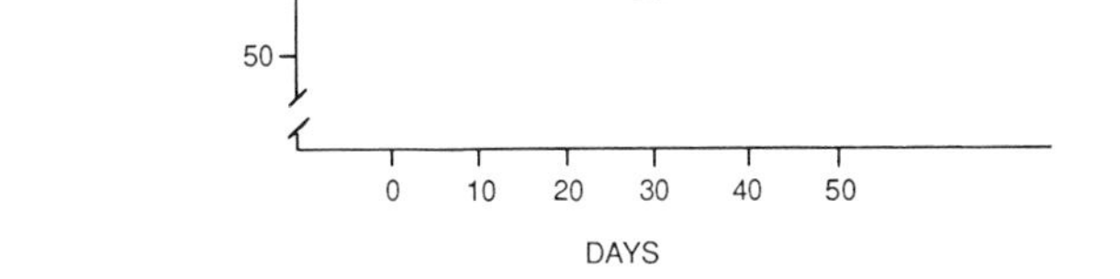

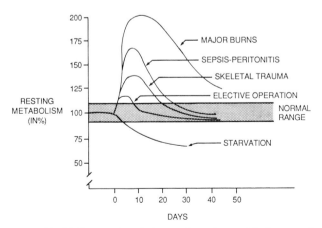

Figure 14–15. Stress-induced changes in resting metabolic expenditure. (Adapted from Long CL, Schaffel N, Geiger JW, et al: Metabolic response to injury and illness: Estimation of energy and protein needs from indirect calorimetry and nitrogen balance. JPEN 3:452–456, 1973. © by Am Soc of Parenteral and Enteral Nutrition.)

Fat is not maximally utilized during the injury response. The reason for this is not clear. The slight rise in insulin secondary to the initial surge of glucose appears to modulate or inhibit triglyceride lipase activity. Fatty acids may however supply a considerable portion of energy requirements in trauma.[22] Lipid metabolism in trauma has not been studied as extensively as glucose or protein metabolism. Some studies suggest increased mobilization, whereas others report impaired FFA oxidation. Shaw and Wolfe[23] report increases in the rate of glycerol turnover, and fat oxidation was double in their study of 43 blunt trauma patients. Similarly, in 1990, Jeevanandam et al[24] studied the nutritional impact on the energy cost of fat free mobilization in polytrauma patients. They concluded that fat mobilization usually exceeds the need for oxidative substrates and the leftover fatty acids are reesterified, resulting in a "futile" triglyceride-FFA cycle. They quantified the energy cost of this cycling to be 1.34 per cent of resting energy expenditure. See Table 14–4 for a summary of the metabolic response to injury.

The consequences of sustained hypermetabolic injury states are as follows:

1. Lean body mass sacrificed
2. Immune system blunted
3. Delayed wound healing
4. Increased basal energy needs

TABLE 14–4. METABOLIC RESPONSE TO INJURY

Metabolic rate	Increase
Body temperature	Increase
Blood glucose levels	Increase
Serum insulin	Increase or no change
Glucagon levels	Increase
Catecholamines	Increase
Cortisol levels	Increase
Blood lactate	Increase
Free fatty acids	Increase
Urine nitrogen excretion	Increase
Interleukin-1	Increase

5. Increased oxygen consumption ($\dot{V}_{O_2}$)
6. Increased carbon dioxide production ($\dot{V}_{CO_2}$)

As stated previously, the time of peak metabolic rate due to injury ranges from 5 to 10 days. The peak response varies in relation to the severity of injury- and/or disease-related metabolic processes. Controversy exists over the exact increases in metabolic rate or calories associated with the critically ill trauma population. Long[25] cites the general increases in basal metabolic rate (BMR) after multiple fractures as 10 to 30 per cent; after sepsis, 25 to 45 per cent; and after major burns, 40 to 100 per cent. The Wilmore nomogram (Fig. 14–16) shows patients with multiple trauma and infection as having estimated increased demands that range from 30 to 54 per cent above BMR, and a multiple-trauma patient on a ventilator exhibiting a need of 52 to 75 per cent above BMR. Recent studies of critically ill patients suggest needs ranging between 12 and 20 per cent above BMR.[26–28] Stress-induced changes in metabolic rate appear to return to normal within about 20 days as long as complications are prevented. Measuring metabolic rate and BMR, and energy prediction equations are discussed later in this chapter.

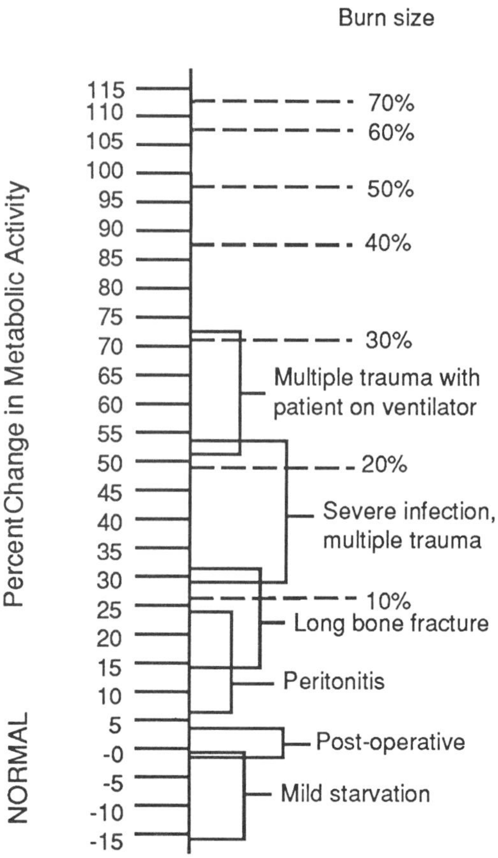

Figure 14–16. Estimate of increased energy needs with stress. (Adapted from Wilmore DW: The Metabolic Management of the Critically Ill. New York, Plenum Medical Book Co, 1977, p 36.)

NUTRITIONAL ASSESSMENT ACROSS THE CYCLES

Nutritional assessment involves subjective and objective data as well as laboratory or biochemical data. Subjective data usually are obtained by self-report through an interview process. Examples of this include the dietary and medical history. Objective data are obtained by direct measurement and include physical examination, height, weight, anthropometric measures, and skin antigen testing. Additionally, biochemical or laboratory data are gathered, analyzing composition of blood and urine. A critical summary of the most widely utilized measures is given.

Nutritional indices may be significantly influenced by nonnutritional factors, and standards derived from epidemiological studies may not always be applicable to evaluation of a given person. Nutritional assessment should not depend on a single parameter but should involve the determination of multiple parameters, the interpretation of which must take into account the entire medical status of the patient.[29]

Critical Care Phase Assessment Strategies

Medical and Dietary History

On admission, a medical and dietary history should be taken. Medical and dietary histories are focused on items that help to determine patients at risk for nutritional deficiency before hospitalization. These items include observations such as the following:

1. Change in eating habits with rationale
2. Recent weight loss or gain with rationale
3. GI disorders with rationale
4. Past diet history, special diets, types of foods eaten
5. Chronic illness with rationale

These items help to direct the assessor to potential dietary or medical imbalances that might result in nutrient deficiencies. Important clues include recent weight loss of greater than 10 per cent of body weight, chronic illness, food faddism, substance abuse, and GI disorders. These factors may further complicate recovery. The susceptibility of malnourished patients to infection is well known. Combine this scenario with a hypermetabolic trauma state, and the risk for complications increases.

In an intensive care unit (ICU) setting, a family member is often the one who provides information; therefore, the validity of this information is questionable. One might give greater value to a spouse's interview (if a close relationship exists) than to a distant sister. This process, however, serves as an initial screening. For instance, there are a number of nutritional deficiencies associated with specific disease processes. Therefore, knowledge of the disease alcoholism might lead one to suspect related nutritional deficiencies (e.g., protein, folate, niacin, thiamine, and riboflavin).

The nurse is frequently the person who obtains this information by way of a nursing data base. Prior height and weight estimates, when available, provide baseline information on current body weight. These indicate nutritional risk when compared with the patient's usual weight, desirable weight, or both. For the most part, serial weights are not valid as an indicator of nutritional status in the acute phase.

Special attention must be paid to the obese patient, who commonly is labeled as overnourished. For example, an elderly obese woman was admitted to the trauma unit with severe protein-calorie malnutrition. Her calorie intake was excessive; however, she had visceral protein depletion due to a deficient protein intake. This patient's course was complicated by multiple infections, which typically are present in visceral protein depletion.

The traumatic event itself is critical to the history. This important information may help to determine which patient is at risk for developing protein-calorie malnutrition. A close relation exists among urea nitrogen excretion, resting metabolic expenditure, and magnitude of injury. The greater the magnitude of injury, the greater the risk for nutritional deficiencies. Prolonged protein catabolism results in muscular weakness (contributing to inadequate pulmonary ventilation and cardiac insufficiency), reduced immune system potency, and eventually loss of wound strength and improper healing.[30]

In summary, a history (both dietary and medical) is important to use in assessing a trauma victim. The advantage of this method is its ability to identify preexisting dietary or disease processes that could complicate recovery. A physical examination can contribute to identification of nutrient deficits.

Physical Examination

A physical examination is of limited use in assessing nutritional status in most trauma patients. This is due, in part, to overt mechanical disruptions in total body integrity. Additionally, information derived from this examination can be determined more accurately through anthropometric and laboratory values. For example, changes in color (i.e., paleness), which might indicate anemia, can be tested more accurately by a complete blood count. Similarly, overt body wasting can be detected visually, but quantification and confirmation are done with anthropometric measures. In an initial evaluation of the trauma patient, physical examination as a nutritional assessment strategy is of limited value. One might, however, rely on this method for detecting vitamin deficiencies in a different clinical setting or at a later stage of trauma recovery.

Weight and Height

Weight relative to height is a measure of gross body composition and a valuable indicator of nutritional risk when compared with the patient's usual weight, desirable weight, or both. Weight is the most widely used measure of nutritional status. According to Jensen et al,[5] weight is a valuable general indicator of malnutrition. In contrast, Grant et al[31] state that "percentage ideal body weight will incorrectly detect malnourishment in the normally ectomorphic patient and overlook possible depletion in the obese patient." They recommend using "usual body weight instead of ideal body weight avoiding the use of the Metropolitan Life Insurance tables."[31] This assumes that the patient and/or family knows his or her best or usual weight. The utility of weight/height measures can be seen as an adjunct in nutritional evaluation.

In the trauma assessment, one would look at the total clinical picture; therefore, weight would be viewed as one small piece of the clinical puzzle. The main concern is evaluation of trends. For instance, a 10-lb weight loss in a patient 2 days after admission might not be significant in view of edema and fluid overload.

The early postadmission weight of the multiple-trauma or thermally injured patient may be elevated 12 to 15 per cent above the patient's preinjury weight as a consequence of massive fluid resuscitation. In contrast, the cachectic patient with anasarca may lose body weight during the introduction of nutritional therapy in response to an increase in colloid osmotic pressure and subsequent diuresis.[5] Additionally, weights are falsely elevated owing to body casts, braces, Hoffman apparatus, and other devices. Utilize weights to note trends. Preweight/height ratios provide a baseline index or general comparison of nutritional reserves. If the patient is hemodynamically stable with adequate osmolarity, trends of small weight increases with specific nutritional support serve as an indication of adequate support. Anthropometric measures offer a more accurate assessment of body composition; however, they also have significant drawbacks for use during the acute phase with this population.

Anthropometric Measures

Each of the body's basic fuels can be evaluated using anthropometric, biochemical, and immunological parameters. Anthropometric measures include triceps skin fold, midarm circumference, and midarm muscle circumference. Precise measurement technique (for triceps skin fold) is mandatory because the fat distribution in the upper arm is not uniform and limitations in accuracy depend primarily on location of the skin fold and intraobserver variability; utilization of defined procedures may be impossible in patients with orthopedic, neurologic, burn and other injuries who are unable to sit or stand upright because of limitations imposed by traction, mental status, massive injury or other common impediments.[5] Additionally, owing to time and equipment required, these methods are of little clinical use.[31] In comparison, mid–upper arm circumference and arm muscle area are more easily measured and require little time and training.

Although still subject to intrarater reliability, midarm circumference measures could be used as an adjunct in noting trends in nutritional status. Mid–upper arm circumference and arm muscle area are indicators of skeletal muscle protein mass and, therefore, are extremely important in assessing losses due to catabolic processes identified in trauma patients. Improved accuracy could be obtained by marking position of measurement directly on the skin, thus also improving reliability. One must discontinue use in the presence of body edema.

In general, interpretation of anthropometric data derived from a given individual is confused by the variability of "normal" values obtained from different populations. In addition, the magnitude of "malnutrition" is ill-defined, and suggested criteria have not been rigorously validated.[29] Further, variations in height, weight, extent of obesity, sex, age and the presence of edema contribute to error in these bodily measurements. Standard tables for age, sex, and fat pad have not been adequately developed for this population. In light of these findings, anthropometric measures should be used cautiously, if at all, during this phase of trauma. Their use may be more appropriate during the intermediate and/or rehabilitation phases of recovery. Biochemical measures provide a more reliable means of assessing skeletal muscle mass.

Creatinine/Height Index

It is debatable whether creatinine/height index (CHI) should be utilized. Creatinine/Height Index provides another estimate of skeletal mass since urinary levels of creatinine are dependent principally upon the extent of skeletal muscle catabolism, particularly during protein depletion.[5] Muscle is the largest protein-containing tissue in the body, and therefore, the CHI provides a useful measure for evaluating the degree of protein depletion. To maintain serum levels constant as protein catabolism occurs, there is an increase in creatinine excretion. Forbes and Bruining[32] "found an excellent reported correlation ($r = 0.988$) between lean body mass and urinary creatinine excretion."

Accurate interpretation of the test requires normal kidney function and effective collection of urine. "Since the calculations of CHI are, in part, dependent on ideal body weight, creatinine/height index is subject to the same errors of interpretation as the latter."[29] Excretion is dependent on age, sex, and height and can be affected by multiple medications. Additionally, although serial tests detect further depletion, positive responses to nutritional therapy during short-term hospitalization may not be detected, since some physical activity is essential to the synthesis of lean body mass.[5] Excretion is not affected by fluid shifts and is therefore more sensitive than height and weight comparisons. Three consecutive 24-hour urine collections must be obtained and averaged to obtain a high reliability.[32] Errors frequently result from incomplete collections. In addition, creatinine may rapidly elevate secondary to crushing musculoskeletal injury and thus not reflect nutritional status. Comparison tables use weight and height for medium-frame young adults and ignore the wide normal variations in healthy body types.

Creatinine/height index appears to be of some value in the long-term critically ill trauma patient in that protein depletion over time could be measured.

Additionally, many trauma patients have adequate renal function; therefore, validity is improved. In the long run, urea nitrogen might be a better assessment alternative, since it affords the ability to measure anabolism as well as catabolism of proteins.

Serum Proteins

An assessment of serum proteins helps to estimate the degree of visceral protein depletion. Albumin, transferrin, prealbumin, and/or retinol-binding protein have varying sensitivity in estimating visceral protein depletion. Fibronectin and somatomedin-C have been studied as potential serum visceral protein markers.[33, 34] "During protein deprivation, albumin levels in the serum may require days or weeks to decrease; as a result, redistribution of extravascular albumin into the plasma pool occurs."[5] This occurs because the total albumin pool is large and the liver continues to synthesize new albumin; therefore, serious, prolonged deficits may exist before they are obvious. Additionally, various nonnutritional factors appear to be associated with a decrease in serum albumin. The critically ill trauma patient has hypoalbuminemia for multiple reasons: excessive loss by way of the GI tract, skin, and kidneys; hemodynamic instability; steroid administration; injury; sepsis; and blood loss. "For example, expansion of the extracellular fluid compartment will result in a reduction in serum albumin."[29] Further, "corticosteroids cause a change in the distribution of albumin into the intravascular spaces."[5] The administration of albumin for osmotic purposes can falsely elevate albumin levels. Repeated studies have correlated hypoalbuminemia with increased morbidity and mortality at levels below 3 g/dl, and albumin is used in clinical practice because of this correlation.[35, 36] Studies of this nature have not been done in the trauma population. Albumin levels below 3 g/dl are not uncommon in this population. Other serum proteins, such as transferrin, retinol-binding protein, prealbumin, somatomedin-C, fibronectin, and C-reactive protein, are either controversial or drastically altered in the acute phase of trauma. Their measure often does not reflect nutritional status or adequacy of nutrition supplementation, especially in the acute stress period.[37] These are, however, still to be studied.[16] An excellent review of albumin's use in nutritional support, its synthesis, and use as an assessment strategy exists.[38, 39]

In conclusion, although albumin, like all other parameters, has limitations, its value as a correlate of morbidity and mortality trends offers clinical significance in the trauma setting.[40]

Nitrogen Balance

"Since nitrogen is the primary component that differentiates protein from other basic nutrient moieties and since protein status reflects overall state of nutrition, nitrogen balance is also employed as an index of protein nutritional status."[5] Nitrogen balance reflects homeostasis if it is approximately zero. During stresses such as severe trauma and sepsis, the balance between anabolism and catabolism in terms of protein is altered. Nitrogen balance in this case would be negative owing to the greater degree of protein catabolism. Therefore, nitrogen balance serves as an indication of the magnitude of injury because daily nitrogen losses from catabolism can be estimated through use of 24-hour urine collections. Accurate collection is a must. Although a 24-hour collection is ideal, reliability has been reported with shorter collection time (i.e., 12 hours and greater).[41] Although, in theory, nitrogen balance studies are ideal, in practice, accurate collection is difficult because of numerous variables. This appears to be the greatest problem with this test. Serial use of this assessment tool also allows for evaluation of nutrient adequacy. In general, the extent of nitrogen losses depends on prior nutritional status. For example, nitrogen losses usually are lower in nutritionally depleted people. According to Long,[42] during stress, nitrogen depletion cannot be prevented during the body's peak catabolic response. It can be significantly replenished with vigorous nutritional support. Therefore, maximum nutritional replacement corresponds with maximum nitrogen loss in most patients. An example is the patient with a spinal cord injury, who will have losses in nitrogen that reflect protein loss due to denervation and disuse of paralyzed muscles. Other sources of protein must also be assessed in determining this balance.

Determination of nitrogen balance requires meticulous evaluation of all nitrogen intake (oral, enteral, parenteral) and of all nitrogen-excreting routes (urinary, fecal, dermal).[5] Renal diseases and identification of specific medications must be considered when interpreting results. The nurse must accurately collect urine and maintain intake and output records. Additionally, because calculations do not account for abnormal nitrogen losses, nitrogen excretion is underestimated in those patients with burns, diarrhea, vomiting, fistula drainage and other abnormal nitrogen losses.[5] Reporting potential nitrogen losses, such as diarrhea and large draining wounds, to the dietitian contributes to valid results from this study. When utilizing nitrogen balance in the trauma patient, one must consider these occult losses. The formula for nitrogen balance is as follows:

Nitrogen balance =
nitrogen intake − (nitrogen output and obligatory losses)

Nitrogen balance equals the nitrogen intake minus the nitrogen output as urine urea nitrogen plus obligatory nitrogen losses from skin, feces, drains, and menstrual losses. The factor for obligatory losses is about 3. Total amount of nitrogen intake is calculated from the protein intake from enteral and/or parenteral routes in the 24-hour study period. For every 6.25 g of protein, there is 1 g of nitrogen.

$$\frac{\text{protein (grams)} = \text{nitrogen intake (grams)}}{6.25}$$

Nitrogen output is calculated from a 24-hour urine collection and sent to the laboratory for urine urea nitrogen. Nitrogen balance calculations become more complex if there is renal dysfunction with significant changes in blood urea nitrogen.

Nutritionists utilize C-reactive protein as a modulator of stress and compare it with nitrogen balance to assist in determining if energy needs are being met. For example, if C-reactive protein is elevated and nitrogen balance is negative, the goal is to provide calories relative to measured or calculated needs, keeping in mind that if stress levels are high, it may be impossible to reach positive nitrogen balance. Conversely, if C-reactive protein is not elevated and nitrogen balance persists, then it is clear that energy expenditure is exceeding energy intake and adjustments must occur in caloric intake.

In conclusion, nitrogen balance should be determined in patients who are free from renal disease and in patients in whom nutritional support is to be evaluated. In trauma patients, this evaluation must also consider potential occult losses. These balances can be followed serially, thus indicating effectiveness of nutritional support.

Additionally, of utmost importance in traumatically injured patients is an intact immune system. Although numerous clinical observations and epidemiological data document close association between protein-calorie malnutrition and increased susceptibility to infection, the exact relation between nutrition and host defense mechanisms remains unclear.[5] Immune functions are influenced by multiple factors, including one's nutritional status; therefore, evaluation of such parameters are of nutritional importance.

Total Lymphocyte Count

Protein-calorie malnutrition is recognized as the most common cause of immune dysfunction. Total lymphocyte count (TLC) is one way to assess immune functioning. Multiple factors can alter TLC and must be considered before low counts are used to reflect the degree of visceral protein losses. For example, lymphocytopenia has been observed in well-nourished patients following anesthesia and operations; such depressed counts usually return to normal within 48 hours.[29] Lewis and Klein[43] found that preoperative lymphocytopenia was associated with depressed albumin levels. This association was found to be significant. Additionally, if both parameters were depressed, an increased rate of postoperative sepsis was observed. In contrast, leukocytosis may be caused by a number of factors including tissue necrosis or infection.[5] Therefore, the utility of total lymphocyte count as a nutritional parameter is dependent upon excluding the influence of many possible non-nutritional factors.[29] In general, this assessment parameter would be collected and utilized for noting trends in relation to the patient's clinical picture. Potential research also exists in this area. Considering the influence of non-nutritional factors such as sepsis, necrosis, and surgical interventions evident in most trauma patients, TLC is of limited use in this phase of trauma. Loss of immune competence can also be evaluated by skin antigen testing.

Inability to respond (anergy) is related to visceral protein depletion. Delayed-type hypersensitivity reactions to common skin test antigens evaluate function of the cellular immune system.[31] To date, no universal standards for interpretation have been developed.

It has been stated that serial testing can serve as a sensitive guide to prognosis and adequacy of clinical management. However, most subjects who are tested repeatedly exhibit accelerated reactions which start within several hours post-injection, peak within 24 hours and subside quite rapidly,[5] thus indicating increased response without any nutritional treatment associated. After trauma, skin tests are almost always unresponsive and remain so for at least 10 days.[16] Because there are no conclusive reports or clinical standards, this test should not be utilized in the trauma setting.

Metabolic Rate

Historically, the study of human energy metabolism, or metabolic rate, has undergone periods of great activity as well as periods of relative disinterest. The classic investigations during the first 25 years of this century include Lusk, DuBois, and Benedict. They applied both direct and indirect calorimetry to the study of nutrition, exercise, and certain disease states.[44] There has been a resurgence of interest in the measurement of energy expenditure. Special populations of patients have stimulated much research in this area, such as those patients with cancer, malnutrition-starvation syndromes, obesity, and critical illness. There is general acceptance that these acute conditions are associated with alterations in energy expenditure that favor weight loss, protein catabolism, and immunosuppression. There is still controversy over the extent to which increased energy expenditure plays a role in tissue depletion.[44] In addition, the development of TPN and new attempts at prophylactic nutritional regimens have prompted many new questions regarding energy expenditure and utilization by acutely ill or injured patients.

Multiple factors underline the body's metabolic rate. BMR is the amount of energy required to carry on the involuntary work of the body, which includes the functional activity of various organs, such as the brain, heart, liver, kidneys, lungs; secretory activities of glands; peristaltic movements of the GI tract; oxidation occurring in resting cells; and maintenance of muscle tone and body temperature.[45] BMR is the measurement of caloric expenditure (heat production) in a person under specific controlled conditions, such as supine, at rest, with some muscle tone, and fasting a minimum of 12 hours in a thermally neutral environment.[46] BMR can be considered a baseline energy reading in the normal, healthy person. It is calculated as the energy expenditure minus the effect of food (specific dynamic effect) above basal activity and specific disease processes. In normal people, the BMR is primarily dependent on several factors—body size (body surface area), age, and sex. Body surface area represents the metabolically active cellular component in the BMR. Studies show that females with the same body size have a lower BMR than males. This is believed to be due to a smaller body proportion of lean mass and, therefore, less active metabolic tissue.[2]

The type of food ingested has been noted to alter the heat production observed. This phenomenon, known as the specific dynamic effect (SDE) of food, was first described by Rubner in 1902 (cited in Wilmore[2]). The SDE represents the energy required for digestion and absorption as well as the stimulating effect of nutrients on metabolism.[45] Studies in normal people demonstrate that the SDE of protein is about 12 per cent, carbohydrate (CHO) is 6 per cent, and fat is 2 per cent.[2] Later, studies from Glickman et al[47] and Bradfield and Jourdan[48] indicated a smaller change in energy production after food ingestion in febrile, critically ill patients and obese females. Wilmore[2] concludes that failure to account for the SDE of food in critically ill hypermetabolic patients will lead to a small error. A major variable of energy expenditure in normal people is activity.

Energy expenditure is directly proportional to body size and the intensity and duration of the activity. On a fixed caloric intake, activity level determines energy balance in normal people. In contrast, traumatically injured patients' temperature is a more significant factor in altering metabolic rate.

Wilmore[2] reported that as body temperature increases, there is a rise in the rate constant for chemical reactions and that for each 10°C increase there is a twofold to threefold increase in the reaction rate. Kinney and Roe[49] observed energy expenditure values that exceeded DuBois' formula of a 7 per cent increase in metabolic rate associated with each 1°F rise in a severe trauma and septic population. Clowes, O'Donnell, and Blackburn[50] postulate the following reasons for the apparent discrepancy: increased work of respiration and elevated metabolic rate as well as possible uncoupling of phosphorylation.

Wilmore[2] also described a 10 to 13 per cent increase in heat production for each 1°C rise in body temperature and noted a wide variation in clinical practice (Fig. 14–17). Temperature alone, without increased metabolic demands due to trauma or sepsis, may have a predictable increase in energy expenditure. The question still remains as to its cumulative effect or lack thereof when concomitant conditions exist (e.g., systematic infection along with trauma and febrile conditions). Aulick[51] suggests that energy demands independent of temperature are detrimental and must be treated appropriately with nutritional support. Aulick[51] emphasized the distinction between thermal and nonthermal demands in severely ill patients because thermal demands are best treated by environmental control and nonthermal metabolic needs can only be satisfied by providing exogenous

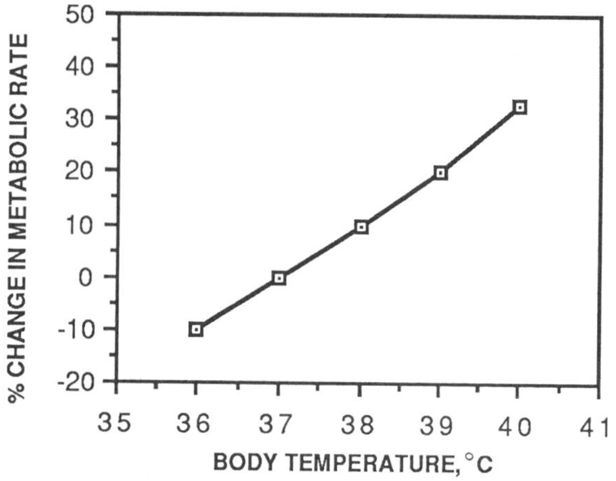

Figure 14–17. Body temperature and metabolic rate. (From Wilmore DW: The Metabolic Management of the Critically Ill. New York, Plenum Medical Book Co, 1977, p 29.)

substrates. A decrease in body temperature signals a proportional decrease in metabolic demands. In addition, as people age, their metabolic rate decreases (Fig. 14–18). The decreased metabolic rate among older people as well as with female subjects is thought to be related to a decrease in lean body mass.

Variables that have been noted to affect a person's metabolic rate and that are not accounted for by most energy prediction equations are disease processes, therapeutic regimens, acute events, and temperature changes. In addition, if weight is significantly below ideal, as in semistarvation states, the energy prediction that relies on weight is falsely low. Similarly, the needs of obese people are overestimated. Further, if one is older, despite a traumatic injury, he or she receives less caloric replacement, since age becomes a negative factor in the equation. BMR decreases with increasing age and must be considered when predicting caloric needs. The exact relation between age variation and degree of metabolic response to injury has yet to be described. Historically, studies that look at metabolic rate utilize direct and

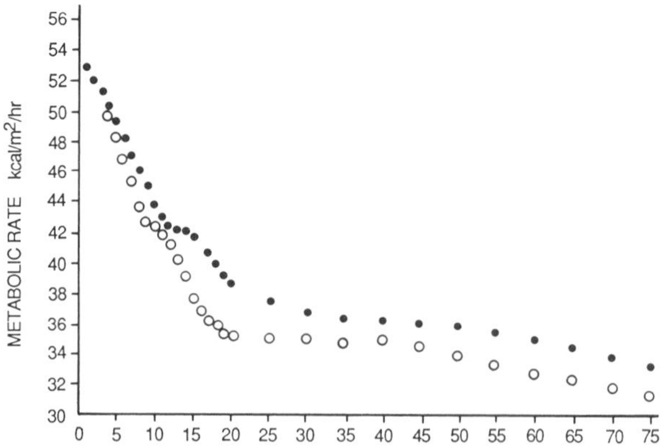

Figure 14–18. Age and metabolic rate. (From Wilmore DW: The Metabolic Management of the Critically Ill. New York, Plenum Medical Book Co, 1977, p 28.)

indirect calorimetry as a means of measuring energy expenditure.

Measuring Energy Expenditure

A kilocalorie is the amount of heat required to raise the temperature of 1 g of water 1°C at a pressure of 1 standard atmosphere. Heat loss from the body can be measured by direct calorimetry, which is the measurement of energy expenditure. This process of direct calorimetry requires standard conditions. The patient must be in a relatively steady state and enclosed in a carefully controlled chamber environment designed for calorimetry measurement. The process involves heat measurement through surface thermocouples located inside and outside the calorimeter, which measures heat as it is produced by the subject.[2] These techniques seldom are utilized in the clinical setting. Indirect calorimetry is the method of choice in the clinical setting and serves as a standard for other methods of determining caloric requirements.

Indirect calorimetry is the measurement of the integral component of heat production during oxidative processes, that is, $\dot{V}_{O2}$, $\dot{V}_{CO2}$, and nitrogen excretion.[52] A standard amount of oxygen is consumed for each mole of glucose oxidized; that is, the amount of O_2 consumed and CO_2 produced is quantified and related to heat production. Indirect calorimetry has been widely accepted because of its close correlation to direct calorimetry.[2] Therefore, indirect calorimetry determines energy expenditure based on quantification of gas exchange. Metabolic carts are probably one of the best, widely available measurement tools. Both direct and indirect calorimetry were utilized to develop the energy prediction equations used in practice. Problems associated with the metabolic carts are primarily related to short duration of sampling periods, expense, and the need for trained personnel. Frequently, the patient is monitored for 15 to 30 minutes, and values obtained are projected for a 24-hour period.

Only a few studies exist that utilize indirect calorimetry as a means for determining energy needs in the critically ill trauma population. Short-duration sample periods do not reflect normal changes that occur in the critical care environment during, for example, multiple anxiety-provoking or painful procedures. Weissman and associates[53] examined the effect of routine nursing and medical interventions on metabolic rate. Their results support the need for continuous 24-hour metabolic measurements to provide a composite view of variables that alter metabolic rate throughout the day. Chest physiotherapy was cited as causing the most sustained increase in metabolic rate. This study demonstrated that routine daily ICU activities can significantly alter metabolic rate and must be observed and reported. The measurement of the respiratory quotient (RQ) is an additional gas exchange parameter obtained from a metabolic chart that helps to assess nutritional status.

Respiratory quotient or ratio is the volume of CO_2 produced divided by the volume of O_2 consumed during the same period of time ($\dot{V}_{CO2}/\dot{V}_{O2}$). This ratio varies, depending on the primary substrate being utilized. A respiratory quotient (RQ) of less than 0.70 has been associated with oxidation of ketones or synthesis of carbohydrate from fat. A mixed diet results in an RQ of about 0.82. When excess carbohydrate loads are given, lipogenesis (production of fat) occurs, resulting in increased CO_2 production and an RQ of greater than 1.00. Excess carbohydrates may precipitate respiratory failure, which is of particular interest in patients who have difficulty being weaned from mechanical ventilation.

When interpreting energy expenditure and RQ from indirect calorimetry, one must be careful, since hyperventilation can cause an inaccurate test situation. Readings taken over time help to minimize respiratory variation. An RQ in septic hypermetabolic patients may remain below 1.00 even with excessive glucose loads because endogenous fat (RQ 0.70) is preferentially used and glucose is stored as glycogen.[54] In addition, values significantly below 0.70 may reflect methodological error and should be regarded with skepticism.[2]

The mass spectrometer and light spectrometer are also multiple gas analyzers that have been utilized in a multibed computerized capacity.[55] The latter is used in one of the major trauma centers to assess minute-by-minute gas exchange readings in several patients at the same time.[56] It is connected to a large central computer that calculates RQ, energy expenditure, and various other ventilatory parameters by way of a computer program.[57] This valuable information can be plotted over time. Such a sophisticated monitoring system is of aid in both nutritional and ventilatory management. Equations that are routinely used in the healthy and hospitalized need further validation by way of indirect calorimetry for use in the critically ill trauma population.

Predicting Energy Expenditure

Multiple energy prediction equations, nomograms, and tables exist and are utilized in practice. The Harris and Benedict equation (HBE) is the most widely used equation.[58] This is a basal energy prediction equation, which was developed by Harris and Benedict in 1919. They used indirect calorimetry technique to develop their multiple linear regression formula (Fig. 14–19). The fact that it is a basal energy equation implies the need for modification related to various activities, diseases, or variables that might increase or decrease the metabolic rate. In this equation, weight, height, and age are included in the calculations. Because of gender differences, metabolic rates for women and men are determined by separate regression equations. Other approaches exist, each with varying accuracy, such as those by Fleisch[59] and Boothby et al.[60] The HBE appears to be the most popular because of its historical use, availability, cost-effectiveness, and perceived accuracy.

The accuracy of the HBE as a technique for determining

Men	BMR = 66 + (13.7 x W) + (5 x H) - (6.8 x A)
Women	BMR = 655 + (9.6 x W) + (1.7 x H) - (4.7 x A)

W = actual weight in kilograms

H = height in centimeters

A = age in years

Figure 14–19. Harris-Benedict equation.

energy needs has been scrutinized by several researchers. Long and associates[61] disputed its accuracy with specific patient populations. They studied a group of 39 patients in various states of health and added an activity and injury factor to be multiplied by the HBE (Fig. 14–20). Although various institutions utilized these factors, their small sample size necessitates replication for continued validation and thus limits the ability to generalize these results to other samples. Despite problems, many health professionals are utilizing these factors for lack of other ways to adjust equations for the critically ill population. In addition, several more recent studies suggest that these factors overestimate energy needs.

McCamish et al[62] compared the HBE with Long's various injury factors and the HBE without additional factors to indirect calorimetry as measured by a metabolic cart. Their study indicates that Long's stress factor adjustments to the HBE significantly overestimated energy needs in their critically ill sample of 102 subjects when compared with indirect calorimetry.

Rutten et al[63] conducted a study designed to determine the protein and calorie requirements associated with a favorable response to TPN using a fixed nitrogen-calorie ratio. They concluded that in mild to moderate catabolism, energy repletion from 1.75 to 2.0 times the calculated BMR from HBE would afford a positive nitrogen balance.

In contrast, two more recent studies as well as several others suggest that the HBE needs only modest increases to afford better accuracy of prediction. Baker and associates[64] indicated a small difference between mean HBE value and mean indirect calorimetry values; that is, indirect calorimetry means equal 1609 ± 105 Kcal per day, and HBE mean equals 1580 ± 57 Kcal/day (N = 10).

Stanek[26] studied 35 traumatically injured patients and compared the HBE with and without Long's[61] activity and injury factors and a simple kilocalorie per kilogram ideal body weight formula with indirect calorimetry. Measurements were taken at frequent intervals throughout a 24-hour period (about two gas exchange readings per hour). The HBE was closest to predicting energy needs with a mean difference of 251 Kcal/day (underestimation), while the simple formula and the HBE with Long's factors overestimated energy needs by 1589 and 824 Kcal/day, respectively. Although continued research is necessary, the 15.5 per cent above basal energy needs found in this study are consistent with several recent studies that suggest needs ranging from 13 to 20 per cent above basal for the critically ill population.[28, 65]

Recently,[66] a predictive equation was developed for use in mechanically ventilated critically ill patients. Fifty-two trauma patients were included out of 112 total patients. Although no difference was found in energy expenditure for trauma and nontrauma patients, this may be due to the small sample size.[66] Studies of patients with head injuries seem to indicate extreme variability in metabolic rates.[66, 67] Studies note ranges between 26 and 200 per cent above BMR. This variability has been proposed to relate to increased motor activity, including posturing, which has been shown to increase metabolic rate.[67] Similarly, central fevers, coma states, brain death, neurosweats, and shivering could contribute to this variance. Barbiturate use has been studied and shown to decrease metabolic rate in patients with head injuries.[68] Indirect calorimetry is ideal for use with this population. The need to define operationally the degree of injury and/or to develop standard definitions for various factors cannot be overemphasized. Similarly, these factors and equations need to be compared with more sophisticated gas analysis techniques, which allow for multiple automatic gas samples taken over a 24-hour period.[69]

Nomograms such as the one developed by Wilmore[2] (see Fig. 14–16) assess the multiple-trauma patient on a ventilator as having energy needs between 52 and 72 per cent above basal. Data that support such large energy needs are lacking.

Activity Factor

Confined to bed	= 1.2
Out of bed	= 1.3

Injury Factor

Surgery	
Minor	= 1.1
Major	= 1.2
Infection	
Mild	= 1.2
Moderate	= 1.4
Severe	= 1.6
Trauma	
Skeletal	= 1.35
Head with Steroid	= 1.6
Blunt	= 1.35
Burns	
40% BSA	= 1.5
100% BSA	= 1.9

BSA = Body Surface Area

Figure 14–20. Activity and injury factor for the Harris-Benedict equation. (From Long CL: Nonseptic Stress Metabolism. Nutritional Management of Metabolic Stress. Monograph 97-1530-20-6. Abbott Laboratories, 1983, p 11.)

Health professionals need to evaluate energy/caloric needs carefully, since serious complications can occur with overfeeding.

The HBE appears to need a more modest multiplication factor, such as 1.15 to 1.16,[70, 71] to improve its accuracy in trauma patients. The patient who is severely burned, head injured, or septic with above-average energy needs may need an additional or larger factor used with the HBE. In contrast, the spinal cord–injured patient with paralysis may have needs that are slightly overestimated by the HBE[71] because of the loss of functional muscle tissue related to neuromuscular disruption. Metabolic demands seem to increase within the first week of spinal cord injury and then decrease relative to denervation of muscle tissue and associated loss of lean body mass. It is possible to have less than basal requirements based on the HBE in the quadriplegic population. Weight shifts in the spinal cord–injured population require adjustments to the Metropolitan Life tables of 10 to 15 lb for the paraplegic patient and 15 to 20 lb for the quadriplegic patient.[72] The importance of accurately assessing energy needs will be mentioned because complications can be serious and prolong recovery.

Excess Nutritional Replacement

Multiple complications can occur if energy needs are overestimated or underestimated. Wolfe and Chock[73] summarize the detrimental effects of excess intake as it relates to two major body systems, the liver, and the pulmonary system. For example, liver function test elevations, such as alkaline phosphatase, serum glutamic oxaloacetic transaminase (SGOT), and, occasionally, bilirubin, are a complication associated with overzealous parenteral carbohydrate (CHO) feeding.[74] Biopsies have shown fatty infiltration and increased glycogen stores within the hepatocyte. Many authors suggest excessive glucose administration (CHO loads) as the causative factor for the changes indicated.[75]

In addition, excess CHO loads associated with TPN are a physiological stress due to an increase in minute ventilation (V_E), oxygen consumption ($\dot{V}_{O_2}$), and carbon dioxide production ($\dot{V}_{CO_2}$).[76] RQ represents the oxidative properties of a given substrate. For example, mixed substrate utilization yields an RQ of about 0.85.[52] When available glycogen is depleted, there is a gradual shift to oxidation of fat, which is indicated by an RQ of 0.70.[42] When the intake of CHO exceeds the requirements, excess CHO is converted to fat, which yields more CO_2 than O_2, as represented by an RQ higher than 1.[73] Consequently, this increase in $\dot{V}_{CO_2}$ could play a role in patients who are difficult to wean from a ventilator.[77] The increased $\dot{V}_{CO_2}$ contributes to an increased workload, which may precipitate respiratory failure in the compromised host.[78] Patients with low cervical and upper thoracic spinal cord injuries are particularly vulnerable to being overfed due to their decreased energy needs combined with their inability to utilize intercostal, abdominal, and diaphragm muscles to compensate for increased $\dot{V}_{CO_2}$.

Gieske et al[79] showed an increase in $\dot{V}_{CO_2}$ and V_E and $\dot{V}_{O_2}$ means in a group of 13 patients with chronic obstructive pulmonary disease (COPD) after ingestion of a high-carbohydrate meal. In this relatively healthy group of COPD patients, only seven had an increase in Pa_{O_2} that was significant; more important, the increase in Pa_{CO_2} was not significant. They concluded that in this population, an increase in endogenous CO_2 load due to a high-carbohydrate diet is well tolerated.

In contrast, Covelli et al[80] studied patients who needed ventilatory support. Acute respiratory failure developed in three patients within hours after TPN was started. They concluded that excessive carbohydrate loading may precipitate acidosis in patients unable to adequately improve their alveolar ventilation when compensating for increasing $\dot{V}_{CO_2}$. The trauma population frequently consists of patients with pulmonary contusions, rib fractures, and hemopneumothoraces, which can alter the ability to compensate for increased $\dot{V}_{CO_2}$. Excessive carbohydrate loads are therefore an important consideration for this population of patients.

Burke et al[81] studied 18 severely burned patients and showed that there is a physiological cost of exceeding the optimal glucose infusion rate as indicated by increased rates of $\dot{V}_{CO_2}$ as well as large fat deposits in the liver at autopsy in patients infused with great amounts of glucose. It was concluded that there appeared to be a maximal rate of glucose infusion beyond which physiologically significant increases in protein synthesis and direct oxidation of glucose cannot be expected.

Similarly, other authors suggest that high intakes of glucose in a hypermetabolic patient may constitute a physiological stress as well as nutritional support.[28] Askanazi et al[28] examined 18 nutritionally depleted patients who had undergone prior weight loss versus 14 patients classified as septic or injured (febrile patients who had positive blood cultures and/or evidence of localized intra-abdominal infection). TPN with hypertonic glucose amino acid solutions given to the depleted group resulted in a rise in the RQ. This suggests little change in the metabolic rate; $\dot{V}_{O_2}$ only increased 3 per cent. Excess glucose in depleted patients was converted to fat as evidenced by an RQ of greater than 1.0. Administration of similar glucose solutions in hypermetabolic patients resulted in a smaller rise in the RQ, whereas $\dot{V}_{O_2}$ increased 29 per cent. They concluded that when glucose is administered in quantities above energy expenditure in hypermetabolic patients, fat is still being utilized for energy, resulting in an RQ significantly less than 1.0. Although further studies are indicated, excess nutritional replacement appears to increase metabolic rate.

Wolfe et al[82] support the concept that increasing a glucose solution beyond energy needs does not increase the rate of oxidation of glucose (its utilization) and therefore will contribute to an RQ of greater than 1.0, such as that found with lipogenesis. In other words, there is a point at which excess fuel sources may be of no obvious value and potentially detrimental to a person's preexisting metabolic status.

Similarly, a case study by Askanazi et al[83] indicated a rise in temperature (37.6° to 39°C) and an associated increase in BMR up to 23 per cent when the patient was changed from a 5 per cent dextrose solution to TPN. This patient, when studied clinically, showed no other evidence that would account for this increase, since the white blood cell count remained within normal limits and blood cultures were negative. After 4 days, the TPN was discontinued with a coincidental prompt drop in body temperature. These authors have previously documented an increase in energy expenditure and norepinephrine excretion in association with the administration of hypertonic glucose in hypermetabolic patients.[28, 78] In contrast to excessive energy replacement, inadequate caloric replacement has been associated with other complications.

Inadequate Nutritional Replacement

Multiple complications can occur if energy needs are underestimated. For example, somatic protein loss, impaired wound healing, and diminished resistance to infection are characteristics of inadequate nutritional replacement. Birkhahn et al[84] studied nitrogen losses in 14 patients, 8 of whom were normal and healthy and 6 of whom were trauma patients. Both groups had received 5 per cent dextrose as their only nutritional source for 72 hours. The control subjects lost an average of 6 g of nitrogen per day, whereas trauma patients lost 25 g of nitrogen per day. Trauma patients also had a 50 per cent increase in whole-body protein synthesis and a 79 per cent increase in protein breakdown. One interesting aspect of their data was the indication that women exhibit a dampened response compared with men. The nitrogen excretion, plasma flux, and leucine oxidation of the women studied were closer to those of the control group, indicating that much less protein destruction and turnover occurred. Despite the small sample size, their work suggests that metabolic differences between sexes merits further investigation.

Similarly, Long et al[85] studied the contribution of skeletal muscle protein in elevated rates of whole-body protein catabolism in trauma patients. The breakdown rates were 187 and 163 per cent (male and female, respectively) greater than those of eight control subjects. This protein loss, if sustained, may affect the respiratory musculature, leading to a decrease in effective ventilation as well as affecting other vital organs.

Bassili and Dietel[86] studied 47 patients who required mechanical ventilation. Group A received calories far below required amounts (400 Kcal/day), whereas group B received optimum caloric replacement (1300 to 1600 Kcal/day). Of group A, only 54.4 per cent could be weaned from the ventilator, whereas 92.8 per cent in group B were successfully weaned. Semistarvation states have also been explored in relation to alteration in hypoxic ventilatory drive.

A study by Doekel et al[87] examined the effect of depressed hypoxic ventilatory response due to the decreased metabolic rate noted in semistarvation states. By the 10th day of a 500-calorie CHO diet with vitamin and mineral supplements, metabolic rate was significantly decreased and hypoxic ventilatory response decreased to 47 per cent of that for controls. In addition, they noted that this hypoxic response was virtually abolished in two subjects. Their findings point to the potential complication malnutrition has on the hypoxic ventilatory response in humans.

Bartlett et al[88] looked at the metabolic rate of 15 patients with the most extensive chest trauma injuries from a group of 44 patients admitted to a surgical ICU. Indirect calorimetry readings were used to assess $\dot{V}_{O2}$, $\dot{V}_{CO2}$, RQ, and daily energy balance. There was a moderate increase in metabolic rate, which usually returned to normal within the first week. A late increase in $\dot{V}_{O2}$ was associated with sepsis, large energy deficits, and death in three patients. These authors also noted CO_2 overload due to excessive feeding, which resulted in weaning difficulty in three ventilator patients. The correlation between measured and predicted metabolic rate was only 0.52 using Wilmore's[2] formulas for energy prediction. Their report supported the need for direct measurement of $\dot{V}_{O2}$ and $\dot{V}_{CO2}$ by way of indirect calorimetry in traumatically injured patients. Inadequate caloric replacement can also alter the body's reparative processes.

Multiple nutrient deficits can inhibit wound healing in trauma patients. Adequate quantities of the macronutrients, CHO, and fats are necessary to meet the energy requirements of cells such as leukocytes and fibroblasts.[89] Similarly, arginine is necessary for the synthesis of collagen[90] and supplementation with it promotes wound healing and enhanced immune function (by decreasing T-cell dysfunction) in animal models.[91] If these cells are not adequately nourished, resistance to infection as well as collagen synthesis is impaired.[89] Immunosuppression and the inability to react to skin antigen testing is an additional negative consequence associated with malnutrition.

The inability to respond to skin testing of standard antigens (anergy) has been associated with increased sepsis and mortality in general surgical patients.[92] Protein malnutrition is associated with an impaired host defense mechanism, specifically cell-mediated immunity, as evidenced by the skin antigen recall testing.[93] Similarly, other immune dysfunctions, such as depressed antibody production, function of phagocytic cells, and levels of complement, occur in malnutrition.[94] Viral and fungal infections are associated with depressed T-cell–mediated immunity, which is affected by malnutrition. Protein-calorie malnutrition is common in patients with a combination of severe catabolic stress and low nutrient intake.

Protein-calorie malnutrition (PCM) is an imbalanced diet that is inadequate in calories or protein. These patients have a normal somatic compartment but visceral proteins (i.e., albumin and total protein) are low. In contrast, the patient may have normal visceral proteins and low somatic proteins, typical of balanced deficit diets.[95] Many traumatically injured patients exhibit low visceral proteins, whereas initially, their somatic compartments are normal.[5] The population with chronic illness is most susceptible to the end-stage nutritional classification in which there is a combination of low visceral and somatic stores. This seldom is seen in the average trauma patient.

PCM has been shown to result in poor wound healing, decreased resistance to infection, decreased ability to tolerate surgery, and decreased sense of well-being.[96] A decrease in visceral proteins is considered severer than a decrease in somatic proteins because it is associated with a deficient immune response combined with loss of other vital functions associated with visceral proteins. The trauma patient is at serious risk for development of PCM, which could drastically alter recovery. Accurate nutritional assessment of energy and protein needs and delivery of necessary nutrients can positively influence the prognosis of the trauma patient. Therefore, it is essential to find the most accurate means for estimating metabolic needs in this patient population.

In addition to determining energy requirements, fluid and electrolyte status must be closely monitored in this acutely ill group. The physician, dietitian, and nurse should monitor serum glucose levels as well as urine glucose and acetone

TABLE 14–5. GUIDELINES FOR METABOLIC MONITORING DURING STRESS

VARIABLE	SUGGESTED FREQUENCY*
Serum glucose concentration	Daily
Insulin resistance	Daily
Serum lactate concentration	Initially and every 3 days
BUN and serum creatinine concentration	Daily until condition is stabilized, then every 3 days
Serum triglyceride concentration	Initially and twice weekly
Serum transferrin concentration	Initially and weekly
Prealbumin or retinol-binding protein levels	Initially and weekly
Creatinine clearance	Every 3 to 4 days
Urinary nitrogen (urea) excretion and balance	Initially and weekly
Urinary 3-methylhistidine excretion	Initially and weekly
Liver enzymes	Twice weekly
Coagulation screen	2 to 3 times weekly
Vitamin and trace element levels	As needed
Zinc and magnesium levels	Weekly

*Actual frequency is dictated by clinical need. (From Cerra FB (consultant): The Trauma Patient. Abbott Laboratories Monograph, 1982, with permission.)

levels in all patients on TPN. If lipids are being given, special attention should be given to triglyceride levels. Suggested guidelines for metabolic monitoring during stress as well as variables to be monitored during TPN are provided in Tables 14–5 and 14–6, respectively. Appendix 14–1 provides a synopsis and critique of nutritional assessment parameters in the trauma patient.[97] Appendix 14–2 provides an example of a nutritional flowsheet used to document nutritional intake and specific metabolic assessment parameters ($\dot{V}_{CO_2}$, $\dot{V}_{O_2}$, RQ, urine urea nitrogen) in the critical care phase of trauma.

TABLE 14–6. VARIABLES TO BE MONITORED DURING STANDARD TPN

	SUGGESTED FREQUENCY
Growth Variables	
Weight	Daily
General Measurements	
Volume of infusate	Daily
Oral intake (if any)	Daily
Urine output	Daily
Clinical Observations	
Vital signs	Daily
Fluid balance	Daily
Cardiovascular status	Daily
Metabolic Variables	
Fractionated urine samples for glucose and acetone levels	Every 6 hours
Serum glucose and electrolyte (sodium, potassium, and chloride) values	Twice weekly, initially; later at least weekly
Blood urea nitrogen, creatinine, calcium, phosphate, magnesium values, and complete blood count	Twice weekly
Total protein values	Weekly
24-hour urine determinations for urea nitrogen levels	Weekly
24-hour determinations for creatinine values	Weekly

From Cerra FB (consultant): The Trauma Patient. Abbott Laboratories Monograph, 1982, with permission.

Intermediate-Phase Assessment Strategies

Physical Examination

Although not quantitative, the physical examination may give clues to nutrient deficiencies. Table 14–7 offers an overview of substrate and nutrients, assessment parameters, physical assessment findings, patients at risk, and related wound and healing alterations seen with specific deficiencies. This table is not exhaustive but offers some guidelines to the relation between nutrient deficiencies, function, and potential alteration in physical assessment findings. Astute observation of physical assessment findings may lead to changes in patient management. Patients who continue to have muscle wasting, despite what appears to be adequate caloric replacement, may need nitrogen balance studies or metabolic cart evaluation. Similarly, a patient whose level of consciousness improves may be ready to convert from enteral to oral feedings. Signs of fluid overload may require a more concentrated form of calories.

Height-Weight Ratios

Height-weight ratios may be a little more appropriate at this time if the patient is hemodynamically stable and without edema. Use of ideal body weight has been criticized because a patient may have a stable body weight that is below ideal and not be considered malnourished. Similarly, an obese person may lose large amounts of weight, still be overweight, and not be considered malnourished. Serial weights can, however, note trends that can be helpful when viewed in relation to other factors. Patients whose nutritional status is improving with increased visceral proteins may have an initial decrease in weight secondary to the subsequent diuresis. Grant[7] as well as others suggests utilizing usual body weight divided by actual body weight and determining the percentage of usual weight. Although it too must be interpreted carefully, it would avoid missing recent weight loss as a clinical parameter.[7]

Anthropometric Measures

Most nutrition experts agree that anthropometric measurements, despite accurately reflecting total body fat when compared with densitometry in stable populations,[95] should be interpreted with caution, if interpreted at all.[2, 7, 29] A more recent technique, discussed in the next section, studying body composition holds promise for more accurate assessment of body protein and fat compartments.

Radiographic Measurements

Radiographic measurement of midarm compartment composition is possible by means of computed tomographic (CT) scans. This method allows for direct visualization and quantification of bone, fat, and muscle tissue. The value of this test is its ability to assist in establishing more precise standards for arm anthropometric measurements. Institutions that rely on anthropometric measurements may be able to use this technique on patients who are edematous or obese.

TABLE 14–7. NUTRITIONAL ASSESSMENT AND WOUND HEALING

SUBSTRATE, VITAMIN, MINERAL, TRACE ELEMENT	WOUND AND HEALING ALTERATION/NEEDS	ASSESSMENT PARAMETER	PHYSICAL ASSESSMENT AND PATIENT AT RISK
General			
Protein status	Decreased wound healing, decreased resistance to local infection, decreased protein synthesis	Albumin, transferrin, MAMC,* nitrogen balance, CHI*	Delayed wound healing; muscle wasting; edema; protein-calorie malnutrition; dull, dry, sparse, depigmented hair; moon face; hepatosplenomegaly; psychomotor changes
CHO status	Energy requirements of specialized cells, e.g., leukocytes, fibroblasts; therefore, resistance to infection decreased and collagen synthesis impaired. Adequate CHO and fats prevent metabolism of protein-amino acids from being used to meet caloric needs[89]	RQ, indirect calorimetry, Harris and Benedict equation, nomogram, anthropometric	Local infection, slowed wound healing, muscle wasting (amino acids used for energy), marasmus (somatic stores low, visceral normal)
Fats	Questionable role in wound healing; however, constituent of cell membrane Possible inhibition of reparative process Adequate CHO and fat necessary to prevent metabolism of amino acids	Triglyceride level, triceps skin fold, RQ	Decreased fat stores
Specific			
Vitamin C	Fibroblastic function and collagen formation, resistance to infection. Metabolic oxidation of specific amino acids. Formation of norepinephrine from dopamine	Vitamin C levels	Fragility and rupture of capillaries; slowed capillary formation; poor wound healing; infection; spongy, bleeding, receding gums
Vitamin B complex (pyridoxine, pantothenic acid, folic acid)	Alteration in cofactor in variety of enzyme systems necessary for normal protein, fat and CHO metabolism Possible mechanism by which B complex affects wound healing. Major effect on antibody and WBC formation[89]	Serum levels	Dry, thickened, inflamed cornea or conjunctiva; fissures at corners of mouth; swollen, beefy tongue; papillary atrophy with smooth appearance; listless, apathetic, mental confusion, depression, nausea
Vitamin A	Maintains epithelial integrity and retinol pigments. Animal studies show deficiencies retard epithelialization, closure of wounds, rate of collagen synthesis, and cross-linking of newly formed collagen. Appears to modify response to stress and infection in patients and animals	Carotene levels	Malaise; dermatitis; peripheral edema; dry, rough inflamed skin; bruising; dry thickened, inflamed cornea or conjunctiva
Vitamin K	Synthesis of prothrombin and clotting factors II, VIII, IX, X; indirect effects on wound healing—bleeding and hematoma formation that can impair wound healing and predispose to infection	Decreased PT	Potential deficiencies seen with antibiotics: bile fistula; obstructive jaundice; bleeding; liver disease and disorders of fat digestion and absorption; bleeding, and hematoma formation
Zinc	Low levels (< 100 mg/100 ml) likely to see problems in wound repair. In animals, wound strength impaired	Serum levels	Possible slowed wound healing; possible dehiscence; seborrhea dermatitis; glossitis
Iron	Collagen formation	Iron levels	Collagen deposition on wounds; angular stomatitis; glossitis
Copper	Two functions in wound healing: (1) erythrocyte output (together with iron)—deficiencies interfere with oxygen transport and therefore collagen synthesis; (2) formation of lysyl oxidase, which leads to inadequate collagen cross-linking and diminished wound strength	Copper levels	Pale wound with decreased strength—possible dehiscence; decreased pigmentation, alopecia
Manganese	Affect formation of connective tissue	Serum levels	

*MAMC, midarm muscle circumference; CHI, creatinine/height index. Prepared by G. L. Stiver Stanek.

Creatinine/Height Index

As previously stated, the CHI must be utilized with caution, with special emphasis on accurate collection and normal renal function. An overall trend may be useful when analyzed in conjunction with multiple nutritional parameters.

Serum Proteins

Serum proteins, specifically albumin, similarly assist in noting trends. Albumin does not reflect rapid changes in visceral protein status. Transferrin, because of its short half-life, is thought to reflect more rapid changes in protein status. Similarly, trends are the key to appropriate interpretation, keeping in mind that values can be altered with even minor stresses.

Nitrogen Balances

Nitrogen balances, as previously mentioned, have assumed a greater priority in most nutritional assessment plans. In the intermediate phase, one would expect the patient to be moving toward a neutral or more positive balance. Persistent negative nitrogen balance studies or studies that are not showing progress toward a positive balance reflect failure of the prescribed nutritional plan, necessitating reassessment of energy and protein requirements. Recent efforts to clarify nitrogen balance in relation to protein flux with the use of isotope technology may provide even more promise for future interpretation of this parameter. Both TLC and skin antigen testing are utilized in the ambulatory setting. (Refer to Appendix 14–1 for the advantages and disadvantages of their use in trauma patients.)

Energy Expenditure

Determining energy or caloric requirements is essential in this phase, as in any other phase of trauma recovery. The HBE continues to offer guidelines for energy needs in this phase. The activity level is a much greater variable than it has been in the critical care phase. Although energy requirements due to the metabolic effects of injury may be gradually decreasing, activity level is probably increasing. Long's[61] research offers two activity levels to be multiplied by the HBE. The factor 1.2 is utilized for a patient who is confined to bed, and 1.3 is used for a patient who is out of bed. Caution must be exerted when using these factors because they have not been rigorously tested. Tables that present the energy costs of different types of activity may also be helpful in adjusting basal needs to actual needs (Table 14–8). The nurse is responsible for relaying information that updates the dietitian's records on activity level.

Similarly, altered wound status and temperature are important factors that might alter the patient's energy expenditure. Infections frequently can occur with associated temperature elevations. As previously mentioned, a 1°C temperature elevation is associated with a 13 to 14 per cent increase in basal energy requirements. If this goes unnoticed and is sustained, it could lead to inadequate caloric requirements with associated complications. Similarly, an open wound that is infected and in need of débridement may contribute to significant elevations in metabolic rate because of endogenous mediator release. Open communication regarding changes in activity, infection, and wound status assist in accurately assessing the patient's energy requirements. In addition, if available, indirect calorimetry helps to quantify these changes in metabolic rate more accurately.

Intake and Output Records

Intake and output records are an essential aspect of nutritional assessment. The dietitian reviews records when determining nitrogen balances as well as calculating actual substrate intake. The nurse has total control of this record and must make sure intake of all oral, enteral, and parenteral nutrition is documented. Similarly, ensuring that the patient has received prescribed feedings is a must. Feedings may be held because of chest physiotherapy, but attempting to minimize this loss of intake is an important responsibility. Information regarding excessive diarrhea, vomiting, or drainage from other sources assists in determining adequacy or complications that relate to prescribed nutritional regimens.

TABLE 14–8. ENERGY REQUIREMENTS OF A PATIENT (65 kg) IN THE HOSPITAL WARD

	AVERAGE ENERGY EXPENDITURE	
	KCAL/MIN	KJ/MIN
Sitting	1.4	6.0
Standing	1.7	7.0
Walking	3.0	13.0
Washing and dressing	3.5	15.0

From Moghissi K, Boone JRP: Parenteral and Enteral Nutrition for Nurses. Rockville, MD, Aspen Systems, 1983, p 93, with permission.

Calorie Counts

Calorie counts are another assessment tool used to assess the amount of protein, carbohydrate, fat, and caloric intake. The nurse, patient, and, possibly, a family member may participate in accurately recording type of food and quantity ingested. These records are analyzed by the dietitian or technician to determine whether an adequate intake exists. Recommendations are made based on this record keeping. For example, adequate calories may be consumed; however, protein intake may be below ideal levels. In this case, protein supplements are ordered to improve dietary intake.

Protein Requirements

Protein requirements may vary significantly, depending on degree of stress and amount of tissue loss and healing. As with the acute phase, requirements range from 1 to 2 g/kg/day. The critical care phase usually requires a protein intake closer to 2 g/kg/day, whereas protein intake in the intermediate phase is between 1 and 1.5 g/kg/day. The calorie-nitrogen ratio is about 120 to 200 calories to 1 g of nitrogen. The calorie-nitrogen ratio and actual caloric intake are frequently assessed by the dietitian. These parameters are adjusted by utilizing other assessment measures (e.g., nitrogen balance studies and albumin and transferrin levels).

Rehabilitation Assessment Strategies

Weight

Nutritional assessment parameters are taken less frequently, if at all, in some patients. Weight measurements are much more valid in this stage of recovery and provide a gross assessment of body composition. Similarly, anthropometric measures may also assist in determining fat and protein stores. These are best utilized to note trends over time. The spinal cord–injured population will have a weight shift from protein muscle loss due to atrophy and disuse. The range for paraplegics and quadriplegics is about 10 to 15 lb and 15 to 20 lb, respectively, below the Metropolitan Life tables.[72]

Serum Protein/Nitrogen Balance

Adequate visceral proteins should also be evidenced by normal serum protein levels and by albumin and transferrin levels. If a patient's protein and caloric needs do not appear adequate, nitrogen balance studies may still be performed and are probably more reliable, since occult losses are minimal. Similarly, total lymphocyte count and skin antigen testing may confirm adequate immune system functioning. However, little in the way of assessment is performed in this style unless the patient does not appear to be progressing rapidly or exhibits frequent infections.

Less emphasis is placed on determining specific energy requirements because the patient is responsible for his own dietary requirements. Teaching patients appropriate selection of food groups assists in a balanced diet. Diet instruction is done by the nurse and/or dietitian before discharge. The focus is on foods high in calories and protein if the patient's nutritional status is not adequate. The neurotrauma population, especially the spinal cord–injured patient, needs extensive health teaching because of their tendency to be malnourished and their increased risk for pulmonary infection and pressure ulcerations. Similarly, patients are reminded of the importance of dietary calcium to assist in bone healing and maintenance of bone structure.

During this phase of trauma recovery, assessment strategies focus on teaching and assessing the patient's ability to be independent in his care.

NURSING CONSIDERATIONS THROUGH THE CYCLES

Special nursing considerations as they relate to the critical care, intermediate, and rehabilitation phases of the trauma patient's recovery are addressed in this section. An overview of patient characteristics, overall nutritional goals, and feeding modalities are presented for all phases of trauma. Nutritional assessment and interventions occur as a process and are multidisciplinary in nature.

Figure 14–21 shows the process of nutritional assessment and intervention. Ideally, the entire process begins with a basic understanding of metabolism and nutrition. Initial baseline data are obtained from the patient and/or family. When this information is obtained early, it helps to predict whether or not the patient is at risk (phase I). Once the level of risk is established, appropriate referrals must be made. Assessment strategies are determined individually, and nutritional goals and interventions are established. Nurses play a role in referral and planned intervention (phase II). More important, the nurse at the bedside provides constant surveillance and feedback, such as tolerance of tube feeding, adequacy of central line to achieve goals, and complications of planned regimen. The evaluation process (phase III) involves subjective, objective, and biochemical data. In Figure 14–21, dotted lines represent potential choices and solid lines are mandatory steps. Failure of a specific plan or intervention requires a new plan that incorporates rationale for failure as well as collection of additional data necessary to intervene appropriately. Once the goal is achieved, continued assessment by the health care team provides ongoing evaluation for goal maintenance and revisions as necessary. This process is dynamic as goals change throughout the trauma patient's recovery.

Critical Care Phase

Patient Characteristics

Catabolism is the most striking characteristic of the critical care phase of injury. "The excretions of nitrogen, creatinine, sulfur, phosphorus, and potassium increase immediately, signifying a substantial breakdown of tissue."[98] The muscle protein compartment appears to suffer the most, and losses exceed what might be expected in relation to the decrease in food intake. This hypermetabolic response is thought to peak at about 5 to 10 days and then gradually decreases (see Fig. 14–15). The degree of catabolism and hypermetabolism and the duration of negative nitrogen balance depend on the extent of injury and the nutritional status of the patient at the time of injury.[99] Multiple hormonal as well as humoral factors have been identified as responsible for this response.

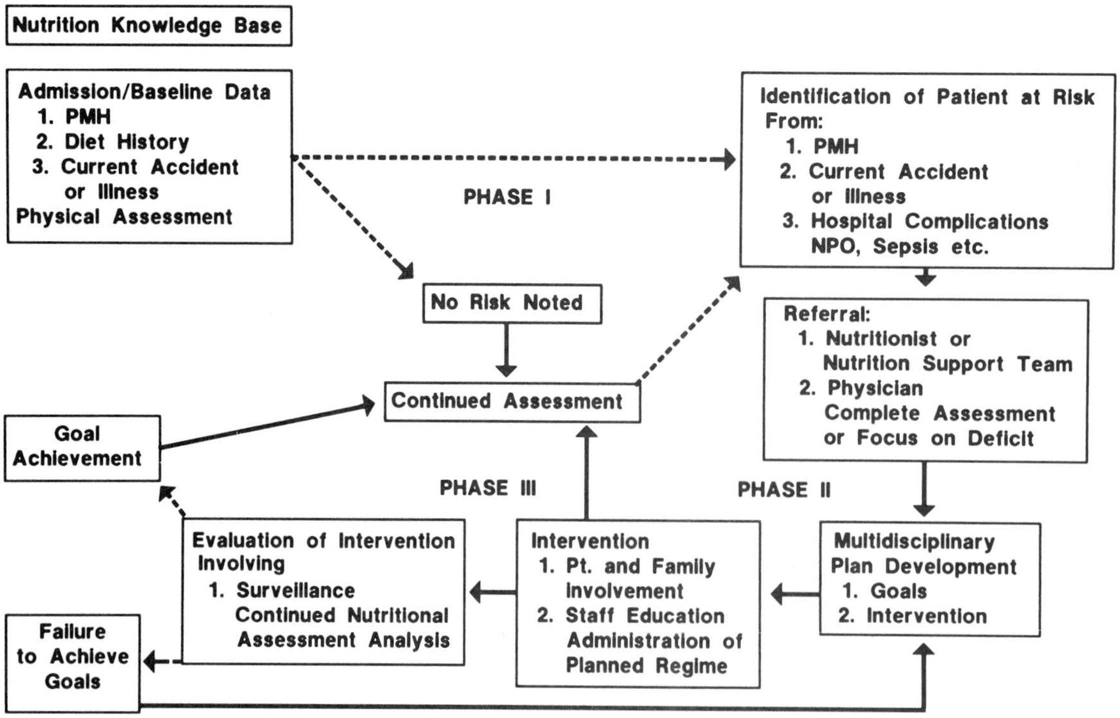

Figure 14–21. Nutritional assessment process.

The trauma patient frequently has multiple systems affected and has undergone extensive surgical interventions. Massive blood loss results in coagulopathies and hemodynamic instability. Mechanical ventilation is usually required for several days to weeks, depending on the extent of head injury and/or pulmonary involvement. The GI tract is rendered useless for the first 42 to 48 hours owing to extensive surgeries. In addition, abdominal trauma with bowel surgeries frequently eliminate the GI tract as a route for nutrient intake. A severe head injury with altered levels of consciousness and gag reflex may prevent oral intake for long periods of time.

Similarly, paralytic ileus is common initially in the spinal cord–injured population. This is due to autonomic disruption and ischemia at the time of injury.[72, 100] There is an increased incidence of GI ulceration related to unopposed vagal stimulation in the spinal cord–injured population.[101]

The neurologically injured patient has exhibited increased energy requirements that are greater than those of the general multiple-trauma patient, but they are extremely variable. Multiple nutritional assessment parameters need to be obtained and reviewed in relation to the total clinical picture to make an appropriate assessment and intervention. The overall goal for nutritional intervention at this stage is provision of nutrients and energy requirements for maintenance during this catabolic phase. As stated previously, it appears difficult, if not impossible, to halt the metabolic response due to injury that results from a complex combination of neurohormonal, endocrine, and humoral factors. This response is self-limiting, providing wounds are closed, infections are prevented or treated, wounds are debrided, and supportive nutritional measures are maintained.

Feeding Modalities

The type of feeding modality used depends largely on the severity and type of injury and the expected recovery period. The physician usually has some idea how long patients will need to be NPO and which feeding modality is preferred. "The accepted practice in most routine surgical procedures is to restrict intravenous intake to 5 per cent dextrose and water, amounting to 500 to 760 Kcal/day (120 to 190 g of glucose/day), in patients who are well nourished, whose surgical trauma or injury is moderate and uncomplicated, and in whom it is anticipated that oral feedings will be resumed within 5 to 7 days."[98] This amount is thought to be adequate for the glucose requirements of the brain and formed blood elements.[102] In most serious trauma requiring critical care management, the critical care phase is lengthy, with multiple potential complications. The least invasive and most natural feeding approach is ideal.

There is increasing evidence that the route of nutritional support is important in the early care of multisystem trauma.[103] Infection and sepsis remain the primary cause of death in patients who live at least 5 days but eventually die of their injuries. Recent studies[11, 12, 104–108] indicate that immediate enteral feedings reduce septic complications and improve survival compared with parenteral nutrition. Central to this concept is the documentation of bacterial translocation from the GI tract of stressed patients. As stated previously, bacterial translocation occurs when gut organisms migrate through the epithelial mucosa into mesenteric lymph nodes, other organs, and the bloodstream. This, in conjunction with reduced hepatic detoxification, is the basis for irreversible postinjury shock.

In addition, some theorize that the damage that occurs to the gut related to delayed enteral feeds may be one of the main precipitating factors for multiple system organ failure (MSOF).[108] Bacterial translocation is widely accepted; however, its role in the development of postinjury MSOF is not completely clear.[11] In the Moore et al study[12] comparing enteral and parenteral feedings, the authors noted greater general complications (57 versus 34 per cent), septic complications (37 versus 17 per cent), and major infections (20 versus 3 per cent) in the TPN group compared with the enteral group. In addition, Meyer et al[11] data suggest that neutrophil function is affected by route of feeding. They found significant differences in the number, function, and plasma complement level of neutrophils in parenterally fed patients.[11] In general, the gut is not a dormant organ and, therefore, needs to be considered vital to the patient's nutritional plan of care. Small bowel motility and absorption remain intact despite surgery or injury stress and should be considered even if gastric or colon motility or peristalsis is impaired.

Assuming that the patient is unable to utilize the oral route voluntarily, nutritional replacement should start as soon as the GI tract is functioning; that is, when it has recovered from the initial posttraumatic paralytic ileus.[109] The nurse plays a key role in assessing bowel sounds and in reporting these findings to the physician and dietitian so enteral feedings may begin. If for some reason there is a long delay before bowel sounds are present, an alternative route is utilized. Most sources agree that in serious injury, a nutritional regimen should be initiated no later than 3 to 4 days after injury. Fluid and blood product resuscitation and control of any major fluid, electrolyte, and acid–base disturbances should be achieved before nutritional support.

Enteral Tubes and Feedings. The physician or nurse passes a flexible, weighted Silastic feeding tube through either an orogastric or a nasogastric route. Frequently, an orogastric route may be chosen because of facial trauma or potential sinusitis and/or sinus infections, which may occur with the nasogastric route. Postpyloric feedings are usually preferred over stomach feedings if the patient is at risk for aspiration and/or needs frequent chest physiotherapy. Before administering any tube feeding by way of a small-bore, weighted Silastic tube, a radiograph should be taken to confirm proper placement. Frequently, the trauma patient has pulmonary contusions, atelectasis, and pneumonia, which necessitate chest physiotherapy and postural drainage. During the critical care phase, most patients are intubated, thus the endotracheal tube cuff serves to protect the airway from aspiration. The nurse is responsible for proper endotracheal tube cuff inflation. Aspiration is particularly a concern in elderly, head-injured, and unconscious patients when feedings are introduced too rapidly as a bolus or when gastric motility is a problem. Similarly, if tube placement is not frequently checked and/or the tube is not securely taped, displacement of the tube into the esophagus may increase the risk for aspiration. If gastric motility is a problem, the drug metoclopramide (Reglan) may be effective in increasing gastric motility.[110] Discontinuing tube feedings 1 hour before and during chest physiotherapy make aspiration less likely. If

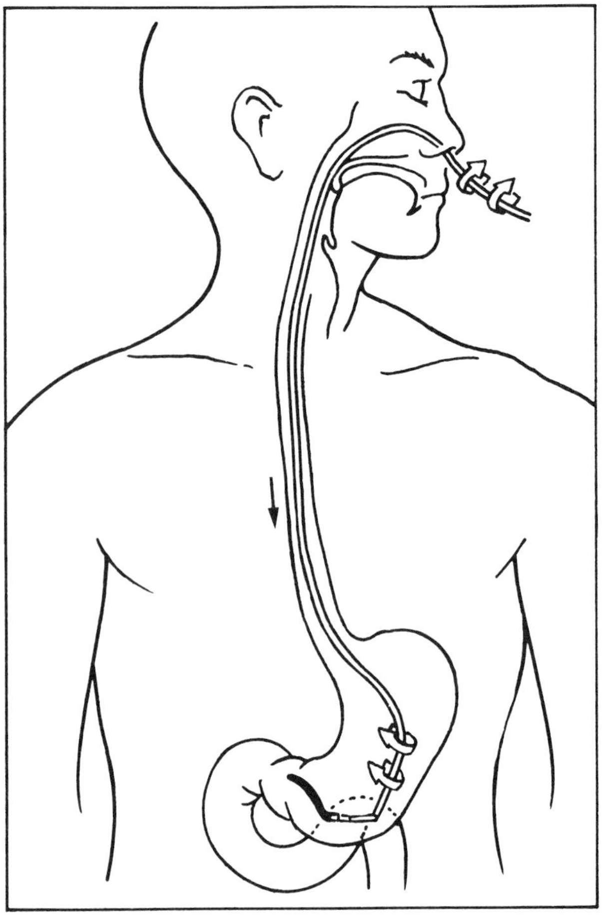

Figure 14–22. Enteral tube passage through the pylorus. (Reprinted with permission from Thurlow DM: Bedside enteral feeding tube placement into the duodenum and jejunum. JPEN 10:104–105, 1986. © by Am Soc of Parenteral and Enteral Nutrition, 1986.)

Several methods exist for placing feeding tubes in specific anatomical positions. Surgical placement for jejunostomy and gastrostomy can be done initially when surgical repairs are being performed at admission. Endoscopic examination and placement of the feeding tube in the duodenum or percutaneous gastrostomy can be effective in certain patients. In addition, tubes can be placed under fluoroscopy. However, fluoroscopy usually requires patient transport, which is difficult in a critically ill patient. Thurlow[112] described a bedside method of inserting a soft, weighted feeding tube into the duodenum. His method requires 2 to 15 minutes and utilizes gravity and corkscrewing of the feeding tube past the pylorus (Fig. 14–22). Another set of authors describe a simple, economic method for placing a postpylorus feeding tube.[113] Auscultating and injecting air verify tube position from the location and character of transmitted sounds to the stethoscope.[102] In most cases, simple placement of soft, weighted feeding tubes is adequate. Figure 14–23 reviews feeding tube placement. Monturo[111] offers a thorough review of enteral access device selection and placement.

Various tube feeding solutions are available, and their use is determined based on the nutritional assessment. It is the nurse's responsibility to ascertain whether or not the patient is tolerating the prescribed formula and amount. If the patient can communicate any abdominal discomfort or if there is distention, diarrhea, nausea, or vomiting, the feeding should be discontinued for further evaluation. If the patient cannot communicate, an abdominal girth measurement can be taken every 4 hours, with assessment for abdominal distention. In addition, attempts should be made to access residual GI contents every 2 to 4 hours and PRN. Residual volumes greater than 100 to 150 ml consistently or gastric distention and/or vomiting may signify the need to change feeding route.[111, 114] The head of the bed should remain at a 30- to 45-degree angle during the feeding.

postpylorus tubes are in place, there is no need to turn off the tube feeding. If there is any reason to doubt placement, radiographic verification is required to ensure patient safety. In most cases, the risk of aspiration is small relative to the benefit of feedings when appropriate nursing interventions are instituted.

If the risk of aspiration is high, the patient has a marginal pulmonary status, and GI tract feedings are desired, efforts should be made to feed into the duodenum or the jejunum.[111] The benefits of early enteral jejunal feedings were studied in head-injured patients. The increased caloric and nitrogen intake and improved nitrogen retention markedly reduced infections and days of stay in the ICU.[107] If long-term feeding is expected, soft, small-bore Silastic tubes should be used. The rigid large-bore tubes have several potential problems. The trachea and esophagus are close anatomically, which can predispose the patient to a tracheoesophageal fistula. Thus, the two rigid tubes create pressure, with eventual necrosis and fistula formation. Similarly, gastritis and esophagitis are not uncommon complications of rigid nasogastric tubes. The rigid tube may also prevent complete closure of the cardiac sphincter and therefore permit reflux of acid gastric contents into the esophagus. Chronic esophagitis can lead to esophageal strictures.

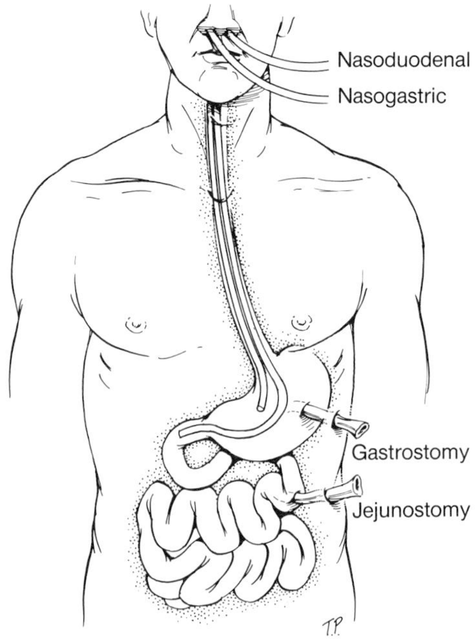

Figure 14–23. Feeding tube placement. (From Moghissi K, Boorne JRP: Parenteral and Enteral Nutrition for Nurses. Rockville, MD, Aspen Systems, 1983, p 168.)

A recent study of tube feeding complications in 50 patients identified inadequate gastric emptying (33 per cent), profuse diarrhea (13.3 per cent), vomiting (11.1 per cent), and nausea (8.9 per cent) as the most common GI complications.[115] The incidence of tube dislodgment or obstruction was 22.2 per cent of reported mechanical complication.[115] No metabolic complications were reported. Continued assessment and dissemination of findings regarding vomiting, bowel sounds, residual volume, flatus, and amount and consistency of stools assist in evaluating the adequacy of the nutritional regimen.

Nurses should be aware of the osmolality of the formula. In general, tube feedings vary in osmolality from 300 (isotonic) to 850 mOsm (hypertonic). Standard tube feeding solutions are usually 300 to 450 mOsm with about 1 calorie per milliliter. The concentrated formulas range from 1.5 to 2.0 calories per milliliter, with an osmolality of 600 to 700 mOsm. The elemental formulas that utilize amino acids rather than protein tend to have osmolalities that range from 550 to 650 mOsm and have a caloric content of 1 calorie per milliliter. Beginning with a formula that is isotonic or diluting a hyperosmolar solution to 1/4 or 1/2 strength is usually the preferred method of initiating tube feedings. Gradually increasing the strength and then the volume is usually better tolerated. Total nutrient requirements are met with about 1500 to 2000 ml of full-strength solution. A concentrated hyperosmolar nutrient solution introduced into the GI tract is probably the most common cause of diarrhea.[116]

Controversy exists regarding whether or not one should use continuous or bolus feedings. Although continuous feedings appear to be the method of choice, bolus feedings have worked equally well in some patients. One cause of diarrhea has been cited as a too-rapid administration of nutrients; if this occurs, absorption can be reduced.[116] Continuous feeding reduces this risk and can save time. Microbial contamination can also cause diarrhea. Changing the feeding bag every 24 hours and utilization of clean technique during administration helps to minimize microbial growth. Similarly, feedings should be hung in no greater than a 4-hour supply.[115] Two other causes of diarrhea include concurrent antibiotic therapy, GI tract infections, and lactose intolerance. When diarrhea occurs, all potential sources (amount, composition, osmolality, and method of administration) must be considered.

Gastrostomy tube feedings may be the choice for long-term feeding. As stated previously, this tube may be placed using the percutaneous endoscopic technique or may be placed during laparotomy. Because these tubes exit from the stomach through a small external opening, there is increased risk of infection. Care should be given each day to the exit site. Checking for redness, edema, exudate, and leakage of acidic stomach contents that break down the skin barrier is important. Dry sterile dressings and antimicrobial ointments should be applied to protect the exit site. Because the tube feeding goes into the stomach, if the patient becomes nauseated or vomits, he is at risk for aspiration. Keeping the head of the bed elevated during the infusion of tube feeding, getting the patient out of bed, and activities that encourage peristalsis help to reduce this risk.

Jejunostomy tube feedings usually are indicated when it is expected that a patient will have long-term feeding problems. A jejunal feeding tube is placed at the time of laparotomy and can be used several hours later. Some practitioners are reluctant to utilize this approach in the early postinjury period. A recent study of jejunostomy feeding (n = 71) after major abdominal trauma supports that the vast majority tolerate full-scale needle catheter jejunostomy feedings in the early postoperative period.[117] Elemental diets are available and need only a small amount of small bowel for absorption. They do not have a residue, so stools should be minimal and mainly due to the normal sloughing of the GI tract. Because there is an opening where the catheter exists in the abdomen, this area needs special care to prevent infection and accidental removal. A clean, dry dressing and antimicrobial ointment at the exit site are usually recommended. Careful taping to prevent tugging or traction on the tube should be done and checked frequently. The site and tube should be protected from restless, agitated patients who could accidently pull the tube out. Continuous versus bolus feedings are preferred, and no attempt should be made to aspirate contents. If the jejunum becomes overdistended, it can rupture, with peritonitis possibly occurring as a serious complication. Watching for signs of distention and intolerance is important. These catheters are also at risk for clogging.

Obstruction results from residual tube feedings and medications caking on the inner lumen.[118] Several methods of unclogging[118, 119] as well as tubes designed to decrease clogging[120] have been described in the research literature. The techniques are as follows: flushing with cold to hot tap water, pancreatic enzymes, cola, cranberry juice, reintroducing an introducer, and utilizing newly designed tubes. The newest technique calls for utilizing a pancreatic enzyme, for which this study claimed a 96 per cent success rate.[119] The nurse should never attempt to force a clog through the tube because the tube may rupture. Prevention remains the best solution to clogged tubes.

Many drugs, such as potassium chloride, are hyperosmolar and, when given through the feeding tube, can cause diarrhea. Control of peristalsis may be drug-related. Tincture of opium or a more natural fiber bulk form (such as Metamucil) may be prescribed to slow down GI motility and diarrhea. "One of the more controversial areas in the field of nutrition has been the use of fiber-containing diets to control diarrhea."[121] Fiber works by bacterial fermentation in the gut and in turn short-chain fatty acids are generated, which leads to increased sodium and water absorption.[121] This theory has not been well supported. Frankenfield and Beyer[122] studied the effect of soy-polysaccharide fiber on diarrhea in tube-fed head-injured patients and found no significant difference in diarrhea. Palacio and Rombeau[123] review the use of dieting fiber in enteral nutrition. The registered dietitian is an integral part of the team and should be consulted on the type of formula each patient needs rather than a decision being made arbitrarily based on availability.

Parenteral Feedings. Parenteral feeding modalities include peripheral or partial parenteral nutrition (PPN) and TPN. Parenteral nutrition should be considered as either primary or adjunctive therapy. GI trauma, paralytic ileus, small bowel fistulas, partial or complete bowel obstructions, and peritonitis are just a few of the problems that might prevent the use of enteral nutrition. In these cases, the primary therapy would be parenteral nutrition. Patients with head, respiratory, and multisystem injuries may initially need parenteral nutrition as the primary source but should soon be able to progress partially or completely to enteral feedings. Parenteral nutrition as adjunctive therapy may be needed by burn and multisystem trauma patients who have extremely high calorie and protein needs but are unable to have all their needs met by the enteral route.

The use of TPN has become controversial. Twenty patients were studied to determine whether TPN influenced the recovery of neutrophil locomotory dysfunction in blunt trauma.[103] TPN appeared to worsen and delay the recovery of neutrophil locomotory responses.[103] Meyer et al[11] suggest that neutrophil number, function, and plasma complement level are greater in enteral- versus parenteral-fed patients.

Alverdy et al[124] studied the effect of parenteral nutrition on GI immunity in the rat model. They established that TPN caused a marked reduction in the amount of intestinal secretory immunoglobulin A (S-IgA). S-IgA is the principal defense that protects the mucosal wall of the intestine against bacteria. Further, these authors indicate that parenteral nutrition promotes bacterial translocation from the gut by increasing the cecal bacterial count and impairing intestinal defense.

Peterson et al[104] studied total enteral nutrition (TEN) versus TPN after major torso injury. They found that both were tolerated well and that serum proteins increased over time in the TEN group while decreasing in the TPN group. In addition, septic complications were greater, however not significantly different, in the TPN group. They concluded that TEN attenuates reprioritization of hepatic protein synthesis in patients sustaining major torso injury.

Long-term TPN patients who have had small bowel biopsy have shown dramatic changes in the microvilli height mass and absorptive area. In addition, glutamine plays an important role in GI tract metabolism. Glutamine deficiency is associated with prolonged parenteral nutrition leading to atrophy of the intestinal mucosa.[125, 126] The enterocyte uses glutamine as a fuel. More recent work indicates that glutamine may be an essential dietary component.[20] Further study is necessary to determine the exact role glutamine plays in parenteral and enteral nutrition. It is clear that although TPN can be life-saving, its use must be carefully considered. Similarly, discontinuing TPN use as soon as possible and transitioning to an enteral feeding should be considered. Lastly, it has been estimated that TPN is 5 to 10 times more expensive than an equal amount of enteral feeding.[127]

PPN has several advantages. It can be given in peripheral veins, thereby avoiding the potential complications of central venous access. It can be given fully from the first day, since the dextrose content is 5 to 10 per cent. There are fewer metabolic complications associated with hypoglycemia, hyperglycemia, hypophosphatemia, and increased CO_2 production, since the major calorie source is fat emulsions, which are isotonic.

There are several disadvantages in considering PPN therapy. A limited amount of protein and calories can be infused into the small peripheral veins. Veins can rapidly thrombose due to the hypertonic PPN solutions, causing pain and frequent rotation of sites. Anabolism usually cannot be promoted unless the patient is also receiving enteral feedings. It requires more volume to deliver fewer calories and protein than does TPN. Many patients are on fluid-restricted regimens or require diuresis during PPN infusions. It was designed for short-term therapy versus long-term therapy.

A complete nutritional assessment should be made before initiating PPN therapy. Those patients who can tolerate about 3 liters of fluid each day, have peripheral access, have no history of hyperlipidemia, have adequate platelet counts, have no serious history of malnutrition, and will be able to eat in less than 1 week are potential candidates for PPN therapy. PPN is used in conjunction with lipids, and hence the rationale for no history of hyperlipidemia. Similarly, controversy exists over whether lipids decrease platelet adhesiveness and thus increase the risk of bleeding. Some laboratory studies suggest that lipids may alter immune function; thus far, no studies have shown an effect on outcome.[127] Lipids have been given without complications in the trauma population.

Nursing responsibilities include careful observation of sites to prevent infusion into the subcutaneous space; application of heat to painful or swollen sites; and using other peripheral sites to infuse medications such as antibiotics rather than stopping PPN, flushing the tubing, and infusing antibiotics and other medications in the same site. Coinfusing intralipids with PPN solutions may help to save the veins. Lipids have been shown to protect venous endothelium from injury due to hypertonic dextrose solutions.[128] Rotating sites every 48 hours helps to decrease vein thrombosis.

Nitrogen balance studies and fluid and electrolyte status are also important to monitor. Fluid and electrolyte imbalances can occur because of the large volumes of fluids being administered. Special attention to intake and output records, particularly in patients who are prone to fluid overload, is required. Patient and family teaching should also be done. Many patients may think that they are starving when in fact they are receiving maintenance nutrition until they can eat.

TPN is instituted early in the course of recovery and is indicated throughout the acute catabolic phase in patients in whom GI intake is not anticipated for more than 5 days. TPN can provide enough calories and protein to promote anabolism in patients who are unable to use the GI tract. It must be infused into the superior vena cava because of the hyperosmolar glucose content, preferably by the subclavian route. Each liter of TPN usually contains 4 to 10 per cent amino acids, 20 to 35 per cent glucose, electrolytes, trace elements, and, sometimes, insulin and heparin. It is important to prepare both the patient and the family before initiating TPN.

If the patient is awake and oriented, the Valsalva maneuver should be taught to prevent air emboli during line insertion. The patient should practice taking a deep breath, holding it, and bearing down. Explain to the patient that the head of the bed will be in a slight downward position and a towel roll will be placed between the neck and shoulder blades to fill the superior vena cava for easy access. Insertion should not be painful but somewhat uncomfortable owing to the position and pressure the physician will need to use to locate landmarks. The entire procedure takes about 15 minutes. A chest radiograph should be taken to ascertain that the tip of the catheter is in the superior vena cava before infusion of TPN. Any isotonic solution such as D_5W, 0.9 NS, or 0.45 NS, can be infused at a minimal rate until line placement is confirmed. This line should be used only for TPN and lipids to maintain a closed system with minimal chance for contamination. Tubing should be changed every 24 to 48 hours,[129, 130] and dressing changes should vary from every 24 hours to once every 7 days, depending on patient population, dressing type, and hospital policy. This will assist in reducing infection rate. An occlusive dressing change using aseptic technique is essential. The use of in-line filters remains somewhat controversial. Most hospitals that use in-line filters do so to trap air and particulate matter or coring from TPN bottles. There has been no published conclusive evidence that there have been detrimental effects from this particulate matter, and all intravenous solutions contain varying amounts of it. Pediatric patients would be the exception, and in-line filters are usually used not only with TPN but with most intravenous solutions.

Complications during line insertion can be serious, but with proper preparation of the patient and good surgical techniques, these complications should be minimal. Because the superior vena cava is so close to the lungs, the needle may nick the lung and cause a pneumothorax, requiring insertion of a chest tube. Close observation of the patient for signs of respiratory distress during line insertion are important. If a chest tube is needed, this can cause added discomfort and pain to the patient. Supportive care and reassurance that he will be all right should be a priority. If the artery is severed, bleeding may occur, requiring firm pressure for at least 5 to 10 minutes. TPN lines should be considered as life lines and used only for TPN except in an emergency that could be life-threatening. $D_{10}W$ peripherally can prevent rebound hypoglycemia if there is sudden cessation of TPN. Sepsis is a major complication in the trauma patient, and the TPN line is especially susceptible to contamination due to the hyperosmolar glucose. If the patient has sudden onset of temperature, blood cultures from the TPN line and site cultures should be done along with peripheral blood cultures. If the TPN line blood cultures are positive, changing the line over a guidewire and culturing of the catheter should be done. If this culture is positive, the line should be removed, and a new line should be inserted at a new site after 48 hours of appropriate antibiotic therapy.

A nutritional assessment before initiating TPN and close monitoring during therapy are important. Trauma patients are already stressed, and TPN can add to that stress if close monitoring is neglected. Careful recording of intake and output, fluid and electrolyte status, kidney and liver function tests, serum glucose levels, and nitrogen balance studies should be done and evaluated on a regular basis. Intake and output records are extremely important. Fluid overload can occur if renal and cardiac function are not adequate. Similarly, infusing hyperosmolar solution can lead to osmotic diuresis and potential dehydration and fluid shifts. Serum and urine osmolality are routinely measured to assess fluid status. The volume and type of TPN should be clearly recorded so that calculations for intake of energy, nitrogen, and other nutrients can be done. An accurate record is critical to calculating nitrogen balance correctly.

Testing the patient's urine for glucose and acetone every 4 to 6 hours initially as well as serum glucose daily and PRN detects glucose intolerance. Insulin can then be appropriately administered. The frequency of specific laboratory tests varies, depending on the patient's clinical status (see Tables 14–5 and 14–6). In general, daily tests of electrolyte status should be done, since alterations can be serious. For example, intravenous feedings that have high glucose and amino acid content frequently cause hypokalemia. Correction is necessary to avoid cardiac arrhythmias. Similarly, hypophosphatemia may occur with long-term TPN. This results in generalized muscle weakness and fatigue due to the reduction in red blood cell ATP content.

Metabolic acidosis can occur because TPN solutions tend to have a lowered pH. In addition, solutions with high chloride content may cause excess chloride retention and subsequent acidosis. High glucose loads cause a rise in CO_2 levels, another potential source of acidosis. This is not usually a problem unless the patient has a poor pulmonary status. High arterial CO_2 levels in patients who fail to be weaned may indicate excessive carbohydrate administration. This may have specific implications for the spinal cord–injured patient, especially those with high thoracic and cervical injuries. These patients may have a difficult time ridding the body of CO_2 due to lost respiratory muscle function. Further, they may have a decreased metabolic demand related to muscle denervation. Uremia may also occur because of the kidneys' inability to clear nitrogen.

In situations in which kidney function is poor, special low-nitrogen formulas are available. In contrast, high blood urea nitrogen (BUN) levels can also occur in patients who have an intact renal system. BUN levels may be elevated owing to insufficient caloric intake in relation to nitrogen. In this situation, increasing the calorie-nitrogen ratio decreases the BUN. The preferred calorie-nitrogen ratio is usually 1:150.

TPN can induce alterations in liver function tests as well as fatty liver; therefore, liver function testing should be done routinely. Initially, liver function tests should be done every 3 to 4 days. Important physical assessment strategies include assessing skin and sclera for jaundice, palpating the liver for tenderness or enlargement, and assessing urine color. An alteration in liver function tests may signal the need to decrease or change TPN solutions. A study by Robertson and associates[131] indicates that most patients who had normal liver function tests on commencing TPN developed abnormalities during their feeding period. The incidence of abnormal tests was almost double in septic patients when compared with nonseptic patients, strongly suggesting that sepsis plays an important role in the development of liver function test abnormalities. Robertson et al[131] found that the most sensitive biochemical test of liver dysfunction during their study was γ-glutamyltransferase, which was usually elevated by week 4. Although most abnormalities were transient, the elevation of alkaline phosphatase persisted beyond week 9 of the study. The clinical significance of these abnormalities is uncertain, as long-term adverse clinical effects appear to be rare. In addition, their results indicated that patients who were malnourished to begin with were more likely to develop abnormalities, suggesting the need to provide nutritional support cautiously in this group.

Most researchers are in agreement that both lipids and carbohydrates are important sources of nonprotein calories and that too much glucose can be hazardous. Lipid is recommended in patients who receive long-term TPN and have COPD and to meet the essential fatty acid (linoleic acid) requirements while avoiding the physiological effects of glucose overloading. Lipids provide fat to the TPN regimen. Fat calories should be about 30 to 40 per cent of the total calorie intake. It is clear that lipid metabolism and mobilization are increased after trauma. Ten per cent lipids provide 500 Kcal, whereas 20 per cent lipids provide 1000 Kcal. Both solutions are 500 ml, and this concentrated caloric source should be given twice a week to prevent essential fatty acid deficiency or daily as a caloric source for ventilator-dependent and fluid-restricted patients.

Initial triglyceride levels should be drawn, and if mildly elevated, a trial dose of 10 per cent lipids should be given, with serial triglyceride levels drawn before infusion, 4 hours after infusion is initiated, post infusion, and 8 hours post infusion. Levels should return to normal 8 hours post infusion. If not, lipids should be held. Lipids should be given cautiously if platelet counts are low, since there has been some controversy over lipids decreasing platelet adhesiveness and increasing the risk of bleeding, unless platelet count is above 80,000. This appears to be a rare problem in practice. There have been some reports of patients developing cramping, tachypnea, and tachycardia and becoming diaphoretic during lipid infusions. This remains a rare occurrence, and the cause is still under investigation. Infusing lipids over a 12-hour period appears to be well tolerated by most patients with minimal, if any, adverse effects. In addition, lipids should be infused about 4 to 6 hours before morning blood work because triglyceride and other routine plasma analyses may be altered.

New reports indicate that it is safe to administer a mixture of amino acids, glucose, and lipids concurrently.[132] Some evidence suggests that TPN with lipid given continuously over a 24-hour period is preferred because oxidation of the lipid is sustained, thus minimizing carbohydrate utilization.[133] In addition, as previously mentioned, lipid has been shown to protect the venous endothelium from injury due to hypertonic glucose solutions.[128]

Administration of branched-chain amino acid-enriched TPN solutions has been studied. Branched-chain amino acids have been associated with a nitrogen-sparing effect in septic and traumatized patients.[134, 135] Data suggest that it reduces proteolysis and urea nitrogen production.[134] It appears to decrease urine urea nitrogen by depressing proteolysis.[135] The use of branched-chain amino acid solutions is based on the findings that these amino acids are reduced in plasma after sepsis and injury. The septic trauma patient, with and without MSOF, utilizes branched-chain amino acids when other amino acids cannot be utilized. This appears to support potential use of these specific types of TPN in this population.[136] Although further studies are indicated, results suggest that survival rates may be improved in patients with MSOF who received branched-chain amino acid solutions.[137] It appears that septic,[134] multisystem trauma,[135, 138] and surgical patients[139] may potentially benefit from branched-chain amino acids; however, the exact role in trauma patients remains unclear as indicated by other literature.[16, 140]

An important but often neglected aspect of nursing care evolves around range-of-motion activities. To build muscle, one must exercise. Similarly, the disuse phenomena causes bones to demineralize and muscles to weaken and atrophy. Only giving protein does not increase muscle mass. Therefore, promoting muscle activity, whether it is passive initially or active later, improves muscle function and growth. Patients who have been on long-term controlled mechanical ventilation because of extensive trauma need encouragement to increase their respiratory muscle activity. Similarly, frequent passive and active range-of-motion exercises should be incorporated into one's daily assessment activities. Patients are often fearful of various tubes and drains and need to be encouraged to exercise as tolerated. The physical therapist should be consulted at the earliest possible date to assist in planning extensive activity. Nursing personnel should provide ongoing range of motion to assist in rebuilding the muscle mass lost because of the catabolic processes associated with severe trauma.

Intermediate Phase

Patient Characteristics

The intermediate phase of the trauma patient's recovery is characterized by an overall gradual decrease in metabolic rate. Severe septic complications have occurred; however, bacteremia and wound infections are still potential problems that can increase metabolic rate. Skeletal muscle wasting has occurred despite nutritional support and requires continued support as well as physical therapy. A generalized weakness is apparent owing to multiple factors. Prolonged bed rest, anemia, muscle wasting, and psychosocial alterations contribute to this general malaise. Most patients have been extubated and are capable of maintaining adequate oxygenation and ventilation. Similarly, patients have exhibited hemodynamic and fluid and electrolyte stability. Chief nutritional concerns are the transition to intermediate phases of nutritional support, quantification of energy expenditure with new activity levels, improvement of muscle and visceral protein compartments, and maintenance of immune functioning. Frequently, patients are ready to begin learning more about nutritional requirements and interventions. Family members play an integral role in the total patient recovery. Psychological sequelae of a traumatic illness can cause stress, anger, dependence, and depression that could potentially alter the success of the prescribed nutritional regimen. Similarly, neurological and physical deficits may prevent independent feeding. Interdisciplinary assessment, planning, and interventions are critical to successfully achieving goals.

Feeding Modalities

Feeding modalities may be similar to those in the critical care phase if the rationale behind using a specific route has not been resolved. For example, if a patient receiving parenteral nutrition is still undergoing multiple surgical interventions that require an NPO status, parenteral nutrition will continue. In contrast, if a patient has been extubated and major wound problems resolved, enteral or oral nutrition may be initiated. Similar rationale for the utilization of various feeding routes exist in any phase.

Enteral feeding is gradually decreased or changed in relation to time schedules as the patient's mental status improves. The head-injured patient requires a creative approach to nutritional interventions for multiple reasons. Altered levels of consciousness, cranial nerve damage, and general weakness and/or paralysis may alter the patient's ability to take in food voluntarily. Maintaining caloric needs is imperative to avoid negative nitrogen balances and associated complications; therefore, feeding modalities must be tailored to each patient's specific needs. If cranial nerve damage exists, swallowing ability must be assessed. Frequently, special consultants, such as occupational therapists and/or speech and language specialists, evaluate this function. The ideal foods to test this ability are those with the consistency of gelatin, mashed potatoes, or ice cream. Soft foods pose less risk of aspiration and test swallowing ability better. Once swallowing ability has been confirmed, the patient can be switched to regular meals as tolerated. Tube feeding is not stopped completely until calorie counts confirm an adequate intake.

Several methods have been utilized to help ensure an appetite when meals are delivered. Using enteral feedings at night, while the patient is sleeping, and discontinuing them during the day is one method of ensuring adequate intake. Calorie counts provide information on the patient's ability to take in adequate nutrients on his own. When several days are surveyed that consist of adequate oral intake, enteral feeding may be decreased or discontinued. If appetite problems persist because of continued enteral feedings, a trial period in which enteral feedings are discontinued may help. The nasogastric tube may stay in place for several days just to ensure consistent feeding behaviors. Similarly, some institutions continue tube feeding throughout the day, turning it off 2 hours before meals and reinstituting it 1 to 2 hours after a meal. These methods are individualized to meet the patient's personal as well as metabolic demands. Negotiating feeding schedules when appropriate may help the patient gain control over feedings and increase motivation. Patients who have marginal intake receive supplements that are high in calories as well as protein between meals. Families may be encouraged to bring in special foods the patient may desire. Psychosocial or cultural implications must be considered. Eating while family members visit may be helpful from a psychological as well as physical standpoint. Family members may also be included to help feed or encourage the patient during mealtimes. Their input may be valuable with regard to special likes, dislikes, and psychological or cultural considerations.

Patients who are being changed from parenteral to enteral or oral feedings may also need some special consideration. It is generally agreed that as use of the new nutrition route increases, parenteral nutrition will be gradually decreased. Discontinuing TPN abruptly can lead to significant metabolic alterations, such as hypoglycemia. Similarly, it may take several days before the gut can be used optimally. As stated previously, studies have shown a marked reduction in the mass of the large intestine during TPN.[9, 10] If for some reason the patient had preexisting malnutrition, loss of absorptive surface and decreased enzyme concentrations of the GI lining may contribute to malabsorptive problems. Endoscopic biopsy may be helpful in determining the cause of malabsorption problems. In addition, some findings suggest a thinning of the microvilli structure in the intestine during TPN. The reason for this situation is unclear. Two possibilities have been suggested: disuse of the GI tract when the bowel is put to rest and lack of a vital gut amino acid (glutamine) in standard TPN solutions.[7, 20, 125] Based on these hypotheses, utilizing the gut to some extent (when possible) during TPN is being considered as a future treatment modality. When a patient is making a transition from TPN to enteral feeding, high residuals due to decreased peristalsis may occur. Reglan has proved effective in some cases in increasing GI motility and decreasing problems with high residuals. If TPN or enteral support are still required, assessment strategies, as previously described, should be continued. Similarly, ongoing nursing, dietary, and medical assessment is necessary to determine the earliest possible transition to the oral or enteral nutrition route.

Rehabilitation Phase

Patient Characteristics

The rehabilitation phase of recovery is characterized by a stabler metabolic rate. The patient's basal needs are closer to normal. The type of rehabilitation necessary greatly affects the patient's overall metabolic needs. For example, a patient who has sustained major pelvic fractures requires weeks to months of rigorous physical therapy, necessitating high caloric intake. This period is characterized by muscle building or anabolic processes. Physical and occupational therapists are actively involved in assisting the patient to greater levels of independent functioning. Teaching the patient to overcome handicaps and understand the rationale behind proper nutritional intake is essential. The patient may have been transferred to a rehabilitation facility, which usually promotes greater freedom and independent functioning. The patient has usually begun to adjust psychologically to his situation, although depression may still be present. Boredom may exist, and the patient may be eager to return home. Most patients have advanced from parenteral or enteral nutritional support to a complete oral diet.

Feeding Modalities

As stated previously, the patient is usually on a regular diet. Some patients still require dietary supplements. Patients who require continued enteral or parenteral support are rare. If that situation exists, a long-term care facility may be indicated. These situations represent the extreme. Extensive teaching and home health care assistance must be provided for those who are going home with either enteral or parenteral support.

Home Parenteral Support. Home parenteral nutrition (HPN) is an effective nutritional support system for patients who have compromised GI function.[141] Preparing the patient and/or significant other for HPN requires multidisciplinary coordination. Social workers, nursing staffs, pharmacologists, and a home health agency are required for an adequate transition to home. Preparing for discharge requires teaching about technical aspects of material storage, line care, site care, dressing changes, infusion pump functions, physical activities, catheter complications, metabolic assessment (intake and output, urine testing, daily weights), and solution preparation if premixed solutions are not utilized. Before teaching begins, assessment of the patient's and/or support person's cognitive and motor skills must be completed. Similarly, psychological concerns related to life-style changes must be discussed. Insurance coverage should also be discussed to decrease financial concerns.

Once the team has determined the patient to be an appropriate candidate, the teaching process begins. Time frames should be mentioned, since the entire process probably takes 2 to 3 weeks. Most patients are anxious to go home but may be frustrated if all procedures are not mastered. Therefore, adequate time for preparation is a must. The following should be done:

1. Identify patient learning needs.
2. Determine readiness to learn.
3. Establish mutual goals and objectives.
4. Choose the appropriate method/plan for teaching.[141]

Health personnel teach by demonstration, utilizing a return demonstration by the patient to indicate acquisition of skills. In addition, written instruction is necessary. The nurse should document all aspects of the educational process. Keeping lines of communication open by reinforcing the need to communicate questions and concerns may prevent major problems.

Home Enteral Support. Patients who go home with enteral nutrition need similar educational and preparative efforts. Patients referred for home enteral nutrition (HEN) are those whose diagnoses prohibit oral intake of normal foodstuffs.[142] The HEN experience of Nelson and associates[142] indicates that 6 per cent of their referrals in 1985 were patients diagnosed with traumatic injury. Clinicians must teach techniques related to tube care, nutrient delivery system, and site care (with gastrostomy and jejunostomy). Complications such as diarrhea, dehydration (due to inadequate free water), and tube blockage should be discussed. Patients must be taught to report nausea, vomiting, and abdominal distention because these may indicate feeding intolerance. A coordinated approach to HEN requires appropriate selection, training, and follow-up for effective and safe application.

PREVENTION AND RESEARCH IMPLICATIONS

Independent and collaborative opportunities exist for nursing research. Therefore, pairs of researchers such as nurse-physician and nurse-dietitian or a combination of these could produce valuable contributions for improved patient care in this area. The ultimate goal is to prevent malnutrition by identifying patients at greatest risk and intervening before serious functional losses appear. Additionally, the demand to determine and select the most beneficial, risk-free nutrition for the trauma population cannot be underestimated.

One area of primary research is in the field of education: What types of nutritional assessments are known to trauma nurses? What is their general knowledge base? Future workshops could aim their content at identified weaknesses in nutritional knowledge. To participate effectively in a team approach, nurses as well as physicians need a sound knowledge base in nutrition.

Nurses are in a strategic position for identifying high-risk trauma patients or patients in need of further nutrition evaluation. A study could be designed to evaluate an assessment technique, with the purpose of determining special risk patients. This technique or tool could be implemented by a primary nurse and/or nutrition support nurse. If this technique were successful, case findings would determine initial nutritional interventions. Hypothetically, patients could be classified according to the following:

1. Immediate need for nutritional support (1 to 2 days)
2. Early nutritional support (2 to 3 days)
3. Normal nutritional support (3 to 4 days)

Such studies may ultimately help to reduce complications such as sepsis, wound dehiscence, and altered healing.

In addition, special antisepsis techniques or protocols could be examined for use with the patient who has been determined to be at greater risk for infection due to nutritional assessment findings. For instance, a patient who is determined to have a 50 per cent or greater increase in metabolic expenditure may need special respiratory or dressing protocols. Similarly, an index could be developed that quantifies a person's metabolic status on admission. This index could be correlated with morbidity and mortality incidence.

If nutritional status is quantified in a comprehensive way, it could be utilized as a predictor of the ability to be weaned from a ventilator, thus testing a similar hypothesis. There is a relation between the ability to be weaned from a ventilator as evidenced by increased negative inspiratory force and vital capacity and nutritional indices as measured by albumin, transferrin, and nitrogen balance. What nursing or collaborative measures could be instituted to improve a patient's ability to be weaned?

Another potential study might examine the effect of body temperature increases on nutritional demand. It is known that there is a linear relation between a 1°C increase and oxygen consumption.[2] The question is what effect does this increase have on nutritional demand in critically ill trauma patients? Can we quantify this effect and project the increased energy expenditure associated with it? Most studies looking at the effects of temperature elevation are done on healthy people with normal metabolic rates. Is temperature a big contributor to a person's metabolic rate when it is already elevated because of other variables?

Similarly, we are aware that increased CO_2 production occurs with increased glucose loads in patients on ventilators. Further, this increase in CO_2 can be detrimental when attempting to wean certain patients from the ventilator. Are there other specific actions due to fuel substrate utilization that hinder the trauma patient's recovery? What nursing assessment strategies might be necessary?

Energy prediction equations with various factors need to be further validated. Standard operational definitions need to be developed so that various institutional settings can consistently utilize a formula and factors accurately based on objective criteria. Nurses' input regarding use of various activity factors and the objective criteria is essential because nurses are in the best position to validate these factors. Similarly, we need to validate the characteristics in trauma patients that have a high correlate with metabolic rate alterations. Existing trauma severity scores might be helpful in this endeavor. Further, studies that quantify energy expenditure with sophisticated 24-hour gas analysis techniques such as the one developed by Dr. S. Z. Turney need to be used on large samples of critically ill trauma patients.

Subgroups of trauma patients need further consideration. For example, elderly and premorbidly obese people have greater complications when traumatically injured. Are there specific metabolic or nutritional interventions that might improve prognosis? Are there differences in metabolic rate and injury response in specific subgroups that necessitate different nutritional interventions? As our population ages, we may see more traumatic injuries in elderly people.

Studies indicate that anesthesia can dampen the metabolic response to injury. Is there any benefit from modifyng the response to injury? What types of nursing and medical interventions increase catecholamine release? Can specific environmental conditions decrease a person's metabolic rate? Can therapeutic touch or communication decrease anxiety and therefore decrease metabolic rate? Is sedation an effective, safe way to decrease metabolic rate, or is the teleologic response to injury necessary for survival?

What are the most effective measures to decrease abdominal distention and/or diarrhea in patients being tube fed? Is there a greater incidence of diarrhea in patients who have been on long-term TPN once enteral feedings are initiated? Is it best to stop tube feedings completely before oral feedings are tolerated? What are the patient's subjective feelings related to his first oral intake? There is a need for more studies with the head- and spinal cord–injured population. Although studies exist in the acute phase of injury, further research needs to focus on the subacute and rehabilitation population. The head-injured population appear to have a variable metabolic rate. Can subgroups be identified that will help practitioners individualize nutrition support? Similarly, further studies are needed that evaluate the benefits of early enteral support.

Can the nurse and/or physical therapist improve nitrogen retention and increase muscle mass in patients who are non–weight bearing and receiving nutrition support, by an active or passive range-of-motion program?

Finally, further studies such as the one by Weissman et al,[53] which examines the effects of routine nursing and medical care interventions on metabolic rate, need to be performed. Results from these studies will help to improve energy prediction when indirect calorimetry is not available. All studies should look at metabolic rate as it compares with theoretical attributes of the metabolic response to injury over time.

In conclusion, previous research emphasized the need to prevent underfeeding. Although this is an extremely important finding, recent studies suggest equally significant consequences related to overfeeding. It is possible that because of the emphasis on hospital malnutrition in the past, distorted findings from unreliable energy measurements are being utilized without significant validation. It is hoped that future research will reveal ways in which to assess nutritional status accurately and to improve nutritional intake and energy prediction uniformly, thus improving overall outcome and reducing excessive costs due to overfeeding in this critically ill population.

SUMMARY

This chapter has provided an overview of normal metabolism, substrates in humans, and nonstressed starvation metabolism. In starvation, the body adapts by lowering the metabolic rate and metabolizing fat, the fuel substrate that has the greatest availability and the least functional consequences. In contrast, various hormonal and humoral factors that favor catabolism are present in injury. Combined with the inability to take in food, the trauma patient utilizes endogenous substrates to provide for the high-magnitude energy needs present during the hypermetabolic response. The protein compartment, the most functional compartment, is the most seriously depleted during injury. Complications related to depletion of this compartment have serious sequelae.

Nutritional assessment, at best, is an art rather than a science. Assessment parameters acceptable in healthy people are of questionable validity in a critically ill trauma population. Various factors need to be assessed and viewed in relation to a patient's clinical picture to be meaningful. A multidisciplinary approach that involves a close relation among the nurse, dietitian, and physician is necessary to achieve goals. Prescribed nutritional regimens need accurate assessment and evaluation by an astute nursing staff.

Multiple nutritional modalities exist and are utilized, depending on specific patient criteria. Multiple complications can occur related to excessive or deficient calories. The entire team must provide continuous monitoring of nutritional assessment parameters, as well as fluid and electrolyte status. This continued monitoring provides data necessary to institute different nutritional modalities as the patient progresses through the critical care, intermediate, and rehabilitation phases of recovery. Teaching patients and/or families about nutritional modalities as well as the rationale and/or consequences associated with inadequate intake is essential.

Multiple research implications have been presented that emphasize the need for individual and collaborative studies. We must continue to evaluate our current practices to provide the best possible comprehensive metabolic and nutritional care for this seriously injured population.

REFERENCES

1. Kudsk KA, Stone JM, Sheldon GF: Nutrition in trauma and burns. Surg Clin North Am 62:183–192, 1982.
2. Wilmore DW: The Metabolic Management of the Critically Ill. New York, Plenum Medical Book Company, 1977.
3. Delmi M, Rapin CH, Bengoa JM, et al: Dietary supplementation in elderly patients with fractured neck of the femur. Lancet 335:1013–1016, 1990.
4. Tweedle D: How the metabolism reacts to injury. Nurs Mirror Nov 23:34–36, 1978.
5. Jensen TG, Englert DM, Dudrick SJ: Nutritional Assessment—A Manual for Practitioners. Norwalk, CT, Appleton-Century-Crofts, 1983.
6. Butterworth CE, Weinsier RL: Handbook of Clinical Nutrition. St. Louis, C. V. Mosby, 1981.
7. Grant JP: Nutritional assessment in clinical practice. Nutrit Clin Practice 1:3–11, 1986.
8. Windmueller HG: Glutamine utilization by the small intestine. Adv Enzymol 53:202–237, 1982.
9. Cameron IL, Pavlat WA, Urban E: Adaptive responses to total intravenous feeding. J Surg Res 17:45–52, 1974.
10. Koga Y, Ikeda K, Inokuchi K, et al: The digestive tract and total parenteral nutrition. Arch Surg 110:742–745, 1975.
11. Meyer J, Yurt RW, Duhaney R, et al: Differential neutrophil activation before and after endotoxin infusion in enteral versus parenterally fed volunteers. Surg Gynecol Obstet vol 167, December 1988.
12. Moore FA, Moore EE, Jones TN, et al: TEN versus TPN following major abdominal trauma-reduced septic morbidity. J Trauma 29(7):916–923, 1989.
13. Stanek GLS: Nutrition: A Concept Paper (unpublished manuscript), 1984, p 3.

14. Guyton AC: Textbook of Medical Physiology. 5th ed. Philadelphia, WB Saunders Co, 1976.
15. Kaminski MV, Ruggiero R, Mills CB: Nutritional assessment—A guide to diagnosis and treatment of the hypermetabolic patient. J Flor Med Assoc 66:390–395, 1979.
16. Bynoe RP, Rudsk KA, Fabian TC, Brown RO: Nutrition support in trauma patients. Nutr Clin Pract 3:137–144, 1988.
17. Pomposelli JJ, Flores EA, Bristrain BR: Role of biochemical mediators in clinical nutrition and surgical metabolism. JPEN 12(2):212–218, 1988.
18. Boosalis MG, McCall JT, Solem LM, et al: Serum copper and ceruloplasm in levels and urinary copper excretion in thermal injury. Am J Clin Nutr 44:889–906, 1986.
19. Jeevanandam M, Young DH, Schiller WR: Endogenous protein-synthesis efficiency in trauma victims. Metabolism 38(10):967–973, 1989.
20. Ruderman NB, Berger M: The formation of glutamine and alanine in skeletal muscle. J Biol Chem 17:550–556, 1974.
21. Cerra FB, Siegel JH, Coleman B, Border JR, McMenamy RR: Septic autocannibalism: A failure of exogenous nutritional support. Ann Surg 192:570–581, 1980.
22. Hurst JM, Koetting CA, Lang CE: Multiple trauma. Trauma Quarterly 4(4):67–78, 1988.
23. Shaw JH, Wolfe RR: An integrated analysis of glucose, fat, and protein metabolism in severely traumatized patients. Ann Surg 209(1):63–72, 1989.
24. Jeevanandam M, Young DH, Schiller WR: Nutritional impact on energy cost of fat fuel mobilization in polytrauma victims. J Trauma 30(2):147–154, 1990.
25. Long CL: Energy balance and carbohydrate metabolism in infection and sepsis. Am J Clin Nutr 30:1301–1310, 1977.
26. Stanek GLS: Predicting energy expenditure in critically ill trauma patients. JPEN Supplement 10:45, 1986.
27. Quebbeman EJ, Ausman RK: Estimating energy requirements in patients receiving parenteral nutrition. Arch Surg 117:1281–1284, 1982.
28. Askanazi J, Carpentier YA, Elwyn DH, Nordenstrom J, Jeevanandam M, Rosenbaum SH, Gump FE, Kinney JM: Influence of total parenteral nutrition on fuel utilization in injury and sepsis. Ann Surg 191:40–46, 1980.
29. Silberman H, Eisenberg D: Parenteral and Enteral Nutrition for the Hospitalized Patient. Norwalk, CT, Appleton-Century-Crofts, 1982.
30. Ryan NT: Metabolic adaptations for energy production during trauma and sepsis. Surg Clin North Am 56:1073–1087, 1976.
31. Grant JP, Custer PB, Thurlow J: Current techniques of nutritional assessment. Surg Clin North Am 61:437–463, 1981.
32. Forbes GB, Bruining GJ: Urinary creatinine excretion and lean body mass. Am J Clin Nutr 29:1359, 1976.
33. Mattox TW, Brown RO, Boucher BA, et al: Use of fibronectin and somatomedin-C as markers of enteral nutrition support in traumatized patients using a modified amino acid formula. JPEN 12(6):592–596, 1988.
34. Buonpane EA, Brown RO, Boucher BA, et al: Use of fibronectin and somatomedin-C as nutritional markers in the enteral nutrition support of traumatized patients. Crit Care Med 17(2):126–132, 1989.
35. Forse AR, Shizgal HM: Serum albumin and nutritional status. JPEN 4:450–454, 1980.
36. Law DK, Dudrick SJ, Abdou NI: Immunocompetence of patients with protein-calorie malnutrition. The effects of nutritional repletion. Ann Intern Med 79:543, 1973.
37. Boosalis MG, Ott L, Levin AS, Slag MP, et al: Relationship of visceral proteins to nutritional status in chronic and acute stress. Crit Care Med 17(8):741–747, 1989.
38. Andrassy RJ, Durr ED: Albumin: Use in nutrition and support. Nutr Clin Pract 3:226–229, 1988.
39. Tayek JA: Albumin synthesis and nutritional assessment. Nutr Clin Pract 3:219–221, 1988.
40. Wolfe BM: On-going controversies regarding albumin and nutrition support. Nutr Clin Pract 3:217–218, 1988.
41. Sorkness R: The estimation of 24-hour urine urea nitrogen excretion from urine collections of shorter duration in continuous alimented patients. JPEN 8:300–301, 1984.
42. Long CL: Nonseptic stress metabolism. Nutritional Management of Metabolic Stress Monograph, 97-1530-20-6. Abbott Laboratories, 1983, pp 5–19.
43. Lewis RT, Klein H: Risk factors in postoperative sepsis: Significance of preoperative lymphocytopenia. J Surg Res 26:365–371, 1979.
44. Kinney JM: The application of indirect calorimetry to clinical studies. In Kinney J (ed): Assessment of Energy Metabolism in Health and Disease. Columbus, Ross Laboratories, 1978, pp 42–48.
45. Robinson CH, Lawler MR: Normal and Therapeutic Nutrition. New York, Macmillan, 1977.
46. MacBurney MM: Enteral nutrition—Part 1: Determination of energy and protein needs in the hospitalized patient. Am J Intravenous Ther Clin Nutr Feb:18–27, 1983.
47. Glickman N, Mitchell HH, Lambert EH, Keaton RW: The total specific dynamic action of high protein and high-carbohydrate diets in human subjects. J Nutr 36:41, 1948.
48. Bradfield RB, Jourdan MH: Relative importance of specific dynamic action in weight-reduction diets. Lancet 2:640, 1973.
49. Kinney JM, Roe CF: Caloric equivalents of fever; patterns of postoperative response. Ann Surg 156:610–618, 1962.
50. Clowes GH, O'Donnell TF, Blackburn GL, Maki TW: Energy metabolism and proteolysis in traumatized and septic men. Surg Clin North Am 56:1169–1184, 1976.
51. Aulick LH: Studies in heat transport and heat loss in thermally injured patients. In Kinney J (ed): Assessment of Energy Metabolism in Health and Disease. Columbus, Ross Laboratories, 1978, pp 141–151.
52. Clinical applications of indirect calorimetry. Clin Nutr Newsletter Apr 1–2, 1983.
53. Weissman C, Kemper M, Damask MC, Askanazi J, Hyman AE, Kinney JM: Effect of routine intensive care interventions on metabolic rate. Chest 86:815–818, 1984.
54. Kaufman CS: Nutritional support of the trauma patient. Nutr Support Services 1:11–13, 1981.
55. Turney SZ: Computerized multibed respiratory monitoring. Comput Crit Care Med 3:9–25, 1983.
56. Fraser RB, Turney SZ: A new method of respiratory gas analysis: The light spectrometer (unpublished manuscript), 1985.
57. Turney SZ, McCluggage C, Blumenfeld W, McArkin TC, Cowley RA: Automatic respiratory gas monitoring. Ann Thorac Surg 14:161, 1972.
58. Harris JA, Benedict FG: A Biometric Study of Basal Metabolism in Man. Washington, DC, Carnegie Institute of Washington, Publication No. 279, 1919.
59. Fleisch A: Le metabolisme basal standard et sa determination au moyen du metabocalculator. Helv Med Acta 18:23, 1951.
60. Boothby WM, Berkson J, Dunn HL: Studies of the energy of metabolism of normal individuals: A standard for basal metabolism with a nomogram for clinical application. Am J Physiol 116:468–484, 1936.
61. Long CL, Schaffel N, Geiger JW, Schiller WR, Blakemore WS: Metabolic response to injury and illness: Estimation of energy and protein needs from indirect calorimetry and nitrogen balance. J Parenteral Enteral Nutr 3:452–456, 1979.
62. McCamish MA, Paauw JD, Dean RE: Re-evaluation of caloric needs in the clinical setting. Am J Clin Nutr 35:18, 1982.
63. Rutten P, Blackburn GL, Flatt JP, Hallowell E, Cochran D: Determination of optimal hyperalimentation infusion rate. J Surg Res 18:477–483, 1975.
64. Baker JP, Detsky AS, Stewart S, Whitwell J, Marliss EB, Jeejeebhoy KN: Randomized trial of total parenteral nutrition in critically ill patients: Metabolic effects of varying glucose lipid ratios as the energy source. Gastroenterology 87:53–59, 1984.
65. Quebbeman EJ, Ausman RK, Schneider TC: A re-evaluation of energy expenditure during parenteral nutrition. Ann Surg 195:282–286, 1982.
66. Swinamer DL, Grace MG, Hamilton SM, et al: Predictive equation for assessing energy expendation in mechanically ventilated critically ill patients. Crit Care Med 18(6):657–661, 1990.
67. Fruin AH, Taylor C, Pettis MS: Caloric requirements in patients with severe head injuries. Surg Neurol 25:25–28, 1986.

68. Dempsey DT, Guenter P, Mullen JL, Fairman R, Crosby LO, et al: Energy expenditure in acute trauma to the head with and without barbiturate therapy. Surg Gynecol Obstet 160:128–134, 1985.
69. Turney SZ: The American Pharmaseal Respiratory Monitoring System Operating Manual. American Pharmaseal Respiratory Products, 1980.
70. Mann BS, Westenskow DW, Houtchens BA: Measured and predicted caloric expenditure in the acutely ill. Crit Care Med 13:173–177, 1985.
71. Stanek GLS: Predicting energy expenditure in critically ill trauma patients. Masters Thesis, University of Maryland at Baltimore, 1985.
72. Zejdlik CP: Promoting optimal nutrition. In Management of Spinal Cord Injury. Monterey, CA, Wadsworth Health Sciences Division, 1983, ch. 11.
73. Wolfe BM, Chock E: Energy sources, stores and hormonal controls. Surg Clin North Am 61:509–527, 1981.
74. Sheldon GF, Petersen SR, Sanders R: Hepatic dysfunction during hyperalimentation. Arch Surg 113:504–508, 1978.
75. Brown RO: Total parenteral nutrition-induced liver dysfunction: A review. Nutr Support Services 2:14–16, 1982.
76. Askanazi J, Rosenbaum SH, Hyman AI, Silverberg PA, Milic-Emili J, Kinney JM: Respiratory changes induced by the large glucose levels of total parenteral nutrition. JAMA 243:1444–1447, 1980.
77. Hunker FD, Braton CW, Hunker EM, Durham RM, Krumdieck CL: Metabolic and nutritional evaluation of patients supported with mechanical ventilation. Crit Care Med 8:628–632, 1980.
78. Askanazi J, Elwyn DH, Silverberg PA: Respiratory distress secondary to the high carbohydrate load of TPN: A case report. Surgery 87:596, 1980.
79. Gieske T, Gurushanthaiah G, Glauser FL: Effects of carbohydrates on carbon dioxide excretion in patients with airway disease. Chest 71:55–58, 1977.
80. Covelli HD, Black JW, Olsen MS, Beekman JF: Respiratory failure precipitated by high carbohydrate loads. Ann Intern Med 95:579–581, 1981.
81. Burke JF, Wolfe RR, Mullany CJ, Mathews DE, Bier DM: Glucose requirements following brain injury. Ann Surg 190:274–285, 1979.
82. Wolfe RR, O'Donnell TF, Stone MD, Richmond DA, Burke JF: Investigation of factors determining the optimal glucose infusion rate in total parenteral nutrition. Metabolism 29:892–900, 1980.
83. Askanazi J, Rosenbaum SH, Michelsen CB, Elwyn DH, Hyman AI, Kinney JM: Increased body temperature secondary to total parenteral nutrition. Crit Care Med 8:736–737, 1980.
84. Birkhahn RH, Long CL, Fitkin D, Geiger JW, Blakemore WS: Effects of major skeletal trauma on body protein turnover in man measured by L-[1, ^{14}C]-leucine. Surgery 83:294–300, 1980.
85. Long CL, Birkhahn RH, Geiger JW, Blakemore WS: Contribution of skeletal muscle protein catabolism in trauma patients. Am J Clin Nutr 34:1087–1093, 1981.
86. Bassili HR, Dietel M: Effect of nutritional support on weaning patients of mechanical ventilators. J Parenteral Enteral Nutr 5:161–163, 1981.
87. Doekel RC, Zwillich CW, Scoggins CH, Kryger M, Weil JV: Clinical semi-starvation—Depression of hypoxic ventilatory response. N Engl J Med 295:358–361, 1976.
88. Bartlett RH, Dechert RE, Mault JR, Clark SF: Metabolic studies in chest trauma. J Thorac Cardiovasc Surg 87:503–508, 1984.
89. Keithly JK: Wound healing in malnourished patients. AORN 36:1094–1099, 1982.
90. Seifter E, ReHura G, Barbul A, et al: Arginine: An essential amino acid for injured rats. Surgery 84:224–230, 1978.
91. Barbul A, Fishel RS, Shimazu S, et al: Intravenous hyperalimentation with high arginine levels improves wound healing and immune function. J Surg Res 38:328–334, 1985.
92. Pietsch JB, Meakins JL, MacLean LD: Delayed hypersensitivity response: Application in clinical surgery. Surgery 82:349, 1977.
93. Jensen TG, Englert DM, Dudrick SJ: Interpretation of nutritional assessment data. Nutr Support Services 1:14–20, 1981.
94. Bower RH: Nutrition and immune function. Nutr Clin Pract 5:189–195, 1990.
95. Durnin JV, Womersley J: Body fat assessed from total body density and its estimation from skin fold thicknesses: Measurements on 481 men and women aged from 16 to 72 years. Br J Nutr 32:77–97, 1973.
96. Gray DS, Kaminski MW: Nutritional support of the hospitalized patient. Am Fam Pract 28:143–150, 1983.
97. Siler M: Laboratory tests to monitor fluid status/nutritional/metabolic lab assessment. (unpublished manuscript), 1986.
98. Gilder H: Parenteral nourishment of patients undergoing surgical or traumatic stress. JPEN 10:88–99, 1986.
99. Cuthbertson DP: The disturbance of metabolism produced by bony and non-bony injury, with notes on certain abnormal conditions of bone. Biochem J 24:1244–1266, 1930.
100. Blissitt PA: Nutrition in acute spinal cord injury. Crit Care Clin North Am 2(3):375–384, 1990.
101. Kuric J, Lucas CE, Ledgerwood AM, et al: Nutritional support: A prophylaxis against stress bleeding after spinal cord injury. Paraplegia 27:140–145, 1989.
102. Cahill GF Jr: The physiology of insulin in man. Diabetes 20:785–799, 1971.
103. Maderazo EG, Woronick CL, Quercia RA, et al: The inhibitory effect of parenteral nutrition on recovery of neutrophil locomotory function in blunt trauma. Ann Surg 208(2):221–226, 1988.
104. Peterson VM, Moore EE, Jones TN, et al: Total enteral nutrition versus total parenteral nutrition after major torso injury: Attenuation of hepatic protein reprioritization. Surgery 104(2):199–207, 1988.
105. Alverdy JC, Aoys E, Moss GS: Total parenteral nutrition promotes bacterial translocation from the gut. Surgery 104(2):185–190, 1988.
106. Border JR, Hassett J, LaDuca J, et al: The gut origin septic states in blunt multiple trauma (ISS = 40) in the ICU. Ann Surg 206(4):427–448, 1987.
107. Grahm TW, Zadrozny DB, Harrington T: The benefits of early jejunal hyperalimentation in head-injured patients. Neurosurgery 25(5):729–735, 1989.
108. Moore EE, Jones TN, Moore FA: Immediate postinjury enteral feeding: Reducing gut bacterial translocation. Panam J Trauma 1:31–41, 1989.
109. Curreri PW: Nutritional replacement modalities. J Trauma 19:906–908, 1979.
110. Jackson DM, Davidoff G: Gastroparesis following traumatic brain injury and response to metoclopramide therapy. Arch Phys Med Rehabil 70:553–555, 1989.
111. Monturo CA: Enteral access device selection. Nutr Clin Pract 5:207–213, 1990.
112. Thurlow PM: Bedside enteral feeding tube placement into duodenum and jejunum. JPEN 10:104–105, 1986.
113. Caulfield KA, Page CP, Pestana C: Technique for intraduodenal placement of transnasal enteral feeding catheters. Nutr Clin Pract 6:23–26, 1991.
114. Bookus S: Troubleshooting your tube feedings. Am J Nurs 91(5):24–30, 1991.
115. Breach CL, Saldanha LG: Tube feedings: A survey of compliance to procedures and complications. Nutr Clin Pract 3:230–234, 1988.
116. Moghissi K, Boore JRP: Parenteral and Enteral Nutrition for Nurses. Rockville, MD, Aspen Systems, 1983.
117. Jones TN, Moore FA, Moore EE, McCroskey BL: Gastrointestinal symptoms attributed to jejunostomy feeding after major abdominal trauma—a critical analysis. Crit Care Med 17(11):1146–1150, 1989.
118. Bommarito AA, Heinzelmann MJ, Boysen DA: A new approach to the management of obstructed enteral feeding tubes. Nutr Clin Pract 4:111–114, 1989.
119. Marcuard SP, Stegall KS: Unclogging feeding tubes with pancreatic enzyme. JPEN 14(2):198–200, 1990.
120. Benson DW, Griggs BA, Hamilton F, et al: Clogging of feeding tubes: A randomized trial of a newly designed tube. Nutr Clin Pract 5:107–110, 1990.

121. Brinson RR: Fiber-containing enteral formulas: Clinical importance. (Editorial) Nutr Clin Pract 5:97–98, 1990.
122. Frankenfield DC, Beyer P: Soy-polysaccharide fiber: Effect on diarrhea in tube-fed, head-injured patients. Am J Clin Nutr 50:533–538, 1989.
123. Palacio JC, Rombeau JL: Dietary fiber: A brief review and potential application to enteral nutrition. Nutr Clin Pract 5:99–106, 1990.
124. Alverdy J, Chi SH, Sheldon GF: The effect of parenteral nutrition on gastrointestinal immunity. Ann Surg 202(6):681–684, 1985.
125. Furst P, Albers S, Stehle P: Evidence for a nutritional need for glutamine in catabolic patients. Kidney Int 36(Suppl 27):287–292, 1989.
126. Turner WW: Postoperative nutritional support of patients with abdominal trauma. Surg Clin North Am 70(3):703–714, 1990.
127. Martindale RG, McCarthy MS: Enteral and parenteral nutrition in the trauma patient. Trauma Quarterly 4(4):47–58, 1988.
128. Fujiwara T, Kawarasaki H, Fonkalsrud EW: Reduction of post-infusion venous endothelial injury with intralipid. Surg Gynecol Obstet 158:57–65, 1984.
129. Simmons BP: CDC guidelines for the prevention and control of nosocomial infection—guidelines for prevention of intravascular infection. Am Infect Control 11:183–195, 1983.
130. Band J, Maki P: Safety of changing intravenous delivery systems of longer than 24-hour intervals. Ann Intern Med 91:173–179, 1979.
131. Robertson JF, Garden MB, Shenkin A: Intravenous nutrition and hepatic dysfunction. JPEN 10:172–183, 1986.
132. Jacobson S, Christenson I, Kager L: Utilization and metabolic effects of a conventional and a single-solution regimen in postoperative total parenteral nutrition. Am J Clin Nutr 34:1402–1409, 1981.
133. Abbott WC, Grakauskas AM, Bristrian BR, Rose R, Blackburn GL: Metabolic and respiratory effects of continuous and discontinuous lipid infusions. Arch Surg 119:1367–1371, 1984.
134. Chiarla C, Siegel JH, Kiddy S, et al: Inhibition of post-traumatic septic proteolysis and ureagenesis and stimulation of hepatic acute phase protein production by branched-chain amino acid TPN. J Trauma 28(8):1145–1172, 1988.
135. Cerra FB, Mazuski J, Teasley K, et al: Nitrogen retention in critically ill patients is proportional to the branched-chain amino acid load. Crit Care Med 11(10):775–778, 1983.
136. Pittiruti M, Siegel JH, Sganga G, Wiles CE, Belzberg H, Wedel S, Placko R: Increased dependence of leucine in posttraumatic sepsis: Leucine/tyrosine clearance ratio as an indicator of hepatic impairment in septic organ failure syndrome. Surgery 98:378–386, 1985.
137. Moyer ED, Border JR, Cerra FB: Multiple system organ failure: IV balances in plasma amino acids associated with exogenous albumin in the trauma-septic patient. J Trauma 21:543–547, 1981.
138. Mori E, Hasebe M, Kobayashi K, et al: Immediate stimulation of protein metabolism in burned rats by total parenteral nutrition enriched in branched-chain amino acids. JPEN 13(6):484–489, 1989.
139. Cerra FB, Mazuski J, Chute E, et al: Branched-chain metabolic support. A prospective, randomized, double-blind trial in surgical stress. Ann Surg 199(3):286–292, 1984.
140. Kuhi DA, Brown RO, Vehe KL, et al: Use of selected visceral protein measurements in the comparison of branched-chain amino acids with standard amino acids in parenteral nutrition support of injured patients. Surgery 107(5)504–510, 1990.
141. Marein C, Misny B, Paysinger J, O'Neill M, Srp F, Galledge AD, Holpit L, Matarese L, Steiger E: Home parenteral nutrition. Nutr Clin Pract 1:179–192, 1986.
142. Nelson JK, Palumbo PJ, O'Brien PC: Home enteral nutrition: Observations of a newly established program. Nutr Clin Pract 1:193–199, 1986.

15

PAIN MANAGEMENT IN THE TRAUMA PATIENT

JOYCE S. WILLENS

Definition of Pain

Pain, long recognized as a subjective experience, was at one time considered undefinable because of individual variations.[1] In a classic study that paved the way for providing information about pain, to decrease patient anxiety, pain was defined as "an experience which can be described as having two components: sensory and reactive."[2] This definition was based on work by Melzack and Torgerson,[3] who had begun to classify words descriptive of pain for use in what later became known as the McGill Pain Questionnaire.[4] Melzack conceptualized pain as a phenomenon that has three components: sensory-discriminative, motivational-affective, and cognitive-evaluative.

The sensory-discriminative component of pain is the neurophysiological aspect concerned with the transmission and processing of pain impulses. The motivational-affective component is the emotional response to the sensory component of pain. Anxiety, fear, panic, and suffering are automatic responses to pain. The cognitive-evaluative component involves thinking, judging, interpreting, and deciding on the meaning of the pain and includes cultural determinants of pain.

Curro[5] used categories similar to Melzack's but made more of a distinction between them. Curro defines pain as "a multidimensional experience consisting of motivational, cognitive, affective, and discriminative components." The motivational component manifests in the form of action or escape, which often is reflexive. Past memory of the painful experience is the cognitive component. Examples of the affective component include fear, anxiety, and stress that is associated with the painful experience. The discriminative component is derived from the response of the peripheral nervous system to the noxious stimulus. This component includes the onset, duration, intensity, and location of the pain.

Pain is defined by the International Association for the Study of Pain as "an unpleasant sensory and emotional experience associated with actual or potential damage or described in terms of such damage."[6]

McCaffery describes pain as "whatever the experiencing

person says it is and existing whenever he says it does."[7] This broad definition emphasizes the subjective nature of pain.

All the definitions mentioned here recognize the multidimensional nature of pain. Johnson and Rice[2] recognized the sensory component as physiological and that the reactive nature to pain involves a psychological emotional aspect. They included the intensity and magnitude of pain in the reactive component. Melzack[4] expanded the definition of pain to include past experience with pain, the meaning of pain, and cultural determinants of pain. Curro[5] added greater specificity to the components. Basically, all the definitions recognize the highly subjective nature of a multidimensional experience.

The multiple dimensions combined with the highly subjective nature of pain contribute to the difficulty in effectively assessing and managing pain. When pain is not relieved or well managed, it can affect a patient's physiology, his behavior, and his emotional state. Poorly managed pain can lead to negative patient outcomes.

PATHOPHYSIOLOGY OF NOCICEPTION AND PAIN

Peripheral Nervous System

Nociception refers to the body's reaction to a noxious stimulus. Pain describes the perception of the event. Nociception is induced as a result of tissue damage that results in the liberation of *algogenic* or pain-producing substances such as bradykinin, leukokinins, serotonin, norepinephrine, histamine, potassium, acids, acetylcholine, proteolytic enzymes, and prostaglandins.[8] The tissue damage causes the release of algogenic substances such as bradykinin and cholecystokinin, which are released from the plasma, and substance P, which is released from nerve terminals. These algogenic substances are released into the extracellular fluid that surrounds nociceptors. Pain is produced directly by excitation of the nociceptor membranes. The release of algogenic substances may exert an excitatory action by altering local microcirculation. Depending on the substance, vasodilation, vasoconstriction, or an increase in capillary permeability results. The increase in capillary permeability disturbs the microenvironment of the nociceptors and contributes to an increase in the excitability, which results in sensitization of the fibers. The nociceptive-producing substances activate the peripheral nerve endings.[8, 9]

The activated nerve endings, called *mechanoreceptors, thermoreceptors,* and *chemoreceptors,* respond to mechanical, thermal, or chemical stimuli, respectively. Most receptors are sensitive to all these stimuli and are called *polymodal receptors.* Others respond only to specific stimuli. Pain receptors, called nociceptors, are located throughout the body. They are widespread in the skin, periosteum, joint surfaces, arterial walls, subcutaneous tissue, muscle, fascia, and viscera. Most other deep tissues have fewer pain receptors.[10]

Nociceptors seldom adapt to a painful stimulus. It is possible, however, to sensitize nociceptors by repeated exposure to noxious stimuli. Repeated exposure to noxious stimuli enhances sensitivity, lowers the threshold to stimulation, and enhances the response to stimulation. Threshold is defined as the intensity and quality of a stimulus that are adequate to produce a response. Thus, when nociceptors are sensitized, smaller than usual amounts of algogenic substances may stimulate nociception, which may go on to be perceived as pain.

Central Nervous System

After tissue injury, which causes the release of algogenic substances and the stimulation of nociceptors, nociception is conducted on one or two types of peripheral nerve fibers. Figure 15–1 shows the transmission of nociceptive information. The A-delta or C fibers conduct the information of nociceptors. Well-localized, sharp pain is conducted by the fast A-delta fibers, whereas dull, poorly localized pain is conducted by the slower C fibers.

A-delta, acute, pricking pain travels the neospinothalamic pathway and arrives in the ventrobasal complex of the thalamus. From here it travels to other areas in the thalamus and to the somatosensory cortex. Figure 15–2 depicts the transmission of nociceptive information along neospinothalamic and paleospinothalamic tracts to the cortex. Sensory information arrives quickly by these pathways and permits localization, perception of intensity, and duration of the pain stimulus. The ventrobasal complex of the thalamus is also the area of termination for tactile sensation fibers from the spinothalamic and dorsal-lemniscal systems. Localization of pain may result from simultaneous stimulation of tactile receptors and pain receptors. Other sensory information also travels the neospinothalamic pathway and other sensory tracts contribute to pain.[8]

C fiber sensations, or the slow, burning, aching pains, are transmitted on the paleospinothalamic tract. These slow pain fibers terminate in the reticular area of the brainstem and in the intralaminar nuclei of the thalamus. Both these areas are part of the reticular activating system. Impulses are projected to all parts of the brain—upward through the thalamus, laterally to the hypothalamus, and to all areas of the cerebral cortex. These fibers excite the entire nervous system; they affect ventilation, endocrine function, and circulation. C fiber pain sensations are poorly localized, and gradations of intensity are poor. They function primarily to alert the person to harmful processes in the body. They are responsible for the feeling and behavioral components of the pain experience. Other sensory information, such as crude touch, tickle, heat, and cold, are also transmitted by this pathway.[8]

Regulation of Pain

Before pain signals reach the higher brain centers, they are modified in various ways. Pain-producing substances, spinal reflexes, descending modulation systems, and neurotransmitters may influence the pain signals before they reach the higher brain structures.

Pain-Producing Substances

Stimuli that provoke pain receptors are mechanical, thermal, and chemical, with chemical stimuli being most common. When tissues are injured, serotonin, histamine, and

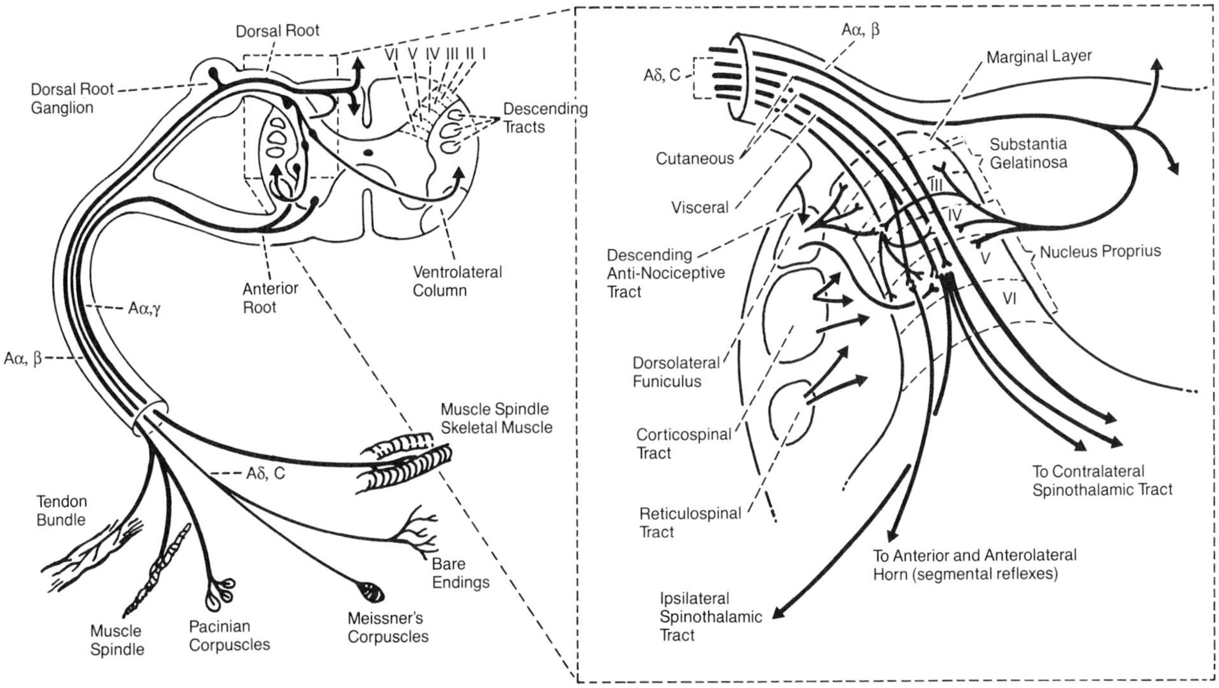

Figure 15–1. Transmission of nociceptive information in the A-delta and C fibers with projection onto the laminae. (From Bonica JJ: Management of Acute and Chronic Pain–An Introduction. Proceedings: Recent Advances in the Management of Acute and Chronic Pain, a symposium held in conjunction with the Second World Congress on Pain, Montreal, Canada, August 26, 1978. New York, HP Publishing Co., 1979. Sponsored by Pfizer Laboratories Division, Inc., New York, p. 6, Fig. 2.)

bradykinin are released, causing stimulation of chemoreceptors. This process triggers the formation of prostaglandins, which in turn further sensitizes the receptor to the effects of bradykinin. Potassium ions are also released. The pain of inflammation is thought to be associated with the effects of these chemicals on pain receptors. Release of these chemicals in the body decreases the threshold of all receptors, not just pain receptors. These substances convert all receptors functionally to nociceptors. This may be one of the mechanisms associated with the hyperalgesia experienced in an undamaged area surrounding the area of injury.

Spinal Reflexes

Traumatic injury may stimulate efferent and sympathetic reflexes, producing muscle spasm in the area of injury. The muscle spasm stimulates chemoreceptors, generating more pain. The pain of muscle spasm is generated by ischemia and an increased metabolic rate. Ischemia stimulates nociception by liberating pain-producing substances such as lactic acid when metabolism takes place without sufficient oxygen. Ischemia may also cause tissue damage, with injured cells releasing toxic substances.

Descending Modulation Systems

Although the nervous system is organized for the caudal-rostral ascending flow of impulses, it is evident that descending neural systems significantly influence the transmission and processing of nociceptive information. It is apparent that the selection, modulation, and control of ascending sensory information is influenced by fibers that descend from the nucleus raphe magnus.[8] The rubrospinal, reticulospinal, and raphespinal tracts have synaptic terminations to several laminae of the spinal cord. Figure 15–3 shows the descending modulation systems.

Electrical stimulation of periaqueductal gray areas in the brain can produce analgesia.[10] This stimulation-produced analgesia (SPA) depends on impulses being transmitted on descending nerve fibers from the brain to the spinal cord. The descending pathways in the dorsolateral funiculus of the spinal cord carry signals from the raphe magnus to inhibit pain impulses at the first synapse in the dorsal horn. The substantia gelatinosa in the dorsal horn of the spinal cord contains projections from the raphe magnus.

Opiate analgesia and SPA may share a similar mechanism of action. Electrical stimulation of certain raphe nuclei enhances morphine analgesia. Naloxone, a narcotic antagonist, reverses the analgesic effect of SPA and opiate medications. Opiate receptor sites are found throughout the brain and in heavy concentration in the periaqueductal gray areas.

THEORIES OF NOCICEPTION AND PAIN

Theories of nociception and pain assist in the explanation of how pain occurs and why treatments modulate it. Many theories have been proposed. The two presented here, the gate control theory (GCT) and the opioid receptor theory, frequently are cited and provide explanatory purposes.

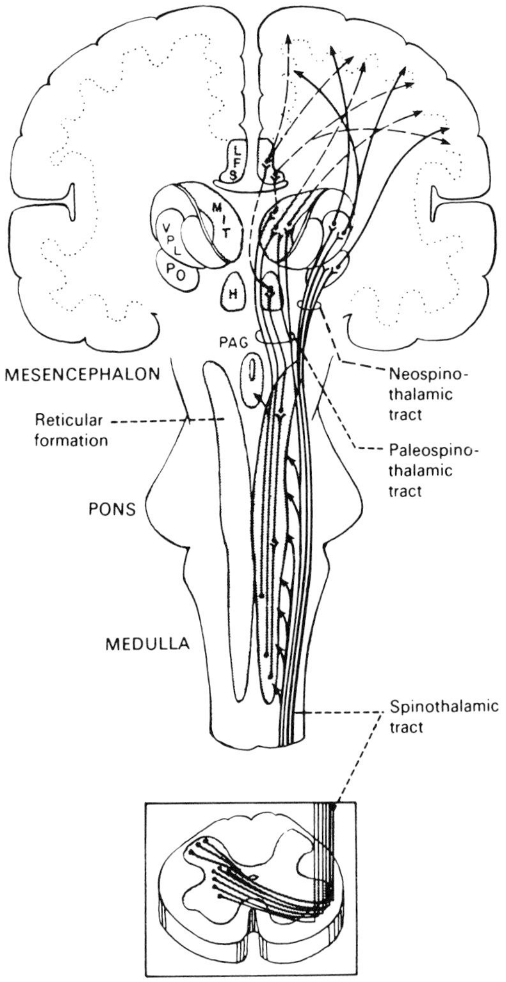

Figure 15–2. Simple diagram of the course and termination of the spinothalamic tract. Most of the fibers cross to the opposite side and ascend to the brainstem and brain, although some ascend ipsilaterally. The neospinothalamic (nSTT) part of the tract has cell bodies located primarily in laminae I and V of the dorsal horn, whereas the paleospinothalamic tract (pSTT) has its cell bodies in deeper laminae. The nSTT fibers ascend in a more superficial part of the tract and project without interruption to the caudal part of the ventroposterolateral thalamic nucleus (VPLc), the oral part of this nucleus (VPLo), and the medial part of the posterior thalamus (POm). In these structures, they synapse with a third relay of neurons, which project to the somatosensory cortex (SI, SII, and retroinsular cortex) *(solid lines)*. Some of the fibers of the pSTT pass directly to the medial/intralaminar thalamic nuclei (MIT), and others project to the nuclei and the reticular formation of the brainstem and thence to the periaqueductal gray (PAG), hypothalamus (H), nucleus submedius, and MIT. In these structures, these axons synapse with neurons that connect with the limbic forebrain structure (LFS) by way of complex circuits and also send diffuse projection to various parts of the brain *(dashed lines)*. (From Bonica JJ: The Management of Pain. 2nd ed. Philadelphia, Lea & Febiger, 1990, p. 54.)

Gate Control Theory

The GCT, first proposed by Melzack[11] and later modified, encompasses the physiological and psychological aspects of nociception but does not clearly elucidate its neurochemical nature. This theory proposes that stimulation of the skin evokes nervous impulses that are transmitted by three systems located in the spinal cord. The substantia gelatinosa in the dorsal horn of the spinal cord, the dorsal column fibers, and the central transmission cells act to stimulate or inhibit nociceptive impulses. The transmission of noxious impulses from the afferent fibers to the spinal cord transmission cells is modulated by a spinal gating mechanism in the dorsal horn. This gating mechanism is influenced by the amount of

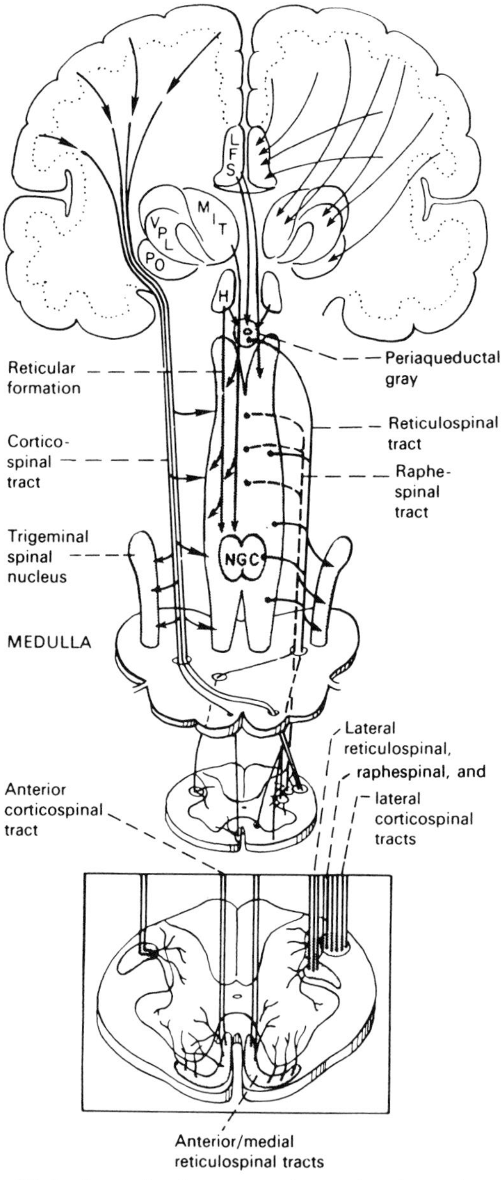

Figure 15–3. A simple diagram to depict the descending control systems. Note that the thalamus and the limbic system (LFS) receive afferents from the cerebrum and they, in turn, send descending systems to the brainstem and spinal cord. The corticospinal tracts modulate (excite or inhibit) various structures in the brainstem, the trigeminal spinal nucleus, and the dorsal and ventral horns. The raphespinal and the medullary reticulospinal tracts from each side project bilaterally, descend in the dorsolateral funiculus, and send terminals to laminae I, IIo, and V–VII, except that the reticulospinal fibers originating in the nucleus gigantocellularis (NGC) have their terminals in laminae VII–VIII. The pontine reticulospinal tracts project ipsilaterally and descend in association with the medial longitudinal fasciculus in the anterior funiculus and terminate in laminae VII and VIII. (From Bonica JJ: The Management of Pain. 2nd ed. Philadelphia, Lea & Febiger, 1990, p. 106.)

activity in the large-diameter fibers. Stimulation of the large-diameter fibers inhibits the transmission of pain, thus "closes the gate," whereas stimulation of the smaller fibers facilitates transmission, or "opens the gate." The gating mechanism is influenced by nervous impulses that descend from the brain. The theory proposes a specialized system of large-diameter fibers that activate selective cognitive processes that then influence, by way of descending fibers, the modulating properties of the spinal gate. Figure 15–4 shows a schematic representation of the GCT.

Researchers have uncovered much evidence to support the GCT. This theory is useful in explaining how pain interventions such as cutaneous stimulation, heat, massage, and hypnosis work to modulate pain. Emotional influences are depicted by the cognitive control box, which has direct input into the gate control system. This theory prophetically hints at the importance of the spinal cord in the biochemical modulation of pain.

Opioid Receptor Theory

The opioid receptor theory, solely biochemical in nature, serves to emphasize the role of the descending system that acts to inhibit nociception. The first evidence of an endogenous analgesic system stemmed from reports that electrical stimulation of the periaqueductal gray area produced potent analgesia, which became known as SPA.[12, 13] Pert and Snyder[14] first reported the discovery of endogenous opiate receptors. Hughes and coworkers[15] reported the discovery of endogenous opiate substances in the brain. These substances are now known as enkephalins, meaning *in the head,* and endorphins, meaning *endogenous morphine.* Once these substances were found in the brain, spinal cord, blood, and intestines, much research was directed at ascertaining the role these substances play in nociception.

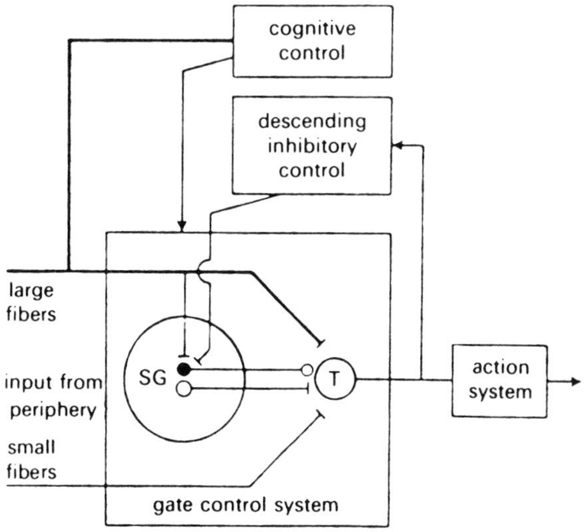

Figure 15–4. The gate-control theory (Mark II). The new model includes excitatory *(white circle)* and inhibitory *(black circle)* links from the substantia gelatinosa (SG) to the transmission (T) cells as well as descending inhibitory control from brainstem systems. The round knob at the end of the inhibitory link implies that its actions may be presynaptic, postsynaptic, or both. All connections are excitatory, except the inhibitory link from SG to T cell. (Modified from Melzack R, Wall PD: The Challenge of Pain. New York, Basic Books, 1983.)

Three distinct classes of endogenous opioids are known: enkephalins, dynorphins, and β-endorphins, which represent three chemically distinct families of opioid peptides and different precursors.[10, 16, 17] Later, the opiate binding sites were discovered and named. The opiate binding sites, also known as receptors, are classified as mu (μ), kappa (κ), delta (δ), and sigma (σ). Each receptor responds in a different manner when activated. Table 15–1 summarizes the effects of each receptor on stimulation. The function of the d-receptor in humans is unclear; however, it is thought that this receptor may modulate μ-receptor activity.

The opiate receptors are found in high concentrations in the spinal and medullary dorsal horn, caudate nucleus, substantia nigra, periaqueductal gray area, hypothalamus, and amygdala as well as other parts of the central nervous system. These areas, when stimulated, inhibit the perception of pain. The enkephalins, dynorphins, and β-endorphins are concentrated in areas involved in the descending inhibitory system. Figure 15–5 shows the role of enkephalins in pain modulation.

It is thought that the enkephalins and β-endorphins, when released, modulate nociception presynaptically and postsynaptically by interfering with calcium or potassium channels.[10, 18, 19] When exogenous opioids are administered, it is believed that they bind with the same opiate receptors to modulate nociception. A given opioid may interact to a different degree with one or more opiate receptors. The opioid may act as an agonist, a partial agonist, or an antagonist. The scientific understanding of opioid pharmacodynamics is in its infancy.[20]

The information regarding neuronal transmission of nociception continues to evolve. Each neuron is no longer considered to act as a single relay unit that responds to one type of stimulus. It is proposed that a neuron may receive information from many neurotransmitters and that each neurotransmitter may have multiple actions.

In summary, the existence and location of endogenous opiates are well documented.[10, 14–17, 21] Endorphins and enkephalins bind to opiate receptor sites to modulate pain. What eludes scientists is the exact biochemical mechanism involved in the inhibition of pain when the stimulation of endogenous opioids occurs and when exogenous opioids are administered.

PHYSIOLOGICAL RESPONSE TO NOXIOUS STIMULI FROM TRAUMA AND SURGERY

Knowledge of the transmission and modulation of painful impulses is useful in understanding why pain is problematic for trauma patients. The physiological response to pain suffered as a result of trauma provides a basis for understanding the importance of effective analgesia for the prevention of complications that result from poor management of pain.

Trauma initiates a myriad of physiological responses that are responsible for many deleterious effects. Crushing injuries produce local tissue damage that results in the release of algogenic substances. The release of algogenic substances produces a barrage of noxious stimuli that results in nocicep-

TABLE 15–1. OPIATE RECEPTOR CLASSIFICATION AND ACTION

ORGAN EFFECT	μ	κ	σ	δ
Pupil	Miosis	Miosis	Mydriasis	Mydriasis
Respiratory rate	Stimulation, then depression	No change	Stimulation	Stimulation
Heart rate	Bradycardia	No change	Tachycardia	Tachycardia
Body temperature	Hypothermia	No change	No change	Unknown
Affect	Indifference	Sedation	Delirium	Dysphoria
Gastrointestinal	Constipation	No effect	No effect	Nausea

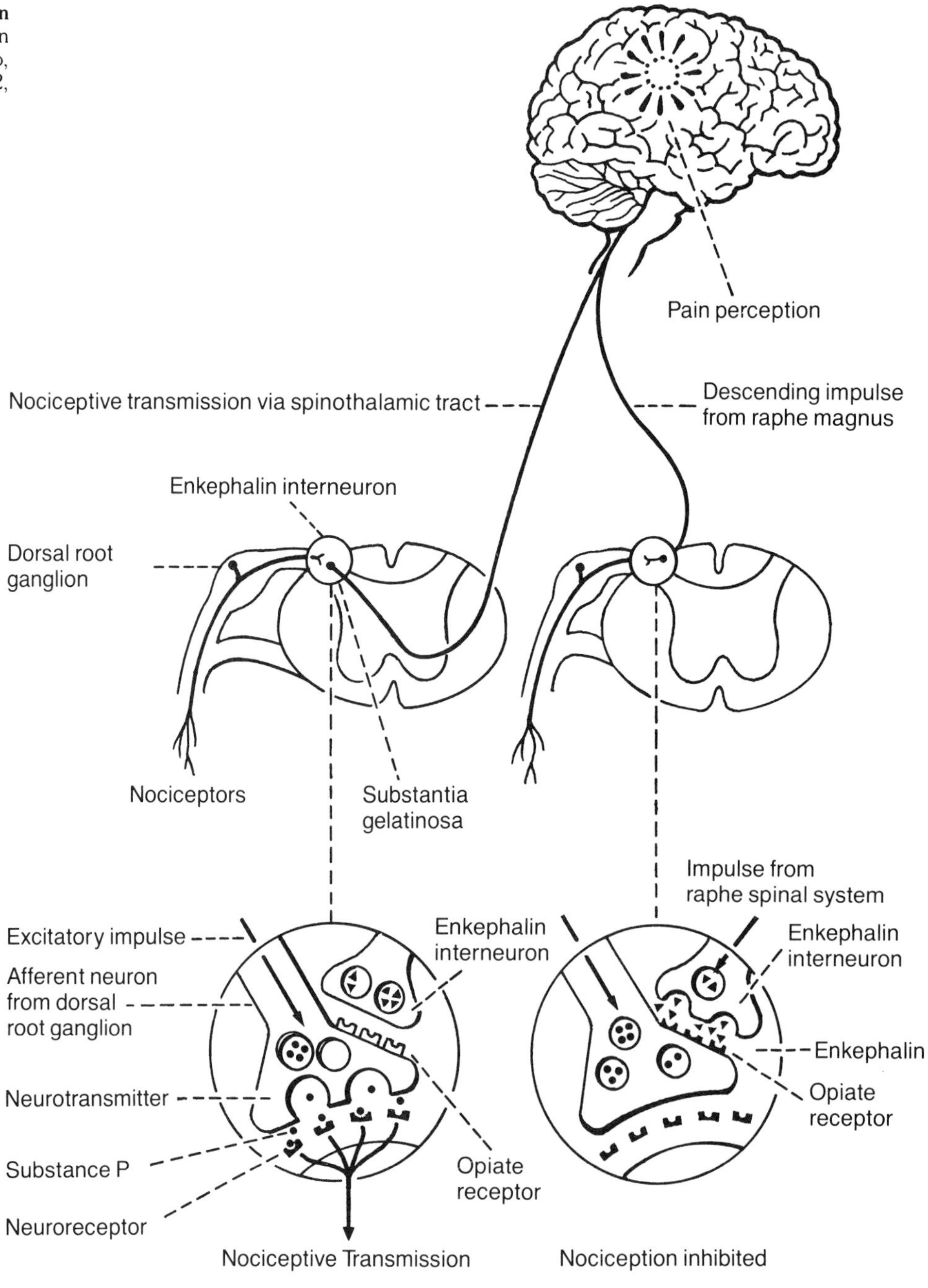

Figure 15–5. Role of enkephalin in pain modulation. (From Chapman CR, Bonica JJ: Acute Pain. Kalamazoo, Upjohn Company, 1983, pp. 9, 12, and 15.)

tion. The patient perceives the nociception as pain.[22, 23] Some of the algogenic substances sensitize the nerves that carry the noxious impulse. The sensitization leads to a decreased threshold. The sensitization can persist for days after the initial trauma. Some of the noxious impulses are carried on fibers that pass through the anterolateral horn of the spinal cord, which in turn stimulate segmental, suprasegmental, and cortical reflex responses. Figure 15–6 shows the body's response to abdominal trauma induced by surgery. The spinothalamic tract and the descending control systems are depicted along with the cortical, suprasegmental autonomic, segmental autonomic, and local responses. This figure shows how the body responds to a planned and controlled trauma, which means that the response to traumatic injury involving many body systems may be greater.

The stimulation of these reflex responses results in skeletal muscle tension and a concomitant decrease in chest wall compliance that sets into motion the circular response of pain and muscle spasm, followed by more pain and muscle spasm.[22, 24] The circle of muscle spasm and pain contributes to difficulty for the patient in mobilizing after trauma or surgery. Figure 15–7 shows this cycle for a patient who has undergone surgery, but the same cycle applies to the trauma patient.

After trauma, the liberation of algogenic substances continues, which sensitizes nociceptors. This sensitization results in tenderness and pain from seemingly innocuous stimulus such as touch. A number of complications can be directly or indirectly attributed to pain after trauma. In addition to enhancing nociception, segmental (spinal) reflexes alter ventilation and circulation as well as the functioning of the genitourinary and gastrointestinal systems. Stimulation of sympathetic preganglionic neurons in the anterolateral horn of the spinal cord results in an increase in heart rate and stroke volume, which in turn increases cardiac work load and myocardial oxygen demand. Severe pain causes the

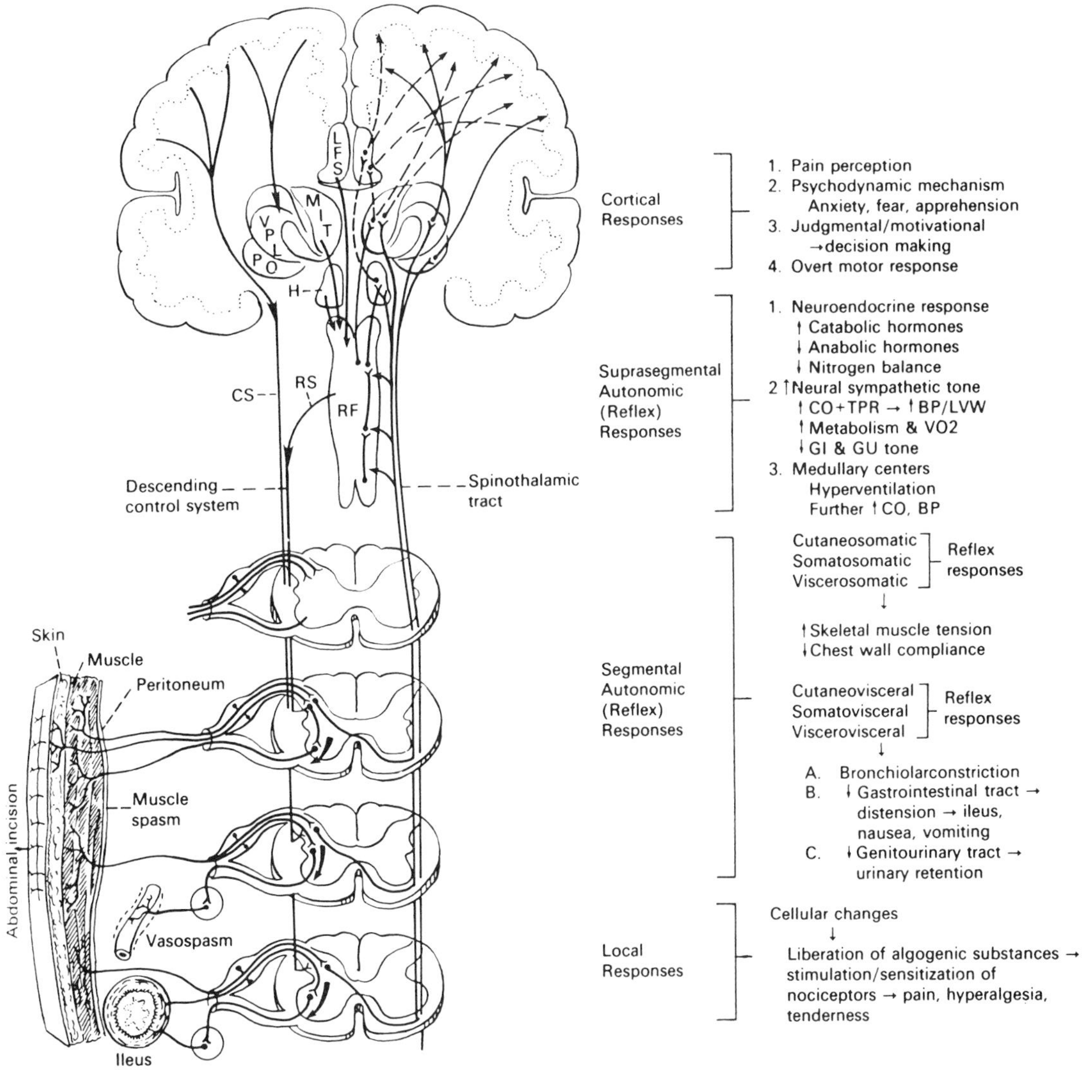

Figure 15–6. Schematic depiction of the responses to noxious stimuli induced by trauma during intra-abdominal surgery. LFS, limbic forebrain structure; MIT, medial and intralaminar thalamic nuclei; VPL, ventroposterolateral nucleus; PO, posterior group of thalamic nuclei; H, hypothalamus; CS, central gray substance; RS, rubrospinal tract; and RF, reticular formation. (Modified from Bonica JJ: Introduction to recent advances in the management of acute and chronic pain. Hosp. Pract. (Special Report), January 1979, pp. 4–10.)

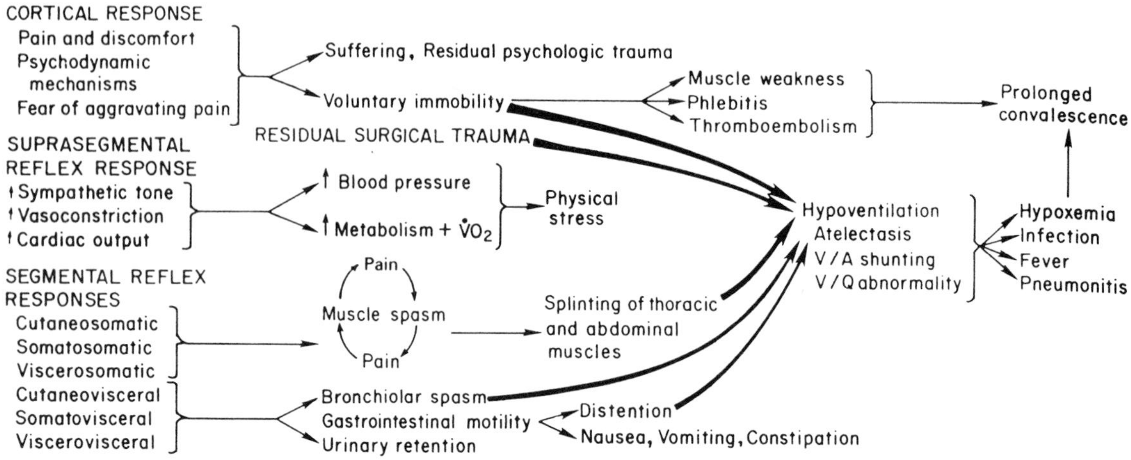

Figure 15–7. Schematic depiction of the pathophysiology of postoperative pain. (From Bonica JJ: The Management of Pain. 2nd ed. Philadelphia, Lea & Febiger, 1990, p. 466.)

release of catecholamines, which can cause dysrhythmias that may become serious.[25] Gastrointestinal (GI) tone can decrease to the point of an ileus, and a decrease in renal function manifests as a decrease in urine output.

The suprasegmental reflex responses seen after trauma result from the stimulation of medullary centers of ventilation and circulation, the hypothalamic neuroendocrine function, and some structures of the limbic system. Table 15–2 summarizes these and other bodily responses to injury.

Hyperventilation, increased hypothalamic neural sympathetic tone, and increased endocrine secretions are the reflex responses seen. Increased sympathetic tone along with increased catecholamine secretion add to the segmental reflex response, which results in an increase in cardiac output, peripheral resistance, blood pressure, cardiac work load, and myocardial oxygen consumption. The endocrine response, similar to the stress response, is marked by catecholamine release; an increase in the secretion of cortisol, corticotropin, glucagon, cyclic adenosine monophosphate, antidiuretic hormone, growth hormone, and renin; and a decrease in insulin and testosterone secretion. The widespread metabolic effects can result in a negative nitrogen balance. The degree and duration of the endocrine and metabolic changes are related to the degree of tissue damage.

Intense anxiety and fear are the cortical responses seen in conscious patients. Patients who suffer from a traumatic injury may develop an abnormal neuroendocrine response to stress. Markedly elevated neural sympathetic tone and elevated catabolic hormones may act to initiate and maintain shock. The conscious patient who is capable of emotional arousal undoubtedly experiences distress as a result of the trauma. This distress is heightened by pain. The emotional arousal enhances nociception at the periphery. The release of norepinephrine combined with sympathetic reflexes and arousal exacerbate the release of algogenic substances associated with tissue damage. Anxiety is also accompanied by reflex skeletal muscle tension or spasm that can initiate a vicious cycle of increased muscle tone near the site of injury followed by activation of nociceptors, which in turn causes an increase in muscle tone and so forth. The meaning given to the traumatic event and the resultant suffering affect how the patient responds to the pain.

Physiological Effects of Pain After Surgery

Because many trauma patients undergo surgery, it is important to mention the physiological effects of pain after surgery. Furthermore, because surgery is considered a "controlled" trauma, the same mechanisms do apply after traumatic injury.[25] The most prominent problems that are directly or indirectly related to postoperative pain include dysfunctions of the pulmonary, circulatory, GI, and urinary systems and impairment of muscle function and metabolism.

Pulmonary Dysfunction. A number of factors are responsible for pulmonary dysfunction, which especially occurs after thoracic or abdominal surgery. Reflex muscle spasm and involuntary splinting of the abdominal muscles lead to ventilation and perfusion abnormalities.[22] The pulmonary effects may be worsened by ileus and subsequent abdominal distention.[26] The experience of pain or the fear of pain when suctioned or during coughing causes patients to breathe shallowly and resist coughing. Bronchiolar spasm may result from activation of cutaneovisceral reflexes. The pain-induced stimulation of the respiratory center produces hyperventilation, which is offset by a decrease in chest wall compliance and bronchiolar spasm. When these effects are combined with the previously mentioned effects, a decrease in vital capacity (VC) and functional residual capacity (FRC) is seen. The reduction in VC and FRC may cause hypoxemia. Unless preventive therapeutic measures are performed, pulmonary dysfunction may progress to atelectasis and pneumonitis.[22]

Circulatory and Metabolic Dysfunction. The circulatory and metabolic dysfunctions that result from postoperative pain have been discussed with the suprasegmental responses. In addition to the aforementioned problems, the trauma patient is at high risk for circulatory problems that result from immobility. See Chapter 21 for a discussion of complications related to immobility.

Gastrointestinal and Urinary Dysfunction. Segmental sympathetic hyperactivity, discussed earlier, is responsible for similar postoperative GI problems commonly

TABLE 15–2. NEUROPHYSIOLOGICAL, ENDOCRINE, AND METABOLIC RESPONSE TO INJURY

I. Segmental and suprasegmental reflex responses
- A. Increase in general sympathetic tone due to increases in hypothalamic activity, segmental sympathetic reflexes (norepinephrine), and adrenal medullary secretion (epinephrine and norepinephrine), which results in:
  1. Vasoconstrictions in skin, splanchnic region, and nonpriority organs → increase in peripheral resistance and decreased venous capacitance
  2. Increased stroke volume and heart rate → increased cardiac output
  3. Increased blood pressure and consequent increased myocardial work load
  4. Increased metabolic rate and oxygen consumption
  5. Decreased gastrointestinal tone → decreased gastric emptying that may progress to ileus
  6. Decrease in urinary tract tone → urine retention
- B. Increased skeletal muscle tone that may progress to spasm
  1. Increased tone of skeletal muscles of the trunk → decrease in chest wall compliance and increased intra-abdominal pressure → alveolar/arterial mismatch → hypoxemia and possibly pneumonitis

II. Endocrine response
- A. Catabolic: Increases in corticotropin, cortisol, antidiuretic hormone (ADH), growth hormone (GH), cyclic adenosine monophosphate, catecholamines, renin, angiotensin II, aldosterone, glucagon, interleukin-1
- B. Anabolic: Decreases in insulin, testosterone

III. Metabolic response
- A. Carbohydrate: Hyperglycemia, glucose intolerance, insulin resistance due to increases in hepatic glycogenolysis (epinephrine, glucagon), gluconeogenesis (growth hormone, cortisol, free fatty acids, epinephrine, glucagon), and decreases in insulin secretion/action
- B. Protein: Increased muscle protein metabolism provides alanine for gluconeogenesis due to increases in cortisol, glucagon epinephrine, interleukin-1
- C. Fat: Increased lipolysis and oxidation of tissue fat provides increases in free fatty acids, gluconeogenesis due to increases in catecholamines, glucagon, cortisol, GH

IV. Water and electrolyte flux
- A. Retention of water and sodium and increased excretion of potassium due to increases in aldosterone, ADH, cortisol
- B. Decreased functional extracellular fluid as it shifts to vascular and cellular compartments due to increases in catecholamines, ADH, angiotensin II, prostaglandin

V. Respiration

Suprasegmental stimulation of respiratory center with consequent hyperventilation counteracted by hypoventilation caused by the skeletal spasm, reflex bronchiolar constriction, etc.

VI. Diencephalic and cortical responses
- A. Anxiety and fear increase hypothalamic response → further increase in general sympathetic tone, catecholamines, etc.
- B. Cortically induced increased blood viscosity, clotting time, fibrinolysis, and platelet aggregation → risk of thromboembolism and other dysfunction
- C. Pain and suffering → psychological mechanisms → deleterious psychological effects

From Bonica JJ: The Management of Pain. 2nd ed. Philadelphia, Lea & Febiger, 1990, p. 177.

seen after trauma. The administration of epidural anesthesia, compared with general anesthesia, provides a more rapid return of bowel function and decreases the incidence of urine retention.[26]

Effects on Muscle Metabolism and Mobility. Persistent pain and reflex responses (vasoconstriction) and consequent limitation of movement cause muscle atrophy and prolong the return of normal muscle function.[22] Patients who have adequate pain relief may have more comfort with mobility, which may decrease the degree of atrophy.

PAIN PREVENTION

Knowledge of the extent of the pain problem and factors that contribute to the inadequate treatment of pain are important to consider before the proposal of solutions for the problem.

Incidence of Inadequate Treatment

The existence of inadequate treatment of pain in hospitalized patients was brought to light in the early 1970s by Marks and Sachar.[27] These researchers conducted structured interviews regarding the adequacy of pain treatment for patients admitted to a medical service with pain as a primary diagnosis. The results indicated that 32 per cent of the patients suffered severe distress and 41 per cent suffered moderate distress from pain. In addition, pain interfered with sleep in 78 per cent of patients who had marked to moderate distress scores. Forty-nine per cent of the patients in the same category stated that the pain interfered with eating and caused them to be anxious, depressed, or irritable or to cry.

An additional part of this study[27] consisted of a questionnaire and vignettes that were completed by house physicians regarding their attitudes, beliefs, and knowledge about the treatment of pain, pharmacological properties of opioids, and drug addiction. The results of the survey revealed that physicians had an exaggerated concern about addiction that contributed to their ordering subtherapeutic doses. Furthermore, physicians who prescribed lower initial doses were more likely to prescribe lower maximal doses and less inclined to increase the dose of an analgesic to relieve oncologic pain in a terminal patient. Although it is recognized that the population for this classic study was not postoperative, the results point to the severity of the problem of inadequate treatment of pain.

Keeri-Szanto and Heaman[28] interviewed patients about postoperative pain and the dose and timing of analgesics administered. Forty per cent of the patients reported some degree of pain, and 21 per cent admitted that they suffered significant (self-defined) pain despite receiving medication for it.

Of the postoperative patients questioned by Cohen,[29] 79.8 per cent stated that pain relief was adequate. When asked specifically whether pain interfered with sleep, 66.9 per cent responded affirmatively. In addition, when the nurses caring for these patients were asked about the goal of pain relief in the first 2 postoperative days, 3.3 per cent said that the goal was to relieve pain completely, 57 per cent said that the goal was to relieve pain as much as possible, and 38.3 per cent replied that it was to relieve pain just enough for the patient to function. Patients asked about their ideal goal for pain relief replied 25.7 per cent, 42.2 per cent, and 16.5 per cent in the same categories.

In recent studies,[30, 31] researchers interviewed patients regarding their expectations of postoperative pain and relief. The results showed a disparity between patients' and nurses' expectations about the degree of pain relief.[30] One fourth of the patients had effective pain relief and more than one half had pain most or all of the time.[31] Seventy-five per cent of the patients expected to receive an opioid immediately after requesting it.

These and other studies point to the extent of the postoperative pain problem. Researchers have demonstrated that postoperative analgesia is inadequate. Low doses of opioids ordered by physicians, health care professionals' and patients' fear of addiction, waiting too long to request or receive analgesics, and inaccurate pain assessment contribute to the problem. The studies summarized here and in Table 15–3 refer to postoperative pain patients who were able to respond to the researchers' questions. The application of these results can be applied with confidence to trauma patients; however, one hopes that the health care professionals' expectation that trauma patients suffer from severe pain leads to adequate treatment of pain.

The intramuscular as-needed (IM-PRN) injection, until recently the mainstay for the treatment of pain, has been inadequate. Many nurses interpret PRN as *when the patient requests it* rather than *as necessary*.[23] When the patient requests pain medication, the nurse first assesses the patient's level of pain. Nursing assessments of pain have been demonstrated to be less than optimal.

Using vignettes to describe a patient's illness or injury, age, sex, and race, Holm and colleagues[35] investigated the relation between a nurse's experience with pain and her assessment of pain. Two main factors were noted to influence a nurse's pain assessment: the nurse's experience with pain and the nurse's religious preference. The intensity of the nurse's experience with pain significantly predicted perceptions of the patient's suffering. Nurses who reported a religious preference (no definition given for this) inferred less pain than those who reported no religious preference.

Other researchers used vignettes to determine the influence of the duration of pain, presence of psychological and physical symptoms, and diagnostic category on nurses' estimates of patient suffering.[36] Nurses attributed significantly less pain to patients without physical pathology than to patients with physical pathology and significantly more pain to patients suffering from acute conditions than to those suffering from chronic conditions. A disturbing finding was the nurses' unwillingness to perform pain-relieving interventions for patients who were depressed.

Once the nurse decides to give the IM-PRN medication, the fear of addiction plays a role in the amount of narcotic that is prescribed by the physician and administered by the nurse.[37] Physicians order inadequate amounts of opioids,[27] which is compounded by nurses who administer these doses, when given a choice, in lesser amounts or by extending the time between doses beyond what has been ordered.[29, 38]

When the injection finally is given, the variability in the rate of absorption becomes a problem. The varied rate of absorption contributes to peaks and troughs in the patient's level of opioids. The patient begins at a level of pain when the opioid is first administered. As the opioid level rises, the patient moves to a level of no pain until the opioid level approaches its peak. If a large dose of opioid has been given, the patient then reaches a level of mental clouding until the drug is metabolized. The patient reverts to a level of analgesia followed by a level of pain. The cycle is repeated when another IM-PRN opioid is requested. The IM-PRN method is not problematic if adequate doses are given frequently. To relieve pain, larger doses typically are ordered, so that pain is reduced for a 3- to 4-hour period. The larger doses of opioid produce mental clouding.

The final problem regarding the IM-PRN method of analgesia is the adverse effects. Systemic opioids cause respiratory depression, nausea, vomiting, and central nervous system depression. Respiratory and central nervous system effects are of special concern.

Misconceptions About Pain

Misconceptions interfere with effective assessments and lead to ineffective management of pain. That patients become tolerant of pain is one such misconception. Tolerance is defined as the greatest level of pain a person is willing to tolerate. The decision to endure a certain amount of pain changes with many variables: time of day, fatigue, presence of others, and stress. The patient may become less tolerant as the pain continues. The pain level may increase as the nociceptors become sensitized from continued stimuli. There is a cumulative effect from the struggle, and the patient may become fatigued.

Nurses frequently report that patients must not be having much pain because they were able to fall asleep or sleep through the night. Instead, many patients sleep owing to exhaustion from their struggle with pain. Patients sleep to escape from their pain. Other patients, if they did not receive an analgesic, awaken from extended sleep with uncontrolled pain. This indicates that the painful process continues even while sleep occurs.

Clock-watching often is misinterpreted. Many patients do become preoccupied with their pain medication. They may know exactly when their next dose is due and may try to bargain for an earlier delivery. This behavior may be interpreted as a sign of addiction rather than as a sign of the patient's receiving inadequate doses or doses at too lengthy intervals. This commonly occurs with one of the most frequently prescribed opioids, meperidine. Meperidine usually is prescribed at 75 to 100 mg IM every 4 hours. The duration of action is about 2 to 3 hours. Patients report that the pain subsides in 1 hour and is relieved for about 1 hour. This leaves 2 hours of varying degrees of pain. Thus, the patient is interested in receiving the next dose.

Solving the Problem of Inadequate Analgesia

Factors that contribute to the inadequate treatment of pain are inadequate pain assessment, lack of knowledge of the pharmacodynamics and pharmacokinetics of opioids, and different expectations between patients and health care professionals. The treatment of pain is a responsibility shared by the patient, nurse, and physician. The effective treatment of pain is accomplished by an accurate assessment, development and execution of planned interventions, and evaluation of the results. Many of the problems in the treatment of pain stem from a lack of clarity in the shared responsibility.

The nurse must coordinate the care performed by all members of the trauma service. She must organize the patient's care to avoid exposure to multiple procedures that may potentiate the pain experience by tiring the patient. Her knowledge of the pharmacokinetics and pharmacodynamics

TABLE 15–3. SUMMARY OF RESEARCH CONCERNING INADEQUATE POSTOPERATIVE ANALGESIA

AUTHOR	METHOD	INCIDENCE	CONTRIBUTING FACTORS	RECOMMENDATIONS
Donovan (1983)[32]	Survey	31% insufficient analgesia; 62% had pain, but were satisfied with analgesia; 75% expected pain	Patients expect pain. Insufficient amount of opioids prescribed. Doses not individualized. Problem with IM injections.	Continuous infusion of IV opioids. Decrease fear of addiction.
Sriwatanakul et al (1983)[33]	Patient interview survey of nurses and physicians caring for patients interviewed	41% complained of at least moderate pain; 90% reported pain interfered with sleep. Patients received 70% of maximum prescribed dose during 1st 24 hours, 43% during 2nd 24 hours. Average dose given was 30% < prescribed.	Patients failed to request PRN opioid even when suffering. Physician prescribed traditional doses instead of individual doses. Lack of knowledge of pharmacokinetics and pharmacodynamics. IM injections are a problem.	Educate the patient and health care professionals. Individualize analgesia. Frequent pain assessment.
Cartwright (1985)[34]	Survey of nurses and patients	26% fear contributing to patient addiction; 11% thought that respiratory rate was most affected by opioids; 79% thought BP was most affected; 29% thought it was OK to give IM opioids to patients receiving epidural opioids; 52% feared IM injections	Deficiencies in communication between physicians, nurses, and patients. Lack of nursing involvement in pain management. Lack of preoperative education for patients.	Prescribe opioids in therapeutic range. Assess the effectiveness of analgesia. Use the IV route. Educate patients and health care professionals.
Kuhn et al (1990)[30]	Patient interview after IM dose; survey of nurses and physicians	40% stated postoperative period was painful. Patients average pain intensity was 60% of maximum.	Lower level of pain was expected by patients. Staff underestimated pain. Fear of addiction by 20% of nurses.	Educate patients. Assess pain relief. IV-PCA Decrease fear of addiction.
Owen et al (1990)[31]	Patient interview	66% said they would wait until in severe pain before requesting analgesia; 75% expected IM injection immediately after requesting it	Nurses underestimate lag time between request and injection. All parties expect some degree of unrelieved pain.	Increase knowledge. Increase priority of pain control.

of analgesics must be sufficient to provide adequate analgesia. The nurse frequently is in a position to influence the selection of the drug and its route of administration.

Anticipating the patient's pain rather than waiting for the patient to request an analgesic is the key principle in good pain management. Administering analgesics before the patient experiences pain can decrease not only future pain but also the patient's anxiety and fear of future pain. Excellent assessment techniques are also critical to the treatment of pain. Once an analgesic has been given, it is imperative that the nurse assess its effectiveness by noting any changes in the characteristics of pain.

Part of adequate pain management is to determine the best route and timing for delivering the analgesics. Intermittent dosing is appropriate for occasional short episodes of acute pain. For example, a short-acting opioid could be given by the IM or intravenous (IV) route before the insertion of a chest tube. Enough time should be allowed for the analgesic to act before the painful treatment or diagnostic test is begun. It is incumbent on the nurse to request that a physician wait until the analgesic exerts an effect before the painful treatment. When the pain is more constant and predictable, more frequent doses, use of longer-acting agents, or constant infusions are necessary to keep the level of pain as low as possible. The key to adequate pain management is the administration of an analgesic at doses and intervals appropriate for that patient and drug.

NURSING ASSESSMENT AND DIAGNOSIS OF PAIN

The Trauma Pain Data Base that follows is divided into two sections. The accident data base and history are first; assessment factors in the critical, intermediate, and rehabilitation stages of the trauma cycle are second.

Refer to Appendix 15–1 for the accident data base and history guidelines. Gathering facts about the accident is helpful in acquiring a broad perspective of the person's situation. The accident situation itself, accident responsibility, others involved in the accident, relationship of others to the patient, deaths, loss of consciousness, rescue events, and alcohol and other drug involvement are important factors that may affect a person's emotional state and, thus, the level of pain. Positive drug test results complicate the patient's treatment and recovery. Many trauma patients test positive for alcohol and other drugs.

Refer to Appendix 15–2 for the critical care assessment factors. The pain factors most important in the critical care stage are those associated with stabilizing the patient physically. The patient's report of pain, past experience with pain, and social functioning cannot be collected when the patient is unconscious or physiologically unstable. The information is not necessarily collected in any order but varies according to each individual case. The information obtained should be used to plan the pain care of the patient and to be built on for use in later stages.

The assessment of pain without the subjective report of the patient is difficult. The anxiety, fear, panic, and suffering may not be apparent. Withdrawal from a painful stimulus, grimacing or groaning while turning, inconsistent reports of pain, and autonomic signs of arousal may indicate that the patient is experiencing pain.

A general nursing assessment of a patient in pain is presented in the next section. The questions the nurse uses during a pain assessment varies with the type and duration of pain. The assessment of acute pain differs in some respects from the assessment of chronic pain. For example, the patient in chronic pain may have tried different interventions to find relief and suffered greater negative life-style effects compared with a patient who is experiencing acute pain. The guidelines presented are intended as a baseline for a global pain assessment. Appendix 15–3 contains sample tools for pain assessment. How the pain assessment changes during the trauma cycle is discussed in a separate nursing assessment section for each phase of the cycle.

Nursing Assessment

A comprehensive pain assessment requires evaluation of the sensory, perceptual, and response aspects of the pain. The nurse begins by asking the patient specifically about pain. Some patients are reluctant to discuss pain because they need to be in control and use the stoic behavior as a method of coping.[39] Other patients are unwilling to acknowledge pain because they fear injections or the adverse effects of opioids. Careful attention must be paid not only to what the patient says but also to what is not said. Gaining insight into the perception of pain is difficult in the unconscious patient.

The nurse must rely on observations of the patient. Behaviors in response to pain may be helpful but often are unreliable. The patient may grimace, cry, or exhibit tachycardia or elevated blood pressure. In the unconscious patient, the only response to painful stimuli may be decerebrate or decortical posturing. An accurate pain assessment in the unconscious patient is an educated guess at best, but the nurse should assume that the patient feels pain, regardless of the presence or absence of behaviors that are indicative of pain.

Location. Inquire about the location of pain by asking the patient to point to the area involved. A drawing of painful areas may be helpful, especially if the pain radiates. The location of the pain can be represented by a circle with shaded areas used to indicate areas of referred pain. The location of the pain may indicate the underlying cause or give clues about the type of pain the patient is experiencing.

Intensity. The intensity of pain ranges from mild discomfort to excruciating. It is important to remember that there is no correlation between the stimulus and the patient's perception of pain. The patient's rating of the intensity is influenced by his threshold and tolerance for pain. Threshold refers to the least amount of pain a person recognizes. Tolerance is the greatest level of pain a person can stand. Both threshold and tolerance vary from person to person.

The patient should be asked to rate the intensity of his pain on a scale that is used consistently. (Appendix 15–3 contains several types of rating scales.) The consistent use of a rating scale enhances the patient's ability to communicate the level of pain as well as the effectiveness of analgesics. A frequently used, easy method is to ask the patient to verbally rate the intensity of the pain on a scale of 0 to 10. Zero usually represents no pain and 10 represents the worst possible pain. The patient can rate the pain intensity on a visual analog scale to produce a record of the pain.

Some patients have difficulty translating their pain intensity into a number. For these patients, the words in the pain intensity portion of the McGill Pain Questionnaire are useful (see Appendix 15–3).

Quality. Ask the patient to describe the quality of the pain without offering cues. For example, "What does the pain feel like?" should elicit a descriptive answer. If the patient is unable to state words that describe the quality of the pain, the nurse can offer words listed in the McGill Pain Questionnaire. The exact words the patient uses should be documented for future reference.

Onset and Chronology. Questions that pertain to the onset, duration, time-intensity relation, and changes in the rhythmic patterns help to determine the cause of pain. It is important to determine whether the pain occurred suddenly or increased gradually. Pain of a sudden nature that rapidly reaches maximum intensity often is indicative of tissue rupture. Ischemic pain increases gradually and becomes more intense over time. The time-intensity relations are useful in detecting diurnal correlations that may occur with chronic pain. For example, arthritic pain is most intense in the morning or after periods of inactivity.

Aggravating and Alleviating Factors. Ask the patient what makes the pain worse. This can lead to detection of factors associated with the pain. For example, chest pain only on deep inspiration may be a symptom of a pulmonary embolus. Ask specific questions about the relation between pain and activity. Also obtain data about what environmental influences affect pain, such as temperatures and noise levels. Last, determine whether the pain affects or is affected by sleep deprivation and anxiety.

Knowledge of the alleviating factors is helpful in planning treatment of the pain. Ask the patient what medications—prescription and over-the-counter—have helped to relieve the pain. Inquire whether nonpharmacological interventions have decreased the pain. Examples of nonpharmacological interventions include guided imagery, massage, warm baths, rest, and position changes.

Effects of Pain on Life-Style. Determine what the pain means to the patient. This helps in understanding what the patient thinks may happen because of the pain. If the patient thinks that the pain is a sign of impending death, the nurse

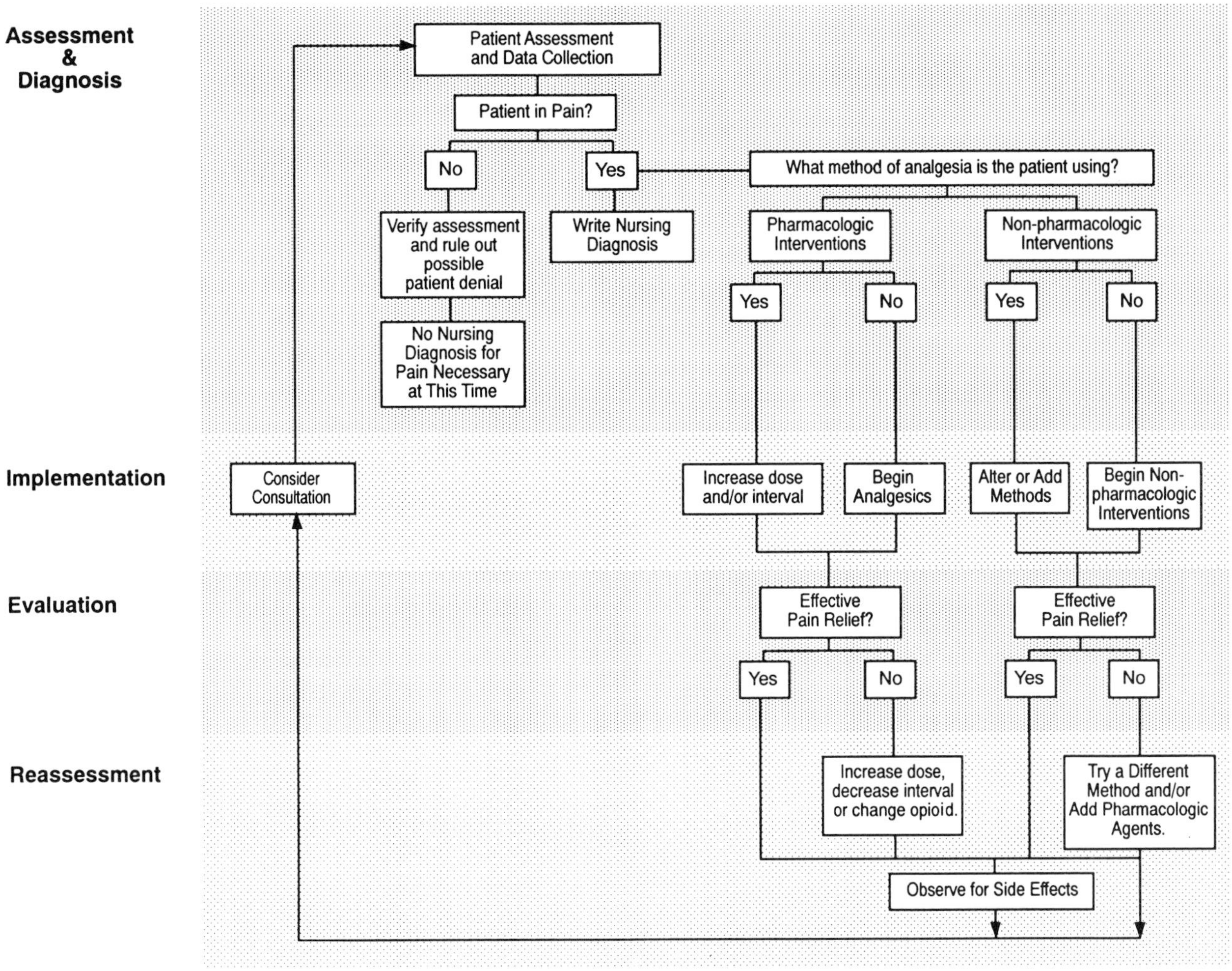

Figure 15–8. Use of the nursing process to manage the patient in pain.

can anticipate that the patient requires education and psychological interventions to help him cope with the pain. Knowledge of how well the patient copes with pain is useful when planning interventions and evaluating their effectiveness. If the pain is chronic, ask whether and how it interferes with activities of daily living, relationships, nutritional needs, and sleep.

Other Observations. Observe the nonverbal ways a patient expresses pain. Some may grimace, cry, or withdraw. When a patient is nonresponsive, rely on physiological observations to indicate pain. The physiological responses mentioned earlier are not reliable indicators. The body adapts to the stress response over time. Trauma patients may have responses from injury that mask indications of pain. For example, a patient who is bleeding into the tissues from a large bone fracture exhibits tachycardia from the blood loss. This tachycardia related to blood loss may mask the existence of pain. It is essential to look for and note any observations of pain; however, it is equally important not to assume that the absence of clinical signs indicates that there is no pain.

Nursing Diagnosis

The categories for pain accepted by the North American Nursing Diagnosis Association (NANDA) are *pain* and *chronic pain*.[40] The first diagnostic category applies to the resuscitation, critical care, and intermediate phases of the trauma cycle. The NANDA category of chronic pain may apply in the same phases if the patient suffered from chronic pain before the traumatic injury but is more appropriate in the intermediate and rehabilitation phases of the cycle.

Using the nursing process involves more than writing a nursing diagnostic statement. A decision tree for the nursing management of the patient in pain is presented in Figure 15–8. This figure incorporates the nursing process, from the assessment step to evaluation of interventions aimed at pain relief.

EFFECT OF EXOGENOUS OPIOIDS ON NEUROMODULATION

Nurses routinely administer opioids for the effective management of pain. Knowledge of the effect of exogenous opioids on the modulation of pain is essential for the nurse to administer such a drug and to monitor and treat adverse effects.

When opioids are administered, analgesia is thought to be

the result of activation of the μ- and κ-receptors; the σ-receptors may also be involved. All opioid receptors are thought to exert an inhibitory modulation effect on the synaptic transmission of nociception. The receptors typically are found on presynaptic nerve terminals, where they act to decrease the release of neurotransmitters.

It is thought that morphine produces analgesia through stimulation of the μ-receptor. Consequences of activation of the μ-receptor include respiratory depression, miosis, reduced gastric motility, and euphoria. Two types of μ-receptors have recently been isolated and are classified according to their relative affinities for agonists.[20] The μ_1-receptor has a higher affinity and is thought to mediate supraspinal analgesic actions. The μ_2-receptor has a lower affinity and is thought to mediate respiratory depression and GI actions. The lack of selective agonists that cross the blood–brain barrier is responsible for the uncertainty of the results of stimulating the δ-receptor. In animals, stimulation of the δ-receptor produces analgesia and antinociception for thermal stimuli at spinal sites.[20] The δ-receptor may be responsible for modulating the activity of the μ-receptor.

Even though evidence indicates that the μ-, δ-, and κ-receptors are distinct molecular entities, they share common characteristics. All appear to exert their effect by inhibitory modulation of synaptic transmission in the central nervous system. Even though their locations may differ slightly, all the receptors are located on presynaptic nerve terminals. When stimulated, there is a decrease in the release of excitatory neurotransmitters.

Opioids produce their major effects on the central nervous and GI systems. Some of these effects are analgesia, sedation, mood changes, respiratory depression, decreased intestinal motility, nausea, and vomiting[41] (Table 15–4).

Opioids produce analgesia and mood changes and decrease the level of consciousness.[28] A significant feature of opioid analgesics in therapeutic doses is that analgesia occurs without loss of consciousness.

Meperidine may produce excitation with muscle twitching and convulsions if large doses (400 mg/24 hr) are given. These effects are probably caused by the active metabolite normeperidine. Normeperidine has a half-life of 14 to 21 hours and accumulates with prolonged administration.

Opioids have a direct effect on the brainstem respiratory centers with the primary mechanism being a reduction in the responsiveness of the respiratory centers to increases in carbon dioxide tension. The mechanism also involves depression of pontine and medullary centers involved in regulating respiratory rhythm. Maximal respiratory depression occurs within 10 to 20 minutes after IV administration of morphine.[41] Voluntary control of respiration may also be altered. After large doses of opioids, patients will breathe if told to do so. Without such instruction, patients may remain relatively apneic. The respiratory depressant effect may be exaggerated in patients who have suffered traumatic head injuries. The effects of opioids and sleep on respiration are additive. Natural sleep apparently produces a decrease in the sensitivity of the medullary centers to carbon dioxide. Opioids also depress the cough reflex by affecting the cough center in the medulla.[41]

Respiratory depression and sedation occur after initial administration. Tolerance to the analgesic effect of the opioid develops with repeated doses; tolerance to the sedation and respiratory depression occurs as well. Naloxone, an opioid antagonist, can be used to reverse severe respiratory depression. It should be titrated in small doses, slowly, so as not to reverse all the patient's analgesia. A suggested method of titration is to dilute 0.4 mg in 10 ml of diluent and give 1 ml at a time, waiting 2 minutes between doses. This can be continued until respirations return to 10 per minute. If the respiratory rate does not improve after 10 mg of naloxone, the respiratory depression is probably not narcotic-induced. Because the half-life of naloxone is considerably shorter than that of the narcotics, continued observation is important after naloxone is administered and respirations improve. Respiratory depression may recur when the naloxone is excreted.

ROUTES OF ADMINISTRATION FOR OPIOIDS

Knowledge of the various methods used to administer opioids and of how opioids are absorbed is helpful in understanding why one method of analgesia may be superior to another in certain phases of the trauma cycle. The methods discussed include by mouth (*per os;* PO) and the IM, IV, neuraxial, transdermal, and rectal routes.

TABLE 15–4. COMPARISON OF OPIOID ADVERSE EFFECTS

DRUG	ANALGESIC	CONSTIPATION	RESPIRATORY DEPRESSION	SEDATION	EMESIS
Morphine	+ +	+ +	+ +	+ +	+ +
Hydromorphone	+ +	+	+ +	+	+
Oxymorphone	+ +	+ +	+ + +	+	+ + +
Meperidine	+ +	+	+ +	+	+
Methadone	+ +	+ +	+ +	+	+
Levorphanol	+ +	+ +	+ +	+	+
Fentanyl	+ +	–*	+	+	+
Codeine	+	+	+	+	+
Oxycodone	+ +	+ +	+ +	+ +	+ +

*No effect reported.

Adapted from Kastrup E: © 1992 by Facts and Comparisons. Used with permission from Facts and Comparisons, 1992 ed. St. Louis, Facts and Comparisons, a Division of JB Lippincott Company. p 242.

Per Os Route

The oral route usually is chosen because it is the easiest and most convenient route of administration. Drugs administered by mouth are well absorbed by the GI tract but may also irritate the gastric mucosa or cause nausea and vomiting. The onset of action is slower with a prolonged duration of effect compared with the IM or IV routes. Absorption by the GI tract of orally effective opioids usually is complete, but the rate of absorption varies. Many drugs undergo significant first-pass hepatic metabolism after absorption. First-pass hepatic metabolism is the effect seen after drugs are absorbed by the GI tract and then enter the portal venous blood, thus passing through the liver before entering the systemic circulation for delivery to tissue receptors. While in the liver, the drugs are metabolized, which may explain the large discrepancy between IV and PO doses.[41]

This route is not suitable for severe pain because of the slower onset of action and the variability of absorption. In addition, it is not useful during the early phases of the trauma cycle if patients are to receive nothing by mouth or unable to swallow. Oral analgesics are used in the intermediate and rehabilitation phases of the trauma cycle, when the pain is less severe and the patient is able to take oral medications.

Intramuscular Route

The traditional method of analgesia for postoperative patients has been the IM injection. This route enables the patient to receive a faster effect from strong opioids. The IM route avoids the interference of the digestive system, which makes this route more predictable compared with the oral route. The rate of absorption after injection, however, is limited by the surface area of the capillary membranes, the circulation to these capillaries, and the solubility of the drug in the interstitial fluid.[41] Austin and colleagues[42] cite the variability as a problem for individualizing analgesic orders for postoperative pain. After the administration of 75 mg of meperidine every 4 to 6 hours, minimum effective analgesic levels were exceeded as little as 35 per cent of the time.

There is a longer waiting period for the opioid to exert an effect, which is related to the rate of absorption. Other factors, such as the time of administration of the injection relative to the amount of pain and anxiety the patient is experiencing, contribute to the relative insufficient nature of the IM route to provide adequate analgesia. The negative aspects of the IM route are responsible for the development and increased use of continuous IV infusion of opioids and patient-controlled analgesia (PCA), which may soon replace the IM injection in all clinical areas.

Intravenous Route

When morphine and other opioids are given IV, they quickly exert an effect. IV opioids are absorbed first by the highly perfused vessel-rich tissues. As the plasma concentration of the opioid decreases below the level found in the vessel-rich tissues, the drug leaves these tissues and is consequently distributed in the less well perfused sites, such as the skeletal muscles and fat. In addition to tissue perfusion, the physicochemical properties of the opioid govern its ability to be absorbed by certain tissues. For example, only small quantities of morphine, a relatively hydrophilic opioid, pass the blood–brain barrier compared with more lipid-soluble opioids, such as fentanyl, codeine, meperidine, and heroin.[20] Administration of IV opioids allows for more rapid access to the site where they exert an effect, the central nervous system and the opioid receptors. Shafer and Varvel,[43] through manipulation of secondary pharmacological data, relate that the concentration at the effect site, rather than the plasma concentration, is what determines the drug effect.

The IV route is used during the resuscitation, critical care, and early part of the intermediate phase of the trauma cycle. By the time the patient reaches the intermediate phase, the pain is manageable by other routes.

Neuraxial Route

The administration of opioids into the neuraxis (intrathecal and epidural space) places the drug closer to the receptor site compared with the IM and IV routes. When opioids are injected into the neuraxis, they bind with presynaptic and postsynaptic receptors in the substantia gelatinosa of the dorsal horn.[44] Smaller doses are used, which have a longer duration of action compared with systemic administration. The onset of action of epidural morphine is 20 to 35 minutes. Intrathecal morphine has a shorter onset of action—10 to 20 minutes. Fentanyl, given in the epidural space, has an onset of action from 4 to 6 minutes.

The administration of opioids into the intrathecal or epidural space is not without effects similar to those that occur when opioids are given by other routes. The pharmacokinetics and pharmacodynamics of epidural and intrathecal opioids compared with those of the IV route are shown in Table 15–5.

The neuraxial route is used in the critical care phase of the trauma cycle. Pain relief by this route may also be used in the rehabilitation phase if a patient is suffering from intractable pain. Neuraxial opioids are used more for chronic pain from cancer than for chronic pain caused by traumatic injury.

Transdermal Route

The transdermal route is appealing because it provides steady, therapeutic plasma levels without the peaks and troughs seen with intermittent dosing. Characteristics of a drug that make it effective for transdermal use include mixed water and lipid solubility, molecular weight less than 1000, pH between 5 and 9 in a saturated aqueous solution, absence of histamine-releasing effects, and fairly low dose requirements for a 24-hour period. The advantages of transdermal application include the avoidance of the first-pass effect, prolongation of effect, and its ability to be used when swallowing is a problem.

Fentanyl is the only opioid that possesses the characteristics that make it suitable for transdermal use. The fentanyl patch comes in 25-, 50-, 75-, and 100-μg doses. Steady-state concentrations are reached in 8 hours, and concentrations decrease slowly over time after removal.[45] Latasch and Luders[46] recommend application of the patch 5 hours before surgery. The long period of time necessary to reach analgesic concentrations and the apparent deposition of drug beneath the skin (which is responsible for the slow decline of fentanyl)[46] are two disadvantages of using this drug for acute pain.

The transdermal route is more effective in the latter part of the intermediate phase and in the rehabilitation phase of

TABLE 15–5. COMPARISON OF OPIOID AGONIST AND AGONIST-ANTAGONIST ANALGESICS

DRUG	ROUTE	USUAL DOSE (mg)	DURATION (hr)	HALF-LIFE (hr)	NURSING CONSIDERATIONS
Opioid					
Morphine	PO	30	Up to 6	2–3	GI absorption not reliable.
	IM	10			30 mgm dose is used for q 3–4° administration. 60 mgm should be used for single or intermittent doses.
	IV	10			Inject over 4 to 5 minutes.
	IT	0.1–0.5	8–24	1.1–2.83	Variable time of absorption. Possible early or late respiratory depression.
	E	2–5	8–22	2.88	Same as intrathecal route.
Meperidine (Demerol)	IM	100	2–4	3–8	Significantly less effective compared with IV route. May cause local irritation at injection site. Reduce dose when given with a phenothiazine or other tranquilizers. With renal dysfunction or high doses, normeperidine (toxic metabolite) may accumulate and cause seizures.
	IV	100	2–4	3–7	Inject slowly.
	IT	35–70			
	E	25–50	7–10	1.5	
Hydromorphone (Dilaudid)	PO	7.5	4–5	2–4	
	IM	1.5		Up to 5	
	IV	1–2	4–6		
	IT	NA			
	E	1	6–19		Early and late respiratory depression reported.
Codeine	PO	15–60	4–6	3–4	Rapid onset–15 min.
	IM	130			
Oxycodone	PO	5–10	4–5		
Fentanyl (Sublimaze)	IM	0.1	1–2	1.5–6.0	Respiratory depression may be delayed.
	IV	0.1	1	2–4	
	E	0.1	2–3	4	Continuous infusion recommended.
Sufentanil (Sufenta)	IV	0.02	1	2.41–2.75	Rapid onset.
	IT	0.02	1		
	E	0.01–0.05	6	2.83	High doses and rapid injection have caused respiratory depression.
Alfentanil (Alfenta)	IM	15–30 μg/kg	1.5		Short duration makes drug useful for short-term pain only.
	IV	0.5–1.0	0.5	1.1–1.8	
	IT	0.5–1.0	0.5		
	E	0.5–1.0	1.5	1.5	
Opioid Agonist/Antagonists					
Pentazocine (Talwin)	PO	50	5		May cause hallucinations, confusion, and delusions. Maximum dose 600 mg/day.
	IM	30–60	3	2–3	May cause hallucinations, confusion, and delusions. Maximum dose 360 mg/day.
	IV	30	3–4	2–4	Weak antagonist.
Nalbuphine (Nubain)	IM	10	3–6	5	May cause withdrawal in patients receiving opioid agonists. Antagonist effect 10 times that of pentazocine.
Butorphanol (Stadol)	IM	2	3–4	2.5–3.5	May cause withdrawal. Antagonist effect is 30 times that of pentazocine. May cause dysphoria.
Dezocine (Dalgan)	IM	5–20	3–6		Antagonist activity is less than that of nalorphine but greater than that of pentazocine.
	IV	2.5–10.0	2–4	1.2–7.4	Respiratory depression is similar to the effects of morphine. Upper limit to magnitude of respiratory depression seen with increased doses. Pediatric studies not conducted. Studies suggest 15 mg IM may be optimum dose.

PO, by mouth; IM, intramuscular; IV, intravenous; IT, intrathecal; E, epidural; NA, not applicable.

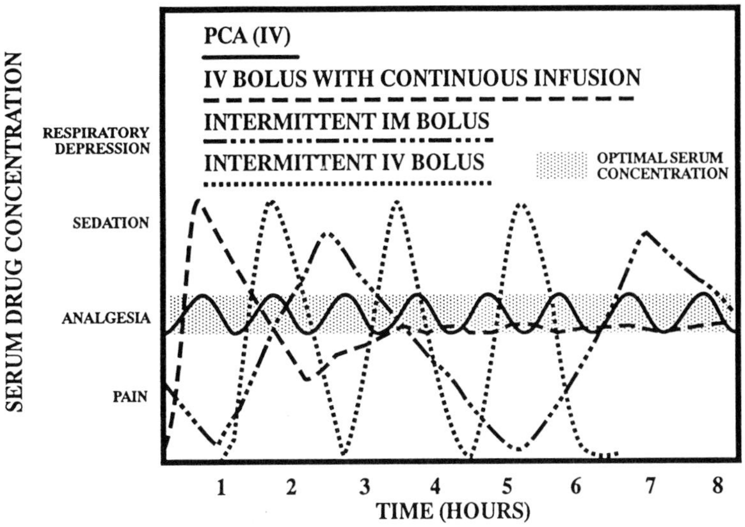

Figure 15–9. Effects of narcotics according to increasing serum levels versus time. (From Lubenow TR, Ivankovich AD: Patient-controlled analgesia for postoperative pain. Crit Care Clin North Am 3:35, 1991.)

the trauma cycle. Transdermal opioids have been used successfully in patients who suffer chronic pain from cancer, and the use of transdermal opioids for the trauma patient is not widely publicized.

Rectal Route

The effectiveness of drugs administered rectally depends on whether the drug is inserted into the proximal or the lower rectal area. Drugs inserted into the proximal rectum are absorbed by the hemorrhoidal veins and then go to the portal circulation (first-pass effect). Drugs absorbed in the lower rectal area go directly to the general circulation without undergoing the first-pass effect. The unpredictable nature of drug absorption in the rectal area along with possible local mucosal irritation make this route one that is less desirable.

Aspirin, acetaminophen, and some opioids (oxymorphone and hydromorphone) are available in suppository form. Aspirin and acetaminophen relieve mild pain, and the opioids are used for severe pain. The difficulty in using rectal analgesics is due to the variable absorption rate. Rectal suppositories occasionally are used in the intermediate phase of the trauma cycle.

METHODS OF ANALGESIA

Many different methods of analgesia are used during the phases of the trauma cycle. The IM-PRN injections, scheduled intermittent IM injections, PCA, patient-controlled epidural analgesia (PCEA), and continuous epidural analgesia are discussed in this section. Nonpharmacological interventions are included in the discussion of the rehabilitation stage.

Intramuscular Pro Re Nata Injections

Misinterpretation of the IM-PRN order, inadequate pain assessment, fear of addiction, administration of inadequate doses of opioids, and variable absorption rates are factors cited for the ineffectiveness of the IM-PRN method of postoperative analgesia.

The patient may be suffering so much pain and anxiety by the time the IM-PRN medication arrives that there is little chance the medication will effectively relieve the pain.[47, 48] This is the rationale for scheduled or regular IM injections.

Regular IM injections given every 4 hours achieve serum levels that are equal to or exceed the minimum effective analgesic concentration for a short period in the 4-hour time frame.[48] Large doses given at longer intervals result in higher peak concentrations and lower trough levels. The larger doses cause undesirable effects and make the IM route less than desirable. For these reasons, practitioners have begun to use constant infusions because lower doses are given to provide a steady plasma concentration of opioid and avoid the adverse effects seen with large doses. Figure 15–9 compares the effects of opioids according to serum levels produced by different methods of administration.

Patient-Controlled Analgesia

The inadequate treatment of postoperative pain coupled with advances in computers has led to the placement of pain-relieving technology in the hands of the patient. PCA is thought to provide superior analgesia because the plasma levels of opioids are kept at a more constant level compared with the IM-PRN method.[49] With PCA, a computerized pump device is programmed to deliver a constant dose of drug. A microcomputer within the pump allows the clinician to easily program any combination of opioid delivery method to suit the needs of the individual patient. (Table 15–6 shows common PCA settings.) Most PCA pumps allow the administration of a bolus dose as well as deliver the opioid at a constant rate, called a background dose. The bolus dose is administered on request by the patient's pressing a button on a cord attached to the pump. The patient is instructed to self-administer the opioid when the constant background dose is insufficient or when the patient anticipates the need for more opioid to ambulate or perform pulmonary preventive measures. Some practitioners do not program the pump to deliver a background dose, so that the only time the patient receives the opioid is when the button is pushed. An advantage to the use of a constant background infusion is

TABLE 15–6. COMMON PCA SETTINGS

ANALGESIC	BOLUS DOSE (mg)	MAINTENANCE DOSE	LOCKOUT INTERVAL (min)
Agonists			
Fentanyl	0.02–0.1	15–60 μg/hr	3–10
Hydromorphone	0.1–0.5	0.1–0.3 mg/hr	5–15
Meperidine	5–30	5–20 mg/hr	5–15
Morphine	0.5–3.0	0.5–3.0 mg/hr	5–20
Sufentanil	0.003–0.015	2–8 μg/hr	3–10
Agonist-antagonists			
Buprenorphine	0.03–0.2	NA	10–20
Nalbuphine	1–5	NA	5–15
Pentazocine	5–30	NA	5–15

NA, Information not available.
Adapted from Lubenow TR, Ivankovich AD: Pain and post anesthesia management. Crit Care Nurs Clin North Am 3:35, 1991.

that it allows the patient to sleep without waking in pain. Programmed into the pump are time and dose lockout features that do not allow delivery of a bolus dose even if the patient requests it. The lockout feature prevents delivery of a dose of opioid before the prior dose has had time to exert an effect. The lockout feature also prevents overdosing. In some pumps, the computer records how often the patient requests a bolus dose and how often the request is honored. This feature helps to assess the effectiveness of PCA.

It is postulated that by allowing patients to control their own pain and suffering, they titrate the amount of opioids they want to receive with the degree of discomfort and adverse effects from the opioids they are willing to tolerate.[50] Egan[50] proposed that the belief in the controllability of pain, whether true or not, influences the patient's appraisal of the situation. Having control over one aspect, the level of pain, may have a far-reaching influence on the patient's emotional and cognitive appraisal. The end result is that by allowing patients to control their level of pain, they suffer less and have less anxiety and distress. Patients can participate in therapeutic regimens, which decreases the likelihood of developing postoperative complications that are a consequence of pain.

The effectiveness of PCA is only as good as the doses that are provided. The same problems inherent with other methods of analgesia occur with PCA if the doses or time frames used are inadequate. Figure 15–9 shows the importance of appropriate doses and timing in producing adequate serum levels without the unwanted effects.

Neuraxial Analgesia

The discovery of enkephalins and endorphins spurred research into the efficacy of epidural and intrathecal opioids. The epidural space, the part of the spinal canal that lies outside the dura mater, is enclosed by the connective tissues covering the vertebrae. Moving inward, between the arachnoid mater and the pia mater lies the intrathecal space. A cross section of the spinal cord in which the intrathecal (subarachnoid) and epidural spaces are labeled is shown in Figure 15–10.

In little more than a decade since Wang and colleagues[51] first reported the use of intrathecal opioids and Behar and his associates[52] reported the use of epidural morphine for the treatment of pain, the use of epidural and intrathecal opioids has become commonplace in clinical and research arenas.

The advantages of neuraxial opioids stem from what Cousins and Mather[44] called selective spinal analgesia. This term emphasizes the difference between analgesia that occurs after the administration of nonselective blockade by anesthetic agents and the antinociceptive effects of opioids. Drugs administered in the epidural and intrathecal spaces, proximal to opioid receptors, relieve pain with minimal effects on other body systems. This is the rationale for the main advantage of opioids administered near the vertebral column. The avoidance of large doses of opioids in the central circulation prevents depression of the central nervous system. Epidural and intrathecal opioids have an advantage over anesthetic agents, since the latter produce sympathetic blockade, which is responsible for postural hypotension, cardiovascular collapse, and prolongation of ambulation for the first time.[53]

The adverse effects of intrathecal and epidural opioids stem from the specific opioid receptors that are occupied. Morphine is a pure μ-agonist, and stimulation of this receptor causes respiratory depression, miosis, euphoria, and bradycardia. Respiratory depression occurs with the intrathecal administration of morphine and more rapidly with the epidural route. The uptake of epidural morphine varies because of the fatty lining of the epidural space. The hydrophilic nature of morphine causes the absorption rate to be varied. This causes respiratory depression to occur as soon as 30 minutes after injection[44, 54] and as long as 22 hours after a single intrathecal injection.[44] The former, termed early respiratory depression, is not as problematic as the latter, termed late respiratory depression. Early respiratory depression is thought to be caused by vascular absorption into epidural veins and is similar to an equal IM dose. Late respiratory depression is thought to be caused by the slow rate of absorption from the site of injection.

Opioids initially were administered repeatedly into an epidural catheter. Now, postoperative epidural analgesia is administered by a PCEA pump or through a low-volume pump that gives a constant dose of opioid on a continuous basis. This allows the use of shorter-acting, lipophilic opioids, such as fentanyl. The use of fentanyl for PCEA has nearly eliminated the problem of respiratory depression.[55]

Sometimes bupivacaine is added to the opioid being ad-

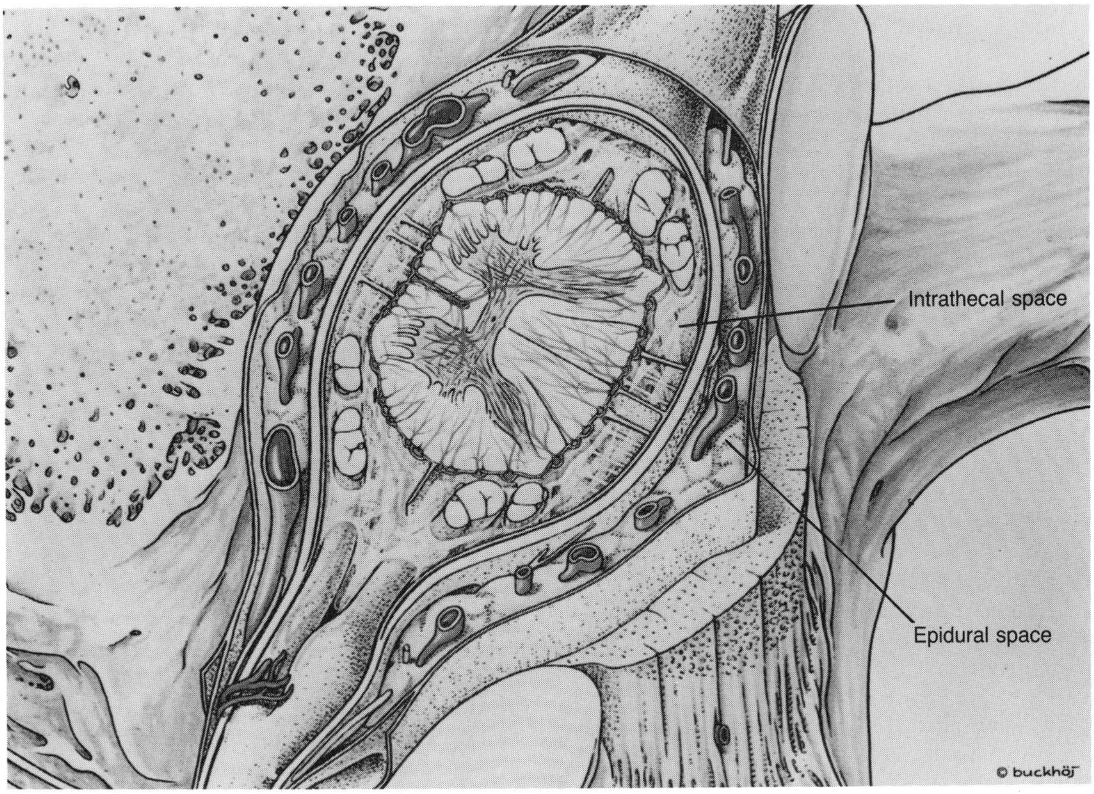

Figure 15–10. Oblique view of a cross section of the thoracic spine showing the contents of the epidural space. (From Covino BG, Scott DB: Handbook of Epidural Anaesthesia and Analgesia. Orlando, Grune & Stratton, 1985, p. 26.)

ministered into the epidural space to decrease the amount of opioid needed. Comparing epidural morphine with epidural bupivacaine and epidural morphine combined with bupivacaine, researchers noted that the average pain score was lower for patients who received morphine combined with bupivacaine.[56] Other researchers[55] compared continuous epidural infusions of fentanyl with bupivacaine given continuously or by PCEA. The pain scores were similar for both groups. The patients who received PCEA used less fentanyl compared with patients who received fentanyl and bupivacaine by continuous epidural infusion.

NURSING MANAGEMENT DURING THE TRAUMA CYCLE

Pain in the Resuscitation Phase

Pain in the resuscitation phase is classified as acute pain, which is pain that lasts from the time of injury to 6 months after the injury. After 6 months, pain is classified as chronic.[1] Pain in the resuscitation phase is severe and sharp and associated with autonomic arousal. The suprasegmental responses play a large role in the resulting stress response. The objectives for pain management in the resuscitation phase are to quickly and accurately complete a pain assessment and to initiate interventions to minimize the pain.

Nursing Assessment

To accurately assess pain during the resuscitation phase is difficult, considering the myriad of other activities and lifesaving interventions that rapidly are taking place. Information from rescue personnel regarding the nature of the injury and the extent of trauma helps the nurse to know the severity of pain to expect. Refer to Appendix 15–1 for the accident data base and history guidelines.

If the patient is conscious and somewhat cooperative, the pain assessment can be completed. A picture of how the patient copes with pain can be gleaned from any family members who are present. If the patient is not conscious, the pain assessment must be based on other indicators, such as grimacing, withdrawal, and body posturing. The main concern should be for the nurse to perform the pain assessment as accurately as possible.

Nursing Management

The patient often is frightened and confused. Steps toward orienting the patient to reality and providing psychosocial support assist in decreasing fear and anxiety. Decreased anxiety helps in the control of pain.

Although the relief of pain is paramount to minimizing autonomic arousal and the resulting suprasegmental responses, medications must be administered with caution. Opioids can make accurate neurological assessment difficult. They frequently are withheld when a patient's hemodynamic status is unstable. In a patient who is hemorrhaging and maintaining a normal blood pressure, the administration of morphine causes vasodilatation, which in turn causes hypotension.

Morphine in doses of less than 5 mg IV does not result in a release of histamine and the associated hypotension.[41] When morphine is given rapidly or in doses greater than 5 mg IV, significant decreases in systemic vascular resistance and blood pressure result. The nurse is in an excellent position to remind the physician that a small dose of morphine will relieve pain and probably have little effect on the patient's blood pressure. Fentanyl and sufentanil do not evoke the release of histamine.[41] These agents have the added advantage of a shorter duration of action compared with morphine.

On other occasions, pain may be complicated by a combative, agitated patient. The patient may require sedation to allow control of the airway and a thorough examination. The sedative may allow the nurse to perform an adequate pain assessment to determine the need for analgesics.

The decision to medicate a patient who is unstable is problematic for many health care professionals. Some practitioners believe that the most important factor is to stabilize the patient and treat pain after the patient is stable. Others believe that the administration of an amnestic when opioids cannot be given is justified. Still other health care providers have difficulty knowing that a patient has suffered. It is important for the nurse to explore these issues with coworkers before encountering this dilemma.

Two types of medications, opioids and benzodiazepines, are indicated in this phase of trauma. Opioids, given for severe pain, must be administered judiciously. If hypotension is not a problem, a small IV dose of morphine or fentanyl is appropriate. Both drugs are antagonized by IV naloxone. Morphine has a longer duration of action compared with fentanyl. Table 15–5 shows the duration of action of these and other opioids. The choice of drug should be based on the pharmacodynamics and the duration of action.

If the patient is receiving mechanical ventilation, opioids can be given to control pain. When the patient is not mechanically ventilated or if increased intracranial pressure is a consideration, opioids may be withheld. This becomes a challenging nursing situation to keep the patient calm and as pain-free as possible. Nonpharmacological interventions, such as massage, guided imagery, and touch, may be used.

It is important for the nurse to treat pain with the appropriate agent and treat anxiety with an antianxiety medication. Benzodiazepines, such as diazepam and midazolam, are excellent antianxiety agents. Diazepam may be difficult to administer in the hurried resuscitation phase, since it precipitates when given with most IV solutions. Midazolam has advantages over diazepam, in that it does not precipitate and has the added benefit of producing amnesia (the production of amnesia is an indication for its use).[57] A dose of 1 mg may be sufficient for the average adult. It may be better to titrate the drug, using 1 mg/ml of normal saline solution or dextrose 5 per cent in water. These agents, diazepam or midazolam, should be given by slow IV push. The nurse should remember that the concomitant use of sedatives with opioids increases the adverse effects of each agent.

If the administration of opioids is contraindicated because the patient is unstable, the use of amnestics should be considered. Midazolam should be given when possible. Scopolamine also produces amnesia, but when it is given alone (without opioids), agitation and disorientation may result.

Anesthesia may be necessary for the emergent treatment of some injuries. Although the administration of anesthesia is not the responsibility of the registered nurse, knowledge of the agents used and their duration of action is essential. The nurse is responsible for monitoring the postoperative effects of anesthesia as well as collaborating to determine the best method of pain control to use when the anesthetic effects subside. In some cases, if an epidural catheter has been used for anesthesia, epidural analgesia should be considered.

Pain in the Critical Care Phase

Nursing Assessment

Patients in the critical care phase of trauma are typically in the intensive care unit (ICU). They are admitted to the ICU at least several hours after the initial injury. The prominent complaint is severe pain.[58] As in the resuscitation phase, physiological indicators may be the only behaviors that form the basis of a pain assessment. The presence of tachycardia, hypertension, and restlessness may be the result of pain if other causes, such as hypoxemia, have been ruled out. When it is possible to communicate with the patient, a thorough pain assessment should be performed. Although it is important not to provide the patient with adjectives that describe pain, it may be necessary for the patient on mechanical ventilation. In this instance, it is the gathering of information by the best means possible that is most important. The nursing assessment not only provides a picture of the patient's pain but also serves as means of communicating a caring attitude to the patient. The caring attitude can help to decrease a patient's anxiety, which serves to lessen pain.

Nursing Management

Nursing interventions in critical care are classified as pharmacological and nonpharmacological.

Pharmacological Interventions

For the severe, predicted pain that is characteristic of the critical care phase of the trauma cycle, the route of choice is the IV route. Continuous opioid infusions provide a consistent level of analgesia that serves to enhance the rest that is essential for healing in this patient population. Methods that can be used to achieve consistent plasma levels of opioids are continuous IV infusions, PCA, continuous epidural infusions, and PCEA.

The continuous IV opioid infusion must be individually tailored to each patient. To determine the dose necessary to effectively relieve pain, consider the patient's physical condition and other medications, including sedatives and previous response to opioids. If a patient is receiving mechanical ventilation, the concern about respiratory depression is lessened. The patient who has received opioids for several days may have developed a tolerance to the opioid and the dose may need to be increased.

A loading dose of opioids provides rapid pain control when the continuous infusion is first started. It is preferable to a bolus because of the adverse effects associated with a large bolus. A loading dose provides pain control while the continuous infusion reaches the effective blood concentration. Without a loading dose, it may take several hours to reach an effective blood concentration. The loading dose and the continous infusion rate can be adjusted up or down, depending on the patient's response.

Regardless of the type of continuous infusion given—IV, PCA, epidural, or PCEA—loading doses are necessary. These doses typically are given in the postanesthesia recovery room. If the patient should be admitted directly to the ICU from the operating room, it is incumbent on the nurse to make certain that an initial loading dose is given. Table 15–6 shows commonly ordered doses and parameters for PCA.

When the patient is more alert and able to comprehend how to use the pump, PCA should be started. The use of PCA enables the patient to titrate the opioid to achieve the desired level of comfort. Most patients who receive PCA use less opioids compared with patients who receive opioids by the IM-PRN route. Researchers have also demonstrated that patients use PCA to keep pain at a tolerable level rather than ablate it.[59] The issue of patient control serves to decrease anxiety and increase patient satisfaction with treatment. When patients are more satisfied about their care, the outcome may be enhanced.[58]

Continuous epidural infusions have four distinct advantages over the IV route. The opioid is administered neuraxially, thus pain relief is achieved with minimal effects on other body systems. Smaller doses of opioids provide analgesia and with less drug in the central circulation compared with IM injections.[60] The patient's pulmonary function improves, and he is less sedated.

As with continuous IV opioid infusions, continuous epidural infusions are used when the patient is unable to effectively use a PCA pump. When the patient is able, PCEA should be used for reasons similar to those for using PCA.

Pharmacological Agents Used in Continuous Opioid Infusions. Morphine, fentanyl, and meperidine are appropriate opioids to be used with continuous infusion because of their medium to high rate of systemic clearance. Meperidine is used infrequently because of the accumulation of normeperidine.

Table 15–5 compares several opioids that are used for the relief of pain. A comparison of the duration of action and effective single dose shows what dose the nurse can anticipate will be given.

Morphine has traditionally been the drug of choice for continuous opioid infusions. It is slowly being replaced by fentanyl because less pruritus occurs with the latter agent. Although fentanyl is a more potent opioid, produces less pruritus, and has a higher index of safety, it is not a panacea. It is absorbed by vascular organs, skeletal muscles, and fat. When fentanyl is released from the skeletal muscles and fat, the opioid is redistributed to the central circulation, which may cause delayed respiratory depression.[61] This delayed respiratory depression is more likely to occur when fentanyl is given repetitively or in high doses. It is speculated that fentanyl undergoes gastric secretion and is sequestered in the gastric fluid and that secondary peaks of plasma fentanyl levels are the result of the recycled fentanyl between the gastric fluid and plasma.[62]

Other disadvantages include apnea when fentanyl is given with midazolam[61] and prolongation of the half-life to 15.8 hours in elderly patients, thus necessitating a decreased dose.

Advantages of fentanyl over other opioids are that the hyperglycemic response to surgery is abolished, release of plasma cortisol and growth hormones in response to surgery is decreased, and histamine seldom is released, which means fewer complaints of pruritus.[62]

Sufentanil has a high affinity for the μ-receptor that is about ten times that of fentanyl.[63] The high affinity for the μ-receptor contributes to its potency, which is five to ten times that of fentanyl. Sufentanil has the same advantages as fentanyl. Researchers compared intraoperative morphine, meperidine, fentanyl, and sufentanil. Intraoperative plasma norepinephrine levels were lower in patients who received sufentanil and meperidine compared with patients who received fentanyl and morphine.[64]

Nursing care of patients receiving continuous opioid infusions includes accurately assessing pain, caring for the catheter, monitoring the patient for adverse effects, and making certain the machinery used to provide analgesia is operating correctly. Table 15–4 compares the adverse effects of commonly used opioids.

The nurse should frequently evaluate the effectiveness of the opioid as well as the method used to deliver it. If pain relief is inadequate, the nurse must first determine whether the catheter (IV or epidural) is in the right place and whether the pump is working properly. Operator errors such as incorrectly loading or programming the pump may occur. The nurse must make certain that the tubing from the pump to the catheter has not become disconnected. If the IV is infiltrated and it will take longer than 30 minutes to restart it, an IM dose of opioid should be given. If the epidural catheter becomes disconnected from the pump tubing, the nurse must decide collaboratively with the physician who is prescribing the pain control whether to cut and repair the catheter or discontinue this method of analgesia.[65] When the catheter is intact and the pump is working properly but the pain relief is inadequate, the dosing parameters must be changed.

The patient's mental status should be monitored. When a decreased sensorium is detected, a decrease in the elimination of opioid must be suspected. The dose should be adjusted. Ampules of naloxone should be ready for use if the patient's respiratory rate decreases to less than eight breaths per minute accompanied by shallow respirations and increased sedation. The nurse should consult the patient's order sheet or nursing protocol for guidelines to treat respiratory depression and other adverse effects.

Oxygen (O_2) saturation monitors commonly are used in the presence of continuous opioid infusions. Their use provides another measure of sedation caused by a decrease in oxygenation. The nurse must be cautioned against increasing the percentage of O_2 delivered in the presence of respiratory depression. The decline in O_2 saturation may be temporarily corrected, but the cause of the declining O_2 is not. The physician must be called when O_2 saturation drops in the presence of respiratory depression. If the nurse continues to increase the amount of O_2 given without performing a complete respiratory assessment and collaborating with the physician to treat the cause, respiratory arrest could result.

When bupivacaine is added to the epidural opioid infusion, the nurse must assess the level of sensation and document by dermatome level. If the level of anesthesia rises, the rate of infusion may need to be adjusted. The patient must also be observed for postural hypotension. This is especially important when the patient is getting out of bed.

Infection from an IV catheter is serious; infection from an epidural catheter is disastrous. Strict sterile technique must be followed during catheter insertion and in preparing and administering neuraxial opioids. When alcohol or povidone-iodine (Betadine) is used to wipe injection ports or during catheter repair, the nurse must make certain that the catheter is thoroughly dry before injection or connection, since alcohol and Betadine are known to be toxic to the spinal cord.

The nurse must make certain that the patient does not receive other doses of opioids without the knowledge of the physician managing the continuous opiate infusion. The administration of opioids in addition to the continuous infusion may cause respiratory and central nervous system depression. Similar to the concomitant administration of opiates, the nurse should make certain that no sedatives are administered unless first cleared by the physician managing the continuous opioid infusion. When sedatives are combined with opiates, the dose of each agent should be reduced to avoid deleterious effects.

The nurse must take every precaution to avoid the administration of other drugs into an epidural line. Medications such as antibiotics and vasopressors can permanently damage the spinal cord.

For severe pain, regular IM injections of opioids can be used. The use of regular IM injections is not recommended for longer than one to two days for several reasons. Beyond 24 to 36 hours, the injection sites become sore. No matter how diligent nurses are about charting the IM site used and rotating sites, the likelihood of repeatedly using the same injection sites is high. Most trauma patients have limited mobility, which decreases the number of sites available. Also, the presence of multiple sites of injury limits the area suitable for injections and affects the rate of absorption, making it unpredictable. Even though the injections are ordered regularly, the same problems that occur with IM-PRN injections come into play with the administration of regular IM injections. An accurate pain assessment is necessary to evaluate the effectiveness of this method.

Nerve Blocks. The direct application of a local anesthetic to nerves can control pain by chemical blockage of neural transmission. Nerve blocks are aimed at modifying or blocking the painful impulses. Local anesthetics may be given IV or by infiltration or administered directly to a nerve.[66] Nerve blocks have a role in the treatment of pain and chest trauma, in which rib fractures are common. In addition, nerve blocks may be indicated in the treatment of certain posttraumatic pain syndromes, such as the pain of reflex sympathetic dystrophy.[66]

Interpleural Analgesia. First used as a method of analgesia for patients undergoing cholecystectomy and renal or unilateral breast surgery, interpleural analgesia is now used for postoperative analgesia, rib fractures, and pain in the upper extremities from reflex sympathetic dystrophy.[67, 68] An epidural catheter is carefully inserted through the parietal pleura into the interpleural space. Complications include pneumothorax, tension pneumothorax, intrapulmonary catheter placement, and local toxicity to anesthetics. The intercostal vessels can be lacerated.

Twenty to 30 ml of bupivacaine 0.25 per cent or 0.5 per cent commonly is used as a bolus dose to begin interpleural analgesia. Sometimes epinephrine is added to prolong the duration of analgesia. Continuous infusions of 0.25 per cent or 0.5 per cent bupivacaine are given at rates between 5 and 10 ml/hr.[53, 67]

The nursing care of a patient who receives interpleural analgesia involves assisting the physician during insertion, maintaining sterility during insertion and afterward, and clearly labeling the injection ports to prevent injection of other medications into the interpleural space. The nurse should assess the amount of pain relief and report ineffective analgesia. The patient must be observed for signs of pneumothorax.

Individual institutional policy directs which health care professional, the physician or the nurse, injects medications into the catheter. After the anesthetic is given, the patient should be observed for local toxicity. The signs and symptoms appear and escalate over time approximately in the following order: tinnitus, metallic taste, light-headedness, somnolence, visual and auditory disturbances, restlessness, delirium, slurred speech, nystagmus, muscle tremors, convulsions, dysrhythmia, and cardiovascular collapse.

Similar to drug administration, individual institutional policy directs which health care professional removes the catheter. No matter who removes the catheter, the nurse should inspect the insertion site for signs of infection, apply a sterile dressing to the site, and inspect the tip of the catheter to ensure that the entire catheter has been removed.[65, 67]

Adjuvants to Opioid Analgesia[69]

Benzodiazepines. These medications are used to promote sleep in the critically ill patient, with diazepam the most commonly used of this class. Besides promoting sleep, it reduces anxiety, relaxes muscles, and prevents convulsions. Diazepam has a long half-life. With high doses over several days, recovery of consciousness in the ventilated patient may take several days. In the critically ill patient, diazepam may have greater respiratory and cardiovascular effects than in a healthy patient.

Chlorpromazine. Chlorpromazine is used to decrease motor restlessness and acute confusional states. It is given until the desired effect is achieved and is followed by single or twice-daily doses to maintain the desired effect. Its adverse effects are α-adrenergic receptor blockade and hypotension. Its elimination half-life is 16 to 30 hours.

Butyrophenone. Butyrophenone is used to decrease motor restlessness and acute confusional states. It is thought to produce less sedation and hypotension than chlorpromazine. It is administered in a manner similar to that for chlorpromazine but in smaller doses. Two milligrams of butyrophenone is about equal to 100 mg of chlorpromazine. The elimination half-life is similar to that of chlorpromazine.

Nitrous Oxide. Inhalation of nitrous oxide is primarily used for physiotherapy and wound dressings, especially with burn patients. It is used in addition to other methods of analgesia. It is administered in concentrations of up to 70 per cent by an anesthesia device or as 50 per cent nitrous oxide in conjunction with other anesthetic agents.[68] Prolonged use may be associated with bone marrow depression.

Nonpharmacological Interventions

Nonpharmacological interventions include measures to decrease anxiety, massage, relaxation exercises, guided imagery, and cognitive preparation. These interventions can be used alone or in conjunction with the methods of analgesia presented earlier.

The prevention and control of anxiety are the prime objectives for any psychological intervention with pain. Preventing anxiety, fear, panic, and suffering, the usual responses to pain, markedly increase a patient's tolerance for pain.

The first step is the prevention of anxiety. An important aspect of preventing anxiety in a patient is preventing anxiety in oneself. Presenting a calm and thoughtful manner helps the patient and his family stay calm. Answering questions simply and honestly and being unhurried gives the patient and family a sense that they are being heard. Avoid stereotypes of patients and families, which allows the nurse to present an attitude of helpfulness to the family and patient. Some of the most agitated patients can respond positively to the simple question "How can I help you?"

Although difficult to accomplish in critical care units, it is important to have a family member stay with the patient as much as possible. The contact helps to calm the patient. The patient who is intubated and cannot voice his needs and who is fearful and confused may continually initiate the stress response.

Memories of pain, thinking they are in places other than the hospital, and wrongly identifying doctors, nurses, and family have been reported by trauma patients several weeks after transfer from critical care.

Controlling pain may prevent the memories of pain that patients verbalize in later stages of trauma. It may also prevent some of the dysphoria and nightmares that patients experience with trauma.

Massage and passive exercise are effective interventions for pain in the critical care phase of trauma. Massage can help to relax and decrease the tension in muscles, thus decreasing another stimulus for pain. There are no adverse effects, and the family can easily be included to assist with massage two or three times a day. Back massage and foot massage are relaxing to most people. The frontalis muscle is one of the muscles that is more sensitive to stress. Massaging the forehead, temple area, scalp, and base of neck usually produces significant relaxation. Passive or relaxation exercises are helpful in relaxing the muscles and preventing pain caused by stiffness and immobility. Discussing the types of exercises with the physician and the physical therapist is appropriate. The cumulative effect of massage and exercise may allow the patient to rest and sleep better and perhaps to use less medication.

The use of relaxation exercises, imagery, distraction, and cognitive preparation depend on the ability of the patient to focus and think clearly. Because of the critical nature of the patient, mental fatigue and the inability to concentrate for any length of time are common. Relaxation, imagery, and distraction are presented in the intermediate phase of trauma, but if the patient can mentally focus, it would be most appropriate to use these interventions in this phase of the trauma cycle. Cognitive preparation reduces the anxiety associated with pain, thus reducing the intensity of the pain. Cognitive preparation is based on research that shows that when patients are given information about the sensations to expect, they report less pain.[2] Cognitive preparation may also allow the patient to use less pain medication.

When a patient indicates that he is beginning to understand his situation, some preparation regarding pain can take place. Informing the patient about the occurrence of pain and its onset and duration and providing information about what the pain may feel like, its underlying causes, and what is being done to relieve it are appropriate interventions. Frequent evaluation of pain effectiveness with the patient is helpful. It assists the patient to maintain control and to feel less anxious.

This may also be the time to begin to assist the patient with the reconstruction of trauma events. It is best to answer the patient's questions honestly. If possible, family members can give most of the information and answer his questions. Sometimes the family needs support and reassurance in this process. This is especially true if a death is involved. Informing a patient of a death is likely to produce anxiety in some nurses and doctors as well. When a patient asks a few times about a person who died in the accident, it is best to be honest. Many patients resent information being withheld from them and have some inner sense that a person has died and are asking the question to confirm the fact.

Reconstruction of trauma events takes place through all stages of care. Many patients want to see pictures and talk with police officers and rescue workers as well as visit the trauma units where they initially received care. Some patients may have no recall for any of the events of the trauma. These patients are not usually bothered by dreams or nightmares of the accident. They may feel somewhat anxious though because they have no memory of the event.

Nursing Evaluation

It is important for the nurse to evaluate the effectiveness of interventions used to relieve pain. The involvement of the patient and family with the health care team in the plan for pain control is tantamount. Therefore, the patient and family should be involved in the evaluation. Consultation with the patient and family communicates a caring attitude and enhances the feeling of control. When patients perceive control over their care, anxiety can be reduced. Because anxiety plays a role in pain perception, all possible measures to reduce it should be taken.

The subjective report of pain is the most important method of evaluation. If the patient cannot communicate, the nurse must use the presence or absence of behaviors to assess the level of pain. As stated earlier, these behaviors are not reliable. The nurse can, however, note a change in behavior, such as a decrease in restlessness, after the administration of opioids. If the decrease in restlessness occurs at the time the drug is expected to exert its peak effect, one could conclude that the drug was effective.

Observations for effective pain relief and adverse effects from therapy should be carried out continuously. The evaluation of pain-relieving interventions is part of a continuous process in which the patient is assessed, changes are made, and the patient reevaluated. Accurate evaluation is equally as important as accurate assessment.

Pain in the Intermediate Care Phase

Pain in the intermediate phase of the trauma cycle is also within the definition of acute pain. The nature of pain and

TABLE 15–7. EQUIANALGESIC DOSES OF COMMONLY USED ANALGESICS*

DRUG	ROUTE	EQUIANALGESIC DOSE (mg)	NURSING CONSIDERATIONS
Codeine	IM	75	GI adverse effects occur more often with increased doses.
	PO	130	Frequently combined with acetaminophen or aspirin.
Meperidine (Demerol)	IM	100	
Hydromorphone (Dilaudid)	IM	1.5	
	PO	7.5	
Methadone (Dolphine)	IM	10	Duration of action is 4–8 hours.
	PO	20	
Levorphanol (Levo-Dromoran)	IM	2	Duration of action is 4–8 hours.
	PO	4	
Morphine	IM	10	Can be given rectally or in sustained-release 30–60-mg tablets.
	PO	30–60	30 mgm dose is used for q 3-4° administration. 60 mgm for single dosing.
Oxymorphone (Numorphan)	IM	1–1.5	Available in 5-mg rectal suppositories.
	Rectal	10	
Oxycodone	PO	30	Usually combined with acetaminophen or aspirin. Plain tablets and oral solution available in 5-mg/ml strength.
Dezocine (Dalgan)	IM	10	5 mg IV is equivalent to 1 mg IV butorphanol

*All doses are equal to 10 mg of IM morphine.

its underlying causes are changing. It may range from the sharp pain associated with immediate injury and surgery to a more aching pain associated with inflammation. The intensity of pain may fall within a severe to moderate category. Pain usually begins to decrease in intensity, waxing and waning at various times of the day. However, there may be increases in intensity of pain with repeated surgery, procedures, or infection.

The objectives of pain management become more broad than those in critical care. Pain management is directed toward controlling the pain so the patient can eat and drink, eliminate, rest and sleep, move, cough and deep breathe, and interact with others more independently. The goals regarding the prevention of stress response and other complications as well as the suffering and memories of pain are independent of the phases of trauma.

The interaction among the patient, the family, nursing staff, physicians, and other patients plays an important part in pain perception and pain behavior in this phase. Because the patient probably is alert and aware in this phase of the trauma cycle, pain perception and behavior become modified by interactions with others.

Nursing Assessment

The characteristics of this phase of the trauma cycle may be a patient with an increased ability to communicate but with some residual cognitive dysfunction. The patient may have an increased ability to participate in his care. (Refer to Appendix 15–2 for assessment factors in the intermediate phase.)

The most important factors for pain assessment for the intermediate phase are those that would affect the patient's independent functioning. The patient's past health history is important. This often is the time when one learns that the patient has had a previous back injury and regularly took medication. This may also be the time when an alcohol problem is revealed. The signs and symptoms of alcohol withdrawal that were delayed by opioid administration may now surface.

The continuous pain assessment helps the nurse recognize changing causes of pain and plan treatment accordingly. Without reassessment, one may fail to recognize increased pain from an infection and inappropriately treat it with only a change in analgesic administration.

Nursing Management

Pharmacological Interventions

With the changing nature of pain, not only may the route of medications change but also the selection of the analgesic compound. The patient may now benefit from IM injections or oral medications. The common pitfalls in controlling pain when changing medications, doses, and routes of administration can be avoided by using sound pharmacological principles.

Equianalgesia. Equianalgesia refers to the dose and route of one medication that produces about the same analgesic effect as the dose and route of another medication. Knowledge about equivalent doses of opioids is necessary when changing from one opioid, route, or dose to another. Equianalgesic doses are guidelines to be used in consideration with the individual's response to a particular analgesic. Equianalgesic doses are shown in Table 15–7.

Variation of Analgesic Response. Variability of an individual patient's response to analgesics is influenced by the patient, characteristics of the analgesic, mood, stress, other drugs, and pathophysiology. The patient's age, culture, and tolerance to pain as well as the site and intensity of pain affect the response to interventions for the relief of pain. The pain tolerance or response to interventions between patients should not be compared. Each patient should have his analgesic individually ordered and assessed for the degree of relief achieved.

The initial elimination of drugs can be enhanced by fluid

loss from blood, plasma, or burn areas.[70] The later stages of drug elimination can be slowed in patients who have altered liver or kidney function. This delays the excretion of analgesics, which prolongs their effect. The metabolism of analgesics may be increased in burn patients because of increases in ribosomal activity.

Protein binding of analgesic agents varies. Patients in the intermediate phase of trauma may have hypoproteinemia, and thus exhibit an increased sensitivity to analgesics. If the patient's total body fat and total body mass are also decreased, an increased sensitivity to analgesics occurs.

Guidelines for Changing Routes of Administration. Patients fear changing their routines when they have a medication that works. There may be a lack of trust related to previous experiences, they may have observed another patient's negative response to a change in medication, or they may have had experience with different analgesics and have formed their own opinions about the quality of analgesia.

Most patients quickly become aware that an oral opioid does not relieve pain as quickly as an opioid delivered by the IM route. In the transition from an IM dose to an oral dose, the analgesia often is not ordered in an equivalent dose. As a result, patients may report ineffective pain relief from an oral analgesic. It is essential that the oral dose be equivalent (see Table 15–7). In some instances, if the patient has been in severe pain or if he questions the effectiveness of oral opioids, McCaffery[7] recommends starting with a higher dose than the equivalent one.

Medicating a patient before pain becomes severe may allow for pain control with smaller doses of opioids, and thus with fewer adverse effects. Giving the oral opioid on a regularly scheduled basis rather than on an as-needed basis may also prevent the peaks of pain. This can help prevent the patient from feeling anxious and out of control.

Scheduled multiple dosing provides an accumulated therapeutic effect; the opioid is not completely metabolized before the next dose is administered. Scheduling of multiple dosing allows smaller doses of opioid to be effective. See Table 15–8 for a list of guidelines when changing routes of administration.

Oral Opioids. Although oral opioids typically are used for mild to moderate pain, severe pain can also be managed orally if doses are adequate.

Oral morphine is metabolized during absorption, which can be erratic, depending on the individual patient. Methadone, hydromorphone, and levorphanol are more reliably absorbed. Oral hydromorphone is shorter-acting than morphine. Oral methadone and levorphanol are longer-acting than morphine (6 to 8 hours and 4 to 6 hours, respectively).

Rectal Suppositories. Although aspirin and acetaminophen suppositories are available, the rate of absorption is slow and the extent of absorption varies. These drugs do relieve mild pain. Oxymorphone (Numorphan) appears to be the most potent agent in suppository form (see Table 15–7). Hydromorphone suppositories have been found to be less effective. Ten milligrams of oxymorphone given rectally is about equivalent in analgesic effect to 10 mg of morphine given IM. Rectal oxymorphone has a slower onset of action but a longer duration in comparison to IM-administered opioids. It is important to remember that an empty rectum facilitates absorption, whereas a full rectum may hinder absorption. In addition, patients may consider suppositories invasive and distasteful.

Nonsteroidal Anti-inflammatory Medications. Inflammation greatly contributes to trauma pain. The nonsteroidal anti-inflammatory drugs (NSAIDs) can offer pain relief to the trauma patient able to tolerate oral medication (Table 15–9). Infection, a high risk in trauma patients, may be masked by anti-inflammatory drugs. However, it is important to begin introducing them as soon as possible because of the anti-inflammatory effect and additive effects of these peripheral-acting compounds to the central-acting opioids.

Ketorolac tromethamine (Toradol) is the only NSAID that can be given by the IM route. Two similar studies[71, 72] were conducted in postoperative pain comparing 30 mg IM ketorolac tromethamine with morphine 6 and 12 mg. The average pain relief and average pain intensity were not significantly different between 12 mg of morphine and 30 mg of ketorolac tromethamine. Less nausea, vomiting, and sedation were associated with 30 mg of ketorolac tromethamine compared with 12 mg of IM morphine. Spindler and colleagues[72] reported only 3 of 185 patients complained of injection related adverse events.

The manufacturer[73] suggests a 60-mg loading dose followed by regular IM injections every 6 hours. This would produce steady plasma levels for optimal pain relief. A lower dose (30-mg loading dose and 15-mg maintenance dose) is recommended for patients who weigh less than 50 kg or are over age 65 and for those with impaired kidney function.

The specific mode of action of NSAIDs is unknown but may be inhibition of prostaglandin biosynthesis. Their effect is to afford symptomatic relief. Clinical indications for using one agent over another are not clear, but concomitant use of aspirin offers no therapeutic advantage and may decrease the blood level of these compounds and increase adverse effects. With NSAIDs, there may be fewer GI adverse effects

TABLE 15–8. GUIDELINES FOR CHANGING IM TO ORAL OPIOIDS

1. The oral opioid should have good GI absorption, be capable of relieving moderate to severe pain, and have a relative long duration of action.
2. As a general rule, make the oral dose equivalent to the IM dose using the equivalency table.
3. Titrate the dose according to the individual patient's response. Two factors that might alter the initial dose are variable oral absorption and tolerance.
4. Supplement the oral opioid with IM doses during the initial transition period if necessary for effective pain relief.

TABLE 15–9. SOME COMMON NONSTEROIDAL ANTI-INFLAMMATORY MEDICATIONS

Salicylates	**Indoles**
Acetylsalicylic acid (aspirin)	Indomethacin (Indocin)
Diflunisal (Dolobid)	Sulindac (Clinoril)
Para-aminophenols	Tolmetin (Tolectin)
Acetaminophen (Tylenol)	**Fenamates**
Propionic acids	Meclofenamate (Meclomen)
Ibuprofen (Motrin)	**Oxicams**
Naproxen (Naprosyn)	Piroxicam (Feldene)

than with aspirin, and some may increase steady-state lithium levels. Central nervous system effects such as insomnia, confusion, inability to concentrate, depression, and emotional lability may be seen.[74]

Patient-Controlled Analgesia. PCA is useful during the intermediate phase of the trauma cycle as long as the patient's mental status is clear. As the intensity of pain decreases over time or the number of pain-producing treatments (such as dressing changes) decreases, PCA is discontinued and the patient is switched to oral analgesics. The use of the oral route depends on the patient's GI motility.

Patient-Controlled Epidural Analgesia. Like PCA, PCEA is useful during this phase of the trauma cycle. The epidural catheter can be used as long as it provides adequate analgesia. Catheter migration has been reported and is detected by the sudden onset of severe sedation and central nervous system depression if the catheter has moved into the intrathecal space or adjacent blood vessels. If the catheter has migrated out of the epidural space and into adjacent tissues or has moved out of the body, the patient will complain of pain that is not relieved by requests from the pump for more opioids.

Transdermal Fentanyl. Transdermal fentanyl may be useful in the intermediate phase. The patch should be applied about 8 to 10 hours before discontinuing PCA or PCEA. The parameters of PCA and PCEA should be changed to avoid negative effects from too large a dose of opioid as the level of fentanyl from the patch begins to rise. Researchers[75] compared the two strengths of fentanyl patch (70 to 80 μg/hr and 90 to 100 μg/hr) with a placebo patch. All patients in the study used PCA with 20 to 40 μg/kg morphine on demand. There was no significant difference between the amount of morphine used by PCA for patients who used the low-dose patch and those who used the placebo patch. Those patients who used the high-dose fentanyl patch used significantly less morphine by PCA compared with patients who received the placebo patch. These differences were not seen until 12 and 24 hours after placement of the patches.

Both PCA and PCEA are tapered gradually before discontinuing, which allows for adequate analgesia during the switch from one method of analgesia to another. If PCA or PCEA should be discontinued before adequate blood levels of fentanyl are reached, the patient will not only experience pain but also become anxious and have little confidence in the patch. More research is necessary to determine whether the fentanyl patch can adequately relieve pain when used alone rather than in conjunction with other methods of analgesia.

Tolerance. Tolerance to opioid analgesics is characterized by decreased duration of action followed by a decrease in the intensity of the analgesic, sedative, and other central nervous system depressant effects. As a result, large doses can be given without harm to the patient.[41]

Tolerance should not be confused with addiction or physical dependence; it may occur in the absence of either. Tolerance may involve, among other mechanisms, an adaptation of the cells to the action of the drug. Tolerance to the analgesic effect or the respiratory depressant effect is not a permanent state; it usually subsides within 2 to 4 weeks, and tolerance to opioids largely disappears when withdrawal is completed.

It is not clear whether tolerance develops in all people who are taking opioids or, if it does develop, whether it presents a practical clinical problem. In most patients, pain becomes less severe as healing takes place; thus, the need for higher doses does not develop.

The development of tolerance is apparently related to the rate of use. With intermittent use of a narcotic, it is possible to obtain adequate analgesic effect for an indefinite period. Tolerance more commonly develops with continuous use of an opioid.[41]

Using opioids to control pain, even for as short a period as 10 days on a regularly scheduled basis, may allow some degree of tolerance to develop. The nurse must be prepared to use higher doses to control the pain and then decrease the dose slowly as pain lessens.

Tolerance does not develop equally to all effects of opioids. It occurs primarily to the respiratory, analgesic, sedative, and euphoric effects, not to the miotic and constipative effects. If a patient is tolerant to the analgesic effect, then he is also tolerant to the respiratory depressant effect of the opioid. Thus, increasing the opioid dose does not decrease respirations significantly.[41] Cross-tolerance between opioids may develop. As a result, a patient who is tolerant to one opioid may also be tolerant to another.

If pain medication becomes ineffective, the nurse must consider whether the patient may have developed a condition that is causing either increased pain or new pain unaffected by the analgesic. A combination of these factors may contribute to inadequate analgesia.

Patients who have received IV opioids long enough to develop a tolerance before being switched to neuraxial opioids should be observed for signs of withdrawal. The longer time necessary before the onset and peak effect are noted may be sufficient for the patient to exhibit signs of withdrawal. The patient may need an IV dose of opioid sooner than anticipated to prevent withdrawal.

Addiction and Physical Dependence. There is concern among health care professionals regarding addiction. It is frequently the reason given for withholding opioids or giving less than adequate doses. Withholding opioids, giving opioids at longer intervals than they are pharmacologically active, and giving less than adequate doses are not methods thought to prevent addiction.[7] Addiction to various drugs is far more complex than merely being exposed to opioids.

Addiction is a term commonly used incorrectly for dependence. Physical dependence is a predictable normal response to repeated doses of an opioid. Dependence demonstrates itself through withdrawal symptoms when the opioid is not taken. Physical dependence is easily treated.[41] Withdrawal could occur in many patients in the hospital if opioids were stopped abruptly, but this is not often seen because patients usually decrease the amount of opioid they are taking as their pain decreases. Some patients require IM opioids throughout their hospital stay. They may go through withdrawal at home and be unaware of what they are experiencing. The aches and pains they experience may be considered part of recovery and may be treated with acetaminophen or aspirin.

Addiction, on the other hand, involves a pattern of excessive preoccupation with obtaining and using the drug for psychological rather than medical reasons.[41] It is true that those who are addicted are probably physically dependent, but it is not a fact that patients who become physically dependent are or will become addicted. Studies indicate that addiction occurs in less than 1 per cent of the hospital population.[75] Porter and Jick[76] reported that 4 out of 11,000 patients, with patients already addicted excluded, became addicted to opioids during a hospital stay.

There is a subset of patients who are addicted and abuse opioids. This abuse may present itself in many different variations, from those who use opioids intermittently to the person who uses opioids daily. There are scarce references on working with an addicted patient in a medical setting. Some clinical guidelines are given for consideration here. (Refer to Chapter 30 for additional information.)

Working with a person who abuses opioids chronically is a challenging experience. Feeling manipulated, angry, and out of control and fear of contributing to the addictive process by giving opioids are all predictable responses of those working with the addicted patient. The anxiety inherent in this type of situation is high. The memories associated with the situation once it has passed remain vivid for many nurses and physicians. This situation contributes to the fear of using opioids and leads to the undertreatment of pain with opioids.

It is important to obtain information about drug use and possible addiction through a thorough history. Any addicted patient should have a psychiatrist working with him from the time of admission. In addition, consultation for the staff from the psychiatrist as well as a psychiatric liaison nurse may be helpful. If drug use is suspected but cannot be verified, a psychiatric consultation to aid in the diagnosis is appropriate. One psychiatrist and one nurse on each shift should be the primary decision makers to prevent the confusion and manipulation that occur around opioid administration.

The patient must be maintained on the level of opioid used on a daily basis or another one substituted to prevent withdrawal. Untreated withdrawal may be life-threatening. Treatment of the patient's drug problem is not the goal of the patient's stay in the trauma setting. Drug treatment and withdrawal can be carried out in the medical setting if drug treatment staff are actively involved in the patient's care. The patient should be involved in the decision to withdraw, if possible. The patient may also voluntarily enter a drug treatment program at the time of discharge to resolve his addiction problem.

If a patient is in a drug treatment program, a coordinated effort with the staff from that program is helpful. Written permission must be obtained from the patient to contact the treatment program. Most patients who are seriously addressing their addiction problem give permission. Already existing routines set up in the drug program can be modified to work in the hospital setting. This coordinated effort provides continuity of care and helps to prevent the patient and the nurses from feeling manipulated. Enlisting the family or significant others to promote motivation, consistency, and continuity may be helpful to the patient and staff.

Opioids given in a liquid form make observation of ingestion easier. This task is necessary to prevent the patient from saving the medication and taking it all at once or administering it by a different route. As with any other patient, documenting the effect of opioids on the patient's respiratory and pulse rates and blood pressure is necesary. A patient who has had a previous addiction problem with one opioid may not want to use the same one for his current pain. This request should be respected, and every effort should be made to find a substitute.

Nonpharmacological Interventions

Alternative pain management techniques are sometimes referred to as noninvasive techniques. Noninvasive techniques originate externally but have internal effects. These techniques do not involve penetration or physical invasion of the body, as surgery or medication administration does. Exceptions to this would be the use of medicated cream to massage a patient.

These techniques are not new. Nurses and patients have been using them for years, but there is now an increasing interest in more medically untraditional, self-reliant methods. Noninvasive physical or sensory techniques appropriate for use in the intermediate phase of trauma are cutaneous stimulation with pressure, massage, cold, heat, contralateral stimulation, and breathing exercises. Again, other techniques, such as the transcutaneous nerve stimulator, can be used, depending on the characteristics of the injury, pain, and patient. These are discussed in the rehabilitation phase of the trauma cycle.

The use of alternative techniques for pain control raises many unanswered questions about how and when to use these techniques and with what kind of injuries.[77] Although there are guidelines for general practice, research has not been done to dictate specific use with the trauma patient. These techniques present opportunities for innovation and creativity. They can be modified for the nurse's and patient's style and for the patient's preference, ability, and degree of pain.

The use of noninvasive physical techniques presents a low risk to the patient. Adverse effects are minimal and can be managed by changing or stopping the strategy. These techniques can be used by themselves or in conjunction with analgesics and may reduce the patient's requirement for analgesics. Given the current knowledge of pain, using several interventions to achieve control is the most effective approach.

It is important to ask the patient what usually is done for pain relief. Sometimes patients use effective methods at home but may not use these while in the hospital. Patients can be supported in continuing their efforts and can be taught additional, supplemental methods. Learning about a patient's interest can be helpful in selecting a method.

Patients may need time to develop confidence in these pain-relief measures, especially if they focus on medication as the primary source of pain relief. As a result, patients may need assurance that the validity of their pain is not being questioned and that their pain medication will not be taken away. Some methods, such as breathing exercises and massage, can be used without much prior explanation. Other methods require explanation and cooperation. The degree to which the patient can cooperate and is willing to try other pain-relief measures affects the method chosen and, usually, its success.

The patient learns more easily if the noninvasive techniques are tried or taught when his pain is at a lower level. Preventive teaching is a good idea. However, if the opportunity to teach the patient a noninvasive technique does not arise until pain is experienced, the technique should still be demonstrated. We have had some good results in teaching patients with considerable pain. Although pain may distract from learning, it can also contribute to a patient's motivation and willingness to learn.

Pressure. It is an instinctive reaction to use pressure in response to pain. Applying pressure is useful for procedures and activities that produce pain and for painful conditions such as headache. Pressure may be applied with the finger, the heel of the hand, or the entire hand to the painful site or a nearby location. Pressure can help relieve pain in procedures and activities such as giving IV medications and injections, changing dressings, and respiratory care. With headache, applying pressure and massage to the temple areas in headache sometimes reduces pain.

Pressure can decrease the blood supply to the area, diminishing the accumulation of fluid. However, when the pressure is released, there may be a quick return of pain with increased blood flow.

Massage. Massage, or rubbing, frequently is a natural reaction to an injury. It can be done with or without ointments, mentholated or nonmentholated. The hands may be used in various ways—firmly, lightly, slowly, or briskly—to promote relaxation and sedation. Sleep can be induced by massaging a hand, an arm, or a foot.

Cold. The use of ice for pain relief is an old method. Melzack and associates[78] have reported on the use of ice massage on the Hoku acupuncture point, the web between the thumb and the index finger, to relieve mouth pain. This is a good example of how several noninvasive methods can be combined. Ice massage should be limited to sessions lasting about 10 minutes.

Cold packs can be helpful in reducing the swelling, and thus the pain, of trauma or surgery. Quick relief from headache, muscle sprain, sore throat, joint pain from immobility, and muscle spasm can also be obtained with cold. Although heat has long been used for muscle spasms, some patients find that cold provides longer-lasting pain relief.

Cold may be contraindicated or should be used with caution with vascular compromise or cold sensitivity. Patients may report a return of the throbbing pain, which initially may be quite severe, after the numbing sensation produced by the cold wears off.

Heat. Although cold may be more effective for certain pain, some patients prefer heat. With both heat and cold, pain is perceived as less intense. Because heat may produce an inflammatory response, an increase in blood flow, and edema, it may not be the best choice in the initial stages of pain control for the trauma patient. It may be more beneficial in the later stages.

Contralateral Stimulation. Contralateral stimulation is cutaneous stimulation to a site opposite that of the pain. This method can be especially useful when the painful site cannot be stimulated directly because it is too painful, the limb is missing (as in phantom pain), or the site is covered by a cast or dressing. There are hypotheses regarding the mechanism of contralateral stimulation. One is that the substantia gelatinosa is affected by fibers from both sides of the body, so that stimulation of either side of the body might have similar effects.[79] Another is that a simple spinal reflex may modulate a stimulus going from one side of the body to the other.[80]

Patients may express disbelief at the prospect of applying an intervention to an area other than the pain site. With a simple explanation, most patients are willing to try. For many, the area becomes slightly numb, and the painful area is described as a feeling of pressure rather than pain.

Breathing Exercises. Breathing exercises produce both distraction and relaxation. Relaxation presumably is produced by a decrease in skeletal muscle tension. McCaffery[7] offers excellent examples of different breathing exercises. The following are some guidelines for using breathing exercises. Breathing from the abdomen is associated with relaxation. Breathing in through the nose and out through the mouth is suggested. Slow, regular breathing produces relaxation, whereas fast, short breaths are distracting and take energy. Fast, short breaths are useful if done for a short period, to get a patient through a limited painful procedure. This technique should only be used for brief periods to prevent hyperventilation, although with practice, patients can use it for longer periods without experiencing hyperventilation.

Distraction. Distraction is simply focusing on something else unrelated to the pain. McCaffery[7] describes it as sensory shielding. Cutaneous stimulation and relaxation exercises may provide distraction. Activities such as talking, reading, watching TV, and listening to music may serve as good distractions. Patients and the health care team frequently use distraction successfully.

When the distraction is removed, the painful sensation can flood back, appearing more intense. The nurse should explain that this is an expected occurrence. This phenomenon may be occurring when the patient who was smiling 5 minutes before suddenly calls for pain medication after the visitors leave.

Progressive Relaxation. Progressive relaxation is a form of distraction. Progressive relaxation teaches the patient to contract and relax muscle groups in a logical sequence, from head to toe, for example. This allows the muscles to relax and let go of tension, which results in a decrease in the sympathetic nervous system response. To produce deep relaxation, progressive relaxation should be encouraged for 10 to 20 minutes twice a day. The reader is referred to an excellent article by Doody and colleagues[81] for a sample script that could be used by a nurse to direct the patient to perform progressive relaxation.

Guided Imagery. Guided imagery is using the imagination to alter a physical or an emotional state. This intervention may not be useful for the head-injured patient if mental functioning is compromised. It is reported to strengthen the immune system, to provide mental relaxation, and to decrease sensations of pain. This technique relies on mental processes and images that invoke the senses.[81] One patient envisioned pouring cool water over a searing, hot pain. Another patient pictured tubes with faucets leading to painful areas. Mentally turning off the faucets turned off the sensation to the pain in his chest.

To effectively use guided imagery, the patient must have a thorough understanding of his illness and treatment.[81] Imagery should be performed when the patient is totally relaxed. Thus, guided imagery should be used after progressive relaxation exercises. The nurse can guide the patient to gain a more positive attitude about his trauma and gain hope for recovery. The patient should be instructed to use his own image. If the patient is unable to think of his image, he can be instructed to think of a warm, comfortable place.

Placebo Response. Administration of placebos and use of the placebo response are two different techniques. The use of a placebo as a pain medication has no place in the treatment of acute pain. It should never be used to validate the authenticity of a patient's pain.

In clinical drug trials, a placebo group is used to determine as best as possible the effects caused by the active drug and those caused by the placebo response. All medications as well as any nursing or medical intervention have a placebo effect.

It is impossible not to influence the patient in some way. If the patient perceives the caretaker to be caring, the patient may experience greater benefit from an intervention. If a patient is informed of the adverse effects of a medication, he may develop those effects, not from the active drug, but because he was aware of the adverse effects. If a respected caretaker suggests to the patient that he will obtain relief from a certain intervention, the patient may obtain relief from the suggestion and not the intervention. There are many other examples of placebo responses. The important point is that there is a placebo response to some degree for any intervention. Taking advantage of this naturally occurring phenomenon can create an environment for a positive rather than a negative response.

Cognitive Sensory Preparation. Several studies have reported a reduction in stress levels when a patient received information about what his senses will experience.[77, 82] The patient usually is provided with technical information about what will be done to him but not necessarily what sensations he may feel. The patient feels more in control and less anxious when given knowledge of what will be experienced with all the senses. Sensory information and explanation of the procedure before the procedure may allow the patient time to prepare mentally. Achterberg[83] believes in the powerful influence of the prepared mind, or mental rehearsal, on a healing body. Some patients may become more anxious as a result of information. Asking the patient if he would like to know some of the sensations that other patients have experienced is an effective way of trying to assess how the patient may respond. Asking if he would like to know about procedures ahead of time or just a few minutes before they are performed also allows the patient some choice and, therefore, control.

Pain in the Rehabilitation Phase

Patient characteristics that may be represented in the rehabilitation stage of trauma are varying degrees of dysfunction to normal ability to communicate, think, and concentrate. The patient's memory and ability to pay attention may or may not be intact. Attention from the nursing and medical staff is now on the patient's ability to function independently. Care may be given on an inpatient or outpatient basis. An inpatient probably is out of bed most of the day, possibly dressed in street clothes, and receiving various therapies in other parts of the hospital.

Acute and Chronic Pain

Some traumatic injuries take a long time to heal, such as deep, open wounds and infected, large broken bones. These conditions may continue to produce pain for months as they heal. Pain associated with injuries with a lengthy healing time is still considered to be acute pain. Acute pain may progress to chronic pain; the conditions delineating this progression are not clear.

Chronic pain is defined as pain that lasts longer than 6 months.[6] Bonica[1] argues that this definition often is not appropriate because many acute injuries heal in 2 to 6 weeks, and if pain is still present a month afterward, it must be considered chronic. Bonica's definition—"pain which persists a month beyond the usual course of an acute disease or reasonable time for an injury to heal, or pain that recurs at intervals for months to years"—allows the clinician to suspect reflex sympathetic dystrophy at a time when the immediate therapy of sympathetic blockade could prevent the development of such a painful chronic condition. Regardless of the definition used, it is imperative to consider how long the pain has continued despite interventions and whether the chronicity of pain is related to the original injury or could be the result of causalgia or other reflex sympathetic dystrophies.

The mechanisms of chronic pain are more complex than those of acute pain. The lack of scientific data on chronic pain makes it necessary to rely on theories that help to explain the cause and guide treatment. Chronic pain is thought to be caused by peripheral mechanisms or the combination of peripheral and central mechanisms.

Peripheral mechanisms are thought to be responsible for the chronic pain associated with arthritis, myofascial syndromes, chronic tendinitis, headache, coronary artery disease, and peripheral vascular disease. It is thought that the chronic pain is the result of persistent noxious stimulation of nociceptors or their sensitizations or a combination of both. Chronic inflammation or damage to a nerve or blood vessel may change the microenvironment in which the release of algogenic substances sensitize nociceptors to nonnoxious stimuli.

Peripheral–central mechanisms are thought to be the cause of chronic pain syndromes associated with reflex sympathetic dystrophy, phantom limb pain, and cancer pain. In these conditions, the central nervous system is damaged and the dysfunction also involves the peripheral nerves.

Examples of chronic pain seen in trauma patients include causalgia, reflex sympathetic dystrophy, phantom limb pain, osteomyelitis, and stress-related posttraumatic chronic pain syndrome. Discussed in this section are causalgia, reflex sympathetic dystrophy, and stress-related posttraumatic chronic pain syndrome. Phantom limb pain is a complex phenomenon that requires treatment by a host of health care professionals who specialize in the treatment of pain. Osteomyelitis, a painful musculoskeletal disorder, is not discussed here (refer to Chapter 21).

Causalgia. The term causalgia is used to refer to the syndrome of sustained, diffuse, burning pain, allodynia, and hyperpathia after traumatic nerve lesions. Allodynia is pain caused by a stimulus that normally does not produce pain. Hyperpathia refers to an increased reaction to a stimulus, especially a repetitive stimulus, as well as an increased threshold.[1] Thus, causalgia is a specific type of pain syndrome that should be suspected in patients who have received injury to a nerve as a result of a high-velocity missile. Pain usually develops promptly or soon after the injury and is characterized by burning that is located in the distal part of the limb. The pain is almost always aggravated by physical and emotional factors. Interruption of all sympathetic pathways to the affected limb early in the course of the disease produces prompt and complete pain relief. Thus, detection through an accurate pain assessment is essential. Causalgia is mentioned here to differentiate it from reflex sympathetic dystrophy, which, if not detected and treated early, can become chronic.

Reflex Sympathetic Dystrophy. Clinically, reflex sympathetic dystrophies are more important than causalgia because they typically cause pain and disability. The precipitating factor is accidental or surgical trauma. Reflex sympathetic dystrophy is characterized by varying degrees of pain, vasomotor and other autonomic disturbances, delayed recovery of function, and trophic changes.[84] Trauma is a common cause. It occurs after sprains, dislocations, and fractures of the hand, foot, or wrist. There is no correlation between the severity of the injury and the incidence, severity, and the course of symptoms.

Like causalgia, reflex sympathetic dystrophy is characterized by allodynia, hyperalgesia, and hyperesthesia. Hyperesthesia is an increased sensitivity to stimulation, excluding special senses. Vasomotor and sudomotor disturbances and skeletal muscle hypotonia are frequently seen in reflex sympathetic dystrophy. In later stages, weakness, atrophy, and trophic changes of the skin, muscles, bones, and joints are seen.

Reflex sympathetic dystrophy is classified into grades 1 to 3, with the first being the severest, or into stages, which are used when it is not diagnosed and progresses without treatment from an acute stage to the atrophic stage. Some mild, early cases may subside spontaneously in a few weeks, whereas some moderately severe cases have healed spontaneously within a year. In most cases, without proper treatment, reflex sympathetic dystrophy can progress to irreversible trophic changes and psychological disturbances that severely impair the patient's ability to function. Thus, the importance of an accurate assessment for the development of this syndrome cannot be overemphasized.

Preventive measures include treatment at the site of injury, early and adequate relief of pain with analgesic blocks, and psychological support for the patient and family. A series of sympathetic blocks may be necessary. When sympathetic blockade provides only transient relief, a sympathectomy may be done. Transcutaneous nerve stimulation and systemic corticosteroids have also been reported as effective modes of treatment.[84]

Stress-Related Posttraumatic Chronic Pain Syndrome. Stress-related posttraumatic chronic pain syndrome, coined by Muse,[85] includes anxiety, apprehension, fear, and emotional suffering, which serves to enhance the pathophysiological effects of the injury. Muse[85] emphasizes that patients with stress-related posttraumatic chronic pain syndrome experience psychological trauma because in addition to coping with the discomfort and functional disabilities that are a result of the trauma, they must cope with terrifying phobic reactions to the traumatic event. These phobic reactions threaten the patients' self-confidence. Patients who are diagnosed with stress-related posttraumatic chronic pain syndrome show some of the following signs and symptoms: impaired ability to sleep, difficulty with concentration, impaired memory, exaggerated startle response, and sudden acting or feeling as if the traumatic event were happening again in response to an environmental stimulus.

This syndrome is treated by deconditioning the patient by pairing relaxation with the original anxiety associated with the trauma. Success has been noted through the use of narcosynthesis with sodium amytal.

Nursing Assessment

Some trauma patients arrive at the hospital with preexisting chronic pain. A thorough history is necessary to discover this. The patient may not volunteer the information, thinking that it is not important, or may have forgotten because the new pain has overridden awareness of the old pain. (See Appendix 15–2 for assessment factors in the rehabilitation phase of trauma.)

The assessment for the presence of chronic pain syndromes is important at this phase of trauma. The progression from acute pain that is now considered chronic should be well documented in the medical record. Assessment in the rehabilitation phase centers on the changes in the characteristics of pain and the patient's response to interventions to relieve pain.

Nursing Management

The objectives for acute pain management in the rehabilitation phase of trauma are similar to those in the intermediate phase of trauma. Although there is greater emphasis on the patient using oral analgesics along with other nonpharmacological interventions to control pain, there is also greater emphasis on the patient functioning independently.

The nature of the pain may not have changed dramatically from that in the intermediate phase. It may fall within a moderate to mild range of intensity, occasionally becoming severe, may be absent, may be an aching pain or pain with spasm, or may burn or be a pinching kind of sensation. If left untreated or inadequately treated, the pain could fatigue the patient. At this stage, some symptoms of depression may be seen. Using many interventions for pain relief is more effective than reliance on any single method.

The chronic pain discussed in this section is not that associated with a fatal illness and is different from acute pain. Chronic pain often is aching and burning in nature. It may be pinching but seldom is sharp. Muscles feel tight and tense. A great deal of fatigue is associated with chronic pain. There are many mood alterations, ranging from irritability to depression. There is an acceptance of the condition, which is necessary in taking measures to care for oneself, much as with any chronic disease.

The management of chronic pain is different from that of acute pain. The objectives of treatment are to assist the patient to function as fully and independently as possible. Treatment goals are aimed at helping the patient to be pain-free or to reduce the pain to tolerable limits. Opioids are not used. Antidepressants are given if depression exists, and antidepressants in smaller doses may also be used to affect the pain in the absence of depression. Daily exercise is strongly recommended as well as regular use of relaxation exercises to prevent tense muscles from causing pain. Warm, moist heat, cold packs, transcutaneous nerve stimulators, adequate rest, and a healthy diet are all helpful.

Pharmacological Interventions

Opioid Use With Acute and Chronic Pain. Acute pain in the rehabilitation phase of trauma should be treated in the same pharmacological manner as acute pain in any other phase of trauma. The use of opioids in this phase may be more complex. Physical dependence and tolerance may have developed. When pain is long-term, switching to different opioids and using longer-acting oral opioids are appropriate. Most patients with long-standing pain but whose pain is expected to end when healing occurs can use oral opioids or, at times of severe pain, injectable opioids to control their pain. The use of peripheral and centrally acting pain medications either combined in one formula or given separately is most helpful in this phase. It is important to continue to reassess pain to rule out new sources of pain, such as the development of an abscess, inflammation, or osteoarthritis.

Adjuvant Analgesics. Adjuvant analgesics include antidepressants, some phenothiazines, and hydroxyzine (Vistaril).

The antidepressants amitriptyline (Elavil) and doxepin (Adapin, Sinequan) have been studied for their analgesic effects associated with an increase in serotonin activity in the central nervous system. Drugs that increase the serotonin level in the brain may reduce pain threshold and improve sleep.[87] Antidepressants such as desipramine (Norpramin, Pertofrane) and imipramine (Tofranil) are controversial because they enhance noradrenaline levels.

Although the antidepressant effect may take from 2 to 4 weeks to occur, pain relief may occur in 1 or 2 days. Drowsiness, a side effect of antidepressants, can reduce sleeplessness, a common problem for a patient in pain. Pain relief from antidepressants can be obtained with smaller doses (25 to 75 mg/day) than are needed to produce an antidepressant effect.[41]

Hydroxyzine is classified as a minor tranquilizer with antiemetic, antispasmodic, antihistaminic, and sedative effects. When it is given with an opioid, the dose of the opioid may be reduced.[88] Doses higher than those recommended may cause anticholinergic effects, such as dry mouth and jitteriness. Hydroxyzine frequently is ordered with an opioid on an every-4-hour-prn basis.[88] This may result in the patient's getting higher than the recommended dosage of hydroxyzine.

Promethazine (Phenergan), long used as a potentiator, has been found to have pronounced antianalgesic properties.[41] Other phenothiazines, such as prochlorperazine (Compazine) and trifluoperazine (Stelazine), also produce some antianalgesic effects.

Muscle Relaxants. Muscle spasms from injury, traction, and immobility can contribute significantly to pain in the trauma patient. Muscle relaxants can be useful in interrupting the tension–muscle spasm–pain cycle. (See Table 15–10 for some common muscle relaxants.) Muscle tension reduces the circulation of blood, which results in reduced oxygen to the muscles and nerves. Oxygen deprivation appears to be a direct cause of muscle and nerve pain.[89] Adverse effects with many of the muscle relaxants involve a central nervous system depressant effect and GI irritation. Phenothiazines, antihistamines, opioids, barbiturates, monoamine oxidase inhibitors, tricyclic antidepressants, and alcohol may potentiate their effects. They have some anticholinergic effects.

TABLE 15–10. COMMON SKELETAL MUSCLE RELAXANTS

Single agents
Cyclobenzaprine HCl (Flexeril)
Metaxalone (Skelaxin)
Methocarbamol (Robaxin)
Carisoprodol (Soma)
Chlorzoxazone (Paraflex)
Diazepam (Valium)
Combination skeletal muscle relaxants
Methocarbamol with aspirin (Robaxisal)
Carisoprodol with aspirin (Soma Compound)
Chlorzoxazone and acetaminophen (Parafon Forte)

Nonpharmacological Interventions

The nonpharmacological interventions for the rehabilitation phase of the trauma cycle include transcutaneous nerve stimulation, spinal cord stimulation,[90] physical exercise, psychological interventions for depression, stress management, and patient education.

Transcutaneous Nerve Stimulation. The transcutaneous nerve stimulator (TENS) is a small, battery-operated device that transmits an electric impulse through electrodes placed on the body. It is uncertain how TENS decreases the sensation of pain, but there are several theories, including the production of endorphins as one mechanism of action.[91] Although initially used for chronic pain, TENS has been effective for the relief of acute postoperative pain. Some patients report that pain returns as soon as the stimulator is turned off, whereas others report that relief lasts for a few to many hours. In many hospitals, the physical therapy department is responsible for evaluating the patient for the use of the units and for treatment and follow-up. Clearly, the trauma nurse must facilitate a team approach to provide effective pain management for the trauma patient.

Spinal Cord Stimulation. Spinal cord stimulation, based on the gate control and the opioid receptor theories of pain, involves implanting electrodes in the spinal cord. Spinal cord stimulation is also thought to produce analgesia by stimulation of endogenous opioids. The patient's fibers or tracts that are involved in the activation of pain suppression mechanisms are identified.[92] When the electrodes are implanted, the spinal cord is stimulated with energy just sufficient to produce paresthesia. The patient provides stimulation several times a day, similar to that produced by a TENS unit, according to orders from the physician. Spinal cord stimulators use technology similar to that used in cardiac pacemakers that can be programmed and reprogrammed transcutaneously to alter the amount of energy necessary to produce the desired effect. The electrodes can be placed surgically or percutaneously. Spinal cord stimulation is a relatively new complex technique that is undergoing much research. It has been effective in relieving reflex sympathetic dystrophy, postamputation pain, and pain from spinal cord lesions.

Physical Exercise. Some form of regular exercise that

is specifically planned for the injured part may be necessary for the control of chronic pain. Exercise, leading to increased circulation and oxygenation of the muscles, can promote pain relief. The physician needs to decide when the patient can begin to exercise. With injuries that cause neck and shoulder pain, such as a whiplash injury without any specific injury to other tissue, exercise can begin in a few weeks. Damaged tissue usually heals within this period. The physical therapist can work out a program with the patient.

Psychological Interventions. Some patients with chronic pain have hysterical and hypochrondriacal characteristics. These were once thought to be preexisting personality traits but are now viewed by some experts as adaptive responses to pain. Patients with chronic pain may begin to focus their entire lives around their pain. These patients can be helped to learn strategies to gain control of their pain and their lives.

Depression is common with chronic pain. Patients with chronic pain feel hopeless and out of control and may think that they have no means to end the pain and must live with it forever. Feeling cornered and trapped, they become depressed.

Depression may have preceded the chronic pain because it is the most common type of emotional illness. It affects women more often than men and can occur at any age. Regardless of which came first, chronic pain cannot be effectively treated without concomitantly treating the depression.

Bowen[93] describes chronic physical, emotional, and social dysfunction as a phenomenon that occurs with high levels of anxiety cemented in place by continuous feedback from the family system. Chronic pain may be one of the many symptoms that may continue to persist in families that are less resilient and have a more limited repertoire of coping responses. The continuation of chronic pain may be influenced to a greater extent by the family emotional issues than by the physical and structural damage from the injury.

Work with patients who have chronic pain indicates that many appear to be disconnected from the emotional pain and issues in their lives. To the extent that issues are not expressed or recognized emotionally, it may increase the likelihood that issues get expressed in physical symptoms. Some families express anxiety predominantly in either physical, emotional, or social symptoms, whereas other families demonstrate a mixture of symptoms. Knowledge about a patient's history, including information about the resiliency of the patient and his family and how his family expresses anxiety, may prove useful in anticipating the susceptibility to chronic pain. Early identification may increase the opportunity for a positive response to treatment.

Stress Management. External events in a person's life often cause stress. Stress is associated with increased anxiety, and anxiety is associated with increased pain. Patients with pain need to pay particular attention to the level of stress in their lives. They can achieve some control over their pain by increasing their awareness of how they react to stress and by acquiring some control over their reactivity.

People respond to stress with automatic reactions activated by the sympathetic nervous system. These automatic responses are spontaneous. For survival, humans were genetically programmed with the fight-or-flight response. The ability to return to a normal resting or unstressed physiological state once the need for arousal passes is of particular importance in the control of stress. Some people, after being aroused many times, cannot return to their normal base. Over the years, a person's normal base state may have been raised considerably, so that there is continually some degree of arousal. Hypertension, ulcers, depression, irritability, pain, and an increased use of drugs and alcohol are some of the illness states that may develop.

People may begin to understand and take control of their reactivity through biofeedback,[81] psychotherapy, and progressive relaxation exercises.

Patient Education. The meaning of pain can increase or decrease a patient's perception of its intensity. Patients with chronic pain need to learn that their pain does not mean that they have some fatal illness or that some kind of destructive tissue damage is taking place at the site of pain. The facts pertaining to the existence of chronic pain are not understood, but certainly there is interaction with all three components of pain.

The treatment of chronic pain differs considerably from treatment of acute pain. Patients with chronic pain must take an active role in their treatment. Dealing with one's pain involves more than taking a pill or staying in bed for a few days; it involves a permanent change in life-style. Treatment in the form of physical and relaxation exercises must be continued for the rest of their lives. Chronic-pain support groups may be helpful.

Education includes teaching patients with jaw, neck, and shoulder pain not to lean their heads on their hands. When sitting, people often prop their arms on the arm of a chair and lean their heads on their hands. This position puts pressure on the temporomandibular joints and cervical vertebrae, pulling on muscles and ligaments. Patients with jaw pain should not chew ice, pencils, or their nails. Those with neck and shoulder pain should not carry heavy purses over their shoulders. In addition, people with neck and shoulder pain should not hold the hand set between their ears and shoulders when talking on the phone.

Nursing Evaluation

The evaluation of the patient in the rehabilitation phase of trauma differs little from that in other phases, except that the nurse should be suspicious of any new pain or pain that does not respond to interventions. The early detection and treatment of chronic pain are the major reasons for recommending such diligence in this phase. Of special importance is the early recognition of reflex sympathetic dystrophy, since it responds well to treatment when given early and can be debilitating when the diagnosis is delayed.

Any new intervention should be evaluated to ascertain its effectiveness. An intervention that does not relieve pain should be evaluated for accuracy in administration. The evaluation includes patient input because the patient may have lost faith in the treatment's effectiveness. Careful documentation is crucial because the patient may be transferred to another unit or institution as recovery progresses. Accurate documentation allows for adequate treatment when other nurses are involved in caring for the patient.

SPECIAL ISSUES IN PAIN MANAGEMENT

Pediatric Pain

The pediatric population often receives inadequate pain control. Historically, it was thought that the neurological system in pediatric patients was immature and, consequently, no pain was perceived. Therefore, little or no interventions were instituted for painful procedures or after injury. Moreover, extant research based on the mature animal and human populations was applied to the child. When opioids are ordered, they are given in subtherapeutic doses or at intervals too long to adequately manage pain.[94]

Knowledge of child development is essential in the assessment and management of the pediatric patient. Infants do not have fully developed cerebral cortexes, and their cortical function is minimal. They are unable to localize painful stimuli, and a painful experience may not be remembered. Children aged 2 and under have limited verbal skills and use magic to explain events. Children of this age respond to pain according to past experience. They describe illness in terms of the visual effects; thus, injuries that are visible are also described as being more painful.[95]

Children between the ages of 7 and 11 have developed the ability to provide a more logical explanation for events. Despite their increased ability to reason compared with younger children, their logic is simplistic, and they may still use magical thinking. Children aged 7 to 11 may see pain as a punishment for breaking a rule and are likely to regress to an earlier developmental stage when suffering from pain.

Adolescents aged 12 to 18 years are more likely to conceptualize pain in abstract terms compared with younger children. They are concerned with body image and integrity. Thus, if adolescents are anxious about a possible alteration in their body image, the increased anxiety causes the perceived pain to be more intense than that experienced by an adult.

Researchers must be able to accurately assess pain before interventions can be evaluated and recommendations made based on objective findings. Pain assessment in the pediatric population has recently received attention. Pain research has uncovered much knowledge about the transmission of nociception and factors that influence the perception of pain in the adult. These same factors—expectation of pain, ability to control the painful event, coping abilities, fear, and anxiety—affect a child's perception of pain. Other factors unique to the pediatric population include parental response, the child's ability to predict what will happen, the child's behavior, and attention.[96] Most children who are more distressed experience stronger pain. To optimally manage pain, an accurate pain assessment is essential.

An accurate pain assessment for a child involves the use of tools similar to those used for the adult, with an emphasis on practicality and versatility. Tools should be easy to use in various settings and should be adaptable to children of all ages, cognitive levels, and cultural backgrounds. Pain assessment in the pediatric patient includes the use of behavioral, physiological, projective, and direct response methods.

Behavioral methods for the infant are based on the assumption that the overt response seen is related to the noxious stimulus and perception of pain. The presence or absence of any one or combination of behaviors does not necessarily indicate the quality, intensity, or duration of pain.[96] Typical behaviors in response to noxious stimuli include body movements of the torso and limb, facial expressions, and cries. Behavioral measures of pain in children focus on crying, facial expressions, verbal expressions, torso position, touch behaviors, and position of the legs. These behaviors were included as part of the Children's Hospital of Eastern Ontario Pain Scale, which was developed by McGrath and colleagues.[97] (See Appendix 15–3 for the specific behaviors.) A disadvantage in measures that rate the number and frequency of behaviors is that they do not provide adequate information about the total pain experience. Without more global information, successful interventions are difficult to plan and implement.

Like behaviors, physiological responses do not necessarily indicate the quality, intensity, or duration of pain.[96] The physiological responses, similar to those seen in adults, include an increase in heart and respiratory rates and in blood pressure. Large fluctuations in transcutaneous O_2 levels below 50 and above 100 mm Hg have been noted.[98] Other physiological indices include changes in cortisol levels and palmar sweating.[96] Problems with physiological measures are similar to those in the adult; the response does not necessarily indicate the presence of pain or yield information about the intensity, quality, or duration of the pain. Some of the physiological changes seen in children are directly correlated to the behavioral change of overt distress. The physiological changes occasionally are correlated with the child's subjective report. Changes in endorphin levels are an additional physiological measure used in children.

In addition to behaviors and physiological responses, pain measures for children include projective and direct response methods. Projective methods include colors, shapes, drawings, and cartoons. Much can be learned about a child's pain experience through these measures.

Direct response methods to assess pain in children include the visual analogue scale, pain thermometers, and the Oucher scale.[96] Children aged 5 or older reliably rate pain using a traditional visual analogue scale (see Appendix 15–3). Pain thermometers consist of a vertical or horizontal visual analogue scale with 0 designated *no hurt* and 10 or 100 representing *most hurt possible.* Children point to the level that indicates the severity of pain. These measures have had varied success. Children may not be able to recall the abstract application of numbers to represent the degree of pain. Another problem is that different orientations may be better for different children.[96]

The Oucher scale consists of six photographs of a child's face in different expressions of pain. These photographs are positioned at regular intervals along a vertical numerical scale. This scale is reliable and valid, but there is not sufficient evidence that each face shows an equal degree of pain that increases in intensity.[96]

The management of pain in children involves both pharmacological and nonpharmacological interventions. The pharmacological interventions are the same as for the adult. Morphine and fentanyl are given by both the IM and the IV route. Meperidine is not recommended because of the metabolite normeperidine and the associated central nervous system excitability.[99] The recommended dose of morphine is

0.1 to 0.2 mg/kg and for fentanyl, 2 μg/kg. The adverse effects are the same. PCA (IV and epidural) has been successfully used with children aged 9 or older. It can be used in a younger child who is accustomed to surgical or painful procedures and is what Moyer and Howe[99] call "medically wise."

Nonpharmacological interventions for the infant include holding, rocking, sucking, and providing a position of comfort.[99] The side-lying position is best when possible, since it promotes sleep. The child should be given as much control as possible over the painful experience.[96] If possible, allow the child to choose the time of the painful intervention or the preferred site for an injection. Distraction by reading to the child or talking about a pleasant subject may also be helpful. Another measure the nurse can try to institute is relaxing the parent. The child is less likely to become anxious in the presence of a calm parent.

Pain in the Elderly Patient

Myths concerning the decreased perception of pain in elderly people contribute to misdiagnosis and adverse outcomes. Some elderly patients have decreased sensation to noxious stimuli.[100] A decrease in the transmission of noxious impulses should be associated with disease states rather than age. The affective and cognitive aspects of pain do not change with age.

Accurate pain assessment can be difficult if the patient is confused. This is not to say that all elderly patients are confused, but that nurses should strive to obtain an accurate neurological assessment to determine the best methods to use in the assessment of pain.

Elderly patients are more sensitive to opioids than are other adults. They may respond to a dose of morphine as if it were a fourfold dose. The clearance rate of morphine is also slower in elderly patients. Thus, morphine (and other opioids) must be carefully titrated according to effect. The individualization of dosing is important for this population.

Similar to opioids, the range between therapeutic and toxic effects from NSAIDs is narrower compared with other adults. Because NSAIDs are bound to protein, they can displace drugs from protein binding sites. The elderly patient can be prone to toxic effects of NSAIDs when serum albumin levels are low. Thus, NSAIDs may cause confusion in the predisposed elderly person.[100] Table 15–11 summarizes the drugs used for pain and special considerations for dosing in elderly patients.

Pain in the Head-Injured Patient

Assessing pain in the patient with a head injury is complicated because there is limited access to the subjective self of the patient. The unconscious patient is thought not to perceive pain, but the patient may perceive pain at the earliest level of return of cognitive functioning. This level is characterized by inconsistent and nonpurposeful responses to stimuli of a nonspecific nature. The patient with severe head injury who wakes up a few weeks after the injury usually reports amnesia for the initial few weeks of hospitalization. Most patients with mild concussion to severe head injury report headache pain on awakening.

The patient who has suffered a head injury presents a challenge to the nurse. Pain can be caused by neurological changes alone or, in the case of multisystem injuries, can originate from many sites.

Adequate pain control is essential to prevent the patient from becoming anxious, agitated, or uncooperative. Nonpharmacological interventions should be tried during the resuscitation and critical care phases in the patient for whom drugs would negatively affect neurological assessment. The patient should be stroked or massaged in noninjured areas to promote relaxation and provide distraction. Analgesics that do not affect the central nervous system, such as acetaminophen, can be useful if the pain is not severe. Acetaminophen has the added advantage of being available in rectal suppositories for use in patients who are to receive nothing by mouth.

When nonpharmacological interventions are insufficient, the choice of drug used depends on the patient's neurological status. If the patient is being observed for signs of neurological deterioration, analgesics may be withheld or given in small, frequent doses to avoid central nervous system effects that mask signs of neurological deterioration. In a situation where a mechanically ventilated patient is agitated and appears to be in pain and opioids are contraindicated because of the need to monitor the patient's neurological status, paralytic agents with sedation may be the best choice. Paralytic agents do not alter the perception of pain or interfere with the transmission of noxious impulses. This is the rationale for the use of sedatives with the paralyzing agent. In this situation, the sedatives act to decrease the patient's anxiety. If the patient still appears to be suffering from pain, the nurse should administer a small dose of opioid. The nurse should have naloxone at the bedside in the event that this small dose of opioid does mask neurological indicators.

If the patient has negative neurological findings, pain is not as difficult to manage. An accurate assessment is still necessary, but it may be hampered in patients with a head injury. If the patient's blood pressure is stable and the pain is severe, the opioid of choice is fentanyl or morphine. These opioids can be titrated in small amounts and have the advantage of rapid reversal with naloxone. Fentanyl is a short-acting opioid and may be preferred over morphine. No matter which drug is given, the patient should be carefully observed for signs of respiratory depression.

As soon as feasible, when vital signs are stable and the danger of neurological deterioration has passed, patients with a head injury should be medicated similar to other trauma patients. It is important to continue careful monitoring for adverse effects from analgesics.

CURRENT RESEARCH IN PAIN AND IMPLICATIONS FOR THE FUTURE

The major areas of research include the use of α_2-adrenergic agonists, transdermal clonidine, selective opiate receptor agonists, and pain in the trauma patient.

α_2-Adrenergic Receptors

The α_2-adrenergic agonists reduce the need for opiates during the induction of anesthesia and reduce the dose of

TABLE 15–11. DRUGS USED IN TREATMENT OF PAIN IN ELDERLY PATIENTS

DRUG	DOSAGE CONSIDERATIONS	ADVERSE EFFECTS	SPECIAL CHARACTERISTICS
Narcotic analgesic	Reduce dosage to 25%–50% that of younger patients; clearance reduced; fixed time interval preferred to ad lib or prn dosing	Respiratory depression with excessive doses, especially in patients with chronic obstructive pulmonary disease or sleep apnea; constipation more frequent; bowel regimen needed concurrently; mood alterations, psychomimetic effects, and delirium more frequent	More useful for acute pain than chronic pain; more useful for dull pain than for sharp or colicky pain
Antidepressants	Low doses to avoid frequent adverse effects; single dose at half-strength sufficient because of long half-life	Constipation, postural hypotension, urine retention more frequent; more sensitive to anticholinergic effects, delirium	Drug of choice for chronic deafferentation pain; amitriptyline and trazodone have independent analgesic action useful in nondepressed patients
Carbamazepine	100 mg bid; increase slowly to tolerance	Nausea and sedation can limit compliance; bone marrow depression, hepatic failure, rash, CNS depression can limit use	Effective for trigeminal neuralgia and denervation neuropathy
Benzodiazepines	Increased half-life; lorazepam and oxazepam have shorter half-lives and are more easily metabolized	Sedation, drowsiness, and decreased cognitive performance can persist for some time after drugs are withdrawn.	Education and counseling should be preferred means of reducing anxiety; more useful in patients with musculoskeletal pain; can paradoxically increase pain in some.
Nonsteroidal anti-inflammatories	Higher serum levels because of lowered albumin binding	Salt and water retention; GI bleeding; allergic reactions; blood dyscrasia	Should be administered with meals; should be avoided in patients who are anticoagulated; because ibuprofen and aspirin are nonprescription drugs, patients should be cautioned against excess use
Phenothiazine	Low doses for pain	Sedation, constipation, orthostatic hypotension, urine retention, tardive dyskinesia, extrapyramidal syndromes	Useful for denervation pain, thalamic pain; synergistic with antidepressants; tardive dyskinesia a special risk
Corticosteroids	Use in dose required to treat underlying medical condition (e.g., arthritis, polymyalgia rheumatica)	Osteoporosis; hypothalamic-pituitary suppression; decreased resistance to infection; diabetes mellitus	Not to be used for symptomatic treatment but as needed for medical indication

From Bonica JJ: The Management of Pain. 2nd ed. Philadelphia, Lea & Febiger, 1990, p. 556.

opiate necessary to maintain an adequate depth of anesthesia. The intrathecal administration of α-adrenoceptor agonists produced a significant increase in pain thresholds of rats.[101] Opioid analgesics exert a direct action on the spinal cord and modulate responses to nociceptive stimuli through activation of descending serotonergic and noradrenergic inhibitory pathways. Clonidine, given systemically, suppresses nociceptive reflex and sensory neuronal responses.[102]

In addition to studying the effects of the administration of α-adrenergic agonists alone, others[103] have researched the interaction between α_2-adrenergic agonists and opiate subtypes. These investigators examined the effects of combining low doses of clonidine, an α_2-adrenergic agonist, with the selective μ-agonist DAGO, the less selective μ-agonist morphine, the selective agonist DPDE, and the less selective δ-agonist DADL. All combinations were administered directly onto the spinal cord of 68 cats. The combination of 25 mg of intrathecal morphine and 5 mg of intrathecal clonidine produced synergistic inhibition of noxious stimuli. A similar synergism was noted when an apparent ineffective dose of clonidine was combined with ineffective doses of DPDE and DADL. The synergism between clonidine and opiates appears to involve mediation through δ-receptors.

The authors conclude their study with an important clinical application. If α_2-adrenergic receptors and opiates are synergistic at doses that are ineffective when given alone, the actual dose of opiate can be lower. The lower dose of intrathecal opioid would lessen the adverse effects and still provide adequate analgesia when combined with the α_2-adrenergic receptors.

Other researchers[104] studied the additive and synergistic effects of medetomidine, an α_2-adrenergic agonist, with fentanyl, morphine, and meperidine in rats. The systemic combination of medetomidine and opioids produced an additive effect. The intrathecal administration of morphine and meperidine combinations with medetomidine produced synergistic effects. The authors concluded that the antinociception effects of medetomidine and opioids are the result of spinal mediation.

The synergistic and additive effects of medetomidine and α_2-adrenergic receptor agonists were studied in six healthy male volunteers.[101] Dental pain thresholds, cutaneous thermal sensitivity, and ischemic pain induced by the inflation of a blood pressure cuff were measured. There was no significant change in the intensity of pain induced by dental pain, cutaneous heat, or ischemia. The medetomidine did, however, significantly decrease the unpleasantness produced by the ischemia. The authors conclude that because postherpetic neuralgia has been successfully treated with single doses of oral clonidine, more studies should be conducted. They question whether higher doses would produce analgesia without hypotension. Also, because medetomidine has been shown to produce synergistic effects with opioids in animals, additional studies with humans are warranted.

Transdermal Clonidine Patch

Kirkpatrick[105] studied the effects of a clonidine patch (systemic dose of 0.1 mg) on nine patients with reflex sympathetic dystrophy. Five patients were considered to have sympathetically mediated pain and the others had sympathetically independent pain. The patch was applied to hyperalgesic skin near a joint and changed every 3 days. In patients whose pain was sympathetically mediated, clonidine eliminated or reduced hyperalgesia to mechanical stimuli, improved range of motion, and increased strength of the affected extremity. A reduction in hyperalgesia to mechanical stimuli was reported within 24 to 48 hours after the patch was applied. The pain returned 2 to 3 days after the patch was removed. Clonidine had no effect on patients who were considered to have sympathetically independent pain. Kirkpatrick[105] concluded that the clonidine is acting locally by blocking the release of norepinephrine by activation of the α_2-receptor located on sympathetic terminals. A placebo effect is considered unlikely because of the selective response seen between patients whose pain is and those whose pain is not sympathetically mediated.

Larger clinical trials that are prospective and double-blind need to be conducted to determine the safety and efficacy of the clonidine patch for the treatment of reflex sympathetic dystrophy. The reduction in pain and functional improvements seen in the Kirkpatrick[105] study hold promise for the treatment of this syndrome.

Selective Opiate Agonists

The search for the perfect opioid continues. The perfect opioid would be such that the negative effects from stimulating opiate receptors are avoided while the positive, analgesic effects remain. The μ-receptor has two subtypes, μ_1 and μ_2. The former is responsible for supraspinal analgesia and the latter is responsible for the negative effects of respiratory depression, bradycardia, and physical dependence.[41] Meptazinol is a relatively selective μ_1-agonist that does not produce the effects seen with stimulation of the μ_2 subtype. One hundred milligrams is equivalent to 8 mg of morphine (both given IM). Meptazinol has a rapid onset of action, but the short duration of action (less than 2 hours) is a disadvantage in using this agent.[41] Nausea and vomiting are common adverse effects. Neither physical dependence nor constipation occurs. Miosis is slight. More research is necessary to develop similar agents that would have a longer duration of action.

Trauma Pain Research

The body of research about pain in the trauma population is sparse. Much knowledge has recently accumulated regarding the pathophysiology of pain and the consequences of inadequate pain control, and this knowledge is applicable to the trauma patient. Areas for future research include pain experienced during routine care and diagnostic procedures such as the insertion of central lines or chest tubes, the characteristics of trauma pain, and nursing interventions designed to decrease pain.

Health care professionals inflict pain almost daily while providing patient care to the trauma patient. The insertion of IV and arterial lines, for example, is painful. Because this type of pain is unavoidable and short-lived, some nursing care professionals become accustomed to the pain and may not think about methods to avoid or decrease the suffering. Research regarding this area could pave the way for the clinical application of measures that would alleviate the pain of routine or diagnostic procedures.

Research into the common characteristics of trauma pain is inadequate. Researchers[106] have recently categorized the characteristics of pain reported by burn patients. Using the McGill Pain Questionnaire, visual analogue scale, and measures of depression and anxiety, these researchers noted wide variations in the intensity of pain experienced from patient to patient. The variations in pain were unrelated to demographic characteristics, length of time since injury, or the amount of analgesics that was given. The extent of burns was a significant predictor of pain for the first week after injury. Patients who were more anxious or depressed tended to report greater pain at rest, but higher anxiety and depression levels were not associated with higher pain scores during therapeutic procedures. The authors concluded that more research should be done to further understand the role of anxiety in burn patients.

Common characteristics such as the intensity, timing, and relation of anxiety and pain should be considered in future research. The findings could be applied clinically to assist in the reduction of pain for the trauma patient.

Nursing intervention studies could include specific interventions to decrease pain and the effect of psychological and educational programs for the patient and family on the level of pain. Specific nursing interventions that could be investigated include the administration of small doses of anesthetics before the insertion of IV or arterial lines. Does a small dose of lidocaine (Xylocaine) decrease pain and anxiety during arterial or venous catheterization?

The specific psychological and educational programs used in trauma centers for patients and families could be tabulated and described by a survey. The interventions that health care professionals have found useful could be researched. If specific interventions are widespread, research could be done to document the commonalities, which could then be implemented clinically by others.

REFERENCES

1. Bonica JJ: Definitions and taxonomy of pain. In Bonica JJ (ed): The Management of Pain. 2nd ed. Philadelphia, Lea & Febiger, 1990, pp 18–27.
2. Johnson JE, Rice VH: Sensory and distress components of pain. Nurs Res 23:203–209, 1974.
3. Melzack R, Torgerson WS: On the language of pain. Anesthesiology 34:50–59, 1971.
4. Melzack R: The McGill Pain Questionnaire: Major properties and scoring methods. Pain 1:277–299, 1975.
5. Curro F: Assessing the physiologic and clinical characteristics of acute versus chronic pain. Dent Clin North Am 31:xiii–xxiii, 1987.

6. International Association for the Study of Pain (IASP) Subcommittee on Taxonomy. Pain 6:249–252, 1979.
7. McCaffery M: Nursing Management of the Patient with Pain. 2nd ed. Philadelphia, JB Lippincott, 1979, pp 11, 92, 150, 223, 236.
8. Bonica JJ: Anatomic and physiologic basis of nociception and pain. In Bonica JJ (ed): The Management of Pain. 2nd ed. Philadelphia, Lea & Febiger, 1990, pp 28–94.
9. DeCastro J, Meynadier J, Zenz M: Regional Opioid Analgesia. Dordrecht, Netherlands, Kluwer Academic, 1991.
10. Bonica JJ: Biochemistry and modulation of nociception and pain. In Bonica JJ (ed): The Management of Pain. 2nd ed. Philadelphia, Lea & Febiger, 1990, pp 95–121.
11. Melzack R: Pain mechanisms: A new theory. Science 150:971–979, 1965.
12. Mayer DJ, Wolfle TL, et al: Analgesia from electrical stimulation in the brainstem of the rat. Science 174:1351–1354, 1971.
13. Reynolds DV: Surgery in the rat during electrical analgesia induced by focal brain stimulation. Science 164:444–445, 1969.
14. Pert CB, Snyder SH: Opiate receptor: Demonstration in nervous tissue. Science 179:1011–1014, 1973.
15. Hughes J, Smith TW, Kosterlitz HW, et al: Identification of two related pentapeptides from the brain with potent opiate agonist activity. Nature 258:577–579, 1975.
16. Akil H, Watson SJ, Young E, et al: Endogenous opioids: Biology and function. Annu Rev Neurosci 7:223–255, 1984.
17. Goldstein A: Opioid peptides (endorphins) in pituitary and brain. Science 193:1081–1086, 1976.
18. Millan MJ: Multiple opioid systems and pain. Pain 27:303–347, 1986.
19. Yaksh TL: Spinal opiate analgesia: Characteristics and principles of action. Pain 11:293–346, 1981.
20. Jaffe JH, Martin WR: Opioid analgesics and antagonists. In Gilman AG et al (eds): Goodman and Gilman's The Pharmacological Basis of Therapeutics. 8th ed. New York, Pergamon Press, 1990, p 487.
21. Hughes J: Isolation of an endogenous compound from the brain with pharmacological properties similar to morphine. Brain Res 88:295–308, 1975.
22. Bonica JJ: Postoperative pain. In Bonica JJ (ed): The Management of Pain. 2nd ed. Philadelphia, Lea & Febiger, 1990, pp 461–480.
23. Wild L: Pain management. Crit Care Clin North Am 2:357–547, 1990.
24. Woolf CJ, Wall PD: Relative effectiveness of C primary afferent fibers of different origins in evoking a prolonged facilitation of the flexor reflex in the rat. J Neurosci 6:1433–1442, 1986.
25. Bonica JJ: General considerations of acute pain. In Bonica JJ (ed): The Management of Pain. 2nd ed. Philadelphia, Lea & Febiger, 1990, pp 159–196.
26. Modig J: Respiration and circulation after total hip replacement surgery. Acta Anaesthesiol Scand 20:225–236, 1976.
27. Marks RM, Sachar EJ: Undertreatment of medical inpatients with narcotic analgesics. Ann Intern Med 78:173–181, 1973.
28. Keeri-Szanto M, Heaman S: Postoperative demand analgesia. Surg Gynecol Obstet 134:647–651, 1972.
29. Cohen FL: Postsurgical pain relief: Patients' status and nurses' medication choices. Pain 9:265–274, 1980.
30. Kuhn S, Cooke K, Collins M, et al: Perceptions of pain relief after surgery. Br Med J 300:1687–1690, 1990.
31. Owen H, McMillan V, Rogowski D: Postoperative pain therapy: A survey of patients' expectations and their experiences. Pain 41:303–307, 1990.
32. Donovan BD: Patient attitudes to postoperative pain relief. Anaesth Intensive Care 11:125–129, 1983.
33. Sriwatanakul K, Weis OF, Alloza JL, et al: Analysis of narcotic analgesic usage in the treatment of postoperative pain. JAMA 250:926–929, 1983.
34. Cartwright PD: Pain control after surgery: A survey of current practices. Ann R Coll Surg Engl 67:13–16, 1985.
35. Holm K, Cohen F, Dudas S, et al: Effect of personal pain experience of pain assessment. Image: Journal of Nursing Scholarship 21:72–75, 1989.
36. Taylor AG, Skelton JA, Butcher J: Duration of pain condition and physical pathology as determinants of nurses' assessment of patients in pain. Nurs Res 33:4–8, 1984.
37. Melzack R: The tragedy of needless pain. Sci Am 262:27–33, 1990.
38. Oden RV: Postoperative pain: Incidence and severity. In Ferrante FM, Ostheimer GW, Covino BG (eds): Patient Controlled Analgesia. Boston, Blackwell Scientific, 1990, pp 10–16.
39. Fuller J, Schaller-Ayers J (eds): Pain assessment. In Health Assessment: A Nursing Approach. Philadelphia, JB Lippincott, 1990, pp 286–291.
40. Carpenito LJ: Nursing Diagnosis—Application to Clinical Practice. 4th ed. Philadelphia, JB Lippincott, 1991, pp 227–248.
41. Stoelting RK: Pharmacology and Physiology in Anesthetic Practice. 2nd ed. Philadelphia, JB Lippincott, 1991, pp 1–32.
42. Austin KL, Stapleton JV, Mather LE: Relationship between blood meperidine concentrations and analgesic response: A preliminary report. Anesthesiology 53:460–466, 1980.
43. Shafer SL, Varvel JR: Pharmacokinetics, pharmacodynamics and rational opioid selection. Anesthesiology 74:53–63, 1991.
44. Cousins MJ, Mather LE: Intrathecal and epidural administration of opioids. Anesthesiology 61:276–310, 1984.
45. The promise of transdermal drug delivery. Br J Anaesth 64:7–10, 1990.
46. Latasch L, Luders S: Transdermal fentanyl against postoperative pain. Acta Anaesthesiol Belg 40:113–119, 1989.
47. Belatti RG: Patient-controlled analgesia. Nebr Med J March:49–54, 1989.
48. Lubenow TR, Ivankovich AD: Patient-controlled analgesia for postoperative pain. Crit Care Clin North Am 3:35–41, 1991.
49. Tamsen A, Hartvig P, Fagerlund C, Dahlstrom B: Patient-controlled analgesic therapy. II. Individual analgesic demand and analgesic plasma concentrations of pethidine in postoperative pain. Clin Pharmacokinet 7:164–175, 1982.
50. Egan KJ: What does it mean to be "in control"? In Ferrante FM, Ostheimer GW, Covino BG (eds): Patient Controlled Analgesia. Boston, Blackwell Scientific, 1990, pp 17–26.
51. Wang JK, Nasuss LA, Thomas JE: Pain relief by intrathecally applied morphine in man. Anesthesiology 50:149–151, 1979.
52. Behar M, Olswang D, Magora F, Davidson JT: Epidural morphine in the treatment of pain. Lancet 1:527–529, 1979.
53. Scott DB: Acute pain management. In Cousins MJ, Bridenbaugh PO (eds): Neural Blockade in Clinical Anesthesia and Management of Pain. 2nd ed. Philadelphia, JB Lippincott, 1988, pp 861–881.
54. Bromage PR, Camporesi EM, Durant PAC, Nielsen CH: Nonrespiratory side effects of epidural morphine. Anesth Analg 61:490–495, 1982.
55. Boudreault D, Brasseur L, Samii K, Lemoing JP: Comparison of continuous epidural infusion or patient-controlled epidural injection of fentanyl for postoperative analgesia. Anesth Analg 73:132–137, 1991.
56. Logas WG, El-Baz N, El-Ganzouri A, et al: Continuous thoracic epidural analgesia for postoperative pain relief following thoracotomy: A randomized prospective study. Anesthesiology 67:787–791, 1987.
57. Versed brand of midazolam HCL/Roche. Nutley, NJ, Hoffman-LaRoche, Inc, Product Information, 1987.
58. Murray MJ: Pain problems in the ICU. Crit Care Clin North Am 6:235–254, 1990.
59. Ferrante FM, Orav EJ, Rocco AG, Gallo J: A statistical model for pain in patient-controlled analgesia and conventional intramuscular opioid regimens. Anesth Analg 67:457–461, 1988.
60. Crews JC: Epidural opioids. Crit Care Clin North Am 6:315–342, 1990.
61. Bailey PL, Pace NL, Ashburn M, et al: Frequent hypoxemia and apnea after sedation with midazolam and fentanyl. Anesthesiology 73:826–830, 1990.
62. Wood M: Opioid agonists and antagonists. In Wood M, Wood AJJ (eds): Drugs and Anesthesia—Pharmacology for Anesthesiologists. 2nd ed. Baltimore, Williams & Wilkins, 1990, pp 152–153, 156.

63. Sufenta information. JPI-SU-040. Piscataway, NJ, Janssen Pharmaceutica, 1990.
64. Flacke JW, Bloor BC, Kripke BJ, Flacke WE, Warmeck CM, VanEtten AP, Wong DH, Katz RL: Comparison of morphine, meperidine, fentanyl, sufentanil in balanced anesthesia: a double-blind study. Anesth Analg 64:897–910, 1985.
65. Willens JS: Action stat: Disconnected epidural catheter. Nursing91 21:33, 1991.
66. Cousins MJ, Bridenbaugh PO (eds): Neural Blockade in Clinical Anesthesia and Management of Pain. 2nd ed. Philadelphia, JB Lippincott, 1988.
67. Bragg CL: Interpleural analgesia. Heart Lung 20:30–38, 1991.
68. Lee VC: Non-narcotic modalities for the management of acute pain. Crit Care Clin North Am 6:451–481, 1990.
69. Mather L, Phillips G: Opioids and adjuvants: Principals of use. In Cousins M, Phillips G (eds): Clinics in Critical Care Medicine. Acute Pain Management. New York, Churchill Livingstone, 1986, pp 73–103.
70. Teeple E: Pharmacology and physiology of narcotics. Crit Care Clin North Am 6:255–282, 1990.
71. Brown CR, Mazzulla JP, Mok MS, et al: Comparison of repeat doses of intramuscular ketorolac tromethamine and morphine sulfate for analgesia after major surgery. Pharmacotherapy 10:45S–50S, 1990.
72. Spindler JS, Mehlisch D, Brown CR: Intramuscular ketorolac and morphine in the treatment of moderate to severe pain after major surgery. Pharmacotherapy 10:51S–58S, 1990.
73. Toradol (ketorolac tromethamine). Prescribing information. Palo Alto, Calif, Syntex Laboratories, March 1990.
74. Insel PA: Analgesic-antipyretics and antiinflammatory agents: Drugs employed in the treatment of rheumatoid arthritis and gout. In Gilman AG et al (eds): Goodman and Gilman's The Pharmacological Basis of Therapeutics. 8th ed. New York, Pergamon Press, 1990, pp 638–681.
75. Newman R: The need to redefine "addiction." N Engl J Med 308:1096–1098, 1983.
76. Porter J, Jick H: Addiction rare in patients treated with narcotics. N Engl J Med 302:123, 1980.
77. Vandalfsen PJ, Syrjala KL: Psychological strategies in acute pain management. Crit Care Clin North Am 6:421–431, 1990.
78. Melzack R, Guite S, Gonshor A: Relief of dental pain by ice massage of the hand. Can Med Assoc J 122:189, 1980.
79. Melzack R, Schecter B: Itch and vibration. Science 26:1048, 1965.
80. Marckovich S, Giula M, Beal J: Electrophysical aspects of the pain response: Relating TNS to skin resistance and bioelectric impedance measurements. Paper presented at Conference on Pain Management, Des Plaines, Ill, May 14, 1977.
81. Doody SB, Smith C, Webb J: Nonpharmacologic interventions for pain management. Crit Care Clin North Am 3:69–76, 1991.
82. Johnson J: Stress reduction through sensory information. In Sarason I, Speilberger C (eds): Stress and Anxiety, Vol 2. New York, John Wiley & Sons, 1975, pp 361–378.
83. Achterberg J: Imagery and Healing: Shamanism and Modern Medicine. Boston, New Science Library, 1985, pp 3, 293, 205.
84. Muse M: The stress-related post-traumatic chronic pain syndrome: Criteria for diagnosis and preliminary report on prevalence. Pain 23:295, 1985.
85. Muse M: Stress-related post-traumatic chronic pain syndrome: Behavioral treatment approach. Pain 25:389, 1986.
86. Wenger G: Antianxiety drugs. In Craig C, Stitzel R (eds): Modern Pharmacology. Boston, Little, Brown, 1982, p 530.
87. Hendler N: Diagnosis and Nonsurgical Management of Chronic Pain. New York, Raven Press, 1981, pp 121–133.
88. Crippen DW: The role of sedation in the ICU patient with pain and agitation. Crit Care Clin North Am 6:369–392, 1990.
89. Bonica JJ, Teitz CC: Pain due to musculoskeletal injuries (including sports injuries). In Bonica JJ (ed): The Management of Pain. 2nd ed. Philadelphia, Lea & Febiger, 1990, pp 368–386.
90. Mackersie RC, Karagianes TG: Pain management following trauma and burns. Crit Care Clin North Am 6:433–449, 1990.
91. Sjoluand BH, Eriksson M, Loeser JD: Transcutaneous and implanted electric stimulation of peripheral nerves. In Bonica JJ (ed): The Management of Pain. 2nd ed. Philadelphia, Lea & Febiger, 1990, pp 1852–1861.
92. Meyerson BA: Electrical stimulation of the spinal cord and brain. In JJ Bonica (ed): The Management of Pain. 2nd ed. Philadelphia, Lea & Febiger, 1990, pp 1862–1877.
93. Bowen M: Theory and the practice of psychotherapy. In Guerin P (ed): Family Therapy Theory and Practice. New York, Gardner Press, 1976, pp 42–89.
94. Foster R, Hester N: The relationship between assessment and pharmacologic intervention for pain in children. In Funk SG, Tornquist EM, Champagne MT, et al (eds): Key Aspects of Comfort: Management of Pain, Fatigue, and Nausea. New York, Springer, 1989, pp 72–79.
95. Tyler DC: Pain in infants and children. In Bonica JJ (ed): The Management of Pain. 2nd ed. Philadelphia, Lea & Febiger, 1990, pp 538–551.
96. McGrath PA: Pain assessment in children—a practical approach. Advances in Pain Research and Therapy 15:5–30, 1990.
97. McGrath P, Johnson G, Goodman JT, et al: CHEOPS: A behavioral scale for rating post-operative pain in children. Advances in Pain Research and Therapy 9:395–402, 1985.
98. Eland JM, Coy JA: Assessing pain in the critically ill child. Focus Crit Care 17:469–475, 1990.
99. Moyer SMR, Howe CJ: Pediatric intervention in the PACU. Crit Care Clin North Am 3:49–58, 1991.
100. Harkins SW, Kwetus J, Price DD: Pain and suffering in the elderly. In Bonica JJ (ed): The Management of Pain. 2nd ed. Philadelphia, Lea & Febiger, 1990, pp 552–560.
101. Danzebrink RM, Gebhart GF: Antinociceptive effects of intrathecal adrenoreceptor agonists in a rat model of visceral nociception. J Pharmacol Exp Ther 253:698–705, 1990.
102. Kauppila T, Kemppainen P, Tanila H, Pertovaara A: Effect of systemic medetomidine, an $alpha_2$ adrenoceptor agonist, on experimental pain in humans. Anesthesiology 74:3–8, 1991.
103. Omote K, Kitahata LM, Collins JG, et al: Interaction between opiate subtype and alpha-2 adrenergic agonists in suppression of noxiously evoked activity of WDR neurons in the spinal dorsal horn. Anesthesiology 74:737–743, 1991.
104. Ossipov MH, Harris S, Lloyd P, et al: Antinociceptive interaction between opioids and medetomidine: Systemic additivity and spinal synergy. Anesthesiology 73:1227–1235, 1990.
105. Kirkpatrick AF: Treatment of reflex sympathetic dystrophy by local application of the clonidine patch. Reg Anesth 17:64, 1992.
106. Choiniere J, Melzack R, Tondeau J, et al: Pain of burns: Characteristics and correlates. J Trauma 29:1531–1539, 1989.

16

THE DEMAND FOR TRAUMA REHABILITATION

KAREN J. KLENDER HEIST

The specialty of trauma has evolved over the past 20 years along with great strides in medical technology. Emergency services have become highly sophisticated, creating the ability to save lives of even the most severely injured people. The introduction of rapid transport from the scene of injury, often involving air transportation, along with our increasingly mobile and active society have resulted in a new population of injured people, those who probably would have died one or two decades ago.

Without fully realizing the impact of saving the lives of the severely injured, emergency and critical care services have created a demand in health care for services that restore the quality of life to those people who have been salvaged from injury. The result is the specialty practice of trauma rehabilitation. In recent years, the ramifications of recovery from injury have been fully realized. Health care providers are recognizing that the long-term needs of the injured are not being met. Needs continue to be identified and services designed to complete the cycle of trauma care.

Trauma rehabilitation begins the instant health care services are provided to a trauma patient. At first, the focus is preventing further injuries by thorough assessment and stabilization. As the patient stabilizes, the focus changes to restoring and maximizing function. Rehabilitation provides for physical, intellectual, and psychosocial needs at each point throughout the trauma cycle.

This chapter provides an explanation of the relation between the concept of rehabilitation and the trauma patient and describes the rehabilitation process at various points in the cycle. The philosophy of rehabilitation is essential to any practicing nurse, from emergency and critical care to rehabilitation hospitals and transitional and home care. Nurses must think as rehabilitation professionals throughout the trauma cycle.

As the specialty of trauma rehabilitation evolves, political, ethical, societal, and professional issues emerge. Some of the issues are presented in this chapter, but for an in-depth understanding of rehabilitation legislation and political issues, the reader is referred to other texts and resources that are available through politically active advocacy groups.[1]

Definition of Rehabilitation

Rehabilitation is a dynamic process of maximizing an impaired person's potential by utilizing competencies and altering deficits to achieve the best quality of life possible.[2] It involves prevention of further injury, stabilization and restoration of function, and compensation and adaptation to disability.

Among the factors that affect the success of patients' rehabilitation, the most influential are the goals set by the patients for themselves. It is the role of the rehabilitation professional to assist and support patients until they take full responsibility for themselves.[3]

History of Trauma Rehabilitation

The focus of trauma rehabilitation has changed in its short existence. In the early stages, it was defined as "physical medicine," primarily referring to restoration of physical ability and compensating for and adapting to physical disability.[4] This remains the current perception in much of society. Most early strides in rehabilitation occurred through work with patients with chronic diseases such as polio and with disabled veterans, many of them spinal cord–injured patients and amputees. Other types of rehabilitation, such as psychiatric, substance abuse, learning disability, and mental retardation, received far less attention and understanding from society. Therefore, most of the early rehabilitation programs were geared to the treatment of the physically diseased, injured, and disabled.

Vocational rehabilitation grew out of this physical illness perception. Once adaptation to a physical disability had occurred, the next step was return to work. Vocational rehabilitation programs involve extensive evaluation of the patient's physical capabilities followed by job testing, training, and placement. It is important to understand the beginnings of rehabilitation in physical medicine and vocational services to recognize the deficits in today's rehabilitation systems. The need for physical, cognitive, and psychosocial rehabilitation is poorly understood by professionals, patients, families, society, legislators, and third-party payers.

The introduction of the severely head-injured person into the rehabilitation population has forced society and health care professionals to become aware of all the needs of the trauma patient. More than any other population, head-injured people require a focus on the cognitive as well as the physical and psychosocial issues by all disciplines working with them. It is impossible for a physical therapist to work only with the patient's spasticity and ignore a shortened attention span and memory loss. It is impossible for a speech pathologist to isolate concentration tasks and ignore motor control problems. The head-injury population has expanded rehabilitation from the limited focus of physical and vocational goals to comprehensive physical, cognitive, and psychosocial goals. Additionally, the knowledge gained and techniques learned from the treatment of mental illness, learning disability, and substance abuse have been integrated into trauma rehabilitation. These improvements in rehabilitation programming better meet the needs of all trauma patients, not just those who have head injuries.

There has been a proliferation of rehabilitation services in the past decade. According to the National Association of Rehabilitation Facilities (NARF), the number of beds allocated for use by rehabilitation patients has increased from 15,204 in 1985 to 29,544 as of September 1991.[5] Even with this rate of growth, the availability of services has not kept pace with the recognition of needs. Appropriate services are not conveniently available to all trauma patients because of the specialized services required and the level of reimbursement provided for that specialized service. It is not unusual for patients to go out of state or across the country for rehabilitation programs that meet their needs. This does not easily support continuity from the rehabilitative setting to the patient's home and family. It also interferes with the patient's return to social and family roles, since visitors and home visits are few. For the patient to be rehabilitated, it is important that the rehabilitation program be part of the patient's community.

TRAUMA POPULATIONS THAT REQUIRE REHABILITATION

All trauma patients require some degree of rehabilitation. It may be as simple as patient and family education done by the emergency department staff to identify complications and the need for follow-up services for a patient with a minor head injury. The omission of this rehabilitative teaching can result in devastating neglect of critical rehabilitative concerns. The severely injured require rehabilitation that is specially designed for diagnostic groups. Patterns of patient needs evolve with each type of injury. The most common diagnostically differentiated rehabilitation programs in trauma are for spinal cord injury, brain injury, orthopedic and soft-tissue injury, and multiple trauma. Sometimes the latter two groups are combined. Pediatric and adult rehabilitation are also seen as distinct subspecialties in rehabilitation. Each of these groups require different rehabilitation program components, including facilities, equipment, mix of professionals, and approaches to treatment. The Commission on Accreditation of Rehabilitation Facilities provides and evaluates standards for comprehensive inpatient rehabilitation, spinal cord injury, brain injury, post acute rehabilitation, comprehensive outpatient rehabilitation, pain rehabilitation, and various other specialized rehabilitation programs. These standards are considered the expected level of practice by today's rehabilitation providers.[6]

Spinal cord–injury programs focus on life-changing physical disability. A great deal of focus is on relearning physical activities, using compensatory methods and adaptive devices. A large portion of the program involves patient teaching. It requires a motivated patient with enough self-directedness to become independent and avoid complications. Psychosocial support is a major component. The patient must learn to adapt to the disability physically and psychologically to be successfully rehabilitated.[7] Advances in computer technology, electrical muscle stimulation, and research in nerve cell growth are shaping the future of spinal cord–injury rehabilitation. (See Chapter 18 for additional information.)

The head-injured population requires a different focus. The type of rehabilitation is related to the degree of deficit resulting from the injury.[8] Patients in coma require multisensory stimulation and prevention of physical complications caused by immobility. Confused patients or those with inappropriate behavior need specific behavioral modification and therapeutic behavioral approaches, including secured settings for some cases. Cognitive functioning and social awareness are treated by all team members. The physical effects of brain injury are as varied as the cognitive deficits. (See Chapter 17 for information specific to the head-injured patient.)

The teaching component of brain injury rehabilitation is also different. Because of cognitive and behavioral deficits in the patient, most of the teaching about the injury, its effects, and management of problems is done with the patient's family and support systems. As the patient recovers enough insight to learn and use the information, more teaching is done with the patient. This is also true in the provision of psychosocial support. Rehabilitation research relates on-going support to improved long-term outcome.[9] Societal acceptance and community reintegration are key areas of brain injury rehabilitation programming for the future.

Patients with orthopedic or soft-tissue injuries or those with multiple system trauma need a rehabilitation program with both medical and surgical emphasis. These patient populations need an extended period for multiple reconstructive surgeries and the corresponding healing process. Attention is given to prevention of infection and other complications during tissue healing. Physical changes, such as amputations, may require the use of prosthetic or adaptive devices. Psychosocial support addresses changes in body image, loss of independence and control, self-esteem, and associated concerns. The teaching emphasis commonly is on the patient's physical care needs.

COMPONENTS OF REHABILITATION

Although certain trauma populations require a specialized program for the best rehabilitative success, several components are common to all rehabilitation programs, regardless of the setting. Two key elements are a team approach to maximizing the patient's potential and the development of an individualized rehabilitation plan.

Rehabilitation Team

Like other specialties in health care, trauma rehabilitation requires teamwork. The concept of a team being a group of people working toward a common goal is simplistic but taken quite literally in the rehabilitation setting. Inherent in team philosophy is congruency in goals, consistency in approach, and communication among all team members.[10] Most teams exclusively treat a set group of patients and meet frequently to discuss the patients' progress.

Early rehabilitation teams were called multidisciplinary, with each specialty having separate goals and approaches. This method offered the benefit of input from many specialties to the patient's plan of care, but each discipline had individual goals. Fragmentation of care became a major problem.

The interdisciplinary team has alleviated fragmentation. Each member of the team focuses on a particular area of expertise, which is brought to the team to be blended with the expertise of other team members. Patient goals are developed by the team rather than by each discipline. An example of this is the cooperative development of behavior modification strategies. A consistent approach to patient behavior enhances the program's success.

The latest evolution in team dynamics, the transdisciplinary team, is similar to the interdisciplinary team in the method in which mutual goals are formed. Team members bring their special expertise to the team. The distinguishing characteristic in this model is that each member is responsible for sharing observations about all aspects of the patient's rehabilitation. An observer of the team would find it more difficult to determine each member's primary discipline, based on their verbal input in a team meeting. Disciplines may approach therapeutic treatments together rather than individually, as in the past. Physical and occupational therapists have joint therapy sessions with the patient to establish the most appropriate custom wheelchair for proper positioning. A speech pathologist, occupational therapist, and rehabilitation nurse may schedule a mealtime session with the dysphagic patient for assessment and establishment of approaches to feeding.

Each team specialist has the ability to step beyond his or her own discipline into the overall functional goals for the patient. It takes mature and secure team members to let go of the traditional realm associated with each discipline, allowing others to make observations in their discipline, while stepping into the perspective of fellow team members.

Composition of the Team

The team is composed of everyone who has input to the rehabilitation plan. The number can range from 3 to 25 persons. Team membership is determined by two factors: the diagnosis and the phase of the trauma cycle (Table 16–1). Different injuries require a set complement of appropriate specialists who are able to meet the comprehensive needs of the patient. In many cases, the mix of team members reflects more physical rehabilitation emphasis in the early phases, and the cognitive and psychosocial components are brought into play further along in the cycle. By the time the patient is in the reintegration phase, the physical issues may have been resolved, leaving a team mix focused primarily on psychosocial adaptation after injury.

All members of the team are essential to the patient's success. Some disciplines, such as nursing and social services, remain involved with the patient throughout the cycle, but the focus of their involvement changes over time. Other primary team members are involved for limited periods, working with the patient through the intermediate and rehabilitation phases, where most of the traditionally understood rehabilitation occurs. For example, physical, occupational, speech, and respiratory therapies are intensively active during these times.

The essential member of the rehabilitation team is the patient. It is the responsibility of the professionals on the team to help the patient understand his or her active role on the team. In many rehabilitative settings, patients are called clients to indicate the cooperative investment in recovery between the injured person and the rehabilitation professionals. As the patient moves through the cycle, he or she

TABLE 16–1. CHANGES IN TEAM MEMBERSHIP AND FOCUS THROUGHOUT THE TRAUMA CYCLE

	CRITICAL CARE PHASE	INTERMEDIATE PHASE	REHABILITATION PHASE	REINTEGRATION PHASE
Rehabilitation Focus	Life saving is priority. Focus on prevention of further injury or debilitation.	Prevent complications of injury and immobility.	Restoration of function and compensation for disability.	Adaptation to abilities and disabilities in community/home life.
Team Member and Role				
Patient, family, significant others	Passive and dependent role (may be in crisis), provide data base for patient.	Support physical healing; learn about injury, potential problems, and process of rehabilitation; psychosocial support system; more active input to plan of care.	Determine goals with team; process of learning skills, practicing and testing new situations; make realistic plans for future.	Selfdetermining, utilize team as resource consultants, establish lifelong plan.
Medicine	Emergency stabilization and treatment.	Promote physical healing, may involve many specialists, introduce physiatrist as consultant.	Physiatrist primarily, with medical consultants.	Follow-up as indicated, lifelong physical adaptation.
Nursing	Stabilization, physical treatment, support in crisis.	Promote healing, holistic assessment of recovery process, patient/family teaching.	Integrates therapy gains into 24-hour daily routine, patient and family teaching.	Screening, assessment for areas of difficulty in adaptation.
Social worker	Crisis intervention, collect psychosocial data base.	Psychosocial support—grieving, financial process, referral planning.	Planning for reintegration process, resources for family and patient.	Support and referral during adaptation, peer support groups.
Physical therapy		Initial assessment of rehabilitation potential, prevent immobility problems.	Active restoration, compensation, and adaptation.	Consultant role or single service provider.
Occupational therapy		Initial assessment of rehabilitation potential, prevent immobility problems, begin self-care.	Active restoration, compensation, and adaptation.	Consultant role or single service provider.
Cognitive, speech, and audiology specialists		Initial assessment of rehabilitation potential, alternative communication, swallowing, cognitive remediation.	Active restoration, compensation, and adaptation.	Consultant role or single service provider.
Vocational counselor		May be consultant, early assessment.	Assessment, retraining, and job placement.	Consultant role.
Therapeutic recreation		May be consultant.	Integration of new skills into a quality leisure life-style.	Consultant role.
Possible consultants	Variety of medical specialists, clergy, respiratory therapy.	Respiratory therapy, psychologist-neuropsychologist, financial planner, medical and nursing specialists, dietitian.	Same as for intermediate phase plus prosthetics, orthotics, biomedical engineering.	Potentially any health care provider based on long-term patient and family need.
Payer	Informed of initial injury.	Insurance specialist may plan for transfer to acute and other rehabilitation programs.	Find most cost-effective rehabilitation gains.	Lifelong plan for finances, responsibility shifted to patient.

releases the sick role and returns to a status of self-responsibility.[11]

To ensure that the most appropriate and individualized team is created, someone must have the global view of the patient. The team leader sets the tone for the team's interactions and ability to function. The team leader usually determines which specialists will be part of the team.

Team Leadership

Another aspect of team dynamics is leadership style. Various models of leadership exist. The physician-dominated team, the multidisciplinary team, the rehabilitation coordinator role, and the case manager role are discussed in this section.

Early models of team leadership involved a physician-led team. In these situations, the physician would request specific input from therapists to formulate medically stated patient goals. The advantage of this system was consistency of goals for all members. But with limited input and impact by a variety of disciplines, the goals were based on one person's perspective. Most rehabilitation goals were focused on physical medicine, often neglecting cognitive and psychosocial needs.

The disciplines gradually took on a stronger role. Members of each discipline would report their own observations and treatment plans to the physician and the other team members. Goals were formulated by each discipline. This provided greater input to treatment for the patient, but the problem of fragmentation became apparent. At times, the goals of two disciplines were completely opposite.

In an effort to create a more congruent plan, the role of the rehabilitation coordinator was created. Rehabilitation teams established this new role to pull together the fragmented, multidisciplinary efforts of the team. The team meetings are led by either the physician or the rehabilitation coordinator, blending the goals of all team members into overall functional goals for the patient. A rehabilitation plan is established that addresses physical, cognitive, and psychosocial issues as well as defined rehabilitation potential and a discharge plan. The rehabilitation coordinator has only informal influence over the other members of the team while having the responsibility to ensure a quality and individualized rehabilitation program for the patient.

The role of the case manager was introduced when the focus in health care switched from predominantly quality of care issues to cost-effective quality care. The role of the case manager initially began in the health care insurance industry.[12] Facility-based case management has become the standard of practice for many rehabilitation programs.

The case manager, who typically is a registered nurse, oversees the ongoing progress and treatment of patients who have experienced catastrophic events, which are known to be extremely expensive. They coordinate a rehabilitation plan that not only is clinically advantageous to the patient but also extends the patient's health care funding to the maximal benefit projected over the long-term course of recovery. Some case managers, often those hired by the third-party payer, follow the case over the patient's lifetime, spanning multiple-provider settings.[13] Case managers working for an individual provider do not follow the patient over the life-span; however, a responsible case manager considers the future impact of decisions made in a single-provider setting.[14]

In an age when numerous diagnostic evaluation methodologies and specialized treatments exist, the case manager coordinates the most appropriate rehabilitation strategies based on the assessment of the patient and the experience of the clinical team. When an order for a custom wheelchair is requested, the case manager tries to project the cost against the length of time the chair would be appropriate for the patient. For a patient who is making successive physical gains, an adaptable chair might be the wiser choice. On the other hand, a physically stable or nonprogressing patient might maximize the use of a custom chair designed for his current status. An analysis of purchase versus rental may enter into the decision. By selectively using funds, the patient actually receives more effective rehabilitation because it is given at the most appropriate time for the patient's maximum gain. In this way, the patient's funds are stretched over a long-term plan as opposed to an intensive short-term program that exhausts funds and leaves the patient with no long-term support.

The case manager functions similarly to the rehabilitation coordinator, improving on the ability to effect change in the patient's therapeutic plan. A typical facility-based case management work load is 8 to 12 patients, depending on the severity and complexity of the cases. A rehabilitation program would have a number of case managers, each leading team conferences for their case load. Although in other models the physician was the team leader, case management changes the physician's role. In a truly collaborative approach, the physician, providing specialized medical input, is an equal partner in developing a rehabilitation plan.

Both the case manager and the rehabilitation coordinator roles are excellent career ladder opportunities for rehabilitation nurses. These roles demand a rehabilitation professional who can step beyond his or her own discipline and into a holistic clinical and financial perspective as the patient's advocate. The nursing profession lends itself easily to support a role of this nature; however, case managers and coordinators practice with a variety of professional backgrounds. In settings without case management, nursing may identify this as a new opportunity, resulting in improved patient care, cost savings, and an elevated level of function for the nurse.

Regardless of team leadership styles, one goal is paramount: As the patient becomes more physically, cognitively, and psychosocially independent, he or she gradually becomes the case manager. A fully independent person uses the resources and consultation of the health care system but makes his or her own decisions.

Rehabilitation Plan

Rehabilitation Potential

Thorough assessment and evaluation of rehabilitation potential are the first steps toward rehabilitation. Although it is difficult to predict a final outcome after trauma, there are parameters that help to determine the amount and rate of a patient's potential progress. These factors represent the patient's strengths and weaknesses in the areas of physical, cognitive, and psychosocial functioning.[3, 15] Other factors that influence rehabilitation potential are the patient's age, length of time since injury, and availability of resources.

Physical Factors. For some injuries, there are well-established physical limits owing to normal anatomy and physiology. These limits change as technology and expertise increase. Twenty years ago, a C6 quadriplegic patient would not have been able to become functionally independent. Today this is possible. Perhaps in the future, there will be no physical limits because medical technology will be able to replace, rebuild, or stimulate the growth of a new spinal cord. It is important that rehabilitation professionals maintain their awareness of current research in rehabilitation outcomes so that their patients can achieve maximum physical outcomes. Concurrent diagnoses are an influencing factor in rehabilitation potential. Many trauma patients have multiple injuries, pre-existing conditions, or complications of trauma that significantly impact on their potential to recover.

Cognitive and Psychosocial Factors. If physical limitation were the only factor determining rehabilitation potential, then two similar injuries would result in the same outcome. Cognitive and psychosocial factors influence rehabilitation outcome as well. Cognitive factors include the patient's affinity for learning, ability to process and understand information, ability to make appropriate judgments and decisions, educational level, readiness to learn, and prior experiences and many other complex factors. Psychosocial supports, including income, family system, outside stressors, roles, relationships, personal identity, and coping ability, affect the patient's potential. A motivated patient with sufficient financial resources and a supportive family living nearby is thought to be the ideal rehabilitation candidate. This is not the common scenario in trauma rehabilitation, however.

Evaluating Rehabilition Potential. The evaluator first defines the rehabilitation outcome that would be typical for the patient's injury. Then the potential is further defined by assigning a probability factor or percentage of predicted success to the estimated outcome. A candidate who has had a typical below-the-knee amputation may have excellent potential for return to work and former life-style with a prothesis. However, when the evaluator factors in that the candidate is 53 years old and mildly mentally retarded, lives alone, and has sustained multiple infections and stump revisions during the acute phase, the candidate's potential for success may drop to 70 per cent of the typical outcome. Recognizing these probability factors provides rehabilitation professionals with a clearer picture that the candidate either will need significantly greater resources or may not be able to reach the standard desirable outcome.

Rehabilitation potential should not be a question of yes or no or good or poor. The rehabilitation assessment summarizes the positive aspects that will support rehabilitative efforts and considers strategies to work with or around the negative aspects to prevent a failure. Nearly every patient has some potential for improvement, but the potential must be weighed against what is both cost-effective and a reasonable expectation for patient success.

Rehabilitation was traditionally defined as a return to work and home life. This outcome was expected to occur in the time constraints of the relatively few rehabilitation program options—acute physical rehabilitation and vocational counseling and training. There has been a change in thinking. Current desired outcome is the improvement of the quality of life. Time frames are subject to patient needs. From the quality of care perspective, individual expected outcomes and rate of recovery dictate the type of rehabilitation program that is best for the patient. As health care costs increase and treatment options multiply, cost-benefit analysis is a critical element in the evaluation of rehabilitation potential. The ability of the rehabilitation industry to measure its success and failure in outcomes will greatly influence future decisions.

Realistic goals are set for the patient and an estimated time for achievement is established. If these goals are individualized and sensitive to the patient's strengths and weaknesses, any patient should have good rehabilitation potential for his or her unique goals.

Goal Development

The development of long- and short-term goals is a flexible process. The goals are adjusted with progress and influencing factors. Long-term goals reflect a period of the patient's life or even a lifelong goal. Short-term goals are the achievable steps toward the overall long-term goal. Goals have a functional outcome in the patient's life, rather than the achievement of a singular skill that does not alone improve quality of life. This can even be true of a patient who is in a persistent vegetative state after a severe brain injury. Increased range of motion alone is not a functional goal. However, the resulting improved chair positioning to provide increased variety of stimulation, improved ability for hygiene, or decreased spasticity, allowing heightened awareness to stimuli, are functional goals that are benefited by increased range of motion. To establish a functional goal, the team considers the realistic and appropriate outcomes for the individual patient. Ambulation for 20 feet is not a functional goal, but the patient's ability to get to and from the bathroom is functional. Ambulation becomes part of that goal.

For rehabilitation to be successful, there must be mutuality of goals between the patient and the rehabilitation specialists.[11] Mutuality is defined as a unified acceptance and agreement by both parties of what will be achieved. It should be based on the patient's value system, not that of the professional. Initially, after the trauma occurs, the patient takes a fairly passive position in the plan of care. The patient usually agrees to follow the regimen or to allow treatments without much thought or question. As the crisis period subsides, the patient becomes more actively interested and involved in decision making.

Working with a compliant patient often is considered an ideal situation. This assumption is extremely misleading. Even the term *compliance* suggests that the decision and plan are created and enforced by outside sources. It is the patient, not the staff, who has the ultimate responsibility for outcome. The patient should be included as an equal partner in the decision-making process. Values play a major role in the functional goals set by both the staff and the patient. A values conflict should be recognized openly, and mutual goals agreed on. Education in values clarification is helpful to staff members working in rehabilitation to prepare for these conflicts.

Implementation of the Plan

Individualized strategies for the implementation of the rehabilitation plan are developed for all functional goals.[6] Any strategy to be used should be understood by all team members to avoid incongruent techniques that ultimately will deteriorate functional gains in both areas. Strategies used to achieve restoration of function are different from those used to compensate for disability.

Therapy implementation is traditionally thought to be a one-on-one session. Therapists have recently changed their approach and work with a group of patients or convene a mix of disciplines to work with one patient. This frequently occurs in the rehabilitation or reintegration phases of the cycle.

In the first option, functional goal groups are created, such as social skills group, mobility group, and self-care skills group. Patients with common goals are organized to work through a specific program to achieve that goal with the benefit of group dynamics and peer feedback. The use of group technique improves application of rehabilitation strategies in the real world. Society revolves around interactions with others in one-on-one, small-group, and large-group situations. To approximate society, various interactive strategies are used. This prepares the injured patient to function in society, builds coping skills, and allows the patient to test out his adaptation to injury in a supportive group setting. It is appropriate for the rehabilitation nurse to participate in this therapy and, in some situations, direct it.

In interdisciplinary therapy sessions, several specialists work with one patient at the same time. An example might be a daily lunchtime session with the occupational therapist, speech pathologist, and nurse to improve self-feeding of a dysphagic patient. The team members become more integrated as they focus on functional rather than disciplinary goals. Because of the interactive evaluation and treatment process, the resulting outcome is more comprehensive than the benefit of individual sessions with each of the component disciplines. Members of the disciplines who find the consistent need to work together should set up routine joint therapy sessions in anticipation of these needs. Goal achievement through rehabilitation intervention is measured by outcome data systems.

Rehabilitation Outcome

One of the most sorely lacking components of rehabilitation is the accurate comprehensive and universal measurement of patient outcome.[15, 16] Literally hundreds of assessments of function exist. Most rehabilitation programs collect data relevant to their own program. It is difficult to compare programmatic outcomes because the evaluation tools collect data by different methods and at varying times.

What constitutes a quality outcome? Functional gains that are not retained over time initially may give the appearance of higher outcome. An example of good outcome measurement would include measures of function done at rehabilitation admission and discharge followed by measures at 6 months and 1 year after discharge. Postdischarge interval measurements are used to document sustained function post rehabilitation. Exorbitant costs to achieve a slightly higher outcome may not be the wisest use of the patient's financial resources. Comparison of cost with functional outcome needs to be documented.

Third-party payers are driving the rehabilitation system toward more cost-effective alternatives. To demonstrate effectiveness or efficiency of the rehabilitation options available, a national data system is being implemented. The Uniform Data System (UDS) is designed to collect outcome data on all rehabilitated patients, including trauma patients (Fig. 16–1).

The National Association of Rehabilitation Facilities recognizes that some additional measures are required, particularly a cognitive outcome component for the head-injured population. The UDS and other standard functional measures can be easily performed at varying intervals, before and after discharge. It also has the ability to measure sustained outcome over time.

The simplicity of such measures provides a basis for comparison of programs in terms of quality, cost-effectiveness, time efficiency, and development of lasting outcomes. These measures create a better match between the individual patient and the most appropriate rehabilitation option at each point along the cycle.

AVAILABILITY OF REHABILITATION TO THE TRAUMATIZED POPULATION

The available rehabilitation options have become widely varied. Traditional medical inpatient rehabilitation is now just one of many types of programs. As the complex needs of trauma patients have been recognized, a full range of rehabilitation programs and services has developed. One of the confusing aspects in understanding what rehabilitation options exist is clearly understanding the difference between rehabilitation programs and rehabilitation services. It is also necessary to recognize when each option is most appropriate to the patient's rehabilitation goals.

Programs and Services. A rehabilitation service is a single component that could exist in a full rehabilitation program. A simple example would be physical therapy services on an outpatient basis to a posttraumatic amputee for long-term follow-up. In this case, the patient does not require other therapy or rehabilitative services, so the single service of physical therapy meets the patient's needs.

In comparison, a rehabilitation program is much more than a cumulative effect of multiple rehabilitation services. It is the coordination and blend of multiple disciplines, which provide a true rehabilitation program to the patient. A program can exist in either an inpatient, outpatient, or residential (home care) setting if the services are coordinated and if the approach is a team effort.

A rehabilitation program must provide for cooperation and communication by all who work with the patient. An inpatient setting that provides for nursing and medical care of the patient and offers physical, occupational, and other therapies is not necessarily a rehabilitation program. If those multiple disciplines integrate their efforts toward mutual functional goals and there is carryover from therapy to nursing care, then the essence of program is offered to the patient.

Discharge planning for the trauma patient involves understanding if the patient requires a single service or the multiple and coordinated services of a rehabilitation program. Fragmentation of care is one of the primary causes for failure of rehabilitative efforts. The match of patient needs and goals to appropriate programs and services maximizes the patient's outcome. When evaluating potential programs for patient placement, it would be important to determine whether there is adequate coordination of services to provide integration rather than fragmentation of goals.

Severely injured patients in the late rehabilitative phase and reintegration phase of the trauma cycle could appropriately have their follow-up needs met by single rehabilitation services. This depends on the complexity of injury, psychosocial supports, and intellectual ability of the patient and family to carry out the plan.

Centers of Excellence. Over the past two decades, some rehabilitation programs have elevated themselves to distinction through continual research in the specialty of rehabilitation as well as application of that research to practice. Often these facilities are known for a subspecialty in rehabilitation, such as spinal cord injury, head injury, or burn rehabilitation. Some of them are known regionally, whereas others have a reputation established nationwide. Patients with extremely complex or unique injuries may require a facility of this expertise. The determination usually is made by the referring medical and acute care treatment team and a payer representative (often a case manager) along with the family and patient.

Influence of Managed Care. The availability of resources continues to be shaped by the growth and influence of managed care. Managed care is a group of "systems that integrate financing and the delivery of appropriate health care services through: selected health care providers furnishing services to members, explicit standards for provider selection, quality assurance and utilization review programs, and financial incentives for members to use selected providers."[17] A payer selects preferred providers in rehabilitation to deliver services to the patient at different points in the

UNIFORM DATA SYSTEM FOR MEDICAL REHABILITATION

Appendix C

INPATIENT CODING SHEET

SIDE 1

IF DATA ON THIS FORM ARE REVISED, WRITE DATE HERE: ___/___/___, AND CIRCLE NEW DATA.

COMPLETE BOTH SIDES

1. **Rehab Facility Code** ☐☐☐
2. **Patient Number** ☐☐☐ ☐☐ ☐☐☐☐
3. **Admission Date** ☐☐ MONTH ☐☐ DAY ☐☐☐☐ YEAR
4. **Discharge Date** ☐☐ MONTH ☐☐ DAY ☐☐☐☐ YEAR
5. **Program Interrupted** ☐ 1-Yes 2-No

   1st Interruption
   a. **Transfer Date** ☐☐ ☐☐ ☐☐
   b. **Return Date** ☐☐ ☐☐ ☐☐

   2nd Interruption
   c. **Transfer Date** ☐☐ ☐☐ ☐☐
   d. **Return Date** ☐☐ ☐☐ ☐☐

   3rd Interruption
   e. **Transfer Date** ☐☐ ☐☐ ☐☐
   f. **Return Date** ☐☐ ☐☐ ☐☐

6. **Admission Class** ☐

   1-First Rehab 2-Evaluation
   3-Readmission

7. **ZIP Code** (home) ☐☐☐☐☐ ☐☐☐☐
8. **Birthdate** ☐☐ MONTH ☐☐ DAY ☐☐☐☐ YEAR
9. **Sex** ☐ 1-Male 2-Female
10. **Race/Ethnicity** ☐

    1-White 2-Black 3-Asian
    4-American Indian 5-Other 6-Hispanic

11. **English Language** ☐

    1-Yes 2-No 3-Partial

12. **Marital Status** ☐

    1-Single 2-Married 3-Widowed
    4-Separated 5-Divorced

13. **Living Arrangement**

    a. **Setting** PRE HOSPITAL ☐☐ ADMIT FROM ☐☐ DISCHARGE ☐☐

    01-Home 02-Board and Care 03-Transitional Living
    04-Intermediate Care 05-Skilled Nursing
    06-Acute Unit-your own facility 07-Acute Unit-another facility
    08-Chronic Hospital 09-Rehab Facility 10-Other 11-Died

    b. **Living With** PRE HOSPITAL ☐ DISCHARGE ☐

    1-Alone 2-Family/Relatives 3-Friends 4-Attendant 5-Other

14. **Vocational Status**

    a. **Category** PRE HOSPITAL ☐

    1-Employed 2-Sheltered 3-Student 4-Homemaker
    5-Not working 6-Retired-age 7-Retired-disability

    b. **Effort** PRE HOSPITAL ☐

    1-Full-time 2-Part-time 3-Adjusted workload

IMPAIRMENT GROUP CODES

01 Stroke:
01.1 Left Body (Right Brain)
01.2 Right Body (Left Brain)
01.3 Bilateral
01.4 No Paresis
01.9 Other Stroke

02 Brain Dysfunction:
02.1 Non-Traumatic
02.2 Traumatic
02.21 Open Injury
02.22 Closed Injury
02.9 Other Brain

03 Neurologic Conditions:
03.1 Multiple Sclerosis
03.2 Parkinsonism
03.3 Polyneuropathy
03.4 Guillain-Barré
03.9 Other Neurologic

04 Spinal Cord Dysfunction:
04.1 Non-Traumatic SC
04.110 Paraplegia
04.111 Incomplete
04.112 Complete
04.120 Quadriplegia
04.1211 Incomplete C1-4
04.1212 Incomplete C5-8
04.1221 Complete C1-4
04.1222 Complete C5-8
04.130 Other Non-Trauma
04.2 Traumatic Spinal Cord
04.210 Paraplegia
04.211 Incomplete
04.212 Complete
04.220 Quadriplegia
04.2211 Incomplete C1-4
04.2212 Incomplete C5-8
04.2221 Complete C1-4
04.2222 Complete C5-8
04.230 Other Traumatic SC

05 Amputation:
05.1 Single Upper AE
05.2 Single Upper BE
05.3 Single Lower AK
05.4 Single Lower BK
05.5 Double AK/AK
05.6 Double AK/BK
05.7 Double BK/BK
05.9 Other Amputation

06 Arthritis
06.1 Rheumatoid
06.2 Osteoarthritis
06.9 Other Arthritis

07 Pain Syndrome
07.1 Neck Pain
07.2 Back Pain
07.3 Extremity Pain
07.9 Other Pain

08 Orthopaedic Conditions
08.1 Status Post Hip Fracture
08.2 SP Femur (Shaft) Fracture
08.3 SP Pelvic Fracture
08.4 SP Major Multiple Fracture
08.5 SP Hip Replacement
08.6 SP Knee Replacement
08.9 Other Orthopaedic

09 Cardiac

10 Pulmonary:
10.1 Chronic Obstr. Pulm. Disease
10.9 Other Pulmonary

11 Burns

12 Congenital Deformities:
12.1 Spina Bifida
12.9 Other Congenital

13 Other Disabling Impairments

14 Major Multiple Trauma:
14.1 Brain + Spinal cord
14.2 Brain + Mult. Fx./Amp.
14.3 Sp. Cd. + Mult. Fx./Amp.
14.9 Other Mult. Trauma

 UDS Code-1 3/2/90

A-4

Figure 16–1. National Data System for medical rehabilitation inpatient coding sheet. (From Granger CV: Advances in functional assessment for medical rehabilitation. Top Geriatric Rehabilitation 1:59–74, 1986.)

COMPLETE BOTH SIDES

UNIFORM DATA SYSTEM FOR MEDICAL REHABILITATION INPATIENT CODING SHEET

SIDE 2

Patient Number ___/__/_____

15. Followup: Use separate Followup Coding Sheet

16. Impairment Group (complete on discharge) ☐☐.☐☐☐☐

Put condition requiring admission to rehabilitation here, using Impairment Group Codes listed at the bottom of page 1. Be as specific as possible.

17. Date of Onset (of impairment) ☐☐ MONTH ☐☐ DAY ☐☐☐☐ YEAR

18. Principal Diagnosis (complete on discharge) ☐☐☐.☐☐ ICD 9 Code

Use ICD code related to Impairment Group here.

19. Other Diagnoses (complete on discharge)

ICD Code for other impairments, etiology, co-morbidity, and complications

1 ☐☐☐.☐☐
2 ☐☐☐.☐☐
3 ☐☐☐.☐☐
4 ☐☐☐.☐☐
5 ☐☐☐.☐☐
6 ☐☐☐.☐☐
7 ☐☐☐.☐☐

20. Payment Source (complete on Discharge)

a. **Primary** ☐☐

b. **Secondary** ☐☐

01-Blue Cross 02-Medicare 03-Medicaid/Welfare
04-Commercial Insurance 05-HMO 06-Worker's Comp.
07-Crippled Child. Serv. 08-Regional Ctr. Devel. Disab.
09-State Voc. Rehab. 10-Private Pay 11-Employee Courtesy
12-Free 13-Champus 14-Other 15-None

21. Charges (Rehab only) (Dollars only)

a. **Total Rehab. Hospital $** ☐☐☐☐☐☐

b. **Include Physician?** ☐ 1-Yes 2-No

22. Functional Independence Measure (FIM)

LEVELS		
	7 Complete Independence (Timely, Safely) 6 Modified Independence (Device)	NO HELPER
	Modified Dependence 5 Supervision 4 Minimal Assist (Subject = 75%+) 3 Moderate Assist (Subject = 50%+) Complete Dependence 2 Maximal Assist (Subject = 25%+) 1 Total Assist (Subject = 0%+)	HELPER

	ADMIT	DISCH
Self Care		
A. Eating	☐	☐
B. Grooming	☐	☐
C. Bathing	☐	☐
D. Dressing-Upper Body	☐	☐
E. Dressing-Lower Body	☐	☐
F. Toileting	☐	☐
Sphincter Control		
G. Bladder Management	☐	☐
H. Bowel Management	☐	☐
Mobility		
Transfer:		
I. Bed, Chair, Wheelchair	☐	☐
J. Toilet	☐	☐
K. Tub, Shower	☐	☐
Locomotion		
L. Walk/wheel Chair	w/c ☐	w/c ☐
M. Stairs	☐	☐
Communication		
N. Comprehension	a/v ☐	a/v ☐
O. Expression	v/n ☐	v/n ☐
Social Cognition		
P. Social Interaction	☐	☐
Q. Problem Solving	☐	☐
R. Memory	☐	☐
Total FIM	☐	☐

NOTE: Leave no blanks; enter 1 if patient not testable due to risk.

COPY FREELY - DO NOT CHANGE

 UDS CODE-2 3/2/90

A-5

Figure 16–1 *Continued*

cycle. These systems may limit alternatives for the patient at times. However, the coordination of services often is greatly improved. Case management, discussed earlier, can be a component of a managed care system. Trauma nurses may find themselves providing referral documentation to utilization review nurses, case managers, and other payer representatives to plan for transfer to a rehabilitation facility or services.

CURRENT AND FUTURE REHABILITATION ALTERNATIVES

The future of rehabilitation delivery offers a spectrum of programs and services ranging from acute inpatient rehabilitation to outpatient and residential settings. Quite a variety of rehabilitation alternatives presently exist. As the number of alternative rehabilitation programs increases, the number of acute patients served by acute inpatient programs will stabilize or decrease.

Programs are carried out in three general locations: inpatient, outpatient, and home-based. Traditional rehabilitation has predominantly been inpatient. Today's rehabilitation programs function in various settings but continue to provide the essential components of team approach and long-term rehabilitation planning. Individual therapy services provide follow-up on an outpatient basis if needed.

The following sections describe program options that may be provided to the trauma population. It is not an all-inclusive list; rather, it is an attempt to demonstrate the variety of programming available throughout the country. Not all these options are reasonably accessible to all patients.

Inpatient Rehabilitation

Comprehensive acute inpatient rehabilitation units may be found in hospitals, freestanding facilities, and skilled nursing facilities. Included in the Commission on Accreditation of Rehabilitation Facilities (CARF) criteria for comprehensive inpatient rehabilitation[6] (often referred to as acute rehabilitation) is the requirement that functional patient gains must be demonstrated at least every 2 weeks and patients must be active in therapy for 3 or more hours per day. This is an extremely active program. Typically, patients are in various individual and group therapies for the bulk of the day, with rehabilitation carryover on the nursing unit, as well as specific therapeutic evening and weekend programs. Patients who are ready to begin transition to home and community use a therapeutic leave of absence (TLOA). Each TLOA has specific individual goals and preeducation and post-TLOA conferencing to evaluate the success of the transition.

Subacute rehabilitation is a growing alternative inpatient program. It meets the needs of patients who are not able to tolerate the daily intensity of an acute inpatient program and those who are making slower progress but still require the coordinated services of an interdisciplinary team. This second level of inpatient rehabilitation could exist in hospitals, freestanding units, and skilled nursing facilities if the components of rehabilitation programming are provided.[18] A critical differentiation of subacute rehabilitation from long-term care is that the subacute patient requires an active rehabilitation program by a coordinated team as opposed to residential placement with maintenance rehabilitation services.

The similarities between acute and subacute inpatient rehabilitation cause a great deal of confusion. This is due to the fact that the programs can be found in the same types of buildings with the same list of services being provided. The key difference is the intensity of service provided and the expected rate of patient recovery. CARF is giving some consideration to standards for subacute rehabilitation to assist in clear definition and evaluation of such programs. This would provide for more appropriate referrals to each program type.

Transitional living programs focus specifically on community reintegration. The patient lives in a structured home environment, often with other rehabilitative patients. Social and behavioral adaptation are stressed in addition to the adjustment to physical disabilities in a home and community setting. The home environment usually is paired with a modified work or school setting in either the same or an alternative location. Transitional living provides inpatient rehabilitation for a specific length of time and to achieve identified goals.[19] It is not a long-term residential placement, as the name may indicate.

Nonmedical residential rehabilitation, on the other hand, is an extended placement that provides structured living and rehabilitation support services. It may also be called a group home or supervised living situation.

Outpatient Rehabilitation

Comprehensive outpatient rehabilitation facilities (CORFs) are among the new alternatives in outpatient programs. A CORF provides a wide range of therapeutic services and approaches by a coordinated team in both individual and group sessions. The patients require less medical and nursing care and are functionally independent enough to live in another setting and commute to their rehabilitation program. Depending on the intensity of need, the patients are seen on a daily or intermittent basis. CARF has established a separate set of accreditation criteria to ensure consistency of comprehensive outpatient rehabilitation programs.[6] The number of work hardening programs has grown in the past few years. Work hardening commonly is associated with a CORF and provides physical and cognitive strengthening of the client. The program simulates the clients' work components and increases the complexity and repetition of tasks until clients are prepared to return to their work setting.

Another outpatient program for specific patient needs is a day treatment program. Patients in these programs are more functionally independent than those in inpatient settings. The focus of the rehabilitation program is geared to a specialized aspect of reintegration, such as social behavior, cognitive rehabilitation, and prevocational training. Day hospitals provide nursing, medical, and therapy services to a patient during daytime hours to improve the level of patient function or, in a day-care model, to relieve the family from 24-hour care. Vocational programs may provide highly specialized services, including in-depth patient evaluation, work assessment, trial work settings, work hardening, supervised and assisted work settings, and training for new employment skills. A sheltered workshop is a supervised and structured work setting that is used as either a short-term rehabilitation approach or a somewhat permanent job placement, depending on the rehabilitation potential of the patient.

Home-Based Rehabilitation

Home-based rehabilitation programs are possible if there is full coordination of the therapeutic services involved. The patient lives and participates in the program at home. Potentially, the patient does not have to be independent and can require up to 24-hour-a-day nursing care. Home-based programs are an especially therapeutic approach if the family feels strongly about the patient being at home and if there are limited accessible inpatient and outpatient programs. It is also a good alternative if the patient's nursing care needs preclude the patient from benefiting from a more aggressive inpatient rehabilitation setting or if a transportation problem interferes with outpatient rehabilitation. Improved family input and involvement often result from home-based programs, although the lack of social and behavioral rehabilitation because of isolation from the patient's peer group can be a drawback. A combination of home-based and outpatient programs is an effective option, especially when an inpatient program would be inappropriate. Home-based rehabilitation often is not a cost-effective option and is not used as frequently as other alternatives.

With such a variety of rehabilitation settings, it becomes more complex to match the patient's needs to services and programs. The increased options require rehabilitation providers to better distinguish between the types of programs offered to identify the most appropriate setting.

What factors really determine placement now? In theory, we match the patient needs to program goals. In reality, the factors of local program availability and funding play major roles in decision making. As availability improves and funding issues settle, more appropriate placement can occur. Program distinction could be made through an analysis of the population best served, including such factors as the patient's medical stability, types and intensity of services needed, functional ability, and social and psychological considerations.

FOCUS OF REHABILITATION THROUGHOUT THE CYCLE

Rehabilitation is the momentum that moves the patient through the cycle, although it often is identified as an isolated period within the cycle. Maximized patient function is the common goal of all health care providers.[2]

As the patient proceeds through the cycle, the focus of rehabilitation shifts. After the initial crisis of injury, the patient is stabilized. At this early stage, the severely injured patient depends on family and professionals to anticipate complications and plan for future progress. Later, the patient takes on a much more active role in the rehabilitation team, eventually to determine all individual goals.

No clear distinction or key event marks the patient's departure from one phase and entry into the next. Depending on the complexity of the injury, complications, and the psychosocial system into which the patient tries to reintegrate, movement through the cycle may be at varying pace and intensity. Patients may need to return to earlier phases in the cycle over the course of recovery. Most rehabilitation protocols are diagnoses-specific. These specialties are delineated in other chapters of this book.

Critical Care Phase

From the scene of the injury through resuscitation and immediate stabilization, the rehabilitation focus during the critical care phase is to prevent further injury. Delay in treatment, unidentified injuries, and unintended injury caused by emergency procedures can cause additional physical damage, resulting in a lengthened or increasingly complicated rehabilitation process. Decreased functional recovery may be a result of preventable problems during the critical phase.

Life-threatening injury is the greatest concern in an emergency setting. The long-term effects of a seemingly minor injury may be the most devastating to the patient's daily life. For example, in a patient with a multisystem injury, including multiple fractures, a pneumothorax, and abdominal bleeding, the presence of a brachial plexus injury may go relatively unnoticed. But as the other injuries are resolved, loss of motor function or chronic pain from the brachial plexus injury could interfere with the patient's productive return to work and home life. A patient with a cervical spinal cord injury is likely to have an associated minor head injury. It may easily go undetected. But the cognitive effects, such as poor concentration and memory loss, and the behavioral effects, such as inappropriate judgment and apathy, could greatly interfere with the learning process required in spinal cord injury rehabilitation. The patient could be labeled as noncompliant or unmotivated, when he or she actually is in need of specific head injury rehabilitative techniques.

The severity of injury must be considered in context. A minor injury may have severe consequences. This is not to say that stabilizing the most life-threatening injury is not the priority. Rather, it infers that the emergency practitioner needs to have an awareness of all the patient's injuries, the potentially unidentified injuries associated with the patient's condition, and the potentially lifelong consequences of all injuries. This awareness can foster prevention of further injury and appropriate follow-up of less life-threatening injuries.

Another rehabilitation focus in the critical care phase is the establishment of baseline information about the patient's response to the injury. Rehabilitation is an individualized process that depends on the perspective of the patient and family. People respond to injury in terms of the loss or potential loss that is perceived. A construction worker may potentially be more devastated by the loss of a limb than might a computer data processor because a source of income is threatened. A fashion model may be more concerned about a facial laceration than a moderate head injury. Generalizations cannot be made, but a perceptive emergency practitioner can anticipate these priorities. Those who have initial contact with the family or with the patient, if appropriate, should note the initial reaction to suspected diagnosis. Documentation of such responses provides valuable insights to patient and family values and to the impact each injury potentially has on the patient. Early assessment of baseline social history provides another indicator of the type of psychosocial and rehabilitative support the patient will need in the future. Even at this early critical phase, this information can become the basis for an individualized rehabilitation plan.

Intermediate Phase

For the purpose of rehabilitation, the intermediate phase includes the period of medical stabilization, which may occur in critical care, intensive care, step-down, and medical-surgical units. During this period, the patient requires major treatment of injuries, including surgery, multiple procedures, medications, and other complex care. Even though most energy is spent treating the patient, the necessary rehabilitation focus for this phase is the prevention of complications. The critical care nurse must combine technical treatment expertise with a return to nursing fundamentals such as positioning for proper body alignment, providing psychosocial support, teaching, and minimizing the complications of immobility.[20]

Prevention of physical complications can avoid interruption or delay of progress toward rehabilitation as well as additional cost to the patient.[21] Although it is only one of many complications, decreased mobility is common in severely traumatized patients. All body systems are at risk for complications from immobility (Table 16–2).[22] Specific nursing measures that merit noting include positioning to prevent pressure sores and contractures, and enhanced nutrition for healing and prevention of skin breakdown.

Regardless of how complex the trauma, the nurse can apply mobilization techniques and compensatory strategies to prevent complications. The trauma nurse needs a thorough understanding of normal body mobilization and physiology of body systems. Many prevention techniques result from approximating normal body function. Intervention at this point may prevent or minimize the consequences of immobility. Avoidance of immobility altogether is the best strategy. For example, many new surgical treatments for serious fractures promote early weight-bearing and ambulation. The trend is to eliminate the need for unnecessary immobilization and to promote a normalization of activity even through the intermediate phase of trauma.

In addition to physical complications, immobility has a number of psychosocial effects on the patient. Sensory deprivation, loss of control, and changes in body image and self-esteem are all related problems of the immobilized patient. An acute reaction could alter the patient's ability to adapt and to recover from the injury.

Support from the trauma nurse as a round-the-clock caregiving professional prevents or minimizes psychological reactions of the patient. The nurse can use empathy and receptive listening to allow the patient to ventilate stress. Support of communication and visitation by family and significant others helps to prevent social isolation. Encouragement of independence in daily activities as well as decision making and in making choices whenever possible promotes improved feelings of self-esteem and worth, which increases the patient's motivation and determination to progress toward recovery. The trauma nurse should apply principles of adaptive and maladaptive coping and the process of grieving loss into the assessment of the patient's psychosocial status.[23] This same supportive role is required from the nurse by the patient's family.

Patient and family teaching begins in the intermediate phase. The nurse, as a readily accessible member of the trauma team, may be bombarded with questions by the patient and family. An understanding of readiness for learning helps the nurse to recognize the purpose behind these questions. Many families and patients in the early phases of trauma care are not ready to learn fully about the injuries and the consequences. They are more specifically searching for comfort and support. This is evidenced in the situation in which a family asserts several weeks later that "no one ever told me this" in regard to information that was supposedly taught in response to questions. When the family or patient is under stress, they are not able to maximize their learning potential. Readiness for learning includes the right environment and motivation for learning and the ability to retain the presented material. When a family asks a question to find support and comfort, the technical answer often is lost, whereas the feeling of comfort is retained. With this in mind, the trauma nurse prepares to teach, reteach, and review necessary learning consistently with the family and patient. The trauma nurse can be a key resource to the patient and family to prepare them for the cycle of care ahead and the prospective outcome of the injury.[24]

Rehabilitation specialists are introduced to the patient's treatment team early in the intermediate phase.[25] The decision of which rehabilitation specialties should be added to the team depends on the diagnosis and effects of injury. The trauma nurse, as a holistically focused professional, coordinates the multiple specialties for an individual patient and makes appropriate recommendations for rehabilitation referrals.

Physical, occupational, and respiratory therapists are among the first rehabilitationists to evaluate and treat the patient. Largely focused on physical aspects of disability, they may follow the patient even in the critical care unit. Until the patient is medically stable enough to be seen in therapy departments or treatment areas, they provide bedside interventions.

Physical therapists increase mobility of the patient through range-of-motion exercises, positioning techniques, and active exercise programs. Their musculoskeletal evaluation provides a multitude of suggestions for movement and positioning in daily care. Physical therapies may also begin early transfer to a chair or to weight-bearing activity.

Respiratory therapists or, in some instances, physical therapists work on mobilization of respiratory secretions by percussion, vibration, and postural drainage. Physiological monitoring of respiratory status through blood gas analyses and pulmonary function testing provides indicators for treatment of further effects of immobility.

Assessment of the performance of activities of daily living by the occupational therapist can begin while the patient is still bedridden. In addition to establishing functional goals, it promotes improved self-esteem in the patient. For patients who are less functionally responsive, the occupational therapist may focus on maintaining upper-extremity position and mobility, which will allow for functional use of limbs or muscle groups, including splinting of the extremities for therapeutic positioning. The occupational therapist may also

TABLE 16–2. PHYSICAL COMPLICATIONS RELATED TO IMMOBILITY COMMONLY SEEN IN TRAUMA PATIENTS

BODY SYSTEM	COMPLICATIONS	PATHOPHYSIOLOGY	PREVENTION
Neurological	Potentially affects all body systems.	Due to decreased LOC; injury to cortex, motor, or sensory systems.	Neurological assessment, specific focus to the effects seen in other body systems; understand neurological basis of complication.
Respiratory	Fatigue, decreased productivity; infection, pneumonia, respiratory acidosis.	Decreased respiratory movement, unable to mobilize secretions, alterations in blood gases, eventual depression of respiratory center in brainstem.	Assessment of respiratory status and changes in LOC; mobilization of secretions by turning, coughing, and deep breathing; postural drainage, percussion, vibration, early ambulation, humidification.
Cardiovascular	Orthostatic hypotension, fatigue, increased cardiac work load, thrombosis, embolus.	Increased heart rate, cardiac output, stroke volume in supine position; loss of supporting muscle tone resulting in venous stasis; orthostatic neurovascular receptors cannot adjust to position changes; hypercoagulability and external pressure to vessels.	Cardiovascular assessment; encourage mobilization, exercise, ROM, positioning, antiembolitic stockings; provide adequate hydration; avoid Valsalva maneuver.
Gastrointestinal	Anorexia, fatigue, malnutrition, constipation, impaction, bowel obstruction, diarrhea, dehydration.	Negative nitrogen balance and protein deficiency; stress; decreased appetite, creates bowel intolerance; muscle weakness, diminished ability to apply abdominal pressure needed for evacuation; psychological factors and position for defecation may increase difficulty.	Assessment of GI functioning, including baseline history of nutrition, exercise, and bowel habits; coordinate bowel plan with nutrition, hydration, positioning, privacy, and gastrocolic reflex timing factors and use of digital stimulation, stool softeners, and suppositories for stimulation; adjust tube feedings to avoid constipation or diarrhea; small, frequent feedings to increase tolerance and decrease anorexia; encourage intake of protein, fluids, bulk foods; encourage exercise.
Urinary	Urinary reflux, incontinence, urinary stasis, renal calculi, urinary tract infection.	Loss of effect of gravity, urinary stasis in renal pelvis; increased calculi formation from urine sediment in renal pelvis; diminished coordination of sphincters and muscles in supine position; bladder distention, overflow incontinence.	Assessment of urinary tract function; promote movement and exercise, use prone position; maintain fluid intake, decrease calcium intake; monitor distention and voiding patterns, prevent incontinence; use upright or sitting position for voiding if possible; intermittent catheters preferred to indwelling.
Musculoskeletal	Muscle atrophy, contractures.	Muscles shorten and atrophy; loss of ROM as supporting ligaments, tendons, and capsule lose mobility; ROM becomes permanent; spasticity of antagonistic muscle, with weakness of opposing muscle creates contracture also.	On-going assessment; passive, active, and active-assisted ROM exercises; appropriate positioning and body alignment in both bed and chair.
	Osteoporosis, stress fractures, heterotrophic ossification.	Normal bone-building activities are dependent on weight bearing and movement; increased destruction of bone, release of calcium; bone becomes porous and fragile; abnormal calcification over large joints may also occur.	Calcium supplement to diet is not recommended; promote weight bearing.
Integumentary	Skin breakdown; stage I to IV skin ulcers; secondary infection of skin ulcers, sepsis.	Prolonged pressure to skin diminishes capillary blood supply and stops flow of nutrients to cells; necrosis of cells results in skin breakdown, allowing infection to enter body.	Assessment of skin integrity, nutritional status, and risk factors for breakdown; reposition; shift pressure and patient weight frequently; "every 2 hours" rule may not be adequate; check for changes in blanching, sustained redness; keep off all red areas; massage at-risk areas to promote circulation, teach patient to inspect own skin and shift weight; increased protein in diet; take immediate, consistent action on any areas of breakdown.

LOC, level of consciousness; ROM, range of motion.

suggest specific adaptive equipment and techniques to the nursing staff.

A speech pathologist is an appropriate early rehabilitation referral for trauma patients with head injury, high cervical spinal cord injury, and facial injury. Any patient with an artificial airway, such as tracheal or endotracheal tubes, also may benefit from a speech or communication specialist. A speech pathologist can offer various techniques to promote stimulation from coma, cognitive rehabilitation, communication through alternative methods and devices, and improvement of perceptual deficits.

Dysphagia is a specific area of disability that may need to be evaluated and treated in the intermediate phase as the patient is ready for a regular diet. Video fluoroscopy can be used to assess the exact nature of a swallowing problem.[26] Treatment of swallowing disorders often includes consultation by a speech pathologist, an occupational therapist, a rehabilitation nurse, and a respiratory therapist.

An early referral to a physiatrist, if available, would expedite the implementation of rehabilitation principles during the intermediate phase. In some settings, a rehabilitation clinical nurse specialist or nurse practitioner can begin to plan and implement the rehabilitation process. Early assessment by rehabilitation specialists permits a projection of rehabilitation potential and an active plan for maximal recovery.

The subject of rehabilitation may be a new concept to the patient and family. They may not realize that acute medical stabilization is just the beginning. Preparation for transfer to a rehabilitation program includes education about potential patient functional goals, identification and selection of appropriate programs, and support during the upheaval of the transfer process.

It can be a shock to the patient and family when he is transferred from the atmosphere of the intensive care unit, where the patient is given total care, to a rehabilitation unit. There is a point in the patient's hospital course when the emphasis of care should begin to change, with encouragement for the patient to be independent. Implementing strategies to promote independence as early as possible better prepares the patient for rehabilitation.

Rehabilitation Phase

A great deal of rehabilitative effort is necessary during the rehabilitation phase, especially for severely injured patients. However, it is only one portion of rehabilitation during the trauma cycle. If rehabilitation were ignored in the other phases, functional outcomes would be severely decreased.

Most restorative rehabilitation occurs in an inpatient setting, including a rehabilitation unit of an acute care hospital or a freestanding rehabilitation facility. Depending on the type and severity of disability, the frequency and type of medical monitoring, family support systems, and patient motivation, an outpatient or home-based rehabilitation program could be appropriate if a comprehensive team approach is provided.

Key themes throughout the rehabilitation phase are restoration, compensation, and adaptation. The rehabilitation team evaluates each individual case for (1) the ability to recover normal function, (2) appropriate areas to replace normal function with other strategies (compensation), and (3) areas in which the patient must change his or her lifestyle, roles, and expectations to adapt to disability. This evaluation results in a rehabilitation plan, with setting of both long- and short-term goals. Depending on the patient's progress, these goals may need periodic adjustment.

Active rehabilitation includes learning new skills, practicing them, and testing skills in the environment. This is why the rehabilitative process takes weeks to months to complete. Some patients may be in and out of rehabilitation hospitals for years, learning and further improving skills with each admission. Few people have the capacity for learning all that is necessary to adapt to injury at one time. Many goals spill over into the reintegration phase. Progress with each short-term goal may vary.

As medical stability and functional independence increase, the patient asserts his or her rights for self-determination. This issue is extremely frustrating at times to the trauma team, whose values conflict with those of the patient they worked so hard to save.

For example, a patient who had sustained a C4-5 injury with resulting quadriplegia was transferred to a rehabilitation hospital from an acute care setting. The acute care staff had made every effort to maintain function of all body systems. Specifically, the patient's upper extremity range of motion was outstanding. About 8 weeks after transfer, the rehabilitation hospital provided the acute trauma nurses with a progress report on the patient. He was taking notably more control of his life and responsibility for his own actions. But the presence of upper-extremity contractures was shocking. At first, the acute care staff blamed the rehabilitation staff for neglect. It was difficult for them to understand that this severely injured young man chose to maintain enough range of motion to scratch his nose for comfort. He did not share the rehabilitation team's goal of self-feeding. His goal was control of his comfort and reserving his energy for activities other than self-feeding.[27]

The patient's values guide the course of rehabilitation. The challenge is understanding when a traumatized patient is ready to be released from the sick role and considered competent and sufficiently informed to make self-determining judgments. The trauma nurse strives to provide as many options for maximized function, but the injured person makes the ultimate decision.

Reintegration Phase

Reintegration strategies usually begin during the rehabilitation phase. One strategy is the use of a TLOA from an inpatient setting, which allows the patient to test the adapted function in the real world. This also occurs in modified reintegration settings that involve home care and outpatient programs. Of all areas in trauma rehabilitation, the reintegration process is most limited in resources and yet rapidly growing. Our society values a return to a productive life.

Reintegration is the process of applying therapeutic adaptation and compensation to the patient's premorbid lifestyle. A difficult question facing rehabilitationists today is "When does rehabilitation end and lifelong health management begin?" Trauma patients stay in the health care system for extended periods. Functional gains are achieved even years after injury. Rehabilitation professionals target maximized patient potential. Who determines when a patient has reached his or her potential?

One of the most difficult barriers in rehabilitation is that the services that are provided are limited by what services are funded. Many patients are kept in the rehabilitation system for inappropriately long periods. This has both a positive and a negative effect. Positively, some achieve continual goals at a slower pace, therefore reaching a higher outcome. Others remain in the rehabilitation system for a lifetime without making appreciable gains. Not enough lifelong care options exist. The patient either remains in the rehabilitation system or receives no services because there are no alternative settings or funding.

For the trauma cycle to end with a positive outcome, society needs to put the following pieces into place: (1) awareness and acceptance of the posttraumatically injured patient in society, (2) provision of a complex variety of services that meet the specific reintegration needs of the trauma patient, and (3) financial support for the most appropriate alternatives at each phase of rehabilitation. It is only with these ingredients that each person who experiences injury can realize quality of life.

ISSUES IN TRAUMA REHABILITATION

Funding for Rehabilitation

The most pressing issue in trauma rehabilitation is the lack of available funds to pay for rehabilitation programs and services.[17] Most health care professionals would probably find that they are not covered for rehabilitation by their own health insurance. The prospect of paying out of pocket for rehabilitation is highly unrealistic for the average citizen. Because of inadequate private funding and limited federal and state reimbursement systems, many traumatized patients never receive the rehabilitation that is appropriate for their disability. This creates an ethical dilemma. Emergency and life-saving services are provided to many who are not then able to return to a fully functional role in society.

Private insurance has defined rehabilitation in terms of physical and vocational services. Rehabilitation services in an acute care hospital may be funded, but such services provided in a freestanding rehabilitation facility or in the home, long-term rehabilitation, and transitional living may not be. The available coverage often does not provide for what could be the most appropriate and cost-effective program for the patient. Often the insurance benefits are exhausted and the patient and family bankrupted early in the rehabilitative care of a catastrophic injury.

Rehabilitation professionals are providing support, data, and education to third-party payers to improve the availability of funding to the injured person. Several insurers have made a separate catastrophic coverage plan available for purchase that protects patients from some expenses. Insurers are also using the expertise of rehabilitation nurses as case managers to enhance cost-effectiveness and appropriateness of rehabilitation admissions. Administrative waivers, in which third-party payers agree to a cost-effective plan of care not covered by the patient's policy, are an alternative that sometimes is negotiated on a case-by-case basis. Alternatives in private funding will increase as the public becomes more educated about what is covered by their insurance benefits and as insurers recognize the potential for overall cost reduction.

Federal and state funds for rehabilitation are reimbursed based on a projection of costs. Such cost reimbursement does not always recognize all the complex costs associated with the patient's rehabilitation, particularly those who are catastrophically injured. This creates a financial deficit for the rehabilitation provider. As a result, many rehabilitation programs limit their admission of government-funded patients. This issue is particularly true of government funding for the nontraditional rehabilitation alternatives and for programs that support the patient's late-stage rehabilitation and reintegration. It is a vicious cycle that forces the increased utilization of less appropriate and costlier rehabilitation options, especially in the later stages of the cycle.

One option for future federal and state funding would be the negotiation of a higher rate of reimbursement that is more in line with the true cost of care and services required by traumatically injured patients. Compilation of cost-comparison factors, specific treatment plans, functional goals, and expected outcomes can assist in the lobbying of funding sources for an alternative rate. An incentive needs to be developed by the government payment systems to encourage cost-effective, quality alternatives. Managed care is likely to be initiated throughout various government payment settings.

Catastrophic health care insurance is an issue that is repeatedly discussed by the U.S. Congress. Mandatory contributions by all citizens would be made into a pool of funds, which would then be available for rehabilitation and long-term services for those who sustain severe disability. The public, however, may not be willing to pay the economic cost, as evidenced by the rescinding of the Medicare catastrophic care provision in 1990. A number of advocacy groups for the disabled continue to support the development of a model of funding that eventually will include catastrophic care for all. At this point, there does not appear to be an indication of change in reimbursement in the near future.

Until the funding issues are resolved, professionals will experience continued frustration as injured people fail to receive the most appropriate and state-of-the-art rehabilitation. Many injured people are not able to reach their full potential of recovery without this financial support.

Acceptance of the Trauma-Disabled Person in Society

Societal awareness of trauma and its long-term effects is minimal, considering it is the leading cause of death and disability for young adults.[28, 29] Long-term disability in such a young population leads to an ever-increasing percentage of traumatically life-altered people in our society. The media have helped to enlighten society about physical disability. Parking spaces reserved for handicapped people, curb ramps, and other accessibility-related standards, such as those defined in the Americans with Disabilities Act of 1990, are accepted and expected in daily life. Society's acceptance of the physically disabled person is becoming a reality.

Not as much progress has been made in the acceptance of the cognitive and psychosocial ramifications of injury. Cognitive and behavioral disability caused by head injury or injury related psychological trauma is poorly understood by the public. People who do not comprehend the nature of the problems and the needs of the cognitively and behaviorally disabled are frightened of and reject them. There is an attempt to label people with behavior problems as mentally retarded, crazy, or rude. Mental illness has a long history of poor acceptance in society.

As the mentally disabled population grows, more people will have contact with these problems in the work, home, and community settings. Efforts at public education and sensitization enhance the true reintegration of intellectually and behaviorally disabled people. This process is necessary for trauma-disabled people to return to a contributing role in society. However, it is unrealistic to think that all catastrophically injured people will return to the community, whether because of limited function or societal resistance.

Trauma Prevention

The multiple issues of trauma rehabilitation would not exist if the initial trauma were prevented. Initiation of media exposure and legislation by advocacy groups, such as Mothers Against Drunk Driving, has created nationwide support for the prevention of trauma. The greatest focus has been placed on prevention of traffic accidents and drug- and alcohol-related trauma. Recent changes in child car seat safety, seat belt, and air bag legislation reflect a growing consciousness of prevention. Punitive drug, alcohol, and handgun laws represent attempts to deter a person's actions that may result in severe trauma to others.

Trauma prevention is an educational process. As in any preventable problem, it is not that society does not want to prevent the trauma, but rather that it recognizes the potential for injury. As an awareness of trauma increases, so will legitimate public support for those actions that can prevent the injuries from occurring.

It is the responsibility of all rehabilitationists to support education through individual and family teaching, media exposure, community interest groups, churches, schools, and every setting in society. The public also expects health care professionals to act as role models of healthier and safer living.

Total prevention of traumatic injury is a worthy challenge to professionals and society. It is a reasonable goal for society to work toward reduced incidence and severity of injury and disability in the immediate future.[29]

SUMMARY

Role of the Trauma Rehabilitation Nurse

Trauma rehabilitation presents many exciting and expanding opportunities for nurses. New roles for expert rehabilitationists benefit from nursing's holistic approach to the physical, cognitive, and psychosocial components of rehabilitation programming. Rehabilitation liaison and discharge planning roles in trauma centers effectively link the intermediate and rehabilitation phases.[2] Clinical nurse specialists and nurse practitioners support early initiation of rehabilitation techniques by awareness of potential rehabilitation outcomes. In the rehabilitation and reintegration phases, nursing makes significant contributions to the roles of rehabilitation coordinator and case manager.[13, 30, 31]

In addition to clinical practice, many nurses have blended rehabilitation specialization with administration, public relations, and research to provide a wealth of expertise and skill to health providers and the trauma population. Nurses are effective in program development, direction, marketing, and consulting roles.

Regardless of the trauma rehabilitation nurse's distinct role, it is essential that all members of the profession involve themselves in the issues that rehabilitation faces in the future. Active participation in professional and disability-related organizations such as the Association of Rehabilitation Nurses, the American Congress of Rehabilitation Medicine, the American Association of Spinal Cord Injury Nurses, the Case Management Society of America, the National Association of Rehabilitation Professionals in the Private Sector, the American Spinal Cord Injury Association, and the National Head Injury Foundation, or their local networks offers an opportunity for nurses to work creatively and constructively toward improved legislation and guidelines for practice, community awareness, and community support for the disabled population. Involvement in rehabilitation issues may occur on an individual basis or through activities by the employing facility or organization. Nurses in clinical practice with direct interaction with patients and families have the vital role of educating those most directly affected about rehabilitation issues. Through this comprehensive effort, issues are resolved.

A wealth of personal and professional growth is available to nurses in trauma rehabilitation. The specialty is at such a stage of development that it welcomes new ideas and expertise. For the person who longs to create an advanced role in nursing, trauma rehabilitation may offer this opportunity.

Future Research

A great deal of research still needs to be conducted on the steps involved in rehabilitation after traumatic injury. Trauma rehabilitation has borrowed therapeutic approaches from many other specialties, including stroke and neurological disease rehabilitation, psychiatry, normal and abnormal child development studies, and mental retardation. The areas in which clinical research can be conducted over the next decade are unlimited.

The cost-effectiveness of rehabilitation poses both ethical and pragmatic concerns. In 1985, the estimated cost for the first year of rehabilitation after a severe head injury was $500,000.[32] Recent analysis by the House Subcommittee on Small Business, including private rehabilitation facilities, cited lifetime care costs for a severely brain-injured person to be more than $4 million.[33] Does society have the funds to rehabilitate everyone? The cost could be cut by close scrutiny of rehabilitation provided on a case-by-case basis, or the funds might be made available only to those injured people who meet specified criteria, having the greatest potential outcome. How would society decide who has the greatest potential outcome?[34]

It is the responsibility of every rehabilitation practitioner and facility to closely examine and study the cost-effectiveness of treatments and practices. Sometimes health care professionals assume that more is better. Future research could be directed toward identifying minimal standards that still result in high-quality outcomes. How often is an equipment change or a treatment needed? Could it be done half as often with the same result, therefore cutting the cost in half? Beginning with the simplistic adjustments and practice based on clinical research will level the skyrocketing costs of rehabilitation.

Because the specialty of trauma rehabilitation is young, adequate data are not yet available to evaluate the long-term and lifelong needs of the traumatized population. Beyond rehabilitation outcome studies, usually only 1 to 5 years after rehabilitation, the study of effects of aging and life-style in people who have experienced a catastrophic illness will help the rehabilitation profession provide appropriate education, adaptation, and follow-up for lifelong support.

Clinical research in the direction of heightened potential for recovery is a most exciting prospect. Current physiologic studies of central nervous system tissue support the theory that nerve cells are able to regenerate. Studies of "sprouting" in damaged brain tissue offer great possibilities for future brain recovery.[35] Electrical stimulation of muscle groups supports the use of previously ineffective limbs. Rehabilitationists are slow to accept these new alternatives, but the potential for improved recovery is becoming a reality.

The field of trauma rehabilitation and its patient population benefit from the research, education, expert clinical practice, and leadership of professional rehabilitation nurses.

REFERENCES

1. NARF Issue Brief. Washington, DC, National Association of Rehabilitation Facilities, membership publication.
2. Role of the Rehabilitation Nurse in the Trauma Care System. Skokie, Ill, Association of Rehabilitation Nurses, 1991.
3. Sbordone RJ, Howard ME: Pre-Injury Predictors of Rehabilitation Potential and Outcome from Head Injury (A Scale). Dallas, Dallas Rehabilitation Institute, 1986.
4. Stryker R: Rehabilitation Aspects of Acute and Chronic Nursing Care. 2nd ed. Philadelphia, WB Saunders Co, 1972, pp 5–11.
5. Statistics on Rehabilitation Hospitals, Units and Number of Beds Excluded from Medicare Prospective Payment System. Washington, DC, National Association of Rehabilitation Facilities, February 2, 1992.
6. Standards Manual for Organizations Serving People with Disabilities. Tucson, Commission on Accreditation of Rehabilitation Facilities, 1989.
7. Krueger DW: Psychological rehabilitation of physical trauma and disability. In Krueger D (ed): Rehabilitation Psychology. Rockville, Md, Aspen Systems, 1984, pp 6–8.
8. Cobble N, Bontke C, Brandstater M, Horn L: Rehabilitation of brain disorders; intervention strategies. Arch Phys Med Rehabil 4-S:324–331, 1991.
9. White MJ, Holloway M: Patient concerns after discharge from rehabilitation. Rehabil Nurs 6:316–318, 1990.
10. Keith RA: The comprehensive treatment team in rehabilitation. Arch Phys Med Rehabil 5:269–274, 1991.
11. Byrne ML, Thompson LF: Key Concepts for the Study and Practice of Nursing. 2nd ed. St. Louis, CV Mosby, 1978, pp 103–126.
12. Wiener SM: Rehabilitation nursing in the private sector. Rehabil Nurs 8:31–32, 1983.
13. National Association of Rehabilitation Professionals in the Private Sector: Professional performance criteria for medical case management. NARPPS Journal & News 6:111–115, 1990.
14. Jaffe K: Facility Based Case Managers: The Evolution Continues. Case Manager, April 1991, pp 39–42.
15. Rondinelli RD, Murphy JR, Wilson DH, Miller CC: Predictors of functional outcome and resource utilization in inpatient rehabilitation. Arch Phys Med Rehabil 7:447–453, 1991.
16. Granger CV, Hamilton BB, Keith RA, et al: Advances in functional assessment for medical rehabilitation. Top Geriatric Rehabilitation 1:59–74, 1986.
17. Masso AR: Trends in managed care. Presentation at the Medical Case Management Conference III, Individual Case Management Association, held in Dallas, July 18, 1991.
18. Rehabilitation: Facilities target service to a changing market. Provider, November 1990, pp 8–14.
19. Jones M, Evans RW: Rating outcomes in post-acute rehabilitation of aquired brain injury. Case Manager, January 1991, pp 44–47.
20. Sherburne E: A rehabilitation protocol for the neuroscience intensive care unit. J Neuro Nurs 18:140–145, 1986.
21. Deutsch PM, Sawyer HW (eds): A Guide to Rehabilitation. New York, Matthew Bender, 1986, chaps. 7 and 13.
22. Mobility, Rehabilitation Nursing: Concepts in Practice. A Core Curriculum, Evanston, Ill, Rehabilitation Nursing Foundations, 1981, pp 95–126.
23. Campion L: The nurse's role in the management of emotional problems. In Krueger D (ed): Rehabilitation Psychology. Rockville, Md, Aspen Systems, 1984, pp 213–220.
24. Campbell CH: Needs of relatives and helpfulness of support groups in severe head injury. Rehabil Nurs 6:320–325, 1988.
25. Boughton A, Ciesla N: Physical therapy management of the head injured patient in the intensive care unit. Top Acute Care Trauma Rehabilitation 1:1–18, 1986.
26. Ulrey BJ, Woods NM: The role of video fluoroscopy in the diagnosis and treatment of mealtime dysfunction in the brain injured patient. Top Acute Care Trauma Rehabilitation 1:19–31, 1986.
27. Ridley B: Tom's story: A quadriplegic who refused rehabilitation. Rehabil Nurs 5:250–253, 1989.
28. Baker SP, O'Neill B, Karpf RS: The Injury Fact Book. Lexington, Lexington Books, 1984.
29. Parsons KC, Lammertse DP: Epidemiology, prevention and system of care in spinal cord disorders. Arch Phys Med Rehabil 4-S:290–292, 1991.
30. Standards of Rehabilitation Nursing Practice. Kansas City, Mo, American Nurses Association and the Association of Rehabilitation Nurses, 1986.
31. Role Description of Case Managers. Skokie, Ill, Association of Rehabilitation Nursing, 1990.
32. Massive Injury Medical Management Reserve Projection Guidelines. New York, American Re-insurance Company, 1985.
33. Office of United States Congressional Representative, Ron Wyden (D-OR), Memo of 2/1/92 to House Subcommittee on Small Business on "Silent Epidemic"—Brain injury rehabilitation costs. Long-Term Care Management, February 27, 1992, p 1.
34. Wennberg JE: Outcomes research, cost containment and the fear of health care rationing. N Engl J Med 323:1202–1204, 1990.
35. Bach-y-Rita P: Central nervous system lesions: Sprouting and unmasking. Arch Phys Med Rehabil 62:413–417, 1981.

PART III

Single System Injuries

17

CENTRAL NERVOUS SYSTEM I: CLOSED HEAD INJURIES*

PAMELA H. MITCHELL

Head injury is the leading cause of all trauma-related deaths. Head injuries occur every 15 seconds, and someone dies from a severe head injury every 12 minutes. Head injury mortality is almost 50 per cent, but equally significant is the high incidence of long-term disability in survivors and the annual societal costs totaling almost $5 billion. In terms of incidence, mortality and morbidity, economic costs, and use of medical resources, head injury constitutes a major health problem in the United States today.

Once injured, the brain remains in jeopardy of further insult, unlike other system injuries. Subsequent events such as hypoxia, hypercarbia, hypotension, and intracranial hypertension promote brain ischemia and are frequently responsible for worsening the initial event and causing secondary injury to viable brain tissue. Many head-injured patients who would otherwise recover with only mild neurological deficits are left with major disability as a result of these secondary events. The prevention, recognition, and immediate treatment of these complications in the prehospital, resuscitation, and critical care cycles of head injury management are of utmost importance. The intermediate care and rehabilitation cycles of head injury management present unique problems as well. Patients who have sustained severe injury are often in coma for weeks to months and manifest innumerable multisystem complications secondary to immobility and central nervous system disarray. Recovery is often a lifelong process beset with physical, mental, emotional, and social obstacles. Optimal nursing care, aggressive rehabilitation, and continuance of family support are essential.

The purpose of this chapter is to provide the trauma nurse with a comprehensive review of traumatic brain injury and its sequelae from prevention through rehabilitation. Trauma nursing is not "system selective"; it requires proficiency in assessment and management of all system injuries, including the central nervous system. A basic understanding of correl-

*Revised from a chapter in the first edition written by Gerri Spielman McGinnis, with contributions from Karen McQuillan.

ative neuroanatomy, neuroassessment, and treatment modalities provides a strong foundation for the trauma nurse caring for brain-injured patients.

EPIDEMIOLOGY

We do not know the incidence of head injury in the United States because such data are not collected centrally and because varying types of injuries may be included in the category "head injury." However, extrapolations of a few systematic studies estimate the annual incidence at 400 to 600 per 100,000 people.[1–4] These injuries account for 2 to 5 per cent of all hospital admissions and result in 17 deaths per 100,000 persons.[5] The vast majority of head injuries occur in motor vehicle accidents, with 15- to 24-year-old males outnumbering females 3 to 1.[3, 5] Falls account for the majority of head injury deaths in people older than age 65, with older males outnumbering older females 2 to 1. Overall rates of head injury death are similar for all races; however, the death rate from motor vehicle accidents is nearly 40 per cent higher for 15- to 34-year-old whites than for blacks. In contrast, the death rate from firearm-caused head injuries is higher for blacks than for whites aged 15 to 44.[5] About two-thirds of head injury deaths occur prior to hospitalization, thus emphasizing the importance of prevention and prehospital treatment. Of those admitted to hospitals with severe head injury, defined as a Glasgow Coma Score of 8 or less, 50 per cent die. Overall mortality varies from 9 to 74 per cent, depending on type of injury.[4, 6]

Economic costs of head injury are staggering. According to the National Head and Spinal Cord Survey, updated to current dollars, direct and indirect costs total more than $6 billion.[7] *Direct costs* include initial and follow-up diagnosis, treatment, and rehabilitation. *Indirect costs* include societal losses secondary to restricted productive activity. One state estimated individual costs, which, if updated to current dollars, are nearly $11,000 per person, or $50 million annually, 41 per cent of which are paid from public funds.[8]

ETIOLOGY

The major causes of head injury are, respectively, motor vehicle accidents, falls, and assaults. Most traffic accidents and fatalities occur in the summer, on weekends, and during normal weather conditions. Falls are more common in the elderly, and assaults are more prevalent in urban areas.[9] All major causes of head injury have one commonality—they are all highly associated with coexisting alcohol usage.

Alcohol

In a comparison study of intoxicated versus nonintoxicated injured patients, intoxicated patients were found to have a higher incidence of head injury, total body injury, and mortality.[10] Several factors contribute to increased mortality and morbidity in this population: (1) alcohol-impaired drivers are less likely to wear seat belts, rendering them more prone to both head and extracranial injuries, (2) acute and chronic alcoholism increases susceptibility to aspiration, seizures, and metabolic complications, and (3) alcohol masks neurological injury and decreases the chances of accurate diagnosis and prompt initiation of treatment. The magnitude of the alcohol problem is evident by the fact that approximately 40 per cent of all individuals sustaining trauma and 60 per cent of head-injured persons are under the influence of alcohol at the time of hospital admission.[9, 11, 12]

Other Factors

Other population subgroups noted to be at increased risk for traffic injury are individuals who fail to use a safety restraint system; cyclists without protective helmets; those under stress; those who surpass recommended speed limits; the illiterate, the senile, and the drug user; and those with limited vision, convulsive disorders, or medical conditions that involve loss of neuromuscular control.[12–14] After an initial head injury, the relative risk of having a second injury is tripled, and after a second injury, the risk increases to eight times that of the general population. It is felt that the increased risk of repeated injury is due to behavioral characteristics such as alcohol abuse.[1] The reader is referred to Chapters 1 and 7 for detailed discussion of causative factors and prevention of head injury.

CORRELATIVE NEUROANATOMY

The Central Nervous System

The central nervous system (CNS) consists of the brain and spinal cord. The brain provides most of the control functions for the entire body. Like a computer, the brain receives thousands of bits of information from the different sensory organs and then integrates them to determine the response to be made by the body. In general, the brain maintains the quality and uniqueness of human life and behavior. The major divisions of the brain are the cerebrum, cerebellum, and brainstem (Fig. 17–1). The following section focuses on the correlative anatomy of major cerebral and brainstem structures and systems that are essential to nursing assessment of the head-injured patient.

Cerebrum

The cerebrum includes the two cerebral hemispheres and the diencephalon. It is capped by gray cortex (neuronal cell bodies), under which lies extensive white matter (axons). The cerebral hemispheres are responsible for sensory and motor processes of the contralateral side of the body. Sensory information entering the spinal cord from the right side of the body crosses over to the left before reaching the cortex. Similarly, motor impulses originating from the right cerebral cortex cross over to the left before synapsing in the cord. This accounts for one of the fundamental principles of motor assessment; i.e., structural lesions causing compression of descending motor tract fibers will almost always result in contralateral motor signs.

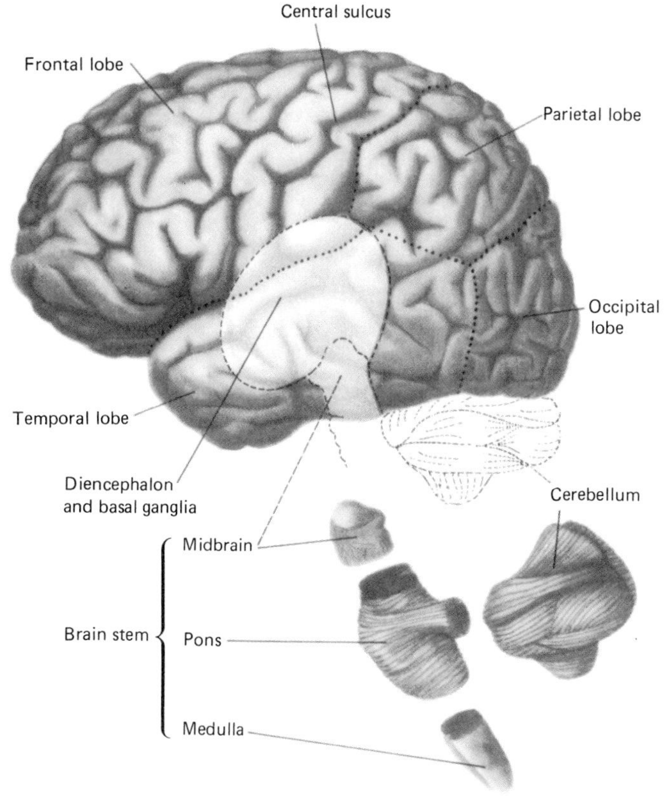

Figure 17–1. Major parts of the central nervous system. (Reprinted by permission of the publishers from Kandel E, Schwartz J: Principles of Neural Science, 3d ed. New York, Elsevier/North-Holland, 1991. Copyright 1991 by Elsevier Science Publishing Co., Inc.)

Cerebral Hemispheres

The cerebral hemispheres are divided into four lobes: frontal, temporal, parietal, and occipital (Fig. 17–2). Knowledge of the primary functions of the lobes (Table 17–1) and lesion location can provide the nurse with relevant information that can be applied more specifically to the neurological assessment. For example, it can be anticipated that a lesion in the prefrontal region may result in altered behavior, whereas a lesion in the posterior frontal region of the dominant hemisphere may result in language dysfunction. Accordingly, the assessment and nursing care plan anticipate and focus on these actual or potential problems.

The Diencephalon

The diencephalon is a complex of structures consisting of the epithalamus, thalamus, hypothalamus, and subthalamus. The hypothalamus, situated deep within the brain and just above the brainstem, is the most notable of the diencephalic structures. The hypothalamus is the primary regulator of autonomic function and controls numerous visceral and metabolic activities, including regulation of temperature, blood pressure, pupils, shivering, sweating, gastrointestinal stimulation, and water balance. Through its connection with the pituitary gland via the hypophyseal stalk, the hypothalamus directly influences pituitary hormonal activities and, in con-

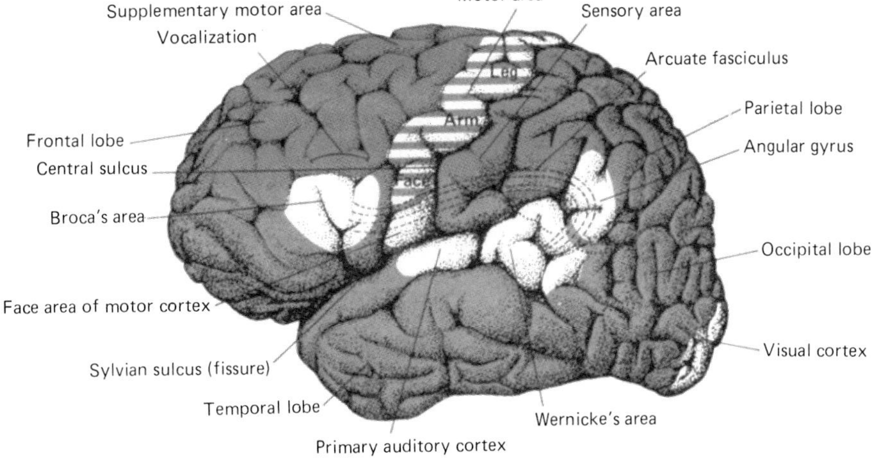

Figure 17–2. Lobes of the brain. (From Kandel E, Schwartz J: Principles of Neural Science, 3rd ed. New York, Elsevier North-Holland, 1991. (Copyright 1991 by Elsevier Science Publishing Co., Inc.)

TABLE 17–1. PRIMARY FUNCTIONS OF THE CORTEX BY LOBES

LOBE	FUNCTION
Frontal	Prefrontal
	Short-term memory
	Emotional responsiveness
	Abstract thinking
	Foresight/judgment
	Behavior/tactfulness
	Primary motor cortex
	Broca's speech area (dominant hemisphere)*
	Expressive speech/vocalization
	Intellect
	Personality
Temporal	Primary auditory cortex
	Visual task learning
	Dominant hemisphere*
	Wernicke's speech area
	Receptive speech/comprehension
	Interpretive area
	Intellect
	Emotion
	Long-term memory
	Dominant hemisphere: verbal
	Nondominant hemisphere: sensory
Parietal	Primary sensory cortex
	Sensory interpretation
	Tactile and kinesthetic sense
	Body awareness
	Body image
	Spatial orientation/relations
	Dominant hemisphere
	Language
	Object perception/recognition
	Nondominant hemisphere
	Neglect syndrome
Occipital	Primary visual cortex
	Visual association

*Dominance: The majority (80 per cent) of both right- and left-handed people have left hemispheric dominance for speech. A small percentage of left-handed people have both right and left hemispheric speech control. The preponderance of left cerebral dominance is felt to be due to anatomical asymmetry of the human brain. Sixty-five per cent of people have a larger speech area (Wernicke's) surface on the left hemisphere; in 11 per cent the right is larger, and in 24 per cent the right and left sides are equal in size. Hemispheric lateralization or dominance is also found in functions related to mood and affect as well as verbal, auditory, and visuospatial tasks.

junction with the pituitary, mediates the body's stress/adaptation response.

The stress response can be seen immediately following cerebral or extracranial injury and consists of hypothalamic stimulation of the autonomic nervous system (ANS) and adrenals to increase circulating corticoids and catecholamines. This results in increased levels of cortisol, aldosterone, epinephrine, and norepinephrine (Fig. 17–3). The systemic responses resulting from elevation of these hormones and the alterations they produce are listed in Figures 17–4 to 17–6.

The stress response generally lasts for 72 hours, with the degree of response and level of circulating corticoids and catecholamines being directly proportional to the injury severity. In patients with severe injury, the response can be prolonged and exaggerated and result in major metabolic complications. The most frequently encountered metabolic complications associated with severe traumatic brain injury are listed in Table 17–2.

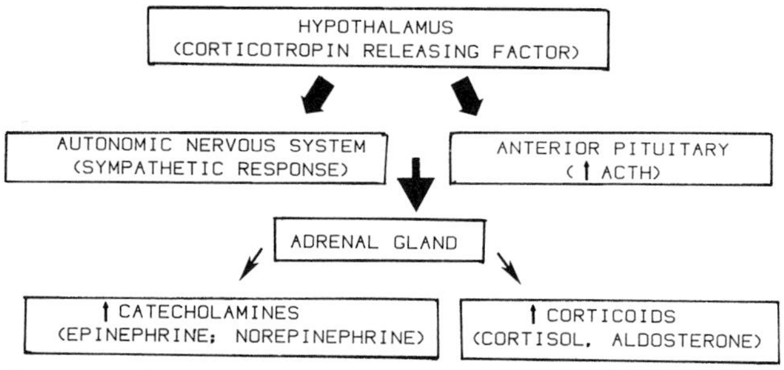

Figure 17–3. Normal physiological response to injury/stress. (From Spielman G: Metabolic complications associated with severe diffuse brain injury. J Neurosurg Nurs 2:83–88, 1985.)

The hypothalamus is also vulnerable to direct cerebral trauma, increased intracranial pressure, edema, and compressive lesions. Hypothalamic dysfunction is most frequently associated with severe diffuse axonal injury (DAI) and complicates the recovery process.[16, 17]

Brainstem

The brainstem is a midline structure located within the center of the brain. It is situated between the diencephalon and the spinal cord, which descends directly downward from the lowest segment of the brainstem, the medulla. The brainstem is surrounded by the temporal lobes on either side and the fourth ventricle and cerebellum to the rear. The brainstem has three sections: the midbrain, the pons, and the medulla (see Fig. 17–1).

A variety of activities are assigned to the brainstem. It is the vegetative center of the brain that controls basic and reflexive activities like sleep and wakefulness, breathing, blood pressure, and heart rate. It is the pathway used by sensory fibers as they ascend from the cord to the cortex. Corticospinal motor tract fibers on their descent from the cortex also traverse the brainstem and cross over (decussate) in the medulla before exiting the spinal cord. The reticular activating system responsible for consciousness originates in the brainstem. The brainstem also controls many of the special senses that are mediated by the cranial nerves, which arise and exit from this structure.

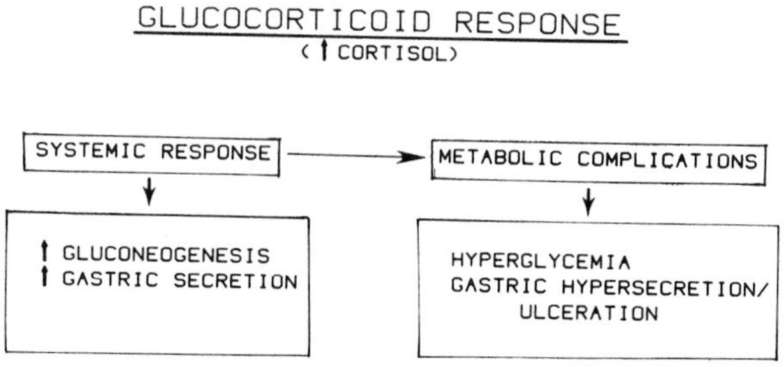

Figure 17–4. The systemic response to elevated glucocorticoids. (From Spielman G: Metabolic complications associated with severe diffuse brain injury. J Neurosurg Nurs 2:83–88, 1985.)

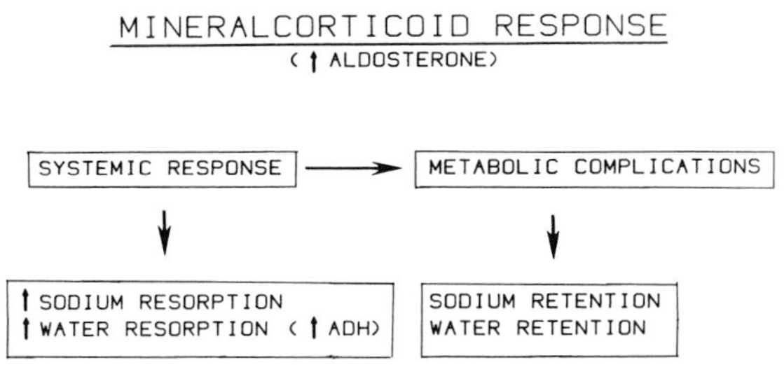

Figure 17–5. The systemic response to elevated mineral corticoids. (From Spielman G: Metabolic complications associated with severe diffuse brain injury. J Neurosurg Nurs 2:83–88, 1985.)

TABLE 17–2. METABOLIC COMPLICATIONS ASSOCIATED WITH SEVERE TRAUMATIC BRAIN INJURY

Hyperglycemia
Sodium retention
Water retention
Anemia
Immunosuppression
Intravascular thrombosis
Fat embolus
Coagulopathy
Hypermetabolism
Hypercatabolism
Gastric hypersecretion

From Spielman G: Metabolic complications associated with severe diffuse brain injury. J Neurosurg Nurs 2:83–88, 1985.

GENERAL RESPONSE TO CNS INJURY

Central Nervous System Cellular Response

The nervous system contains two classes of cells: the neuroglial or glial cell and the nerve cell or neuron. Glial cells outnumber neurons 9 to 1 and are generally classified as astrocytes, oligodendrocytes, microglia, ependymal cells, or Schwann cells. Glial cells lack axons and function primarily as connective tissue by providing support for nerve cells and vasculature.

In response to CNS disease or injury, glial cells have both beneficial and deleterious effects. Following neuronal injury, glial cells mobilize and proliferate at the injury site. They act as scavenger cells and aid in the healing process by phagocytosing cellular debris and toxic products left by injured degenerating neurons. This proliferation of glia at the zone of trauma also results in obstructive scar tissue formation, which can block the course of regenerating axons and prevent the formation of new synaptic connections.

The neuron consists of a cell body, dendrites, axon, and presynaptic terminals of the axon (Fig. 17–7). Each component of the cell has a distinctive function. The cell body synthesizes and packages the products of neuronal metabolism and transports them to other regions of the cell. It exchanges nutrients, ions, and other metabolically active substances with the extracellular environment through the cell membrane. This lipid bilayer membrane is crucial to depolarization of the neuron through such mechanisms as Na^+, K^+, and ATPase pumps, ion-selective channels, and voltage-sensitive channels. The cell membrane is the mediator of CNS metabolism that serves the basic cellular function of synaptic transmission (activation metabolism) and which is required to maintain the integrity of the nerve cell itself (residual metabolism).[18] The myelin-covered axon, a tubular extension of the cell body, is responsible for rapid nerve conduction. The presynaptic terminals are specialized endings at the distal portion of the axon that transmit information by chemical or electrical means to other neurons or effector cells. The specialized contact zone between the transmitting (presynaptic cell) and the receiving (postsynaptic cell) neuron is the synapse. The cell body and its fine arborizing extensions, the dendrites, are the receptor surfaces that receive the incoming impulses. The physiological and anatomical properties of the nerve cell account for its ability to communicate with other cells, a function unique to the neuron. In general, the neuron is a signal cell, responsible for processing, analyzing, and acting on all incoming and outgoing information that ultimately culminates in all our behavioral responses. Neurons differ from other cells not only in their communicative ability but also in their lack of mitotic ability. Without mitosis, neurons cannot multiply. With CNS maturity, the number of neurons is fixed at approximately 10^{12}, and no new neurons are added.

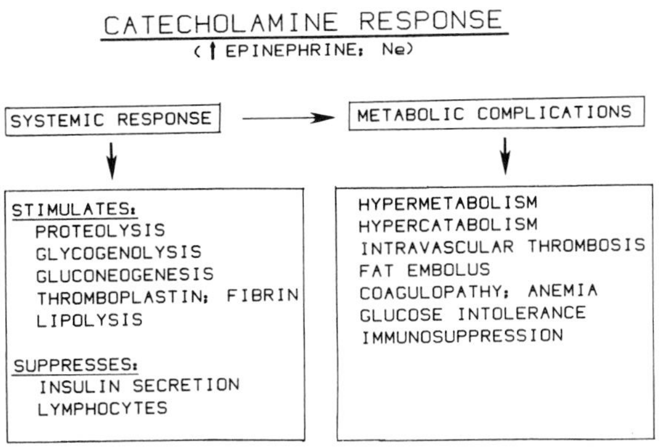

Figure 17–6. The systemic response to elevated catecholamines. (From Spielman G: Metabolic complications associated with severe diffuse brain injury. J Neurosurg Nurs 2:83–88, 1985.)

Loss of neurons normally occurs with aging, and it is estimated that 1000 nerve cells are lost each day after age 40. This rate may be markedly accelerated by alcohol, the most common cause of cortical atrophy in the fifth and sixth decades of life. A substantial reduction in neurons occurs in CNS disease states, particularly in severe traumatic brain injury.

Injury to neurons is significant because it results in cell loss with no new cell replacement. This causes permanent structural changes in the nervous system with subsequent neurological deficits and disability.

Cerebral Metabolism

The average brain weighs 3 pounds and accounts for 2 per cent of the adult body weight. Despite its size, the brain receives almost a quarter of the body's total oxygen and glucose requirements. The primary energy source for the brain is glucose, which is converted by oxidative metabolism into a high-energy phosphate form, adenosine triphosphate

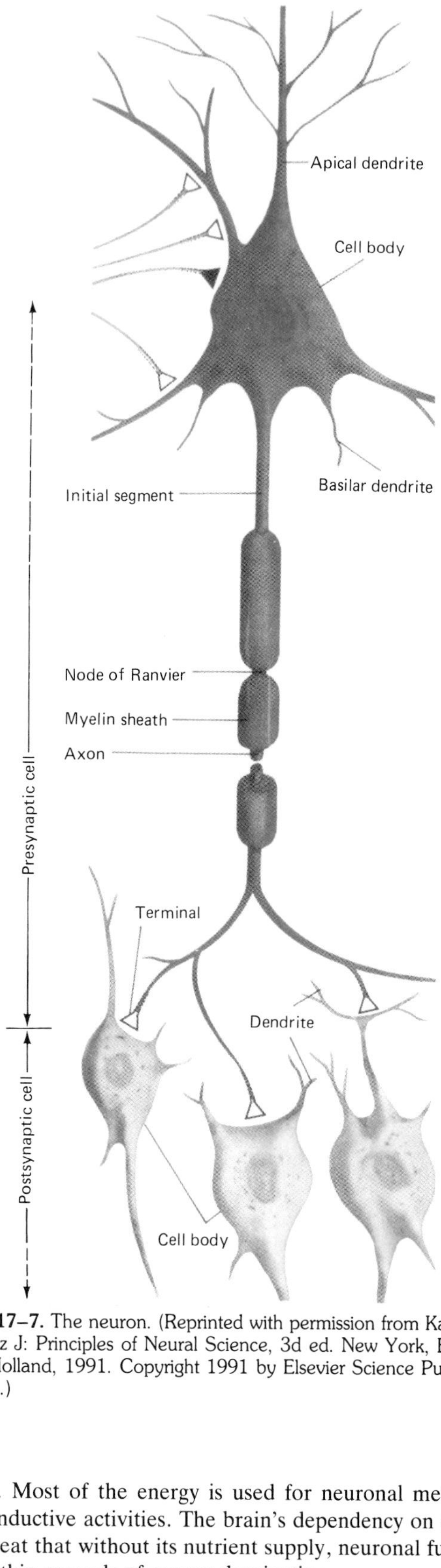

Figure 17–7. The neuron. (Reprinted with permission from Kandel E, Schwartz J: Principles of Neural Science, 3d ed. New York, Elsevier/North-Holland, 1991. Copyright 1991 by Elsevier Science Publishing Co., Inc.)

(ATP). Most of the energy is used for neuronal metabolic and conductive activities. The brain's dependency on energy is so great that without its nutrient supply, neuronal function fails within seconds of energy deprivation.

The need for glucose and its rate of production depend on the degree of metabolic activity coupled with the rate of oxygen consumption. If metabolism is increased, as occurs in seizures, hyperthermia, or decerebration, oxygen requirements increase; when metabolism is decreased, as in coma or hypothermia, oxidative requirements are reduced.

Oxygen and glucose are in continuous demand, since the brain has minimal storage capacity for either substrate. Following severe head injury, oxygen availability can easily be jeopardized when hypoxemia or ischemia is present. Hypoxemia has detrimental effects on cerebral metabolism and function when the level of O_2 in arterial blood is less than 50 mm Hg. For this reason, airway management and oxygen delivery are priorities in the prehospital and resuscitation management of comatose head-injured patients. During critical care head injury management, frequent monitoring of arterial blood gases is essential to maintain the PaO_2 at 100 mm Hg or greater.

Cerebral ischemia results in hypoxia and causes neuronal death and injury. Ischemia is present in 90 per cent of head injury deaths and is a primary factor in head injury morbidity. Attempts have been made to protect the brain from ischemia with barbiturates and hypothermia. The use of these agents is based on the premise that by depressing cerebral metabolism, overall energy and oxygen requirements will be reduced. Brain cells will then be more likely to survive the ischemic assault because their nutrient requirements are minimized.

Other causes of cerebral ischemia are increased intracranial pressure and hypotension. For these complications, current treatment modalities are employed to maintain intracranial pressure (ICP) less than 20 mm Hg and systolic blood pressure greater than 100 mm Hg with pressors as needed. Too aggressive hyperventilation also has been cited as an ischemia-producing factor, and higher levels of $PaCO_2$ (27–30 mm Hg) are advised to prevent overwhelming constriction of cerebral vessels.[4]

Primary versus Secondary Injury

Damage to neurons is either primary or secondary. Primary injury results in tissue and/or vascular disruption and occurs at the time of injury. Once primary injury occurs, the damage is done, and it cannot be reversed. Secondary neuronal injury is generally associated with the acute phase of head injury and results from subsequent events or complications that accompany the initial injury. The major events associated with secondary neuronal injury are hypoxia, hypotension, hypercarbia, ischemia, edema, and increased intracranial pressure.[4] The major goal of prehospital, resuscitation, and critical care management is prevention, early recognition, and prompt treatment of these secondary injury mechanisms.

Reaction of the Neuron to Injury

In head injury, as in any type of injury, hypoxia/ischemia is the fundamental initiator of cellular injury. Ischemia may occur either by direct damage or occlusion of local brain blood supply or by systemic loss of pumping or aerating capacity of the heart and lungs. Thus both primary and secondary injury, as described above, operate by producing cellular hypoxia. This hypoxia sets in motion a cascade of cellular events that not only compromises the ability of the cell to maintain its metabolic functions but also may affect noninjured cells by damaging the microvasculature and thereby increasing CNS ischemia. The hypothesized cellular injury cascade is shown in Figure 17–8. Injury initiates cellular hypoxia, producing loss of Ca^{2+} channel regulation and subsequent influx of Ca^{2+} into the cells. In turn, this influx of Ca^{2+} activates phospholipases which hydrolyze membrane phospholipids and result in accumulation of free fatty acids, such as arachidonic acid. These events disrupt both mitochondria and the plasma membrane, creating a vicious cycle with further influx of extracellular ions. Such damage to the membrane of the microvasculature induces further ischemia, which results in lactic acidosis and generation of free radicals (substances such as oxygen and hydroxyls that have an unpaired electron and thus an electric charge). These events further disrupt cell membranes and thus synaptic transmission.[19–21]

Once a neuron has been injured, distinct morphologic changes occur throughout the cell in reaction to the injury. Proximal to the site of injury, the cell body undergoes chromatolysis. These chromatolytic changes result in cessation or impairment of cellular metabolism. Degenerative changes (wallerian degeneration) occur distal from the zone of trauma and involve the axon and terminals. This results in lost or impaired nerve conduction. Depending on the severity of injury, the neuron has two options.

1. When injury is extensive and the damage is irreversible, progressive degeneration of the nerve cell occurs, followed by glial cell phagocytosis. A void is created by the vanished cell, and neuronal loss results. The loss of relatively few neurons may be insignificant, but substantial loss results in marked cortical atrophy as brain cells literally disappear. The degree of functional disability correlates with the extent of neuronal loss.
2. When neuronal injury is less extensive, the nerve cell has the potential to restore its functional capabilities. Restoration of function is believed to occur through neuronal rearrangement of the injured neurons themselves or of neighboring uninjured neurons.

Neuronal Rearrangement: Axonal Repair and Regeneration

Injury to the neuron results in loss of synaptic contact or denervation. Since previous sites of synaptic contact are no longer innervated, the cell must receive innervation from new synaptic connections. The generation of a new synapse is termed *synaptogenesis.* If reinnervation and synaptogenesis are successful, then return of function is possible.

The recovery process of injured neurons involves rearrangement or "rewiring" of the injured nerve cells. This "reprogramming" process is thought to play a major role in promoting recovery of function after CNS injury. Two types of rewiring are theorized to occur following neuronal injury: axonal regeneration and sprouting.

Axonal regeneration occurs in response to neuronal injury or axotomy and consists of neurite outgrowths or axonal sprouts that extend from the proximal segment of the injured axon. The neurites eventually form axons and nerve terminals if an appropriate target cell membrane is contacted. Growth of neurites appears to be directed by protein substances called *tropic,* or *nourishing, factors.*

Sprouting involves the outgrowth of neurites from adjacent uninjured neurons in response to loss of neighboring injured neurons. These new branches or axon collaterals establish new sites of innervation in close proximity to the denervated site. When synaptogenesis is accomplished, the injured nerve cell has regained the potential for receiving and transmitting messages. Whether sprouting is always functional is still questionable, since sprouting fibers may arise from a different location and react in a different manner from the original nerve cell. Sprouting has been observed within a few days following injury and continues over several months. Sprouting appears to occur more readily in the immature nervous system, an observation that is reinforced by the fact that children make better recoveries than do adults following CNS injury. Mechanical barriers such as scar tissue formation, hematomas, and infection are thought to hamper sprouting by inhibiting or blocking effective regrowth or causing misdirected growth away from the target area.

The existence of CNS sprouting in humans is still inconclusive, but based on evidence from mammalian research, the reality of repair and regrowth is supported by the fact that functional loss associated with cerebral lesions is not always permanent and irreversible. Following CNS insult, many patients who initially have severe functional losses go on to make dramatic recoveries with only minimal neurological deficits. Immediately after a stroke, for example, a patient may have marked aphasia and paralysis, but over time, significant improvement in speech and motor function occurs.

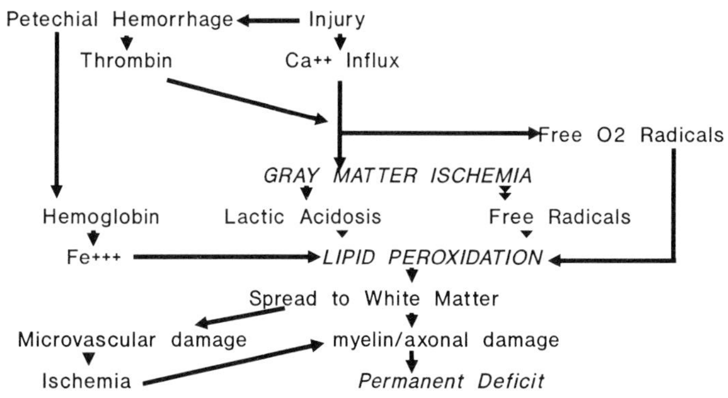

Figure 17–8. Hypothesized mechanisms by which ischemia and petechial hemorrhage create secondary injury in the brain already injured brain. (Redrawn from Hall ED: Free radicals and CNS injury. Crit Care Clin 5:793–805, 1990.)

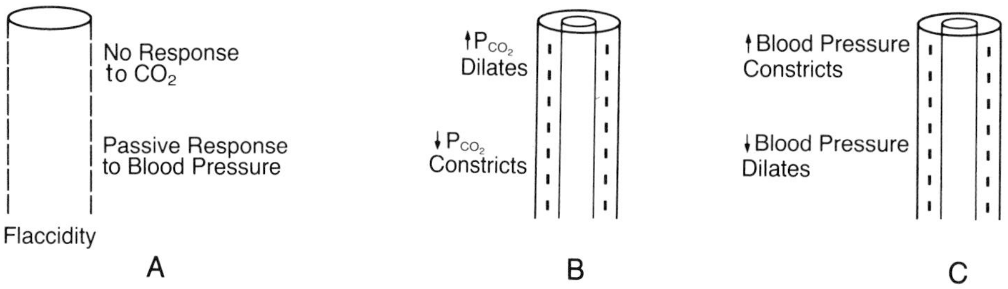

Figure 17–9. Autoregulation. Effect of blood pressure (*A*) and carbon dioxide (*B*) on cerebral arterioles with intact autoregulation. *C*, Loss of vasoconstrictor tone and autoregulatory response.

Both neuronal repair and axonal sprouting have significant potential for CNS recovery and as such have become major foci of CNS research. Current research includes investigation of (1) neurotropic agents such as NGF (nerve growth-promoting factor) to enhance sprouting by stimulating and guiding outgrowing neurites, (2) enzymatic substances to block scar formation, (3) hormones to enhance neuronal growth, and (4) tissue graft implantation to bridge regenerative peripheral nervous system (PNS) cells to injured CNS tissue.[22–24]

CEREBROVASCULAR RESPONSE

Cerebral Blood Flow

The normal brain receives a total of 750 ml of blood per minute or 50 ml/100 gm/minute. The disproportionate amount of flow is necessitated by the brain's incessant need for oxygen and glucose delivery. The rate of flow depends on neuronal activity. Gray matter, which contains the metabolically active cell bodies, normally receives three times more flow than white matter. Cerebral blood flow (CBF) decreases globally in coma and increases regionally with activation (hand movement) or specific activities (seizures, mental processing). In pathological deprivation states, blood flow reduction below 20 ml/100 gm/minute results in complete failure of neuronal electrical activity. In coma, both cerebral metabolism and blood flow are normally depressed. Even with a blood flow reduction of as much as 40 per cent, neuronal integrity can still be maintained as long as metabolism is equally reduced.

In comatose head-injured patients, especially those with elevated intracranial pressure (ICP), it is useful to know the metabolic rate and CBF so that treatment can be geared toward maintaining the correct balance of flow and metabolism. To determine coupling of CBF and metabolism and adequacy of cerebral perfusion, studies such as cerebral blood flow (CBF), cerebral metabolic rate for oxygen ($CMRo_2$), and arterial-jugular venous differences in oxygen ($a\text{-}vDo_2$) are sometimes performed. Obtained values indicate whether flow is sufficient, abnormally low, or in excess of metabolic needs. Cerebral blood flow studies indicate that 45 per cent of severely head-injured patients have subnormal flows, whereas 55 per cent demonstrate a hyperemic response. Those with supernormal flows are more likely to have intracranial hypertension than are patients with reduced flows.[25, 26]

Autoregulation

Pressure autoregulation is the brain's ability to maintain a constant rate of blood flow over a wide range of perfusion pressures despite changes in arterial blood pressure and ICP. The cerebral arterioles or resistance vessels are the primary agents of pressure regulation because of their ability to change diameter in response to certain metabolic and pressure variations (Fig. 17–9). These vessels have an inherent "self-regulatory" (autoregulatory) mechanism contained within their muscular walls which allows them to respond to changes in transmural pressure. As a result, an increase in arterial pressure causes vasoconstriction of the vessels, and a decrease in arterial pressure causes vasodilation (see Fig. 17–9). It is this mechanism that keeps cerebral blood flow essentially constant for a range of mean arterial pressures (MAP) from approximately 50 to 170 mm Hg.

Within the normal autoregulatory range there is a close relationship between cerebral perfusion pressure (CPP) and CBF, but once outside this range, CBF becomes passively dependent on the cerebral perfusion pressure, and delivery of metabolites is impaired. Exceeding the lower limits (MAP of 50 mm Hg or less) causes a decrease in flow and perfusion and results in ischemia; surpassing the upper limits (MAP greater than 160 to 170 mm Hg) causes a breakthrough in vasoconstriction with disruption of the blood–brain barrier, followed by passive dilation and increased flow.

Intact autoregulation safeguards the brain from fluctuations in arterial pressure and ICP. Normally, ICP increases during coughing and sneezing, blood pressure falls during a syncopal attack or shock, and arterial pressure rises in hypertensive individuals. In these instances, there is a compensatory increase or decrease in the vascular resistance to offset the change in the perfusion pressure. CBF remains adequate despite fluctuations as long as autoregulation is functional. In addition to the previously described myogenic pressure response, several metabolic factors have a marked effect on cerebral blood flow, namely, Pao_2, pH, and $Paco_2$. A decrease in Pao_2 below 50 mm Hg increases cerebral flow and volume. Extracellular reduction in pH or cerebral acidosis, caused by hypercarbia or lactic acid accumulation in ischemic brain tissue, causes vascular dilation and increases cerebral flow and volume. It must be kept in mind that in the presence of intracranial hypertension or impaired autoregulation, the addition of increased (blood) volume has deleterious effects. Of the metabolic factors, the regulation of Pco_2 is the most important for blood flow regulation. Carbon dioxide is the most potent vasodilator known to cerebral vessels, and an increase in CO_2 will cause vasodilation with an increase in cerebral flow and volume. Inversely, a decrease in CO_2 will constrict cerebral vessels, decrease flow, and decrease volume (see Fig. 17–9). This mechanism is the underlying principle for the number one treatment modality for increased ICP, i.e., hyperventilation. Hyperventilation, in effect, constricts cerebral vessels, which in turn reduces cerebral volume and subsequently decreases intracranial pressure.

The brain's ability to autoregulate becomes impaired or lost when critical parameters of perfusion are exceeded. This occurs as the result of (1) brain injury, (2) prolonged elevations of ICP greater that 35 mm Hg, and (3) sustained elevation or reduction in arterial pressure (greater than 160 or less than 60 mm Hg). Failure of the autoregulatory mechanism (see Fig. 17–9*C*) signifies that reactivity and responsivity of the resistance vessels is lost, and cerebral blood flow is now harmonious with changes in blood pressure and cerebral perfusion pressure.[4] The nurse may recognize this loss of autoregulation when ICP rises in parallel with increases in systemic blood pressure.

Cerebral Perfusion

The normal range for cerebral perfusion is 50 to 130 mm Hg, with an average of 80 to 100 mm Hg. Values less than 50 mm Hg are indicative of decreased perfusion or ischemia; values greater than 130 mm Hg are associated with hyperemia. Hyperemia is an increase in cerebral flow over and above the brain's metabolic needs. The hyperemic response can be just as detrimental to cerebral tissue as ischemia, since the increased blood flow results in increased volume and, subsequently, increased ICP. Hyperemia is seen most frequently in pediatric head injuries and in adults with acute subdural hematoma.

The rate of blood flow actually delivered to the brain depends on the pressure difference between its arteries and veins (cerebral perfusion) and the resistance vessels, or arterioles (cerebral vascular resistance). Since pressure in the cerebral veins is the same as ICP, cerebral perfusion pressure (CPP) can be determined by calculating the difference between the mean systemic arterial pressure [MSAP = ⅓ (systolic − diastolic) + diastolic] and ICP. The formula is CPP = MSAP − ICP. For example, if the MSAP is 90 and the ICP is 15, the CPP is 75 and the brain is being sufficiently perfused. If MSAP is 60 and ICP is 30, then CPP is 30 and the brain is being deprived of adequate flow. In this particular situation, treatment may consist of increasing systemic pressure with vasopressors as well as lowering the ICP. When MSAP is 80 and ICP is 80, there is no flow, and brain death is imminent. The critical point of CPP is reached when ICP is within 40 mm Hg of MSAP.

Based on CPP values, treatment modalities may be manipulated, especially for patients who fall in the extremes. For example, cerebral perfusion may be increased for ischemic hyperventilated patients by decreasing their respiratory rate and elevating their PCO_2. In patients who are hyperemic, blood flow may be lessened by increasing their hyperventilation and lowering the PCO_2. Calculation of CPP should be a routine nursing procedure when caring for patients with ICP problems.

In summary, blood is the nutrient carrier of glucose and oxygen, which the brain must receive continuously to sustain neuronal functioning. Blood that flows to the brain (CBF) and the amount or volume that the brain receives (CBV) are dependent on the cerebral perfusion pressure (CPP), which ultimately determines how much flow is delivered to the brain. Cerebral perfusion is dependent on pressure (CPP) within the resistance vessels and the influential effects of oxygen, pH, and carbon dioxide on these vessels (autoregulation).[4, 27, 29]

Cerebrospinal Fluid

Cerebrospinal fluid (CSF) supports and cushions the central nervous system during traumatic impact. It is theorized that CSF also has nutritive qualities and aids in the removal of waste products of neuronal metabolism. Of primary importance in head injury is the role that CSF plays in intracranial dynamics and ICP monitoring and management.

Cerebrospinal fluid is a clear, colorless liquid that is produced intrinsically within the choroid plexuses of the ventricles. CSF contains small amounts of protein, glucose, and potassium and relatively large amounts of sodium chloride. The total daily production of CSF is 480 ml produced at a rate of 20 ml/hr. The volume of CSF is 150 ml, with 15 to 25 ml contained within each lateral ventricle and the remainder circulating in the third and fourth ventricles and about the cortex and spinal cord. The CSF pathway (Fig. 17–10) is a free-flowing system whereby CSF passes from the lateral ventricles (hollow cavities within each cerebral hemisphere) through the foramina of Monro into the third ventricle. From here it flows into the fourth ventricle via a small, narrow opening, the aqueduct of Sylvius, then through the foramina of Magendie and Luschka into the subarachnoid space (SAS). Within the SAS, the CSF flows upward over the convexity of the brain and downward into the spinal canal.

Since there is continuous synthesis of CSF, it is essential that both a functional outlet system and a patent pathway are maintained to facilitate absorption and prevent fluid buildup. The arachnoid granulations or villi provide the outlet system for CSF absorption into the venous system. Arachnoid granulations are outpouchings of the arachnoid membrane that herniate through the dura and into the large venous sinuses where brain metabolites are subsequently emptied into the jugular system. These structures are pressure-dependent one-way valves that open at 5 mm Hg to allow unidirectional flow of CSF from the subarachnoid spaces into venous blood. Flow ceases when pressure is less than 5 mm Hg and increases with elevated ICP.

Impairment of CSF absorption is seen following head injury and is primarily due to obstruction of the absorption outlet (villi) or the pathway (aqueduct) by blood, protein, or bacterial contaminants that have escaped into the circulating subarachnoid CSF. When outflow impediment is significant, acute hydrocephalus and increased ICP develop, and fluid must be removed by a ventriculostomy or shunt procedure.

CSF volume reduction plays a major role in ICP management. When brain volume and ICP are increased, a reduction in CSF volume can afford additional room for the compressed brain and subsequently reduce ICP. CSF volume reduction occurs intrinsically by compensatory displacement of CSF

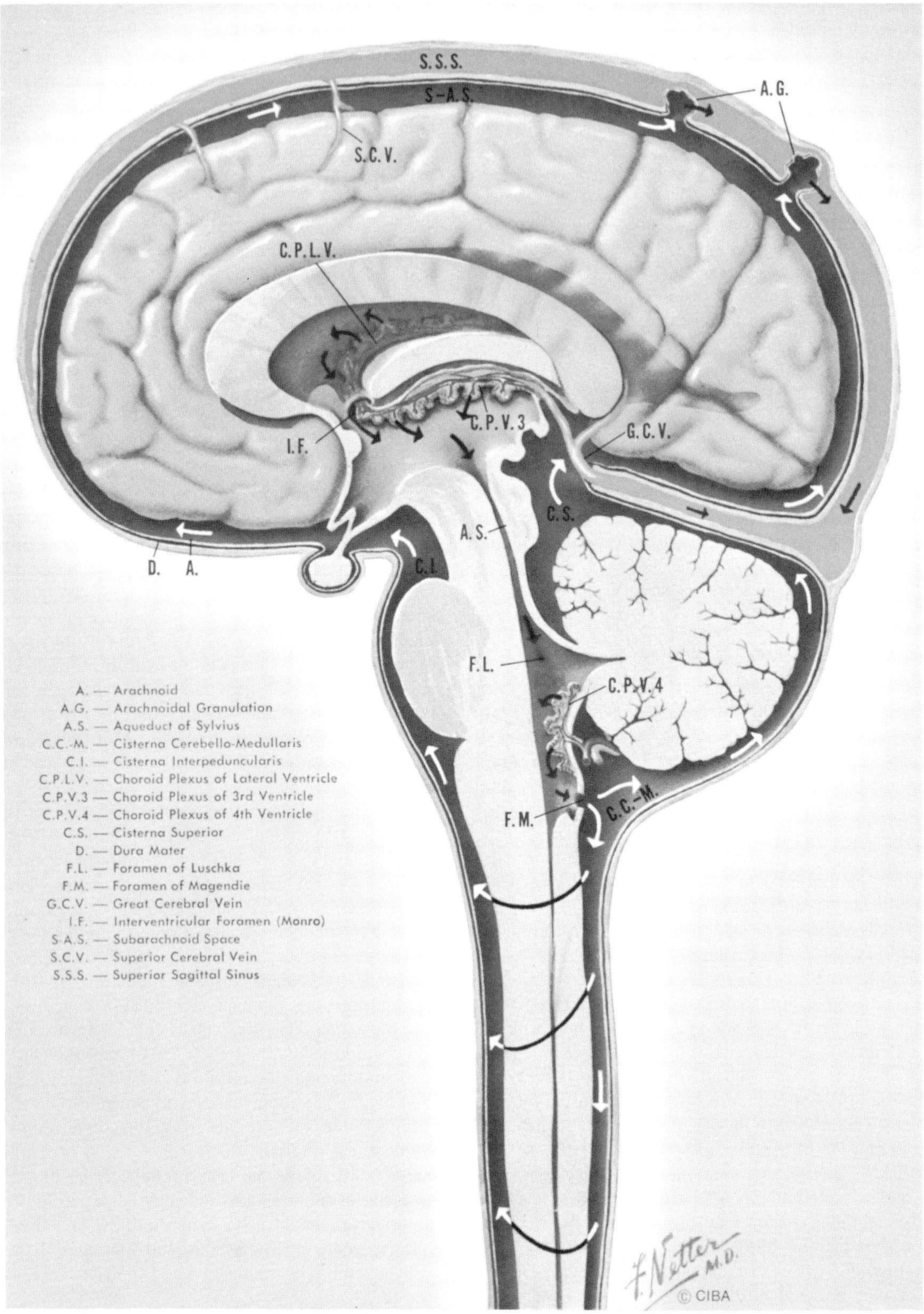

Figure 17–10. Cerebrospinal fluid pathway. (From Netter F: The Nervous System, Vol 1. The CIBA Collection of Medical Illustrations, 1975, © 1975, CIBA-GEIGY Corporation. Reproduced with permission from the CIBA Collection of Medical Illustrations by Frank Netter, M.D. All rights reserved.)

into the spinal subarachnoid space and by the increased rate of CSF absorption through the arachnoid villi. Extrinsic reduction of CSF volume is the basis of many therapeutic modalities, as discussed in the section on management of intracranial hypertension.

INTRACRANIAL PRESSURE RESPONSE

The normal range of intracranial pressure (ICP) is 0 to 15 mm Hg (or torr). Sustained pressures greater than 15 mm Hg are considered increased ICP, or intracranial hypertension. Intracranial hypertension is the leading cause of death following severe head injury and the primary cause of morbidity in head injury survivors. Death usually results from sustained pressure elevations that terminate in brainstem compression and herniation. In survivors, neurological disability is presumed to result from decreased cerebral perfusion and neuronal cell death during sustained pressure elevations.[29] The best clinical predictors of head-injured patients who will develop sustained ICP > 20 mm Hg include admission CT scan evidence of brain swelling, midline shift, and subarachnoid blood.[28]

Physiology

The intracranial cavity is the space within the skull that is filled with three components: brain tissue, blood, and CSF (Fig. 17–11*A*). Brain tissue comprises approximately 80 per cent of the volume, with blood and CSF taking up an additional 10 per cent, respectively. Intracranial volume is fixed externally by the rigid skull, which restricts expansion of the intracranial contents. Internally, volume expansion is relatively fixed. This means that a change in volume is possible within the individual compartments as long as the total volume remains the same. This is the basis of the modified Monro-Kellie hypothesis, or box theory, which states that an increase in one volume compartment must be offset by a reciprocal decrease in one or both of the remaining compartments so that the total volume remains constant (Fig. 17–11*B*). For example, a patient sustains a fall and develops an intracerebral hematoma. As the clot begins to

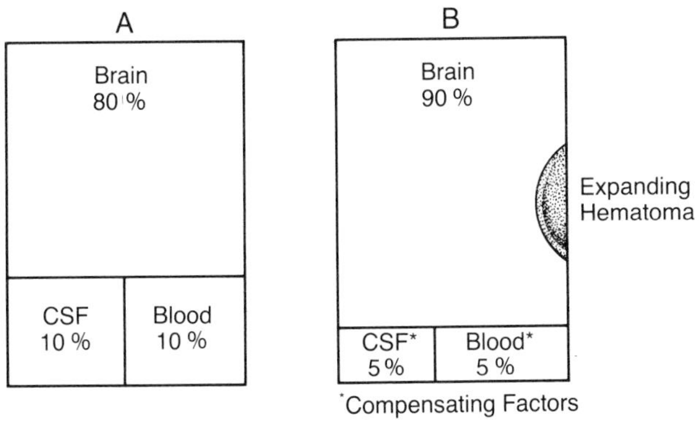

Figure 17–11. *A*, Intracranial contents as a volume percentage. *B*, The box theory predicts that any change in one intracranial compartment is offset by a reciprocal change or decrease in another compartment. Therefore, the volume remains constant.

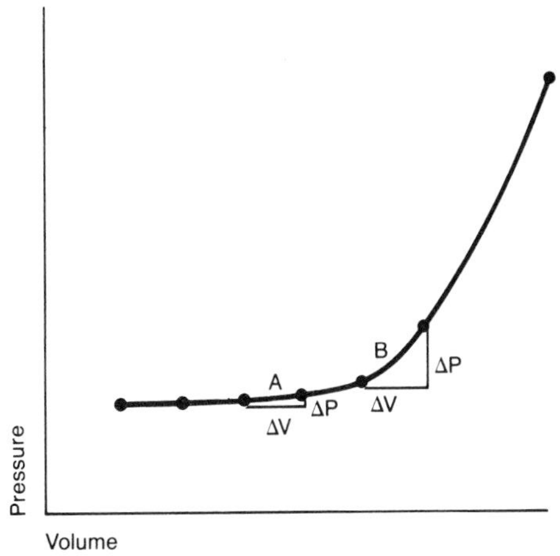

Figure 17–12. Pressure-volume curve. *A*, A change in volume (ΔV) causes only a small change in pressure (ΔP), and so elastance ($\Delta P/\Delta V$) is small. *B*, The elastance is high and the same ΔV causes a much greater ΔP. (From Bruce D: The Pathophysiology of Increased Intracranial Pressure. Upjohn Pharmaceutical, Current Concepts, 1978.)

expand, the brain tissue volume compartment increases from 80 to 90 per cent. In order to compensate for this increase, the CSF and blood compartments must give up some of their volume so that total intracranial volume remains unchanged. Blood from the compressed vasculature is displaced into the venous sinuses, and ventricular CSF is displaced into the more distensible spinal subarachnoid space. Once compensatory displacement of CSF and blood has been exhausted and the hematoma continues to increase in size, a critical point is reached at which the total volume is finally exceeded. When this occurs, even a small increase in additional volume will cause a dramatic increase in ICP with brain tissue displacement and herniation.

This relationship between pressure and volume is best illustrated by the intracranial pressure–volume curve, an exponential curve that reflects the growth rate of ICP in response to volume increase (Fig. 17–12). The flat portion of the curve represents the compensatory phase, or the buffering effect of vascular and CSF volume displacement. During this period, intracranial homeostasis is maintained. The inflection point indicates that the displaceable volume has been exhausted, and now a sharp rise in ICP is precipitated by a minimal increment in volume.

The brain's ability to yield under pressure is exceeded as volume and pressure rise. This decreased ability to yield is called *decreased compliance,* and the brain is said to be "tight." In the clinical setting, decreased compliance can be assessed by the pressure–volume index (PVI), a mathematical model that correlates changes in volume with changes in pressure in response to a small bolus injection into the CSF space. A large PVI indicates a soft, compliant brain, whereas a small PVI indicates a tight system of decreased compliance. The normal adult PVI is approximately 25, with values of 18 or less considered to be pathological.[4]

In addition to the mathematical index (PVI), compliance is measured clinically by an infusion test in which the ICP response is observed following the rapid addition of volume (usually 0.25–1 ml saline) to the intracranial space. A pressure increase of 5 mm Hg or greater per 1 ml of saline indicates intracranial decompensation.[4] Patient observation can provide a rough approximation for these invasive measures of compliance. Head-injured patients who show substantial or sustained pressure deviations in response to changes in head position, turning, suctioning, or other noxious stimulation should be suspected of having decreased compliance or adaptive capacity and should be treated accordingly.[4, 48]

Causes of Intracranial Hypertension in Head Injury

Since the intracranial cavity is filled to capacity with brain, blood, and CSF, an increase in the volume of any one of these will cause intracranial hypertension once the compensatory mechanisms described earlier are exhausted. An increase in the brain compartment volume occurs with the addition of mass or bulk, most often in the form of a blood clot or hematoma, a suppurative process, or a tumor. Brain volume is also increased when there is an excess in cerebral water content, or edema.

An increase in cerebral blood flow with subsequent increase in cerebral blood volume is associated with hypercarbic and hyperemic responses to head injury. Any obstruction of venous outflow, including simple neck flexion or rotation, also can transiently contribute to increased blood volume.

The CSF compartment increase is almost always due to obstruction of the CSF pathways or absorption of CSF by the villi. Foreign particulate matter (primarily blood) plugs the narrow openings in the aqueducts or foramina, or the absorption sites at the villi. Conditions other than head injury in which blood can escape into the subarachnoid space include hypertensive stroke, ruptured arteriovenous malformations, or ruptured cerebral aneurysms. Increased rate of CSF formation is not a causative factor of increased CSF volume in head injury.[30–32] Rapid changes in the volume of cranial contents can link intracranial hypertension and cerebral herniation.

CEREBRAL HERNIATION

Cerebral herniation is the distortion and displacement of brain from one compartment to another within the intracranial cavity. Expanding mass lesions or hematomas are the primary causes of brain shift and herniation. The location of the lesion often determines the direction in which the brain will be forcibly moved and, consequently, the type and pattern of herniation that will occur. The majority of mass lesions are hemispheric or supratentorial (located within the cerebral hemispheres above the tentorium). Infratentorial or posterior fossa mass lesions are less common in head injury. Clinical signs of infratentorial herniation include coma, abnormal eye signs, vomiting, cranial nerve dysfunction, and changes in respiratory pattern that correspond to low brainstem compression.

There are three types of herniation: cingulate (or subfalcine), central, and transtentorial. Supratentorial lesions can produce all three herniation patterns simultaneously as pressure gradients shift the brain laterally and eventually downward through the foramen magnum (Fig. 17–13).

In *cingulate,* or *subfalcine, herniation,* the cingulate gyrus (a convolution of brain tissue in the medial aspect of the hemispheres) is distorted beneath the falx cerebri (the segment of dura that separates the cerebral hemispheres longitudinally into paired lateral compartments). Although cingulate herniation has been thought to be relatively asymptomatic, CT scanning has clearly shown that early decrease in consciousness occurs with a lateral brain shift of 3 to 4 mm.[33, 34]

Central herniation consists of downward displacement of portions of the temporal lobes, diencephalon, and midbrain through the tentorium into the posterior fossa (infratentorial compartment). Clinical signs of central herniation are a reflection of compression and dysfunction of the displaced structures. These include impaired consciousness, bilateral motor dysfunction, and upper cranial nerve deficits. Diffuse brain swelling, bilateral lesions, and lesions located in the midline have the greatest probability for causing central herniation.

In *transtentorial herniation,* the medial aspect of the temporal lobe (the uncus) is shifted toward the midline and then over the edge of the tentorium cerebelli. The tentorium is the horizontal dural partition that hangs over the posterior fossa and separates it from the cerebral hemispheres. Synonyms for transtentorial herniation are *uncal herniation, midbrain herniation,* and *tentorial conus.* Transtentorial herniation is most commonly associated with a unilateral hemispheric lesion, particularly epidural and subdural hematomas. The clinical signs are discussed in the section on assessment.

SPECIFIC TYPES OF BRAIN INJURY

The primary types of head injury are focal brain injury, diffuse brain injury, and skull fracture. Focal brain injuries

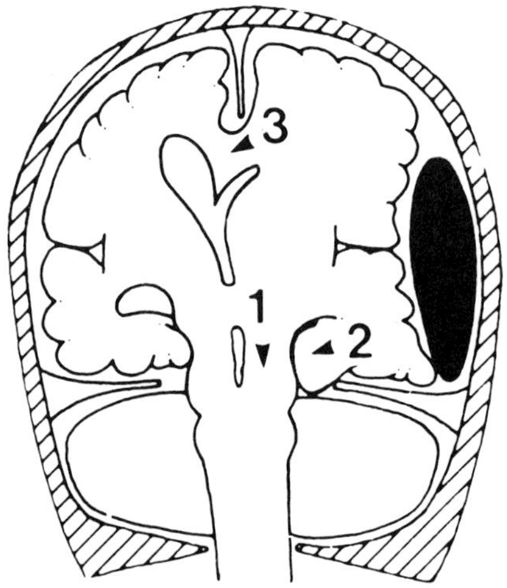

Figure 17–13. Brain displacement from supratentorial hematoma: (1) Central: downward displacement of brainstem. (2) Transtentorial: herniation of uncus of temporal lobe into tentorial notch. (3) Cingulate: herniation of cingulate gyrus below falx. (From Jennett B, Teasdale G: Management of Head Injuries. Philadelphia, FA Davis, 1982.)

include cerebral contusion and hematomas—epidural, subdural, and intracerebral. The diffuse brain injury category includes concussion and diffuse axonal injury. Skull fracture types are linear, depressed, or basilar.

Focal Brain Injuries

Focal injuries, also known as *expanding mass lesions,* are responsible for 50 per cent of all head injuries and account for 60 per cent of all deaths. Focal lesions create havoc by taking up brain volume space, increasing ICP, and causing brain shift and herniation. These lesions cause local brain damage at the site of injury and are associated with focal, lateralizing, or localizing signs. Pupillary dilatation, hemiparesis, decerebration, cranial nerve dysfunction, and speech deficit are all focal signs that help in localizing the site of injury. Focal injuries are produced by (1) contact or nonmovement forces (an object striking or struck by the head) or (2) acceleration–deceleration forces (the head is forcibly moved or stopped from moving). Since most head trauma involves both contact and movement, an isolated head injury is rare.[35] Focal injuries include cerebral contusion and hematomas—epidural, subdural, and intracerebral.

Cerebral Contusion

Contusions involve cortical bruising and, at times, laceration of vessels and brain tissue with subsequent tissue necrosis, pulping, and infarction. They are the most common head injury lesions and are significant because of associated hemorrhage, edema, and brain swelling. Contusions are sometimes classified as coup (those occurring at the site of the impact), contrecoup (those occurring opposite the site of impact), gliding, and petechial. The latter two types are characteristic of shearing effect or diffuse axonal injury.[36, 37]

The primary sites of brain contusion are the frontal and temporal lobes, deeply embedded within the base of the skull. In forward acceleration, the frontal lobe is thrust against the inner table of the frontal skull bone and the temporal lobe is forced against the sphenoid bone. Contusions are most often multiple and occur in association with other lesions. Depending on the degree of acceleration, contusions can be mild or severe, superficial or deep. Superficial contusions involved the cortical and subcortical tissue, whereas deep contusions penetrate the underlying white matter.[36–38]

Signs, symptoms, and severity depend on the site and extent of contused brain. Isolated contusions do not generally produce immediate loss of consciousness. When coma is present, it is usually the result of associated concussion or diffuse injury. Since the majority of contusions occur in the frontal and temporal lobes, patients usually present with localizing personality, behavior, motor, and speech deficits. Sorting the effects of alcohol-related behavior from frontal and temporal lobe dysfunction is problematic in patients with significant alcohol levels. Patients with temporal lobe contusion are in particular danger because of the proximity of the lesion to the tentorium and midbrain. Progressive edema formation can cause abrupt mass effect, ICP elevation, and herniation.

Management. Treatment consists of monitoring the patient with a small (<5–7 mm of brain shift on CT) lesion and evaluating for signs of increased ICP. Special attention should be paid to patients with temporal lobe contusions, especially during the period of maximum brain edema (3–5 days after injury). Monitoring is directed toward the appearance of subtle neurological changes rather than toward ICP values. More extensive contusions with mass effect will require surgical evaluation as early as possible. Mortality from contusion ranges from 25 to 60 per cent. As is true for all head injuries, patients who do best are those who are not in coma and those under 50 years of age.[4, 35–38]

Epidural Hematoma

An *epidural hematoma* is a blood clot situated between the dura and the skull (therefore extradural), most commonly located in the temporal region. The predominant mechanisms of injury are falls, assaults, and traffic accidents. In the majority of patients, a linear fracture of the temporal bone lacerates the underlying middle meningeal artery or veins, and the accumulating bleeding forms the hematoma (Fig. 17–14). The presence of a temporal fracture on skull films in association with clouded consciousness or focal deficit on assessment warrants a CT scan and probable hospital admission to rule out epidural hematoma.[50]

Epidural hematoma is a potentially fatal lesion because of its rapid expansion (within minutes if is its arterial rather than venous in origin) and resultant brain displacement and herniation. Signs and symptoms depend on the source and rapidity of the bleeding, with almost 60 per cent of patients demonstrating clinical manifestations within 6 hours or less. Pupillary dilation, hemiparesis, and decerebration are common manifestation of an expanding hematoma with brainstem compression. About 33 per cent of epidural hematomas are associated with a lucid interval—initial unconsciousness followed by lucidity with subsequent unconsciousness.[39] The initial loss of consciousness is due to concussion, with the patient awakening within several minutes only to deteriorate from the effects of the expanding hematoma. The lucid interval is therefore not pathognomonic of epidural hematoma but may be present with other expanding mass lesions as well.

Management. Treatment consists of surgical evacuation as soon as possible. If this is not possible and a neurological emergency is in progress, a burr hole is often placed ipsilateral to the side of the dilated pupil or contralateral to the side of motor deficits, and the hematoma is evacuated through the burr hole. Outcome depends on the initial severity. Patients with Glasgow Coma Scale (GCS) scores of 3 to 5 and signs of brainstem compression have a 40 per cent mortality compared with 9 per cent mortality when the GCS is 6 to 8. In general, the better the neurological function as reflected in the GCS, the better is the outcome.[40, 49]

Subdural Hematoma

A *subdural hematoma* is a collection of blood within the subdural space. Causative factors are falls, assaults, and motor vehicle accidents. Subdural hematomas may be acute, subacute, or chronic. However, it is often difficult to differentiate acute and subacute forms. Some define subdural hematomas as acute when clinical manifestations are present within 48 to 72 hours after injury, whereas others classify them as acute if symptoms are present immediately after

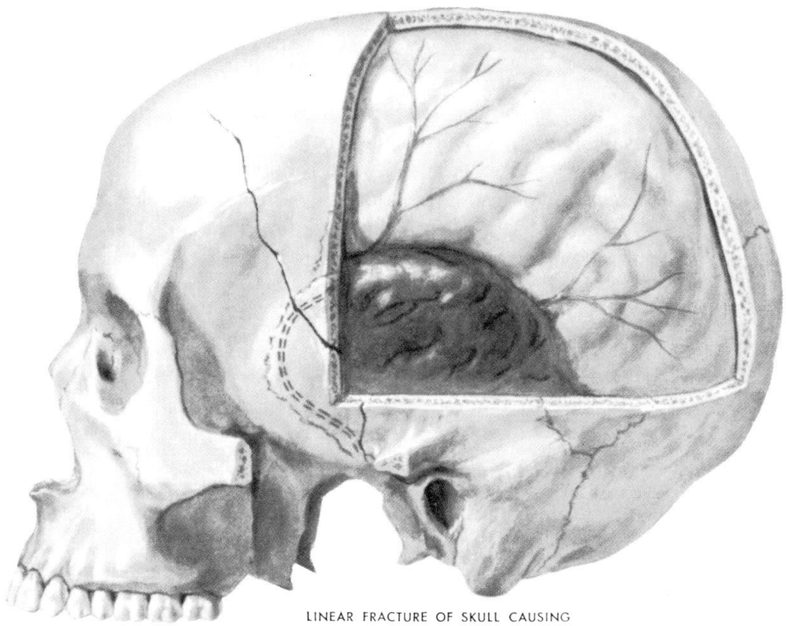

Figure 17–14. Epidural hematoma resulting from temporal vault fracture with laceration of middle meningeal artery. (From Netter F: The Nervous System, Vol 1. The CIBA Collection of Medical Illustrations, 1975, © 1975, CIBA-GEIGY Corporation. Reproduced with permission from the CIBA Collection of Medical Illustrations by Frank Netter, M.D. All rights reserved.)

injury. In general, symptoms appearing within 2 to 10 days are considered subacute, and symptoms appearing within weeks to months are considered chronic. This discussion is directed to the acute subdural hematoma population with the gravest prognosis—those who manifest symptoms immediately and have GCS scores of 8 or less.

The acute subdural hematoma develops as the result of a rapid accelerative mechanism that tears the veins bridging the subdural space. These bridging veins extend from the cortical surface of the brain and connect with the dural sinuses. Beneath the clot, which may extend the length of the entire hemisphere, the underlying brain tissue is damaged by contusion and ruptured veins and arteries. The term *burst lobe* is also associated with subdural hematomas and describes an intracerebral hematoma that is in continuity with a subdural hematoma.

The acute subdural hematoma carries the highest mortality of all head injuries (60 to 90 per cent). The poor survival has been attributed to several factors: (1) the primary brain damage underlying the clot, (2) vascular injury (lacerated bridging veins), (3) hyperemic response leading to increased cranial blood volume, (4) ipsilateral hemispheric or total brain swelling, and (5) intracranial hypertension. Factors predictive of functional recovery are (1) evaluation of clot within 4 hours after injury, (2) a postoperative ICP of less than 20 mm Hg, (3) normal postoperative evoked potentials, and (4) a GCS score greater than 5.[35, 51]

Patients who sustain a severe acute subdural hematoma are comatose on admission with low GCS scores (8 or less). They are more likely to have neurological deficits that reflect extensive bleeding, primary brain injury, and compressive effects of a mass lesion (i.e., motor deficit, pupil abnormality, and cranial nerve dysfunction). Patients with acute subdural hematomas of lesser severity may be conscious or unconscious or have a lucid interval.

Management. Surgical treatment of acute subdural hematoma consists of evacuation of the clot (if it is 3 mm or more thick), control of hemorrhage, and resection of contused, nonviable brain. Clot size can vary from 10 to 400 ml. The operative procedure generally involves initial trephines or burr holes for clot identification, followed by conversion to a craniotomy flap for optimal evacuation. A soft drain, frequently a Jackson-Pratt drain, may be left in the subdural space for 24 to 48 hours. Postoperative complications include brain swelling with subsequent increased ICP, clot reaccumulation, delayed intracerebral hemorrhage, and seizures.

Intracerebral Hematoma

An *intracerebral hematoma* is a well-defined blood clot that is deep within the brain tissue or parenchyma. Similar to contusions, 90 per cent of intracerebral hematomas occur in the frontal and temporal lobes.[52, 53] Small, deep hematomas within the periventricular, medial, or paracentral areas are associated with shear forces and generally indicate a diffuse axonal injury.[35] Intracerebral hematomas may be multiple and associated with other lesions, particularly contusions. An intracerebral hematoma is generally a closed head injury, but it can result from an open or penetrating injury or from embedding of the skull into the brain, such as occurs with a depressed skull fracture. The most common mechanism is the accelerating head being stopped by a fixed object.

The signs and symptoms of intracerebral hematoma are similar to those of contusions, with course and outcome dependent on the size and location of the hematoma. Dominant hemispheric lesions are frequently associated with motor and speech deficits.

Intracerebral hematomas are complicated by progressive focal edema and mass effect, which leads to neurological deterioration. Deterioration can occur soon after injury or as long as 7 to 10 days after injury, but the majority of deterioration occurs in the first 48 to 72 hours. An additional complication is the occurrence of delayed hemorrhage—clot formation in areas of brain that were injured at the time of impact but appeared normal on the initial CT scan. Thus determining the onset of neurological deterioration in a patient with an initially normal scan requires reimaging. This late deterioration and clot formation are associated with poor outcome and a high incidence of intracranial hypertension. Other risk factors include disseminated intravascular clotting disorders, hypoxia, hypotension, and alcohol abuse.[54, 55]

Diffuse Brain Injuries

Diffuse brain injury includes concussion and diffuse axonal injury (DAI). Diffuse injuries account for 50 per cent of all head injury hospital admissions and 35 per cent of all head injury deaths. Resulting almost exclusively from motor vehicle accidents, they are the leading cause of major neurological disability in survivors. Most patients who are unconscious from severe head injuries are assumed to have diffuse injury, often in combination with specific focal injuries.[4]

Unlike focal injury, diffuse injuries produce widespread damage that is scattered throughout the brain. The focal injury is well demarcated and could be seen with the naked eye or on CT scan. In contrast, the diffuse injury involves microscopic damage to cells deep in the white matter and may be impossible to visualize. Often, the only visible evidence is brain shift and swelling that are secondary evidence of this widespread damage.

Diffuse brain injuries are created as lateral head motion produces angular movement of the brain over a 45- to 60-degree arc within the skull. This type of motion causes shearing or stretching of axonal nerve fibers. Damage is variable and dependent on the amount of accelerative force transmitted to the brain. Diffuse brain injuries lie on a continuum of severity ranging from mild concussion with little or no brain dysfunction to diffuse axonal injury that produces disabling deficits.[17, 56–57]

Cerebral Concussion

Concussion causes a temporary disturbance of neurological function and results from rapid acceleration–deceleration or a sharp sudden blow to the head. Temporary alteration in function is theorized to result from transient ischemia, neural depolarization following sudden acetylcholine release, or microscopic axonal disruption.[41, 57]

Mild concussion is the most common head injury, but individuals are not usually admitted to the hospital because of the benign nature of mild concussion. The injury produces confusion, disorientation, and, at times, retrograde amnesia (inability to recall events just preceding the injury) or posttraumatic amnesia. The confusion and disorientation last only minutes, and there are usually no permanent deficits, although some individuals suffer many months with dizziness, headache, and difficulty concentrating. Preservation of consciousness is the feature that distinguishes mild from classic concussion.[58, 59]

Classic concussion involves temporary loss of consciousness, retrograde and posttraumatic amnesia, and sometimes mild neurological impairment. Unconsciousness is usually less that 5 minutes and no longer than 6 hours. The duration of posttraumatic amnesia is often a predictor of the severity of injury. Classical concussion is an extension of mild concussion but requires greater mechanical stress to the brain, suggesting a degree of neuronal damage.[57, 59] Although these patients have normal CT scans and neurological examinations, they are often admitted to a hospital for a short observational period in order to detect delayed intracranial bleeding, should an epidural or subdural hematoma masquerade as a concussion.[60]

The typical subjective experiences associated with both mild and classic concussions have been termed *postconcussive syndrome* and consist of headache, dizziness, and vertigo that may be attributed to vestibular dysfunction. Subtle changes in personality, difficulty in concentration, and poor memory are also part of the syndrome and are attributed to cerebral cortical dysfunction. Persistence of these problems in some persons may be related to a greater degree of neuronal damage, a quest for secondary gain, psychological reaction to the injury, or a combination of these factors.[57, 61–62]

Diffuse Axonal Injury (DAI)

DAI is the severest form of brain injury and differs from concussion in degree rather than kind of brain injury. Severity and outcome depend on the extent and degree of structural damage—mild, moderate, or severe. The hallmark of DAI is immediate and prolonged coma (greater than 6 hours' duration). The prolonged coma results from severe, widespread damage to conducting white matter (axons) that functionally disconnects the cerebral hemispheres from the brainstem reticular activating system. Since DAI is microscopic in nature, the severity of the injury is not determined radiographically, but by the patient's clinical characteristics and duration of coma. Mild DAI is associated with coma of 6 to 24 hours. Decerebration or decortication is transiently present in a small percentage (about 30 per cent); mortality is 15 per cent, with 80 per cent having a good recovery. Moderate DAI is more common and is distinguished by coma lasting more than 24 hours and abnormal posturing. As injury severity increases, the percentage of those attaining good outcome lessens, and mortality increases to 24 per cent.[35, 38, 59]

Severe Diffuse Axonal Injury. Severe DAI occurs almost exclusively as a result of high-speed motor vehicle collisions. Rotational acceleration forces cause the nonrigid brain to move forcibly within the skull. The point of maximal stress occurs in areas where tissues of different density interface (i.e., between gray and white matter). Since cortical gray matter is less dense than white matter, the gray matter is thrown forward while the more dense white matter lags behind. As a result, axonal fibers are stretched, sheared, and sometimes literally torn apart.[35, 59, 64] The concept is easily appreciated when illustrated with a deck of cards (Fig. 17–15). The top card represents the cerebral cortex or gray matter, and the underlying cards represent the more dense white matter. When energy or acceleration is applied to the rectangular pack, it is transformed into an obliquely angled stack. The top card (gray matter: cell bodies) is thrown forward, whereas the heavier underlying cards (white matter: axons) lag behind.[63] This mechanism is applicable to all types of diffuse brain injury but is more severe with the highest degree of acceleration causing the injury.

The most severe form of DAI results in extensive anatomical disruption of axonal white matter fibers throughout both hemispheres, the diencephalon, and the brainstem[17, 35, 59, 64]

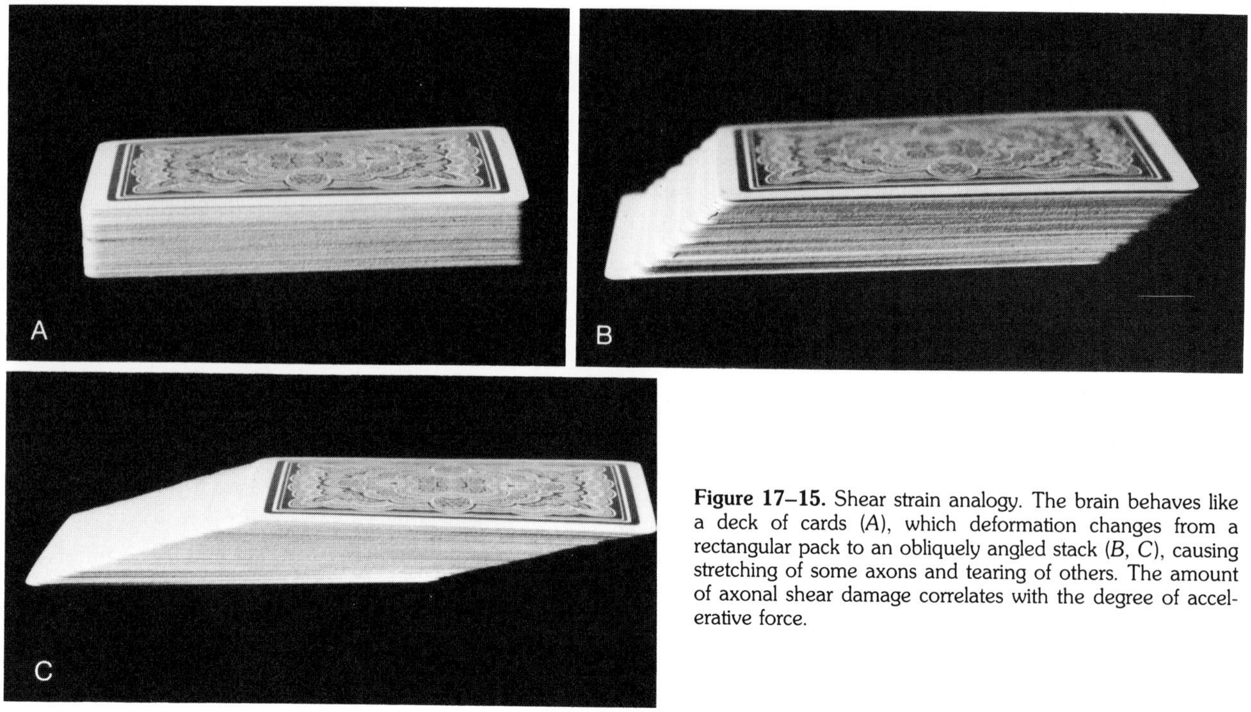

Figure 17–15. Shear strain analogy. The brain behaves like a deck of cards (*A*), which deformation changes from a rectangular pack to an obliquely angled stack (*B, C*), causing stretching of some axons and tearing of others. The amount of axonal shear damage correlates with the degree of accelerative force.

Small tissue and vessel tears appear on CT as small hemorrhagic lesions in the corpus callosum, superior cerebellar peduncles, basal ganglia, or periventricular regions. Because these hemorrhages are small, they may be missed on the initial CT scan, and their early resolution makes detection difficult on subsequent scans. Magnetic resonance imaging (MRI) appears to be more effective than CT in visualizing these small lesions. Additionally, diffuse cerebral edema is found with severe DAI.[65, 66]

Clinically, severe DAI is manifested by deep and prolonged coma (weeks or months). Those who emerge from coma usually do so within the first 3 months.[67] Signs of severe cerebral and brainstem dysfunction, such as decortication and decerebration, are often present on admission or develop with 24 hours of injury. Hypertension, hyperthermia, and hyperhidrosis are manifestations of diencephalic involvement. Abnormal motor activity and diencephalic signs are associated with a higher rate of nonrecovery of consciousness.[67, 68]

Hypertension is usually moderate, with a systolic pressure of 140 to 160 mm Hg, and does not require therapy. Hyperthermia, with temperature as high as 104 to 105°F (40–40.5°C), is due to dysfunction of the hypothalamic temperature-regulating mechanism. Hyperthermia can be present on admission or appear within the first few days following injury and subsides periodically only to sporadically reappear throughout the recovery process or until hypothalamic control is reestablished. Hyperthermia can be problematic because of the uncertainty of its origin. One should never assume that fever in a deeply comatose, severely head-injured patient is of cerebral origin, since such a patient is prone to many infectious sources for that fever. A search for an infectious source should always be conducted.

Hyperhidrosis, or excessive sweating, is a sympathetically mediated disorder. In severe DAI, patients are observed to have beads of sweat continuously covering the face and less frequently the neck and upper thorax. This condition, like fever of central origin, seems to subside with stabilization and clinical improvement.

Because of the extensive structural damage to neurons, the majority of DAI survivors have major residual disabilities reflecting varying degrees of damage to almost every part of the brain. Extensive neuronal loss literally results in brain shrinkage. Follow-up CT scans typically show cerebral atrophy, as evidenced by enlarged sulci and ventricular dilatation. The major sequelae of severe DAI are deficits in cognition, memory, speech and motor function, and personality. Mortality in severe DAI is 51 per cent, second only to acute subdural hematoma. Although approximately half of those with coma persisting past 1 month recover, this constitutes only about 15 per cent of the total DAI victims who have a good outcome, with 27 per cent significantly disabled and 7 per cent in persistent vegetative state.[59, 67–68]

Associated Injuries

Fractures

An estimated 111,000 skull fractures occur annually in the United States. These fractures occur most commonly in the cranial vault or at the base of the skull. Linear (as opposed to depressed) fractures are the most common, occurring with greatest frequency in children and the elderly.[63] Severe head injuries can occur with or without skull fractures. Even when present, the fracture is seldom the cause of neurological disability. The type of fracture that occurs depends on the amount and direction of force of the object striking the skull, the size of the object, and the thickness of the skull at the impact site.[35]

A *linear fracture* is a discontinuity of the skull bone that dissects both the outer and inner table. Linear fractures are essentially benign and require no treatment. The fracture line usually disappears within 6 months in children and within 3 to 4 years in adults. However, a linear vault fracture that is accompanied by neurological signs warrants CT scanning to rule out an epidural hematoma or other intracranial lesion. This is particularly true of linear fractures in the temporal and occipital regions, since arteries lie particularly close to bone in these regions. Such linear vault fractures increase the risk of hematoma about 400 times.[69]

Depressed fractures result from high-velocity contact sustained over a small surface area. The most common depressed fractures are (1) closed, with scalp intact; (2) compound, with scalp open but intact dura; and (3) complex, with scalp and dura lacerated by bone fragments. The fragmented bone particles often proceed to embed themselves into brain tissue, resulting in cortical laceration and hemorrhage. Treatment consists of debridement, evacuation of clots and bone fragments, elevation of depressed bone, and repair of lacerated dura. Complications of depressed fractures are infection and seizures, both of which are treated prophylactically with antibiotics and anticonvulsants.

Basilar fractures are fractures located at the base of the skull. The five bones that form the base of the skull are the occipital bone, the cribriform plate of the ethmoid bone, the orbital plate of the frontal bone, the sphenoid bone, and the petrous and squamous portions of the temporal bone. Because basilar fractures are seldom detected radiographically, diagnosis is made by clinical examination. A patient who has any one of the following clinical manifestations has a basilar fracture: (1) periorbital ecchymosis (raccoon's eyes), (2) mastoid ecchymosis (Battle's sign), (3) rhinorrhea (CSF or blood leading from the nose) or otorrhea (CSF or blood leaking from the ears), (5) hemotympanum, and (6) conjunctival hemorrhage without evidence of direct trauma.

The presence of otorrhea or rhinorrhea indicates a dural laceration with increased risk of meningitis. Although 80 per cent of CSF leaks stop spontaneously, those which persist after 7 to 14 days may require dural repair. Medical management is variable, but current practice includes bed rest, antibiotics, head-up position, and occasionally, lumbar subarachnoid drainage of CSF for 3 to 4 days. An additional complication of basilar fracture is cranial nerve injury. Because of their location at the base of the brain, the cranial nerves are in jeopardy of direct injury when a fracture line crosses the base of the skull. The most frequently injured cranial nerves are the olfactory, facial, and acoustic.[36, 69]

Gunshot Wounds

Gunshot wounds (GSWs) are classified as perforating missile injuries. A *perforating brain wound* is one in which a bullet passes through the brain but does not exit the skull. When the bullet exits the skull, it is called a *perforating head wound.* The extent of gunshot damages depends on the velocity and mass of the missile. Low-velocity missiles tend not to exit the skull but are inclined to ricochet within the cranial cavity and create multiple destructive missile tracts within the brain. Many patients remain conscious following gunshot wounds to the head only to deteriorate rapidly with the onset of edema that surrounds the entire missile tract. Death is due to extensive structural brain damage that causes massive brain swelling and uncontrollable ICP. Surgical treatment consists of debridement of the missile tract with evacuation of associated hematoma and bullet fragments when accessible.

Overall mortality from GSWs to the brain is approximately 50 per cent. Outcome depends on the site of the missile tract, the presenting neurological status, and the extent of brain tissue destruction. A missile tract through the frontal lobes is generally survivable with residual focal deficits from local brain damage. Multiple missile tracts are generally fatal, and a missile tract through the brainstem is always fatal.[38, 70] The initial level of consciousness following a GSW is considered the best indicator of prognosis, with reported mortality of 11.5 per cent in awake patients, 33.3 per cent in lethargic patients, and 100 per cent in comatose patients.[71] Anticonvulsant therapy is commonly used, based on the 45 per cent incidence of posttraumatic epilepsy developing within 5 years of missile injury.[69]

NEUROLOGICAL ASSESSMENT IN TRAUMA

Neurological assessment following head injury includes a thorough baseline evaluation followed by on-going reassessment for changes. As in all types of traumatic injury, the assessment includes an initial accident data base that provides information about the events of the accident or assault, the probable mechanism of injury, and subsequent injury patterns. The previous health history is obtained from family members or others significant to the patient. The assessment process for the head-injured patient includes the physical examination, neurodiagnostic technologies, and the use of tools such as the Glasgow Coma Scale.

Clinical Examination

Cerebral and brainstem function is the principal focus of the examination. Cranial nerve function and sensory-motor capabilities are carefully assessed and monitored over time. The following section highlights key areas of the neurotrauma examination; the reader is referred to other sources for review as needed for general neurological physical diagnosis. All suspected head injuries from mild to severe are evaluated in terms of level of consciousness, vital signs, and pupillary, sensory, and motor responses.

Level of Consciousness

The most important sign of CNS dysfunction is deterioration in level of consciousness. The Glasgow Coma Scale (GCS) is internationally recognized as the accepted tool for evaluation and determination of this function. The components of the GCS are described in detail within the section on assessment tools. There are two components of consciousness: arousal, which depends on the brainstem, and cognition or awareness, which depends on the cerebral hemispheres. Arousal is mediated by nerve cells within the reticular formation, which is a network or "reticulum" of fine fibers that originate in the brainstem (spinal cord–medulla junction) and then project upward to the cortex where awareness is realized. Since consciousness has both cortical and brainstem control, patients who are in a depressed conscious state must have either bilateral cerebral hemispheric dysfunction or a primary lesion in the brainstem.

Generalized cerebral edema, increased ICP, and expanding masses that cause brain shift, brainstem compression, and infarction are the primary agents responsible for hemispheric or brainstem dysfunction and depressed consciousness.

The most common causes of coma fall into three categories and are due to either (1) structural brain lesions, (2) metabolic dysfunction, or (3) psychiatric disorders.[41, 42] The mnemonic "vowel tipps" is a helpful guide for etiological determination of coma, especially for emergency department personnel (Table 17–3). Head injuries are considered structural lesions and may be supratentorial or infratentorial in location.

The very fact that a head-injured patient is comatose indicates the presence of substantial injury and significant brain damage. The longer the patient remains in coma, the greater the likelihood of extensive, severe neurological deficit. Duration of coma is longest in patients with severe diffuse axonal injury (DAI), with coma averaging 1 to 3 months. The *majority* of patients who emerge from coma generally do so by 3 months. After a coma duration of 3 months, the chances of remaining vegetative increase daily.

Confusion often results when altered states of consciousness are described as lethargy, stupor, or obtundation. By objectively describing assessment findings and utilizing the Glasgow Coma Scale, the ambiguity of subjective terms is avoided.

Cranial Nerve Function

There are 12 pairs of cranial nerves. With the exception of cranial nerves 1 and 2, which lie right above the midbrain, all remaining cranial nerves originate and exit from the brainstem (Fig. 17–16). Cranial nerve assessment not only gives the evaluator information regarding the function of the specific nerve being tested but also, and more important, yields vital information on general functioning of the brainstem itself. In head injury, cranial nerve dysfunction often provides substantive evidence of impending or actual brain herniation. An expanding intracranial hematoma, for example, can cause brain shift, herniation, and brainstem compression. A classic sign that frequently accompanies this event is pupillary dilation and unreactivity due to brain compression of the third cranial nerve (oculomotor) and the parasympathetic fibers as they exit from the upper brainstem region.

Assessment of cranial nerves consists of several components. First, knowledge of the 12 cranial nerves and their respective functions is essential. Although some shortcuts do exist, the best way to learn the cranial nerves and their respective functions is by memorization and routinely performing cranial nerve assessments. A helpful mnemonic for naming the nerves is "*O*n *O*ld *O*lympics *T*owering *T*ops, *A* *F*inn and *G*erman *V*ied *A*t *H*ops," in which the first letter of each word represents the ordered sequence of each cranial nerve. Locating the cranial nerves within the brainstem is simplified by sectioning the brainstem into three parts, dividing the cranial nerves into three groups, and then placing each cranial nerve group within its respective brainstem segment (Fig. 17–17). For example, group I (cranial nerves 1, 2, 3, and 4) lies within the first segment of the brainstem, the midbrain; group II (cranial nerves 5, 6, 7, and 8) within the second segment of the brainstem, the pons; and group III (cranial nerves 9, 10, 11, and 12) within the third segment of the brainstem, the medulla. With the exception of cranial nerves 1 and 2, which lie right above the midbrain, any dysfunction of cranial nerves 3 through 12 can be localized to a specific region of the brainstem. Table 17–4 lists the cranial nerves, their function, and anticipated deficits in the presence of altered function.

When peripheral injury to a cranial nerve can be excluded, the identification and localization of an intracranial or central cranial nerve deficit is significant because it may represent brainstem compression and neurological deterioration. Documentation of cranial nerve dysfunction is included as part of the nursing record so that deficits requiring nursing intervention (e.g., loss of the gag reflex, visual field deficits, or impaired hearing) receive appropriate planning and follow-up.

Cranial nerve injuries, especially those involving the optic, abducens, facial, and acoustic nerves, are not uncommon in head injury. Cranial nerve injuries result from direct mechanical trauma, herniation, increased ICP, ischemia, missile injuries, and fractures of the face, temporal bone, or base of the skull.[36, 38]

Eye Signs

Frequent pupil checks and recognition of early signs of pupillary dysfunction are vitally important in the nursing assessment of the head trauma patient. A brief review of pupillary innervation and oculomotor function will provide a better understanding of pathological eye signs.

The oculomotor nerve is situated at the midbrain level and performs the following functions: (1) innervates the inferior oblique and medial rectus muscles to move the eye in the inferior oblique plane and medially (toward the nose), (2) innervates the levator palpebrae muscle to elevate the upper eyelid, and (3) provides ipsilateral parasympathetic constrictor innervation to the pupil. Compression of the nerve will cause partial or complete loss of related functions. A patient with a complete third nerve deficit will have an eye that does not move medially, an eyelid that droops, and a pupil that is dilated and does not react to light or accommodation.

The site of parasympathetic innervation to the pupil is the midbrain (Fig. 17–18). Parasympathetic influence normally causes pupillary constriction, but with midbrain compression, the parasympathetic innervation is blocked, and the sympathetic fibers act unopposed, causing pupillary dilation (mydriasis). Inversely, if sympathetic innervation is interrupted,

TABLE 17–3. VOWEL TIPPS: COMMON CAUSES OF COMA

A lcohol	T rauma
E pilepsy	I nfection
I nsulin	P sych
O piates	P oison
U rates	S hock

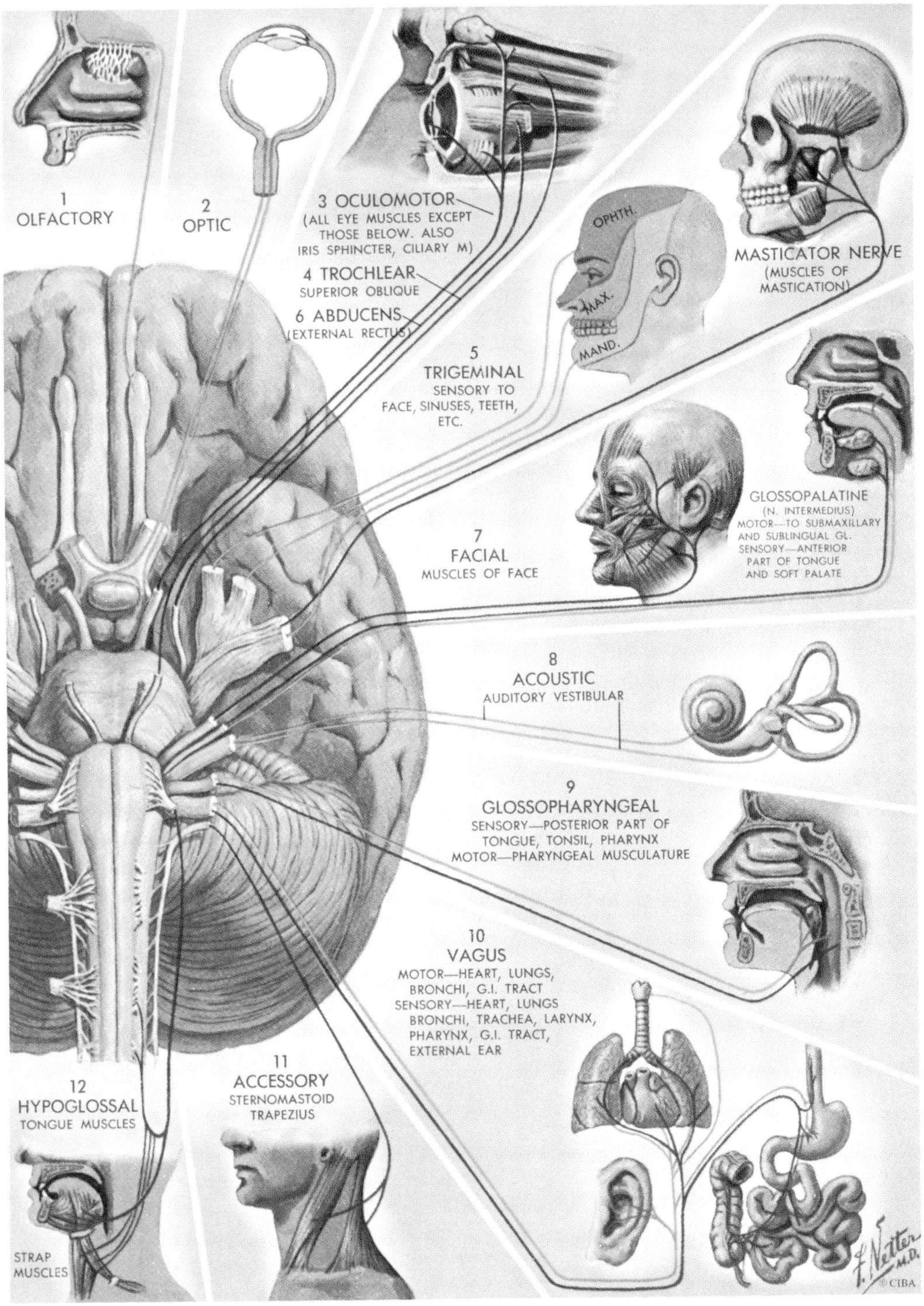

Figure 17–16. Cranial nerves: origin and innervation. (From Netter F: The Nervous System, Vol 1. The CIBA Collection of Medical Illustrations, 1975. © 1975, CIBA-GEIGY Corporation. Reproduced with permission from the CIBA Collection of Medical Illustrations by Frank Netter, M.D. All rights reserved.)

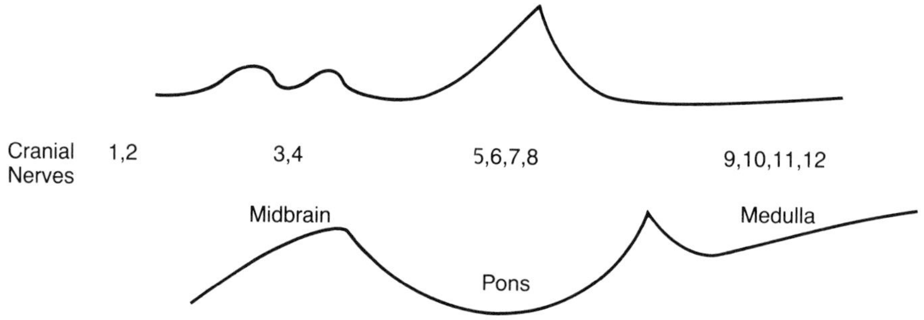

Figure 17–17. Cranial nerve localization.

the parasympathetic fibers act unopposed, and the result is small (miotic) pupils. There are three nuclei or points of origin for sympathetic innervation—the hypothalamus, the pons, and the cervical ganglion (Fig. 17–19). A lesion at any one of these sites can result in pupillary constriction. Since the cervical ganglion is an extracranial site, miosis of intracranial origin is due to pontine or diencephalic dysfunction. An interruption of innervation at either one of these sites can result in pupillary constriction. Constricted pupils secondary to hypothalamic or metabolic dysfunction retain reactivity to light, whereas pontine pupils are unreactive or fixed to light.

Causes of unilateral pupillary dilation in addition to midbrain compression are seizures and postictal states, direct orbital trauma, and optic nerve injury. Bilateral dilation is seen following mydriatic instillation (scopolamine/atropine) and anoxic episodes. The most common causes of pupillary miosis are pontine dysfunction, hypothalamic dysfunction, lesions of the cervical ganglion (brachial plexus injury), and opiates (street drugs, high-dose barbiturates).

Pupil Assessment

The three components of pupil assessment are size, shape, and reactivity. Depending on the amount of light that is entering the eye, pupils can vary in diameter from 1.5 to 8 mm but generally average about 3 mm. Variation in light source should be taken into consideration when assessing pupil size. A nurse who judiciously turns off the lights will have completely different results from the nurse who does pupil checks with bright overhead lighting. Consistency in assessment must be kept in mind. Variation in size is generally not significant as long as both pupils are the same diameter. Of pathological importance is pupillary inequality, asymmetry, or anisocoria. A small percentage of people (approximately 11 to 16 per cent) normally have anisocoria (inequality of the pupils in diameter), but the pupil difference is generally less than 1 mm. *Pupillary asymmetry of 1 mm or greater is significant* and often forewarns of subsequent progressive dilation.

Pupils are normally round and regular. An early warning sign of a pupil that will progress to become "fixed or dilated" is a change in the shape from round to oval. *An irregularly shaped or oval pupil is significant.*[43]

Pupillary reactivity to light consists of the direct and indirect or consensual response. When light is shined in one eye, both pupils constrict. The constriction of the pupil with the direct light source is the direct response, and the constriction of the contralateral pupil is the indirect response. Absence of the direct response indicates either midbrain compression of the third nerve or an optic nerve lesion resulting in blindness. A third nerve lesion will cause loss of both direct and consensual responses. A blind eye will have no direct reaction to light but the consensual response will remain intact.

The normal pupillary light response is brisk constriction of the pupils to light stimulus. The response is especially brisk in the young and in people with blue eyes. Pupil size as well as reactivity normally decreases with age, especially in those over age 60. The smaller the pupil, the smaller the amplitude of light reaction, so miotic pupils should be carefully assessed in a dim or darkened environment to determine optimal reactivity. The early foreboding sign of a pupil that will go on to become fixed to light is a delayed response to the light reflex. *Sluggishly reacting pupils are significant.*

Abnormal pupils are important because of their localizing value. Fixed, dilated pupils are associated with upper brainstem (midbrain) compression. Small pupils that retain reactivity are due to either metabolic or hypothalamic dysfunction, the latter associated with the mass lesion. Small and unreactive pupils are associated with lower brainstem dysfunction at the level of the pons.

Pupillary changes in shape, size, or reactivity can be ominous signs of neurological deterioration, especially in the presence of concomitant motor and sensorium changes, and warrant physician notification. The prognostic importance of pupil abnormalities is exceeded only by age and GCS score in predicting survival after head injury. Unilateral fixed pupils are associated with 30 per cent mortality, whereas 95 per cent of patients who die have bilaterally fixed pupils at 6 hours after injury.[36, 41, 42, 44]

Vital Signs

Vital signs are routinely monitored in all critically ill neurotrauma patients. Blood pressure and heart rate are assessed to determine if pressure is adequate to meet brain tissue perfusion requirements. The Cushing phenomenon[45–47] is a late sign of rising ICP and brain herniation. Changing blood pressure and heart rate without an accompanying change in level of consciousness indicates a nonneurological source of difficulty.

Respiration, unlike blood pressure and pulse, has several centers of regulatory control scattered throughout the cerebral hemispheres and brainstem, with each center responsible for its own unique respiratory pattern (Table 17–5). Because of the dissemination of centers and patterns, respiration has localizing value and serves as an early indicator of neurolog-

TABLE 17–4. CRANIAL NERVES: LOCATION AND FUNCTION

CRANIAL NERVE	LOCATION	FUNCTION	DEFICIT
1. Olfactory	Anterior cranial fossa	Smell	Anosmia/hyposmia
2. Optic	Retina to chiasm	Vision	Visual loss • blindness • field cuts
3. Oculomotor	Midbrain	Moves eye (medially/inferior obliquely)	Loss of medial eye movement Eye "down and out" Diplopia (double vision)
		Elevation of upper eyelid	Ptosis
		Pupil constriction (parasympathetic innervation)	Pupil: dilated unreactive to light
4. Trochlear	Midbrain	Moves eye (superior oblique direction)	Impaired downward gaze Diplopia
5. Trigeminal	Pons	Sensation to face, scalp, nasal and oral cavities	Loss of sensation
		Corneal reflex	Absent blink
		Chewing muscles (masseter/temporalis)	Muscle atrophy
6. Abducens	Pons	Moves eye laterally	Eye fails to abduct Diplopia
7. Facial	Pons	Facial muscles	Lower motor neuron • Ipsilateral weakness • Entire side of face • Loss of corneal reflex Upper motor neuron • Contralateral weakness • Lower half of face
		Taste, anterior two thirds of tongue	Lost, delayed, or metallic taste
		Lacrimation/salivation	Impaired/excessive salivation and lacrimation
8. Acoustic	Pons	Vestibular, balance	Dizziness
		Cochlear, hearing	Hearing loss
9. Glossopharyngeal	Medulla	Taste, posterior third of tongue	Loss of taste and sensation in posterior third of tongue
		Pharyngeal reflex	Loss of gag reflex
		Carotid sinus reflex	Impaired blood pressure regulation
10. Vagus	Medulla	Innervation to palate, pharynx, larynx, thoracic and abdominal viscera Conveys sensory impulses from digestive tract, heart, and lungs	Unilateral lesion Ipsilateral paralysis of soft palate, pharynx, and larynx • Impaired gag • Impaired palatal reflex • Dysphagia • Vocal cord impairment • Hoarseness Bilateral lesion • Complete paralysis of pharynx and larynx • Death due to asphyxia • Vocal cord paralysis • Atonia of stomach and esophagus—vomiting • Dysphagia
11. Accessory (spinal)	Medulla	Sternocleidomastoid and trapezius muscles	Weakness and atrophy
12. Hypoglossal	Medulla	Tongue musculature	Ipsilateral tongue paralysis and atrophy • Tongue deviation to side of lesion • Dysphagia • Dysarthria

ical deterioration. The earliest and most common alteration in the respiratory pattern is Cheyne-Stokes, a consequence of hemispheric compression. As rostral to caudal deterioration becomes evident, progressively worse patterns of respiration are seen as the pons and medulla become dysfunctional. Lower brainstem respiratory patterns are characterized by slower rates and longer periods of apnea. It is not as important to know the name of a specific pattern as it is to recognize the pattern as abnormal and prepare for ventilatory and neurological support.[41]

Temperature monitoring is essential. Elevations may indicate an infectious process or hypothalamic dysfunction secondary to a lesion or rising ICP. Patients can have rapid alterations in body temperature and may quickly move from a hyperthermic to a hypothermic state. Continuous temperature monitoring via rectal probe is indicated.

Motor and Sensory Function

The range and complexity of the sensory-motor examination is directed by the overall clinical status of the patient.

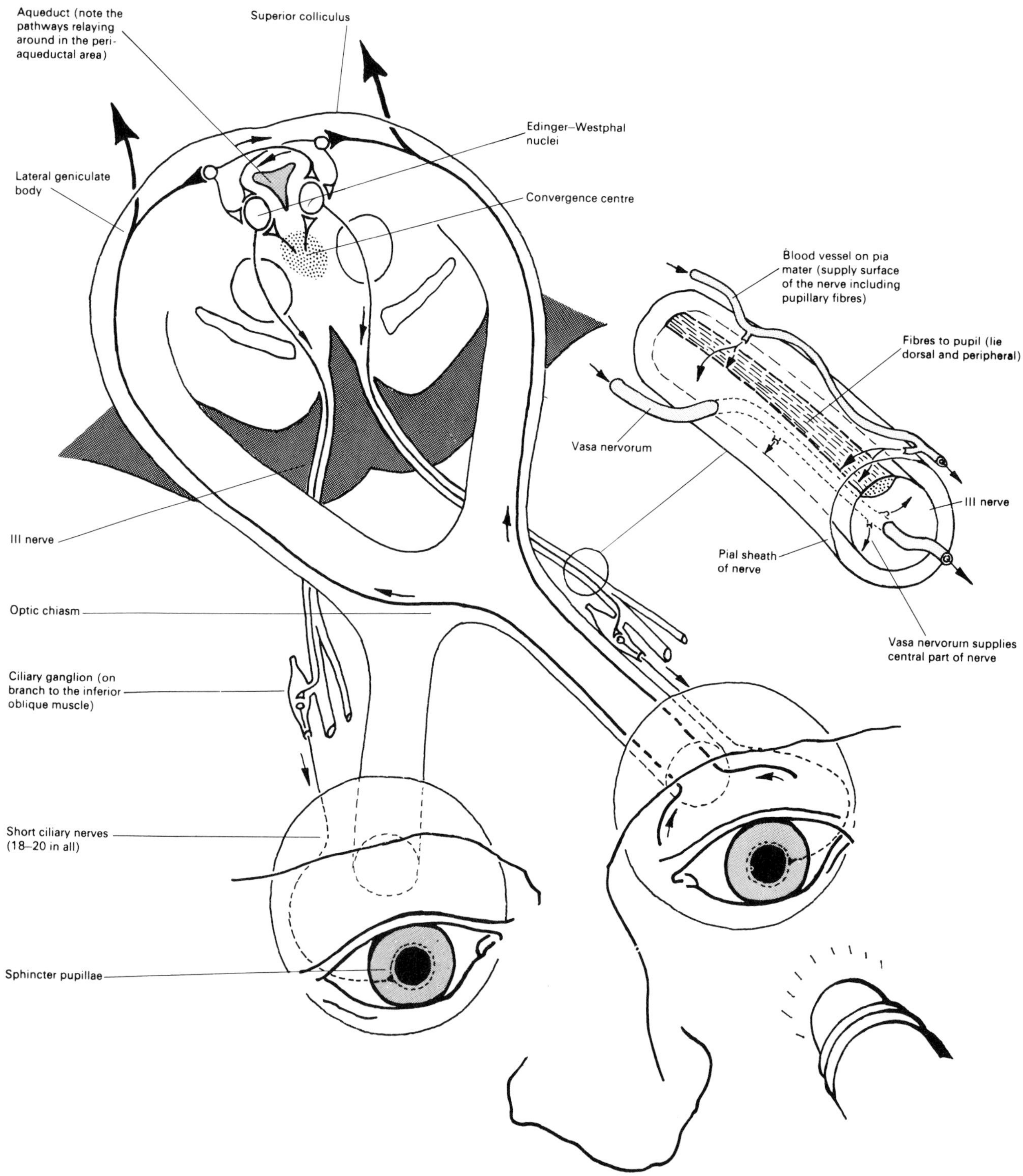

Figure 17–18. Parasympathetic pupillary innervation. (From Patten J: Neurological Differential Diagnosis. New York, Springer-Verlag, 1978.)

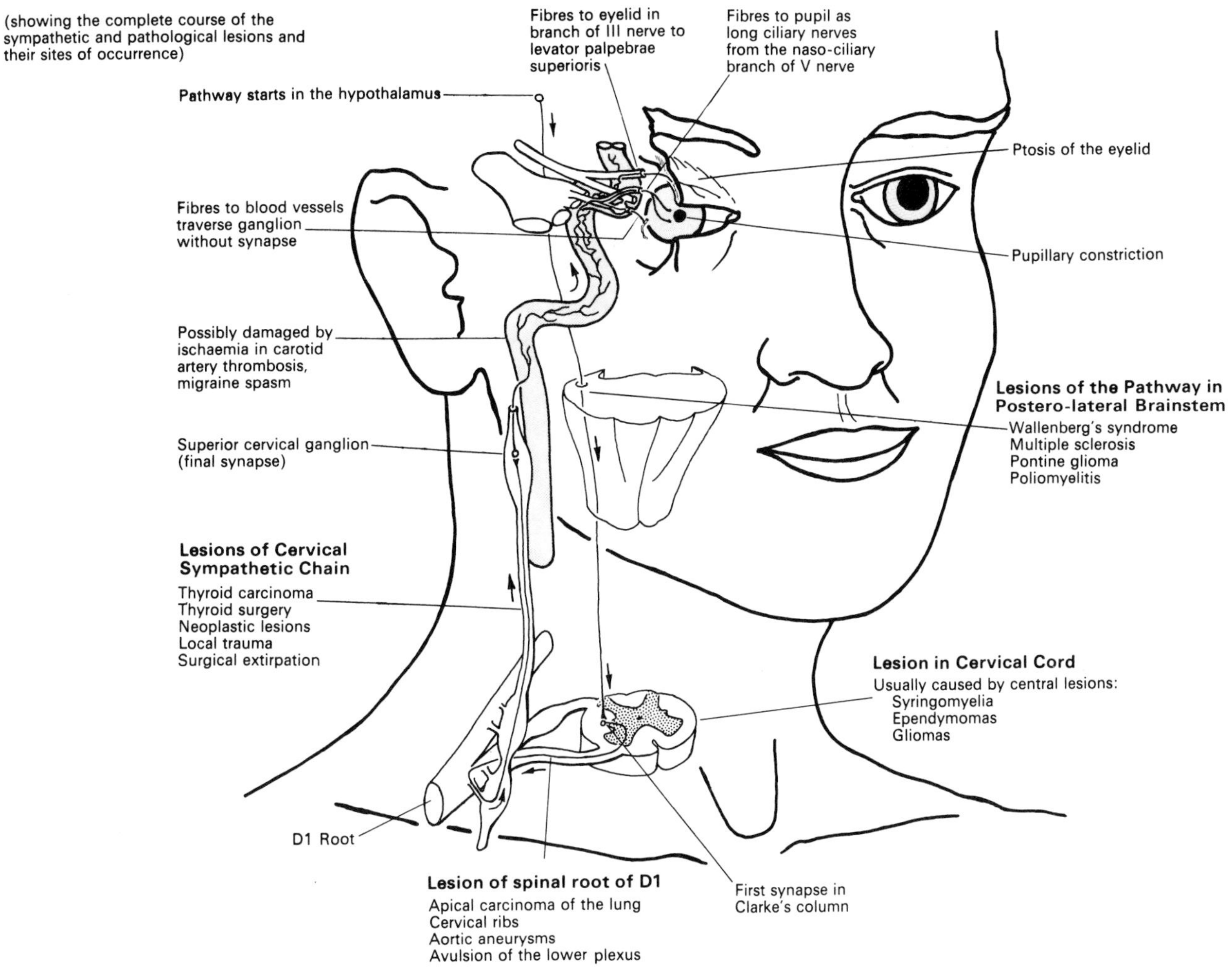

Figure 17–19. Sympathetic pupillary innervation. (From Patten J: Neurological Differential Diagnosis. New York, Springer-Verlag, 1978.)

If the patient is alert, complete testing of sensory function is carried out. In most situations, the sensory component of the examination is conjunctive with motor testing.

Motor abnormalities in the head trauma population are primarily due to upper motor neuron dysfunction, i.e., compression of the descending pyramidal or corticospinal pathways (Fig. 17–20). Corticospinal fibers normally descend from the cortex through the cerebral hemispheres, where, arranged in bundles, they pass through the cerebral peduncles and into the brainstem. At the level of the medulla, the fibers decussate and terminate in the opposite side of the spinal cord. Their "crossing over" at the medullary level to synapse in the opposite side of the cord results in contralateral motor dysfunction. Occasionally, the motor deficit is on the same side as the lesion. This occurs when the medial temporal lobe shifts the brainstem and compresses the opposite cerebral peduncle against the opposite edge of the tentorium. This is referred to as *Kernohan's notch phenomenon.*[36, 41]

The corticospinal tract terminates in the spinal cord. It is a long tract in comparison with other descending motor tracts that terminate above the cord. Signs of hemispheric corticospinal tract compression are sometimes called *long tract* signs and consist of weakness, hypertonicity, hyperreflexia, spasticity, and the extensor plantar response.

Considerably worse motor signs are abnormal flexion (decortication), abnormal extension (decerebration), and flaccid

TABLE 17–5. RESPIRATORY CONTROL CENTERS AND PATTERNS OF BREATHING

RESPIRATORY PATTERN	CHARACTERISTICS	LOCATION
Cheyne-Stokes	Regular Waxing and waning hyperpnea alternates with period of apnea	Hemispheric/ diencephalic
Central neurogenic hyperventilation	Sustained; rapid hyperpnea	Midbrain/pons
Apneustic	Prolonged inspiratory pauses	Pons
Cluster	Irregular groups of breaths with irregular pauses in between	Low pons/high medulla
Ataxic	Irregular depth Irregular pauses	Medulla

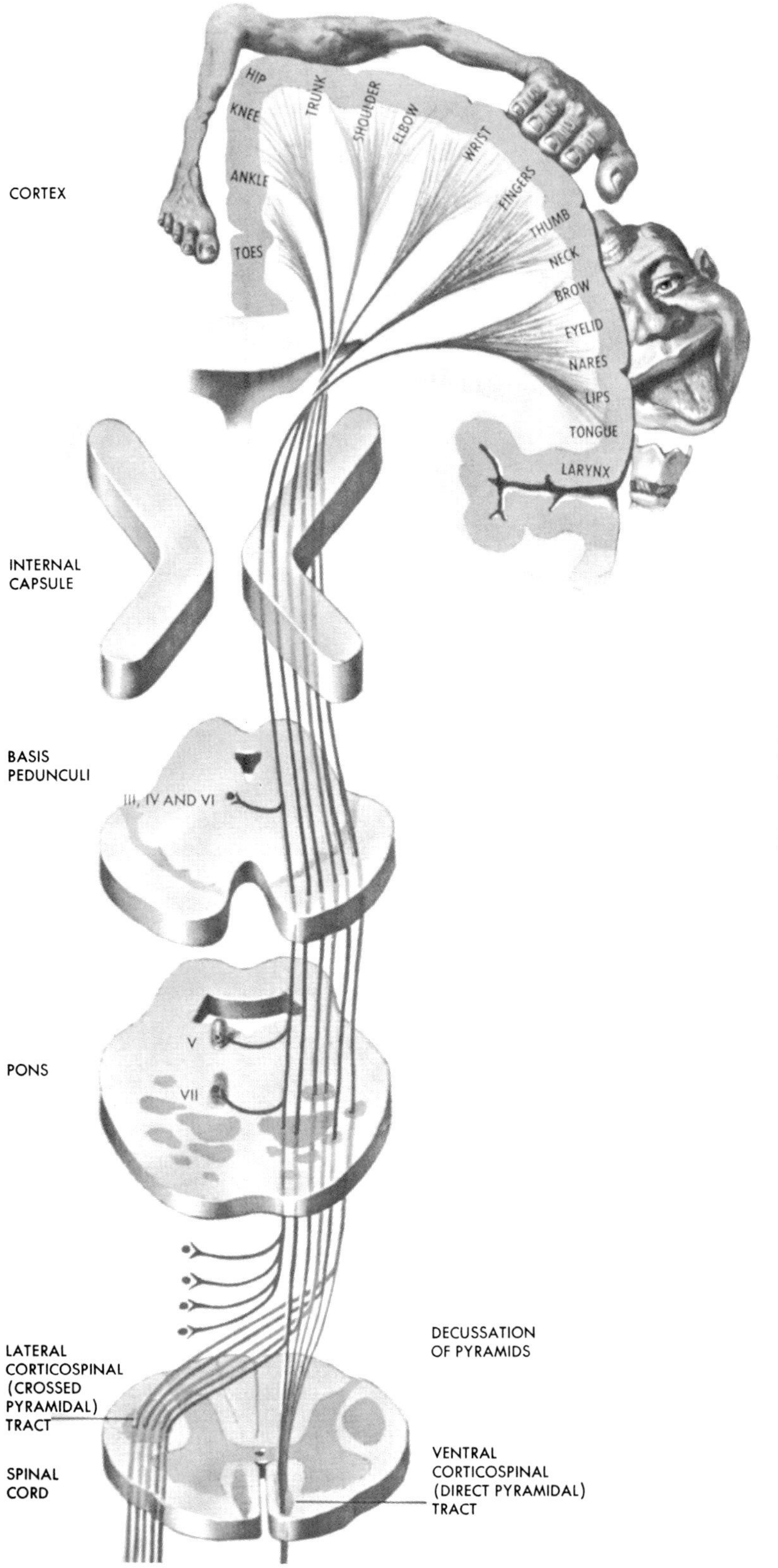

Figure 17–20. Descending pyramidal corticospinal motor tracts. (From Netter F: The Nervous System, Vol 1. The CIBA Collection of Medical Illustrations, 1975. © 1975, CIBA-GEIGY Corporation. Reproduced with permission from the CIBA Collection of Medical Illustrations by Frank Netter, M.D. All rights reserved.)

motor responses. Decortication is associated with hemispheric dysfunction, whereas flaccidity and most forms of decerebration are indicative of brainstem compression at the level of the pontomedullary junction and midbrain, respectively. There are varying patterns and degrees of decortication and decerebration, some with a better prognosis than others. Patterns that carry the worst prognosis are those associated with brainstem involvement or characterized by fixed pupils or impaired/absent oculomotor activity. Because of the varying types of decorticate and decerebrate motor responses, it is best to classify these movements as "abnormal flexor" and "abnormal extensor." In general, decortication is better than decerebration and decerebration is better than flaccidity.[36, 41]

In the awake patient, the signs of corticospinal tract compression are best evaluated by testing motor tone and strength. Tone can be normal, increased, or decreased. Patients with upper motor neuron lesions will have increased tone. Muscle strength is best evaluated by resistance measures and hand grasp. Resistance testing consists of asking the patient to pull his limb in opposition to the examiner. Hand grasp is tested by placing the examiner's index and third fingers inside the patient's hand and asking him to squeeze while attempting to withdraw the inserted fingers. The best determiner and earliest indicator of motor weakness is "pronator drift." Asking a patient to extend his arms outward with palms up and eyes closed will initially cause hand pronation and then downward drift of the weak or hemiparetic limb when motor tract compression is present. Comparison of both sides of the body is essential to determine equality or laterality; i.e., is one side of the body weaker than the other? The extensor plantar or Babinski reflex is a pathological reflex that consists of dorsiflexion of the big toe in the presence of long tract compression. This classic response can be elicited in awake or comatose patients.

In patients who are unable to follow commands, the initial evaluation consists of standing back and looking for spontaneous movement. If movement is present, are both sides moving equally well? If no spontaneous movement is present, a noxious stimulus is presented to each limb to determine type and consistency of response on both sides of the body. In the impaired patient, the motor examination is based on GCS criteria, as described in the subsequent section, and the following responses are possible:

1. Pain localization: Patients in lighter stages of coma are aware of pain, and they attempt to remove the painful stimulus.
2. Flexion withdrawal: The patient is in a deeper state of unconsciousness, and although aware of the stimulus, he is no longer able to reach it and withdraws or pulls the limb away with a normal flexor movement.
3. Abnormal flexion (decortication) and extension (decerebration): These are abnormal posturing responses associated with deep coma (Fig. 17–21). They reflect significant brain dysfunction, frequently with initial herniation and increased ICP. These responses may be elicited by noxious stimuli or occur spontaneously, and they may be transient or prolonged. Increased tone and spasticity of the involved limbs also precipitate additional complications, such as flexor/extensor deformities and contractures. Spasticity has been implicated as an inciting factor in the development of crippling heterotopic bone formation in head-injured patients. Continuous decerebration increases metabolism and oxidative requirements, causing massive weight loss and protein depletion with catabolism and negative nitrogen balance. Continuous abnormal muscle activity must be eliminated. This can be achieved by hyperventilation, mannitol, pentobarbital, or muscle blockade.
4. Flaccidity or lack of any motor response following resuscitative measures is associated with lower brainstem dysfunction, and death is usually imminent.

Of greatest significance in the motor assessment of head trauma patients is a worsening change in the clinical examination, which indicates neurological deterioration. A patient who has been exhibiting decortication and is found to be decerebrating is definitely worse, and physician notification is warranted.

Assessment of Transtentorial Herniation

Transtentorial herniation is an immediately life-threatening event in patients with mass lesions and rapidly increasing intracranial hypertension. Serial "neurochecks" are intended to detect early signs of incipient transtentorial herniation, as evidenced by the following classic signs of herniation:

1. Deterioration in the level of consciousness
2. Pupillary abnormality
3. Motor abnormality
4. Brainstem dysfunction
5. Alteration in vital signs, especially respiratory patterns

The following section reviews the cause, significance, and nursing implications of each of the classic signs of transtentorial herniation resulting from a supratentorial mass lesion.

Level of Consciousness. Deterioration in the level of consciousness is the earliest indicator of neurological deterioration. Dysfunction is due to compression or ischemia of the reticular activating system fibers or projections at either the hemispheric or brainstem level. Hemispheric compromise is caused by brain swelling, increased ICP, mass lesions, or widespread axonal shearing. Horizontal shift of the pineal gland of 4 mm or more visualized on CT scan is associated with a decrease in the level of consciousness with focal head injury masses. Although postmortem examination has led us to believe that transtentorial herniation was the basis for progressive loss of consciousness with mass lesions, more recent studies correlating CT scans with examined level of consciousness show that interference with the reticular activating system through lateral displacement of the hemispheres rather than transtentorial herniation is the basis for decreasing level of consciousness in focal mass lesions.[72, 73] In diffuse injury or vascular occlusion, focal brainstem or widespread hemispheric axonal damage is presumed to be the source of coma.

The state of consciousness is best assessed with a standardized scale, such as the Glasgow Coma Scale. Since a change in the level of consciousness is an indicator of acute improvement or deterioration, it is essential that all head-injured patients have an accurate baseline as well as continued assessment.

Pupillary Abnormality. The classic pupil abnormality associated with transtentorial herniation is the ipsilateral fixed and dilated pupil. The abnormal pupil is found on the same side (ipsilateral) as the hematoma in 90 per cent of patients. The cause is an expanding mass with midline shift, uncal herniation, and compression of the third cranial nerve (oculomotor) and the parasympathetic fibers that innervate the pupil.

Transtentorial herniation can produce two types of changes

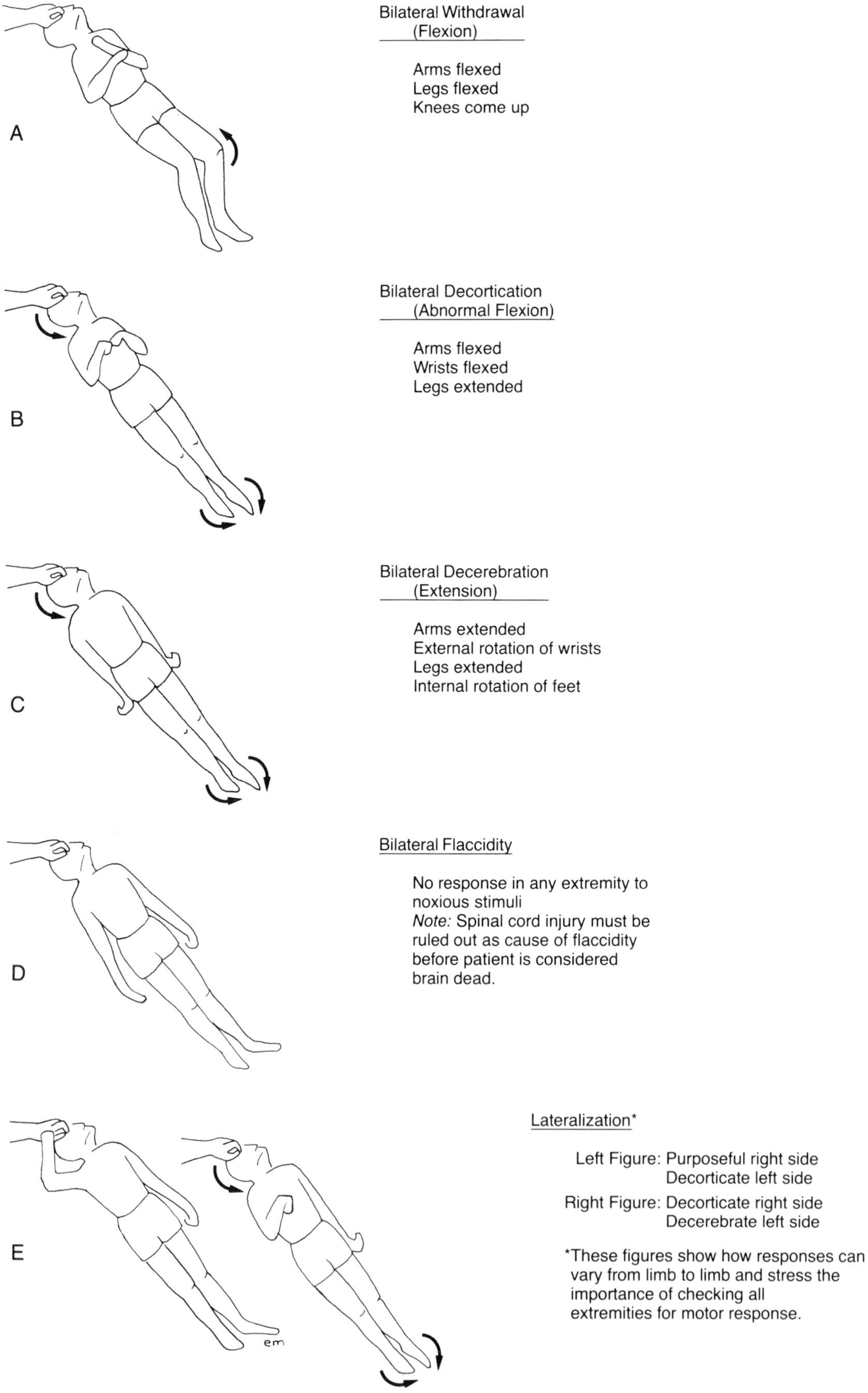

Figure 17–21. Abnormal motor responses. *A*, Bilateral withdrawal (flexion). *B*, Bilateral decortication (abnormal flexion). *C*, Bilateral decerebration (extension). *D*, Bilateral flaccidity. *E*, Lateralization. (From Marshall SB, et al: Neuroscience Critical Care. Philadelphia. WB Saunders Co, 1990.)

in pupil size—dilation or constriction. The most consistent response is dilation from compression of the ipsilateral oculomotor nerve at the midbrain level. This results in larger than normal or midposition pupils (4 to 6 mm in diameter) that are fixed to light and often irregular, with the larger pupil generally on the same side as the lesion. Symmetrical constriction of the pupils with retained reactivity has been known to precede dilation when the upper diencephalic region is involved during the initial stages of downward brain displacement. Nursing assessment includes frequent pupil checks with recognition of early and subtle changes in pupil size and shape.

Motor Abnormality. Motor abnormalities associated with transtentorial herniation syndrome are due to dysfunction of the upper motor neurons and their descending corticospinal pathways. The most common motor abnormalities are weakness, decortication, and decerebration. Motor signs are more variable and depend on the site and severity of brain involvement. The classic motor abnormality is *contralateral hemiparesis,* or weakness of the side opposite the lesion, due to compression of the corticospinal fibers at the level of the cerebral peduncle, temporal lobe, and midbrain region.

Cranial Nerve Dysfunction. The cranial nerves exit from the brainstem, with the exception of cranial nerves 1 and 2. During the initial course of transtentorial herniation, the upper portion of the brainstem (midbrain) and accompanying cranial nerves 3 and 4 undergo displacement and compression. As herniation progresses, there is downward displacement and compression of the lower segment of the brainstem and corresponding cranial nerves. Brainstem compression at the level of the pons results in dysfunction of cranial nerves 5, 6, 7, and 8, and medullar involvement causes abnormalities of cranial nerves 9, 10, 11, and 12.

Of most significance in cranial nerve evaluation is a good baseline assessment with documentation of cranial nerve dysfunction. Since brainstem herniation is a rostral-to-caudal (head-to-tail/midbrain-to-medulla) event, sequential progression of cranial nerve deficits is significant and can be a manifestation of progressive herniation. Because the brainstem is a relatively small structure, such progression also signals that time is critical to reverse the process when this is possible.

Changes in Vital Signs. As early as 1901, Cushing demonstrated the occurrence of arterial hypertension, bradycardia, and slowed respirations associated with increased ICP and cerebral compression. He concluded that these signs were a compensatory mechanism that facilitated brainstem perfusion.[45, 46] This classical widening of pulse pressure (increased systolic, decreased diastolic pressure) and bradycardia became known at *Cushing's triad* and was subsequently used as the criterion for detecting early intracranial decompensation. Later studies disputed this conclusion and determined that the changes in blood pressure and pulse were late, exhaustive, and ominous manifestations of medullary compression.[47]

Since blood pressure and pulse are regulated by the medulla, changes in these parameters are localizing signs of lower brainstem dysfunction and indicate impairment of the vasopressor mechanism. Altered respiratory patterns become progressively apparent as the pons and medulla become dysfunctional.

Standardized Assessment Tools

Use of standardized assessment tools is an important adjunct to performing a clinical neurological examination. These tools were often created during clinical research to consistently document one or more aspects of the patient's initial condition, overall neurological status, and trends during therapy and to permit comparison among groups of patients. Two such tools with widespread use in care of the head injured are the Glasgow Coma Scale (GCS) and the Rancho Los Amigos Levels of Cognitive Functioning Scale (Rancho).

Glasgow Coma Scale

Assessment of head injury severity and degree of coma is most commonly determined by the internationally recognized Glasgow Coma Scale (GCS) shown in Table 17–6.[74] The overall score ranges from 3 to 15 and is the sum of the best response in three subscales: eye opening, motor response, and verbal response. The total GCS score has been used as a descriptor to classify the severity of head injuries, with a score of 13 to 15 defined as mild injury, a score of 9 to 12 as moderate, and a score of 8 or less as severe head injury and coma.[75] The ability to score the tool has enabled clinicians and researchers to make meaningful comparisons between series of patients and more accurately predict head injury outcome.

GCS Components

In general, the lower the GCS score, the deeper is the coma and the higher are the associated mortality and morbidity. The presence of alcohol, aphasia, or an endotracheal tube and the use of paralyzing agents during ventilator therapy all interfere with accurate interpretation of the patient's verbal and motor responses and should be noted.

Eye Opening Category. The eye opening component, as a measure of spontaneous arousal, is most accurate when

TABLE 17–6. GLASGOW COMA SCALE

Eyes	Open	Spontaneously	4
		To verbal command	3
		To pain	2
		No response	1
Best motor response	To verbal command	Obeys	6
	To painful stimulus	Localizes pain	5
		Flexion—withdrawal	4
		Flexion—abnormal (decorticate rigidity)	3
		Extension (decerebrate rigidity)	2
		No response	1
Best verbal response		Oriented and converses	5
		Disoriented and converses	4
		Inappropriate words	3
		Incomprehensible sounds	2
		No response	1
Total			3–15

From Teasdale G, Jennett B: Assessment of coma and impaired consciousness: A practical scale. Lancet 2:81, 1974.

TABLE 17–7. REACTION LEVEL SCALE (RLS85)

LEVEL	LABEL	OPERATIONAL DESCRIPTION OF BEHAVIOR
1	Alert	Oriented; if intubated, reacts quickly; if sleeping, arouses quickly
2	Drowsy or confused	Responds to light stimuli; reactions are delayed; may be disoriented to time and place
3	Very drowsy or confused	Responds to strong stimuli such as loud noise, shaking, or pain; may respond verbally or by attempting eye contact, warding off pain, or obeying commands
4	Unconscious, localizes	On painful stimulation of fingertips, other hand moves to push stimuli away
5	Unconscious, withdraws	On painful stimulation of fingertips, pulls stimulated hand away
6	Unconscious, flexion response	Does not localize or withdraw; flexes arms and wrists to stimuli
7	Unconscious, extensor response	Does not localize or withdraw; arms and legs extend to stimuli (if both flexion and extension are noted, best response is recorded)
8	Unconscious, no response to pain	With repeated strong stimulation, no movement noted in face, arms, or legs

From Starmark JE, Stalhammar D, Holmgren E: The Reaction Level Scale (RLS85): Manual and guidelines. Acta Neurochir (Wien) 91:12–20, 1988.

used within the first 5 to 7 days following head injury. Thereafter, many patients have return of the normal sleep–wake cycle with associated spontaneous eye opening. Crediting a patient with this reflexive type of eye opening will erroneously increase the GCS score by 3 points despite lack of true neurological improvement.

Verbal Category. The question posed most frequently in this category is whether it is accurate to score an intubated patient for lack of verbal response. Head-injured patients are generally intubated because they have sufficiently decreased level of consciousness to maintain effective breathing patterns and require hyperventilation therapy for increased ICP. They are usually unable to speak because they are comatose, not because they are intubated. However, some systems that score multisystem indicators of severity of illness do allow giving at least 3 points for patients who through head nods and other behaviors indicate that they would talk if not intubated.[76]

Motor Response Category. When patients exhibit two different motor responses, they are graded for the "best" response both because it correlates more closely with outcome and because there is greater interrater reliability about best response. For example, a patient with abnormal flexion (decorticate-type response) of the right upper extremity and abnormal extension (decerebrate-type response) of the left upper extremity would receive a score of 3.

Motor responses can be ambiguous, particularly when an initial flexion response becomes an extension response. Some investigators suggest that this type of alternating response is significantly affected by the initial limb position and the type of stimulus used. For example, an abnormal extension response (decerebrate) is more likely to be elicited when the stimulus is supraorbital pressure and the limb is already extended. In contrast, abnormal flexion responses (decorticate) predominate when nailbed pressure is used and the limb is already flexed.[77] Therefore, examiners need to be consistent in both the type of painful stimulus used and in maintaining a consistent initial limb position.

Other Coma Scales

While the GCS has been the dominant scale internationally, with demonstrated usefulness in predicting outcome from initial severity of head injury, there have been many criticisms of its relative insensitivity to significant clinical change in the early period and to the subtleties of neurological function in recovering patients.[78] The developers of the GCS emphasized that it cannot stand alone in evaluating overall neurological function in the acute period but must be supplemented with neurologic evaluation of brainstem and overall motor function. The Glasgow–Pittsburgh Coma Scoring Method incorporates bedside evaluation of brainstem function as well as responsive level.[76] Several scales have been proposed that integrate components of evaluation of consciousness and general neurological function, including the Pinderfield Scale,[78, 86] the Glasgow–Liege Scale,[79] the Edinburgh-2 Coma Scale,[80] the Reaction Level Scale (RLS85),[81] and the Clinical Neurologic Assessment Scale (CNA).[82] The RLS85 (Table 17–7) has been the most extensively evaluated of these tools and has been recommended to replace the GCS in Sweden. This scale creates eight mutually exclusive categories based on behavioral manifestations of arousal and motor response to stimuli. International comparisons among the RLS85 and other scales have shown its scores to have high correlation with other scales, greater agreement across examiners, and greater ability to classify all patients compared with the GCS.[83, 84] Infant and pediatric versions of the GCS and Pinderfield scales have been developed and validated.[85, 86]

Rancho Los Amigos Cognitive Scale

The Rancho Scale is a multidisciplinary tool developed for use with head-injured patients in intermediate care or rehabilitative settings.[87] The scale has standardized evaluating criteria leading to a numerical description of patients at each of eight levels, ranging from nonresponsive to independent functioning (see Appendix 17–1). The scale infers behavior that stems from brainstem to higher cortical functioning and can be used throughout all phases of head injury management. Since other disciplines frequently use the Rancho Scale, implications of the scale levels for care can be coordinated among speech, occupational, and physical therapists as well as among nursing staff.

Neurodiagnostics: Technologies

The neurodiagnostic evaluation of head injury incorporates radiographical procedures, imaging procedures, and neural monitoring techniques.

Radiographic Evaluation: CT and Angiography

Computed tomographic (CT) scanning provides anatomical localization of space-occupying lesions and is the definitive diagnostic procedure for evaluation of patients following head trauma. Because of its rapidity, a diagnosis can be obtained within several minutes of scanning, and rapid diagnosis via CT scan has been a significant factor in reducing mortality from mass lesions. The greatest advantage of CT is identification of blood clots, intracranial shifts, and cerebral herniation, but it falls short in detecting vascular lesions.[4, 85, 86]

The use of angiography in the initial evaluation of head injury has virtually been eliminated by CT. Angiography is essential in identifying posttraumatic vasospasm and in trauma-related vascular injuries such as vertebral laceration or carotid artery occlusion. However, the ability of magnetic resonance imaging to detect movement of blood through vessels promises to supplant standard angiography with magnetic resonance angiography (MRA).

Imaging Procedures: Magnetic Resonance Imaging

Magnetic resonance imaging (MRI) utilizes the interaction of atomic nuclei placed in a static magnetic field that is moved about by radiowaves to produce excellent-quality anatomical composites of the brain. This method differs from CT, which uses ionizing radiation or x-rays. The most distinctive feature of MRI, compared with CT, is the clear differentiation between gray and white matter. MRI also exceeds CT in visualization of the small midline hemorrhages associated with severe DAI, in detection of posterior fossa/brainstem lesions, and in detection of nonhemorrhagic contusions and shearing injuries.[88–90]

There are several technical disadvantages to MRI that hinder its use in the unstable severe head trauma patient who requires ICP monitoring and mechanical ventilation. Some of the problems encountered include (1) longer study time than CT (MRI study takes approximately 45 to 60 minutes), (2) the magnetic field does not accommodate ferrous-containing compounds in the imaging suite (this excludes most ventilators and ICP monitoring devices), and (3) the radiofrequency waves cause interference with hemodynamic monitoring devices (blood pressure, heart rate, and ICP). Although MRI is costly and requires much coordinative effort, the technical problems can be circumvented by purchasing special monitoring and ventilator (Monahan) equipment that is not sensitive to the magnet or radiofrequency interference. Once technical problems have been solved, patient safety must be addressed. The clinical status and specialized needs of these patients require constant attendance and monitoring by the primary nurse and the neurosurgical, anesthesia, and respiratory therapy staff throughout the imaging procedure.

If these needs cannot be met, MRI should be reserved for stable head-injured patients and those who have neurological deficits with a negative CT scan. Patients excluded from MRI are those with electronic implant devices such as an insulin pump, pacemaker, or hearing aid and those with metallic prostheses or aneurysmal clips.

In head injury management, CT still surpasses MRI in two vitally important areas: the initial emergency scan when time is a critical factor and the evaluation of the critically ill head-injured patient requiring ICP monitoring.

Positron-Emission Tomography

Positron-emission tomography (PET) differs from CT and MRI in its ability to detect brain function rather than brain anatomy. Similar to CT, PET yields tomographic images, but they are physiological rather than anatomical. Where CT detects transmitted x-rays, PET detects emission of photons from a previously injected isotope-labeled biochemical compound that "traces" a specific biological process.

The isotopes (radionuclides) used in PET are oxygen-15 (half-life 2.05 min), carbon-11 (half-life 20.4 min), nitrogen-13 (half-life 9.96 min), and fluorine-18 (half-life 110 min). Because of the short half-life of these isotopes, there is minimal patient radiation exposure per study. Decay of these isotopes results in the emission of a subatomic particle called a *positron.* An emitted positron collides with an electron, resulting in annihilation. Each positron decay sends a two-directional signal that is picked up by the tomograph detectors; the data are computerized and analyzed, and an image is reconstructed. The reconstruction shows the distribution of the compound containing the positron-emitting atom or, in the case of head-injured patients, the distribution and utilization of glucose in the various regions of the brain.

PET is used primarily in head injury research to measure local glucose metabolism. The positron-emitting agents generally used are (^{18}F) fluoro-2-deoxyglucose (FDG) or ^{11}C. The tracer is given intravenously and taken up by the brain, and scanning is begun. Since glucose and oxygen metabolism vary with the state of neuronal activity, any areas of depressed metabolism secondary to injury are identified by reduced glucose uptake.

Although PET is still in its early stage of development, this research tool holds much promise for the future. Preliminary studies in head injury have demonstrated PET's ability to visualize areas of depressed brain metabolism and cerebral dysfunction that neither CT nor MRI have been able to identify as areas of injury.[91, 92]

Single-Photon-Emission Computed Tomography (SPECT)

Cost, scanning time, and the need for on-site creation of the radioisotopes have made PET a research tool used in only a few centers. A more clinically useful development is single-photon-emission computed tomography (SPECT), which uses readily available isotopes and a rotating gamma camera to measure regional cerebral blood flow (RCBF). Since metabolism is directly linked to regional blood flow, this method provides a reasonable estimate of brain metabolic activity.[4, 93, 94]

Doppler Ultrasound

Extracranial Doppler ultrasound techniques are well established in noninvasive imaging of the carotid vasculature at the base of the brain and in the neck. More recently, the development of transcranial Doppler techniques provides the ability to measure cerebral blood flow velocity in intracerebral arteries. The technique has received most extensive use in identifying vasospasm in patients with subarachnoid hemorrhage but is also stimulating interest in evaluating interaction of changes in blood flow velocity with intracranial hypertension in head-injured patients.[95–97] Because the skull is very thin at the temporal bone, it is possible to transmit an ultrasonic signal that is reflected from the moving red cells in the target intracranial artery. Velocity is inferred from the time required for the probe to receive the emitted pulsed signal. The reflected echoes are transformed to electric signals and graphically displayed via spectral analysis of the sound waves.

Neurophysiological Monitoring: Evoked Potentials

Evoked potentials (EP) have become a valuable aid in head injury management for lesion localization, as an early predictor of deterioration, and for prognosis. Unlike the EEG, which reflects spontaneous brain activity, evoked potentials reflect brain activity in response to a specific sensory stimulus. Three types of EPs are used in the clinical setting: visual evoked potentials (VEPs), which use light stimulus; somatosensory evoked potentials (SEPs), which use touch; and auditory evoked potentials (AEPs), which use click or sound stimulus. Although stimuli vary, they all evaluate brainstem integrity.

The auditory stimulus is used most often in head injury. It is a noninvasive bedside study that takes a relatively short time to administer and essentially does not interfere with patient care. A series of click stimuli delivered to the patient via earphones or a small sensor device activates the eighth cranial nerve. The impulse then travels up and through the auditory regions of the brainstem to the cortex. As the sound stimuli make their ascent to the cortex, specific regions or "generator sites" within the pathway produce a waveform that corresponds to that region (Fig. 17–22*A* and *B*).

The normal auditory brainstem response (ABR) is a series of five to six positive-voltage waves occurring within 1 msec following presentation of a brief click stimulus (Fig. 17–22*B*). Each wave is thought to represent synchronous firing of groups of neural units as the impulse ascends the auditory pathways of the brainstem. Wave I corresponds to activation of the eighth nerve. Waves II through V correspond to activation of the proposed generator sites. The presence of wave II indicates that the stimulus has reached the medullary–pontine junction of the auditory pathway. The presence of waves III, IV, and V indicates that ascending levels of the midbrain auditory pathway are intact. A normative value exists for the time it takes the stimulus to travel from site to site and to complete its course, i.e., the latency. When the intensity of the acoustic stimulus is increased, ABR amplitude increases and latency decreases. ABRs are considered normal and indicative of brainstem integrity when all waves are present with normal amplitude and latency.

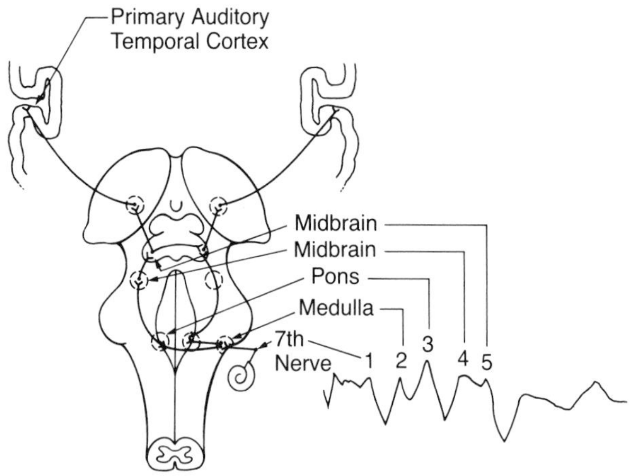

Figure 17–22. Neural generator sites of the auditory brainstem response and its corresponding waveform.

The most common ABR abnormalities are (1) absence of all waves, which is consistent with brain death, (2) prolonged relative or interwave latency, indicating a problem in conduction and some degree of brainstem dysfunction, and (3) absence of a wave or waves, indicating brainstem dysfunction at that particular level. For example, if waves I, II, and III are present but waves IV and V are absent, this may be indicative of midbrain dysfunction.[98, 99]

The AEP is not influenced by CNS depressants or barbiturate-induced coma, which makes this diagnostic tool useful for monitoring the clinical status of otherwise unexaminable patients.

NURSING MONITORING AND THERAPEUTICS

Care of the head-injured patient is a multidisciplinary team effort from the resuscitation phase through the rehabilitation phase. Therefore, nursing monitoring and therapeutics must always be seen in the context of medical, nutritional, physical, and social therapies, for example. Further, in a well-orchestrated team it is often not possible to distinguish the contributions of one discipline from another at any phase of the patient's care. The following sections discuss the primary focus of nursing care at each of three phases, resuscitation, critical care, and rehabilitation, in full recognition of the interdependency, with care and direction provided by other disciplines involved in overall management of the head-injured patient.

Nursing Monitoring and Therapeutics in Resuscitation

The initial priorities of care during resuscitation of the head-injured patient are the same priorities used for any trauma patient, that is, ensuring adequate airway, breathing, and circulation. It is essential that airway patency, effective ventilation, and adequate circulation be established as soon as possible in order to ensure adequate oxygen transport to the brain. Hypoxia from airway obstruction, ventilatory insufficiency, or inadequate cerebral perfusion related to circulatory collapse serve to exacerbate the magnitude of neuronal damage. Preliminary efforts to prevent or minimize secondary brain injury should therefore focus on maintaining sufficient oxygenation and perfusion by restoring airway and cardiopulmonary stability. Once these initial care priorities are accomplished, efforts are directed toward neurological assessment and continued treatment of the patient's head injury.

Accident Data Base

As with any injury, an accident data base should be obtained from the field care providers. This data base includes all possible information about the onset and cause of the injury as well as significant events such as drug ingestion that occurred prior to the traumatic episode. It is important to determine the patient's neurological status while in the field and changes that have occurred during transport to the hospital. This is best accomplished by utilizing the Glasgow Coma Scale. The patient's initial responses to field resuscitation efforts are noted.

Potential or Actual Airway Obstruction

An obstructed airway with inadequate ventilatory exchange can transform a potentially mild head injury into a severe head injury as a result of hypoxia. The sequelae of head injury may inhibit normal reflexes that maintain an effective airway and diminish the patient's natural airway defense mechanisms. Decreased sensorium associated with head injury and depression of protective gag, swallow, and cough reflexes result in an inability to clear the pharynx of normal secretions or foreign material. All head injury patients with a depressed level of consciousness are at risk of vomiting and pulmonary aspiration. Loss of consciousness leads to relaxation of jaw muscles and a subsequent backward prolapse of the tongue, which impair airway patency. Associated maxillofacial injuries heighten the predisposition for airway obstruction. However, since 10 per cent of head injuries also have a spinal cord injury, great care must be taken to maintain cervical spine alignment during any attempt to reestablish the airway.[4]

As soon as impaired airway patency is recognized, interventions to alleviate the problem take precedence and are instituted immediately. The chin-lift or jaw-thrust maneuver may be all that is needed to open the airway, and the oropharynx is suctioned to clear foreign debris. A curved oropharyngeal airway can then be inserted by the nurse to position the tongue and avoid obstruction. If a basilar skull fracture is suspected, the use of a nasopharyngeal airway should be avoided owing to the risk of penetration into brain tissue. Nasotracheal emergency intubation is preferred in patients suspected of a spinal cord injury or unconscious patients until cervical spine fracture is ruled out, in order to avoid manipulation of the cervical spine.

If protective airway reflexes are depressed and/or a decreased level of consciousness impairs airway control, the patient is intubated endotracheally, by cricothyroidotomy, or by tracheostomy.[4] Any patient with an initial GCS score of 8 or less generally requires immediate endotracheal intubation.[4] Mortality is significantly improved in severe head injury when intubation and ventilation are accomplished within 1 hour of trauma (22 per cent) as compared with those patients in whom intubation is delayed for 1 hour or more (38 per cent).[100] The risk of aspiration is greatly reduced by early tracheal intubation and gastric decompression using an orogastric tube.[101]

Sedatives or paralytic agents are frequently required to facilitate intubation and prevent intracranial hypertension. A rapid neurological assessment of the patient's level of consciousness, sensory-motor capabilities, and eye signs should be done prior to the administration of these pharmacological agents. Since spinal cord injury is present concurrently in 10 per cent of head injuries, cervical spine alignment must be maintained during all airway interventions.[4] Cervical spine injury precautions are maintained until injury is definitively ruled out by radiological examination.

Alterations in Ventilation and Oxygenation

Central nervous system injury frequently results in abnormal breathing patterns characterized by shallow, rapid, or irregular respirations and/or periods of apnea. These respiratory patterns impair effective ventilation and result in inadequate oxygenation and retained carbon dioxide. Since both hypoxia and hypercarbia potentiate intracranial hypertension, prevention or immediate resolution of these conditions is a priority in head injury management. Even when ventilatory patterns appear normal, it is estimated that 65 per cent of all severely head-injured patients are hypoxic upon hospital admission.[4] In addition to CNS dysfunction, other factors such as depressant drugs and associated chest injuries may cause early impairment of ventilation.

It must be emphasized that until it is proved otherwise, all head trauma patients are assumed to have a spinal cord injury prior to the initiation of ventilatory management. Neck stability must be provided before the airway is manipulated. Once a patent airway has been secured, effective ventilation must be established. The nurse rapidly assesses the patient's respiratory status, particularly rate, rhythm, chest excursion, and breath sounds. Supplemental oxygen should be administered at high flow levels starting at an inspired concentration of 100% to ensure adequate cerebral oxygen supply. The head-injured patient should ideally maintain a PaO_2 of 100 mm Hg. Hyperventilation producing moderate hypocarbia of 25 to 30 mm Hg is desirable and initially achieved by manual inflation followed by mechanical ventilation. Serial arterial blood gases are essential to guide oxygen and ventilatory therapy. Preoxygenation and hyperventilation precede and follow intermittent suctioning through the established airway.[4, 101, 102]

Alterations in Systemic and Cerebral Perfusion

Once adequate ventilation and oxygenation have been attained, the priority is circulatory stabilization and maintenance of oxygen-carrying capacity. Circulatory instability resulting in hypotension rarely occurs secondary to head injury itself unless there has been prolonged medullary compression and brain death is imminent. It must be emphasized that hypovolemic shock secondary to blood loss from extracranial injury is the primary cause of hypotension and consequent cerebral hypoperfusion during head injury resuscitation. Shock, present in approximately 30 per cent of head injury admissions, is predictive of intracranial hypertension and an overall less positive outcome.[103]

In order to restore circulatory stability, cardiac pump function must be optimized and intravascular volume restored. External and internal hemorrhage are controlled, and intravenous fluids and blood components are administered. Isotonic crystalloids, colloids, and blood products should be infused to maintain the mean arterial blood pressure at levels sufficient to keep the cerebral perfusion pressure above 50 mm Hg. Special care should be taken during fluid resuscitation to prevent fluid overload, which may exacerbate cerebral edema. If the patient's hypotension is unresponsive to fluid therapy, other causes, such as spinal shock, must be ruled out. Further discussion of shock causation in the trauma patient is found in Chapter 9.

Monitoring Neurological Status

During the interventions discussed previously, it is imperative that neurological status be continually monitored and evaluated for responses to therapy. The neurological examination techniques described earlier in this chapter are used to determine if brain function is deteriorating or improving over time. Although head injury should always be suspected when a trauma patient presents with an altered level of consciousness, other causes must be ruled out. For example, if the sensorium improves as oxygenation and perfusion deficits are corrected, cerebral hypoperfusion and hypoxia may be the cause of altered mentation. Hypoxia, as well as an increasing intracranial lesion, should be suspected when increasing agitation is assessed in a trauma patient.[103]

A toxicology screen should be part of the admission laboratory testing in order to evaluate substance abuse as a possible cause of abnormal neurological findings. Alterations in mental status due to drug use usually improve after a few hours as the drugs are metabolized.[104] A 2.0-mg dose of the narcotic antagonist naloxone is given intravenously during resuscitation to rapidly reverse possible drug effects.[105] It is also important to distinguish organic disease that may account for alterations in neurological function. For example, if blood glucose measurement establishes hypoglycemia, a 50-ml dose of 50% dextrose is given intravenously to promptly reverse cerebral symptoms. However, glucose should not be administered routinely and indiscriminately to unconscious patients, since there is growing evidence that it may worsen cerebral ischemic lactic acidosis, which in turn leads to further damage via free-radical release.[106, 107]

The technological diagnostic procedures described earlier in this chapter are used to determine the source of the neurological deficit. These include skull films, cervical spine radiographs, and CT scan. The CT scan is obtained as soon as possible. If an operable lesion is confirmed, the patient is immediately prepared for surgery. Delay in surgical intervention can escalate mortality and morbidity in patients with intracranial hematomas.[51, 108]

Patient and Family Psychological Support

During resuscitation, emphasis is placed on treating and maintaining the patient's physical being, but his psychological, emotional, and spiritual welfare must not be overlooked. Even the patient who is confused or partially responsive may be aware of his surrounding environment and treatment events. The nurse, as well as other trauma team members, should take the time to explain procedures in simple terms, offer emotional support, and reorient the patient at frequent intervals.

The family is in crisis and also requires support and information.[109, 110] Repeated simple and clear explanations of the patient's condition and progress must be provided at timely intervals. Family coping mechanisms and support systems should be evaluated and mobilized whenever possible.

Analgesia, Sedation, and Control of Agitation

Pain and agitation must be controlled in order to decrease cerebral metabolic requirements, reduce ICP, facilitate effective ventilation, and provide patient comfort. Severe pain is most likely from extracranial sources, since the brain tissue itself lacks pain receptors. Agitation places the head-injured patient at risk of self-inflicted injury. When initial attempts to calm the patient by offering reassurance and reorientation are unsuccessful, pharmacological therapy may be required. Prior to administration of sedatives or analgesia, a complete baseline neurological examination is completed. Precise anatomical areas of pain or tenderness are identified when possible.

Agitation frequently accompanies the emergent state of coma. However, other causes such as hypoxia or electrolyte imbalance must be ruled out prior to attributing the altered mental status solely to craniocerebral trauma. Pharmacological agents that reduce agitation should complement, but not replace, other nursing measures designed to protect the patient from harm. Side rails are padded, and soft extremity restraints are used. (In some institutions, a physician's order must be obtained prior to applying restraints.)

Sedatives and analgesics must be administered judiciously in head-injured patients, since their use eliminates many clinical signs and findings that are predictive of neurological deterioration. Management of pain and/or agitation in head injury is based on individual patient assessment. For example, a stable, awake, and oriented patient with a mild concussion, negative CT scan, and negative neurological findings who is complaining of severe pain from an open femur fracture is quite different from the comatose head-injured patient who is extremely agitated, resisting the ventilator, and manifesting ICP waves. Analgesia is required in the first situation, whereas the latter demands sedation and muscle paralysis.

The first-choice drug for pain relief should be a non-CNS depressant, i.e., a mild analgesic such as Tylenol. Codeine, a short-acting analgesic with minimal CNS effects, is used on occasion in the stable, awake patient with severe pain of extracranial origin. Muscle paralysis with pancuronium bromide and sedation are used for intubated patients with severe agitation. Morphine (2 to 3 mg/hr intravenously) is one preferred agent for pain and sedation because it is easily reversed with a narcotic antagonist such as naloxone, has minimal effect on cardiac output, and does not interfere with pupillary dilation if midbrain/oculomotor compression were to occur. Other agents such as fentanyl, thiopental, or pentobarbital may be used to control agitation and intracranial hypertension in the mechanically ventilated patient.

Extreme caution should be exercised when administering sedation or analgesics to patients with mild or moderate head injuries who lack ventilatory support or ICP monitoring capabilities. Small doses of short-acting analgesics or medications to reduce agitation are preferred. The threat of respiratory depression inherent in the use of these agents contraindicates rapid intravenous administration in the spontaneously breathing patient.[111]

Nursing Therapeutics in Critical Care

In the critical care setting, nursing care continues to focus on preventing or minimizing secondary brain injury in order to optimize functional recovery. Avoidance of hypoxemia, hypercarbia, hypotension, and intracranial hypertension is the key physiological priority for nursing management of the patient with craniocerebral trauma.[4, 101] In collaboration with the trauma team, the critical care nurse is responsible for recognition and prevention of intracerebral and systemic complications associated with head injury. Complications also may arise in response to nonneurological injuries and associated treatment modalities. Early, aggressive treatment directed toward prevention of these secondary complications reduces mortality and morbidity in the head-injured patient.[4, 108, 112]

Expansion of new or previously identified space-occupying lesions (e.g., contusion, subdural hematomas) may necessitate emergency surgery during the critical care stay. Nursing responsibilities preoperatively include readying the patient for immediate craniotomy, stabilizing vital signs, ensuring adequate oxygenation via ventilation and adequate brain compliance via hyperventilation, assessing for progressive neurological deterioration, and treating raised ICP as per institutional protocol.

Postoperatively, the most common complication is increased ICP. Patients with brain swelling will be extremely sensitive to any stimuli and will react with abrupt increases in ICP. These patients tend to have the highest levels of ICP and are often refractory to treatment. Patients with acute subdural hematoma constitute the largest population of those placed on high-dose barbiturates to control ICP. Nursing responsibilities include management of intracranial hypertension, frequent assessment and physician notification of neurological deterioration, monitoring Jackson-Pratt or catheter drainage for signs of hematoma reaccumulation, prophylactic administration of anticonvulsants, and family contact for support, education, and explanation.

Continued meticulous monitoring is essential to detect clinical changes and guide treatment appropriately. Physical examination, technological studies such as evoked potential monitoring and postresuscitation CT, and clinical monitoring of cerebral perfusion pressure and ICP are all used to appraise neurological recovery. ICP is usually monitored in any patient who is at risk for intracranial hypertension. Postoperative patients who are nonpurposeful and at risk of mass lesion reaccumulation or development of cerebral edema also require ICP monitoring. Data are documented on a time-oriented flow sheet to facilitate rapid recognition of changes in patient status. Analysis of clinical findings permits the development of nursing diagnoses and a plan of care appropriate for the individual.

Monitoring and Treating Increased ICP

The detection and control of intracranial hypertension is a central activity of nursing and medical management in the critical care phase. Therefore, this aspect of nursing care is described extensively below. There is currently no approved nursing diagnosis in the North American Nursing Diagnosis Association (NANDA) nomenclature that specifically guides the nursing interventions commonly used in patients with increased ICP (intracranial hypertension). Many nurses use the general category of altered cerebral tissue perfusion related to increased ICP or decreased adaptive capacity, intracranial.[4, 48]

ICP Monitoring. Electronic ICP monitoring provides the only direct measurement of ICP. Its usefulness is unsurpassed in (1) providing early identification of patients with escalating ICP and impending brain herniation, (2) determining the need for therapy, (3) determining the effectiveness of therapy, and (4) predicting outcome. The criteria for ICP monitoring depend on the individual patient, but in general, head-injured patients who are comatose with a GCS score of 8 or less should be monitored.[113]

Presumptive evidence of increased ICP can be obtained from clinical examination and diagnostic studies, but frequently only after a neurological disaster has occurred and the brain has herniated from rapidly increasing ICP. Compressed ventricles, absent or compressed cisterns, brain shift, and vessel displacement as demonstrated on CT, MRI, and arteriography indirectly support the diagnosis of increased ICP but do not tell the level of pressure increases, nor are they useful in hour-to-hour management and reduction of pressure.

ICP Monitoring Systems. The two systems currently employed for monitoring ICP are hydraulic and fiberoptic. The *hydraulic,* or fluid-filled, system has been used almost exclusively during the past 30 years for monitoring hemodynamic cardiac, pulmonary, and intracranial parameters in critically ill patients. Critical care nurses are familiar with the inherent problems of the fluid-filled system, which include kinked tubing, air bubbles within the tubing or transducer, movement of the catheter, loose connections, and catheter occlusion from blood clots or herniated brain tissue. These problems result in damping (smoothing) of the waveform characteristics, artifacts, and distorted waveforms. Each of these problems may result in inaccurate information. Other components of the system, such as the external transducers, stopcocks, flushing devices, and pressure tubing are also prone to technical malfunction.[114] Even when the system is functioning well, changes in the patient's position relative to the reference level of the transducer may produce inaccurate readings and require frequent releveling of the transducer unless it is secured to the patient's body at the reference point.

Since accuracy of ICP values is of utmost importance, it is essential that fluid-filled systems be optimally maintained. When a damped waveform exists, occlusion, air bubbles, or system leak is suspected. If no obvious leak is detected, the tubing and stopcock are checked for moisture, which would indicate a microleak. The system distal to the patient is flushed, and air bubbles are removed, if present; all connections are tightly wedged, and the transducer is rebalanced. If there is no improvement in the waveform and occlusion of the measuring tip seems likely, the physician should be notified. The physician may then elect to irrigate the intracranial device with a small amount of nonbacteriostatic saline to open the proximally clogged system. In contrast to hemodynamic pressure measuring systems, one never hangs a bag of irrigating fluid for routine flushing of the measuring device within the patient's cranium because of the danger of inadvertently introducing a large volume of fluid into the cranial cavity.

In contrast, the *fiberoptic* ICP monitoring system is nonhydraulic. This system incorporates the transducer or pressure-sensing device with the distal tip of the intracranial device or catheter. This eliminates the need for a fluid-filled system to carry pressure waves to an external transducer and thus eliminates the problems inherent to an hydraulic system. Measurements are accurate when compared with simultaneous standard intraventricular hydraulic system values, and the waveforms are excellent.[114–116] The major problems stem from the inability to recalibrate the measuring sensor after implantation and an increasing drift of measured values over several days. The optical fibers within the system are relatively fragile, but breakage can be avoided by carefully securing the tubing and avoiding kinking.[111]

Location of Monitoring Device. ICP is monitored from the extradural (epidural), subdural/subarachnoid, or ventricular spaces (Fig. 17–23). The advantages and disadvantages of each system are discussed below.

Epidural Monitoring. Epidural sensors are placed between the skull and the dura. Since the dura is not penetrated, this method is considered relatively noninvasive, reduces the risk of infection, and renders the risk of intracranial hematoma and brain injury negligible; however, CSF cannot be drained with this system. Because the sensor may not achieve perfect placement with the plane of the dura (applanation), the measurements obtained from an epidural transducer may provide falsely high or low readings when compared with intraventricular monitoring.[114, 117] For this reason, the epidural route remains the least used monitoring technique.

Subdural Monitoring. The subarachnoid bolt or screw is the device most often used to record pressures from the subdural space. The device was originally intended for subarachnoid use, but it has been found to work best in subdural application with an intact arachnoid membrane. Since the

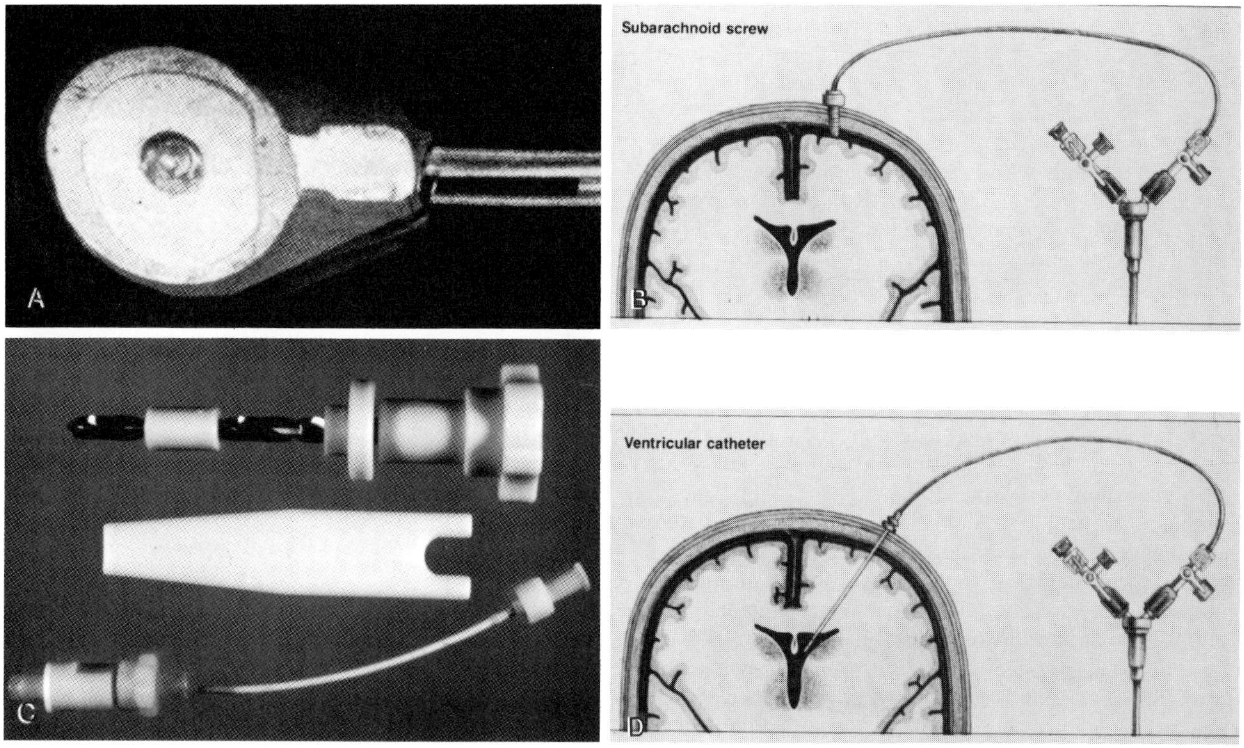

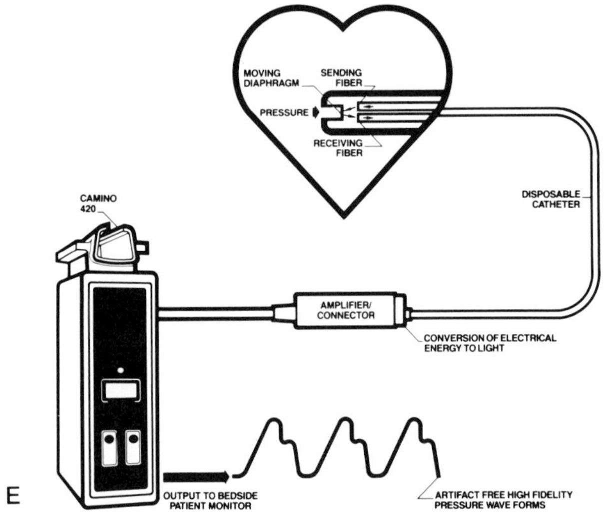

Figure 17–23. ICP monitoring devices. *A,* Epidural sensor device. *B,* Subarachnoid screw. *C,* Plastic model of Philly Bolt with ventricular catheter adaptability. *D,* Ventricular catheter. *E,* Fiberoptic transducer-tipped.

development of the first hollow device, known as the *Richmond screw*, several modified versions have emerged, including the Philly bolt, the Leeds screw, and the Landy screw.[118–120]

The screw is inserted via a twist drill hole through the skull. The dura of the nondominant hemisphere is pierced, and the bolt is projected onto the arachnoidal surface of the brain. Pressure changes in the CSF are transmitted to the fluid-filled bolt and monitoring system. The advantages of the system are the relative ease of insertion and relatively accurate recordings. Disadvantages include the potential for infection (which increases with the length of monitoring beyond 3 days), obstruction of the bolt by tissue, and inability to withdraw CSF and to measure cerebral compliance.[114, 121, 122] The latter problem is overcome by the design of the Philly bolt, which permits access to the CSF. The metal screws cause excessive artifact on CT and are not compatible with PET or MRI. This problem can be overcome by using a plastic model of the Philly bolt. However, the increasing use of intraparenchymal and subarachnoid fiberoptic monitoring may greatly diminish use of the subarachnoid screw in the next decade.

Intraventricular Monitoring. Monitoring ventricular fluid pressure involves inserting a catheter through brain tissue into the anterior horn of the lateral ventricle, preferably the nondominant hemisphere. Insertion can be difficult, particularly when there is brain shift and ventricular displacement. Each repeated attempt to pass the catheter or needle through brain tissue increases the risk of injury to cerebral vessels and intracranial bleeding.

The ventricular method is used for both diagnostic and therapeutic purposes. As a diagnostic tool, it is the most reliable of the monitoring devices. As a therapeutic modality, it is used to drain CSF from the ventricular cavity to decrease CSF volume and thus reduce ICP. Ventricular drainage may be continuous or intermittent. The continuous drainage system is open at all times to facilitate the automatic egress of CSF when ICP exceeds a predetermined value. The intermittent method is essentially a closed system that is opened periodically for drainage when ICP rises. The physician determines the ICP value that will promote drainage as well as the amount to be drained at any one time. Excess drainage with ventricular collapse is the major complication of a continuous system.[38]

Nursing prevention of ventricular collapse includes proper securing and positioning of the CSF collection bag. The bag can be secured with a safety pin or other attachment device and is generally placed at the level of the foramen of Monro. The lateral canthus of the eye and the tragus of the ear are commonly used anatomical landmarks for the foramen of Monro. Ventricular collapse may occur with the intermittent method if the system is inadvertently left open after perfunctory drainage has occurred.

The risk of infection (ventriculomeningitis, brain abscess) is highest with intraventricular monitoring, with the rate as high as 27 per cent in some studies. The duration of monitoring is important in that 33 per cent of patients who develop infection do so by day 5, and nearly 100 per cent do so by day 10.[122] The infection rate may be reduced by replacing the intraventricular catheter with a less invasive device when CSF withdrawal is no longer needed, but continued monitoring is necessary by relocating the monitoring device after 3 to 5 days. Prophylactic systemic or local antibiotics do not appear to alter the infection rate.[122] Nursing measures to maintain a closed system with all portals of entry covered and the use of aseptic technique when changing full drainage bags are essential.

ICP Waveforms. The ICP tracing reflects CSF pressure and has characteristic components that reflect systemic blood volume changes and respiration. Normally, a rapid biphasic oscillatory wave accompanies each heart beat, accompanied by a slow respiratory component. The upward sweep of the wave reflects cardiac systole followed by the diastolic slope and dicrotic notch (Fig. 17–24). Natural fluctuations in the ICP/CSF pulse wave are due to a small amount of blood that is added to the intracranial blood volume with each systolic ejection. This natural volume stress causes the ICP to increase minimally by 2 mm Hg within each cardiac cycle. Respiratory intrathoracic pressure is transmitted to the CSF pressure waves via central venous pressure. As a result, ICP normally fluctuates a few millimeters of mercury during the respiratory cycle as well.

Synchronous pulsations with cardiac systole and diastole indicate filling and emptying of the cerebral vessels. An increased in cerebral blood volume with each systole increases the amplitude or difference between systolic and diastolic pressures of the first wave. The pulse-wave amplitude is an estimate of cerebral compliance or the slope of the pressure–volume curve. As cerebral blood volume increases, compliance decreases, amplitude increases, and the waveform becomes more rounded. When CSF disequilibrium occurs, it is reflected in the CSF pressure wave.[123]

Wave abnormalities associated with decreased compliance (and therefore decreased adaptive capacity) are (1) an increase in the height of the wave (amplitude), (2) rounding of the wave, (3) loss of the dicrotic notch, and (4) increase of the relative height of the second wave component (P_2) compared with the first component (P_1). This change in relationship of P_2 relative to P_1 is the earliest change observed prior to a rise in the mean level of ICP.[123–127] Figure 17–25 shows this progression in loss of waveform as mean ICP rises.

In addition to the characteristic shape of each waveform, there are three patterns of collected waves: C waves, B waves, and A or plateau waves. C waves are rapid, rhythmic (4 to 8 per minute), small in amplitude, and correspond to changes in blood pressure of the Traube-Hering-Meyer type (Fig. 17–26). No clinical significance has been ascribed to C waves.

B waves are sharp, rhythmic elevations to levels of ap-

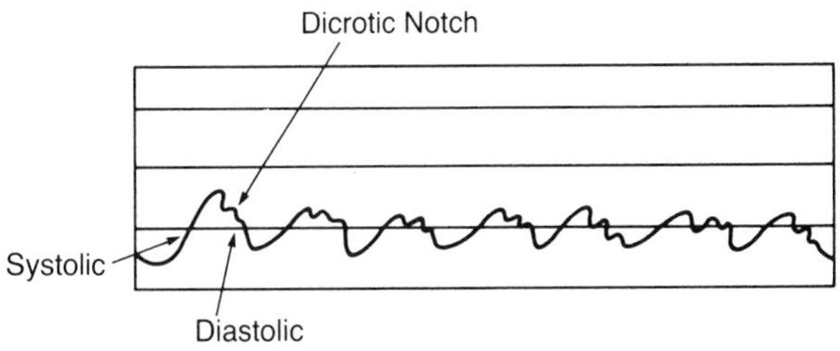

Figure 17–24. Cerebrospinal fluid pressure/intracranial pressure waveform.

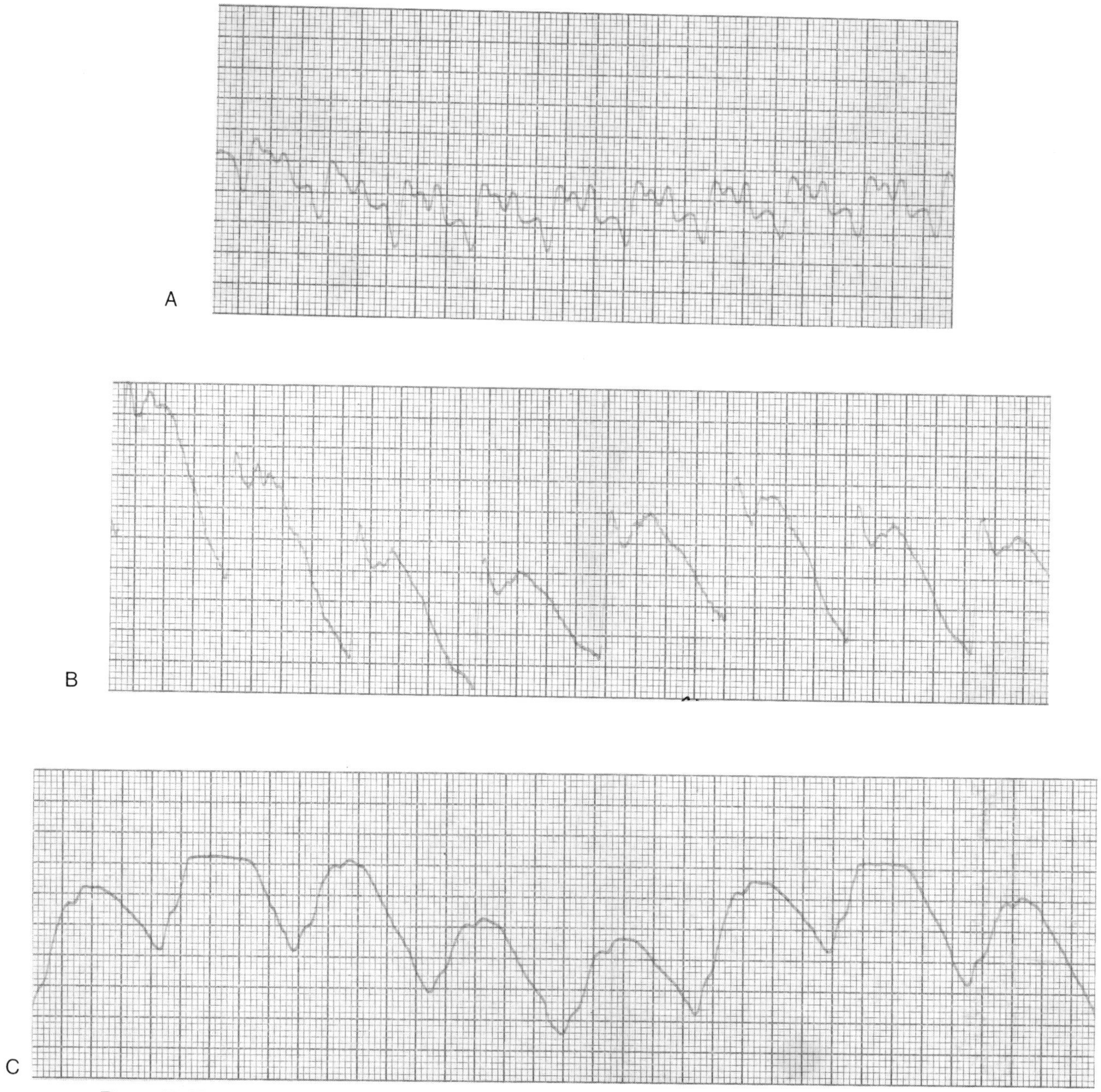

Figure 17–25. Pressure wave. Progressive deterioration in intracranial pressure waveform formation. *A*, Second wave component becoming larger than the first. *B*, Increase in height of wave. *C*, Rounding and loss of dicrotic notch.

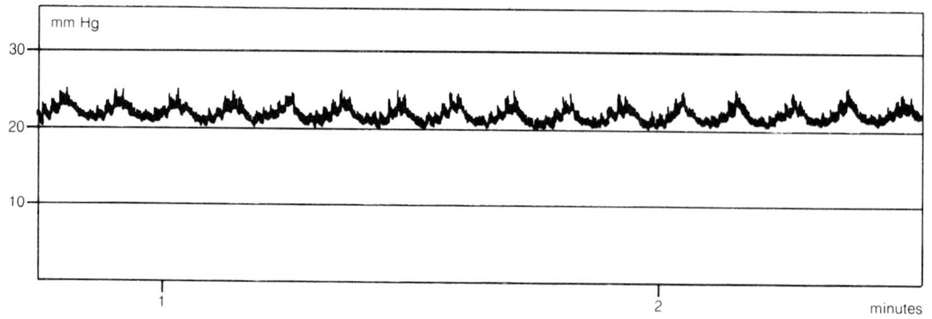

Figure 17–26. C waves.

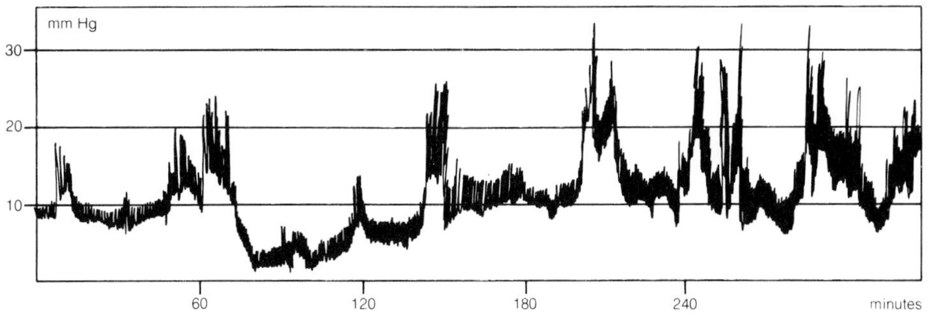

Figure 17–27. B waves.

proximately 50 mm Hg that occur at 1/2- to 2-minute intervals (Fig. 17–27). The elevations occur from a normal baseline (less than 15 mm Hg) and are only a few seconds in duration. They have been known to accompany Cheyne-Stokes breathing and to precede plateau (A) waves. They are clinically important and indicate decreasing intracranial compensation. Patients exhibiting B waves should be monitored frequently and carefully assessed for changes in their neurological status.

A waves are also known as plateau or pressure waves and indicate severe cerebrovascular decompensation (Fig. 17–28). A waves are characterized by the following:

1. Steep pressure rises to 60 mm Hg or greater
2. Duration of 5 to 15 minutes or longer
3. Initiated from an elevated baseline (mean greater than 15 mm Hg)
4. Varying in intervals
5. Precipitated spontaneously or by physiological alteration (e.g., changes in PaO_2, noxious stimulation)
6. Frequently accompanied by neurological deterioration
7. Generally terminate in a return to baseline pressure but may continue indefinitely or fall in concert with blood pressure as brain death ensues
8. Often herald impending brain herniation[4, 36, 128]

The presence of A waves demands immediate intervention. During the course of a plateau wave, there is limited brain perfusion. For example, if ICP is 80 mm Hg and MAP is 90 mm Hg, then CPP is only 10 mm Hg. In an acutely injured brain, depending on the degree and duration of inadequate perfusion, further neurological damage or even brain death may result. Patients with preexisting orders for treatment of ICP elevations should receive therapy without delay. If a prescriptive protocol is not in force, the initial treatment is manual hyperventilation and simultaneous notification of the physician.

Understanding the significance of each ICP waveform, recognizing clinically important changes, and providing therapeutic intervention are vital components of the nursing management of patients whose ICP is being monitored.

SURGICAL AND MECHANICAL THERAPIES FOR INCREASED ICP. ***Surgical Intervention.*** Mass lesions are the primary cause of increased ICP and brain herniation in head-injured patients. Their evacuation is often a lifesaving measure, with speed of treatment being crucial. A study of comatose patients with acute subdural hematoma showed that those undergoing surgical evacuation within 4 hours of injury had a mortality of 30 per cent compared with 90 per cent mortality in those with surgical intervention after 4 hours.[51]

CSF Drainage. Reduction of CSF volume effectively but temporarily reduces raised ICP. Use of a ventriculostomy catheter allows both measurement of ICP and continuous or intermittent drainage. Such therapy does not alter intracerebral compliance, however, and is thus likely to be helpful primarily when there is blockage of the CSF system.

Hyperventilation. Hyperventilation remains the most frequently used modality of ICP management. Hyperventilation decreases $PaCO_2$, which causes constriction of cerebral blood vessels. This, in turn, decreases cerebral blood volume and thus ICP. Its effectiveness is apparent within 2 to 3 minutes. When cerebral autoregulation is intact, a reduction in $PaCO_2$ from 40 to 20 mm Hg can cause a 30 per cent reduction in ICP through reduction in cerebral blood flow. Since marked reduction in cerebral blood flow could worsen cerebral ischemia in an already injured brain, $PaCO_2$ values below 20 mm Hg should be avoided, and most authorities recommend keeping the level between 27 and 30 mm Hg. Hyperventilation also can lower the seizure threshold by producing respiratory alkalosis.[4, 69, 102]

PHARMACOLOGICAL THERAPIES FOR INTRACRANIAL HYPERTENSION. ***Nonosmotic Diuretics.*** Furosemide is the pri-

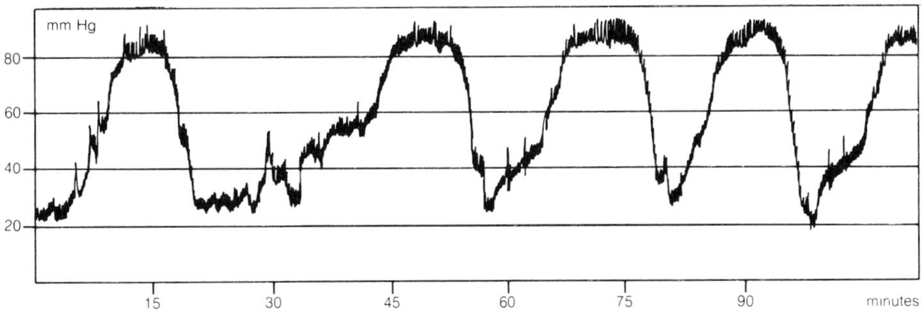

Figure 17–28. A waves.

mary nonosmotic diuretic used for ICP reduction. It is a potent loop diuretic that has been reported to reduce ICP by several possible mechanisms. It decreases sodium transport into the brain, reduces body fluid volume by renal tubular diuresis, and inhibits CSF production. The advantage of furosemide over hyperosmotic agents is minimization of electrolyte and osmolarity disturbances.[128, 129]

Osmotic Diuretics. Osmotic diuretics are the most common pharmacological agents used to control intracranial hypertension. Mannitol is the most frequent agent used because of its rapid onset and effectiveness, with lesser use of urea and glycerol. Osmotic diuretics create an osmotic gradient between the blood and brain, leading to translocation of fluid from the cerebral extracellular space into the intravascular compartment with subsequent reduction of overall brain volume.

Mannitol is given intravenously, by bolus or continuous infusion. Since it causes skin sloughing when extravasated from a vein, a central line is preferred. Dosage often starts with 0.25 to 0.5 gm/kg, with a second dose if no response is seen in 10 to 15 minutes. Total dosage varies according to physician preference (0.25–1.5 gm/kg), but authorities agree that the smallest dose that reduces ICP is the optimal dose.[102, 129–131]

Nursing responsibilities include frequent monitoring of serum sodium level and osmolality because hyperosmolarity and renal dysfunction are the prime complications of hyperosmolar therapy. Serum osmolarity should be maintained between 305 and 315 mOsmol/l (normal range 275–300 mOsmol/l). Osmolarity greater than 315 mOsmol/l necessitates a reduction in frequency or termination of the therapy.

Barbiturates. Intravenous barbiturates have been used for the past decade in the management of severe head injury to reduce elevated ICP and to provide brain protection against hypoxia and ischemia. Barbiturates are thought to reduce ICP by reducing cerebral metabolism and cerebral blood flow while stabilizing cell membranes. Although there was initial hope that the documented effectiveness of barbiturates in reducing ICP would translate to overall outcome improvement through use of high-dose barbiturate therapy, this hope has not been realized in controlled studies to date.[132–134] Some authorities believe that barbiturate therapy has a place for the 10 per cent of patients whose ICP cannot be controlled by standard measures.[4, 135]

Current recommendations are for high doses of pentobarbital, with an initial loading dose of 5 to 10 mg/kg by slow intravenous injection. Additional boluses may be given until the ICP is reduced below 20 mm Hg and preferably below 15 mm Hg, with total dosage up to 20 mg/kg during the first 4 hours. Thereafter, a maintenance dose of 100 to 200 mg/hr is used until the ICP is well controlled. Further maintenance doses are titrated against the ICP.

Because barbiturates are cardiac depressants, it is essential to measure pulmonary artery wedge pressure and arterial pressure prior to and during the course of therapy. Mean systemic arterial pressure should be maintained at 90 mm Hg or greater, and barbiturates should be stopped if MAP falls below 70 mm Hg. The accuracy of serum barbiturate levels varies with laboratories. Some advocate maintaining daily pentobarbital serum levels at 3 to 4 per cent if accurate laboratory assays are assured[4]; others recommend monitoring with continuous EEG. EEG burst suppression and isoelectric (flat) tracings reflect pentobarbital serum levels of 3 to 4 per cent and allow dosage adjustments based on the degree of cortical depression.

The neurological examination is nearly lost when patients are on high-dose barbiturates because there is no motor, eye opening, or verbal response to stimuli. Most brainstem and motor reflexes are also effectively suppressed. Contrary to popular opinion, the pupillary dilatation response to brainstem compression is *not* lost. Therefore, pupil measurements should continue, and the patient should be sent for CT scanning to rule out compression if one or both pupils dilate. Suppression of most motor and sensory reflexes means that the patient is completely dependent on nursing care to protect eyes, skin, and airway.

Steroids. Glucocorticoids most commonly used in head injury are dexamethasone and methylprednisolone. They have been shown to be quite effective in reducing the edema surrounding brain tumors and were introduced into head injury treatment based on the hope of reducing cerebral edema and thus ICP. Steroids also stabilize cell membranes and prevent lysosomal rupture. Although these agents have been effective in animal models, much controversy surrounds their clinical effectiveness. Uncontrolled clinical studies claimed effectiveness in improving outcome in head injury, but randomized, controlled trials have not been able to substantiate any long-term benefit to corticosteroids, and many centers have abandoned their use.[136–138] The recent dramatic success of immediate high-dose methylprednisolone in improving outcome after spinal cord injury[139] has renewed enthusiasm for corticosteroids in CNS injury care.

NURSING THERAPIES FOR INTRACRANIAL HYPERTENSION. Nursing measures to reduce ICP and prevent further increases in ICP are predicated on judicious use of medical protocols to reduce baseline ICP in conjunction with individualized care planning that includes (1) managing caregiving activities and the environment to minimize and reduce noxious stimuli and (2) maximizing interpersonal strategies that reduce ICP in given individuals.

Minimizing Noxious Stimuli. ICP elevations routinely occur in all persons from coughing, straining, sneezing, or variations in head and body position. These elevations are secondary to increased intrathoracic pressure and increased cerebral blood volume. Under normal conditions, these physiological elevations are transient (last only seconds) and are well tolerated. However, in patients with decreased adaptive capacity (decreased intracranial compliance), such transient elevations of ICP may provoke prolonged increases that threaten cerebral perfusion. Clinical research has not clearly identified patients who are most at risk for these sustained elevations over baseline; however, patients with elevated baseline ICP, wide amplitude tracings, and elevation of the P_2 portion of the ICP waveform are suggested to be at highest risk.[48, 125, 126] In patients with decreased adaptive capacity or intracranial decompensation, activities associated with respiratory care procedures, positioning, and specifically noxious stimuli are most often responsible for abrupt increases in ICP. The effects of such activities should be anticipated and reduced whenever possible by nursing intervention.

Respiratory Care Procedures. Pulmonary infections rank second only to intracranial hypertension in leading causes of head injury death. Accordingly, optimal pulmonary toilet

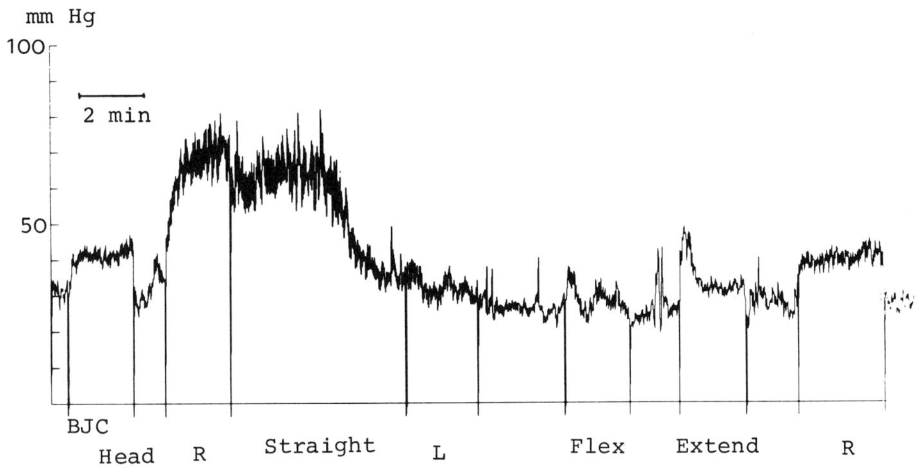

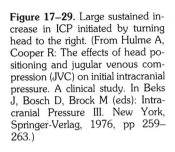

Figure 17–29. Large sustained increase in ICP initiated by turning head to the right. (From Hulme A, Cooper R: The effects of head positioning and jugular venous compression (JVC) on initial intracranial pressure. A clinical study. In Beks J, Bosch D, Brock M (eds): Intracranial Pressure III. New York, Springer-Verlag, 1976, pp 259–263.)

and suctioning of intubated patients are mandatory. Endotracheal suctioning is known to cause hypoxia and hypercarbia, both of which increase cerebral blood volume and ICP. In addition, stimulation of the carina by the suction catheter is a potent stimulus to coughing, which can increase ICP by increasing intrathoracic pressure.[140] In a within-subject controlled study comparing levels of preoxygenation and number of suction passes, Rudy and colleagues[144] found that suctioning caused significant, although usually transient, rises in ICP with maintenance of adequate CPP regardless of level of preoxygenation. Further, there was a cumulative increase in ICP with each 10-second suction pass.[141] Consequently, current suctioning recommendations to minimize the mechanical and biochemical stimuli associated with suctioning include limiting suctioning to no more than 10 seconds per pass, limiting the number of suction passes, hyperventilating and preoxygenating for 1 minute prior to and between each catheter insertion, administering prophylactic medication such as topical lidocaine prior to suctioning (in those patients whose cough is strong), and providing at least 10 to 15 minutes of recovery time between suctioning and other potentially noxious activities.

Fulminating infection and other hypoxic pulmonary disorders such as adult respiratory distress syndrome (ARDS) and aspiration often necessitate the use of positive end-expiratory pressure (PEEP). Whereas PEEP does improve oxygenation, it has the potential to impede cerebral venous return and thus increase ICP, especially in patients with reduced intracranial compliance. However, studies have shown that PEEP will not usually increase ICP if the patient is maintained in the head-up position (most commonly 30 degrees).[143, 144] Since chest physiotherapy can be administered with controlled increases in ICP, it is incorporated in the plan of care as tolerated, even with head-down positioning for postural drainage.[145, 146]

Positioning. Patients with increased ICP have been positioned with the head elevated 15 to 30 degrees for decades, based on the belief that this position facilitates venous return and reduces ICP. Recent studies have challenged this belief by demonstrating that some patients have lower ICP when recumbent and that head elevation reduces CPP more than it does ICP in others. The Trendelenburg position has been avoided for fear of increasing ICP but has been shown not to harm CPP, even when ICP does rise.[97, 146–148] Therefore, backrest elevation of the bed should be based on the individual patient's response rather than on standing protocols. The goal is to maintain optimal CPP; therefore, both ICP and MAP must be considered in order to calculate CPP. It is important to remember that elevating the backrest raises the cerebral circulation higher than the heart; therefore, arterial pressure at the head can be as much as 20 mm Hg lower than arterial pressure referenced to heart level, depending on the cardio- and cerebrovascular reactivity of the patient in response to position change.

Head flexion, extension, or rotation increases intracranial volume by causing mechanical compression of veins in the neck or base of the skull. This results in temporary increase in overall intracranial blood volume when the venous return is thus trapped. Asymmetry of the venous outflow system, with 65 per cent of the outflow from the right, probably accounts for the greater increase in ICP with right head rotation compared with left (Fig. 17–29). Lateral neck flexion while the patient is being passively turned may account for much of the increase in ICP often associated with turning the patient in bed.[149–151]

The deleterious effects of positioning can be prevented or eliminated by ensuring head and neck immobilization both at rest and during position changes. This can be accomplished with bilateral rolled towels, small sandbags, or other immobilizing devices. Some use soft cervical collars, but others find them to be a potent stimulus for neck rotation in patients who have decerebrate posturing.

Specific Noxious Stimuli. The most common sources of noxious stimulation associated with increases in ICP are the painful stimuli in the neurological examination, clinical procedures such as those requiring needle puncture or tube insertion, suctioning, shivering, and decerebrate posturing. Excesses in temperature change due to intrinsic causes, such as fever and hypothermia, or extrinsic sources, such as cooling blankets, are also noxious stimuli. Nursing responsibilities include evaluation and elimination or reduction of these sources whenever possible.

For the most part, patients who react negatively to nursing care procedures, positioning, or noxious stimuli are those with an established elevated baseline or a lower baseline but evidence of decreased compliance. In these situations, it may be useful to pretreat with protocol-based prophylactic medications (such as morphine, mannitol) prior to initiating groups of care procedures.

Maximizing Interpersonal Strategies. Several reports have suggested a beneficial effect on ICP of parental voice, tape recordings, or stroking in both children and adults.[153–155] However, larger systematic studies of these stimuli have been inconclusive, often due to limitations in design or measurement. These studies have supported the conclusion that there is a wide variation in patient responsiveness to interpersonal and tactile stimuli and that such responses could form the basis for adjunctive therapy in patients with less severe intracranial hypertension.[156–158]

Inadequate Gas Exchange Related to Airway Obstruction and Insufficient Ventilation

Respiratory complications are inherent to severe head injury. Head-injured patients with a decreased level of consciousness frequently have suppressed protective airway reflexes with consequent increased susceptibility to secretion retention and aspiration. A decreased level of consciousness, in concert with immobility and potentially abnormal respiratory patterns, can lead to small airway closure, atelectasis, and pulmonary infection. Prolonged immobility and venous stasis pose the threat of pulmonary emboli. Fat embolism in the head-injured population is frequently overlooked as a cause of pulmonary deterioration. The two contributing factors are the hypercoagulable state and associated long bone fractures.[158, 159] Detailed discussion of fat embolism and the complications associated with immobility is found in Chapter 21. Complications of neurogenic pulmonary edema, adult respiratory distress syndrome, or thoracic trauma also can lead to impaired pulmonary function. All these pulmonary conditions increase the likelihood of hypoxia and hypercarbia and account for a large share of the mortality and morbidity in head injury.[4, 160]

Airway patency is maintained by selection of the most appropriate airway device (i.e., endotracheal tube or tracheostomy), use of aspiration precautions, and vigorous pulmonary toilet. The spontaneously breathing patient with a natural airway is carefully monitored for signs of airway insufficiency. All needed equipment for emergency intubation is kept in close proximity. The patient who is beginning to localize stimuli but is not yet ready for removal of the artificial airway should have soft restraints or mittens in place to avoid self-extubation.

Aspiration Precautions. Aspiration precautions are always employed in caring for a head-injured patient. The cuff of the endotracheal or tracheostomy tube remains inflated with a minimal air leak to prevent tracheal erosion. An oropharyngeal gastric tube is placed for gastric decompression. Patients who receive enteral alimentation require assessment of gastric residual contents before each feeding, and feedings are withheld if residuals exceed a predetermined amount. Enteral feeding is discontinued at least 30 minutes prior to and during chest physiotherapy in the head-dependent position. A swallowing evaluation is performed prior to initiating feedings by mouth.

Respiratory Care. Meticulous pulmonary toilet is essential, including positioning, suctioning, and chest physiotherapy (CPT). However, all these interventions are instituted while remaining cognizant of their effect on cerebrovascular status. Elevations in ICP are associated with respiratory care procedures. Therefore, neurological status, including ICP and CPP, is closely monitored during these activities. Pulmonary care measures are discontinued if ICP exceeds 20 mm Hg or CPP falls below 50 mm Hg beyond the brief spikes during suctioning and are reinstituted when ICP has been controlled.

The patient should be turned frequently to reduce secretion accumulation and segmental or lobar consolidation. Chest physiotherapy, inclusive of percussion, vibration, and postural drainage, is performed as tolerated by the patient's cerebrovascular status.

Recent research has demonstrated that CPT in the head-down position can be safely performed on head injury patients without detrimental effects as long as ICP, MAP, and CPP are adequately monitored. Continuous monitoring throughout the treatment enables rapid recognition of clinically significant ICP elevations or a decline in CPP, and the treatment can be immediately aborted.[146, 160] The patient's ability to tolerate the treatment is greatly facilitated by premedication with a short-acting sedative and maintenance of neck alignment throughout the procedure. The nurse should confirm with the neurosurgeon that the Trendelenburg position is not contraindicated.

Suctioning is performed via the established airway as necessary. Nasopharyngeal suctioning should be avoided until the possibility of a basilar skull fracture has been ruled out. As previously discussed in the treatment of intracranial hypertension, endotracheal suctioning is preceded by sedation, hyperoxygenation, and hyperinsufflation. The suctioning interval is limited to less than 10 seconds.

Ventilator Management. Most patients with significant head injury require mechanical ventilation to provide arterial carbon dioxide reduction and to ensure optimal oxygenation. Hyperventilation, generally implemented during resuscitation to reduce cerebral blood volume and subsequently decrease ICP, is generally continued in critical care for patients with intracranial pathological processes. The nurse must carefully monitor the effects of hyperventilation on respiratory gases, pH, and neurological status. Sedatives and paralytic agents are used to maintain controlled hyperventilation.

Intermittent removal of mechanical ventilation is contraindicated in the head-injured patient with poor cerebral compliance and inadequate pulmonary function mandating support with high levels of PEEP. These patients are best managed with portable mechanical ventilators rather than manual "bagging" if transport for diagnostic studies or surgery is required. When evaluating the neurologically impaired patient for removal from the ventilator, several factors are considered: the need for therapeutic hyperventilation, the spontaneous ventilatory pattern, the presence of pulmonary complications, and the patient's ability to protect his own airway.[160]

Monitoring Gas Exchange. Monitoring includes serial arterial blood gas analysis as well as evaluation of venous blood gases, oxygen extraction, and other cardiopulmonary parameters when available. Continuous evaluation of oxygenation is facilitated by the use of intra-arterial electrodes, fiberoptic oximetry catheters for jugular bulb measurement, ear or digital pulse oximeters, or transcutaneous or transconjunctival oxygen sensors. End-tidal CO_2 can be continuously monitored with a capnometer that fits in line with the ventilator system.

Alterations in Fluid and Electrolytes

Diuretics and the fluid restrictions used in the treatment of increased ICP potentially create fluid and electrolyte imbalance. Head injury also can induce imbalance by causing increases or decreases in antidiuretic hormone (ADH) output by the hypothalamic–neurohypophyseal system.[161] Nursing therapeutics include evaluation of key clinical parameters and precise fluid administration.

Serial monitoring includes serum and urine electrolytes and osmolarity, urine specific gravity, intake and output records, body weight, hourly urine output, and hemodynamic variables such as central venous pressure and pulmonary artery pressures. With these trends in mind, the nurse carefully administers diuretics and fluids as prescribed. The goal is to titrate the patient's hydration status to reduce cerebral edema while maintaining adequate fluid and electrolyte levels. Severe dehydration leading to hypotension and diminished cardiac output must be avoided in order to maintain cerebral and systemic tissue perfusion. Extreme hyperosmolarity (greater than 320 mOsmol/l) can potentially cause renal failure.

Maintenance fluid in head injury management is preferably half-normal saline solution. Normal saline (causing sodium overload) and the more hypotonic dextrose and water solutions (implicated in edema formation and lactic acidosis in injured brain tissue) are contraindicated. The amount of fluid delivery is somewhat controversial. The practice of keeping patients dehydrated and in a hyperosmolar state to prevent intracranial hypertension is currently being challenged. Studies indicate that extreme dehydration (less than 1 l/day) may compromise cardiac output. Dehydration also may jeopardize cerebral and other organ perfusion in isolated head injury and in multiply-injured patients. In the presence of decreased intravascular volume, cerebral blood flow has been shown to be more dependent on cardiac output than on systemic arterial pressure.[162] In lieu of these findings, current recommendations are to provide adequate fluid to maintain normal blood pressure, CVP, and greater than 30 ml/hr urine output.[4] This is usually 2 l/day.

The most common alterations in fluid balance associated with head injury are water and sodium retention, diabetes insipidus (DI), and the syndrome of inappropriate antidiuretic hormone release (SIADH). Table 17–8 summarizes the key aspects of assessment and treatment of DI and SIADH.[4, 161–164]

Sodium Retention. Posttraumatic sodium retention is the result of the metabolic response to stress and injury and the consequent release of adrenocorticotropic hormone (ACTH) and aldosterone. Sodium retention averages 3 days in duration, but both duration and degree of response are directly proportional to the severity of injury. Despite the excess of retained total body sodium, serum sodium values falsely reflect a mild hyponatremia (130 to 135 mEq/l). This relative or dilutional hyponatremia is due to intracellular shift of sodium in conjunction with simultaneous water retention. Serum sodium level is closely monitored, anticipating mild hyponatremia and recognizing that the relative hyponatremia is not indicative of sodium loss. Salt replacement is not indicated unless sodium values fall below 125 to 130 mEq/l.

TABLE 17–8. CLINICAL MANIFESTATIONS AND TREATMENT OF NEUROGENIC DI AND SIADH

PARAMETER	NORMAL	DIABETES INSIPIDUS	SYNDROME OF INAPPROPRIATE ADH
Urine specific gravity	1.010–1.030	Less than 1.005	Elevated
Urine osmolality	50–1400 mOsmol/l Avg: 500–800 mOsmol/l	Less than 300 mOsmol/l (usually 50–100 mOsmol/l)	Increased (usually greater than 900 mOsmol/l)
Serum osmolality	275–300 mOsmol/l	Elevated if thirst is impaired	Decreased (usually less than 275 mOsmol/l)
Serum sodium	135–145 mEq/l	Greater than 145 mEq/l	Usually below 130 mEq/l
Clinical manifestations		Hypovolemia, dehydration Intensive thirst (if mechanism is not impaired) Poorly concentrated urine when fluids are restricted Aqueous Pitressin administration causes urine osmolality increase of 9% or more	Overhydration Increased urine sodium Fatigue, headache, restlessness, muscle cramps Weight gain without edema Lethargy, confusion, personality change, irritability, sluggish deep tendon reflexes Anorexia, nausea/vomiting, diarrhea, abdominal cramps Severe signs—coma, seizures, death
Treatment		Repletion of fluid volume • Hypotonic fluids are usually indicated • Use rate to replace urine output and insensible losses Administer exogenous ADH • Aqueous Pitressin—commonly used in the critical phase • Pitressin tannate in oil • L-Desamino,8-D-arginine vasopressin (desmopressin) • Nasal lysine vasopressin	Fluid restriction • 400 to 800 ml/day • Based on replacement no greater than urine output For severe symptoms • Give 3% saline (500 ml over 6–8 hr) • Diurese with Laxis Declomycin (600–1200 mg/day) to produce renal resistance to ADH

Sources: Rice[164]; Nelson[163]; Barrow and Tindall[161]; Marshall et al.[4, 130]

Water Retention. Posttraumatic water retention is a consistent response to injury and stress as the result of hypothalamic stimulation of ADH, also known as arginine vasopressin (AVP). ADH is released in response to injury in order to maintain volume and osmolarity, but it simultaneously causes water accumulation and hypotonicity. The result is positive water balance, which generally subsides in diuresis within 3 to 4 days of injury. Clinical signs include low urine output with high specific gravity and urine concentration. During the 72-hour period of posttraumatic water retention, the low urinary output will not accurately reflect the patient's true state of hydration or volume requirements. The use of urinary output as a single indicator of hydration can lead to fluid overload and water intoxication. Prolonged mechanical ventilation increases water retention susceptibility by stimulating ADH release through positive pressure sensed by left atrial and pulmonary artery volume receptors. Hypotonic fluid administration is avoided, and a mild fluid restriction is instituted (not greater than 2 l/day intake).

Neurogenic Diabetes Insipidus. Neurogenic DI is caused by the disruption or decreased secretion of antidiuretic hormone (ADH) or arginine vasopressin (AVP) from the posterior pituitary gland. This hormone is normally released in response to hyperosmolarity, hypovolemia, the stress response, or any stimulus that signals the body to conserve water. AVP acts on the kidney to stimulate water reabsorption and consequently increase urine specific gravity and decrease urine output. Head injuries that affect the hypothalamic–pituitary axis cause partial or complete cessation of AVP, resulting in diabetes insipidus.

Diabetes insipidus is diagnosed clinically when urinary output exceeds 200 ml/hr for two consecutive hours and urine specific gravity is less than 1.005. Treatment varies according to the patient's mental status and the degree of DI. Patients who are alert with mild DI can preferably regulate themselves by drinking in response to thirst. More severe degrees of DI and patients with altered consciousness unable to self-regulate are treated pharmacologically with aqueous vasopressin or vasopressin tannate in oil. For severe or chronic DI, intranasal or parenteral forms of DDAVP (desmopressin acetate) are recommended.

Syndrome of Inappropriate ADH. SIADH is a complication of CNS trauma that results in the abnormal secretion of ADH without appropriate inducement by osmoreceptor or volume stimulation. This inappropriate increase in ADH secretion causes continuous reabsorption of water from the renal tubules, resulting in hypotonicity (less than 280 mOsmol/kg of water) and hyponatremia (serum sodium less than 125 mEq/l). The ultimate consequence of SIADH is water intoxication with cerebral edema. Additional signs of SIADH include weight gain with absence of edema, neurological deterioration, increase in urinary sodium, and increase in urine osmolality. Treatment depends on severity and may include fluid restriction to approximately 800 ml/day, demeclocycline to produce renal resistance to ADH, induced diuresis with furosemide, and, when severe, judicious use of hypertonic fluids, usually 3% sodium chloride. Isotonic solutions are preferred initially, since saline administration causes sodium excretion with water retention and worsening of the hypotonicity.

Altered Temperature Regulation

Hyperthermia, frequently seen in patients with injury to the diencephalon, increases cerebral metabolic rate and subsequently aggravates increased ICP. The nurse should closely monitor the patient's body temperature and avoid elevations above 38°C (100.4°F). Once hyperthermia is recognized, measures to reduce body temperature, such as acetaminophen administration, cool baths, ice packs, and cooling blankets, should be implemented. Rapid cooling of the patient or prolonged use of hypothermia blankets may precipitate shivering, which also increases ICP. Shivering can be controlled by reducing body temperature slowly, discontinuing hypothermia use when the temperature is reduced to 100°F, and, in severe cases, administering sedatives such as Thorazine.

Sedation and Control of ICP

As in the resuscitation cycle, pain and agitation must be adequately controlled in the head-injured patient by the appropriate use of sedation and analgesia. Sound, accurate judgment is required in managing sedation and analgesia. The patient's neurological and cerebrovascular status should be closely monitored to recognize the need for sedation when acute intracranial hypertension arises (e.g., during abnormal posturing). Recognition of the need to withhold sedation when the patient must be evaluated clinically is equally important. The nurse continually evaluates the effectiveness of the sedatives and analgesics ordered and works interdependently with the physician to find the drug and dosages that best meet the patient's needs.

The use of barbiturate therapy to reduce cerebral metabolism and ICP presents a major challenge to the nurse. Most of the patient's body systems are affected by the drug. Due to the adverse depressant effects on cardiovascular status, hemodynamic monitoring via a Swan-Ganz catheter is imperative. Continual assessment of arterial blood pressure and hemodynamic parameters permits early recognition of hypovolemia and hypotension that can precipitate CPP reductions. Vasopressors, namely dopamine and dobutamine, are frequently necessary to support the hemodynamic state of the patient receiving barbiturates.

The gastrointestinal depression caused by barbiturates may negate the use of enteral alimentation; thus parenteral nutrition is necessary. Barbiturate-induced respiratory depression makes the patient ventilator-dependent. Meticulous pulmonary care must be provided, recognizing that the patient's spontaneous protective airway reflexes are completely suppressed. Potential immunosuppression caused by barbiturate administration mandates strict aseptic technique and careful assessment for the presence of infection. When monitoring body temperature for signs of a septic process, the nurse should be aware that barbiturate coma commonly induces hypothermia. Warming blankets may be necessary to keep the patient's body temperature above 33°C (91.4°F).

Potential for Injury Related to Seizure Activity

Prevention and treatment of seizures are imperative in the head-injured patient to avoid increases in cerebral metabolic rate and ICP. Anticonvulsants are administered both as prophylaxis and as treatment of seizure activity, although there is growing evidence that prophylactic Dilantin reduces the incidence of seizures only in the first week.[165] Precautions are instituted in all head-injured patients, particularly those with previous history of seizure. An airway and appropriate anticonvulsants are located at the bedside. Side rails should be kept upright and padded as needed to protect the patient from injury.

In the event of a seizure, the nurse should observe and document the onset, characteristics, and duration of the abnormal activity. Maintenance of a patent airway is always the first treatment priority. Any objects in the patient's physical proximity are removed to prevent injury, but no attempt is made to hold him still or in any one position. Diazepam, 5 to 10 mg IV, is commonly used to stop a seizure if the patient is already on phenytoin. Patients not already receiving phenytoin who have a seizure should be given a 15- to 18-mg/kg loading dose intravenously at a rate no greater than 50 mg/min.[4]

Nutrition less than Body Requirements: Hypermetabolic State

Trauma increases the basal metabolism up to twice the normal rate. Thus the nutritional needs of these patients are markedly increased even though they have essentially no activity other than resting metabolic needs. Immune suppression and delayed tissue healing are concomitants of the catabolic state. Early parenteral and enteral feedings have become standard in trauma units because of this catabolic response to injury. While there is no question that head-injured patients experience the hypermetabolism of general injury, opinion is mixed regarding the wisdom of early hyperalimentation in these patients.[4, 168, 169]

Hyperglycemia that precedes the ischemic insult worsens ischemic brain damage in animal models, probably by increasing lactic acidosis. However, there is inconclusive evidence that hyperglycemia subsequent to injury affects the extent of ischemic brain injury.[106, 166, 167] In addition, some neurosurgeons feel that the volume and tonicity of enteral and parenteral feedings make ICP difficult to control if initiated early. Keeping these concerns about hyperglycemia and increased fluid volume in mind, many centers begin small amounts of hyperalimentation enterally or parenterally within the first 24 hours and replacement feedings within the first week following severe head injury.[4, 168, 169]

Nutritional assessment and management are multidisciplinary, involving nutritionist, physician, and nurse. The nutritionist's assessment involves serial monitoring of weight; fluid intake and output; serum levels of sodium, albumin, glucose, and lymphocytes; and urine creatinine and urea as markers of protein loss. The nutritional prescription is a collaborative effort of nutritionist and neurosurgeon, taking into account management of ICP. Nursing responsibilities include administering the feedings parenterally or enterally, monitoring for infection if alimentation is parenteral, and preventing aspiration if an enteral feeding tube is used. In early head injury enteral feedings, a duodenal tube is most commonly used, and its placement must be verified by x-ray. The nurse is critical in monitoring the patients residual abdominal distention and any evidence of gastrointestinal discomfort as the quantity and rate are increased. Diarrhea can be treated with Metamucil and withheld for a time if intolerance is evident.

Impaired Physical Mobility

When sedatives and pharmacological paralytic agents are required, the patient with severe brain injury is at risk for complications associated with immobility. Meticulous skin care and frequent turning aid in prevention of skin breakdown. Antiembolic hose and pneumatic compression devices decrease venous stasis and the incidence of embolus formation.[170] Daily measurements of calf and thigh girths aid in recognition of a lower extremity thromboembolism. Frequent passive range of motion is needed and may be provided by nursing or by physical or occupational therapy.

Serial lower extremity casting and upper extremity splints may be initiated in the critical care setting to treat spasticity.[171] Neck and head alignment should be maintained at all times with the use of a cervical collar or cloth rolls. Proper alignment and elevation of the head of the bed 30 to 45 degrees may facilitate cerebrovenous and CSF outflow in selected individuals but may increase the shearing forces on the sacrum. Therefore, the patient must be turned regularly to relieve this pressure. Sharp hip flexion is avoided if the patient has increased ICP.[172]

Potential for Gastrointestinal Bleeding

Gastrointestinal bleeding has long been associated with intracranial disease, although the pathogenesis of the ulcerative process as it relates to intracranial hypertension is currently unclear. Prevention is best accomplished by careful monitoring of gastric pH and administration of enteral or parenteral antacids to maintain pH above 4.5. The character of gastric drainage and stool, particularly the overt or chemical presence of blood, provides early clues to the development of this complication.[4, 173]

Potential for Intracranial Infection

Intracranial infections may take the form of meningitis or brain abscess. Patients with open head injuries are at greatest risk, but contamination of invasive intracranial monitoring devices predisposes any patient to CNS infection. Therefore, strict aseptic technique is imperative when manipulating monitoring devices in any way. In addition to the nursing responsibilities in ICP monitoring described earlier, the patient must be repeatedly evaluated for signs of infection. It is important to assess trends in body temperature and total and differential white cell count and to note the length of time an ICP monitoring device remains in place.

ICP elevations, focal neurological deficits, and development of brain shift are symptomatic of brain abscess. Meningitis is a more diffuse intracranial process characterized by signs of systemic infection, nuchal rigidity, positive Brudzinski's and Kernig's signs, deteriorating neurological status, and evidence of an infective organism in the CSF.[4, 174] Antibiotics sensitive to the cultured organism, temperature control, seizure precautions, and management of ICP elevation are all indicated. If drainage of an abscess is required, the patient and family are prepared for the upcoming surgery.

Alteration in Cognitive Function Related to Brain Injury

Cognitive retraining begins during critical care once the patient is stabilized and ICP has been controlled.[171] The goal at low levels of function is to solicit behavioral responses that move the patient toward early environmental awareness and development of prefunctional skills.[171, 175] One approach to cognitive retraining is the use of the Rancho Los Amigos Cognitive Scale to evaluate the patient's level of function and plan therapies appropriate to that level. The patient in the critical care cycle of recovery is best typified by the first three levels of the Rancho Los Amigos Cognitive Scale. This means that the patient usually has no response to stimuli, a nonpurposeful and inconsistent generalized response, or an inconsistent localized, purposeful response (see Appendix 17–1).

Nursing, in collaboration with speech, physical, and occupational therapy, begins cognitive retraining by providing meaningful stimuli to all five senses. Sensory stimulation and all components of brain rehabilitation are based on the theory that repetition and consistency of stimuli strengthen recessive or alternate pathways through which function may be regained. Sensory stimulation therapy is designed to arouse only one sense at a time, and it is administered in a controlled fashion in order to minimize confusion.[176] Little well-controlled research exists regarding the effect of sensory stimulation on recovery. However, one well-controlled study has shown a more rapid recovery of awareness in patients with a post-ICU sensory stimulation program.[177]

Most stimulation occurs naturally during routine nursing interventions. For example, tactile stimulation can be provided when performing hygiene measures. Soft, smooth speech patterns during reorientation or explanation of needed procedures, as well as intermittent music, provides auditory stimuli. Taste can be stimulated during mouth care with the use of flavored mouth swabs or by touching the tongue with a popsicle. Placing substances with pleasant odors near the patient provides an olfactory stimulus. The family is asked to bring photographs and familiar items that are shown to the patient as visual input.

The nurse should identify particular stimuli that best elicit a patient response. These stimuli are presented to the patient at intervals as part of the plan of care. The period of stimulation should be brief, followed by a rest period. The stimuli are varied and presented one at a time to prevent sensory overload.[175]

The family is included in the early cognitive retraining program. Family members and significant others are instructed on how to interact with the patient and are encouraged to do so. Their ability to provide familiarity for the patient is invaluable. If the family members are unable to visit, they are encouraged to make audiotapes and to supply personal items that have pleasant associations for the patient.

Nursing Therapeutics in Intermediate Care/Rehabilitation

Active rehabilitation begins as soon as the patient is stabilized. Whether a head-injured patient is admitted to a medical–surgical floor or to the intensive care unit, a rehabilitation consultation should be placed on admission for all patients with neurological deficits, especially those in coma and those with abnormal motor movements. Physical and occupational therapy will ensure splinting to abnormal flexor or extensor limbs within 24 hours of injury and help to minimize secondary contractures and deformity. Motor problems must be addressed promptly to prevent complications that can retard the recovery process, prolong the rehabilitation course, and potentially result in functional loss of the involved limb or limbs. In addition to splinting and other therapeutic interventions, occupational therapy plays a major role in cognitive therapy and provides sensory stimulation to patients with depressed levels of consciousness. Speech therapy focuses on communicative disorders, swallowing deficits, and associated memory deficits.

Neurological disability after traumatic brain injury varies according to the degree of brain damage incurred. Disability ranges from a mild deficit to irreversible coma. The consequences of head injury are more than the sum of the deficits, since a myriad of dynamic psychosocial phenomena needs to be considered to complete the picture. The individual must be viewed within the context of his or her life, with age-specific goals and tasks and unique personality traits, since all these will affect the rehabilitation process.

Ineffective Airway Clearance

Maintaining a patent airway remains a priority during the intermediate/rehabilitation cycle. The patient's airway can be partially or completely obstructed by improper positioning and/or by the collection of secretions in the respiratory tree. The patient should be positioned so that the upper airway is completely open. A sidelying or upright position is advisable. The comatose patient will require frequent repositioning, since there is a tendency to slump forward, which results in neck flexion. A cervical collar may need to be applied to facilitate maintenance of effective head position.

Postural drainage and suctioning should continue to be incorporated into the plan of care to assist in clearing secretions from the lungs and airways, thereby preventing atelectasis and the possibility of pneumonia in immobile patients.

Impaired Physical Mobility

The comatose patient relies on the nurse for all activities of daily living. With severe self-care deficits, the patient is dependent on the nurse for all hygiene, grooming, and mobilization. The patient requires meticulous attention to skin care and range-of-motion exercises to prevent breakdown and contractures. Getting the patient out of bed, properly supported in a chair at least twice a day, is essential to prevent complications of immobility. Not only is it important to monitor the patient's tolerance for sitting in a chair, but the patient must be adequately restrained for his safety if alterations in level of consciousness are present, and pressure areas must be adequately padded to prevent skin breakdown.

Therapies for Motor Deficits. The most common motor problems in head injury are loss of power (extremity weakness) and increased tone (hypertonicity). Hypertonicity varies in degree from a mild increase in motor tone, to rigid states of decortication and decerebration, to spasticity. In comatose patients, extremity weakness is treated with passive range of motion (PROM). Strengthening exercises are limited until the patient is actively involved in therapy. Flexor or extensor rigidity requires frequent PROM and splinting of the affected extremity.

Spasticity is the most severe form of hypertonicity. It

frequently, but not always, appears in concert with decorticate or decerebrate rigidity, hyperreflexia, and clonus. It is characterized by "clasp-knife" response to passive stretch. The complications of prolonged spasticity are secondary contractures and heterotopic ossification.[61] Heterotopic ossification (HO) is the deposition of bone about the major joints with the potential of causing complete ankylosis of the affected joints and functional loss of the limb.[177] Spasticity lessens at times and worsens with inciting stimuli such as a bed bath, rectal temperature probe, infection, the presence of HO, decubitus ulcers, and fecal impaction.

Spasticity implies destruction of one or more of the descending motor tract pathways. Patients who develop this complication are those who have sustained severe head injury, generally a GCS of 6 or less. If spasticity is unrelenting and involves the entire limb, functional use of the extremity is limited and ambulation is often impossible.

The presence of early spasticity does not always imply persistent spasticity. In patients who make substantial improvement, early rigidity and spasticity become diminished as their recovery progresses. Prolonged and functionally incapacitating spasticity is treated to prevent secondary contractures and deformities, to improve limb position, and to facilitate physical therapy. Treatment consists of (1) physical modalities such as cold application, stretching techniques including serial casting and splints, and electrical stimulation, (2) antispasticity drugs (diazepam, baclofen, dantrolene), (3) orthopedic procedures such as myotomy/tenotomy or muscle/tendon release, (4) neurosurgical procedures such as peripheral neurotomy or peripheral nerve stimulator implantation, and (5) chemical neurolysis or nerve block.[178]

Sensory-Cognitive Alterations

The patient in the intermediate care or rehabilitative cycle of recovery can be frequently described by the last two levels of the Rancho Los Amigos Cognitive Scale.[179] The level IV patient is confused and agitated, whereas the level V patient is confused and inappropriate. Stimulation and informational input must be drastically reduced during this period, since the ability to process information is severely impaired and the sensory overload point is rapidly reached. Short-term memory is severely impaired, which means that the patient is unable to ground himself with information about people, places, and events in the environment. Bizarre behavior, such as screaming outbursts, aggression, disinhibition, delusions, hallucinations, or incoherent verbalizations, may be evident. The patient has a limited attention span. Confabulation and perseveration also may be present.

Sensory stimulation programs are continued from the critical care cycle into the intermediate care and rehabilitative phases for all patients with a depressed level of consciousness. Patients with alterations in perception and cognition are candidates for cognitive therapy. Nursing interventions for the brain-injured patient with cognitive dysfunction should be based on the premise that cognitive deficits impair information processing. In order to optimize the patient's cognitive processing, the nurse must provide a structured environment with controlled stimulation, order, repetition, and consistency.

A *structured environment* can be defined as one that is predictable, with an ordered sequence of activities and events that minimally change. In the cognitively disabled patient, a break in routine can precipitate rebellious or negative behavior. This can often be avoided by adequately preparing the patient for change as far in advance as possible and providing frequent reinforcement. These patients also have difficulty in deciphering stimuli, and when bombarded, their behavior becomes erratic and confused. Stimuli should not be excessive. Music and television may be productive for short periods of time but may become overbearing if misused. Visitors should be limited to one or two persons, and conversation should include only one person at a time. Giving a patient two-step commands when he is only capable of handling one can result in confusion and inability to effectively carry out either step.

Stimuli should be meaningful, and repetition should be encouraged. When patients need to relearn previous skills, it is most productive to use meaningful objects. For example, when assessing a patient's ability to grasp and release, it is beneficial to use practical objects such as a spoon or cup. Simple mnemonics, visual imagery, association, and organizational strategies are helpful to cue patients with memory deficits. Patient teaching should be simple and concrete with an ordered and positive reinforcement. Since the purpose of rehabilitation is to make patients as independent as possible, nurses must be prepared to expend considerable time and patience in assisting a disabled patient to attain this goal.[180, 181]

Psychomotor activities, such as ambulation, are encouraged to help decrease agitation. A quiet environment, a room with padding to prevent injury, and one-to-one supervision may be necessary during periods of extreme agitation. Antipsychotic drugs such as benzodiazepines (e.g., Ativan) and haloperidol (Haldol) may sometimes be helpful in calming the patient.[182]

Participation on the part of the patient can be limited during this phase. A calm, quiet atmosphere supports information processing. Specific, brief directions and explanations should precede any activity. Choices must be restricted so as not to increase confusion in the patient. A strict schedule of therapies and activities should be established, accompanied by intermittent rest periods. Interdisciplinary goals are established on a priority basis to ensure that the patient is not overwhelmed.[171]

Disruptive and, at times, aggressive behavior are common during this time. The nurse needs to be cognizant of the potential for self-injury and injury to others. This type of behavior can be handled by distracting tactics, capitalizing on the patient's short attention span and impaired processing skills.

By the time the patient is at a Rancho cognitive level VI (confused and appropriate), he is ready for transfer to a rehabilitation facility. Although confusion is still present, the person is able to accomplish tasks with supervision. Information processing has improved by this time, although memory deficits persist. Behavior modification programs can be utilized to control disinhibited, disruptive behavior. Cognitive remediation at this point in the patient's recovery addresses five core deficit areas: (1) arousal and attention, (2) skill structures, (3) memory, (4) language and thought processes, and (5) emotion. Cognitive remediation is based on assessment of deficits and strengths, remedial cueing interventions, and the patient's ability to respond to the interventions.

As the patient reaches the appropriate levels, self-care responsibilities are increased and ability to complete activities is assessed. Cue cards can be utilized to jog the patient's memory regarding daily activities and times.

Alterations in Bowel and Bladder Function

The patient in a vegetative state has persistent problems with bowel and bladder incontinence. Female patients with urinary incontinence may require an indwelling catheter or intermittent catheterization, whereas male patients can be managed with an external condom device for collection of urine. Prevention of urinary tract infection is critical for these patients.

Constipation is common in the immobilized patient. Diarrhea is commonly associated with intolerance of tube feedings or drugs that alter the normal flora of the bowel. A goal of nursing care is to prevent constipation and incontinence. Bowel retraining can be done even when the patient is comatose. It is usually initiated during the intermediate care cycle, the goal being to establish an effective bowel evacuation pattern for the patient.

Long-Term Problems

The changes in intellect and personality that accompany traumatic brain injury have a lifelong impact on the patient and family. Support groups for both families and patients can be helpful in adaptation to these sequelae. For example, the goal of the National Head Injury Foundation is to act as advocate for the needs of persons with head injury. Most states have a chapter of the foundation, and health care professionals are encouraged to participate in their programs. Discharge from the rehabilitation facility may be only the start of a lifelong program for the head injury survivor.[183]

The Family and Resources

Families are often in a state of disbelief when they realize that their relative has sustained brain damage. This may be due to emotional shock, lack of comprehension of what is said during the acute phase, denial, or lack of sufficient information, which has been cited as the greatest source of stress for relatives.[184] Miscueing severe injuries by reference to "head injury" rather than "brain injury" also can foster disbelief and confusion on the part of the family.

The head trauma patient may never be the same again as a result of extensive and irreversible neuronal damage. The resulting changes are difficult for families to understand. Some families never quite come to grips with the realization of permanent disability.

Families of severely injured patients seem to pass through stages: anxiety, denial and isolation, anger, remorse, guilt, and hope.[185] When the head-injured patient is severely disabled or vegetative, families often continue in the denial phase for many years. Denial is often necessary to hold the family together but becomes a negative factor when reality and the implications of extensive brain damage are obscured. For some, acceptance comes reluctantly when years of stasis have passed and all available resources have been tapped to no avail. For others, acceptance never comes, and they continue to hope that some day a "cure" will be made available to restore the function and personality of their child or spouse.[186] Families of patients remaining in a vegetative state often cope by partially disengaging themselves from the unresponsive patient so that they can continue with the practicalities of everyday life.[187] It is extremely important that nurses establish a daily communication system with the family, provide direct support throughout each phase of adjustment, and assist in identifying other resources that will enable the family to cope more effectively with the catastrophic event.

Families should be made aware of all head injury support services within the institution, the community, and the nation. Sources of referral within the acute care setting may include social services, nursing psychiatric specialties, pastoral care, neuropsychological consultations, and an in-house head injury support group, if available. Community and national support service referrals include a local head injury support group, the National Head Injury foundation (NHIF), and the state chapter of NHIF.

The National Head Injury Foundation, established in 1980, is the only advocacy organization concerned exclusively with the unique problems faced by head-injured persons and their families. The NHIF and its state associations act as a central clearing house for all information and resources pertinent to head injury. Some of the activities of the NHIF include lobbying at the state and federal levels to ensure the rights of head-injured individuals, distribution of educational materials for professionals and families, active support of head injury prevention and research programs, sponsoring local and national head injury conferences, and providing assistance in the development of state and local support groups.

Eligibility for benefits and possible sources of financial assistance can be investigated at the state or federal level. These may include Social Security, Medicare, veterans benefits, vocational rehabilitation, Supplemental Security Income (SSI), Medicaid, and social services block grants. In addition to these programs, local organizations such as Goodwill Industries, YMCA/YWCA, National Easter Seal Society, Catholic Social Services, and various denominational organizations also may prove helpful to families in need.

OUTCOME FROM SEVERE HEAD INJURY

Glasgow Outcome Scale

The Glasgow Outcome Scale (GOS) is the internationally accepted method of grading outcome from head injury (see Table 17–9).[187] Four categories of survival are recognized. Good recovery implies the ability to participate in normal social activities and return to work. Mild physical or psycho-

TABLE 17–9. GLASGOW OUTCOME SCALE

Good recovery (GR)
Moderate disability (MD)
Severe disability (SD)
Vegetative state (VS)
Death (D)

From Jennett B, Bond MR: Assessment of outcome after severe brain damage. Lancet 1:480, 1975.

logical impairment may be present. Moderate disability implies the patient is independent but disabled by memory or personality deficits, hemiparesis, dysphasia, or major cranial nerve deficits. Those who are severely disabled are conscious but dependent on others for at least some of their needs on a daily basis. These patients have more marked personality or motor deficits. Patients in a vegetative state show no evidence of meaningful activity because the cerebral cortex is irrefutably damaged.

Death from head injury occurs early or late. Early deaths are biphasic: (1) those occurring within minutes of injury due to massive structural brain damage incompatible with survival and (2) those occurring within hours or days due to uncontrolled intracranial hypertension. Some patients of the first group are maintained for hours or days by life-support systems, and their eventual mortality is reported as part of the "hours to days" category. The primary causes of late death are pulmonary complications and sepsis. The majority of patients who succumb from intracranial pathological processes die a cerebral or brain death. The primary focus of caring for the brain dead patient is to support the family and assist them in understanding the concept and finality of brain death. The nurse should recognize that the patient may be a candidate for organ donation and contact the appropriate organ procurement personnel. The nursing management of potential or actual donor candidates is discussed in Chapter 31.

Outcome is generally assessed at 6 months after injury, since maximum recovery occurs in most patients during this period. This is not to say that recovery does not continue for years after the injury. It appears that physical deficits improve more quickly than cognitive ones, with the latter showing slow improvement over the years.

Predictors of Outcome

Although some patients with a poor prognosis do well and others who should conceivably do well make poor recoveries, the outcome of the majority of severe head injuries can be fairly well predicted from injury and clinical data. The most reliable predictors of outcome after severe head injury are depth of coma (based on postresuscitation GCS score), pupil reaction, eye movements, motor response, age, and type of head injury lesion.

Depth or degree of coma indicates the severity of brain damage; in general, the worse the GCS, the poorer is the prognosis. For example, a GCS of 3 to 5 is associated with 60 to 80 per cent mortality, whereas a higher GCS of 6 to 8 decreases mortality to 18 to 25 per cent.[188, 189] Since nonreactive pupils indicate compression at the midbrain level, it is not surprising that 95 per cent of patients who manifest this sign have poor outcomes. When eye movements are impaired (determined by oculocephalic or oculovestibular testing), 64 per cent of patients remain vegetative or die; when they are absent, 95 per cent of patients do poorly. In the motor category, mortality is 100 per cent with flaccidity, approximately 85 per cent with bilateral decerebration, and almost 60 per cent with classic decortication.[190] About half the patients with prolonged unconsciousness (greater than 60 days) do subsequently awaken. Early motor reactivity, absence of hydrocephalus, and adequate ventilatory status were the best predictors of recovery from prolonged unawareness.[191]

Other parameters such as type of lesion, hypoxia, hypotension, associated injuries, age greater than 60 years, duration of posttraumatic amnesia, ICP greater than 20 mm Hg, abnormal evoked potentials, and elevated enzymes [lactic dehydrogenase (LDH), aspartate aminotransferase (AST), and creatine phosphokinase (CPK)] also have been found to correlate with outcome.[192–194] Of additional interest and worth further investigation are the social indices that relate to outcome. It is said that after a head injury, "it is not only the kind of injury that matters, but the kind of head."[195] It is believed that premorbid IQ, education, and occupation also influence outcome potential.

Sequelae of Head Injury

Neurological disability after head injury varies according to the degree of brain damage incurred. Deficits may be subtle and subjective when the injury is of a mild nature or totally disabling when injury is severe. Even though the disability is mild, it may be extremely troublesome and the source of great anxiety to the individual. When deficits are severe and cognitively disabling, the family often bears the burden of the disability.

Disability results from motor, sensory, cognitive, and personality (behavioral) deficits. The most common motor deficits following head injury are hemiparesis, plegia, spasticity, secondary contractures, aphasia, dysphasia, dysarthria, and cranial nerve dysfunction. Sensory deficits are less common and primarily involve visual disturbances such as field cuts (hemianopia), diplopia, and blindness. Blindness is a less frequent occurrence and generally results from occipital lobe infarction. Most motor and mild sensory deficits do improve over time. Some patients have complete functional recovery, and the majority of those with permanent deficits generally learn to compensate or adapt to their loss. Cognitive and personality deficits, however, tend to persist even after focal deficits have resolved; they are the major cause of chronic disability following head injury, and they are the chief cause of concern to families of head-injured persons.

The primary cognitive deficits associated with severe head injury include problems in information processing; inability to plan, initiate, or complete tasks; diminished attention span; and marked impairment in short-term memory. Short-term memory impairment is the most persistent of all deficits. In severe disability, it generally does not return to any functional extent. This presents a major problem in recovery because new information cannot be retained sufficiently for relearning to take place. Behaviorally, patients may be disinhibited, aggressive, apathetic, depressed, impatient, easily fatigued, and generally socially inappropriate. The list is limitless, with the type and degree of deficits depending primarily on the site and severity of the injury.[180] There is growing evidence that formalized rehabilitation programs produce improvement in vocational and social function beyond that expected from spontaneous recovery alone.[183, 196, 197]

COMMUNITY REINTEGRATION

Disposition of patients following head injury depends on the extent of neurological disability. The majority of mildly head-injured patients without neurological deficiency are discharged home with follow-up instructions. Depending on the degree of disability, patients with obvious deficits are either discharged with plans for outpatient rehabilitation or discharged directly to an inpatient rehabilitation facility. Patients in a vegetative state or too severely disabled to actively participate in a structured rehabilitation program are discharged to extended-care facilities or to facilities that have special coma management programs.

Historically, the presence of motor deficits has been the criterion for rehabilitation center admission. Some head-injured patients are without motor deficit but do have cognitive disability; these patients were not considered for inpatient therapy. Only recently, with an increase in specialized head injury rehabilitation programs, have the concerns of this population been addressed in the form of cognitive remediation programs. Today there are specialized head injury programs to meet every need of the head-injured patient. In addition to acute rehabilitation and coma management, other programs include behavioral, transitional living, independent living, community reentry, prevocational, vocational, and sheltered work training.

REFERENCES

1. Frankowski FR, Annegers JF, Whitman S: Epidemiology and descriptive studies: I. The descriptive epidemiology of head trauma in the United States. In Becker DP, Povlishock JT (eds): Central Nervous System Trauma: Status Report 1985 (Pub. No. 1988-520-149/00028). Washington, DC, US Government Printing Office, 1988, pp 33–48.
2. Jagger J, Levine J, Jane J, Rimel R: Epidemiologic features of head injury in a predominately rural population. J Trauma 24:40–44, 1984.
3. Krause JF, Black MA, Hessol N, et al: The incidence of acute brain injury and serious impairment in a defined population. Am J Epidemiol 119:186–201, 1984.
4. Marshall SB, Marshall LF, Vos HR, Chesnut RM: Neuroscience Critical Care: Pathophysiology. Philadelphia, WB Saunders Co, 1990.
5. Sosin DM, Sacks JJ, Smith SM: Head injury-associated deaths in the United States from 1979 to 1986. JAMA 262:2251–2255, 1989.
6. Krause JF: Epidemiology of head injury. In Cooper P (ed): Head Injury, 2nd ed. Baltimore, Williams & Wilkins, 1987.
7. Kalsbeek WD, McLaurin RL, Harris BS, et al: The national head and spinal cord injury survey: Major findings. J Neurosurg 53(suppl):19–31, 1981.
8. State of Washington: Traumatic Brain Injury in the Washington State: Report of the Health Promotion and Chronic Disease Prevention Branch. Olympia, WA, Department of Health, 1990.
9. U.S. Department of Transportation. National Highway Traffic Safety Administration: Fatal Accident Reporting System, 1989. Washington, DC, US Department of Transportation, 1990.
10. Luna GK, Maier RV, Sowder L, et al: The influence of ethanol intoxication on outcome of injured motorcyclists. J Trauma 24:695–700, 1986.
11. Brismar B, Engstrom A, Ryberg U: Head injury and intoxication: A diagnostic and therapeutic dilemma. Acta Chir Scand 149:11–14, 1983.
12. Reyna T, Hollis H., Hulsebus R: Alcohol-related trauma. Ann Surg 201:194–197, 1984.
13. Haddon W: Conference on the prevention of motor vehicle crash injury. Proc Isr J Med Sci 16:45–68, 1980.
14. Sosin DM, Sacks JJ, Holmgreen P: Head injury-associated deaths from motorcycle crashes: Relationship to helmet-use laws. JAMA 264:2395–2399, 1990.
15. Thompson RS, Rivara FP, Thomson DC: Prevention of head injury by bicycle helmets: A field study of efficacy. N Engl J Med 320:1361–1367, 1989.
16. Spielman G: Metabolic complications associated with severe diffuse brain injury. J Neurosurg Nurs 17:83–88, 1985.
17. Adams JH, Doyle D, Ford I, Gennarelli, TA, et al: Diffuse axonal injury: Definition, diagnosis and grading. Histopathology 15:49–59, 1989.
18. Astrup J: Energy-requiring cell functions in the ischemic brain: Their critical supply and possible inhibition in protective therapy. J Neurosurg 56:482–497, 1982.
19. Hall ED: Free radicals and CNS injury. Crit Care Clin 5:793–805, 1990.
20. Murdoch J, Hall R: Brain protection: Physiological and pharmacological considerations: I. The physiology of brain injury. Can J Anaesth 37:663–671, 1990.
21. Willmore LJ, Triggs WJ: Iron-induced lipid peroxidation and brain injury responses. Int J Dev Neurosci 9:175–180, 1991.
22. Davis J: Neuronal rearrangements after brain injury: A proposed classification. In Becker D, Povlishock J (eds): Central Nervous System Trauma: Status Report 1985 (Pub. No. 1988-520-149/00028). Washington, DC, US Government Printing Office, 1988.
23. Freed WJ, deMedinaceli L, Wyatt RJ: Promoting functional plasticity in the damaged nervous system. Science 227:1544–1552, 1985.
24. Cadelli DS, Bandtlow CE, Schwab ME: Oligodendrocyte and myelin-associated inhibitors of neurite outgrowth: Their involvement in lack of CNS regeneration. Exp Neurol 115;189–192, 1992.
25. Obrist W. Langfitt TW, Jaggi J, et al: Cerebral blood flow and metabolism in comatose patients with acute head injury. J Neurosurg 61:241–253, 1984.
26. Lou HC, Edvinsson L, MacKenzie ET: The concept of coupling blood flow to brain function: Revision required? Ann Neurol 22:289–297, 1987.
27. Walleck CA: Controversies in the management of the head-injured patient. Crit Care Clin North Am 1(1):67–74, 1989.
28. Eisenberg HM, Gary HE, Aldrich EF, et al: Initial CT findings in 753 patients with severe head injury. J Neurosurg 73:688–698, 1990.
29. Brown JK: The pathological effects of raised intracranial pressure. In Minns RA (ed): Problems of Intracranial Pressure in Childhood. New York, Cambridge University Press, 1991, pp 38–76.
30. Brown JK: Mechanisms of production of raised intracranial pressure. In Minns RA (ed): Problems of Intracranial Pressure in Childhood. New York, Cambridge University Press, 1991, pp 13–37.
31. Miller JD: Basic intracranial dynamics. In Minns RA (ed): Problems of Intracranial Pressure in Childhood. New York, Cambridge University Press, 1991, pp 1–12.
32. Kosteljanetz M: Acute head injury: Pressure-volume relations and cerebrospinal fluid dynamics. Neurosurgery 18:17–24, 1986.
33. Ropper AH: Lateral displacement of the brain and level of consciousness in patients with acute hemispheral mass. N Engl J Med 314:953–958, 1986.
34. Ross DA, Olsen WL, Ross AM, et al: Brain shift, level of consciousness and restoration of consciousness in patients with acute intracranial hematoma. J Neurosurg 71:498–502, 1989.
35. Gennarelli TA, Thibault L: Biomechanics of head injury. In Wilkins R, Rengachary S (eds): Neurosurgery. New York, McGraw-Hill, 1985, pp 1531–1536.
36. Jennett B, Teasdale G: Management of Head Injuries. Philadelphia, FA Davis, 1982.
37. Adams JH, Doyle D, Graham DI, et al: The contusion index: A reappraisal in human and experimental non-missile head injury. Neuropathol Appl Neurobiol 11:299–306, 1985.
38. Cooper, PR: Post traumatic intracranial mass lesions in head injury. In Cooper PR (ed): Head Injury. Baltimore, Williams & Wilkins, 1987.

39. Bricolo AP, Pasut LM: Extradural hematoma: Toward zero mortality. A prospective stud. Neurosurgery 14:8–12, 1984.
40. Reale F, Deflin R, Mencattini G: Epidural hematomas. J Neurosurg Sci 28:9–16, 1984.
41. Plum F, Posner, J: The Diagnosis of Stupor and Coma, 2nd ed. Philadelphia, FA Davis, 1982, pp 1–70.
42. Spielman G: Coma: A clinical review. Heart Lung 10:700–707, 1981.
43. Marshall L, Barba D, Toole B, Bowers S: The oval pupil: Clinical significance and relationship to intracranial hypertension. J Neurosurg 58:566–568, 1983.
44. Narayan RK, Greenberg RP, Miller JD, et al: Improved confidence in outcome prediction of severe head injury: A comparative analysis of the clinical examination, multimodality evoked potentials, CT scanning, and intracranial pressure. J Neurosurg 54:751–762, 1981.
45. Cushing H: The blood pressure reaction of acute cerebral compression, illustrated by cases of intracranial hemorrhage. Am J Med Sci 125:1017–1045, 1903.
46. Cushing H: Concerning a definite regulatory mechanism of vasomotor center which controls blood pressure during cerebral compression. Johns Hopkins Hosp Bull 12:290–292, 1901.
47. Langfitt T, Weishein J, Kassell N: Cerebral vasomotor paralysis produced by intracranial hypertension. Neurology 15:622–641, 1965.
48. Mitchell PH: Decreased adaptive capacity, intracranial: A proposal for a nursing diagnosis. J Neurosci Nurs 18:170–175, 1986.
49. Lobato RD, Rivas JJ, Cordobes AE, et al: Acute epidural hematoma: An analysis of factors influencing the outcome of patients undergoing surgery in coma. J Neurosurg 68:48–57, 1988.
50. Miller JD, Murray LS, Teasdale GM: Development of a traumatic intracranial hematoma after a "minor" head injury. Neurosurgery 27:669–673, 1990.
51. Selig J, Becker D, Miller D, et al: Traumatic acute subdural hematoma. N Engl J Med 304:1511–1518, 1981.
52. Jamison KG, Yelland JDN: Traumatic intracranial hematoma: Report of 63 surgically treated cases. J Neurosurg 37:528–532, 1972.
53. Rivano C, Barzone M, Carta F, et al: Traumatic intracerebral hematoma: Seventy-two cases surgically treated. J Neurosurg Sci 24:77–84, 1980.
54. Ninchoji T, Uemura K, Shimayama I, et al: Traumatic intracerebral hematomas of delayed onset. Acta Neurochir 71:69–90, 1980.
55. Cooper P: Delayed brain injury: Secondary insults. In Becker D, Povlishock J (eds): Central Nervous System Trauma: Status Report 1985 (Pub. No. 1988-520-149/00028). Washington, DC, US Government Printing Office, 1988.
56. Gennarelli TA: Cerebral concussion and diffuse brain injuries. In Cooper P (ed): Head Injury, 2nd ed. Baltimore, Williams & Wilkins, 1987, pp 108–123.
57. Jane JA, Steward O, Gennarelli TA: Axonal degeneration induced by experimental noninvasive minor head injury. J Neurosurg 62:96–100, 1985.
58. Binder LM: Persisting symptoms after mild head injury: A review of the postconcussive syndrome. J Clin Exp Neuropsychol 8:323–346, 1986.
59. Gennarelli TA: Cerebral concussion and diffuse brain injuries. In Cooper P (ed): Head Injury, 2nd ed. Baltimore, Williams & Wilkins, 1987, pp 108–123.
60. Miller JD, Murray LS, Teasdale GM: Development of a traumatic intracranial hematoma after a "minor" head injury. Neurosurgery 27:669–673, 1990.
61. Rimel R, Giordani M, Barth J, et al: Disability caused by minor head injury. Neurosurgery 9:222, 1981.
62. Alves W, Jane J: Mild brain injury: Damage and outcome. In Becker D, Povlishock J (eds): Central Nervous System Trauma: Status Report 1985 (Pub. No. 1988-520-149/00028). Washington, DC, US Government Printing Office, 1988.
63. Holbourne A: The mechanics of brain injury. Br Med Bull 3:147, 1945.
64. Adams JH, Graham DI, Gennarelli TA: Head injury in man and experimental animals: Neuropathology. Acta Neurochir 32(suppl):15–30, 1983.
65. Hadley DM, Teasdale GM, Jenkins A, et al: Magnetic resonance imaging in acute head injury. Clin Radiol 39:131–139, 1988.
66. Adams JH, Graham DI, Murray LS, Scott G: Diffuse axonal injury due to non-missile head injury in man. Ann Neurol 12:557–563, 1982.
67. Sazbon L, Groswasser Z: Outcome in 134 patients with prolonged posttraumatic unawareness: I. Parameters determining late recovery of consciousness. J Neurosurg 72:75–80, 1990.
68. Grosswasser Z, Sazbon L: Outcome in 134 patients with prolonged posttraumatic unawareness: II. Functional outcome of 72 patients recovering consciousness. J Neurosurg 72:81–84, 1990.
69. Cooper PR (ed): Head Injury, 2nd ed., Baltimore, Williams & Wilkins, 1987, pp 89–107.
70. Parkinson J: The ballistics of craniocerebral gunshot wounds. J Neurosurg Nurs 14:232–238, 1982.
71. Crockard HA, Brown FD, Calica FB, et al: Physiologic consequences of experimental cerebral missile injury and use of data analysis to predict survival. J Neurosurg 46:784–794, 1977.
72. Ropper AH: Lateral displacement of the brain and level of consciousness in patients with an acute hemispherical mass. N Engl J Med 314:953–958, 1986.
73. Ross DA, Olsen WL, Ross AM, et al: Brain shift, level of consciousness, and restoration of consciousness in patients with acute intracranial hematoma. J Neurosurg 71:498–502, 1989.
74. Teasdale G, Jennett B: Glasgow coma scale. Lancet 2:81–84, 1974.
75. Marshall SB, Cayard C, Foulkes MA, et al: The Traumatic Coma Data Bank: A nursing perspective, part I. J Neurosci Nurs 20:253–257, 1988.
76. Teasdale G, Safar P, Smyder J, et al: Brain resuscitation clinical trial II, 1984–1989 (Glasgow-Pittsburgh coma scoring method). In Safar P, Bircher NG (eds): Cardiopulmonary Cerebral Resuscitation, 3d ed. Philadelphia, WB Saunders Co, 1988, p 262.
77. Barolat-Romana G, Larson S: Influence of stimulus location and limb position on motor responses in the comatose patient. J Neurosurg 61:725–728, 1984.
78. Price DJ: Factors restricting the use of coma scales. Acta Neurochir 36(suppl):106–111, 1986.
79. Born JD, Hans P, Albert A, Bonnal J: Interobserver agreement in assessment of motor responses and brainstem reflexes. Neurosurgery 20:513–517, 1987.
80. Sugiura K, Muraoka K, Chishiki T, Baba M: The Edinburgh-2 coma scale: A new scale for assessing impaired consciousness. Neurosurgery 12:411–415, 1983.
81. Starmark JE, Stalhammar D, Holmgren E: The Reaction Level Scale (RLS85): Manual and guidelines. Acta Neurochir (Wien) 91:12–20, 1988.
82. Crosby L, Parsons LC: Clinical neurological assessment tool: Development and testing of an instrument to index neurologic status. Heart Lung 18:121–129, 1989.
83. Tesseris J, Pantazidis N, Routsi CR, Fragoulakis D: A comparative study of the Reaction Level Scale (RLS85) with Glasgow Coma Scale (GCS) and Edinburgh-2 Coma Scale (Modified)($E_2CS(M)$). Acta Neurochir (Wien) 110:65–76, 1991.
84. Stalhammar D, Starmark JE, Holmgren E, et al: Assessment of responsiveness in acute cerebral disorders: A multicentre study on the Reaction Level Scale (RLS85). Acta Neurochir (Wien) 90:73–80, 1988.
85. Reilly PL, Simpson DA, Sprod R, Thomas L: Assessing the conscious level in infants and young children: A paediatric version of the Glasgow Coma Scale. Childs Nerv Syst 4:30–33, 1988.
86. Williams J: Assessment of head-injured children. Br J Nurs 1(2):82–84, 1992.
87. Hagen C, Malkmus D, Dunham P: Levels of Cognitive Functioning in Rehabilitation of the Head-Injured Patient: Com-

prehensive Physical Management. Downey, CA, Professional Staff Association of Rancho Los Amigos Hospital, 1979, pp 87–88.
88. Livingston DH, Loder PA, Koziol J, Hunt CD: The use of CT scanning to triage patients requiring admission following minimal head injury. J Trauma 31:483–487, 1991.
89. Hadley DM, Teasdale GM, Jenkins A, et al: Magnetic resonance imaging in acute head injury. Clin Radiol 39:131–139, 1988.
90. Hans JS, Kaufman B, Alfidi RJ, et al: Head trauma evaluated by magnetic resonance and computed tomography: A comparison. Radiology 150:71–77, 1984.
91. Ginsberg MD: Positron emission tomography. In Wilkins R, Rengachary S (eds): Neurosurgery. New York, McGraw-Hill, 1985, pp 255–264.
92. Langfitt, TW, Obrist W, Alavi A, et al: Applications of CT, MRI, and PET to the study of brain trauma: Preliminary observations. J Neurosurg 64:760–767, 1986.
93. Roper SN, Mena I, King WA, et al: An analysis of cerebral blood flow in acute closed-head injury using technetium-99m-HMPAO SPECT and computed tomography. J Nucl Med 32:1684–1687, 1991.
94. Newton MR, Greenwood RJ, Britton KE, et al: A study comparing SPECT with CT and MRI after closed head injury. J Neurol Neurosurg Psychiatry 55:92–94, 1992.
95. Newell DW, Aaslid R: Transcranial Doppler. New York, Raven Press, 1992.
96. Gomez, CR, Backer RJ, Bucholz RD: Transcranial Doppler ultrasound following closed head injury: Vasospasm or vasoparalysis? Surg Neurol 35:30–35, 1991.
97. March K, Mitchell, PH, Winn HR, Grady S: Effect of backrest position on intracranial and cerebral perfusion pressures. J Neurosci Nurs 22:375–381, 1990.
98. Hall JW, Spielman GM, Gennarelli TA: Auditory evoked response in acute severe head injury. J Neurosurg Nurs 14:225–231, 1982.
99. Barelli A, Valente MR, Clemente A, et al: Serial multimodality-evoked potentials in severely head-injured patients: Diagnostic and prognostic implications. Crit Care Med 19:1374–1381, 1991.
100. Gildenburg PL, Makela ME: The effect of early intubation and ventilation on outcome following head injury. In Ratcheson RA (ed): Neurosurgical Critical Care. Baltimore, Williams & Wilkins, 1987, pp 1–50.
101. Nikas DL: Resuscitation of patients with central nervous system trauma. Nurs Clin North Am 21:693–704, 1986.
102. Walleck CA: Controversies in the management of the head-injured patient. Crit Care Nurs Clin North Am 1(1):67–74, 1989.
103. Eisenberg H, Weiner R, Tabaddor K: Emergency care: Initial evaluation. In Cooper P (ed): Head Injury, 2nd ed. Baltimore, Williams & Wilkins, 1987, pp 20–33.
104. Lewis FR: Initial assessment and resuscitation. Emerg Med Clin North Am 2:733–748, 1984.
105. Jackimczyk KC, Roberts MR: Approach to the intoxicated patient. Top Emerg Med 6:9–13, 1984.
106. Siesjo BK: Acidosis and ischemic brain damage. Neurochem Pathol 9:31–88, 1988.
107. Kraft SA, Larson CP, Shuer LM, et al: Effect of hyperglycemia on neuronal changes in a rabbit model of focal cerebral ischemia. Stroke 21:447–450, 1990.
108. Marshall LF, Toole BM, Bowers SA: The national traumatic coma data bank: 2. Patients who talk and deteriorate: Implications for treatment. J Neurosurg 59:285–288, 1983.
109. Mauss-Clum N, Ryan M: Brain injury and the family. J Neurosurg Nurs 13:165–169, 1981.
110. Rogers PM, Kreutzer JS: Family crisis following head injury: A network intervention strategy. J Neurosurg Nurs 16:343–346, 1984.
111. Thal E: Initial management of the multiply injured patient. In Cooper P (ed): Head Injury, 2nd ed. Baltimore, Williams & Wilkins, 1987, pp 34–50.
112. Butterworth JF, DeWitt, DS: Severe head trauma: Pathophysiology and management. Crit Care Clin 5:807–819, 1989.
113. Saul TG: Is ICP monitoring worthwhile? Clin Neurosurg 34:560–571, 1986.
114. McQuillan KA: Intracranial pressure monitoring: Technical imperatives. AACN Clin Iss 2:623–636, 1991.
115. Crutchfield JS, Narayan RK, Robertson CS, et al: Evaluation of a fiberoptic intracranial pressure monitor. J Neurosurg 72:482–487, 1990.
116. Tasker RC, Matthew DJ: Cerebral intraparenchymal pressure monitoring in nontraumatic coma: Clinical evaluation of a new fiberoptic device. Neuropediatrics 22:47–49, 1991.
117. Coroneos N, McDowell D, Gibson R, et al: Measurement of extradural pressure and its relationship to the other intracranial pressures: An experimental and clinical study. J Neurol Neurosurg Psychiatry 36:514–522, 1973.
118. Vries J, Becker D, Young H: A subarachnoid screw for intracranial pressure monitoring: Technical note. J Neurosurg 39:416–419, 1973.
119. Landy H, Villanueva P: An improved subarachnoid screw to intracranial pressure monitoring: Technical note. J Neurosurg 61:606–608, 1984.
120. Deardon NM, McDowell DG, Gibson RM: Assessment of Leeds device for monitoring intracranial pressure. J Neurosurg 60:123–129, 1984.
121. North B, Reilly P: Comparison among three methods of intracranial pressure recording. Neurosurgery 18:730–732, 1986.
122. Aucoin P, Kotilainen H, Gantz N, et al: Intracranial pressure monitors: Epidemiologic study of risk factors and infections. Am J Med 80:369–376, 1986.
123. Adolph RJ, Fukusumi H, Fowler NO: Origin of cerebrospinal fluid pulsation. Am J Physiol 212:840–846, 1967.
124. Cardoso ER, Rowan JO, Galbraith S: Analysis of the cerebrospinal fluid pulse wave in intracranial pressure. J Neurosurg 59:817–821, 1983.
125. Germon K: Interpretation of ICP pulse waves to determine intracranial compliance. J Neurosc Nurs 20:344–349, 1988.
126. Rauch ME, Mitchell PH, Tyler ML: Validation of risk factors for the nursing diagnosis decreased intracranial adaptive capacity. J Neurosci Nurs 22:173–178, 1990.
127. Doyle DJ, Mark PWS: Analysis of intracranial pressure. J Clin Monit 8:81–90, 1992.
128. Bakay R, Wood J: Pathophysiology of cerebrospinal fluid in trauma. In Becker D, Povlishock J (eds): Central Nervous System Trauma: Status Report 1985 (Pub. No. 1988-520-149/00028). Washington, DC, US Government Printing Office, 1988, pp 89–122.
129. Pollay M, Jullenwider C, Roberts PA, Stevens FA: Effects of mannitol and furosemide on blood-brain osmotic gradients and intracranial pressure. J Neurosurg 59:945–950, 1983.
130. Marshall L, Smith R, Rauscher L, Shapiro H: Mannitol dose requirements in brain injured patients. J Neurosurg 48:169–172, 1978.
131. Muizelaar J, Lutz H, Becker D: Effect of mannitol on ICP and CBF and correlation with pressure autoregulation in severely head injured patients. J Neurosurg 61:700–706, 1984.
132. Ward JD, Becker DP, Miller JD, et al: Failure of prophylactic barbiturate therapy in severe head injury. J Neurosurg 62:383–388, 1985.
133. Brain Resuscitation Clinical Trial I Study Group: Randomized clinical trial of thiopental loading in comatose survivors of cardiac arrest. N Engl J Med 314:397–403, 1986.
134. Piatt JH, Shiff SJ: High-dose barbiturate therapy in neurosurgery and intensive care. Neurosurgery 15:427–44, 1984.
135. Eisenberg HM, Frankowsi RF, Contant CF, et al: High-dose barbiturate control of elevated intracranial pressure in patients with severe head injury. J Neurosurg 69:15–23, 1988.
136. Bremer A, Yamada K, West C: Ischemic cerebral edema in primates: Effects of acetazolamide, phenytoin, sorbitol, dexamethasone and methylprednisolone on brain water and electrolytes. Neurosurgery 6:149–154, 1980.
137. Braughler JM, Hall ED: Current applications of "high-dose" steroid therapy for CNS injury J Neurosurg 62:806–810, 1985.
138. Cooper P, Moody S, Clark K, et al: Dexamethasone and severe head injury: A prospective double-blind study. J Neurosurg 51:307–316, 1979.
139. Bracken MB, Shephard MJ, Collins WF, et al: A randomized,

controlled trial of methylprednisolone or naloxone in the treatment of acute spinal cord injury. N Engl J Med 322:1405–1411, 1990.
140. Fisher DM, Frewen T, Swedlow DB: Increase in intracranial pressure during suctioning: Stimulation vs. rise in $Paco_2$ Anesthesiology 57:416–417, 1982.
141. Rudy EB, Turner BS, Baun M, et al: Endotracheal suctioning in adults with head injury. Heart Lung 20:667–674, 1991.
142. Donegan M, Bedford R: Intravenously administered lidocaine prevents intracranial hypertension during endotracheal suctioning. Anesthesiology 52:516–518, 1980.
143. Cooper KR, Boswell PA, Choi SC: Safe use of PEEP in patients with severe head injury. J Neurosurg 63:552–555, 1985.
144. Londrini S, Monofolivo MD, Pluchino F, Borroni B: Positive end-expiratory pressure in supine and sitting positions: Its effect on intrathoracic and intracranial pressure. Neurosurgery 24:873–877, 1989.
145. Boughton A, Ciesal N: Physical therapy management of the head-injured patient in the intensive care unit. Top Acute Care Trauma Rehabil 1:1–18, 1986.
146. McQuillan KA: The effects of the Trendelenburg position for postural drainage on cerebrovascular status in head-injured patient. Heart Lung 16:327, 1987.
147. Kenning JA, Toutant SM, Saunders RL: Upright positioning in the management of intracranial hypertension. Surg Neurol 15:148–152, 1980.
148. Feldman Z, Kanter MJ, Robertson CS, et al: Effect of head elevation on intracranial pressure, cerebral perfusion pressure and cerebral blood flow in head-injured patients. J Neurosurg 76:207–211, 1992.
149. Mitchell PH: Intracranial hypertension: Influence of nursing care activities. Nurs Clin North Am 21:563–576, 1986.
150. Parsons LC, Wilson M: The cerebrovascular status of severe closed head injured patients following passive position changes. Nurs Res 33:68–75, 1984.
151. Mitchell PH, Johnson FB, Habermann-Little B, et al: Nursing and ICP: Studies of two clinical problems. In Miller JD, Teasdale GM, Rowan JO (eds): Intracranial Pressure VI. Berlin, Springer-Verlag, 1986, pp 702–705.
152. Walleck C: The effects of purposeful touch on intracranial pressure. Heart Lung 12:428, 1983.
153. Pollack LD, Goldstein GW: Lowering of intracranial pressure in Reye's syndrome by sensory stimulation. N Engl J Med 304:732, 1981.
154. Mitchell P, Habermann-Little B, Johnson F, et al: Critically ill children: The importance of touch in a high-technology environment. Nurs Adm Q 9:38–46, 1985.
155. Hendrickson S: Intracranial pressure changes and family presence. J Neurosurg Nurs 19:14–18, 1987.
156. Johnson SM, Omery A, Nikas D: Effects of conversation on intracranial pressure in comatose patients. Heart Lung 18:56–63, 1989.
157. Sisson R: Effects of auditory stimuli on comatose patients with head injury. Heart Lung 19:373–378, 1990.
158. Kaufman HH, Moake JL, Olson JD, et al: Delayed and recurrent intracranial hematomas related to disseminated intravascular clotting and fibrinolysis in head injury. Neurosurgery 7:445–449, 1980.
159. Irska E, Myllynen P: Fat embolism in patients with multiple injuries. J Trauma 22:891–894, 1982.
160. Giesler FH, Salcman M: Respiratory system: Physiology, pathophysiology and management. In Wirth FP, Rateheson RA (eds): Neurosurgical Critical Care. Baltimore: Williams & Wilkins, 1987, pp 1–50.
161. Barrow DL, Tindall GT: Neuroendocrine physiology, pathophysiology, and management. In Wirth FP, Rateheson RA (eds): Neurosurgical Critical Care. Baltimore: Williams & Wilkins, 1987, pp 109–131.
162. Davis DH, Sundt DM: Relationship of cerebral blood flow to cardiac output, mean arterial pressure, blood volume and alpha and beta blockage in cats. J Neurosurg 52:745–754, 1980.
163. Nelson PB: Fluid and electrolyte physiology, pathophysiology and management. In Wirth FP, Rateheson RA (eds): Neurosurgical Critical Care. Baltimore: Williams & Wilkins, 1987, pp 69–80.
164. Rice V: Problems of water regulation: Diabetes insipidus and syndromes of inappropriate antidiuretic hormone. Crit Care Nurs 3:63–81, 1983.
165. Temkin NR, Dikmen SS, Wilensky AJ, et al: A randomized, double-blind study of phenytoin for the prevention of post-traumatic seizures. N Engl J Med 323:497–502, 1990.
166. Chopp M, Welch K, Tidwell B, et al: Global cerebral ischemia and intracellular pH during hyperglycemia and hypoglycemia in cats. Stroke 19:1383–1387, 1988.
167. Helgason CM: Blood glucose and stroke. Stoke 19:1049–1053, 1988.
168. Clifton GL, Robertson CS, Contant CF: Enteral hyperalimentation in head injury. J Neurosurg 62:186, 1985.
169. Deutschman CS, Konstantinides FN, Raup S, et al: Physiological and metabolic response to isolated closed-head injury. J Neurosurg 64:89–98, 1986.
170. Gardner D: Acute management of the head-injured adult. Nurs Clin North Am 21:555–587, 1986.
171. Baggerly J: Rehabilitation of the adult with head trauma. Nurs Clin North Am 21:577–587, 1986.
172. Nornes H, Magnaes B: Supratentorial epidural pressure recorded during posterior fossa surgery. J Neurosurg 35:541–549, 1971.
173. Muwaswes M: Increased intracranial pressure and its systemic effects. J Neurosurg Nurs 17:238–243, 1985.
174. Hoff JT, Schaberg D, McGillicuddy J: Infection: Prevention and management. In Wirth FP, Rateheson RA (eds): Neurosurgical Critical Care. Baltimore: Williams & Wilkins, 1987, pp 151–168.
175. Hagen C: Planning a therapeutic environment for the communicatively impaired post closed head injury patient. In Shanks SJ (ed): Nursing and Management of Adult Communication Disorders. San Diego, College Hill Press, 1983, pp 137–169.
176. Mitchell S, Bradley VA, Welch JL, Britton PG: Coma arousal procedure: A therapeutic intervention in the treatment of head injury. Brain Injury 4:273–279, 1990.
177. Sazbon L, Majenson T, Tartakovsky M, et al: Widespread periarticular new-bone formation in long-term comatose patients. J Bone Joint Surg 63-B:120–125, 1981.
178. Griffith ER: Spasticity. In Rosenthal M, Griffith E, Bond M, Miller JD (eds): Rehabilitation of the Head Injured Adult. Philadelphia, FA Davis, 1983, pp 125–143.
179. Hagen C, Malkmus D, Durham P: Levels of Cognitive Functioning in Rehabilitation of the Head-Injured Adult: Comprehensive Physical Management. Downey, CA, Professional Staff Association of Rancho Los Amigos Hospital, 1979, pp 87–88.
180. Ben-Yishay Y, Diller L: Cognitive deficits. In Rosenthal M, Griffith E, Bond M, Miller JD (eds): Rehabilitation of the Head Injured Adult. Philadelphia, FA Davis, 1983, pp 167–183.
181. Snyder M: Abnormally increased behavioral arousal. In Mitchell PH, Hodges LC, Muwaswes ML, Walleck CA (eds): AANN's Neuroscience Nursing. East Norwalk, CT, Appleton & Lange, 1988, pp 85–97.
182. Rac N, Jillmick HM, Wooston D: Agitation in closed head injury: Haloperidol effects on rehabilitation outcome. Arch Phys Med Rehabil 66:30–34, 1985.
183. Uomoto JM, McLean A: The care continuum in traumatic brain injury rehabilitation. Rehabil Psychol 34(2):71–79, 1989.
184. Oddy M, Humphrey M, Uttley D: Stresses upon the relatives of head injured patients. Br J Psychiatry 133:507–513, 1978.
185. Kleeman KM: Families in crisis due to multiple trauma. Crit Care Clin North Am 1(1):23–31, 1989.
186. Habermann B: Cognitive dysfunction and social rehabilitation in the severely head injured patient. J Neurosurg Nurs 14:220–224, 1982.
187. Jennett B, Bond MR: Assessment of outcome after severe brain damage. Lancet 1:480, 1975.
188. Gennarelli TA, Spielman GM, Langfitt TW, et al: Influence of

the type of intracranial lesion on outcome from severe head injury: A multicenter study using a new classification system. J Neurosurg 56:26–32, 1982.
189. Jaggi JL, Obrist WD, Gennarelli TA, Langfitt TW: Relationship of early cerebral blood flow and metabolism to outcome in acute head injury. J Neurosurg 72:176–182, 1990.
190. Bricolo A, Turazzi S, Feriotti G: Prolonged posttraumatic unconsciousness: Therapeutic assets and liabilities. J Neurosurg 52:625–634, 1980.
191. Sazbon L, Fuch C, Costeff H: Prognosis for recovery from prolonged post-traumatic unawareness: Logistic analysis. J Neurol Neurosurg Psychiatry 54:149–152, 1991.
192. Eisenberg HM: Outcome after head injury: General considerations and neurobehavioral recovery. In Becker D, Povlishock J (eds): Central Nervous System Trauma: Status Report 1985 (Pub. No. 1988-520-149/00028). Washington, DC, US Government Printing Office, 1988, pp 271–299.
193. Marshall LF, Becker DP, Bowers SA, et al: The national traumatic coma data bank: 1. Design, purpose, goals and results. J Neurosurg 59:276–284, 1983.
194. Gianotta S, Weiner JM, Karnaze D: Prognosis and outcome in severe head injury. In Cooper P (ed): Head Injury, 2nd ed. Baltimore, Williams & Wilkins, 1987, pp 464–487.
195. Symonds C: Mental disorder following head injury. Proc R Soc Med 30:1081–1094, 1937.
196. Brooks N: The effectiveness of post-acute rehabilitation. Brain Injury 5:103–109, 1991.
197. Cope DN, Cole JR, Hall KM, Barkans H: Brain injury: Analysis of outcome in a post-acute rehabilitation program: I. General analysis. Brain Injury 5:111–125, 1991.

18

CENTRAL NERVOUS SYSTEM II: SPINAL CORD INJURY

CONSTANCE A. WALLECK

A spinal cord injury (SCI) resulting in loss of motor or sensory function is one of the most catastrophic medical conditions.[1] The damage from this injury not only changes the entire life-style of the patient but also affects the family, friends, community, and society in general. The potential for SCI exists for everyone at all times. It can result in permanent paralysis and total loss of sensation. The ability to breathe can be destroyed or diminished. It also may affect the bowel, bladder, and sexual functioning of the individual. In addition to physical dysfunctions, there are significant psychological, social, and economic ramifications as well.

SCI and its effect on patients are the subjects of this chapter. The purpose is to review the nature and effect of injuries to the spinal cord, particularly in the cervical region and in regard to the alterations in functions throughout the cycles of trauma recovery. Included are the epidemiology and mechanisms of SCI, the state-of-the-art medical and nursing management, and the nursing diagnoses associated with the alterations in physiological functions. The final section of the chapter focuses on the long-term potential complications for the patient who has suffered a severe SCI with deficit.

The care of the person with SCI can be very complex and demanding. Although many problems and needs of these patients are common through all the cycles of trauma care, they will be discussed individually under the cycle in which their occurrence is a main focus of care.

EPIDEMIOLOGY

The incidence of SCI is relatively low, being approximately 40.1 per 1 million persons, but it is considered a high-cost disability.[1] About 250,000 people in the United States today have traumatic SCIs, and 10,000 people are newly injured each year.[2] Average lifetime care costs are estimated at $400,000 for a person with quadriplegia and $225,000 for a paraplegic.[3] The economic impact of spinal cord injury in the United States is estimated to be $4 billion per year.[4]

SCI most frequently occurs in younger age groups, with 80 per cent of the injured under 40 years of age and 50 per cent between the ages of 15 and 25 years. The "typical" individual sustaining an SCI is a young male (82 per cent male versus 18 per cent female), who is most frequently injured in a motor vehicle accident. Analysis of data on these patients reveals that 57 per cent possess at least a high school education and that most were either working or were full-time students at the time of their injury.[3]

Motor vehicle accidents account for 55 per cent of SCIs, followed by falls (21 per cent) and sports injuries (14 per cent).[5] Penetrating wounds are responsible for about 15 per cent of all SCIs, but children experience a higher percentage of these types of injuries.[2]

Mortality and morbidity have drastically changed for SCI patients over the past 65 years. During World War I, the life expectancy for the victim of SCI was 6 to 12 months following injury. In the past 15 years, improvements in critical care and in the treatment and prevention of complications encountered by spinal cord–injured patients have allowed these patients to live a near-normal life expectancy. Factors that affect the survival rate include the level of the lesion, extent of the paralysis, age at the time of the injury, and ability to survive the first 3 months following the injury.[6] Statistics show that 10 per cent of those who survive the initial resuscitation period die within 3 months from cardiopulmonary complications. Forty per cent of all spinal cord–injured patients have associated injuries, including closed head injuries and thoracic and abdominal injuries (Table 18–1).

Quadriplegic patients with complete lesions are prone to multiple complications throughout their lives. Respiratory compromise, diminished mobility, and infection account for significant numbers of the complications (Table 18–2).

As stated earlier, although the incidence of spinal cord injury is low (40.1 per million), the financial and personal costs are very high. An increase in the number of SCIs has been noted, and a trend has developed of increased survival of severely disabled patients with this type of trauma. Providing nursing care that is aimed at ensuring physiological stability and the prevention of complications through all the cycles is the major goal when caring for these patients.

PREVENTION

The term *prevention* as used here refers to the overall program to lower the number of persons suffering SCI. Since the majority of these persons are young (15 to 25 years of age), it seems reasonable to focus prevention programs at the middle-school and high-school populations. In these age groups, there is a sense of invulnerability and great peer pressure for risk-taking behavior, especially in males. Males are also allowed greater latitude in exploration during the preteen and early teen years. Public education regarding the consequences of actions involving drug and alcohol abuse combined with driving or other high-risk activities can be effective in reducing SCIs. Specific protection to be stressed in discussing prevention includes law enforcement for use of passenger restraints. One aggressive public education program in Florida has focused on the prevention of SCI from diving accidents. The program, *Feet First, First Time,* has focused on prevention of diving headfirst into shallow water, and has resulted in a 50 per cent decrease in the incidence of SCI in Florida over a 1-year period.[7]

Today's challenge, in terms of preventing spinal cord injury, is to motivate the general public to apply safety practices and to minimize risk situations. Widespread public education supported by media coverage is very effective in disseminating the information needed to prevent this usually preventable trauma.

Two other levels of prevention are also of concern to nurses. Secondary prevention focuses on early diagnosis and prompt intervention in the disease process. Prehospital management of the potentially spinal cord–injured patient is an example of secondary prevention.[8, 9] Tertiary prevention occurs throughout the trauma cycles of care to prevent further complications and to restore the patient to his or her fullest potential.[9] The remaining sections of the chapter incorporate aspects of secondary and tertiary prevention.

TABLE 18–1. INCIDENCE OF INJURIES ASSOCIATED WITH SPINAL CORD TRAUMA

DIAGNOSIS	PARAPLEGIA (%)	QUADRIPLEGIA (%)
Girdle, long bone fracture	27	11
Closed fracture: ribs, sternum	25	47
Pneumothorax, hemothorax	16	2
Injury to intrathoracic organs	15	4
Injury to visceral organs	14	3
Major head injury	8	6

Table 18–2. INCIDENCE OF SELECTED MAJOR COMPLICATIONS DURING INITIAL HOSPITALIZATION

DIAGNOSIS	PARA-PLEGIA (%)	QUADRI-PLEGIA (%)
Urinary tract infection	66	>0
Pressure sores	20	26
Pneumonia	8	19
Atelectasis	11	17
DVT, phlebitis, thrombophlebitis	15	14
Respiratory arrest	3	13
Anemia	11	11
Heterotrophic ossification	5	7
Septicemia	4	6
Gastrointestinal ulcer	2	5
Pulmonary embolus	4	5
Cardiac arrest	1	5
Calculus, kidney, ureter	1	0

DVT, deep vein thrombosis.

SPINAL CORD ASSESSMENT IN TRAUMA

All persons with traumatic injury have the potential for SCI. The index of suspicion is particularly high in individuals involved in high-speed vehicular accidents, in the unconscious patient, and in patients with penetrating injury to the neck, back, chest, or abdomen.

Accident Data Base

The events of the accident itself can provide a great deal of information regarding the potential for the patient to have

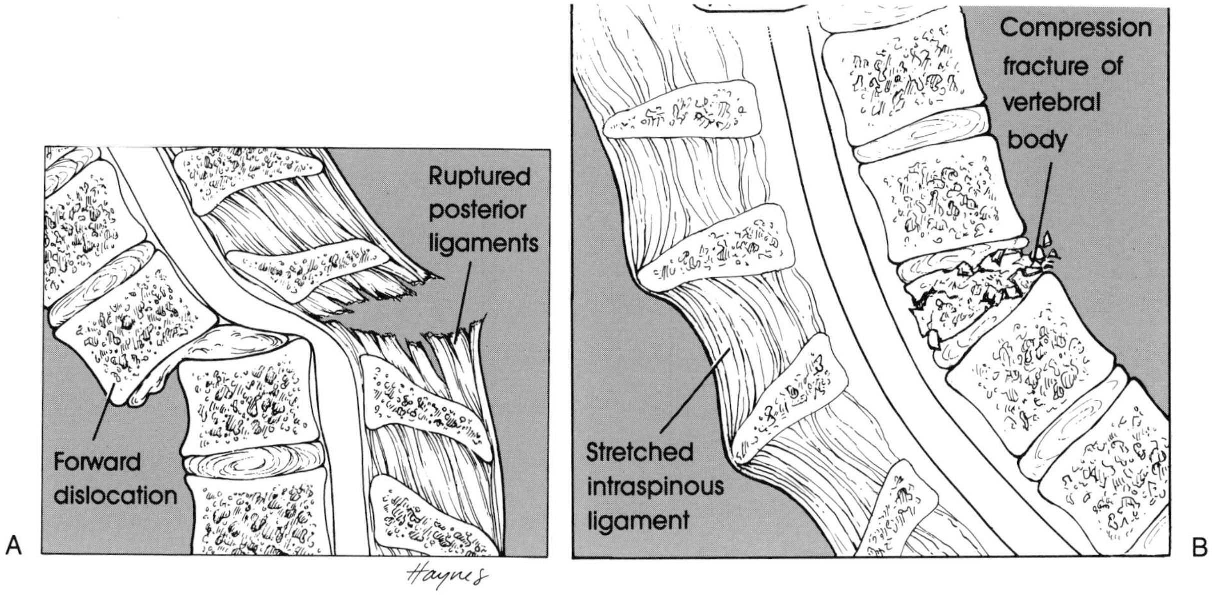

Figure 18–1. *A* and *B*, Flexion injury. (Reprinted by permission of Jones and Bartlett Publishers, Inc, from Management of Spinal Cord Injury by Cynthia Zejdlik, p 84, 1983.)

SCI. The overall goals of prehospital management are to anticipate the possibility of SCI in the trauma patient, to initiate appropriate treatment, and to prevent further neurological damage to the patient with SCI. The accident data base will guide not only the prehospital management of the patient but also subsequent resuscitative plans.

The type of accident, e.g., motor vehicle, motorcycle, diving, gunshot wound, or fall, can provide information as to the mechanisms of injury (see Chapter 7). The most common mechanisms of injury that result in SCI include forced flexion, flexion with rotation, hyperextension, and vertical compression (axial loading).[8–10] Flexion injuries (Fig. 18–1) are most often associated with motor vehicle accidents when the head is thrown violently forward. Flexion injuries also can occur if the head is struck from behind. Flexion and rotational forces (Fig. 18–2) occurring simultaneously are associated with fracture-dislocations and may be related to any number of accident situations. Falls are the most common causes of hyperextension injuries (Fig. 18–3) in which the chin is struck, causing violent extension of the neck. Burst fractures are associated with vertical compression injuries (Fig. 18–4) from a high-velocity blow to the top of the head, as seen in diving accidents. These mechanisms can occur singularly or in combination. Penetrating wounds can directly pierce the spinal cord or cause a concussion of the cord.

The status of the person at the time of injury and at the

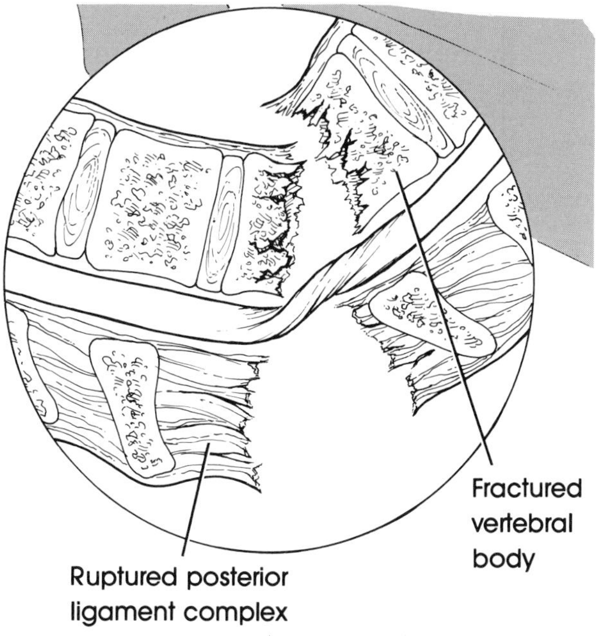

Figure 18–2. Flexion-rotation injury. (Reprinted by permission of Jones and Bartlett Publishers, Inc, from Management of Spinal Cord Injury by Cynthia Zejdlik, p 85, 1983.)

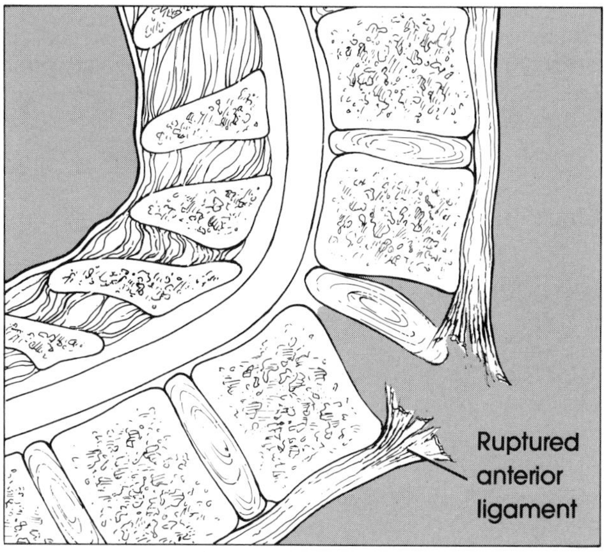

Figure 18–3. Hyperextension injury. (Reprinted by permission of Jones and Bartlett Publishers, Inc, from Management of Spinal Cord Injury by Cynthia Zejdlik, p 85, 1983.)

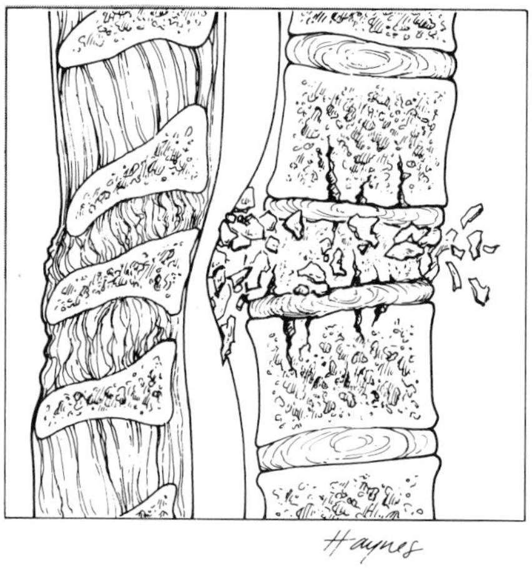

Figure 18–4. Vertical compression injury. (Reprinted by permission of Jones and Bartlett Publishers, Inc, from Management of Spinal Cord Injury by Cynthia Zejdlik, p 86, 1983.)

time of admission is important to note. The ability to move the extremities and the sensory ability of the patient need to be clearly documented, because all other motor and sensory assessments will be compared with the initial data base to determine if the patient is deteriorating or improving neurologically. Any complaints of neck or back pain or muscle spasms also need to be documented, because these signs may indicate an injury without deficit.

Previous Health History

A number of preexisting conditions can increase the risk of SCI. Conditions such as ankylosing spondylitis (a disease characterized by calcification and ossification of soft tissue and ligamentous structures and rigidity of the vertebral column) and rheumatoid arthritis (a chronic inflammatory condition causing osteoporosis, ligamentous damage, and abnormal mobility of the spine) can increase the chances of incurring spinal cord damage with only minor trauma. The elderly are particularly prone to hyperextension injuries from a simple fall because of the preexisting degenerative and osteoporotic changes that are often seen with aging that narrow the spinal canal. This type of injury typically results in the central cord syndrome (to be discussed later in this chapter), with minimal or no actual bony displacement.[11, 12]

Anatomical Considerations

The vertebral skeletal system is composed of bony elements, ligaments, and disks. The bone structure of the vertebrae consists of two sections: an anterior body and posterior arch (Fig. 18–5). The vertebral arch is a series of fused bony parts composed of two pedicles (which attach the arch to the disk body), two laminae (which form the roof of the arch), and seven bony protrusions (two superior and inferior facets, two transverse processes, and one spinous process) (Fig. 18–6). The surfaces of facets and processes articulate with other vertebrae. The spinal cord passes through this bony ring. The vertebrae vary in size but have similar structure except for C1, the atlas, and C2, the axis. C1 is a ringlike structure that articulates with the occiput and provides 50 per cent of the normal flexion and extension of the neck. C2 is also a ring structure with a special process called the *odontoid process* that articulates with the anterior arch of C1 to provide 50 per cent of the normal rotation of the head. The vertebrae increase in size as they descend. There are 7 cervical, 12 thoracic, 5 lumbar, 5 fused sacral, and 4 fused coccygeal vertebrae.

The function of the spinal column is to provide vertical stability for walking and to protect the spinal cord.[13] The rib cage and trunk muscles aid in maintaining spinal balance and control.

Disks are located between the vertebrae to act as shock absorbers during weight-bearing. They are composed of a cartilaginous outer ring and a gelatinous center. Disks and vertebral bodies are held in position by the anterior and posterior longitudinal ligaments, major ligaments that run the length of the spine (Fig. 18–7).

Ligaments are designed to prevent the spine from undergoing excessive flexion and extension.[14] The ligamentum flavum connects the laminae, whereas supraspinous and interspinal ligaments join the spinous processes. The transverse processes are connected by intertransverse ligaments. These ligaments are shorter and thicker than the anterior and posterior longitudinal ligaments.

Spinal Cord

The adult spinal cord is a gelatinous, cylindrical structure that travels through the vertebral canal from the level of the foramen magnum to the lumbar bony level 1 or 2, where it terminates as the conus medullaris. Although cylindrical, it

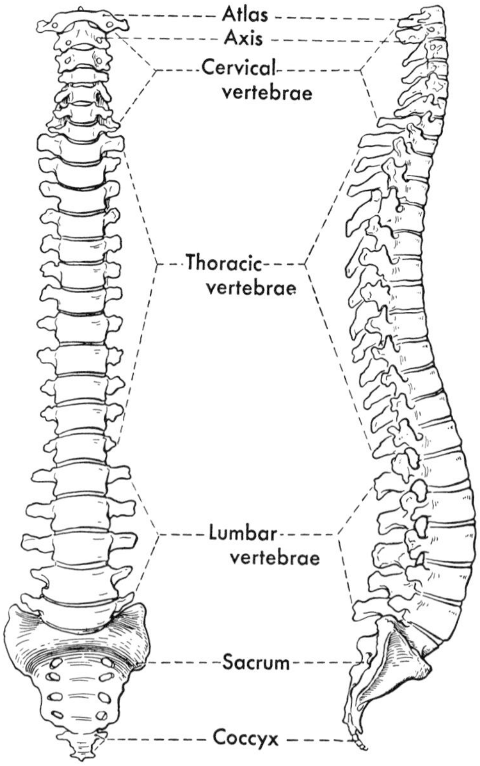

Figure 18–5. Anterior and lateral views of the vertebral column. (From Hollinshead WH, Jenkins DB: Functional Anatomy of the Limbs and Back, 5th ed. Philadelphia, WB Saunders Co, 1981.)

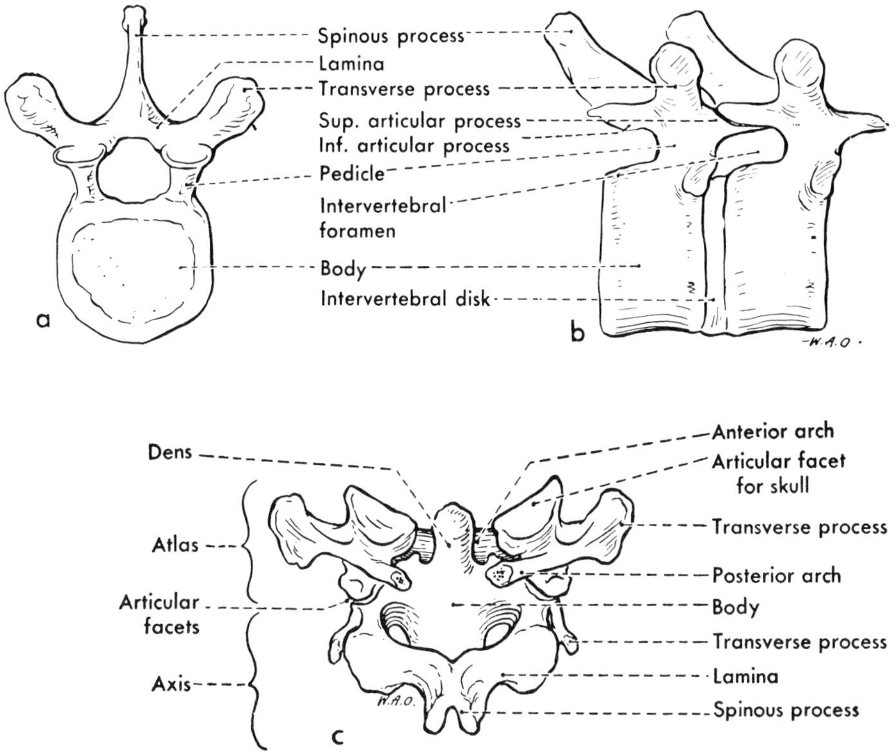

Figure 18–6. Structure of the vertebrae. *A*, Thoracic vertebra viewed from above. *B*, Two adjacent vertebrae, lateral view. *C*, The first two cervical vertebrae, posterior view; the posterior arch of the atlas has been partially cut away, and the ligaments that hold the dens in place are not shown. (From Hollinshead WH, Jenkins DB: Functional Anatomy of the Limbs and Back, 5th ed. Philadelphia, WB Saunders Co, 1981.)

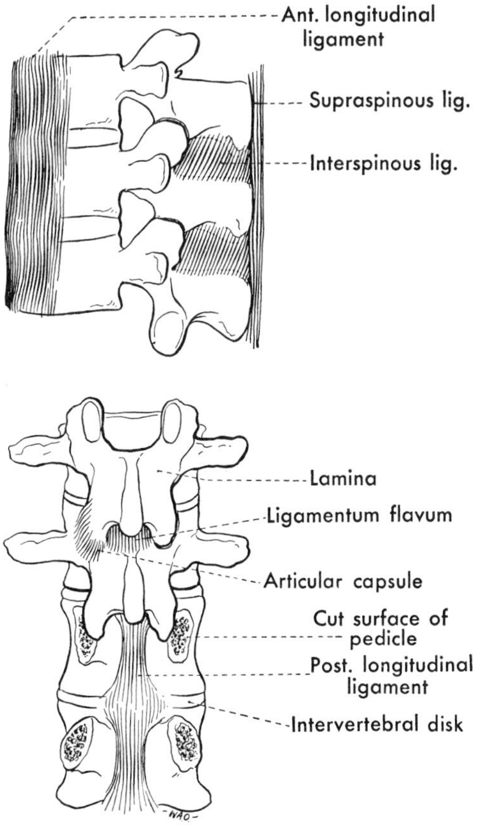

Figure 18–7. The chief ligaments of the vertebral column. (From Hollinshead WH, Jenkins DB: Functional Anatomy of the Limbs and Back, 5th ed. Philadelphia, WB Saunders Co, 1981.)

is slightly flattened in the anteroposterior diameter and is approximately 40 cm (18 in) in length and 9 mm (1/2 to 3/4 in) in diameter. It is continuous with the medulla oblongata and contains two areas of enlargement corresponding to the large nerve supplying the upper and lower extremities: cervical (from C3 to T2) and lumbar (from T9 to T12).

The spinal cord is enveloped by the dura mater, the arachnoid, and the pia mater. External to the dura is the epidural space, which is filled with a layer of fat, areolar tissue, and veins. The subarachnoid space is filled with cerebrospinal fluid (CSF), as is the central canal that pierces the central gray matter of the cord. The central canal is continuous with the fourth ventricle. CSF provides a cushioning effect for the spinal cord as well as providing the cord with the optimal physiological fluid environment for nerve function. Removal of some metabolic waste products also occurs through the CSF, where they are carried to the arachnoid villi in the brain for return to the venous sinuses.

Gray Matter

The spinal cord consists of nerve cell bodies and their processes and fibers. The cell bodies together with some unmyelinated fibers are massed into columns, which in cross section resemble the letter H and are known as the *gray matter.* The gray matter is divided in two ways: into columns (posterior, horizontal, and anterior) and into nine laminae counting from posterior (dorsal) to anterior (ventral). The posterior gray column is sensory, and incoming sensory impulses terminate in laminae 4, 5, and 6. Lamina 6 contains the end point for incoming proprioception messages; lamina 5 is the terminating point for protopathic messages. Messages regarding position sense, pressure sense, vibratory sense, movement, and stereognosis terminate in lamina 4. The horizontal gray matter contains interconnecting neurons between the posterior and anterior columns that form the first part of a two-neuron pathway for the sympathetic nervous system in the thoracic and lumbar regions. The horizontal gray matter is also pierced by the central canal. The anterior portion of the gray matter contains the motor cell bodies that form the final common pathway of all impulses going to the skeletal muscles. Their axons pass out of the spinal cord by way of the ventral root to end in the motor end plates at muscles.

White Matter

The surrounding white matter of the spinal cord is formed by the axons of the cells within the gray matter of the spinal cord; axons of the sensory cells in the dorsal ganglia either directly or by way of relay interneurons; and descending tracts from the brain, brainstem, or cerebellum. The myelination of most of the axons gives the white matter its color. The fibers in the white matter are organized into tracts that are oriented parallel to the vertical axis of the spinal cord (Fig. 18–8). The tracts ascend to and descend from the brain and other levels of the spinal cord. There are many tracts in the spinal cord, but only those of clinical importance will be discussed here.

White Matter Tracts. The major ascending tracts include the posterior columns, the spinocerebellar tracts, and the spinothalamic tracts. The posterior columns are composed of sensory pathways for muscle and joint sensations, vibration sense, two-point discrimination, deep pressure, touch, and position sense. These columns decussate in the medulla and ascend through the thalamus to the cerebral cortex.

The spinocerebellar tracts transmit impulses from the muscles of the extremities and trunk to the cerebellum. These impulses contain information on position sense and body movement and are necessary for coordinated movement.

The two spinothalamic tracts carry vital sensory information from the periphery to the thalamus. The ventral spinothalamic tracts transmit impulses of touch, whereas the lateral spinothalamic tracts mediate most of the pain and temperature sensations. These tracts are formed by axons of cells in the ventral gray horns that cross in the ventral white commissure to ascend on the opposite side of the spinal cord to the thalamus.

The major descending tract of clinical concern is the corticospinal tract. Originating in the motor cortex of the brain, this tract crosses in the medulla to innervate the opposite side of the body. This tract carries impulses to primary motor neurons for voluntary motor movement.

Spinal Nerves

The spinal nerves provide pathways for automatic reactions or involuntary movement in response to stimuli. They also innervate voluntary striated muscle. Spinal nerves have efferent fibers that transmit outgoing motor messages and afferent fibers that transmit incoming sensory data. The spinal nerves occur in pairs and correspond to the 31 seg-

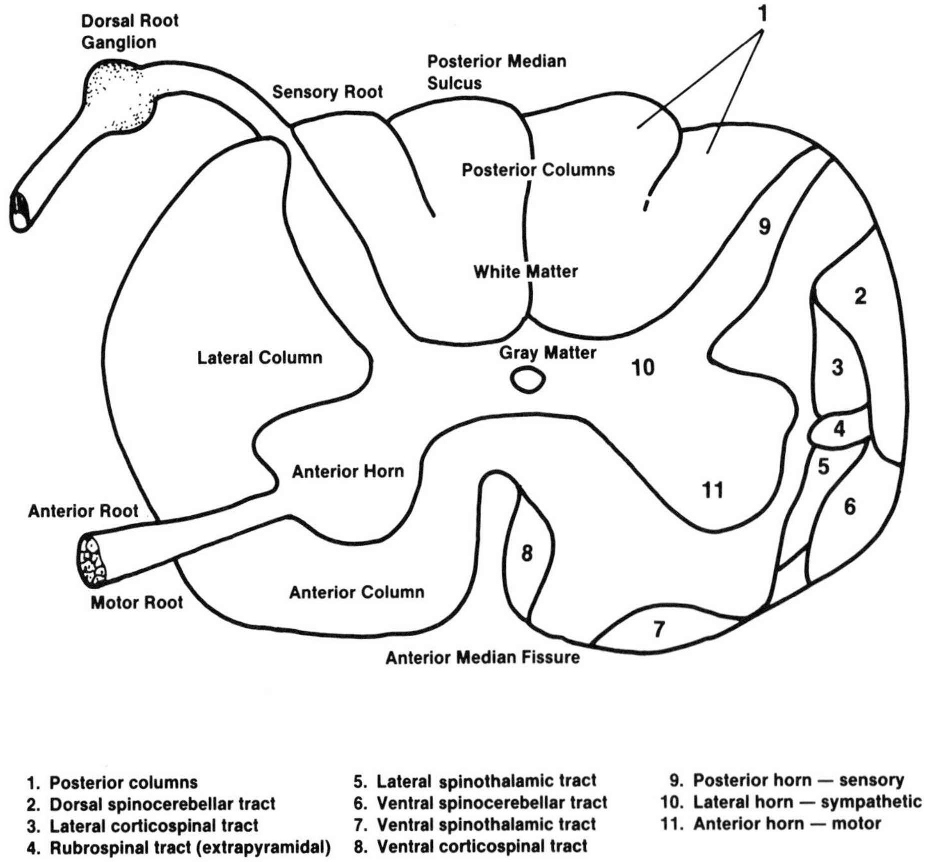

Figure 18–8. Cross section of spinal cord.

ments of the spinal cord: 8 cervical nerves, 12 thoracic nerves, 5 lumbar nerves, 5 sacral nerves, and 1 coccygeal nerve. These nerves originate as an anterior (motor) root and a posterior (sensory) root as they exit the spinal cord. Beyond the spinal dorsal root ganglion, the roots are enclosed in a common dural sheath where they form the spinal nerve.

The spinal nerves lie horizontally in the cervical region, but below these segments the spinal nerves assume an increasingly oblique and downward direction as they approach the lumbar region, where they are almost vertical, forming the cauda equina.

Blood Supply

The spinal cord derives its blood supply from the vertebral artery and from a series of spinal rami that enter the intervertebral foramina at various levels[14] (Fig. 18–9). The anterior spinal artery is formed by the union of the two branches of the terminal portion of the vertebral artery at the level of the foramen magnum. The artery descends as a single trunk along the anterior aspect of the spinal cord behind the vertebral body. It supplies blood to two-thirds of the spinal cord. The remaining third of the blood supply is carried by the two posterior spinal arteries, which are branches derived from the vertebral arteries. The posterior spinal artery on each side receives a succession of small arterial branches that enter the spinal canal through the intervertebral foramina. These vessels and their branches anastomose freely around the posterior roots and with corresponding vessels on the opposite side. The venous system parallels the arterial system.

Autonomic Nervous System

The autonomic nervous system (ANS) provides automatic control at a subconscious or involuntary level of vital functions such as blood pressure, heart rate, body temperature, appetite, fluid balance, gastrointestinal motility, and sexual functioning (Fig. 18–10). Most organs innervated by the ANS receive a double supply of nerves, one set originating from neurons in the craniosacral regions of the central nervous system that form the parasympathetic nervous system, the other from the thoracolumbar region of the spinal cord that forms the sympathetic nervous system. Although the parasympathetic and sympathetic nerves often have opposite effects on an organ, their activity is integrated to ensure the appropriate response of that organ. The ANS is governed by the hypothalamus and other recently identified cortical and medullary structures and, to a certain extent, by local reflex activity. [The ANS is an efferent (outflowing) system of fibers.]

The parasympathetic division of the ANS controls those activities concerned with everyday body functioning. It initiates functions such as digestion or elimination and conserves body energy. Stimulation of this system results in specific responses, such as increased peristalsis and slowing of the heart rate. The chemical transmitter for this system is acetylcholine. The long nerve fibers of the parasympathetic system synapse directly on the effector organs innervated by them. Parasympathetic stimulation is not extended to the voluntary muscles, skin, sweat glands, adrenal glands, and spleen; these muscles, organs, and glands receive only sympathetic input.

The sympathetic nervous system allows maximum energy for stress defense, which is commonly called the "fight or flight system." Stimulation of the sympathetic system causes a generalized response that includes an increased heart rate and respirations, a shunting of blood from the viscera to the cardiopulmonary circulation, a decreased gastrointestinal motility, a release of red blood cells from storage in the spleen for additional energy, and a release of epinephrine. The structure of this system is different from the parasympathetic system. The central gray matter in the thoracolumbar spinal cord contains the neurons of the sympathetic outflow. All the preganglionic fibers leaving the spinal cord at those levels enter a chain of ganglia that lie on either side of the spinal cord. These sympathetic ganglia are linked together to form the sympathetic chain. Two neurotransmitters are used in carrying messages in this system. Acetylcholine carries the message to the sympathetic ganglia, and

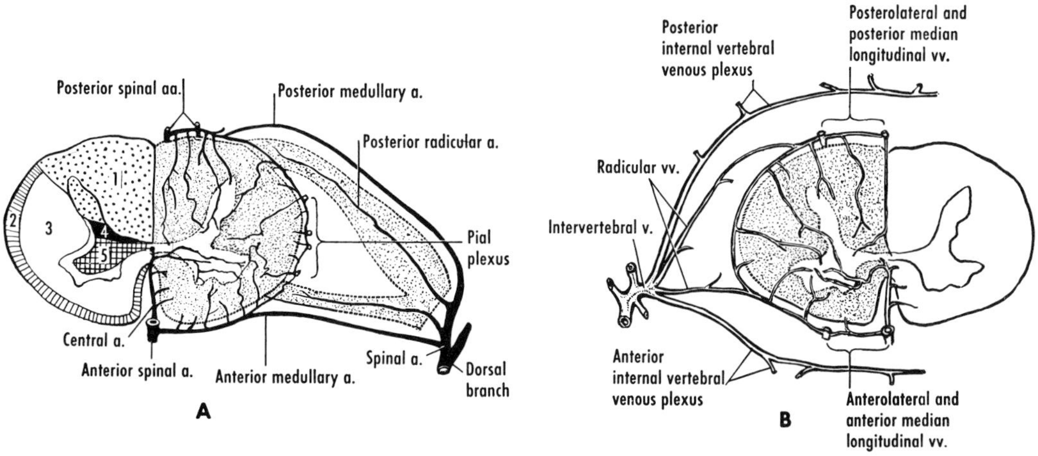

Figure 18–9. The arterial (*A*) and venous (*B*) drainage of the spinal cord. (1) The area supplied by the posterior plexus; (2) the area supplied by the lateral and ventral parts of the pial plexus; (3) the area of common supply by the central artery and by the lateral and ventral pial parts of the pial plexus; (4) the area of common supply by the central artery and the posterior plexus; (5) the area supplied by the central artery. (Based on Gillian.) (From O'Rahilly R: Gardner, Gray and O'Rahilly Anatomy: A Regional Study of Human Structure, 5th ed. Philadelphia, WB Saunders Co, 1980.)

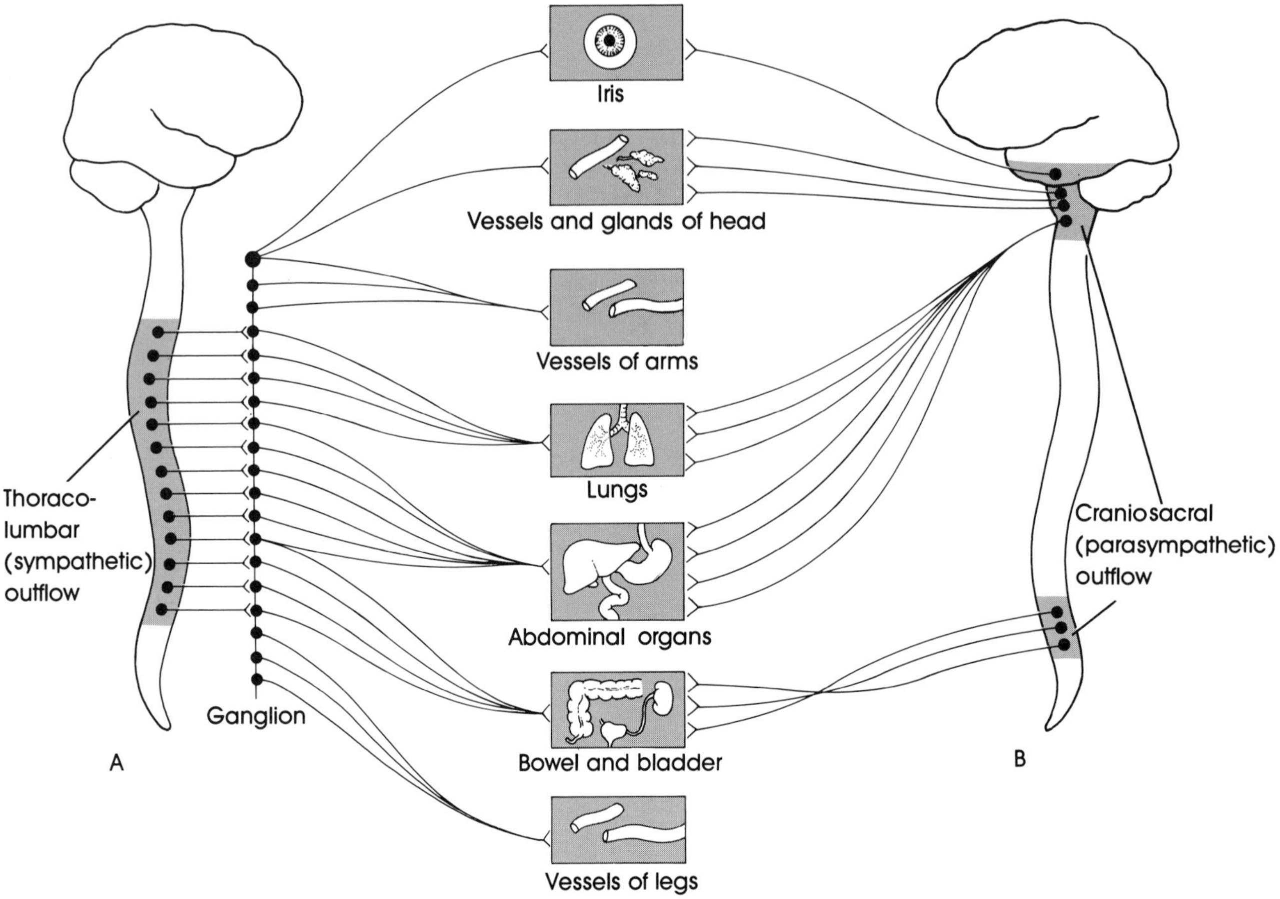

Figure 18–10. Sympathetic nervous system, composed of the thoracolumbar outflow (*A*) and of the parasympathetic nervous system, composed of the craniosacral outflow (*B*). (Reprinted by permission of Jones and Bartlett Publishers, Inc, from Management of Spinal Cord Injury by Cynthia Zejdlik, p 80, 1983.)

epinephrine or norepinephrine is the transmitter between the sympathetic ganglia and the structures they innervate.

Neurological Assessment

Field

Initial assessment of the traumatically injured person with actual or potential SCI involves ensuring the patency of the airway, adequate breathing, and circulation. If the patient is breathing spontaneously, check the rate and depth of respirations to ensure adequate oxygenation. If the person is unconscious and without an adequate airway, the jaw thrust maneuver or chin lift should be utilized in attempts to establish an airway. Care must be taken to prevent movement of the head and neck, especially flexion and hyperextension. A brief neurological assessment at the scene should include a motor and sensory assessment. Beginning at the shoulders and working down, all major muscle groups should be evaluated for motor function (Fig. 18–11). Pinprick over all dermatome levels is used to assess the sensory level[7] (Fig. 18–12). The initial motor and sensory determination will form the baseline for all subsequent examinations to determine deterioration or improvement in sensorimotor status.

The neck should be examined for any obvious signs of deformity or hematoma formation especially near the trachea. The entire spine should be examined, if possible, for deformity or localized pain.[8, 15]

A rapid examination of the chest, abdomen, and long bones for injury should be done to ascertain injuries to these systems. Patients with cervical spine injury, if deficit is present, will not be able to tell if they are injured elsewhere.

At the scene of the accident, acute immobilization of the neck is imperative. Of major concern is the form of cervical spine immobilization used in the field prior to transporting the person. Studies have reported the potential for neurological deterioration during transport to be 3 to 25 per cent.[8, 13, 16] One of the major goals during field management is to reduce the risk of neurological deterioration.

Several studies have compared various forms of pre- and posthospital immobilization devices.[8, 17] These reports indicate that in the acute situation, sandbags and adhesive tape across the forehead, taped to the backboard, are far superior to the cervical hard collar in preventing cervical motion. However, the combined use of sandbags, tape, and a cervical hard collar best restricts flexion, extension, rotation, and lateral bending[8, 17, 18] (Fig. 18–13). The person may need additional hand and body restraints to prevent restless movement during transport.

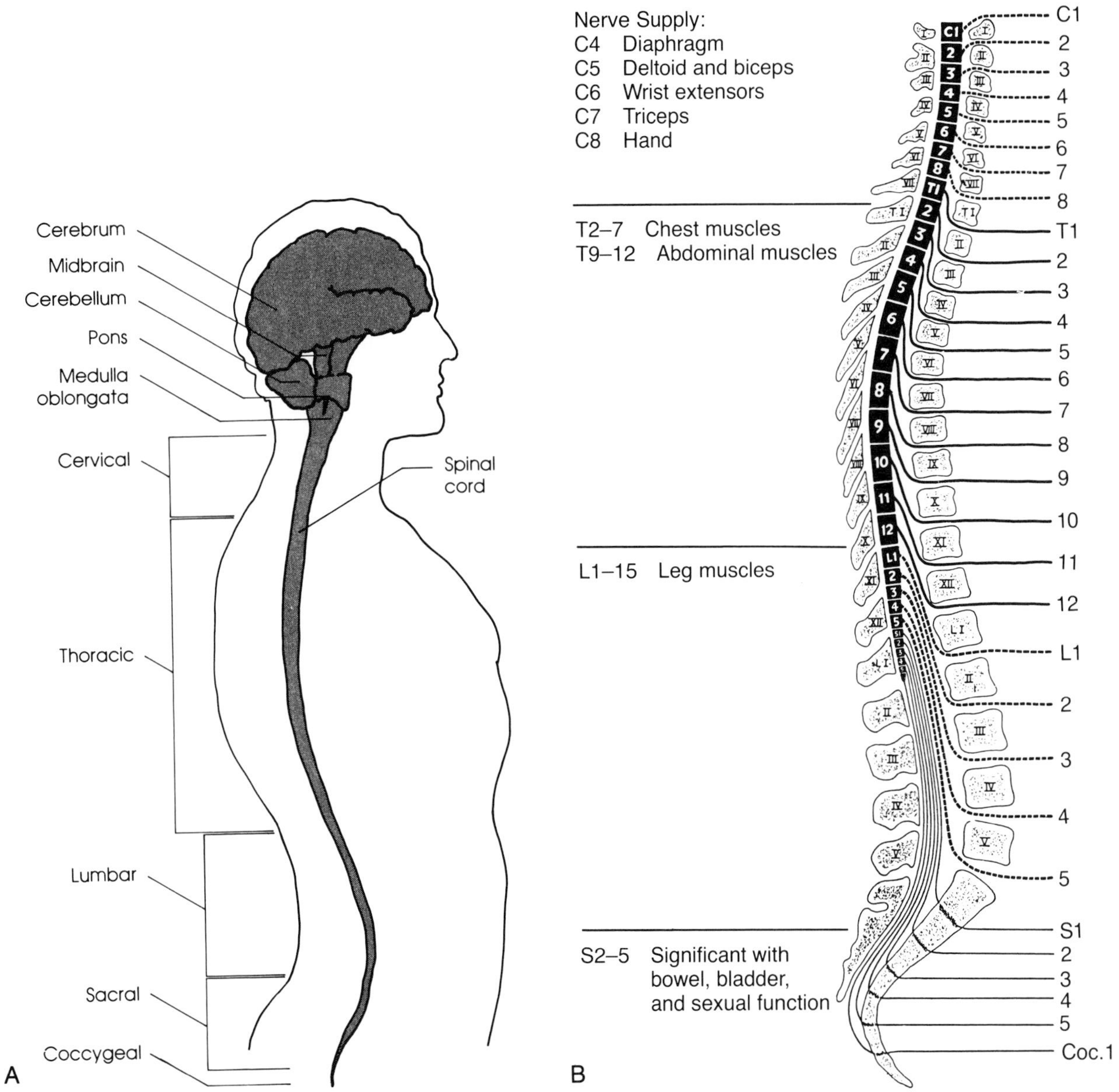

Figure 18–11. *A,* Major anatomical divisions of the central nervous system. (Reprinted with permission from Keane CB: Essentials of Medical-Surgical Nursing, 2nd ed. Philadelphia, WB Saunders Co, 1986.) *B,* Relation of the spinal cord and nerve roots to the vertebral column. Vertebral bodies and spinous processes bear Roman numerals; spinal nerves and the segments of the cord from which each arises bear Arabic numerals. Note that the cord segments are shorter than the vertebral ones so that even in the lower cervical and upper thoracic region the nerve roots run downward to their exits. The lumbar and sacral segments of the cord are especially short, and the nerves arising here run markedly downward; below the end of the cord, these nerves constitute the cauda equina. (From Haymaker W, Woodhall B: Peripheral Nerve Injuries, 2nd ed. Philadelphia, WB Saunders Co, 1953.)

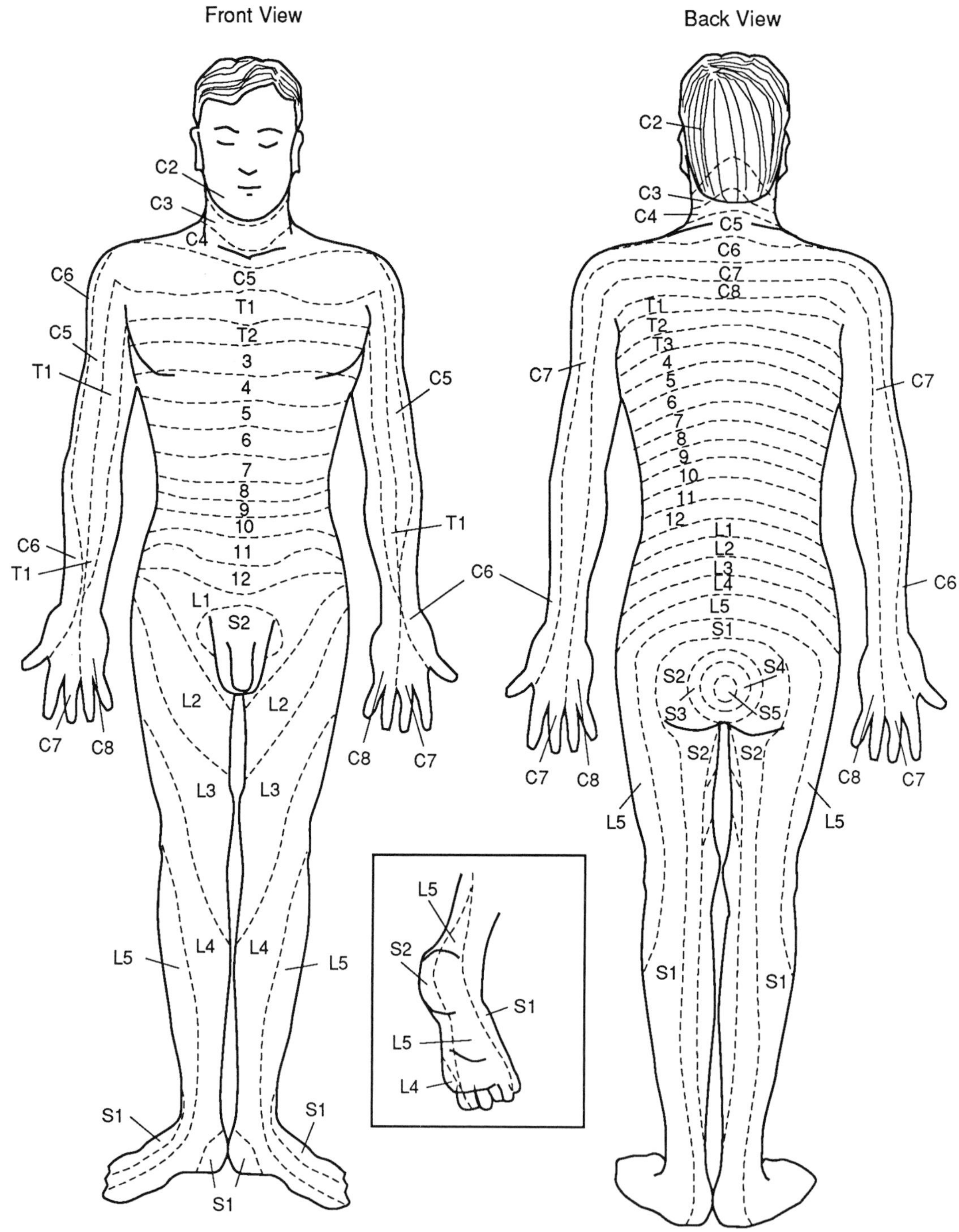

Figure 18–12. Dermatomes.

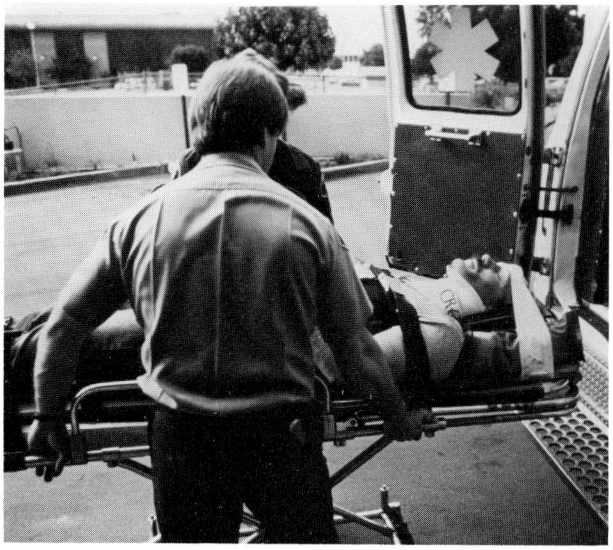

Figure 18–13. Combined use of sandbags, tape, and a cervical hard collar for transport.

On-going Assessment

Once the patient has been stabilized, a more in-depth spinal cord assessment can be completed (Fig. 18–14). The *motor assessment* is performed by asking the patient to move all the major motor groups, beginning with the deltoids and biceps (C5). The patient is asked to attempt to move each group, and a five-point scale is used to grade the strength in each of the groups tested: 5 means normal strength and 1 indicates trace movement.

In addition to assessing the motor abilities, a complete sensory examination is done. Using a pin and beginning in an area where the patient has sensation, such as on the side of the face, all dermatomes are tested to determine if dull versus sharp pinprick sensation can be differentiated. Proprioception, the ability to sense the position of body parts, should be evaluated in each hand and foot by moving the finger or toe up or down and having the patient state the direction of the digit movement. Rectal tone also should be tested to determine sacral sparing.[8, 16] Reflexes also should be tested at this time, including superficial and deep tendon reflexes to determine sensory or motor sparing and approximate level of SCI.

The focus of the more thorough assessment after stabilization is to look for occult injuries, missed injuries, or complications of the original injury such as airway obstruction, aspiration, or spinal shock. It is extremely important that all assessments be well documented so that any subsequent changes in function can be readily identified.

Physiological Approach

The monitoring of blood pressure, heart rate and rhythm, respirations, fluid intake, urine output, and blood gases is important during and after resuscitation. With the loss of the sympathetic output, most patients will be hypotensive and bradycardic, representing a neurogenic shock state. Arterial line, pulmonary artery catheter, and electrocardiogram (EKG) are helpful and in many cases vital for monitoring and assessing treatment of the patient, especially during the spinal (neurogenic) shock state associated with cervical and upper thoracic cord injuries.[8, 19] Temperature also must be monitored very closely, because the patient may be hypothermic owing to peripheral vasodilation and loss of temperature-regulating capacity. *Spinal shock* refers to the loss of all reflexes below the level of a complete physiological spinal cord injury beginning immediately with the injury and resolving within 2 to 16 weeks.[18, 20, 21] With the resolution of spinal shock, reflexes below the level of injury return and are hyperreflexic. The motor tone is markedly increased as the upper motor neuron injury becomes evident clinically.

A patient with an injury above the C5 level will usually require ventilatory support. Monitoring arterial blood gases and measuring respiratory parameters are important to assess oxygenation. If a ventilator is not necessary, as is generally the case in patients with injury below C5, vital capacity, tidal volume, pulse oximetry, and other respiratory parameters should be measured frequently during the first 3 days following injury, since this will be the time of peak spinal cord edema, which may produce temporary decrease and/or loss of respiratory function.

Integrating Other Data Sources

The information gained from cervical spine films and other neuroradiological tests, such as the computed tomographic (CT) scan, permits rational therapeutic decision making. Cervical spine films are obtained on admission. The film-taking process must be performed carefully with the neck maintained in the neutral position so as not to cause further damage to the spinal cord. All seven cervical vertebrae should be seen on the plain x-ray films; this typically requires that someone pull the patient's shoulders down in order to visualize C7, or else the lower cervical spine is obscured by the shoulders. X-ray examination should be repeated until all vertebrae are visualized. If they cannot be visualized, a swimmer's view is often helpful. If a major neurological deficit is present, then a myelogram may be performed on admission to determine the presence or absence of pressure on the spinal cord. A C1–2 level puncture is made, and the dye, either iophendylate (Pantopaque) or a water-soluble dye such as metrizamide (Amipaque) or iohexal (Omnipaque), is injected while the patient is supine.[22] A myelogram can be performed alone or in combination with a CT scan. The nurse as well as a physician should accompany the patient to the radiology department where the myelogram and CT scan are performed. Tomography with or without flexion and extension movement of the neck may be used to obtain cross sections of the vertebral column to better define the extent of bony injury. Based on the findings of the neuroradiological studies, the type of injury, and the condition of the patient, the patient will be transferred to the operating room for acute spinal cord decompression or the intensive care unit for hemodynamic monitoring and stabilization. Magnetic resonance imaging (MRI) also may be done to better visualize the location, nature, and extent of spinal cord injury. However, critically ill, unstable patients on vasoactive drips administered by pump may not be able to be evaluated with this test, since no metallic equipment can accompany the patient.

UNIVERSITY OF MARYLAND

MIEMSS—UMMS

SPINAL CORD INJURY FLOW SHEET

Muscle Strength

5 Normal
4 Active movement through range of motion against resistance
3 Active movement through range of motion against gravity
2 Active movement through range of motion with gravity eliminated
1 Palpable or visible contraction
0 Total paralysis
U Unable to test strength of extremity

Rectal Tone, Proprioception, Diaphragm

P–Present A–Absent U–Untestable

Medication	Sensation
S—Sedation	N—Normal
PL—Paralytic	ABN—Abnormal
T—Tranquilizer	A—Absent
P—Pain	U—Untestable

Level of bony/ ligamentous injury	
Anatomical Classification	

MOTOR LEVEL *Circled entry means to refer to nurses note*

Date													
Time													
Medications													
Diaphragm (R/L)	C_4												
Deltoid (raise arms) (R/L)	C_5												
Biceps (elbow flexion) (R/L)	$C_{5.6}$												
Wrist extensors (R/L)	C_6												
Triceps (elbow extension) (R/L)	C_7												
Flexer digitorum profundus (finger flexion) (R/L)	C_8												
Hand intrinsics (finger abduction) (R/L)	T_1												
Iliopsoas (hip flexion) (R/L)	L_2												
Quadriceps (knee extension) (R/L)	L_3												
Tibialis anterior (dorsiflex foot) (R/L)	L_4												
Extensor hallucis longus (great toe extension) (R/L)	L_5												
Gastrocnemius (ankle plantar flexion) (R/L)	S_1												
Function	Level												
Proprioception (finger) (R/L)													
Proprioception (toe) (R/L)													
Rectal Tone (P/A)													
Initials													
Initials/signature													

Medical Records No.

Figure 18–14. SCI assessment tool.

SENSATION

DATE												
TIME												
C_2 (R/L)												
C_3 (R/L)												
C_4 (R/L)												
C_5 (R/L)												
C_6 (thumb and forefinger) (R/L)												
C_7 (middle finger) (R/L)												
C_8 (ring and little finger) (R/L)												
T_1 (R/L)												
T_2 (R/L)												
T_3 (R/L)												
T_4 (nipple) (R/L)												
T_5 (R/L)												
T_6 (R/L)												
T_7 (R/L)												
T_8 (R/L)												
T_9 (R/L)												
T_{10} (umbilicus) (R/L)												
T_{11} (R/L)												
T_{12} (R/L)												
L_1 (R/L)												
L_2 (R/L)												
L_3 (R/L)												
L_4 (R/L)												
L_5 (R/L)												
S_1 (R/L)												
S_2 (R/L)												
$S_{3,4,5}$ (sacral sparing) (R/L)												
Sensory function												
Initials												

Figure 18–14 *Continued*

Another diagnostic tool available for use in spinal cord–injured patients is the somatosensory evoked potentials. The testing of evoked responses may be useful in establishing the prognosis. A peripheral nerve in the arm or leg, below the level of the injury, is stimulated, and the response of the cerebral cortex is recorded through scalp electrodes. When the injury is complete, the somatosensory evoked potentials are absent, since no messages can be conducted through the damaged cord. In the case of an incomplete injury, an altered response is noted. Early persistence and progressive normalization of evoked potentials generally precedes any clinical evidence of improvement.[7]

Laboratory data should be evaluated to give additional information on the status of the trauma patient. Arterial blood gases, hematocrit, hemoglobin, complete blood count, coagulation studies, serum electrolytes, serum glutamine oxaloacetic transaminase (SGOT), serum glutamic pyruvic transaminase (SGPT), lactic dehydrogenase (LDH), creatinine phosphokinase (CPK), alkaline phosphatase, bilirubin, blood urea nitrogen (BUN), amylase, and typing and crossmatch should be included in the initial evaluation.[11]

Classification of Injury

Vertebral Injuries. Fractures can occur in any part of the vertebra. The irregular shape of the vertebra allows this bony structure to fracture easily. Fractures are caused by either direct or indirect trauma.

Vertebral injuries can be classified into major divisions: simple fractures, compression fractures, comminuted fractures, teardrop fractures, special fractures (involving the atlas and axis), dislocations, subluxations, and fracture-dislocation.[5, 10, 11]

Simple fractures usually occur at a spinous or transverse process, facets, or pedicles. Alignment remains intact and neural compression is usually not present.

A wedge fracture or compression fracture is one in which the vertebral body is compressed anteriorly due to a hyperflexion injury. Neural compression may or may not be present.

A comminuted fracture, also known as a *burst fracture,* results in a shattering of the vertebral body. Bone may be driven into the spinal cord with this type of fracture. These fractures are associated with vertical (axial) loading forces and generally result in a serious spinal cord injury.

As the result of a hyperflexion fracture-dislocation, a small fragment of bone from the anterior edge of the vertebrae can break off and may lodge in the spinal canal. This is known as a *teardrop* fracture. Neurological deficits will result if the fragment penetrates the cord.

If the cervical fracture occurs at the level of the first cervical vertebra (atlas) and the second cervical vertebra (axis), specialized fractures occur. A Jefferson fracture is a bursting of the ring of C1 as a result of axial loading on C1. There is usually no immediate damage to the cord, although if there is displacement of the fracture, the injury is fatal.

Atlanto-occipital dislocations are produced by an avulsion of the atlas from the occipital bone. Death is usually immediate with this type of injury, but if the patient does survive, there is usually no neurological deficit.[8]

Odontoid fractures involve the odontoid process (dens) of vertebra C2. There are three types of fractures at this site. Death occurs if the odontoid process is driven into the spinal cord. Most injuries of this type do not result in death or neurological deficit. The hangman's fracture results in a fracture through the arch of vertebra C2. The patient is usually asymptomatic. Dislocation of a vertebra occurs when one vertebra overrides another and there is unilateral or bilateral facet dislocation. This injury usually results in ligamentous injury. A subluxation is a partial or incomplete dislocation of one vertebra over another.

A descriptive term used to convey the idea that the injury involves both a fracture and a dislocation is *fracture-dislocation.* Ligament injury and cord injury are usually present.

Spinal Stability. Vertebral fractures are classified as *stable* and *unstable.*[10] Models have suggested that stability of the cervical spine is maintained if all the anterior and posterior ligaments plus one additional structure are intact.[8] Even though an injury may be described as acutely unstable, delayed stability can occur depending on the relative presence of bony and ligamentous injury. Injuries with significant bony injury may be acutely unstable; however, bony healing can result in stability of the injury. This is in sharp contrast to injuries in which ligamentous damage predominates. These fractures are chronically unstable.

Type of Injury. Spinal cord injury occurs secondary to concussion, contusion, hemodynamic changes, transection, or damage to blood vessels supplying the cord and biochemical derangements.

A concussion of the spinal cord causes a temporary loss of function lasting 24 to 48 hours. It is due to a severe shaking of the cord. No identifiable neuropathological changes are noted on examination of the cord.[21]

Contusion of the spinal cord is a bruising of the cord that includes bleeding into the cord with subsequent edema and possible necrosis from cord compression. The extent of neurological deficit depends on the severity of the contusion and the presence of necrosis.[10, 23]

A transection is a severing of the cord and can be complete or incomplete. Complete physical transection of the cord is rare, but complete physiological transection is frequently seen.

Damage to the anterior spinal artery or the two posterior spinal arteries results in cord ischemia and necrosis. This type of injury can be likened to a "stroke" of the spinal cord. Episodes of ischemia can cause temporary deficits; prolonged ischemia and the resultant necrosis will cause permanent deficits.

The hemodynamic changes that occur in the spinal cord are a major factor in the evolution of spinal cord damage. An acute spinal cord injury produces instantaneous as well as prolonged systemic and local cord hemodynamic changes that have a profound effect on the outcome of the lesion. Autoregulation is lost during the acute phase of injury, resulting in a profound decrease in blood flow.[23–26] The hemodynamic changes seen in the spinal cord cause an ischemic injury to the cord.[8, 26, 27]

The biochemical derangements following acute cord injury are quite diverse. Initially, lactic acid accumulates in the injured tissue. This lactic acid accumulation sets in motion a series of events involving the release of prostaglandins leading to vasoconstriction and vasospasm.[8] The end result is further cord ischemia.

Classification by Functional Changes. Neurological injuries are described as complete, partial (incomplete), or root injury. A complete injury reflects total loss of conscious motor and sensory function below the level of injury. An incomplete injury spares some motor or sensory function. A root lesion impairs function of the motor ability and sensation in the distribution of one nerve root. Incomplete injuries occur more often than complete injuries. The incomplete injuries result in particular syndromes (Table 18–3).

The *anterior spinal cord syndrome* is most often associated with a flexion injury and most commonly with cervical cord injuries.[11, 28] The patients present with loss of motor, pain, and temperature function below the level of injury, with dorsal column function preserved. This syndrome is associated with injury to the anterior spinal artery causing ischemia, and infarction to the anterior two thirds of the spinal cord.[9]

The *Brown-Séquard syndrome* is generally associated with a physiological hemisection of the spinal cord, causing ipsilateral loss of dorsal column function and motor function and a contralateral loss of pain and temperature sensation.[11, 12, 28] This syndrome is often associated with penetrating injuries or a rotational type of closed injury.

Commonly associated with the hyperextension injury is the *central cord syndrome.*[11, 12, 28] It is often seen in middle or older age groups. The picture presented by the patient is one of motor and sensory deficit that is greater in the upper than in the lower extremities.

RESUSCITATION CYCLE

Resuscitation of the patient with SCI begins with prehospital care and continues until a definite treatment plan is determined. The sophistication of prehospital management in the past decade has been the single most important factor in the improved prognosis of patients with SCI.[7, 23]

The cardinal principle in moving a patient with a suspected spine injury is to prevent any motion of the spine that can further damage the cord or nerve roots. It is also important to provide reassurance at this time to attempt to decrease anxiety so that the patient will remain still.

After stabilization, a patient should be transported quickly to an appropriate medical facility, preferably a trauma center. Respiratory and cardiovascular stabilization and the maintenance of immobilization remain the priorities initially. The neck must be immobilized throughout transport. If the patient is extremely agitated or restless, restraints may be utilized to prevent the patient from self-injury. (Psychosocial priorities are discussed elsewhere in this text.)

Respiratory insufficiency, further deterioration of vertebral stability, alteration in tissue perfusion, and alteration in temperature regulation are potential problems during the prehospital and resuscitation phases of care.

Respiratory Insufficiency

Respiratory insufficiency is one of the most serious threats to the patient with SCI. In fact, all quadriplegics and most paraplegics should be considered to have some degree of respiratory insufficiency until proven otherwise.[30] The insufficiency may be related to airway obstruction, intercostal or diaphragmatic respiratory muscle paralysis, associated thoracic or tracheal trauma, or aspiration.

Assessment of the patient's respiratory function is ongoing throughout all cycles of trauma care, since respiratory

TABLE 18–3. SPINAL CORD SYNDROMES

SYNDROME	ETIOLOGY	SYMPTOMS	
Brown-Séquard	Transverse hemisection of cord	Ipsilateral spastic paresis, loss of proprioception, touch and press sense Contralateral loss of pain and temperature Tracts involved: LPT—lateral pyramidal tract—descending motor tracts LST—lateral spinothalamic tract—ascending pain and temperature AST—anterior spinothalamic tract—ascending like touch PC—posterior cord	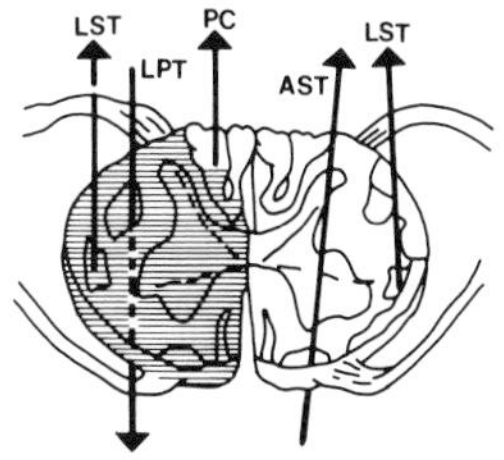
Central cord	Hyperextension injuries Disruption of blood flow to cord Swelling in the center of cord	Quadraparesis—greater in arms than legs	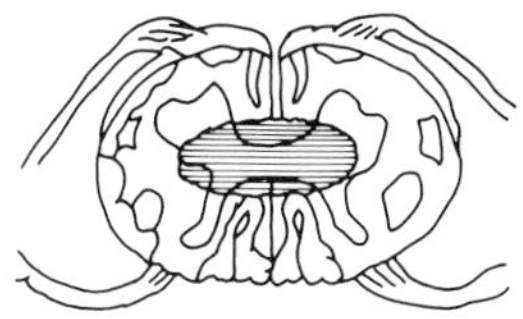
Anterior cord	Acute anterior cord compression or mechanical destruction of anterior cord Disruption of blood flow to anterior cord	Immediate, complete paralysis below lesion with loss of pain and temperature sensation below lesion; light touch, position, and vibration senses remain intact	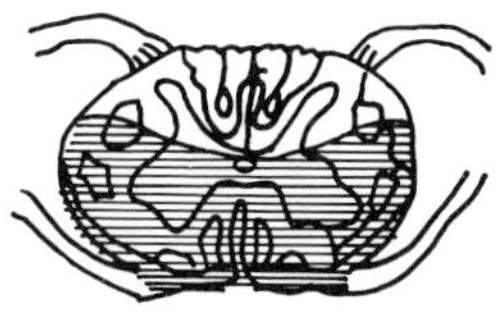

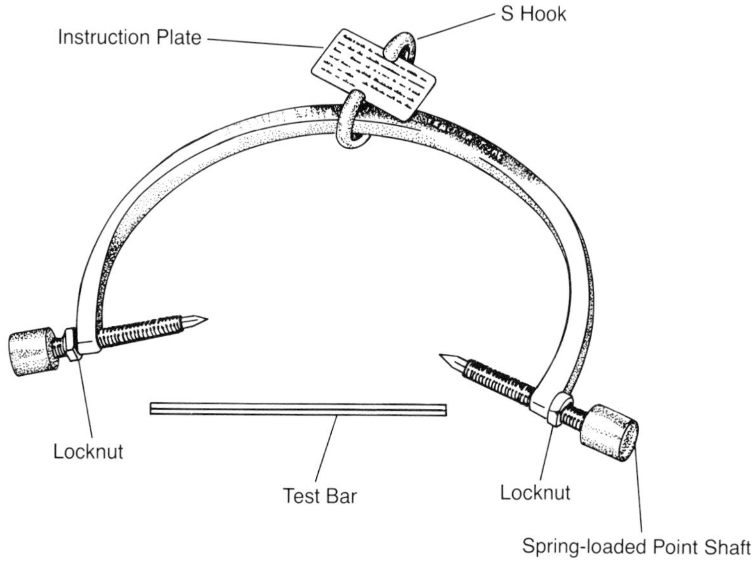

Figure 18–15. Gardner-Wells tongs.

failure is the leading cause of death for the quadriplegic patient. Arterial blood gases, continuous pulse oximetry, physical assessment of the chest, and chest films are all part of the assessment strategy for determining the respiratory status of the patient. It might be normal for a quadriplegic to have a chronic Pa_{O_2} in the range of 60 to 70 mm Hg and a high Pa_{CO_2} (45 to 60 mm Hg) due to the compromised respiratory musculature; however, during the few days immediately following the injury, this is not acceptable.[7, 11] Hypoxemia can only compromise the injured neurons and lead to an increased neuronal death at the injury site. A Pa_{O_2} of at least 80 mm Hg in conjunction with normalization of other parameters such as Pa_{CO_2} and saturation is the goal of treatment.

If the patient is experiencing respiratory insufficiency and ventilatory difficulty, immediate action needs to be taken to prevent hypoxemia, which can increase the extent of the neural damage. The establishment of an airway in a patient with SCI requires special consideration. Initially, the jaw-thrust or chin lift technique is used in an attempt to open the airway. Care must be taken not to manipulate the neck during establishment of the airway. Nasotracheal intubation is preferred by some, but oral intubation can be done if intubation is needed. The intubation can be performed relatively safely with the patient in Gardner-Wells tongs and with the neck aligned.[29] Tracheostomy or cricothyroidotomy is usually avoided initially, because it compromises the ability to do an anterior cervical procedure should one be needed.

Patients with an injury at the C4 level and above will definitely require intubation and ventilation owing to the loss of phrenic innervation and useful respiratory function. Patients with a C5 injury may or may not require ventilatory support, depending on arterial blood gases and respiratory parameters. An injury below C5 usually allows the patient to be managed with supplemental oxygen via a natural airway.

An understanding of the great potential for respiratory insufficiency guides the need for repeated respiratory assessment. Observation of the patient's breathing is essential. The presence of diaphragmatic breathing indicates a high cervical injury. Close attention to the arterial blood gases is essential to ensure adequate oxygenation. The nurse needs to be available to assist with the intubation of the patient if required. Frequent respiratory assessment during the resuscitation phase is critical.

Further Deterioration of Vertebral Stability

During resuscitation, there is always the potential to cause further neurological injury from movement of the vertebral column. Immobilization must be maintained throughout the resuscitation phase. Generally a hard collar, such as a Philadelphia collar, Stiff Neck, or Nec-Lok, will be maintained on the patient throughout this cycle. Cervical traction is applied to assist in immobilizing the spine, to pull the bones into alignment, and to relieve spinal cord compression. Several devices can be used in applying cervical traction, e.g., Gardner-Wells tongs (Fig. 18–15) or the halo ring (Fig. 18–16). With the Gardner-Wells tongs, a 50-cent-piece-size area is shaved above the anterosuperior aspect of both ears. The area is prepared with povidone-iodine (Betadine) and infiltrated with a local anesthetic. The tongs are placed and tightened with pliers or a calibrated torque or pressure wrench to ensure that they will not become dislodged. With the halo ring, the anterior pin sites are placed one fingerbreadth above the eyebrows. The posterior pins are placed behind the ear. The posterior pin sites are shaved. All sites are cleaned with Betadine and infiltrated with a local anesthetic. The pins are then placed and tightened with a torque wrench. All equipment for tong insertion or halo ring application should be readily available in the emergency department. In cases of cervical cord injury without obvious spinal disruption, usually 10 lb of traction is applied to prevent flexion or turning of the neck. If vertebral subluxation is apparent on plain films, then the usual rule of initiating traction is to start with 5 lb per vertebral level to initially reduce the injury.[7, 8] Once reduction is attained, weights are slowly reduced to a minimum holding weight. In spite of traction and reduction, surgical intervention may be indicated to stabilize the vertebral column and/or relieve neural compression.

Frequent spinal cord assessment (as outlined previously) of motor and sensory function is necessary, particularly immediately after any manipulation of the patient (such as x-ray examination or tong insertion) to determine if the patient is changing neurologically. Changes noted at this time may be due to vertebral instability or to early spinal cord edema, although changes related to cord edema are generally not seen until about 12 hours after the injury. Careful recording of the assessment is also necessary so that accurate comparisons can be made. Neuroradiological studies, as outlined in the assessment section, are done to determine the location, nature, and degree of neurological injury and to ensure that the appropriate treatment plan is instituted. There are multiple devices available that enable traction to be maintained when transporting the patient to diagnostic tests. These include the Scoop stretcher, the Suc-off board, and the Tactical Alignment Cervical Immobilization Transport (TACIT) Vest by Minto Research and Development (Redding, CA).

Assisting with the application of traction devices is a major role for the nurse during this phase. All necessary equipment, including traction rope and weights, must be ready. Preparing the patient for diagnostic testing and surgery, if needed, is also part of the nurse's role. Explaining the procedures being done and the neuroradiological tests to be performed will help allay the patient's anxieties.

The patient will be frightened during this phase. Reassurance and information giving are important nursing interventions during this time. Psychological numbness (refer to Chapter 10) also may occur.

Alteration in Tissue Perfusion

Spinal Shock

Bony compression of the spinal cord and the severe hypotension and bradycardia seen with patients in neurogenic shock contribute to decreased spinal cord perfusion. This decrease in perfusion causes ischemia and can lead to necrosis of the injured spinal cord segment.[8] Rapid initiation of traction to reduce the bony compression is used in an attempt to improve circulation to the injured spinal cord by reducing the pressure caused by an impinging bone fragment. Other experimental methods that have been studied to deal with the decreased blood flow and reduced oxygenation to the damaged area include hyperbaric oxygenation therapy[31–33] and spinal cord cooling to reduce the metabolic demand of the cord.[34–38] Unfortunately, these interventions have not improved outcome as much as hoped.[39]

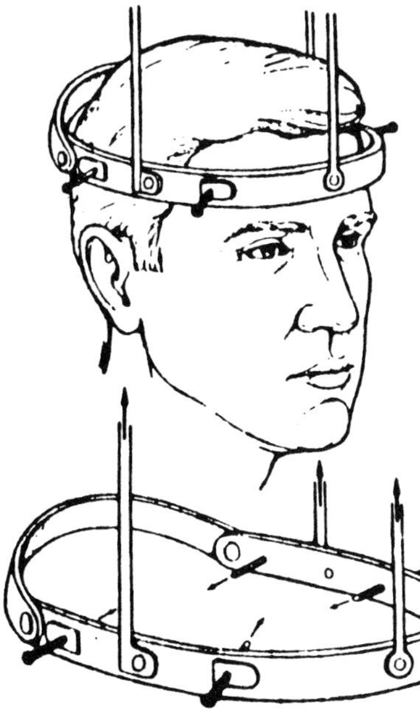

Figure 18–16. Halo ring.

Treatment

Recently, the focus of treatment has turned to preventing the secondary damage related to the release of endogenous factors stimulated by ischemia and hypoxia of the cord. Antagonism of these factors could limit the extent of the secondary injury and improve the ultimate clinical outcome. Various factors have been identified as potential contributors to this secondary injury: free radicals, catecholamines, arachidonic acid metabolites, and changes in glucose utilization, oxygen utilization, or calcium flux. Opiate antagonists have been shown to improve spinal cord blood flow and ultimate neurological recovery in animal studies.[40, 41, 43] Naloxone is currently being studied in a multicenter trial. The drug is given within 6 hours of injury.[40, 41, 43] Another experimental agent being studied is thyrotropin-releasing hormone (TRH).[42, 43] These drugs are given to block the activation of endorphins and encephalins, which are postulated to have an effect on the circulation in the injured cord, causing further ischemia. It is felt that these drugs can improve spinal cord blood flow in the injured area.[40–43]

In 1990, the National Acute Spinal Cord Injury Study Group II released the findings of a study that compared three treatments—placebo, high-dose naloxone, and high-dose methylprednisolone—administered to acutely injured patients. The data demonstrated that high-dose methylprednisolone (i.e., a bolus of 30 mg/kg followed by a 23-hour infusion of 5.4 mg/kg per hour) started within 8 hours of the injury resulted in measurable improvement in both motor and sensory function. Naloxone was shown to be ineffective in this study.[44]

Another recently released study by Geisler and associates[23] demonstrated that monosialotetrahexosylganglioside (GM I), a protein that causes axonal sprouting, enhances the functional recovery of damaged neurons. More studies with GM I need to be done to determine its true efficacy in treating spinal cord injury.

Other agents being evaluated in the immediate intervention for spinal cord injury include calcium channel blockers and lazaroids (a synthetic corticosteroid). Research continues to be done to find the best treatment during the acute phase of care.

Another advance in the resuscitative management of the spinal cord–injured patient is treatment of the neurogenic shock that results in severe hypotension, bradycardia, and thermoregulatory dysfunction. Vasopressor agents, such as dopamine, isoproteronol (Isuprel), or dobutamine, are administered to stabilize the cardiovascular status and increase the blood pressure. The goal of this therapy is to maintain a mean arterial blood pressure of 80 mm Hg or greater. Vasopressors are titrated to attain the goal mean pressure.

Continual monitoring of the vital signs with special attention to the blood pressure is critical. Hemodynamic monitoring utilizing a pulmonary artery catheter is preferred during the neurogenic shock period. Determining the cause of hypotension in these patients is very important. If the hypotension is related to poor systemic vascular resistance, then vasopressor agents will be effective, but if the hypotension is related to hypovolemia from other injuries, fluid replacement is essential. Hemodynamic monitoring enables appropriate fluid replacement and guides vasopressor titration. Hourly reports of the mean arterial pressure, pulmonary artery pressure, and central venous pressure should be documented. Cardiac output measurements should be obtained at least every 12 hours. A cardiac output in the high normal range up to 1.5 to 2 times normal is desirable. Monitoring of the arterial blood gases is also important to ensure adequate oxygenation to meet the increased tissue demand at this time.

The key role of the nurse is assessment and monitoring of the overall patient status during this phase of care. Accurate documentation of the vital signs, hemodynamic parameters, and neurological status is critical in the first few hours after the injury to assess for trends that might indicate deterioration of the patient's condition.

Alteration in Temperature Regulation

Injury above the thoracolumbar outflow of the sympathetic nervous system results in a loss of the hypothalamic thermoregulatory function. The patient experiences a lack of internal temperature control below the level of the lesion, mainly from an absence of vasoconstriction and loss of the abilities to shiver, to conserve heat, and to sweat to dissipate heat. There is a continual loss of body heat, and the patient exhibits poikilothermia, a condition in which the patient tends to assume the temperature of the environment. Depending on the time of the year that the trauma is experienced, a patient can present in severe hypothermia with a temperature less than 35°C (95°F). The higher the injury level, the more severe are the effects of this loss of thermoregulation.

Continual monitoring of the temperature via a rectal probe or pulmonary artery catheter is important. The goal is to attain and maintain normothermia in these patients. Adequate measures must be taken to warm the patient. Placing the patient on a warming blanket, adding blankets, giving warm baths, applying heat lamps, using warmed IV fluids, and using heat-conserving materials such as space blankets can be effective in warming the patient. Occasionally, the problem may be that the patient is too warm, especially in the summer or in warm areas of the country. The goal then is to help the patient dissipate body heat. A fan can be used to cool a warm patient. Providing moisture to the body also can help: water vapor sprayed on the skin can act as perspiration to promote heat loss through evaporation.

Anxiety

If the patient is awake, fear may be the patient's biggest problem and can be aggravated by the shock state. Continual reassurance by the nursing staff is important to help allay anxiety and fear. Touch is an important way to reassure the patient and provide a feeling of caring. The patient with SCI has limited sensory input, so the parts of the body with sensation should be the focus of the touch, such as the face. Maintaining eye contact when speaking to the patient is also important. The nurse should take time to adequately prepare the patient for transfer to the operating room or the intensive care unit.

Throughout the immediate postinjury phase, physiological stabilization of the patient is the major goal. The neuroradiological diagnosis made at this time will determine if the patient is transferred to the operating room or the intensive care unit following resuscitation.

OPERATIVE CYCLE

Although the decision to operate on the patient lies with the neurosurgeon, certain general guidelines in the decision-making process are listed here:[7]

1. Patients with no evidence of external pressure being exerted on the spinal cord and who are stable in traction are transferred to the intensive care unit.
2. Patients with no evidence of external pressure but with radiological evidence of spinal instability are transferred to the intensive care unit, where they are immobilized on a special bed such as a Stryker frame or kinetic treatment table. (The choice of bed will depend on the degree of bony instability, location of injury, associated injuries, patient tolerance and safety, nursing experience, and physician preference.) Seven to 10 days after injury, surgery will be done to either fuse the bones of the neck or place the patient in a halo apparatus.
3. Patients with neuroradiological evidence of extrinsic spinal cord compression that traction and/or manipulation has failed to relieve are taken immediately to the operating room. Surgery is performed to reestablish the integrity of the spinal column by realigning the column, decompressing the spinal cord and/or its nerve roots, and stabilizing the column by fusion. The procedures are more commonly done in thoracic and lumbar injuries and in the case of cervical bilateral locked facets, which are intractable to realignments.
4. Patients with penetrating wounds primarily involving the spinal column and its surrounding soft tissues without any other system damage may or may not be surgical candidates. Cervical level injuries are explored if a bullet is in the spinal canal and impinging on the cord or its nerve roots. Patients with incomplete thoracic and cervical gunshot wounds are considered surgical candidates, as are those with lumbar wounds. Most often, complete lesions will not be explored, since surgery does not generally result in an improvement of neurological function.

Surgical procedures performed on patients with acute SCI include spinal cord and nerve root decompression by means of spinal column realignment and, when necessary, removal of bone, soft tissue, or foreign bodies from the canal. These procedures are generally combined with spinal column stabilization with the use of one or more of the following: bone grafts, wire, or metal instrumentation.[7] The overall goal of the operative intervention is to provide early stabilization, permitting early mobilization, thus preventing or minimizing the risks of secondary neurological injury as well as the systemic complications associated with prolonged immobility.[45]

Routine care during the operative procedure is really no different for a patient with SCI than for any other surgical patient. Throughout the operative phase the hemodynamic status should be monitored carefully, since the potential for hemodynamic instability remains a constant problem. Hypotension, low cardiac output, and bradycardia will compromise perfusion to the injured spinal cord as well as to other vital organs. During surgical procedures for thoracic and lumbar injuries, large volumes of blood loss also contribute significantly to cardiovascular instability. Invasive monitoring throughout the operative procedure is required via a pulmonary artery catheter and an arterial line. Fluid intake and output must be assessed frequently to prevent fluid overload and ensure adequate urinary output. Attention to the patient's temperature to prevent further hypothermia is also a priority.

CRITICAL CARE CYCLE

Once stabilization has occurred, with or without surgery, the patient with neurological deficit is transferred to the intensive care unit for management. Prior to the 1970s, cord-injured patients were seldom cared for in the intensive care unit. It was generally felt at that time that there was little to be done for the acutely injured patient and that intensive care would not make a difference. Now with the concern over the cardiovascular and pulmonary complications associated with SCI, initial critical care management has become routine.

Every system of the body is affected by SCI, and a holistic approach to care throughout the critical care cycle is essential. Cardiopulmonary complications remain the major causes of death in the critical care phase of treatment.[7] These complications tend to be more profound in patients with cervical injuries.

The focus of attention during the critical care cycle is on the cardiovascular and respiratory systems. The goal is to prevent any life-threatening complications while maximizing the functioning of all systems. The cardiovascular complications are those seen during the resuscitative cycle, i.e., hypotension, bradycardia, and poikilothermia.

Alteration in Cardiac Output

Hypotension

The hypotension seen in these patients is related to the loss of the sympathetic outflow. Vasodilation and decreased venous return are responsible for the decreased cardiac output, not a hypovolemic state, unless the patient has other injuries. Judicious fluid replacement must be done to prevent pulmonary edema and congestive heart failure in patients who are unable to handle the additional fluid load. As mentioned in the resuscitation cycle, the use of vasopressors such as dopamine has been recommended to treat the cardiovascular instability. The patient will remain hypotensive and bradycardic throughout his lifetime, but cardiovascular stability will usually return within 72 hours.

Hemodynamic monitoring with a pulmonary artery catheter should be instituted. Parameters should be corrected as needed so as not to overtreat the patient. This monitoring is maintained for at least 72 hours or until cardiovascular stability is attained.

Bradycardia

The sympathetic blockade is also responsible for the bradycardia seen in the cervical spinal cord–injured patient. In addition to bradycardia, junctional escape beats, atrioventricular blocks, supraventricular tachycardia, and premature atria and ventricular complexes may be seen.[45] The dysrhythmias also may be aggravated by hypothermia and hypoxia. If the patient is symptomatic from the bradycardia, atropine, which should be at the bedside, may be given.[7,8,11] Prolonged therapy is required in rare instances and may include temporary transvenous pacing.[45]

Constant cardiac monitoring is maintained in all patients with acute SCI. Auscultation of the heart is also important. Blood work analysis to examine serum enzyme levels can be useful in detecting ischemic heart problems, which may be preexisting or due to other injuries.

Vasovagal Response

A vasovagal response may occur in these patients in addition to the bradycardia already discussed. Stimulation, such as rapid position changes or deep tracheal suctioning, is believed to trigger the vasovagal reflex. Massive activation of the parasympathetic nervous system unchecked by the sympathetic nervous system can lead to cardiac arrest.[46,47]

To ensure adequate cardiovascular function in the preceding three disorders, nursing care focuses on preserving adequate pumping action of the heart, maintaining desirable blood volume and composition, and promoting blood flow in the peripheral vascular system.[9,21]

Preventing hypoxia and minimizing the workload of the heart will preserve cardiac function. Attention to the respiratory status to ensure adequate oxygenation in the face of a low cardiac output is critical. Allowing the patient frequent rest periods and minimizing the patient's stress will help to reduce the heart workload.

Close observation of the fluid and electrolyte balance in the patient and prompt treatment of imbalances will assist in maintaining desirable blood volume and composition and prevent further cardiac compromise. Intravenous fluid administration and electrolyte replacement therapy are important components of management in the critical care phase.

Promoting blood flow through the paralyzed limbs will increase the venous return to the heart. The immobility of the patient imposed by the injury and the intensive care unit environment contribute to poor venous return from the extremities. Dependent edema also may be noted in these patients. Range-of-motion exercises should be started as soon as possible after admission. Antiembolic stockings and alternating pressure devices on the legs (see Chapter 21) can be used to promote venous return and prevent the pooling of blood in the periphery. Measurement of thighs and calves should be done every shift for the first 72 hours and then every day to detect swelling in the extremities, which may indicate lower extremity deep vein thrombosis from venous pooling of blood. Once it is determined that there is no internal bleeding from other injuries, the patient may be started on prophylactic heparin to prevent clot formation. Kinetic therapy that keeps the patient in constant motion for 16 to 20 hours per day also has a positive effect on the cardiovascular status of the patient.[49] Early mobilization of the patient from the bed to a chair is still seen as the best way to decrease the cardiovascular sequelae from immobility.

The patient must be adequately oxygenated prior to suctioning to help prevent the vasovagal response. Changing the position of the patient in bed should be done slowly. The rectum should be checked frequently for stool, which also can trigger a vasovagal response.

Alteration in Respiratory Function

Altered respiratory function is a major problem for the patient with a cervical or high thoracic injury. If the injury is at or above the level of C4, the patient will be ventilator-dependent with loss of all ability to breathe spontaneously because of the loss of diaphragmatic action due to phrenic nerve disruption. Even if the injury occurs below C4, spinal cord edema and hemorrhage can affect the upper cervical cord and interfere with normal respiratory effort, causing ineffective breathing patterns. Prophylactic endotracheal intubation is utilized, especially in quadriplegics.[7, 29, 30] Paralysis of abdominal and intercostal muscles will aggravate the respiratory insufficiency and lead to an ineffective cough and retention of secretions. The respiratory management of these patients must be very aggressive. Even if the patient is able to breathe spontaneously, pulmonary toilet remains very aggressive.

Complications

Aspiration and pneumonia are two common complications in the patient with acute SCI. Aspiration may occur at the time of trauma. Pneumonias tend to develop within the first few weeks of hospitalization and are usually related to immobilization, aspiration, and placement of an artificial airway. Adult respiratory distress syndrome may follow the onset of aspiration or pneumonia and may also be attributed to the presence of a shock state. Pulmonary edema in this patient population can be attributable to fluid overload during initial management. Pulmonary emboli are also frequently seen in the first few weeks following injury in these patients. They generally arise from dislodgment of a deep vein thrombosis in the lower extremities or pelvis.[30]

Physical assessment of the chest, including observation, inspection, palpation, percussion, and auscultation, should be done frequently during the first 72 hours following injury. It is important to note the rate, depth, and type of respiration (i.e., abdominal, diaphragmatic). Chest expansion and abdominal movement should be observed to determine the muscle groups being used for respiration. Diagnostic procedures can be used to assist in determining actual respiratory function. Pulmonary function tests performed at the bedside can help to guide ventilation support. Tidal volume, inspiratory and expiratory reserve volumes, residual volume, total lung capacity, and functional residual capacity, as well as vital capacity, should be assessed routinely. Serial blood gas analysis and continuous pulse oximetry also will assist in guiding required supplemental oxygen or ventilatory support, if any is needed. Initially, the $Pa{O_2}$ should be maintained at or above 80 mm Hg, since systemic hypoxemia may increase the severity of the SCI.[47] In addition to observing the $Pa{O_2}$ closely, one must also monitor the $Pa{CO_2}$ carefully. The quadriplegic patient will tend to retain carbon dioxide because of hypoventilation. Chest films should be obtained daily to rule out pulmonary complications and to initiate treatment early.

Prevention of pulmonary complications is the major role of nursing in the critical care cycle. Initiating and maintaining aggressive pulmonary toilet, including frequent chest physiotherapy, is critical in the first 72 hours after injury and ongoing throughout hospitalization. Chest physical therapy is performed every 4 hours whether the patient is on a ventilator or not and regardless of the type of bed on which the patient is being maintained. Patients with spinal cord injury may be safely placed in the Trendelenburg position to facilitate postural drainage during chest physical therapy. A patient in a halo vest can be turned onto his side, and one side of the vest can be loosened to perform the therapy. Prevention of retained secretions is a priority of care. The subtle signs of respiratory insufficiency may include a decreased level of consciousness, increased confusion and restlessness, increased rapid, shallow breathing, and tachycardia.

The loss of intercostal and abdominal muscles affects the patient's ability to cough. The quad-assist cough is used to replace the abdominal muscles of the patient during the expiratory phase of a cough. The patient is asked to take three or four breaths. On the expiratory phase of the last breath, the nurse places a fist or the heel of the hand between the umbilicus and xiphoid process and pushes very hard upward during the cough. Performed correctly and frequently, this maneuver can be very effective in assisting the patient to clear secretions. It generally needs to be repeated several times and eventually will be effective enough to replace tracheal suctioning.

The patient with a C5 or lower motor level of injury is generally able to successfully wean off the ventilator. Weaning a patient with a unilateral or partial C5 motor level can be a very slow and tedious process and requires a multidisciplinary approach. Physical therapists and respiratory therapists can assist in doing exercises with the patient to build up tolerance for breathing without the assistance of the ventilator. Abdominal binder use can enhance effective diaphragm movement and improve the patient's respiratory capability. Anxiety is common during the weaning process, because the patient fears dying due to an inability to breathe. The nurse must remain with the patient during weaning periods and attempt to allay the fears. Weaning generally occurs during the intermediate cycle of care.

Throughout the hospitalization, the nurse must observe for the signs and symptoms of pulmonary infection, e.g., temperature elevation and increased sputum production. A respiratory infection may represent a setback to the patient being weaned or cause increased muscle fatigue related to the need to cough frequently.

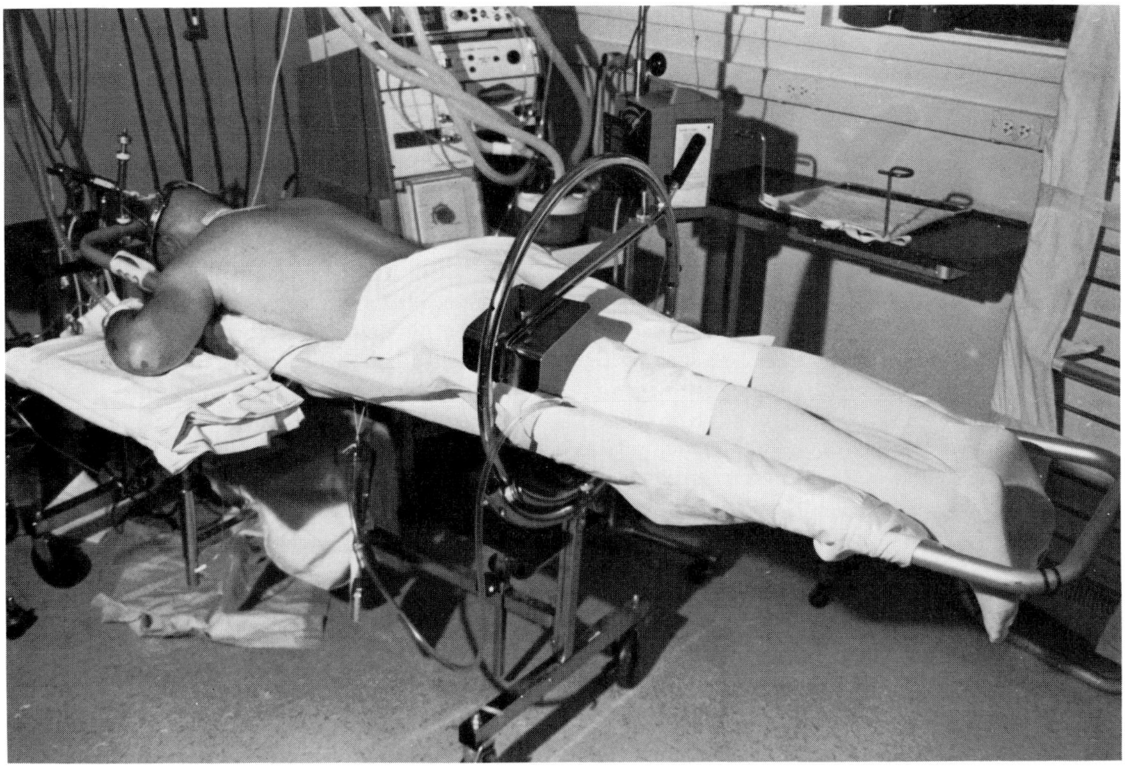

Figure 18–17. Stryker frame.

Alteration in Nutrition

The gastrointestinal system undergoes physiological change as a result of the SCI during the critical care cycle. Gastrointestinal paralysis is often combined with a state of relative ischemia. This can precipitate gastrointestinal ulceration and hemorrhage. Without treatment, gastrointestinal paralysis routinely causes constipation with possible subsequent obstruction.[47, 48] Placement of a Salem sump nasogastric tube and gastric suction are done initially to prevent the accumulation of gastric secretions, allow monitoring of the gastric pH, and enable instillation of antacids. Spinal cord–injured patients generally present with a paralytic ileus, which allows fluid and gas to accumulate in the bowel, a condition that is usually alleviated by decompression with low suction. These individuals are also especially prone to stress ulceration because of the increased acidity of the gastric contents related to the unopposed vagal outflow. Antacids are recommended if gastric pH is less than 4 and may be combined with routine doses of hydrogen ion blocking agents such as cimetidine or the use of glycopyrrolate (Robinul). Another complication encountered in the spinal cord–injured patient is acute pancreatitis. Patients with pancreatitis are maintained with constant low suction and are supported with hyperalimentation until their serum and urine amylase levels return to normal.[7]

As soon as bowel sounds return, the gastric tube is removed and a diet is started. The presence or absence of bowel sounds should be assessed on admission and at least once per shift until bowel sounds return. Patients with high spinal cord injury should have their swallowing ability evaluated when oral feedings are started. Measurement of the abdominal girth can document increasing distention due to occult bleeding or gas. Laboratory values, including serum albumin, hemoglobin, hematocrit, and creatinine, should be obtained routinely to assess nutritional status. Caloric intake should also be recorded to ensure adequate nutrition.

Checking the gastric pH as ordered and treating low pH can prevent gastrointestinal hemorrhaging. If hemorrhaging does develop, gastric lavage and/or intra-arterial infusion of vasopressin may be necessary to control gastric bleeding.[50, 51] Adequate metabolic support must be provided during the critical care phase. The caloric needs of the patient are increased during the catabolic phase of injury. Total parenteral nutrition or tube feedings can be used during the critical care phase of injury to provide the needed nutritional requirements.

Further Deterioration of Vertebral Stability

Although the patient is stabilized and immobilized during the resuscitation cycle, there always remains the potential for a loss of vertebral alignment and additional mechanical insult to the spinal cord. Early immobilization is most often accomplished by the application of Gardner-Wells tongs or a halo ring with online cervical traction. Upon entering the intensive care unit, the patient is usually cared for on a specialized bed that helps to maintain spinal stability. Stryker frames and kinetic treatment tables are two beds commonly used to manage the spinal cord–injured patient in traction. The recently introduced Bremmer in-line-traction board allows the patient to be cared for in a regular bed while traction is maintained.

The Stryker or wedge turning frame (Fig. 18–17) is the

most widely used bed at the present time. It consists of an anterior and a posterior frame so that the patient can be turned supine and prone. One advantage of this frame is the simplicity of operation: Only one person is required to turn it even though another person must function as a spotter for safety purposes. The bed also allows accessibility to all body areas for good skin care, and the patient can be placed in the Trendelenburg position for pulmonary toilet.[52] (See SCI Master Care Plan, Appendix 6–1.)

The kinetic treatment table (Fig. 18–18) was introduced in the United States in the late 1970s. A patient on this bed is rotated slowly in a 60- to 60-degree arc from left to right almost continuously (16 to 20 hours per day). The continuous motion decreases the complications associated with immobility. A system of hatches and flaps permits access to all areas of the body without compromising spinal stability.[49, 52]

At the Neurotrauma Center of the Maryland Institute for Emergency Medical Services Systems, Dr. Fred Geisler devised a traction maintenance system that can be utilized on a regular bed. The Bremmer in-line-traction board (Fig. 18–19) is used in patients with unstable neck fractures requiring prolonged traction. The major advantage of this device is that the patient can be cared for in a regular bed and can feel more "normal." The patient can be turned side to side, and the head of the bed may be elevated without compromising the traction stability. This allows better sensory input. (*Note:* The number of degrees for side-lying and head-of-bed elevation using this device must be specified for each patient by the neurosurgeon.)

Continued neurological assessment of the motor and sensory status of the patient remains of prime importance. The patient's tolerance of the bed on which he is being cared for should also be assessed. Many patients are anxious when turning on the Stryker frame, and a few patients are unable to tolerate the constant motion of the kinetic treatment table.

Frequent checking of the placement of the tongs or pins is important to ensure that they are not displaced. Pin sites are inspected and cleaned at least every shift. Traction must be maintained at all times. The traction knot should always rest 1 to 2 in below the pulley, and the weights should hang freely.

When caring for a patient on the Stryker frame in the critical care unit, extreme care must be taken not to dislodge any monitoring devices, intravenous lines, or tubes. It is best to drape all cable lines and tubes over the top frame before turning the patient. Potential pressure areas such as the chin and shoulders should be inspected frequently and padded to prevent skin breakdown.[53]

The patient on a kinetic treatment table will benefit most from the bed if it can be in almost continual motion.[49, 52] Care should be scheduled in blocks of time so that the turning of the bed is minimally interrupted. The skin along the side pads must be checked for reddening, and all potential pressure points must be monitored for breakdown.

Fear Related to the Psychological Impact of the Injury

Fear is one of the overriding emotions during the critical care cycle. Acute SCI is not only a devastating physiological injury but also an equally devastating psychological trauma. The sudden onset of paralysis does not allow time for any preparation by the patient. The fear the patient experiences at this time about the injury may be accompanied by anxiety generated by the environment of the intensive care unit, the lack of familiarity with the people delivering care, the feelings of total dependence and total helplessness, and the unknown future. Fear can be further intensified by sensory deprivation and an inability to communicate if the patient is intubated and on a ventilator. Managing the physical state of the patient does not always allow time for meaningful interpersonal conversations between the medical or nursing staff and the patient. In lieu of long conversations, use of touch, good eye contact, and patience can be very reassuring to the patient. The patient should be informed about the injury, the diagnosis, and the prognosis as soon as possible after the injury. The family and/or significant other also should be a part of these early discussions. This information will not ease the fears of the patient but will provide the patient with some reality so that he can begin to deal with those fears.

Questioning the patient and family about the patient's ability to cope with stress can be helpful in planning care. Past history of psychological functioning also can provide information about the present state of the patient. (See Chapter 10 for further assessment strategies.)

In order to help reduce the patient's fear, he must learn to trust the people who are administering care. Care givers who follow a consistent plan of care can help to establish early trust.[53–55] Patients who are able to talk should be allowed to verbalize their fears. Mechanisms that enable the intubated patient to communicate effectively (i.e., Passy-Muir tracheostomy, "talking" track, blink writer, or artificial larynx) should be tried as soon as possible. The nurse should be a receptive listener and be careful not to appear to be in a hurry. Time should be spent talking with patients to reinforce their feelings of self-worth and to allow them to ventilate their feelings.

During the critical care cycle, verbal communication is often not possible for the patient on a ventilator. The patient may resort to "clicking" to bring the nurse to the bedside and to call attention to himself. Clicking frequently becomes excessive, which can become annoying to the staff to the point where it becomes tuned out. The cause of clicking is multidimensional. It is used to alert the nurse of patient needs but also can be linked to fears and anxieties. It can be used to ventilate anger. The underlying cause for the clicking must be adequately assessed by the nurse. Attempts to alleviate the patient's fears and anxieties also can decrease the amount of clicking. Contracting is a useful tool for determining mutually agreed on situations when clicking is appropriate, e.g., severe shortness of breath or popping off of the ventilator.[53]

During the critical care phase, and indeed throughout the rest of the quadriplegic patient's life, many other problems that require nursing intervention are encountered. Since each patient is a unique individual, the priorities of care for each patient are also unique. In the critical care cycle, the priority of care is focused on the hemodynamic and pulmonary aspects, but the nurse also must provide holistic care during this phase of care. Impaired physical mobility, potential impairment of skin integrity, potential for infection, alteration in bowel elimination, and impairment of urinary elimination are all nursing diagnoses associated with the spinal

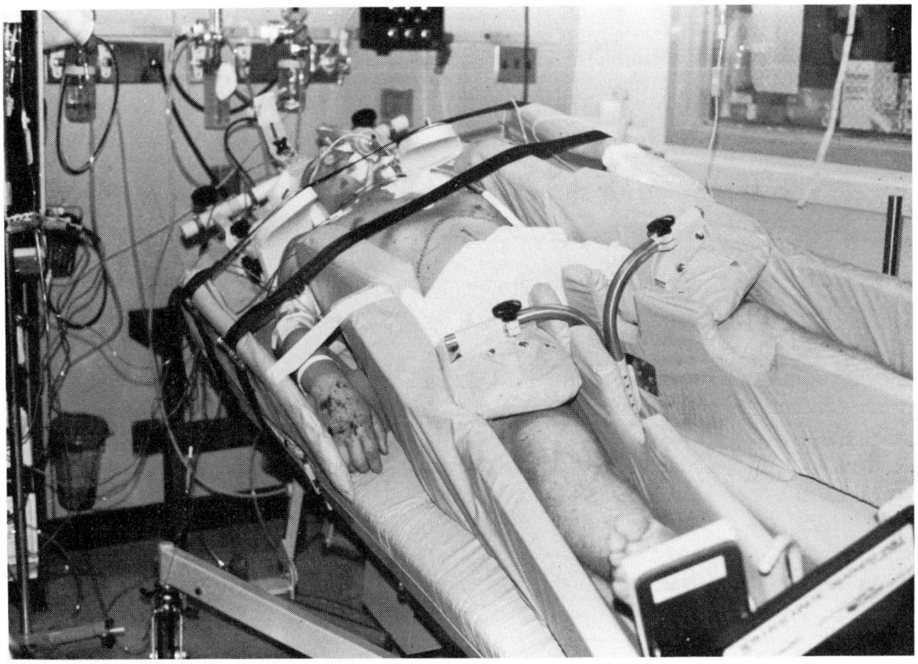

Figure 18–18. Kinetic treatment table.

cord–injured patient that occur at the time of the injury due to spinal shock and generally last throughout the patient's life. All these problems will require planning and intervention throughout the hospitalization. They will be discussed in more depth in the intermediate and rehabilitation phases of care, when these diagnoses emerge as priorities.

The critical care cycle of treatment is directed toward stabilizing the patient, treating life-threatening sequelae of the injury, and preparing the patient for intermediate care and rehabilitation. Rehabilitation is actually started during the critical care phase. Physical therapy, occupational therapy, and even speech therapy consultations can be obtained in the critical care unit, and plans for a rehabilitation program begun. This contact with the members of the rehabilitation

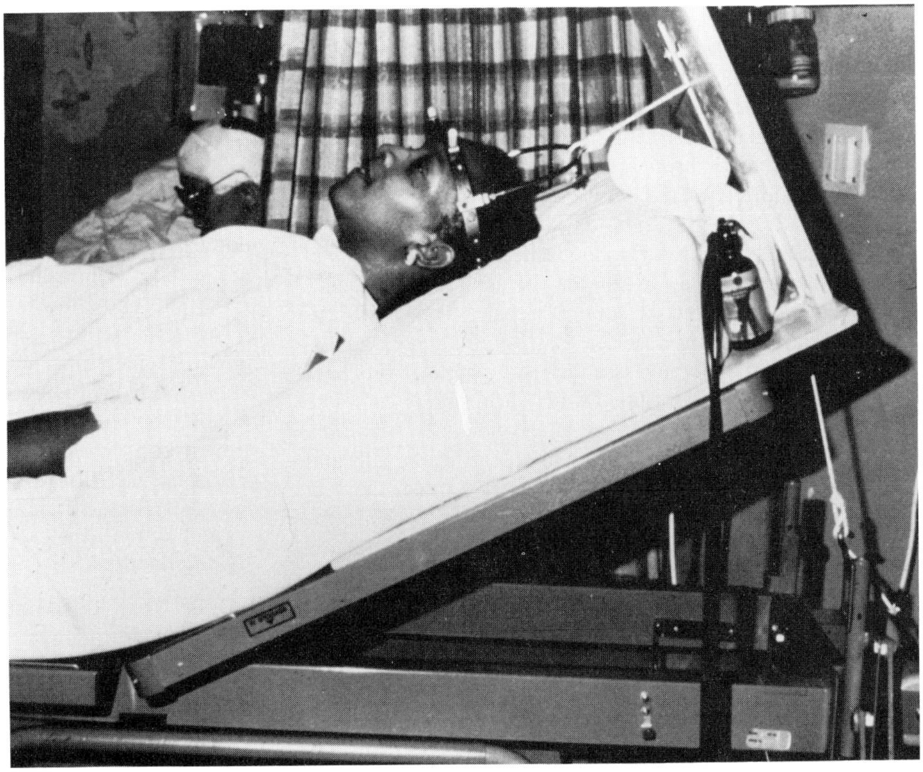

Figure 18–19. Bremmer in-line traction board.

team can help to make the transition from the intensive care unit to intermediate care a little easier, since a relationship will have been started between the patient, the patient's family, and the therapists.

INTERMEDIATE CARE/REHABILITATION CYCLE

The patient who is hemodynamically stable and able to maintain a mean arterial pressure between 60 and 80 mm Hg is ready to be transferred to intermediate care. This usually occurs approximately 1 to 2 weeks following the injury. Of course, patients with minimal neurological deficit may progress earlier to this stage. A patient with high cervical cord injury may be maintained with ventilatory support at this time but does not require the critical care unit. Tracheostomies are usually performed on this group of patients to enable them to eat and to maximize the use of their mouths. To enhance communication with these patients, a "talking" tracheostomy may be utilized.

The focus of care in the intermediate care unit is to begin to foster independence and to help the patient begin to adapt to the disability. The transition from critical care to intermediate care can be very frightening to the totally dependent patient. This fear can be exhibited by anger, frequent calling of the nurse, and/or withdrawal. Constant reassurance will be needed in the first few days following the transfer to a less intense environment.

Impaired Physical Mobility

Impaired physical mobility is really the basis for other patient problems. Mobilization is introduced on a gradual basis to minimize the effects of postural hypotension. X-ray examination may be ordered as the patient is mobilized 15 to 30 degrees at a time to ensure that the surgical repair or brace immobilization of the original injury site is stable. In patients with thoracic and lumbar injury, bracing is done to assist in stabilizing the fracture site. Range-of-motion exercises are continued throughout this phase of care to help retain and restore joint and muscle function. Muscle strengthening exercises are also begun, because atrophy and muscle weakness usually occur during the critical care cycle.

A halo apparatus (Fig. 18–20) may be applied as a primary treatment or to protect a surgical repair. This is a self-contained immobilization device that permits increased patient mobility. A halo ring is attached by metal struts to a fiberglass or plastic vest lined with sheepskin.[10, 56, 57] The patient is placed on a regular bed at this time (see Appendix 6–1). The pin sites should be cleaned at least every shift and inspected for any signs of infection. The skin under the vest should be checked at least daily for possible breakdown. Every nurse caring for the patient in a halo vest should know the proper procedure for removing the front of the vest should CPR be necessary.

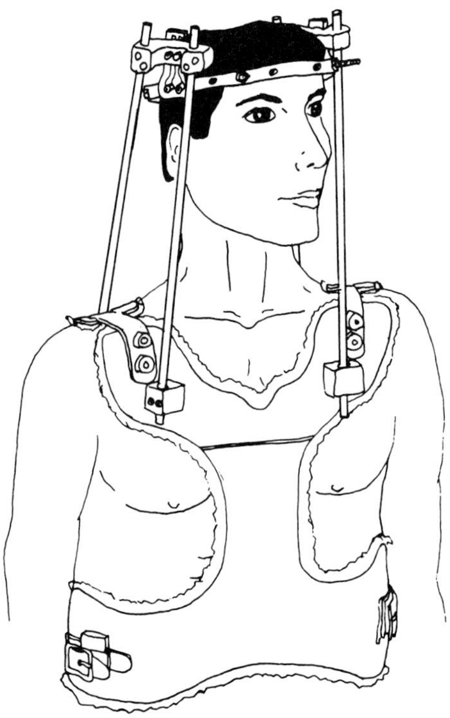

Figure 18–20. Halo vest. (From Patient Care Guide for the PMT Halo System. Chanhassen, MN, PMT Corp., Copyright, 1990.)

During the first phase of activity, pain may be experienced by the patient. Although some patients complain of bone pain or severe spasms during the critical care phase, pain can become a major problem during the intermediate care and rehabilitation cycle of care. If the patient does not receive adequate relief from pain and muscle spasms, he will not be willing to actively participate in the mobilization program. The sudden onset of severe pain during this time may indicate subluxation of the spine at the injury site and indicate that the spine is not stable enough to withstand the stress of movement.[7] Analgesia should be provided to the patient as needed prior to the beginning of physical activity.

The onset of hyperreflexia, increased muscle tone, and muscle spasms indicates that spinal shock is over. The injury that had been a lower motor neuron injury, with a flaccid paralysis, now converts to an upper motor neuron injury, reflecting the loss of cerebral control over muscle activity. Active rehabilitation begins when spinal shock is over. The spasms may be so severe at times that they interfere with mobilization of the patient. Antispasmodics such as dantrolene sodium (Dantrium) or baclofen are useful to minimize the spasms and allow mobilization to proceed.[58]

The spinal cord assessment will give information about muscle strength and sensory function. Muscle tone must also be assessed. Position sense and body coordination are important components of assessment in this phase. Patients with intact position sense and body awareness do better when performing activities of daily living, such as moving in bed or transferring to a chair.

Complications

Deep Vein Thrombosis. One major complication that can result from impaired physical mobility is deep vein thrombosis (DVT). The clinical incidence of DVT following injury to the spinal cord is about 15 per cent.[11, 57, 58] A significant precipitating factor in the patient with SCI is sluggish venous return to the heart. Impairment of vasomotor

TABLE 18–4. FUNCTIONAL GOALS FOR SPINAL CORD–INJURED PATIENTS

SPINAL CORD LEVEL	MUSCLE FUNCTION	FUNCTIONAL GOALS
C3–4	Neck control Scapular elevators	Manipulate electric wheelchair with mouth stick Limited self-feedings with ball bearing feeders Dress upper trunk Turn self in bed with arm slings
C5	Fair to good shoulder control Good elbow flexion	Propel wheelchair with handrim projections Self-feeding with handsplint Assist getting to and from bed
C6	Good shoulder control Wrist extension Supinators	Transfer from wheelchair to bed and car with or without minimal assistance Self-feeding with tenodesis hands Assist getting to and from commode chair
C7	Weak shoulder depression Weak elbow extension Some hand function	Independent in transfer to bed, car, and toilet Total dressing independence Wheelchair without handrim projections Self-feeding with no assistance devices
C8 to T4	Good to normal upper extremity muscle function	Wheelchair to floor and return Wheelchair up and down curb Wheelchair to tub and return
T5 to L2	Partial to good trunk stability	Total wheelchair independence Limited ambulation with bilateral long leg braces and crutches
L3 to L4	All trunk-pelvic stabilizers intact Hip flexors Adductors Quadriceps	Ambulation with short leg braces with or without crutches, depending on level
L5	Hip extensors, abductors, knee flexors, ankle control	No equipment needs if plantar flexion is enough for push off at end of stance

Boston University School of Nursing.

control, loss of muscle tone, and prolonged immobilization contribute to poor circulation in the lower extremities.

Prevention of DVT is a goal of care in these patients. Active and passive range-of-motion exercises, minidose heparin, antiembolization stockings, and alternating compression devices are used routinely as preventive measures. Venous punctures should be avoided in the lower extremities. Clotting factors and hemoglobin and hematocrit levels should be measured at least twice a week. Dehydration must be prevented or corrected. Prophylactic anticoagulant therapy may be ordered when the patient is no longer at risk for hemorrhage. Heparin (5000 units every 12 hours subcutaneously) has been shown to be a good prophylactic agent, although no definitive studies with spinal cord–injured patients have been published to date. Calf and thigh measurements should be documented daily to detect swelling in the lower extremities, which would indicate venous obstruction. The nurse should look for signs of redness, warmth, or swelling of veins in the legs. The temperature curve of the patient should be monitored: A low-grade fever without any apparent cause can be indicative of DVT.

If DVT is present, the patient is placed on bed rest and anticoagulation is begun with heparin. If anticoagulation is contraindicated, placement of a vena cava filter may be indicated. The goal then becomes prevention of pulmonary embolism, which can be fatal.

Heterotropic Ossification. Another complication of immobilization is the abnormal deposit of calcium in the joints known as *heterotropic ossification.* This deposit causes pain as well as difficulty moving the extremity involved. This complication occurs in 16 to 53 per cent of all SCI patients. Etidronate disodium (Didronel) can be used to prevent hypercalcemia and may be effective in preventing heterotropic ossification.

During patient mobilization, the nurse is constantly monitoring the patient's vital signs and observing for signs of cardiovascular insufficiency. Participation in active and passive range-of-motion exercises is important, as is knowing the entire mobilization plan, so that activities can progress even though a physical therapist may not be present.[10] Encouraging independence in the patient as skills are attained is important. An increase in the nurse's patience may be necessary, since the patient may take an extremely long time to perform an activity that the nurse could do quickly. Realistic activity goals should be set for the patient, depending on the level of injury (Table 18–4), to decrease the patient's as well as the nurse's frustration.

Potential Impairment of Skin Integrity

Patients with complete SCI lose all sensory appreciation and voluntary motor ability below the level of their lesion. The injury also causes alteration of the autonomic nervous system mechanisms that control blood vessels, which affects hemostasis and circulation. The lack of sensory warning mechanisms, inability to move freely, and circulatory changes pose the major threats to the skin integrity of the patient with SCI at any level. With poor blood flow to the skin, any prolonged pressure will cause skin breakdown, which is difficult to heal when circulation is poor. Along with pressure, shearing forces to the skin, such as those caused by pulling a patient across a sheet, also can cause a disruption in the skin integrity.

Evaluation of the skin combines visual observation and palpation. The skin should be observed for developing reddened pressure areas, especially over bony prominences. Orthotic devices such as the halo brace, thoracic braces, and splints can cause pressure on selected areas of the skin; thus it is important to remove these devices routinely and inspect the area under them carefully. A thorough nutritional assessment should be done to ensure that enough protein is included in the diet. An assessment of the patient's understanding of the potential for skin breakdown is essential, since the patient will have to give attention to skin care for the rest of his or her life (see Appendix 6–1).

Complication

Decubitus Ulcers. The development of a decubitus ulcer can create a long-term problem for the patient with SCI. These ulcers may lead to rehospitalization for sepsis or debridement of the area to promote healing. Plastic surgery may be necessary to close the wound. A severe ulcer may hinder the patient's rehabilitation, since the patient may have to be placed on bed rest and will not be able to participate in various therapies.

The overall goal of nursing care is to prevent a disruption in skin integrity. It has been demonstrated that localized changes from microscopic ischemic alterations in capillary blood flow due to pressure can be reversed if the pressure is relieved every 2 hours.[11, 59] Regular turning and bridging of bony prominences remain significant in prevention and treatment of pressure sores.[9, 59] Correct positioning of the patient is important. The patient should be moved carefully by lifting to avoid shearing and friction forces. When patients are sitting up in a wheelchair, they need to be encouraged to lift weight off their buttocks every 15 minutes. Specialty seat cushions that reduce pressure to the buttocks during sitting should be used when possible. Routine skin inspection should be done, and patients and their families should be taught how to inspect the skin routinely. Since this is a lifelong problem for the patient, patient education should focus on prevention techniques.

Alteration in Bowel Function

The location and completeness of the SCI determine the extent to which bowel function is altered. Generally, a few days after injury, bowel sounds return to normal, but bowel function does not. The level of the injury will dictate the type of alteration in bowel elimination the patient will experience. A cervical or thoracic injury is associated with spastic paralysis and an inability to feel the urge to defecate; the reflex activity for defecation remains intact. With an injury to the sacral cord segments in the conus medullaris or cauda equina, the reflex center for defecation is destroyed, and there is a loss of anal tone. Fecal retention and oozing of stool through the flaccid anal sphincter are associated with this type of injury (lower motor neuron damage).

This problem carries many psychological implications with it. The loss of bowel control causes a regression in patients who are forced to return to an earlier developmental time. Bowel control is generally achieved by the age of 3 years, and now patients must face this developmental task again. Many patients exhibit great difficulty in learning and adhering to a bowel program. This aspect of the injury is a true reflection of the loss of control the patient has experienced. Teaching the importance of regaining control and the tasks needed to achieve the control will help the patient to adapt to this dysfunction.

Establishment of a bowel program as soon after admission as possible is important to prevent constipation and to enhance psychological control. The use of stool softeners daily with every-other-day suppositories is a common program. If the patient has a high cervical or thoracic injury, digital stimulation is used to initiate a reflex bowel evacuation. With a flaccid bowel, digital stimulation is of no value. The goal is to set up a reliable and convenient bowel program that the patient will be able to perform or teach others involved in his care to manage.

A history of elimination patterns and problems is important in designing an appropriate bowel program for the patient. Routine physical assessment of the abdomen and rectal area also should be performed.

Complications

Constipation. Constipation is a common problem in patients with SCI. This complication is related to sluggish movement of the stool through the bowel. It may be aggravated by insufficient bulk in the diet, immobility, and low fluid intake. Manual evacuation of the stool from the rectum may be necessary. The established bowel program should be followed, and its effectiveness should be evaluated regularly. The patient should be checked for impaction daily (see Appendix 6–7).

Autonomic Dysreflexia. Autonomic dysreflexia or hyperreflexia is a life-threatening complication for the patient with an SCI above the T6 level.[60, 61] The onset of autonomic dysreflexia can occur any time after spinal shock is resolved. This complication can be caused by a variety of stimuli in the anesthetic area, including a full rectum, an overdistended bladder, or a decubitus ulcer. The stimuli create an exaggerated response of the sympathetic nervous system below the level of the lesion due to lack of control from higher centers. Autonomic dysreflexia is characterized by a sudden severe headache secondary to an uncontrolled elevation in blood pressure, which, if untreated, may progress to cerebral hemorrhage or myocardial infarction.[10, 61, 62] Although autonomic dysreflexia is more likely to occur during the first year after injury, it is considered a lifelong problem. Patients and their families should be taught that autonomic dysreflexia is a medical emergency. Besides the headache and the severe hypertension, the patient also may experience bradycardia or tachycardia, sweating and flushing above the level of the lesion and pallor and coolness below the level, nasal stuffiness, and unusual apprehension.[9, 10, 61] Nursing intervention is aimed at prevention of the syndrome. If the syndrome occurs, the patient should be placed in a sitting position in bed. The blood pressure and pulse must be monitored closely. The physician should be notified immediately. The source of the causative stimuli should be removed immediately; e.g., if the bladder is overdistended, an intermittent catheterization should be performed immediately, or if a Foley catheter is in place, it should be checked for kinks or plugging. Ganglionic blocking agents are required to disrupt the hyperreflexic state. Apresoline (hydralazine hydrochloride), 20 mg, may be given cautiously so as not to cause abrupt hypotension. Hyperstat (diazoxide), Procardia (nifedipine) or atropine sulfate also may be used.[61] Patients may be sent home with oral ganglionic blocking agents to be used in case of emergency. If the onset of the autonomic dysreflexia was during bowel evacuation, a local anesthetic applied to the rectum may decrease the chance of the syndrome's recurring.[9, 65, 68]

Alteration in Urinary Tract Function

Micturition is controlled by voluntary and autonomic means. Autonomic control is mediated by the sympathetic and parasympathetic systems. *Sympathetic* innervation is a result of afferent (sensory) fibers from the detrusor muscle to the hypogastric plexus to the spinal cord at the T9 to L2 region. Pain and proprioception travel via this circuit. Efferent fibers (motor) exit from T11 to L2 via the hypogastric plexus to the detrusor muscle and internal sphincter. The motor fibers provide movement to the internal sphincter and inhibition to the detrusor muscle during bladder filling.

The *parasympathetic system* receives afferent fibers from the bladder via the pudendal nerve to the S2, S3, and S4 spinal cord segments. The sensory fibers carry muscle stretch sensation, pain, touch, and possibly temperature. The efferent fibers exit from the spinal cord at S2 to S4 by way of the pelvic nerves to provide the detrusor muscle with motor action. The efferent fibers facilitate bladder emptying through contraction of the detrusor muscle and relaxation of the internal sphincter.

Voiding results from a series of events, culminating in the micturition reflex. Stretch receptors in the proximal urethra and bladder wall are stimulated by bladder fullness. This causes contractions of the detrusor muscle of the bladder wall. Afferent fibers carry signals to the sacral area of the spinal cord through the pelvic nerves and then return parasympathetic motor stimulation to the bladder. As the detrusor muscle contracts, relaxation of the internal and external sphincters occurs. The perineal musculature also relaxes to begin voiding. The pelvic musculature relaxation allows the urethra to fill with urine. The detrusor muscle continues to contract until the bladder empties. In conjunction with contraction of the bladder, the abdominal muscles and diaphragm contract as the glottis closes to cause an increase in intra-abdominal pressure. These actions enhance urination. Following urination, the bladder is closed off by reflex and voluntary contraction of the internal and external sphincters. The cycle repeats as the bladder fills to a volume of approximately 400 ml or 7 to 8 cm water pressure.

Following SCI, the bladder is areflexic-flaccid during the spinal shock phase. This is related to loss of reflexes and voluntary control after cord injury. As spinal shock resolves, bladder dysfunction can be evident in several areas. The detrusor muscle and sphincters can be individually affected, resulting in uncoordinated opening and closing of the sphincters and loss of contractibility of the detrusor muscle.[63]

The two most common types of neurogenic bladder are the flaccid bladder and reflex emptying type. *Reflex bladder* means that the reflex arc is intact, and once filling occurs in the bladder, then the detrusor is stimulated to contract, initiating nonvoluntary voiding. A *flaccid bladder* lacks the motor innervation to contract; therefore, the bladder continues to fill until urine overflows, but it never completely empties. There also can be bladder emptying problems due to asynchrony in the complex functions necessary for urinary elimination.

Inspection, palpation, and percussion of the abdomen with particular attention to the suprapubic area should be performed to determine the presence of bladder distention. Observation of urine color, odor, and concentration as well as measurement of urine output is important in determining the adequacy of the urinary system function. Diagnostic tests can give further information about bladder function. Urinalysis should be done routinely, particularly for the patient on an intermittent catheterization program (see Appendix 6–1). Urine culture and sensitivity are used at frequent intervals to monitor for urinary tract infections. An intravenous pyelogram may be performed early in the patient's hospital course to obtain information about the urinary system. Urodynamic tests, such as the cystometrogram, are used to diagnose the nature and extent of the neurological impairment to the bladder.

Initially following SCI, the patient is managed with an indwelling catheter. Accurate measurement of intake and output is needed during that time. Prior to removing the catheter, a fluid restriction of 2000 ml/day is imposed on the patient. The purpose of this restriction is to prevent large quantities of urine from remaining in the bladder between catheterizations, which would make the patient more at risk for UTI or autonomic dysreflexia. The ultimate goal of intermittent catheterization programs is for the patient to become catheter free. In some cases, this may not be possible, so the goal changes for these patients. Patients with a permanent indwelling catheter are at higher risk for UTI and calculi formation, so the goal becomes prevention of complications.

Complications

Urinary Tract Infection. The most common complication in the spinal cord–injured patient is urinary tract infection (UTI).[10, 62–64] Although the use of intermittent catheterization has reduced the incidence considerably, the bladder remains very susceptible to UTI. The predisposition to UTI remains throughout the patient's life. A UTI is indicated by the following:[9]

- A systemic illness with pyrexia.
- An oral temperature of 37.5°C (99.5°F) or a rectal temperature of 38°C (about 100°F) for more than 8 hours.
- A white blood cell count greater than 10,000/mm^3.
- Presence of one or two pathogenic organisms in the urine greater than 100,000 organisms per milliliter.
- Presence of 20 or more pus cells in the urine.
- A low urinary output of concentrated, cloudy, or foul-smelling urine.
- An increase in muscle spasticity.

UTIs are treated with the appropriate antibiotics. Intermittent catheterization need not be stopped if the patient has an infection, unless an increase in fluid intake is required.

Calculi Formation. Calculi formation is another complication associated with the alteration in urinary function. Patients with SCI experience hypercalciuria when calcium is mobilized from the bones and concentrated in the urine. Other predisposing factors include metabolic imbalances, urinary stasis, and infection. Adequate fluid intake of 2000 ml/day, up to 4000 ml/day if the patient has an indwelling catheter, is encouraged. The use of intermittent catheterization also seems to decrease the risk of stone formation.

Sexual Dysfunction

Sexuality is a complex concept composed of physical and emotional components.[64] After a complete SCI, the brain becomes isolated from the sensory signals arising in the genitalia.

Disruption of the autonomic nervous system results in partial or complete loss of motor/sensory functions of the sexual act. Individuals with complete upper motor neuron lesions are unable to psychogenically cause male erection or female lubrication; however, nipple erection, increased pulse, and increased blood pressure can occur. Direct stimulation of the genitals in this group will produce vaginal lubrication and pelvic engorgement in females as well as erections in males. The majority of males in this group are able to have erections. Autonomic dysreflexia can be triggered by genital stimulation. Orgasm in patients with complete lesions can occur on a subjective sensory level in genital and nongenital erotic zones. Ejaculation occurs rarely.

Psychogenic erection can occur in patients with lower motor neuron complete lesions. This is due to intactness of the thoracolumbar sympathetics. Approximately 25 per cent of males with complete lesions are able to have reflexogenic erections. Men with partial lesions have a higher incidence of reflexogenic erections. Ejaculation occurs to a greater degree in this group.

The effects of incomplete lesions on the sexual response depend on the damage to the specific pathways. In patients with central cord lesions, the sexual response might not be disturbed. Sensory or motor sparing may occur in some lesions, and some aspects of the sexual response remain intact.[65]

Fertility in spinal cord–injured males is low as a result of difficulty with erection/ejaculation, decreased sperm count, abnormal sperm motility, and morphological changes. Female fertility is unchanged after SCI although menses may cease for several months. Therefore, birth control measures are an important concern for females of childbearing age. Oral contraceptives and IUDs should not be used, since oral contraceptives can cause blood clots and the possible infection caused by IUD placement may go unnoticed in the patient without sensation. Females with SCI can become pregnant and carry the fetus to full term. However, patients with complete lesions have difficulty identifying the onset of labor. Autonomic dysreflexia also can be triggered by uterine contractions.

There are two tests of value to determine if male or female orgasmic reactions might occur in response to genital stimulation: the pain or heat/cold sensation test and the contracting of the anal opening on command.[65] The first test determines if the sensory pathways between the genitalia and brain are intact, whereas the second test provides information about the motor fibers going to the genitalia from the brain. If either one or both of these tests are negative, the patient will be unable to experience orgasm or ejaculation.

A sexual history should be obtained to determine sexual interest, sexual activities, and sexual behavior prior to the injury. This information can be used to assist in sexual counseling when the patient is ready.

The major nursing intervention in the intermediate care cycle is the recognition of the sexuality of the patient. Granting the patient permission to talk about his or her sexual concerns is also an important part of the care. A qualified counselor should be provided if needed. The sexual partner should be involved in conversations as much as possible. Overt sexual advances or sexual language may be the patient's way of testing his or her sexuality with a "safe" person rather than toward the sexual partner.

Sexual counseling by an appropriate individual should focus on emotional adaptation and providing information on the physical changes of sex and ways of coping with various problems, such as urinary devices, positioning, and spasticity. Nursing goals of sexual counseling are to provide education on normal sexual functioning, assist the patient in understanding and defining his or her own sexuality, and provide specific interventions for dealing with problems associated with sex. Social interactions and weekend passes provide the opportunity for the patient to explore sexual functioning.

Ineffective Coping

Once the patient realizes that the life-threatening crisis is over and is transferred to the intermediate care area or rehabilitation facility, he begins to face the realities of disability. Patients and families experience a normal grieving process. The first phase is characterized by denial of the paralysis and/or its permanency. This denial persists even with daily frank communications with physicians and other health care team members. This phase can persist for a few days or several months. The second phase is anger, which is often indiscriminately directed toward staff and family or friends. The patient generally refuses to discuss the disability and may actually verbally or physically abuse others. Feelings of powerlessness, helplessness, fear, and humiliation are common. The patient may refuse medical and nursing interventions and express a desire to die.

Depression eventually replaces anger. The patient may become withdrawn and nonverbal and refuse to eat. During the depressive stage, staff support is extremely critical, as is support from family and friends. Mood elevators such as amitriptyline or Xanax can be used to help the patient during this time.[3] Often given at night to help the patient sleep, these drugs seem to assist the patient in getting through this depressive phase.

As the individual begins to incorporate previous coping behaviors, he decides to try to "cope" with the present disability. A period of bargaining is initiated in which the patient attempts to change the disability to one of a lesser extent. "Wishful thinking" and hope of changing the disability by participating in the care occurs during this stage of recovery. As the disabled person begins active physical and occupational therapy, physical limitations are identified. Depression may return as feelings of dependency and helplessness return.

The process of adaptation occurs as the individual begins to deal with the reality of disability and decides to make the best of the situation. Successful rehabilitation is dependent on the person's ability to adapt to the disability. Some spinal cord–injured patients never adjust. Slow suicide through immobility and the use of alcohol and drugs is the choice for a few. Generally, this behavior is related to a severe depression and continued ineffective coping. Active psychiatric intervention is the only way to prevent death in these patients. The majority of the disabled hope for a miracle cure or technological advance, and this hope becomes the motivation to complete rehabilitation.

Recognition of the stages of grieving that the patient is experiencing will help in planning appropriate interventions. Assessment of previous appropriate coping behaviors to be supported can assist the nurse in identifying ways for the patient to handle anger and frustration. Determining the needs of family members and where they are in the grieving process will allow appropriate support to be provided to them.[66, 67]

Approaching the situation using a crisis intervention model can help to make nursing management more successful and less stressful.[54] Being attentive to the psychological needs of the patient is part of the overall plan of care. Behavior modification and limit setting may be needed as well as giving the patient some control over his care. (See Chapter 10 for more interventions.)

The goal of the rehabilitation phase is to return the patient to the community as a productive person. In many instances, the patient does indeed return home and to the community even if the patient must go home with special equipment such as a ventilator.

Discharge planning requires not only preparing the patient to go home but also determining what the home environment is like and what changes in the home will be needed to accommodate the patient. Home remodeling may be needed to accommodate the wheelchair and other needed equipment. Loans are available to help families with remodeling. A community assessment for needed resources that may be utilized by the patient and family also should be done, and a list should be made for future reference. Generally, weekend visits prior to discharge are helpful in determining how the patient and family will function in this new situation.[66]

Reintegration of the quadriplegic patient into the community can be very difficult. The ability to return to work can be complicated by the length of time it takes for the patient to perform activities of daily living. Often specialized equipment is needed to perform simple tasks. The cost of this equipment may be more than the patient can afford. In discharge planning, all aspects of the patient's life must be considered, including desire to return to work and mechanisms to allow that to happen.

Another aspect of reintegration involves the psychological adaptation the patient has accomplished regarding the enormous physical disability accompanying the injury. If the patient has demonstrated good adaptation, the ability to "carry on" is easier. Support groups are often helpful in the early stages of reintegration even if good adaptation has occurred. Life outside the rehabilitation center will be different, and another readaptation may need to occur. Support during this period is important for patient and family.[66, 67]

SUMMARY

The state of the art in the care of the patient with SCI has changed dramatically over the past 25 years. The recognition that this injury requires intervention throughout the entire continuum of health care—from prehospital to long-term follow-up—was the most important factor in reducing the morbidity and mortality of spinal cord–injured patients. Research into the exact causes of disability in these patients has led to rapid transport of these patients to definitive care centers and aggressive critical care management of the hemodynamic and respiratory status. Research is now focusing on pharmacological interventions aimed at preserving neurological structures or enhancing neural regeneration. Other studies are aimed at improved rehabilitation techniques with computer-assisted biomedical technology. The future does look a little brighter for the spinal cord trauma patient.

The role of nursing in the management of the patient with SCI is multifaceted. Accurate assessments throughout the cycles of trauma care, management of life-threatening emergencies, prevention of complications, assisting in psychosocial adjustments, and education of the patient and family are all part of the nurse's role. The physiological effects and hemodynamic effects of turning a patient on a Stryker frame versus a kinetic bed, the management of fever or hypothermia in a spinal cord–injured patient, the nursing interventions needed to prevent complications and optimize functioning, and validation of selected nursing diagnoses associated with SCI are a few topics on which nursing studies are needed. Research into nursing's role in the psychological care of these patients is also needed.

The trauma nurse caring for the patient with SCI is faced with a complex challenge. This chapter establishes a framework to be used in planning care for the patient with SCI to assist the nurse in facing this challenge.

REFERENCES

1. Krauss JF: Epidemiological aspects of acute spinal cord injury: A review of incidence, prevalence, causes and outcome. In Becker D, Povlishock J (eds): Central Nervous System Trauma Status Report 1985. Bethesda, MD, NINCDS/NIH, 1985, p 314.
2. Walker MD: Acute spinal cord injury. N Engl J Med 324(26):1885, 1991.
3. Young JS, Northrup NE: Statistical Information Pertaining to Some of the Most Commonly Asked Questions About Spinal Cord Injury. Phoenix, National Spinal Cord Injury Data Research Center, 1981, p 8.
4. Stripley TE: The cost of SCI: The economic consequences of traumatic spinal cord injury. Paraplegic News August:50, 1990.
5. Buchanan LE: An overview. In Buchanan LE, Nawoczenski DE (eds): Spinal Cord Injury: Concepts and Management Approaches. Baltimore, Williams & Wilkins, 1987, pp 1–19.
6. Kurtzke JF: Epidemiology of spinal cord injury. Exp Neurol 48:165, 1975.
7. Green BA, Klose KJ, Goldberg ML: Clinical and research considerations in spinal cord injury. In Becker DP, Povlishock J (eds): Central Nervous System Trauma Status Report 1985. Bethesda, MD, NINCDS/NIH, 1985, p 342.
8. Carol MP, Ducker TB: Spinal cord injury and spinal shock syndrome. In Siegel JH (ed): Trauma: Emergency Surgery and Critical Care. New York, Churchill Livingstone, 1987, pp 947–981.
9. Zejdlik CP: Management of Spinal Cord Injury. Monterey, CA, Wadsworth Health Sciences Division, 1983.
10. Hickey JV: The clinical practice of neurological and neurosurgical nursing. 2nd ed. Philadelphia, JB Lippincott, 1986, pp 378–423.

11. Marshall SB, Marshall LF, Vos HR, Chesnut RM: Acute spinal cord injury. In Neuroscience Critical Care: Pathophysiology and Patient Management. Philadelphia, WB Saunders Co, 1990, pp 307–349.
12. Bose B, Northop BE, Osterholm JL, et al: Reanalysis of central cord injury management. Neurosurgery 15:367, 1984.
13. Panjabi M, White A: Basic biomechanics of the spine. Neurosurgery 7:76, 1980.
14. Bucy PC: Acute cervical spinal injury. Surg Neurol 20:427, 1983.
15. Buchanan LE: Emergency care. In Buchanan LE, Nawczozenski DE (eds): Spinal Cord Injury: Concepts and Management Approaches. Baltimore, Williams & Wilkins, 1987, pp 23–34.
16. Swain A, Grundy D, Russell J: ABC's of spinal cord injury at the accident. Br Med J 291:1558, 1985.
17. Padolsky S, Baroff LJ, Simon RR, et al: Efficacy of cervical immobilization methods. J Trauma 23:461, 1983.
18. Granzian AF, Scheidel EA, Cline JR, et al: A radiographic comparison of prehospital cervical immobilization methods. Ann Emerg Med 16:1127, 1987.
19. Cowley RA, Dunham CM: Shock Trauma Critical Care Manual. Baltimore, University Press, 1983.
20. Walleck CA: Neurologic considerations in the critical care phase. In Sullivan J (ed): Spinal Cord Injury, Critical Care Nursing Clinics of North America. Philadelphia, WB Saunders Co, 1990, pp 357–361.
21. Adelstein W, Watson P: Cervical spinal injuries. J Neurosurg Nurs 15:65, 1983.
22. Carol M, Ducker TB, Byrnes DP: Minimyelogram in cervical spinal cord trauma. Neurosurgery 7:219, 1980.
23. Geisler FH, Dorsey FC, Coleman WP: Recovery of motor function after spinal cord injury: A randomized placebo-controlled trial with GM-I ganglioside. N Engl J Med 324(26):1829, 1991.
24. Senter HJ, Venes JL: Loss of autoregulation and posttraumatic ischemia following experimental spinal cord trauma. J Neurosurg 50:198, 1979.
25. Senter HJ, Venes JL: Altered blood flow and secondary injury in experimental spinal cord trauma. J Neurosurg 49:569, 1978.
26. Ducker TB, Assenmacher DR: The pathologic circulation in experimental cord injury. VA Clinic Spinal Cord Injury Conference 18:10, 1969.
27. Ducker TB, Kindt GW: The effect of trauma on the vasomotor control of spinal cord blood flow. Curr Top Surg Res 3:163, 1971.
28. Kidd PS: Emergency management of spinal cord injury. In Sullivan J (ed): Spinal Cord Injury. Critical Care Nursing Clinics of North America. Philadelphia, WB Saunders Co, 1990, pp 349–356.
29. Geisler FH, Salcman M: Respiratory system physiology, pathophysiology, and management. In Wirth FP, Ratcheson PA (eds): Neurosurgical Critical Care. Baltimore, Williams & Wilkins, 1987, p 40.
30. Carter ER: Medical management of pulmonary complications of spinal cord injury. Adv Neurol 22:267–268, 1979.
31. Jones RF, Unsworth IP, Marosszcky JE: Hyperbaric oxygen and acute spinal cord injuries in humans. Med J Aust 2:573, 1978.
32. DeJesus-Greenburg DA: Acute spinal cord injury and hyperbaric oxygen therapy: A new adjunct in management. J Neurosurg 12:155, 1980.
33. Gamache FW, Myers RAM, Ducker TB, Cowley RA: The clinical application of hyperbaric oxygen therapy in spinal cord injury: A preliminary report. Surg Neurol 15:85, 1981.
34. Albin MS, White RJ, Locke GE: Treatment of spinal cord injury by selective hypothermic perfusion. Surg Forum 16:423, 1965.
35. Tator CH: Acute spinal cord injury in primates produced by inflatable extradural cuff. Can J Surg 16:22, 1973.
36. White RJ: Current status of spinal cord cooling. Clin Neurosurg 20:400, 1973.
37. Rubini L, Columbo F: Modified technique for local cooling in spinal cord injuries. Spine 6:417, 1981.
38. Hansebout RR, Tanner JA, Romero-Sierra C: Current status of spinal cord cooling in the treatment of acute spinal cord injury. Spine 9:508, 1984.
39. Hansebout RR: A comprehensive review of methods of improving cord recovery after acute spinal cord injury. In Tator CH (ed): Management of Acute Spinal Cord Injury. New York, Raven Press, 1982, pp 181–196.
40. Faden AI, Jacobs TP, Mongey E, Holaday JW: Endorphins in experimental spinal injury: Therapeutic effect of naloxone. Ann Neurol 10:326, 1981.
41. Faden AI, Jacobs TP, Holaday JW: A possible pathophysiologic role for endorphins in spinal cord injury. Science 211:493, 1981.
42. Faden AI, Jacobs TP, Smith MT, Holaday JW: Comparison of thyrotropin releasing hormone (TRH), naloxone, and dexamethasone treatments in experimental spinal injury. Neurology (NY) 33:673–678, 1983.
43. Faden AI: Recent pharmacological advances in experimental spinal injury: Theoretical and methodological considerations. Trends Neurosci 6:375, 1983.
44. Bracken MD, Shepard MJ, Collins WF, et al: A randomized, controlled trial of methylprednisolone or naloxone in the treatment of acute spinal cord injury. N Engl J Med 322(20):1405, 1990.
45. Schwenker D: Cardiovascular considerations in the critical care phase. In Sullivan J (ed): Spinal Cord Injury: Critical Care Nursing Clinics of North America. Philadelphia, WB Saunders Co, 1990, pp 363–367.
46. Flesh JR, Leider LL, Erickson DL, et al: Harrington instrumentation and spine fusion for unstable fractures and fracture dislocations of the thoracic and lumbar spine. J Bone Joint Surg 59A:143, 1977.
47. Lehmann KG, Lane JG, Prepmeier JM, et al: Cardiovascular abnormalities accompanying acute spinal cord injury in humans—Incidence, time course and severity. J Am Coll Cardiol 10:46, 1987.
48. Tyson GW: Acute care of the spinal cord injured patient. Crit Care Q 2:45–60, 1979.
49. Blissett PA: Nutrition in acute spinal cord injury. In Sullivan J (ed): Spinal Cord Injury: Critical Care Nursing Clinics of North America. Philadelphia, WB Saunders Co, 1990, pp 375–384.
50. Green BA, Green KL, Klose KJ: Kinetic therapy for spinal cord injury. Spine 8:224, 1983.
51. Nikas DL: Acute spinal cord injuries: Care and complications. In Nikas DL (ed): The Critically Ill Neurosurgical Patient. New York, Churchill Livingstone, 1982.
52. Nikas DL: Pathophysiology and nursing interventions in acute spinal cord injury. Trauma Q 4(3):23, 1988.
53. Brockett TO, Condon N: Comparison of the wedge turning frame and kinetic treatment table in the acute care of spinal cord injury patient. Surg Neurol 22:53, 1984.
54. Richmond T: The patient with a cervical cord injury. Focus Crit Care 12:32, 1985.
55. Richmond TS: Spinal cord injury: A family centered approach to assessment and management. Trauma Q 4(3):58, 1988.
56. Sullivan J: Individual and family response to acute spinal cord injury. In Sullivan J (ed): Spinal Cord Injury: Critical Care Nursing Clinics of North America. Philadelphia, WB Saunders Co, 1990, pp 407–414.
57. Chan RC, Schweigel JF, Thompson GB: Halo thoracic base immobilization in 188 patients with acute cervical spine injuries. J Neurosurgery 58:508, 1983.
58. Toth L: Spasticity management in spinal cord injury. Rehabil Nurs 8:14–17, 1983.
59. Buchanan LE, Ditunno JF: Acute care: Medical/surgical management. In Buchanan LE, Nawoczenski DE (eds): Spinal Cord Injury: Concepts and Management Approaches. Baltimore, Williams & Wilkins, 1987, pp 37–60.
60. Nawoczenski DE: Pressure sores: Prevention and management. In Buchanan LE, Nawoczenski DE (eds): Spinal Cord Injury: Concepts and Management Approaches. Baltimore, Williams & Wilkins, 1987, pp 101–121.
61. Manson R: Autonomic dysreflexia: A nursing challenge. Rehabil Nurs 6:18–19, 1981.
62. Finocchiaro DN, Herzfeld ST: Understanding autonomic dysreflexia. Am J Nurs 90:56, 1990.
63. Wahlquist G: Regaining urinary continence through intermittent catheterization. J Neurosurg 12:73, 1980.

64. Kraft C: Bladder and bowel management. In Buchanan LE, Nawoczenski DE (eds): Spinal Cord Injury: Concepts and Management Approaches. Baltimore, Williams & Wilkins, 1987, pp 83–98.
65. Hahn MA: Elimination concerns with spinal cord trauma: Assessment and nursing interventions. In Sullivan J (ed): Spinal Cord Injury: Critical Care Nursing Clinics of North America. Philadelphia, WB Saunders Co, 1990, pp 385–398.
66. Solomon J: Sex and the spinal cord injured patient. J Neurosurg Nurs 15:306, 1983.
67. Hart G: Spinal cord injury: Impact on client's significant others. Rehabil Nurs 6:11–15, 1981.
68. Woodbury B, Redd C: Psychosocial issues and approaches. In Buchanan LE, Nawoczenski DE (eds): Spinal Cord Injury: Concepts and Management Approaches. Baltimore, Williams & Wilkins, 1987, pp 187–217.

19

THORACIC INJURIES

PATRICIA D. HURN and ROBBI L. HARTSOCK

Thoracic injuries are diverse yet include much of the immediate life-threatening trauma encountered in the field or in the hospital setting. These injuries usually require rapid and skilled responses by nurses and considerable clinical judgment and experience. They are frequently the "glamorous," frightening injuries to which the public is exposed via the press and visual media. Trauma patients occasionally have some knowledge, and many misconceptions, about chest injuries and how they are treated. Yet the pervasive chest pain, the inability to breathe, and the growing weakness of hypovolemic shock are unexpected. Such a situation is terrifying and different for each person.

Chest injuries and their effect on patients are the subject of this chapter. The purpose is to educate the nurse about the most common injuries sustained in the thoracic region and about complications of these injuries throughout the cycles of trauma recovery. This chapter includes specific organ injuries: the heart, lungs, lower airways, major vascular structures, and bony thorax itself. Each of these organs comprises a part of what we know as the cardiopulmonary system or the thoracic cardiovascular system. Nursing diagnoses in thoracic trauma encompass both the anatomical injury and an alteration in the physiological function. Therefore, injuries and posttraumatic thoracic complications are grouped according to the relevant nursing diagnosis. The chapter also includes airway management, since this topic is traditionally included in a review of thoracic injuries. Esophageal injuries are treated as a unit and are contained in Chapter 20. The remainder of this chapter deals with general problems that all thoracic trauma patients experience and is organized according to the cycle or phase of trauma recovery in which the patient is most likely to have the problem.

This injury- or problem-based approach is used to organize and simplify much detailed information. The discussion of each injury begins with a description not only of the injury's symptoms, pathophysiology, diagnosis, and treatment but also of the patient's pain and fear of treatment and death. The analysis of each intervention begins with the nurse's action in explaining the procedure, treating the pain and fear, and supporting the patient and family through medical and nursing therapies. The reader will not find these statements written over and over again but must understand that they are implied in each injury, each complication, and each outcome. There is time to assist in treating the pneumothorax *and* to change the uncomfortable position *and* to explain what a chest tube will be like as a constant companion for several days. Each of these three therapeutic actions is done in the appropriate order of priority assessed for the individual patient.

EPIDEMIOLOGY OF THORACIC INJURIES

Thoracic injuries are responsible for 25 per cent of all trauma-related deaths[1–4] and are second only to central nervous system injuries as the leading cause of all trauma deaths. At least half of all fatalities, regardless of primary etiology, involve significant chest trauma. An estimated 70 per cent of motor vehicular crashes result in thoracic injury.[5] Fortunately, sophisticated prehospital care and expeditious air transportation have improved the detection and treatment of injuries that were previously found only on postmortem examinations. Of those patients admitted to a hospital, 15 per cent require thoracotomy as definitive management. These patients have sustained severe, life-threatening injuries that necessitate complex postoperative care and experience numerous complications. However, the remaining 85 per cent are treated successfully with general resuscitative measures and ventilatory management.[4]

The epidemic of societal violence has changed the patterns of chest injuries that dominated previous decades. One-seventh of all deaths by injury now involve violent interpersonal exchanges.[6] A significant number of these interactions result in penetrating chest trauma from shootings or stabbings. Likewise, growth in the aging segment of the population has an impact on the changing pattern of thoracic injury. Approximately 10 per cent of all blunt chest trauma patients are now 65 years of age or older. Significant morbidity, specifically pneumonia and respiratory distress syndrome, is associated with 50 per cent of aging patients who sustain thoracic injury.[7]

THORACIC ASSESSMENT IN TRAUMA

The assessment for thoracic injury is based, as in any type of trauma examination, on a series of diagnostic clues obtained from directed data collection. Initially, the data are used to form a diagnostic set known as the *index of suspicion*. In other words, given the specific details of the incident and the initial, rapid assessment, what injuries are most likely to be present? The total assessment is frequently completed after the initial resuscitation but always includes the initial data base.

Injury Data Base. The injury data base is the most immediate part of the patient history and helps to identify patterns of thoracic injury. It is the first component of the thoracic assessment process. There are at least four major areas of essential information.

1. *Type of incident.* Information about the type of incident or injury provides clues as to the etiology of injury. Was the patient involved in a motor vehicle crash? Was the injured person wearing a seat belt or shoulder harness? Driver or passenger? Was the patient a pedestrian? Was the patient shot or stabbed?
2. *Events of the incident.* Field care providers, police, or witnesses may provide information about what occurred during the incident. In penetrating chest trauma, highly useful details include the type of weapon used, the design and range of the weapon, and an estimate of missile velocity. How fast was the car traveling on impact in the motor vehicle crash? Did the person travel within the car? What types of deceleration forces were involved?
3. *Mechanism of injury.* Mechanism information is critically important to obtain as part of the injury history. No detail is unimportant. Is the injury a result of blunt force? What part of the thorax received the initial impact? Did the anterior chest hit the steering wheel, or was the patient thrown forward against a shoulder harness? Or is the injury a result of a penetrating force such as a stabbing? Does the apparent mechanism correlate with the initial examination and resuscitation?
4. *Events of the extrication or transport.* How long did it take the rescuers to extricate the person from the car? Were there special problems in freeing the torso from surrounding metal? What were the events of transporting the patient from the field? How long did it require? Airway problems? Vital signs?

Previous Health History. In addition to the injury history, the personal health history gives insight into the individual's unique response to shock and thoracic injury. Whether the historian is the patient or, more likely, a family member, the nurse attempts to identify the previous respiratory, cardiac, or vascular status. Previous cardiopulmonary problems are uncovered through the usual "review of systems" approach as well as selective and directed questioning. The injured person is frequently young and presents an unremarkable cardiopulmonary or vascular history. Nevertheless, ask specifically about the presence of persistent upper or lower respiratory infections, asthma, chronic sinus problems, and a smoking, alcohol, or drug abuse history. Any of these problems may affect the patient's tolerance of nasal or oral endotracheal tubes or the response to mechanical ventilation. Is there a history of chest pain, heart disease, cardiac surgery, or vascular implantation? It is particularly important to inquire if there have been any previous incidents or injuries.

Physical Examination. The physical assessment always begins with a primary survey of the ABCs: airway status with cervical spine control, breathing, and circulation. This basic principle holds for all trauma patients from resuscitation to rehabilitation. For example, during the resuscitation phase, airway status assessment includes tongue position; the presence of blood, vomitus, or foreign bodies; and upper or lower airway edema. In later phases of the patient's trauma course, the examination may focus on evaluating maxillofacial restraining devices that affect airway status, tracheostomy cuff pressure, or simply the patient's ability to manage oral secretions. The ABCs imply that the nurse must always know at any point in time whether a patient's cervical spine has been cleared radiographically. Breathing, whether spontaneous or mechanically assisted, and circulation are rapidly evaluated to complete the primary survey. Only at this point does the detailed examination begin.

Thoracic Anatomy. Correlation of underlying anatomy and surface landmarks is imperative in the trauma examination. The examiner must be able to identify key structures in the true thorax as well as the cervicothoracic inlet and boundaries of the thoracoabdominal cavity (Fig. 19–1). Key structures include the trachea, carotid arteries, carina, lung fields, diaphragm, cardiac borders, aorta, subclavian arteries, and pulmonary artery (Table 19–1). External landmarks and knowledge of the relationships between internal structures assist in identifying injuries (Figs. 19–2 and 19–3).

Secondary and Detailed Examinations. The traditional physical examination techniques (inspection, palpation, percussion, and auscultation) are used in the thoracic assessment of the trauma patient, usually in an *adapted* form. The key word is *adapted,* not *deleted.* Visual inspection of the thorax requires a clean field for the examination. The removal of debris and blood wherever possible helps to avoid overlooking wounds or subtle signs of trauma. Hair-covered

TABLE 19–1. THORACIC SURFACE ANATOMY

STRUCTURE	LANDMARKS
Aorta	
Root	Angle of Louis, midsternal line
Arch	First rib, sternal border
Pulmonary artery	Within and below aortic arch
Subclavian artery	First rib, clavicle
Cardiac borders	
Apex	5th left ICS, midclavicular line
Base	2nd left ICS, substernal
Carina	Angle of Louis
Diaphragm	Right dome superior to left
Full inspiration	10th–11th rib posteriorly, 6th–8th rib anteriorly
Full expiration	10th thoracic vertebra posteriorly, 4th–5th rib anteriorly

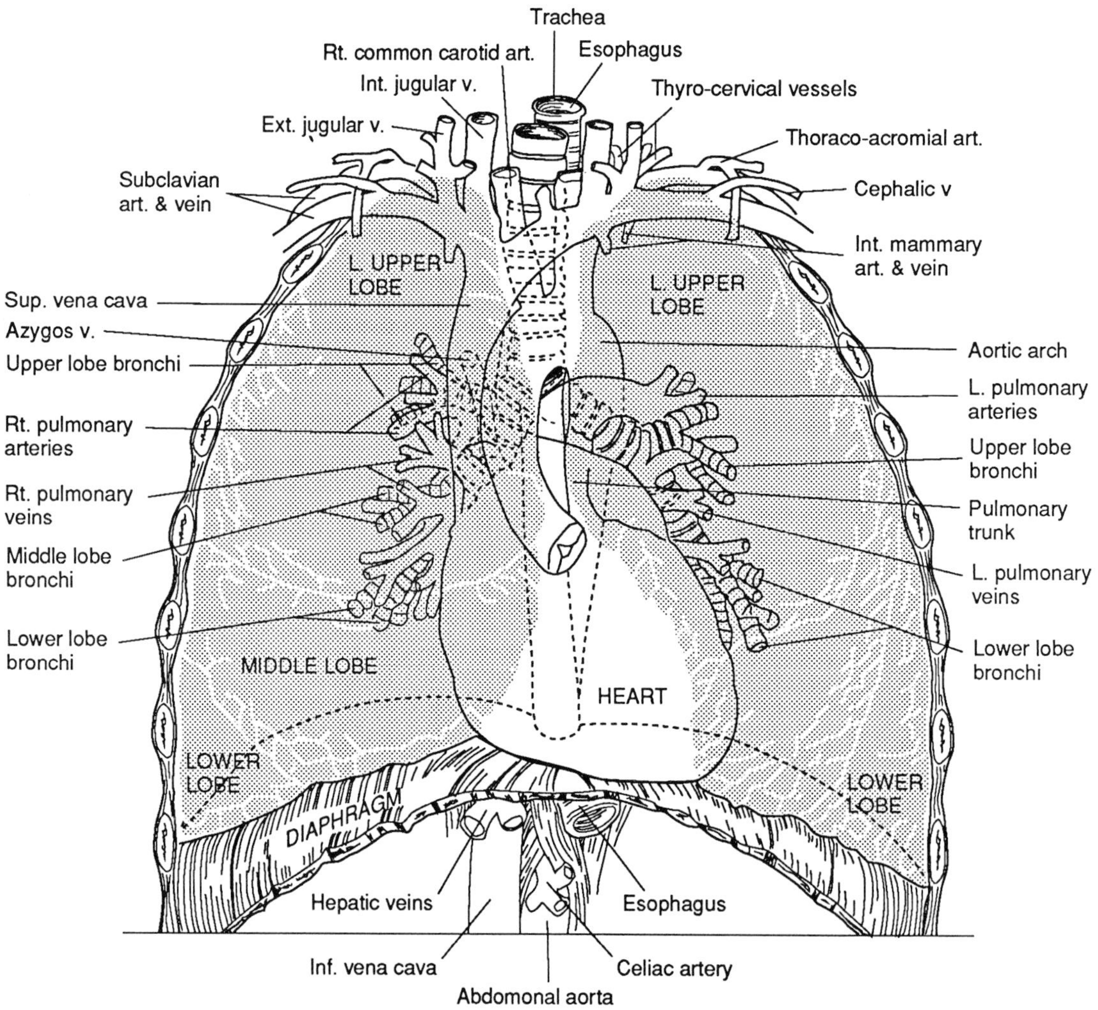

Figure 19–1. Anatomy of the thorax and its contents. (From Shires GT: Care of the Trauma Patient. New York, McGraw-Hill, 1985.)

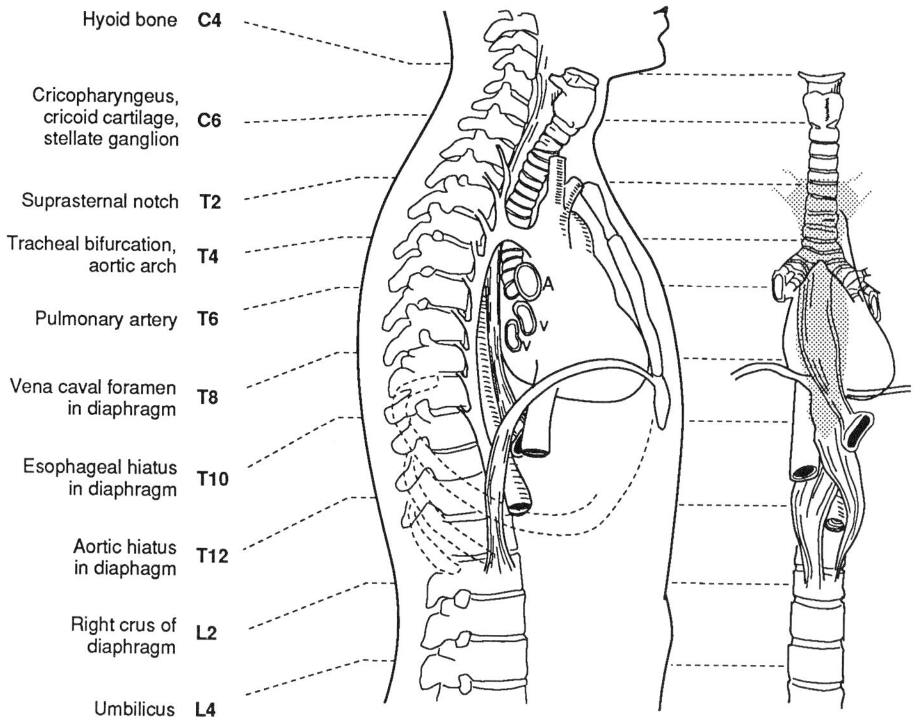

Figure 19–2. The cervical, thoracic, and lumbar vertebrae correspond with specific anatomical structureships. These landmarks are helpful in determining different thoracic levels. Palpation of the spinous processes proves helpful in ascertaining the level of the wound and the structures that may be involved. (From Naclerio EA: Chest Injuries. Orlando, Grune & Stratton, 1971.)

areas are carefully inspected. The examiner must be particularly alert to contusions, steering wheel marks, and sites of a penetrating wound's entrance and exit. Palpation and percussion are difficult to perform in the patient with numerous tubes, dressings, and traction. Yet each anatomical area must be palpated for crepitus, hematomas, and unstable bone fragments. Percussion is used to locate blood and air by identifying inappropriately dull or tympanic notes over the chest wall. Chest auscultation may be difficult over the noise of a ventilator or bubbling chest tubes. However, each of these techniques can and must be used in examining the thoracic region.

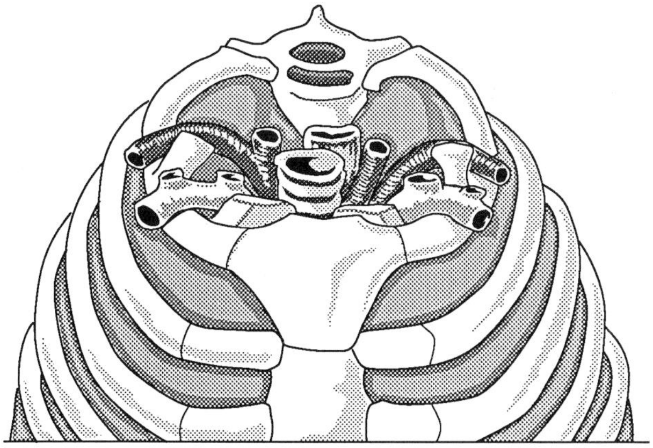

Figure 19–3. The root of the neck is actually the cervicothoracic region, which forms a boundary between the neck and the thorax. It is occupied by a number of vital structures that enter or leave the thoracic cavity. As shown, the apex of the lung rises above the level of the anterior part of the first rib. The subclavian artery lateral to the subclavian vein is separated from the lung by the membranous cervical diaphragm and the pleura. (From Naclerio EA: Chest Injuries. Orlando, Grune & Stratton, 1971.)

During the initial evaluation and resuscitation phase of care, each technique is applied rapidly and specifically. Treatment may precede diagnostic examination in life-threatening injuries such as tension pneumothorax or cardiac tamponade. In the critical care phase of recovery, the examination may be much more detailed and is assisted by a variety of invasive technologies. The focus of the assessment is slightly different, centering on occult injuries, overlooked injuries, and later complications of serious injury and shock. A great deal of additional data is available through electromechanical monitoring and extensive laboratory and radiographic procedures. These additional data are always correlated with the history and physical examination. As the patient progresses through each cycle of care, the thoracic assessment builds on the findings of the preceding cycle. What is learned during resuscitation must be communicated and reassessed during critical, intermediate, and rehabilitative care.

Anatomical Approach to Thoracic Examination. The anatomical examination component in thoracic trauma assessment includes the neck, cervicothoracic region, and upper abdomen, as well as the true thorax. Each area is examined for injuries and abnormalities. Focal points in the neck examination include the trachea, neck veins, and carotid arteries. The trachea is inspected and palpated to identify any deviation in position from the midline indicative of mediastinal shifting. Neck veins are examined for distention or flatness as an indication of intrathoracic pressure. The carotid arteries are separately palpated for decrease or loss of pulse and then are auscultated for bruits (Fig. 19–4).

Note the overall size and shape of the patient's true thorax. The thoracic cavity size provides clues as to underlying lung disease and how well a specific injury may be tolerated. For example, a large male will tolerate a considerably greater volume of intrathoracic bleeding without signs of lung or

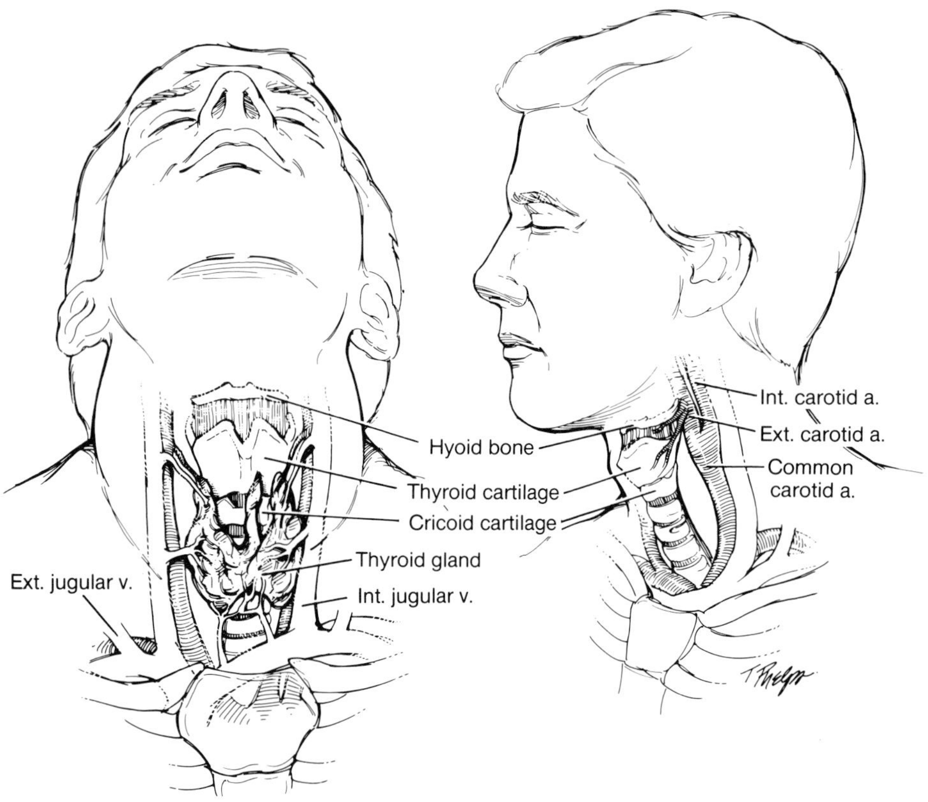

Figure 19–4. Important structures in the neck component of thoracic assessment.

mediastinal compression than will the patient with a small or inflexible chest. This may be the difference between 4000 and 1000 ml of air and fluid.

The entire surface of the chest is inspected for signs of trauma. The bony points of the thorax and intercostal spaces provide references in localizing internal thoracic structures (Fig. 19–5). All supporting structures (clavicles, sternum, ribs, and the thoracic spine) are palpated for fractures and observed for symmetry. Percussion of the chest begins at the apices and moves downward across both the lateral and anterior aspects. Examination of the back must not be delayed, although it is frequently limited to palpation until the patient can be safely moved for a more complete assessment. The examiner searches for changes in normal resonance on percussion or loss of normal diaphragmatic excursion. Breath sounds are auscultated over the anterior and lateral chest wall in order to identify air entry in each lobe of the lung. Heart sounds are evaluated for overall loudness or distance of the sounds and for the presence of murmurs across the right ventricle and septum.

Finally, the thoracoabdominal area is carefully examined for evidence of trauma. This is particularly of concern in penetrating injuries which may have had an upward trajectory with possible diaphragmatic tears and involvement of the pleural space. The position of the diaphragm is located on inspiration and expiration (Fig. 19–6).

Physiological Approach. Clinical monitoring of blood pressure, cardiac rate and rhythm, respirations, urine output, and arterial blood gases is always considered to be part of the thoracic assessment process. However, it is generally recognized that blood pressure is frequently unaffected until a 15 to 20 per cent loss in blood volume has been sustained. Although invasive monitoring of central venous pressure may be helpful, it is not routinely initiated during the initial fluid replacement and management of significant thoracic injuries. The time required to insert a central venous catheter cannot be afforded during initial resuscitation; therefore, large-bore (14-gauge) peripheral intravenous catheters are preferable for volume repletion.

Definitive management in the operative and critical care phases requires a practical yet comprehensive approach to systemic cardiopulmonary monitoring. The nurse must be familiar with an extensive array of cardiopulmonary variables and accompanying monitoring technology. For example, a number of parameters are used in forming the diagnosis of impaired gas exchange related to posttraumatic respiratory distress or inadequate cardiac output in myocardial contusion. The patient–ventilator system is monitored as a unit and is an important source of data about the patient's pulmonary status. For example, one important mechanical parameter, static pulmonary compliance, can be monitored in intubated patients via the ventilator system. The measurement is accomplished by noting the tidal volume, the airway pressure at end inspiration after inflation of the lung has stopped, and the end-expiratory pressure. Static compliance is the ratio of tidal volume to the change in pressure from end inspiration to end expiration. Normal values are approximately 60 to 80 ml/cm H_2O; however, in patients with

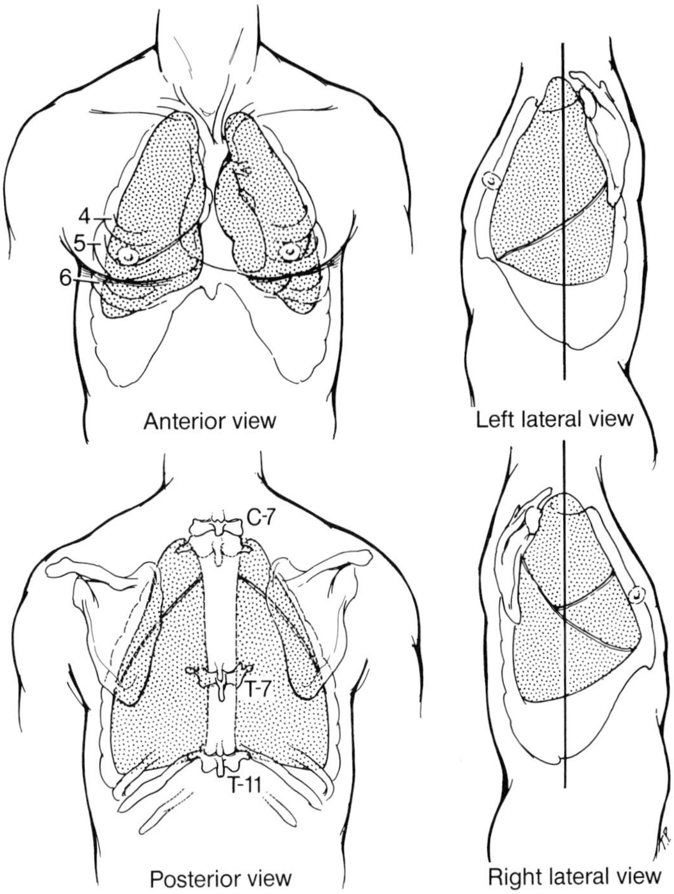

Figure 19–5. Correlation of surface to underlying thoracic anatomy. *Anterior view.* Note the relationship of the heart, great vessels, and lungs to bony thorax. *Posterior view. Right lateral view.* Major and minor interlobar fissures. *Left lateral view.* Note single interlobar fissure.

respiratory distress syndrome, the value commonly drops to 30 ml/cm H_2O.

The insertion of peripheral arterial and pulmonary artery catheters provides much of the needed information for assessment of extensive injuries, their complications, and the effect of therapies such as mechanical ventilation and positive end-expiratory pressure (PEEP). When available, mixed venous oxygen tension (Pvo_2) and saturation (Svo_2) monitoring is a useful tool in determining circulatory sufficiency and tissue oxygenation. Table 19–2 is a summary of physiological parameters that are often obtained via invasive monitoring and are part of comprehensive thoracic trauma assessment. The reader is referred to one of many excellent references to ensure understanding of the variable, its importance, and measurement.[8]

Noninvasive Monitoring. The oxygenation status of the patient can be assessed using noninvasive monitoring via pulse oximeters and transcutaneous, conjunctival, or tissue oxygen tension monitors. Pulse oximetry is well accepted as a convenient, portable, and cost-effective monitor of peripheral arterial oxygen saturation. In general, oximetry estimates fractional hemoglobin saturation by determining the maximum light absorbances of the different hemoglobin species. In pulse oximetry, multiple arteriolar beds may be used (e.g.,

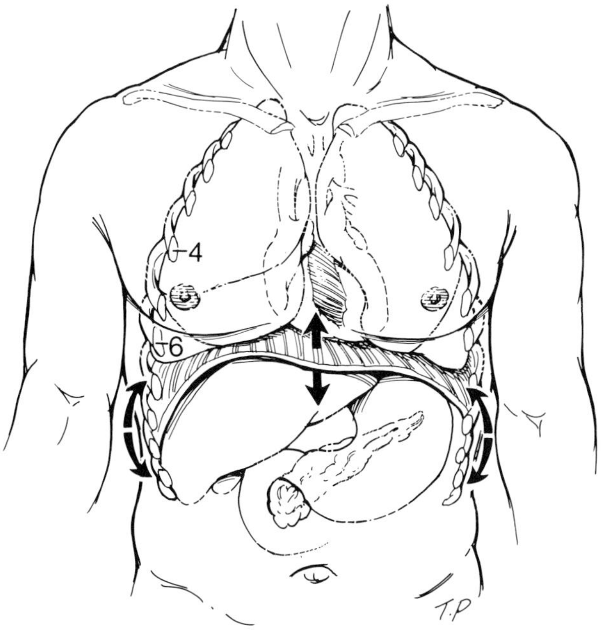

Figure 19–6. The thoracoabdominal region in thoracic assessment. Note the variation in diaphragm and lung position during respiration.

TABLE 19–2. CARDIOPULMONARY PARAMETERS IN THORACIC ASSESSMENT

VARIABLE	ABBREV.	MEASUREMENTS OR CALCULATION	NORMAL RANGE		
			LOW	HIGH	UNITS
Heart rate	HR	Direct measurement	70	90	bpm
Mean arterial pressure	MAP	Direct measurement	80	100	mm Hg
Central venous pressure	CVP	Central venous catheter Direct measurement	1	9	mm Hg
Pulmonary capillary wedge pressure	PCWP	Pulmonary artery catheter Direct measurement	4	12	mm Hg
Mean pulmonary artery pressure	$\overline{PA}$	Pulmonary artery catheter Direct measurement	11	16	mm Hg
Cardiac output	Q_T	Fick method or thermodilution Direct measurement	Varies with size		
Cardiac index	CI	Q_T/body surface area	2.8	3.6	l/min/m^2
Stroke index	SI	CI/HR	30	50	ml/m^2
Left ventricular stroke work	LVSW	SI × $\underline{MAP}$ × 0.0144	44	68	g-m/m^2
Right ventricular stroke work	RVSW	SI × $\overline{PA}$ × 0.0144	4	8	g-m/m^2
Systemic vascular resistance	SVR	79.92 × ($\underline{MAP}$ − CVP)/CI	1700	2600	dyne-sec-cm^{5}m^2
Pulmonary vascular resistance	PVR	79.92 × ($\overline{PA}$ − PCWP)/CI	45	225	dyne-sec-cm^{5}m^2
Arterial blood gases	ABGs	Direct measurement			
$Pa{O_2}$			80	100	mm Hg
$Pa{CO_2}$			35	45	mm Hg
pH			7.35	7.45	
HCO_3			22	26	mEq/l
Oxygen saturation	$Sa{O_2}$		>95		per cent (%)
Base excess			−2	2	
Mixed venous blood gases	MVBGs	Direct measurement			
$Pv{O_2}$			35	40	mm Hg
$Pv{CO_2}$			41	51	mm Hg
pH			7.31	7.41	
HCO_3			22	26	mEq/l
Oxygen saturation	$Sv{O_2}$		70	75	per cent (%)
Base excess			−2	2	
Arterial O_2 content	$Ca{O_2}$	$Sa{O_2}$ × (1.39 × Hgb) + 0.003 × $Pa{O_2}$	20 ml O_2/100 ml		
Mixed venous O_2 content	$Cv{O_2}$	$Sv{O_2}$ × (1.39 × Hgb) + 0.003 × $Pv{O_2}$	15 ml O_2/100 ml		
Arterial–mixed venous O_2 content	Ca-vO_2	$Ca{O_2}$ − $Cv{O_2}$	4	5.5	ml/dl
Oxygen delivery	O_2 del	$Ca{O_2}$ × CI × 10	500	700	ml/min-m^2
Oxygen consumption	$\dot{V}O_2$	Ca-vO_2 × CI × 10	100	180	ml/min-m^2
Respiratory rate	RR	Direct measurement	12	20	bpm
Tidal volume	V_T	Spirometry	Varies with size 200	550	ml
End inspiratory pressure	P_i	Direct measurement	Volume-dependent e.g., 7 cm H_2O for V_T = 600 ml		
Vital capacity	VC	Spirometry	65	75	ml/kg
Inspiratory force	IF	Direct measurement	−100	−75	cm H_2O
Dead space to tidal volume ratio	$\dot{V}_D/\dot{V}_T$	($Pa{CO_2}$ − $Pe{CO_2}$/$Pa{CO_2}$)	0.2	0.4	
Respiratory compliance	C	$V_T/(P_i$ − PEEP)	60	100	ml/cm H_2O
Physiological shunt fraction	Q_s/Q_t	$(C_{end\text{-}cap}O_2 - CaO_2)/(C_{end\text{-}cap}O_2 - CvO_2)$	3	5	per cent (%)

Adapted from Shoemaker WC: Pathophysiology and therapy of shock states. In Berk J, Sampliner J (eds): Handbook of Critical Care. Boston, Little, Brown, 1982.

fingers, toes, nasal septum). The accuracy is approximately 3 to 5 per cent at true saturations > 70 per cent, assuming that the only hemoglobin species present are reduced and oxyhemoglobin.[9] Accuracy falls in the presence of significant amounts of carboxyhemoglobin, hypothermia, severe anemia, and hypovolemia with mean arterial blood pressure < 50 mm Hg.[9] Since the technique depends on pulse transmission, intense peripheral vasoconstriction also may be associated with loss of or inaccurate readings.

Noninvasive assessment of carbon dioxide (CO_2) is more difficult, especially in critically ill patients with significant ventilation–perfusion abnormalities, increased physiological dead space, and hemodynamic instability. When these intervening factors are stable, changes in end-tidal CO_2 can be assumed to reflect changes in alveolar ventilation and arterial CO_2 tension ($Pa{CO_2}$). End-tidal CO_2 monitoring by mass spectrometry or infrared analyzer correlates reasonably well with $Pa{CO_2}$ in normal patients and is used in a variety of environments, including the resuscitation, operating, and recovery areas.[10] Analysis of trends over time rather than individual values is most useful, since there is considerable breath-to-breath variability in all patients.

PATIENT–VENTILATOR SYSTEM. The integrity and effectiveness of the ventilator equipment is part of thoracic assessment. There is no one preferred ventilator system or mode. Volume-cycled ventilators are by far the most commonly used, since the minute volume, flow, and resultant airway pressure can be manipulated. Specialized methods of ventilation such as high-frequency ventilation may be useful in specific types of airway or chest trauma. In addition, several modes of conventional mechanical ventilation are used:

1. *Control mode (CMV).* CMV allows total control of the patient's rate and tidal volume. It is generally used in patients for short-term ventilation when no inspiratory effort is desired or in multiply injured patients without spontaneous ventilatory efforts because of accompanying neurological injury or drug overdose.

2. *Assist/control.* This mode is also known as *continuous mandatory ventilation* on newer generation ventilators. The patient can initiate spontaneous ventilation, and each breath is assisted by the ventilator to a preset volume. Infrequently used in thoracic trauma or multiply injured patients, assist/control can allow an inappropriately high minute ventilation as well as increase the work of breathing.

3. *Intermittent mandatory ventilation (IMV).* IMV allows the patient to receive a baseline minute volume but also breathe spontaneously at a fast or slow rate and variable tidal volume. *Synchronized intermittent mandatory ventilation* (SIMV) provides the additional advantage that the IMV mandatory breaths are triggered when the ventilator senses inspiratory effort by the patient. SIMV is generally well tolerated in most patients and diminishes the risk of barotrauma, since there is less chance of ventilator breaths imposed over spontaneous inspiration (stacking). All IMV modes provide several key advantages: The individual patient's respiratory efforts are utilized, weaning begins at the outset of ventilation, and mean intrathoracic pressure is decreased (and therefore venous return and cardiac filling are increased). The last advantage is particularly important in hypovolemic patients and in those with myocardial injury.

4. *Continuous positive airway pressure (CPAP).* This mode generally refers to a patient breathing spontaneously at an elevated baseline airway pressure. The objective, as with PEEP, is to increase functional residual capacity (FRC) and, therefore, the surface area available for gas exchange. During inspiration, the ventilator provides gas flow as a function of the patient's inspiratory effort. Exhalation is passive to the level of the preset baseline pressure. CPAP can be used to support the patient during weaning and allows ventilation at a lower inspired oxygen concentration. Conversely, CPAP does not provide mandatory breaths via positive-pressure mechanical ventilation; it only supports the patient's spontaneous alveolar ventilation.

5. *Pressure-support ventilation.* This modality is a newer, less well studied technique. Pressure support allows spontaneous breathing at a set airway pressure (like CPAP); however, the pressure is provided only during inspiration, not continuously. The patient initiates a breath, and the ventilator delivers gas flow to the patient while maintaining a preset inspiratory pressure. In theory, pressure support increases the pressure gradient across the airway, therefore reducing resistance.[11] The effect can be useful in patients with high airway resistance related to underlying pulmonary pathology or a small artificial airway. Pressure support decreases the work of breathing and can prevent fatigue when combined with IMV. These factors can be critical in solving weaning difficulties. However, pressure support does not ensure an adequate minute ventilation; neither rate nor tidal volume is guaranteed.

Ventilatory modes may be used singly or in combination (i.e., IMV with pressure support). It is impossible to overemphasize the importance of a thorough understanding of ventilatory modalities and their physiological and psychological effects. A detailed review of these therapies is available elsewhere.[11]

Integrating Other Data Sources. Laboratory and radiographical data provide the final components of the total thoracic trauma assessment. Essentials include arterial blood gases, hematocrit and hemoglobin, complete blood count, clotting studies, serum electrolytes and osmolarity, and a recent sputum or transtracheal aspirate culture.

Thoracic evaluation includes a chest roentgenogram in order to visualize any significant bone, vascular, or pulmonary injuries. Figure 19–7 provides a review of normal roentgenographical anatomy as a foundation for interpretation of abnormal findings. A comprehensive discussion of chest film interpretation in trauma is available elsewhere.[12]

The angle of the film (supine, upright, or lateral) is chosen for best exposure of specific structures yet must consider any restrictions in positioning the patient. A supine anteroposterior film is selected for the patient who is being evaluated for cervical spine injury or whose hemodynamic instability makes an upright position impossible.

One of the most valuable assessment tools in thoracic trauma is a clear, *true upright* chest radiograph. The patient faces the x-ray beam at a 110-degree angle so as to avoid unnecessary distortion of underlying structures on the radiograph (Fig. 19–8). The true upright film allows better visualization of vascular injuries within the chest and some estimation of the amount of blood or fluid in the chest cavity. Cardiac and aortic borders are also less distorted. Prior to obtaining an upright film, cervical spine injury must be ruled out. Thoracic and lumbar spine pathology also must be excluded before removing the patient from a long backboard to enable a sitting position. If the patient is intubated, suctioning may be necessary before the procedure. When the patient is pharmacologically paralyzed and sedated, support of the head and neck is necessary. The agitated patient must be protected from inadvertent dislodgment of an endotracheal tube or vascular catheters.

Additional diagnostic information is provided through thoracic computed axial tomography (CT scan). The CT scan is more sensitive in detecting air and fluid in the pleural space than is the radiograph. Evaluation of underlying lung, cardiac, and mediastinal structures is also enhanced by the use of CT scans.[13] Mirvis[13] advocates the addition of aortography to detect great vessel injury in patients who have a history of blunt, decelerating thoracic trauma.

The use of magnetic resonance imaging (MRI) provides detailed visualization of blood vessels with rapid flow rates. Contrast dye is not required. Although its accuracy makes MRI a valuable diagnostic tool, its use in the acutely injured patient is somewhat limited by the difficulties encountered in hemodynamic monitoring and ventilatory support within the field around the magnet.[13]

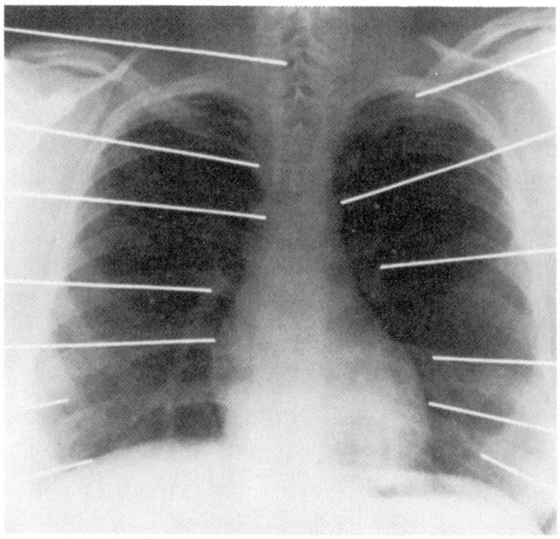

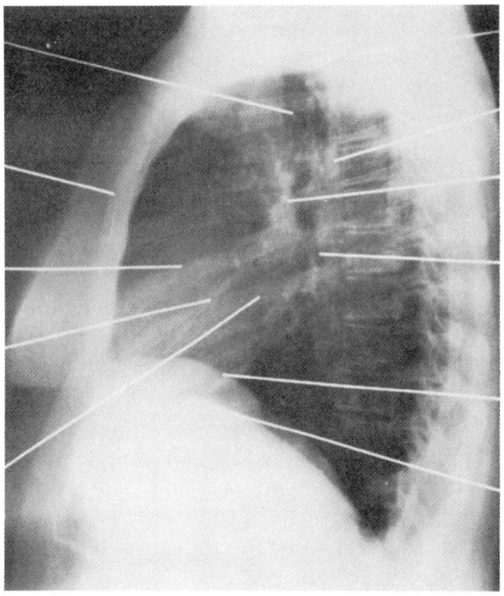

Figure 19–7. Normal posteroanterior and lateral films of the chest. (From Naclerio EA: Chest Injuries. Orlando, Grune & Stratton, 1971.)

Reassessment and Early Thoracotomy. Repeated thoracic assessment is the key to determining missed or progressive injuries. Should the patient's condition deteriorate or result in cardiac arrest, immediate exploratory thoracotomy may be performed. The indications for the procedure have historically been the subject of considerable controversy. Dunham and Cowley[14] maintain that the point at which a youthful myocardium arrests usually represents an irreversible insult and recommend specific indications for emergency thoracotomy. These include arrest in a young patient, an arrest time of less than 5 minutes' duration, and positive neurological signs such as reactive pupils and spontaneous movement of the extremities.

THE INJURIES

Ineffective Airway Related to Obstruction

Every injured patient is at risk for developing some form of airway problem. Airway obstruction occurs frequently in trauma both as a primary problem or as the result of some other injury. The source of an obstruction and the therapeutic approach are slightly different in the patient with a natural airway or one with an artificial airway already in place. However, the principles of basic and advanced life support are fundamental in management of all obstructions. Specific airways procedures are described in Appendix 19–1.

The Patient with a Natural Airway. The most common sources of obstruction are the tongue and foreign bodies such as teeth, blood clots, and bone fragments. The unconscious patient in shock or one with central nervous system, maxillofacial, or neck injuries is particularly at risk. Assessment begins with rapid determination of level of consciousness and mental status, followed by observation of rate and pattern of respiration. Air movement through the airway, if any, is noisy. Respiratory distress may or may not be immediately evident, and arterial blood gases are measured as the most certain method of assessing oxygenation and ventilation.

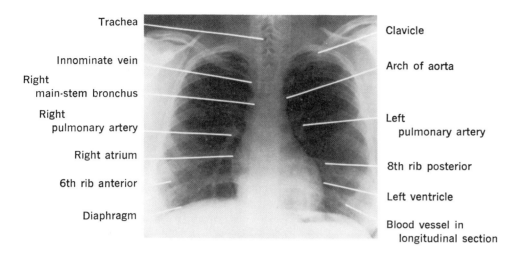

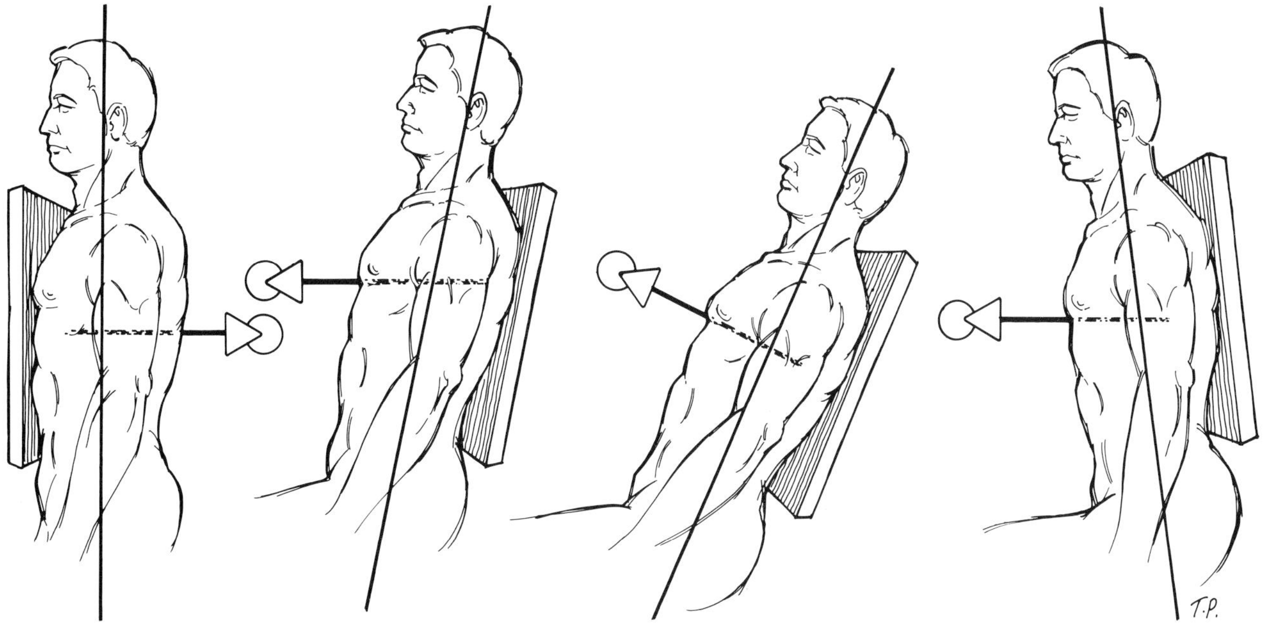

Figure 19–8. Positioning for the true erect anteroposterior chest radiograph. *A,* Normal position for posteroanterior film. *B,* Most common position for portable anteroposterior chest film. *C,* Unacceptable position for erect anteroposterior film. *D,* True erect position.

Initially, the airway is opened by a chin lift or jaw thrust, and the oropharynx is cleared by suction and digital exploration. Each step is performed with great care to maintain immobility of the cervical spine unless injury to the spine has been ruled out clinically and radiographically. Initial airway maneuvers may be inadequate or only temporary solutions; therefore, more definitive airway control is often required.

The simplest of adjuncts includes an oral or nasal airway. Both are generally for short-term use in trauma and have restricted use in facial trauma such as nasal fractures, cribriform plate fractures, or oropharyngeal injury. When positioning does not relieve the obstruction, endotracheal intubation is the management technique of choice in most types of trauma. An esophageal obturator airway (EOA) or esophageal gastric tube airway (EGTA) are ineffective adjuncts in maintaining the airway[15] but may still be encountered in patients received from the prehospital setting. Complications such as inadvertent tracheal intubation, esophageal trauma from excessive cuff inflation, and vomiting with aspiration upon removal are common (Fig. 19–9).

In general, oral endotracheal intubation with rapid-sequence induction is the preferred method for securing an airway. This may be done safely after cervical spine injury has been ruled out or even in cases of unknown cervical spine status provided the neck does *not* require aggressive manipulation to visualize the vocal cords. Cricoid pressure is routinely applied during the procedure. The rationale is that the trauma patient is likely to have a full stomach and is therefore at risk for aspiration of gastric contents.[14]

However, orotracheal intubation constitutes the preferred airway management with several caveats. If the patient is unstable but breathing and the urgency of airway management does not allow preliminary cervical spine clearance, blind nasotracheal intubation is attempted (Fig. 19–10). Conversely, an orotracheal route is used if the patient is apneic and the cervical spine is manually immobilized in a neutral position. Lastly, fiberoptic endoscopy may be useful in facilitating difficult intubations in stable patients, particularly in those individuals with maxillofacial or cervical spine trauma or in patients with short necks.[15]

If the patient cannot be intubated successfully, emergency cricothyroidotomy is recommended.[15] There are two cricothyroidotomy procedures currently in use. The first is a

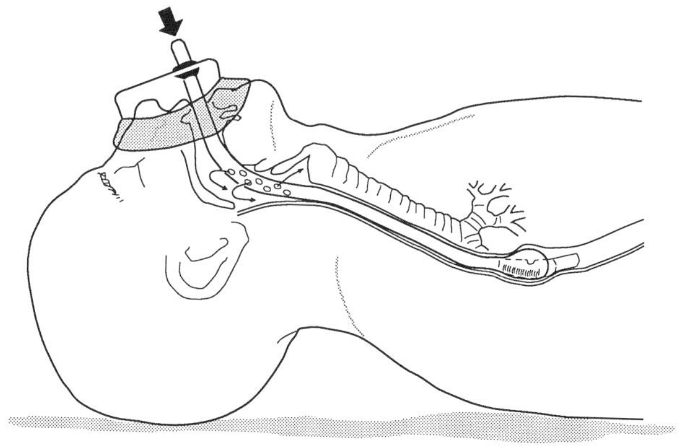

Figure 19–9. Schematic representation of esophageal obturator airway in proper position. Air *(thick arrow)* is blown into proximal end and exits via small holes into the trachea. (From Schofferman J, Oill P, Lewis AJ: The esophageal obturator airway: A clinical evaluation. Chest 69:67, 1976.)

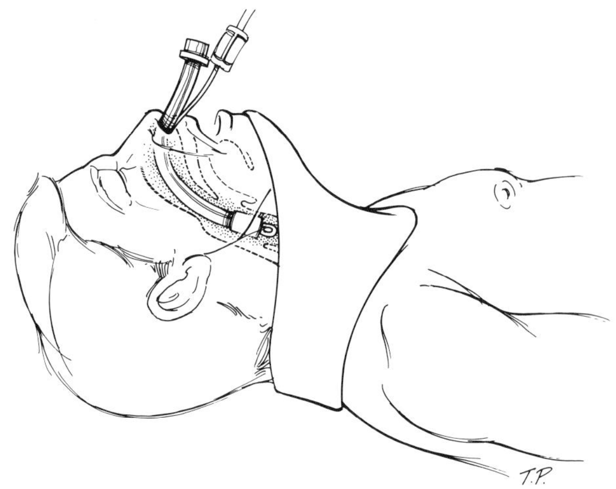

Figure 19–10. Blind nasotracheal intubation in a patient with potential cervical spine injury.

surgical technique in which a transverse incision is made through the skin and cricothyroid membrane located below the thyroid prominence of the neck. A standard tracheostomy tube is then inserted into the exposed airway (Fig. 19–11). A second approach, needle cricothyroidotomy or percutaneous transtracheal ventilation, is initiated by insertion of a 14-gauge needle into the trachea at the cricothyroid membrane below the level of obstruction. Pressurized oxygen is intermittently insufflated through the needle into the trachea. Which method is used is dependent on the injury present, available equipment, and the capability of the resuscitating health professional.

The choice of appropriate airway requires consideration not only of available equipment and personnel but factors specific to the patient, the injury, and the short- and long-term management of the patient. For example, early intubation may be indicated not only for airway management but also for intraoperative or critical care management of thoracic injuries. Table 19–3 summarizes the advantages of the different artificial airways, restrictions, and potential complications.

The Patient with an Artificial Airway. Consider the trauma patient who has an artificial airway in place, routinely an endotracheal or tracheostomy tube. Obstructions or partial obstructions occur in these patients usually in an insidious and subtle fashion. Assessment of airway patency and effectiveness includes an on-going evaluation of the strategic component. Is the reasoning behind originally placing this airway still valid? Is this still the right airway for the patient? The following factors should be considered as part of the assessment:

1. Evaluate the level of consciousness at this phase of trauma care. What is the patient's ability to guard his own airway and manage oral and nasal secretions?
2. Evaluate the prophylactic aspects of the airway. Is there a future risk of obstruction, as in glottic edema from airway burns or maxillofacial trauma?
3. Examine for complications apparent from the present airway. Is the intubation time prolonged beyond 2 weeks and tracheostomy a better alternative? Is there purulent nasal drainage due to a developing sinusitis while a nasal tube is in place? Does a previously overlooked injury such as intraoral lacerations or tracheal tear change the choice in airway management?
4. Evaluate the patient's response to the airway. Are head and neck movements rapid and agitated, endangering tube position or creating further airway damage? What is the probability of self-extubation?

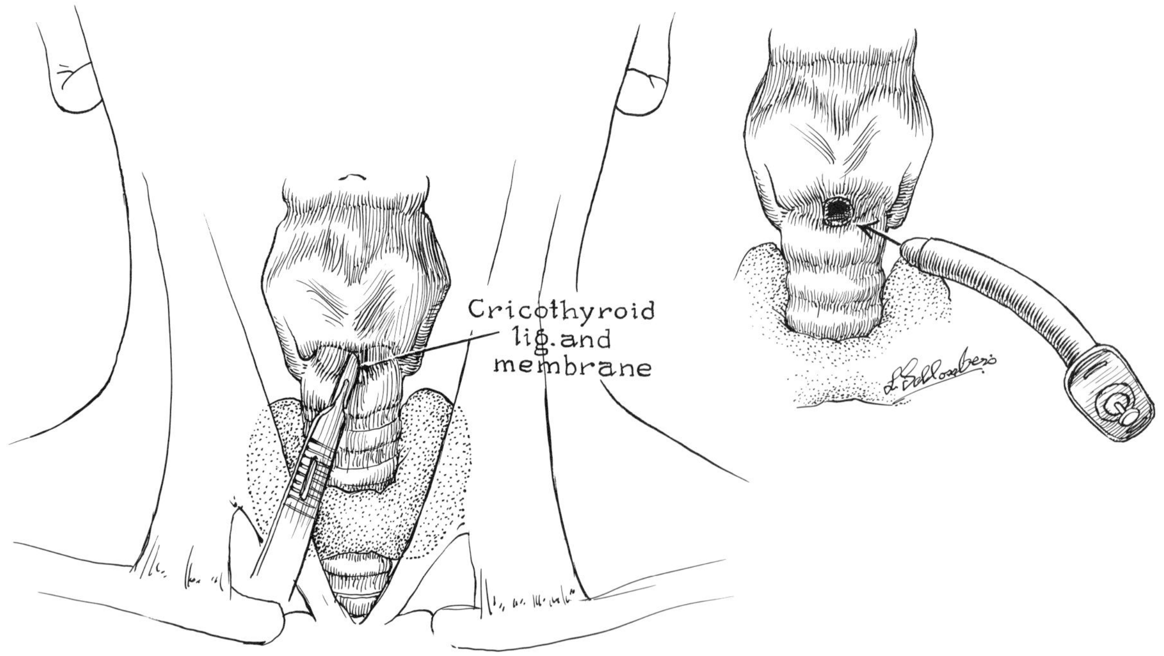

Figure 19–11. Cricothyroidotomy technique. (From Zuidema GD, Rutherford RB, Ballinger WF: Management of Trauma, 4th ed. Philadelphia, WB Saunders Co, 1985.)

TABLE 19–3. AIRWAY ADJUNCTS IN TRAUMA

OROPHARYNGEAL AIRWAY	
INDICATIONS:	Unconscious patients without gag reflex; short-term use
ADVANTAGES:	Holds tongue away from posterior pharynx
RESTRICTIONS:	Oropharyngeal injuries
COMPLICATIONS:	Intraoral injury; induction of vomiting and aspiration; increased obstruction if positioned incorrectly by pushing the tongue back into pharynx
NASOPHARYNGEAL AIRWAY	
INDICATIONS:	Semicomatose or arousable patients with decreased control of upper airway; prevention of tissue trauma during frequent nasotracheal suctioning
ADVANTAGES:	Better tolerated in awake patients than oral airway; easily secured
RESTRICTIONS:	Maxillofacial trauma such as nasal, nasoethmoid fractures
COMPLICATIONS:	Nasopharyngeal injury; nasal bleeding
ESOPHAGEAL OBTURATOR AIRWAY (EOA)	
INDICATIONS:	As an alternative when endotracheal intubation is technically not feasible.
ADVANTAGES:	Can be positioned quickly, with minimal manipulation of cervical spine; allows oxygen to be delivered through exit holes at laryngeal level of esophageal tube; proper face mask seal prevents escape of air through nose and mouth
RESTRICTIONS:	May produce retching and esophageal tears when used in awake or semiconscious patients; posterior pharyngeal bleeding; esophageal injury
COMPLICATIONS:	Tracheal compression on inflation of cuff above the level of the carina; inadvertent insertion of tube into trachea; induction of vomiting and aspiration upon removal; esophageal rupture from excessive cuff inflation
ENDOTRACHEAL TUBE	
INDICATIONS:	Preferred method of airway control
ADVANTAGES:	Stable airway; provides protection from aspiration; permits mechanical ventilation to be carried out; decreases gastric distention associated with bag-mask ventilation; nasal intubation preferred in the awake patient or when cervical spine integrity is unknown
RESTRICTIONS:	Used with caution in presence of laryngotracheal injuries (glottis, subglottis, and upper trachea)
COMPLICATIONS:	Esophageal intubation leading to hypoxia; right mainsteam bronchus intubation; induction of vomiting and aspiration; vocal cord injury; pharyngeal injury; tracheal lacerations; conversion of cervical spine injury without neurological deficit to injury with deficit; dislodged tube
CRICOTHYROIDOTOMY	
INDICATIONS:	When intubation does not relieve obstruction or the trachea cannot be intubated
ADVANTAGES:	More rapid, greater ease of accessibility, and lower incidence of bleeding than tracheostomy
RESTRICTIONS:	Children under 12 years; laryngeal injury or inflammation
COMPLICATIONS:	Subglottic stenosis; vocal cord injury; aspiration; hemorrhage; tracheal or esophageal laceration; mediastinal emphysema; dislodged tube
STANDARD TRACHEOSTOMY	
INDICATIONS:	When intubation does not relieve obstruction or in significant laryngeal or tracheal trauma; used for prolonged ventilatory support
ADVANTAGES:	Bypasses upper airway and glottis; stable airway with low resistance to airflow; easily suctioned
RESTRICTIONS:	Limited use as an emergency procedure due to time requirements and potential for bleeding
COMPLICATIONS:	Early or delayed hemorrhage; aspiration; mediastinal emphysema with or without pneumothorax; tracheoesophageal fistula; tracheal stenosis; tracheomalacia; tracheoarterial fistula; dislodged tube

Assessment for partial or impending obstruction is initiated as often as required. Frequent signs include increasing level of agitation, increasing airway pressures during mechanical ventilation, difficulty in advancement of a suction catheter, and frequent evacuation of bloody clots or mucous plugs. Proper airway position and cuff pressure are determined by clinical and radiographical examinations.

General nursing management begins by documentation of airway tolerance, complications, length of intubation, or date of tracheostomy. The specific plan of care is based on such factors as a history of any airway problems, difficulty in intubation, and patient behavior, such as attempts at self-extubation or bronchospasm on suctioning. An identical spare airway is located at the bedside for rapid management of obstruction. Airway hygiene is implemented on the basis of assessment findings. Tracheostomy care is patient-specific depending on the newness of the tract, type of secretions or peritracheal drainage, and any signs of infection. A record is maintained at the bedside of all tube changes, tube size, and any difficulties encountered in tube placement. The need for long-term airway management is apparent in the intermediate care setting if not before. Substitution of a fenestrated or "talking" tracheostomy will help communication, and speech therapy consultation is required for patients recovering from laryngeal or vocal cord injury. As soon as the patient and family indicate readiness, a teaching plan is begun that covers long-term and home management of secretions and tracheostomy care.

Ineffective Airway Related to Tracheobronchial Trauma

Description. The tracheobronchial tree may be injured at any level; most commonly, injury involves the mainstem bronchi within an inch of the carina (Fig. 19–12). Injuries may be complete or incomplete, and total separation of the tracheobronchial tree can occur. However, continuity of the airway may be maintained by the fascia surrounding the trachea and bronchi.[14] The lower airway injuries are of interest to nurses in all phases of trauma care because injury discovery may occur dramatically during intubation and ventilation or surprisingly late into the patient's posttrauma course. The injury is usually caused by blunt forces, the common denominator being violent injury. An example is a frontal crush injury, a vertical stretching of the trachea or bronchus, or any impact creating suddenly increased pressure within the airway against a closed glottis. Tracheobronchial tears due to penetrating injury also occur, frequently seen in association with esophageal, carotid artery, or jugular vein trauma.

Resuscitation/Critical Care Assessment. The index of suspicion is initiated by the history of violent trauma, particularly in patients with fractures of the upper five ribs. The rupture may be immediately symptomatic through dyspnea, hemoptysis, and/or difficulty in intubation. Severe injuries are frequently fatal. In other cases, the tear may be suspected in the patient with mediastinal and subcutaneous emphysema accompanied by a persistent pneumothorax which resists reexpansion. More commonly, the rupture develops in two stages. The patient shows almost no symptoms until 3 or 4 days after admission, when pneumothorax or subcutaneous emphysema develops. Should the patient already have chest tubes in place, a persistent pleural air leak is evident, possibly with continued extravasation of air into tissues. An additional clinical picture may evolve, one that is particularly difficult to diagnose and requires the correlation of nursing and medical observations. Early atelectasis appears and persists due to occlusion of the bronchus with blood and secretions. Bloody secretions are evident on coughing or during suctioning as pleural fluid is drawn back through the damaged airway.

In assessing for tracheobronchial tears, one must consider possible location, size, and involvement of bronchial vessels or the mediastinal pleura. The patient may demonstrate significant hemoptysis, airway obstruction, pneumothorax, tension pneumothorax, or massive atelectasis. Any one of these characteristic findings raises the possibility of tracheobronchial injury. The diagnosis is confirmed through tracheobronchoscopy, an emergent procedure for the highly unstable patient.

Management. Initial management is dependent on the severity of the symptoms described above. An airway is secured in the patient with significant hemoptysis and airway obstruction either by insertion of an endotracheal tube or tracheostomy. If present, pneumothorax, tension pneumothorax, and any mediastinal compression are treated by tube thoracostomy and evacuation of pleural air by suction. The rate and amount of air evacuated by the chest tube are continuously monitored, as is the adequacy of air intake into the lungs. Immediate thoracotomy is indicated in the presence of massive air leak that prevents adequate air intake.

More commonly, the initial tube thoracostomy is followed by definitive diagnostic bronchoscopy and plans for injury repair. If the tear is large and irregular or a complete rupture, early surgical repair is accomplished by a cervical or thoracic approach. The tear is resected and closed by end-to-end anastomosis. A small tear may be treated conservatively solely through airway management. The airway chosen for management is dependent on the location and leaking effect of the tear. A standard endotracheal tube or tracheostomy may be used. Selective endobronchial intubation with a

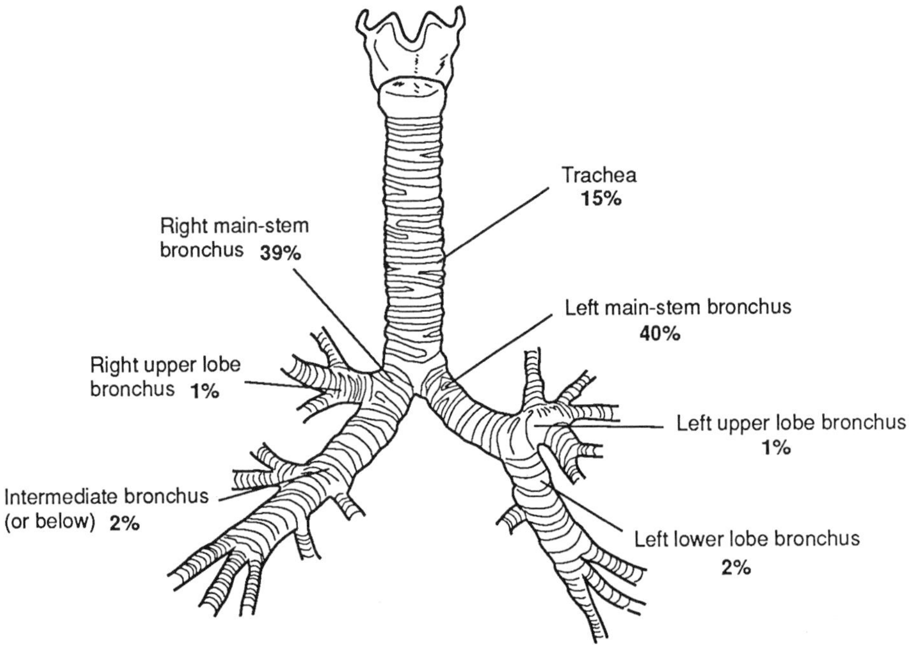

Figure 19–12. Tracheobronchial ruptures: General localizations based on literature review. (From Besson A, Saegesser F: Chest Trauma and Associated Injuries. Oradell, NJ, Medical Economics, 1983.)

biluminal tube also can be accomplished if there is a need for independent lung ventilation; this technique is discussed within the critical care therapeutics section of this chapter. As the inflammation and edema due to injury subside, the area can potentially heal with complete sealage.

Specific Nursing Management. The nurse must know the location of the tear and repair status to create an appropriate plan of care. In all cases, the existing airway must be carefully secured and protected from dislodgment or inadvertent repositioning. It may be technically difficult to reposition a dislodged tube, exposing the patient to needless risk of hypoxia, asphyxia, or extension of the tear. If surgical repair has been completed, airway protection remains critical while the suture line heals. Careful suctioning and neck positioning to avoid increased suture tension protect the area of surgical repair.

An additional management focus is measurement of the quantity and effect of any air leak on ventilation and oxygenation. Pleural drainage is inspected regularly for sudden air evacuation and increases in a known leak. Thoracic examination is repeated to appreciate changes in subcutaneous air and the development of pneumomediastinum or pneumothorax (Fig. 19–13). Nursing care is directed toward avoiding sudden rises in the patient's airway pressure, which will delay sealage of the injury.

Bronchial injury may be accompanied by lung injury and tears in surrounding small blood vessels, allowing air to enter the pulmonary venous circulation. Monitoring for signs of air embolism is important, particularly prior to repair or for the patient who is conservatively managed without repair. A sudden cardiovascular deterioration after endotracheal intubation, without signs of bleeding, may be indicative of air embolism. Focal neurological signs in the non–head–injured patient are also significant. Placing the patient in the head-down position (Trendelenburg position) is presumably optimal to trap air in the apex of the left ventricle. Immediate cardiocentesis may be indicated to evacuate the air, and thoracotomy may be required to control the air leak.[16]

Intermediate Care Assessment and Management. Late diagnosis of tracheobronchial tears is frequent, and thoracic assessment for occult or missed injury continues during intermediate care. An additional focus of the assessment is the identification of posttraumatic complications such as bronchial stenosis. The initial tracheobronchial tear results in a stenosed airway obstructed by granulation tissue and prone to repeated inflammation and infection. Delayed atelectasis appears as granulation tissue obstructs the bronchus. Resection of the area of stricture and reanastomosis may be required to prevent repeated infections and heightened scar tissue formation below the level of the stenosis. Nursing management is directed toward specific chest physiotherapy for the affected areas and airway clearance. The patient's vital capacity, chest x-ray, and secretions are monitored. Assistance in coughing is a priority because the injury frequently leaves a residual decrease in bronchial sensitivity and a diminished cough reflex.[17]

Tracheal injury or, less commonly, tracheostomy may result in tracheal stenosis apparent by a hoarse unproductive cough, wheezing, and periodic dyspnea on exertion. Occasionally, assessment may reveal signs of tracheomalacia, which is a softened tracheal wall. This is the outcome of damage and loss of tracheal cartilage from tissue ischemia, necrosis, infection, and long exposure to an overinflated cuff. The patient's trachea expands and collapses during respiration. Repair of both types of complications is achieved by surgical resection and anastomosis or graft insertion.

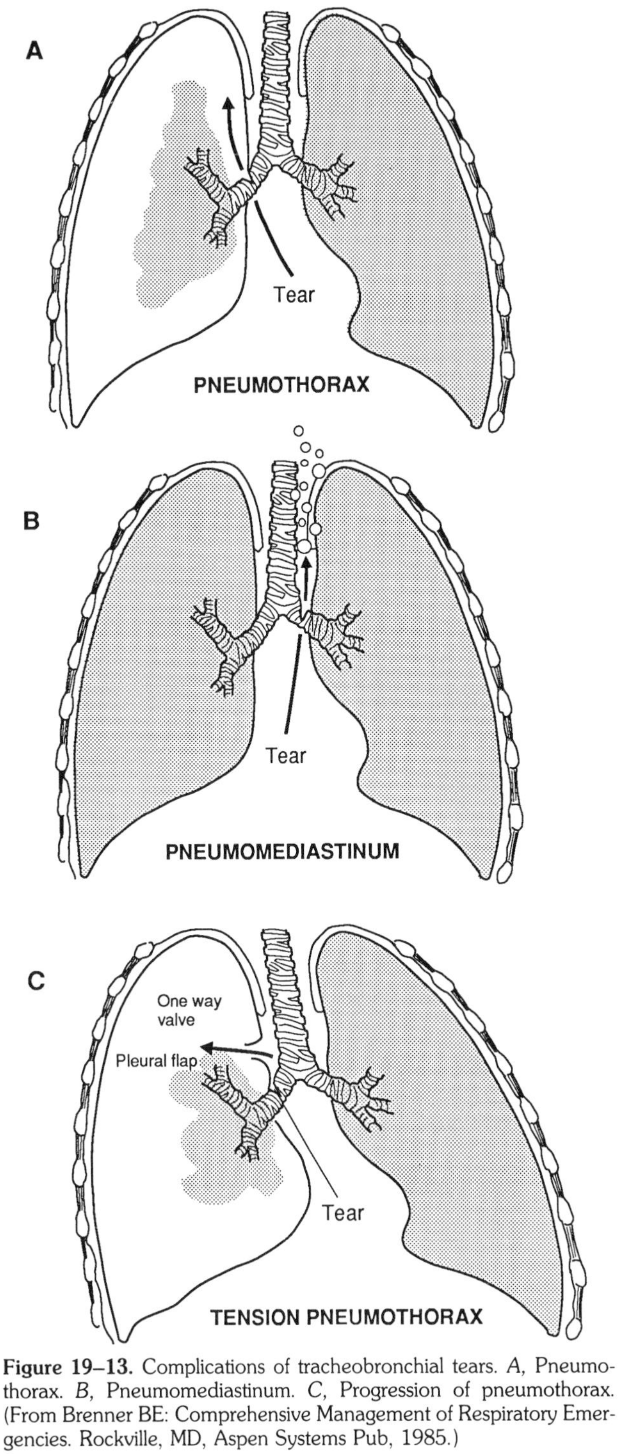

Figure 19–13. Complications of tracheobronchial tears. *A,* Pneumothorax. *B,* Pneumomediastinum. *C,* Progression of pneumothorax. (From Brenner BE: Comprehensive Management of Respiratory Emergencies. Rockville, MD, Aspen Systems Pub, 1985.)

Ineffective Airway Related to Posttraumatic Tracheal Fistula

Description and Etiology. Tracheoarterial or esophageal fistula may be the result of blunt injury in much the

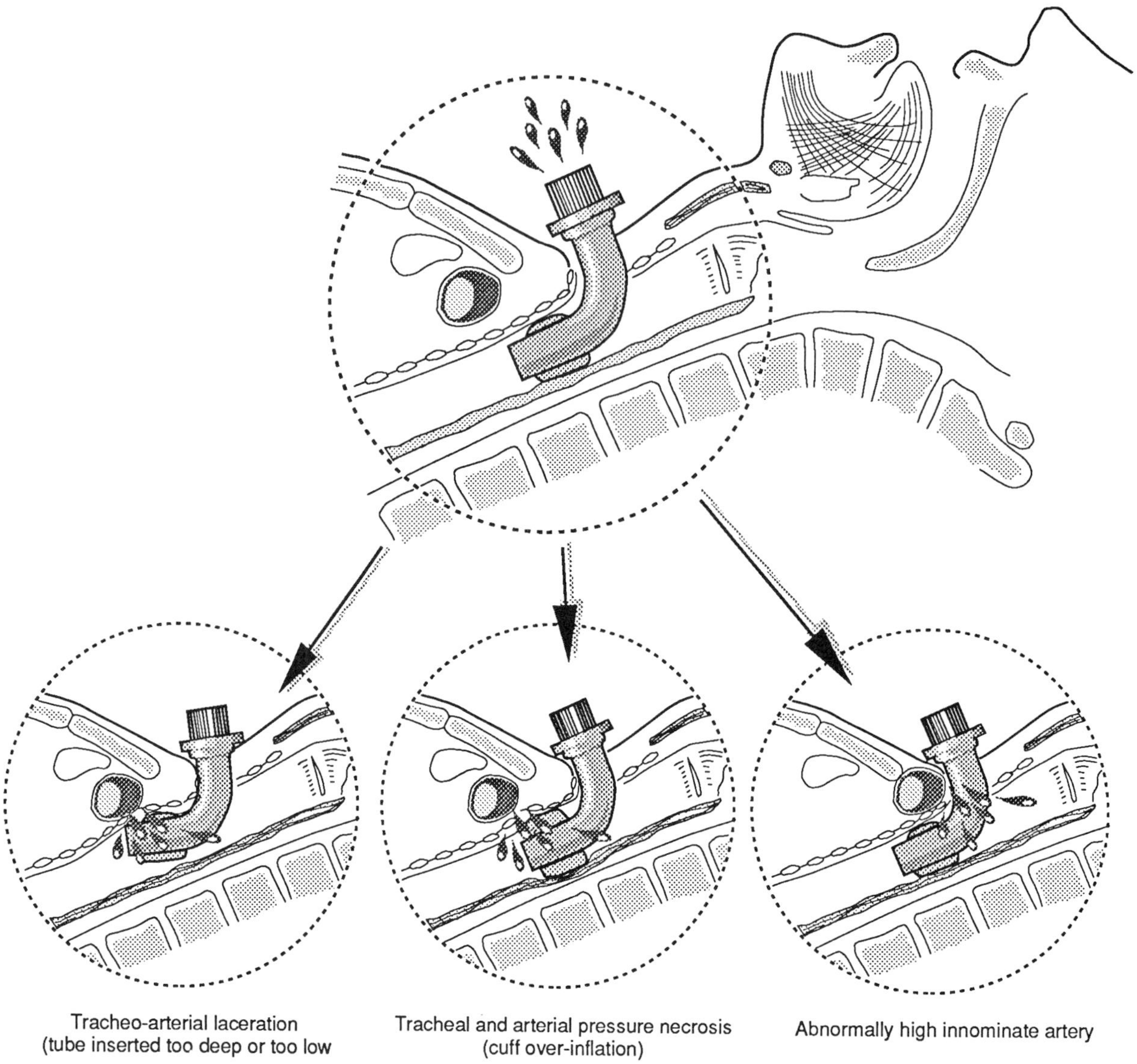

Figure 19–14. Tracheoarterial fistula. (From Besson A, Saegesser F: Chest Trauma and Associated Injuries. Oradell, NJ, Medical Economics, 1983.)

same fashion as tracheobronchial tears. More commonly, it is a form of "tube trauma." Although the association between high pressure or overdistended cuffs and tracheal fistulas is well known, cuff pressures and position can be difficult to manage and require special consideration and cooperation from the trauma team. Significant airway pathology can occur after as little as 6 hours of intubation and mechanical ventilation.[18] Tube trauma can be a sequela of a difficult intubation or tracheostomy. During these procedures, a retropharyngeal or tracheal wall nick or tear can occur. The area becomes infected with upper airway secretions, erodes, and becomes a fistula. Successful repair of tracheoarterial (TA) and tracheoesophageal (TE) fistulas is reported with increased frequency. Discussion of surgical repair and its complications is found elsewhere.[19]

Tracheoarterial Fistula. The vessel involved may be the innominate, right carotid, or a lower thyroid artery which has been exposed to pressure from an overinflated cuff or a poorly positioned airway. As the tracheal wall erodes, the vessel is perforated and suddenly bleeds into the airway. The patient may die immediately from hemorrhage through the tracheostomy. Figure 19–14 shows how poor tube positioning and cuff overinflation cause a hemorrhage.

Prevention. Physiological cuff pressure is maintained at less than mean mucosal capillary pressure of 20 to 25 mm Hg.[20] The different commercially available tracheostomy and endotracheal tubes all exert varying tracheal wall pressures, including the soft, large-volume cuffs and foam cuffs which are autoregulated by air valve. Proper inflation of the cuff according to product recommendations is useful; however, the actual cuff pressure must be systematically and regularly measured. Measurement is made by a special cuff pressure gauge or, if necessary, by a simple stopcock and manometer apparatus. The current standard of continuous inflation to a minimal leak is discussed within the nursing research literature.[21, 22] If there is reason to believe that the patient is at risk for TA fistula, a shorter or longer tube of appropriate diameter may be inserted to relieve the immediate pressure. A pulsating tracheostomy tube is evidence of such risk but does not confirm fistulization. Any patient at high risk can be examined by tracheoscopy for evidence of fistula formation.

Immediate Management of the Disaster. An attempt is made by immediate maximal cuff inflation to stem the bleeding. If cuff overinflation fails, the tracheostomy tube is removed, and a translaryngeal tube is inserted. The cuff is again inflated at the level of the fistula to control the bleeding, or the tube may be positioned so as to allow direct finger pressure and control. The finger is inserted along the anterior trachea and compresses the blood vessel against the sternum.[14] The patient is ventilated and prepared for immediate transport to the operating room. If transport is not possible, the surgical equipment necessary for artery ligation is readied. A standard thoracotomy tray or a complete cutdown preparation tray contains the needed equipment. Suction must be immediately at hand.

Definitive Management. Should the patient survive the initial hemorrhage and artery ligation, ventilation is provided by a long transtracheal tube with the cuff positioned below the necrotic area. Delayed repair of the trachea and arterial reconstruction are accomplished once the risk of infection is lessened. The repair includes resection and anastomosis or grafting, if necessary. Every effort should be made to wean the patient from the ventilator and remove the tracheostomy tube as soon as possible.

Tracheoesophageal Fistula. The tracheoesophageal fistula also can be life-threatening, although not in the sense of the vascular fistula. It is not an emergency, yet it threatens life through respiratory insufficiency and infection. The injury is a pressure necrosis of the trachea and the anterior esophageal wall. Rarely is it a primary injury from blunt trauma. Figure 19–15 shows how fistulas occur from tube placement and cuff inflation.

Prevention. The techniques described for prevention of vascular fistulas are also appropriate in this case. The most likely pressure site is between the airway cuff and nasogastric tube. Frequent evaluation of the need and use of these tubes is a primary preventive action. Each tube is viewed as a risk factor and is eliminated as soon as possible. For example, a gastrostomy tube can be placed for long-term gastric decompression and permit the removal of a nasogastric tube. The risk of a fistula continues into the rehabilitative phase for the trauma patient who requires long-term tracheostomy.

Assessment. Most symptoms are usually identified by the observing nurse. The patient coughs on swallowing, or pulmonary secretions appear contaminated by gastric contents. The usual amount of tracheal secretions increases, and gastric distention may consistently be evident. The appearance of swallowed methylene blue dye in tracheal aspirate is a classic bedside test. Visualization of the fistula is accomplished by endoscopy or bronchoscopy. Contrast studies are associated with a high risk of aspiration and are not recommended.

Management. The fistula must be closed surgically, generally through a cervical incision, but the timing of surgical repair depends on the patient's general condition. The patient may require considerable pulmonary care and nutritional support via parenteral nutrition and jejunostomy before repair is attempted. A large-volume, low-pressure cuff airway is used during the period of supportive preoperative therapy and after the surgical repair. The airway cuff is positioned at a different site within the trachea if possible.

Alteration in Ventilation Related to Bony Thorax Fractures

Description and Fracture Sites. The triad of pain, ineffective ventilation, and secretion retention is consistently observed in patients with rib fractures, sternal fractures, or flail chest. It is from this perspective that the patient with thoracic cage fractures presents the greatest demand for creative and effective nursing care. The first two ribs are generally protected by the surrounding muscles, clavicle, scapula, and humerus. Fractures of these ribs signal high-impact trauma and are generally accompanied by injury to lungs, the aortic arch, or vertebral column. Ribs 3 through 9 are most commonly fractured in blunt trauma and are frequently associated with underlying lung injury. The lower rib has a similar anatomical association with liver tears or other abdominal injuries. Sternal fractures are also generally associated with considerable blunt trauma (Table 19–4).

Flail Chest. Flail chest is an injury of multifocal fractures, whether anterior, lateral, or posterior. Generally, multiple rib fractures and a sternal fracture are present. The continuity of the thorax is destroyed, and the rib cage no longer moves evenly and in unison. The injured parts of the bony thorax do not respond to the action of the respiratory muscle but move according to changes in intrapleural pressure. The flail segments appear to move paradoxically, and from this appearance, the term *paradoxical breathing* has been used traditionally to describe the patient's respiratory efforts. Gas flow within the lungs may or may not move paradoxically, but it is significantly diminished. The bellows effect of the chest is lost, intrapleural pressure is less negative than normal, and ventilation is compromised. The decreased gas flow and increased respiratory dead space are evident in lowered patient tidal volumes, increased respiratory effort, and varying degrees of hypoxia.

Resuscitation Assessment of Flail Chest. The best assessment is simply to carefully observe the patient's breathing and chest wall. Breathing is rapid and labored, and the chest wall moves in an asymmetrical and uncoordinated manner. The flail will be evident by inspection and by palpation of the crepitus from bony fragments. The amount of dyspnea and initial hypoxia is dependent on the size of the flail and associated pulmonary parenchymal injuries, as well as the patient's ability to exert the needed respiratory effort in compensation for the flail. The injury causes great chest wall pain and patient fatigue. The initial chest film identifies the general extent of the flail and additional thoracic injuries.

It is difficult to characterize a specific profile for the patient with flail chest because the injury is so often accompanied by either a pneumothorax or some degree of pulmonary contusion. Both these injuries are discussed in detail later in this chapter. It is essential to associate flailing thoracic injuries with a high probability of underlying parenchymal damage. Serial blood gases and continuous observation of patient tidal volume and respiratory effort should be initiated, particularly in the patient who is not immediately intubated and mechanically ventilated. Flail chest and associated injuries frequently also produce upper and lower airway obstruction from blood, mucus, or vomit.

Initial Management. All patients with flail chest injury will require appropriate airway management, some type of analgesia, and oxygen therapy to maintain the Pao_2 at levels of 80 to 100 mm Hg. The flail must be stabilized so as to reestablish the thoracic bellows effect and promote air exchange. Prehospital use of sandbags, tape, straps, or belts to splint the flail is of questionable utility. If these measures promote patient comfort, and therefore ventilation, they cannot be categorically excluded.[23] Positioning the patient with the injured side down may improve oxygenation, but it is generally precluded by the need for immobilization of the spine and supine positioning for transport. In-hospital management includes internal "splinting" through positive-pressure ventilation for as much as 3 weeks.[24] External skeletal traction has been used but is associated with high risk of infectious complications (Fig. 19–16). Surgical internal stabilization of rib and sternal fragments also has been recommended, especially if thoracotomy is required for some other reason. Internal fixation has been shown to significantly improve patient outcomes, as well as avoid the complications associated with prolonged ventilatory support.[24]

Ventilatory Therapy. There are several ways to support ventilation in patients with significant flail chest. Nonventilator support with oxygen therapy may be successful in patients who can follow commands and do not have underlying parenchymal damage. In other patients, mechanical ventilation offers specific advantages, including airway and ventilatory control for pulmonary hygiene, functional positioning of flail segments, decreased muscular work, and a decrease in painful, paradoxical chest wall motion. Specific patients who benefit from mechanical ventilation in some mode include nonambulatory or disoriented patients, those

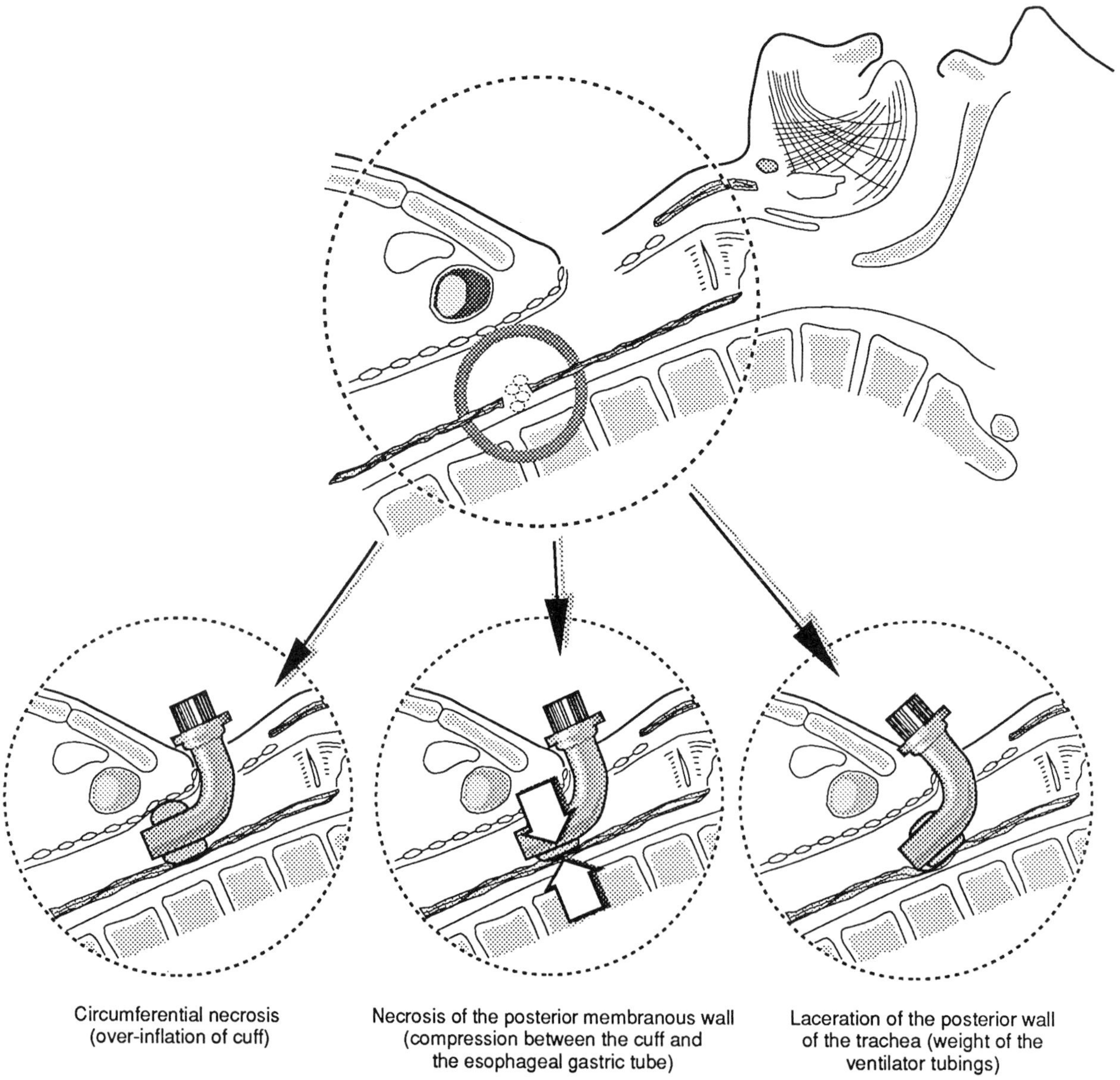

Figure 19–15. Causes of tracheoesophageal fistula in patients with tracheostomy. (From Besson A, Saegesser F: Chest Trauma and Associated Injuries. Oradell, NJ, Medical Economics, 1983.)

TABLE 19–4. CLASSIFICATION OF RIB FRACTURES

INJURY	MAJOR MANIFESTATIONS, RELATED INJURIES, AND COMMON COMPLICATIONS
Fractures of one rib	
Simple	Pain aggravated by deep breathing, coughing Localized tenderness Roentgenograms may or may not demonstrate fracture
Complicated	Pneumothorax, hemothorax Pulmonary infection or atelectasis
Multiple rib fractures	
With stable chest wall	Severe chest wall pain Underlying lung contusion or contusion of opposite lung Decreased cough and accumulation of secretions Acute gastric dilation Hemothorax, pneumomediastinum, and pneumothorax
With instability of chest wall	Generally involves fracture of each rib in two sites Panel of chest wall moves independently of thoracic cage (paradoxical respiration) Severely impaired cough and airway clearance Contusion of underlying lung Hemothorax and pneumothorax
Fractures of first rib	Usually associated with fractures of clavicle and upper ribs May involve neurovascular structures of neck Intrathoracic injuries
Fractures of lower ribs (seventh to twelfth)	Injuries to liver and spleen Acute gastric dilation

Reprinted with permission from Guenter CA, Welch MH: Pulmonary Medicine, 2nd ed. Philadelphia, JB Lippincott, 1982.

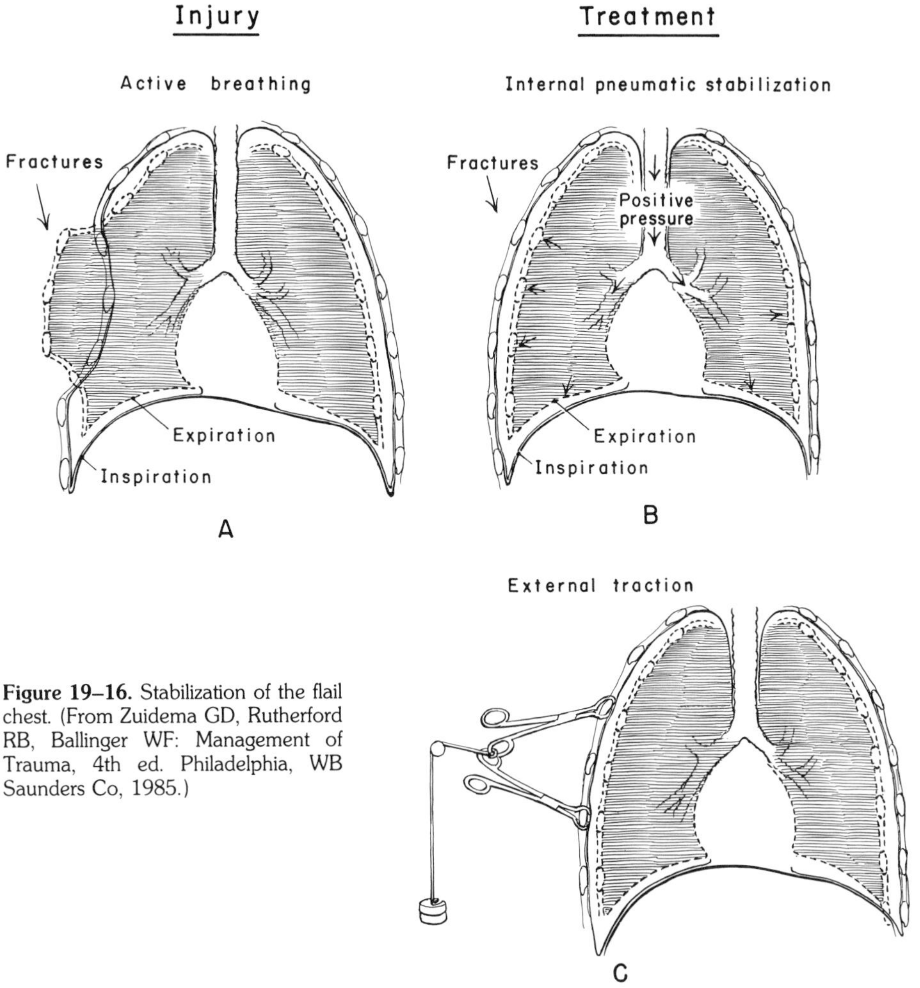

Figure 19–16. Stabilization of the flail chest. (From Zuidema GD, Rutherford RB, Ballinger WF: Management of Trauma, 4th ed. Philadelphia, WB Saunders Co, 1985.)

with significant lung pathology, and those with consistently diminished tidal volume (i.e., <15 ml/kg) due to fatigue and other injuries. Critics of mechanical ventilation cite disadvantages such as increased risk of barotrauma, pulmonary contamination, and a potentially longer need for therapy. A reasonable approach to ventilatory therapy in flail chest injuries is to individualize ventilatory support for the patient. The choice of therapy is dependent on the size of the flail; immediate degree of pulmonary dysfunction; work of breathing and fatigue; the presence of other thoracic injuries, particularly underlying pulmonary contusion; the need for general anesthesia and surgical procedures related to associated traumatic injuries; and the risk of posttraumatic respiratory insufficiency. Intubation/tracheostomy and mechanical ventilation are indicated if there is a respiratory rate greater than 35 breaths per minute, PaO_2 below 60 mm Hg on supplemental oxygen, or $PaCO_2$ above 50 mm Hg.[24]

Critical Care Assessment and Management. The choice of intubation and ventilator therapy may not be made until admission to the critical care unit. In addition to the preceding criteria, the choice may depend on equipment and available nursing management. The patient with significant flail and underlying lung contusion is frequently a long-term patient in the intensive care unit. Management of the injuries and weaning from ventilator support may require as many as 10 to 25 days. Appropriate equipment and effective nursing management must be available throughout the period. As stated earlier, the common triad in flail chest is ineffective ventilation, accumulation of secretions, and chest pain. Specific nursing care includes management of the patient–ventilator unit, pulmonary care, and pain control.

Managing the Patient–Ventilator Unit. Whichever ventilator therapy is selected, the patient must be closely monitored through pulse oximetry, blood gases, and pulmonary function studies such as vital capacity, inspiratory force, tidal volume, and a measure of the work of breathing in order to determine therapy results. Most frequently, the patient is treated and later weaned by IMV or SIMV with pressure support with rate, pressures, tidal volume, and oxygen concentration adjusted to maintain acceptable blood gases. Repeated clinical examination and daily chest films trend respiratory complications such as respiratory distress syndrome or atelectasis and progress toward chest wall stability. Chest wall rigidity is apparent at approximately 3 weeks, and a full 6 weeks are usually required before the fractures are consolidated.

Pulmonary Care. As ventilation is stabilized, pulmonary care begins to clear the airways and lung fields. Aggressive chest physiotherapy consisting of postural drainage, gentle percussion, vibration, and suctioning are used at varying intervals, usually every 4 hours. The quality and quantity of secretions are monitored for infection. A plan for patient position change is based on observation of which position provides greatest chest wall stability (such as lying on the flail segment) and best ventilation/oxygenation. These treatments are discussed in more detail in the section on critical care therapeutics.

Pain Control. Detailed discussion of pain assessment and management is covered in Chapter 15. Pain control is critically important and may be the primary problem for patients with bony thorax fractures. A variety of useful treatments have been reported for thoracic pain which include intercostal nerve blocks and intrapleural administration of narcotics. Patient-controlled administration (PCA) of both intravenous and epidural narcotics is supported by nursing research as a safe and effective modality for pain control.[25, 26] Continuous intravenous narcotics which are titrated by the nurse according to the patient's respiratory status, level of consciousness, and level of pain also constitute a well-accepted method of pain control, especially in patients who are not candidates for PCA. Regardless of the method or route of administration, appropriate dosage ranges are established for the patient and then are trended by nursing observation and management. Nonpharmacologically, the application of a transcutaneous electrical nerve stimulator (TENS) may be successful in relieving pain associated with thoracic injuries and is described elsewhere.[27]

Intermediate/Rehabilitation Care Assessment and Management. At this point in the trauma recovery, new complications of bony thorax fractures begin to be evident. The normal healing of the fractures may be altered, and deformities may be evident to the patient and family. Some deformities, from flail chest in particular, are permanent, unattractive, and difficult for the individual to accept. Others may create ventilatory impairment leading to chronic disability and changes in life-style. Attempts at surgical reconstruction may dominate the patient's recovery experience.

The plan of care for the patient is built around assessment of the emerging complications and disability as well as previously described needs for pulmonary care, control of retained secretions and infection, and continued chest pain. The goal of pulmonary care is support of spontaneous ventilation and weaning from oxygen therapy. Chest physiotherapy and incentive spirometry are continued in order to clear problem areas in the lungs and improve respiratory mechanics such as thoracic muscle strength. The patient continues to experience chest pain to some degree, for some, an intractable, intercostal pain or neuralgia. Chest pain can be managed pharmacologically. However, other methods must be initiated if they have not previously been in progress, since pain relief is frequently a lengthy and complex problem. TENS, massage, and positioning are only a few of the possibilities.

Complications of Fracture Healing. Rib fractures usually heal within 6 weeks. Occasionally, malunion or a failure to consolidate fractures, even an entire flail segment, does occur. Inspection and palpation as previously described will identify the unstable chest segment and can be confirmed radiographically. Internal fixation can be achieved by the wiring of bone fragments or insertion of metal plates.

Abnormal healing also results in excessive or hypertrophic callus formation, which may be gradually reabsorbed or surgically excised. The callus rubs on surrounding tissue and muscle and creates considerable pain. An abnormal union of adjacent ribs, intercostal synostosis, may proceed over months after injury. Clinical and radiographical examinations identify the abnormal healing in a patient who continually experiences pain and restricted chest wall movement.

Surgical intervention may be needed for definitive management of these healing abnormalities. As with any surgical patient, preoperative teaching is required, with detailed discussion of the procedure, anticipated experiences, and outcomes. The initial trauma did not allow for such preoperative preparation, and the current surgery may have a unique and special meaning for the patient.

Posttraumatic Respiratory Disability. Observation and interview identify dyspnea, shortness of breath, and a feeling of chest tightness in some patients. Blood gas analysis and chest film findings are frequently unchanged. The long-term sequelae of significant bony thorax trauma are unclear, and published case reports are few. Restrictive defects in ventilation have been identified in patients with flail chest and accompanying pleural or lung injury, as evidenced by moderate or severe dyspnea, abnormal spirometry, and lessened overall activity levels. The current nursing approach includes trending the patient's unique problems, instituting measures that provide comfort, ensuring appropriate physical therapy referrals, and providing a great deal of psychological support.

Alteration in Ventilation Related to Pleural Space Injuries

All the pleural space injuries have both blunt and penetrating etiologies. The force of injury, whether from blunt impact against the steering column or from a knife wound, produces laceration or perforation of an intrathoracic structure, usually a lung or blood vessel. Blood and/or air collect between the pleural layers, and the normal negative intrathoracic pressure is lost. All or part of the lung on the affected side collapses due to its unopposed elasticity. The result may be a pneumothorax (intrapleural air collection), hemothorax (intrapleural blood collection), or, very commonly in trauma, a hemopneumothorax (mix of both air and blood). If intrapleural air continues to increase within the constraints of the closed intrathoracic cavity, internal structures are compressed, and tension builds. The result is a tension pneumothorax. In all cases, the pleural space injury may be unilateral or bilateral.

General Pleural Space Injury Assessment. Examining for any type of pleural space injury follows the thoracic assessment procedure described earlier. It is useful to remember that the clinical findings are determined by the severity of all thoracic injuries as a whole as well as the severity of the pleural space injury. In addition, the signs of injury may change over the period of examination and resuscitation. A small hemothorax may become massive if bleeding resumes at some point after the patient's admission. The apparently small pneumothorax can evolve into a tension pneumothorax.

There are several classic assessment findings which are seen in all the significant pleural space injuries. Some degree of respiratory difficulty or dyspnea is evident. Since the primary problem is altered ventilation, there is evidence of poor gas exchange. There is frequently a loss of breath sounds on the affected side or sides. Diminished or absent breath sounds are evident with a collapsed lung and when blood loss into the thoracic cavity is significant (generally > 350 ml). There is a loss of normal resonance on percussion of the affected side. A dullness is audible in hemothorax, and there is hyperresonance when significant pneumothorax is present.

Early analysis of blood gases is useful only in the context of the patient's clinical examination and response to trauma. The patient who is breathing rapidly because of shock and pain may have relatively normal initial blood gases. Alternatively, there may be the "expected" rise in $Paco_2$ and fall in Pao_2 that is normally associated with poor ventilation.

Chest x-ray findings assist in documenting the injury and must be obtained as rapidly as possible. Small amounts of blood may not be visible, but in an average-sized chest, blood which fills the costophrenic angle on an upright film is usually over 300 ml in quantity. An air–fluid level which extends 5 cm above the diaphragm contains at least 1000 ml, while the volume of air in the chest can only be estimated. The film may reveal not only blood in the intrathoracic cavity but a segment of spleen or liver which has been displaced through a ruptured diaphragm.[28]

Closed Pneumothorax or Hemothorax. The simple, closed pneumothorax is usually the result of a lung laceration by a fractured rib or penetrating wound (Fig. 19–17). In more complex injuries, a diaphragmatic tear allows abdominal contents to protrude into the chest cavity, causing a compressive pneumothorax or hemopneumothorax. In many instances, the intrapleural air leak is self-limiting in that the progressive collapse and decreasing ventilation of the affected lung seal the leak. In other cases, depending on the size and location of the injury, the lung may collapse completely.

Common sources of bleeding in hemothorax include systemic chest wall vessels, internal mammary arteries, and intercostal arteries and accompanying veins. Penetrating wounds may involve major pulmonary vessels, any of the mediastinal structures, or the diaphragm. Although the pulmonary parenchyma is a common source of bleeding, major blood loss is generally not from parenchymal vessels. The lung is a low-pressure vascular system capable of tamponading sources of bleeding[29] (Fig. 19–18).

Resuscitation Management. As always, appropriate airway, ventilatory, and oxygen therapy begins the management process. Moderate pneumothorax or hemothorax requires the correct placement of a chest tube for the purposes of lung reexpansion and drainage of air, blood, and clots from the pleural space. Inadequate drainage creates short- and long-term complications, including intrapleural infections and adhesions. Insertion of a chest tube also reduces the risk of tension pneumothorax, which may develop as blood and/or air fill the chest cavity. Explanations of the injury and treatment are offered to the patient in a manner most appropriate for his emotional state and level of consciousness. The patient's pain must be recognized and treated.

A large-bore chest tube, such as a no. 40, is inserted generally in the fourth or fifth intercostal space in the midaxillary line so as to drain both air and blood. Alternatively, but less optimal in traumatic injuries, a tube may be placed in the second intercostal space in the midclavicular line to drain a simple pneumothorax. As soon as the tube is connected to the underwater seal system and suction drainage, the effects of the treatment are assessed by analysis of blood gases, chest x-ray, and physical examination. The bleeding is frequently self-limiting, and estimated blood loss is replaced at a rate consistent with the patient's overall status. Small to moderate air leaks will usually seal over in the first few posttrauma days. Occasionally, a major air leak persists, requiring more negative pressure in the suction drainage system or an additional chest tube. Bronchoscopy and open thoracotomy may be required to determine if

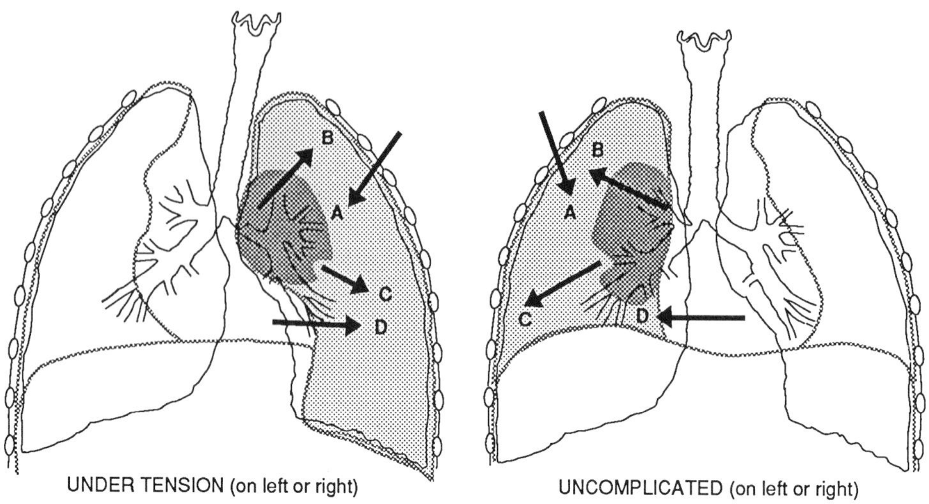

A	7%	Perforating or penetrating wound	20%
B	13%	Tracheobronchial injury (including barotrauma)	5%
C		Pulmonary laceration	
	71%	{ 27% probable 36% }	73%
		{ 44% documented 37% }	
D	9%	Oesophageal injury	3%
	33%	Accompanied by haemothorax	54%
	26%	Accompanied by subcutaneous emphysema	33%

Figure 19–17. Origins of pneumothorax. (From Besson A, Saegesser F: Chest Trauma and Associated Injuries. Oradell, NJ, Medical Economics, 1983.)

major bronchial injury is responsible for the continued air leak.

Critical Care/Intermediate Care Management. A simple pneumothorax or moderate hemothorax will not necessarily require critical care for the patient. However, this type of injury may be one of several thoracic injuries or frequently a symptom of more life-threatening injuries.

Monitoring the Injury and Drainage. The nurse evaluates the functioning of the chest tube system and the progress of the injury. Repeated physical assessment and follow-up chest films will determine if the lung has reexpanded and ventilation has returned to the patient's normal baseline. Pulse oximetry is utilized, and blood gases and a chest film are obtained whenever problems arise or the clinical status changes. Blood loss through or around the chest tube is measured and evaluated for further progression of bleeding. Drainage of more than 200 ml/hr for 2 successive hours may indicate additional or missed injuries and the need for exploratory thoracotomy. The patient's tidal volume and air evacuation through the chest tube system are trended for significant air leaks and loss of ventilatory volume. Nursing management of pleural drainage is discussed in more detail later in this chapter.

Massive Hemothorax. Massive hemothorax is defined as a 1.5- to 4-l intrathoracic blood loss and is truly a life-threatening injury. Frequently, there are severe associated thoracic injuries, and the source of bleeding is a large systemic blood vessel or mediastinal structure. Since the chest cavity is large enough to contain most of the patient's circulating blood volume, the bleeding slows only when the pressure within the pleural cavity is equal to or greater than the pressure within the damaged vessel. A left massive hemothorax is more common than a right one and is often associated with aortic rupture.

Resuscitation Assessment and Management. Thoracic assessment is initiated after basic life-support needs are managed. The patient may arrive in cardiopulmonary arrest and in need of immediate thoracotomy to control bleeding. Assessment findings in massive hemothorax differ from the moderate pleural injuries in degree. The immediate clinical picture includes signs of hypovolemic shock, dyspnea, tachypnea, and cyanosis. Shock is the predominant picture evident before or concomitantly with impaired ventilation. Ventilation problems are due to lung compression and collapse, and signs of mediastinal shift with cardiac compression also may be evident. The initial chest film identifies the extent of the hemothorax as a predominantly opaque chest cavity.

Hypovolemic shock is managed immediately by insertion of large-bore intravenous lines and rapid administration of resuscitation fluids. The next step is dependent on the amount of anticipated or apparent intrathoracic bleeding. The truly massive injury requires emergent exploratory thoracotomy with rapid control of bleeding. Delay of thoracotomy and initial insertion of a chest tube may provide an avenue for exsanguination by eliminating any tamponade effect of the closed chest injury (Fig. 19–19). Assuming that one or more chest tubes are in place and signs of exsanguination occur, the chest tube is clamped as an interim measure pending

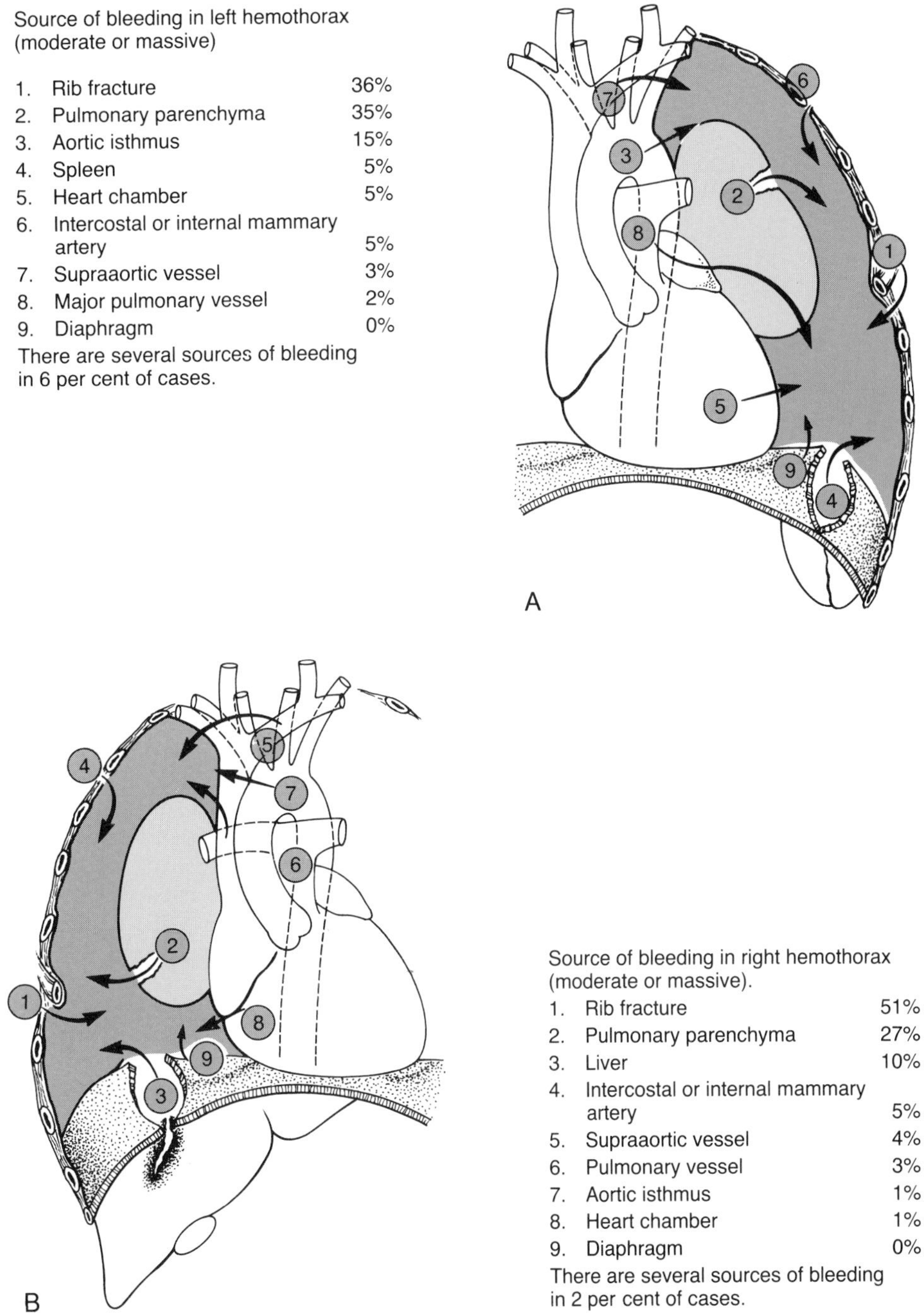
Source of bleeding in left hemothorax
(moderate or massive)
1. Rib fracture 36%
2. Pulmonary parenchyma 35%
3. Aortic isthmus 15%
4. Spleen 5%
5. Heart chamber 5%
6. Intercostal or internal mammary artery 5%
7. Supraaortic vessel 3%
8. Major pulmonary vessel 2%
9. Diaphragm 0%
There are several sources of bleeding in 6 per cent of cases.
A
B
Source of bleeding in right hemothorax
(moderate or massive).
1. Rib fracture 51%
2. Pulmonary parenchyma 27%
3. Liver 10%
4. Intercostal or internal mammary artery 5%
5. Supraaortic vessel 4%
6. Pulmonary vessel 3%
7. Aortic isthmus 1%
8. Heart chamber 1%
9. Diaphragm 0%
There are several sources of bleeding in 2 per cent of cases.

Figure 19–18. Sources of bleeding in hemothorax. (From Besson A, Saegesser F: Chest Trauma and Associated Injuries. Oradell, NJ, Medical Economics, 1983.)

emergency thoracotomy. In general, urgent thoracotomy is performed if there is:

1. Greater than 1500 ml of blood evacuated upon initial chest tube insertion
2. Continued bleeding of more than 300 ml/hr for 3 consecutive hours
3. Bleeding of more than 150 ml/hr for 3 consecutive hours in an elderly patient
4. Any of the preceding in the face of hemodynamic instability[24]

Autotransfusion. Autotransfusion is useful in the management of hemothorax and intrathoracic sources of bleeding. The reinfusion of blood aspirated from the chest as a thoracic trauma management method was reported by military surgeons as early as 1916.[30] A variety of techniques and commercially available autotransfusion devices are available for resuscitation of the injured patient. The technique's advantages and contraindications are well described in the literature.[31–37]

Advantages. The increasing use of autotransfusion in resuscitative, operative, and critical care attests to the numerous advantages of autologous blood administration. These include the following:

1. The blood is readily available and particularly useful in

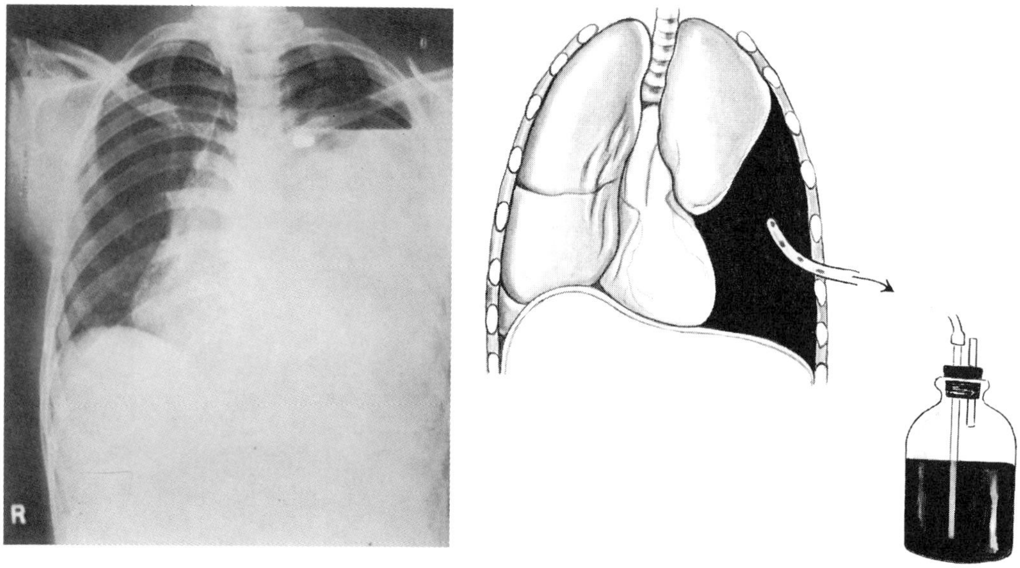

Figure 19–19. Radiograph of a young man in profound shock from gunshot wound of the chest. Bullet entry was in sixth intercostal space in midaxillary line. Hemothorax and shock were treated by chest tube drainage and fluid administration. Film (R) shows the central position of the bullet. The patient was transported to the operating room but died there from continuing hemorrhage from injury to the pulmonary hilar vessels. In massive hemothorax, exsanguination may occur following chest tube drainage. (From Naclerio EA: Chest Injuries. Orlando, Grune & Stratton, 1971.)

the patient with massive hemorrhage that exhausts or severely taxes the bank blood availability.

2. Autologous blood requires no cross-matching and should be free of pyrogens, avoiding allergic and febrile reactions.

3. Autotransfusion avoids the risk of hepatitis, AIDS, or exposure to homologous antigens.

4. Platelet counts and 2,3-diphosphoglycerate (2,3-DPG) levels essential to normal oxygen delivery to tissues are reported to be near normal in rapidly autotransfused blood. No warming is required.

5. Autologous blood may be acceptable to patients with religious backgrounds such as Jehovah's Witnesses who would normally refuse bank blood.

6. Savings in cost are generally appreciated depending on institutional pricing of equipment, operation, and packaging.

Techniques. Current autotransfusion devices range in cost, sophistication in function, and requirements for special technical assistance. One system separates out red cells and washes and resuspends them before patient infusion as a means of removing any plasma contaminants or debris while retaining red blood cells. More simple techniques can be employed rapidly in blunt and penetrating chest trauma. A thoracostomy tube inserted by standard technique and connected to suction provides an avenue for retrieval of shed intrathoracic blood. The blood is aspirated through sterile tubing, collected in a plastic reservoir with liner, filtered, and returned to the patient intravenously. The retrieval bag may contain citrate phosphate dextrose (CPD), although other types of anticoagulants or *no* anticoagulant are successfully used. Details of the autotransfusion procedure are contained in Appendix 19–2.

Contraindications. Specific contraindications to autotransfusion include known malignancy, inadequate renal or hepatic function, wounds greater than 3 hours old, and significant contamination due to bowel, stomach, or esophageal wounds. Clinical judgment is required as to the degree of contamination and risk of septic complications.

Management Concerns. Precautions and implications for nursing management center on the procedure's effect on the blood and risk of coagulopathy and microembolism. The primary effect on the blood is hemolysis leading to a reduced hematocrit and increased urine and serum hemoglobin. Typical falls in hematocrit of 10 to 15 per cent and increases in serum hemoglobin of 5 to 10 times normal have been reported. The hemolysis appears to occur at the blood–tissue and blood–plastic interfaces if roller pumps are used during collection and infusion.[38] Autologous blood from serosal cavities such as the thorax is without fibrinogen, contains elevated levels of fibrin split products, and shows prolonged prothrombin (PT) and partial thromboplastin (PTT) times.[39] Microembolism on infusion of shed blood is of concern due to hemolytic cell debris or platelet aggregation. Air embolism is also a concern, especially when the shed blood is reinfused using a surrounding pressure bag. Extraordinary care must be used to expel all the air within the reservoir bag prior to application of the pressure bag.

In view of these concerns, the patient who is or has recently been autotransfused is monitored through coagulation profiles, including a complete blood count and urine hemoglobin. Platelets and fresh-frozen plasma are given if clotting factors need to be replaced. If an anticoagulant accompanied the autotransfused blood, the same concerns are present as for bank blood. Serum calcium level is measured due to the chelating effect of citrate on calcium. Filters are used during the collection of autologous blood and as part of the blood administration protocol. If contaminated shed blood is reinfused, the patient is monitored for symptoms of emerging sepsis.

Use of an autotransfusion system may be episodic in many hospital units. The entire team, particularly nurses who assume responsibility for the use of equipment and monitoring the patient's response to treatment, must maintain their knowledge and skills. Methods and equipment need to be the subject of periodic inservice training, with the goal that all trauma team members can initiate autotransfusion rapidly, safely, and without complications.

Tension Pneumothorax. Immediate recognition of this life-threatening injury is required of nurses who manage patients in any phase of trauma care. Tension pneumothorax may be the immediate result of the primary traumatic injury, a delayed complication of an occult injury such as bronchial tear, or the undesirable result of necessary therapies such as mechanical ventilation. Air (and possibly blood) that has entered the pleural space is trapped without exit, creating a one-way-valve closed system (Fig. 19–20). One or more internal thoracic structures (most notably the trachea, lung, heart, and great vessels) are progressively compressed and fail to function adequately. The compression/failure mechanism may affect one or both sides of the chest cavity simply because pressure is transmitted through the chest as a whole. The patient outcome is a failure in ventilation, venous return, and eventually cardiac output. Assessment and treatment deal with the problem in ventilation and/or cardiovascular performance.

Initial Assessment. Systematic assessment and diagnosis are not always simple in the trauma patient. Classic signs of tension pneumothorax may be obscured by shock and other injuries or treatments until the patient is badly compromised. Under these circumstances, the initial assessment begins by identifying the high-risk patient, such as one with an inadequately resolved pneumothorax, bronchial tear, lung contusion, or pulmonary cyst. The use of moderate to high levels of PEEP also creates a risk of tension pneumothorax. Discovery of the injury at times does not occur until the patient presents a rapid and steep fall in oxygenation. The patient is ventilated with difficulty yet appears to have an open airway.

The patient is carefully and rapidly examined for clues as to the failure in ventilation and/or cardiac output. One focus of the assessment is for signs of increased intrathoracic pressure, the compression/failure effect. Chest wall movement is observed for asymmetry, and the chest wall is percussed for the characteristic hypertympanic note of trapped air. Tracheal shift is a classic finding but may be difficult to determine in the intubated patient except by chest radiograph. Unless the patient is severely hypovolemic, neck veins may be distended reflecting downstream intrathoracic pressure. Breath sounds are carefully compared from one side to the other and are diminished. Blood gases, if available, show a sudden drop in PaO_2. Finally, cardiac output is quickly assessed through decreases in blood pressure, tachycardia, or a general shock state that is unexplained by other injuries.

Immediate Management. Supplemental oxygen is provided, and then the chest must be decompressed by release of the trapped air. Decompression is achieved in three phases. Initial relief can be accomplished by inserting a 14- to 16-gauge needle into the pleural space, usually at the second to fourth anterior intercostal space. The needle is inserted over the rib and only 1 cm beyond to avoid puncturing the lung or injuring intercostal nerves and vessels.[14] As air is released, ventilation should improve. The pleural space equilibrates with atmospheric pressure, and the tension pneumothorax is temporarily converted to an open pneumothorax. The next phase of treatment occurs as one or more chest tubes are inserted both to reexpand the lung (or both lungs in bilateral tension pneumothorax) and as prophylaxis for any repeated episodes. Third, the cause of the injury must be explored and managed appropriately. The chest film, blood gases, hemodynamic measurements, and clinical examination are repeated to reassess the patient's posttreatment state.

Open Pneumothorax. Penetrating chest trauma which opens the pleural space to the atmosphere creates an open pneumothorax or sucking chest wound (Fig. 19–21). Historically described as early as the 13th century, the open pneumothorax is a common combat injury. It is most likely seen in civilian life as the result of penetrating injury or impalement. A number of factors have been proposed in explanation for the ventilatory difficulty present in open pneumothorax. If the size of the chest wall defect is approximately two-thirds the tracheal diameter, air will preferentially enter the chest wall during respiration. This "false airway" allows intrathoracic and atmospheric pressures to equalize, losing the essential pressure gradient required for normal ventilation.[15] Loss of normal intrathoracic negative pressure reduces venous return and cardiac performance, which is aggravated by mediastinal shift and compression of the vena cava and heart.

Resuscitation Assessment and Management. The first step

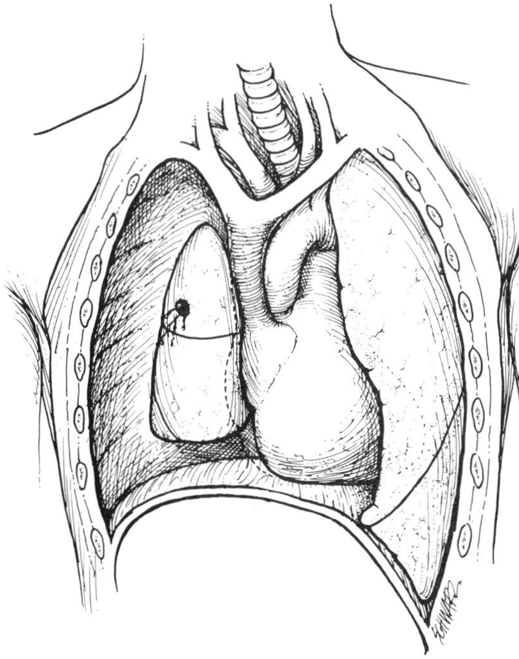

Figure 19–20. Tension pneumothorax. A bullet or knife wound to the lung can create a check-valve perforation, resulting in a tension pneumothorax. Pressure builds in the right hemithorax, impeding venous return, shifting the mediastinum to the left, and depressing the diaphragm. The great vessels become twisted and distorted. This decreases cardiac output and leads to shock with cyanosis, dyspnea, and neck distention. Atelectasis of an entire lobe leads to shunting, with cyanosis and tachypnea. Insertion of a venting needle or chest tube can be life saving. (From Weiner SL, Barrett J: Trauma Management for Civilian and Military Physicians. Philadelphia, WB Saunders Co, 1986.)

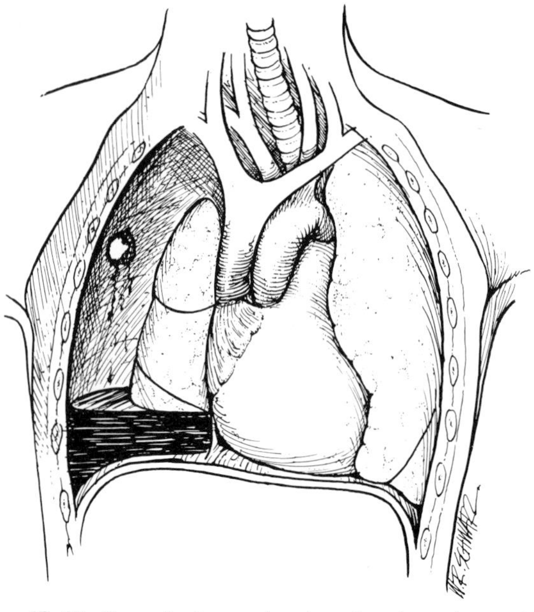

Figure 19–21. Open chest wound and resulting hemothorax. (From Weiner SL, Barrett J: Trauma Management for Civilian and Military Physicians. Philadelphia, WB Saunders Co, 1986.)

is locating the wound. Careful inspection of the entire thorax, including the patient's back, reveals the injury. Once the wound has been found, the sucking action is readily apparent. Not infrequently, there are gas bubbles at the wound site, and abnormal gas exchange may be audible. Not all penetrating chest wounds create an open pneumothorax; some are superficial although menacing in appearance. Conversely, a small and unassuming wound may be responsible for the pneumothorax and other threatening injuries. The previously described thoracic assessment techniques are used to detect difficulty in ventilation and hypoxia.

The management objectives are to restore ventilation and to debride and close the wound. Ventilation is, as always, the priority. Extensive open wounds, such as from a close-range shotgun blast, will require intubation and mechanical ventilation. In all cases, the false airway must be sealed and the lung allowed to reexpand. A sterile occlusive dressing is immediately applied over the entire wound, the effects of which are repeatedly reassessed. An old but still useful method is three-sided taping of dressing materials to the chest wall. This creates a flutter effect as the dressing is sucked down to the chest wall on inspiration yet allows air to escape on expiration. After the dressing is applied, a chest tube is inserted at another site to treat the pneumothorax. Should the occlusive dressing seal off the wound without a means of escape for the trapped air, barotrauma and a tension pneumothorax are possible. Therefore, the effect of the dressing on ventilation is observed over time, particularly while waiting for effective placement of the chest tube. The treatment effect is monitored without removing the dressing by noting changes in breath sounds and signs of intrathoracic pressure.

After ventilation has been adequately managed, the wound will require cleansing and debridement. The need for definitive surgical exploration and closure is dependent on the wound and on the presence of additional injuries requiring high-priority treatment.

Impaired Gas Exchange Related to Pulmonary Contusion

Mechanism and Pathophysiology. Essentially a compression/decompression injury, lung contusion occurs as the chest wall hits an object such as a steering wheel or is impacted on by an outside force such as an explosion. The force against the chest wall is transmitted to the lung, rupturing tissue, small airways, and alveoli. The pressure wave abates, and the chest wall springs back, pulling the lung with it and causing additional injury. It is a bruising process possibly accompanied by pulmonary tear or laceration. This injury occurs most often in young people because the chest wall is more flexible than in older individuals. Whereas the older person might sustain multiple rib fractures, the young patient may sustain more contusion.[40] Those individuals with thin chests sustain greater contusion because there is less protection provided by extensive muscle and adipose tissue.

Contusions may be mild and go unnoticed in the treatment of associated injuries such as flail chest or hemopneumothorax. However, unilateral or bilateral contusion can be severe, even life-threatening, and can seriously interfere with gas exchange. The contusion process is hemorrhagic but is also a process of interstitial and alveolar edema as a response to injury. Hemorrhage and edema occur within the area of contusion and gradually involve surrounding tissue in general inflammation. Damaged or closed alveolar–capillary units produce ventilation and perfusion abnormalities and shunt. If no further lung injury occurs, the areas of infiltrate begin to clear, and healing occurs. More commonly, however, the injured area evolves into areas of atelectasis due to secretion retention and infection. Blunt trauma that produces significant lung contusion is frequently associated with pulmonary hematoma or laceration. Severe lacerations which bleed into the pleural space or airway require thoracotomy and pulmonary resection.

Resuscitation Assessment. During the initial resuscitation, respiratory distress may be evident. Accompanying rib fractures are common but not universal. If the contusion is clinically significant, the Pa_{O_2} is frequently less than 60 mm Hg on room air. Lung infiltrates may be seen on the admission chest film. Bloody sputum may be present.[14]

Critical Care Assessment. In the first 24 hours, the patient shows progressive clinical and radiographical changes which correlate with underlying alveolar capillary injury. Patchy infiltrates persist on subsequent chest films. Bloody sputum continues to be evident on suctioning either as fresh blood or as old blood and clots in the mature contusion. Local areas of wheezing are a common finding. Patients with significant contusions show progressive evidence of stiff, wet lungs and increased work at breathing. Measured pulmonary compliance falls. Peak airway pressure increases. The degree of deterioration in Pa_{O_2} and pH is usually a function of failure to recognize the extent of the contusion and to institute early ventilatory support and pulmonary hygiene. The presence of associated injuries, including shock, produces secondary changes within the lung. Posttraumatic respiratory distress syndrome may be superimposed on the evolving lung contusion.

Critical Care Management. ***Managing Gas Exchange.*** Supportive oxygen therapy and pulmonary care to mobilize and clear bloody secretions are required in every patient as the contusion resolves over the first few posttrauma days. The need for early intubation and mechanical ventilation in blunt chest trauma remains a controversy, as discussed in the section on flail chest injuries. Support of spontaneous ventilation with supplemental oxygen may be adequate for some patients. Others required controlled ventilation or SIMV at the least. Criteria for instituting mechanical ventilation are available.[24] The implication for nurses is that several forms of ventilatory management can be effective in individual patients provided the benefits and risks of that therapy are monitored. In all cases, adequate gas exchange is observed over time by frequent blood gas analysis and parameters such as Q_s/Q_t and compliance.

Managing the Patient–Ventilator Unit. Massive contusions may require pharmacological paralysis and controlled mandatory ventilation or high-frequency ventilation in an effort to aerate the poorly compliant, damaged lungs. This poses considerable risk of pneumothorax or tension pneumothorax if chest tubes are not in place and adequately positioned. Barotrauma also can be reduced by maintaining adequate sedation and analgesia levels. Further discussion of barotrauma is found in the section on critical care therapeutics.

Airway Management. Airway management is problematical and requires careful monitoring for obstruction. Many of these patients have an endotracheal or tracheostomy tube in place. The airway lumen may become partially obstructed with bloody mucus, clots, and pieces of dead tissue. Frequent suctioning may be required to avoid obstruction. Meticulous technique is essential because these procedures always increase the risk of contamination and infection. Locating a spare airway at the bedside is an essential precaution, since airway obstruction may occur even with apparently adequate irrigation and suction.

Pulmonary Hygiene. This is particularly important in managing patients with significant lung contusion. Early institution of chest physiotherapy, postural drainage, and percussion assists in avoiding or treating postcontusion atelectasis. The treatment should be specific to the lung segment involved. Monitoring the quality of pulmonary secretions provides an important outcome criteria. By 48 to 72 hours, the bloody mucus should become thinner and darken, eventually clearing to normal appearance. Routine cultures and daily chest films are helpful in monitoring infection.

Fluid Administration. There remains considerable debate over the therapeutic range for fluid administration.[41] Some investigators have found that aggressive crystalloid administration is associated with pulmonary insufficiency and interstitial edema following pulmonary injury.[42–44] Conversely, others propose that crystalloid infusion in volumes necessary to restore and maintain preload and hemodynamic stability is not detrimental.[45] Regardless of the controversy, volume administration is guided by the monitoring of oxygen saturation and invasive hemodynamic parameters. Typically, the contusion begins to clear radiographically within 72 hours of injury. The presence of one or more persistent infiltrates suggests pulmonary complications such as pneumonia, aspiration, or posttraumatic respiratory distress syndrome.[14, 24]

Intermediate/Rehabilitation Management. The focus of nursing management continues to be pulmonary hygiene and restoration of respiratory reserve. Weeks after injury, the patient may develop a traumatic cyst, a further concern for pulmonary infectious sequelae. Most patients appear to recover from significant lung contusion with minimal respiratory disability. However, this area has not been the source of systematic study.

Impaired Gas Exchange Related to Posttraumatic Respiratory Distress Syndrome

Severe respiratory insufficiency has been observed following trauma as early as World War II, and during the Vietnam era it came to be viewed as the point beyond which severely injured patients did not survive. Although originally known as "wet" or "shock" lung, it has become apparent over the years that hypotensive shock per se is not the sole etiology or mechanism of the syndrome. Numerous traumatic and biochemical insults produce apparently similar responses in the lung and a characteristic clinical picture. Mortality from posttraumatic respiratory insufficiency remains high despite prolific research that has identified specific risk factors, described the pathology, and evaluated clinical management strategies.

Terminology used in describing posttraumatic respiratory distress can be confusing. In addition to older literature centered on "shock" lung, one encounters references to "traumatic respiratory insufficiency," "wet" lung, and the ubiquitous "adult respiratory distress syndrome" (ARDS). ARDS was first described by Ashbaugh and Petty[46] in 1967 as a cluster of clinical features with apparent similarities in pathology and pathophysiology. Of the dozens of etiologies or related factors, ARDS is clearly linked with severe traumatic injury, sepsis, and shock. For the purposes of specificity, the term *posttraumatic respiratory distress syndrome* (RDS) is used in this chapter. This does not imply a unique pathology in trauma. On the contrary, the lung may respond in a common manner to any number of causative agents or injuries.

Description and Risk Factors. RDS is not a primary disease. It is a syndrome that is always secondary to some other insult or combination of injuries. Major risk factors or conditions associated with the development of RDS in trauma include shock of any type (septic, hemorrhagic, cardiogenic, or anaphylactic), multisystem trauma with extensive tissue destruction, direct pulmonary contusion, multiple orthopedic injuries (particularly long bone or pelvic fractures), massive transfusions, thoracic trauma (such as pulmonary contusions, bacterial pneumonia, sepsis, near-drowning, and gastric aspiration), and major head injuries.[47, 48] There is a higher incidence of the syndrome in those patients with multiple risk factors than in those with a single risk condition[47, 49, 50] (Table 19–5). It is well recognized that RDS is not a natural sequela of hemorrhagic shock and hypotension but develops in hypovolemic patients with other insults or predisposing problems. The presence of sepsis is a key factor leading to RDS, usually from a nonpulmonary source. The risks asso-

TABLE 19–5. INCIDENCE OF ARDS AFTER JUST ONE OF THE SPECIFIED CLINICAL CONDITIONS AND THE INCIDENCE WHEN SIMULTANEOUSLY COMBINED WITH ONE AND TWO OTHER OF THESE CONDITIONS

	ALONE		WITH ONE OTHER CONDITION		WITH TWO OTHER CONDITIONS		TOTAL	
CLINICAL CONDITION	*n*	%	*n*	%	*n*	%	*n*	%
1. Sepsis syndrome	5/13	38	2/4	—	2/2	—	9/19	47
2. Aspiration of gastric contents	7/23	30	3/9	33	0/0	—	10/32	31
3. Pulmonary contusion	5/29	17	7/12	58	7/9	78	19/50	38
4. Multiple emergency transfusions	4/17	24	3/11	27	12/14	86	19/42	45
5. Multiple major fractures	1/12	8	4/10	40	10/12	83	15/34	44
6. Near-drowning	2/3	—	1/1	—	0/0	—	3/4	—
7. Pancreatitis	1/1	—	0/0	—	0/0	—	1/1	—
8. Prolonged hypotension	0/1	—	0/1	—	2/2	—	2/4	—

From Pepe PE et al: Clinical predictors of the adult respiratory distress syndrome. Am J Surg 144:126, 1982.

ciated with sepsis and multiple organ failure are discussed in detail in Chapter 8.

The varied insults result in a final common pathway of lung responses which are clinically evident 2 to 48 hours after injury.[51] The major problem is respiratory insufficiency, evidenced by hypoxemia, noncardiogenic pulmonary edema, pulmonary hypertension, and intrapulmonary shunting. A description of the major clinical features helps to define the syndrome[51, 52] (Table 19–6). One prospective study emphasizes the need to exclude other pulmonary or cardiac pathology and uses four broad but statistically powerful components in describing the syndrome: presence of (1) a severe defect in oxygenation, (2) new, diffuse bilateral infiltrates on chest x-ray, (3) a pulmonary wedge pressure less than 18 mm Hg, and (4) the absence of other clinical explanation for these findings.[53]

Pathophysiology. Whatever the precipitating insults, the central pathophysiological component is damage to the alveolar–capillary interface, both endothelial and epithelial. The architecture and degree of alveolar–capillary disruption varies. Studies with CT scans demonstrate considerable regional variability within the lung fields; normal areas are adjacent to areas of severely injured tissue.[50] Early stages of the syndrome's pathophysiology are explained by this primary loss of microvascular and alveolar membrane integrity, resulting in noncardiac pulmonary edema, hypoxemia, pulmonary hypertension, $\dot{V}/\dot{Q}$ mismatching, and decreased pulmonary compliance. Progressive alveolitis and fibrosis occur in later stages of RDS, accompanied by respiratory infection and pneumonia.

RDS has often been described as "high-permeability" pulmonary edema; however, the characteristic edema is due in part to increased capillary permeability and in part to increased hydrostatic pressure secondary to pulmonary hypertension. The effect within the lung includes formation of interstitial then alveolar edema, abnormal surfactant action, and nonuniform collapse of functional lung units. The lung edema may not necessarily correlate well with the clinical findings, particularly with the severity of the early oxygenation deficit.[54, 55] The apparent lack of correlation is related to the ability of the pulmonary lymphatics to compensate for increases in microvessel permeability. It is also related to the concept that edema, although a hallmark of RDS, is a consequence of lung injury, not a causative agent.

One of the most significant problems is hypoxemia which is relatively resistant to supplemental oxygen. The increased work of breathing associated with the underlying inflammatory process and edema may rapidly consume a large portion of available oxygen and energy stores.[56, 57] Eventually, the inflammatory exudate overwhelms lymphatic drainage, and the lung interstitium can no longer act as a reservoir, leading to alveolar flooding. Compensatory hypoxic pulmonary vasoconstriction is lost,[58, 59] and pulmonary hypertension occurs. There is significant intrapulmonary shunting and a lack of response to oxygen.

RDS produces stiff lungs, resulting in reduced functional residual capacity and high airway pressures required to inflate the lungs. A decrease in pulmonary compliance is present, due to the interstitial and alveolar edema and cellular infiltration initially and then fibrosis later in the patient's course. The efficacy of surfactant is decreased, perhaps due to metabolic abnormalities in the alveolar type II cells which retain the capability to produce surfactant.[60] Peribronchial edema can lead to airway constriction with wheezing, decreased $\dot{V}/\dot{Q}$ ratio, and increased airway pressures.

The etiology of the underlying alveolar–capillary lesion is unclear. It is the subject of extensive research, primarily through several different animal models of lung injury that employ biochemical agents, microembolism, acid aspiration, and hemorrhagic or septic insults. A single injury mechanism or pathophysiological cascade has not been identified; how-

TABLE 19–6. CLINICAL FEATURES OF POSTTRAUMATIC RESPIRATORY DISTRESS SYNDROME

History compatible with known risk factors
Respiratory distress
Tachypnea (>30 breaths per minute)
Dyspnea
Hypoxemia
Pa_{O_2} <50 mm Hg when FI_{O_2} >0.6)
Pa_{O_2}/FI_{O_2} <200 mm Hg with mechanical ventilation
Increased shunt fraction (Q_s/Q_t > 15–20%)
Increased dead space ventilation ($\dot{V}_D/\dot{V}_T$ >0.6)
Decreased static compliance (<30 ml/cm H_2O)
Pulmonary hypertension ($PAP_{systolic}$ >30 mm Hg)
Diffuse pulmonary infiltrates on chest film (interstitial then alveolar)

ever, numerous substances have been implicated (Table 19–7). In general, leukocyte aggregation is an important factor in producing lung injury, potentially involving several types of phagocytic cells (i.e., neutrophils, eosinophils, monocytes, and macrophages). Neutrophils are present in large numbers within the lungs of patients with RDS[61] and are well known as a source of toxic oxygen radicals and proteolytic enzymes. A number of studies have indicated that activation of the complement system creates lung injury by leukocyte stimulation and chemotaxis.[62–64] More recent data suggest that although complement activation may initiate injury in some forms of lung pathology, it is not a necessary or sufficient condition in trauma-related RDS.[65]

However, a large body of experimental evidence supports the hypothesis that white cells elaborate mediators which contribute to alveolar–capillary pathology and pulmonary edema. The importance of these mediators is in the future potential for pharmacological therapies and interventions with blocking agents to interrupt the pathophysiological cascade and improve patient outcomes. Leukocyte products include oxygen free radicals (e.g., superoxide anion, hydrogen peroxide, and hydroxyl radicals), proteases which can destroy the vascular basement membrane (e.g., elastase, cathepsin G, and collagenase), and arachidonic acid metabolites.[66] Phagocytic cells such as pulmonary alveolar macrophages are able to synthesize various products of endogenous and exogenous arachidonic acid via the cyclooxygenase or lipooxygenase pathways. Which metabolites are released at what time point in RDS pathology is not known. Nevertheless, these lipid mediators have potent effects on pulmonary vascular and airway smooth muscle and on cell membrane permeability.[67] For example, prostaglandin I_2 (PGI_2) is a potent pulmonary vasodilator and may affect inflammatory cell function. PGF_2 and thromboxane are vasoconstrictors with effects on both microvascular and large-vessel smooth muscle. Thromboxane also enhances platelet aggregation. Platelets play an important role in ARDS pathology in some experimental models.[68]

Much of the clinical evidence for the role of neutrophils is dependent on their presence and that of their products in the lungs of patients with differing forms of the disease process. A cause-and-effect relationship has not been established, and it is possible that leukocyte activation only aggravates pathology from some other mechanism. Furthermore, it has recently been suggested that it is the failure of neutrophilic defense mechanisms which is important in ARDS pathology.[69] Neutrophils have key protective and reparative functions, e.g., the production of oxidant scavengers and bactericidal agents. Loss of these functions may have important consequences in these patients, particularly in preventing pulmonary infections.[69]

Other factors may act as mediators or markers of injury. Platelet-activating factor (PAF) is a phospholipid mediator produced by numerous cell types, e.g., platelets, vascular endothelium, and leukocytes. PAF is associated with a variety of important effects on pulmonary and systemic vascular tone, vessel permeability, and other RDS-linked mediators such as cyclooxygenase and lipoxygenase products.[70, 71] Its role in RDS, if any, is inconclusive. Monokines, protein mediators of inflammation released by macrophages and monocytes, are currently under investigation in late-stage RDS and multiple organ failure. Interleukin 1 (IL-1) may be important in attracting phagocytic cells and lymphocytes and in promoting cell adherence to injured endothelium.[72] A second monokine, tumor necrosis factor (TNF), produces acute lung inflammation in a manner similar to that of endotoxin when injected into animals, and it also increases capillary protein leakage.[73–75]

Resuscitation Assessment. Clinical evidence of the syndrome is not apparent during the initial resuscitation period. A major requirement is to assess and document the risk of posttraumatic respiratory insufficiency for each patient. It remains unclear if the type and volume of resuscitation fluids have implications for the pulmonary edema of posttraumatic RDS. However, fluids are administered and documented carefully with pulmonary sequelae in mind.

Critical Care Assessment. Patients who are at risk for RDS after major trauma should be observed closely for signs of respiratory difficulty. There are four clinical phases based on clinical findings and pathophysiological changes: impending insufficiency, clinical insufficiency, and severe failure or resolution.[75]

Impending Insufficiency. The physical examination may be essentially normal. Lungs are dry to auscultation, and secretions are minimal or explained by other injuries. However, the patient is dyspneic, even though $Pa{O_2}$ is relatively normal. Arterial blood gases also reveal decreased $Pa{CO_2}$ and respiratory alkalosis, as either a new finding or as a continuation of the tachypnea observed during initial resuscitation. Changes in the chest film which are characteristic of RDS are rarely evident. Lung pathology is poorly defined in this early phase, except that neutrophil sequestration and some degree of interstitial edema are apparent. Knowledge of the patient's set of risk factors and these early assessment

TABLE 19–7. PROPOSED MEDIATORS OR MECHANISTIC MARKERS OF INJURY IN RDS

Leukocyte chemotaxins
Complement fragments (C5a, C5a des arginine, C3a)
Complement complexed proteins (C5b,6,7,8,9)
Platelet-activating factor
Bacterial products
Leukotriene B_4 and HETE
Fibrin degradation products
Platelets and platelet factors (PAF)
Monokines
Tumor necrosis factor (TNF) or cachectin
Interleukins
Interferons
Arachidonic acid metabolites
Prostaglandins (PGE_1, PGE_2, PGD_2, PGF_{1a}, PGF_{2a}, PGI_2 or prostacyclin)
Leukotrienes (LTB_4, LTC_4, LTD_4, LTE_4)
Thromboxane (TxA_2)
Oxidants and oxygen free radicals
Hydrogen peroxide
Superoxide anion
Hydroxyl radical
Peroxide radical
Phospholipase products
Neutral proteases (elastase, β-glucuronidase, cathepsin D, E, and G, collagenase)
Vasoactive substances
Bradykinin
Serotonin
Histamine

findings form the basis for supportive oxygen therapy and pulmonary care.

Clinical Insufficiency. Within the first 24 hours there are both clinical and pathological signs of acute lung inflammation. Oxygenation is markedly depressed in relation to the delivered concentration. The patient is markedly dyspneic and in respiratory distress with hypoxemia. Increases in physiological dead space and pulmonary vascular resistance are measurable (see Table 19–6). Patchy lung infiltrates are evident on the chest film, particularly in dependent areas. With appropriate ventilatory management and control of underlying infection or unresolved trauma, the RDS process can be resolved at this point.

Some patients continue to experience progressive respiratory failure over the next 2 to 3 days and require prolonged ventilatory and hemodynamic support. Physiological dead space continues to increase, and the shunt fraction is high. The patient requires a high concentration of inspired oxygen, despite PEEP. Characteristic bilateral infiltrates are recognizable on the chest radiograph. The lungs are heavy and wet, with continued white cell infiltration, alveolar edema, and microvascular congestion. Many individuals are in a hyperdynamic state with elevated cardiac index, regional perfusion shifts, and peripheral defects in oxygen utilization.[52, 76, 77] The hyperdynamic state may be due to the same processes, trauma and sepsis, which originally produced the respiratory dysfunction.

Severe Failure. Usually irreversible, respiratory pathology includes fibrosis, atelectasis, and recurrent pneumonia. Hypoxemia is refractory to continued increases in delivered oxygen concentration. Despite careful ventilator adjustments, impaired gas exchange and a progressive decrease in compliance are accompanied by impaired peripheral O_2 extraction and acidosis.

Despite advances in ventilatory support, posttraumatic RDS mortality remains high. Mortality has been reported at 41 per cent in blunt trauma[52] and 65 per cent in a mixed critically ill population.[49] Deaths associated with RDS can occur within 72 hours of the initial insult; however, early deaths are not as common as delayed mortality secondary to sepsis.[49] Typically, the patient dies within 2 weeks of the onset of the syndrome not because of hypoxemia or complications of respiratory support but due to an inability to eliminate the underlying disease or infectious process. Multiple organ failure is associated with high patient mortality.[48, 49]

Resolution. Some patients do not progress into the severe failure stage. If complications such as infection are contained and the functional lung tissue appropriately supported over time, the alveolar–capillary injury heals, and clinical abnormalities abate. Most studies indicate that there is little or no permanent respiratory disability in survivors of RDS. It is toward this end that nursing management is directed.

CRITICAL CARE MANAGEMENT. Despite early identification of patients at high risk for RDS and knowledge of the progressive disease pattern, there are no clearly preventative agents or procedures. Similarly, there is no one cure for the syndrome. Therapies which are designed to intervene in the process of mediator activation may ultimately be useful in ameliorating the disease process. Studies of RDS pathophysiology have led to trials of numerous therapeutic agents: PGE_1, ibuprofen, indomethacin, prostacyclin, free-radical scavengers, and fibronectin, to name a few. However, none of these agents is recommended for clinical use at present. Early and effective ventilatory and hemodynamic support remains the foundation of critical care management. Equally important is the treatment of underlying trauma and infection (Fig. 19–22). The patient with RDS requires sedation and analgesia which balance both comfort and desired ventilatory status, consistent emotional support, and planned periods of rest and sleep. Explanation of the patient's injury and expected outcomes of ventilatory therapy are needed not once, but many times throughout the changing events and the patient's perceptions of events.

Ventilatory Support. Patients with known risk factors are monitored closely for signs of respiratory deterioration. Alternative causes of respiratory dysfunction such as atelectasis or pulmonary contusion should be considered and treated appropriately. Most patients require mechanical ventilation once dyspnea, tachypnea, and hypoxemia are evident. Numerous criteria must be analyzed in selecting the right ventilatory method and equipment, including work of breathing, compliance, airway resistance, and possible complications of the therapies. The ventilatory mode chosen for the patient should be one that provides adequate minute volume at the lowest possible airway pressure and does not exacerbate existing ventilation–perfusion abnormalities. In general, the inspiratory volume is set so as to maintain the desired Pa_{CO_2} (e.g., 12–15 ml/kg body weight) at a flow rate that is comfortable for the patient. The inspired oxygen concentration is chosen to establish a physiological Pa_{O_2} at a nontoxic F_{IO_2}. An inspiratory-to-expiratory time (I/E) ratio of 1:2 is commonly used, although longer inspiratory times can reduce mean airway pressure and increase Pa_{O_2}.[78] A number of techniques have been recommended, including control mode, IMV or SIMV with or without pressure support, inverse I/E ratio ventilation, and in selected cases, simultaneous independent lung ventilation or HFV.

Use of CMV with PEEP. Controlled ventilation can be used in patients with marked compliance problems and difficulty in achieving adequate gas exchange by other ventilatory methods. A common example in trauma is the individual with severe pulmonary contusion and progressive respiratory distress syndrome. One goal of nursing management is to synchronize patient–ventilator gas exchange so as to avoid barotrauma and further lung injury. This is a much greater problem for the patient with CMV and significant PEEP levels than with IMV or SIMV therapy. Pharmacological paralysis is usually required for total control of patient ventilation. Intravenous pancuronium or vecuronium can be administered at regular intervals. Both sedation and analgesia must accompany these agents. Heavy sedation may be used

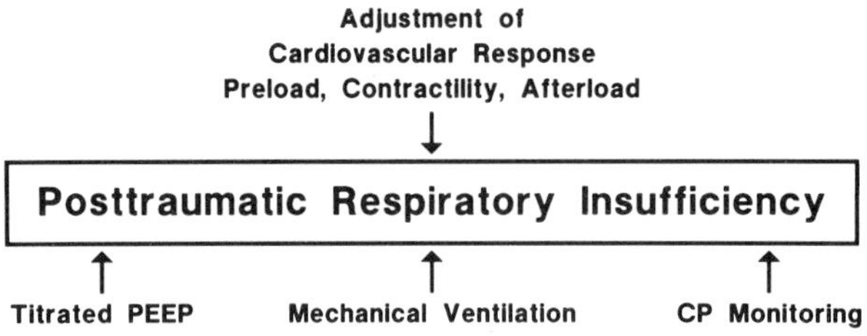

Figure 19–22. Posttraumatic respiratory distress syndrome.

alone for ventilatory control but is not reported to be as effective as therapeutic paralysis. The nurse maintains a schedule of administration and assesses for the desired level of paralysis and ventilatory control. Frequently, the patient will display a subtle change in at least one parameter which indicates loss of therapeutic ventilatory control. This parameter may be an increase in peak airway pressure or particular chest wall movements which are significant for the individual patient.

Supported Ventilation. There is an on-going controversy concerning the advantages of IMV or SIMV modes versus CMV in RDS patients. At the least, these modes are commonly used in weaning the patient from ventilatory support.[79] Advantages include the decreased need for sedation or muscle relaxants to promote ventilator synchrony and decreased barotrauma. Pressure-support ventilation also has been employed in and is reportedly more comfortable for the semialert patient than IMV.[80]

Appropriate Application of PEEP. One of the most essential treatment components is PEEP titration to the desired physiological endpoints. One obvious benefit of appropriate PEEP in posttraumatic RDS is an increased Pa_{O_2} at lower inspired oxygen concentrations. The mechanisms of improved Pa_{O_2} are increased functional residual capacity, prevention of alveolar collapse, and recruitment of closed alveoli. PEEP can be applied regardless of the mode of ventilation selected for the patient. Low- or moderate-level PEEP (under 15 cm H_2O) is used widely; however, higher levels may be required in refractory hypoxemia.

PEEP has no prophylactic value in RDS.[81] However, it does have well-recognized adverse effects on cardiovascular function, specifically cardiac output, and may contribute to selected alveolar overdistention and physical lung injury. Unfortunately, the adverse effects of PEEP are neither uniform nor predictable. Compliance may be increased or decreased by PEEP, and effects on dead-space volume are also variable.[52] In view of the benefits and negative effects of PEEP, it is essential to define the optimal level for the individual patient and the time to initiate the therapy. A rational management approach includes the use of patient PEEP trials, a series of systematic assessments of changes in cardiopulmonary parameters as PEEP is increased in small increments, 2.5 to 5 cm H_2O or less.[51, 82] Changes can be made rapidly, allowing 15 to 20 minutes for evaluation of the effect of the new PEEP level. All parameters related to tissue oxygen delivery should be assessed when PEEP levels are adjusted.[51, 52]

Nonconventional Ventilatory Techniques. Conventional methods of ventilation with generalized PEEP may worsen ventilation–perfusion relationships in patients with severe RDS. Consequently, several modified ventilation modes can be useful. Simultaneous independent lung ventilation can be used in patients with asymmetrical lung disease. HFV may provide improved gas exchange with lower peak airway pressures and less barotrauma in RDS than conventional ventilation. Both techniques are discussed in the critical care therapeutics section. In addition, inverse-ratio ventilation has been used in both infants and adults with severe respiratory dysfunction. This technique employs conventional volume or pressure-cycled ventilation with I/E ratios of up to 4:1.[83, 84] The maneuver extends inspiratory time, which theoretically can improve gas exchange at lower PEEP levels and airway pressures. There are no current studies which compare patient outcomes in inverse-ratio and conventional ventilation; a review of favorable and adverse case reports is available elsewhere.[52, 78] Patients must be monitored for adverse hemodynamic effects of the therapy, since venous return and cardiac filling can be altered. In addition, most patients require sedation, since the long inspiratory time can produce discomfort and anxiety.[11]

Positioning. In many cases, the interstitial and alveolar infiltrates of RDS appear to be distributed uniformly throughout the lung fields on chest radiograph. However, CT scans emphasize that the pathology is nonuniform in nature, and the most involved segments of the lung are those in dependent positions.[50] Changes in body position affect blood gases by altering $\dot{V}/\dot{Q}$ within the lung. Therefore, it is clearly important that no one segment of the lung remain constantly in a dependent position. In addition, oxygenation can be manipulated by therapeutic positioning, i.e., positioning the patient so as to achieve an improved Pa_{O_2}.[85] If the patient is monitored with pulse or transcutaneous oximetry, arterial oxygen saturation is used as the therapeutic endpoint when the patient is moved from the supine to the lateral decubitus position.[52] The semiprone position also has been advocated for patients with acute RDS.[86]

Cardiovascular Therapies. It is imperative to remember that most patients who develop posttraumatic RDS may have compromised cardiovascular function or underlying hypovolemia due to their injuries and injury complications. Frequently, the patient's physiological reserve is insufficient to maintain cardiac output when additionally stressed by the hemodynamic consequences of mechanical ventilation and PEEP. In addition, the net surface area for gas exchange is reduced in the alveolar–capillary lesion of RDS. Therefore, optimizing cardiac function and ventricular output supports pulmonary perfusion and, therefore, gas exchange. Preload, contractility, and afterload can be manipulated to support hemodynamic performance while respiratory failure is treated.

Appropriate fluid management is directed toward (1) decreasing the intrapulmonary edema that is a great part of the syndrome's pathology without compromising intravascular volume and cardiac performance and (2) maximizing the blood's oxygen-carrying capacity. Actual or effective intravascular volume depletion is corrected with the fluid of choice, whether balanced electrolyte solutions, colloids, or blood, and is titrated to the desired ventricular filling pressure. The type of fluid administered remains a subject of debate and conflicting reports as to effect on pulmonary function. There is universal agreement, however, that careful monitoring of responses to therapy is essential to avoid overhydration and increased pulmonary lung water. Sequential measurements of pulmonary artery pressure, wedge pressure, and cardiac output and construction of ventricular function curves are useful in guiding fluid management. Periodic transfusion of red cells may be required to support oxygen delivery. In all cases, accurate fluid balance intake and output recording and daily weights, whenever possible, help to trend fluid needs.

Pharmacological agents also can be used. Specific vasodilator therapy with low-dose isoproterenol has been reported to be helpful in reducing right heart afterload, as well as dobutamine to provide inotropic support.[52] Afterload-reducing agents such as nitroprusside are at times included in the therapy to improve stroke volume and left ventricular filling pressure. The goal of using such agents is to improve cardiac output and pulmonary blood flow without greatly increasing pulmonary shunt fraction or myocardial work.

Intermediate/Rehabilitation Care. Published reports of respiratory abnormalities in recovering patients differ in the patterns and severity of dysfunction.[87–91] These differences may be partially explained by the variability in RDS etiology, in the patient's previous health history, and in the length of time over which patients were studied. Pulmonary function is abnormal in 40 per cent of survivors at 6 months after recovery.[51] Measurable aberrations in vital capacity and FRC, respiratory mechanics, and arterial oxygenation, particularly during exercise, have been described in patients recovering from ARDS of varying etiologies.[90, 91] There is general agreement that lung function is restored in most survivors by 1 year. Most interestingly, there is no apparent correlation between severity of the syndrome, duration of ventilatory support, and degree of residual respiratory impairment.

Nursing management is directed toward weaning the patient from ventilatory support and protecting the patient from further respiratory complications, particularly retained secretions and infection. Weaning from mechanical ventilation may begin at varying points in the patient's recovery course. In general, weaning is initiated once the patient is alert, with a stable hemodynamic status, and respiratory drive and muscle strength are sufficient for spontaneous ventilation. Withdrawal of support will be unsuccessful if there is a persistent septic focus or major organ insufficiency of some type. Most patients are successfully weaned. However, it has been reported that up to 19 per cent of spontaneously breathing patients require reinstitution of mechanical support during recovery from ARDS.[92] Weaning strategies are discussed in both the critical and intermediate care therapeutics sections.

Once the patient no longer requires ventilatory support, blood gases and/or pulmonary function tests are evaluated daily or on a routine basis. The patient is observed for dyspnea and shortness of breath both at rest and during exercise, and the plan of care is modified accordingly. The survivor of posttraumatic RDS needs considerable support and information to integrate the events of his recovery and to understand any current limitations in respiratory function and exercise tolerance.

Alteration in Cardiac Output Related to Cardiac Tamponade

Description. Both a symptom and an injury, cardiac tamponade is life-threatening and requires immediate treatment. Injury to the pericardium and/or heart results from a penetrating wound or from blunt anterior chest wall trauma. Hemopericardium, bleeding into the pericardial sac, or a small pericardial rupture may or may not be accompanied by cardiac tamponade depending on intrapericardial pressure.[93] The pericardial sac, a tough and nondistensible structure, normally holds approximately 25 ml of fluid that serves to cushion and protect the heart. Usually, the addition of small amounts (50–100 ml) of blood or air from traumatic injury into the sac produces only a small rise in intrapericardial pressure. Continued bleeding sharply increases this pressure and produces the symptoms of cardiogenic shock. Cardiac output falls as the increased intrapericardial pressure interferes with venous return into the right atrium. Decline in cardiac performance is directly related to the speed with which the pericardial sac must accommodate blood and fluid, as well as the total amount. The slower the leak, the longer the increased pressure can be tolerated (Fig. 19–23). This characteristic is important because injury recognition and treatment may not occur immediately on the patient's admission to the emergency department or critical care unit.

Resuscitation Assessment and Management. Diagnosis can be difficult, since some of the classic symptoms may be obscured by hypovolemic shock. The index of suspicion is used in discovery of the injury. The patient with an inappropriately low cardiac performance in relationship to his injuries falls within the index. Evidence of precordial trauma, such as a wound along the lateral sternal border from second to seventh intercostal space or an injury history that indicates the possibility of myocardial injury, also leads to the diagnosis. The patient experiences midthoracic pain and dyspnea.

Classic symptoms include the presence of Beck's triad: systemic hypotension, muffled heart tones, and elevated venous pressure reflected in neck vein distention. The latter may not be evident in the injured patient who is already hypotensive and volume-depleted. Distant or muffled heart tones are difficult to assess in noisy patient care areas. Pulsus paradoxus of greater than 15 mm Hg during inspiration is significant but difficult to measure reliably unless an arterial line is in place. Useful parameters include an elevated central venous pressure (CVP), narrowed pulse pressure, and pre-

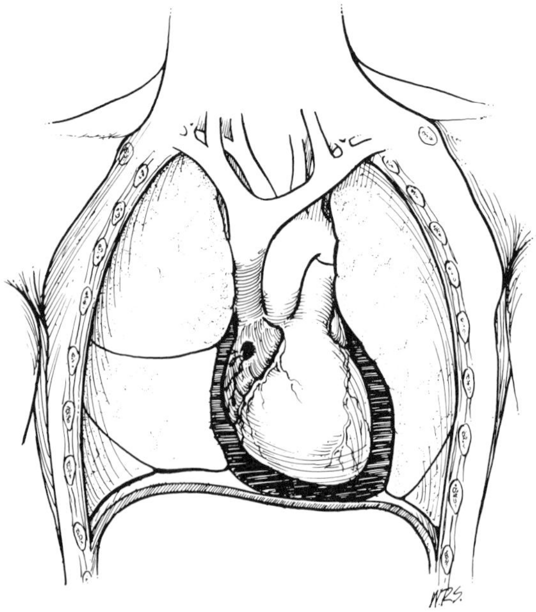

Figure 19–23. Cardiac tamponade resulting from a knife wound. Such wounds may bleed slowly enough to permit survival for several hours. The heart becomes compressed by blood, and cardiac output decreases resulting in shock. Removal of blood by pericardiocentesis can restore cardiac output and allow time for definitive repair. (From Weiner SL, Barret J: Trauma Management for Civilian and Military Physicians. Philadelphia, WB Saunders Co, 1986.)

cipitously falling cardiac output. The EKG may demonstrate low-voltage complexes, particularly in the precordial leads.

The diagnosis and immediate treatment may occur simultaneously through pericardiocentesis or pericardial tap (Fig. 19–24). One method is as follows: a long (6-in) 18-gauge over the needle catheter attached to a stopcock is inserted below or along the left side of the xiphoid process into the pericardial sac. The fluid present in the sac is aspirated, usually with some immediate improvement in cardiac performance. Since the pericardium is self-sealing, the tamponade may recur. Therefore, the catheter is left in place and secured for possible repeated aspiration. The procedure and needed equipment are described in Appendix 19–3.

Pericardiocentesis may be falsely negative, often because the needle becomes obstructed by tissue or clots during the procedure. The correctly performed procedure will aspirate the pericardium without cardiac puncture. One indication that the heart has been entered is rapid clotting of aspirated blood. Pericardial blood should not clot because it is defibrinated by cardiac motion within the pericardium.

Cardiac tamponade is an injury yet also a symptom. The underlying cause of the cardiac tamponade must be determined, and thoracotomy may be required to identify and repair the source of bleeding. The choice of management by pericardiocentesis alone or by thoracotomy is an area of historical debate among resuscitating physicians. Factors that influence management include the mechanism of injury (ice pick wound versus gunshot wound), hemodynamic status, and response to pericardiocentesis. The resuscitation nurse needs to be aware of these factors, monitor the patient's response to pericardiocentesis, and make preparations for rapid thoracotomy should it be required.

Alteration in Cardiac Output Related to Myocardial Contusion

Description. Blunt cardiac injuries may include cardiac wall rupture, valvular disruption, coronary artery dissection, and ventricular contusions. Cardiac contusions are the most common result of injury, with dysrhythmias being of greatest concern. The contusion itself is rarely fatal, except in relationship to other traumatic injuries.

Identification During Resuscitation. The index of suspicion is established in the patient with chest wall contusions, severe anterior blunt trauma, and fractures of sternum and ribs. A standard 12-lead EKG is obtained, since nearly half the patients suspected of having myocardial contusion have EKG abnormalities upon admission.[94] Continuous EKG monitoring is initiated, and blood is analyzed for cardiac isoenzymes. Of special interest is an elevation in the myocardial band of the creatinine phosphokinase (CPK-MB). Standard antidysrhythmic agents are administered if EKG changes become clinically significant.

Critical Care Assessment. Current literature contains an exhaustive debate over the standard of care for myocardial contusion patients.[94–104] There is no diagnostic method that is universally accepted; therefore, the postresuscitative management is equally controversial. The patient is continuously surveyed for symptomatic dysrhythmias, specifically ventricular irritability and conduction defects. Two-dimensional echocardiography (ECHO) and multigated angiography (MUGA) may be useful in determining abnormalities in ventricular wall movement and ejection fraction. Serial monitoring of cardiac isoenzymes is supported by some authors.[98]

Critical Care Management. The patient with a clinically significant contusion chiefly requires nursing observation. Myocardial oxygenation is maintained through appropriate ventilatory support. Continuous EKG and hemodynamic monitoring is needed to detect and manage dysrhythmias. Intravenous fluid administration is guided by hemodynamic parameters. Low stroke volume and ejection fraction are treated pharmacologically with inotropic agents such as dopamine, dobutamine, and digitalis. Cardiovascular data are correlated with the effect of drugs, fluids, and any treatments the patient receives for associated injuries. Chest

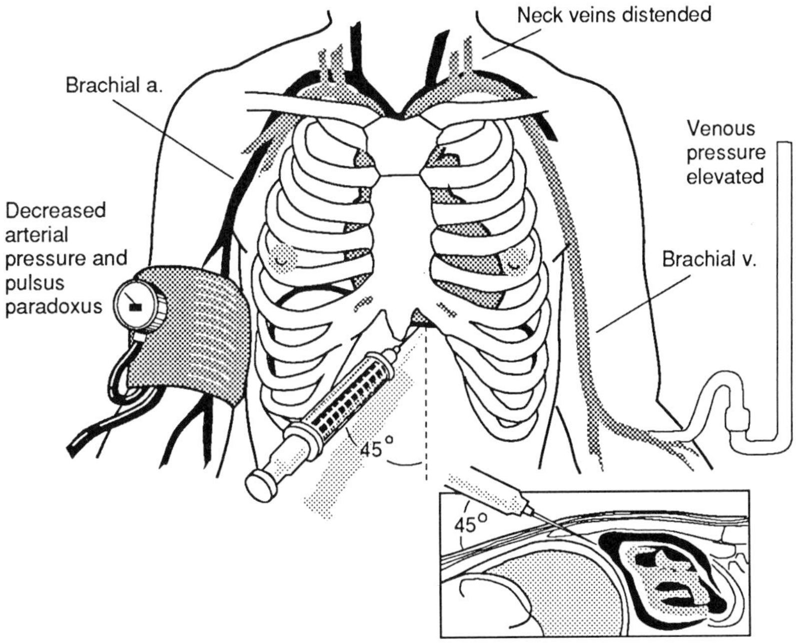

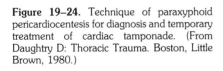

Figure 19–24. Technique of paraxyphoid pericardiocentesis for diagnosis and temporary treatment of cardiac tamponade. (From Daughtry D: Thoracic Trauma. Boston, Little Brown, 1980.)

pain that mimics angina but does not respond to nitrates is managed by other pain-control modalities.

Nurses are caring for the equivalent of a cardiac patient in the busy environment of a surgical intensive care unit or general medical–surgical floor. This implies that nursing care should be targeted toward eliminating unnecessary stressors and preventing needless myocardial work or increases in oxygen consumption until the injury has healed. However, currently few studies have been done that could help to direct the nursing care of these patients or to compare patient outcomes with those of patients with primary cardiac disease.

Altered Blood Transport Related to Aortic Disruption

Disruption of the thoracic aorta due to blunt trauma is a leading cause of immediate death in patients involved in motor vehicle crashes and falls.[105] A recent comprehensive study within a sophisticated trauma system revealed that 22 per cent of patients who sustained a ruptured aorta died prior to reaching the trauma center, while another 37 per cent died during initial resuscitation or in the operating room. An additional 14 per cent died postoperatively. Of the remaining survivors, 19 per cent developed paraplegia or paresis.[106] The lethality of this injury demands that nurses be familiar with the injury and its difficulties in diagnosis, operative repair, and postoperative care.

Description. In survivors of blunt trauma, there are three common locations of vessel rupture. The thoracic aorta is relatively mobile, and the tears occur at points of anatomical fixation. The most common is at the aortic isthmus, just distal to the left subclavian artery, where the vessel is attached to the chest wall by the ligamentum arteriosum. Two other sites of rupture are in the ascending aorta, where the aorta leaves the pericardial sac, and at the entry to the diaphragm (Fig. 19–25). On deceleration from impact, the inner layers of the vessel (intima and media) tear. Only the outer layer, the adventitia, remains intact and balloons out into a pseudoaneurysm. Alternatively, a partial circumferential hematoma may be tamponaded by surrounding tissue (Fig. 19–26). Either mechanism prolongs the survival of the patient, but it is clearly a time-limited effect.

Resuscitation Assessment. The injury or assault history and associated injuries raise the question of aortic disruption. Penetrating mediastinal injuries or thoracic injuries sustained by the occupant of a car wearing a shoulder harness are examples of the index of suspicion. First or second rib fractures, high sternal fracture, left clavicular fracture at the sternal margin, and massive left hemothorax are associated with aortic injury.

The underlying physiological problem is loss of effective blood transport due to major vessel disruption. The goal of assessment is to seek evidence of poor perfusion beyond the aortic lesion. Although many patients are surprisingly free of symptoms, certain findings are associated with the injury:

1. Pulse deficit in any area, particularly lower extremities
2. Hypotension unexplained by other injuries
3. Upper extremity hypertension relative to lower extremities
4. Sternal pain or interscapular pain

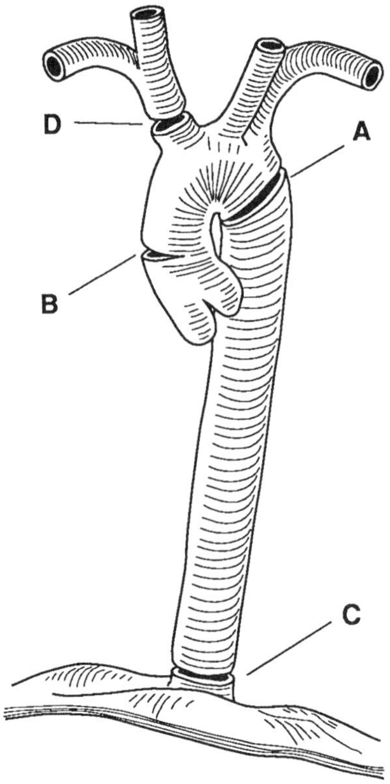

Figure 19–25. Sites of aortic rupture in order of frequency. *A,* Distal to left subclavian artery at the level of the ligamentum arteriosum. *B,* Ascending aorta. *C,* Lower thoracic aorta above diaphragm. *D,* Avulsion of innominate artery from aortic arch. (From Frey C: Initial Management of the Trauma Patient. Philadelphia, Lea & Febiger, 1976.)

5. Precordial or interscapular systolic murmur due to turbulence across the disrupted area
6. Hoarseness due to hematoma pressure around the aortic arch
7. Dyspnea or respiratory distress
8. Lower extremity neuromuscular or sensory deficit

The initial chest film is done with the patient in the supine position for reasons related to spine immobilization and hemodynamic instability. A widened mediastinum and/or obscured aortic knob is highly suggestive of aortic disruption and demands further evaluation. As soon as it is safe to do so, a true upright (110-degree erect) chest film is obtained. This position greatly enhances radiographical power to reveal the characteristic findings of great vessel disruption. However, up to a 50 per cent error has been reported on the basis of chest film findings. A supine or semierect chest film distorts the mediastinum and makes it appear widened.[107]

Unless the patient is deteriorating rapidly, the definitive diagnosis is made by aortography, a retrograde dye study via the femoral artery which allows visualization of the aneurysm or hematoma (Fig. 19–27). Although this study is essential for identifying the site or sites of the life-threatening rupture, there is risk of aneurysm rupture during transport to the angiography suite or during the procedure. The risk of rupture is greatest on catheter insertion and dye injection.

Transport. Transporting the patient must be approached by preparing for every eventuality, including full cardiopulmonary arrest. An emergency cart accompanies the patient and transport team. All equipment and supplies required to manage an arrest, including a thoracotomy tray, chest tube apparatus, and additional resuscitation fluids, are immediately available. Vital signs and baseline physical findings are monitored intensively during transport and the aortogram procedure. Aortography is a priority procedure. Any needless delays in transport or the procedure must be anticipated and eliminated.

Resuscitation Management. The rupture will require surgical resection and repair. The initial resuscitation includes establishing an appropriate airway (frequently endotracheal intubation), securing large-bore intravenous access, and treating other immediately life-threatening injuries. Treat-

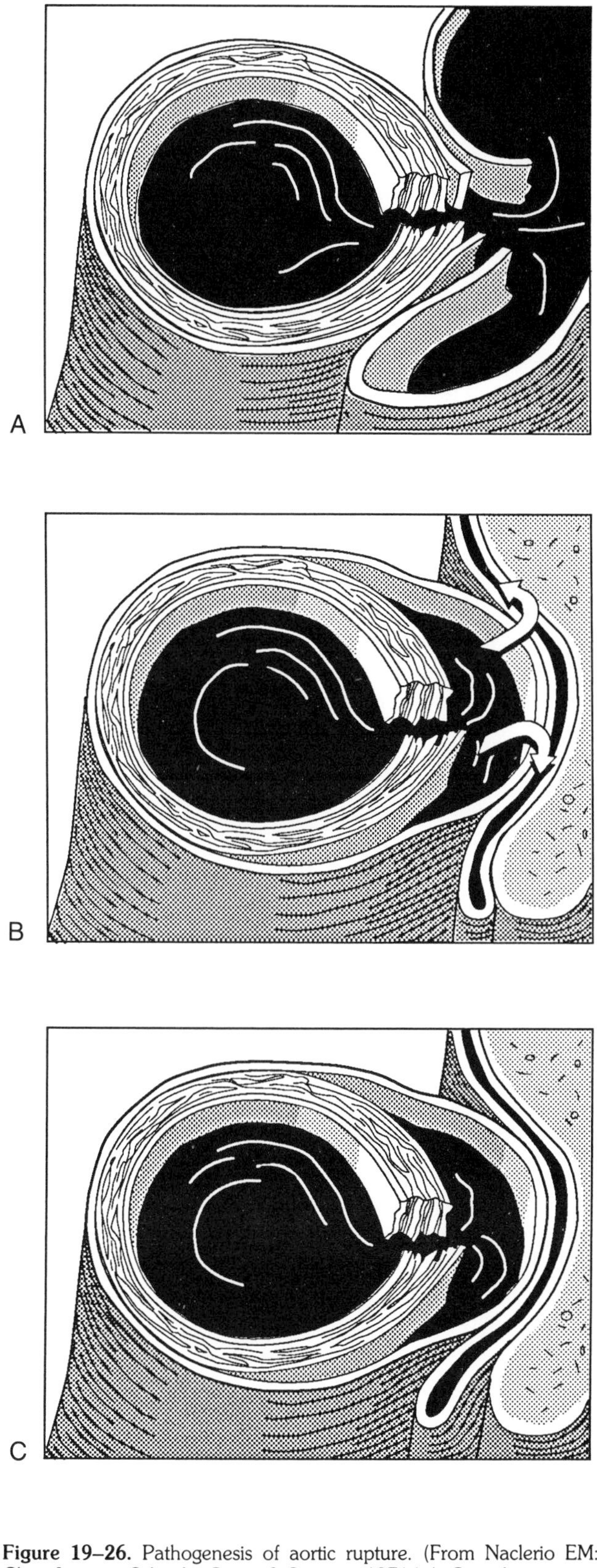

Figure 19–26. Pathogenesis of aortic rupture. (From Naclerio EM: Chest Injuries. Orlando, Grune & Stratton, 1971.) *A*, Complete rupture and death. Transection of all layers of thoracic aorta and mediastinal pleura, with death occurring within minutes. *B*, Lethal delayed rupture. Hematoma is tamponaded temporarily by adventitia or aorta and mediastinal pleura. These structures are torn completely, usually within the first 24 to 48 hours. *C*, Chronic aneurysm formation. A chronic aneurysm results when the adventitial layers remain intact.

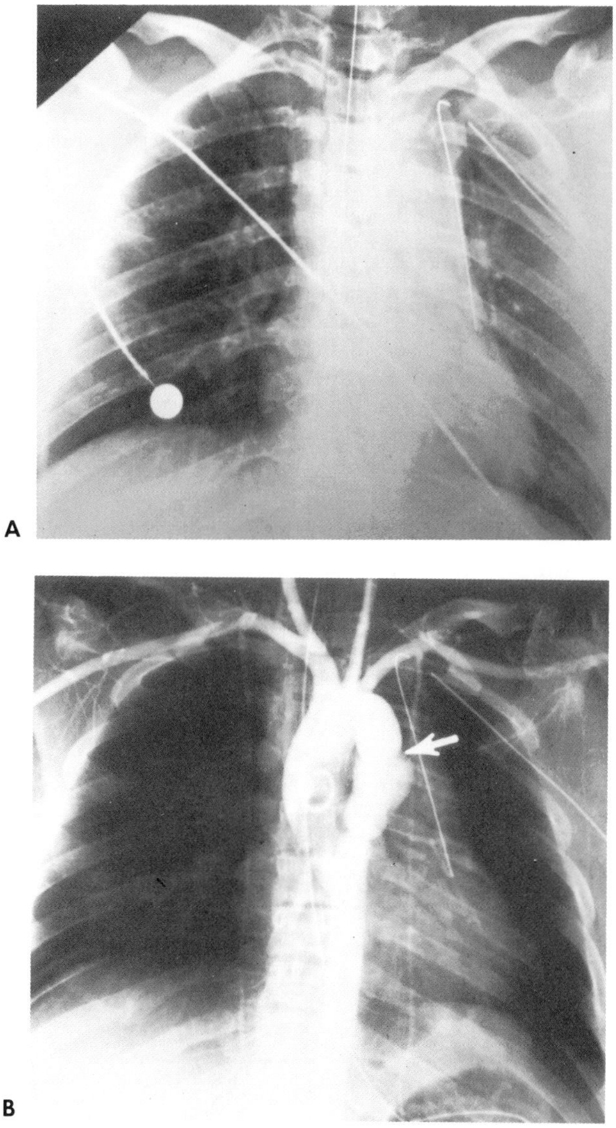

Figure 19–27. Aortic disruption in a 19-year-old person involved in a motor vehicle accident. Initial chest radiograph shows opacification of the left hemithorax. Widened mediastinum is evident (*A*). Aortography (*B*) demonstrates transection of the thoracic aorta distal to the left subclavian artery with pseudoaneurysm formation (arrow). (Copyright 1985. Urban & Schwarzenberg, Baltimore-Munich. Reproduced with permission from Diagnostic Imaging of the Acutely Injured Patient, edited by T. Berquist. All rights reserved.)

ment of other injuries may occur in the operating room or be assigned a lower priority than the disrupted aorta. Should delay in repair occur (e.g., awaiting transport to a trauma center), the resuscitation nurse keeps the patient as quiet and comfortable as possible. A major focus of care is directed toward maintaining the blood pressure within a specified range. Patients with aortic isthmus lesions are usually hypertensive due to baroreceptor stimulation within the cardiac plexus at the isthmus. Since vessel stress must be minimized, mean blood pressure is maintained under 90 mm Hg with antihypertensive agents. An indwelling arterial catheter is essential in monitoring pressures. Blood is typed and cross-matched, and 10 units of packed red blood cells are made available.

Operative Management. The operative procedure is determined by the site or sites of rupture and the choice of the surgical team. Cardiopulmonary bypass is used, although the need for anticoagulation presents difficulties in the multiply injured patient. More commonly, a shunt bypass technique is used, allowing perfusion of the distal aorta while resection and repair are completed (Fig. 19–28). A left thoracotomy incision is made for best visualization of the aorta, and the vessel is cross-clamped to control bleeding. A heparinized shunt is placed proximally and distally, the rupture site is resected, and a Dacron graft is inserted with anastomosis to the vessel edges. Flow through the grafted vessel is observed, the shunt is removed, and insertion sites are closed with patch grafts. Chest tubes are placed for drainage, and the chest is closed.

One disadvantage of the shunt technique is the time for insertion prior to repair. This may be an additional 1.5 hours before effective aortic blood flow is restored. An alternative and faster approach is a cross-clamp repair without shunt. The aorta is clamped proximally and distally to the tear, the rupture site is resected, and the graft is inserted as previously described. Cross-clamp time must be as short as possible, generally less than 30 minutes, since flow to the distal aorta is occluded. The concept of a "safe" cross-clamp time is difficult to define due to individual variation in tolerance. Long cross-clamp times are associated with markedly increased postoperative complications resulting from poor perfusion to the spinal cord, kidneys, and mesentery. All repair techniques described hold the risk of perfusion-related complications.[105, 106, 108]

Intraoperative Problems. Blood pressure control remains a focal point of concern. An antihypertensive agent is administered by continuous intravenous infusion, if not already in progress, to regulate mean arterial pressure. Reducing vessel and graft anastomosis stress is the primary objective. An additional intraoperative objective is replacement of blood loss with blood, colloids, and crystalloids. Autotransfusion, as previously described, is highly useful in fluid management.

Critical Care Assessment and Management. Many of the individuals who survive the operative period die in the first week after injury. Repair of the thoracic aorta requires similar postoperative monitoring and management as for any patient recovering from major chest surgery. Systematic assessment for residual injury effects and complications of tissue hypoperfusion is an additional and primary concern for these patients. Any organ system below the level of aortic tear may be damaged during the period of hypoperfusion. This period extends from the time of injury until reestablishment of adequate blood transport through the vessel. It is

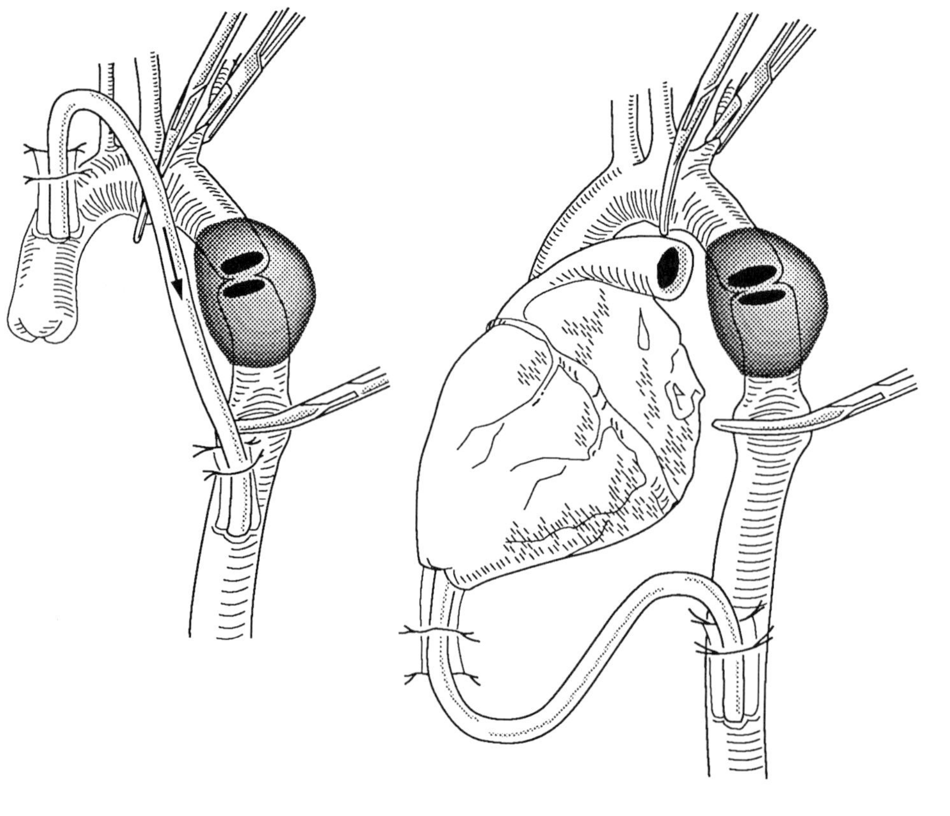

Figure 19–28. Shunt bypass technique in aortic repair. (From FW Blaisdell MD, DD Trunkey MD: Cervicothoracic Trauma. New York, Thieme Medical Publishers, Inc, © 1986.)

important for the nurse to determine the hypoperfusion time, particularly the length of cross-clamp time, in order to predict postoperative problems. The patient's age, previous cardiovascular status, preexisting diabetes or pulmonary and renal disease, and additional injuries are factors that influence the incidence of postoperative problems.[105] The most serious postoperative problems are transient or permanent hypertension, paraplegia, bowel infarction, renal failure, graft leaks, and infection.

Hypertension. Patients with aortic isthmus repairs frequently remain hypertensive postoperatively. Continuous hemodynamic monitoring is essential to trend systemic and pulmonary pressures. Once clear postoperative parameters for acceptable systolic, diastolic, and mean blood pressure have been established with the surgeon, antihypertensives are titrated to those parameters. The nurse correlates the effect of the drugs with not only mean arterial pressure but also the effect on tissue perfusion. Dosages are carefully balanced to protect the integrity of the fresh graft and the tissue needs of the brain, spinal cord, kidneys, and other organs.

Postoperative Paraplegia. Evidence of paraplegia due to interruption of spinal cord blood supply may have been apparent during the initial resuscitation. More often, critical care assessment reveals the effect of hypoperfusion of the spinal cord. Lower extremity weakness, loss of reflexes, spasticity, or overt paralysis may be evident. Spinal cord perfusion can be compromised by preoperative hypotension or lengthy cross-clamp time. The anterior spinal arteries and intercostal vessels are significant sources of spinal cord blood supply and can be damaged as a consequence of the injury or the reparative surgery. The use of antihypertensives as described above can maintain mean arterial blood pressure at a level incompatible with spinal cord perfusion. Once the paraplegia has been identified, every effort is made to maximize possible recovery of function. A comprehensive discussion of spinal cord injuries is contained in Chapter 18.

Bowel Ischemia. The bowel is at risk for ischemia and infarction if mesenteric arterial perfusion is compromised. Older patients with primary vascular disease are particularly at risk. The nurse assesses for delayed return of bowel sounds, fever, abdominal pain, and distention. Surgical removal of dead or diseased bowel segments will be required for definitive management.

Renal Failure. Hypoperfusion of the kidneys may result in poor renal function or outright failure. A comprehensive discussion of renal injuries is contained in Chapter 24.

Graft Leaks and Infection. Graft leaks are possible, since there is little permanent bonding of graft to the aorta. Chest tube drainage is carefully monitored for signs of rebleeding as long as the tubes are in place, since delayed leakage is possible. Intermittent leakage and fever of unknown origin are particularly concerning, since these are some of the first signs of graft infection. Prophylactic antibiotics and rigorous precautions are employed to prevent bacteremia which could seed the graft site.

INTERMEDIATE/REHABILITATION CONCERNS. The patient's specific plan of care will depend on the resulting disabilities. For example, if postinjury paraplegia persists, spinal cord injury care and rehabilitation protocols are implemented. Frequently, these patients are able to regain much lower extremity function with the help of exercise and physical therapy. Postoperative hypertension also may be encountered in the long-term survivor of a ruptured aorta. It can persist for months following aortic repair and is treated with standard antihypertensive agents if necessary.[105, 106]

There are also a number of general considerations for the patient during the intermediate and rehabilitative stages. Surveillance for graft leaks and infection continues throughout this part of the trauma recovery. Intermittent, small leaks may occur at the graft–vessel anastomosis resulting in chronic aneurysm formation that is dangerous because of the risk of delayed hemorrhage into the pleural cavity or pericardium. Additionally, thrombus formation within the aneurysm presents a risk of embolism.

The patient must always be protected from bacteremias. Continuing assessment includes systematic inspection of all wounds, old chest tube sites, and incisions. Temperature, white cell count, and fluid and electrolyte status are all monitored for signs of infection and sepsis. The patient and family become part of an instructional plan about the vascular prosthesis, the risk of infection, concern for long-term aneurysm formation, and need for long-term follow-up in a thoracic clinic.

The degree of continued chest pain is individual and is related to any additional thoracic injuries. Pulmonary care is directed toward the goal of preventing retained secretions and atelectasis. More detailed discussion of this area is contained in the section on intermediate care therapeutics.

NURSING THERAPEUTICS IN THE CRITICAL CARE CYCLE

The previous survey of thoracic injury management includes actions and strategies specific to a given injury and highlights therapeutics common to all chest trauma and its complications. The following sections are intended to provide greater detail concerning these therapies as used in critically ill patients.

The Patient–Ventilator Unit

A great many patients with significant chest trauma require mechanical ventilation during their critical stay and, less commonly, into the intermediate care phase. The rationale for initiating some form of mechanical ventilation may be either as definitive management, as in the case of flail chest, or as a supportive therapy, as in posttraumatic RDS. It is useful to keep the well-known goals for ventilatory therapy in mind: to improve oxygenation, correct hypoventilation and acidosis, and ease the work of breathing. Although the decision to commit the trauma patient to any given form of ventilatory therapy is based on individual history, type of injury, and injury complications such as sepsis, some general criteria for initiating mechanical ventilation are listed in Table 19–8.[109, 110]

Common ventilatory techniques used in managing thoracic injuries were summarized in the section on thoracic assessment. The nurse must be familiar with the benefits, disadvantages, and complications of several different ventilator modes and settings, as well as unique system features. IMV

Table 19–8. CRITERIA FOR INITIATION OF MECHANICAL VENTILATION

	NORMAL RANGE	FAILING FUNCTION
Respiratory rate	12–20/min	>35/min
Vital capacity	65–75 ml/kg	<15 ml/kg
Tidal volume	10–15 ml/kg	<7 ml/kg
Inspiratory force	−75 to −100 cm H_2O	>−25 cm H_2O
$Paco_2$	35–45 mm Hg	>50 mm Hg
$\dot{V}_D/\dot{V}_T$	0.2–0.4	>0.6
Pao_2	80–100 mm Hg	<70 mm Hg (on oxygen therapy)
A − aDo_2	50–75 mm Hg	>300 mm Hg (on 100% O_2)
$\frac{Pao_2}{Fio_2}$ (P/F ratio)	>280	<200

or SIMV is most commonly used in the acute injury phase because it allows the patient to stabilize while preserving respiratory muscle function and minimizing barotrauma.

Close communication among nurse, physician, and respiratory therapist is essential in determining which specific equipment and therapies are to be used. This communication is particularly important when complicated techniques such as independent lung ventilation or some form of high-frequency ventilation is in progress. Whatever the type of ventilator or mode chosen, the nurse monitors not only the patient's responses to therapy but also the functional status of the patient–ventilator unit. Disconnections or leaks within the breathing circuit may or may not be obvious and must be included as part of continuous monitoring. Checking to see that all alarms are functional at all times is one of the simplest and most essential nursing actions. The bedside nurse and respiratory therapist are the most likely persons to note high resistance or obstruction in the endotracheal tube, increased resistance in the inspiratory and expiratory circuits, or improper function of the exhalation valve. Changes in equipment or ventilatory technique are explained to even the semialert patient who may panic at sudden changes in his airflow or work of breathing.

In addition to the common types of ventilation, nurses may be required to develop a plan of care for the thoracic trauma patient who requires more unusual respiratory therapy.

Independent Lung Ventilation (ILV). In limited instances, a patient with a tracheobronchial tear or asymmetrical pulmonary contusion with massive air leak may not respond well to conventional mechanical ventilation and PEEP. Volume delivered by the ventilator will go to the more compliant lung, particularly when there are large differences in compliance between lungs. The good lung can then be at risk of hyperinflation and barotrauma, while the stiffer lung receives inadequate volume. Under such circumstances, intubation of each bronchus with a double-lumen tube and ILV provide an alternative ventilatory therapy. The endotracheal tubes are connected to (1) separate, synchronized ventilators, (2) a modified circuit allowing independent but synchronized ventilation, or (3) separate ventilators without synchronization.[111] ILV is most frequently used to manage the patient with high peak inspiratory pressures and a persistent, large air leak.[112]

Nursing management can be unusually demanding depending on the complexity of ventilator setup and the cardiopulmonary stability of the patient. Blood gases, ventilatory parameters (including end-tidal CO_2 monitoring), and hemodynamic status are closely observed. Air leak through the chest tubes is trended and measured if appropriate volumetric equipment is available. The patient may have large amounts of pulmonary or bloody secretions requiring careful airway hygiene and suctioning. It is rarely necessary to remove the patient from the ventilator system for suctioning or changing body position, but it is useful to have two manual resuscitation bags and spare double-lumen endotracheal tubes at the bedside. Pharmacological paralysis is generally required, accompanied by sedatives and analgesia. Family members will need some explanation of the therapy before entering the patient care area, since it may appear complex and frightening.

High-Frequency Ventilation (HFV). This form of ventilation is identified by the use of high respiratory rates and small tidal volumes which are less than the patient's anatomical dead space volume. *High-frequency ventilation* is a general term used to include different types of mechanical systems, specifically high-frequency oscillation (HFO) and high-frequency jet ventilation (HFJV). HFJV is the most commonly used and delivers small pulses of gas through a cannula in either an endotracheal tube or tracheostomy tube or via a specialized jet endotracheal tube. The pulses can be delivered under high pressure at rates of 30 to as many as 1000 per minute. In practice, the rate is limited to less than 150 per minute due to current regulations from the Food and Drug Administration.[11, 113] The major advantage of HFJV for trauma patients is that ventilation can be effectively accomplished at reduced peak airway pressures.

HFV has been used successfully during bronchoscopy, laryngoscopy, and tracheal reconstruction; as a weaning procedure; and in the treatment of bronchopleural fistula, acute RDS, and flail chest.[114, 115] It also has demonstrated utility in a variety of thoracic surgical procedures. Neurosurgical patients also may benefit from HFV; however, further study is warranted.[11, 111, 113]

Since HFV is used in patients who also may suffer multiple injuries and system failure, intensive patient monitoring is essential and complex. Tidal volume, system pressures, inspired oxygen concentration, and ventilator frequency are difficult to measure accurately unless specialized equipment is available. Bilateral breath sounds and chest wall movements are carefully assessed to identify potential cannula dislodgment and barotrauma. In some systems, the lack of conventional ventilator safety features such as alarms requires constant nursing vigilance and the immediate availability of a respiratory therapist. Humidification is problematic and has not been uniformly successful in HFV. Increased mobilization of pulmonary secretions may be evident and may require increased suctioning and airway care. To avoid decreases in Pao_2, the patient is not disconnected from the ventilatory system during suctioning.[116] Decreased sedation needs have been reported during HFV as opposed to conventional ventilation; however, the need for analgesia and sedation in trauma patients is difficult to predict and should be determined by individual evaluation. A more detailed discussion of general critical care nursing considerations in HFV management is contained elsewhere.[11, 117–119]

Barotrauma

Defined broadly as injury resulting from alveolar overdistention and rupture, barotrauma is a complication of conventional mechanical ventilation and PEEP. As controlled mechanical ventilation has frequently been replaced by the widespread use of SIMV and pressure support, barotrauma is less common and usually less severe. However, patients with significant lung damage are particularly susceptible to the effects of pressure-induced injury regardless of the type of mechanical ventilation used in management of respiratory sequelae.

Clinical Syndromes. There are a variety of mechanisms that produce barotrauma. Secretions trapped in the lower airways may produce a ball-valve obstruction effect as, on inspiration, the ventilator cycles gas past the partial obstruction into the alveoli. When expiration of the gas is blocked, the lung unit remains inflated. As the cycle is repeated, the alveolus ruptures. Air escapes through the ruptured area into surrounding structures.

Regional hyperinflation also may cause alveolar rupture. Unstable lung units resulting from contusion, RDS, or necrotizing pneumonia are unable to tolerate high pressure and appear to "blow out," leaking air into surrounding tissue or potential space. The end result is subcutaneous emphysema, pneumomediastinum, pneumothorax, or tension pneumothorax with a Macklin-type effect evident on chest film. The patient most likely to experience the complication has poor total compliance or high airway pressures or requires high levels of PEEP and tidal volumes. The patient with lung injury is also at risk because the injured areas vary in level of damage and healing. Regional hyperinflation or obstruction may occur within the injured region. These patients warrant particularly careful monitoring for sudden increases in airway pressure, changes in air leak through or around chest tubes, subcutaneous emphysema, and changes in vital signs or oxygenation level. Changes in breath sounds can be difficult to appreciate because referred breath sounds from ventilated areas may be audible across the lung fields.

Nursing management is directed toward controlling events that cause increased intrathoracic pressure. Pulmonary care prevents an accumulation of secretions, which leads to extensive coughing, "fighting the ventilator," and periods of preventable bronchospasm. Sedation is not administered randomly but given in early response to a rising level of patient discomfort or agitation. The source of discomfort or agitation is controlled or eliminated by appropriate positioning, massage, or pleasurable diversion such as a favorite tape recording, family visits, and conversation.

Ventilator Dependence

Ventilator dependence has not been studied extensively in singly or multiply injured patients. The trauma patient may be difficult to wean from ventilatory support for many of the same reasons present in any group of critically ill individuals. Previous respiratory disease complicates the recovery from injury and can be anticipated from the patient's health history. Psychophysiological factors have a profound effect on weaning success and are discussed extensively in the literature.[120–123] Chapter 10 also examines psychological responses in detail.

Ventilator dependence can arise from direct thoracic injury or be a function of central nervous system injury, RDS, or the enormous metabolic demand of sepsis or healing. The patient may be unable to protect his airway and may sustain numerous, yet difficult to detect, episodes of aspiration. Failure to fully manage the patient's underlying trauma and requirements for healing is the most common cause of weaning failures.

Weaning Methods. Owing to the multisystem influences on the trauma patient's need for mechanical ventilation, a weaning plan is established by the primary nurse, trauma surgeon, or intensivist and respiratory therapist. There are currently four weaning techniques in use: (1) T-piece weaning, (2) IMV protocols, (3) CPAP weaning, and (4) pressure support or PSV. T-piece weaning alternates periods of full ventilator support with progressively prolonged periods of spontaneous ventilation. IMV protocols employ a gradual reduction of the mechanical breaths delivered per minute while allowing the patient to breathe spontaneously. CPAP weaning allows the patient to breathe entirely without machine-delivered breaths but with continuous positive airway pressure. Lastly, PSV allows the patient to control the length, depth, and frequency of inspiration while augmenting each breath with a predetermined positive pressure from the ventilator.[121–123] Weaning criteria and desired endpoints are adapted to the unique demands of the patient's injuries, previous delivered oxygen concentration, and level of PEEP/CPAP. Each change in ventilatory support or oxygen therapy is evaluated by repeated clinical examinations, end-tidal CO_2 monitoring or capnography, and blood gas analyses. In some patients, on-line evaluation of peripheral oxygen saturation is particularly helpful. Explanations of the weaning process and daily progress are reviewed with the patient and family members. Table 19–9 serves as an example of weaning criteria.[14]

Table 19–9. WEANING CRITERIA IN TRAUMA

Underlying trauma and septic complications are resolved
Oxygenation
P/F ratio is >250 at all times
Q_s/Q_t is <15%
Ventilatory mechanics
VC is >15 ml/kg
Total compliance is >35 ml/cm H_2O
Ventilatory drive is sufficient
Sedation and analgesia are tapered
Evidence of electrolyte balance
No evidence of overventilation, pH >7.35
Work of breathing is not excessive
Appropriate size airway is in place
Bony thorax is intact or stabilized
Adequate pain management is in progress
Muscle strength is adequate
Nutritional deficits are eliminated
Maximum inspiratory force is < −20 cm H_2O
Ventilatory demand is reasonable
$Paco_2$ is <45–50 mm Hg
CO_2 production through carbohydrate intake is not excessive
Maximum temperature is reasonable
$\dot{V}_D/\dot{V}_T$ is <0.5
Spontaneous respiratory rate is <30 per minute
Airway remains intact and protected
Plan for psychological and family support is in place

Weaning criteria have limited value under some circumstances, particularly in the trauma patient with preexisting pulmonary disease. In one case, the patient may be successfully extubated who does not meet the usual criteria. Such a patient must be repeatedly reevaluated and all equipment readied for rapid reintubation and continued ventilatory support, if needed. In another case, the patient does not progress beyond a given level of support. This type of weaning failure is likely due to incomplete resolution of underlying trauma or an emerging sepsis. Clearly, there are no general solutions for weaning difficulties. One or more strategies may be required, e.g., changing the patient from T-piece weaning to an alternative such as pressure support.

Pulmonary Therapeutics

Procedures that effectively clear the airways at all anatomical levels and remove retained secretions are the foundation of thoracic injury management. Pulmonary care is frequently a difficult and time-consuming process in trauma patients. How can the repetitive clogging of the endotracheal tube or tracheostomy with bloody secretions and tissue clots be avoided? How can a piece of tooth be removed from the posterior lung segment? How does one maximize overall oxygenation and ventilation in a patient with edematous or hemorrhagic lung segments? Problems such as these are frequently encountered in traumatic injuries and are treated with chest physiotherapy, suctioning, and injury-specific positioning.

Chest Physiotherapy. A plan for chest physiotherapy (CPT) includes selection and evaluation of several treatment components. Postural drainage, percussion, and vibration are used to mobilize intrapulmonary secretions, accompanied by suctioning or coughing to clear the larger airways. Effective postural drainage, i.e., positioning the patient so that the affected segmental bronchus is uppermost, assists movement of secretions from the lung by gravity and requires knowledge of which lung segments are abnormal. Percussion, a rhythmical clapping with a cupped hand, is performed directly on the chest wall throughout the respiratory cycle. Vibration intermittently compresses the involved area during expiration. Percussion can be used over fractures or painful areas, carefully and gently.

Each selected component, its frequency, and the length of a therapeutic session are planned in relation to the patient's total injuries as well as specific respiratory abnormalities. The frequency of treatment, usually every 4 hours in critically ill patients, is evaluated every 12 to 24 hours on the basis of desired endpoints such as the appearance of the daily chest film, trends in total lung compliance, stability of blood gases, and clinical examination. Patients with copious secretions or high-risk injuries such as flail chest with significant lung contusion may require more frequent or longer treatments. The length of a treatment is determined by clinical parameters such as improved breath sounds and changes in airway pressures and lung volumes. The amount of sputum or suctioning aspirate is rarely an indicator of the therapy's effectiveness and does not serve as the sole criterion for ending a therapy session. The duration of a treatment also may be determined by adverse effects on intracranial pressure or hemodynamic stability.[124]

CPT may be performed by the nurse, physical, or respiratory therapist. Frequently, positioning for therapy requires several assistants to avoid inadvertent extubation, disconnection of intravenous or arterial lines, or physical trauma to the patient. Appropriate positioning and use of restraints need to be planned for in treating agitated patients. The therapy session is coordinated with the patient's analgesia and sedation requirements. In all cases, the nurse's role includes planning the treatment schedule and evaluating both desirable and undesirable effects during and after treatment. Desired effects include improvement in sequential chest films, blood gases, total compliance, and airway resistance. Undesired effects on arterial oxygenation and hemodynamic parameters occur but are difficult to predict. The use of prone, head-down, and/or lateral positions during CPT may be responsible for the adverse effects as well as benefits.[125]

Suctioning. The optimal method of endotracheal suctioning has been the subject of considerable nursing research[126–133] as well as clinical reviews.[134, 135] Controversy remains regarding the use and amount of hyperinflation and hyperoxygenation prior to and following suctioning. The value of instilling sterile saline into the endotracheal tube is also debated but not proven to be effective. However, it is well accepted that there are risks associated with suctioning, including hypoxemia, aspiration, hypertension, and serious dysrhythmias. Suctioning in the multiply injured individual has not been well studied, particularly in the patient with preexisting lung disease or significant physiological instability. Lookinland and Appel[133] conclude that three hyperoxygenation breaths are adequate to prevent the hypoxemia associated with endotracheal suctioning in young and hemodynamically stable trauma patients. However, further study is needed before rational protocols can be developed. The need for suctioning, as well as the technique used, is best determined by the patient's injuries, clinical presentation, and assessment findings.

Positioning. Another form of pulmonary therapy is therapeutic positioning, the use of specific body positions to maximize oxygenation and ventilation despite lung abnormalities. Turning the patient has long been accepted as the treatment for the complications of immobility, and the effect of position on gas exchange must be considered in clinical management. The usefulness of positioning techniques is based on the effect of gravity on the lung fields, specifically on gravity-dependent ventilation–perfusion matching in particular respiratory segments. Recognizing that perfusion is greatest in the dependent lung or dependent portions of the lung, it is possible to position the patient so that specific lung areas receive a greater or lesser proportion of blood flow. Position is manipulated so that the healthy portion of the lung is dependent and, therefore, receives greatest perfusion. In a similar way, lung areas that are compromised by injury and poor ventilation are positioned uppermost, thus receiving a gravity-dependent reduction in blood flow. The end result is increased blood flow to areas of best ventilation, decreased flow to poorly ventilated areas, and overall improved matching of perfusion and ventilation. Therefore, altering body position can be used to improve arterial oxygenation in some patients.[135, 136]

Positioning becomes part of pulmonary care in many patients with respiratory abnormalities and significant thoracic trauma. Thoracic assessment and knowledge of the most recent chest film are used to choose positions: sitting, prone, and, most commonly, lateral decubitus. Immediate effects of the position are noted, such as change in airway position, respiratory rate, and chest excursion and increased airway pressures and hemodynamic parameters. The effect of body position is also evaluated at 30 minutes to determine changes in blood gases, cardiac output, and subsequent oxygen transport to tissues.[137] In all cases, body alignment, support of head and neck, and comfort are evaluated. Part of the positioning protocol is planning for pain relief and removing secretions that are mobilized by turning. Frequency of position change is determined by the results of this ongoing evaluation, not by an arbitrary recommendation for turning every 2 hours.

Pleural Space Drainage

Most thoracic injuries are treated by the insertion of one or more chest tubes, often under emergent conditions. While the management of pleural space drainage systems is common to all types of critical care nursing, there are some special concerns for the thoracic trauma patient. For example, how can nursing management decrease the persistently high incidence of chest tube–related infections? A chest tube may be inserted in close proximity to fractures, wounds, and large skin abrasions. What can be done to prevent chest tubes from aggravating other injuries? Fragile, damaged lung tissue may be in close proximity to the lumen of the tube. What is the best way to milk the chest tube of drainage without further damage? Major considerations for nursing are maintaining an effective and infection-free chest tube system, protecting associated injury sites, and avoiding damage to underlying lung tissue.

Choice of Drains. The chest tube chosen for trauma management is large bore, e.g., a no. 40 French, so as to evacuate a mixture of air, blood, and tissue fragments. The usual insertion site is the fourth intercostal space at the midaxillary line. Multiple tube insertion sites may be necessary to capture drainage and evacuate air.

Removal of the Drainage Tube. Daily chest radiographs and physical examination assist in determining the need to reposition the chest tube or to insert additional drains. The decision to remove the tube is frequently a matter of balancing the risk of infection and the possibility of a secondary pleural space injury. Generally, a chest tube that drains liquid exudate is removed 3 or 4 days after insertion. Chest tubes that drain primarily air are removed 2 to 10 days after insertion, depending on the amount of continued air evacuation and the degree of lung reexpansion. Partial lung reexpansion does not necessarily imply that a previous leak has sealed. The gradual absence of air in the tube or water seal, as well as clinical and radiographical examination for subcutaneous or mediastinal air, provides assurance that the leak has sealed.

Adequate Suction. Suction through the drainage system is generally maintained at 20 cm H_2O, a continuous and gentle bubbling. The suction must be adequate to facilitate drainage of air and blood but not high enough to entrap tissue or delay healing of the injury. Occasionally, the suction level is inadequate to properly evacuate air and seal an existing air leak. Additional suction may be provided by adding water to the suction chamber. The new level of suction is clinically and radiographically evaluated.

Conversely, low suction levels may be required in selected patients managed with controlled mechanical ventilation to avoid increasing the gradient between positive airway pressure and negative intrapleural suction. The increased gradient may delay healing, create additional air leak, and potentiate a bronchopleural fistula.

Examining the Drainage. The pleural drainage system must be checked regularly to determine if it is fully functional. This is generally determined by fluctuation or bubbling of the water seal as negative pressure is transmitted during inspiration. A seemingly obstructed drain that continues to evacuate large amounts of fluid or air is likely to still be functional. Liquid drainage through the system is easily measured and is correlated with the patient's injury and recovery. The amount of blood initially evacuated from the pleural cavity is a criterion for estimation of blood loss and replacement need. The hourly blood loss is useful as an indicator of an overlooked or occult injury, particularly a vascular injury. The trend of drainage over time, both air and fluid, provides information about the resolution of underlying injury. For example, bleeding visibly slows from a small pulmonary laceration as the lung reexpands, sealing off the injury.

Maintaining Patency. The drainage system is positioned below the level of the chest to facilitate the flow of bloody fluid, and the drainage tubing is milked in small segments to remove clots. Patency of the drain is always a concern, since a residual intrathoracic clot will require thoracotomy for removal and not a simple chest tube reinsertion. It is well known that high intrathoracic pressures can be generated by compressing or pulling on the chest tube to the point of collapse (stripping).[138] In order to minimize the stress on underlying tissue, a sequential short-segment squeezing motion is used. The frequency of tube milking is determined by the difficulty in maintaining a clear lumen.

Protecting Against Infection. An initial pleural space injury may become infected by a break in the drainage system or by inadequate dressing techniques. Several nursing therapeutic measures can minimize this risk or prevent infection. Skillful and careful assistance during insertion or removal of the drainage system is essential. Even under emergent conditions, skin disinfection is employed. Surveillance of aseptic technique is required on the part of all individuals during insertion, repositioning, or removal of the chest tube. Ensure the sterility of all parts of the drainage system that connect to the pleural space. Every connection is taped or secured with chest tube bands. Collection containers, whether glass or disposable underwater seal systems, are replaced when contaminated. It is important to date the drainage system and to document when it was initiated or changed. Many patients have large amounts of drainage and require several changes of the collection system. Under these circumstances, disposable systems that allow replacement of only the collecting canister are particularly useful.

The chest tube is sutured in place, dressed, and carefully secured to the chest wall. The objective is to avoid slippage of the tube back and forth, which increases local injury and the possibility of infection. Cloth adhesive tape is used for greatest security. Underlying skin can be protected by commercial skin preparation or by the use of sterile stoma care materials.

The dressing procedure is sterile, requiring a small sterile field, mask, and gloves. It can be done economically and quickly without compromising sterile technique. The site and the surrounding skin are cleansed with separate sponges and antiseptic solution. The use of an antibiotic ointment at the site has not been shown to decrease infection. The final dressing is closed to the environment by adhesive tape and changed whenever it is wet or contaminated. It is useful to establish a standard for routine changing, such as every 2 days, and to systematically document the date of dressing change, the appearance of the site, and drainage apparent on the dressing.

Wounds around the chest tube site are dressed separately whenever possible. These wounds may require frequent dressing changes, such as every 4 hours, to avoid contamination of the chest tube site.

NURSING THERAPEUTICS IN THE INTERMEDIATE/REHABILITATION CARE CYCLES

Not all patients with thoracic injuries require critical care nursing. Many need subacute postresuscitation or postoperative care and progress into rehabilitation and return to the community. Alternatively, numerous patient problems identified and initially managed in the critical care cycle persist into intermediate care and rehabilitation. The following sections focus on such specific nursing therapeutics.

Ventilator Dependence

In some instances, a patient will remain dependent on mechanical ventilation even though the causes of weaning failure have been considered and considerable management has already been directed toward the problem. The causes of extended ventilatory dependence are not usually complications of thoracic injury per se but are related to central nervous system injury or previous chronic respiratory disease. Under these circumstances, weaning therapies are continued into the patient's intermediate trauma phase, and the problem of ventilator dependence is incorporated into the plan of care. If continued dependence on some form of mechanical ventilation is preventing the patient from hospital discharge, home respiratory therapy may be considered.[139]

Table 19–9 lists criteria for weaning based on experience with trauma patients. The most valid predictors of successful weaning have not been determined in the multiply injured population. It seems reasonable to use well-studied predictors obtained in general surgical patients to evaluate readiness for spontaneous breathing with supplemental oxygen: tidal volume > 5 ml/kg, forced vital capacity > 10 to 15 ml/kg, maximal inspiratory pressure > −20 cm H_2O, and an acceptable $Pa_{O_2}/F_{I_{O_2}}$ ratio.[140] However, a large survey of weaning practices indicated that "clinical assessment" rather than pulmonary function tests formed the basis for weaning decisions.[141] Furthermore, there is no clear consensus on the value of measurements or predictors in ventilator dependence.

More is known about the mechanisms of ventilator dependence. One principal factor is respiratory muscle failure after terminating mechanical ventilation. Muscle contractility is diminished in the presence of low plasma phosphate, magnesium, and calcium levels, as well as hypercapnia and acidosis.[141] Respiratory performance is decreased by infections. For example, muscle performance as measured by maximum inspiratory and expiratory mouth pressures falls by approximately 30 per cent of control values during an upper respiratory infection.[142] Atrophy has been demonstrated to be associated with septic processes, and weaning failure has been reported to occur in the presence of positive blood cultures.[92]

Once causative factors have been corrected, ventilator dependence may be reversed. At this point, an appropriate weaning protocol is used to gradually strengthen respiratory muscles through exercise. The basic strategy is to allow the patient to breath spontaneously for gradually longer periods of time with interspersed rest periods. The means by which this strategy is put into operation are similar to those described in the critical care therapeutics section. Traditional methods include (1) the familiar T-piece technique with or without CPAP, in which the patient breathes spontaneously for periods of increasing duration and is mechanically ventilated between periods, and (2) IMV, in which the mechanical breaths are progressively reduced in number. Numerous studies have explored the relative efficacy of T-piece or IMV; however, the data do not support the superiority of either technique. A recent review summarizes these data and appropriately emphasizes that the merits of a weaning technique must be suited to the individual patient circumstances.[123] For example, the patient with exercise dyspnea can be supported during ambulation with ventilation via a self-inflating bag. The sleep-deprived patient can receive SIMV during rest periods and night hours. The SIMV periods are gradually shortened and eliminated as the patient gains strength and vitality. Newer techniques have been advocated for weaning such as pressure-support ventilation or airway pressure-release ventilation. Both techniques deliver positive pressure when needed, reportedly without causing excess patient discomfort or increased mean airway pressure and work of breathing. Further details are available elsewhere.[11, 52]

Weaning is a great burden both physically and mentally for the patient who has been ventilated for many days or weeks. Anxiety and fear can prolong ventilator dependence in some patients.[143] A number of studies in medical–surgical patients have demonstrated that biofeedback, relaxation, and imagery can reduce negative emotional responses to weaning.[144–146] These therapies have not been well studied in the multiply injured at the present time.

Pleural Space Infections

The previous discussion of critical care nursing management of pleural space drainage is pertinent to intermediate care settings. The risk of posttraumatic empyema remains high and is frequently a product of initial treatment and stabilization. Discussion of the etiology, diagnosis, and pathogens of empyema can be found in Chapter 12.

Management of Empyema. Once the pathogens have been identified, specific antiobiotic treatment is initiated and based on the results of the Gram stain. The contents of the infected pleural space are drained, and the underlying lung is allowed to reexpand. Closed or open drainage techniques can be used depending on the number of infectious pockets and organization of the infected material. Each requires lengthy and persistent medical and nursing management. Decortication may be chosen as definitive management as opposed to prolonged drainage or as a method to remove thickened pleura that entraps the lung and prevents healing.

In closed techniques, a chest tube is inserted or an existing thoracostomy tube is converted to an "empyema tube." Although the general management of the closed system is as previously described, frequent cultures of drainage fluid are needed. The nurse avoids milking the chest tube or positioning the drainage collection container in a manner that allows reflux of contaminated material back into the pleural space. The drainage initially appears as a purulent fluid but may change to a thicker, more fibrous material. After 2 or 3 weeks, the closed system may be converted into open drainage of the most dependent part of the cavity. Should open drainage be required, nursing care includes a specific protocol for irrigation, absorbent wound dressing, and protection of surrounding skin. As the infection clears and healing begins, the drainage tube is slowly advanced and removed as the cavity closes behind it.

Paraplegia

Spinal cord injury is the most serious complication encountered in patients who survive the critical care phase of ruptured thoracic aorta. Whether the paraplegia results from cord ischemia during aortic cross-clamping or from direct injury to the spinal arteries, spinal cord injury is a devastating condition that occurs in nearly 20 per cent of survivors.[105, 106] The considerable physical and psychological nursing care needs of these patients persist throughout the intermediate and rehabilitative cycles and are described in detail in Chapter 18.

Pericarditis

Posttraumatic pericarditis may become symptomatic weeks or months following myocardial contusion. Bleeding into the pericardial sac irritates the epicardium and pericardium, producing inflammation and edema. Three types of pathology have been associated with blunt chest trauma.[97] These include pericarditis with or without effusion and constrictive pericarditis. Individuals with effusion slowly develop signs of cardiac tamponade, while those without effusion demonstrate a significant pericardial rub, fever, and retrosternal pain. The patient with constrictive pericarditis shows signs which mimic right-sided heart failure. Heart sounds are diminished, and a third heart sound may be heard. Nursing care includes careful physical examination, including auscultation of heart sounds. Identification of a friction rub as well as a change in the quality and quantity of chest pain are important findings.[96]

Persistent Pain

Chronic chest wall pain has been described in nearly half of all long-term survivors of flail injuries. Likewise, the same percentage of patients are unable to return to full-time employment after 5 years owing to continued and significant pain.[147–150] The nurse must be able to differentiate between acute and chronic pain in order to provide appropriate therapy. A detailed discussion of pain control modalities is contained in Chapter 15.

Dyspnea

Shortness of breath, decreased chest expansion, and compromised exercise tolerance have been demonstrated in 50 per cent of patients who survive significant chest wall injury.[147–150] Nursing care seeks to minimize respiratory effort by planning rest periods for the patient and supporting ventilatory functioning with proper positioning and supplemental oxygen.

Nutritional Deficiencies

Restoration of optimal nutritional status is a problem common in trauma patients (see also Chapter 14). The individual with insufficient or excessive caloric and protein intake is likely to experience respiratory disability and difficulty in weaning from supplemental oxygen. Consultation with nutritional support services, as well as the patient's family, is essential to ensure adequate nutritional intake.

Delayed Wound Healing

Healing difficulties are not common in chest tube sites or thoracic soft tissue wounds due to a rich, muscular blood supply. Deformities, diminished sensation due to intercostal nerve damage, and soft tissue defects are more common and may be associated with higher morbidity and longer hospital stays for the trauma patient. Although some chest wall and related musculoskeletal deformities may require surgical intervention, others can be prevented and treated by exercise. Wound assessment and management are detailed in Chapter 13.

Pulmonary Therapeutics

All trauma patients, particularly those with thoracic injuries, require care directed toward removal of retained pulmonary secretions from the airways and protection from aspiration and associated pneumonia. Chest physiotherapy is used extensively as described in critical care therapeutics. Airway clearance may be accomplished by suctioning through an existing airway such as tracheostomy, by nasotracheal route, or by directed coughing. Breathing exercises are added to the plan of care, particularly in postoperative patients or those with neuromuscular or chronic pulmonary disease. A clear rationale for therapy, as well as simple-to-follow instructions, is particularly important because the patient may not remember prior therapies employed in his early recovery course.

Directed Coughing. Coughing remains the most rapid and effective method for clearing the larger airways. It is generally a reflex under control of the afferent vagus nerve triggered by mechanical stimulation of laryngeal and bronchial receptors. However, both involuntary and voluntary cough suppression occurs in trauma patients as a result of decreased inspiratory or expiratory effort, poor glottic function, or fear and pain.

Directed coughing techniques are accompanied by monitoring for cough suppression and treating its cause. For example, the unhealed stoma left after tracheostomy tube removal can reduce the effectiveness of coughing and should be sealed with an airtight dressing. The patient is taught to put light pressure on the dressing during coughing. If the patient has difficulty mobilizing secretions toward the primary bronchi, coughing is less effective as a means of removing mucus. In this case, directed coughing is preceded by postural drainage, percussion, or vibration as one way of centralizing secretions and increasing the cough's effectiveness. Effective pain relief must be in progress before the majority of patients can even attempt to breathe deeply and cough. Although many patients naturally "splint" injured or postoperative areas during coughing, the majority benefit from a demonstration of effective splinting that does not impair chest wall movement.

Several methods can be used to stimulate coughing. "Huff coughing" is a single, large inspiration followed by short, forceful exhalations producing rapid changes in airflow and an improved cough.[151] External tracheal stimulation by gentle pressure above the sternal notch can stimulate coughing. Gentle oropharyngeal stimulation with the end of a suction catheter or direct suction aspiration may be necessary when the patient has difficulty clearing secretions in this area. Directed coughing takes place over short time periods alternating with rest. Repetitive and strained coughing is tiring and can precipitate bronchospasm.

Breathing Exercises. The main goals of breathing exercises are improved tidal volume, chest wall mobility, mobilization of secretions, and relaxation. Muscle training may increase respiratory strength and endurance. Specific exercises include diaphragmatic breathing, pursed-lip breathing, forced expiration, costal excursion exercises, and summed breathing. Exercise techniques and patient instruction plans are available elsewhere.[152]

Adjuncts Used to Improve Lung Expansion. Numerous devices are available to augment chest physiotherapy, directed coughing, and breathing exercises. Most are types of incentive spirometry. Blow bottles are expiratory incentive devices; most commercial equipment packages are inspiratory incentive spirometers. Although published reports of the relative benefits and complications of these devices are abundant, the effectiveness of these adjuncts in reducing postoperative or posttraumatic pulmonary complications remains in question.[153–155]

Should such devices be incorporated into the plan of care, they are considered an addition to, not a substitute for, the pulmonary therapeutics described earlier. How frequently and for what length of time the patient uses the device are determined by its effectiveness in improving lung volumes and respiratory status. The patient should be clearly instructed and supervised periodically to determine if the device is used properly and if benefits or problems are present. If incentive spirometry is a consistent part of the patient's pulmonary care, the nurse and/or respiratory therapist trends the achieved volumes and maintains a record of volume change over time.

Active Exercise Programs

Muscular exercise and range-of-motion programs are appropriate for the thoracic trauma patient even in unusual situations when other injuries restrict the patient to bed. In consultation with a physical therapist, an exercise program for involved joints or muscles is included in the plan of care. Patients are likely to avoid moving trunk and upper extremities following thoracotomy or significant chest wall injury. As a result, they can develop deformities, most commonly frozen shoulder syndrome. Range-of-motion exercises include passive stretch of the affected area or active contraction of opposing muscle groups. Repeated exercises with weights can improve strength and endurance.

The presence of chest tubes and even ventilatory or oxygen delivery equipment does not commit the patient to bed rest. After reviewing all tubes, drains, and oxygen requirements with the trauma physician, progressive ambulation is planned with the patient as part of the exercise program. Chest tube drainage systems can be temporarily disconnected from suction, and oxygen tanks, if needed, are attached to a rolling pole or walker.

SUMMARY

This chapter outlines nursing knowledge of chest trauma, yet it must be emphasized that a great deal is unknown about the physiological and psychological effects of our nursing therapies. In solving these "unknowns," we do the greatest service for our patients.

It is also evident from this chapter that thoracic injuries can be highly lethal, and nursing management must be rapid, technically flawless, and comprehensive. Many chest injuries do not threaten life or create permanent disability, again in large part due to nursing expertise. The trauma nurse's expert care is based on a thorough understanding of thoracic anatomy, respiratory physiology, injury mechanics, and the techniques of cardiopulmonary assessment. Management of chest injuries revolves around individualized ventilator support, exquisite airway care, objective pain-control strategies, and intensive pulmonary hygiene.

Trauma nursing care is built from experience, consultation with nursing specialists and other disciplines, as well as from research. We have much to offer the patient with thoracic injuries. We offer *relief* from the pervasive chest pain, the inability to breathe, and the growing weakness of hypovolemic shock. We also offer *support* in tolerating chest tubes, positioning and coughing, and the endless days until it is possible to go home.

REFERENCES

1. Peitzman AB, Udekwu AO, Pevec W, Albrink M: Transection of the inferior vena cava from blunt thoracic trauma: Case reports. J Trauma 29(4):534–536, 1989.
2. Fulda G, Brathwaite CEM, Rodriquez A, et al: Blunt traumatic rupture of the heart and pericardium: A ten-year experience. J Trauma 31(2):167–173, 1991.
3. Howanitz EP, Buckley D, Galbraith TA, et al: Combined blunt traumatic rupture of the heart and aorta: Two case reports and review of the literature. J Trauma 39(4):506–508, 1990.

4. Rodriquez A: Initial patient evaluation and indications for thoracotomy. In Turney SZ, Rodriquez A, Cowley RA (eds): Management of Cardiothoracic Trauma. Baltimore, Williams & Wilkins, 1990.
5. Jurkovich GJ, Moore EE: Thoracic trauma. Trauma Q 11:37–51, 1984.
6. Wolfgang ME: Interpersonal violence and public health care: New directions, new challenge. In Surgeon General's Workshop on Violence and Public Health Report (DHHS Publication No. HRS-D-MC86-1). Washington, DHHS, 1986, pp 9–18.
7. Shorr RM: Blunt chest trauma in the elderly: The MIEMSS experience. In Turney SZ, Rodriquez A, Cowley RA (eds): Management of Cardiothoracic Trauma. Baltimore, Williams & Wilkins, 1990.
8. Varon AJ, Civetta JM: Hemodynamic monitoring. In Berk J, Sampliner J (eds): Handbook of Critical Care. Boston, Little, Brown, 1990.
9. Ralston AC, Webb RK, Runciman WB: Potential errors in pulse oximetry: I. Pulse oximeter evaluation. Anesthesia 46:202–206, 1991.
10. Schuster DP: Bedside evaluation of respiratory function. In Parrillo JE (ed): Current Therapy in Critical Care Medicine. Philadelphia, BC Decker, 1991.
11. Richless CI: Current trends in mechanical ventilation. Crit Care Nurs 11:41–50, 1991.
12. Ayella RJ: Radiologic Management of the Massively Traumatized Patient. Baltimore, Williams & Wilkins, 1978.
13. Mirvis SE: Imaging of thoracic trauma. In Turney SZ, Rodriquez A, Cowley RA (eds): Management of Cardiothoracic Trauma. Baltimore, Williams & Wilkins, 1990.
14. Dunham CM, Cowley RA: Shock Trauma/Critical Care Manual. Gaithersburg, MD, Aspen Publishers, 1991.
15. Committee on Trauma, American College of Surgeons: Advanced Trauma Life Support Care Course, 1989.
16. Guernsey JM, Blaisdell WB: Pulmonary injury. In Blaisdell F, Trunkey D (eds): Cervicothoracic Trauma. New York, Thieme, 1986.
17. Besson A, Saegesser F: Chest Trauma and Associated Injuries II. Oradell, NJ, Medical Economics, 1983.
18. Burns HP, Dayal VS, Scott A, et al: Laryngeal trauma. Laryngoscope 89:1316, 1979.
19. Elkins RC: Complications of intubation, tracheal surgery, and trauma. In Greenfield LJ (ed): Complications in Surgery and Trauma. Philadelphia, JB Lippincott, 1984.
20. Berlauk JF: Prolonged endotracheal intubation vs tracheostomy. Crit Care Med 14:742–745, 1986.
21. Bostick J, Wendelgass ST: Normal saline instillation as part of the suctioning procedure: Effects on PaO_2 and amount of secretions. Heart Lung 16(5):532–537, 1987.
22. Elpern EH, Jacobs ER, Bone RC: Incidence of aspirations in tracheally intubated adults. Heart Lung 16(5):527–531, 1987.
23. Smith TR, Ramzy AI: Prehospital care of thoracic trauma. In Turney SZ, Rodriquez A, Cowley RA (eds): Management of Cardiothoracic Trauma. Baltimore, Williams & Wilkins, 1990.
24. Rodriquez A: Injuries of the chest wall, the lungs, and the pleura. In Turney SZ, Rodriquez A, Cowley RA (eds): Management of Cardiothoracic Trauma. Baltimore, Williams & Wilkins, 1990.
25. Lange MP, Dahn MS, Jacobs LA: Patient-controlled analgesia versus intermittent analgesia dosing. Heart Lung 17(5):495–498, 1988.
26. Puntillo KA: Pain experiences of intensive care patients. Heart Lung 19(5):526–533, 1990.
27. Puntillo KA: The phenomenon of pain and critical care nursing. Heart Lung 17(3):262–271, 1988.
28. Besson A, Saegesser F: Chest Trauma and Associated Injuries I. Oradell, NJ, Medical Economics, 1983.
29. Blaisdell FW: Pneumothorax and hemothorax. In Blaisdell F, Trunkey D (eds): Cervicothoracic Trauma. New York, Thieme, 1986.
30. Henry H, Elliott T: The morbid anatomy of wounds of the thorax. J Army Med Corps 27:520–555, 1916.
31. Jacobs LM, Hsieh JW: A clinical review of autotransfusion and its role in trauma. JAMA 251(24):3282–3285, 1984.
32. Merlotti G: Penetrating thoracic trauma. Trauma Q 1:42–53, 1985.
33. Beckwith N, Carriere SR: Fluid resuscitation in trauma: An update. Journal Emergency Nursing JEN 11(6):293–299, 1985.
34. Dawson RB: Transfusion: Volume expansion, oxygen transport, hemostasis, transfusion reactions, autotransfusion. In Cowley RA, Conn A, Dunham CM (eds): Trauma Care Medical Management II. Philadelphia, JB Lippincott, 1987.
35. Martin E, Harris A, Johnson N, et al: Autotransfusion systems. Crit Care Nurs 9(7):65–73, 1989.
36. Holler DL: Autotransfusion. In Welton RH, Shane KA (eds): Case Studies in Trauma Nursing. Baltimore, Williams & Wilkins, 1990.
37. Ullman K: Demystifying autotransfusion. Cardiovasc Nurs 1:8–9, 1991.
38. Glover JL, Broadie TA: Autotransfusion in trauma. Crit Care Q 6:33–43, 1983.
39. Broadie EF, Indeglia RA, Shea RM, et al: Clotting competence of intracavitary blood in trauma patients. Ann Emerg Med 10:127–130, 1981.
40. Ruth-Sahd L: Pulmonary contusion: The hidden danger in blunt chest trauma. Crit Care Nurs 11(6):46–57, 1991.
41. Luchtefeld WB: Pulmonary contusion. Focus Crit Care 17(6):482–488, 1990.
42. Sheehy SB, Marvin JA, Jimmerson CD: Manual of Clinical Trauma Care the First Hour. St. Louis, CV Mosby, 1987.
43. Fulton RL, Peter ET: Compositional and histological effects of fluid therapy following pulmonary contusion. J Trauma 14:783–790, 1974.
44. Richardson JD, Franz JL, Grover FL, et al: Pulmonary contusion and hemorrhage: Crystalloid versus colloid replacement. J Surg Res 16:330–336, 1974.
45. Carrico J: Lung contusion. In Matlon KL, Moore EE, Feliciano DV (eds): Trauma. East Norwalk, CT, Appleton & Lange, 1988.
46. Ashbaugh DG, Bigelow DB, Petty TL, et al: Acute respiratory distress in adults. Lancet 2:319–323, 1967.
47. Pepe PE: The clinical entity of adult respiratory distress syndrome: Definition, prediction and prognosis. Crit Care Clin 2:377–387, 1986.
48. Montgomery AB, Stager MA, Carrico CJ, et al: Causes of mortality in patients with the adult respiratory distress syndrome. Am Rev Respir Dis 132:485–489, 1985.
49. Fowler AA, Hamman RF, Good JT, et al: Adult respiratory distress syndrome: Risk with common predispositions. Ann Intern Med 98:593–597, 1983.
50. Maunder RJ: Clinical prediction of the adult respiratory distress syndrome. Clin Chest Med 6:413–415, 1985.
51. Horn JK, Lewis FR: Respiratory Insufficiency. In Moore EE, Mattox KL, Feliciano DV (eds): Trauma. Norwalk, CT, Appleton & Lange, 1991.
52. Siegel JH, Stoklosa JC: Physiologic diagnosis and management of the acute pulmonary insufficiency in the adult respiratory distress syndrome. In Berk JL, Sampliner JE (eds): Handbook of Critical Care. Boston, Little, Brown, 1990.
53. Pepe PE, Potkin RT, Reus DH, et al: Clinical predictors of the adult respiratory distress syndrome. Am J Surg 144:124–130, 1982.
54. Sivak ED and Wiedemann HP: Clinical measurement of extravascular lung water. Crit Care Clin 2:511–512, 1986.
55. Brigham KL, Kariman K, Harris T, et al: Lung water and vascular permeability surface area in humans during respiratory failure. Am Rev Respir Dis 121:121–125, 1980.
56. Aubier M, Viires N, Syllie G, et al: Respiratory muscle contribution to lactic acidosis in low cardiac output. Am Rev Respir Dis 126:648–650, 1982.
57. Gelb AW: Pulmonary dysfunction in trauma. Can Anaesthesiol Soc J 32:235–237, 1985.
58. Fishman AP: Hypoxia in the pulmonary circulation: How and where it works. Circ Res 38:221–224, 1976.
59. Newman JH: Pulmonary vascular reactivity in primary pulmonary edema. Semin Respir Med 4:296–300, 1983.
60. Fein AM, Wiener-Kronish JP, Niederman M, et al: Pathophysiology of the adult respiratory distress syndrome. Crit Care Clin 2:429–433, 1986.

61. Weiland JE, Davis WB, Holter JF, et al: Lung neutrophils in the adult respiratory distress syndrome: Clinical and pathophysiological significance. Am Rev Respir Dis 133:218–225, 1986.
62. Hammerschmidt DE, Weaver LJ, Hudson LD, et al: Association of complement activation and elevated plasma-C5a with adult respiratory distress syndrome: Pathophysiologic relevance and possible prognostic value. Lancet 1:947–948, 1980.
63. Jacobs H, Craddock P, Hammerschmidt D, et al: Complement-induced granulocyte aggregation: An unsuspected mechanism of disease. N Engl J Med 302:789–791, 1980.
64. Parsons PE, Fowler AA, Hyers TM, et al: Chemotactic activity in bronchoalveolar lavage fluid from patients with adult respiratory distress syndrome. Am Rev Respir Dis 132:490–499, 1985.
65. Tennenberg SD, Jacobs MP, Solomkin JS, et al: Complement-mediated neutrophil activation in sepsis- and trauma-related adult respiratory distress syndrome. Arch Surg 122:26–31, 1987.
66. Fantone JC, Feltner DE, Brieland JK, et al: Phagocytic cell-derived inflammatory mediators and lung disease. Chest 91:428–429, 1987.
67. Hechtman HB, Weisel RD, Vito L, et al: Role of humoral mediators in adult respiratory distress syndrome. Chest 86:623–626, 1984.
68. Heffner JE, Sahn SA, Repine JE: The role of platelets in the adult respiratory distress syndrome. Am Rev Respir Dis 135:482–486, 1987.
69. Martin TR, Pistorese BP, Hudson LD, et al: The function of lung and blood neutrophils in patients with the adult respiratory distress syndrome. Am Rev Respir Dis 144:254–262, 1991.
70. Mojarad M, Hamasaki Y, Said SI: Platelet-activating factor increases pulmonary microvascular permeability and induces pulmonary edema. Clin Respir Physiol 19:253, 1983.
71. Braquet P, Touqui L, Shen T, et al: Perspectives in platelet activating factor research. Pharmacol Rev 39:97–145, 1987.
72. Dinarello CA: Interleukin-1 and the pathogenesis of the acute phase response. N Engl J Med 311:1413–1418, 1984.
73. Stephens K, Ishizika A, Larrick J, et al: Tumor necrosis factor causes increased pulmonary permeability and edema. Am Rev Respir Dis 137:1364–1370, 1988.
74. Tracey K, Beutler B, Lowry S, et al: Shock and tissue injury induced by recombinant human cachectin. Science 234:470–474, 1986.
75. Demling RH: Current concepts on the adult respiratory distress syndrome. Circ Shock 30:297–309, 1990.
76. Pepe PE, Culver BH: Independently measured oxygen consumption during reduction of oxygen delivery by positive end-expiratory pressure. Am Rev Respir Dis 132:788–792, 1985.
77. Ronco JJ, Phang PT, Walley KR, et al: Oxygen consumption is independent of changes in oxygen delivery in severe adult respiratory distress syndrome. Am Rev Respir Dis 143:1267–1273, 1991.
78. Marcy TW, Marini JJ: Inverse ratio ventilation in ARDS. Chest 100:494–504, 1991.
79. Weisman IM, Rinaldo JE, Rogers RM, et al: Intermittent mandatory ventilation. Am Rev Respir Dis 127:641–650, 1983.
80. Boysen PG, McGough E: Pressure-control and pressure-support ventilation: Flow patterns, inspiratory time and gas distribution. Respir Care 33:126–130, 1988.
81. Pepe PE, Hudson LD, Carrico CJ: Early application of PEEP in patients at risk for the adult respiratory distress syndrome. N Engl J Med 311:281–283, 1984.
82. Craig KC, Pierson DJ, Carrico CJ: The clinical application of PEEP in the adult respiratory distress syndrome. Respir Care 30:184–202, 1985.
83. Tharratt RS, Allen RP, Albertson TE: Pressure controlled inverse ratio ventilation in severe adult respiratory failure. Chest 94:755–760, 1988.
84. Gurevitch MJ, Van Dyke J, Young ES, et al: Improved oxygenation and lower peak airway pressure in severe adult respiratory distress syndrome: Treatment with inverse ratio ventilation. Chest 89:211–213, 1986.
85. Zack MB, Pontippidan H, Kazemi H: The effects of lateral positions on gas exchange in pulmonary disease. Am Rev Respir Dis 110:49–51, 1974.
86. Schmitz TM: The semi-prone position in ARDS: Five case studies. Crit Care Nurs 11:22–33, 1991.
87. Lakshminarayan S, Hudson LD: Pulmonary function following the adult respiratory distress syndrome. Chest 74:489–490, 1978.
88. Klein JJ, van Haeringen JR, Sluiter HJ, et al: Pulmonary function after recovery from the adult respiratory distress syndrome. Chest 69:350–355, 1976.
89. Yahav J, Lieberman P, Molho M: Pulmonary function following the adult respiratory distress syndrome. Chest 74:247–250, 1978.
90. Rotman HH, Lavell TF, Dimcheff DG, et al: Long-term physiologic consequences of the adult respiratory distress syndrome. Chest 72:190–192, 1977.
91. Elliott CG, Morris AH, Cengiz M: Pulmonary function and exercise gas exchange in survivors of adult respiratory distress syndrome. Am Rev Respir Dis 123:492–495, 1982.
92. Tahvanainen J, Salmenpera M, Nikki P: Extubation criteria after weaning from intermittent mandatory ventilation and continuous positive airway pressure. Crit Care Med 11:702–704, 1983.
93. Cardona VD: Trauma Reference Manual. Bowie, MD, Brady Communications, 1985.
94. Fabian TC, Cicala RS, Croce MA, et al: A prospective evaluation of myocardial contusion: Correction of significant arrhythmias and cardiac output with CPK-MB measurements. J Trauma 31(5):653–660, 1991.
95. McLean RF, Devitt JH, Dubbin J: Incidence of abnormal RNA studies and dysrhythmias in patient with blunt chest trauma. J Trauma 31(7):968–970, 1991.
96. Chyun D: Myocardial contusion: The hidden menace in chest trauma. AJN 11:1459–1462, 1987.
97. Sommers MS: Nursing care of patients with blunt cardiac trauma. Crit Care Nurs 5(6):58–66, 1985.
98. Rodriquez A, Turney SZ: Blunt injuries of the heart and pericardium. In Turney SZ, Rodriquez A, Cowley RA (eds): Management of Cardiothoracic Trauma. Baltimore, Williams & Wilkins, 1990.
99. Kumar SA, Puri VN, Mettal VK, et al: Myocardial contusion following nonfatal chest trauma. J Trauma 23:327–331, 1983.
100. King RM, Mucha P Jr, Seward JB, et al: Cardiac contusion: A new diagnostic approach utilizing two-dimensional echocardiography. J Trauma 23:610–614, 1983.
101. Frazee RC, Mucha P Jr, Farnell MB, et al: Objective evaluation of blunt cardiac trauma. J Trauma 26:510–520, 1986.
102. Fabian TC, Mangiante EC, Pattern CR, et al: Myocardial contusion in blunt trauma: Clinical characteristics, means of diagnosis, and implications in patient management. J Trauma 28:50–57, 1988.
103. Miller FB, Shumate CR, Richardson D: Myocardial contusion: When can the diagnosis be eliminated? Arch Surg 124:805–808, 1989.
104. Mooney R, Niemann JT, Bessen HA, et al: Conventional and right precordial ECGs, creatine kinase, and radionuclide angiography in post-traumatic ventricular dysfunction. Ann Emerg Med 17:890–894, 1988.
105. Turney SZ, Rodriquez A: Injuries to the great thoracic vessels. In Turney SZ, Rodriquez A, Cowley RA (eds): Management of Cardiothoracic Trauma. Baltimore, Williams & Wilkins, 1990.
106. Cowley RA, Turney SZ, Hankins JR, et al: Rupture of thoracic aorta caused by blunt trauma. J Thorac Cardiovasc Surg 100:652–661, 1990.
107. Gundry SR, Burney RE, MacKenzie JR, et al: Assessment of mediastinal widening associated with traumatic rupture of the aorta. J Trauma 23:293–299, 1983.
108. Mattox KL: Evolving concepts in the management of decelerative injury to the thoracic aorta. In Najarian JS, Delaney JP (eds): Trauma and Critical Care Surgery. Chicago, Year Book Medical Publishers, 1987.
109. Selivanov V, Sheldon GF: Principles of monitoring the injured patient. In Gardner B, Shaftan G (eds): Reference to Surgical Emergencies. Philadelphia, JB Lippincott, 1986.

110. Holcroft JW, Boyle WA: Assessment and treatment of cardiopulmonary dysfunction. In Blaisdell F, Trunkey D (eds): Cervicothoracic Trauma. New York, Thieme, 1986.
111. Benumof JL: Anesthesia for Thoracic Surgery. Philadelphia, WB Saunders Co, 1987.
112. Dodds CP, Hillman KM: Management of massive air leak with asynchronous independent lung ventilation. Intensive Care Med 8:287–290, 1982.
113. Kirby RR: The use and misuse of mechanical ventilators. In Najarian JS, Delaney JP (eds): Trauma and Critical Care Surgery. Chicago, Year Book Medical Publishers, 1987.
114. Carlon GC, Guy YG, Ray C: Comparison of high-frequency jet ventilation and volume-cycled ventilation. Chest 86:194–197, 1984.
115. Sjostrand UH, Herrera-Hoyos JO, Smith BB: New anesthetic techniques for intrathoracic operations. In Kittle C (ed): Current Controversies in Thoracic Surgery. Philadelphia, WB Saunders Co, 1986.
116. Guntupalli K, Sladen A, Klain M: High-frequency jet ventilation and tracheobronchial suctioning. Crit Care Med 12:791–792, 1984.
117. Warren TE, Howell C: High-frequency jet ventilation: A nursing perspective. Heart Lung 12:432–437, 1983.
118. Gruden M: High-frequency ventilation: An overview. Crit Care Nurs 5:36–40, 1985.
119. Loder BJ, Guy Y, Carlon GC: Critical care nurse and high-frequency ventilation. Crit Care Med 12:798–799, 1984.
120. Mendel JG, Khan FA: Psychological aspects of weaning from mechanical ventilation. Psychosomatics 21:465–471, 1980.
121. Norton LC, Neureuter A: Weaning the long-term ventilator-dependent patient: Common problems and management. Crit Care Nurs 9(1):42–52, 1989.
122. Henneman EA: The art and science of weaning from mechanical ventilation. Focus Crit Care 18(6):490–501, 1991.
123. Knebel AR: Weaning from mechanical ventilation: Current controversies. Heart Lung 20(4):321–334, 1991.
124. MacKenzie CF, Ciesla N, Imle PC, et al: Chest Physiotherapy in the Intensive Care Unit. Baltimore, Williams & Wilkins, 1981.
125. Tyler ML: Complications of positioning and chest physiotherapy. Respir Care 27:458–466, 1982.
126. Parsons LC, Shogan JS: The effects of endotracheal tube suctioning/manual hyperventilation procedure on patients with severe closed head injuries. Heart Lung 13(4):372–380, 1984.
127. Harris RB, Hyman RB: Clean vs sterile tracheotomy: Care and level of pulmonary infection. Nurs Res 33(2):80–85, 1984.
128. Buchanan LM, Baum NM: The effect of hyperinflation, inspiratory hold, and oxygenation on cardiopulmonary status during suctioning in a lung-injured model. Heart Lung 15(2):127–134, 1986.
129. Bostick J, Wendelgass ST: Normal saline instillation as part of the suctioning procedure: Effects on PaO_2 and amount of secretions. Heart Lung 16(5):532–538, 1987.
130. Preusser BA, Stone KS, Gonyon DS, et al: Effects of two methods of preoxygenation on mean arterial pressure, cardiac output, peak airway pressure, and postsuctioning hypoxemia. Heart Lung 17(3):290–299, 1988.
131. Stone KS, Vorst EC, Lanham B, et al: Effects of lung hyperinflation on mean arterial pressure and postsuctioning hypoxemia. Heart Lung 18(4):377–390, 1989.
132. Rudy EB, Turner BS, Baum M, et al: Endotracheal suctioning in adults with head injury. Heart Lung 20(6):667–674, 1991.
133. Lookinland S and Appel PL: Hemodynamic and oxygen transport changes following endotracheal suctioning in trauma patients. Nurs Res 40:133–138, 1991.
134. Barnes CA, Kirchhoff KT: Minimizing hypoxemia due to endotracheal suctioning: A review of the literature. Heart Lung 15(2):164–178, 1986.
135. Bradley RB: Adult respiratory distress syndrome. Focus Crit Care 14(5):48–59, 1987.
136. Robichaud AM: Alteration in gas exchange related to body positioning. Crit Care Nurs 10(1):56–58, 1990.
137. Norton LC, Conforti CG: The effects of body position on oxygenation. Heart Lung 14:45–51, 1985.
138. Duncan C, Erikson R: Pressures associated with chest tube stripping. Heart Lung 11:166–171, 1982.
139. Splaingard ML, Frates RC, Harrison GM, et al: Home positive-pressure ventilation: Twenty years' experience. Chest 84:376–382, 1983.
140. Nacht A, Kahn RC, Miller SM: Adult respiratory distress syndrome and its management. In Capan LM, Miller SM, Turndorf, H (eds): Trauma Anesthesia and Intensive Care. Philadelphia, JB Lippincott, 1991.
141. Goldstone J, Moxham J: Weaning from mechanical ventilation. Thorax 46:56–62, 1991.
142. Mier-Jedrzejowicz A, Brophy C, Green M, et al: Respiratory muscle weakness during upper respiratory tract infections. Am Rev Respir Dis 138:5–7, 1988.
143. Grossbach-Landis I: Successful weaning of ventilator-dependent patients. Top Clin Nurs 2:45–65, 1980.
144. Corson J, Grant J, Moulton D, et al: Use of biofeedback in weaning paralyzed patients from respirators. Chest 76:543–545, 1979.
145. LaRiccia P, Katz R, Peters J, et al: Biofeedback and hypnosis in weaning from mechanical ventilators. Chest 87:267–269, 1985.
146. Holliday J, Hyers T: The reduction of weaning time from mechanical ventilation using tidal volume and relaxation biofeedback. Am Rev Respir Dis 141:1214–1220, 1990.
147. Tammelin BR: Long-term sequelae of blunt respiratory trauma. Trauma Q 2:71–77, 1986.
148. Davidson IA, Bargh W, Cruickshank AN, et al: Crush injuries of the chest. Thorax 24:563–567, 1969.
149. Hanning CO, Ledingham E, Ledingham I: Late respiratory sequelae of blunt chest injury: A preliminary report. Thorax 36:204–207, 1981.
150. Landercasper J, Cogbill TH, Lindesmith LA: Long-term disability after flail chest injury. J Trauma 24:410–414, 1984.
151. Hietpas BG, Roth RD, Jensen WM: Huff coughing and airway patency. Respir Care 24:710–712, 1979.
152. Ciesla N: Postural drainage, positioning, and breathing exercise. In MacKenzie CF, Ciesla N, Imle PC, et al (eds): Chest Physiotherapy in the Intensive Care Unit. Baltimore, Williams & Wilkins, 1981.
153. Lederer DH, Van de Water JM, Indech RB: Which deep breathing device should the postoperative patient use? Chest 77:610–613, 1980.
154. Craven JL, Evans GA, Davenport PJ, et al: The evaluation of the incentive spirometer in the management of postoperative pulmonary complications. Br J Surg 61:793, 1974.
155. Iverson LI, Ecker RR, Fow HE: A comparative study of IPPV, the incentive spirometer, and blow bottles. Ann Thorac Surg 25:197–200, 1978.

20

ABDOMINAL INJURIES

PAULA J. BASTNAGEL MASON

Trauma is the leading cause of death in the first three decades of life. In 1973, blunt abdominal injuries accounted for approximately 1 per cent of all trauma-related hospital admissions.[1] In 1991, Trunkey and associates noted that abdominal trauma accounted for 13 to 15 per cent of trauma deaths.[2] Penetrating injuries account for nearly 25 per cent of all traumatic injury in the United States. Mortality rates reported for abdominal trauma have been less than 5 per cent for penetrating injury and between 10 and 30 per cent for blunt injury.[1] As one would expect, single system versus multisystem trauma significantly affects the morbidity and mortality associated with abdominal injury. Numerous authors have noted the rise in mortality based on the length of time from initial injury to treatment and the number of systems involved.[1–4] Intra-abdominal trauma is seldom a single organ injury or single system injury; therefore, patients experience the concomitant rise in morbidity and mortality.

There are two classifications of abdominal trauma: blunt and penetrating. Blunt trauma represents the greatest diagnostic challenge, since the specific injury to the abdomen remains ill-defined 60 per cent of the time until a laparotomy is performed. Multiple organ involvement or central nervous system depression due to injury or drug effect presents such a complex series of symptoms or so clouds normal assessment parameters that definitive diagnosis becomes more difficult. Still, the presence of abdominal tenderness or guarding, circulatory instability, a lumbar spine injury, a pelvic fracture, retroperitoneal or intraperitoneal air, and unilateral loss of the psoas shadow on radiographical examination should raise the question of visceral damage.

Penetrating injuries occur from a number of sources, such as gunshot, stabbing, or impalement. The signs and symptoms cover a spectrum from slight cardiovascular abnormality to asystole yet may be associated with minimal external evidence of trauma. For example, the ricochet effect of a bullet upon entering the abdominal cavity renders multiple organs at risk for injury.

Abdominal trauma challenges even the most experienced nurse. The manifestation of abdominal injury is often subtle, requiring continual assessment and care modification as the patient progresses from the initial injury phase through the rehabilitation cycle. Autopsy studies repeatedly confirm that abdominal injury is the most frequent cause of readily preventable traumatic death.[3] The nurse, as the most constant care provider, is in the best position to assess, define, and reassess abdominal problems early. A high index of suspicion and an organized assessment approach are the keys to early diagnosis and intervention.

THE ABDOMEN: ANATOMY

The abdomen is formally thought of as containing the structures bordered by the diaphragm caudally, the pelvis inferiorly, the vertebral column posteriorly, and the abdominal and iliac muscles anteriorly (Fig. 20–1). For the purposes of discussion of abdominal trauma, the esophagus, which passes through the diaphragm and connects with the stomach, has been added to this chapter.

The peritoneal cavity contains the stomach, small intestine, liver, gallbladder, spleen, transverse colon, sigmoid colon, upper third of the rectum, and, in women, the uterus. Retroperitoneal structures include part of the duodenum, ascending colon, descending colon, kidneys, pancreas, and major vessels.

For purposes of examination, the abdomen is divided into four quadrants: right upper quadrant (RUQ), left upper quadrant (LUQ), right lower quadrant (RLQ), and left lower quadrant (LLQ) (Fig. 20–2). General characteristics of each major organ are highlighted.

Esophagus

This hollow, muscular tube traverses the posterior mediastinum of the thorax through the esophageal hiatus in the central tendon of the diaphragm to join the stomach at the level of the tenth thoracic vertebra. The posterior surface of the intra-abdominal esophagus overlies the aorta, and the anterior surface is covered by peritoneum. The anterior and posterior vagus nerves pass through the esophageal hiatus. There are three areas of narrowing that predispose the esophagus to injury: at the cricoid cartilage, at the arch of the aorta, and as it passes through the diaphragm. The esophageal wall lacks a serosal layer, which may affect the integrity of anastomoses, increasing the chance for leaking postoperatively. In all other respects, it maintains the characteristics of the gastrointestinal tract.

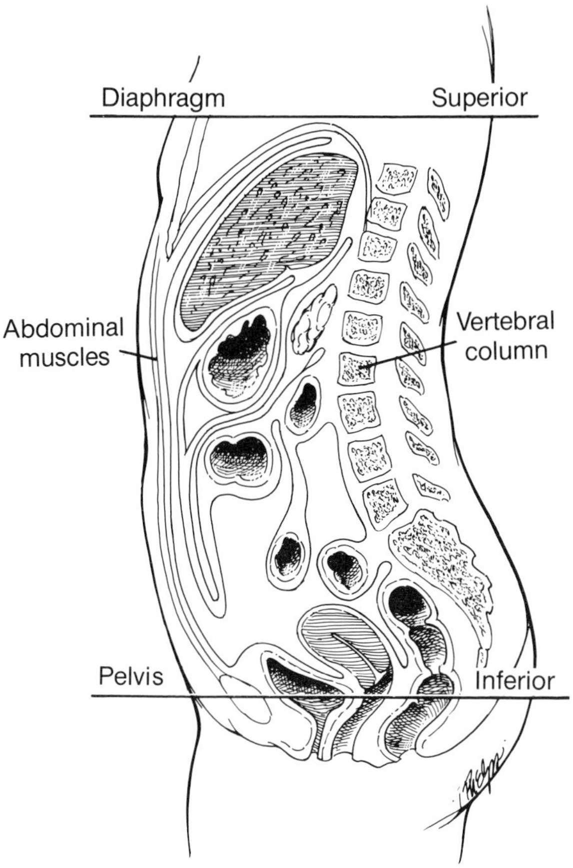

Figure 20–1. The abdominal boundaries.

Diaphragm

The diaphragm is a musculotendinous dome-shaped structure attached posteriorly to the first, second, and third lumbar vertebrae, anteriorly to the lower sternum, and laterally to the costal margins dividing the thoracic and abdominal regions. There are three foramina. The aorta passes through at the T12 level, the esophagus passes through at the T10 level, and the vena cava foramen is at T8. The phrenic nerve, which innervates the diaphragm, passes through the thorax along the posterolateral aspect of the pericardium on both sides and divides into anterior and posterior branches (Fig. 20–3).

Stomach

The stomach joins the esophagus 3 cm below the diaphragm and is located in the left upper quadrant. Suspended by the gastrohepatic ligament superiorly, the gastrocolic ligament inferiorly, and the gastrosplenic ligament laterally, the stomach resides within the peritoneal cavity. It is divided into the cardia, fundus, body, and pyloric antrum (Fig. 20–4). The four-layer stomach wall contains glands that secrete mucus in the cardia; hydrochloric acid (HCl), intrinsic factor, pepsinogen (type I), and serotonin in the fundus and body; and mucus and pepsinogen II in the antrum.[5] The release of these gastric contents into the peritoneal cavity is responsible for the symptoms exhibited following perforating gastric

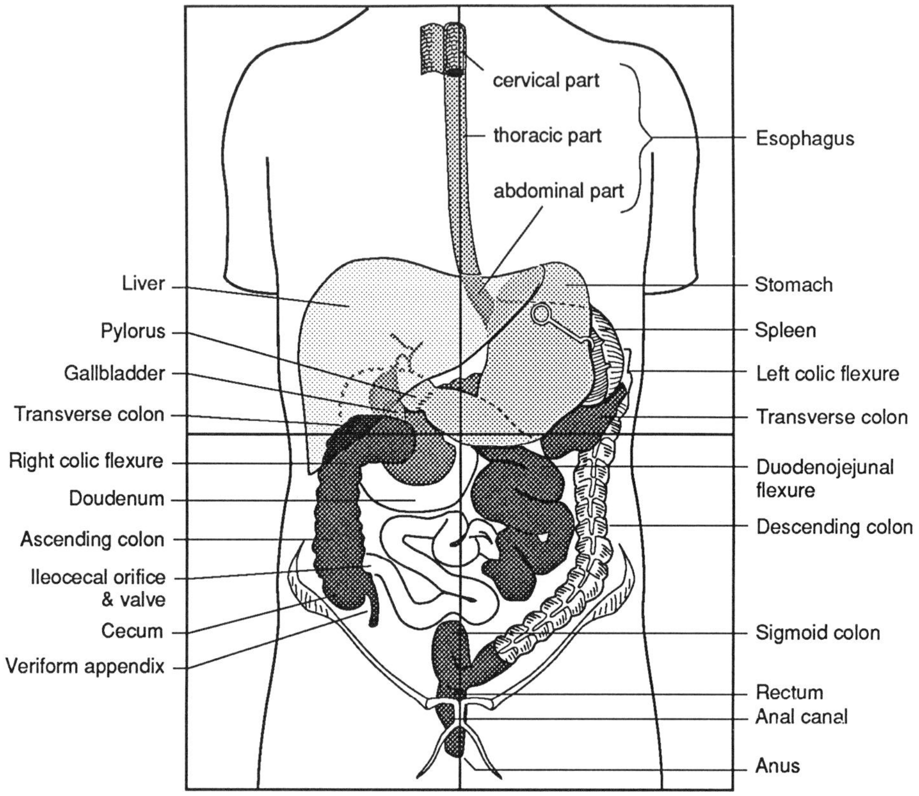

Right Upper Quadrant
Liver and gallbladder
Pylorus
Duodenum
Head of pancreas
Right adrenal gland
Portion of right kidney
Hepatic flexure of colon
Portions of ascending and transverse colon

Left Upper Quadrant
Left lobe of liver
Spleen
Stomach
Body of pancreas
Left adrenal gland
Portion of left kidney
Splenic flexure of colon
Portions of transverse and descending colon

Right Lower Quadrant
Lower pole of right kidney
Cecum and appendix
Portion of ascending colon
Bladder (if distended)
Ovary and salpinx
Uterus (if enlarged)
Right spermatic cord
Right ureter

Left Lower Quadrant
Lower pole of left kidney
Sigmoid colon
Portion of descending colon
Bladder (if distended)
Ovary and salpinx
Uterus (if enlarged)
Left spermatic cord
Left ureter

Loops of small bowel are found in all quadrants

Figure 20–2. Contents of the four abdominal quadrants. (Adapted from GI Series—Physical Examination of the Abdomen. Richmond, Virginia, AH Robins Inc, 1975, p 6.)

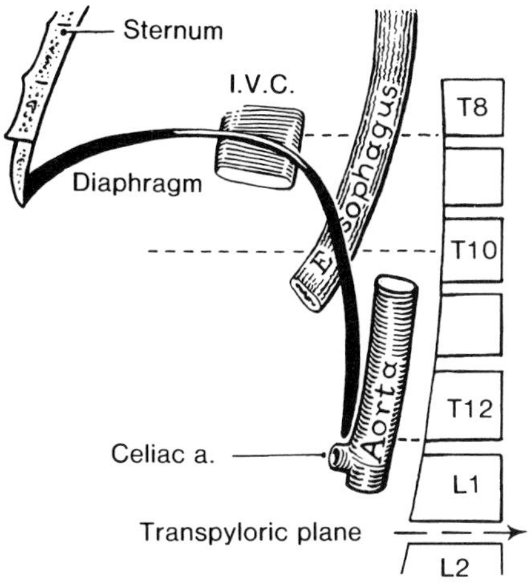

Diagram showing the three openings in the diaphragm and their vertebral levels. Observe that the more superior the vertebral level, the more anterior is the opening in the diaphragm. The vertebral levels are **T8**, **T10**, **and T12** for the inferior vena cava, esophagus, and aorta, respectively.

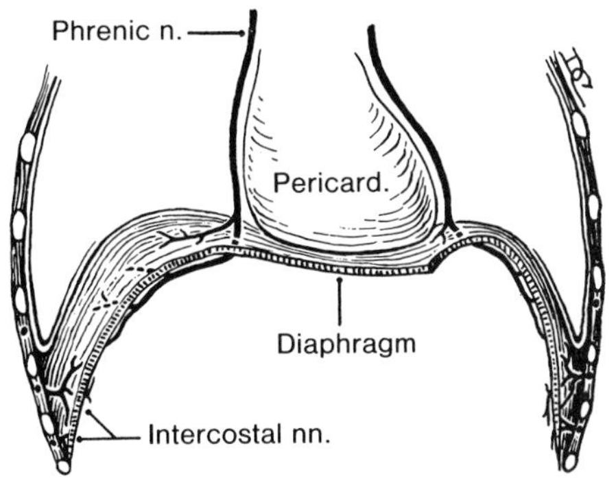

Diagram illustrating the nerve supply to the diaphragm. Note that each phrenic nerve (C3, C4, and C5) is the sole motor nerve to its own half of the diaphragm. It is also sensory to the greater part of its own half of the diaphragm, including the pleura on the thoracic surface and the peritoneum on the abdominal surface. Observe that the inferior intercostal nerves are sensory to the peripheral part of the diaphragm.

Figure 20–3. The diaphragm: Foramina and phrenic innervation. (From Moore K: Clinically Oriented Anatomy. 2nd ed. Baltimore, Williams & Wilkins, 1985, p 272, with permission.)

injury. These same gastric secretions cause stress ulcerations in the stomach.

There is a rich blood supply to the stomach, including the left and right gastric, the left and right gastroepiploic, and the short gastric arteries (Fig. 20–5). Venous drainage occurs through the portal vein for the lesser curvature and the right and left gastroepiploic and short gastric veins for the greater curvature, which also drains into the portal vein.

Gastric emptying is facilitated by peristaltic movement from the antrum, stimulated by stretch receptors. An inhibiting function is controlled in the duodenum.

Omentum

The omentum is a double layer of peritoneum and adipose tissue extending from the greater curvature of the stomach to adjacent abdominal organs. The right and left gastroepiploic arteries supply the omentum. Rupture of these arteries during trauma results in peritoneal irritation or signs of intraperitoneal bleeding.

Liver

The liver is the largest intra-abdominal organ. It is divided into two lobes; the right and left lobes are separated by fissures on the inferior surface. Between these two lobes is the porta hepatis, where veins, arteries, nerves, and lymphatic vessels enter or leave the liver.

Connective tissue fibrous strands partition the liver mass into irregular units termed *lobules*. The hepatic triad, consisting of branches of the hepatic artery, portal vein, and a small bile duct, lies between the lobules (Fig. 20–6).

Approximately three-fourths of the blood to hepatic cells is delivered by the portal vein, which carries a rich supply of nutrients after draining the entire digestive system. The rest is rich in oxygen and enters through the hepatic artery. In a central location within each lobule sits the central vein, which collects the mixture of blood and channels it to sublobular veins, which empty into the hepatic vein and then into the inferior vena cava. This rich vascular supply compromises hemodynamic stability after trauma and complicates surgical repair. Uncontrolled hemorrhage is the primary cause of early mortality following liver trauma.

Liver cells produce bile, which is essential to the digestion of fats. Bile flows from the hepatic cells into bile canaliculi between the cells toward the periphery of the lobule and empties into the interlobular bile ducts of the hepatic triad. The interlobular ducts form the right hepatic duct, which drains the right lobe of the liver, and the left hepatic duct, which drains the left lobe. The ducts join, forming the common hepatic duct, which allows bile to flow into the gallbladder. The gallbladder lies on the inferior surface of

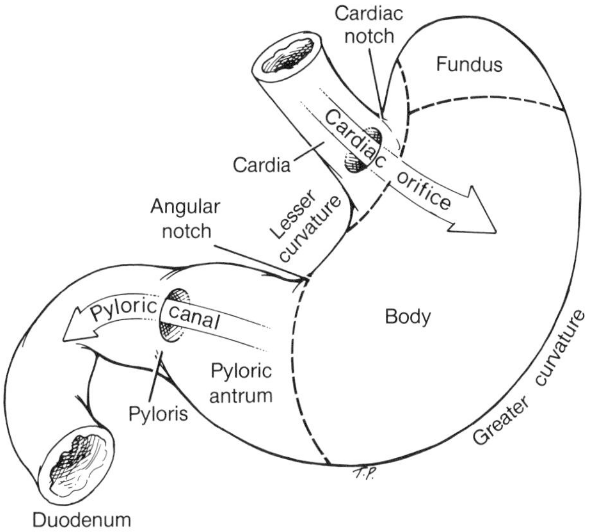

Figure 20–4. The stomach. Four major divisions.

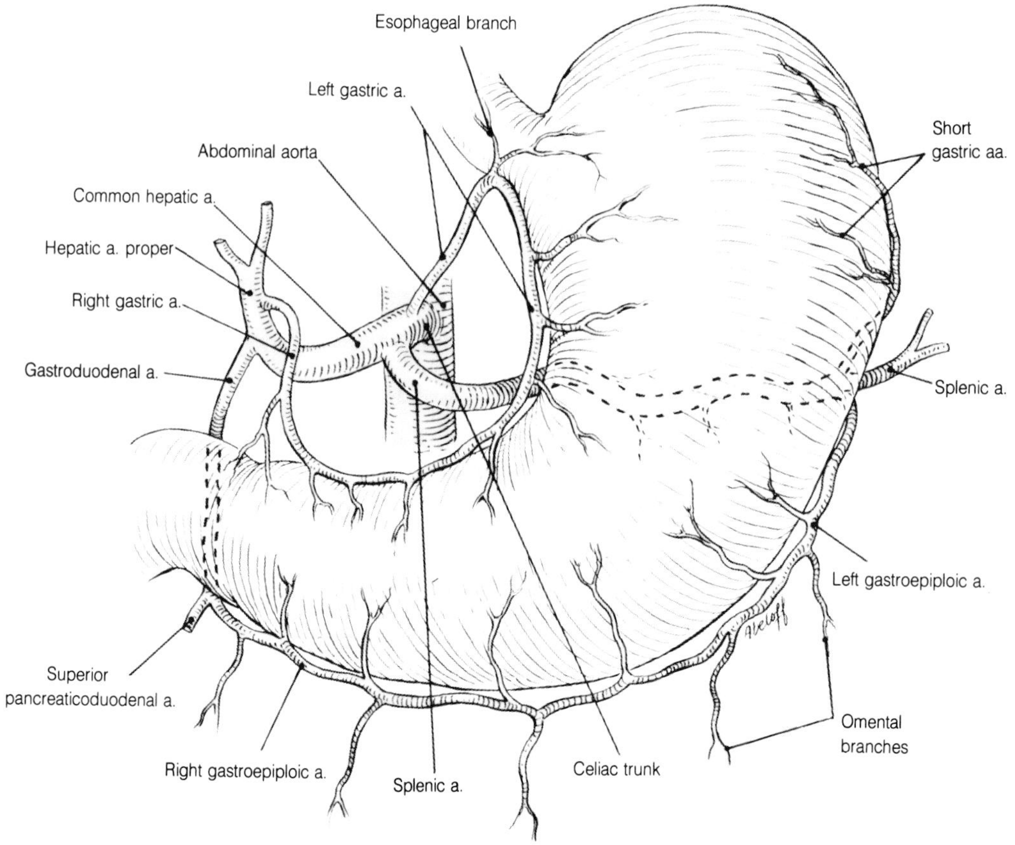

Figure 20–5. The stomach. The blood supply. (Copyright 1985. Urban & Schwarzenberg, Baltimore-Munich. Reproduced with permission from Anatomy as a Basis for Clinical Medicine. Edited by Christopher Hall-Craggs. All rights reserved.)

the liver. Its duct, the cystic duct, meets with the hepatic duct to form the common bile duct, which drains into the duodenum.

Spleen

The spleen is an elongated ovoid body located in the left upper quadrant of the abdomen. It lies beneath the diaphragm, to the left of the stomach, and in immediate proximity to the tail of the pancreas, colon, and left kidney. It is in close proximity to ribs 7 through 10, which makes it vulnerable to injury when ribs are fractured.

Ligamentous attachments include the splenophrenic ligament posteriorly, the gastrosplenic ligament, and the splenocolic ligament. The spleen's blood supply is from the splenic artery, which enters at the hilum and divides into five or six branches before entering splenic pulp. The splenic vein forms outside the hilum and courses along the dorsal pancreatic surface to join the superior mesenteric vein, turning into the portal vein (Fig. 20–7). The vascular nature of the spleen makes it a ready source for profuse bleeding into the peritoneal cavity. Indeed, delayed hemorrhage may occur up to months following an initial splenic injury.[3, 6]

The splenic capsule, 1 to 2 mm thick, encloses the splenic pulp. Lymphoid tissue lies throughout the pulp and is responsible for filtration. The blood supply to the pulp is from arterioles off a central artery. The blood collects in a venous sinus, then moves to trabecular veins coursing to the main splenic veins, and finally to the portal circulation. Arterial blood travels to venous sinuses through splenic cords (connective tissue between sinuses) and "sieves" red cells, destroying many in the process. Five per cent of the body's

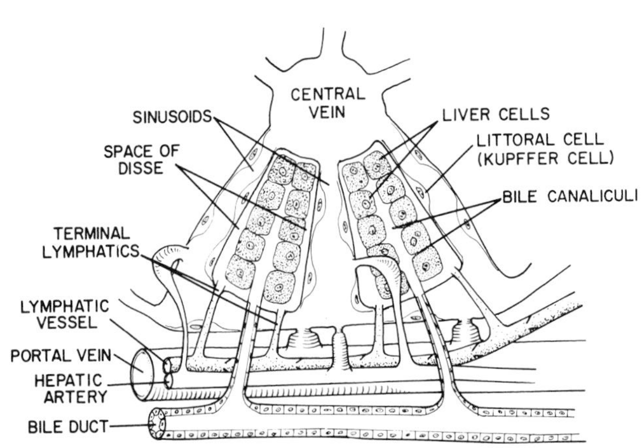

Figure 20–6. Basic structure of a liver lobule showing the hepatic cellular plates, the blood vessels, the bile-collecting system, and the lymph flow system composed of the spaces of Disse and the interlobular lymphatics. (Reprinted from Guyton AC, Taylor AE, Granger HJ [as modified from Elias]: Circulatory Physiology II: Dynamics of Body Fluids. Philadelphia, WB Saunders Co, 1975, p 220, with permission.)

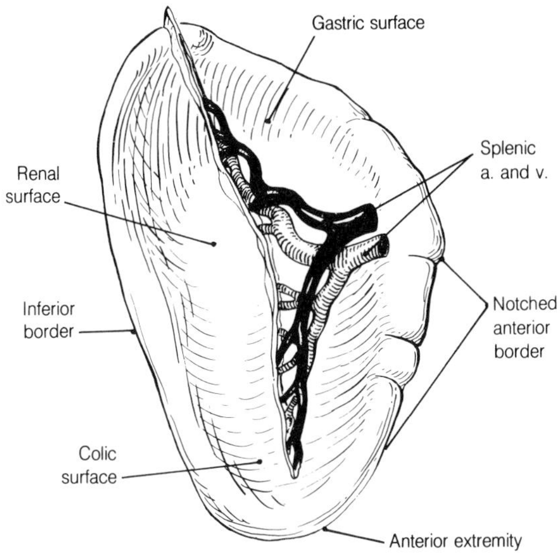

Figure 20–7. The spleen. Vascular supply. (Copyright 1985. Urban & Schwarzenberg, Baltimore-Munich. Reproduced with permission from Anatomy as a Basis for Clinical Medicine. Edited by Christopher Hall-Craggs. All rights reserved.)

total blood flow passes through the spleen each minute, 90 per cent of which participates in this filtering process.[7,8] The spleen's sieving process promotes it as a primary defense organ to remove poorly opsonized bacteria and particulate antigens.

Pancreas

The pancreas lies at the level of the first lumbar vertebra against the posterior abdominal wall. It extends from the curve of the duodenum to the hilum of the spleen. Blunt trauma forcing the pancreas against the vertebral column may rupture the pancreas. The pancreas is divided into lobules that empty into the main pancreatic duct, which passes through the tail, body, neck (uncinate process), and head of the pancreas, emptying into the duodenum at the ampulla of Vater in conjunction with the common bile duct. An accessory duct empties into the duodenum from the head of the pancreas. Rupture of the pancreas frequently tears its ductal system, allowing pancreatic juice (rich in digestive enzymes) to invade pancreatic tissue.

Arterial supply to the head of the pancreas is through the superior and inferior pancreaticoduodenal arteries. The remainder is supplied by the splenic artery. Venous drainage from the body and tail of the pancreas is through the splenic vein to the portal vein; the head empties directly into the portal vein.

Small Intestine

The 21 to 23 feet of small intestine are divided into duodenum, jejunum, and ileum (Fig. 20–8). The major functions are digestion of food and absorption of nutrients and water for the body.

Duodenum

The duodenum is the first part of the small intestine and is a C-shaped loop approximately 25 cm long, molded around the head of the pancreas (Fig. 20–9). Beginning at the pyloric valve junction, the duodenum receives the highly acidic chyme from the stomach as well as fluids, enzymes, and electrolytes from the biliary and pancreatic ducts.

The duodenum is divided into four parts, with only the first portion within the peritoneal cavity. With the exception of the small segment attached to the stomach, the duodenum is anchored to the posterior abdominal wall. Rapid deceleration injuries may lead to rupture between the anchored and free segments of the duodenum. Three-quarters of this organ lies over the vertebral column, which renders it vulnerable to compression injuries (Fig. 20–10).

Blood supply to the duodenum is shared with the pancreas through the superior and inferior pancreaticoduodenal artery. This makes postinjury removal of the entire pancreas impossible without devascularizing the duodenum.

Jejunum and Ileum

From the duodenal jejunal flexure to the ileocecal junction, the jejunum and ileum are responsible for nutrient absorption and fluid and electrolyte shifts. Most of the jejunum lies in the umbilical region of the abdomen, and the ileum is in the hypogastric and pelvic regions. This expansive placement makes the small intestine vulnerable to seat belt injury (from lap belts) as the bowel is crushed between vertebrae and a solid object such as a steering wheel.

Blood supply is from the superior mesenteric artery. Venous drainage is to the portal vein via the superior mesenteric vein. Peristalsis continues through the jejunum and ileum.

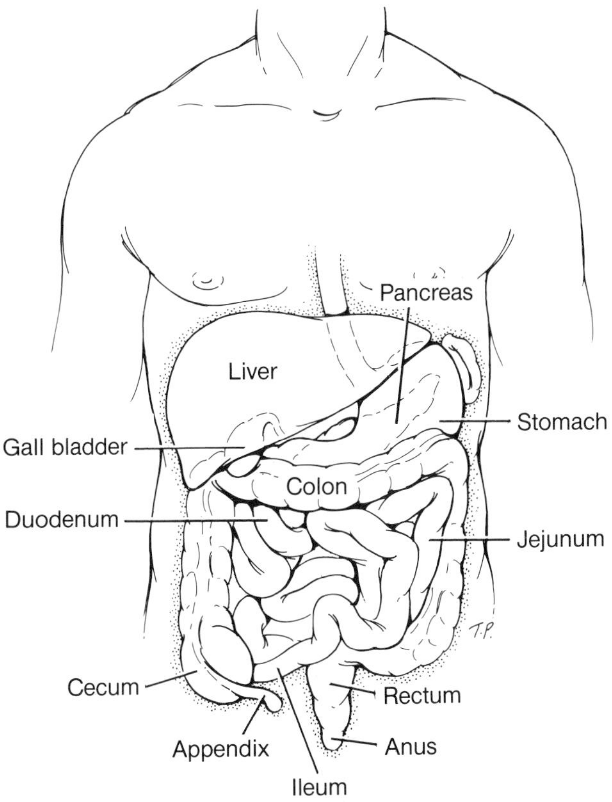

Figure 20–8. The small intestine. Duodenum, jejunum, and ilium in relation to other abdominal structures.

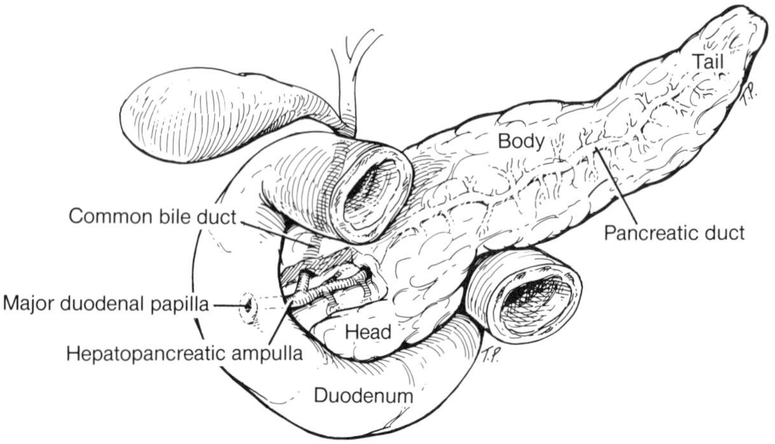

Figure 20–9. Duodenal location in relation to the pancreas.

Most absorption takes place in the jejunum, except for bile salts and vitamin B_{12}, which are absorbed in the terminal ileum. Fluid shifts from gastrointestinal lumen to blood in the duodenum and jejunum, with reabsorption of all but 1/2 to 1 liter of fluid passed to the large intestines.

Large Intestine

The colon, rectum, and anal canal constitute the large intestine. The colon is divided into ascending, transverse, descending, and sigmoid segments (Fig. 20–11). The cecum and ascending colon are continuous from the ileum and rise to the undersurface of the right lobe of the liver, bending to the left at the hepatic flexure and becoming the transverse segment. This segment continues across to the splenic flexure (above the left kidney) and then turns downward to become the descending colon. The sigmoid colon courses from the left iliac fossa to the pelvic cavity, becoming the rectum and terminating at the anal canal. The transverse colon, sigmoid colon, and part of the ascending and descending colon are covered by peritoneum. Blood supply to the colon and rectum is predominantly from the superior and inferior mesenteric arteries arising from the abdominal aorta. Venous drainage of the large intestine is through the portal vein to sinusoids in the liver.

Abdominal Vascular System

Arterial Supply

The descending aorta passes through the diaphragm at the T12, L1 level to become the abdominal aorta. At the L4 level, the aorta bifurcates into the two common iliac arteries. It further divides into external and internal iliac arteries; finally, the external iliac becomes the common femoral artery (Fig. 20–12).

Major branches of the aorta include the celiac axis at the T12 level, which divides into the left gastric artery, splenic artery, and common hepatic artery; the superior mesenteric

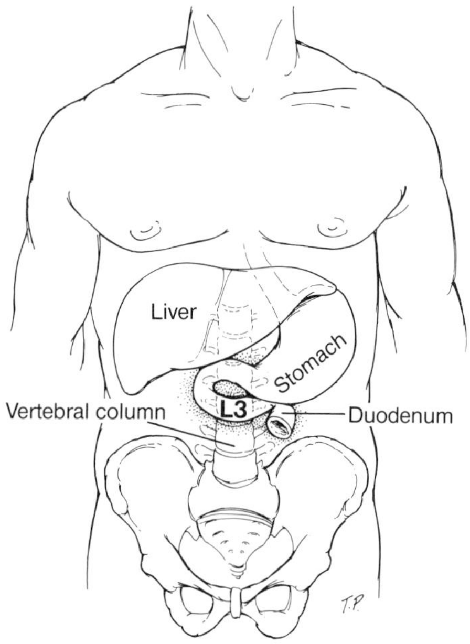

Figure 20–10. Duodenal location in relation to the vertebral column.

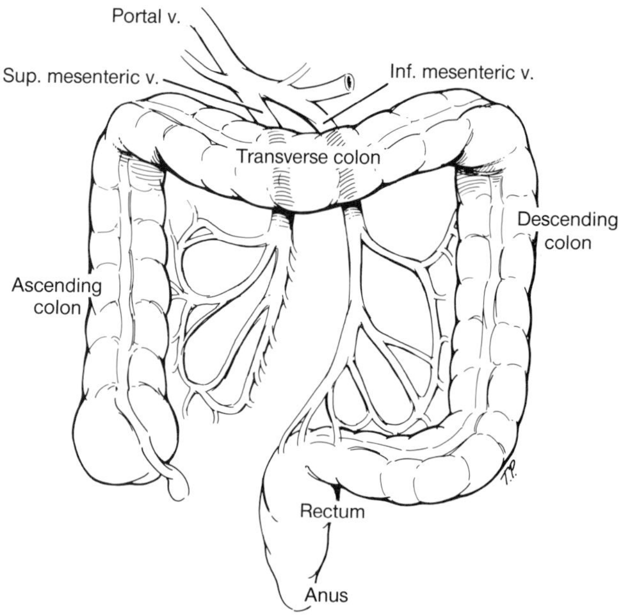

Figure 20–11. Large intestine and rectum.

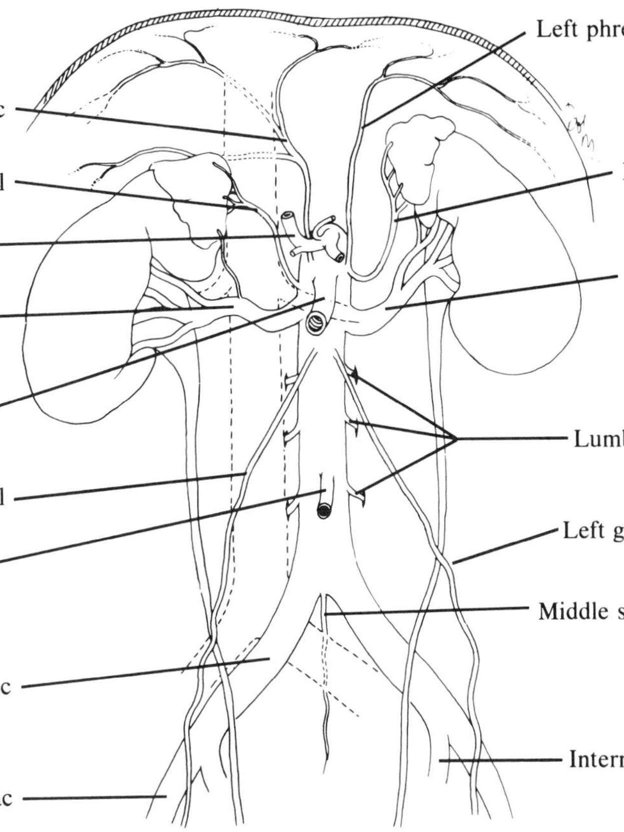

Figure 20–12. Abdominal aorta and branches. (Reprinted with permission from WF Blaisdell, D Trunkey, Abdominal Trauma, Vol 1. New York, Thieme Medical Publishers, 1982.)

artery at the L1 level, dividing later into the middle colic artery and inferior pancreaticoduodenal artery; the renal arteries at the L2 level, which supply the kidneys directly; and the inferior mesenteric artery at the L3–4 level, dividing into the left colic artery and the superior hemorrhoidal artery. Certain of the arteries further subdivide for additional arterial blood supply to abdominal tissue. (See the sections on specific organs for further information.) It is easy to see how any injury to the lower chest or abdomen may include vascular trauma with widespread effects.

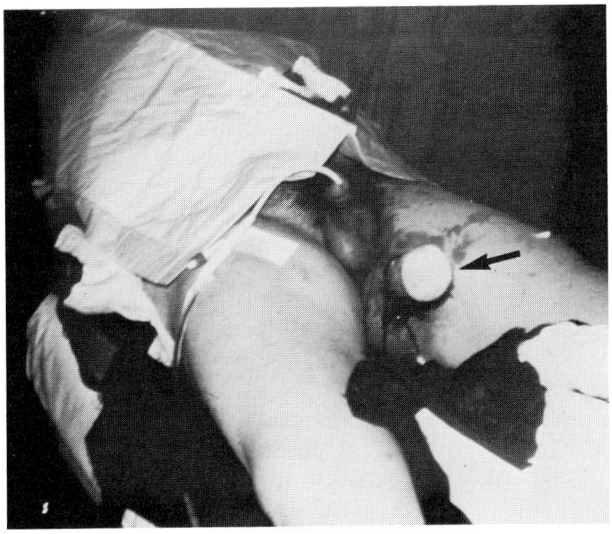

Figure 20–13. Impalement event. Young white male who fell from a tree onto the tree branch, which entered the abdomen through the peritoneum.

Venous Drainage

Venous drainage of the abdomen is more complex than the arterial supply. Blood is drained from the small intestines, stomach, spleen, and pancreas through the superior mesenteric and splenic veins and their tributaries, which join to form the portal vein. This blood then passes through liver sinusoids, supplying nutrients to liver cells before emptying into sublobular veins and then into the hepatic veins, which empty into the inferior vena cava prior to passing through the diaphragm into the right atrium. Traumatic injury to the venous system in this area is complicated by the presence of liver tissue covering the vessel.

Other abdominal venous flow originates in the external iliac veins in the inguinal ligament, which are joined by internal iliac veins to form the common iliac veins, which form the inferior vena cava at the sacral promontory. The renal veins join the inferior vena cava at the L2 level. Other smaller veins join the inferior vena cava as it passes to the superior margin of the liver, through the diaphragm for 2 to 3 cm before entering the right atrium. Much of the inferior vena cava lies in close proximity to the aorta, making injury to one vessel likely to affect the other.

Knowledge of the structure and location of abdominal organs is the first step to understanding the impact of the injury. Potential diagnoses can be developed based on this knowledge.

Initial treatment for abdominal traumatic injury is often directed by protocol without a definitive diagnosis to guide interventions. As soon as possible, a systematic process must begin to collect data to permit definitive diagnosis and care.

The accident data base enhances the picture by supplying information related to the type and mechanism of injury. Together with an understanding of abdominal organ structure and function, the health care team builds a picture of the extent of injury the patient has sustained.

INJURY DATA BASE

The injury data base has many facets and can alert the nurse to damage that may not be readily apparent. The type of injury or forces involved with the injury (rotational, crushing, shearing, deceleration, burst, or penetrating) should be ascertained. A pedestrian struck by a motor vehicle could suffer shearing forces, resulting in a degloving injury of an area as the layers of tissue are torn from their vascular bed. Deceleration injury, the body's hitting a nonmoving object, may cause organs to tear away from attachments or cause crushing of an organ as it is held between the area of impact and the nonmoving object. A direct blow to the abdomen may transmit forces sufficient to rupture an organ from a sudden rise in intra-abdominal pressure.

The mechanism of injury directs attention toward certain organ involvement and should raise the level of suspicion regarding certain injuries. Blunt trauma may be caused by a blow to the abdomen from a moving or nonmoving object, e.g., a baseball bat hitting a stationary individual or a driver hitting a steering wheel. Certain restraining devices, i.e., seat belts, may cause blunt trauma. The more frequent use of restraint devices in motor vehicles has reduced fatal outcomes and serious injury.[9–11] The basic lap belt and the more effective three-point diagonal belt system prevent ejections from the motor vehicle but do not prevent injury entirely. Indeed, seat belts have been associated with blunt cervical, thoracic, abdominal, and extremity injuries.

The classic seat belt injury includes abdominal wall disruption, hollow viscus injury, and flexion-distraction fracture of the lumbosacral spine.[12] Some abdominal wall injuries arise from direct seat belt trauma. Small bowel and colon injuries occur most frequently from a sudden increase in intraluminal pressure or shearing forces due to rapid deceleration. Liver, spleen, and pancreas injuries are reported as well, but with less frequency.

The nursing assessment begins with asking the patient if he was wearing a seat belt. This leads to an inspection of the neck, chest, and abdomen for bruises, abrasions, or discoloration indicative of a seat belt injury. If time permits, the accident record should be checked for any notation concerning seat belt use. Any such indication should raise a suspicion of intra-abdominal injury.

Although utilizing diagnostic peritoneal lavage (DPL) and computed tomography (CT) to evaluate blunt abdominal trauma from seat belt injury remains controversial, the judicious use of both tests is recommended. When ruling out hollow viscus injury, the CT should be performed before the DPL, since important CT signs of intraperitoneal fluid or free air may be related to the DPL itself.[12]

Penetrating trauma may occur from a stab, missile, or impalement event. Stab wounds are straightforward. The size, shape, and length of the stabbing instrument help to estimate intra-abdominal damage. The management is frequently dictated by the degree of penetration into the peritoneal cavity. Nearly one-third of all stab wounds do not penetrate the peritoneal lining.[13] Therefore, some controversy remains regarding the advantage of initial exploration of penetrating trauma wounds, especially without positive physical signs preoperatively. Thal et al. detailed six factors that indicate the necessity for exploratory laparotomy in penetrating abdominal trauma: (1) physical signs suggestive of peritoneal injury, (2) unexplained shock, (3) loss of bowel sounds, (4) evisceration of a viscus, including the omentum, (5) evidence of blood in the stomach, bladder, or rectum, and (6) evidence of visceral injury such as pneumoperitoneum or visceral displacement on x-ray films.[14] Patients without these elements should be admitted for close observation for a 24- to 48-hour period.

Impalement injuries are a dirty form of stab wound that result in high mortality due to bacterial contamination and multiple organ involvement (Fig. 20–13).

Missile injuries are more difficult to evaluate. Mortality depends on major vessel disruption and/or multiple organ involvement. The terminal velocity, or the amount of energy imparted to the tissue by the missile, often determines the extent of injury. The mortality rate from gunshot wounds is 8 to 10 times greater than that for stab wounds.[14] The magnitude of entrance and exit wounds may bear little relationship to the degree of damage or course of destruction from a bullet wound. Bullets may ricochet off organs or bones plus roll or move throughout the body or embolize through the vessels. Organs in proximity to the gunshot wound may be injured through a blast effect. Quick evaluation of the situation is necessary, since hemorrhage and hollow viscus perforation resulting in chemical and bacterial peritonitis are major problems in this type of abdominal trauma. Multiple sources dictate an urgent laparotomy to assess the extent of the damage.[2, 3] Tissue destruction due to velocity, type of weapon or bullet, and tissue characteristics alter the nature of the abdominal wound and its complications. (See Chapter 7 for further information.)

The Penetrating Abdominal Trauma Index (PATI) was developed to quantify the risk of complications after abdominal trauma.[15] A score was assigned to each abdominal organ injured and then multiplied by an estimate of injury severity. The scoring is based on operative findings, with index values greater than 25 correlating with an increased incidence of abdominal septic complications. Although validated for penetrating abdominal trauma only, it also has been used as a scoring system for blunt abdominal injury. Recently, the Abdominal Trauma Index (ATI) was tested as a predictor of abdominal septic complications and proved a valid predictor for both penetrating and blunt abdominal trauma.[16]

Other details of the accident add to the data base. A clean versus dirty or open versus closed injury often dictates medical management and subsequent nursing care (e.g., as indicated earlier, a ballistics injury is considered relatively clean compared with an impalement event). Thus the type of surgery, the necessity for debridement, and even the need for antibiotics can be influenced by these facts.

Changes in the patient's condition alert the nurse to possible abdominal injury. For example, a deterioration in the patient's level of consciousness from the scene to the emergency room may indicate head injury or intra-abdominal bleeding leading to shock. If a patient complains of pain in the lower chest, abdomen, or back at the scene, this may indicate abdominal injury.

Information regarding the history of the accident may be obtained from multiple sources: the patient, witnesses, or the emergency personnel from the scene. This information is vital and is difficult to retrieve later. A member of the health care team should be designated to collect and record necessary information.

The injury data collection and documentation are precursors for the abdominal assessment that follows. This information should direct the nurse's attention toward certain injuries and enhance other clinical data accumulation.

ABDOMINAL ASSESSMENT

Abdominal injury may be insidious, requiring close, systematic assessment by all team members to promote early diagnosis and intervention. Multiple bits of data will be collected during patient assessment, and each has little value when considered alone. Together, however, they will depict a trend or, correlated with information from the injury data base, diagnostic tests, or the patient's physical findings, will direct appropriate interventions.

Although past medical history is gathered as soon as possible on any person who has sustained traumatic injury, these specific issues are particularly significant if abdominal injury is suspected. The directed history includes information such as prior surgery to the abdomen for other trauma or illness. The possibility of the presence of adhesions or altered nutrient absorption or fluid balance must be ascertained. History of allergies, especially to antibiotics or contrast material that may be necessary to diagnose or treat the abdominal injury, is necessary. Any prior or present use of medications that affect abdominal, cardiac, or renal functioning must be ascertained. This includes the use of aspirin or an anticoagulant that may affect the clotting mechanism. Information may be available from the patient, family members, or significant others. Although the family may be too upset to think clearly when detailing such events and the patient may not be able to render the information owing to concomitant injury or the effects of alcohol or other drugs, every attempt should be made to ascertain the patient's previous medical condition.

The physical examination is systematic and continues through all stages of care. Repeated examination by the same nurse or same physician provides the consistency necessary to evaluate changes. The physical examination should be adapted to the patient's present status. Certainly an unstable patient with a penetrating abdominal wound does not need a prolonged, detailed physical examination; rather, prompt appropriate intervention is indicated.

Complaint of abdominal pain from an alert patient is a key indicator of abdominal injury. Peritoneal irritation is described as sharp, localized pain. Referred pain complaints signal damage to the spleen (left shoulder pain), liver (right shoulder pain), or retroperitoneal structures (testicular pain).

Many patients who sustain abdominal injuries may not be able to participate in the physical examination because of alterations in level of consciousness or spinal cord injury; therefore, the four-step abdominal examination is essential.

Inspection

Inspection begins with noting the lower chest wall integrity. Since the last six ribs overlie abdominal structures, disruption to this area may signal organ damage, specifically to the liver, spleen, or diaphragm.

The appearance of the abdomen is documented. Abrasions, contusions, and lacerations are noted. Location, size, shape, and number of entrance and exit wounds will usually indicate the presence of a foreign object within the body.

The abdominal contour, normally flat, slightly rounded, or convex in a heavy patient, may be distended, which is indicative of an accumulation of blood, other fluid, or gas secondary to perforated hollow viscus or rupture of organs (e.g., liver or spleen) or of the vascular supply to the abdomen. Repeated inspection by the same nurse may reveal signs of distention, which, combined with absence of bowel sounds, may be indicative of an ileus or intra-abdominal bleeding.

Involuntary guarding indicates injury to underlying structures. This may be less obvious or not present with retroperitoneal injury. Discoloration, protuberances, peristaltic movement, pulsations, abrasions, and old surgical scars should be noted. Repeated inspection alerts the nurse to new discolorations or other changes indicative of underlying injury. Dissection of blood into the abdominal wall from retroperitoneal tissue (Grey-Turner sign) may occur several hours after the initial injury. Proper inspection includes examining the patient's back and flank area as well as the anterior surface for the signs mentioned. Obvious wounds or ecchymosis of the lumbar area indicates possible damage to abdominal organs below.

Auscultation

Auscultation is often the most difficult part of the abdominal examination during resuscitative or critical care efforts simply because of the noise created by team members performing lifesaving procedures. The absence of bowel sounds is not necessarily an indication of injury. Anderson and Ballinger demonstrated that normal peristaltic sounds can be heard both in the presence of active intraperitoneal bleeding and following rupture of hollow abdominal organs.[1] While auscultating in all four quadrants, the nurse should be alert for the presence of bowel sounds in unlikely locations, e.g., bowel sounds in the chest cavity, which may indicate a diaphragmatic tear. In serial auscultation, diminished or absent bowel sounds may indicate an ileus or peritonitis. The nurse should listen for bruits, especially over the renal arteries, abdominal aorta, and iliac arteries, which may indicate partially obstructed arterial blood flow.

Percussion

Percussion identifies the presence of air, fluid, or tissue intra-abdominally. Tympanic sounds indicate air-filled spaces such as stomach or gut, and a dull sound is present over organ structures such as the liver or spleen.

Dullness throughout the four quadrants indicates free fluid in the abdomen. Fixed areas of dullness (Ballance sign) in the LUQ may suggest a subcapsular or extracapsular hematoma of the spleen or flank. Dullness that does not change with position suggests the presence of retroperitoneal hematoma. Other hollow versus dull tones may represent air in the abdominal cavity indicative of perforated viscus. A diaphragmatic tear or hemothorax may be suspected if a dull sound is elicited over the otherwise tympanic thoracic space.

Palpation

Abdominal tenderness is evaluated by using the whole hand over all four quadrants and progressing from light to deep palpation. This is the most frequent and reliable sign of intra-abdominal injury. Gentle palpation may elicit areas of increased tone or tenderness that suggest underlying injury. Abdominal wall injury produces focal tenderness, which increases on exertion (tensing muscles). Deep palpation is used to elicit guarding, tenderness, and rebound and is associated with parietal peritoneal irritation.

A tender abdomen with guarding, distention, and signs of peritoneal irritation can indicate an organ rupture. RUQ tenderness, guarding, or tenderness over the right lower six ribs may indicate liver damage. Diminished or absent pulses in the femoral arteries may indicate common iliac artery thrombosis, dissecting aortic aneurysm, or chronic vascular disease.

During subsequent examination, symptoms such as rebound tenderness, abdominal rigidity, and guarding suggest peritonitis. An ileus may manifest generalized tenderness or localizing signs.

The patient may experience referred pain. Most common among these is the Kehr's sign, pain in the left shoulder secondary to diaphragmatic irritation by blood following splenic rupture. Right shoulder pain is often indicative of liver injury. The patient must be lying flat or in the Trendelenburg position to elicit this type of shoulder pain.

Rectal examination follows to test for gross blood, indicating hemorrhage, or anterior tenderness, denoting peritoneal irritation. Positive results indicate lower gastrointestinal injury.

During the intermediate care and rehabilitation cycles, the four-step systematic physical examination continues. Inspection includes the same assessment techniques; however, the changes detected in the examination may be secondary to the operative event or late signs of traumatic injury or sepsis. A chemical ileus secondary to late pancreatic rupture or gastric repair leakage will distend the bowel and therefore the abdomen. Either the bowel sounds will be obliterated or a hypertympanic sound appreciated.

Discolorations around a repair site may indicate vessel rebleeding into an area. A wound may appear dark or collect excess cloudy exudate and imply an infection.

Small diaphragmatic tears may be missed during the original operative procedure or simply not manifest until days or weeks after the original injury. Therefore, auscultation of the chest and abdomen should continue periodically; the presence or absence of bowel sounds or the presence of an air leak should be noted.

Physiological and psychological stress from the trauma may induce gastric mucosal erosion over time, leading to gastrointestinal bleeding. Abdominal distention, pain, and tenderness are noticed as the erosion progresses. However, no physical symptoms may be appreciated until bleeding is evident. This event can occur at any time throughout the cycles. Therefore, vigilant, systematic physical assessment is required as the patient advances from admission through rehabilitation.

Although abdominal assessment is not part of the primary survey, the presence of abdominal injury necessitating immediate surgical intervention must be established early. Continual assessment of the abdomen as part of the secondary survey can occur only after life-threatening events have been managed. This allows the nurse to move on to continuous, complete reevaluation and subsequent care.

DIAGNOSTIC STUDIES

Radiographic Films

Chest films as well as abdominal films are ordered to evaluate abdominal trauma if the patient is sufficiently stable. Thoracic injuries are frequently associated with abdominal injury; therefore, chest films provide invaluable information to assess abdominal damage and serve as an aid in establishing a baseline for respiratory care.

Anteroposterior supine abdominal films and left lateral decubitus films may reveal the presence of intraperitoneal fluid or air or alteration in visceral contours. The examiner may note the presence of a foreign body or determine the trajectory of missiles. On an upright film, inspection for free air may disclose a ruptured hollow viscus, such as stomach or colon. Skeletal structure damage should increase suspicion of damage to certain organs; e.g., splenic injury often occurs with left-sided rib fractures. Enlargement or distortion of the outlines of intra-abdominal organs may indicate subcapsular hematoma or hemorrhage confined to an area. In addition, fluid or gas collections may distort outlines.

Negative abdominal films do not exclude significant intra-abdominal injury. Keefe et al. demonstrated that 800 ml of intra-abdominal fluid is the minimum amount detectable radiographically.[17] Water-soluble contrast medium may be used if duodenal perforation or other upper gastrointestinal injury is suspected; this permits localization of the site and extent of injury. In light of a negative "flat" plate and equivocal physical examination, contrast studies assist the physician in making an accurate diagnosis.

Computed Tomography

In 1981, computed tomography (CT) was advanced as an adjunctive diagnostic tool for abdominal injury.[18] Since that time, the benefits of this modality have been debated.[19–22]

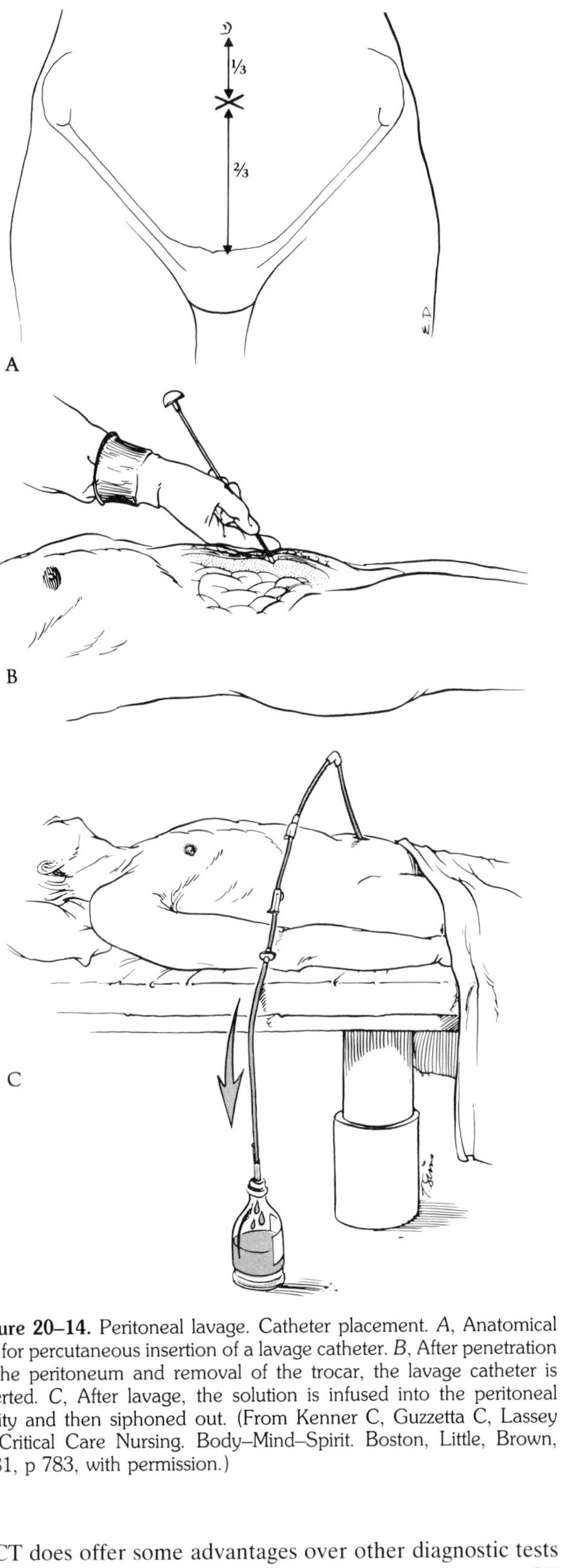

Figure 20–14. Peritoneal lavage. Catheter placement. *A*, Anatomical site for percutaneous insertion of a lavage catheter. *B*, After penetration of the peritoneum and removal of the trocar, the lavage catheter is inserted. *C*, After lavage, the solution is infused into the peritoneal cavity and then siphoned out. (From Kenner C, Guzzetta C, Lassey B: Critical Care Nursing. Body–Mind–Spirit. Boston, Little, Brown, 1981, p 783, with permission.)

CT does offer some advantages over other diagnostic tests for the stable trauma patient. Although noninvasive, a CT still pictures in detail the intra-abdominal and retroperitoneal structures.[23] It can furnish a rough estimate of the amount of bleeding into the peritoneal, retroperitoneal, and pelvic spaces. In addition, the surgeon can use it to grade an injury to determine the need for a laparotomy.[19, 23] However, CT has varying sensitivity, specificity, and accuracy with various intra-abdominal and retroperitoneal organ injuries. Pancreatic injury, for example, is reported with only an 85 per cent sensitivity rate.[2] Diagnostic sensitivity and accuracy may be related to the experience of the radiologist.[2, 24]

Trunkey et al.[2] note these specific indications for CT:

1. A stable patient with equivocal abdominal examination
2. Closed head injury
3. Spinal cord injury
4. Significant hematuria
5. Patients with pelvic fractures, significant bleeding, and a need to rule out intra-abdominal associated injuries
6. Patients lost to physical examination, such as those undergoing operative fixation of extensive orthopedic injuries
7. Patients who have significant dulling of their sensorium by drugs or alcohol

CT, like other diagnostic tests, is an adjunct to performing serial clinical examinations and following the patterns of laboratory data in the assessment of abdominal trauma. CT often requires patient transport from the resuscitation area to the radiology department, complicating the care of an unstable patient. Obviously, adequate staff and materials should be available to ensure the safety of patients when they are transported for testing.

Arteriography

Arteriography is an organ-specific process used with both blunt and penetrating trauma. It is useful in detecting arteriovenous fistulas, false aneurysms, and arterio-biliary fistulas, especially with penetrating trauma.[7] It is the procedure of choice for suspected on-going vascular injury. Selective invasive embolization of a vascular rupture can be accomplished during arteriography.

Diagnostic Peritoneal Lavage (DPL)

Peritoneal lavage is a quick diagnostic procedure that is frequently utilized in the resuscitation phase of care to diagnose intra-abdominal bleeding when the results of the physical examination are equivocal, the patient is unstable and the team is ruling out abdominal injury, or the patient is unable to participate in the abdominal evaluation. DPL is extremely sensitive and relatively accurate but not specific for type or extent of organ injury.

Many techniques have been described. Each includes placement of a Foley catheter to empty the bladder and insertion of a nasogastric tube to decompress the stomach. In the open technique, the skin is prepared and the physician makes a short supraumbilical, paraumbilical, or infraumbilical incision after administering local anesthesia. An opening is made through the rectus sheath or linea alba and into the peritoneum (Fig. 20–14). The lavage catheter is advanced into the peritoneal space, and the contents of the cavity are aspirated with a syringe. If no blood or fluid is aspirated, a liter of balanced saline solution is infused, allowed to equilibrate, and then drained from the cavity. The effluent is evaluated for red blood cells (RBCs), white blood cells

(WBCs), amylase, bile, bacteria, and intestinal contents (Table 20–1).

The nursing role is assistive during the peritoneal lavage procedure (Appendix 20–1). The patient should be informed of what will happen and that some sensation of fullness may be experienced after the solution has been infused. Warmed fluid should be infused to prevent hypothermia. Placing the patient in a slight Trendelenburg position during the infusion of the saline solution facilitates fluid movement to the diaphragm. This position can be reversed when draining the fluid from the abdominal cavity. The lavage catheter may remain in place until the cell counts are received or the patient with equivocal results has a repeat lavage.

Close monitoring of the patient is required following peritoneal lavage. The procedure is not without risk. Forceful catheter placement may result in omental lacerations or visceral and vascular perforations.

Peritoneal lavage is not accurate in diagnosing retroperitoneal injury.[23] Occasionally, injury eludes detection because there is little bleeding, insufficient fluid is retrieved, the injury is isolated by adhesions, or other factors.[25] Therefore, continued close monitoring of vital signs and level of consciousness, serial hemoglobin and hematocrit determinations, and attention to patient complaints of pain are necessary. Changes must be communicated to the physician.

Controversies. The use of DPL versus CT continues to be debated.[19–24] For the unstable patient, DPL is the quickest, most accurate diagnostic tool available to indicate the need for a laparotomy. However, for the stable patient, CT[19, 20, 23] or serial ultrasonography[26] may be utilized to ascertain specific organ injury, thereby assisting the operative decision. Furthermore, DPL is not accurate for all intra-abdominal injuries, specifically those to the retroperitoneal structures such as the pancreas, kidney, and parts of the duodenum. It cannot give information about the specific location, degree of organ injury or diaphragmatic laceration, or fractured spine or pelvis.[19]

Certain criteria eliminate the need for peritoneal lavage.[27] Evidence of hollow organ rupture on radiograph, gross abdominal wall defects, rapidly increasing distention, uncorrectable hypotension, and isolated rigidity on abdominal examination in a cooperative patient are signals for immediate laparotomy. Presence of blood on rectal examination is also a criterion for immediate laparotomy.[28] Peritoneal lavage would only waste precious time. Muncha[29] points out the complementary nature of CT and DPL as diagnostic tools and suggests that there is no need to select one and exclude the other.

Certain authors advocate the use of peritoneal lavage for some penetrating injuries, specifically stab wounds. Although data are being collected for use with gunshot wounds, it appears that this procedure cannot be used for accurate diagnosis of the extent of the injury because of the characteristics of ballistic missiles.

TABLE 20–1. PERITONEAL LAVAGE RESULTS

	RESULT	INDICATION
Aspirant	Gross blood > 20 ml	Positive
	Pink fluid	Intermediate*
	Clean	Negative
Lavage fluid	Bloody	Positive
	Clear	Negative
RBC	>100,000 cells/mm	Positive
	50–100,000 cells/mm	Intermediate*
WBC	>500 cells/mm	Positive
	100–500 cells/mm	Intermediate*
Amylase	>175 U/100 ml	Positive
	75–175 U/100 ml	Intermediate*
	< 75 U/100 ml	Negative
Bacteria	Present	Positive
Fecal material	Present	Positive
Bile	Present	Positive
Food particles	Present	Positive

*Intermediate lavage results require further observation of the patient, possibly repeat lavage, and intervention based on clinical presentation.

MONITORING

Serial blood pressure measurements are a key component of the nursing assessment. Hypotension, especially if it does not respond to fluid replacement, is a sign of intra-abdominal hemorrhage and the need for immediate surgical intervention. Mild volume losses will respond to an infusion of 500 to 1000 ml of solution, but momentary response to fluid therapy followed by return to the hypotensive level is a feature of continuing hemorrhage.

In severe hypotensive states, the central venous pressure permits assessment of response to fluid therapy. Single values are not as significant as is the trend evident in serial readings.

The insidious nature of certain complications of abdominal injury demands continuous monitoring of the patient for signs of late bleeding. The blood pressure is one commonly used assessment parameter through all cycles of care.

LABORATORY DATA

Hemoglobin and Hematocrit

Although samples for hemoglobin and hematocrit determinations are frequently the first obtained, their usefulness is limited during the early resuscitation and critical care stages. They provide a baseline value but do not reflect recent hemorrhage. Several hours are required before equilibration occurs. Serial values, however, offer valuable data regarding the patient's hemodynamic trend.

Leukocyte Counts

Elevated white blood cell (WBC) counts are part of the normal body response to trauma; therefore, this value is of little significance early in the trauma cycle of a patient sustaining abdominal trauma. However, development of neutrophilia on serial evaluations indicates an inflammatory process in the peritoneal cavity.

Amylase Levels

Serum amylase may become elevated as a result of parotid gland, pancreatic, duodenal, or genitourinary injury. However, some patients sustain no rise in amylase level despite injury to these organs. This becomes one more data point which may indicate injury but is not necessarily diagnostic.

Other Laboratory Data

Samples for other laboratory studies such as serum electrolytes, total bilirubin, blood urea nitrogen (BUN), and creatinine are drawn as baseline values for patients sustaining abdominal trauma, especially if surgery is contemplated.

Throughout the cycles, certain laboratory data may indicate posttraumatic complications. An elevated WBC count, for example, could be an initial suggestion of wound infection or abscess formation. Amylase levels rise in posttraumatic pancreatitis. A decreased hematocrit level may demonstrate recurring hemorrhage. Clearly, the nurse should anticipate utilizing laboratory data as a reflection of the patient's clinical status throughout the hospitalization. Specific alterations in these values and their relation to specific organ injury are covered later in the chapter.

ORGAN INJURY

The initial assessment process has been presented, noting the use of a directed history, data base, diagnostic studies, abdominal assessment, and laboratory data. Utilizing nursing diagnoses, specific organ injuries will now be presented. The medical and nursing management of each is discussed.

Loss of Integrity of Thoracoabdominal Cavities Secondary to Diaphragmatic Injury

The diaphragm is partially protected by its anatomical location. It is injured most frequently by penetrating trauma to the chest[30] and is associated with intra-abdominal injuries in 15 per cent of patients with stab wounds and 46 per cent of patients with gunshot wounds to the lower chest.[31] Also, automobile deceleration injury is responsible for blunt diaphragmatic injury because a rapid rise in intra-abdominal pressure creates a burst injury. The forces necessary to create such an injury are so great that other intra-abdominal, orthopedic, or neurologic injury is often present. It has been reported that the incidence of diaphragmatic injury is greater for the left hemidiaphragm due to the buttressing action of the liver on the right.[32] However, with added awareness of the frequency of injury to the diaphragm and the more common surgical practice of searching for a diaphragmatic tear, the reported incidence of right- and left-sided injury has equalized.[33]

Diagnosis. The diagnosis of a diaphragmatic tear is difficult because trauma to the diaphragm, whether blunt or penetrating, usually means multiorgan involvement. On initial examination the physiological instability due to multisystem trauma may render the usual signs of decreased breath sounds and abdominal peristalsis in the thorax indistinguishable for the practitioner. There is a high incidence of late diagnosis or diagnosis upon abdominal exploration secondary to visceral injury. On the right side, the liver may actually plug the defect, making diagnosis impossible until abdominal exploration. Acute herniation resulting in chest pain and shortness of breath signals a diaphragmatic tear.

Chest x-ray can aid diagnosis. However, chest x-rays are often negative unless a substantial injury exists. The presence of abdominal viscera or a nasogastric tube within the chest denotes a perforated diaphragm. An elevated right hemidiaphragm may indicate liver protrusion through a tear.

Team Management. The most accurate diagnosis is made at celiotomy. Operative repair is necessary because visceral herniation can occur through small rents days to years following the traumatic episode. Root[30] discusses the rationale for using either the thoracic or abdominal approach to repair. The abdominal route is preferred for acutely presenting diaphragmatic tears secondary to blunt or penetrating injury. In delayed repair, adhesions are expected between abdominal viscera and intrathoracic structures; therefore, chest exploration is recommended. This approach is also used if there is major hemothoracic involvement or if previous abdominal surgery may interfere with the abdominal approach. Right-sided herniation of the liver into the thorax also requires a thoracic entry, and in certain circumstances a combined abdominothoracic approach is necessary.

Nursing Management. Nursing care in the acute stage begins with raising an index of suspicion concerning any patient who has had blunt or penetrating trauma of the abdomen or thorax as high as the T4 level (the upper limit of diaphragmatic excursion). Assessment focuses on percussion of the abdominothoracic structures for a dull tone and auscultation of the abdomen and the chest for peristaltic sounds in the chest. However, if the patient is splinting the area, even normal sounds may not be appreciated. With gross herniation of visceral contents into the chest cavity, the patient may have a shift of mediastinal structures, resulting in respiratory distress and circulatory instability. Difficulty passing a nasogastric tube also may signal infiltration of abdominal contents into the thorax. Throughout the cycles, unexplained chest pain and increased respiratory rate signal the possibility of acute herniation. In addition, a persistent air leak after chest tube placement may indicate a diaphragmatic tear.

Penetrating trauma can produce a small tear not recognized during the acute stage. A rise in intra-abdominal pressure may cause a small rent to become larger, with the consequent danger of herniation and intestinal strangulation. Patient education must include the possibility of diaphragmatic defect, because evidence of such an injury may occur years after the initial trauma. The patient should understand the necessity of relating the past injury history to the physician if severe epigastric or chest pain is experienced. The symptoms may mimic coronary occlusion and mislead diagnostic efforts.

Loss of Esophageal Integrity Related to Abdominal Trauma

The small portion of the esophagus within the abdominal cavity results in a lower incidence of abdominoesophageal injury compared with the cervical or thoracic locations. Penetrating injury is more common than blunt trauma to the esophagus.

Penetrating trauma to the esophagus may occur from knives, bullets, or foreign body lodgment or removal. Iatrogenic perforation by instrumentation accounts for up to two-thirds of esophageal injuries.[3, 32] This most commonly occurs at sites of narrowing, such as the pharyngoesophageal junction, level of the aortic arch, and cardia. With the rise in penetrating trauma from the use of handguns among civilians, the incidence of esophageal trauma has increased.

Blunt trauma may occur with a blow or blast to the neck, chest, or abdomen, but usually occurs in the distal third of the esophagus. However, rupture of the esophagus from blunt trauma is extremely rare.

Early diagnosis is paramount because damage occurs from the corrosion of tissue by digestive juices and bacterial contamination surrounding the opening. Fluid losses may be massive and affect the thorax as well as the abdomen, leading to respiratory embarrassment. Mediastinitis, paraesophageal abscess, empyema, esophageal fistula, or peritonitis may occur. Mortality is generally due to paraesophageal contamination and infection and has been reported as high as 19 to 27 per cent.[34] The mortality rate increases as length of time from injury to treatment lengthens.

Signs and symptoms are variable according to the site of the rupture and the degree of contamination. Symptoms of perforation include pain at the site of perforation, fever, and dysphagia. The pain may radiate to the neck, chest, or shoulders or throughout the abdomen.

In any cervical injury, esophageal trauma should be anticipated. Cervical perforation is signaled by crepitus, which may be present in patients with intrathoracic perforation as well. Cervical tenderness, pain, resistance of the neck to passive range of motion, dyspnea, hoarseness, bleeding from the mouth or nasogastric tube, cough, and stridor often accompany cervical esophageal perforation. Injury to the thoracoesophageal area or missile penetration crossing the midline should raise the nurse's suspicion of esophageal damage. Intrathoracic perforation is marked by mediastinal emphysema or neck crepitation from extension of air from the esophagus. Mediastinitis is also common. Air may dissect throughout the mediastinum. Rupture of the thoracic esophagus as a result of blunt or blast injury is often associated with pneumothorax.

Tear of the abdominal esophagus may present with the sign of peritoneal irritation from release of gastric contents into the peritoneal cavity. As gastric contents efflux into the pleural space, more fluid than air may be appreciated, producing dyspnea accompanied by pleuritic pain.

Diagnostic Tests. An accurate diagnosis requires correlation of the index of suspicion with physical findings, roentgenographic studies, and endoscopy. Chest and abdominal x-ray films are ordered to document air in the mediastinum or abdomen. Lateral cervical spine films are ordered if cervical esophageal injury is suspected to locate retroesophageal air.

Diagnostic evaluation includes use of esophagoscopy or contrast radiological study (esophagogram). This defines the site of esophageal tear and whether it connects to one or both pleural spaces.

Wilson and Steiger present the controversy over the appropriate contrast medium to use in an esophagogram.[35] Meglumine diatrizoate (Gastrografin) is often used because the extravasated Gastrografin may be less likely to aggravate infection and local inflammation. However, Wilson and Steiger point out that moderate to severe pneumonitis may develop. In addition, Gastrografin fails to show the leak 25 per cent of the time.

Barium is the alternative choice and produces a false-negative result less than 10 per cent of the time, but it may aggravate mediastinitis. Wilson and Steiger note that since the patient will undergo surgery and drainage of the affected area, barium is the contrast medium of choice.

In the unstable, multiply injured patient in whom delay of a diagnostic study such as an esophagogram may increase morbidity or mortality, the abdominal esophagus is examined during surgical exploration.

Team Management. Medical management is directed toward quick assessment and intervention to deter the effects of bacterial contamination or enzyme erosion. Gastric decompression by passing a nasogastric tube, antibiotic therapy, and drainage of the wound site are combined with surgical interventions to treat an esophageal tear. Direct layered closure with drainage of the mediastinum may be possible. However, the extent of injury may dictate defunctionalization, closure of esophagogastric junction, gastrostomy, and drainage of the repair area. The process may be reversed at a later date after healing has occurred. Popovsky describes a process of using absorbable sutures to ligate, thereby allowing a 2-week healing process and negating the need for a second surgery.[36]

Outcome is related to the mechanism of injury, site of perforation, degree of contamination, and delay in treatment. Peritonitis, mediastinitis, intra-abdominal abscess formation, and esophageal fistula are potential complications following esophageal injury and subsequent repair.

Nursing Management. Initial assessment is complicated, since esophageal injuries are rare and are seldom single-system injury events. The index of suspicion must be raised if the patient has had blunt or penetrating trauma to the neck, thorax, or abdomen. Hemodynamic and respiratory stability may be affected by the esophageal injury; therefore, careful monitoring of the cardiovascular and respiratory parameters is necessary.

Since esophageal injury is difficult to diagnose and certain complications can occur later in the cycles, continuous monitoring for signs of peritoneal irritation, respiratory embarrassment, or fistula formation is necessary from resuscitation through rehabilitation.

Postoperative maintenance of the drainage system is necessary. Frequently, Penrose drains will be placed in the paraesophageal space, commencing near the suture repair line. The quantity and quality of drainage should be noted, and dressings should be maintained to guard against further contamination or skin excoriation. Drains are frequently left in place until a follow-up esophagogram is done and oral feedings are tolerated. The repeat contrast studies are usually obtained 1 week postoperatively and prior to commencing feeding.

Skin care presents a challenge to the nurse, especially if the neck is the site of repair. Frequent wound dressing changes are necessary but may cause irritation as tape is applied and removed routinely. A pectin-based wafer applied next to the skin acts as a protection against such irritation. Dressing materials or a bag used to collect copious drainage can be attached directly to this instead of to the skin.

Blunt or penetrating traumatic injury to the esophagus dictates the necessity for alternative nutritional therapy. Total parenteral nutrition or jejunal feedings may be ordered to meet the patient's caloric needs. (See Chapter 14 for specifics of nursing actions with each of these modalities.) Fluid and electrolyte balances as well as caloric demands must be evaluated and maintained as the patient moves from critical care toward rehabilitation.

Complications. Mediastinitis resulting in hemorrhage, necrosis, and acute inflammatory changes can occur in the critical care cycle.[37] This necessitates surgical debridement, drainage, nutritional support, and administration of antibiotics.

Peritonitis from abdominoesophageal leakage causes pain, abdominal tenderness, rigidity, and absent bowel sounds. This is an early complication, and the patient should be observed closely if there has been a delay in surgical repair.

A tracheoesophageal fistula can develop early after traumatic injury and present with subcutaneous emphysema, pneumothorax, or pneumomediastinum.[35] The patient experiences increased bronchial secretions, pneumonia, and severe coughing.

Other fistula formations are later complications and thus may not be evident until the intermediate care or rehabilitation cycle. The symptoms are congruent with the site of fistula formation, whether cervical, thoracic, or abdominal. The patient may experience respiratory distress related to aspiration, gastric reflux, or chemical pneumonitis. When this occurs, a cough, which is aggravated by feeding, develops. Confirmation is established by esophageal swallow of contrast dye. Repair procedures include a tracheostomy, drainage of the fistulous area, and feeding gastrostomy or hyperalimentation to permit sufficient wound healing. Patient and family support is necessary, since this complication has a delayed onset and necessitates prolonged hospitalization. Unresolved feelings regarding the initial trauma may surface at this time and require further intervention.

Esophageal stricture may occur. Patient education prior to discharge should include the signs of such a process and a warning to notify the physician if difficulty in swallowing or alteration in comfort at the cervical, thoracic, or abdominal location of the initial esophageal injury is experienced. Barium studies demonstrate narrowing, and medical intervention depends on the severity of the stricture.

Disruption in Gastric Integrity Secondary to Abdominal Trauma

The location and relative mobility of the stomach protect it from blunt injury. Most stomach trauma is penetrating and accounts for 19 per cent of all intra-abdominal organ injuries.[38] Anderson and Ballinger note that in one-third of all patients experiencing stomach injury, both anterior and posterior walls are perforated.[1] Cardiopulmonary resuscitation can lead to gastric dilation and perforation of the lesser curvature where mucosal elasticity is minimal.[39] The adequate blood supply, relative sterility of the empty organ, and ease in recognition of this single organ injury generally result in a favorable prognosis for those sustaining stomach trauma.

Rapidly developing epigastric pain, tenderness, and signs of peritonitis due to release of gastric contents are symptoms of stomach injury. Blood from the nasogastric tube and free air evident on an abdominal film support the diagnosis. If a posterior wall injury is suspected, an oral gastric study with water-soluble contrast medium will help with the diagnosis because symptoms may be delayed.

Team Management. Medical management includes gastric decompression through placement of a nasogastric tube and surgical intervention, which includes simple debridement and primary closure, resection of devitalized tissue, or partial gastrectomy for extensive injury.[40] Defects may be closed in two layers; the first layer helps to provide hemostasis in the vascular submucosa.

Removal of gastric contents and copious lavage are used to prevent the formation of abscesses if the peritoneal cavity has been contaminated with gastric spillage.[1] No drains are necessary if only the stomach has been injured.[14] Intravenous H_2-blockers or antacid prophylaxis against stress ulceration is maintained until the patient is eating.[38]

Nursing Management. Stomach injury is one of the few organ disruptions that usually presents a clear diagnostic picture. Suspicion is raised in the presence of lower thorax or upper abdominal injuries. Because symptoms appear rapidly, the patient is readied for the operative procedure immediately.

Postoperative care includes maintenance of nasogastric decompression for 3 to 4 days, with prophylactic control of pH to guard against mucosal irritation. Diet is reinstituted when bowel sounds are present and the patient is passing flatus.

Complications such as peritonitis, intra-abdominal abscess formation, or gastric fistulas may occur immediately or during the intermediate care phase of the cycle. Conservative management with nasogastric decompression, antibiotic therapy, and nutritional support is used initially with each of these. Prolonged healing or breakdown of the gastric repair, resulting in further contamination and hemorrhage, necessitates operative stabilization and drainage. Continued nutritional support and nasogastric suction will help healing over time.

Patients normally experience a rapid recovery from stomach injury. Support for the individual and family is necessary if complications arise necessitating further surgery or prolonged hospitalization, although long-term complications are minimal.

Disruption in Liver Integrity Secondary to Abdominal Trauma

The liver's size and location make it particularly susceptible to injury. It is the most commonly injured organ in abdominal trauma from both blunt and penetrating sources. Blunt liver trauma is most often seen at suburban centers, whereas penetrating liver injury has a higher incidence in urban areas. Mortality is affected by associated injuries (e.g., head or chest), the length of time from injury to treatment, and the patient's overall premorbid condition. The highest mortality occurs from blunt hepatic injuries and shotgun wounds.[1, 41] The rate increases with the number of associated injuries. Hemorrhage is the most common cause of death from liver wounds and makes the overall mortality equal 10 to 15 per cent.[42]

Olsen reported that 70 per cent of all liver injuries he studied were due to blunt trauma.[43] Blunt liver injury should be suspected in any patient with a lower chest or abdominal injury, especially on the right side. Motor vehicle accidents—especially those involving deceleration injury encountered when the driver is forced into the steering wheel, thereby crushing the liver between ribs and vertebrae—are responsible for most blunt liver injury.

Penetrating injuries make up the remaining 30 per cent of all liver trauma. The object used to penetrate the abdomen has a significant effect on morbidity and mortality in addition to any vascular injury involvement. Stab wounds of the liver and low-velocity gunshots produce lacerations from which hemorrhage is generally controlled and hemostasis restored. However, high-velocity gunshot wounds are likely to produce widespread damage to liver tissue as well as create massive hemorrhage.

Liver injury can be graded on a scale of I to VI, with type I representing the least severe damage (Table 20–2). This scale,[44] developed by the Organ Injury Scaling Committee of the American Association for the Surgery of Trauma, creates a common classification for comparison in liver injury. From "capsular tear nonbleeding" to "hepatic avulsion," the grading system may be used preoperatively and intraoperatively to categorize the level of injury.[45] Signs of liver damage change depending on the type of injury.

A liver capsule rupture with loss of bile and blood into the peritoneal cavity will produce evidence of peritoneal contamination. A subcapsular hematoma gives no early signs but threatens late hemorrhage. An intrahepatic hematoma causing tissue necrosis, abscess formation, and possible erosion into hepatic vessels may occur. This process may produce hematobilia, presenting symptoms of gastrointestinal bleeding, obstructive jaundice, and colicky abdominal pain.

Lim noted that long-term survivors after liver trauma showed no sequelae from the damaged liver with or without major resection and that liver regeneration will occur if the patient survives the initial postinjury period.[42]

Initial Assessment. Initial assessment is guided by an increased index of suspicion based on the historical evidence of penetrating or blunt trauma to the abdomen or lower chest area. In any patient who presents with persistent hypotension, despite adequate volume replacement, intra-abdominal injury must be suspected, and operative management is required. The specific organ damage may be obvious only upon operative exploration.

Physical examination aids the diagnostic process but is not definitive. Olsen et al., noted that 21 per cent of patients thought to have significant intra-abdominal injury had only trivial injuries.[46] However, 43 per cent who were thought to have "benign" injury were found to have significant injury on laparotomy.

Physical examination may elicit tenderness or guarding over the right lower six ribs or RUQ. Dullness to percussion may exist. If the patient is bleeding into the peritoneal cavity, then signs of irritation and abdominal distention will be evident. Persistent thoracic bleeding or hemothorax associated with abdominal tenderness should raise suspicion of liver injury.

DPN may be used to identify intra-abdominal organ injury; however, CT is increasingly advocated due to its sensitivity and specificity for hepatic injury.[18, 41] Novick and Moylan suggest that CT should be used only for the stable patient, since the test may take up to 45 minutes to complete and a skilled radiologist must be present for interpretation.[47]

Plain radiographs of the abdomen may indicate hepatic injury through presence of right lower rib fractures, elevated right hemidiaphragm, pleural effusion or right hemopneumothorax, loss of normal hepatic outline or increased hepatic shadow, increased opacification of RUQ, and duodenal or intestinal paralytic ileus.[47]

Team Management. Team management includes decid-

TABLE 20–2. LIVER INJURY SCALE

GRADE*	INJURY DESCRIPTION†	ICD-9	AIS 85	AIS 90
I. Hematoma:	Subcapsular, nonexpanding, <10% surface area	864.01 864.11	2	2
Laceration:	Capsular tear, nonbleeding, <1 cm parenchymal depth	864.02 864.12	2	2
II. Hematoma:	Subcapsular, nonexpanding, 10–50% surface Intraparenchymal, nonexpanding, <2 cm in diameter	864.01 864.11	2	2
Laceration:	Capsular tear, active bleeding; 1–3 cm parenchymal depth, <10 cm in length	864.03 864.13	2	2
III. Hematoma:	Subcapsular, >50% surface area or expanding Ruptured subcapsular hematoma with active bleeding; intraparenchymal hematoma >2 cm or expanding		3	3
Laceration:	>3 cm parenchymal depth	864.04 864.14	3	3
IV. Hematoma:	Ruptured intraparenchymal hematoma with active bleeding		3	4
Laceration:	Parenchymal disruption involving 25–50% of hepatic lobe	864.04 864.14	4	4
V. Laceration:	Parenchymal disruption involving >50% of hepatic lobe		5	5
Vascular:	Juxtahepatic venous injuries, i.e., retrohepatic vena cava/major hepatic veins		5	5
VI. Vascular:	Hepatic avulsion			6

*Advance one grade for multiple injuries to the same organ.
†Based on most accurate assessment at autopsy, laparotomy, or radiologic study.
Developed by the Organ Injury Scaling (OIS) Committee of the American Association for the Surgery of Trauma (AAST). From Moore EE, Shackford SR, Pachter HL, et al: Organ injury scaling: Spleen, liver and kidney. J Trauma 29:1664, 1989.

ing whether the patient is a candidate for nonoperative versus operative treatment. Pachter et al. note that increasing success in nonoperative treatment of liver injury in children has spurred an interest in nonoperative treatment in adults.[48] There is some controversary about the role of nonoperative treatment, and several authors state that strict criteria must be met if nonoperative treatment is to be successful.[48–51] The criteria include hepatic injuries of grade I or II or grade III injuries without active bleeding or an expanding hematoma. In addition, the ability to monitor the patient closely with the use of serial CT scans is necessary.[49] Harris et al. caution the use of nonoperative treatment in minor liver injury because it delays treatment of significant concomitant abdominal injury that may need repair.[51] Harris et al. recommend exploratory laparotomy based on positive DPL or clinical findings as the method of choice in treatment of any abdominal injury.

Anderson and Ballinger noted that the goals in the management of liver trauma are control and prevention of bleeding, bile drainage, removal of all severely damaged and nonviable liver tissue, and adequate wound drainage.[1] Medical treatment therefore includes observation for simple liver injury, because the bleeding may be self-controlled. Small lacerations may be treated by suture only or electrocautery or topical hemostatic agents. If there is a distinct possibility of postoperative bleeding or bile leak, closed-suction drainage may be instituted for short periods.[46]

Deep liver lacerations require various interventions to control bleeding, support viable tissue, and prevent postoperative infection. Often wounds will require debridement of nonviable tissue followed by drainage with a combination of Penrose and sump drains.

Hepatic resection carries a high mortality rate.[52] Moore et al. noted an increased interest in options other than resection in complex liver injuries because of the high mortality rates.[53] However, Pachter et al. describe specific indications for hepatic resection.[48] This process is used (1) for total destruction of the normal hepatic parenchyma, (2) if the extent of injury precludes perihepatic packing, (3) in instances in which the injury has virtually performed the resection and completion can be achieved with several additional clamps, or (4) when hepatic resection is the sole mechanism to control exsanguinating hemorrhage.

Other techniques such as perihepatic packing[54, 55] and total mesh wrapping[56] are used in complex liver injuries in an attempt to control hemorrhage. Perihepatic packing requires a second operative procedure to remove the packs and debride devitalized tissue.

The treatment for nonexpanding subcapsular or intrahepatic hematomas is controversial. Certain authors advocate exploration and drainage,[1, 57] while others suggest nonoperative management following the patient with serial CT scans.[48, 58] Operative intervention is required for an expanding hematoma, on-going hemorrhage, signs of sepsis, or deterioration of liver function tests. The complex nature of hepatic injury requires a skillful team using one or many alternative methods to control hemorrhage and prevent postoperative complications.

Twelfth rib resection is necessary, at times, to drain the liver bed adequately. Drainage of all fluid from the area is required to prevent hematoma formation, abscess formation, or creation of a fistula tract. This may include use of large Penrose or Silastic suction drains.

Liver tissue can regenerate, resulting in the return of normal liver function tests. Postoperatively, however, the patient can experience a decreased albumin, since the liver is the body's source of albumin, which is 50 to 60 per cent of the total plasma protein.

In addition, the liver is a key to the regulation of fat, carbohydrate, and protein metabolism. The liver reduces proteins, deaminizing amino acids and releasing nitrogen, which is converted to urea for excretion. It is involved in fat metabolism, oxidizing fats as energy sources and forming lipoproteins and phospholipids. In its role in carbohydrate metabolism, the liver stores glycogen within hepatocytes and later can break down glycogen stores to meet body needs. It converts glucose, fructose, and galactose to glycogen for storage. During starvation states, it can convert protein and fat to glycogen.

After injury, the patient may experience a decrease in blood sugar. The decrease in albumin and glucose is treated with continuous glucose infusion and administration of serum albumin until regeneration or adaptation occurs.

The multiple roles the liver plays in maintaining homeostasis make any liver injury significant. The liver detoxifies substances such as drugs by making them water-soluble and capable of being excreted in the urine or bile. It produces the clotting factors I, II, VI, VII, VIII, IX, and X. It stores vitamin K, which is necessary for the synthesis of certain factors (II, VII, IX, X).

The primary postoperative complication is uncontrolled hemorrhage. Diffuse oozing from the liver surface may represent a consumptive coagulopathy as a result of trauma, shock, or massive transfusions.[42] Treatment includes maintaining vascular volume using fresh blood, platelets, and fresh frozen plasma.

The liver has a role in the body's ability to remain immunocompetent through the removal of bacteria that enter through the portal system from the gut. Kupffer cells lining the liver sinusoids remove foreign debris from the circulation. Sepsis secondary to abscess formation is another complication of liver injury.

Nursing Management. During the resuscitation phase of care for liver injury, the nursing focus is that detailed under "Abdominal Assessment." Although particular signs of hepatic trauma may be elicited, hemodynamic stability is the major goal for these patients after an airway has been ensured. Frequently, the degree of injury is not appreciated until surgical exploration is begun. Hemorrhage is the greatest single cause of mortality during the resuscitation or the critical care cycle.

Certain patients who have sustained blunt trauma to the RUQ may not produce symptoms of liver injury initially. Owing to the possibility of delayed capsular rupture, these patients should be serially assessed over a 48- to 72-hour period for cardiovascular stability and liver function.

Those who have undergone liver resection must have liver function monitored postoperatively: Coagulation profile, ammonia levels, alkaline phosphatase, transaminase, serum protein, and glucose levels are a few. The patient may need albumin replacement until protein synthesis is adequate. Vitamin K supplementation or blood product infusion may be necessary to assist the formation or replacement of clotting factors. Parenteral nutrition is necessary to meet caloric demands until liver and intestinal function is restored.

The patient is observed for signs of hepatic failure secondary to prolonged shock state or extensive tissue damage. Hemorrhage, coagulation disorders, pulmonary insufficiency, and infection are primary concerns postoperatively through each cycle.

Loss of Blood Volume Secondary to Liver Injury

Postoperative hemorrhage may be due to continuous bleeding from liver lacerations, massive blood transfusions causing hemodilution, or an unsecured bleeding point or coagulopathy secondary to liver injury. Increased blood loss can be detected by close serial assessment of drainage sites, increased abdominal distention, hematemesis, certain laboratory values, and vital signs. Hematocrit, platelet count, prothrombin time (PT), and partial thromboplastin time (PTT) should be monitored, with replacement therapy through platelets and fresh frozen plasma transfusion if there is evidence of continuing blood loss.

Vital signs, specifically blood pressure, central venous pressure (CVP), heart rate, and urinary output, are monitored to ensure adequate perfusion and cardiovascular stability. Continual bleeding is suspected if a fluid challenge produces immediate correction of cardiovascular parameters with a subsequent trend downward toward prechallenge level over time.

If altered coagulation persists despite the replacement of clotting factors by infusing fresh frozen plasma and platelets, monitoring PT and PTT, and evaluating vital signs, other specific nursing measures are indicated. Small-gauge needles are used for injections or drawing blood. Prolonged pressure is applied to injection sites. Mouth care is completed with a soft appliance as opposed to a hard toothbrush. Shaving patients with an electric razor minimizes skin irritation and risk of bleeding. Intravenous line insertion sites may ooze blood and need more frequent dressing changes to protect from infection. Monitoring for signs of bleeding continues throughout the cycles.

Subcapsular hematoma may not be evident initially but may be responsible for delayed intraperitoneal bleeding, cause development of an abscess, or decompress into the biliary tree, causing hemobilia. Severe bleeding has been reported when these hematomas are unroofed. If the patient's condition remains stable and subcapsular hematoma is noted on CT, close observation, serial hematocrits, and repeat CT are ordered because the hematoma may resolve spontaneously.[14] As the patient moves from critical care to the intermediate care cycle, the possibility of this hemorrhagic problem should be noted and serial assessments continued. Delayed rupture has been reported, so serial assessment and evaluation should occur from 28 days to 8 weeks after injury.

Potential for Infection Related to Hepatic Abscess Formation

Foreign body fragments, necrotic tissue, blood, or bile remaining at the site of injury and surgical repair may set up an infrahepatic or suprahepatic abscess formation. This localized infectious process may rupture and lead to peritonitis, the formation of fistula tracts, bacteremia, and septicemia.

Signs of abscess formation include fever, chills, abdominal pain in the RUQ, malaise, nausea, and vomiting. Physical examination may reveal hepatomegaly, decreased breath sounds on the right side, and jaundice. Laboratory data show leukocytosis, hyperbilirubinemia, low total protein, and hypoalbuminemia. Diagnostic tests such as CT scan may be utilized to locate the exact site and extent of the abscess. Medical treatment includes surgical exploration, drainage, and use of antibiotics.

Nursing intervention includes assessment for abscess formation throughout the cycle. Hepatic abscesses have been confirmed several days to months following injury. Patients should be educated about the possibility of abscess formation and the symptoms that should be reported to their physician.

Drain maintenance and care include noting color, consistency, and odor of the drainage as well as the presence of necrotic tissue in the exudate. Patency of sump drains must be ensured so that fluid does not collect at the repair site. Because drains are a portal for bacteria to enter the wound, sterile bags or dressings should be used to collect exudate. Meticulous skin care is necessary, since leakage around Penrose or sump drains can cause extensive skin irritation and eventual necrosis. Frequent dressing changes help to maintain a dry area around the drain site. Pectin patches may be cut to fit around drains and permit sterile bags or dressings to be secured and frequently changed without skin irritation.

As drainage decreases and the patient improves clinically, drains are advanced and removed. Wound care may include the application of wet-to-dry saline-soaked dressings to drainage sites to facilitate closure.

Pulmonary Insufficiency Secondary to Liver Injury

Atelectasis, pleural effusion, or pneumonia may occur from hepatomegaly protruding on the right lobes of the lung, chemical irritation of blood or bile on pleural tissue, or inability of the lung to fully expand due to pain from the injury or repair. Pulmonary complications are seen in 20 to 30 per cent of survivors of hepatic injury.[47] Prolonged shock secondary to hemorrhage and sepsis predisposes the patient to the development of adult respiratory distress syndrome. Mechanical ventilation is frequently necessary for days following surgical repair of the liver damage, and respiratory care continues until pulmonary function is restored.

A thorough respiratory care regimen is necessary to maintain adequate ventilation throughout hospitalization. (See Chapter 19 for additional information.)

Involving the patient and family in respiratory care facilitates the patient's sense of control over his situation. Patients who have sustained substantial liver damage may be discharged with drains in place or the need for drain wound care. Education about care procedures and clean technique when changing dressings is necessary. Demonstration of correct technique with return demonstration by the patient or family members allows evaluation of the wound care instruction. Symptoms of infection at the site should be

TABLE 20–3. SPLENIC INJURY SCALE

GRADE*		INJURY DESCRIPTION†	ICD-9	AIS 85	AIS 90
I.	Hematoma:	Subcapsular, nonexpanding, <10% surface area	865.01 865.11	2	2
	Laceration:	Capsular tear, nonbleeding, <1 cm parenchymal depth	865.02 865.12		
II.	Hematoma:	Subcapsular, nonexpanding, 10–50% surface Intraparenchymal, nonexpanding, <2 cm in diameter	865.01 865.11	2	2
	Laceration:	Capsular tear, active bleeding; 1–3 cm of parenchymal depth which does not involve a trabecular vessel	865.02 865.12	2	2
III.	Hematoma:	Subcapsular, >50% surface area or expanding Ruptured subcapsular hematoma with active bleeding Intraparenchymal hematoma >2 cm or expanding		3	3
	Laceration:	3 cm parenchymal depth or involving trabecular vessels	865.03 865.13	3	3
IV.	Hematoma:	Ruptured intraparenchymal hematoma with active bleeding		3	4
	Laceration:	Laceration involving segmental or hilar vessels producing major devascularization (>25% of spleen)	865.04 865.14	3	4
V.	Laceration:	Completely shattered spleen	865.04 865.14	5	5
	Vascular:	Hilar vascular injury which devascularizes spleen		5	5

*Advance one grade for multiple injuries to the same organ.
†Based on most accurate assessment at autopsy, laparotomy, or radiologic study.
Developed by the Organ Injury Scaling (OIS) Committee of the American Association for the Surgery of Trauma (AAST). From Moore EE, Shackford SR, Pachter HL, et al: Organ injury scaling: Spleen, liver and kidney. J Trauma 29:1664, 1989.

written down, and the patient should understand when there is a need to report changes to the physician.

The patient's body image has been altered, and his ability to look at and care for the wounds should be assessed. A family member, a friend, or a visiting nurse may be able to help the individual who has difficulty with caring for the wound.

Disruption of Organ Integrity Related to Splenic Injury

The spleen is the most commonly injured organ in blunt abdominal trauma. Its anatomical location makes it a frequent victim of penetrating trauma to the LUQ. Although the lower ribs in the LUQ provide some protection to the spleen, fracture of these ribs renders it vulnerable to injury. The mortality rate from splenic injury is dependent on the type of trauma (blunt versus penetrating) and the presence of associated injuries. Isolated splenic trauma has little to no mortality associated with it; however, this type of injury accounts for less than 20 per cent of all splenic trauma.[59]

Overall mortality for patients with splenic injury is reported at 11 per cent.[60] Associated injury increases the mortality to 25 per cent. Mortality is related to uncontrolled hemorrhage either initially or in delayed rupture and sepsis.

Initial Assessment. The index of suspicion is based on the description of the accident. Penetrating or blunt injury to the LUQ should immediately signal possible splenic damage. Specific clinical signs of peritoneal irritation, hemorrhage, or tenderness of adjacent chest or abdominal wall may occur but only signal abdominal trauma. They are not considered organ-specific and may be attributed to associated injuries. LUQ pain, Kehr's sign, Ballance's sign (fixed dullness to percussion in the left flank and dullness in the right flank that disappears on change of position), local tenderness, or spasm is elicited frequently after splenic injury.

Signs of hemorrhage may be present, but they vary with the degree of injury and the time from injury to examination. Patients with splenic rupture will often present with signs of profound bleeding, e.g., hypotension, tachycardia, and rapid respiratory rate. Delayed rupture or the slow, hidden hemorrhagic process may not be evident for hours or days following the injury. This process slowly presents with signs of hypovolemia and peritonitis.

Subcapsular hematoma is insidious. Trauma to the splenic tissue causes local bleeding that is encapsulated. The expanding hematoma may force splenic rupture later, producing signs of profound shock.

Diagnostic Testing. Abdominal films are reviewed for signs of increased splenic shadow and loss of normal outline of the spleen, the left kidney, or the left psoas muscle.[3] The most common finding with splenic injury is free blood in the abdomen. At least 800 ml of intraperitoneal blood must be present to show on abdominal x-ray.[61] A CT scan can be the most accurate diagnostic test if the patient is sufficiently stable to have the test completed.[62] Chest films rule out hemothorax as the source for blood loss during suspected hemorrhage and help to focus on the abdomen. The lack of chest wall integrity may lead one to suspect splenic injury. Fractures of the eighth, ninth, and tenth ribs are associated with a 20 per cent chance of splenic rupture.[7]

Laboratory values such as elevated WBC count of 15,000 to 20,000/mm^3 are seen. Falling hemoglobin and hematocrit levels support suspicion of hemorrhage.

Team Management. Management of splenic trauma is dependent on the patient's age, physiological stability, associated injuries, and type of splenic disruption.[61] Splenic injury is graded on an organ injury scale produced by the American Association for the Surgery of Trauma[44] (Table 20–3). Splenic injury is graded from I to V with descriptions for hematoma formation and degree of laceration. Grade V includes a description of vascular injury as well.

Medical management of splenic injury has changed over the years as the role of the spleen in maintaining immunocompetence has been appreciated. Trunkey notes five functions of the spleen.[7] The first four affect the trauma patient's immunocompetence after injury:

1. Filters particulate matter
2. Source of opsonins: tuftsin and properdin
3. Source of immunoglobulin (IgM)
4. Regulates T and B lymphocytes
5. Source of hematopoiesis in utero

Following a splenectomy, the loss of antibody formation, bacterial filtration, and enhanced phagocytosis have led to overwhelming postsplenectomy infection (OPSI). First described by King and Schumacher[63] in children following splenectomy, OPSI has been reported with greater frequency in adults. Therefore, splenorrhaphy and partial splenectomy are recommended methods of treatment.[64–67] Splenorrhaphy is accomplished by generating hemostasis through the use of topical hemostatic agents,[68, 69] direct pressure, absorbable mesh[70, 71] to attain a tamponade effect, the argon beam coagulator,[72, 73] and/or suture repair.

The argon beam coagulator (ABC) is an electrocoagulation device that transmits radiofrequency electrical energy across a jet of argon gas.[72, 73] The gas blows away blood and debris to optimize visualization. Energy transferred through the stream to the tissue surface provides coagulation.[72] The ABC decreases the time required to achieve hemostasis and improves the prospect for successful splenorrhaphy.[72, 74]

Partial splenectomy is necessary for splenic fractures with deep parenchymal involvement.[61] The amount of preserved splenic mass correlates with resistance against infection.[75]

Splenectomy is the procedure of choice for those whose spleen has been separated from its blood supply, those in whom hemostasis cannot be secured, or those with total maceration of splenic parenchyma or multiple concomitant injuries.[76] In all other splenic damage, splenorrhaphy may be attempted.

Drainage of the splenic bed is controversial. Normally, drainage after splenorrhaphy or splenectomy is not necessary unless associated injuries require it.[77] Drainage has been advocated when pancreatic manipulation is necessary to remove pancreatic enzymes released by operative trauma. A higher incidence of subphrenic abscess has been reported with drain use. This has led to the recommendation for active, closed drainage, such as a Jackson-Pratt drain, for 24 hours or less, when necessary. Pachter et al.[78] reported no postsplenectomy complications among patients randomly assigned to groups receiving no drainage or drainage with a Jackson-Pratt tube. Of the group drained with Penrose drains, one produced a subphrenic abscess and one incurred small bowel evisceration through the drain site. Pachter et al. suggested that associated gastrointestinal injuries and duration of drainage play a greater role in influencing infection after splenectomy.

Postoperative complications include abscess formation, bleeding, pancreatitis, thromboembolic phenomena, and infection. These complications may occur immediately or several days to weeks postoperatively.

Nursing Management. Nursing interventions change throughout the cycles. In the resuscitation and critical care stages, the patient is assessed for LUQ pain, Kehr's sign, Ballance's sign, or local tenderness. In addition, signs of hemorrhage or peritonitis are elicited. The patient with any history of chest or abdominal injury is observed closely and at frequent intervals for signs of volume depletion. Changes in blood pressure and heart rate are specifically noted, because hypotension and tachycardia may indicate hemorrhage. Subcapsular bleeding may not be evident for hours to days after trauma. A patient who initially reported some LUQ pain may find this has subsided, only to recur when the bleeding is no longer contained within the capsule. Abdominal pain, rigidity, or rebound tenderness may be evident if bleeding has irritated the peritoneal space.

Loss of blood volume secondary to hemorrhage following splenic repair can be a lethal complication. Postoperatively, the patient is closely monitored for hemodynamic stability, increasing abdominal pain, and distention. Repeated surgical intervention is necessary to drain the blood and prevent abscess formation if rebleeding becomes evident.

Thrombus formation secondary to a rebound elevation of thrombocytes may produce embolic processes following splenic injury and repair. Low-molecular-weight dextran or enteric-coated aspirin may be ordered in the early postoperative period until anticoagulation is feasible.[7] Antiembolism stockings and early mobilization may help to deter thrombus formation.

Infection or sepsis related to the loss of immune support from the spleen is a long-term possibility for those having experienced a splenectomy. More than 50 per cent of these infections are caused by pneumococcus.[79] Therefore, postsplenectomy patients should receive polyvalent pneumococcal vaccine prior to discharge from the hospital. Caplan et al. suggest that splenectomized patients receive polyvalent pneumococcal vaccine within 72 hours of surgery to ensure that all patients are appropriately vaccinated.[79] Continuous antibiotic support is controversial in children and not advocated for adults. (See Chapter 11 for further information.) Patient education should include observation for signs of an infection and the necessity to notify a physician if these symptoms are present. Medic-Alert bracelets noting that the patient is lacking a spleen have been advocated as well.

Disruption of Organ Integrity Related to Pancreatic Injury

Two-thirds of all pancreatic trauma is penetrating injury.[80] The majority are gunshot wounds at close range or high velocity, thereby causing injury to the pancreas and surrounding organs.[81] However, blunt injury is reported with increasing frequency and is associated with the deceleration impact of a steering wheel. Because the pancreas is a retroperitoneal structure, symptoms of injury may not be evident until 12 to 24 hours following the traumatic incident. In addition, the location of the pancreas and its proximity to other organs and vessels make multiorgan injury a frequent occurrence, thereby masking symptoms of pancreatic injury. Injuries to the liver, spleen, and major arteries and veins are associated with pancreatic injury greater than 40 per cent of the time.[82]

Kudsk et al.[83] noted that isolated pancreatic injuries are difficult to detect because pancreatic enzymes may remain inactivated following injury and generate little tissue reaction. Diagnosis of pancreatic injury is complicated by pancreatic spillage confined to the retroperitoneum, therefore not eliciting peritoneal signs; pancreatic secretion is suppressed after trauma to the organ; simultaneous injuries may draw attention away from or mask mild epigastric symptoms; and diagnostic tests to confirm pancreatic injury are unreliable.

Mortality rates are reported as high as 50 per cent for blunt pancreatic injury, 25 per cent for gunshot wounds, and 8 per cent for stab wounds.[1] These frequently reflect injuries to associated organs.[1] Hemorrhage and sepsis are the most frequent causes of death associated with pancreatic injury. Complications include pseudocyst formation, pancreatic abscess, recurrent hemorrhage, and pancreatitis. Pseudocyst and abscess formation are frequently due to inadequate drainage following injury.

Initial Assessment. Abdominal tenderness over the pancreatic area may manifest itself. An ileus and elevated serum amylase and lipase levels may be present. Maintaining an index of suspicion based on the mechanism of injury and drawing serial amylase levels to ascertain elevation over time may be the best means of detecting pancreatic injury. Patients will ultimately develop significant epigastric pain radiating to the back, nausea, vomiting, and tenderness to deep palpation.[81] Peritoneal lavage is of limited usefulness in the detection of pancreatic injury because the presence of amylase in the peritoneal fluid may be due to other visceral damage. CT scans are ordered with increasing frequency.

Medical Management. Medical management depends on the extent of pancreatic injury, which may range from simple lacerations to pancreatic transections. Duct injury complicates repair procedures. Thal et al.[14] classify pancreatic injury into four groups: simple pancreatic contusion without rupture of the capsule or hemorrhage, more severe contusion and disruption of the parenchyma with rupture of the capsule, severe pancreatic injury with disruption of the ductal system, and combined pancreatic and duodenal injury. The goals of surgery are control of hemorrhage, debridement of devitalized tissue, and provision of adequate drainage. Treatment options are dictated by the site and severity of pancreatic injury. Treatment may consist of drainage alone or simple resection to roux-en-Y pancreaticojejunostomy.[1] Occasionally, pancreaticoduodenectomy is necessary for combined extensive pancreatic and duodenal injury.

Regardless of the extent of injury, drainage of the area is necessary. The use of Penrose drains or closed-system sump drains is advocated. Closed-system drainage has been reported to decrease the possibility of pancreatic fistula formation.[84] However, Jordan suggests that this is not the widespread experience and recommends the use of Penrose drains, replaced with a suction drain if a fistula develops.[82]

Drains are left in place to 10 days. When the patient is fed without resulting in increased quantity or change in quality of the drainage, drains can be removed. The drains are advanced slowly over a few days to allow healing of the tract.

Nursing Management. Nursing management in the resuscitation cycle is management of hemorrhage, because this remains the greatest cause of death following pancreatic injury. Maintaining the index of suspicion is necessary, since barring hemorrhage, few signs specific to pancreatic injury may appear initially.

The pancreas has both exocrine and endocrine properties. The exocrine function is the production of fluid rich in enzymes, electrolytes, and bicarbonate used to aid digestion and absorption in the small intestine. Trauma to the pancreatic tissue may affect digestion of fats and fat-soluble substances as well as protein and starches. In addition, these same potent digestive enzymes may work to break down normal tissue if leaked after pancreatic injury. Fistula formation, development of a pancreatic abscess, and pseudocyst formation are complications of pancreatic injury.

Through the resuscitation and critical care cycles, signs of peritonitis become evident as enzymes leak into the peritoneal cavity. Sustained elevated serum amylase levels suggest pancreatic injury. Postoperatively, maintenance of the drainage system and monitoring fluid and electrolyte balance are necessary. Acute pancreatic inflammation can cause fluid sequestration from the intravascular volume to the peritoneal and retroperitoneal spaces. Crystalloid and colloid replacement is necessary to prevent profound dehydration.

The endocrine function of the pancreas includes the secretion of insulin, glucagon, and gastrin involved in the breakdown and increased utilization of glucose in the liver as well as stimulation of the digestive process of the stomach. Injury to the pancreas may alter glucose metabolism in the body significantly.

Glucose intolerance may manifest itself if more than 80 per cent of the pancreas has been removed. Protein and fat metabolism may be altered in the absence of adequate amylase, lipase, and trypsin secretion. Hypocalcemia secondary to calcium binding with fatty acids released from fat necrosis after injury produces symptoms of muscle cramping; tingling fingers, toes, and mouth; hyperactive reflexes; impaired mental functioning; seizures; and positive Chvostek or Trousseau sign. Monitoring the calcium level, observing EKG for electrical changes, and intravenous replacement of calcium as needed may be ordered.

During the intermediate cycle of care, a pancreatic fistula may appear. This is the most common complication of pancreatic injury. Fistulas develop if pancreatic enzymes continue to pour into a tract leading to the peritoneum and/or the abdominal wall. Fistulas are classified by volume of output: Minor fistulas produce less than 200 ml/day, moderate fistulas produce 200 to 700 ml/day, and major fistulas produce greater than 700 ml/day.[85] Output may be as great as 2000 ml/day.[85] Therefore, fluid volume replacement is necessary. Nursing care includes maintenance of the drainage system and removing secretions that may leak around the system and cause skin breakdown. Skin care includes using a protective agent such as a pectin wafer or magnesium paste on the skin at the drain site. When drainage is changed from sump drainage to passive-flow drainage, ostomy bags may be used to collect effluent.

Fluid and electrolyte balance must be monitored due to the high drainage output and the electrolyte-rich nature of this effluent. Bicarbonate replacement may be necessary to keep a chronic acidosis from occurring, since the pancreatic secretions are rich in bicarbonate, enzymes, and electrolytes. In the past, hyperalimentation has been ordered to meet nutritional demands and bypass gastric and intestinal stimulation of the pancreas caused by oral intake. Jordan notes that "although oral intake does stimulate pancreatic secretion, the degree of stimulation is not sufficient to warrant continuous IV hyperalimentation once the patient is able to ingest an adequate diet."[82] Others have recommended jejunal feedings with elemental diet.[86] Certain agents, such as somatostatin, decrease pancreatic secretion and may be ordered as part of the fistula treatment plan.[87] Care of the patient with a fistula is supportive. The patient is placed on bed rest to minimize the metabolic demand for pancreatic output.

Pain management is necessary for patients with pancreatic injury. Patients describe the sensation as "burrowing pain to the back." Meperidine is frequently the drug of choice for pain relief, since it causes less sphincter spasm than does morphine.[88]

Pancreatic pseudocysts may form months after the initial injury, causing release of fluid enzymes and necrotic tissue. This material is contained within a fibrous wall and can become a source of bacterial contamination or abscess formation. Symptoms include pain, nausea, vomiting, and an abdominal mass on palpation. Serum amylase levels elevate and remain elevated. Internal surgical drainage or percutaneous drainage is used to treat pseudocysts.

Nursing management is focused toward early recognition of the pseudocyst to help prevent abscess formation or bacterial contamination. Because pseudocyst formation is most common following blunt pancreatic trauma, the nurse should be alert for this complication when caring for the patient with blunt pancreatic injury.

Pancreatitis Secondary to Organ Disruption

The trauma patient who has experienced injury to the pancreas may develop acute or chronic pancreatitis. Acute pancreatitis is a process of autodigestion brought on by the activation of pancreatic enzymes, causing an inflammatory process. Recurrent episodes of the acute process cause sufficient functional impairment to become a chronic process.

Acute Pancreatitis

Normally, pancreatic enzymes are not activated until they reach the duodenum. The specific cause for activation of these enzymes after trauma is not understood. However, their activation creates an autodigestive state that presents as interstitial edematous pancreatitis or hemorrhagic/necrotic pancreatitis. Interstitial pancreatitis is characterized by edema with exudation. Hemorrhagic pancreatitis occurs when there is tissue necrosis, causing ischemia and bleeding into pancreatic tissue and the retroperitoneal space. Further complications include pseudocyst, abscess development, or pancreatic ascites.

Initial Assessment. Usually occurring on the second to third day after injury, the patient experiences sudden development of pain radiating to the back, which increases if the patient lies flat. The specific location of the pain may indicate which part of the pancreas is involved; e.g., lesions of the tail produce LUQ pain; of the body, epigastric pain; and of the head, RUQ pain. The pain may be accompanied by vomiting and fever, abdominal distention, peritonitis, weakness, and dyspnea.

Vasodilation and an increase in vascular permeability secondary to release of kinins may produce circulatory shock.[5] Diaphoresis, tachycardia, hypotension, and abdominal rigidity may be indicative of shock in acute pancreatitis.[89] This may be accompanied by a paralytic ileus as well. Thompson et al.[5] pointed out that these patients are susceptible to adult respiratory distress syndrome (ARDS) with intrapulmonary shunting and edema due to disruption of the alveolar-capillary membrane. Altered renal function and disseminated intravascular coagulation (DIC) have been noted as well.[5] Hemorrhagic pancreatitis may produce Grey-Turner sign (bluish brown discoloration of the flank) or Cullen sign (bluish discoloration around the umbilicus) as blood extravasates into surrounding tissue.

Diagnostic Tests. Serum and urine amylase levels are elevated. Usually, serum levels rise (greater than 500 U/dl) within 12 hours of onset and decline to normal (60 to 180 U/dl) by 72 hours. The urinary amylase value remains elevated for 72 to 120 hours. Lipase values become elevated as fatty necrosis of the omentum develops. Hyperglycemia due to a decreased release of insulin and hypocalcemia and hypokalemia may occur.

Radiographical studies, CT, and ultrasonography may be ordered to detect calcification of pancreatic ducts, abscesses, pseudocyst, hematoma, or ileus. An EKG to monitor effects of hypocalcemia and hyperkalemia may be ordered.

Team Management. Therapeutic interventions include hemodynamic stabilization, reducing pancreatic stress, and surgical correction if a pseudocyst, abscess formation, or common duct obstruction occurs. Fluid therapy is required to maintain intravascular volume as fluid is lost to the retroperitoneal space, peritoneal cavity, and bowel.

Nasogastric suction is utilized to remove hydrochloric acid that may stimulate release of pancreatic enzymes. Antibiotics are used in hemorrhagic pancreatitis and when an abscess is suspected. Narcotic analgesics are ordered after initial laboratory work has been obtained; many of these compounds elevate amylase and lipase levels. Nutritional therapy in the form of total parenteral nutrition (TPN) or jejunostomy feedings is necessary.

Nursing Interventions. Nursing goals are congruent with medical management as care is planned to deal with potential volume deficits, pain control, alteration in nutrition, electrolyte imbalance, potential for complications such as peritonitis and pseudocyst formation, and patient and family anxiety.

Acute pancreatitis may manifest itself in the critical care or intermediate care cycle. Frequently, the patient has stabilized and begun the recovery process when signs of pancreatitis appear. Therefore, patient and family anxiety often recurs as they recognize the acuity of the situation. Assessment of the patient's and family's anxiety, knowledge of the disease process, and an understanding of diagnostic procedures and treatment regimen will permit development of an adequate plan of care to help them cope with the anxiety.

Pancreatitis can be extremely painful. Nursing measures planned to assist the patient to find a comfortable position and effective analgesia are priorities.

Fluid volume deficits require close monitoring of hemodynamic values such as CVP, pulmonary artery pressure (PAP), blood pressure, and heart rate. Urinary output and daily weights are measured. Replacement fluids, including intravenous fluids, dextran, blood, or blood products, are administered. Hemoglobin and hematocrit are monitored for signs of bleeding. The alteration in nutritional status that occurs as a result of pancreatic dysfunction requires reducing the metabolic demand to a minimum; feeding the patient through TPN or jejunal feedings; and monitoring digestive enzymes, insulin, and glucagon. Bedside glucometers allow the nurse to measure blood glucose levels routinely with a minimal blood sample.

Chronic pancreatitis may develop as an aftermath of multiple bouts with acute pancreatitis following traumatic injury. Jordan notes that chronic posttraumatic pancreatitis occurs in patients who sustained some degree of injury to the major pancreatic duct with resulting obstruction.[82] He recommends endoscopic retrograde pancreatography to identify ductal stricture. Because this condition affects the patient's nutritional status, comfort level, and potential for further complications such as abscess formation, it is imperative that patient education in the intermediate care and rehabilitation phases address this process. The cause of pancreatitis and its relationship to alcohol intake or gallstones should be reviewed. Written dietary instructions and medication instructions should be sent home with the individual. Signs of diabetes mellitus and information regarding insulin therapy, if needed, should be reviewed. The patient is directed to contact the physician if any of the symptoms occur.

Disruption in Organ Integrity Related to Small Bowel Injuries

The small bowel is composed of the duodenum, ileum, and jejunum. It is the hollow viscus structure most frequently injured by penetrating trauma. The incidence of intestinal injury from gunshot wounds alone is 80 per cent.[90]

The spleen and the liver are the only intra-abdominal organs injured more frequently than the small bowel as a result of blunt trauma.[40] In blunt small intestinal trauma, the most common sites of intestinal rupture are the proximal jejunum and the terminal ileum.[40, 81] The mechanism for injury includes direct blows, shearing forces, and pseudo-closed loop obstruction. Direct blows crush the intestine between the force and the spinal column. Shearing forces occur from rapid deceleration, as in a motor vehicle accident. Pseudo-closed loop obstruction occurs when a segment of bowel, partially filled with gas, food, or succus entericus, becomes entrapped between an external force and a firm anatomical object, creating a closed loop. Schwab et al. note in this instance that even a small amount of external force can generate a bursting pressure.[40]

Duodenal Injuries

Because of its location, the duodenum is seldom a single-organ injury. Duodenal injuries frequently occur in association with pancreatic, bile duct, or vena caval trauma. As a predominantly retroperitoneal structure, it provides a diagnostic challenge because peritoneal symptoms may not be immediately evident. The duodenum is generally sterile, and when injured, it does not produce early signs of bacterial peritonitis, as do colon injuries. In addition, morbidity and mortality rise significantly with a delay in treatment. Delay in treatment allows contamination of the retroperitoneal and peritoneal spaces with bile, pancreatic enzymes, and gastric secretions, resulting in peritonitis. This may lead to complications such as fistula formation and wound dehiscence from duodenal wall edema and inflammation. Therefore, it is necessary to maintain an index of suspicion with lower thoracic or abdominal injury. Blunt injury to the duodenum also can produce an intramural hematoma which may cause a partial or complete obstruction.

Jejunum and Ileum

The ileum and jejunum have a neutral pH and, like the duodenum, are bacteria sparse. Therefore, the clinical signs of injury may not be present initially. As bacterial growth occurs, signs of peritonitis become evident.

Assessment and Management of Small Bowel Injuries

Initial Assessment. The index of suspicion should be raised any time the patient presents with upper abdominal or lower chest injury. Testicular pain may indicate retroperitoneal duodenal rupture. Referred pain in the shoulder, chest, or back is also indicative of duodenal injury. The patient may experience mild abdominal tenderness unless a large amount of duodenal contents has spilled. The high alkalinity in the duodenum produces immediate chemical irritation.

Fever, jaundice, high intestinal obstruction, and third-space fluid loss are signs of retroperitoneal duodenal injury. Hyperamylasemia, hyperbilirubinemia, and retroperitoneal air may be seen. Patients with penetrating duodenal injury may present with bile staining of adjacent tissues (appreciated on laparotomy), retroperitoneal hematoma, or crepitation.

Jejunal and ileal injury produce abdominal pain, tenderness, guarding, decreased or absent bowel sounds, and signs of hypovolemia.[91] Because delayed rupture of the small intestine is possible, close observation for such symptoms should be maintained for 48 to 72 hours.

Diagnostic Testing. Diagnostic tests include peritoneal lavage for blood, bile, or small bowel contents. Upright chest film, plain abdominal films, and CT may show free air in the abdomen or stippling of the retroperitoneal space. Lucas and Ledgerwood[92] noted that 90 per cent of the patients sustaining small bowel injury produced nonspecific radiographical findings in the first 12 hours after injury.

Medical Management. Donohue et al.[93] noted that operative management of wounds to the jejunum and ileum is usually straightforward. Simple lacerations receive primary closure, complex or multiple injuries are resected, and ischemic bowel is debrided or resected. It is imperative in any small bowel injury to examine both sides of the bowel carefully to prevent missing a perforation. Compromised blood supply from the mesentery usually dictates resection and anastomosis to guard against perforation secondary to devitalized bowel.[94] Reexploration may be necessary in 24 to 48 hours when there is a question regarding the integrity of the repair.[94] Peritoneal contamination necessitates irrigation prior to closure. Bowel edema may preclude abdominal closure initially. Schwab recommends closing the skin and subcutaneous tissue and repairing the ventral hernia later.[40] In certain situations it may prove beneficial to leave open the subcutaneous tissue and skin.

Management of duodenal injury is not as clear-cut as that described for jejunal or ileal injury. Leak from a duodenal repair may be lethal. Primary repair may be considered. However, complex wounds require resection, serosal patching, end-to-end anastomosis, or diversion of biliary injury.[93] Selection of a surgical procedure depends on the patient's hemodynamic stability and the presence of single-organ injury versus pancreatic or bile duct involvement with the duodenal injury. Postoperatively, decompression through a nasogastric tube is ordered to reduce acid stimulation of the small intestine. This may continue 5 to 7 days postoperatively. Antibiotics may be ordered if peritoneal contamination is present. Oral intake begins when bowel activity returns. Postoperative complications include fistula formation, suture line leakage, wound or intraperitoneal infections, ischemic bowel, bowel obstruction, and abscess formation.

Nursing Management. The lack of specific initial symptoms with small bowel injury directs the nurse to carefully evaluate the information presented as the patient is admitted from the scene of the accident. Any blow to the abdomen or penetrating wound of the lower chest or abdomen should raise the index of suspicion toward possible bowel injury. Spinal injury frequently occurs in conjunction with small bowel trauma and may mask presenting symptoms. Because delayed bowel rupture may occur, assessment should continue for 48 to 72 hours after the initial injury.

Postoperatively, decompression and drainage of the bowel and its contents, secretions, enzymes, blood, and bile are accomplished through use of nasogastric, gastrostomy, jejunostomy, or T-tubes. Assessment of exudate includes recording the character, amount, and odor of drainage and reporting changes in them. Testing drainage for blood or pH may be ordered.

Fluid that may cause abscess or fistula tract formation is drained from the operative area through Penrose or sump drainage. The sump systems require maintenance of drainage and vent portals to prevent occlusion of the drain. Combination jejunostomy tubes may be used to accomplish decompression as well as to act as a feeding port, especially if fistula formation occurs.

The potential for fluid volume deficit, infection, hemorrhage, impaired skin integrity, alteration in comfort, ineffective breathing patterns, altered nutritional status, and altered tissue perfusion are nursing care issues that must be addressed in both the critical care and intermediate care cycles.

Altered breathing patterns related to pain from an abdominal incision and abdominal distention are not unlike the problems experienced by any abdominal surgical patient. Careful monitoring of arterial blood gases and aggressive pulmonary care combined with pain management should be ordered throughout the critical and intermediate care cycles.

Altered tissue perfusion is exacerbated by postoperative complications such as hemorrhage, ischemic bowel with obstruction, or the presence of an infectious process. Monitoring signs of hemodynamic stability such as blood pressure, heart rate, CVP, and cardiac output is routine. Noncorrectable hypovolemia indicates the need to reoperate. Observing for signs of abdominal distention, increased abdominal or referred pain, and changes in incisional integrity may indicate the presence of infection, deterioration of any anastomosis, or blockage of the blood supply to the bowel. Early operative intervention may prevent further deterioration secondary to sepsis or abscess formation resulting from these complications.

The potential for fluid volume deficit related to nasogastric or intestinal suctioning, abdominal wound drainage, fistula formation, or paralytic ileus is present. Postoperatively, fluid shifts to the bowel wall or irritated peritoneum may decrease vascular volume. Continuous gastrointestinal suctioning depletes electrolytes and must be monitored closely, since decompression may be necessary for some time, requiring replacement therapy. Fluid output from wound and fistula tracts is measured to guard against dehydration and to replace necessary electrolytes. The patient's hydration status is monitored through blood pressure, skin turgor, and mucous membranes.

Altered nutritional status may occur if supplemental nutrition is not initiated soon after surgery. Alternate feeding modalities may have to be explored. Moore and Jones point out that liberal use of a feeding jejunostomy with this patient group has eliminated the use of parenteral hyperalimentation in all but a few patients.[95] Malabsorption syndrome may occur if the patient has undergone extensive bowel resection. Loss of greater than 200 cm of small bowel alters bacterial flora and decreases absorptive segments.[96]

Skin integrity may be impaired by the drainage from wound or fistula tracts. Moisture maceration, tape burn, and blocked drainage tubes all irritate the skin surface. Frequently, contaminated bowel injuries are not closed initially and thus require wet-to-dry saline wound care. Moist dressings should remain within the confines of the wound, and Montgomery straps, pectin wafers, or other reusable dressing supports should be evaluated for use. These decrease the skin irritation associated with frequent dressing changes and tape replacement. Blocked sump drainage systems permit intestinal exudate to drain out around the tube itself. Often rich in enzymes, this fluid irritates the skin surface, causing inflammation and breakdown. Adequate maintenance of the tubes includes assessing suction and vent systems to ensure patency.

Wound dehiscence may occur secondary to edema formation in the intestinal wall or peritoneal cavity contamination. Loss of incisional integrity will most often be seen in the early postoperative or critical care cycle. Delayed healing and wound care are dealt with in the intermediate care and rehabilitation cycles. (See Chapter 13 for additional information on wound healing.) Delayed primary closure may be selected if the wound is suspected of being contaminated. Wound infections necessitate reopening the site and permitting secondary closure to occur.

Patient teaching may begin as soon as the patient is capable of understanding the injury and care needs. Active involvement in wound care is one means of permitting the patient to regain control over his situation. The extent of injury and the presence of a complication such as abscess or fistula formation will dictate the length of time needed for an alternate feeding modality and for healing to occur. Involving the patient and family in nutritional assessment and wound care may permit the patient to continue the recuperative period at home. Patients whose injury has necessitated creation of an ostomy, temporary or permanent, will have to demonstrate adequate care technique before discharge is possible. The teaching plan should include information regarding the intestinal injury, extent of repair, and expected outcome. Written instructions include wound care, pain control, activity modification, nutritional needs, and importance of follow-up visits.

Disruption in Organ Integrity Related to Large Bowel Injuries

Trauma to the large bowel is one of the most lethal forms of abdominal injury, owing to the probability of sepsis related to fecal contamination of the abdomen. Five per cent of all abdominal injuries include the colon and rectum, and mortality and morbidity statistics are strongly affected by associated injury. Between 2 and 12 per cent mortality is reported.[14, 97]

In the civilian community, 96 per cent of all trauma to the colon and rectum is penetrating. Missile injuries account for 75 per cent of the injuries in this group, with the remaining injuries being caused by stab wounds or impalement injuries by falls. Rectal perforation from foreign objects may occur, as may iatrogenic injury during colonoscopy or barium enema, although this is uncommon. The ascending and descending colon account for 30 per cent of the perforations, whereas rectal injuries compose 10 per cent of trauma to the large intestines.[98]

Blunt trauma has been related to deceleration injuries involving impact with a seat belt or steering wheel. Pedestrian accidents, assaults, and falls also add to the small percentage of blunt colon/rectal trauma. Rectal laceration secondary to compound pelvic fracture should not be overlooked.

Blunt trauma has been reported to occur most frequently to the mobile transverse and sigmoid segments because their anatomical location makes them most vulnerable. The transverse colon also receives the most penetrating trauma. The majority of injuries are due to contusions, but delayed rupture is also reported.

Associated injuries affect survival. Only 10 to 25 per cent of colon or rectal injuries are isolated trauma. In studies of penetrating trauma, Karanfilian et al.[99] reported that mortality rates rose dramatically with three or more associated injuries. The length of time from injury to surgery affected morbidity and mortality as well.

Initial Assessment. The index of suspicion is raised if blunt abdominal trauma has occurred or if there is a penetrating wound near colon or rectal structures. A history of the event, including the wounding agent and proximity of the patient to the weapon, is helpful in determining the possibility of injury and necessary repair. The history also should include the time elapsed since the last meal, use of alcohol or other drugs, previous tetanus protection, operative procedures in the area, and illness affecting the colon or rectum.

The physical examination includes inspecting the abdomen, flanks, back, buttocks, perineum, and genitalia for signs of penetrating or blunt injury. Palpating for pain or muscle rigidity is necessary. Guarding and rebound tenderness are often present. Bowel sounds may be present initially but disappear over time. The rectal examination is completed to check for evidence of blood, which may further indicate the need for sigmoidoscopy or anoscopy. Certain signs of colon or rectal trauma may not become apparent for hours, and then abdominal pain, tenderness, fever, and leukocytosis become evident.

Diagnostic Tests. A peritoneal lavage may provide evidence of intra-abdominal bleeding and/or the presence of fecal contaminant. However, Nance suggests that most patients with colon injury have sufficient physical findings to warrant a laparotomy without the need for DPL.[97] Abdominal and chest films may show peritoneal free air if the bowel has been ruptured, but this sign is seldom present.

Team Management. Medical intervention is based on early recognition of injury and control of fecal contamination. A laparotomy is performed if colon or rectal perforation is suspected. Preoperative antibiotic therapy is ordered to control the probability of sepsis from enteric contamination.

Operative management includes control of hemorrhage and fecal leakage as well as irrigation to remove fecal material from the abdominal cavity. Anderson and Ballinger[1] outlined five alternatives in operative management: primary closure, primary resection and anastomosis, primary closure and proximal colostomy, resection with colostomy, and exteriorization. Operative technique is selected based on the extent and location of injury, the presence of shock, the extent of peritoneal soilage, associated injuries, and the amount of delay in surgical intervention. Historically, colostomy formation was the only acceptable surgical treatment for penetrating colonic injury.[100] However, in the 1970s, primary repair was advanced as the treatment of choice for all but the most serious colonic injuries.[101] Numerous studies have supported this selection.[97, 100, 102] Extraperitoneal rectal injuries require the use of drainage and copious irrigation to remove fecal material, as well as debridement and diverting colostomy.

Incisional infection is a recognized complication of colon and rectal injury. Therefore, delayed skin closure has been advocated.[81, 98] Nance proposes immediate wound closure unless direct fecal contamination of the subcutaneous tissue has occurred.[97] Drainage of colonic wounds is not necessary, but adequate drainage of rectal wounds with sump or closed-system suction is critical.[81, 97]

Intra-abdominal abscesses, wound infections, intestinal obstructions, colocutaneous fistula, and bowel ischemia may complicate recovery from colon or rectal injury.

Nursing Management. Maintaining an index of suspicion and performing recurrent abdominal examinations may help detect a colon or rectal injury and assist in timely medical intervention. Any impaled object that is present should remain in place and be removed under controlled conditions in the operating room.

Postoperative care demands attention to the possibility of peritoneal or incisional infection. Fluid and electrolyte therapy, nutritional supplementation, wound care, colostomy care, and maintenance of the drainage system are integral parts of the nursing care plan.

Alteration in Skin/Bowel Integrity Related to Colon/Rectal Wound

Wound care includes protection of any exteriorized bowel segments. Petrolatum or moist saline dressings are used, and the bowel is observed for signs of compromised blood supply. The skin surrounding the exteriorized loop should be protected from irritation produced by moisture. A second reconstructive surgery is frequently necessary when the possibility of peritonitis or other infectious process has been reduced, usually in 5 to 7 days.

Incisions made into the abdomen in the presence of fecal

contamination may become infected. For this reason, some wounds are not closed, and the subcutaneous fat and skin are kept open to assist drainage and decrease infection at the site. The wound closes by secondary intention. Dressings are ordered and include gauze moistened with saline and loosely packed in the wound. These are changed multiple times throughout the day to promote granulation of tissue.

Drainage of a wound is necessary when colon injuries include perineal wounds involving the rectum. Anterior or posterior drainage techniques are developed for the particular wound. Soft rubber drains (Penrose) or sump drains are utilized, depending on whether a posterior or anterior drainage site was selected.

Alteration in Elimination Secondary to Creation of a Stoma

Many patients will experience the creation of a temporary or permanent stoma, depending on the degree of tissue destruction and contamination to the area. Stoma care is dictated by the bowel segment that has been exteriorized. The sigmoid colon is the site of most permanent stoma creation and can be trained for systematic evacuation.

In the critical care stage, the stoma is observed for prolapse, retraction, necrosis, or stenosis. Surrounding tissue is observed for parastomal herniation or infection.

In the intermediate care cycle and moving toward rehabilitation, the nurse assesses the patient's self-concept and ability to adapt to the change in body image. Whether the creation of a stoma is temporary (2 weeks to 1 year) or permanent, patients must be encouraged to express their feelings regarding the presence of a stoma and be given the time to adjust accordingly.

The teaching plan outlines instructions for changing appliances, providing skin protection, controlling odor, dietary considerations, and irrigation techniques for sigmoid colostomies. The patient and/or a family member should demonstrate competence in the care of the stoma and surrounding skin prior to discharge.

Alteration in Fluid and Electrolyte Status Related to Intestinal Fistula Formation

Fluid and electrolyte balance is a concern through all aspects of the cycle when colon or rectal trauma occurs. Massive fluid resuscitation may not be necessary if a singular colon or rectal injury occurs. However, postoperative fluid and electrolyte management varies with the location of the injury.

Fistula formation is a recognized complication of colon and rectal trauma and may occur early or late in the postoperative period. Fluid output in a high-output fistula may exceed 200 ml per 24-hour period.[88] Increased metabolic demands that accompany an ensuing fever and local signs of infection make fluid management a challenge.

Assessment of electrolyte and fluid needs with concomitant replacement therapy, including blood products, is necessary. Fluid output from sump drains is measured as part of the intake and output record. The presence of a fistula may not be evident until the intermediate care cycle, but careful fluid and electrolyte management is crucial through all the cycles.

Alteration in Nutritional Status Related to Altered Bowel Integrity Secondary to Trauma

This is a concern after large bowel surgery, as it is following small intestinal injury. Refer to nursing diagnosis in that section for specific information.

Alteration in Organ Perfusion Related to Vascular Injury

Until recently, major vessel injuries were not seen in resuscitation areas or emergency departments because patients exsanguinated prior to transport. With an increase in skilled technicians and emergency resuscitation measures provided at the scene of the accident, more patients with vascular injury are being treated in medical facilities. The reported mortality for all vascular injury ranges from 30 to 60 per cent[1, 3, 103–106] (Table 20–4).

Vessels sustain contusions, lacerations, transections, or avulsion injuries. These occur as a result of penetrating or blunt injury, although the majority of severe damage to the vascular system occurs with penetrating trauma. Blunt injury to the abdominal vasculature by deceleration forces causes avulsion of small branches from major vessels or an intimal tear with secondary thrombosis of the lumen. Direct crush or blow forces cause intimal tears or flaps with secondary thrombosis of a vessel or complete disruption of exposed vessels resulting in intraperitoneal hemorrhage.[107] Penetrating injury causes intimal disruption with secondary thrombosis, lateral wall defects with hemorrhage or pulsatile hematoma, or complete transection with hemorrhage or thrombosis.[108]

Vascular injuries are divided into arterial and venous trauma. Although combination injuries may exist or complications such as arteriovenous fistulas may occur, understanding each system separately helps to direct assessment and intervention strategies.

TABLE 20–4. REPORTED MORTALITY IN VASCULAR INJURY

INJURY TO THE ARTERIAL SYSTEM	
Injured Vessel	**% Mortality**
Superior mesenteric artery	40–50
Aorta	50–70
Renal	25
Iliac	40–53
Celiac	30–60
Inferior mesenteric artery	30–60
INJURY TO THE VENOUS SYSTEM	
Injured Vessel	**% Mortality**
Inferior vena cava	30–53
Retrohepatic	80
Suprarenal	43
Renal	25
Infrarenal	27
Renal	56
Iliac	38
Portal	40–70
Superior mesenteric vein	40–70
Splenic	40–70
Inferior mesenteric vein	40–70

Arterial Injury

The artery, due to its elastic quality, may stop bleeding spontaneously after a clean transection occurs secondary to penetrating trauma. The transected intima curls inward, and the divided media contracts and pulls the adventitia over the end of the vessel. Partially transected vessels are unable to activate this process, and thus bleeding continues. In a partial laceration or transection, hematoma formation may occur, stopping further bleeding or leading to a false aneurysm that may rupture at a later date.

Contusions to the artery are usually secondary to blunt traumatic force or stretching motion on the vessel. Damage may initiate minor bleeding or progress to thrombus formation, occluding the vessel or embolizing distal vessels. Avulsion injury usually occurs with a deceleration event that pulls the artery from its base. In the abdomen, this most frequently occurs at the renal pedicle or the root of the mesentery.

Abdominal arterial injuries are sustained frequently in combination with pelvic, thoracic, or visceral injury. This complicates initial assessment, since specific signs of vascular injury may be obscure. For example, retroperitoneal hematoma, usually found in conjunction with pelvic or spine injury, may cause up to 4 liters of blood to collect in the retroperitoneal space. The presenting symptoms are similar to those of visceral rupture and hemorrhage: abdominal pain, back pain, hypoactive bowel sounds, or tender abdominal mass. Only later will flank discoloration become evident.

Patients presenting in shock of rapid onset without an obvious source of blood loss are suspected of having intra-abdominal injury to a major artery. Patients with abdominal aortic injuries sustained through penetrating trauma present in profound shock and require immediate operative intervention. The presence of a large retroperitoneal hematoma indicates aortic injury.

Team Management. Volume replacement is a priority, but in catastrophic hemorrhage, immediate surgery may be indicated because restoration of hemodynamic stability may be impossible without swift surgical intervention. Anderson and Ballinger[1] noted that exposure and proximal control of blood flow dominate the surgical approach. Primary anastomosis of the lacerated artery is attempted. Grafts may be necessary, and the use of autologous grafts is preferred because these injuries often exist in a contaminated field.

Postoperative care focuses on maintaining an adequate volume status and monitoring for signs of hemorrhage. Coagulopathy and acidosis are major complications following massive transfusion. Millikan and Moore[104] reported a 50 to 70 per cent mortality rate, with outcome affected by the presence of shock upon hospital arrival, associated intra-abdominal vascular injury, and retroperitoneal tamponade of aortic bleeding.

Surgical repair depends on the type and extent of injury. Most major abdominal arterial injuries receive lateral repair, end-to-end anastomosis, or a graft if narrowing of the artery would occur from primary repair. Autogenous tissue grafting, as opposed to use of prosthetic material, is preferred because many abdominal injuries are contaminated. Many major abdominal arteries can be ligated, which often becomes necessary when the site of vascular repair lies within a contaminated field.

Venous Injury

The venous system is a low-pressure system capable of realizing a tamponade effect from the pressure of surrounding tissues. Therefore, profuse bleeding (hemorrhage) must occur into a space at lower pressure, such as an external opening, a body cavity, or a cavity created after injury.

Conti[109] cited five reasons why trauma to the great intra-abdominal veins causes a greater problem than do similar arterial injuries:

1. Proximal control of arterial injuries usually stops hemorrhage, since with shock, distal collateral flow is relatively modest and back bleeding is not a major problem. Venous injuries, conversely, require both proximal and distal control, since distal pressure is raised, causing veins to bleed vigorously in both directions.
2. Whereas cross-clamping of the artery during shock results in very little change in collateral flow, cross-clamping of veins results in a marked increase in pressure, and collateral bleeding is augmented dramatically in all branches entering the injured segment. Proximal and distal control therefore does not necessarily result in control of hemorrhage.
3. Arteries have integrity and hold sutures well. Veins often have the consistency of wet tissue paper and tear with the application of clamps when sutured under tension.
4. Suture lines in large arteries rarely produce thrombotic problems, whereas suture lines in veins that expose raw surface produce a high risk of local thrombosis and embolism. Moreover, suture lines in veins tend to contract and obstruct flow with the passage of time, an unusual occurrence in arteries.
5. Prosthetic substitutes work relatively well in the arterial system and poorly, or not at all, in the venous system. Ligation of veins is a possibility owing to the existence of collateral circulation; however, this may have deleterious effects if the mesenteric, portal, or suprarenal vena cava is ligated.

The inferior vena cava (IVC) may be injured in four areas: juxtahepatic, suprarenal, perirenal, and infrarenal. The juxtahepatic injury carries the greatest mortality owing to its location behind the liver. Exposure of the injury is difficult.

Stewart and Stone[103] reported three factors affecting survival after injury to the IVC: preoperative hypotension, superior location of the injury, and associated vascular or visceral injury increased mortality. Death usually occurs as a result of hemorrhage, although sepsis from visceral damage or abdominal abscess will increase the mortality rate.

Diagnostic Testing. The severity of the vascular injury may not permit multiple diagnostic tests. Patients who appear in the resuscitation area in shock are usually quickly moved to the operating room for definitive diagnosis and treatment. However, in those patients who are more stable, certain diagnostic tests help to define the extent of injury.

Abdominal radiography can show the path of destruction caused by a missile and locate the missile if it has embolized. Doppler flow studies detect flow distal to an obstruction. Pressure differences from the uninjured area direct the need for arteriography. Postoperatively, the Doppler studies show the viability of repair. Angiography is used to rule out injury. In blunt vascular trauma, it localizes the injured area.

Team Management. Venous injury dictates the use of pressure and packing until the extent of injury is identified. Lateral repair, ligation, and venous replacement are used to treat venous injuries. Historically, complicated repairs lead to stenosis of the vessel and increased risk of thrombosis or embolism; therefore, ligation was used as a treatment of choice, except to repair suprarenal or intrahepatic vena cava injuries. More recently, Pasch et al. have advocated the aggressive approach of venous repair for the majority of venous injuries.[110]

Nursing Management. Nursing assessment and intervention in vascular injury demand active involvement in the resuscitation cycle to make the difference in patient outcome. Suspecting vascular injury when a patient has sustained lower thoracic or any abdominal injury will permit guided abdominal assessment and planning.

The patient may arrive in the resuscitation area in pneumatic antishock trousers. However, the use of this garment is controversial. Traverso et al.[111] and Aprahamian et al.[112] documented a positive effect after the use of the pneumatic antishock garment on shock and mortality of major intra-abdominal vascular injury. However, Mattox et al.,[113] in a prospective study, documented greater survival in the group treated without the garment. If the pneumatic antishock garment is in place, volume replacement and close monitoring of blood pressure and heart rate are necessary as the garment is deflated and removed. Hypotension may occur as the garment is removed, releasing the tamponade effect.

The extent of vascular injury may demand quick assessment, massive fluid resuscitation, and transport to the operating room for definitive diagnosis and treatment. Patient response to fluid resuscitation indicates the amount of time available for further diagnostic testing. If the patient becomes alert and produces signs of adequate perfusion, further testing, including arteriogram, may be ordered.

Balanced salt solution is used initially for massive resuscitation because coagulopathy is a significant concern when large quantities of blood are infused. Solutions should be warmed, if possible, to minimize the effects of hypothermia, which often accompanies large volume fluid replacement.

Stewart and Stone suggest the use of available volume expanders (buffered salt solution containing 5% glucose) while a cross-match of blood is completed.[103] Once cross-matched blood is available, it is transfused as rapidly as possible. If more than 8 units of transfused blood is required, then type-specific blood should be given, since there is no longer additional safety gained by a cross-match.

Inspection of extremities may show signs of ischemia, which is rare with single-vessel injury unless the common femoral artery or popliteal is occluded. Lack of ischemia, however, does not mean that vessel injury is absent. Hematoma formation that increases in size may indicate venous damage in the area.

Diminished or absent distal pulses may be detected by palpation. However, collateral circulation or pressure transmitted through an intimal flap or soft clot may permit normal pulses even with a vessel injury.

Auscultation for bruits continues throughout the cycles. Bruits may indicate partial thrombosis or arteriovenous fistula formation, which may be an early or late complication of vascular injury.

Postoperative nursing management is directed toward assessment and maintenance of the vascular repair. Routine monitoring of volume indicators, specifically blood pressure, heart rate, cardiac output, central venous pressure, pulmonary artery pressure, and urinary output, is necessary. Any tachycardia, hypotension, or decreased volume must be noted. In patients with major vascular injuries who have sustained prolonged shock or myocardial damage, pulmonary artery wedge pressure and cardiac output measurements may be necessary. Pressure support medications may be titrated to augment perfusion.

Perfusion should be assessed through pulses, color of skin distal to the repair, and urinary output. Cross-clamp time, when applicable, should be noted in order to assess disruption of flow to the renal system during vascular repair. Fluid challenge, low-dose dopamine infusion, or diuretic therapy may be ordered to assess and augment renal perfusion and function.

Pulse location and character, capillary refill, and signs of cyanosis or mottling are monitored. Pulse volume recordings (PVR) are assessed if pulses are not palpable. Doppler ultrasound may be used to detect blood flow velocity.

Hematocrit, hemoglobin, and coagulation studies are followed for signs of hemorrhage or hemodynamic instability secondary to coagulopathy. Anticoagulants are not routinely ordered following vascular repair; however, a low-molecular-weight dextran solution may be used for its viscosity-lowering effect and antiplatelet aggregating property.[114] Antibiotics are continued postoperatively only if the abdominal cavity has been contaminated through visceral damage.

Later in the cycle, if adequate vascular repair has been accomplished, routine monitoring of vital signs, perfusion, and the wound can ensue; however, infection may manifest itself in the intermediate and rehabilitation stages. Infection associated with vascular injury is usually secondary to peritoneal contamination. This may cause a disruption of the vascular repair, precipitating hemorrhage or thrombus formation at the repair site.

Wilson et al. noted six associated factors that seem to predispose an abdominal vascular injury to infection.[115] They are an initial systolic blood pressure less than 70 mm Hg, five or more organ injuries, initial operative systolic blood pressure less than 70 mm Hg, use of 10 or more units of blood, coincident thoracotomy, or colon injury. A patient who has presented with these signs should be observed closely for signs of infection.

Fever, tachycardia, abdominal tenderness, leukocytosis, increasing fluid demand, glucose intolerance, intravascular coagulation, and progressive failure of the lungs or liver are signs of intra-abdominal infection. Holcroft[114] noted the need for antibiotic therapy and surgical drainage as soon as infection is suspected.

Postoperative nursing management is directed toward assessment and maintenance of the integrity of the repair. This includes inspecting, palpating, and auscultating, as described before, and may include wound care for an exposed vessel. In this situation, specific wound management is directed by the physician and usually includes the use of wet saline dressings. The patient's mobility is constrained to decrease tension to the repair site. Elevation of involved distal extremities facilitates venous return. Antibiotics are administered.

Skin care to an extremity that has sustained vascular compromise includes protecting vulnerable areas such as

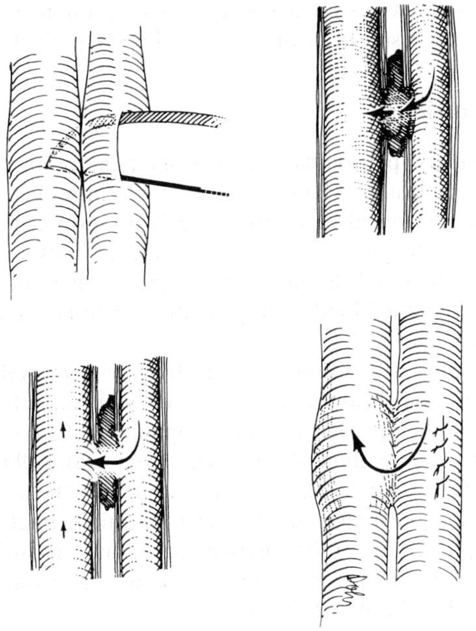

Figure 20–15. Arteriovenous fistula formation. (Reprinted with permission from WF Blaisdell, D Trunkey: Abdominal Trauma, Vol 1. New York, Thieme Medical Publishers, 1982.)

heels, ankles, and elbows from the effects of friction and pressure by using alternating pressure pads or water bags. Frequent position changes, assessment of vulnerable areas, and application of lotion to pressure points are appropriate nursing interventions.

Recognizing the potential for further disruption of the vascular repair secondary to infection that can affect the integrity of the vessel, the nurse must provide meticulous wound care and be alert to changes in quality of pulses in the area. The potential for vessel rupture requires close patient observation and pressure occlusion of the vessel if hemorrhage occurs.

Postoperative Bleeding Secondary to Vascular Injury

Bleeding after vascular repair may occur early or late in the postoperative period. Early hemorrhage is frequently due to the technical inadequacy of the repair or diathesis resulting from shock or dilution of clotting factors.[114] Late onset of bleeding is frequently secondary to the presence of infection.

Medical Management. Medical management is predicated on the source of bleeding. Holcroft[114] mentioned that bleeding that occurs intraoperatively from vessels, muscles, and other areas not previously bleeding denotes some degree of disseminated intravascular coagulopathy. Closing the abdomen may permit a tamponade effect, thus slowing bleeding stimulated by operative hypothermia, cardiac depression, and anesthesia. If this is done, reexploration in 24 hours to remove clots and forestall further bleeding is recommended.

Nursing Management. Nursing management is guided by the most likely cause of the bleeding. Immediate pressure to the repair site is necessary if the vascular repair is disrupted. Volume replacement and transfer to the OR for definitive therapy must be swift to save the patient's life.

Patients with postoperative bleeding secondary to prolonged clotting times require volume and blood component replacement. Close monitoring for signs of acute hemorrhage includes assessing the amount, consistency, and frequency of the bleeding. Laboratory tests should be reviewed to determine the degree of blood loss and effect of therapies. The skin and mucous membranes should be assessed for the presence of petechiae, purpura, or ecchymosis as signs of bleeding into the tissues. The nasogastric aspirate, urine, and stool must be checked for signs of occult or obvious bleeding. Gentle skin and oral care is required to prevent further tissue disruption. Wound care and intravenous site care are performed more often because oozing or dried blood will act as a medium for infectious growth.

Patients are usually fearful and anxious. The nurse must orient the patient and keep him informed. Describe all the therapies and the rationale for them. Encourage patients to express their concerns and let them know they will be monitored closely.

Arteriovenous Fistula Formation Secondary to Vascular Injury

Arteriovenous (AV) fistula formation is a complication of vascular injury which may occur early in the postoperative period or months following the initial injury. AV fistula occurs from a lacerated artery lying adjacent to a lacerated vein and arterial blood decompressing into the venous system (Fig. 20–15). The pressure of arterial blood flow into the vein precludes the tamponade effect in most instances and may produce varicosities in the thin-walled veins.

Assessment. Upon auscultation, a continuous bruit is heard over the fistula. The Nicaladoni-Branham sign, occlusion of the fistula resulting in slowed heart rate due to reduced flow to the right atrium, may exist.

Large shunting may produce ischemic extremities. Perry[116] noted that with the rare AV fistulas between aorta and vena cava, heart failure may result from the recirculation of large quantities of blood.

Treatment. Although spontaneous closure of some AV fistulas occurs, it is more likely that surgical repair will be necessary. This is preceded by arteriography to ascertain the extent of vessel involvement.

Postoperative care is as for other vascular injury repair. Special attention is paid to the presence and quality of pulses as well as the neuromuscular function of the surrounding area or extremity.

The possibility of AV formation for months following injury directs nursing intervention from the resuscitation cycle through discharge. Certainly assessment of vascular integrity should continue during hospitalization and be included in patient and family discharge teaching. The type of vascular injury that the patient has sustained; the possibility of certain late complications; assessing pulses, color, and warmth distal to the site of injury; and reporting any changes to the physician should all be part of the teaching plan.

COMPLICATIONS OF ABDOMINAL TRAUMA

Many individuals may experience abdominal trauma and move through the cycles from resuscitation to rehabilitation with little to no variance from the usual postoperative surgical patient. However, the extent of organ involvement, level of injury, and time from injury until treatment greatly affect the morbidity of these individuals. Injury to any organ or vessel in the abdomen can lead to certain generalized post-traumatic complications. For example, the critical care cycle may evidence development of an ileus, peritonitis, cholecystitis, or stress ulcerations. The intermediate care cycle witnesses abscess formation and wound complications. The rehabilitation period may be the first time that body image alteration, alteration in family coping, or pain control becomes an issue.

The resuscitation cycle for the abdominal trauma patient is straightforward and not unlike that explained in Chapter 6 for all trauma victims. The ABCs of intervention are paramount, with volume replacement or immediate surgery often a priority for the abdominal trauma patient. Afterward, the effects of injury, shock, hemorrhage, and treatment selection begin to affect the physical and psychological adaptation of the patient.

These complications are not specific to a single abdominal organ injury but occur by virtue of damage to the abdominal contents, whether it is single-organ or multiorgan involvement or single-system or multisystem injury. The potential for these complications to occur makes it imperative for nursing assessment to continue throughout the cycles. To some degree they have been arbitrarily placed within a particular cycle, and many overlap between critical care, intermediate care, and rehabilitation cycles. Complications, rationale for therapies, and nursing interventions are described in the following sections.

Ileus

The shock state, sepsis, retroperitoneal hematoma, surgical manipulation of the bowel, premature removal of a nasogastric tube, or even certain medications may aggravate an ileus. Loss of propulsive peristalsis causes abdominal distention, decreased to absent bowel sounds, and diffuse distention of the bowel upon x-ray examination. The patient may begin to experience third-space fluid loss, impaired ventilation, wound disruption, and metabolic alterations.

Gastric decompression and intravenous fluid replacement are used initially following injury and/or surgery when an ileus is anticipated. The patient should experience active bowel sounds or passing flatus prior to removal of the nasogastric tube. Occasionally, an ileus will develop after oral fluid intake has begun. The patient will experience abdominal cramping, nausea, and vomiting.

Early assessment and treatment of infection as well as appropriate pain control with judicious use of narcotics may decrease the incidence of ileus. Appropriate nursing activities include monitoring bowel function, abdominal girth, and weights. Stimulating bowel function by administering suppositories or enemas may be ordered. Patient and family support is necessary, since prolonged ileus or recurring ileus may be viewed as a setback and, depending on the underlying cause, may result in further surgery for the patient.

Peritonitis

Secondary peritonitis occurs from penetrating or blunt abdominal trauma. Penetrating wounds introduce bacteria into the peritoneal space from the injury-producing object, e.g., knife or gun, causing the release of substances from organs penetrated during injury. Blunt trauma may rupture viscera or alter blood supply so that bacterial or chemical irritation ensues.

Peritonitis is a serious complication, with mortality rates reported as high as 50 per cent even with the advances in antibiotic therapy and intensive support. Vascular dilation, hyperemia, and fluid shifts occur from extracellular fluid compartments to the free peritoneal space, the connective tissue, and the lumen of the gastrointestinal tract. This in turn depletes fluid in the vascular space, thus producing signs of shock. Untreated peritonitis leads to septicemia, shock, ileus, and major organ failure.

The patient experiences abdominal pain that increases with movement. Abdominal rigidity, rebound tenderness, and voluntary guarding are evident. Bowel sounds are diminished or absent and accompanied by abdominal distention. Fever with chills, nausea, vomiting, and anorexia occurs. Respiratory status is compromised because pain may decrease excursion, leading to shallow, rapid respirations. The heart rate is rapid although weak and thready, and tissue perfusion as well as cardiac output is diminished.

Laboratory tests will evidence elevated leukocyte counts. X-ray films will show inflammation and edema of the intestinal wall and free air if visceral perforation is the cause.

Team Management. Team management includes supportive as well as surgical intervention. Surgical repair of ruptured viscus, drainage of abscess formation or fistula tract, and removal of foreign material are necessary before supportive treatment can be effective. Peritoneal catheters are placed if local antibiotic irrigation is planned, and systemic antibiotics are ordered as well. Restoration of plasma volume, fluid and electrolyte balance, pain control, respiratory support, and nutritional supplementation are goals of care.

Nursing Management. Monitoring volume status is necessary in the critical care cycle. A Foley catheter is placed to assess urinary output, and a nasogastric tube for decompression removes fluids from the gastrointestinal tract. As fluid is lost to the peritoneum, vascular volume is compromised; therefore, serial measures of blood pressure, heart rate, CVP, pulmonary artery pressure (PAP), and pulmonary capillary wedge pressure are monitored.

Wound care ranging from incisional care to stoma care will be necessary if surgical intervention occurs. Skin maintenance and protection from contamination are priorities in wound care.

Altered patient and family coping may be present as anxiety increases during the disease process. Assessment of the patient's and family's knowledge base regarding peritonitis and its symptoms and treatment is necessary. A planned program of instruction with reinforcement measures is necessary. Time should be provided for verbalization of questions and fears regarding the infection or treatment.

Posttraumatic Acute Cholecystitis

Posttraumatic acute cholecystitis (PAC) has been reported with increasing frequency in patients who have sustained traumatic injury. The majority of reported cases describe an acalculous cholecystitis.[117–119] However, others have reported evidence of calculous disease as well.[120, 121] Although presenting symptoms are similar, acalculous cholecystitis has a higher reported mortality.

PAC has been associated with shock, sepsis, respiratory failure, acute renal failure, parenteral hyperalimentation, multiple transfusions, and the use of high-dose narcotic analgesics. Specifically, bile stasis, bacterial infection, sepsis, activation of factor XII, and the Schwarzman reaction have been proposed mechanisms for developing PAC.

Recently, a prospective study using sonography screened trauma patients for signs of cholecystitis. Using sequential sonography, Raunest et al. found an 18 per cent incidence as opposed to the 0.5 to 4.2 per cent previously reported.[119] Sequential ultrasonography was used to identify subclinical cholecystitis and avoid laparotomy, as well as to survey others for early indication of the need for cholecystectomy.

PAC has been reported from 2 to 60 days after the traumatic event. The patient may have progressed from critical care toward rehabilitation before symptoms are apparent.

Symptoms are nonspecific and make a diagnosis difficult. The patient experiences generalized abdominal pain that localizes in the RUQ. Fever, nausea, vomiting, RUQ tenderness or mass, and leukocytosis are evident.

Radionuclide scanning and ultrasound have received mixed reviews for the diagnosis of PAC.[122, 123] Surgical treatment includes cholecystectomy or cholecystostomy. Flancbaum et al. noted that the mortality rate following cholecystostomy was significantly higher than that for cholecystectomy and therefore recommend only the latter.[118]

Alteration in comfort requires the nurse to assess pain characteristics, location, and severity. The patient should be medicated and the response recorded. Since consistent high-dose narcotics have been associated with the development of PAC, judicious use preoperatively is recommended. In addition, narcotics may cause spasm of the sphincter of Oddi, increasing pain and causing bile stasis.[121]

The potential for fluid volume deficit exists as a result of vomiting or nasogastric drainage. Recording intake and output, observing for signs of dehydration, monitoring serum electrolytes, and providing intravenous fluids are the nursing interventions required.

If a cholecystectomy is performed, maintenance of skin integrity surrounding the drainage tube insertion site is necessary. Pectin wafers cut to fit around the tube protect the skin.

A raised index of suspicion is necessary to diagnose and treat PAC before gallbladder necrosis and subsequent complications occur.

Abscess Formation

Many types of abdominal injury can lead to an abscess formation. Frequently, the signs are not evident until the intermediate care cycle or during a prolonged critical care stage. Organ rupture with release of blood, enzymes, and other fluid sets an appropriate medium for abscess formation unless adequately drained. Peritoneal contamination may render intra-abdominal tissue unable to hold an adequate suture line. With dehiscence, fluid is released into the peritoneal cavity, causing repeated irritation and contamination, leading to abscess formation.

An abscess is a localized infection and inflammatory process. Purulent exudate is walled off by leukocytes and may expand or deepen as leukocytes are drawn to the area, organisms are killed, and necrotic tissue is dissolved.[5] The exudate may be autolyzed and reabsorbed by the body, thereby negating the need for surgical intervention. Rupture of an abscess may occur, causing further contamination. Following rupture, a fistula tract can form to an organ or the skin and spread infectious exudate. Bacteremia, septicemia, cellulitis, or peritonitis may follow.

An abdominal abscess may become manifested through fever, anorexia, weight loss, and abdominal or lower chest pain. A hard mass may be palpable.

Abdominal x-ray or CT scan reveals a displaced diaphragm or organs, indicating the presence of an abscess. The location and extent of the abscess may be defined as well.

Antibiotic therapy and nutritional support are necessary to promote healing. Some abdominal abscesses may resorb, but operative drainage of the abscess may be necessary to promote healing. Early detection of abscess formation decreases morbidity and mortality secondary to a septic response.

Disruption of Wound Healing

Wound healing is affected by many different situations after the patient has sustained abdominal trauma. Certain factors involved with the type of abdominal injury, single versus multiorgan involvement, time from injury to treatment, and the patient's preexisting health status all affect wound healing.

Frequently, traumatically induced wounds are contaminated either through the penetrating injury itself or from viscus rupture following blunt injury. This often dictates the need for healing through secondary closure. When contamination is not evident and the wound is closed, suture line disruption and dehiscence occur later because intra-abdominal tissue is unable to hold the suture.

Initial care of the wound includes monitoring the incision for redness, warmth, edema, or localized pain. The patient may experience a fever if an infection is present. If the wound is open, the drainage amount, color, and odor and the results of culture and sensitivity tests should be noted. Recognizing that most abdominal wounds are considered contaminated, the nurse should be alert to these symptoms so that early treatment can be instituted.

Postoperative care includes use of aseptic technique during dressing changes. Drainage systems should be maintained as closed, sterile systems as much as possible, since these are possible sources of continued contamination. Multiple wounds should be dressed separately to guard against cross-contamination. A culture of the wound and any exudate is obtained if infection is suspected. (See Chapter 13 for further information regarding wound healing.)

Evisceration occurs when pressure or tension on the abdominal suture line is greater than the repair can tolerate. Immediate application of warm, moist saline dressings to the eviscerated organ is necessary prior to any surgical intervention.

The patient can be involved with wound care management as far as he indicates an interest. It is one mechanism for permitting the patient or a family member to regain control. Explanation and demonstration of sterile technique and return demonstration under supervision are necessary before the nurse can permit others to complete the wound care. If the patient is expected to care for the wound at home, ample time should be permitted for discharge instruction and patient evaluation to occur. Signs and symptoms of wound infection should be part of written discharge instructions.

SPECIAL NURSING CONSIDERATIONS

Nursing Diagnosis: Potential Upper Gastrointestinal Bleeding Related to the Stress Response Secondary to Abdominal Trauma

Areas of mucosal breakdown in the stomach or duodenum, with speculated increased acid production, lead to gastrointestinal bleeding. Low gastric pH, "coffee grounds" or frank blood aspirate, decreasing hematocrit, abdominal pain, and melena are indications of mucosal erosion.

The nursing emphasis is on prevention. Controlling gastric pH with antacid administration is a primary intervention. Sedatives may be ordered. H_2-inhibitors are administered. Psychological support through information sharing and the venting of feelings can further decrease the patient's stress response. Relaxation techniques may prove beneficial when the patient is capable of concentration. (See Chapter 15 for a discussion of relaxation techniques.)

If the possibility of stress ulceration is ignored early in the cycles of care, it may lead to active hemorrhage, necessitating iced saline lavage, vagotomy, antrectomy, or even total gastrectomy.

Nursing Diagnosis: Alteration in Body Image Related to Incisional Scarring, Stoma Creation, or Presence of Drains

The trauma patient experiences multiple changes in body image during hospitalization. Patients who experience abdominal injury may be left with permanent or temporary reminders of the traumatic event, such as a colostomy, incisional scar, drains, or drain wounds. The mere lack of abdominal muscle tone or strength following surgical repair of the injury may cause the patient concern during the adaptation process. Those who have sustained certain organ injury are at risk for long-term complications, such as recurrent pancreatitis, abscess formation, or metabolic alterations, that may change the way they view themselves in their social system. The onset of the traumatic event as a sudden illness may accentuate the patient's need for new adaptational strategies.

Nursing interventions begin during the critical care cycle in assessing the patient's understanding of the extent and type of injury and the patient's general adaptation to this. Roberts[124] stated that adaptation to alteration in the body's function and structure depends on the nature of the threat and its meaning, the patient's coping ability, the response from significant others, and the assistance available to the patient as changes occur. Initial nursing goals during the critical care cycle may include simply answering questions regarding the injury and helping the individual maintain a sense of self.

As the person progresses to intermediate and rehabilitation care, some interest should be expressed by the patient in the selected treatments and long-term effects of the injury and treatment. For example, failure of an individual who has sustained intestinal injury that required creation of a stoma as part of the repair to begin to look at and care for the stoma signals difficulty with body image. Information sharing, emotional support, and consultation for formal counseling are all appropriate nursing interventions to help the patient adjust. Informal discussions with former patients who have sustained and survived similar injury often help the patient and family adapt to their situation. (See Chapters 10 and 11 for further information on the patient's coping ability.)

Nursing Diagnosis: Alteration in Comfort Related to Abdominal Trauma

Pain following abdominal trauma may be due to the incision, organ disruption or manipulation, operative procedure, or presence of drainage tubes. The effects of uncontrolled pain are important: Goals such as early mobilization to facilitate peristalsis, to prevent thrombus formation or emboli (especially after a vascular repair), and to assist respiratory excursion are thwarted when the individual cannot become comfortable.

Identification of pain after injury is often the key to locating the type of abdominal injury sustained. Pain postoperatively, especially if it increases over time, is an indication of tissue damage secondary to abscess or fistula formation, delayed viscus rupture, or other process. However, the patient need not experience inordinate discomfort, since this interferes with recovery measures. (See Chapter 15 for specifics of pain control.) The nurse's role is to assess and treat the patient's discomfort adequately. A combination of analgesics, comfort measures such as position change or back rubs, and use of relaxation techniques will help the patient control the pain.

NURSING RESEARCH ISSUES

Research is necessary to refine the art and science of trauma care. In each stage of the cycles, research questions are manifested. Prevention of traumatic injury has increased the nation's awareness of the need for highway safety. Seat belt restraints have been publicized, and statewide restraint laws are in effect. But would an educational plan teaching proper placement of the lap belt decrease abdominal injury related to improper placement? Is there a method of installation of the three-point belt that would ensure proper placement?

Other questions overlap cycles of care. What is the relationship between the adequacy of drainage systems and patient positioning for wound care? How accurate is the four-part abdominal examination in each cycle of care? Which of the alternate feeding modalities best meets nutritional demands following abdominal trauma? How do we adequately measure the patient's pain and pain relief following abdominal injury?

What are the body image changes experienced with abdominal trauma? What nursing interventions have the greatest effect on the patient's ability to adapt to the image changes after experiencing a traumatic event?

Is length of stay decreased when the patient and/or family members are taught routine care procedures early in hospitalization?

These and many other questions remain to be answered as we continue to care for the complex, challenging patient who has sustained abdominal trauma.

SUMMARY

Although each abdominal organ system has been reviewed singularly, the nurse is much more likely to be confronted with a patient who has sustained multiorgan or multisystem trauma. Certain patterns such as pancreaticoduodenal injury and the resultant confusing diagnostic presentation have been described. Quick multisystem assessment is necessary initially, with an emphasis on identifying the life-threatening injuries first. Airway, ventilation, and circulation are initial priorities, with recognition that ventilatory and circulatory control may be affected by the extent of the abdominal injury. The index of diagnostic suspicion cues the nursing assessment and permits early recognition of insidious abdominal injury in each cycle. Delayed rupture or hemorrhage occurs with abdominal trauma. Other consequences of the injury, such as pancreatitis, abscess formation, or wound infection, may become apparent during the intermediate care or rehabilitation cycles. Morbidity and mortality are directly related to the failure to diagnose and treat early. Thus the demand remains for knowledgeable, swift nursing assessment in each aspect of the cycles, focusing on flexible patient care planning to meet the multiple changing needs of abdominal trauma patients and their families.

REFERENCES

1. Anderson C, Ballinger W: Abdominal injuries. In Zuidema G, Rutherford R, Ballinger W (eds): The Management of Trauma, 2nd ed. Philadelphia, WB Saunders Co, 1973.
2. Trunkey D, Hill A, Schecter W: Abdominal trauma and indications for celiotomy. In Moore E, Mattox K, Feliciano D (eds): Trauma, 2nd ed. Norwalk, CT, Appleton & Lange, 1991, p 409.
3. Blaisdell FW, Trunkey D (eds): Trauma Management, vol 1: Abdominal Trauma. New York, Thieme-Stratton, 1982.
4. Moylan J (ed): Principles of Trauma Surgery. New York, Gower, 1992.
5. Broadwell D: Gastrointestinal system. In Thompson J, McFarland G, Hirsch J, et al (eds): Mosby's Manual of Clinical Nursing, 2nd ed. St. Louis, CV Mosby, 1989.
6. Gruenberg J, Horan D: Delayed splenic rupture: The phoenix. J Trauma 23:159–160, 1983.
7. Trunkey D: Spleen. In Blaisdell FW, Trunkey D (eds): Trauma Management. New York, Thieme-Stratton, 1982.
8. McCarthy M, Glover J: Splenic trauma. In Moylan J (ed): Principles of Trauma Surgery. New York, Gower, 1992, pp 8.2–8.20.
9. Orsay E, Dunne M, Turnbull T, et al: Prospective study of the effects of safety belts in motor vehicle crashes. Ann Emerg Med 19(3):258, 1990.
10. Kaplan B, Cowley RA: Seatbelt effectiveness and cost of noncompliance among drivers admitted to a trauma center. Am J Emerg Med 9:4, 1991.
11. Fox M, Fabian T, Croce M, et al: Anatomy of the accident scene: A prospective study of injury and mortality. Am. Surg. 57:394, 1991.
12. Hayes C, Conway W, Walsh J, et al: Seat belt injuries: Radiologic findings and clinical correlation. Radiographics 11:23, 1991.
13. Tomlavich M, Nowak R, Talbert J, et al: Abdominal trauma. In Meislin H (ed): Priorities in Multiple Trauma. Rockville, MD, Aspen, 1981.
14. Thal E, McClelland R, Shires GT: Abdominal trauma. In Shires GT (ed): Principles of Trauma Care, 3rd ed. New York, McGraw-Hill, 1985.
15. Moore EE, Dunn E, Moore J, et al: Penetrating abdominal trauma index. J Trauma 21:439, 1981.
16. Croce M, Fabian T, Stewart R, et al: Correlation of abdominal trauma index and injury severity score with abdominal septic complications in penetrating and blunt trauma. J Trauma 32:380–388, 1992.
17. Keefe EJ, Gagliardi RA, Pfister RC: The roentgenographic evaluation of ascites. AJR 101:388–389, 1967.
18. Federale MP, Goldberg HI, Kaiser JA, et al: Evaluation of abdominal trauma by computed tomography. Radiology 138:637, 1981.
19. McCort J: Caring for the major trauma victim: The role for radiology. Radiology 163:1–9, 1987.
20. Lang E: Intra-abdominal and retroperitoneal organ injuries diagnosed on dynamic computed tomograms obtained for assessment of renal trauma. J Trauma 30:1161, 1990.
21. Day AC, Rankin N, Charlesworth P: Diagnostic peritoneal lavage: Integration with clinical information to improve diagnostic performance. J Trauma 32:52, 1992.
22. Davis J, Hoyt D, Mackersie R, et al: Complications in evaluating abdominal trauma: Diagnostic peritoneal lavage versus computerized axial tomography. J Trauma 30:1506, 1990.
23. Trunkey D: Diagnostic laboratory investigation and diagnostic and interventional radiology. In Champion H, Robb J, Trunkey D (eds): Rob & Smith's Operative Surgery: Trauma Surgery, 4th ed, parts 1 & 2. London, Butterworth, 1989, p 91.
24. Scherck J, Oakes D: Intestinal injuries missed by computed tomography. J Trauma 30:1, 1990.
25. Soderstrom C: Pitfalls of diagnostic peritoneal lavage. In Proceedings of the National Trauma Symposium, Baltimore, 1982.
26. Hoffman R, Nerlich M, Muggia-Sullam M, et al: Blunt abdominal trauma evaluated by ultrasonography: A prospective analysis of 291 patients. J Trauma 32:452, 1992.
27. Bagwell C, Ferguson W: Blunt abdominal trauma: Exploratory laparotomy or peritoneal lavage? Am J Surg 140:372, 1980.
28. Committee on Trauma: American College of Surgeons Advanced Trauma Life Support Course Instructor's Manual, 1984.
29. Mucha P: Intestinal injuries missed by CT (Discussion). J Trauma 30:1, 1990.
30. Root HD: Injury to the diaphragm. In Moore E, Mattox K, Feliciano D (eds): Trauma, 2nd ed. Norwalk, CT, Appleton & Lange, 1991, pp 427–439.
31. Moore JB, Moore EE, Thompson JS: Abdominal injuries associated with penetrating trauma in the lower chest. Am J Surg 140:724, 1980.

32. Rutherford R, Campbell D: Thoracic injuries. In Zuidema G, Rutherford R, Ballinger W (eds): The Management of Trauma, 4th ed. Philadelphia, WB Saunders Co, 1985.
33. Englehardt T: Problem: Blunt abdominal trauma—Diaphragmatic rupture. Emerg Med 20:34, 40, 42, 1988.
34. Glattener M, Toon R, Ellestad C, et al: Management of blunt and penetrating external esophageal trauma. J Trauma 25:784–792, 1985.
35. Wilson R, Steiger Z: Oesophageal injuries. In Champion H, Robb J, Trunkey D (eds): Rob & Smith's Operative Surgery: Trauma Surgery, 4th ed, parts 1 & 2. London, Butterworth, 1989, p 327.
36. Popovsky J: Perforations of the esophagus from gunshot wounds. J Trauma 24:337–339, 1984.
37. Symbos P, Tyras D, Hatcher C, et al: Penetrating wounds of the esophagus. Ann Thorac Surg 13:552–558, 1972.
38. Crass R: Gastric, esophageal, diaphragmatic, and omental injury. In Blaisdell FW, Trunkey D (eds): Trauma Management, vol 1: Abdominal Trauma. New York, Thieme-Stratton, 1982.
39. Register S, Downs J, Febeling B: Gastric mucosal lacerations: A complication of cardiopulmonary resuscitation. Anesthesiology 62:513–514, 1985.
40. Schwab CW, Shaikh K, Talucci R: Injury to the stomach and small bowel. In Moore E, Mattox K, Feliciano D (eds): Trauma, 2nd ed. Norwalk, CT, Appleton & Lange, 1991, p 485.
41. Walt A, Levison M: Hepatic trauma: Juxtahepatic vena cava injury. In Champion H, Robb J, Trunkey D (eds): Rob & Smith's Operative Surgery: Trauma Surgery, 4th ed, parts 1 & 2 London, Butterworth, 1989, p 374.
42. Lim R: Injuries to the liver and extra hepatic ducts. In Blaisdell FW, Trunkey D (eds): Trauma Management, vol 1: Abdominal Trauma. New York, Thieme-Stratton, 1982.
43. Olsen W: Late complications of central liver injuries. Surgery 9:733, 1982.
44. Moore EE, Shackford SR, Pachter H, et al: Organ injury scaling: Spleen, liver and kidney. J Trauma 29:1664, 1989.
45. Croce M, Fabian T, Kudsk K, et al: AAST Organ Injury Scale: Correlation of CT-graded liver injuries and operative findings. J Trauma 31(6):806–812, 1991.
46. Olsen WR, Redman HC, Hildreth DH: Quantitative peritoneal lavage in blunt abdominal trauma. Arch Surg 104:536, 1972.
47. Novick T, Moylan J: Hepatic trauma. In Moylan J (ed): Principles of Trauma Surgery. New York: Gower, 1992.
48. Pachter HL, Liang H, Hofstetter S: Liver and biliary tract trauma. In Moore E, Mattox K, Feliciano D (eds): Trauma, 2nd ed. Norwalk, CT, Appleton & Lange, 1991, pp 465–483.
49. Knudson M, Lim R, Oakes D et al: Nonoperative management of blunt liver injuries in adults: The need for continued surveillance. J Trauma 30:1494, 1990.
50. Bynoe RP, Bell RM, Miles WS, et al: Complications of nonoperative management of blunt hepatic injuries. J Trauma 32:308, 1992.
51. Harris L, McBooth F, Hassett J: Liver lacerations: A marker of severe but sometimes subtle intra-abdominal injuries in adults. J Trauma 31:894, 1991.
52. Pachter HL, Spencer FC: The management of complex hepatic trauma. Controv Surg 2:241, 1983.
53. Moore F, Moore E, Seagraves A: Nonsectional management of major hepatic trauma: An evolving concept. Am J Surg 150:725–729, 1985.
54. Feliciano DV, Mattox KL, Birch JM: Packing for control of hepatic hemorrhage: 58 consecutive patients. J Trauma 26:738, 1986.
55. Carmona RH, Peck D, Lim RC: The role of packing and reoperation in severe hepatic trauma. J Trauma 24:779, 1984.
56. Stevens S, Maull K, Enderson B, et al: Total mesh wrapping for parenchymal liver injuries: A combined experimental and clinical study. J Trauma 31:1103, 1991.
57. Geis WP, Schulz K, Gibschen J, et al: The fate of unruptured intrahepatic hematomas. Surgery 90:689, 1981.
58. Cheatham JE Jr, Smith EI, Tannell WP, et al: Nonoperative management of subcapsular hematomas of the liver. Am J Surg 140:852, 1980.
59. Perry JF: Blunt and penetrating abdominal injury. Curr Prob Surg May pp 3–53, 1970.
60. Naylor R, Coln D, Shires GT: Morbidity and mortality from injuries to the spleen. J Trauma 14:773, 1974.
61. Moore F, Moore E, Abernathy C: Injury to the spleen. In Moore E, Mattox K, Feliciano D (eds): Trauma, 2nd ed. Norwalk, CT, Appleton & Lange, 1991, 465–483.
62. Fisher M: Personal communication, 1992.
63. King H, Schumacher HB: Splenic studies: Susceptibility to infection after splenectomy performed in infancy. Ann Surg 136:239–242, 1952.
64. Cogbill T, Moore E, Jurkivich G, et al: Nonoperative management of blunt splenic trauma: A multicenter experience. J Trauma 29:1312, 1989.
65. Feliciano D, Bitondo C, Mattox K, et al: A four-year experience with splenectomy versus splenorrhaphy. Ann Surg 201:568–575, 1985.
66. Flancbaum L, Dauterive A, Cox E: Splenic conservation after multiple trauma in adults. Surg Gynecol Obstet 162:469–473, 1986.
67. Mucha P: Changing attitudes toward the management of blunt splenic trauma in adults. Mayo Clin Proc 61:472–477, 1986.
68. Kram H, DelJunco T, Clark S, et al: Techniques of splenic preservation using fibrin glue. J Trauma 30:97, 1990.
69. Hauser C: Hemostasis of solid viscus trauma by intraparenchymal injection of fibrin glue. Arch Surg 124:291–293, 1989.
70. Rogers F, Baumgartner N, Robin A, et al: Absorbable mesh splenorrhaphy for severe splenic injuries: Functional studies in an animal model and an additional patient series. J Trauma 31:200, 1991.
71. Lange D, Zaret P, Merlotti G, et al: The use of absorbable mesh in splenic trauma. J Trauma 28:269, 1988.
72. Dunham CM, Cornwell E, Militello P: The role of the argon beam coagulator in splenic salvage. Surg Gynecol Obstet 173:179–182, 1991.
73. Go P, Goodman G, Bruhn E, et al: The argon beam coagulator provides rapid hemostasis of experimental hepatic and splenic hemorrhage in anticoagulated dogs. J Trauma 31:1294, 1991.
74. Dowling R, Ochoa J, Yousem S, et al: Argon beam coagulator is superior to conventional techniques in repair of experimental splenic injury. J Trauma 31:717, 1991.
75. Lucas C: Splenic trauma choice of management. Ann Surg 213:98–112, 1991.
76. Pachter H, Hofstetter S, Spencer F: Evolving concepts in splenic surgery, splenorrhaphy versus splenectomy and postsplenectomy drainage: Experience in 105 patients. Ann Surg 194:266, 1981.
77. Trunkey D, Champion H, Sykes L: Special problems in operative management. In Champion H, Robb J, Trunkey D (eds): Rob & Smith's Operative Surgery: Trauma Surgery, 4th ed, parts 1 & 2. London, Butterworth, 1989.
78. Pachter HL, Hofstetter S, Spencer F: Splenorrhaphy versus splenectomy and postsplenectomy drainage experience in 105 patients. Ann Surg 194:262–269, 1981.
79. Caplan E, Boltansky H, Snyder M, et al: Response of traumatized splenectomized patients to immediate vaccination with polyvalent pneumococcal vaccine. J Trauma 23:801, 1983.
80. Walt AJ (ed): Early Care of the Injured Patient. Philadelphia, WB Saunders Co, 1982.
81. Ferrara J, Curreri PW: Gastrointestinal trauma. In Moylan J (ed): Principles of Trauma Surgery. New York, Gower, 1992, p 9.12.
82. Jordan G Jr: Injury to the pancreas and duodenum. In Moore E, Mattox K, Feliciano D (eds): Trauma, 2nd ed. Norwalk, CT, Appleton & Lange 1991, pp 499–520.
83. Kudsk K, Temizer D, Ellison C, et al: Posttraumatic pancreatic sequestrum: Recognition and treatment. J Trauma 26:321, 1986.
84. Stone HH, Fabian TC, Satiani B, et al: Experiences in the management of pancreatic trauma. J Trauma 21:257, 1981.
85. Jordan G Jr: Pancreatic trauma. In Howard JM, Jordan G Jr, Reber HA (eds): Surgical Diseases of the Pancreas. Philadelphia, Lea & Febiger, 1986, p 875.
86. Cogbill TH, Moore EE, Kashuk JL: Changing trends in the management of pancreatic trauma. Arch Surg 117:722, 1982.

87. Pederzole P, Bassi C, Falconi M, et al: Conservative treatment of external pancreatic fistulas with parenteral nutrition alone or in combination with continuous intravenous infusion with somatostatin, glucagon or calcitonin. Surg Gynecol Obstet 163:428, 1986.
88. Barber J: Gastrointestinal trauma: A review of delayed complication for the critical care nurse. Crit Care Q 5(2):69–80, 1982.
89. Kaldor PK: Pathophysiology and diagnosis of gastrointestinal problems. In Kinney M, Packa D, Dunbar S (eds): AACN's Clinical Reference for Critical-Care Nursing, 2nd ed. New York, McGraw-Hill, 1988.
90. Nance FC, Wennar MH, Johnson LW, et al: Surgical judgment in the management of penetrating wounds of the abdomen: Experience with 2212 patients. Ann Surg 179:639, 1974.
91. Robbs J, Moore S, Pillay S: Blunt abdominal trauma with jejunal injury: A review. J Trauma 20:308, 1980.
92. Lucas CE, Ledgerwood AM: Factors influencing outcome after blunt duodenal injury. J Trauma 15:839, 1975.
93. Donohue F, Crass R, Trunkey D: The management of duodenal and other small intestine trauma. World J Surg 9:904, 1985.
94. Christensen N: Small bowel and mesentery. In Blaisdell W, Trunkey D (eds): Trauma Management, vol 1: Abdominal Trauma. New York, Thieme-Stratton, 1982.
95. Moore EE, Jones TN: Benefits of immediate jejunal feeding after major abdominal trauma. J Trauma 26:874, 1986.
96. Spiro HM (ed): Primary structure disorders, short bowel syndrome. In Clinical Gastroenterology, 3rd ed. New York, Macmillan, 1984.
97. Nance F: Injuries to the colon and rectum. In Moore E, Mattox K, Feliciano D (eds): Trauma, 2nd ed. Norwalk, CT, Appleton & Lange, 1991, pp 521–532.
98. Schrock T: Trauma to the colon and rectum. In Blaisdell W, Trunkey D (eds): Trauma Management, vol 1: Abdominal Trauma. New York, Thieme-Stratton, 1982.
99. Karanfilian R, Ghuman S, Pathad V, et al: Penetrating injuries to the colon. Am Surg 48:104, 1982.
100. Pachter HL, Hoballah J, Corcoran T, et al: The morbidity and financial impact of colostomy closure in trauma patients. J Trauma 30:1510, 1990.
101. Stone HH, Fabian TC: Management of perforating colon trauma. Ann Surg 203:701, 1986.
102. Levison M, Thomas D, Wiencek R, et al: Management of the injured colon: Evolving practice at an urban trauma center. J Trauma 30:247, 1990.
103. Stewart M, Stone H: Injuries to the inferior vena cava. Am Surg 52:9–13, 1986.
104. Millikan JS, Moore E: Critical factors in determining mortality from abdominal aortic trauma. Surg Gynecol Obstet 160:313, 1985.
105. Courcy P, Brotman S, Oster-Granite M, et al: Superior mesenteric artery and vein injuries from blunt abdominal trauma. J Trauma 24:843–845, 1984.
106. Kashuk J, Moore E, Millikan S, et al: Major abdominal vascular trauma: A unified approach. J Trauma 22:672–679, 1982.
107. Feliciano D, Burch J, Graham J: Abdominal vascular injury. In Moore E, Mattox K, Feliciano D (eds): Trauma, 2nd ed. Norwalk, CT, Appleton & Lange, 1991.
108. Feliciano DV: Pitfalls in the management of peripheral vascular injuries. Probl Gen Surg 3:101, 1986.
109. Conti S: Abdominal venous trauma. In Blaisdell W, Trunkey D, (eds): Trauma Management, Vol 1: Abdominal Trauma. New York, Thieme-Stratton, 1982.
110. Pasch A, Bishara R, Schuler J, et al: Results of venous reconstruction after civilian vascular trauma. Arch Surg 121:607–611, 1986.
111. Traverso LW, Lee WP, DeGuzman LR, et al: Military antishock trousers prolong survival after otherwise fatal hemorrhage in pigs. J Trauma 25:1054, 1985.
112. Apprahamian C, Thompson BN, Towne JB, et al: The effect of a paramedic system on mortality of major open intraabdominal vascular trauma. J Trauma 23:687, 1983.
113. Mattox KL, Bickell W, Pepe PE, et al: Prospective MAST study in 911 patients. J Trauma 29:1104, 1989.
114. Holcroft J: Abdominal arterial trauma. In Blaisdell W, Trunkey D (eds): Trauma Management, Vol 1: Abdominal Trauma. New York: Thieme-Stratton, 1982.
115. Wilson R, Wiencek R, Balog M: Predicting and preventing infection after abdominal vascular injuries. J Trauma 29:1371, 1989.
116. Perry M: Vascular injuries. In Shires T (ed): Principles of Trauma Care, 3rd ed. New York: McGraw-Hill, 1985.
117. Fabian T, Hickerson W, Mangiante E: Posttraumatic and postoperative acute cholecystitis. Am Surg 52:188, 1986.
118. Flancbaum L, Majeres T, Cox E: Acute posttraumatic acalculous cholecystitis. Am J Surg 150:252, 1985.
119. Raunest J, Imhof M, Ohmann CH, et al: Acute cholecystitis: A complication in severely injured intensive care patients. J Trauma 32:433, 1992.
120. Kiel M: Posttraumatic acute cholecystitis on the rehabilitation service. Arch Phys Med Rehabil 71:610, 1990.
121. Okada Y, Tanabe R, Mukaida M: Posttraumatic acute cholecystitis. Am J Forensic Med Pathol 8:164, 1987.
122. Deitch E, Engel J: Acute acalculous cholecystitis: Ultrasonic diagnosis. Am J Surg 142:290, 1981.
123. Shumon W, Rogers J, Rudd T, et al: Low sensitivity of sonography and cholescintigraphy in acalculous cholecystitis. AJR 142:531, 1984.
124. Roberts S: Behavioral Concepts and the Critically Ill Patient. Englewood Cliffs, NJ, Prentice-Hall, 1976, p 78.

21

MUSCULOSKELETAL INJURIES

JULIE MULL STRANGE and PAULA M. KELLY

INTRODUCTION

The most basic principles of trauma care stress resuscitation and therapeutic intervention for those life-threatening or potentially lethal injuries most commonly associated with trauma. Musculoskeletal injuries rarely fall into a first-priority category, with the exception of those injuries which significantly alter hemodynamic status such as traumatic amputation and massive pelvic injuries. Musculoskeletal injuries require prompt recognition and appropriate management after stabilization of the cardiopulmonary and neurological systems to maximize the patient's full recovery. Long after the scars of general surgery have healed, the "low-priority" ankle, wrist, or open tibial fracture may continue to affect the patient on a daily basis and cause lifelong disability. This chapter addresses the major musculoskeletal injuries and complications that necessitate early diagnosis and emergency management.

ANATOMY AND PHYSIOLOGY

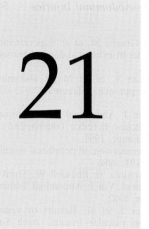

The following brief review of the anatomical structures that constitute the musculoskeletal system is meant only as an overview of the most pertinent information. The reader is directed to any one of the anatomy and physiology texts for a more comprehensive study.[1]

Functions

The musculoskeletal system performs the following five major functions: support, protection, movement and leverage, storage of mineral salts and fats, and hematopoiesis, or blood cell production. Any injury to the musculoskeletal system can cause an alteration in or even cessation of any of these roles, which then produces detrimental and far-reaching effects on the total patient.

Architecture

Figure 21–1 illustrates normal bone architecture, including diaphysis, epiphysis, articular cartilage, periosteum, medullary canal, and endosteum. The diaphysis, or shaft, is composed of a thick layer of compact or dense bone that offers a tremendous degree of support and protection. This most slender part of the bone is slightly curved in long bones to provide added strength and to enable the bone to withstand and absorb stress. The bone shaft can withstand shearing and compression forces but is at risk for injury from tension-producing mechanisms. For example, diaphysis fractures most often occur as a result of tension failure produced by a bending, twisting, and/or pulling mechanism.

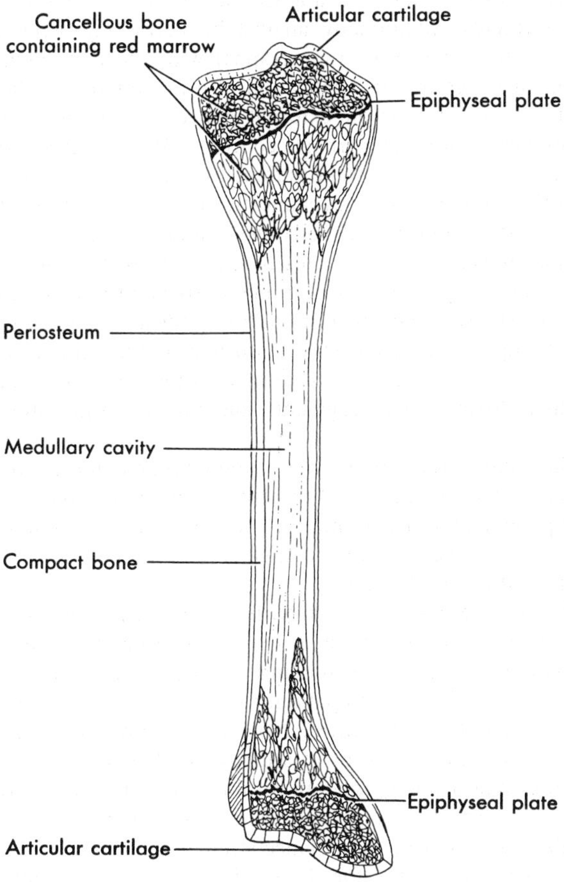

Figure 21–1. Diagram of longitudinal section of a long bone. (From Kimber PC, Gray CE, Stackpole CE: Kimber-Gray-Stackpole's Anatomy and Physiology. New York, Macmillan, 1977.)

The epiphysis, or bone end, is made up primarily of cancellous or spongy tissue that houses red marrow in the large pores. A thin outer layer of compact bone covers the cancellous tissue. This segment of bone is at greater risk for injury from crushing mechanisms, which cause compression or impaction of bone ends. The ramifications of an injury to this area of the bone increase in a prepubescent child because injury to the epiphyseal plate can significantly alter future growth.

The periosteum is a fibrous membrane sleeve that covers the entire bone except over the cartilaginous ends. The inner, osteogenic layer consists of elastic fibers, vessels, and osteoblasts, which are responsible for new bone formation. The outer, fibrous layer is made up of connective tissue and houses blood and lymphatic vessels and nerves. Bone growth, repair, and nutrition all rely on an intact and healthy periosteum. This closely adherent covering is thickest where muscles surround the bone, e.g., the diaphysis of the femur. Because it is a thin and tightly bound membrane in adults, it usually tears at a fracture site rather than separating from the bone. When a fracture occurs, one side of the periosteum usually remains intact (the periosteal hinge). This remaining portion of intact membrane aids fracture reduction and maintenance and serves as an osteogenic covering that promotes healing.

Injuries to the soft tissue, including muscles, nerves, vessels, subcutaneous fat, and skin, occur to some degree in conjunction with all fractures. Often the soft tissue injury may be more serious and have more significant ramifications than the fracture itself. Neglect or underestimation of soft tissue involvement may lead to fracture complications.

Five Stages of Healing

Final healing of an uncomplicated bony injury may take from 6 weeks to 6 months, depending on the bone involved. Table 21–1 lists the five stages that occur from the time of injury until healing is complete. Complications such as infection, vascular compromise, and other associated injuries may prolong the healing process and may even prevent the completion of the process.

EPIDEMIOLOGY

Musculoskeletal injuries found in the trauma patient result from a variety of causes. During a 1-year period from 1989 to 1990, the R. Adams Cowley Shock Trauma Center received 2589 trauma admissions. Sixty-two per cent of these admissions resulted from vehicular crashes. The remaining 38 per cent were related to industrial, home, and farm environments, as well as assaults. From this population, over 3400 musculoskeletal injuries were treated.[2] Frequently, these patients had other system injuries in addition to musculoskeletal injuries.

TABLE 21–1. THE FIVE STAGES OF FRACTURE HEALING

STAGE	ACTIVITY
First: hematoma formation	A hematoma forms at the fracture site.
Second: granulation	Within a few days after the injury, fibroblasts and capillaries invade the hematoma and form granulation tissue.
Third: callus formation	Within 6 to 10 days, plasma and white blood cells enter the granulation tissue and form a thick, sticky substance known as the callus. This material helps keep the bone fragments together.
Fourth: consolidation	Connective tissue and osteoblasts proliferate, bringing the bone ends closer together.
Fifth: remodeling	In this final phase of healing, bone fragments are united, excess cells have been absorbed, the bone is remodeled, and healing is complete.

RESUSCITATION CYCLE

Assessment

Accident Data Base

A wide variety of energy forces can traumatize the musculoskeletal system. Each type of accident exerts a different amount of force on the body. The degree, direction, and duration of that force, along with the patient's age and health history, determine the severity of the injury and its resulting morbidity.

Knowing the type of accident and the mechanism of injury involved should raise the clinician's index of suspicion during the assessment of the musculoskeletal system. A victim of a fall and a driver of a car striking another car head-on may absorb similar amounts of energy from the impact, but the direction of the forces applied to the body, the body surface area involved, and the rate of deceleration that occurs will be different, producing different injuries.

Information concerning the mechanism of injury should be obtained from the patient if possible and from the prehospital care providers. What type of accident caused the injury? Was it a high energy–producing event, such as a road traffic accident, or a low energy–producing event, such as a fall down a few stairs? What was the position of the patient at the time of impact? What was the position of the patient when discovered? What was the environment like where the injury took place? An open fracture that occurs in a farmyard has a greater potential for infection than one that occurs as a result of a fall down stairs in a home. Each injury is the result of energy absorbed and transferred. The fall victim who lands on his feet may have obvious ankle injuries, but other injuries often associated with this type of mechanism, e.g., pelvic and lumbar spine fractures, may be occult (Fig. 21–2*A* and *B*). Other patterns of energy absorption and transfer are demonstrated in Figure 21–3*A*, *B*, and *C*. The patient was an unrestrained front seat occupant who was involved in a head-on collision in which he struck his knee against the dashboard. A minor abrasion of the knee was sustained without any underlying fracture, but the energy transferred to the pelvis resulted in major pelvic ring disruption. Information concerning the events of extrication, immobilization, and stabilization that occurred at the site of the accident is important and should be obtained from the prehospital care providers. Knowing the degree of angulation of a fracture, the attitude of a joint, amount of exposed bone, motor and sensory function, and estimated blood loss heightens suspicion and helps determine the type of treatment necessary (see Chapter 7 for additional information).

Physical Musculoskeletal Assessment

The initial assessment of the musculoskeletal-injured patient must begin with the primary survey, which consists of the standard evaluation of airway, breathing, circulation, and neurological status. Initiation of appropriate interventions to establish or maintain normal cardiopulmonary and neurological function takes precedence regardless of obvious or suspected musculoskeletal injuries.

Attention is directed toward the musculoskeletal system during the secondary survey. Any suspected or obvious musculoskeletal injuries require baseline assessment of the neurovascular and motor status, proper immobilization of affected extremities, and application of sterile dressings to open wounds. Additionally, an unstable pelvic ring disruption (as identified on initial radiographs) with possible vascular injury may require an application of a pneumatic antishock garment (PASG) or an external pelvic fixator during the resuscitation for hemorrhage control. Other interventions should wait until the total patient evaluation is completed and the patient is hemodynamically stable. Throughout the resuscitation process, all personnel should be aware of potential or actual fracture sites to minimize further manipulation or injury. Severe pain from soft tissue or bony injuries may mask symptoms of other more significant injuries; thus a thorough total system evaluation is essential. Conversely, restlessness and agitation caused by other pathology may further disrupt bone fragments and increase the patient's pain.

Suspected areas of injuries should remain immobilized, and their movement should be kept to a minimum. Whenever the patient requires turning or moving, one person should assume responsibility for the affected limb to maintain alignment and immobilization.

Inspection and Palpation. It is important to assess the musculoskeletal system in a systematic fashion, since this decreases the chance of missing an injury. Assessment involves inspection and palpation. Observe the position of the patient and the extremities. Note any deformities such as angulation, shortening, or rotation, as well as open wounds, obviously protruding bone ends, abrasions, and road burns. Estimate external blood loss, calculating what was on the clothes as well as the ambulance stretcher.

Inspect the patient for these additional findings (any of which may indicate musculoskeletal injury):

Ecchymosis: caused by vascular disruption with blood dispersing through soft tissue.

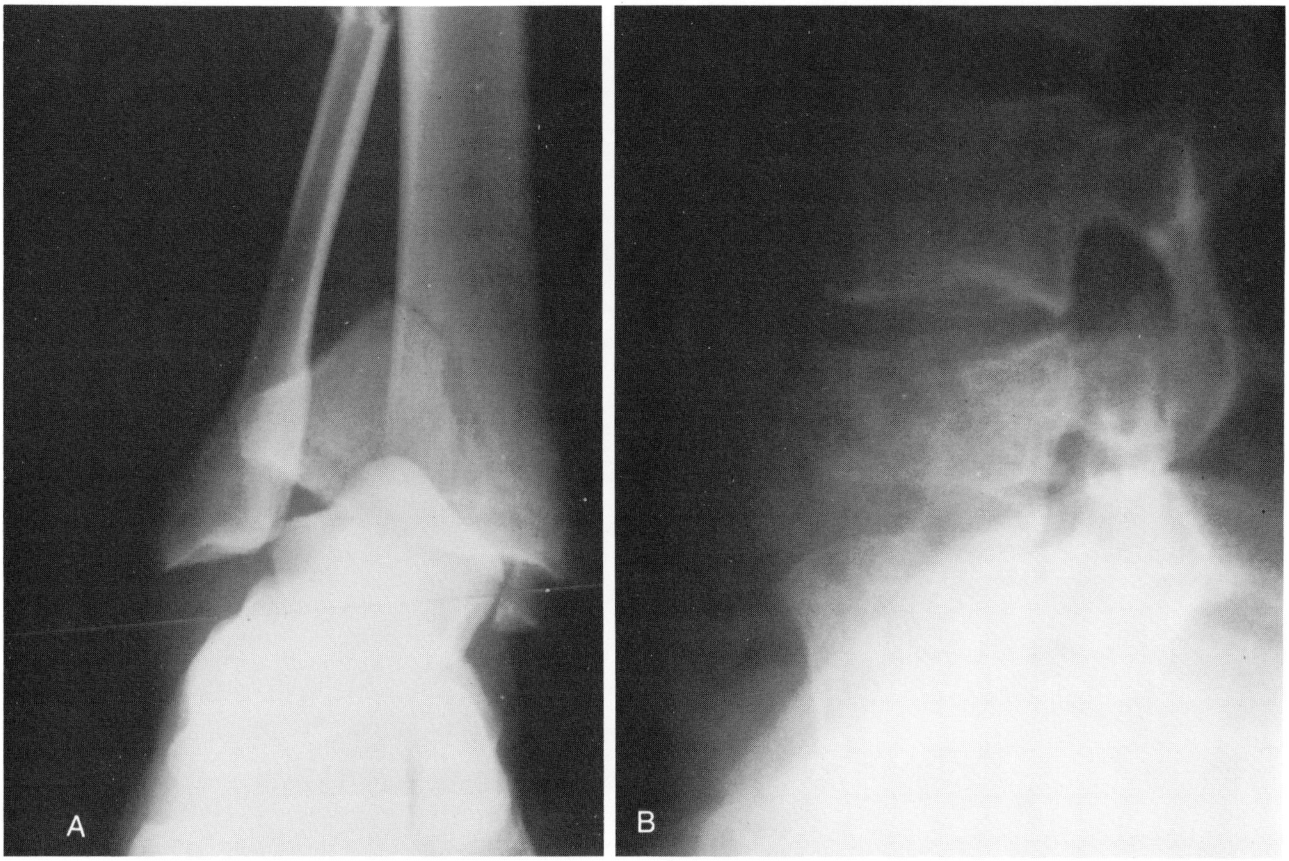

Figure 21–2. Radiographs of a fall victim who landed on his feet. *A*, Fractured ankle. *B*, Associated compression fracture of the lumbar spine.

Muscle spasm: continuous muscle contraction over an injured part; considered a protective mechanism of the muscle to splint the injured part.

Swelling: caused by injury to the soft tissue and interruption of the venous and lymphatic return system.

Extremity color: pale extremity color indicates inadequate arterial blood supply; dusky, bluish color indicates venous congestion.

Palpate each bone, and note any interruptions in the natural integrity. Interruption in bone integrity may be difficult to identify; crepitus, pain, or muscle spasm may be the only indication that an injury exists. Palpation is used to assess the following:

Capillary refill time: a filling time greater than 2 seconds is considered abnormal.

Pulses: check for presence, quality, and equality over the entire length of an extremity and not just distal to an obvious injury.

Crepitus: a grating sound heard, as well as felt, when fractured bone ends move.

Muscle spasm: as noted above.

Movement: range of motion, passive and active. Note any deviation from normal range or limitation of motion or muscle strength. Do not move an obviously injured extremity to test for range of motion.

Sensation: alteration in sensation to sharp and dull pain stimuli and proprioception.

Pain: bones are essentially insensitive. Pain is usually caused by injury to the periosteum (periosteum has sensory innervation), muscle spasms, soft tissue injury, and swelling within fascial compartments.

Zone of Injury. Think of any obvious or suspected injury in terms of the zone of injury, as seen in Figure 21–4. Injuries to the skeletal system are always accompanied by some degree of soft tissue injury. Damage to the soft tissue structures will be greater than what is discovered on clinical assessment and radiological examination. The exact zone of injury is often not fully appreciated until the operative or critical care phase. Because of this, continued physical assessment with a high index of suspicion must include areas both distally and proximally to any obvious or suspected injury.

Diagnostic Studies. Various radiographic studies are utilized to confirm musculoskeletal injuries. For plain radiographic films, at least two views are required to determine the degree of angulation and displacement (Fig. 21–5). Surrounding anatomical structures as well as the structure of the bone/joint in question may reduce the effectiveness of plain films in diagnosing skeletal injuries and necessitate use of other techniques such as computed tomographic (CT) scans, angiography, and CT myelograms. CT scans aid in confirmation of hidden or minimally displaced fractures in areas such as the pelvic ring, the ankle, and the knee. Angiography is necessary for severe fracture/dislocations near the knee joint, in pelvic injuries with persistent hemorrhage, and when distal circulation is compromised. Angiog-

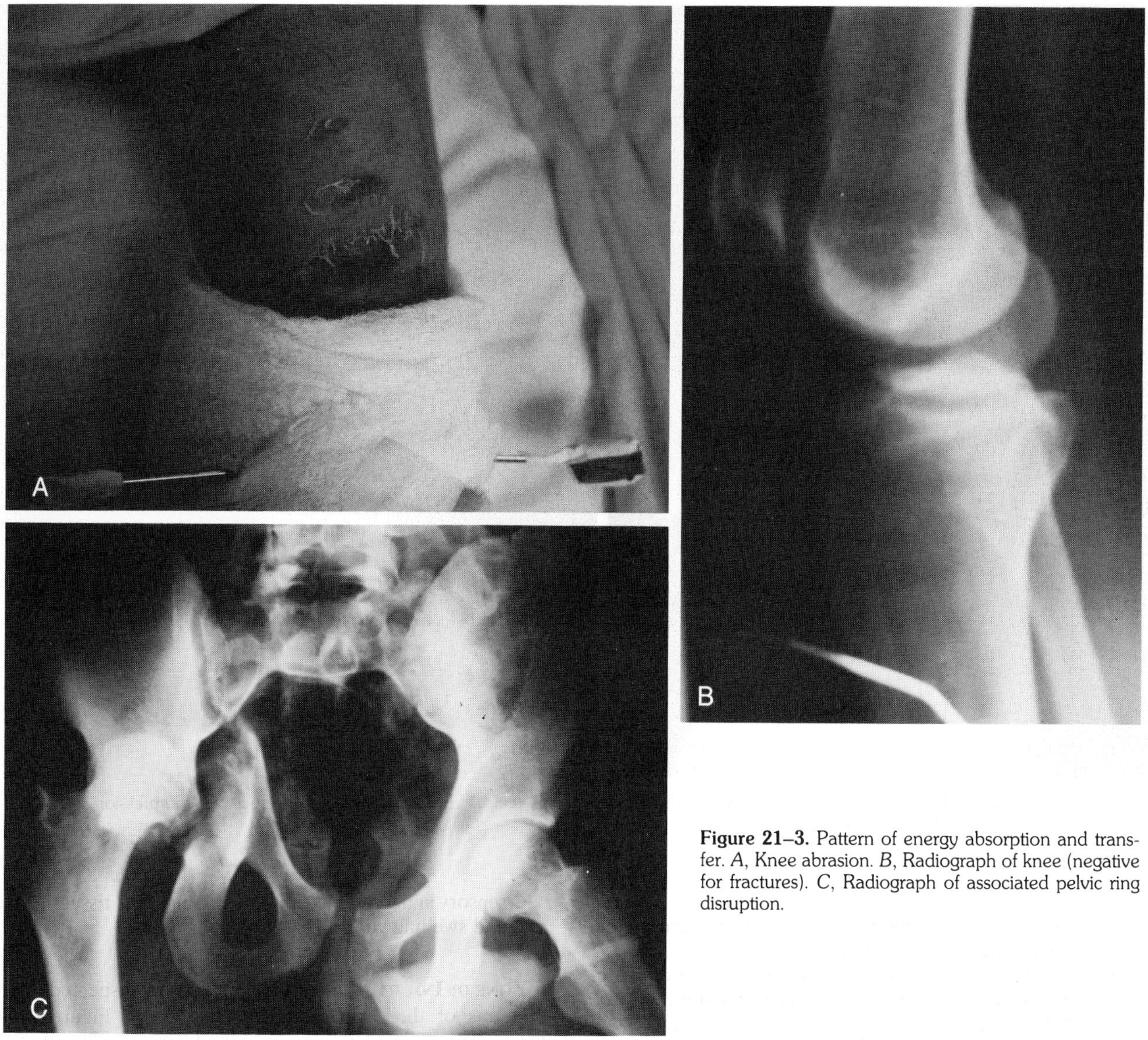

Figure 21–3. Pattern of energy absorption and transfer. *A*, Knee abrasion. *B*, Radiograph of knee (negative for fractures). *C*, Radiograph of associated pelvic ring disruption.

raphy also can provide added information concerning the true zone of injury. Myelography is useful as a delayed diagnostic procedure (at least 2 weeks after the injury) when nerve root avulsion is suspected. If conducted earlier, the study may yield a false-negative result because blood clots can obstruct the meningoceles, which are diagnostic of nerve root avulsion.

During the diagnostic process the nurse is responsible for the following:

1. Assisting with explanation of the procedure to the patient and obtaining consent when necessary.
2. Assisting with safe patient positioning during and after the procedure to prevent further injury- or procedure-related complications. For example, following an angiogram, in which the femoral artery was cannulated, restrict hip flexion for 6 to 8 hours to prevent further bleeding at the insertion site.
3. Protecting the patient from unnecessary radiation exposure by shielding him with a lead-lined apron whenever possible.
4. Constantly monitoring the patient's overall status, including potential reaction to contrast media.
5. Documenting the procedure, patient tolerance, and follow-up evaluation.

Patient Health History. Specific patient health history is an important part of the patient assessment. Information concerning health history can be obtained from the patient or, when necessary, from family members or friends. The nurse should determine whether the patient has ever had an allergic reaction to any medication or contrast material and the type of reaction that occurred. Previous reactions to pharmacological agents can alter the choice of diagnostic studies, e.g., angiograms, or the choice of medications utilized for treatment. The patient should be asked about current or recent use of medication, and its reason, dose, and frequency should be ascertained if possible. It is essential to know whether the patient has taken any anticoagulants, aspirin, or similar medication prior to admission. The patient's tetanus immunization history should be elicited as accurately as possible. It is helpful to know whether the

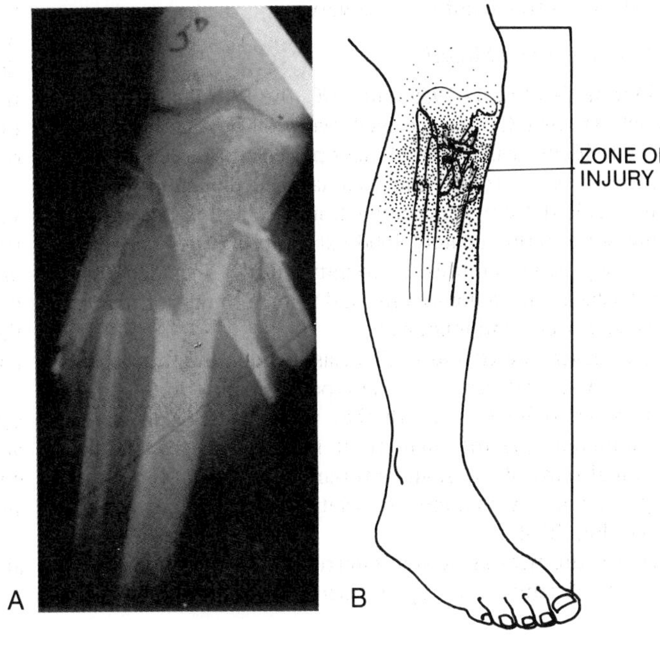

Figure 21–4. The mechanism of injury predicts the zone of soft tissue injury. *A*, Radiograph of a grade III tibia fracture that resulted from a car bumper crush injury. *B*, The zone of injury (stippled) of the leg. The fracture pattern and the mechanism of injury predict the size of this zone. (From Manson PN, Yaremchuk MJ, Hoopes JE: Soft tissue injuries of the extremities. In Zuidema GD, Rutherford RB, Ballinger WF (eds): The Management of Trauma. Philadelphia, WB Saunders Co, 1985.)

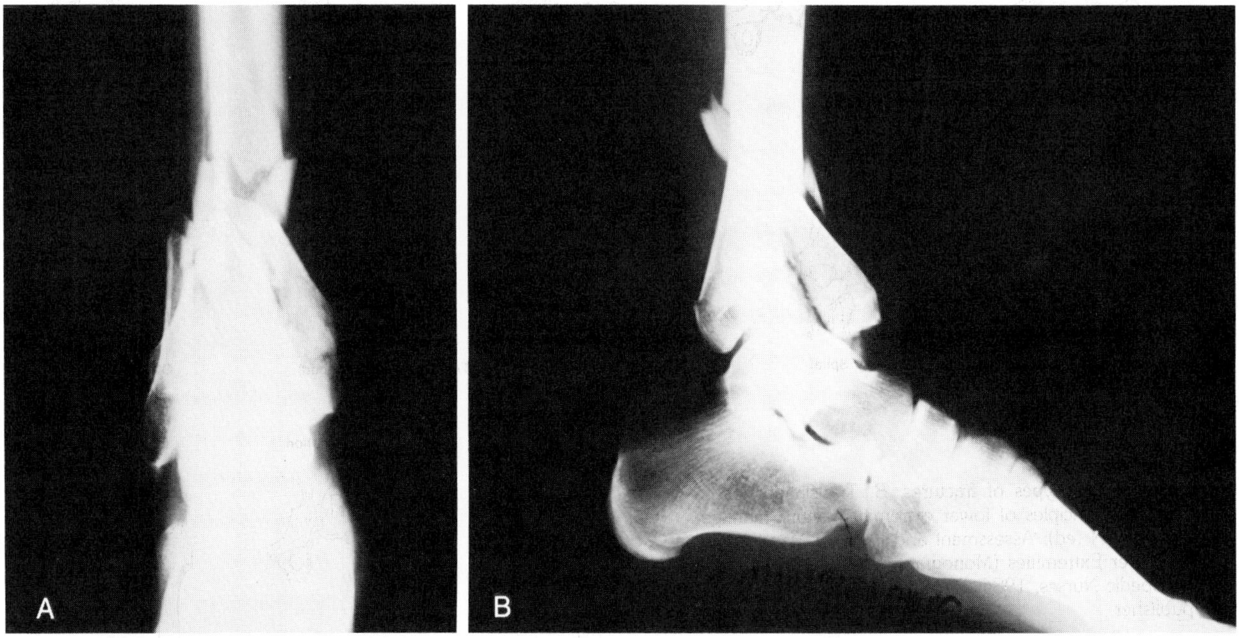

Figure 21–5. Radiographs of a fracture of the distal tibia/fibula and ankle showing the degree of angulation and displacement. *A*, Anteroposterior view. *B*, Lateral view.

patient has ever been hospitalized overnight, has had any previous surgery, and has had (or his immediate family) any specific health problems. Previous fractures, ligamentous or soft tissue injuries, thromboembolic disease, and any problems with infection or delayed healing all potentially affect the patient's treatment and recovery.

Classification of Injuries

During fiscal years 1989 and 1990, the R. Adams Cowley Shock Trauma Center received over 4000 patients directly from accident scenes. Eighty-eight per cent of these patients' injuries resulted from blunt trauma. The remaining 12 per cent resulted from penetrating trauma. In this population there were approximately 1600 extremity injuries and over 320 bony pelvic injuries. Extremity injuries included fracture/dislocations, amputations, and trauma to the soft tissue, nerves, vessels, and tendons.[3]

Extremity Fractures. The classification of a fracture is based on several items: (1) the type of fracture line (spiral, transverse, oblique), (2) whether the fracture is linear or comminuted, (3) the anatomical location (distal, middle, proximal third of the shaft, intra-articular), and (4) type of displacement (angulation, translation, impaction, distraction)[4] (Fig. 21–6).

A fracture with associated interruption in skin integrity is an open fracture. An open fracture is further classified according to the degree of soft tissue involvement and the amount of disruption in skin integrity. A grade I open fracture wound is less than 1 cm in length and is associated with minimal soft tissue damage. A grade II open fracture wound is greater than 1 cm with a moderate amount of soft tissue injury. Criteria for a grade III open fracture include a wound larger than 10 cm with significant avulsion, soft tissue damage, muscle devitalization, or wound flaps, such as fractures caused by gunshot wounds or bumper mechanisms or fractures associated with open segments and neurological or vascular involvement.

The soft tissue injury in a grade I fracture may appear very benign and/or occur some distance from the fracture site. This is attributed to the overriding of fractured bone ends at the time of injury. One end penetrates the skin some distance from the fracture site and then withdraws back through the soft tissue into relatively normal anatomical alignment.

Certain mechanisms of injury will automatically classify an open fracture as grade III, such as a shotgun injury, high-velocity gunshot wound, an open fracture occurring in a farm environment, and a crushing injury from a fast-moving vehicle. An open fracture with diaphyseal segment loss, with associated major vascular injury or segmental fracture, is also classified as a grade III open fracture.

Traumatic Amputations. Traumatic amputations are

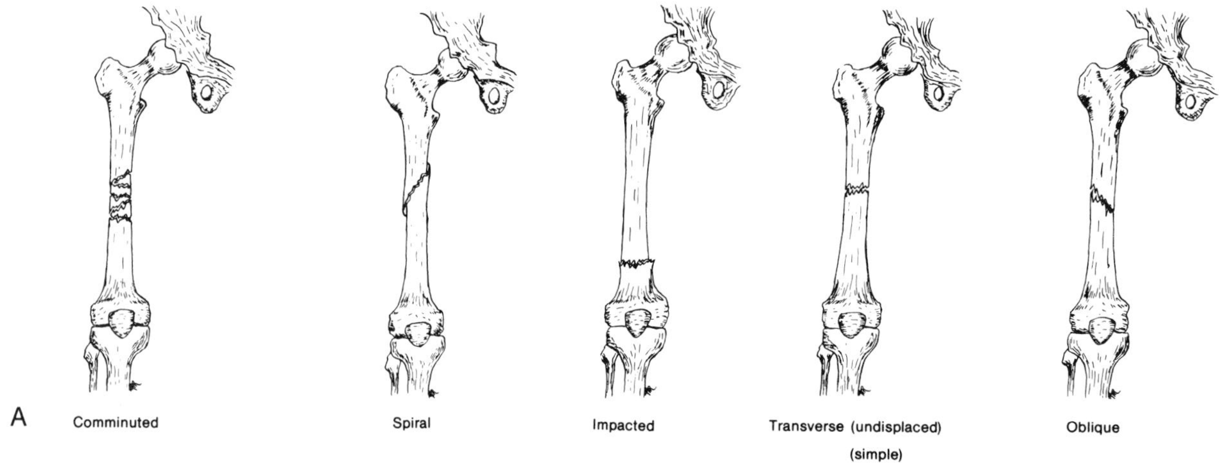

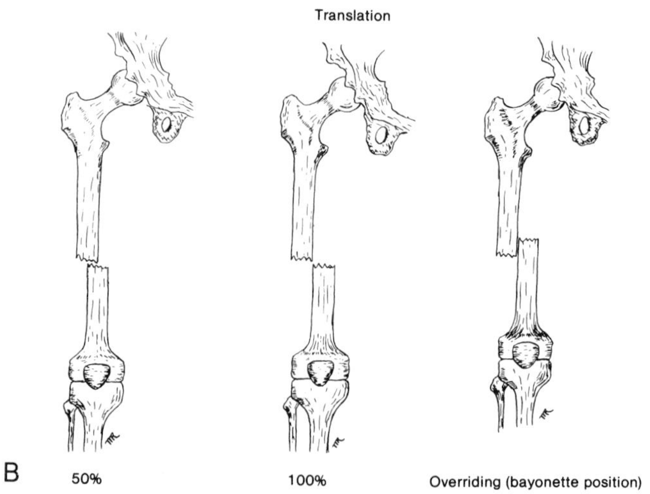

Figure 21–6. *A*, Types of fractures. *B*, Translation. (From Stearns HC: Principles of lower extremity fracture management. In Hilt N (ed): Assessment and Fracture Management of the Lower Extremities (Monograph). National Association of Orthopedic Nurses, 1984. Reproduced with permission of the publisher.

classified according to the degree and extent of soft tissue, nerve, and vascular injury. A *cut* or *guillotine* type amputation has well-defined wound edges and localized damage to soft tissue, nerves, and vessels. A *crush* type amputation wound has more soft tissue damage, especially to the arterial intima. Injury to the soft tissue may be localized or extended some distance from the wound edge. An *avulsive* amputation wound is caused by forceful stretching and tearing away of the tissue. Neural and vascular structures are torn away at levels different from the actual site of the bone fracture.

Dislocations. A dislocation occurs when articulating surfaces are no longer in contact because of joint disruption. Movement can be very limited or impossible. The dislocation is described in terms of the distal component relative to the proximal component. For example, a dislocation of the elbow involving the radius alone can be anterior, posterior, or lateral. Hip dislocations may be classified as anterior, posterior, or central (Fig. 21–7).

Pelvic Ring Disruptions. The pelvis is composed of three bones held together and stabilized by a strong ligamentous network. Anteriorly, the symphysis pubis, a strong ligamentous structure, acts as a strut to prevent anterior pelvic collapse; it has little to do with weight bearing. The major stabilizing force in the pelvis is the posterior tension band that includes the following ligaments: iliolumbar, posterior sacroiliac, sacrospinous, and sacrotuberous (Fig. 21–8). Pelvic ring disruptions are the third most often seen injury in fatal motor vehicle crashes. Pelvic ring disruptions are clinically described as stable or unstable. Two-thirds of pelvic ring disruptions are stable. While lower in incidence, the unstable injury is potentially more life-threatening because it is often accompanied by a myriad of complications. These include massive to exsanguinating blood loss, genitourinary trauma, sepsis, chronic pain, and long-term disability. The injury to the pelvic ring may be closed or open, as with an associated laceration or puncture of the skin, rectum, or

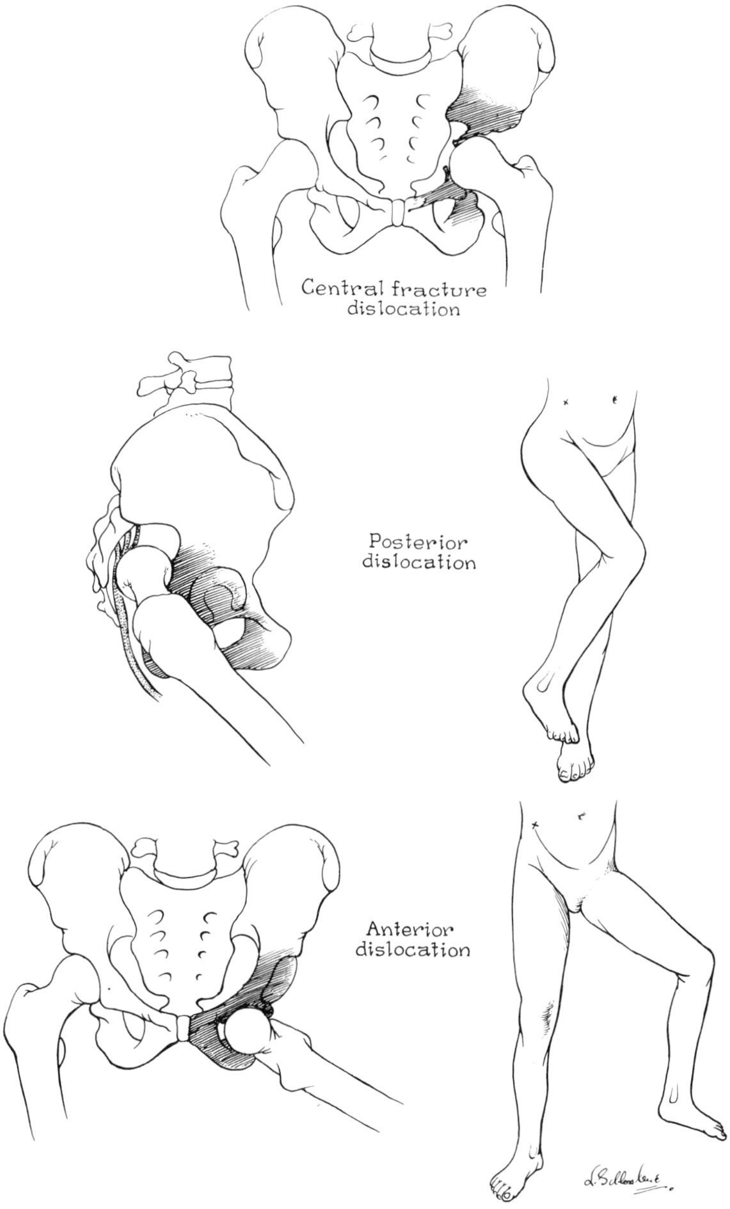

Figure 21–7. Basic types of hip dislocation. (From Thomas Claudia: Fractures of the pelvis and hip. In Zuidema GD, Rutherford RB, Ballinger WF (eds): The Management of Trauma. Philadelphia, WB Saunders Co, 1985.)

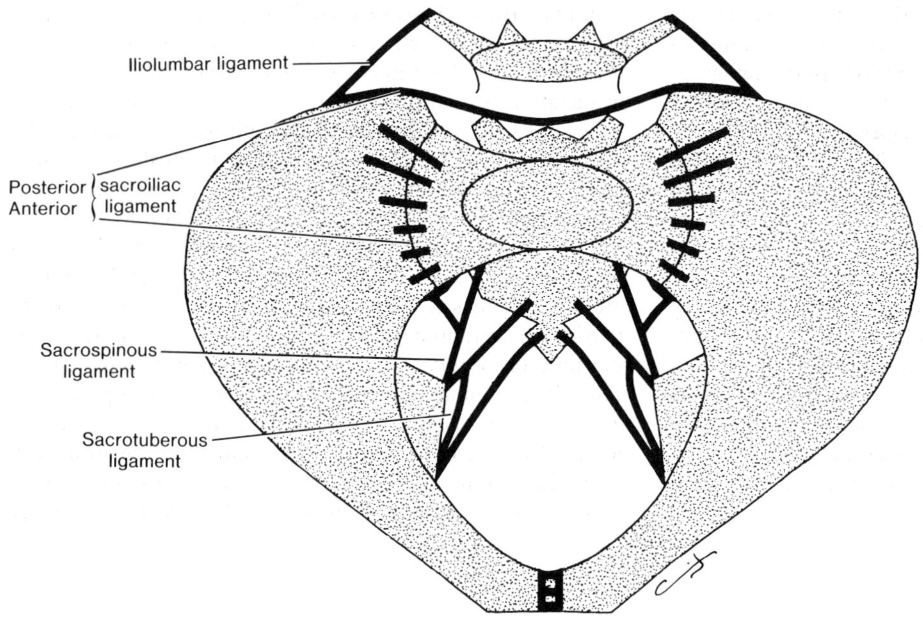

Figure 21–8. Diagramatic representation of the major ligaments of the pelvis: the strong symphysis pubis anteriorly and the posterior tension band of the pelvis, including the iliolumbar, posterior sacroiliac, sacrospinous, and sacrotuberous ligaments. (From Tile M: Fractures of the Pelvis and Acetabulum. Baltimore, Williams & Wilkins, 1984.)

vagina. The mortality rate associated with open pelvic fractures is 40 to 60 per cent.[5]

Various systems exist for classification of pelvic injuries, such as those described by Looser and Crombie,[6] Trunkey et al.,[7] and Pennal et al.[8] The current and most practical classification system, described by Tile,[9] categorizes pelvic ring disruptions by their mechanism of injury and their degree of stability. The four major types of injury are the anteroposterior compression, lateral compression, vertical shear, and complex. Subdivisions exist within all categories; however, this text will address only the four major categories. The reader is referred to the text by Tile[9] for an excellent discussion of this subject.

An anteroposterior compression injury (Fig. 21–9), or external rotation injury, may occur when a crushing force on the posterior superior iliac spines causes the symphysis pubis to spring open anteriorly. Continued external rotation causes rupture of the anterior sacroiliac and sacrospinous ligaments. This disruption is referred to as an "open book" injury. Conversely, direct pressure on the anterior superior iliac spines can disrupt the symphysis pubis and lead to sacrospinous and anterior sacroiliac ligament injury if the compression continues.

Lateral compression (Fig. 21–10), or internal rotation, the most common type of pelvic injury, represents a high-energy injury. Direct pressure to an iliac crest causes an internal rotation injury that crushes the anterior sacrum and displaces the anterior pubic rami. Pressure on the greater trochanter causes the femoral head to disrupt the pubic rami, which can extend into the anterior acetabulum. The ipsilateral sacroiliac complex is also injured by this force. This injury causes bone impaction and may not involve the posterior ligamentous complex.

Most anteroposterior and lateral compression injuries are considered "stable" disruptions because the posterior sacroiliac complex remains intact or because the bone is impacted, thus preventing further disruption. (The magnitude of the injuring force may, however, be so great as to cause extensive soft tissue injury leading to instability.) Because these injuries are generally stable, they are associated with less long-term problems and have low morbidity/mortality rates.

The *vertical shear,* or *Malgaigne fracture* (Fig. 21–11), is an unstable injury associated with bone and soft tissue disruption. Great force, such as that from falls and crush mechanisms, is in the vertical plane and is usually shearing in nature. Fractures may be unilateral or bilateral, the latter representing the most destructive type of unstable disruption. Anterior and posterior ring disruptions are present as well as injuries to the sacrotuberous and sacrospinous ligaments. Anterior injuries may involve disruption of the symphysis pubis and two to four pubic rami injuries. Posterior lesions involve the sacrum, sacroiliac joints, and/or the ilium. Skin and subcutaneous tissue may be torn as well. Vertical shear disruptions impose the greatest risk for associated injuries to the gastrointestinal, genitourinary, vascular, and neurological systems and therefore have the highest morbidity/mortality rates.

Complex pelvic ring disruptions, which result from very powerful forces, cause bizarre fracture/dislocation patterns that do not fit neatly into one of the previously mentioned classifications. These injuries generally represent combinations of applied forces and ligamentous injuries and are usually very unstable.

Pelvic ring disruptions such as the vertical shear and the complex should alert the admitting team to the severity of injury sustained and the need for a comprehensive team approach to resuscitation.

Management

Alteration in Bone/Joint Continuity

Interruption in bone or joint continuity can cause severe muscle spasms that result in pain, angulation, and overriding of bone ends. These complications lead rapidly to decreased venous and lymphatic return, increased soft tissue injury,

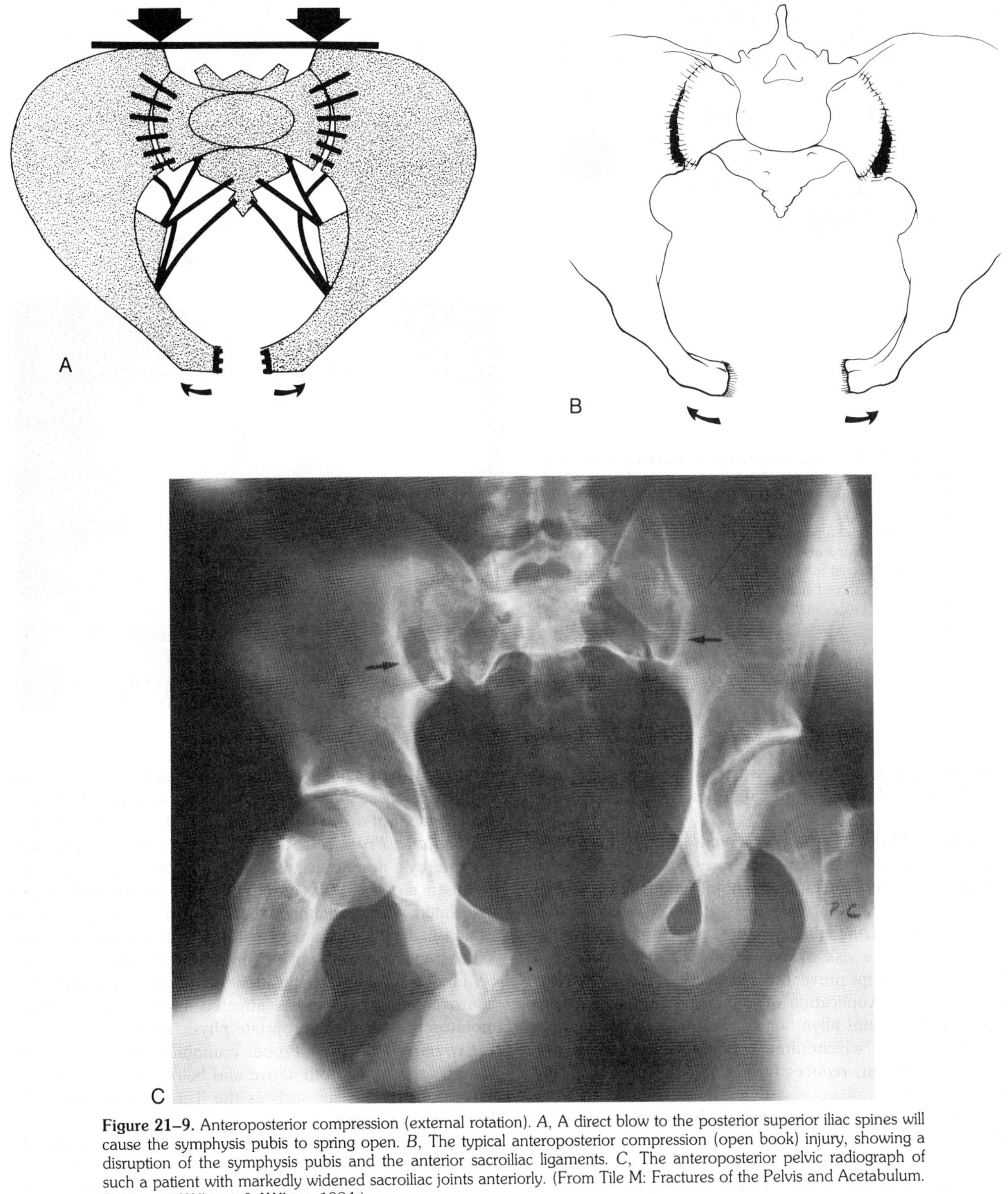

Figure 21–9. Anteroposterior compression (external rotation). *A*, A direct blow to the posterior superior iliac spines will cause the symphysis pubis to spring open. *B*, The typical anteroposterior compression (open book) injury, showing a disruption of the symphysis pubis and the anterior sacroiliac ligaments. *C*, The anteroposterior pelvic radiograph of such a patient with markedly widened sacroiliac joints anteriorly. (From Tile M: Fractures of the Pelvis and Acetabulum. Baltimore, Williams & Wilkins, 1984.)

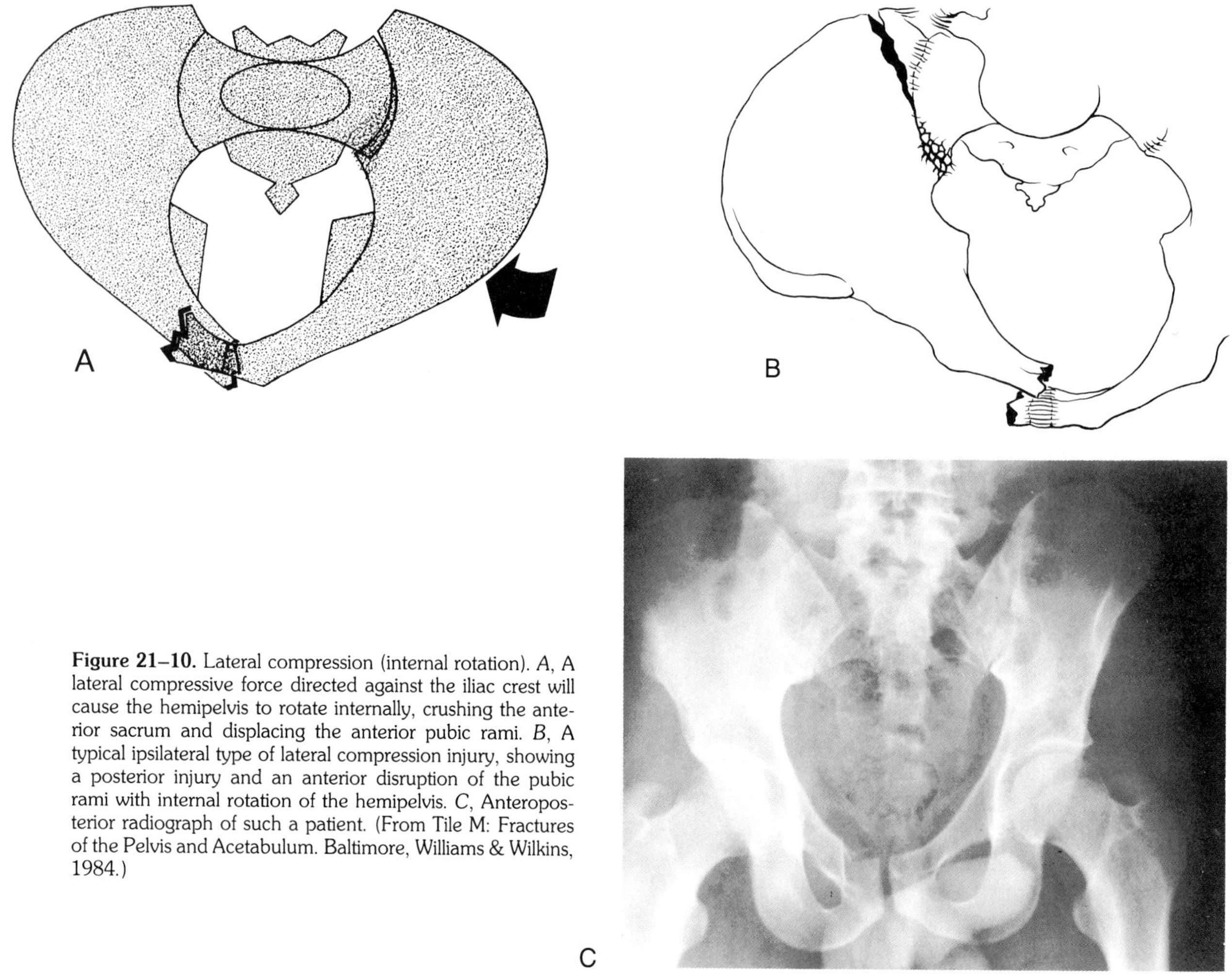

Figure 21–10. Lateral compression (internal rotation). *A*, A lateral compressive force directed against the iliac crest will cause the hemipelvis to rotate internally, crushing the anterior sacrum and displacing the anterior pubic rami. *B*, A typical ipsilateral type of lateral compression injury, showing a posterior injury and an anterior disruption of the pubic rami with internal rotation of the hemipelvis. *C*, Anteroposterior radiograph of such a patient. (From Tile M: Fractures of the Pelvis and Acetabulum. Baltimore, Williams & Wilkins, 1984.)

and swelling. Additionally, persistent bony disruption precipitates further risk for neurovascular injury and fat embolism syndrome.

General Management Principles. Early immobilization at the scene of the accident represents the first step in rehabilitation. Simply stated, immobilization helps to preserve what function currently exists and prevents further injury. By minimizing muscle spasms, proper immobilization also decreases the risk of angulation and of overriding of bone ends and helps prevent closed fractures from becoming open fractures. Application of traction in conjunction with immobilization helps align bone ends in a near-normal anatomical position, which often restores neurovascular and lymphatic function, reduces further soft tissue edema, and decreases pain.

Immobilization techniques and devices applied prior to admission should remain in place until appropriate radiographic studies are done. Continue to frequently monitor neurovascular and motor status despite the presence of an immobilization or traction device. Closely monitor the device itself to ensure proper placement and effectiveness. After radiologic evaluation, more effective or formal methods of immobilization should be applied.

Dislocations. Dislocations should be immobilized in the position in which they are found. Attempting to straighten a dislocated joint usually results in increased pain and potentially may cause further neurovascular damage. Definitive management of dislocations is discussed later in this chapter.

Angulated Fractures. Realignment of a severely displaced fracture by a nonphysician depends not only on the presence or absence of vascular compromise and the amount of pain associated with realignment but, more importantly, on the established policies governing treatment of such an injury. When realignment is not possible, the injured area should be immobilized in the position in which it is found. The neurovascular status of the affected limb should be closely monitored, with the appropriate physician notified.

Extremity Fractures. Proper immobilization of a fracture includes the joints both above and below the site of injury. Manufactured devices such as the Thomas ring splint, the Hare traction splint (Fig. 21–12), or the Sager emergency traction device are useful for fractures of the lower extremity that occur approximately 2 inches proximal to the ankle or above. These devices allow for application of traction while immobilizing the affected area. Positioning of these devices usually requires two people, and established policies should outline the specific procedure to follow to ensure safe, rapid application. The affected extremity must be monitored for swelling, especially with traction, preformed splints, and metal devices. These splints may require loosening of straps

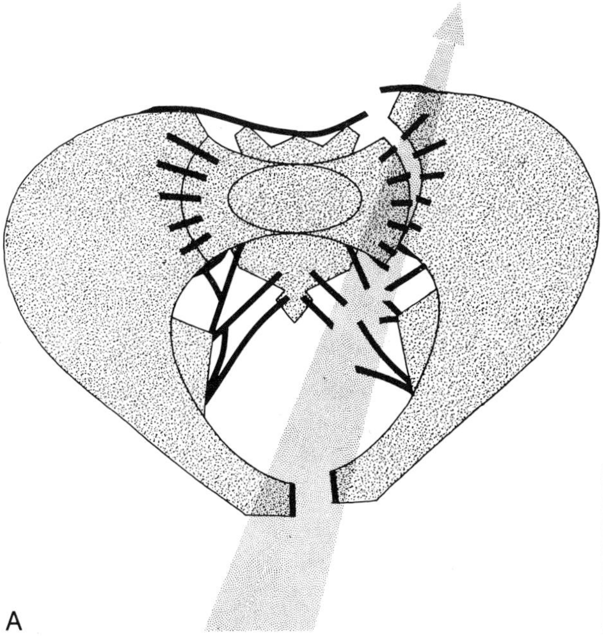

A

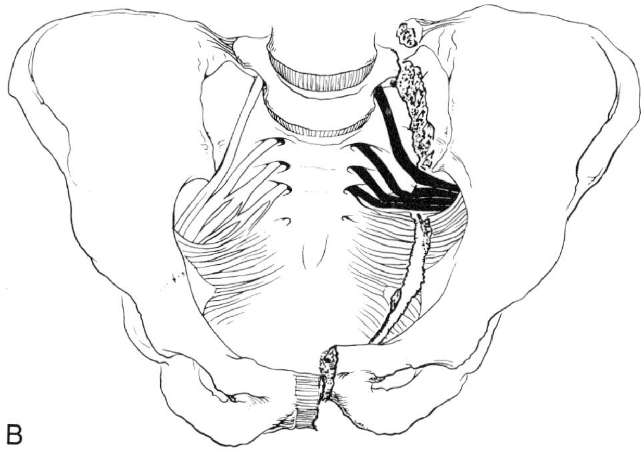

B

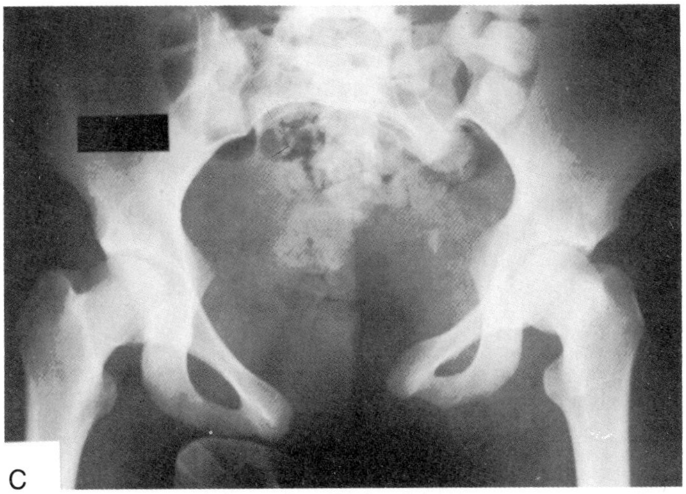

C

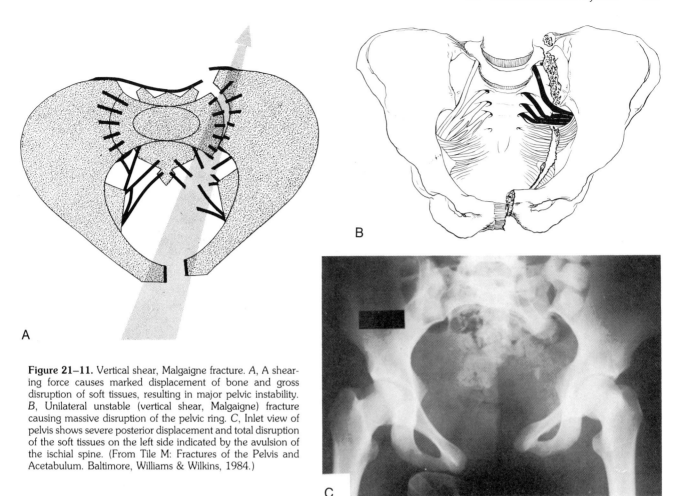

Figure 21–11. Vertical shear, Malgaigne fracture. *A*, A shearing force causes marked displacement of bone and gross disruption of soft tissues, resulting in major pelvic instability. *B*, Unilateral unstable (vertical shear, Malgaigne) fracture causing massive disruption of the pelvic ring. *C*, Inlet view of pelvis shows severe posterior displacement and total disruption of the soft tissues on the left side indicated by the avulsion of the ischial spine. (From Tile M: Fractures of the Pelvis and Acetabulum. Baltimore, Williams & Wilkins, 1984.)

and padding to prevent further injury, such as compartment syndrome, which can occur when edematous tissue meets the resistance of such devices. Air splints or premolded rigid splints are useful for feet, ankles, and upper extremities and decrease edema by applying pressure over the injured area and simultaneously provide tamponade of open, bleeding wounds. Closely monitor the length of time that an inflatable splint has been in place because tissue ischemia can develop if the splint remains on for an extended time and begins to act as a tourniquet. It is impossible to palpate distal pulses with this type of immobilization device in place; therefore, visual assessments are essential. The inflatable splint should be replaced with another device as soon as possible. Pressure changes are common when a splint that has been applied outdoors in a cold environment meets warmer indoor temperatures. Monitor neurovascular status closely, since the warm air will cause the splint to tighten. Direct pressure on an inflatable splint should result in some degree of depression, indicating that the splint is not overinflated.

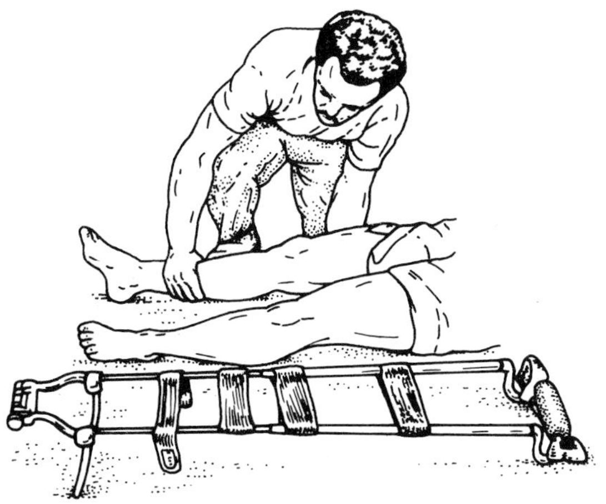

Figure 21–12. Hare traction splint. (From The Maryland Way: EMT—A Skills Manual. Baltimore, MIEMSS, 1985.)

Immobilization should never be prevented or delayed because of a lack of "manufactured" splints. Any rigid material padded with soft material can be used for effective immobilization. A fractured lower extremity can be splinted against the opposite extremity with padding in between when no other resource is available (Fig. 21–13). Injured upper extremities can be immobilized against the torso. Leave ski boots or other heavy protective boots in place until appropriate personnel are available. These types of footwear act as splints and may even cause effective tamponade of underlying vascular injuries.

Pelvic Ring Disruptions. Initial evaluation of the trauma patient may not reveal obvious clinical evidence of a pelvic injury, e.g., extremity rotation or shortening or abnormal

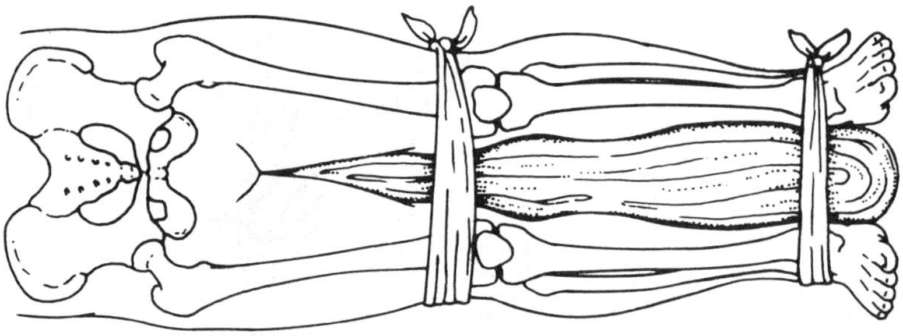

Figure 21–13. Legs immobilized by using blankets and cravats. (From The Maryland Way: EMT—A Skills Manual. Baltimore, MIEMSS, 1985.)

movement on downward or inward compression of the iliac wings. However, any signs or symptoms indicative of pelvic ring disruptions require immobilization prior to patient transport to minimize the risk of further neurovascular injury. Suspected pelvic injuries may be effectively immobilized with a PASG. This garment provides tamponade effects as well as bony immobilization. Obvious pelvic injuries with associated hip dislocations and/or blowout injuries to the acetabulum often require creative techniques to achieve initial immobilization and stabilization. Injuries that cause shortening, rotation, or frog-leg positioning require support and stabilization of the patient's lower extremities in the position in which they are found. The use of a long wooden backboard in conjunction with pillows, rolled sheets, or blankets secured and taped under the patient's knees supports extremity position and ensures immobilization during transport. The patient with an unstable pelvic ring disruption may require formal stabilization (external fixator application) during the early phase of resuscitation to prevent exsanguination and restore hemodynamic stability (Fig. 21–14). Use caution whenever moving a patient with a pelvic injury, since disruption of the retroperitoneal tamponade can rapidly progress to hemorrhagic shock.

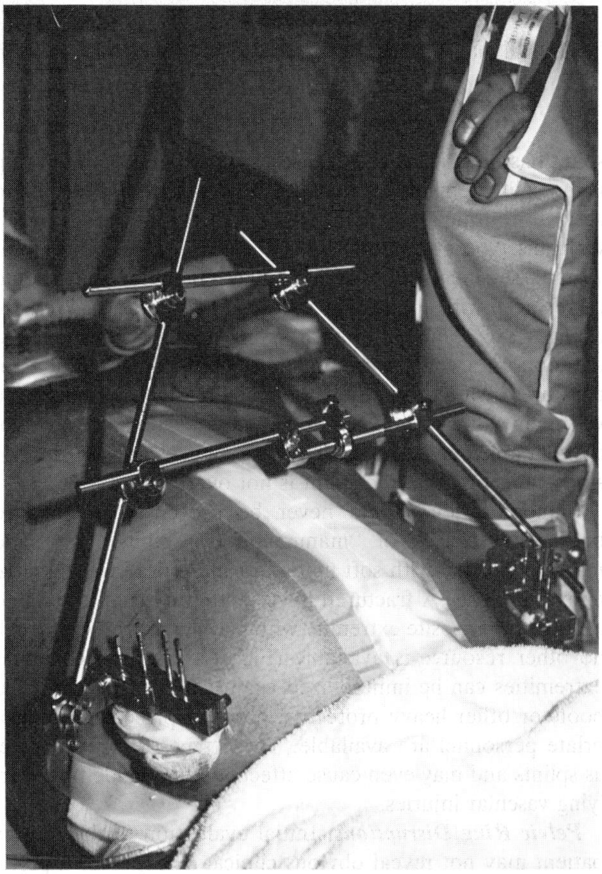

Figure 21–14. Clinical immobilization for pelvic ring disruption.

Potential for Fluid Volume Deficit Related to Blood Loss

Any musculoskeletal injury will result in blood loss. The degree of hemorrhage and its effect on the patient's overall hemodynamic status depend on the type, location, and number of injuries. Generally speaking, musculoskeletal injuries receive attention after stabilization of the cardiopulmonary and neurological systems. However, there are times when musculoskeletal injuries become priorities and necessitate early, aggressive intervention. Two injuries associated with excessive blood loss, traumatic amputations and massive pelvic injuries, require priority care by a coordinated team approach to facilitate restoration and maintenance of cardiovascular stability. Other bony and soft tissue injuries can usually wait for definitive care, but the patient still requires adequate volume replacement to prevent hypovolemia related to blood loss. It is difficult to estimate accurately the actual amount of blood lost, especially with multiple-extremity or pelvic fractures and soft tissue injuries. Hypovolemia should be anticipated in patients with these injuries, and measures to restore and maintain hemodynamics must be instituted. Table 21–2 approximates possible blood loss with open and closed fractures.

GENERAL MANAGEMENT PRINCIPLES

Cardiovascular Status. Any patient with actual or potential circulating volume deficits requires vigilant observation and frequent reevaluation for the clinical indicators of shock. Monitor the patient's EKG rhythm continuously for tachycardia and dysrhythmias and obtain vital signs at least every

TABLE 21–2. BLOOD LOSS CAUSED BY FRACTURES*

FRACTURE	BLOOD LOSS (ml)
Humerus	500–1500
Elbow	250– 750
Radius/ulna	250– 500
Pelvis	750–6000
Femur	500–3000
Tibia/fibula	250–2000
Ankle	250–1000

One unit of whole blood equals approximately 500 ml.
*Data from references 17, 19, and 20.

15 minutes until he is stabilized. Assess generalized perfusion by evaluating skin color and temperature, capillary refill times (which should be no longer than 2 seconds), and the presence, quality, and equality of peripheral pulses. Trend analysis of laboratory data augments the overall assessment of the hemodynamic status. Never leave patients with major musculoskeletal injuries such as traumatic amputations, multiple fractures, and unstable pelvic ring disruptions unattended nor allow them to be transported out of the resuscitation area without qualified personnel. These patients can and do rapidly and unexpectedly deteriorate to a hemorrhagic shock state from massive blood loss. Constant monitoring, especially during transport, is essential. For example, the retroperitoneal hematoma associated with a massive or unstable pelvic ring disruption can break loose during transfer of the patient to the radiography table. This sudden tamponade release precipitates rapid cardiovascular deterioration to shock.

Volume Replacement. Adequate fluid replacement with colloid and/or crystalloid solutions should begin immediately. Blood and/or component therapy is an integral component of successful fluid resuscitation. Early and substantial blood transfusions help prevent deterioration and the sequelae of late shock as a result of massive blood loss (see Chapter 9). The blood bank should be notified early concerning the patient's replacement needs, and updates of changes should be provided as needed. The amount of blood and clotting factors required for a patient with massive pelvic injuries can severely strain the blood bank's supplies. The team may need to consider transferring the patient to a major trauma center for this reason alone.

Pressure Dressing. Obvious sources of external hemorrhage require immediate application of direct pressure and pressure dressings to obtain control. Use a figure eight bandage or a bandage wrapped in a spiral fashion starting at a point distal to the wound, and wrap it proximally to secure the dressing. Pressure dressings minimize damage to soft tissue and neurovascular structures while achieving hemostasis. Properly applied pressure dressings will almost always provide adequate control of hemorrhage, even with traumatic amputations. Closely monitor the dressing for continued bleeding, and reinforce it as necessary. Never use a tourniquet except as a last resort for massive, uncontrollable hemorrhage. Tourniquets increase the extent of the injury to the amputated part by causing ischemic damage to nerves and vessels.[10]

PASG. The benefits from the use of pneumatic antishock garments (PASGs) remain controversial, specifically concerning translocation of blood.[11–17] Their widely recognized values include immobilization and compression effects. PASGs extend the amount of time for resuscitation procedures and provide excellent external tamponade for major hemorrhage, as seen with pelvic injuries and open extremity fractures.

Closed Fractures. Significant blood loss, as indicated in Table 21–2, can occur within an extremity despite the fact that a specific fracture has been classified as closed. The areas surrounding and distal to the fracture site become swollen, and the skin tightens from the accumulation of blood within the soft tissue.

Open Fractures. An open fracture can cause blood loss of at least 1 to 3 or more units, in addition to the amounts listed in Table 21–2. Not only does blood loss become apparent externally, but it also continues internally within the soft tissue.

Traumatic Amputations. Massive blood loss, often potentiating hypovolemic shock, can occur from traumatic amputations. This devastating injury requires priority intervention to restore cardiovascular stability. Emergency measures such as direct pressure and pressure dressings must be initiated immediately during the initial evaluation.

Pelvic Fractures. Exsanguination represents the primary cause of early mortality after an unstable pelvic fracture. As previously mentioned, the pelvis receives a rich blood supply through the arteries and venous plexus of the iliac system (Fig. 21–15). This vascular network can easily sustain injury or disruption because of its close approximation to the bony structures. The retroperitoneal space can hold as many as 4 liters of blood before it spontaneously tamponades, which makes it very difficult to determine actual blood loss.[6, 22] The patient with a pelvic injury is also at increased risk for hemorrhage from common associated injuries, such as intra-abdominal viscera, bladder, and urethra, which compounds the blood loss from the bony and vascular injuries. Hypovolemic shock must be anticipated in patients with massive pelvic injuries, and emergency measures to restore hemodynamics should be instituted early. Refer to Chapter 9 for further discussion.

Potential for Infection

All open orthopedic injuries are considered contaminated and place the patient at risk for developing tetanus, gas gangrene, osteomyelitis, and other infections. These wounds are contaminated by the prehospital environment and are then exposed to very dangerous, resistant hospital organisms. Wound and bone infections represent potentially disastrous and disabling complications associated with increased morbidity. These infections can lead to delayed union, nonunion, or acute or chronic osteomyelitis. These conditions prolong hospitalization, add a tremendous financial burden, and may eventually result in loss of the affected extremity.[23, 24] It is therefore essential that measures aimed at eliminating further wound contamination and preventing microbial growth take precedence early during resuscitation.[25, 26]

GENERAL MANAGEMENT PRINCIPLES

Initial Wound Care. During resuscitation it is important to remove any gross contaminants from the wound and cover any exposed soft tissue and bone with a wet, sterile saline dressing. Prevent reentry of a dirty bone end or soft tissue into the wound whenever possible. Should reentry occur, it is imperative that the orthopedic specialist be notified. Saline-soaked dressings are recommended rather than those saturated with iodine-based solutions.[27, 28] The soft tissue absorbs some of the solution, and iodine has been found to cause local tissue irritation and decrease the tissue's resistance to infection. Additionally, iodine can create cellular toxicity.[27, 29] Saline has replaced iodine solutions intraoperatively and in postoperative wound management as well.[28] Avoid frequent dressing manipulations because the risk of additional pathogens entering the wound increases with each examination. Sterile procedure must be observed by all personnel when handling open wounds and dressings (e.g., use mask, hat, and sterile gloves).

Irrigation. Ideally, the patient should proceed rapidly to

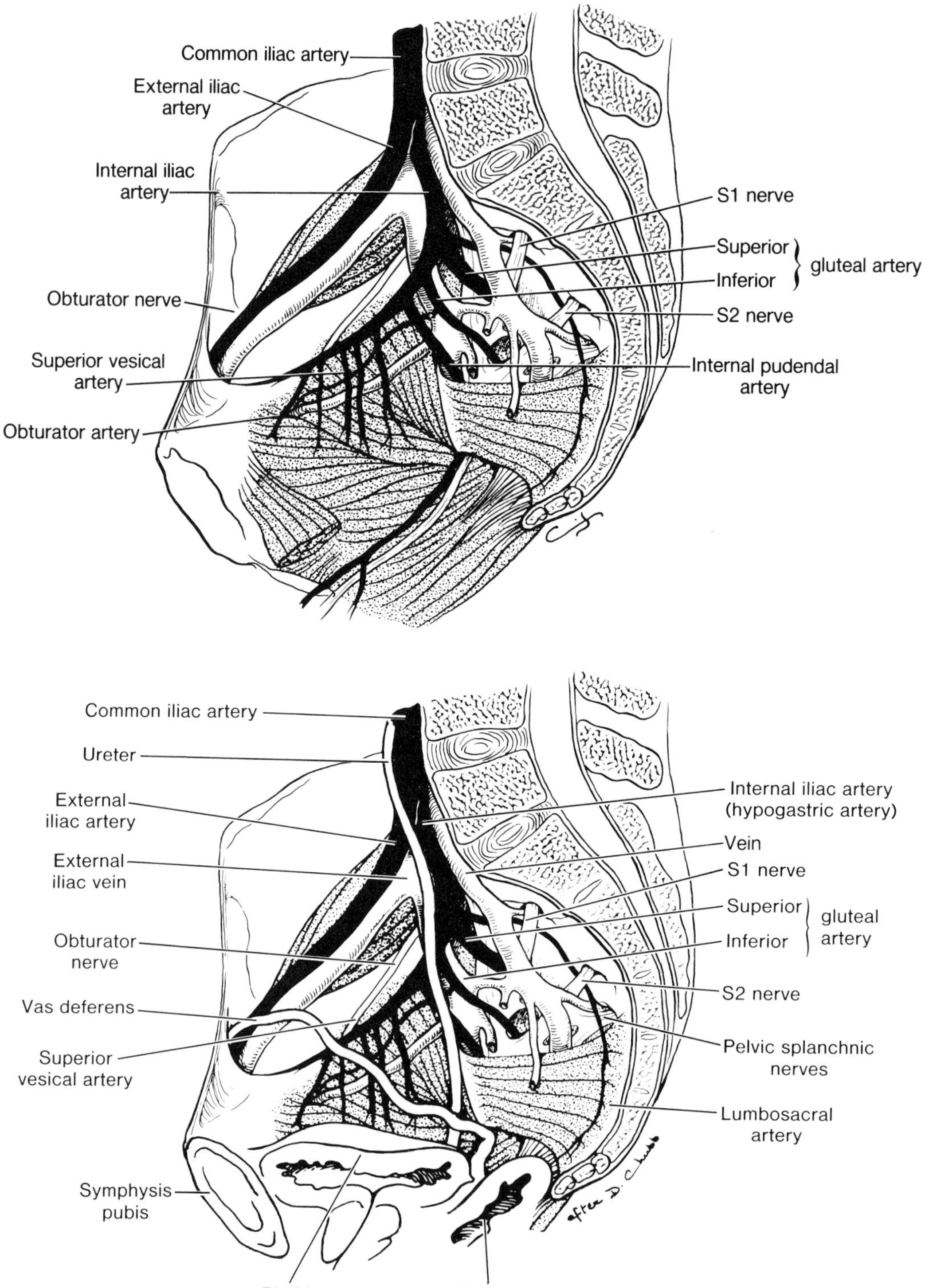

Figure 21–15. The internal iliac system of arteries and veins showing the position of the pelvic viscera. (From Tile M: Fractures of the Pelvis and Acetabulum. Baltimore, Williams & Wilkins, 1984.)

the operating suite for irrigation, debridement, and definitive care. If a delay prevents this transfer from occurring in a timely fashion, the patient should receive early, aggressive wound irrigation in the emergency care area. The optimal method of irrigation includes use of large volumes of saline.

Tetanus Immunization. Tetanus is a preventable yet highly lethal complication caused by anaerobic bacterial growth in necrotic tissue. In an effort to reduce the risk of tetanus, all devitalized tissue must be surgically excised, and the patient must be adequately immunized. Confirm the patient's recent tetanus immunization history, and administer a booster as indicated and ordered. Additional information on tetanus can be found in Chapter 13.

Antibiotic Therapy. Wound contamination may occur from foreign debris such as contaminants that enter at the time of injury, bacteria introduced in the hospital environment, and the products of necrosis. The trauma patient with multisystem injuries and musculoskeletal injuries, especially open fractures and traumatic amputations, is at increased risk for infection from any of these causes and therefore should receive antibiotics during the resuscitative phase.[29–31] Culturing the wound site and the involved soft tissue prior to starting the antibiotics offers a more accurate determination and evaluation of therapy postoperatively. Prevention of microbial growth by antibiotics requires adequate concentrations of the antibiotic at the site of the bone or soft tissue injury or operative site. From the time the antibiotic is administered intravenously, it only takes approximately 20 to 30 minutes to achieve saturation in the interstitial fluid of healthy bone matrix.[33] Antibiotics are most beneficial when they are administered at the peak of bacterial wound contamination, when they satisfactorily invade the bony injury or wound, and when they are chosen specifically for the potential contaminating organisms.[33] For these reasons, administration of intravenous antibiotics should begin in the resuscitative cycle, or approximately 30 minutes prior to an elective operative orthopedic procedure, to achieve maximal antimicrobial effects.[33]

The use of prophylactic antibiotics in open reduction of closed fractures is controversial. The treatment of a specific bacterial organism identified later during the critical care or the intermediate cycle is easier to treat if the organism has not developed a resistance through the administration of prophylactic antibiotics. Many studies on the subject of prophylactic antibiotics report on cases of elective orthopedic surgery and not trauma patients. The trauma patient, although usually young and in relatively good health,[34] may have suffered some degree of shock, may have other associated injuries, and may require long hours of initial operative repair. In the multiple trauma patient, the risk of infection increases as the number of systems involved rises. Studies also have shown that operative procedures lasting longer than 90 minutes have a higher incidence of infection.

Potential for Neurological and/or Vascular Compromise

During the resuscitative cycle, the most imperative initial intervention is early recognition of patients who are at risk for neurological and vascular compromise as a result of musculoskeletal injury. The following mechanisms and injuries are precipitators of neurological and vascular complications:

- Compression or crushing mechanisms
- Open or closed fractures
- Soft tissue injuries
- Arterial involvement/injury
- Dislocations
- Prolonged use of PASG

Essentially any musculoskeletal injury that involves bone and/or soft tissue can potentiate neurological and/or vascular compromise. Muscle and nerve tissues are easily damaged because of several factors, including their close proximity to the bony structures and their extreme sensitivity to impaired circulation and compression. Regardless of the actual cause of the compromise, the same pathology results: When the vasculature becomes impaired, tissue perfusion decreases, which leads to ischemia. If the ischemic process continues, the muscle tissue becomes edematous, as increased permeability occurs at the capillary level. This results in additional edema within the tissues, which adds more pressure on the capillaries and eventually causes their collapse. The progression from ischemia to muscle necrosis occurs rapidly. Within 6 to 8 hours, the nerves, muscles, and vascular structures may experience irreversible damage both locally and distally.[4, 36] Knowing the mechanism of injury and the specific types of injuries that carry the highest incidence of neurovascular compromise is the first step in preventing this common yet serious complication.

Injuries to the brachial plexus and the lumbosacral plexus also may cause altered sensation and mobility. Neither of these injuries ranks high as a priority, nor do they necessitate immediate intervention during the resuscitation and stabilization of the multisystem-injured patient. However, the peripheral nerve involvement associated with both injuries may create an insensate and paralyzed extremity that renders the patient completely disabled in that limb.

General Management Principles

Continuous Monitoring. Potential or actual peripheral nerve or vascular compromise requires continuous, on-going monitoring. Clinical findings commonly seen with dislocations, fractures, or plexus injuries include alteration in pulse quality, edema, change in skin color (pallor, arterial inadequacy, cyanosis, venous congestion), and altered sensory and motor function. On-going motor and sensory assessments are essential even after institution of traction devices, to promote early detection of neurological impairment. Devices such as Buck's skin traction, used, for example, preoperatively for subtrochanteric and hip fractures, can cause peroneal branch nerve compression if improperly applied or maintained. Compression of the peroneal nerve as it passes over the fibular head leads to foot drop, a complication that can extend the patient's hospital stay and increase rehabilitation needs.

Immobilization/Alignment. As discussed previously in this chapter, proper immobilization and alignment are essential elements in preventing further injury to the soft tissue, especially the vessels and nerves. The risk for further injury, such as laceration, continued hemorrhage, and additional impingement or compression, increases if proper immobilization techniques are not employed early after the injury. For example, splinting the entire upper extremity in the position of function is essential for the patient with a brachial plexus injury because further stretching of the deltoid muscle may result in humeral head dislocation. Proper positioning, realignment of fractures, or reduction of dislocations often must take precedence during resuscitation in an effort to reduce extremity morbidity.

Elevation. Maintaining an injured limb in a nondependent position, but not above the level of the patient's heart, may reduce further edema formation and improve venous return. Elevation above the level of the patient's heart may actually impede circulation,[37] since the local arterial pressure decreases 0.8 mm Hg for each centimeter of elevation.[38]

Cooling. Cooling of the injured extremity should begin concurrently with elevation. Prepackaged coolant bags and plastic bags and gloves filled with ice-cooled water all work effectively. Use of frozen products or pure ice bags should be avoided because ice causes vasoconstriction with a resultant decrease in local circulation and venous return and may lead to thermal injuries in areas with decreased sensation.

Protection. Any extremity with neurological impairment should be monitored closely for position and environmental factors. A paralyzed, insensate limb is at increased risk for accidental or secondary injury. Prolonged pressure on bony prominences can quickly lead to skin breakdown and ulceration, which are preventable and very costly complications for the patient.[39] Measures that improve circulation and promote venous return, such as positioning and elevation, should be instituted.

Dislocations. Dislocations are often easily recognized clinically without the aid of diagnostic studies. However, a dislocation may occur at the time of impact and then either reduce spontaneously or during application of an immobilization device at the scene of the accident. For this reason, it is important to obtain a history from either the patient or the prehospital care providers concerning any "popping" or "snapping" of a joint that may have been felt or heard or the presence of an actual dislocation.

Dislocations create orthopedic emergencies when bone impinges on nearby vessels or nerves. For example, dislocations of the elbow or the knee require immediate intervention specifically by the orthopedist because of the extremely high incidence of associated neurovascular disruption. The nerve injury secondary to a dislocation may be actual, as in laceration by a bone fragment, or physiological, as from compression, blast effect, or traction/stretching mechanisms. Clinical findings indicative of a physiological nerve injury may resolve spontaneously after the bones have been reduced and properly aligned. Symptoms may, however, be of a more permanent nature, depending on the severity of the injury and the length of time that elapsed prior to treatment. Vascular involvement may result from laceration, compression, crushing, and traction/stretching mechanisms. The potential resolution of vascular complications depends on the specific injury, the ischemic time, and the ability of collateral circulation to restore and maintain blood flow. Table 21–3 correlates joint dislocations with the potential neurovascular branches involved.[13]

Fractures. Neurovascular compromise associated with fractures results from causes similar to dislocations. Injury to the neurovascular supply of the extremities may result from actual laceration or tearing, compression from bone ends or edematous soft tissue, and stretching by disrupted bone fragments.

TABLE 21–3. NEUROVASCULAR STRUCTURES AT RISK FOR INVOLVEMENT IN JOINT DISLOCATION

JOINT	NERVE/VESSEL
Shoulder	Brachial plexus, axillary artery
Elbow	Ulnar nerve, brachial artery
Wrist	Median nerve
Hip	Sciatic nerve
Knee	Tibial/peroneal nerve, popliteal artery/vein
Ankle	Tibial artery

Pelvic Injuries. The pelvis enjoys a rich vascular supply, as seen in Figure 21–15. Oxygenated blood enters the pelvis via the internal iliac artery. A venous plexus, consisting of valveless, thin-walled veins that allow bidirectional blood flow, drains the pelvic basin. Collateral networks exist on both the arterial and venous sides. The sciatic nerve arising from the lumbosacral plexus innervates the pelvis and the lower extremities. Any disruption of the bones or ligaments of the pelvis or hips can potentially cause severe neurovascular complications. Massive pelvic ring disruptions are considered lethal injuries because of the major vascular complications with which they are associated.

Compartment Syndrome. Compartment syndrome may affect joint compartments throughout the body (e.g., shoulders, upper and lower arms, hands, pelvis, hips, thighs, and feet). Most commonly affected, however, are the lower leg and the forearm, which have two and four muscle compartments, respectively. Sheaths of fascia tightly bind these closed muscle systems, which house neurovascular bundles. Compartment syndrome may result when either internal or external sources increase compartment pressure. Internal causes of increased compartment pressures include increased volumes and increased capillary filtration, which represent increased intracompartment content. External causes of increased compartment pressure, e.g., restrictive devices or procedures and excessive traction, decrease the size of the compartment. Both internal and external causes lead to elevated pressures within the compartments, which result in compression of the microvascular system, leading to ischemia of the muscle tissue (Fig. 21–16). If elevated compartment pressures are not reduced, irreversible damage to the muscle and nerve tissue, including necrosis and scarring, will result within 6 to 8 hours. The following injuries or conditions represent examples of internal and external causes of compartment syndrome:

Internal

- Trauma: compressing or crushing mechanisms, open/closed fractures, soft tissue or vascular injuries
- Burns: thermal, electrical, frostbite
- Bites: spiders, snakes
- Prolonged shock states: tissue ischemia, venous pooling

External

- Prolonged or excessive use of PASGs, splints, traction devices
- Prolonged pressure over compartment: lying or positioning
- Excessive skeletal traction

A common misconception is that open fractures are safe from compartment syndrome because they are open. This is

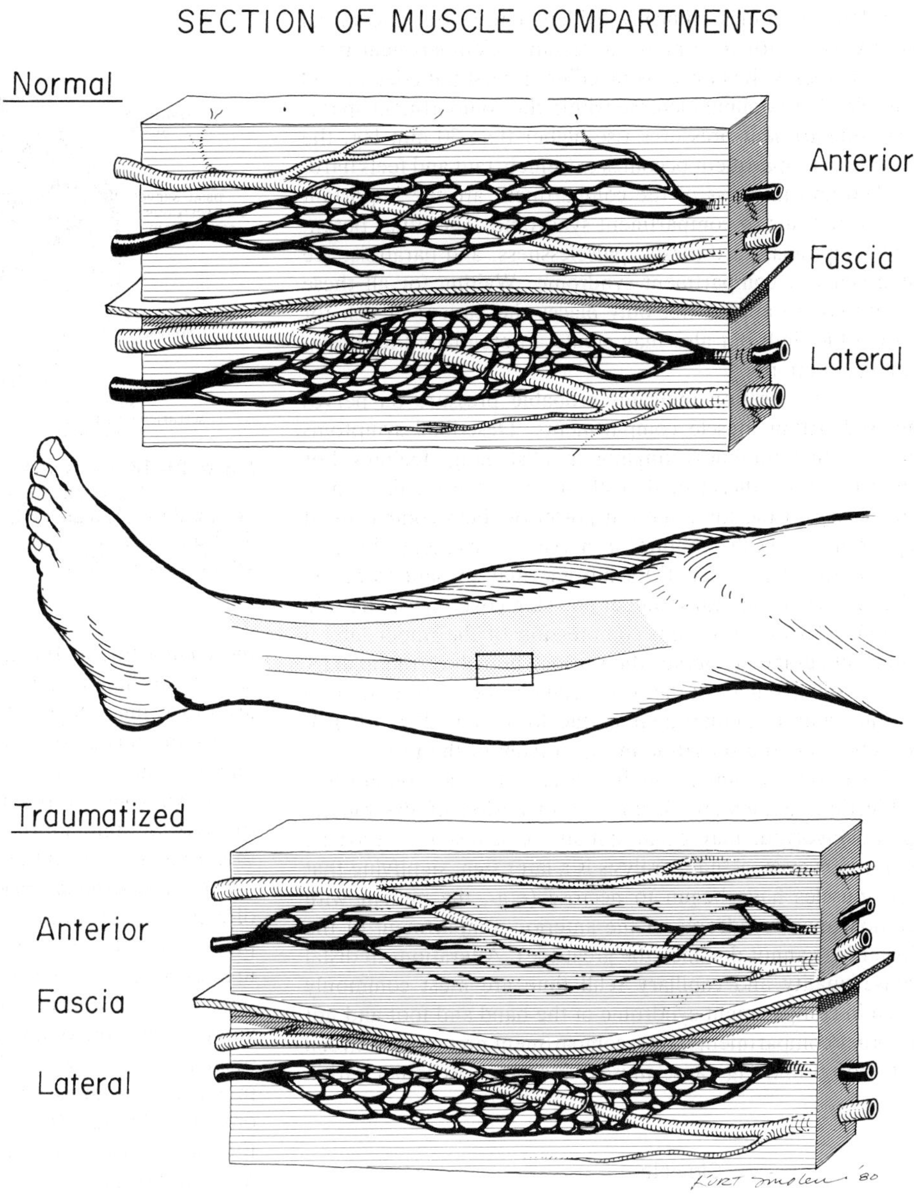

Figure 21–16. Unifying principles of a compartment syndrome. In the enlarged figure above the leg, normal microcirculation is viewed during rest in the anterior and lateral muscle compartments. These two compartments are separated by fascia. During rest, intracompartmental pressure in the anterior and lateral compartments is near zero, and blood flow in all capillaries (network of black vessels) and large arteries (shaded vessels entering figure from the right) is normal. If pressure in the anterior compartment reaches a threshold level near 30 mm Hg (enlarged figure below leg), capillary perfusion is inadequate to maintain tissue viability. It is noteworthy that distal pulses are usually present in the foot primarily because intracompartmental pressure rarely rises above central-artery diastolic pressure. (From Hargens AR, Mubarak SJ: Definition and terminology. In Mubarak SJ, Hargens AR, Akeson WH (eds): Compartment Syndromes and Volkmann's Contracture. Philadelphia, WB Saunders Co, 1981.)

incorrect, however, because even though an open wound may violate a fascial compartment, other compartments remain intact and are at risk for this syndrome. Additionally, traumatic wounds usually occur horizontally and are not large enough to decompress the compartment.[37]

Assessment. Assess the patient frequently for throbbing pain which appears out of proportion to the injury and is localized to the compartment involved and increases on passive muscle stretching; for firmness of the entire compartment; and for paresthesia in the distal distribution of the nerve involved. Paresthesia is a later symptom of compartment syndrome. When these symptoms—pain, firmness, and paresthesia—are found simultaneously as a group, they signal impending extremity morbidity unless appropriate interventions begin immediately. The injured extremity should always be compared with the nonaffected extremity during this evaluation. This assessment must be performed at least every 1 to 2 hours or more frequently, depending on the patient's status and the examiner's clinical observations and judgment. Established protocols or nursing standards provide further guidelines.

The pain associated with neurovascular compromise, often described as burning or searing, results from the ischemic process occurring at the site of injury and in surrounding and distal soft tissue structures. Bleeding and edema within the surrounding soft tissues in addition to the specific injury result in the pain associated with fractures and dislocations. Any type of movement of the extremity will increase pain at the site of injury. Reported compartment syndrome pain usually seems out of proportion to the actual injury. Use of narcotics often cannot provide relief from the pain associated with this syndrome. The pain increases on passive stretching of the muscles. For example, flexion of the ankle and foot or the toes causes increased pain in the lower leg. It is therefore important to monitor and record trends in the patient's pain patterns and effects of medication.

Edema becomes clinically evident early after the initial injury as a normal response to trauma. Compartment pressure increases, however, as bleeding, interstitial edema, and muscle fiber swelling increase within the compartment space. As compartment pressures rise higher than 30 mm Hg, the affected compartment becomes extremely taut and feels hard.

Pain and firmness of the compartment are the important key symptoms of compartment syndrome. The other potential symptoms, paresthesia, pulselessness, and paralysis, are late signs of compartment syndrome. Waiting for all these symptoms to appear not only places the patient at risk for losing the limb but also may create a potentially life-threatening situation.

Altered sensation indicates probable pressure on nerves housed within muscle compartments. Described symptoms may include numbness, tingling, and "sticking" feelings. For example, paresthesia or dysesthesia over the medial aspect of the leg to the knee seen in posterior thigh compartment syndrome indicates obturator nerve involvement. Deltoid compartment (Fig. 21–17) syndrome may present as paresthesia over the lateral shoulder and skin covering the deltoid muscle. This results from compression of the upper lateral brachial cutaneous nerve, the sensory branch of the axillary nerve. Involvement of the superficial peroneal nerve, housed in the lateral compartment of the lower leg (Fig. 21–18), results in altered sensation in the dorsum of the foot.

Decreased voluntary limb movement, e.g., diminished adduction, abduction, flexion, or extension of the muscle group involved, may occur initially as a result of extreme pain. However, actual paralysis is a later sign, signifying that the muscles have begun to necrose (e.g., the patient with compartment syndrome of the anterior compartment of the lower leg cannot dorsiflex the great toe). Alterations in distal pulse quality and capillary refill time are most commonly seen in compartment syndrome of the hand and foot and not in other compartments. Intracompartment pressures between 30 and 60 mm Hg cause muscle and nerve ischemia within the compartment, but these pressures are not usually sufficient to occlude arterial flow (intraluminal pressure in major arteries is much higher than 30 to 60 mm Hg).[40]

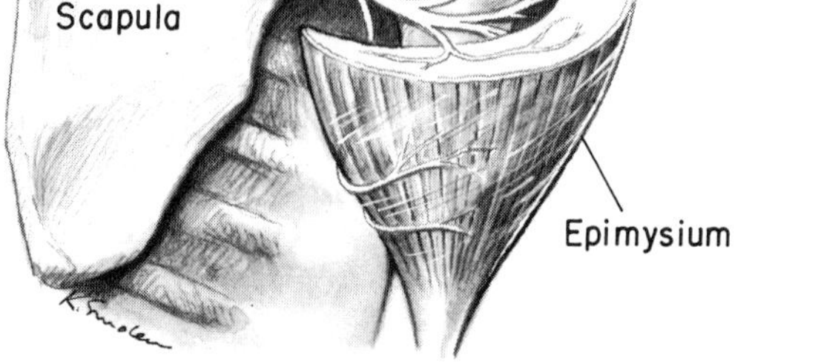

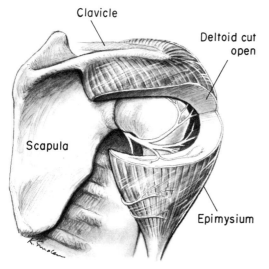

Figure 21–17. Deltoid compartment (posterior view); the epimysium and fascia form one layer enclosing this muscle. (From Garfin SR: Anatomy of the extremity compartments. In Mubarak SJ, Hargens AR, Akeson WH (eds): Compartment Syndromes and Volkmann's Contracture. Philadelphia, WB Saunders Co, 1981.)

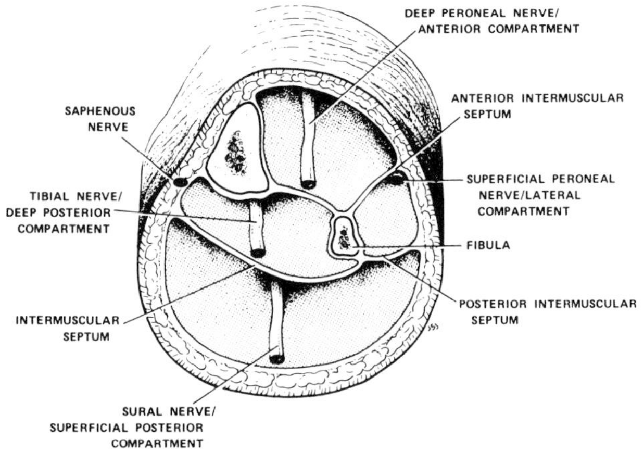

Figure 21–18. Cross section at the junction of the middle and distal thirds of the leg, illustrating the four compartments and their respective nerves. (From Mubarak SJ, Owen CA: Double incision fasciotomy of the leg for decompression in compartment syndromes. J Bone Joint Surg 59A:184, 1977.)

Prompt recognition and early institution of therapeutic measures must occur long before the late signs of compartment syndrome. Early recognition and treatment decrease the risk of limb morbidity and minimize the risk of life-threatening complications.

Intracompartment Pressure Measurements. Clinical signs of compartment syndrome indicate the need to measure the pressures within the muscle compartments. Pressure measurements may be performed prophylactically in the unconscious patient who has signs of increasing pressure. Controversy exists surrounding the upper pressure limits that mandate a fasciotomy, the treatment of choice for elevated pressures; the most aggressive recommendation for fasciotomy uses 30 mm Hg[37, 41, 42] as the determining level, whereas the most conservative recommendation uses 60 mm Hg.[43, 44] Most authorities agree on a gray zone in which the pressure limits may be borderline. If the patient is conscious, can give reliable information, and has the ability to describe pain and other symptoms consistently, close clinical observation should continue, with possible follow-up pressure measurements as indicated. However, if the patient is unconscious and has borderline pressure measurements, fasciotomy is usually recommended. Continuous monitoring is not practical or appropriate in the multisystem-injured patient.[37]

Brachial Plexus Injury. The brachial plexus, which incorporates the roots of the fifth cervical vertebra to the first thoracic vertebra, subdivides to form the following nerves: axillary, musculocutaneous, median, ulnar, and radial (Fig. 21–19). These nerves are responsible for deltoid, biceps, and triceps function as well as innervation of the extensors and flexors of the forearm, wrist, and hand.

Traumatic injury to the brachial plexus may occur from blunt or penetrating mechanisms. Blunt injuries usually result from excessive forces that initially injure the muscle and its fascia and then cause extreme stretching of the nervous network, usually the nerve roots.[45] Associated injuries that often accompany brachial plexus injuries include closed head

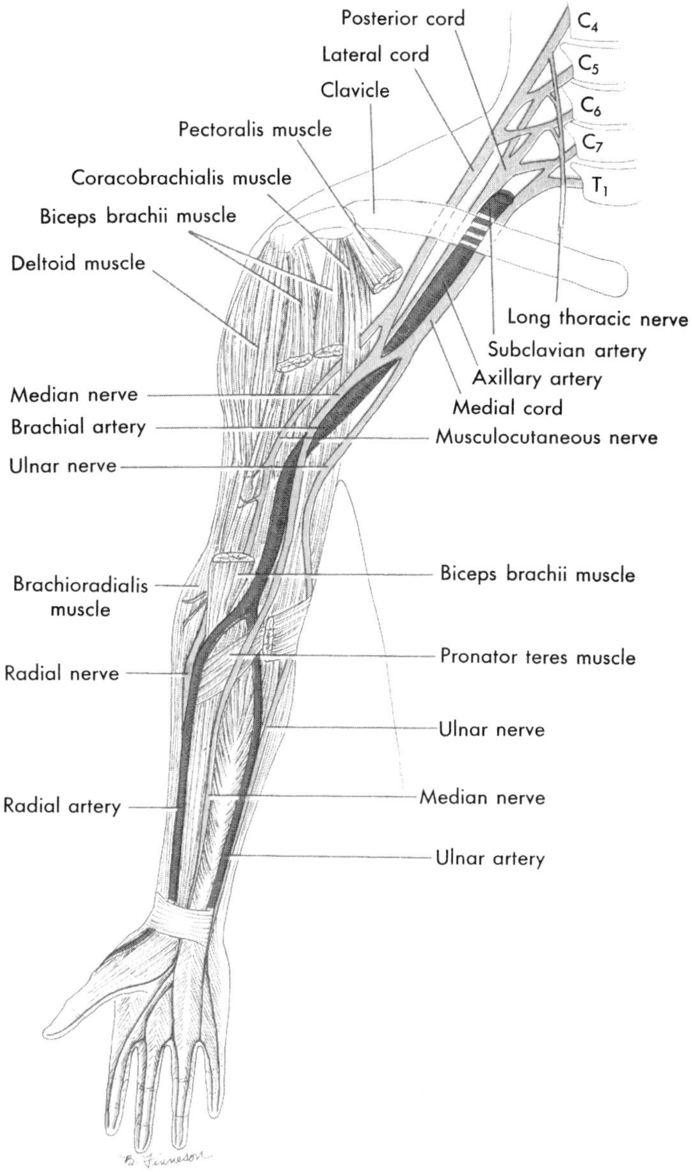

Figure 21–19. Diagram illustrating the brachial plexus and distribution of nerves. Note their relation to arteries and to muscles (right arm). (From Kimber DC, Gray CE, Stackpole CE: Kimber-Gray-Stackpole's Anatomy and Physiology. New York, Macmillan, 1977.)

injuries and shoulder dislocations. Most frequently, the blunt mechanisms that result in a plexus injury involve the patient's ejection from a car or off a motorcycle with a landing such that the head is distracted from the affected shoulder and upper extremity. Blunt brachial plexus injuries may be subdivided into upper root and lower root classifications.[46] The upper roots, C5 to C7, may sustain injury when the head experiences significant lateral bending away from the shoulder and when the shoulder itself is forcefully depressed downward. This upper root injury usually does not affect motor function in the wrist and hand but leaves the patient with a motionless shoulder and elbow. The sensory deficit usually affects the deltoid muscle, arm, and forearm. A lower root injury involving C8 to T1 may occur when the arm is forcefully extended over the head. The shoulder and elbow maintain intact motor function, but the forearm and hand lose sensation and motor function. Any closed or blunt injury to the brachial plexus may be complete or incomplete. Incomplete injuries often present confusing clinical pictures because the patient has inconsistent or unusual patterns of sensory or motor dysfunction. A complete lesion within the brachial plexus results in paralysis and complete sensory loss of the arm and hand.

Penetrating mechanisms such as in missile or blast injuries or stabbings, which cause open wounds near the shoulder or clavicle, may result in injury to the brachial plexus. Associated injuries to surrounding soft tissue and the subclavian vein or artery may precipitate upper extremity ischemia, which further clouds the clinical picture. Motor and sensory deficits could occur from either the ischemic process or the plexus injury. A conclusive differentiation may be difficult.

Neuromotor Assessment. Accurate and complete evaluation of the functional status of the brachial plexus in the critically injured multisystem trauma patient may present a challenge. Often, alterations in the patient's level of consciousness and sensory responses, resulting from concurrent injuries or chemical ingestion, make assessment difficult, if not impossible. It is essential to differentiate this injury from a cervical spinal cord injury and from the flacidity seen with devastating head injuries. The patient should be assessed for Horner's syndrome, or Horner's pupil, which occurs with a preganglionic interruption of the T1 dermatome, causing loss of sympathetic innervation to and constriction of the ipsilateral pupil. The presence of this sign indicates poor chances for limb recovery because of the level of the injury.[47] If the patient cannot abduct the affected arm over the head or extend the elbow against resistance, a brachial plexus injury may have occurred. More specific neuromotor checks to evaluate the nerves in question include the following and are shown in Figures 21–20 and 21–21:

1. The *musculocutaneous* nerve is tested by evaluating the patient's biceps function and sensation over the lateral portion of the forearm.
2. The *radial* nerve primarily serves a motor function. Radial injuries usually result in the inability to extend the wrist.
3. An intact *median* nerve enables apposition of the thumb to the little finger on the affected extremity. Sensory function is evaluated by stimulating the volar surface of the index finger.
4. The motor function of the *ulnar* nerve is assessed by requesting the patient to abduct and adduct the fingers on the extremity.

Intact sensation on the distal volar surface of the little finger represents sensory function.

Interventions. Early care of brachial plexus injuries is generally supportive, including protection of the affected extremity and proper immobilization as previously discussed; these measures must continue during critical care. Early rehabilitation to prevent muscle wasting and joint contractures is essential. Prompt recognition of complications such as causalgia and prevention of secondary disabilities such as skin breakdown (see immobility discussion in the critical care section) are of paramount importance for this patient. Early surgical exploration may be indicated in open injuries; at this time the nerves are "tagged" for later identification. Early primary microsurgical repair of injured nerves is generally not appropriate, however, because of the associated soft tissue injury and the risk of infection.

Causalgia. Brachial plexus injuries that tear sensory nerves at their central attachment may produce causalgia.[46] This altered pain processing is most commonly associated with ulnar and median nerve involvement. Causalgia generally develops within the first month after injury. Changes in the affected extremity reflective of autonomic dysfunction may include alterations in skin color (discoloration, flushing, bluish coloring) and temperature (hot/flushed or cold/clammy, dry, or increased local perspiration). The most severely disabling problem is extreme constant burning pain in the extremity that may be impossible to alleviate. The intractable pain, often leading to behavioral and emotional changes, can interfere with the patient's cooperation and participation and intensify his rehabilitation needs. Early administration of narcotics or sympathetic blocks (with a local anesthetic) may provide pain relief. Dorsal column stimulators that block pain transmissions may be effective. Severe, unrelenting pain may require a sympathectomy. The emotional and behavioral changes generally improve or dissipate after satisfactory pain management. (Refer to Chapter 15 for further discussion.)

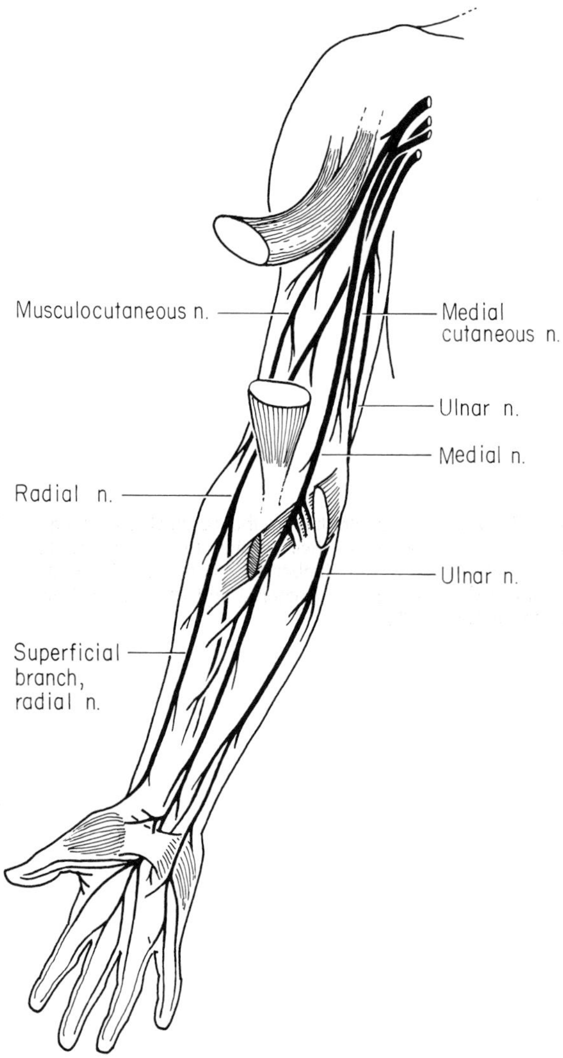

Figure 21–20. Nerves of the arm and forearm. (From Mubarak SJ: Anatomy of the extremity compartments. In Mubarak SJ, Hargens AR, Akeson WH (eds): Compartment Syndromes and Volkmann's Contracture. Philadelphia, WB Saunders Co, 1981.)

Lumbosacral Plexus Injury. The lumbosacral plexus, incorporating the fourth and fifth lumbar spinal nerves and S1, S2, and S3, supplies the sensory and motor function to the lower extremities. The three major nerves arising from the lumbosacral network, as seen in Figure 21–22, include the obturator, the femoral, and the sciatic, which divides into the posterior tibial and the common peroneal nerves.

Injury to the lumbosacral plexus itself, seen much less frequently than injury to the brachial plexus, must be differentiated from spinal injuries and associated root injuries. Lumbosacral plexus injury occurs rarely from blunt forces and more commonly from penetrating mechanisms such as gunshot wounds.[43, 46] Billowitz describes the three types of injuries to the lumbosacral plexus as follows: (1) intradural nerve root avulsion or stretching injury, (2) individual nerve root transection or crushing injury, and (3) disruption or palsy of the plexus.[48] The obturator nerve, protected by its

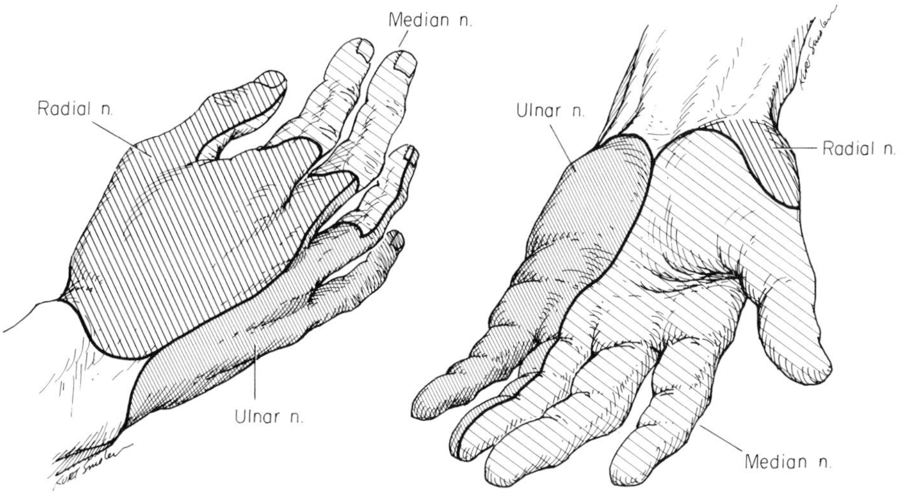

Figure 21–21. Distribution of the cutaneous nerves to the hand. (From Mubarak SJ: Anatomy of the extremity compartments. In Mubarak SJ, Hargens AR, Akeson WH (eds): Compartment Syndromes and Volkmann's Contracture. Philadelphia, WB Saunders Co, 1981.)

position within the pelvis, rarely sustains injury, yet it may be affected by penetrating trauma to the perineum. Any penetrating or blunt forces to the anterior thigh, especially near the inguinal ligament, may produce injury to the femoral nerve. The major trunk of the sciatic nerve lies within the pelvis and therefore remains protected from most external trauma. It is at high risk for injury, however, when pelvic disruption or hip fracture or dislocation occurs. The gluteal folds represent the point of superficial appearance of the sciatic nerve, and any wounds in the area of the buttock or thigh may involve the nerve as well. After the division of the sciatic nerve, the most common site of injury to the peroneal branch is at the head of the fibula, where the nerve is afforded little protection from any type of applied force.

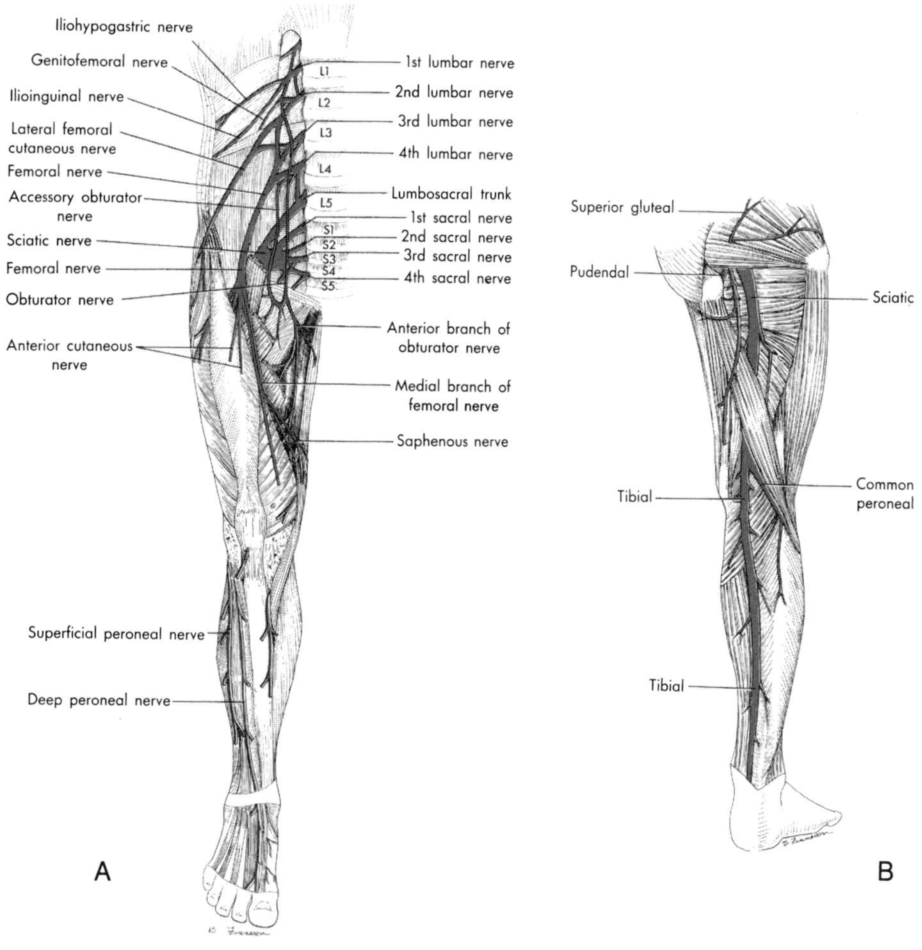

Figure 21–22. *A*, Diagram illustrating the lumbosacral plexus and distribution of nerves. Note their relation to muscles of the leg (right). *B*, Nerve supply to right lower extremity, posterior view. (From Kimber DC, Gray CE, Stackpole CE: Kimber-Gray-Stackpole's Anatomy and Physiology. New York, Macmillan, 1977.)

Blunt or penetrating mechanisms of force may affect the tibial nerve in the popliteal space or in the calf. Elevated pressure within the compartments in the lower leg poses increased risk for tibial nerve damage.

Neuromotor Assessment. Evaluation of the integrity of the nerves that arise from the lumbosacral plexus may present a formidable clinical challenge, as with the brachial plexus, in the multiple trauma patient. It is essential to perform initial and subsequent assessments in the patient suspected of having, or at risk for developing, peripheral nerve involvement. Figures 21–23 and 21–24 show the peripheral nerves of the lower leg and foot, respectively.

The motor function of the *obturator* can be assessed by having the patient adduct the thigh. This examination includes evaluation of the sensory status over the medial aspect of the thigh.

The *femoral* nerve supplies sensation to the medial aspect of the lower leg and foot from the inguinal ligament to the medial malleolus and motor function to the quadriceps. Inability to extend the knee and altered sensation in the medial leg and foot indicate injury to the femoral nerve.

Injury to the *common peroneal* nerve results in foot drop, or the inability to dorsiflex and evert the foot and ankle. Sensory changes in the web space between the first and second toes or over the lateral aspect of the calf indicate peroneal nerve injury.

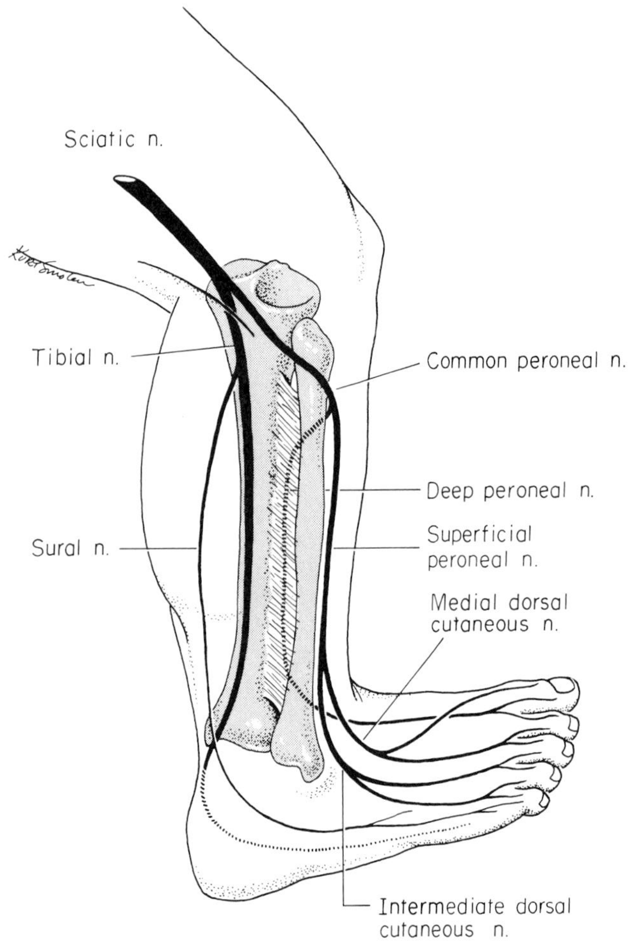

Figure 21–23. Peripheral nerves of the leg. (From Mubarak SJ: Anatomy of the extremity compartments. In Mubarak SJ, Hargens AR, Akeson WH (eds): Compartment Syndromes and Volkmann's Contracture. Philadelphia, WB Saunders Co, 1981.)

If the patient is unable to plantarflex or invert the foot and ankle and experiences sensory changes on the plantar surface of the foot and heel, dysfunction of the *tibial* nerve should be suspected.

Interventions. Often, nerve function can be restored with early reduction (closed or open) of a fracture or dislocation if the angulation or dislocation represents the probable cause of the dysfunction (as with posterior hip dislocation). Actual detection and diagnosis of a lumbosacral plexus injury may not occur until later in the acute care or recovery cycles, as the patient becomes more alert and is permitted more spontaneous movement. Surgical intervention for a lumbosacral plexus or sciatic nerve injury at the hip is generally of no benefit.[43, 49] As previously stated, surgical reduction of a posterior hip dislocation (with associated sciatic nerve involvement) may promote nerve recovery.

Alteration in Comfort

Injury to the musculoskeletal system produces pain of varying intensity depending on the type and location of the injury. Muscle spasms are the major cause of pain associated with fractures. The pain results from fractured bone ends moving, overriding, and passing through soft tissue. Lessening or elimination of muscle spasms by immobilization/stabilization or by reduction of the fracture will often eliminate much of the pain. Cool packs over the site of injury and analgesics will be required.

Pain associated with dislocation is often severe and continuous until the dislocation has been reduced. Additional pain is often caused by intentional or unintentional movement of the joint. Immobilization of the joint in the position in which it is found will help prevent or minimize movement and thereby minimize pain. Muscle relaxants and narcotics will relieve some of the muscle spasms and pain, but complete elimination of the pain associated with dislocations usually can only be accomplished through reduction of the dislocated joint. Because of the time that elapses from injury to attempted reduction (usually greater than 2 hours), increased muscle spasms and pain make muscle relaxants and narcotics necessary to attempt reduction. In severe cases, general anesthesia is required to effect complete muscle relaxation.[50]

Compartment syndrome pain is often described as deep, poorly localized, and continuous and is difficult to control with the usual analgesics required for musculoskeletal pain management. Compartment syndrome is often associated with crush injuries and severe fractures. It is easy to discount the pain as being caused by the original injury and not by compartment syndrome, a complication of the injury. Pain associated with compartment syndrome can only be relieved by eliminating the high fascial compartment pressures, e.g., by removal of constrictive bandages, by elevation of the affected extremity (but not higher than the level of the patient's heart) and application of cool packs to reduce swelling, and by fasciotomies.

The therapeutic plan for acute pain management is often developed and initiated during the resuscitation cycle or the preoperative cycle of care. For example, recognizing the pain associated with a complex acetabular fracture and realizing surgical intervention will be delayed for at least several days, the team may elect to insert an epidural catheter prior to

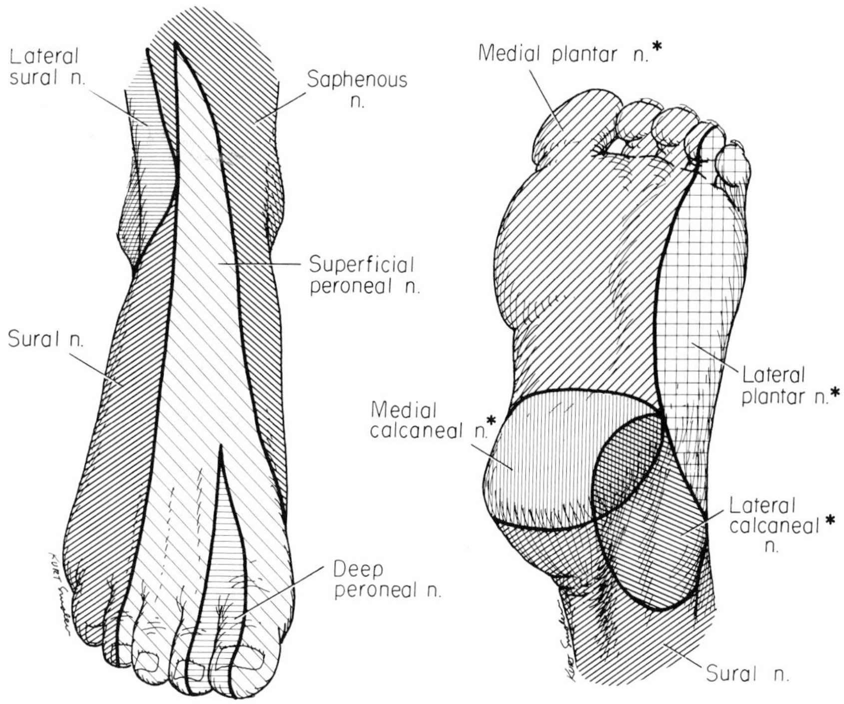

Figure 21–24. Distribution of the cutaneous nerves to the foot. * = Branches of the tibial nerve. (From Mubarak SJ: Anatomy of the extremity compartments. In Mubarak SJ, Hargens AR, Akeson WH (eds): Compartment Syndromes and Volkmann's Contracture. Philadelphia, WB Saunders Co, 1981.)

transferring the patient to the intensive care unit after his resuscitation. Early continuous analgesia given through this type of catheter provides the patient with pain relief, thus enabling him to begin and cooperate with the prescribed physical therapy regimen to prevent muscle wasting. This catheter also may be inserted during the preoperative phase for both intraoperative and postoperative use. Continuous analgesia via an epidural catheter enables early patient mobility and nursing interventions to prevent or minimize complications such as pulmonary problems.

A problem commonly associated with musculoskeletal pain relief regimens is the "peak and valley" effects of physician-ordered, nurse-administered intermittent intramuscular or intravenous analgesics. This pain/pain-free cycle is not only based on the drug's duration of action but also on the usual time delay from when the patient first requests his pain medication to when relief is actually obtained. For example, analgesics are usually ordered to be given every 3 to 4 hours as needed. If the patient in acute pain requires medication before the allotted time has elapsed, he must wait until the prescribed time. Time is then spent in preparing the medication and in waiting for its "administration-to-relief" time span to pass. The patient usually experiences a pain-free interval until the cycle repeats itself—hence the reason for calling this pattern the "peak and valley" effect. Additionally, some patients will wait until their pain is quite severe before they request medication, and then it seems to be forever before the analgesic provides relief. Another component that demands consideration is the likelihood that the nurse will undermedicate the patient for fear of causing adverse reactions or drug dependency.[51]

Analgesics prescribed for the patient with musculoskeletal injuries should be long-acting with minimal side effects and should be provided based on the patient's symptoms and not on a strict timetable designed solely by the health care team. Advances in pain-management programs have shown that patients who have some degree of control over their pain medication provide themselves with more consistent relief and actually require less medication over a 24-hour time period.[52] For example, continuous intravenous drips regulated by the patient (within prescribed limits) enable the patient to increase or decrease his medication based on his symptoms. Morphine sulfate is a popular and very effective drug that can be administered by mouth, intramuscularly, by epidural infusion, or by continuous intravenous or subcutaneous infusions.[53, 54] It blocks pain sensations and dissociates the patient from his pain (and allows him to "feel good"). Morphine and morphine-like drugs cause less burning on administration, less tachycardia, and less myocardial depression than meperidine, a commonly used analgesic.[54] Another consideration when choosing an analgesic is the variation in effectiveness of the drug when given orally as compared with parenterally. For example, oral meperidine has one-third the effectiveness of the same dose of parenteral meperidine.[55] Therefore, the oral dose must be increased accordingly to achieve the same effectiveness of pain control. Pain management, as with all aspects of trauma patient care, requires a comprehensive, team approach for effective, safe results. Management of chronic pain (pain lasting 6 months or longer[56]) is discussed later in this chapter and in Chapter 15.

Potential for Impaired Gas Exchange and Decreased Tissue Perfusion

The multisystem-injured trauma patient is at risk for impaired gas exchange and decreased tissue perfusion from a variety of causes. This section introduces several precipitators for which preventive measures must be initiated during resuscitation: fat embolism syndrome (FES), deep vein thrombosis (DVT), and pulmonary thromboembolism (PTE). Initial preventive management is discussed during this section; more detailed information concerning each entity follows in the critical care section.

Preventive Management Principles

Recognition of At-Risk Patients. Fat embolism syndrome is an ambiguous and controversial process that has been discussed for many years yet still remains not fully understood. FES has been described in association with a variety of injuries and disease processes. The course of the syndrome and the developing symptomatology are often similar, with the end result being a form of adult respiratory distress syndrome (ARDS). FES may develop within hours of to several days after the injury. Close monitoring of patients at high risk for FES should begin upon admission and must continue throughout the early phase of critical care. Although FES is usually discussed in association with musculoskeletal injuries, it also has been described in patients with burns, massive soft tissue injuries, severe infections, and nontraumatic medical problems such as diabetes and pancreatitis.[57, 58] A patient with a long bone fracture, multiple rib fractures, pelvic injury, or a combination of multiple fractures, however, falls into the classic high-risk category.

The three major etiological factors that predispose the patient to DVT and subsequently PTE are (1) venous stasis, such as that from decreased blood flow, decreased muscular activity, and external pressure on the deep veins, (2) vascular damage or concomitant pathology, and (3) hypercoagulation. Clinical situations or injuries within these three categories include the following:

- History of vascular disease
- Previous DVT or PTE episode
- Prolonged bed rest or immobility
- Lengthy surgical procedures
- Shock states
- Sepsis
- Spinal cord injuries
- Long bone, hip, or pelvic fractures
- Soft tissue injuries
- Vessel trauma
- Multiple venous punctures
- Irritating fluid or drug infusion
- Immobilization devices
- Prolonged use of pneumatic antishock garments
- Obesity
- Age (greater than 40 years)
- History of congestive heart failure, acute myocardial infarction, stroke, malignancy
- History of estrogen or anticoagulation therapy

Recognizing DVT/PTE-prone patients early after admission and initiating measures that optimize venous return are integral components of care. For example, patients identified as high risk who require extensive surgery on admission, such as operative stabilization of cervical or thoracolumbar spine injuries or reconstructive plastic surgery, may benefit from preoperative application of graduated elastic stockings or an alternating pneumatic compression device.

Prevention of Further Fracture Site Disruption. Initial care at the accident scene, immediately after musculoskeletal trauma, must include careful, gentle stabilization and immobilization of the suspected or obviously injured extremity. Decreasing the motion at the fracture site not only prevents additional neurovascular injury but also may reduce the injection of marrow components into the circulation through the damaged vasculature. Any further patient movement during resuscitation should be performed with great care to avoid unnecessary disruption in bone alignment and of immobilization devices. Assign one person the responsibility of extremity movement when turning or lifting the patient.

Early Definitive Care. Early operative stabilization and fixation of fractures have many benefits, one of them being reduction of the risk for FES and ARDS.[59, 60]

Restoration and Monitoring of Hemodynamic Stability. This essential component of care also must begin in the prehospital phase at the scene of the accident. Adequate volume replacement via peripheral intravenous access helps reduce the risk of hypovolemic shock, a complication that may increase the potential for and severity of FES.[61] Without an adequate venous return, the heart cannot compensate for the increased pulmonary resistance caused by fat globules, which can obstruct the pulmonary vasculature within seconds to minutes after the injury.[61, 62]

Assessment of Pulmonary Function. One of the earliest signs of FES is a drop in the $Pa{O_2}$, which is indicative of hypoxemia. Administration of supplemental oxygen should begin during the prehospital phase and continue throughout the early cycles to support the pulmonary system.

As with many other trauma-related complications, identification of high-risk patients and institution of preventive measures during resuscitation are essential management principles for quality care. The section on critical care management further addresses the treatment of FES, DVT, and PTE.

Potential for Fluid Volume Deficit, Neurovascular Compromise, Impaired Renal Tissue Perfusion, and Acid–Base Imbalance Related to Crush Syndrome

Crush syndrome results when a patient experiences a prolonged entrapment time or sustains a crushing injury, which may occur with a structural collapse, cave-in, wringer-type industrial or farm accident, motor vehicle accident (as either a vehicle occupant or a pedestrian), or other traumatic mechanism that involves compression. This is a potentially life-threatening syndrome due, in large part, to the number and severity of associated complications.

A predictable series of sequelae develops after a crush injury, as shown in Figure 21–25. Prolonged compression of the involved body part causes ischemia and anoxia of muscle tissue. This ischemia leads to a cycle of events resulting in third-spacing of fluids, increased edema, increased compartment pressures, and impaired tissue perfusion resulting in further tissue ischemia.

Rhabdomyolysis, due to muscle destruction and dissolution from the primary injury and from subsequent ischemia/edema damage, causes a release of myoglobin and potassium. Hypoperfusion from the initial traumatic insult and blood loss, as well as from the relative hypovolemia due to the third-spacing, combines with the myoglobinuria to cause renal dysfunction in the form of acute tubular necrosis and renal failure. Impaired renal function, in the presence of a metabolic imbalance that already exists from the rhabdomyolysis, causes further chemical derangements that may precipitate cardiac dysrhythmias.

Additional complications inherent to crush syndrome in-

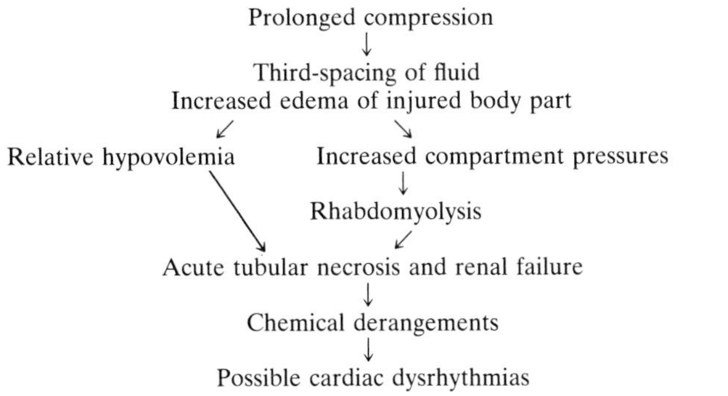

Figure 21–25. Events associated with crush syndrome. (From Peck SA: Crush syndrome: Pathophysiology and management. Orthop Nurs 9(3):33–40, 1990.)

clude neurovascular compromise from compartment syndrome and infection from the original injury and from the subsequent ischemic changes. The major components of crush syndrome are addressed elsewhere in this chapter and also in Chapter 24. See Appendix 21–1 for a sample nursing care plan for the patient with crush syndrome.

OPERATIVE MANAGEMENT

The responsibilities of the perioperative nurse include completing a preoperative patient assessment, which covers a complete systems assessment, confirmed and suspected injuries, potential complications, and therapies instituted. A systematic report from the primary care nurse provides for continuity of care, an essential factor in preventing fragmented therapy. During this preoperative phase, the nurse explains the activities that the awake patient will experience in the operating room. Expected postoperative care is also explained to the patient. The perioperative nurse serves a vital role of coordinator, especially for the multisystem-injured patient with musculoskeletal injuries. This patient may well undergo multiple simultaneous surgical procedures during his first operative visit. General responsibilities, therefore, also would include anticipating the length of stay in the operative suite, patient positioning, use of different operating tables, confirming the sequence of the various planned procedures and equipment needed for each, and ensuring patient safety and monitoring throughout the entire case. During the often lengthy operative procedures, the perioperative nurse may communicate with the patient's family to provide updates and progress reports as requested. Postoperatively, an operative patient report should be given to the receiving nurse whether in the postanesthesia room or in another patient care area. Again, the systematic exchange of patient reports between primary care nurses promotes continuous and consistent nursing therapy.

Potential for Infection

Irrigation/Debridement

Early and aggressive wound irrigation and debridement are two of the most important definitive treatments for an open fracture or traumatic amputation. The most effective irrigation is done with copious amounts of normal saline. Approximately 3 liters is used for grade I open fractures, and as much as 9 to 30 liters for grade III open fractures and traumatic amputations. Debridement of necrotic fascia, devitalized muscle tissue, and bone fragments is necessary to decrease the potential for infection and to promote wound healing.

The risk of infection associated with open fractures depends on the grade and the location of the open fracture.[25] Chapman[64] reported an overall infection rate of 9.3 per cent for open fractures and rates of 1.1 per cent for grade I, 1.3 per cent for grade II, and 14.8 per cent for grade III fractures. A grade III open fracture requires reexploration 24 to 48 hours after the initial debridement to remove any further tissue that has become devitalized.[28] Debridement continues until the wound remains clean and free of any devitalized tissue.

Closure

Closure of an open wound is contraindicated during the initial operative phase. Allowing the wound to remain open promotes drainage of microscopic debris not removed during the initial irrigation. Closure of the wound at this time would impede this drainage, providing the perfect environment for bacterial growth and infection. Delayed primary or secondary closure is performed approximately 5 days later when the wound appears free of infection.

Alteration in Bone Integrity

Timing

Restoring the fractured bone to normal alignment and length is necessary to initiate the healing process. Reduction of the dead space between fractured bone ends decreases the size of hematoma formation, which, in open fractures, can become a site for infection. Restoring the bone to normal alignment improves venous and lymphatic return, which decreases soft tissue swelling and reduces the release of marrow components into the circulation. Early and aggressive operative intervention reduces the overall morbidity and mortality of the multisystem-injured patient.[60, 65, 66] In addition to realizing and comprehending the total clinical picture presented by the patient, including age, number, and severity of injuries, and overall hemodynamic status, members of the trauma team must consider other situational factors when making such decisions, including (1) effectiveness of closed reduction, (2) fractured or displaced articulating surfaces, (3) presence of arterial injury, (4) presence of multiple injuries, (5) contaminated wound, (6) length of time since the injury occurred, (7) contraindication of long-term immobility, and (8) the cost of long-term immobility caused by closed reduction.

Selection of Stabilization Device

The method of stabilization used for an extremity fracture depends on the grade, type, and location of the fracture. The current philosophy of long bone stabilization centers on the use of intramedullary devices.

Recent clinical experience has shown that use of unreamed intramedullary (IM) nails has expanded the indications for nailing to now include grade I and II open fractures. Grade

III open long bone fractures also may be treated with IM nails if debridement was performed within 6 hours of the injury. Modern designs of first- and second-generation IM nails now permit even very complex fracture patterns (i.e., combined femoral shaft and neck fractures) to be treated with a single device.

External fixation (Fig. 21–26) continues to play a very important role in acute fracture management and in limb reconstruction procedures. While an external fixator may be the definitive treatment option for a given fracture, it also can be used as a temporary stabilization device on a critically ill patient who cannot safely undergo a lengthy operative procedure on admission.

External fixation also plays an important role in management of a severely crushed lower leg with significant soft tissue and bone loss. The appropriate use of external fixators allows free access for wound care, soft tissue coverage (free-tissue transfer), and bone transport or transplantation to fill the bony defect.

In unstable pelvic ring disruptions, external fixation provides provisional pelvic fixation and, at times, may be lifesaving. It does not, however, stabilize the posterior bony structures adequately, and therefore, internal pelvic ring fixation must be accomplished as soon as the patient's condition permits. The preferred fixation method for pure sacroiliac joint dislocations is now anterior plating via the retroperitoneal approach rather than posterior screw fixation, which was frequently associated with wound complications.

These recent developments in orthopedic trauma implants and surgical techniques provide better fixation and allow earlier patient mobilization.

Neurological and/or Vascular Compromise

Fasciotomies

Fasciotomies allow for the decompression of fascial compartments that have high pressures due to swelling of tissues. The fascial compartment is opened to allow the increased compartment volume caused by swelling to expand without increasing pressure on the microcirculation. The technique used to open the fascial sheath depends on the compartment(s) requiring decompression. The forearm compartments can be opened with two incisions—one volar, one dorsal—placed at 180 degrees to each other. Similar incisions are ineffective on the lower leg because of the location of its four compartments. The lower leg fasciotomy technique involves an anterolateral incision between the fibular shaft and the tibial crest to relieve pressure in the anterior and lateral compartments. The deep posterior and superficial posterior compartments are approached through a posteromedial incision. The type of incision required for other

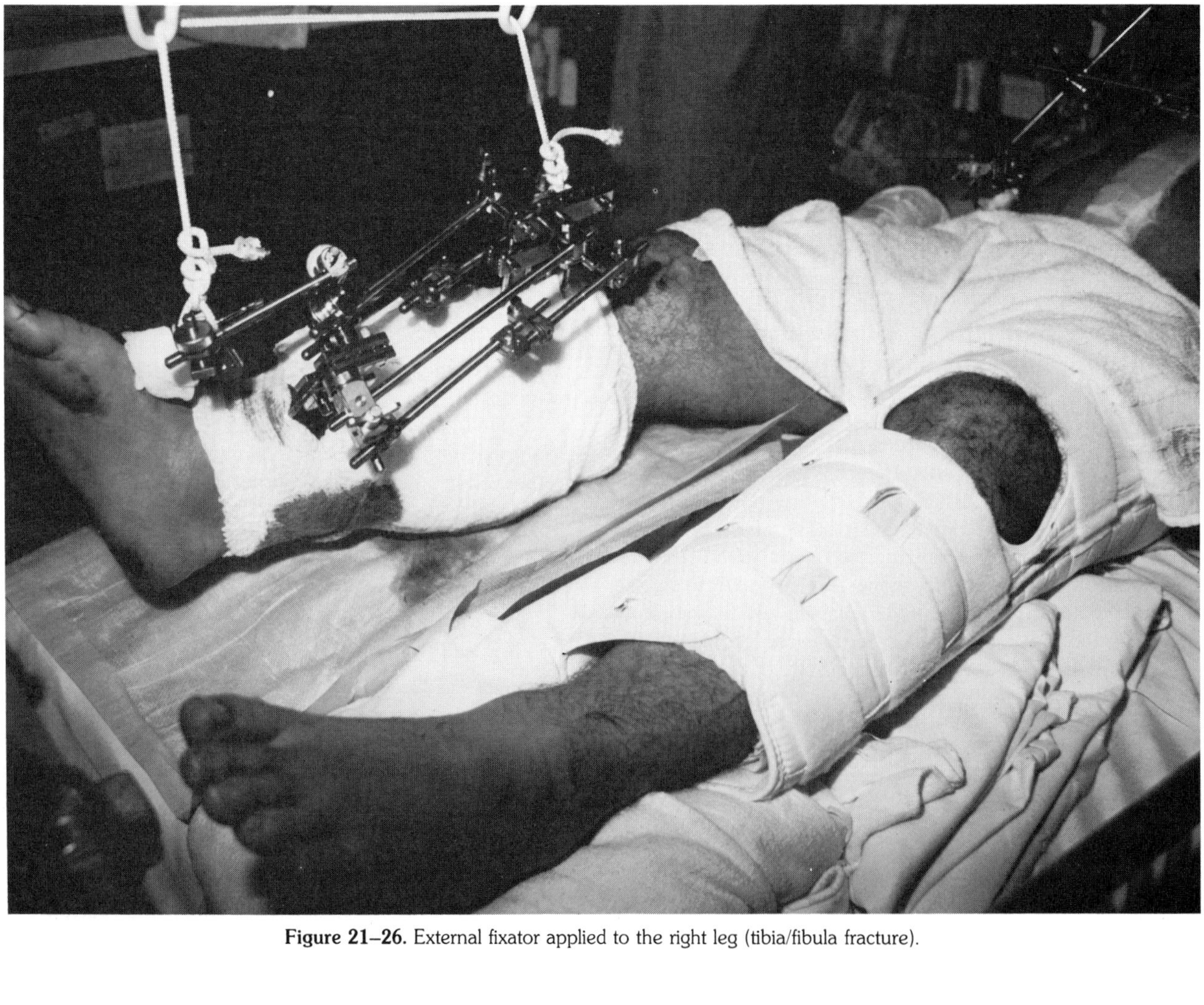

Figure 21–26. External fixator applied to the right leg (tibia/fibula fracture).

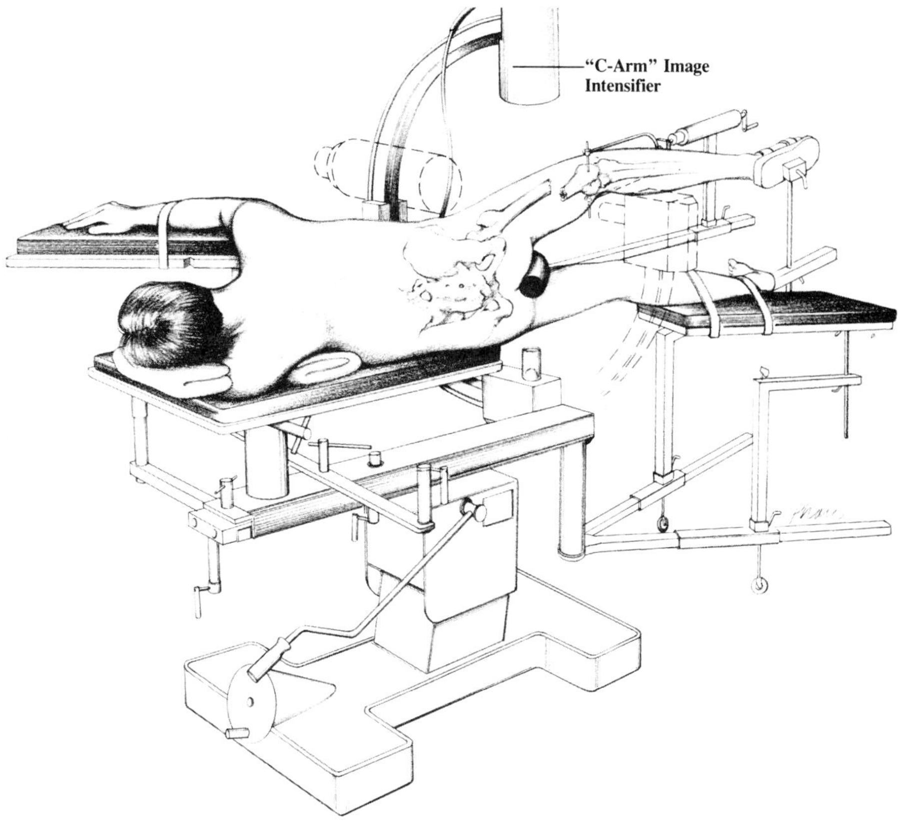

Figure 21–27. Intraoperative patient positioning on a fracture table. (From Boyle M: Grosse and Kempf femoral surgical protocol. In Howmedica Surgical Techniques. Rutherford, Howmedica, 1983.)

compartments, such as those of the hip, thigh, shoulder, pelvis, upper arm, hands, and feet, is determined by the structure and number of fascial compartments involved.

Adequate decompression of the gluteus maximus and the deltoid compartments requires opening of the epimysium as well as the fascial sheath.[41]

The wounds created by the large incisions are left open and covered with wet saline dressings to prevent desiccation. (Wound care and dressing changes are discussed further in the critical care section.) Delayed primary closure or delayed secondary closure by skin grafting is then done when swelling has subsided.

Immobility

One of the fundamentals of perioperative nursing is prevention of immobility-related injuries, most commonly neurological and vascular impairment. The length of the surgical procedure combined with the various positions required for patients with musculoskeletal injuries can increase the risk of iatrogenic injury if proper protection and padding are not provided to prevent compression of neurovascular structures. Figure 21–27 shows just one of the many possible positions required for musculoskeletal surgery. Note extremity positions and the pressure points in contact with the fracture table. Coordinated preoperative planning between nurses, anesthesiologists, and surgeons regarding patient positioning on various types of operative tables, e.g., fracture frame or turning frame, facilitates optimal patient protection.

The potential for a brachial plexus injury as a result of improper positioning and alignment demands strict perioperative attention from the trauma operating room nurse. Postoperative brachial plexus palsy may result from hyperextension or hyperabduction of the upper extremity during surgery.[47] This complication usually represents a temporary alteration in regional or generalized motor and/or sensory function. Healing and full recovery commonly occur within hours to days after the insult.[47, 49]

Pressure sores are another risk for the immobilized patient during surgery. Providing adequate padding over bony prominences and any body area that comes in contact with a rigid surface and keeping such areas dry minimize the risk of these pressure sores developing. Prevention is the primary intervention for these complications.

CRITICAL CARE CYCLE

Potential for Infection

During the critical care cycle, the patient with musculoskeletal injury continues to be at risk for infection. Injuries that require delayed primary or secondary skin closure as well as surgical incisions and pin sites all require close observation and meticulous care. Some of the predisposing factors that will determine whether an infection will develop during the critical care phase include devitalized muscle tissue, dead space, hematomas, and foreign bodies. Other factors include impairment of the immune system as a result of traumatic injury,[59] the patient's age, nutritional status, and presence of any underlying disease.

Continuous Evaluation

Early recognition of the signs and symptoms of infection is important in preventing or minimizing major septic episodes and delayed healing. Trends in vital signs, including temperature, must be monitored, documented, and evaluated. Wound, incision, and pin site drainage should be monitored and documented for amount, consistency, color, and odor.

Dressing Changes

Since primary wound closure is not done during the initial resuscitative/operative cycle of patient care, wounds associated with open fractures, amputations, and fasciotomies require wet-to-wet or wet-to-dry sterile dressing changes. Wet-to-dry dressing changes provide some debridement of the wound. Wounds with exposed bone, veins, tendons, and fat are treated with wet-to-wet sterile dressing changes to prevent desiccation. Continued operative irrigation and debridement are necessary for open fractures, crushing injuries, or traumatic amputations every 24 to 48 hours until tissue granulation becomes apparent and the wound is free of infection.

Drains

Hematomas are avascular and are thus an excellent environment for bacterial growth. Closed-system evacuation drains, such as the Jackson Pratt or the Hemovac, inserted intraoperatively reduce hematoma formation in surgical wounds. These drains require close monitoring for patency and proper function. Specific nursing care includes

1. Emptying and reactivating the suction every 4 to 8 hours (or more frequently with large amounts of drainage)
2. Measuring and documenting the amount and characteristics of the drainage (color, consistency, odor)
3. Recording the drainage amount in output totals
4. Performing dressing changes using aseptic technique every 8 hours (or as ordered) and documenting the status of the skin and tissue surrounding the drain site
5. Preventing accidental drain removal by properly securing them

Drains are generally removed within 3 to 5 days after insertion or earlier if drainage has stopped.

Pin Care

A sample procedure in Appendix 21–2 describes care for percutaneously inserted pins. There are two schools of thought concerning the proper method for carrying out pin site care. The controversy is whether to remove dried exudate from nondraining pin sites or to leave it in place. One school contends that the dried exudate is part of the normal healing process, provides a tight skin–pin interface, and prevents skin flora from entering the bone via the pin tract. The opposing school believes that removing the dried exudate allows the pin holes to drain freely, reducing the bacterial concentration and decreasing the risk of pin tract infection. Generally, pin sites (of simple percutaneous pins for skeletal traction or more complex pins from an external fixator) ooze after insertion. A gently wrapped, loose-fitting 4 × 4 opened gauze dressing (Fig. 21–28) allows free drainage while containing the drainage. Frequent dressing changes and pin site care will be necessary for the first 1 to 2 days postinsertion. Pin care given on every shift will be satisfactory after active drainage has stopped. Cleaning the exterior part of the pins (always wiping from the skin outward) helps prevent retrograde contamination of the pin tract (which leads rapidly to osteomyelitis). This subject is discussed in detail in Chapter 12. The sample pin care procedure listed in the appendix suggests leaving the dried exudate in place.

Antibiotic Therapy

Short-term antibiotic therapy initiated during resuscitation continues during the critical care cycle for any open fracture, crush injury, or traumatic amputation.

Potential for Neurovascular Compromise Related to Compartment Syndrome

As previously discussed, compartment syndrome represents a space versus volume problem. This complication may develop early after the injury during resuscitation, as a result of excessive bleeding into the compartments or the soft tissue. During the critical care cycle, compartment syndrome remains a potential problem for the patient with musculoskeletal injuries. Despite definitive care provided intraoperatively, soft tissue edema can persist owing to sluggish venous return or persistent oozing of smaller injured vessels. This can increase muscle compartment volume, resulting in neurovascular compromise. Additional factors that can lead to compartment syndrome or less acute forms of neurological or vascular impairment include tight-fitting casts, occlusive circular dressings, traction devices, prolonged use of a pneumatic antishock garment, and even improper positioning of the patient when he is lying on his side.

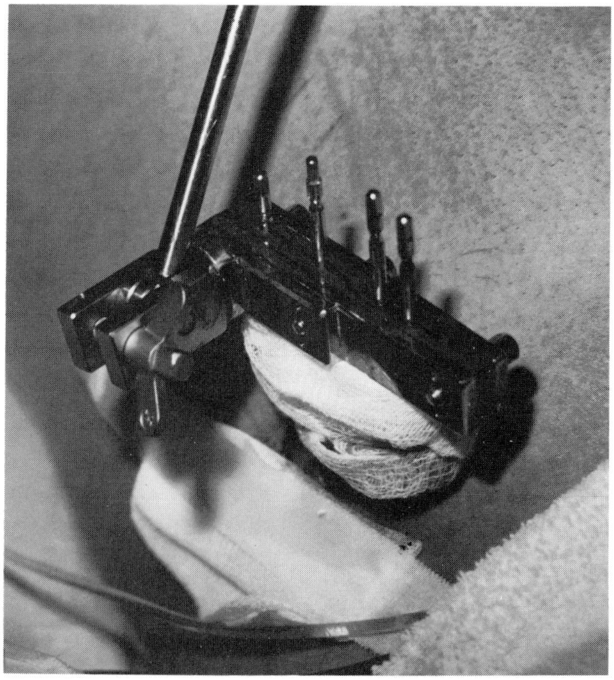

Figure 21–28. Insertion site of a percutaneous pin, with loose-fitting gauze dressing around the pin site.

Management Principles

Assessment. Close monitoring of the neurovascular status of the affected extremity remains the single most important intervention, since prevention is the best therapy for this complication. Evaluation of the compartments must always include comparisons of the injured limb with the noninjured limb. This assessment should be performed, and the findings documented, at least every 1 to 2 hours or more frequently, as warranted by the patient's condition.

Immobilization. Immobilization and stabilization devices must be evaluated to ensure maintenance of proper alignment and to monitor for signs of local or generalized compression. If clinical findings suggest that a tight-fitting cast, for example, may be the causative factor of deterioration in the neurovascular status of the distal extremity, the cast should be bivalved and the top half removed. The posterior portion will continue to serve as a stabilizing device while attention is given to the extremity.

Elevation and Cooling. The interventions described during resuscitation remain essential during critical care. The affected extremity should remain elevated and cooled for the first 24 to 48 hours after injury to promote venous return and minimize further edema. The principles of elevation and cooling apply even when the patient is positioned on one side or out of bed in a chair. An injury that received intraoperative external fixation can be elevated easily with traction apparatus. More conventional methods of elevation include pillows, folded sheets, or preformed foam elevation blocks.

Compartment Pressure Measurements. Clinical signs of increased compartmental pressures will necessitate compartment pressure measurements, as discussed previously.

Potential for Impaired Gas Exchange Related to Fat Embolism Syndrome

The fat embolism syndrome (FES) has been discussed and debated since the 1860s, when it was first described in the literature. Controversy continues surrounding the etiology and appropriate therapy for FES. Two theories have emerged regarding the etiology: active mobilization of fat globules and altered fat metabolism. The mobilization, or mechanical, theory focuses on the actual impact (e.g., the time a bone is stressed and sustains a fracture). The damaged bone and the injured veins, which lie close to the bone itself, allow the release of marrow components, including fat globules, into the circulation. Sauter and Klopper report that increased pressure and longer duration of the externally applied forces result in increased release of fat emboli.[67] The second theory, altered fat metabolism, has been referred to as the "physiochemical theory." The biochemical disturbances that occur after stress or trauma affect the stability and metabolism of fat and other circulating products. Increased catecholamine levels activated by the stressful event cause an increased release of free fatty acids and neutral fats into the circulation. The problem worsens as fibrinolysis, red blood cell aggregation, and platelet adhesiveness increase from the disrupted fat metabolism. The fat globules grow in size as they become coated with platelets.[62, 68, 69]

The subsequent pathology during the syndrome is the same regardless of the etiological theories. The large fat globules are filtered out in the pulmonary system and obstruct the system at the capillary membrane level. This obstruction, in combination with the release of serotonin, causes increased capillary permeability, leading to interstitial fluid leaks, hemorrhage, and finally acute respiratory distress syndrome (ARDS), with alveolar collapse, impaired tissue perfusion, and tissue hypoxia.[68, 70]

A latent period, or the time between the injury and when clinical symptoms of FES appear, has been described and also disputed. Peltier noted that not giving this asymptomatic phase the attention that it warrants causes the early signs to be overlooked or missed.[62] In actuality, acute signs and symptoms of FES have been reported as soon as 1 hour or less after the injury and as long as 96 hours after injury; the average time appears to be between 12 and 48 hours.[68, 70] Mild cases of FES, or the early signs, may be overlooked if high-risk patients are not closely monitored and the syndrome is not anticipated.

General Management Principles

Monitoring of High-Risk Patients. Throughout the postresuscitation phase, high-risk patients must be monitored closely, as during resuscitation. Being acutely aware of the potential for FES and actively looking for suspicious signs facilitate prompt recognition of this syndrome.

Cardiovascular Stability. Efforts to restore normovolemia and sustain hemodynamic stability must continue throughout the early cycles of trauma care. On-going cardiovascular assessments enable trend analysis of the patient's vital signs, cardiovascular status, and response to volume/fluid resuscitation. Insertion of a pulmonary artery catheter may become necessary to evaluate the patient's hemodynamic status critically in an effort to avoid fluid overload.[58] The patient with FES usually develops tachycardia, hypotension, and increased cardiac output in response to increased pulmonary resistance. The patient may complain of chest pain and exhibit signs of right heart strain, as evidenced on serial electrocardiograms. Dysrhythmias, right bundle branch block, inverted T waves, prominent S waves in lead I, prominent Q waves in lead III, and depressed RST segments may all be seen with cardiac strain from FES.[62, 69]

Pulmonary Function. Analysis of serial arterial blood gas determinations aids in early detection of hypoxemia. With the onset and progression of FES, the patient experiences tachypnea and dyspnea and may develop a productive cough. Auscultation of bilateral lung fields may reveal moist rales. Cyanosis, bloody sputum, pulmonary edema, and findings of bilateral fluffy infiltrates on the chest radiograph are all indicative of the ARDS pattern seen with fulminant FES. Pulmonary support is the most important component of care for patients with FES. The patient usually requires therapy similar to the ARDS patient: intubation, mechanical ventilation, and varying levels of positive end-expiratory pressure (PEEP) for adequate alveolar aeration.[68]

Neurological Status. Generally, the first sign that signals the patient's deterioration is an abrupt change in behavior or mentation. A previously awake, alert, cooperative patient without an associated head injury will become restless, agitated, very uncooperative, and even disoriented in the presence of FES. Cerebral embolization may result in localized areas of anoxia because of specific vessel occlusion; generalized anoxia may occur from pulmonary dysfunction–

induced hypoxemia.[62] The patient with cerebral involvement may rapidly deteriorate to a state of unresponsiveness, necessitating close neurological monitoring.

Renal Function. Urine output is a valuable parameter reflecting the effectiveness of volume replacement and tissue perfusion. In FES, oliguria or anuria commonly indicates concurrent problems with hypovolema. Lipuria, fat in the urine, is believed to indicate a serious case of FES.[62] Hematuria also may be present.

Laboratory Data. Progressive analysis of arterial blood gas results usually reveals low $Pa{O_2}$ and elevated $Pa{CO_2}$ measurements indicative of the hypoxemia and carbon dioxide retention seen in FES. Thrombocytopenia with platelet counts as low as $50{,}000/mm^3$ develops as a normal process of the clotting mechanism after injury and also because of platelet aggregation around the fat globules. Platelet levels usually return to normal within 5 to 7 days. Decreases in hemoglobin of 3 to 5 g/dl reflect the sequestration of red blood cells to the fat globules.

Petechiae. A clinical sign of FES that may develop 12 to 96 hours after injury is a petechial rash on the trunk, neck, axillae, conjunctivae, and mucous membranes. The flat red spots usually appear and disappear in waves, often going unnoticed by the unsuspecting observer, and generally cease within 48 hours of onset. Fat globules obstructing the capillaries in the skin and subcutaneous tissue are thought to cause the petechiae.[58, 62, 63]

Body Temperature. A classic sign of FES is a rapid temperature spike to 38° to 40°C (101.4° to 104°F) without other precipitating causes. Altered temperature regulation from cerebral emboli may be responsible for the fever.[58, 69]

Immobility

The degree of physical immobility for the patient with musculoskeletal injuries depends on the type of injury, the pain associated with the injury, the method of treatment chosen, and the presence of other system injuries.

Immobility, the usual common denominator in trauma patients with concomitant musculoskeletal injuries, stresses the body, mind, and spirit in a variety of ways. Not only does it cause altered feelings of self-esteem and a sense of powerlessness, but it also slows anabolic processes and accelerates catabolic activities. Results of immobility often include tissue atrophy, protein catabolism, alteration in intracellular and extracellular exchanges, and fluid/electrolyte imbalances. More specifically, immobility increases the trauma patient's risk for secondary disabilities from pulmonary complications, vascular stasis with thromboemboli formation, skin breakdown, fecal impaction, renal calculi, muscle wasting, and contractures. Appropriate nursing interventions can prevent or minimize the risk of these complications.

Different treatment modalities available for musculoskeletal injuries afford varying degrees of postoperative mobility. State of the art orthopedic management, however, promotes early mobility after surgery.

Immobility-Related Complications

Pulmonary Complications. Ambulation of the trauma patient to prevent pulmonary complications is usually not an option during the critical care phase, but other equally effective measures are possible. Immobilized patients without pulmonary pathology require chest physiotherapy, including turning with postural drainage and percussion every 4 hours, to aid in dislodging secretions from the lung parenchyma. The patient should be instructed and encouraged to cough frequently to further clear any secretions from the tracheobronchial tree. The nurse should instruct the patient in proper deep breathing techniques, concentrating on slow, relaxed, and deliberate expansion of the chest. Use of an incentive spirometer will allow the patient to measure and monitor progress visually while performing deep breathing.

Skin Breakdown. Skin breakdown in the immobilized or insensate patient is a costly complication that can be prevented. It has been estimated that each ulceration can add thousands of dollars to a patient's health care bill in hospital cost, surgical skin repair, and control of infection.[71] Skin ulcerations result from decreased circulation to the localized area. This impaired circulation is secondary to decreased muscle action, which is the result of either general immobility or direct pressure. Other factors that directly or indirectly predispose the patient to skin breakdown include friction from linen or from cast and traction devices, anemia, malnutrition, infection, fever, decreased sensation or paralysis (as with plexus injuries), use of anticoagulants, sedatives, or neuromuscular blocking agents, and increased age (greater than 65 years).[72, 73] All potential breakdown sites must be monitored for redness, burning pain, or itching. Turning and repositioning the patient as frequently as allowed will minimize the length of time that pressure is exerted on any skin area. (See Chapter 13 for further information.)

Fecal Impaction. The frequency of bowel movements in the immobilized patient must be monitored. If allowed, the patient's diet should include juices and roughage to help maintain normal bowel movement. The nurse should check for fecal impaction every 2 to 3 days. Mild laxatives, stool softeners, or enemas may be required to prevent impaction.

Renal Calculi. The patient's urine concentration and intake and output totals must be monitored. Calcium or other crystalline salts can become concentrated in the urine beyond the point of solubility in the immobilized patient with inadequate fluid intake.[74] This high concentration can result in renal calculi formation. An adequate fluid intake level will prevent urine concentration and calculi formation.

Muscle Wasting and Contractures. Immobility, especially of the antigravity muscle groups, precludes normal muscle stresses, which leads to decreased muscle fiber size. Muscle atrophy, or a decrease in muscle mass, begins 3 to 7 days after the onset of immobility.[75] Approximately 3 per cent of original muscle strength is lost each day a muscle remains immobile.[76] Connective tissue fibrosis around immobile joints also begins early after immobilization and progresses to limited range of motion and joint contractures. Muscle wasting, atrophy, and contractures can be prevented or minimized by range-of-motion exercises that are planned appropriately for the patient's degree of dependence or independence. Passive or active-assisted range-of-motion movements should be performed every shift for patients who are unable to carry out independent exercise. This exercise regimen should include noninjured joints required later for ambulation as well as affected joints within physician-ordered restrictions.

This exercise includes moving all possible joints through

their ranges of abduction, adduction, internal and external rotation, pronation, supination, eversion, and inversion and repeating each motion five times successively.[75] Complete range-of-motion exercises help prevent contractures, improve joint function, promote circulation, and build muscle strength. These exercises also increase the patient's tolerance and endurance. Optimal muscle strength, full joint movement, and endurance are all essential components for later mobility and ambulation.[77]

During range-of-motion exercises it is important to monitor and document the degree of each joint's range; any sign of inflammation, spasm, edema, or stiffness; and the patient's complaints of pain. A joint should never be forced to move beyond free range, and the nurse should not persist in performing range-of-motion movements when the patient describes an unusual amount of pain. These actions may precipitate joint or muscle strain or injury, which prolongs rehabilitation.

Some patients, e.g., those with brachial plexus injuries, require splints during prolonged periods of immobility to maintain position of function and reduce the risk of contractures. Properly fitting splints and close monitoring of underlying skin integrity will prevent or minimize skin breakdown. The physician-ordered schedule delineates wearing times.

Deep Vein Thrombosis. Deep vein thrombosis (DVT) is a significant hazard to the trauma patient with musculoskeletal involvement. The March 1986 Consensus Development Conference on Venous Thrombosis and Pulmonary Embolism acknowledged the lack of comprehensive data on DVT/PTE in association with trauma.[78] General data on all general surgery patients over the age of 40 years indicate that DVT occurs in 16 to 30 per cent, significant PTE episodes occur in 1.6 per cent, and fatal PTE occurs in 1 per cent of this patient population. Knee reconstruction or hip surgery increases DVT risk (45 to 70 per cent of these patients develop DVT). Of all hip surgery patients, 20 per cent experience a PTE episode, and 1 to 3 per cent are fatal episodes. As previously mentioned, trauma-related DVT/PTE data are sparse because injuries are commonly multisystem, and tissue trauma can cause false-positive results in some diagnostic studies used for DVT/PTE. Generally, however, 20 per cent of young adult trauma patients develop DVT. More than 40 per cent of elderly trauma patients with hip fractures experience DVT, and 4 per cent have a fatal PTE episode. Data on head- and spinal cord–injured patients reveal a DVT incidence of 40 per cent and fatal PTE of 1 per cent. Prevention of DVT/PTE is emphasized as better than any treatment modality.[78]

Assessment and Monitoring. On-going patient evaluation aids early detection of signs of DVT. The patient should be closely assessed for the following signs and symptoms, and such findings should be reported immediately:

- Calf pain on dorsiflexion of the foot (Homans's sign)
- Subtle to obvious swelling of involved area
- Tachycardia
- Fever
- Distal skin color and temperature changes

An acute pulmonary thromboembolism episode may be the first indication of the presence of a DVT. Any signs or symptoms or combination of these symptoms should arouse suspicions in the high-risk patient.

Patient Education. It is important to consider the patient an essential part of the health care team, especially when discussing DVT prevention and therapy. Patient teaching should include the causes of DVT, common signs and symptoms such as deep leg pain, and self-preventive measures. On-going teaching and reinforcement promote the patient's understanding and ideally his participation and compliance with the preventive regimen.

Mobility. Patient mobility should be encouraged as soon and as much as permitted within the patient's injury limitations because muscle activity optimizes circulation and venous return. Early mobilization may be a primary DVT preventive measure. When ambulation is impossible because of injuries and a critical patient condition, an exercise program should be initiated early after resuscitation. Active range-of-motion and isometric exercises stimulate muscle contraction, which increases venous return. Ambulatory patients should be encouraged to remain as mobile as possible, since walking is beneficial toward preventing DVT. Patients who are allowed out of bed in a chair should be assisted in getting out of bed several times a day even if for short periods, rather than one time a day for a lengthy period. While out of bed the patient should not be permitted to keep the legs in a dependent position for an extended time; rather, the legs should be outstretched and elevated to promote venous return. Pressure areas on the calves or under the knees should be avoided while positioning the patient in the chair. The out-of-bed patient should continue to perform isometric exercises and active dorsiflexion and plantarflexion while in the chair. Awake patients confined to bed rest require encouragement to frequently change positions and perform active range-of-motion and isometric exercises within limitations imposed by their injuries. Specific injuries or alterations in level of consciousness that preclude the patient's participation in an exercise regimen require a team approach to restore and maintain muscle activity and thus venous return. A coordinated, planned exercise program will include active involvement of the physical therapy department, but primary responsibility rests with the bedside nurse. Patient positioning while confined to bed plays an important role in DVT prevention. Frequent changes in the patient's position are beneficial, with close attention being given to extremity placement, positioning, and padding. For example, the lateral recumbent position without adequate padding between the legs increases external pressure on the veins in the lower extremities and increases the risk of intimal damage. Pressure or prolonged flexion of the knees impedes circulation and venous return. The patient's lower extremities should be elevated, for example, by using a slight (30 degree) Trendelenburg position, especially if venous return is further impaired by injury.

Venous Compression Devices. Early recognition of patients who will require prolonged bed rest should lead to early institution of compression devices such as graded elastic stockings or wraps or intermittent pneumatic devices. Elastic bandages wrapped from the toes to the thighs or fitted elastic stockings with a gradual decrease in the amount of compression can be applied early after resuscitation. These wraps or stockings require close monitoring to prevent slippage, wrinkles, and areas of increased compression. The wraps or stockings should be removed once a day for hygiene,

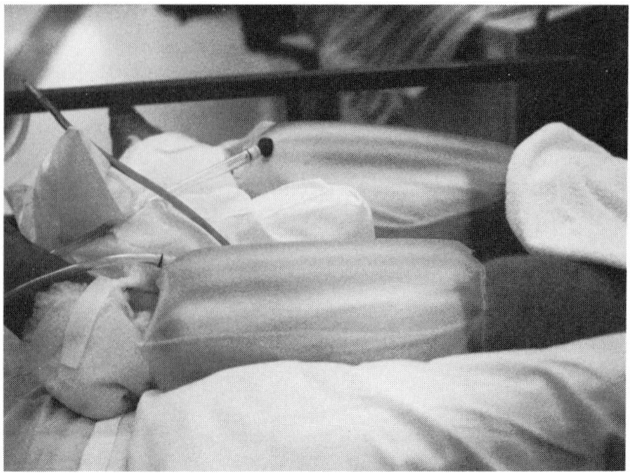

Figure 21–29. Pneumatic compression device applied to the lower legs.

skin inspection and care, and laundering of the stockings as needed.

Pneumatic compression devices (Fig. 21–29) are most beneficial for patients in whom anticoagulation is contraindicated, specifically the newly admitted trauma patient. They are also indicated in patients who are unable to actively perform exercises, e.g., spinal cord– and head-injured patients and patients receiving heavy sedation or neuromuscular blocking agents. Pneumatic compression devices have a tubular section for each leg which is positioned between the ankle and knee. The sections automatically inflate to a predetermined pressure and deflate after a preset length of time. The compartments may inflate alternately or simulataneously and work continuously while in place. Such devices cause no positioning restrictions and should be initiated early after resuscitation, e.g., intraoperatively on patients requiring lengthy operative procedures on admission. Their effectiveness in preventing DVT is related to promotion of venous flow through vein compression and activation of plasminogen activator by distending the vein walls distal to the device.[79]

Prophylactic Anticoagulation. High-risk patients require early prophylactic anticoagulation to aid in prevention of DVT.[78, 79] Aspirin or low-dose heparin, the current drug of choice, also impedes the formation of new clots and may prevent propagation or enlargement of existing clots. Heparin interferes with thromboplastin activity, which leads to prolonged clotting times, decreases platelet agglutination, and prevents formation of additional clots. Subcutaneous injections every 12 hours (used in conjunction with other preventive modalities) or continuous intravenous infusion may be prescribed. Anticoagulation, *performed cautiously in the trauma patient,* can be started after achieving hemostasis and general cardiovascular stability. Semiweekly evaluation of the clotting profile (PT, PTT) and platelet count permits adequate monitoring of anticoagulant therapy. PT and PTT levels should remain within normal ranges during prophylactic anticoagulant therapy. Thrombocytopenia is a complication of anticoagulation which must be recognized promptly. Therapeutic anticoagulation should be avoided during preventive therapy because prolonged PT and PTT clotting times predispose the patient to bleeding episodes. Prophylactic therapy is generally discontinued after the patient is ambulatory.

Diagnosis. To confirm suspected DVT, several diagnostic studies or procedures are available for use, for example:

- Venography
- Radioisotope studies
- Doppler flow studies
- Venous pressure measurement
- Impedance plethysmography (IPG)

Additional research is needed, however, in the area of DVT diagnosis.

Management. After the diagnosis of DVT is confirmed, therapeutic efforts focus on preventing propagation of existing clots and minimizing the risk of new clot formation. Therapeutic measures include the following:

Bed rest: lowers the risk of cloting dislodgment.
Anticoagulation: prevents clot propagation and new clot formation.
Thrombolysis: promotes lysis of thrombus formation.
Surgery: may become necessary to prevent pulmonary embolus.

The primary concern for the patient with DVT is the prevention of a fatal pulmonary thromboembolism.

Pulmonary Thromboembolism. Pulmonary thromboembolism (PTE) is a not infrequent, dangerous complication of musculoskeletal trauma. Injuries or situations that increase the patient's risk were previously cited in the Resuscitation Cycle section. PTE develops when a clot dislodges from a peripheral vein, usually a deep vein in the lower extremity or pelvis.

The clot release is generally precipitated by sudden movement such as rapidly assuming a standing position or by a Valsalva maneuver, which abruptly increases pressure and blood flow. These are examples of mechanical forces that cause clot dislodgment. Spontaneous clot release may occur as well. The mechanical precipitating factors mentioned must be kept in mind when the patient begins to get out of bed, whether in the intensive care unit or later in less acute patient care areas.

The embolus circulates through the body to the heart and eventually lodges in the pulmonary artery or its smaller branches and obstructs blood flow. Both pulmonary and cardiovascular complications may ensue.[73]

Assessment. Sudden-onset dyspnea is the classic signal of a PTE. Additional symptoms of PTE vary according to the size and number of clots, the size of the pulmonary vessels affected, and the presence of lung infarction. Symptomatology is often vague or nonspecific; therefore, a high index of suspicion is essential in high-risk patients.[81] These patients must be monitored closely for the following signs and symptoms:

- Substernal chest pain
- Hypovolemic shock
- Rapid, shallow respirations
- Shortness of breath
- Pale, dusky, or cyanotic skin coloring
- Bronchial breath sounds, rales
- Anxiety

- Altered or decreased levels of consciousness
- Low-grade fever

Signs of a pulmonary infarction, a rare complication of PTE, could include cough and hemoptysis, pleuritic pain, and high fever.

Diagnosis. Diagnosis is often difficult and usually cannot be confirmed by clinical findings alone. Studies that aid in confirmation of PTE are identified in Table 21–4.

Management Principles. Improving gas exchange and tissue perfusion is the basis of all PTE therapy. Cardiopulmonary support, pain control, anticoagulation, and possibly operative intervention may all be necessary in some degree of intensity. The patient experiencing a PTE episode requires support of both cardiovascular and pulmonary systems. The obstructive thromboembolus causes a release of vasoactive substances and an increased pulmonary vascular resistance, leading to right ventricular strain or failure and terminating in a shock state. Simultaneously, the embolus causes a ventilation–perfusion mismatch (ventilation continues, but pulmonary perfusion is impaired), which leads to impaired exchange of O_2 and CO_2 gases. Hypoxia, ischemia, and pain are results of impaired pulmonary circulation.

Atelectasis commonly results after PTE because of the associated alveolar constriction and dead space and the loss of surfactant.[82] Administration of supplemental oxygen provides more oxygen for exchange. Endotracheal intubation and mechanical ventilation with the use of PEEP may be necessary in severe cases (see Chapter 19).

Pain and increased airway resistance can hinder the patient's breathing efforts. Placing the PTE patient in a semi- or high Fowler's position, unless contraindicated, reduces the work of breathing.

TABLE 21–4. DIAGNOSTIC STUDIES FOR PULMONARY THROMBOEMBOLISM

LABORATORY DATA
Arterial blood gases
May be normal initially or show relative hypoxemia
PaO_2 less than 60 mm Hg
Hypocarbia
Decreased arterial saturation
Respiratory alkalosis
CBC
Elevated leukocytes (with pulmonary infarct)
Enzymes
Elevated LDH, CPK, SGOT
EKG
May only show tachycardia (if mild episode of PTE)
Changes with massive PTE reflect right ventricular strain, failure, ischemia
Peaked T waves
Widened QRS
ST and T changes
Right QRS axial shift
CHEST RADIOGRAPH
Initial radiograph usually normal
Later films may reveal atelectasis or infarction pattern
LUNG SCAN (VENTILATION AND PERFUSION)
Not an exclusive diagnostic study for PTE
Normal ventilation—air still enters and expands lungs
Perfusion defect—the clot obstructs the pulmonary circulation distal to the clot, causing underperfused or nonperfused areas
PULMONARY ANGIOGRAM
Most definitive diagnostic study for significant PTE[68]
Reveals clot(s) in the pulmonary vasculature
Identifies areas of impaired perfusion (due to filling defects)

Chest physiotherapy, frequent suctioning, and breathing and coughing exercises all promote alveolar gas exchange and improve arterial oxygen concentrations by clearing and removing secretions, thus preventing or minimizing atelectatic areas.

Analgesic agents reduce the patient's pain and associated anxiety. Pain control promotes the patient's compliance and participation in breathing exercises and pulmonary hygiene, which maximizes breathing efforts and oxygenation.

Cardiovascular collapse from either the vasoactive substances or the right ventricular failure leads to a shock state, necessitating hemodynamic support. Measures such as administration of pressors and inotropes and volume expansion may all optimize cardiac output. Close analysis of vital sign trends, including pulmonary artery pressure measurements, aids in evaluation of resuscitative efforts.

A prolonged clotting time that is 2 to 2½ times normal is the desired elevation. Heparin, the drug of choice, should be administered intravenously. Continuous IV infusion is the recommended route because it reduces the overall amount of heparin needed each day, eliminates the "peaks and valleys" associated with intermittent injections, and minimizes the risks of bleeding episodes.[83] Close monitoring of clotting studies is essential to monitor dose adequacy. Clotting times less than 2 times normal will prove ineffective, and coagulation prolonged beyond 2½ times normal may precipitate bleeding episodes. Platelet counts should be monitored with PT and PTT times, since thrombocytopenia is a complication associated with anticoagulant therapy. Heparin therapy usually continues for 1 week, after which an oral anticoagulant regimen is begun.

Plasminogen activators such as streptokinase and urokinase are used to lyse fresh thrombi and may also inhibit future thrombus formation. These agents, similar to anticoagulants, *should be used judiciously in the trauma patient.* Injuries or situations in which the use of thrombolytics is contraindicated include subdural hematomas and postcraniotomy patients.

Surgical intervention (pulmonary embolectomy) is generally indicated in patients with severe obstructive PTE or in whom the previously mentioned therapy is ineffective or contraindicated. Procedures such as insertion of a caval filter or umbrella or vena caval ligation may be necessary.

INTERMEDIATE CARE REHABILITATION CYCLES

Overview of Rehabilitation

Trauma rehabilitation is the process of restoring the patient to physical, emotional, and economic usefulness. Not all trauma patients with musculoskeletal injuries can return to the level of functioning they enjoyed prior to their accident or illness. New, realistic levels must be defined, and the patient must be assisted through education and therapy to attain these new goals.

Rehabilitation for the patient with musculoskeletal injuries starts at the time of injury. Prehospital care personnel initiate the first stage of rehabilitation by providing the proper care for injuries and preventing further injury. During the resuscitative and operative cycles, injuries are diagnosed, and definitive treatment is initiated. Prevention of secondary disabilities related to immobility during the critical care phase plays an equally important role. Pulmonary hygiene, skin care, and active and passive range-of-motion exercises help maintain the patient's existing capabilities and prevent delays in starting the more active rehabilitation process.

The intermediate and rehabilitative cycles involve the most active efforts in educating and training the patient to adapt to new limitations. Family involvement is greater during these cycles than at any other time since the patient's injury occurred. Both the patient and the family are reeducated and trained in order that the individual may reach the highest possible functioning capability.

Problems During Recovery

Potential for Delayed Healing

Related to Infection. Infection, causing delayed healing of fractures and soft tissue wounds, can postpone the initiation of the active rehabilitative process. Proper nursing care and patient/family education can help prevent or minimize the risk of infection in the patient with musculoskeletal injuries.

Through continuous assessment of wounds, pin sites, and surgical incisions, the nurse can detect early signs of infection and can promptly initiate therapy. The patient and family must be educated in the concept of aseptic technique and the importance and the proper method of pin care and dressing changes for wounds and incisions as necessary. The nurse should ensure that the patient and family can demonstrate their ability to perform these procedures accurately and that they can identify the signs and symptoms of pin tract and wound infections correctly. The education process should be started early so the patient and family have time to become comfortable and competent with this responsibility.

Osteomyelitis, a bacterial invasion of the bone, results from either primary or secondary causes. Primary osteomyelitis results from direct introduction of microorganisms into the bone from trauma, such as open fractures or penetrating injuries, or during surgery. Secondary osteomyelitis results from microorganisms seeded into the bone from soft tissue infections or septicemia.[83] Commonly isolated organisms include *Staphylococcus, Escherichia coli, Klebsiella,* and *Pseudomonas aeruginosa.* Acute osteomyelitis that becomes resistant to therapy can develop into recurring chronic osteomyelitis.

Signs and symptoms of osteomyelitis include local pain with movement, edema, erythema, elevated temperature, chills, diaphoresis, muscle spasms, limited joint movement, weakness, and a direct wound tract with purulent drainage.

Methods utilized to diagnose osteomyelitis include culturing blood, wound drainage, or bone marrow. Results of laboratory tests on serum will show an elevated white blood cell count and erythrocyte sedimentation rate. Approximately 10 to 14 days after onset of the infection in adults, radiographic examination will show elevated periosteum, areas of radiolucency secondary to bone lysis, and areas of density secondary to bone necrosis. Deep bone destruction will be evident on CT scans, and radionuclide scans will demonstrate areas of occult infection.

Treatment for osteomyelitis includes antibiotic therapy and surgical debridement and irrigation to eliminate the causative organism, immobilization to reduce the associated pain and the risk of pathological fractures, nutritional support to optimize healing, and institution of a pain-management regimen. Patients with chronic osteomyelitis may require bone grafting to increase the stability of the bone after extensive bone damage.[83]

Movement of the affected area should be minimized; immobilization, as ordered, is maintained by bed rest, casting, splinting, or traction. If movement of the area is required, full and gentle support must be provided. Analgesia is administered as ordered and the effectiveness is closely monitored. When possible, analgesics should be given prior to dressing changes. Wound drainage monitoring includes a description of its amount, color, odor, and consistency. Wound and skin isolation should be maintained if drainage is present.

Related to Soft Tissue Loss. Soft tissue injuries with significant tissue loss will require tissue grafting to promote healing, provide soft tissue coverage of the bone, and prevent the potential for osteitis. Closing the wound and increasing the vascular supply through grafting can shorten the fracture healing time and decrease the risk of infection.[28] Soft tissue grafting is done when the wound is free of devitalized tissue, which may occur 4 to 7 days after injury. The presence of any wound infection will delay grafting. Dressing changes for soft tissue wounds are done every 4 to 6 hours from the time of injury until the wound is ready for grafting.

Related to Nonunion. Healing times for fractures depend on the location and the type of fracture, associated traumatic injuries, and systemic complications. If healing does not occur within the expected time for the type of fracture present, delayed union is present. The diagnosis of nonunion is made when, after serial patient examinations, motion and pain at the fracture site persist, and when there are no progressive radiologic changes suggestive of healing.[85]

Bone grafting enhances bone formation at the site of nonunion fractures. It is also utilized for fractures in which healing is expected to be delayed because of the severity of the fracture, bone loss, or extensive soft tissue injury. Many fractures with segmental bone loss, significant loss of the cortical diameter, or gross comminution with separation of fracture fragments require bone grafting to aid in bone healing.[86] The grafting may be done in the initial stages of treatment or several weeks after the injury, depending upon the condition of the soft tissue surrounding the area of injury. Bone grafting done during the initial repair or during the first several weeks after injury can significantly decrease the amount of time required for healing.

Potential for Alteration in Bone Integrity Related to Mechanical Failure of Fixators

External fixators are frequently used for stabilization of fractures. The length of time a fixator remains in place depends on the type of injury. The risk of complications increases with the length of time the fixator is in place.

Components of the frame, including the transfixation pins, pin clamps, and couplings, can loosen, causing loss of bone alignment. Regular checks of the frame components are necessary to identify loosened parts. An increase in pain around the pin tract is often associated with pin loosening and may be the first sign that the pin-to-bone contact is decreased. Loose pins also can increase the risk of pin tract infection and need to be removed. The patient and family must be taught prior to discharge how to properly care for the fixator. (See Appendix 21–3 for care of an external fixator.) This includes being able to check for frame tightness and recognition of early signs of pin loosening.

External fixators are adjusted as soon as possible to allow for physiological loading of the bone, which is necessary for healing. The fixator will be removed when soft tissue procedures are completed and adequate wound and skin coverage is achieved.

Metal fatigue from cyclic loading is a problem associated with internal fixators. There is a race between the process of bone healing and implant failure. Healing of *uncomplicated* fractures, however, usually occurs long before the implant fails. With improved operative techniques and metallurgy and increased knowledge of the biomechanics involved in fractures and healing, the incidence of implant failure has been reduced. While implants are usually removed after healing has occurred, removal may be delayed or abandoned if the risk associated with a second surgical procedure outweighs the benefits of hardware removal. Patients who undergo implant removal from weight-bearing bones must be taught to use protected weight-bearing techniques to prevent refracturing.

Protected weight bearing is necessary for a minimum of 6 weeks after implant removal to allow the bone to regain its normal strength.

A fracture is considered completely healed when its strength is equal to that of normal bone and when it tolerates normal stresses without refracturing. Radiographic examination shows dense and continuous bone cortices.[4]

Alteration in Mobility

The effects of immobility caused by fractures, dislocation, plexus injury, or amputation can be disastrous. The nurse must anticipate potential problems and collaborate with the physical therapist to initate actions to prevent these complications.

Pulmonary hygiene must continue with methods such as coughing and deep breathing exercises and use of incentive spirometry. Chest physiotherapy with percussion may be required routinely for patients who are unable to maintain a clear chest through other methods.

Amputations. Amputees require special attention to the residual limb. Active range-of-motion exercises prevent contractures of the joint immediately proximal to the incision. The patient should be taught isometric exercises of the targeted muscle groups if active range of motion is impossible or limited. Activities that promote contracture formation of the proximal joint should be avoided or limited in duration; e.g., a patient with a below-the-knee amputation should not be in a sitting position without extension of the knee joint, and above-the-knee amputees must avoid long periods of sitting and must spend time in the prone position to promote extension of the hip joint. The positioning of the intact extremities and the muscles of the trunk also must be noted. The patient should be taught how to perform active exercises and their importance in promoting mobility. Mobilizing the patient as soon as possible enhances overall recovery and rehabilitation. It will be necessary for the patient with a lower extremity amputation to develop a new sense of balance as new methods of mobility are learned.

Extremity Fractures. Methods of ambulating the patient with a fracture of the extremity will vary according to the type and location of the fracture and whether the bone affected is a weight-bearing or non-weight-bearing bone. Crutch walking for the patient with a single lower extremity fracture and wheelchair transfer for the patient with bilateral lower extremity fractures will facilitate ambulation and reduce the complications of immobility. Active exercises of the upper extremities and trunk are necessary to increase the patient's physical strength and tolerance for these different types of ambulation.

External fixators have greatly increased the mobility of patients with fractures, who at one time were confined to prolonged bed rest with traction. Despite the advantages provided by the external fixator, it can still be intimidating to the patient, resulting in slow acceptance of the device and hesitation to become fully mobilized. Education and emotional support can help the patient understand the function of the external fixator, accept the change in body image, and reduce any fear associated with ambulation with the external fixator.

Patients with tibial plateau, supracondylar, patellar, or acetabular fractures are at risk of formation of joint adhesions and contractures. Limited passive range-of-motion exercises of the joint, according to physician specifications, can help reduce these risks. Use of a continuous passive motion machine (CPMM) has been shown to be effective in restoring or increasing joint extension and flexion, reducing discomfort, and reducing the formation of degenerative bone changes.[87] Lubrication of the articular joint surface is optimized by the production of synovial fluid, which is stimulated by the motion. The CPMM is most effective when applied within the first week after surgery. The nurse must be thoroughly familiar with the operation of the CPMM and any potential complications that it can cause to use it safely. Proper alignment of the CPMM is necessary to reduce contact between skin surface areas and the CPMM. Padding will be necessary to prevent irritation or breakdown of those skin areas which come in contact with the machine. The nurse should be alert for any signs and symptoms of infection around incision sites and for any increased bleeding from surgical drains. Neurovascular checks and skin care should continue while the machine is operating. If the patient needs to get out of bed or requires turning for chest physiotherapy, the CPMM should be removed. Appendix 21–4 shows two types of CPMMs and further describes implications and related nursing responsibilities.

Pelvic Fractures. The degree of mobility permitted following a pelvic fracture depends on the type of fracture, the amount of pain associated with the fracture, and the method of treatment. Extended bed rest may be necessary, with the hip fixed in flexion, extension, adduction, or abduction. Progressive ambulation without weight bearing may be allowed according to the patient's pain tolerance. Internal or external fixation of pelvic fractures can decrease the amount of time required for bed rest.

Plexus Injuries. Functional recovery of a plexus injury depends on several variables, including the type of injury, the specific nerve and level injured, and the patient's age.[88] For example, a patient who sustained nerve impairment after an isolated anterior shoulder dislocation may recover fully within a few days to weeks, whereas a more violent injury, such as from a motorcycle accident with more than one nerve root injured, implies a worse prognosis for recovery. Despite months of intense rehabilitation, the patient with this type of injury may recover minimal function, if any, of the affected extremity.[49]

Rehabilitation must begin early after any type of plexus injury. If, or when, nerve regeneration occurs, the affected limb must be in optimal physical condition to afford function and use of the extremity.

Closed plexus injuries generally require extensive rehabilitation for many months before any significant progress in function is seen. If no improvement develops after a year of rehabilitation, surgical intervention for amputation may become necessary and appropriate. The patient will usually function more fully with a prosthesis than with an insensate, flail extremity.

Open brachial plexus injuries may require early surgical intervention for associated soft tissue, vascular, or bony injuries. Generally, primary nerve repair is performed several weeks after injury when soft tissue wounds are healed and the risk of infection is minimal. Primary repair of more peripheral nerve injuries may be appropriate and indicated for clean injuries in the distal aspects of the extremity. Surgical exploration may also be indicated for the patient who shows little functional improvement after an injury that has a good prognosis for recovery.

Chronic Pain

Chronic pain is a potentially serious complication of musculoskeletal trauma that can delay and intensify rehabilitation. The therapies used for acute pain management are often different from those used in, and sometimes even are contraindicated in, the management of chronic pain. A planned, team approach affords the most effective and comprehensive pain management therapy.

The patient with a musculoskeletal injury may experience any one, or a combination, of the following types of pain:

1. Nociception: tissue damage–induced stimulus to the brain from the periphery, as with degenerative joint diseases.
2. Central pain: abnormal activity along afferent pathways that have been severed from the peripheral connections, as in traumatic amputations.
3. Psychological pain: feelings of anxiety or depression mislabeled as pain sensations.
4. Behavioral pain: for reasons such as attention, sympathy, compensated time off from work, and financial aid the patient continues to behave as if he still has pain.

Because chronic pain can actually be a combination of these pain states, the patient should undergo physical, psychological, and social evaluation. Chronic pain may become the focal point of a patient's life and negatively affect all aspects of his being.[56] Therefore, this patient requires behavioral and psychological therapy in conjunction with analgesic therapy. For example, the patient with chronic pain often experiences depression and may benefit greatly from a combined drug regimen that includes analgesics and antidepressants in addition to psychological therapy. Because pain is often a combination of physical and psychological components, when the pain is relieved, the emotional changes subside and vice versa. When a serious psychological issue is resolved, the pain described by the patient often ceases.

SUMMARY

The future in musculoskeletal trauma promises to provide a continuing challenge to the entire health care team. Four major areas that demand further research and development are trauma reduction and prevention, prehospital trauma care, nursing and medical therapies, and trauma rehabilitation.

The reduction and prevention of musculoskeletal injuries require in-depth research, public education, and, in some cases, state and/or federal legislation. Safety for automobile occupants can be achieved though methods such as proper use of seat restraints. Backaitis and Dalmontas[89] have shown that in head-on collisions, injury severity is reduced for restrained drivers and front-seat passengers compared with unrestrained drivers and front-seat passengers. Rassch[90] stated that a fundamental principle in reducing injury is preventing ejection and the second collision with the hard interior of the vehicle. Siegel and associates demonstrated in a prospective study that a higher incidence of lower extremity injury occurs in frontal crashes, whereas pelvic injuries occur more often in lateral crashes. This study implied a need for improved Motor Vehicle Administration safety design standards based on injury-reduction criteria.[91]

Public education remains the most important aspect in any injury-prevention program. Rothengatter[92] found that children properly educated in road crossing behavior in a traffic environment could demonstrate retention of the skill 4 months after instruction. This alone could help reduce child-related traffic accidents. A study by Mackay[93] of the injuries sustained from motorcycle accidents shows that motorcyclists injured from side impact suffer the most serious lower leg injuries. Ross[94] found that crash bars reduced lower extremity injuries in motorcycle accidents with side impact. This was contrary to Mackay's research, which showed that crash bars had no recognizable influence. Studies such as these suggest that more work is needed in the design of the motorcycle to increase rider protection.

Improvements in prehospital stabilization techniques and in the development of improved immobilization-traction devices for musculoskeletal injuries are essential. Advances need to occur in emergency care of traumatic amputations and partial amputations to optimize replantation efforts.

Research must continue to develop improved assessment techniques and definitive care options. Potential nursing research topics may include acute and chronic pain assessment and management techniques; prevention of secondary injuries and complications, especially those related to immobility; early rehabilitation techniques; patient/family teaching and participation in care; and improved crisis management for families, patients, and staff. Medical issues that require further research and development in the realm of musculoskeletal injury include the stimulation and control of the fracture and soft tissue healing process, management of nonunion, improved microsurgical techniques to optimize replantations, modalities to enable earlier mobility, and development of improved prosthetic and implant devices.

Rehabilitation of both physical and psychosocial injuries must be addressed concomitantly for the musculoskeletal trauma patient. Improved chronic pain management and care of the amputee and management of patients with osteomyelitis, nonunion, and paralysis are all highly worthy areas of potential research.

The future of musculoskeletal trauma patient care will demand a highly collaborative approach by health care providers during all cycles of trauma care. Continued research with an increased emphasis on education and clinical application is essential to the multidisciplinary search for excellence in patient care outcome.

REFERENCES

1. Williams PL, Warwick R, Dyson M, Bannister LH (eds): Gray's Anatomy, 37th ed. New York, Bounty Books, 1989.
2. Maryland Institute for Emergency Medical Services Systems: Annual Report, 1989–1990. Baltimore, MIEMSS, 1990.
3. Maryland Institute for Emergency Medical Services Systems: Clinical Trauma Registry, 1989–1990. Baltimore, MIEMSS, 1990.
4. Stearns HC: Principles of lower extremity fracture management. In NAON Assessment and Fracture Management of the Lower Extremities. Pittman, NJ, Jannetti, 1984.
5. Latenser BA, Gentilello LM, Tarver AA et al: Improved outcome with early fixation of skeletally unstable pelvic fractures. J Trauma 31(1):28–31, 1991.
6. Looser KG, Crombie HD: Pelvic fracture: Anatomic guide to severity of injury. Am J Surg 132:638–642, 1976.
7. Trunkey DD, Chapman MW, Lim RC, Dumphy JE: Management of pelvic fractures in blunt trauma injury. J Trauma 14:912–923, 1974.
8. Pennal GF, Tile M, Wendall JP, Garside H: Pelvic disruption: Assessment and classification. Clin Orthop 151:12–21, 1980.
9. Tile M: Fractures of the Pelvis and Acetabulum. Baltimore, Williams & Wilkins, 1984.
10. Mandelbaum BR, Brooker AS: Trauma to the lower extremities. In Zuidema GD, Rutherford RB, Ballinger WF (eds): Management of Trauma, 4th ed. Philadelphia, WB Saunders Co, 1985.
11. Oxer H: No requiem for the M.A.S.T. Prehosp Disaster Med 6(2):231, 1991.
12. Jameel A, Vanderby B, Purcell C: The effects of pneumatic antishock garment (PASG) on hemodynamics, hemorrhage, and survival in penetrating thoracic aortic injury. J Trauma 31(6):849–851, 1991.
13. Schneider PE, Mitchell JM, Allison EJ: The use of military antishock trousers in trauma—A reevaluation. J Emerg Med 7(5):497–500, 1989.
14. Mattox KL, Bickell W, Pepe PE, et al: Prospective MAST study in 911 patients. J Trauma 29(8):1104–1112, 1989.
15. McSwain NE: Pneumatic antishock garment—Does it work? Prehosp Disaster Med 4(1):42–44, 1989.
16. Mattox K: Blind faith, poor judgment and patient jeopardy. Prehosp Disaster Med 4(1):39–41, 1989.
17. McSwain NE: Pneumatic antishock garment: State of the art 1988. Ann Emerg Med 17(5):506–525, 1988.
18. Eastridge BJ, Burgess AR, Ellison PS, et al: Pelvic ring disruption: Effective classification system and treatment protocols. J Trauma 29(12):1725, 1989.
19. Emerson RH: Fractures of the pelvis and femoral shaft. In Burke JF, Boyd RJ, McCabe CJ (eds): Trauma Management: Early Management of Visceral, Nervous System and Musculoskeletal Injuries. Chicago, Year Book Medical, 1988.
20. Cardona VD (ed): Trauma Nursing. Oradell, NJ, Medical Economics, 1985, p 33.
21. Chipman C (ed): Emergency Department Orthopedica. Rockville, MD, Aspen Systems, 1982, p 8.
22. Yap SNL: The management of traumatic retroperitoneal hemorrhage. Surg Rounds March:34–44, 1980.
23. Pozo JL, Powell B, Andrews BG, et al: The timing of amputation for lower limb trauma. J Bone Joint Surg 72B(2):288–292, 1990.
24. Gurd AR: The repair of bone and fracture healing. In Odling-Smee W, Crockard A (eds): Trauma Care. New York, Grune & Stratton, 1981.
25. Dellinger EP, Miller SD, Wertz MJ, et al: Risk of infection after open fracture of the arm or leg. Arch Surg 123(11):1320–1327, 1988.
26. Merritt K: Factors increasing the risk of infection in patients with open fractures. J Trauma 28(6):823–827, 1988.
27. Block SS: Disinfection, Sterilization and Preservation, 3rd ed. Philadelphia, Lea & Febiger, 1983.
28. Bosse MJ, Burgess AR, Brumback RJ: Evaluation and treatment of high-energy open tibia fracture. Adv Orthop Surg 8:3–17, 1984.
29. Faddis D, Danial D, Boyer J: Tissue toxicity of aseptic solutions: A study of rabbit articular and periarticular tissues. J Trauma 17:895, 1977.
30. Border JR, Hansen ST, Allgower M, Ruedi TP: The management of extremity injuries. In Border JR, Hansen ST, Allgower M, Ruedi TP (eds): Management of Blunt Trauma: Comprehensive Pathophysiology and Care. New York, Marcel Dekker, 1990.
31. Burke JF, Bonco CC: Sepsis folowing trauma: Prevention and control. In Burke JF, Boyd RJ, McCabe CJ (eds): Trauma Management: Early Management of Visceral, Nervous System and Musculoskeletal Injuries. Chicago, Year Book Medical, 1988.
32. Hoyt N: Infection control in trauma care. In Cardona VD (ed): Trauma Nursing. Oradell, NJ, Medical Economics, 1985.
33. Eron L: Prevention of infection following orthopedic surgery. Antibiotic Chemother 33:149–159, 1985.
34. Rice PR, MacKenzie EJ, and Associates: Cost of Injury in the United States: A Report to Congress. San Francisco, Institute for Health & Aging, University of California, and Injury Prevention Center, The Johns Hopkins University, 1989.
35. Stevens DB: Postoperative orthopedic infections. J Bone Joint Surg 46A:92–102, 1964.
36. Bucholz RW, Lippert FG, Wenger DR, Ezaki M: Orthopedic Decision Making. Philadelphia, BC Decker, 1984.
37. Blick SS, Brumback RJ, Polka A, et al: Compartment syndrome in open tibial fractures. J Bone Joint Surg 68A(9):1348–1352, 1986.
38. Slye DA: Orthopedic complications. Nurs Clin North Am 26(1): 113–132, 1991.
39. Committee on Trauma Research, Commission on Life Sciences, National Research Council, Institute of Medicine: Injury in America. Washington, National Academy Press, 1985, p 12.
40. Owen CA: Clinical diagnosis of acute compartment syndromes. In Mubarak SJ, Hargens AR (eds): Compartment Syndrome and Volkmann's Contracture. Philadelphia, WB Saunders Co, 1981, p 102.
41. Roabek CH: The treatment of compartment syndrome of the leg. J Bone Joint Surg 66B:93–97, 1984.
42. Brumback RJ: Early recognition and treatment of compartment syndrome in polytraumatized patients. In Proceedings of the 9th National Trauma Symposium, Baltimore, November 1986.
43. Cowley RA, Dunham CM: Shock Trauma: Critical Care Manual. Baltimore, University Park Press, 1982.
44. Cardea JA: Complications of fractures. In Greenfield RJ (ed): Complications in Surgery and Trauma. Philadelphia, JB Lippincott, 1984.

45. Dula DJ: Trauma avulsion injury of the brachial plexus. Ann Emerg Med 1:45–48, 1981.
46. Clark WK: Trauma to the nervous system. In Shires GT (ed): Care of the Trauma Patient. New York, McGraw-Hill, 1979.
47. Leffert RD: Brachial plexus injuries. N Engl J Med 291:1059–1066, 1974.
48. Billowitz E: Pelvic fractures. Top Emerg Med 1:39–60, 1981.
49. Crockard HA: Peripheral nerve injury. In Odling-Smee W, Crockard A (eds): Trauma Care. New York, Grune & Stratton, 1981.
50. Harkness JW, Ramsey WC, Ahmadi B: Principles in fractures and dislocations. In Rockwood CA, Green DP (eds): Fractures in Adults. Philadelphia, JB Lippincott, 1984.
51. Friedman FB: PRN analgesia: Controlling the pain or controlling the patient. RN 3:67, 1983.
52. Wallace K: Analgesic management of the acute pain patient. In 5th Annual WBAMC Trauma Symposium Combined Skeletal and Vascular Trauma, El Paso, November 1986.
53. Allen PD, Walman T, Concepcion M, et al: Epidural morphine provides postoperative pain relief in peripheral vascular and orthopedic surgical patients: A dose-response study. Anesth Analg 65:165–170, 1986.
54. Briggs GG, Burman ML, Lange S, et al: Morphine: Continous intravenous infusion versus intramuscular injections for postoperative pain relief. Gynecol Oncol 22:288–293, 1985.
55. Jones L: Patient-controlled oral analgesia. Orthop Nurs 6:38–41, 1987.
56. Lamb S, Barbaro NM: Neurosurgical approaches to the management of chronic pain syndromes. Orthop Nurs 6:23–29, 1987.
57. Lehman EP, Moore RM: Fat embolism: Including experimental production without trauma. Am Surg 14:621–662, 1927.
58. Stevenson RCK: Take no chances with fat embolism. Nursing 85 15:58–63, 1985.
59. Burgess A, Mendelbaum BR: Acute orthopedic injuries and critical care. In Seigal JH (ed): Trauma: Emergency Surgery and Critical Care. New York, Churchill Livingstone, 1986.
60. Bone L, Johnson K, Weifelt J, Scheinberg R: Early vs. delayed stabilization of femoral fractures: A prospective, randomized trial. J Bone Joint Surg 71A:336–340, 1989.
61. Pazell JA, Peltier LF: Experience with sixty-three patients with fat embolism. Surg Gynecol Obstet 135:77–80, 1972.
62. Peltier LF: The diagnosis of fat embolism. Surg Gynecol Obstet 121:371–379, 1965.
63. Peck SA: Crush syndrome: Pathophysiology and management. Orthop Nurs 9(3):33–40, 1990.
64. Chapman MW: Open fractures—Future directions. Orthop Nurs 3:46, 1984.
65. Fabian TC, Behrman SW, Kudsk KA, Taylor JC: Improved outcome with femur fractures: An analysis based on injury severity. J Trauma 29(7):1028, 1989.
66. Johnson KD, Cadambi A, Seibert GB: Incidence of adult respiratory distress syndrome in patients with multiple musculoskeletal injuries: Effects of early operative stabilization of fractures. J Trauma 25:375–384, 1985.
67. Sauter AJM, Klopper PJ: Fat embolism after static and dynamic loads: An experimental investigation. Acta Orthop Scand 54:94–100, 1983.
68. Gossling HR, Donohue TA: The fat embolism syndrome. JAMA 241:2740–2742, 1979.
69. Evarts CM, Mayer PJ: Complications. In Rockwood CA, Green DP (eds): Fractures in Adults. Philadelphia, JB Lippincott, 1984.
70. Stenkman B, Stechmiller J: Fat embolism syndrome: Pathophysiology and current treatment. Focus Crit Care 11:26–35, 1984.
71. Krouskop TA, Noble PC, Garber SL, Spencer WA: The effectiveness of preventive management in reducing the occurrence of pressure sores. J Rehabil Res Dev 20:74–83, 1983.
72. Pinchcofsky-Devin GD, Kaminski MV: Correlation of pressure sores and nutritional status. J Am Geriatr Soc 34:435–440, 1986.
73. Van Noy E, Genge ML: Common complications. In Pellino TA, Mooney NE, Salmond SW, Verdisco LA (eds): NAON Core Curriculum for Orthopedic Nursing. Pittman, NJ, Jannetti, 1986.
74. Van Noy E, Genge ML: Nursing care of adults and children with problems of the urinary system. In Saxton DF, Pelikan PK, Nugent PM, Hylane PA (eds): The Addison-Wesley Manual of Nursing Practice. Menlo Park, Addison-Wesley, 1983.
75. Gordon DL, Reinstein L: Rehabilitation of the trauma patient. Am Surg 45:223–227, 1979.
76. Genge NL, Isom VV, Kunz ME: Immobility. In Pellino TA, Mooney NE, Salmond SW, Verdisco LA (eds): NAON Core Curriculum for Orthopedic Nursing. Pittman, NJ, Jannetti, 1986.
77. Trafton PG: Fractures. In Trunkey DD, Lewis FR (eds): Current Therapy of Trauma, 1984–1985. St. Louis, CV Mosby, 1984.
78. Trafton PG: Prevention of venous thrombosis and pulmonary embolism: Proceedings from consensus conference. JAMA 256:744–749, 1986.
79. Gens DR: Venous thromboembolic prophylaxis. Crit Care Rep 1(3):317–322, 1990.
80. Burke CM, Morris AJ: Perfusion scans and pulmonary angiography. Heart Lung 15:357–360, 1986.
81. Glennon SA, Matus VW, Bryan-Brown CW: Respiratory disorders. In Kinney MR (ed): AACN's Clinical Reference Guide for Critical Care Nursing. New York, McGraw-Hill, 1981, pp 518–523.
82. Thoman MN: Acute pulmonary embolism. Focus Crit Care 10:21–28, 1983.
83. Groves MJ: Nursing care of adults and children with problems of the musculoskeletal system. In Saxton DF, Pelikan PK, Nugent PM, Hylane PA (eds): The Addison-Wesley Manual of Nursing Practice. Menlo Park, Addison-Wesley, 1983.
84. Dunnery EL: Infections. In Pellino TA, Mooney NE, Salmond SW, Verdisco LA (eds): NAON Core Curriculum for Orthopedic Nursing. Pittman, NJ, Jannetti, 1986.
85. Arlington RG: Internal fixation of the lower extremity. In Assessment and Fracture Management of the Lower Extremity (NAON Monograph Library). Pittman, NJ, Jannetti, 1984, p 65.
86. Green SA: Complications of external skeletal fixation. Clin Orthop 180:109–115, 1983.
87. Stedman JR, Montgomery JB: Dislocations of the knee in the competitive athlete. In Speigel PG (ed): Techniques in Orthopaedics. Baltimore, University Park Press, 1984.
88. Bartowski HM, Pitts LH: Neurologic injury. In Trunkey DD, Lewis FR (eds): Current Therapy of Trauma, 1984–1985. St. Louis, CV Mosby, 1985.
89. Backaitis SH, Dalmontas D: Injury patterns and injury sources of unrestrained and three-point restrained car occupants in injury producing frontal collisions. In 29th Proceedings of the American Association for Automotive Medicine, Washington, DC, 1985, pp 365–392.
90. Rassch FO Jr: Forensic analysis of trauma. In Nahum AM, Melvin J (eds): The Biomechanics of Trauma. Norwalk, CT, Appleton-Century-Crofts, 1985, p 177.
91. Siegel JH, Mason-Gonzales S, Cushing BM, et al: A prospective study of injury patterns, outcome and cost of high speed frontal versus lateral motor vehicle craches. In Proceedings of the 34th Conference of the Association for the Advancement of Automotive Medicine, Scottsdale, AZ, 1990, pp 289–313.
92. Rothengatter T: A behavioral approach to improving traffic behavior of young children. Ergonomics 27:147–160, 1984.
93. Mackay M: Leg injuries to motorcyclist and motorcycle design. In 29th Proceedings of the American Association for Automotive Medicine, Washington, DC, 1985, pp 169–180.
94. Ross DJ: The prevention of leg injuries in motorcycle accidents. Injury 15:75–77, 1983.

22

MAXILLOFACIAL AND SOFT TISSUE INJURIES

T. CATHERINE BOWER

INTRODUCTION

Effective nursing care for the trauma patient with facial injuries, specifically maxillofacial disruption or soft tissue loss, is complex and challenging. It requires an appreciation of facial beauty and function as well as a broad knowledge of facial injuries and reconstructive techniques. This chapter emphasizes the importance of prevention of facial injuries, reviews assessment skills, and defines nursing problems and interventions specific to the maxillofacially injured patient from resuscitation through rehabilitation.

The face is in an exposed position without protective covering; thus, the incidence of facial injuries is high.[1] A report from Cornell University indicated that 72.1 per cent of those involved in automobile accidents suffered some type of injury to the face.[2] Although this percentage reflects data compiled 20 years ago, other literature reports cite similar percentages for facial injuries. Schultz studied 1042 cases of major facial injuries over a 10-year period (1960 through 1970) and found that 54 per cent of facial injuries resulted from motor vehicle accidents (MVA).[3] Recent epidemiological investigations have reviewed distribution of facial injuries, the incidence of concurrent multisystem injuries, and the effect of increased public awareness of laws and penalties resulting from driving while intoxicated. Cook and Rowe found over a 4-year period that 47.6 per cent of midfacial fractures were a result of automobile accidents.[4] Maxillofacial trauma includes any injury to the bony structure, surrounding tissue, nerves, or vascular supply of the face. Soft tissue injuries can be described as lacerations, contusions, and abrasions.

The author acknowledges the contribution of Sandra L. Deli to this chapter in the first edition.

MECHANISM OF INJURY

Facial trauma can be a result of an MVA, personal assault, accidental fall, or sporting event mishap. Research has revealed much about the cause and mechanisms of facial trauma resulting from MVAs (Fig. 22–1). According to Nahum, when a vehicle strikes an object during a collision, the energy is dissipated by deformation and destruction of the vehicle as it strikes the object.[5] If the force of the blow exceeds the impact tolerance level of the face, injury results. Impacts at relatively lower levels of speed (such as 5 or 10 mph) can result in minor soft tissue injuries. Greater impacts from speeds of 20 mph or greater usually result in facial bone fractures, particularly to the nose, maxilla, and zygoma.

In the case of an MVA, the object that the operator strikes and his position inside the vehicle are important considerations to review in the determination of mechanism of injury. Research has demonstrated that the front-seat passenger often is thrown up and forward toward the windshield at an angle of 45 degrees (Fig. 22–2*A*). During deceleration, the passenger is thrown backward (Fig. 22–2*B*). If the passenger's head penetrates the windshield, avulsion injuries may occur, particularly to the forehead (Fig. 22–2*C*).

A mandate by the National Safety Council in 1966 resulted in a requirement that chemically tempered laminated windshields be installed in automobiles, which replaced glass windshields. The plastic interlayer within the windshield, which has a high penetration resistance, helps to contain the passenger within the automobile. This feature has changed the type of facial lacerations from severe degloving of facial tissue to numerous small superficial lacerations and triangular avulsions (Fig. 22–3). A degloving injury is characterized by avulsion of skin with or without soft tissue from the underlying skeletal or musculoskeletal framework.[6] Repair of such injuries requires the consultation of a plastic surgeon initially, with follow-up surgical revisions if tissue loss is massive.

Excessive loss of soft tissue from the face can be caused by penetrating or blunt forces. Common penetrating injuries directed to the facial region can be those resulting from gunshot, shotgun, or stab wounds. Blunt trauma usually results from MVAs when the face strikes the dashboard or windshield, leaving the passenger contained within the vehicle. Injuries resulting from penetrating or blunt forces commonly are massive and disfiguring. Subsequent tissue cleansing and débridement must occur before approximation can be attempted by the plastic surgeon. Small penetrating injuries require careful examination and observation; a thorough ophthalmologic examination may be indicated to rule out any injury to the globe and surrounding structures.

Other mechanisms of injury can be a result of an assorted array of mishaps (Table 22–1). The 10-year study by Schultz showed several categories of causes of facial injuries.[3] Of particular interest, Cook and Rowe's retrospective study of 225 patients reflected a higher incidence of midfacial trauma resulting from interpersonal violence (Fig. 22–4).[4] Both studies indicate the continued need for ongoing investigation related to the various causes of facial trauma. Facial injuries that occur in the home environment often are secondary to carelessness or other unforeseen circumstances. Most soft tissue injuries are of a shearing nature and are most commonly contaminated. Falling down a flight of steps and missile injuries, such as from a rock thrown by a lawn mower, are two examples of home accidents that may cause facial injuries (Fig. 22–5). Sports injuries, such as baseball injuries resulting from not using face guards, and intended assaults directed to the facial area are other examples (Fig. 22–6). The unhelmeted motorcycle driver who sustains an accident frequently has some type of trauma to the face. Fractures to the upper and midface occur when the driver is thrown forward over the handlebars, striking another vehicle, an object, or the pavement. After this type of injury, soft tissue damage and contamination from environmental dirt and gravel are common (Fig. 22–7).

Prevention of facial trauma resulting from an MVA can best be accomplished through the compulsory use of over-the-shoulder and lap seat restraints (Fig. 22–8). Further studies are needed to demonstrate conclusively the effectiveness of safety belts. Dodson and Kaban's study on the effect of legislation with the mandatory seat belt law in California revealed no reduction in maxillofacial injuries.[7] With the

Text continued on page 593

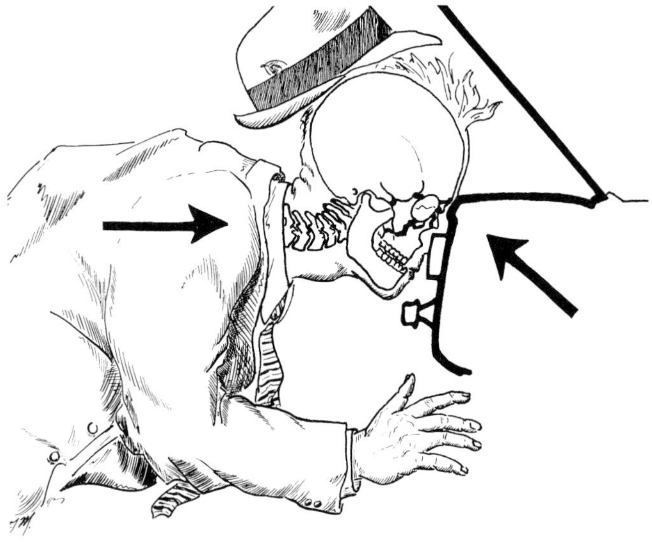

Figure 22–1. Common mechanism of facial fracture in auto accidents. From Schultz RC: Facial Injuries. 2nd ed. Chicago, Year Book Medical Publishers, 1977.)

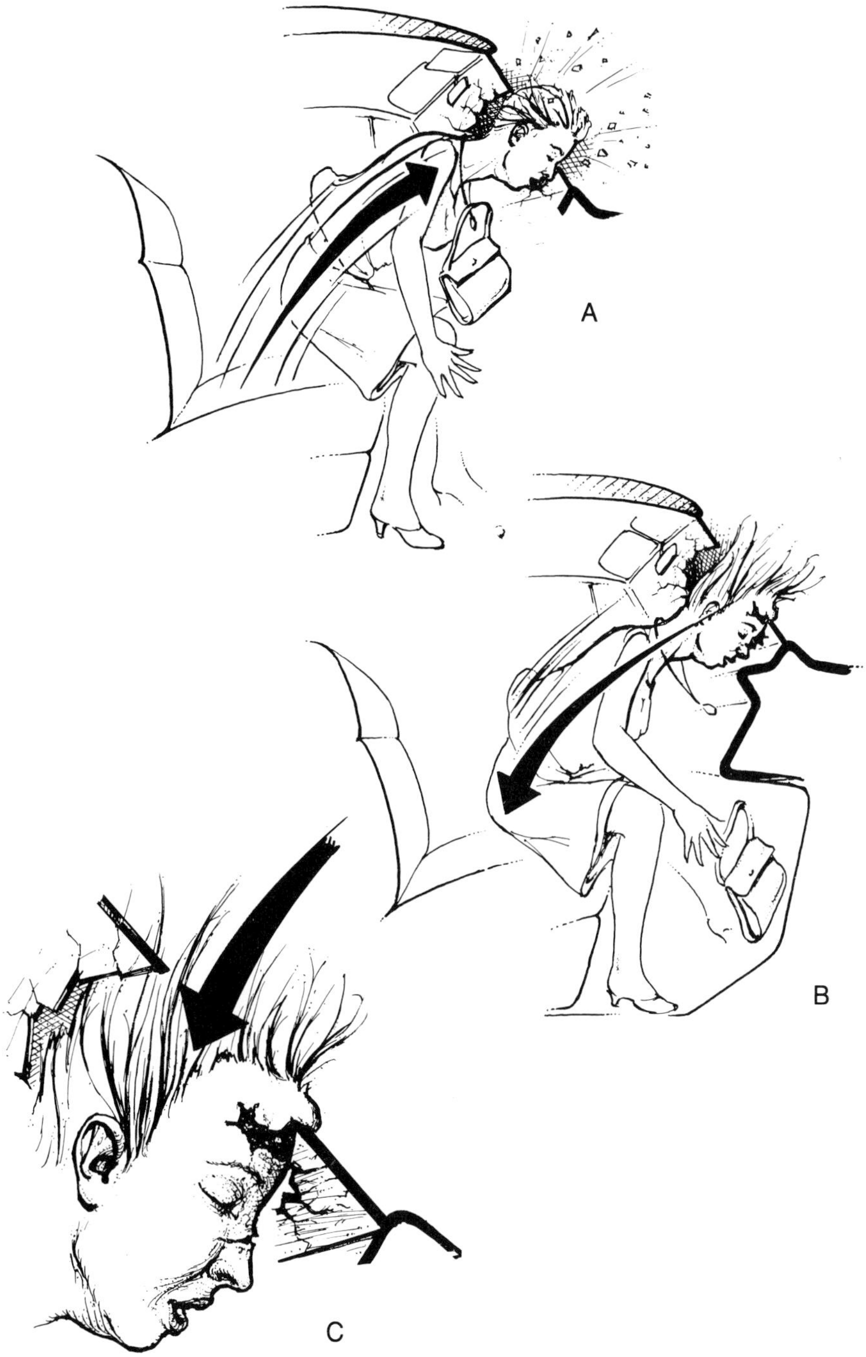

Figure 22–2. Mechanism of soft tissue injury in accidents involving automobile windshields manufactured before 1966. *A*, Passenger thrown up and forward through windshield. *B*, Passenger thrown back and down into front seat after forward momentum has stopped. *C*, Tangential forces create avulsion flaps. (Reprinted with permission from Schultz RC: Facial Injuries. 2nd ed. Chicago, Year Book Medical Publishers, 1977.)

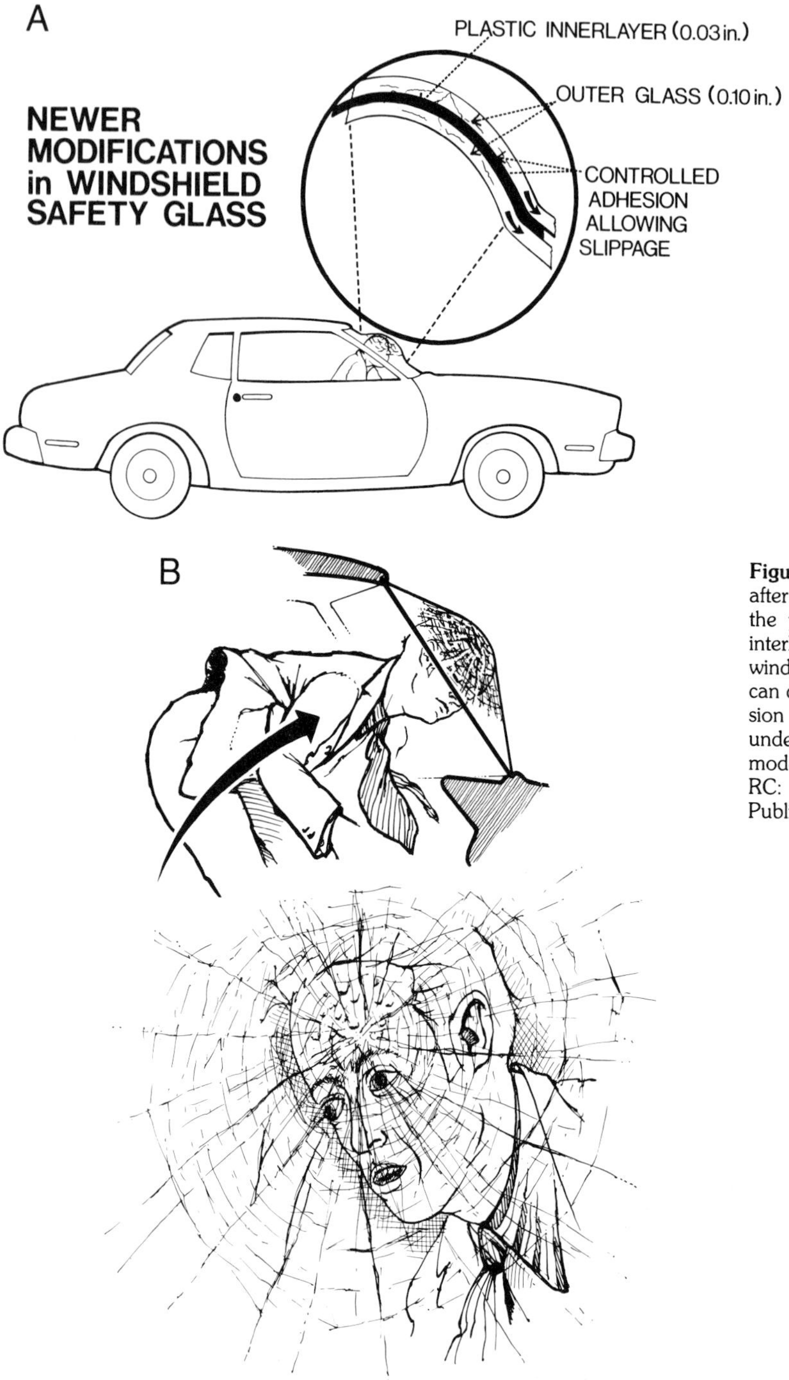

Figure 22–3. The windshields of automobiles manufactured after 1966 and modified again after 1968 help to contain the passenger within the automobile. The thicker plastic interlayer and looser bonding permit ballooning of the windshield on impact (*A*). Multiple small blunt glass particles can cause numerous small lacerations, small triangular avulsion flaps, and tiny avulsion injuries (*B*) but not the deep undermining extensive avulsion flaps sustained on pre-1966 model windshields, as shown in Figure 22–2. (From Schultz RC: Facial Injuries. 2nd ed. Chicago, Year Book Medical Publishers, 1977.)

TABLE 22–1. CATEGORIES OF FACIAL INJURIES BY CAUSE

CATEGORY OF INJURY	AUTO ACCIDENT	HOME ACCIDENT	ATHLETIC INJURY	ANIMAL BITE	WORK INJURY	INTENDED INJURY	OTHER	TOTAL
Soft tissue	556	78	32	63	21	21	36	807
Fractures	598	72	107	0	34	63	61	935
Dental	67	4	12	0	4	3	6	96
Total	1221	154	151	63	59	87	103	1838

Reprinted with permission from Schultz RC: Facial Injuries. 2nd ed. Chicago, Year Book Medical Publishers, 1977.

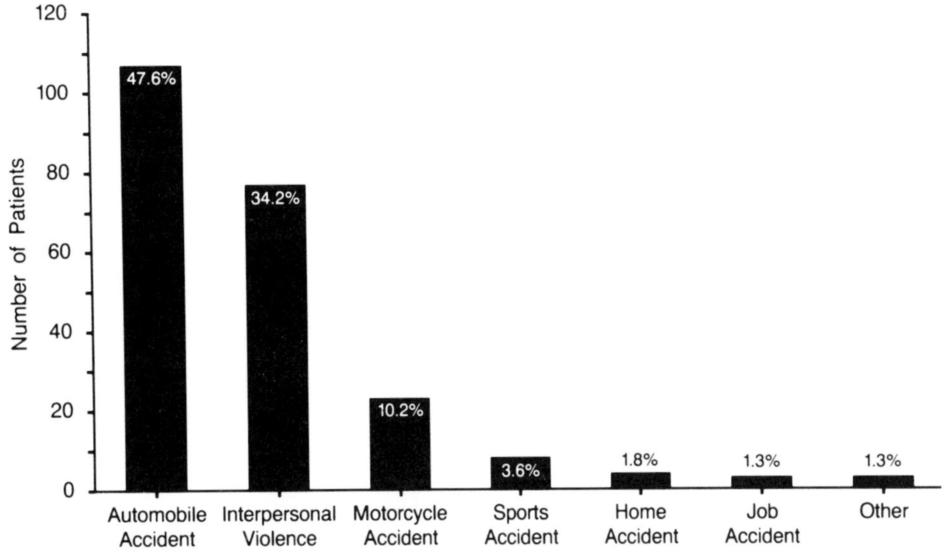

Figure 22–4. Causes of midfacial fractures. (From Cook HE, Rowe M: A retrospective study of 356 midfacial fractures occurring in 225 patients. J Oral Maxillofac Surg 48:575, 1990.)

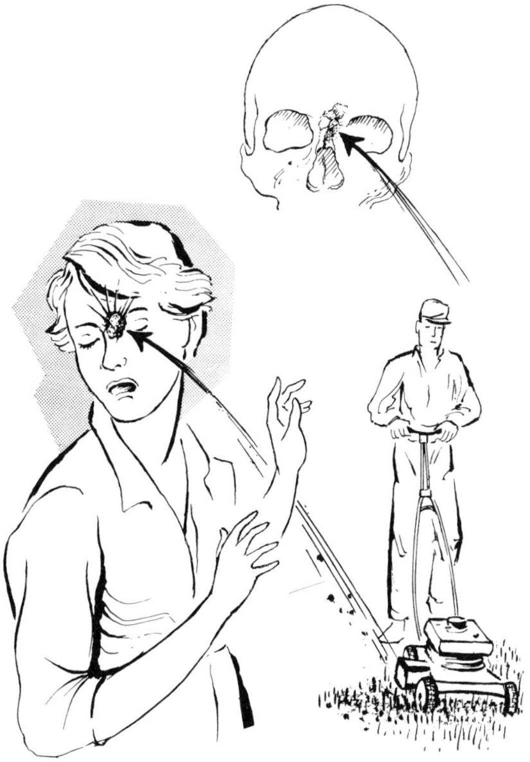

Figure 22–5. Facial injuries that occur around the home can be severe. (From Schultz RC: Facial Injuries. 2nd ed. Chicago, Year Book Medical Publishers, 1977.)

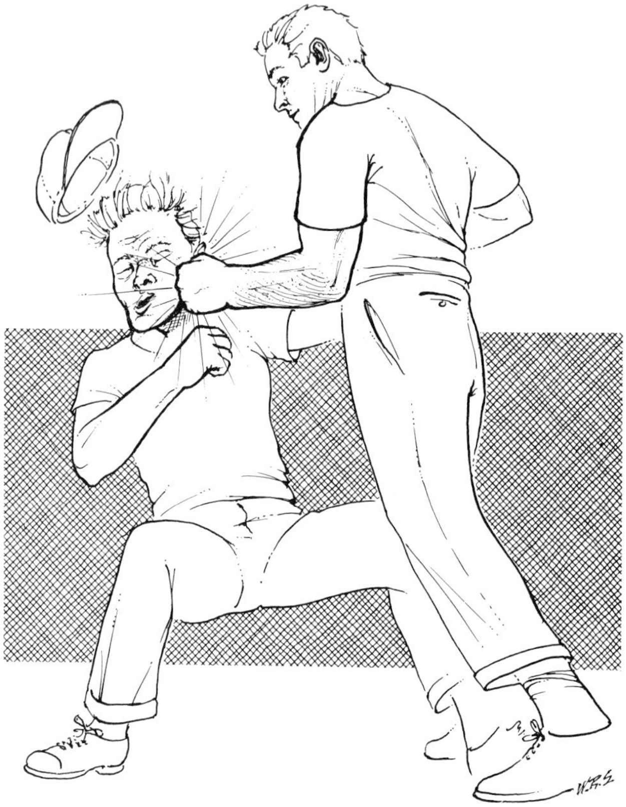

Figure 22–6. Intended injury usually involves the face and can result in fractures and soft tissue injury. (From Schultz RC: Facial Injuries. 2nd ed. Chicago, Year Book Medical Publishers, 1977.)

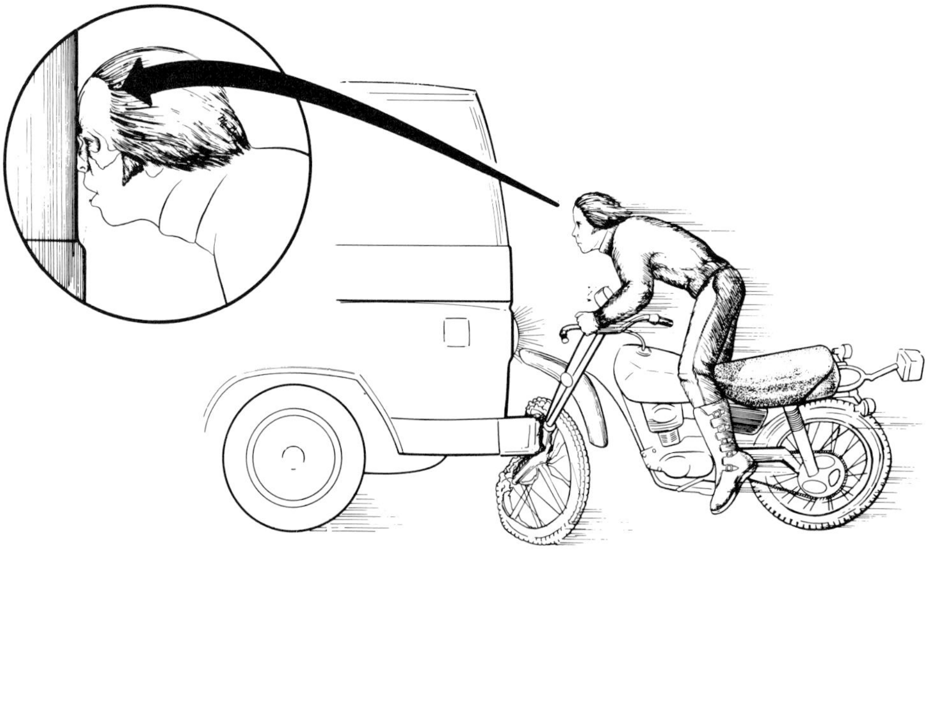

Figure 22–7. Motorcycles provide no protection for the driver. Fractures of the upper face and midface occur when victim is thrown forward. (From Schultz RC: Facial Injuries. 2nd ed. Chicago, Year Book Medical Publishers, 1977.)

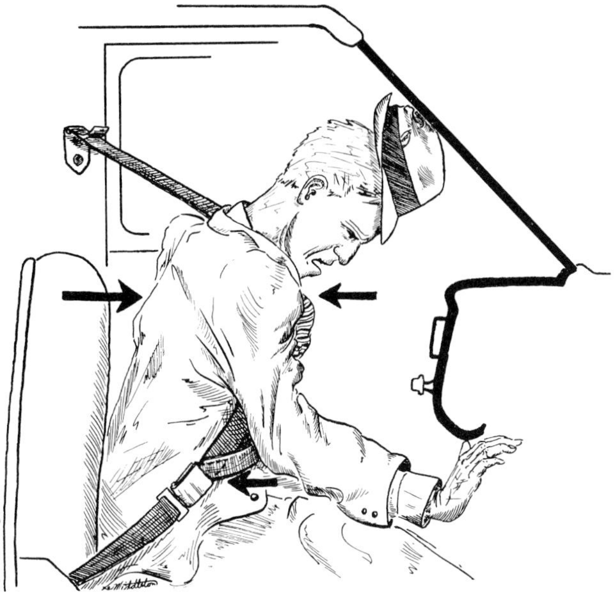

Figure 22–8. In the event of a crash, shoulder-lap–type seat belts tether the driver and the passenger to the car and prevent the face from striking the steering wheel, windshield, or dashboard. (From Schultz RC: Facial Injuries. 2nd ed. Chicago, Year Book Medical Publishers, 1977.)

institution of lower speed limits and the requirement to wear over-the-shoulder seat belts, there has been a relative decrease in the number of facial injuries in countries where mandatory seat belt legislation has been in effect for at least 15 years.[8–10] Reath and coworkers concluded that safety belts are effective in preventing soft tissue injuries and fractures of the mid and upper face. The incidence of mandibular fractures was not decreased with safety restraints (Fig. 22–9).[11] The belted driver continues to move forward and the prominence of the chin impacts on the steering wheel. Air bag restraints may become a standard of the future, and in combination with safety belts, such injuries may be prevented.[12]

Unrestrained rear-seat passengers are less susceptible to facial injury but are thrown forward after impact and sustain other multisystem injuries.

ANATOMY OF THE FACE

An appreciation of basic facial anatomy and structure identification is vital to the understanding of repair and reconstruction after maxillofacial disruption or soft tissue injury. The major bones that form the cranium and face can be divided into three major sections: the upper, middle, and lower portions. The upper third of the facial architecture includes the frontal sinus, frontal bone, glabella, and supraorbital ridge. The middle third, or midface, includes the orbit, maxillary sinuses, nose, vomer, zygoma, maxilla, palate, and maxillary teeth with alveolar process. The lower third includes the mandible and mandibular teeth (Fig. 22–10). The facial bones and other structures give the face its characteristic shape as well as protect the cranial contents and organs of sight.

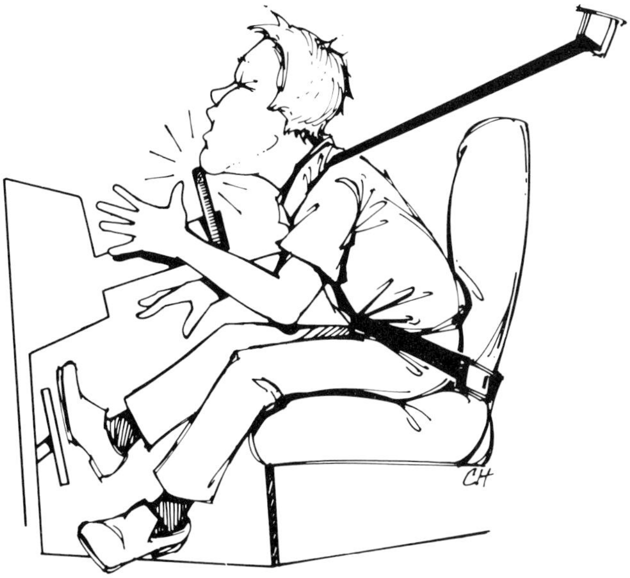

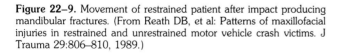

Figure 22–9. Movement of restrained patient after impact producing mandibular fractures. (From Reath DB, et al: Patterns of maxillofacial injuries in restrained and unrestrained motor vehicle crash victims. J Trauma 29:806–810, 1989.)

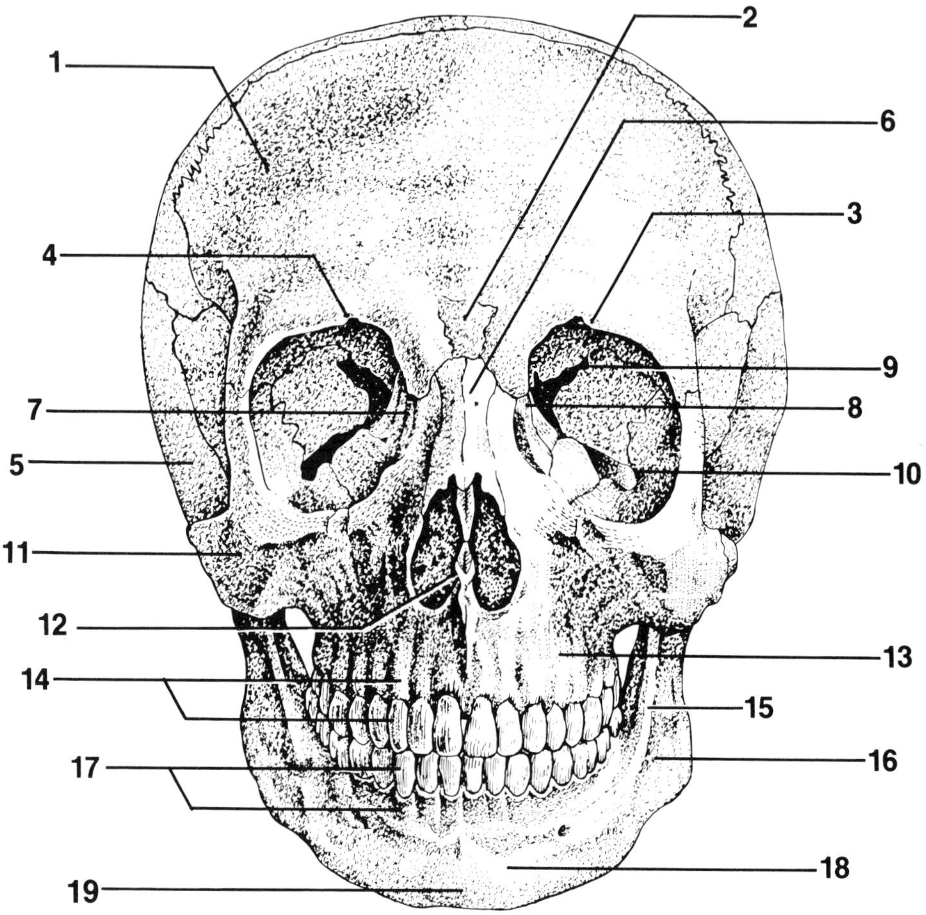

Figure 22–10. Bones of the facial skeleton.

BONES OF UPPER THIRD	BONES OF MIDDLE THIRD	BONES OF LOWER THIRD
1. Frontal bone	9. Superior orbital fissure	15. Ramus of mandible
2. Glabella	10. Inferior orbital fissure	16. Angle of mandible
3. Supraorbital margin	11. Zygomatic bone	17. Alveolar part with teeth
4. Supraorbital notch	12. Nasal septum, vomer	18. Symphysis of mandible
5. Temporal bone	13. Body of maxilla	19. Mental protuberance
6. Nasal bone	14. Alveolar process with teeth	
7. Lacrimal bone		
8. Ethmoid bone		

The mandible (lower jaw) is attached to the skull by the temporomandibular joint and provides the mechanical action needed for chewing. The maxilla (upper jaw) is located at the midface and is immovable. Midface fractures are fairly common after a high-velocity impact because of the immobility of this area.

Muscles

The muscles that cover the bony structures of the face provide movement, as evidenced by facial expressions, and give distinguishing features to each person (Fig. 22–11). Muscles that affect mandibular movement consist of the anterior and posterior groupings. The muscles of the anterior group are the geniohyoid, genioglossus, digastric, and mylohyoid. Their function is the opening of the jaw. When the mandible is fractured anteriorly, these muscles distract the broken fragments inferiorly and lingually. The posterior group are the masseter, temporalis, medial pterygoid, and lateral pterygoid muscles. This group carries out mastication and may displace a proximal fracture laterally and superiorly (Figs. 22–12 and 22–13).

Cranial Nerves

After any type of maxillofacial insult, the cranial nerve functions may be altered secondary to local trauma. The sense of smell (olfactory I) may be affected if the nasal mucosa is irritated or traumatized after blunt trauma to the midface. Vision (optic II) may be altered if the ganglion fibers near the retina have been stretched or contused after any type of impact. Diplopia may be present as a result of orbital floor damage or extraocular muscle dysfunction.[13] Eye movement (oculomotor III, trochlear IV) may be decreased or absent if localized edema develops after the traumatic insult. The nurse must note the light reflex (oculomotor III) in both eyes; a dilated ipsilateral pupil may not be an indication of an intracerebral insult. Residual absence of the light reflex may reflect third cranial nerve damage as well as decreased perception of *light* reflex (optic II) and should be communicated to all team members. Sensory divisions for the entire face and the movement of muscles for mastication are supplied by the trigeminal (V) nerve. The facial nerve (VII) (Fig. 22–14) innervates all the muscles of facial expression for movement and conveys the sense of taste for the anterior two thirds of the tongue. The sensory fibers for the posterior tongue and palate are supplied by the glossopharyngeal (IX) nerve. Trauma to the facial area can affect any of the cranial nerves, and knowledge regarding their innervations can assist one's nursing assessment after injury occurs.

Vascular Supply

Arterial blood supply to the face is provided by the branches of the internal and external carotids (Fig. 22–15). The superficial arterial supply is derived from the external carotid artery. Life-threatening hemorrhage must be controlled quickly, usually by direct pressure, when patients with open wounds of the face are present in the emergency department.

A pterygoid venous plexus is located near the mandibular condyle and temporomandibular joint. Hemostasis, if needed, can be accomplished through direct pressure or pressure dressings. In general, venous bleeding from facial wounds seldom causes life-threatening hemorrhage.

The cervical lymph node chain located under the sternocleidomastoid muscle and the tonsillar, submaxillary, submental lymph nodes below the mandible are important components that contribute to the healing process of facial

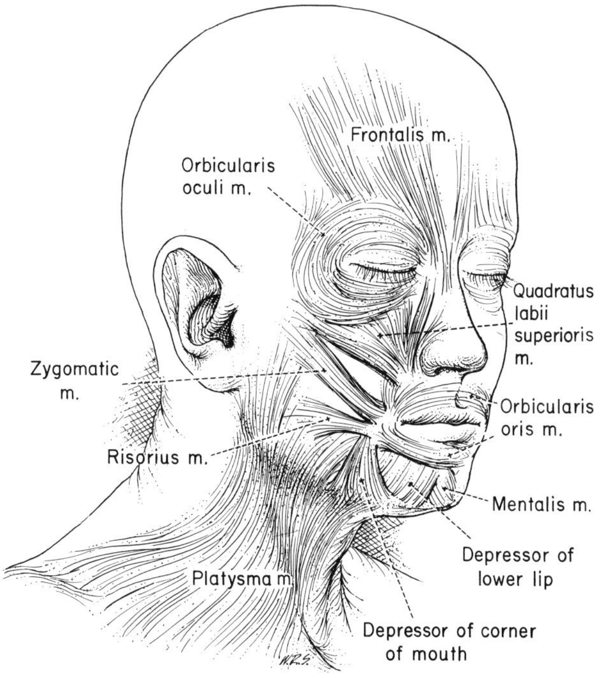

Figure 22–11. Muscles of facial expression. (From Schultz RC: Facial Injuries. 2nd ed. Chicago, Year Book Medical Publishers, 1977.)

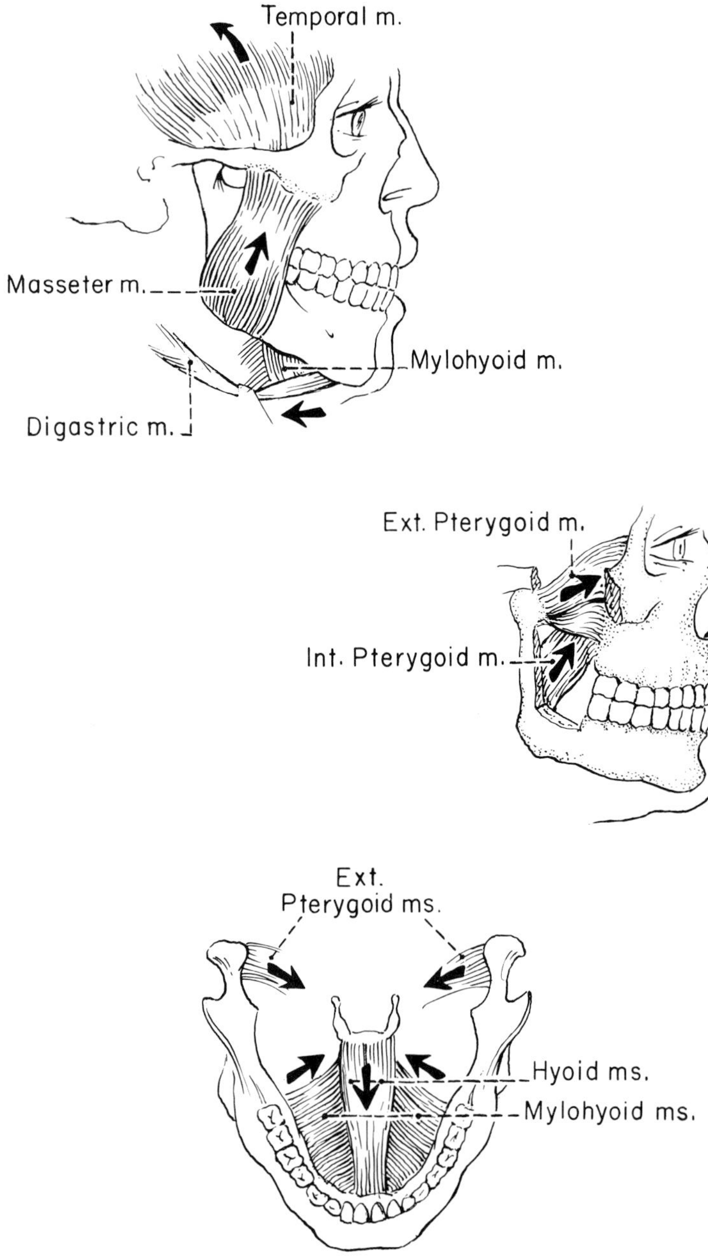

Figure 22–12. Muscles that affect mandibular fractures. (From Schultz RC: Facial Injuries. 2nd ed. Chicago, Year Book Medical Publishers, 1977.)

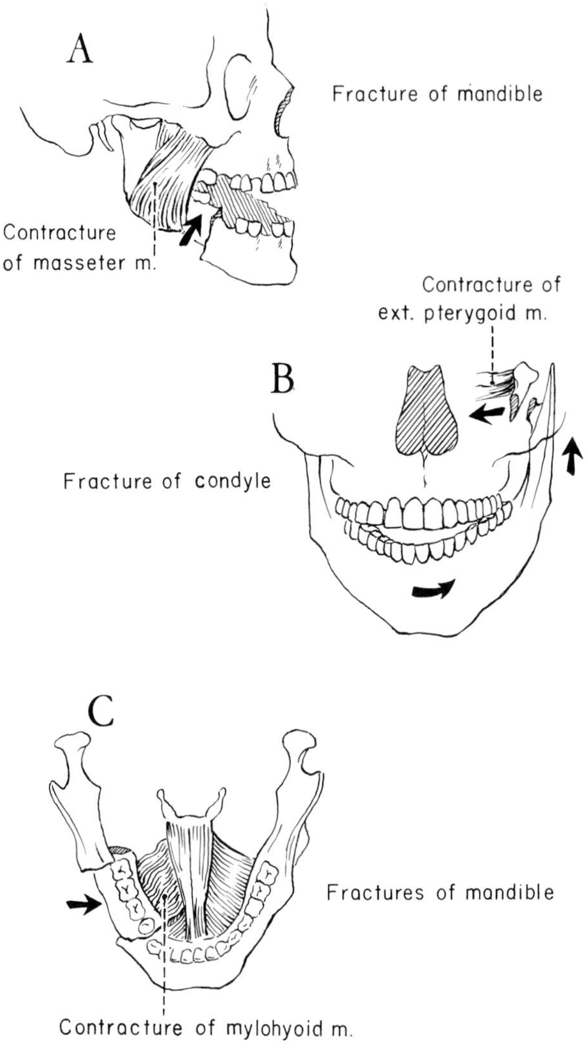

Figure 22–13. Muscle contractures that complicate facial fractures. (From Schultz RC: Facial Injuries. 2nd ed. Chicago, Year Book Medical Publishers, 1977.)

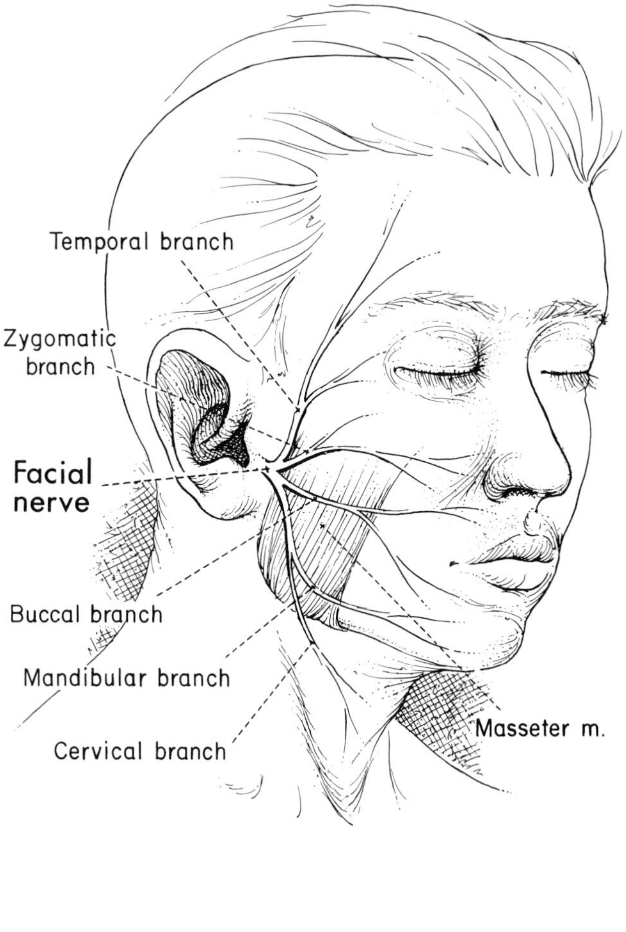

Figure 22–14. Facial nerve and branches. (From Schultz RC: Facial Injuries. 2nd ed. Chicago, Year Book Medical Publishers, 1977.)

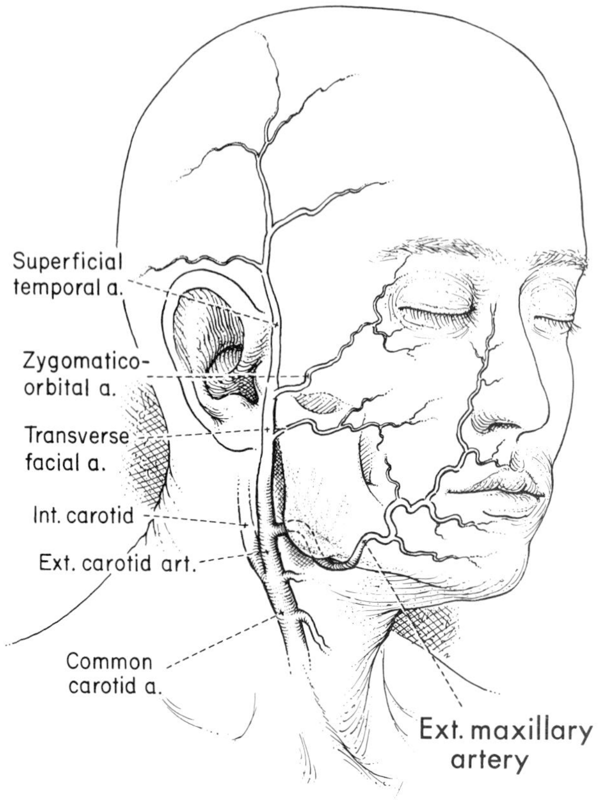

Figure 22–15. Arterial supply of face. (Reprinted with permission from Schultz RC: Facial Injuries. 2nd ed. Chicago, Year Book Medical Publishers, 1977.)

injuries. Functions of the lymphatic system include the return of protein and macromolecules into the systemic circulation, the production of lymphocytes and antibodies, and phagocytosis by the reticuloendothelial cells lining the lymph nodes.[14] If lymphatic drainage is disrupted secondary to massive trauma, residual edema surrounding the disruption occurs. As revascularization and soft tissue healing develop, localized edema subsides.

ASSESSMENT OF FACIAL BONE FRACTURES

A thorough clinical evaluation, combined with radiographic studies and computed tomography, provides enough information for diagnosis and treatment of facial bone fractures. The most frequent radiological examinations are listed in Table 22–2. Three-dimensional computed tomographic and surface imaging provide additional and valuable visualization of bony and soft tissue injuries. Injuries cannot be evaluated accurately with three-dimensional scanning solely.[15] All planes, including axial and coronal views, should be evaluated through the utilization of two-dimensional computed tomography.

Inspecting for symmetry of anatomical features and dental occlusion is one method of identifying certain types of facial injuries during clinical evaluation. Palpation can also be performed in the resuscitative area or emergency department, and the presence of crepitus, tenderness, and irregularity of facial bones can be identified. Clinical evaluation techniques are shown in Figure 22–16. Assessment of cranial nerve function, noting areas of anesthesia or hyperesthesia, and identification of visual abnormalities are other steps to include in the assessment of facial bone fractures.

The presence of an eyelid or periorbital hematoma, laceration, or contusion should initiate examination for penetration of the globe, hyphema, retinal injuries, or underlying orbital fractures. An ophthalmology consultation is highly recommended. Involvement of the lacrimal gland should be suspected if a deep laceration of the outer portion of the upper lid is present or if bones adjacent to the nasolacrimal duct appear disrupted.

Nasal Fractures

The nose, because it is the most prominent structure of the face, acts as the greatest impact absorber and sustains a

TABLE 22–2. RADIOLOGIC EXAMINATIONS FOR FACIAL INJURY

1. Water's view (shows the frontal, supraorbital, orbital floor, zygomaticomaxillary, and nasal areas).
2. Towne's view (shows the condylar and subcondylar regions of the mandible and orbital floor).
3. Lateral and anteroposterior (AP) skull films (show sinuses, roof of the orbits, frontal bone, nasoethmoid area, and zygomatic frontal area).
4. AP and lateral oblique mandible films (show the body, symphysis, condylar, and coronoid).
5. Occlusal and apical films (show symphysis, palate, and roots of the teeth), which are taken when a mandible fracture is suspected.

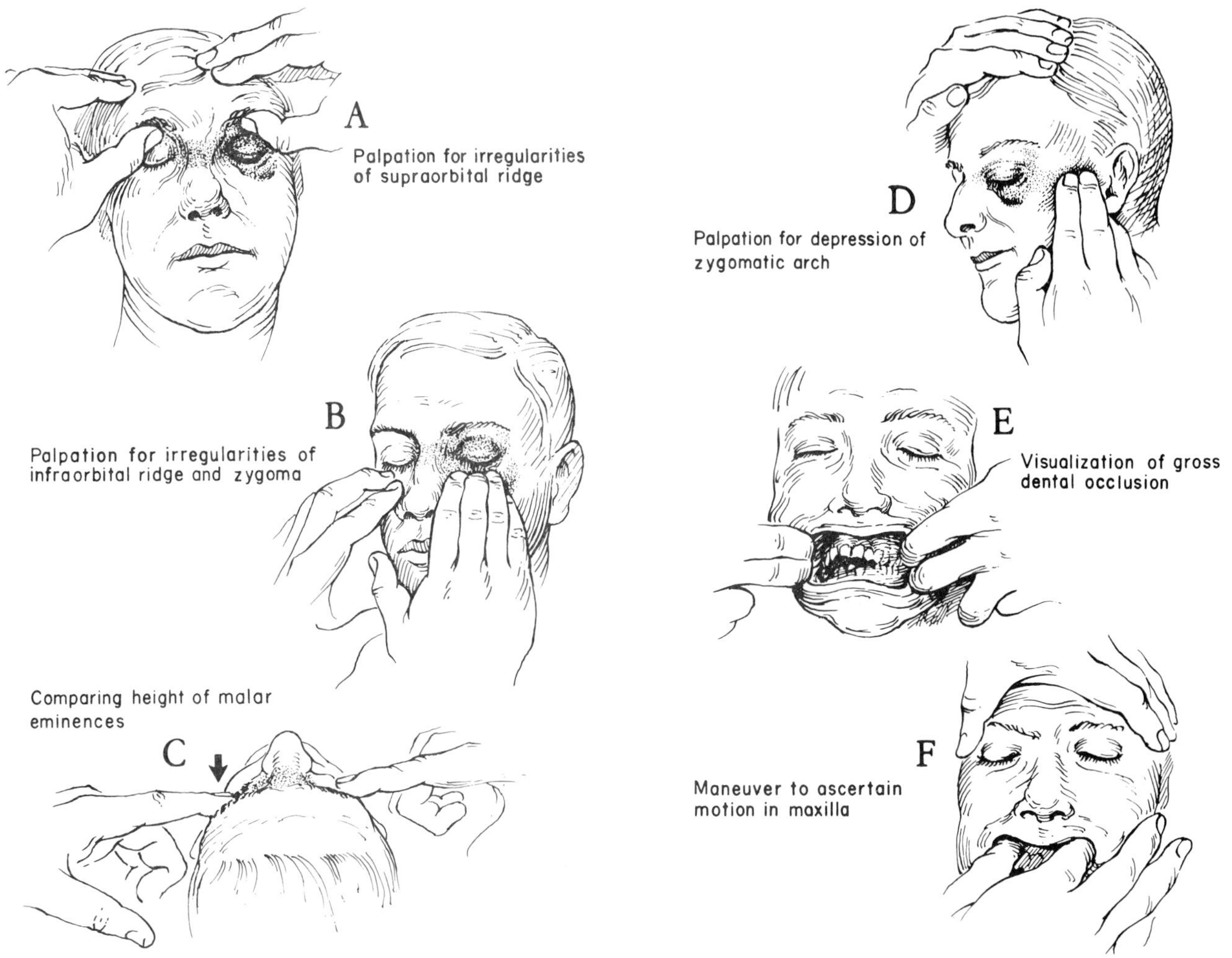

Figure 22–16. Palpation examination techniques for facial injuries. *A*, Palpation for irregularities of supraorbital ridge. *B*, Palpation for irregularities of infraorbital ridge and zygoma. *C*, Comparing height of malar eminences. *D*, Palpation for depression of zygomatic arch. *E*, Visualization of gross dental occlusion. *F*, Maneuver to ascertain motion in maxilla. (From Schultz RC: Facial Injuries. 2nd ed. Chicago, Year Book Medical Publishers, 1977.)

high number of injuries, particularly in the unrestrained operator of a motor vehicle (Table 22–3). Nasal fracture patterns are numerous but may be classified into three major categories: (1) depressed, (2) laterally angulated, and (3) comminuted.[3] Physical examination of the nasal bones is an accurate method for identification of nasal fractures, but radiographic studies are an important part of the assessment after trauma to the face.

Inspection of the nose reveals the major indicators of a nasal fracture: signs of obvious deformity, asymmetry, and inflammation. Specifically, signs of generalized edema and ecchymosis, bleeding from the nasal mucosa, and deviation of the nasal septum alert the examiner that a nasal deformity is present. Palpation of the nose displays crepitus and tenderness.

Zygoma and Orbital Floor Fractures

Zygoma and orbital floor fractures may occur independently or together. Extension of the zygomatic fracture to the orbital floor occurs at the infraorbital foramen, and a Water's view radiographic study is most important in distinguishing the presence of both fractures. Physical examination reveals periorbital ecchymosis as the most common finding in fractures of the zygoma. Areas of anesthesia may be

TABLE 22–3. FREQUENCY OF FACIAL BONE FRACTURES

TYPE	NUMBER	PERCENTAGE
Nasal bones	382	37
Zygoma and arch	159	15
Mandible	112	11
Orbital floor	112	11
Maxilla	84	8
Teeth	71	7
Sinuses	50	5
Supraorbital	36	4
Alveolus	25	2
Total	1031	100

Reprinted with permission from Schultz RC: Facial Injuries. 2nd ed. Chicago, Year Book Medical Publishers, 1977.

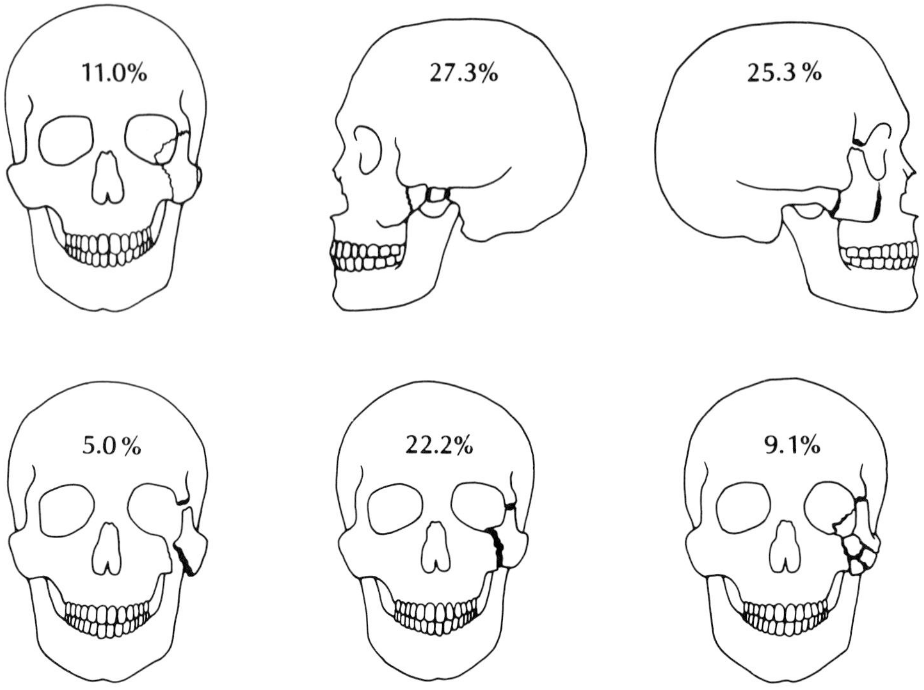

Figure 22–17. Anatomical distribution of zygomatic fractures in 98 patients. (From Haug RH, et al: An epidemiologic survey of facial fractures and concomitant injuries. J Oral Maxillofac Surg 48:927, 1990.)

present as a result of local trauma to the infraorbital nerve. Tenderness along the inferior orbital rim and a decrease in the height of the zygoma may also be present (see Fig. 22–16*D*). Enophthalmos after an orbital fracture often results from edema of the orbital cavity and restriction of eye movement upward because of entrapment of the inferior rectus muscle.[3] Haug and colleagues found in a study of 98 patients that the common site of zygoma fractures was at the arch, resulting from personal assaults and motor vehicle accidents (Fig. 22–17).[16]

Mandibular Fractures

Mandibular fractures usually result from blunt trauma, and because of the mandible's arch shape, the fracture usually occurs in two places. The body of the mandible and the condylar-subcondylar areas are the structures of frequent displacement (Fig. 22–18). On physical examination, dental malocclusion is a common finding (see Fig. 22–16*E*). Pain with jaw movement is present because of the distracting forces of the attached muscles (see Figs. 22–12 and 22–13). The masseter muscle contracts the fracture upward, and the mylohyoid muscle directs forces inward.

Le Fort Classification of Maxillary Fractures

Maxillary fractures occur in various patterns. Classifications of midface trauma after severe impact have been described by Le Fort (1901; Fig. 22–19).[18] A Le Fort I fracture is transverse, involving a horizontal line that separates the maxillary alveolus from the upper fracture. In the Le Fort II fracture, a pyramid-shaped separation involves the nasomaxillary segment of the zygomatic and orbital portions of the midface. The Le Fort III fracture is the most complex type of facial fracture and constitutes a separation of the midface from the cranium. The maxilla, one or both zygomas, and the nose are all involved in this fracture pattern. On physical assessment, malocclusion and elongation of the midface alert the examiner to a possible maxillary fracture. As shown in Figure 22–16*F,* motion of the maxilla is another indicator of a midface fracture, usually Le Fort I.

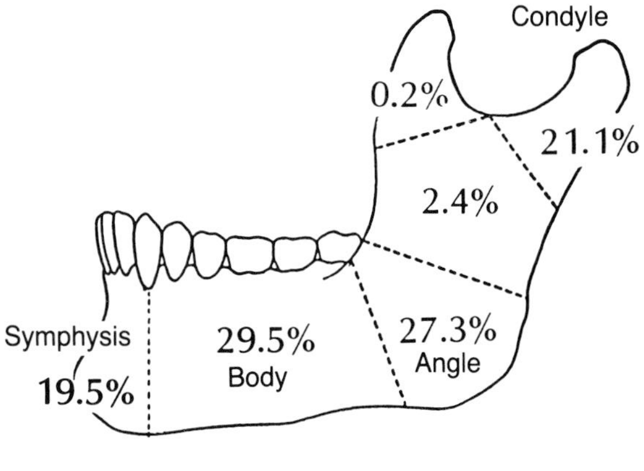

Figure 22–18. Mandibular fracture distribution, classified according to Ivy and Curtis system in 307 patients. (From Haug RH, et al: An epidemiologic survey of facial fractures and concomitant injuries. J Oral Maxillofac Surg 48:927, 1990.)

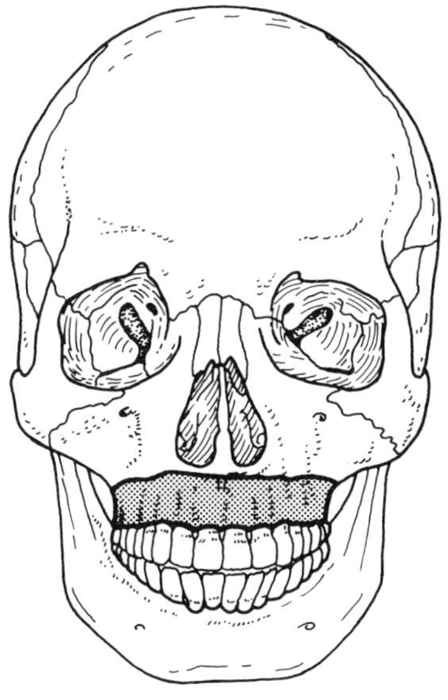

Classical Le Fort I fracture pattern.

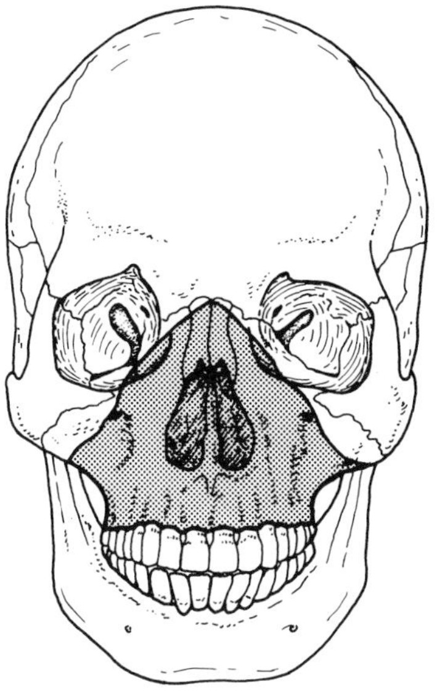

Classical Le Fort II fracture pattern.

Figure 22–19. Classic Le Fort fracture patterns. (From Rowe NL, Killey HC: Fractures of the Facial Skeleton. Baltimore, Williams & Wilkins, 1968.)

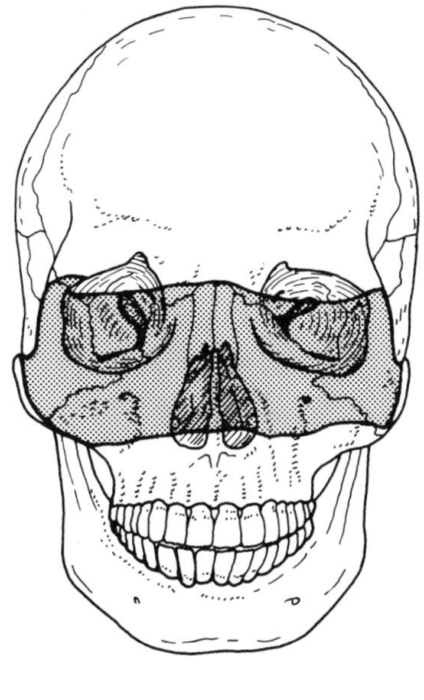

Classical Le Fort III fracture pattern.

Cerebrospinal fluid (CSF) rhinorrhea may be seen in Le Fort II and III fractures, which is indicative of fracture extension through the cribriform plate.

Soft Tissue Injury Assessment

Facial trauma frequently is accompanied by soft tissue injuries, which include lacerations, contusions, abrasions, avulsions, and hematomas. These wounds require meticulous initial evaluation and subsequent management to detect associated injuries, promote healing, and ensure an optimal cosmetic result (Fig. 22–20). A physician performs the initial physical assessment and inspection of soft tissue injuries, including identification of any foreign material and evaluation of the depth of the wound. Bony structures, facial nerve function, and function of adjacent organs (the eye is most commonly injured) should be examined. Facial films confirm the presence of fractures.

The presence of certain soft tissue wounds can be indicative of underlying problems, for which the examiner should retain a high index of suspicion. A fracture should be suspected under any laceration site. Lacerations may transect the branches of the facial nerve. Severe edema and contusions can cause temporary paralysis. Damage should be suspected when lacerations are present over the facial nerve branches. Motor function of the face should be assessed bilaterally.

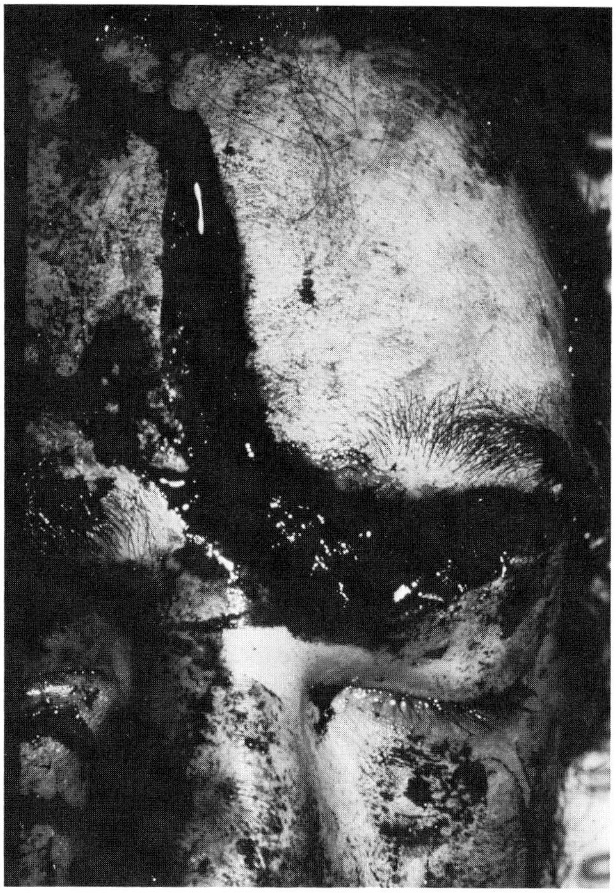

Figure 22–20. Soft tissue injury.

RESUSCITATION CYCLE

After maxillofacial trauma, appropriate management and a definitive plan for surgical intervention can best be accomplished through referral and transport to a trauma center. High-velocity impact injuries to the face are severe and complex. Injury to hidden structures such as bone, sinuses, or nerves may be camouflaged by edema and ecchymosis. Consultation with a plastic surgeon enhances management and, possibly, decreases complications. Airway compromise, aspiration of blood, and hemorrhage are immediate life-threatening problems that must be instinctively and expeditiously addressed during the initial management of the patient with facial trauma. Nursing problems during the resuscitative phase include the potential for alterations in ventilation, fluid volume, consciousness, and skin integrity and the potential for anxiety.

Alterations in Ventilation

The potential for airway compromise and alteration in ventilation results when swelling of the pharynx, occlusion of the pharynx by the tongue or secretions, or excessive bleeding obstructs respirations. Initial attempts to establish a patent airway include the chin lift or jaw-thrust maneuver and removing foreign secretions and debris, such as broken teeth. Hyperextension of the head and neck should not be attempted until a cervical spine fracture has been ruled out. If initial attempts fail to attain a patent airway, emergency intubation or tracheostomy may be necessary. An emergency cricothyroidotomy or tracheostomy may be considered if airway establishment is emergent and if the risk of accidental aspiration of broken teeth and blood is present. Prophylactic tracheostomy may be considered by the plastic surgeon and admitting physician, instead of prolonged endotracheal intubation, when the patient has multiple fractures of the mandible or maxilla, massive soft tissue damage and swelling, and alterations in neurological status.[17]

Once airway management has been established, nursing assessment of the patient's ventilatory status is a priority. Inspecting quality and effort of spontaneous respirations as well as symmetry of chest wall movement and auscultating breath sounds for air exchange are nursing skills necessary to assess ventilation. Because of the high incidence of nasal and intraoral bleeding after direct facial impact, aspiration of blood and oral secretions must be prevented. If endotracheal intubation or tracheostomy is necessary, measurement of intracuff pressure should be performed at least every 8 hours. An intracuff pressure of 20 to 25 mmHg usually prevents aspiration of secretions.[19] Clearing the oral cavity of blood through frequent suctioning and positioning the head of the bed 30 degrees upward (if indicated) are nursing strategies that can prevent aspiration. Indications of aspiration include rales and rhonchi on auscultation, decreased PaO_2, decreased lung compliance, and infiltrates on chest radiographic studies.

Mechanical ventilation usually is the treatment modality after aspiration. Nursing actions during the resuscitative phase include auscultation of breath sounds, arterial blood gas sampling and interpretation, and tracheal suctioning. Collaboration between the physician and nurse ensures that ventilatory trends are managed appropriately. The aforementioned skills are necessary in the emergency department, especially if other body systems need management before disposition to a critical care unit or operating room. Depending on the institution and department protocols, ventilatory management during resuscitation may be the responsibility of the anesthesiologist, respiratory therapist, or nurse. With the introduction of increased invasive and noninvasive monitoring of ventilation, particularly with direct trending of end-tidal carbon dioxide within the ventilator circuit and pulse oximetry application, it is paramount that the resuscitative nurse have the necessary skill and expertise to monitor and interpret data from these modalities.

Alterations in Volume

Hemorrhage after facial trauma is an immediate concern. *The possibility of exsanguination cannot be ignored, especially if one of the facial arteries has been lacerated or contused.* Extensive hemorrhage usually results from injury to the external maxillary artery or the superficial temporal artery (see Fig. 22–15). Direct digital pressure on the lacerated site is the primary method of control. Circumferential pressure bandages can also be used to control hemorrhage. If these measures do not control the bleeding, direct ligation of the vessel may be indicated. The nurse must monitor dressings closely for blood saturation and keep the physician appraised of the estimated blood loss if there is a delay in direct

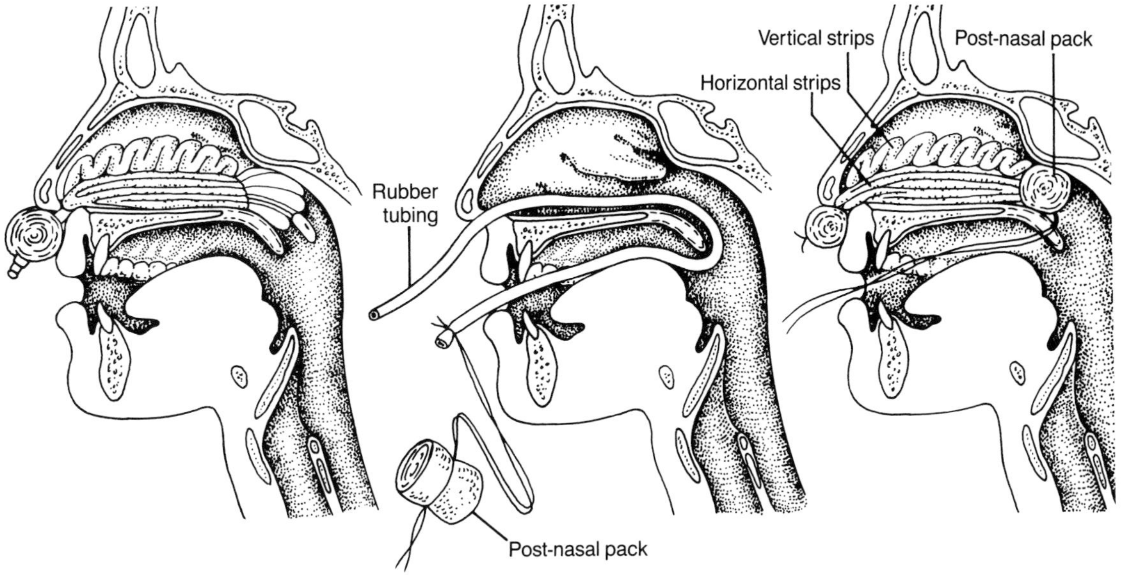

Figure 22–21. Anteroposterior nasal packing. (From Cowley RA, Dunham CM: Shock Trauma Critical Care Manual. Baltimore, University Park Press, 1985.)

visualization of the wound. It is imperative that surgical hemostats, clamps, and suture material be immediately available in the emergency care environment.

Hemorrhage after closed maxillofacial injuries, such as fractures involving the nose, zygoma, frontal sinus, or nasoethmoid, can be controlled by manual reduction. A common method of manual reduction is through the use of anteroposterior nasal packing (Figs. 22–21 and 22–22). Compression of actively bleeding vessels can be accomplished by inserting into each naris either a 30-ml balloon catheter or petrolatum gauze.[20] The packing is removed after 24 to 48 hours. Packing that remains in place longer than 2 days becomes a source of infection and may cause compression necrosis of mucous membranes. Having an emergency nasal packing tray preassembled in the emergency department enhances control of hemorrhage after midface trauma (Table 22–4). The nurse must frequently assess hemoglobin, hematocrit, and coagulation factors after hemorrhage control has been attained to assess the need for blood product replacement and the potential for further bleeding.

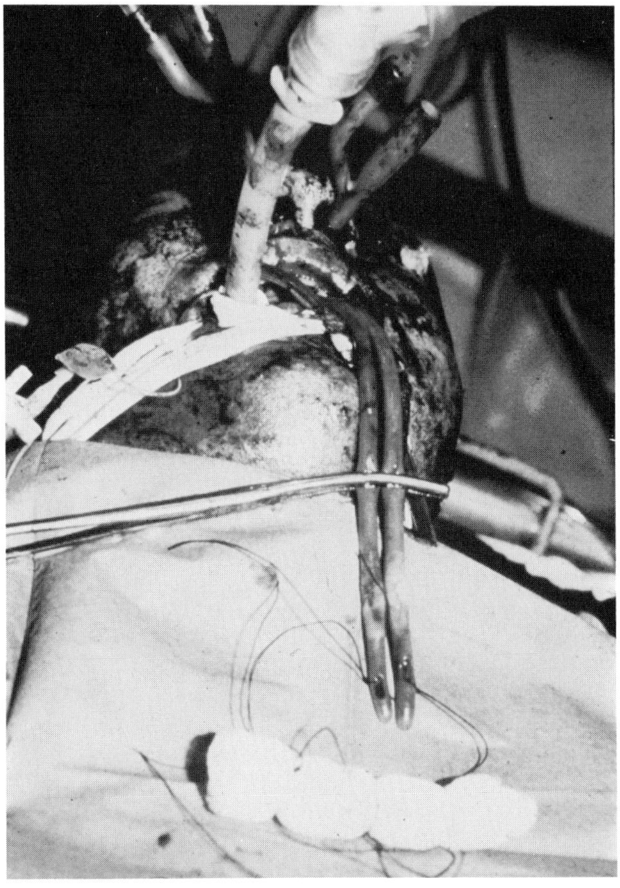

Figure 22–22. Placement of anteroposterior nasal packing in resuscitation area.

Alterations in Consciousness

After maxillofacial trauma, extension of fractures into the cranium with accompanying intracerebral injuries must be assessed. Because of the acceleration-deceleration motion of the cranial contents after sudden impact, brain injury and cervical spine fractures should be suspected until ruled out. A neurosurgical consultation is recommended to evaluate potential neurological injuries completely. Radiographic studies and computed tomographic scanning should be included in the sequence of assessment, especially if alterations in level of consciousness, extremity movement, and sensory

TABLE 22–4. CONTENTS OF ANTEROPOSTERIOR NASAL PACKING TRAY

1. Gauze packing with strings.
2. 30-cc balloon Foley catheter.
3. Oxytetracycline (Terramycin)-coated gauze.
4. Long-smooth pick-ups (forceps).
5. Suture material (silk).

level are displayed by the patient. Nursing responsibilities include frequent neurological monitoring during the evaluation process and immediately reporting any changes to the physician.

An intracranial injury and CSF leak should be suspected in any patient with severe nasal, nasoethmoidal, or Le Fort III fractures. Blood in the nares often increases the difficulty of early recognition of CSF leaks in the recently injured patient. Placing a nasal-drip pad bandage, such as a gauze pad, under the nares and testing the drainage for glucose is a nursing measure that assists in monitoring nasal drainage for the presence of CSF. Accidental perforation of the cranium by tubes and catheters through the cribriform plate is a neurosurgical emergency. This can be prevented by avoiding any insertion of tubes or catheters into the nasal cavity. Oral intubation or insertion of an orogastric tube can be considered as an alternative.

Potential for Anxiety

Nursing priorities during the resuscitative phase must include psychological support. Sudden, disfiguring facial trauma may be perceived as a catastrophe by the professional staff. The nurse must be aware of her own observable actions and behavior, personal feelings, attitudes, and verbal responses while caring for the patient in a busy resuscitative area or emergency department. Facial expressions, eye contact, voice patterns, and behavioral mannerisms should be direct and nonjudgmental. The patient was not prepared for the sudden certainty of facial disfigurement, and actions that convey pity or the inability to look at the wounds are quickly recognized by the patient. Offering clear, concise explanations to the fully awake patient regarding procedures performed during the assessment phase assists in decreasing anxiety caused by lack of information and unfamiliar surroundings. Reinforcing physician explanations regarding diagnosis and treatment of facial injuries is another nursing measure that can be performed during the resuscitative phase to help decrease patient anxiety.

OPERATIVE MANAGEMENT CYCLE

Treatment of Soft Tissue Injuries

In the presence of soft tissue injuries, cleansing and debridement of the wound are priorities during the resuscitative phase when life-threatening problems have been resolved. Small wounds can be irrigated and cleansed with a normal saline lavage and approximated with sutures under a local anesthetic agent. Lidocaine hydrochloride is the most commonly used agent. When epinephrine 1:100,000 is needed in conjunction with the local anesthetic to attain hemostasis, the skin surrounding the wound should be closely observed by the nurse after closure. The vasoconstrictive effects of the epinephrine may cause apparent tissue ischemia and further compromise the soft tissue injury and its healing.

Larger, complex soft tissue injuries, such as degloving or massive penetrating injuries from gunshot wounds, require vigorous irrigation and cleansing before surgical reconstruction can be completed. The best method for irrigation is the utilization of a direct, hydraulic force.[6] Administration of this force is best accomplished with a 30-ml syringe and a 22-gauge plastic needle. The irrigation solution, commonly normal saline solution, is directed into and around the wound to remove foreign debris, such as road dirt, glass particles, and clotted blood. If dirt is not removed within or around the wound, a permanent road tattoo or "traumatic tattoo" results.[21] Direct scrubbing should be limited to dirty wounds not adequately cleansed with irrigation and should not be practiced in the treatment of large degloving injuries. Excess mechanical force may further damage otherwise healthy tissue.

Tissue avulsions of the face and scalp are other types of complex soft tissue injury. Management during the resuscitative or operative phase includes cleansing the avulsed portion with normal saline solution and maintaining external moisture with sterile saline-soaked sponges.

Nasal Fracture Treatment

Treatment may consist of closed reduction by digital pressure and forceps manipulation of the septum under local anesthesia with intravenous sedation given by an anesthetist. Nasal packing allows digital pressure and control of septal hematoma formation. After the reduction and alignment of nasal fragments, external metal splints immobilize the corrected fragments of the nasal septum. The splints usually are padded to prevent pressure necrosis and afford protection to the nose postoperatively (Fig. 22–23). Fibrous bone forms around the aligned segments, and the external splint can be removed within 2 weeks.

Zygoma and Orbital Floor Fracture Repair

Surgical intervention of zygomatic and orbital floor fractures is indicated when there is evidence of inferior rectus muscle entrapment, enophthalmos, or depression or flattening of the zygoma. Surgical reduction of the fracture and internal fixation by wire and bone grafting are performed. The use of miniplates and screws, which can be made of vitallium, titanium, or stainless steel, results in stable fixation

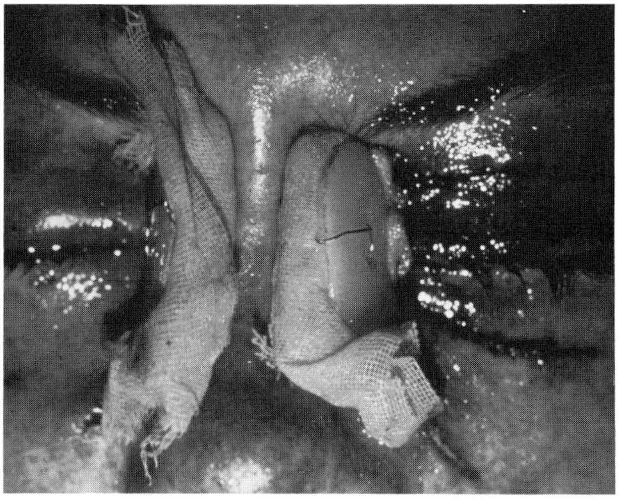

Figure 22–23. Padded metal splints immobilize corrected fragments of nasal septum and prevent pressure necrosis.

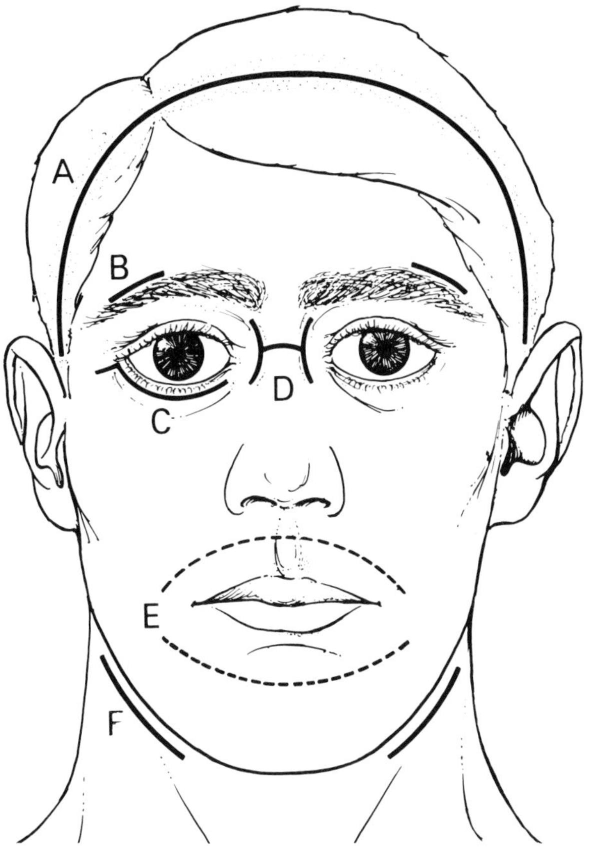

Figure 22–24. Incisions used for the exposure of the facial skeleton. *A*, Coronal incision for the exposure of the upper one third of the face, orbits, nasoethmoid complex, and zygomas. *B*, Brow incisions for exposure of the frontozygomatic area. *C*, Subciliary incision for exposure of the orbital floor. *D*, Transradix incision for exposure of the nasoethmoid complex. *E*, Upper and lower buccal sulcus incisions for exposure of the maxilla and mandible. *F*, Submandibular incisions for exposure of the mandible. (From Marschall MA, et al: Craniofacial approach for the reconstruction of severe facial injuries. J Oral Maxillofac Surg 46:306, 1988.)

of the zygoma and greater chance of regeneration of the infraorbital nerve.[22] Operative incisions to expose the fractures include approaches near the lateral browline and below the lower lid along natural creases and fold lines (Fig. 22–24).

Mandibular Fracture Repair

For traditional repair, intermaxillary fixation with the application of arch bars is performed to immobilize the mandible (Fig. 22–25). This procedure involves the application of hooked metal arch bars to the maxillary and mandibular dentition and wiring or rubber-banding the bars to attain dental occlusion. Intermaxillary fixation is required for 6 to 8 weeks, but serial monitoring through dental impressions may be needed to assess proper healing and alignment of dentition.

With the introduction of plates and screws, open reduction and internal fixation (ORIF) of the mandible has been revolutionized. In combination with wires and bone grafts, mandibular fracture repair usually is performed through the intraoral approach. After reduction and stabilization with compression plates and screws, intermaxillary fixation is shortened or avoided altogether.[23, 24] External fixation may be necessary when fractures are severely comminuted, when open wounds are present with massive soft tissue loss, and when internal fixation is difficult. Highly contaminated wounds, such as those resulting from a gunshot blast to the mandible, may require an external fixator.

The Joe Hall Morris device (Fig. 22–26) is used as an intraoperative biphasic method of external fixation.[25] A metal apparatus is attached externally with two or more transcutaneous intraosseous screws on each side of a stable portion of the fracture. After bony realignment is completed, the metal bar is removed and an acrylic one is placed over the screws, completing the second phase of the fixation. Variations of materials are many, but the principle remains constant. This apparatus usually is left in place for 6 to 12 weeks.

Le Fort Fracture Management

Transverse maxillary fractures (Le Fort I) are managed through intermaxillary fixation, with either elastic bands or

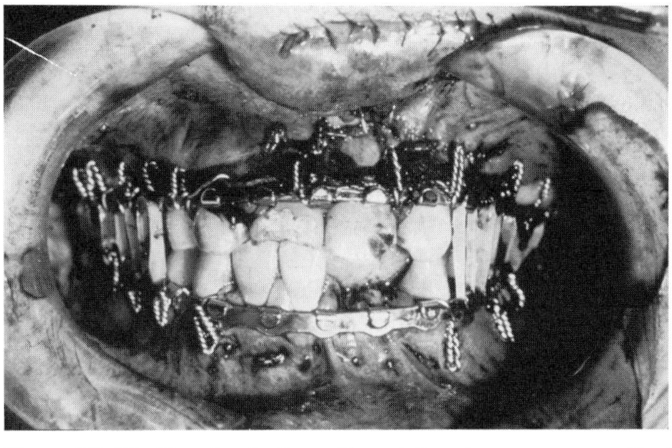

Figure 22–25. Closed reduction with arch bars is a common method of intermaxillary fixation.

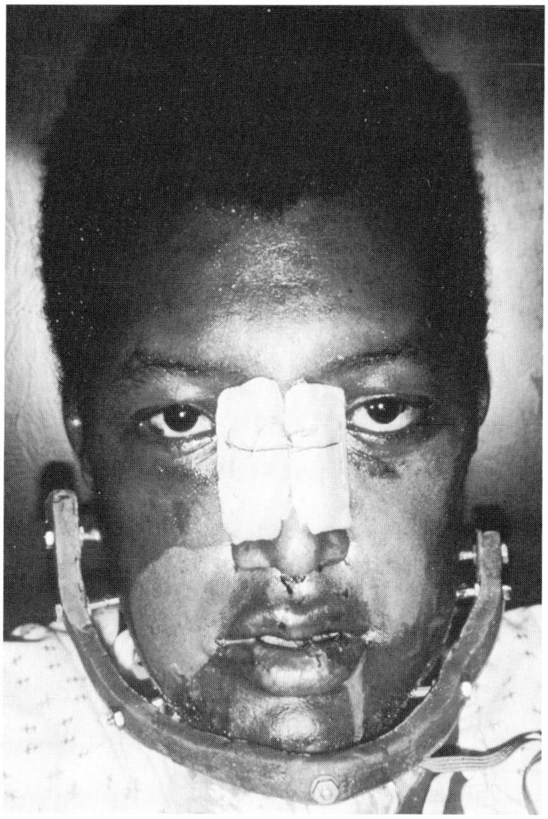

Figure 22–26. Joe Hall Morris device. This is an example of an external fixator device, which usually is placed on the mandible.

metal wires, which are attached to metal arch bars around the patient's dentition. This method aligns the maxilla in its proper relation to the mandible to attain dental occlusion. Intermaxillary fixation may be required until healing has occurred, and release is reassessed in 6 to 8 weeks.

Pyramidal maxillary fractures (Le Fort II) are treated by ORIF with wires, plates, and screws and, if large defects are present, with bone grafts (Figs. 22–27 through 22–29). Incisions are made through the intraoral approach as well as along skin fold lines of the lower eyelids. Closed reduction of the nasal fracture could also be performed and external padded splints applied.

Craniofacial dysjunction (Le Fort III) is the most complex of all facial fractures. Immediate open reduction and bone grafting are recommended to ensure optimal aesthetic results.[26] A coronal approach is used to allow direct visualization of the entire frontal bone, periorbital areas, and nasal region. Neurosurgical repair of dural interruptions may also be accomplished at this time. Fractures are directly exposed, reduced, and internally fixated with plates and screws, wiring, and bone grafting. Each bony fragment may be wired to adjacent fragments to provide structural stability (Figs. 22–27 through 22–29). Severely damaged or absent bone is replaced by primary bone grafting. Common donor graft sites include the rib, skull, and iliac crest. Rib bone grafts are preferred because of their membranous composition. The rib graft can be split and bent to match the exact contour of the cranial defect.[1]

If stability of complex Le Fort fractures is not adequate after internal reduction and fixation, an external fixator device may be required to provide additional stability. External fixation may also be indicated when massive soft tissue injury is present, particularly in the presence of gross contamination, in which case internal wiring cannot be used. The Joe Hall Morris and assorted head frames are used to stabilize the facial bones that have been interrupted.

The internal fixator materials may cause pain or inflammation once underlying bone healing has occurred; this necessitates further operative intervention to remove plates, screws, and wires. Future developments in the field of biocompatible and biodegradable material have been cited in the literature for both orthopedic and maxillofacial repair. Biocompatible agents include metal, alloy, ceramics, and synthetic polymers.[27] Biodegradable materials primarily consist of bone collagen. A preliminary study using resorbable poly (L-lactide) plates and screws for zygomatic repair demonstrated good postoperative results.[28]

Reconstruction of Complex Soft Tissue Injuries

Operative management of complex injuries, such as those resulting in massive tissue loss of the face, is accomplished electively once the area is cleaned and free of infection. The wound may have had serial daily irrigations and debridements before reconstructive techniques could be accomplished. Principles of reconstruction are threefold and are listed here in order of importance: (1) wound closure, (2) restoration of the most aesthetically acceptable form and contour of features, and (3) restoration of function of the missing tissue.[29] Reconstruction may be accomplished through direct primary closure by suturing and tissue approximation. Other methods include delayed primary closure after serial cleansing and

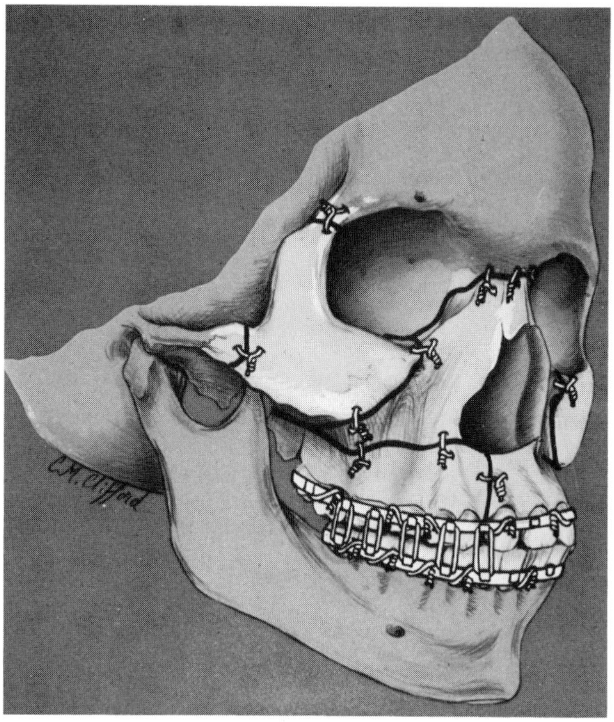

Figure 22–27. Internal wiring of facial fractures.

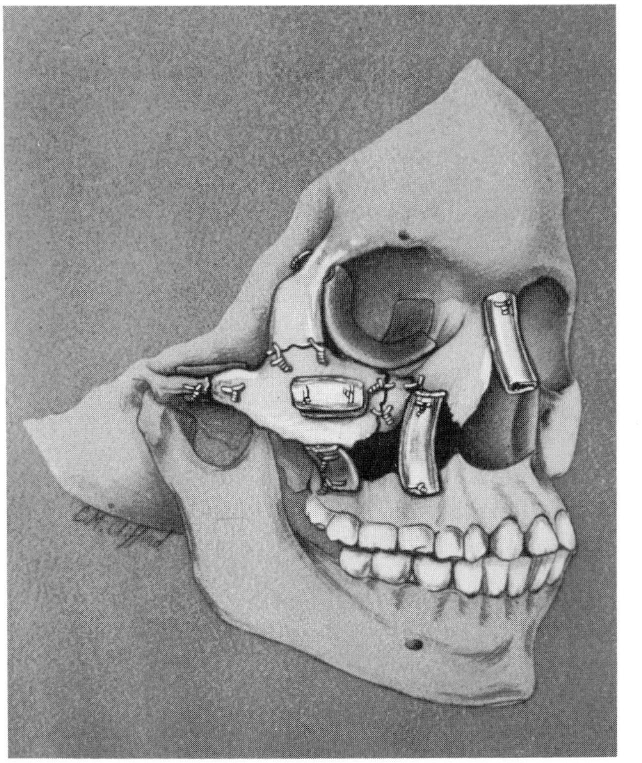

Figure 22–28. Bone grafting of facial fractures.

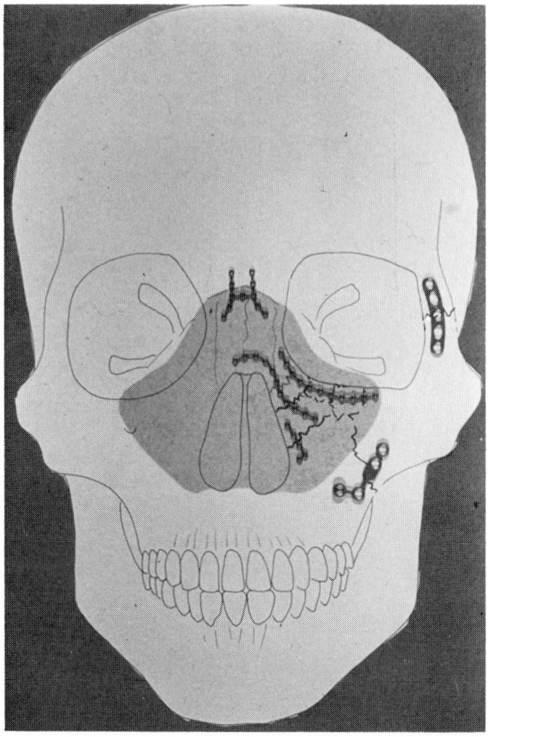

Figure 22–29. Internal fixation of facial fractures utilizing plates, screws and mesh. (From Manson P: Management of facial fractures. Perspect Plast Surg 2:1–41, 1988.)

irrigations, the use of skin grafts, local flaps, and free tissue transfer (distant flaps).

Skin Flaps

According to Kemble, a skin flap differs from a skin graft in that the skin flap retains an attachment and blood supply throughout the transfer from the donor site to the site where coverage is needed.[21] The skin flap consists of skin, its underlying superficial fascia, and perhaps muscle. The base of the skin flap that contains the vascular supply is referred to as a pedicle. Thus, after massive soft tissue loss, a skin flap can be used to cover the defect that was caused by the initial trauma.

The traumatized area can be labeled as the *primary defect.* A skin flap is then transferred to the primary defect, creating a *secondary defect* from the donor area. The secondary defect is then approximated by primary closure or covered with a free skin graft (skin grafts are described in Chapter 28). A *local flap* can be described as the transference of tissue close to or adjoining the primary defect. A *distant flap* involves moving tissue from another site.

Local Flaps to the Face

There are many categories of local flaps. The harvest site is chosen close to the defect or wound to match skin color, contour, and texture closely. Examples of local flaps include rotation, transposition, and Z-plasty. A rotation flap (Fig. 22–30) is described as the rotation of skin and underlying fascia over a defect as part of a circular incision. A defect on the chin can be covered by making a circular incision extending near the temporomandibular region to the defect and rotating the skin over the defect. A transposition flap (Fig. 22–31) is a rectangular skin flap that is moved sideways toward the defect. The secondary defect may then be approximated by primary closure.

Z-plasty is a common procedure performed to cover initial defects as well as to reconstruct scar and thermal contractures during follow-up. Transposition of two interdigitating triangular flaps[30] forms the Z. The overall effect is to lengthen the defect or scar and alter its direction to natural skin folds and lines (Fig. 22–32).

Distant Flaps to the Face

Distant flaps require one or more stages of surgery to allow enough time for revascularization of the distant recipient site. Common skin flaps to the face include the pectoralis major myocutaneous flap and the temporalis fascia flap. The use of a myocutaneous flap is based on the principle that the skin's blood supply is derived from vessels of the underlying muscle. Therefore, if the skin is raised with the muscle and

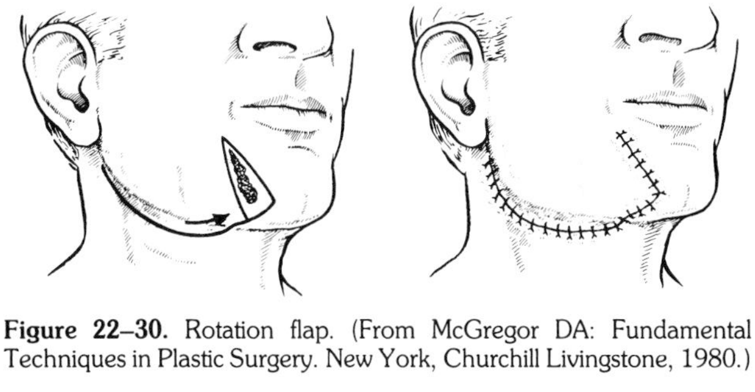

Figure 22–30. Rotation flap. (From McGregor DA: Fundamental Techniques in Plastic Surgery. New York, Churchill Livingstone, 1980.)

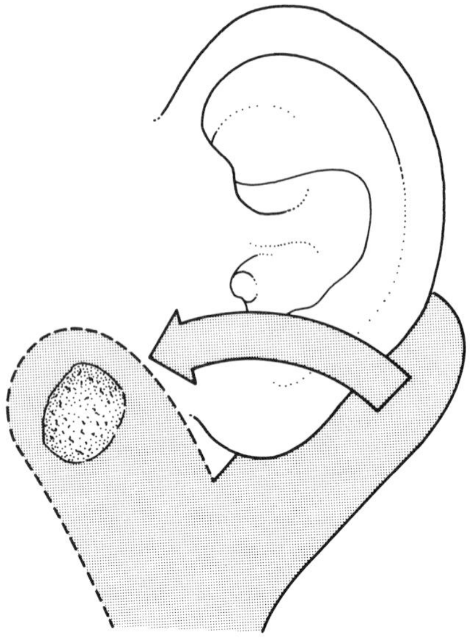

Figure 22–31. Transposition flap. (From Kemble JV, Lamb BE: Plastic Surgical and Burns Nursing. London, Baillière Tindall, 1984.)

vascular supply intact, the viability of the flap is greatly enhanced.[31]

The pectoralis major myocutaneous flap has a vascular supply delivered by the axillary artery and has several segments that can be used to cover face and neck defects (Fig. 22–33). Portions of the muscle may be split in line with muscle fibers to preserve neurovascular structures and motor function of the muscle.[32] Once vascularization has occurred over the primary defect placement area, which can take up to 3 weeks, the pedicle end may be released. Split-thickness skin grafts are applied over the pectoralis major site to cover the secondary defect.

The temporalis fascia muscle is supplied by the anterior and posterior temporal arteries, and this muscle can be used as a distant skin flap for deformities of the upper face (Fig. 22–34). The secondary defect that is left behind can be approximated with sutures, and the suture line can be concealed by the patient's hairline.

Nursing Communication with Family

Intraoperative nursing care directed toward the anesthetized patient is expanded to supportive care of the family or significant other. Facial reconstructive procedures, whether simple or complex, may take several hours of operative time. Identifying one spokesperson for the family and releasing brief updates to that same family member are important means of communication. Brief informative updates may include the estimated time remaining in the procedure as well as postoperative disposition. Specific information regarding the operative procedure should be released by the operating surgeon. If the family member or significant other asks specific questions during a brief update, the perioperative nurse may suggest that the questions be written down so that they can be discussed and answered during a postoperative conference with the surgeon.

Communication with Postoperative Nurse

Verbal communication with the postoperative care nurse is another important intraoperative nursing responsibility. Specific information to be conveyed includes the operative procedure, airway technique, range of vital signs, and location of intravenous lines and catheters. Dressings and drains should also be described. Direct communication with the anesthesiologist or anesthetist can be coordinated by the

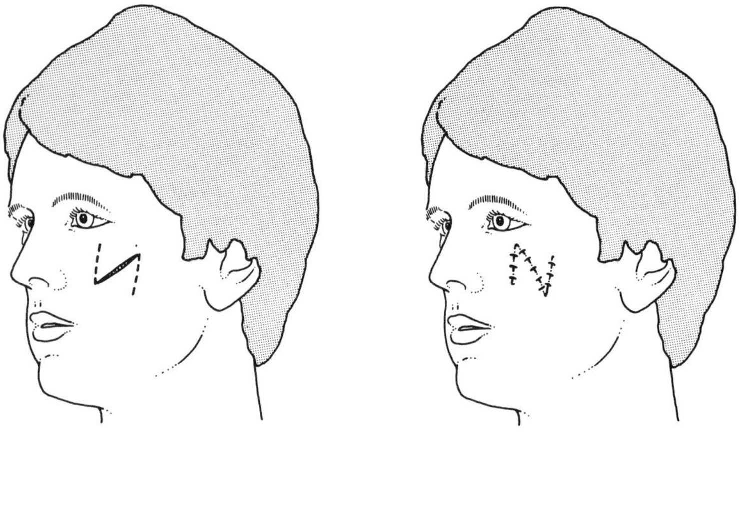

Figure 22–32. Z-plasty. (From Kemble JV, Lamb BE: Plastic Surgical and Burns Nursing. London, Baillière Tindall, 1984.)

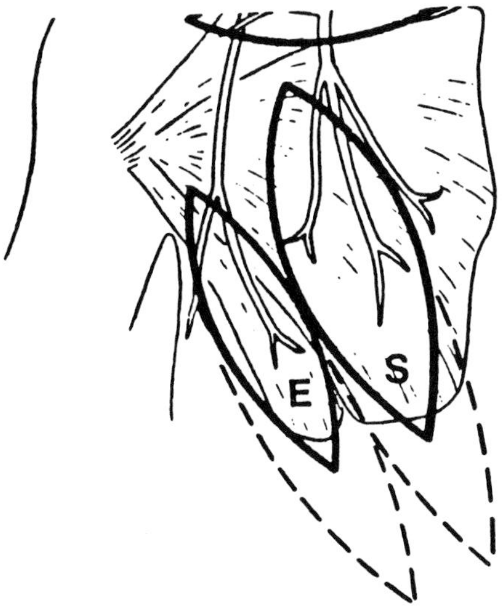

Figure 22–33. Segmental myocutaneous paddle placement on pectoralis muscle segments. Clavicular segment flap (C), sternocostal segment flap (S), and external segment flap (E) are marked. Dashed lines show optional paddle extensions by inclusion of upper abdominal skin and fascia. (From Tobin G: Pectoralis major segmental anatomy and segmentally split pectoralis major flaps. Plast Reconstr Surg 75:814–824, 1985.)

intraoperative nurse for the postoperative nurse to receive specific information regarding intraoperative course and postoperative plan for airway maintenance.

CRITICAL CARE CYCLE

Postoperative critical care nursing management after facial injury and repair is challenging and requires frequent nursing assessment for actual or potential problems related to airway and oxygenation, hydration, neurological status, and skin integrity. A critically ill patient requires rapid, precise nursing interventions that have been prioritized, since other injuries to body systems may have been sustained. Mechanical ventilation, cardiac monitoring, and hourly nursing assessment and treatments are essential components of care (Fig. 22–35).

Potential for Airway Obstruction

Airway management and assurance of adequate oxygenation are nursing priorities after maxillofacial trauma and reconstruction. Because of prolonged anesthesia time required for midface fracture repair or soft tissue reconstruction, postoperative endotracheal intubation or tracheostomy frequently is required during the critical care phase. Patient problems related to edema, ineffective airway clearance, and retained intraoral or pulmonary secretions need special interventions to prevent airway obstruction.

Edema near the trachea may be a result of prolonged intubation or local trauma from the facial injury. Mechanical ventilation and maintenance of an artificial airway are required until edema subsides. Positioning the patient to avoid tension on the artificial airway decreases external forces that

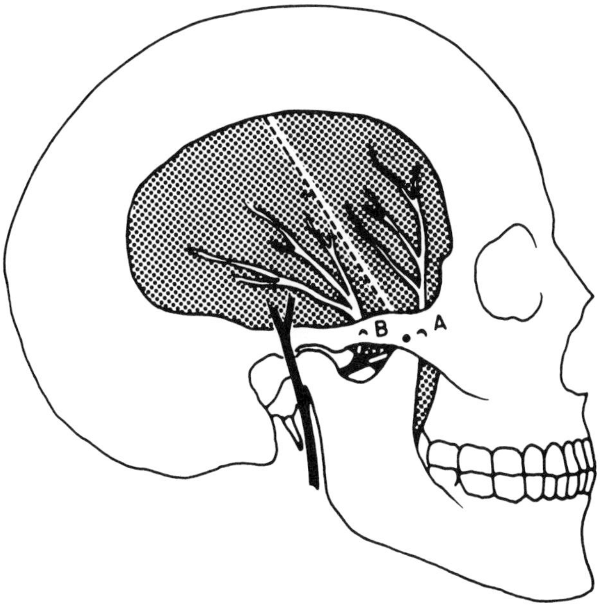

Figure 22–34. *A,* Temporalis muscle vascular supply, showing the anterior and posterior deep temporal arteries entering the muscle on its deep surface. *B,* Temporalis myo-osseous flap. Osteotomy of the zygoma and coronoid process facilitates maximal mobilization of the flap. When tunneled intraorally, the flap is suitable for mandibular reconstruction. (From Antonyshyn O, et al: The temporalis myo-osseus flap: An experimental study. Plast Reconstr Surg 77:406–415, 1986.)

may contribute to airway irritation and edema. Keeping the patient calm through verbal reassurances and mild sedatives aids in decreasing restlessness. Premature self-extubation by the patient with facial edema may be life-threatening, since reintubation may be difficult or even impossible in the presence of massive edema. Every effort must be made to prevent this from occurring. Hand restraints following hospital protocol, usually with a physician's order, or sedation may be required.

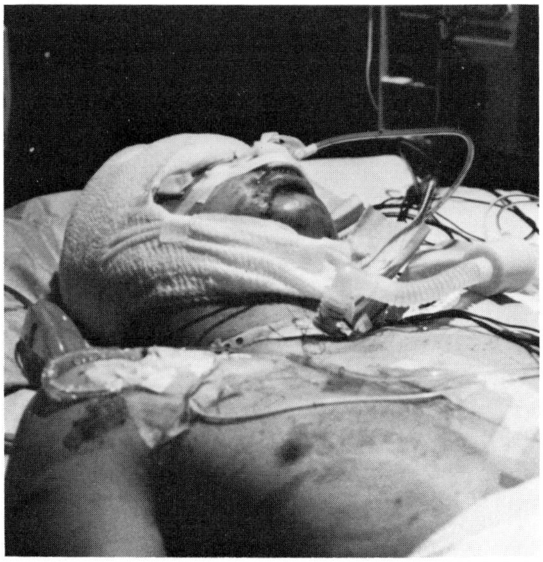

Figure 22–35. Critical care nursing and monitoring after maxillofacial repair is paramount to positive patient outcome.

The patient who is neurologically depressed after facial injury is unable to clear airway secretions effectively. The patient probably has a tracheostomy and requires frequent pulmonary hygiene to prevent airway obstruction. Tracheal lavage with 1 ml of preservative-free normal saline solution may stimulate the cough reflex, followed by tracheal suctioning to remove secretions. If the patient accumulates secretions that are not removed, airway obstruction from mucus plugs may occur.

Intraoral secretions are present after facial injury repair, especially after Le Fort fracture repair and intermaxillary fixation. Special monitoring of the balloon cuff on the endotracheal or tracheostomy tube must be performed to ensure adequate inflation and prevent aspiration of oral secretions into the lungs. Suctioning the oral cavity to remove the secretions must be done as often as necessary and at least every 2 hours for the first 24 hours to decrease the chance of aspiration. Positioning the head to a sidelying position and maintaining elevation of the head at a 30-degree angle or in a semi-Fowler's position may facilitate passive drainage of oral secretions. If intermaxillary fixation is present, means to release fixation is necessary at the bedside in the event of an airway emergency. Wire cutters may be used to release hooked wires around the arch bars.

Alterations in Hydration

Postoperatively in the critical care unit, it is most important to evaluate intraoperative fluid loss and replacement. Surgical intervention for the repair of facial injuries may last as long as 16 to 18 hours, and the patient needs careful hemodynamic monitoring until fluid balance has been stabilized. Replacement of salivary and gastric secretions must be considered part of any apparent deficit in fluid volume.

Alterations in Neurological Status

Neurological assessment, which includes examination of mental status and speech, cranial nerves, motor movement, sensory interpretation, and reflexes, can only be partially performed in the critical care unit after facial reconstruction. It is imperative that the nurse have a baseline report of the patient's neurological status to compare with the postoperative neurological status.

Mental status and speech assessment are hard to establish once the patient has been intubated or has a tracheostomy. Asking simple questions, such as those regarding the patient's name, date, and place, in which the patient can nod his head appropriately may be one strategy to elicit the mental status. Questions answered with head nodding by the patient should not be the only strategy used to determine mental status.

Cranial nerve assessment can be limited owing to facial edema, intubation, and inaccessibility of the pupils because of suturing of the eyelids postoperatively. Thus, motor movement, sensory interpretation, and reflexes are the major components that can be successfully assessed in the awake patient. In the cooperative patient who can appropriately acknowledge simple questions, light perception checks (i.e., flashlight directed over eye patch) are recommended every 2 to 4 hours after zygomatic and orbital repair for at least 24 hours. Asking the patient to move a specific hand or foot to a certain position are simple maneuvers that can assess motor functions, as can asking the patient to write a message on paper or to letter spell in the examiner's hand. For the heavily sedated or unconscious patient, intracranial monitoring and serial computed tomography may be indicated to assess neurological trends of intracerebral edema.

The nurse must monitor the nasal drainage closely in the patient who exhibits CSF rhinorrhea. A nasal-drip pad, usually a folded gauze pad, can be placed under the nose and taped in place. The drainage can be tested for glucose to distinguish CSF from nasal secretions that may be present. Any change in the consistency, color, or odor of the CSF must be reported promptly to the physician.

Alterations in Skin Integrity

Impairment of tissue healing secondary to altered skin integrity from operative incisions, intraoral lacerations, and external hardware apparatus is another nursing problem that needs to be addressed in the critical care phase. Operative incisions as well as facial abrasions should be cleansed at least three to four times daily (Fig. 22–36). Dressings should be moistened with normal saline solution before removal, especially if old blood has crusted near the incision or abrasion, to prevent local trauma. Using cotton-tipped applicators soaked in a 50 per cent solution of normal saline solution and hydrogen peroxide, old serous exudate and blood should be gently removed from any incision or abrasion. A thin layer of antibiotic ointment is then applied over the clean incision line with another cotton-tipped applicator. Special care should be taken when cleansing around eyelid incisional areas. Only a normal saline solution should be used for cleansing incisional lines and sutures, and an ophthalmic antibiotic ointment should be applied. Operative incisional lines may be left open to the air. If serous drainage persists, a gauze dressing may be gently applied.

Intraoral lacerations or incisions may also be present. The operating surgeon should give specific instructions on what type of oral care is required postoperatively. Initially, oral irrigations with a 50 per cent solution of normal saline and hydrogen peroxide may be ordered. A sterile suction catheter tip small enough to reach the sides of the mouth may be needed if intermaxillary fixation with arch bars is present. Depending on the patient's level of consciousness, positioning the head to the side may be required to prevent aspiration during oral lavage. Oral lavage should be performed at least four to six times a day until serosanguineous secretions subside (which could be a minimum of 2 to 3 days). Orthodontic wax may be applied over the metal arch bars to prevent irritation to healthy oral mucosa but should be removed daily by gently lifting the wax away from the teeth to allow thorough cleansing of the mouth. Brushing teeth with a pediatric soft-bristle toothbrush may be performed only with a physician's order; a commercial toothpaste may not be used until intraoral lacerations are healed.

If implant hardware cannot be used, external hardware, such as pins, should be cleansed routinely in the same manner as facial abrasions and operative incisions. Using a 50 per cent solution of normal saline and hydrogen peroxide, old drainage should be gently cleansed away from the pin insertion sites with a sterile cotton-tipped applicator. By physi-

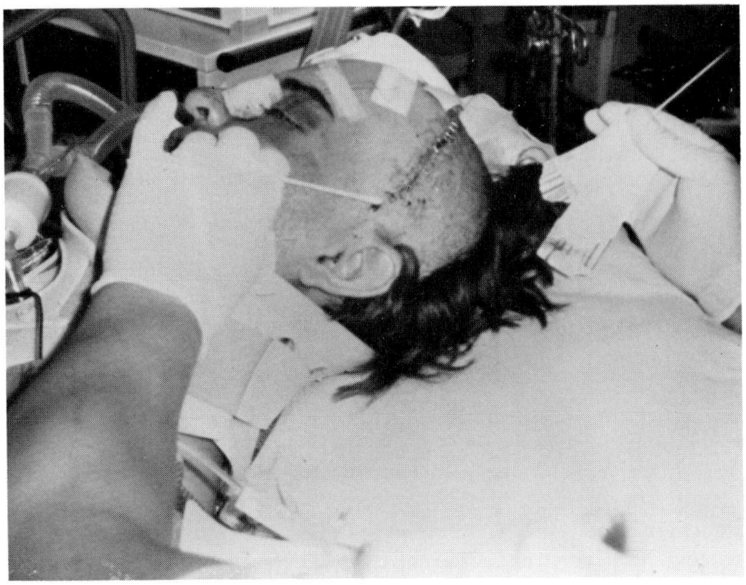

Figure 22–36. A nurse cleanses the coronal suture incision using aseptic technique.

cian's order, an antibiotic ointment should then be applied to the pin sites.

Monitoring of Skin Flaps

Close monitoring of a skin flap and prevention of infection are paramount to the survival and success of a facial skin flap. Nursing care after local flap procedures is designed to decrease postoperative edema. Maintaining the patient's head in good alignment and keeping it immobile as well as elevating the head of the bed to at least 35 to 45 degrees for usually up to 2 weeks postoperatively encourage venous return by gravity. Alignment can be accomplished by placing rolled towels along the side of the head, taking careful consideration not to put any pressure on the operative side.

Nursing care of distant flaps is directed toward preserving the flap's circulation at its new site. Many factors contribute to the cause of a skin flap's circulatory embarrassment, but nursing measures and interventions can diminish the chance of failure and necrosis. Tension, twisting, and eventual kinking of the skin flap's circulatory supply because of improper position can and must be avoided.[20] Tension and pressure directed onto a skin flap can occur in basically two ways: internally and externally. Internal pressure secondary to inflammation and edema can be expected from surgical manipulation of the tissue and lymphatic nodes.[33] Nursing measures that help decrease internal pressure include positioning the head of the bed postoperatively at 35 to 40 degrees for at least 48 hours and frequent checking and deflation of drainage tubes or bulbs that are around and underneath the skin flap and suture lines. If butterfly drains are used, a red-top Vacutainer blood tube is needed to apply some suction to the drainage tube. If the serous drainage has accumulated halfway in the tube, about 4 ml, the Vacutainer is changed. Otherwise, the blood tube should be changed at least every 2 hours. Stripping the plastic butterfly drainage tubing with two pinched fingers may help to dislodge clots.

External pressure that is applied to a skin flap may also embarrass circulation and, ultimately, alter skin integrity. Tracheostomy strings, endotracheal tape, oxygen tubing, electrocardiogram wires, blankets, and curious hands from the patient are examples of external forces that should be diverted away from the skin flap. Hand restraints or constant verbal reminders may be necessary nursing reinforcements until the patient is fully awake from anesthesia and oriented to the environment and his injuries.

Inspection of the skin flap postoperatively and daily after the immediate postoperative period includes assessment of color, capillary return time, temperature, and the presence of a pulse. If a dressing is applied over the skin flap, a portion must be visualized to assess the operative area. Evidence of early flap compromise may include discoloration and inadequate reperfusion after the application of direct pressure on the flap. Sloughing usually is a late sign of flap necrosis. A portable temperature meter may be applied to the skin flap to alert the nurse of acute temperature changes between the body and the skin flap. An audible Doppler ultrasound flowmeter may be needed to assess the presence of an arterial pulse within the flap. Any change in these parameters must be reported to the plastic surgeon immediately, or the flap's viability may be compromised beyond repair.

INTERMEDIATE/REHABILITATIVE CYCLE

Rehabilitative nursing care during this cycle encompasses both physical and psychological support. The potential problems that develop during this cycle are inclusive of those problems previously described. Additional problems that are central to this part of trauma recovery include alterations in comfort, self-concept, nutrition, respiratory patterns, social encounters, self-care activities, sleep and rest, and individual needs for education.

Alteration in Comfort

Patients with maxillofacial injuries may experience postoperative pain and general discomfort the first few days after surgery. If dressing changes or wound irrigations and repacking are required, sedation may be needed to help the patient tolerate these often painful procedures (see Chapter 15).

Once intermaxillary fixation has been discontinued, the patient may experience pain or stiffness when opening the mouth. Jaw exercises and a mild analgesic, such as acetaminophen, may be recommended. A puréed or soft diet usually is suggested until mastication becomes comfortable for the patient.

Alteration in Self-Concept

Body image, self-esteem, role performance, and personal identity are components of self-concept.[34] Any type of facial trauma threatens the concept of self, and each patient's reaction to sudden disfigurement is different, whether the injury involves a small laceration or massive tissue loss. Human interaction usually occurs face to face, and if the appearance of the face is changed, the interaction process also changes.

Maintaining eye contact, avoidance of a hurried overtone, and empathetic communication are all nursing strategies that can be used in this situation. Involving at least one significant other in daily care activities during this phase can also prove beneficial. Reinforcing positive qualities, such as the patient's personality or role as a friend or family member, also enhances his self-worth. Resocialization after facial trauma takes time, and the nurse monitors the patient's interactions with others and responds in a manner appropriate to the patient's responses.

Alteration in Nutrition

During the postoperative phase, enhancement of fracture and soft tissue healing is an important priority for nursing intervention. Adequate hydration and nutrition enhance overall healing and well-being.

In the acute and, possibly, intermediate phases of hospitalization, the patient may require nutritional support by liquid tube feedings. Wound healing requires high-protein, high-carbohydrate intake to prevent negative nitrogen balance, hypoalbuminemia, and weight loss.[34] If the patient has intermaxillary fixation or is restricted in mastication because of a free-tissue transfer, an orogastric or nasogastric tube may be indicated to deliver a commercially prepared liquid feeding. A registered dietitian may be consulted to individualize caloric intake based on calculated needs. Nursing assessment for the presence of bowel sounds as well as monitoring for signs or complaints of nausea or diarrhea are imperative. If nausea and vomiting develop while the patient has intermaxillary fixation, a suction apparatus must be close at hand to remove possible vomitus. If gastric contents cannot be removed by positioning the head to the side and downward while suctioning the oral cavity, wire cutters should be immediately accessible to release the intermaxillary fixation to prevent pulmonary aspiration and eventual respiratory distress. The physician must be notified immediately if this situation develops, and the patient should not be left alone.

Once tube feedings have been discontinued, clear liquids can be introduced with advancement to full and puréed liquids and foods as tolerated by the patient. A dietary consultation can assist the patient in finding attractive and creative ways to enhance caloric intake. Milk shakes fortified with ice cream, cream, or eggs provide calories, protein, and fat-soluble vitamins. Food fibers from blended food that can become trapped between metal arch bars and dentition can be removed by straining the food product through a metal food strainer. Chopping solid food, such as meats, into small portions and liquefying them in a blender with broth, water, or milk is another method of thinning food fibers. Table 22–5 lists cooking recipes for the patient with intermaxillary fixation.

Alterations in Respiratory Patterns

A common posttraumatic complication, alterations in respiratory patterns after facial injuries usually are related to atelectasis after pectoralis major skin flap utilization or adaptation of a tracheostomy once the patient is removed from mechanical ventilatory support. After any type of surgical procedure, deep-breathing and coughing exercises are important. Postoperative splinting on the side of the pectoralis flap may lead to atelectasis secondary to decreased tidal volume and expansion. Pain control and deep breathing

TABLE 22–5. SOLVING THE FOOD PROBLEM

Breakfast Drinks
(Served with juice and coffee, tea or cocoa)

Blended eggnog made with 16 oz milk, 2 eggs, 1 teaspoon vanilla extract, and a scoop of vanilla ice cream to disguise the egg taste for fussy eaters.
Cooked Cream of Wheat thinned and blended with added milk or cream, butter, brown sugar, and 1 tablespoon wheat germ.
Banana shake made with one or two medium bananas, 16 oz milk, 1 teaspoon vanilla extract and a scoop of vanilla ice cream.

Main Lunch Drinks (Fast and simple)	Desserts or Snacks
Canned tomato, chicken, or mushroom soup (creamed and blended)	Jell-O shake
Homemade vegetable soup	Banana shake
Ratatouille	Fruit and milk shakes (peach, pineapple, pear, apple)
Chicken or beef bouillon	Grape juice
Carrot soup	Orange-pineapple juice
Fish chowder	Lemonade
	Cake and milkshake
	Ice cream frappes
	Puddings and sherbet

Hearty Main Dishes
(All are blended and strained)

Chili con carne thinned with tomato juice.
Grilled hamburger or frankfurter with baked beans thinned with V-8 juice.
Spaghetti and meatballs thinned with milk or tomato juice.
Roast turkey or baked chicken with stuffing, green vegetables, and potato thinned with bouillon.
Chop suey with beef or pork thinned with bouillon.
Baked lasagna thinned with milk or tomato juice.
Pot roast and vegetables thinned with bouillon.
Meat loaf and vegetables thinned with V-8 juice.

 Modified from Boucher M: Broken jaw guide and cookbook. AJN May:833–834, 1977.

increase in importance, especially if frequent operative procedures are planned over a short time.

The patient with a long-term tracheostomy requires special teaching while in the hospital setting. Those patients with temporary tracheostomies also need to be instructed in essential safety measures. Safety measures are increasingly important after the tracheostomy is plugged and the client may be allowed to eat and drink by mouth. Reinforcement of instructions to eat and drink slowly, to effectively chew food particles, to use fluids to moisten food, and to clear the throat should be reviewed initially with the client. The patient must know a plan of action if he experiences distress. Within the hospital, the patient must know to press the emergency button and to attract attention to his difficulty immediately. A family member or significant other should know how to perform the antichoking maneuver, especially if the client goes home with the tracheostomy tube in place.

Potential for Social Isolation

The patient may want to isolate himself from social encounters because of the facial injury. Sudden hospitalization and separation from family and friends may also increase the sense of isolation. Offering the patient familiar and secure encounters, such as a visit from a favorite family member or friend, may decrease the patient's isolation. The patient should not be forced into social situations, such as visits from friends, unless he requests such a visit. A familiar person may help to decrease anxiety and apprehension with socialization, but a visit from such a person could also have the opposite effect.

Resocialization into the community should be addressed during the rehabilitation phase. Encouraging the patient to verbalize fears regarding unpleasant comments that may be directed to him by others can be helpful. Role playing a visit to a shopping mall may help to elicit such fears. Offering alternatives to face-to-face encounters with friends and relatives allows the patient to gradually resocialize. Examples include letter writing and telephone conversations with people with whom the patient wants to communicate.

Self-Care Activities

If the patient is ambulatory and capable of self-care activities, safety and wound management should be reviewed with the patient and family. The potential for loss of balance because of the additional weight from a head frame or external fixator must be addressed. Assistance with ambulation or a walker is provided until the patient has adapted to the additional weight and altered sense of balance.

Wound management techniques can also be reviewed in small teaching demonstrations and sessions. The patient must be instructed to perform frequent handwashing, to keep hair clean and styled away from operative incisions, and to avoid air pollutants (such as cigarette smoke and dust). Instruction and demonstration on how to cleanse suture lines and pin sites may be performed in front of a mirror, and the patient's ability to perform suture line care can be evaluated and reinforced as needed. During a teaching session, the signs and symptoms of infection are reviewed. The patient should be able to state at least two symptoms, such as pain and tenderness near the operative site or local erythema with possible temperature elevation. Direct hand contact with suture lines and pin sites must be avoided. Adequate supplies and resources must be arranged for the patient.

Intraoral irrigations and rinses after meals are part of an important regimen during hospitalization, and the continuance of oral hygiene must be stressed as part of the discharge instructions. The physician informs the patient when the use of toothpaste can be started. A small, soft-bristle toothbrush can be used with the oral rinses or a water-jet appliance can be purchased to remove retained food residues in hard to reach areas of the mouth. Orthodontic wax that is used to protect the intraoral mucosa must be changed daily to ensure adequate cleansing of underlying dentition.

The patient should be instructed to avoid direct exposure of incisional lines or skin graft donor sites to sunlight and ultraviolet rays. If sunlight exposure is anticipated, the patient should wear a strong sunscreen over and around the healed facial scar or graft site. Incisional lines will appear red and elevated for about 6 months after repair. Exposure to sunlight will cause that area to become a deeper color.

Information and explanations given to the patient and family should be concise and comprehensible. Conferences with the plastic surgeon should be scheduled regularly so that the patient can understand the choice and rationale for various therapies and procedures.

REINTEGRATION INTO THE COMMUNITY

Patient Education

Patients with maxillofacial trauma or soft tissue reconstruction may require serial operative procedures. Return to the general community may occur before all elective surgery can be performed. It is important to note that a traumatic injury may not be corrected completely to the patient's preinjury appearance. The nurse and the plastic surgeon must reinforce the expected outcomes of reconstruction. Offering false reassurances or reinforcing unrealistic hopes for a new facial appearance is discouraged. Offering clear and frank explanations regarding future surgical procedures and revisions gives the patient a realistic point of reference.

Psychological adjustment and adaptation toward a new facial image may take several weeks to months and the patient should be given this information before returning to the home environment. Frequent reactions encountered outside the hospital setting include altered mood patterns, depression, and, possibly, nightmares in which the patient relives the accident. Follow-up psychiatric consultation or group therapy may be an option that the patient may choose after discharge from the hospital.

In the hospital setting, the patient is somewhat protected from public reactions regarding facial disfigurement. It is imperative that the primary nurse establish a therapeutic rapport with the patient and family to prepare for possible negative reactions once the patient returns to the community. Future judgments regarding employment and social relationships related to attractiveness and disfigurement should be discussed. Studies have proved that physical attractiveness does influence peer acceptance, employability, and motivation to continue rehabilitation.[35]

Other considerations for patient education after skin flaps to the face include certain restrictions. Modification of certain activities should be carefully explained. Avoiding strenuous activities, such as running and weight lifting, and hard foods are considerations to decrease strain on a new flap. Restricting smoking and alcohol intake decreases any vasoconstrictive compromise to the circulation of the flap.[36] All instructions should be reinforced in writing for reference once the patient is home.

Home Health Follow-Up

Home health care may be needed if the facial reconstruction is extensive and the client has a tracheostomy. A visiting nurse may be needed for the first few weeks to reinforce wound care and tracheostomy care and to advise the patient on safety problems in the home.

Cosmetics

A patient may be interested in using makeup to conceal prominent facial scars. The plastic surgeon should be consulted on when various types of makeup can be used during scar healing and maturation. Consultation with a cosmetologist who has experience in extensive scar coverage and concealment is an option that can be presented to the patient.

Techniques to achieve symmetry of color and contour between the scarred areas and natural pigmentation can be practiced by the patient in the home. Through the use of color and outline, reduction of the prominent scar or defect can be accomplished. A yellow or white concealment base over scar tissue can minimize the appearance of a purple or hyperpigmentated defect, followed by a neutral shade base to provide a natural skin color appearance.[37] A cosmetic pencil may add depth and contour around eyebrows and eyelids. Lipstick and rouge can be used to highlight features as needed.

COMPLICATIONS AFTER FACIAL INJURIES

Complications after repair of facial injuries may occur during any phase. Most complications are the result of infectious processes. Cellulitis with subsequent necrotizing fasciitis, meningitis, brain abscesses, and sinusitis may occur, but the incidence of these is extremely low. Bone grafts may also become infected; this, too, is rare and seems to be associated with early grafting. Osteomyelitis may occur but is rare because of the increased vascularity of facial tissue.[38, 39] Nursing therapeutics, specifically proper patient education and reviewing signs and symptoms of infection, may decrease the length of hospital stay and the severity of presenting complications. Patient compliance regarding wound care, reporting incidence of fever or abnormal drainage from incisional lines, and overall follow-up care are considerations that require monitoring.

SUMMARY

We hope nurses are challenged by the previous material to understand the many patient responses after maxillofacial trauma. Reactions and adjustments to sudden hospitalization, disfigurement, and disruption of a normal life-style are varied, depending on the injury and the response of the person experiencing the trauma. Improved facial reconstructive techniques ease the patient toward rehabilitation and reintegration into the community. However, nursing is critically important in assisting the patient in recovering from and adapting to a physically and emotionally serious injury.

The need for continued research in the area of facial trauma is clearly evident. Safety restraint laws and changes in automobile structures have drastically reduced the incidence of facial injury, but further data on the effectiveness of restraint devices such as air bags need to be collected. Further changes in motor vehicle construction and restraining devices may result in changes in the types of maxillofacial trauma experienced by both the driver and the passenger. Clearly, numerous epidemiological studies are needed to determine such changes in injury severity patterns. Much is also unknown about the long-term effects of injuries to the face. Nursing therapeutics designed to prevent infection and promote wound healing must be further evaluated for their efficacy and cosmetic results.

There is much to be learned and studied about maxillofacial injury. It is already known, however, that nursing therapeutics that emphasize meticulous wound care, continuous assessment for possible complications, and strong emotional support are effective in promoting healing and assisting the patient in adjusting to these potentially disfiguring injuries.

REFERENCES

1. Gruss J: Fronto-naso-orbital trauma. Clin Plast Surg 9:577–589, 1982.
2. Cornell University Automotive Crash Injury Research: The Injury Producing Accident: A Primer of Facts and Figures. Ithaca, N.Y., Cornell University Press, 1961.
3. Schultz RC: Facial Injuries. Chicago, Year Book Medical Publishers, 1977, pp 12–40.
4. Cook HE, Rowe M: A retrospective study of 356 midfacial fractures occurring in 225 patients. J Oral Maxillofac Surg 48:574–578, 1990.
5. Nahum AM: The biomechanics of maxillofacial trauma. Clin Plast Surg 2:59, 1975.
6. Cowley RA, Dunhum CM: Shock Trauma/Critical Care. Baltimore, University Park Press, 1982.
7. Dodson TB, Kaban LB: California Mandatory Seat Belt Law: The effect of recent legislation on motor vehicle accident related maxillofacial injuries. J Oral Maxillofac Surg 46:875–880, 1988.
8. Afzeluis LE, Rosen C: Influence of seat belt upon maxillofacial fractures. J Otorhinolaryngol Relat Spec 42:277–287, 1980.
9. Trinca GW, Dooley BJ: The effects of seat belt legislation on road traffic accidents. Aust NZ J Surg 47:150–155, 1977.
10. Ellis DA, Wallace IR: Major facial trauma: The effect of legislation. J Otolaryngol 10:4, 1981.
11. Reath DB, Kirby J, Lynch M, Maull KI: Patterns of maxillofacial injuries in restrained and unrestrained motor vehicle crash victims. J Trauma 29:806–810, 1989.
12. Schultz RC: Facial Injuries. 3rd ed. Chicago, Year Book Medical Publishers, 1988, pp 22–23.

13. Stricker M, et al: Craniofacial Malformations. New York, Churchill Livingstone, 1990, pp 557–570.
14. Luckman J, Sorensen KC: Medical Surgical Nursing. Philadelphia, WB Saunders Co, 1974, pp 829–831.
15. Manson P: Management of facial fractures. Perspect Plast Surg 2:1–41, 1988.
16. Haug RH, Prather J, Indresano T: An epidemiologic survey of facial fractures and concomitant injuries. J Oral Maxillofac Surg 48:926–932, 1990.
17. Manson P: Head and neck injuries. In Cowley RA, Dunham CM (eds): Shock Trauma/Critical Care. Baltimore, University Park Press, 1982, pp 73–98.
18. Tessler P: Experimental study of fractures of the upper jaw (translation from LeFort R: Etude experimentelle sur les fractures de la machoir superieure. Rev Chir 23:479, 1901). In McDowell F (ed): The Source Book of Plastic and Reconstructive Surgery. Baltimore, Williams & Wilkins, 1977, pp 360–377.
19. Bernhard WN, et al: Intracuff pressures in endotracheal and tracheostomy tubes (related cuff physical characteristics). Chest 87:720–725, 1985.
20. Manson P, Hoopes JE, Su CT: Structural pillars of the facial skeleton: An approach to the management of Le Fort fractures. Plast Reconstr Surg 66:54, 1980.
21. Kemble JV, Lamb BE: Plastic Surgical and Burns Nursing. London, Bailliere Tindall, 1984.
22. DeMan K, Bax WA: The influence of the mode of treatment of zygomatic bone fractures on the healing process of the infraorbital nerve. Br J Oral Maxillofac Surg 26:419–425, 1988.
23. Oikarinen K, et al: Treatment of mandibular fractures: Need for rigid internal fixation. J Craniomaxillofac Surg 17:24–30, 1989.
24. Munro IR: The Luhr fixation system for the craniofacial skeleton. Clin Plast Surg 16:41–48, 1989.
25. Strauss HR, et al: External fixation of facial fractures. Am Surg 45:144–50, 1979.
26. Manson P, et al: Midface fractures: Advantages of of immediate extended open reduction and bone grafting. Plast Reconstr Surg 76:1–9, 1985.
27. Hollinger JO, Battistone GC: Biodegradable bone repair materials (synthetic polymers and ceramics). Clin Orthop 207:290–305, 1986.
28. Bos RR, et al: Resorbable Poly (L-lactide) plates and screws for the fixation of zygomatic fractures. J Oral Maxillofac Surg 45:751–753, 1987.
29. Mathes SJ, Nahai F: Clinical applications for muscle and musculocutaneous flaps. St. Louis, CV Mosby Co, 1982.
30. McGregor I: Fundamental Techniques of Plastic Surgery. New York, Churchhill Livingston, 1980.
31. American Academy of Facial Plastic and Reconstructive Surgery: Plastic and Reconstructive Surgery of the Face and Neck. Vol 2. St. Louis, CV Mosby Co, 1984.
32. Tobin GR: Pectoralis major segmental anatomy and segmentally splint pectoralis major flaps. Plast Reconstr Surg 75:814–824, 1985.
33. Stuart MS: Skin flaps and grafts after head and neck surgery. Am J Nurs 78:1368–1374, 1978.
34. Carpenito LJ: Nursing Diagnosis: Applications to Clinical Practice. Philadelphia, JB Lippincott Co, 1983.
35. Elks MA: Another look at facial disfigurement. J Rehabil Jan/Feb/Mar:36–40, 1990.
36. Salasche SJ, Grabsk WJ: Flaps for the Central Face. New York, Churchhill Livingstone, 1990, p 89.
37. Porter AL, Gay WD: Cosmetics as an aesthetic aid to the plastic surgery patient. Cleft Palate J 20:327–330, 1983.
38. Strauss MB: Chronic refractory osteomyelitis: Review and role of hyperbaric oxygen. HBO Review 1:231–256, 1980.
39. Bolton ME: Hyperbaric oxygen therapy. Am J Nurs 81:1199–1201, 1987.

23

OCULAR INJURIES

JAMES KARESH and BARBARA J. KEYES

INTRODUCTION

In 1989, the American Academy of Ophthalmology and the Eye Injury Registry of Alabama estimated that 1.3 million people suffer eye injuries each year in the United States.[1–4] Over 40,000 of these injuries are associated with some degree of visual loss. This may be an underestimation of the true incidence of ocular injury, since the National Institute for Occupational Safety and Health (NIOSH) reported in the *Morbidity and Mortality Weekly Report* that in 1982 work-related ocular injuries alone numbered 900,000 and that 150,000 of these were severe. More recent reports suggest that this is increasing.[2, 3]

The immediate goals in managing ocular injury are (1) protection of the intact portions of the visual system and avoidance of further damage to ocular structures, (2) accurate assessment of the extent of injury and referral of the patient or immediate repair of injured tissue, and (3) institution of therapeutic measures that first achieve optimal function and second, optimal cosmetic results.[4–10] Ocular tissues are frequently more extensively damaged by scar tissue formation than by the original injury. Thus immediate surgical repair following an accurate evaluation of the damage may be required rather than "waiting to see what will happen." Often, a conservative approach may result in permanent scarring, atrophy, loss of tissue, and/or permanent visual disability. Unlike other systems, the function of the eye depends on exact maintenance of anatomical relationships between eyelids, cornea, anterior chamber, lens, retina, extraocular muscles, and nerves. Permanent deficit in any of these components may result in altered visual function and, potentially, loss of the eye.[5–10]

To minimize the incidence of permanent visual loss associated with ocular trauma, it is important that those who come into contact with patients with such injuries understand ocular anatomy and function as well as examination techniques and treatment methods. With this in mind, this chapter is organized to explain the anatomy and physiology of the eye, the ocular examination, the management of a variety of traumatic injuries to the eye, the importance of nursing care, the prevention of ocular injuries, and referral sources for patients with visual loss following trauma.

Upon entrance to a trauma center, a patient will be cared for by a multitude of professionals. The trauma physician and primary nurse will ultimately be responsible for overseeing the patient's hospital course and treatments, while the ophthalmologist usually follows the patient on a consultant basis. Working in conjunction with the trauma physicians, they directly manage and treat ocular injuries. When only ocular injuries are present, the ophthalmologist will primarily direct the treatment of the injured patient.

While physicians diagnose and treat ocular injuries, nurses provide direct bedside care for these patients 24 hours a day. For this reason, they have the potential to have a great impact on the entire recovery process.

The nurse plays a large and important role during the immediate period after a visual handicap is sustained. An understanding of a patient's personal fears, concerns, and anxieties will enable the nurse to individualize the care given to each patient.

ANATOMY AND PHYSIOLOGY[5–10]

Embryologically, the ocular and periocular tissues are derived from surface ectoderm and neuroectoderm, as well as mesoderm. The optic nerve, retina, and portions of the iris and ciliary body are all neuroectodermal structures, as are all components of the central nervous system. Important features of these structures are their inability to regenerate when damaged and their need for a continuous supply of nutrients and oxygen. If that supply is compromised for even a period of minutes, cells will be irreversibly damaged. Injury to these neuroectodermal structures, particularly the optic nerve and retina, is most responsible for permanent visual loss in cases of trauma.

On the other hand, the conjunctiva, lens, corneal epithelium, and eyelid skin are all derived from surface ectoderm. The cells of these tissues are able to regenerate and to repair themselves following injury and can survive a relatively long time without a constant supply of blood and oxygen.

Mesodermal structures include the bony orbit, extraocular muscles, sclera, corneal stroma, ocular and periocular connective tissue, blood vessels, and internal eyelid structures. These tissues are also able to regenerate to varying extents following damage.

Intraocular Structures

The eye and its adnexal structures are as complex anatomically and functionally as they are embryologically. Light rays enter the eye through the cornea, pupil, and lens and fall on the diaphanous retina (Fig. 23–1), thereby activating the retinal photoreceptor elements and the rods and cones. Rods function best in dim lighting and are responsible for night vision. Cones (of which there are three types: red, blue, and green) function best in bright illumination and are responsible for detailed vision. Cones predominate in the macula, which is the site of best visual acuity. Through complex synaptic interconnections between a variety of cell types, the rods and cones transmit the light messages they receive to the 1 million retinal ganglion cells, whose axons

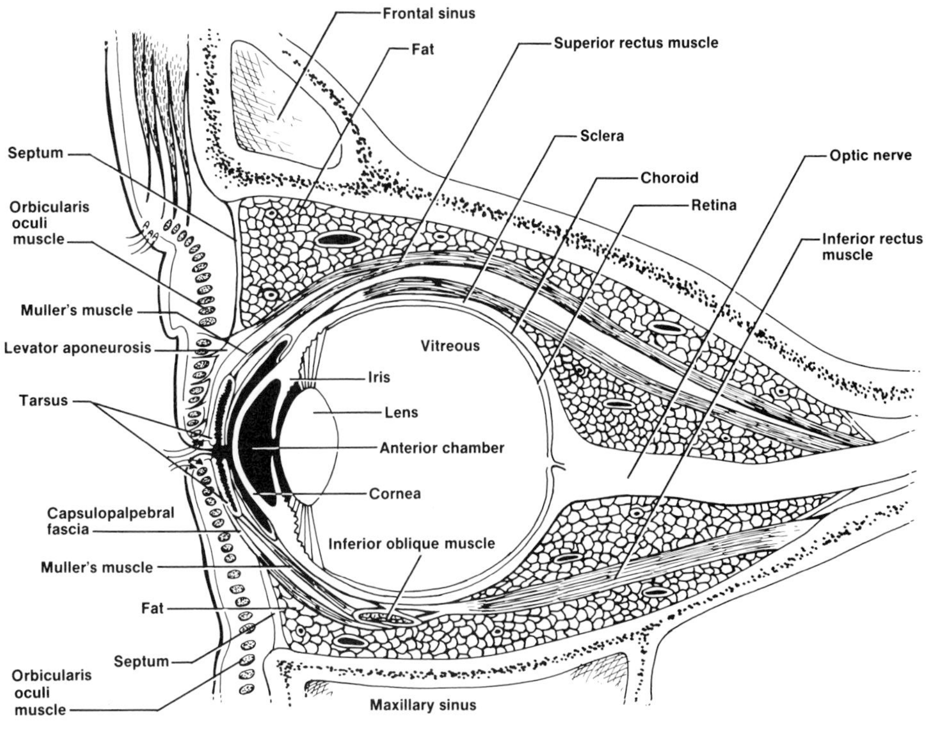

Figure 23–1. Ocular and periocular anatomy, including vascular supply and innervation of ocular structures.

are gathered together at the optic disk and form the optic nerve. The optic disk (Fig. 23–2) measures 1.5 mm in diameter and contains a central depression, or cup, which normally averages one-third the disk diameter. As the axons leave the globe, they travel for approximately 1.0 mm through the sclera. They are then covered by dura and arachnoid while traveling 25 to 30 mm through the orbit, 4 to 9 mm through the optic canal, and 10 mm intracranially before forming the optic chiasm and finally terminating deep in the brain substance.

Anterior to the retina is the vitreous, a gelatinous substance comprising two-thirds the volume of the eye. External to the retina is the choroid, a layer of vascular channels. Surrounding the choroid is the sclera, a tough connective tissue layer that both protects the internal ocular structure and acts as the structural skeleton for the globe.

Anterior to the vitreous lies the lens. This structure is approximately 9 mm in diameter and 4 mm thick. It is suspended just behind the iris by fibers that connect it to the wedge-shaped ciliary body, which consists of muscular, vascular, and epithelial elements. The ciliary body is responsible both for producing aqueous humor and for changing the shape of the lens, which becomes more biconvex for near vision and flattens for distance vision. The iris is an anterior extension of the ciliary body. This flat structure lies just anterior to the lens and contains a central round aperture, the pupil. Contraction of the parasympathetically innervated iris sphincter muscle reduces the pupillary diameter, while contraction of the sympathetically innervated iris dilator enlarges it. These actions control the amount of light entering the eye.

In front of the iris lies the anterior chamber. This contains the aqueous fluid produced by the ciliary body. The total volume of aqueous fluid is approximately 125 μl. It is continuously produced by the ciliary body (although there may be diurnal variations in production) and drains from the anterior chamber via the trabecular meshwork and Schlemm's canal. These structures are located in the angle created by the junction of the iris, cornea, and sclera. The sclera blends into the cornea, an avascular, crystal-clear, concave disklike structure that is 11.5 mm in diameter and ranges in thickness from 0.7 mm peripherally to 0.5 mm centrally. It is covered by a layer of epithelium five to six cells thick. This becomes continuous with the thicker vascularized stratified squamous epithelium of the conjunctiva, the mucous membrane that lines the posterior surface of the eyelids and the anterior portion of the sclera. Overlying the cornea is the tear film, which consists of layers composed of lacrimal, mucinous, and lipid gland secretions. It is produced by the lacrimal and accessory lacrimal glands, conjunctiva goblet cells, and meibomian glands. An adequate tear film that is evenly distributed across the cornea and an intact corneal epithelium are essential factors for achieving clear vision.

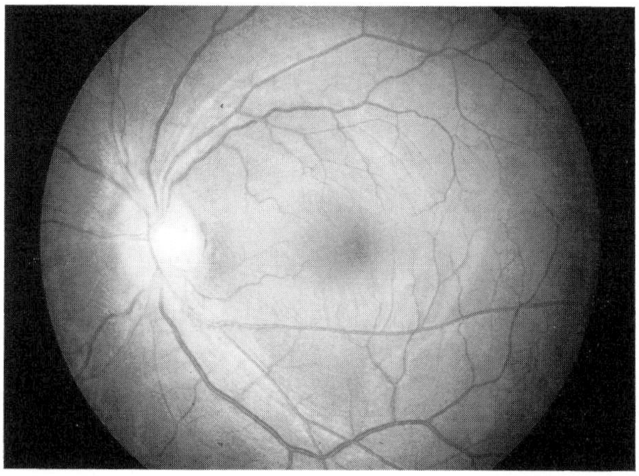

Figure 23–2. Normal ocular fundus with optic disk, retina, macula, and vessels.

Periocular and Orbital Structures

The eyelids cover and protect the globe. In addition, they distribute the tear film evenly across the cornea and aid in the removal of excess tears and tear film debris. The eyelids can be divided into five layers. Most posterior is the conjunctiva. Anterior to this is Müller's muscle, a sympathetically innervated structure that is partially responsible for eyelid elevation. Ptosis is associated with Horner's syndrome because of the absence of Müller's muscle innervation. Müller's muscle is attached to the tarsus, a dense fibrous connective tissue structure containing the meibomian glands. This structure measures 10 mm vertically in the upper eyelid and approximately 3.6 mm in the lower eyelid. It is the structural support element for the eyelid. Anterior to Müller's muscle and tarsus are the levator muscle complex in the upper eyelid and the capsulopalpebral fascia in the lower eyelid. The third cranial nerve innervates the levator muscle, which is responsible for elevating the eyelid. For this reason, ptosis (Fig. 23–3) may be present in third nerve paresis. Since the parasympathetic fibers to the iris sphincter muscle also travel in the third nerve, a dilated (mydriatic) pupil may be associated with third nerve paresis. Anterior to the levator muscle complex is the orbicularis muscle, a structure innervated by the seventh cranial nerve. When this nerve is paretic, as in Bell's palsy (Fig. 23–4*A* and *B*), the eyelids cannot close, resulting in tear film evaporation and corneal epithelial damage. If this is not vigorously treated, the cornea can perforate, and the globe will be permanently and irreversibly damaged. Skin is the final structure covering the eyelid. A component of the eyelid that cannot be overlooked is the orbital septum, which is a continuation of the periosteum covering the bony orbit. This structure extends from the orbital rim and attaches to either the levator muscle complex or the capsulopalpebral fascia and represents the boundary between the orbital and periorbital structures. Violation of this protective barrier exposes the orbital contents to external forces, specifically infectious agents, which can easily involve the entire orbit with subsequent visual loss followed by intracranial spread with meningitis and abscess formation.

The length of the globe from the corneal apex to the point at which the optic nerve exits the sclera is approximately 24.5 mm. The globe weighs 7.5 gm and has a volume of 6.5 ml. The globe lies within the bony orbit, which consists of the maxillary, lacrimal, ethmoid, greater and lesser sphenoid, frontal, palatine, and zygomatic bones. These are joined to form a quadrilateral pyramid with its apex placed posteriorly.

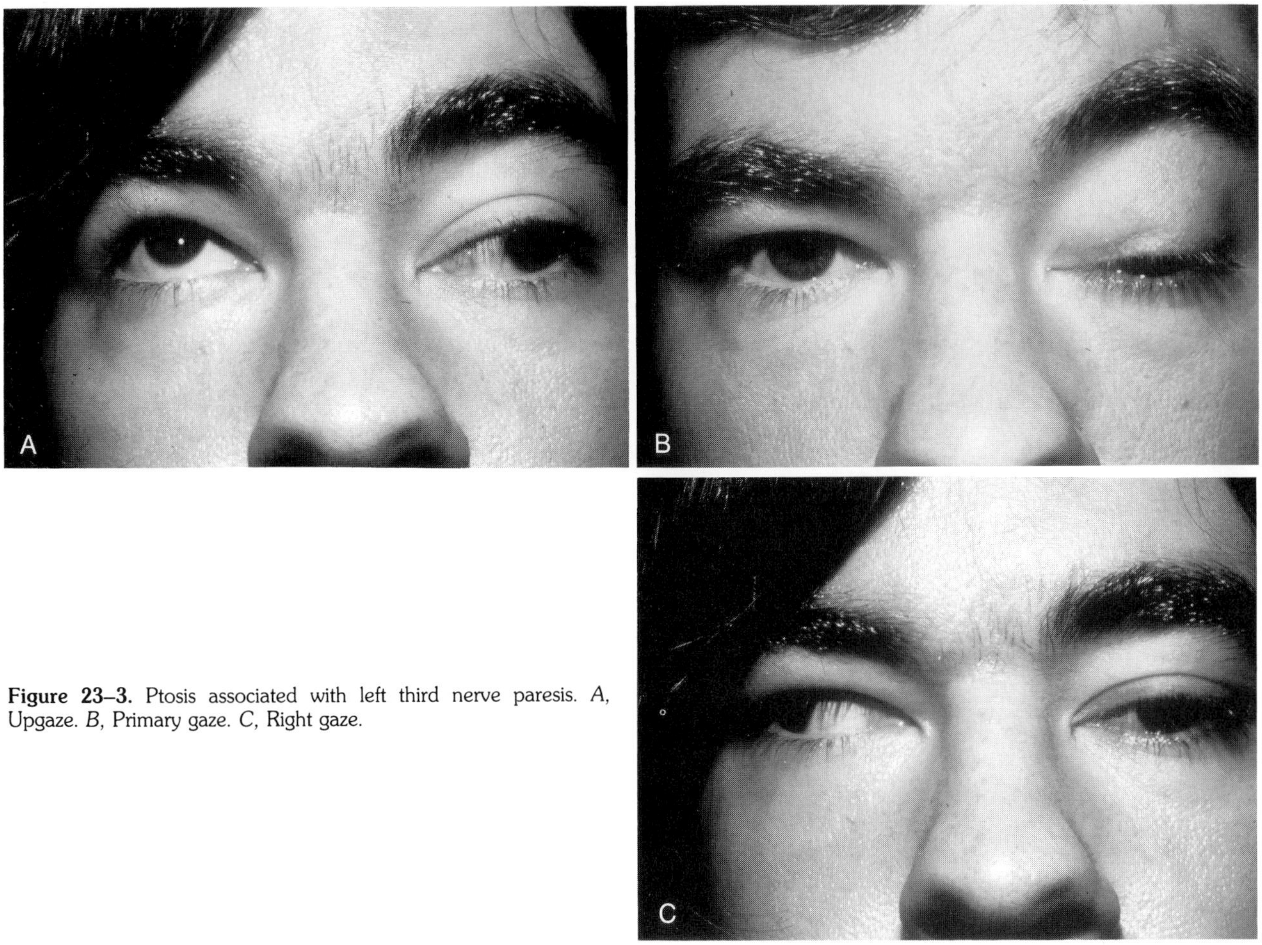

Figure 23–3. Ptosis associated with left third nerve paresis. *A*, Upgaze. *B*, Primary gaze. *C*, Right gaze.

The anterior opening of the orbit measures approximately 35 mm in height and 40 mm in width. The orbit is 40 to 45 mm deep. Superior to the orbit are the frontal sinus anteriorly and the anterior cranial fossa posteriorly. Medial to the orbit are the ethmoid and sphenoid sinuses and the nasal cavity. Inferiorly is the maxillary sinus. Laterally are the temporalis fossa anteriorly and the middle cranial fossa, temporal fossa, and pterygopalatine fossa posteriorly. Posterior to the orbital apex are the clinoid processes, pituitary, cavernous sinus, carotid arteries, middle cranial fossa, and optic chiasm. Since the globe and orbit are in close approximation to many other important nonocular structures, serious ocular injury is often seen in the context of serious nonocular injury.

In addition to many other structures, the orbit contains the extraocular muscles that are responsible for coordinated eye movements. The third cranial nerve innervates the medial rectus, inferior rectus, inferior oblique, and superior rectus muscles, which are respectively responsible for eye movement toward the nose, downward, upward and away from the nose, and upward. The fourth cranial nerve innervates the superior oblique muscle, which moves the eye downward as well as away from the nose. Finally, the sixth cranial nerve innervates the lateral rectus muscle, which moves the eye away from the nose. In paresis of the third cranial nerve, the eye is turned outward, while in paresis of the sixth cranial nerve, the eye is turned inward.

Tear secretions exit through the lacrimal drainage system (Fig. 23–5). Any damage to this system may result in severe and debilitating epiphora as well as infection. Puncta (orifices leading to the lacrimal drainage system) are present in the upper and lower eyelids approximately 5 mm from the medial canthus. These lead to the canaliculi, which are approximately 8 mm long and travel in the medial and superficial eyelid before entering the superior third of the lacrimal sac. This latter structure is attached to the lacrimal fossa and is beneath the medial canthal tendon. Tear secretions flow from the lacrimal sac into the bony nasolacrimal duct within the maxillary bone before entering the nose under the inferior meatus approximately 4 cm from the nasal vestibule.

The arterial supply to the globe and orbit is derived almost entirely from the ophthalmic artery and its branches. This vessel is the first branch from the internal carotid artery after it enters the cranial cavity. This important factor explains the tendency for emboli flowing through this artery to enter the ophthalmic artery, resulting in visual symptoms and deficits. The facial and maxillary arteries, which are branches of the external carotid artery, provide additional blood supply to the lower eyelid, medial canthus, and inferior orbit. The venous drainage of the eye and orbit is via the inferior and superior ophthalmic veins to the cavernous sinus. This is an important route for the intracranial spread of infection. Venous egress also occurs by anastomoses with the angular vein, which drains into the internal jugular system, and by the pterygoid plexus, which drains into the external jugular

A
B
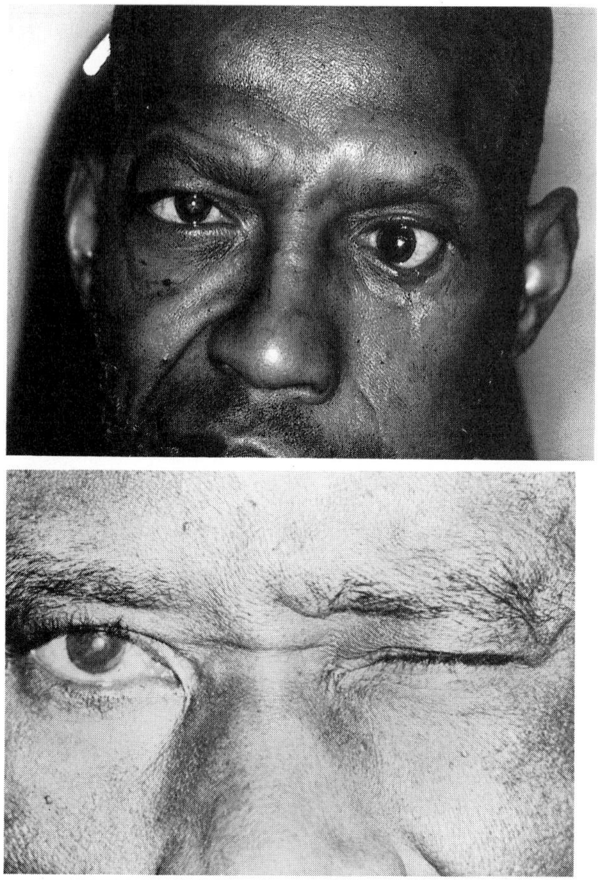

Figure 23–4. *A*, Left-sided Bell's palsy demonstrating facial paralysis and lower eyelid sag. *B*, Right-sided Bell's palsy demonstrating inability to close right eye.

system. There are no lymphatics within the orbit. However, the eyelids have a rich lymphatic system draining into the preauricular nodes and the submaxillary nodes.

Sensory innervation to the ocular structures is via the fifth cranial nerve. The ophthalmic division supplies the forehead, upper eyelid, nose, and cornea. This accounts for the severe ocular pathology often associated with herpes zoster infections involving this nerve. The maxillary division of the fifth cranial nerve supplies the lower eyelid, cheek, medial aspect of the nose, upper lip, gums, and lateral forehead. Portions of this nerve travel beneath the orbital floor. This explains the loss of sensation involving the cheek, lips, and gums following inferior orbital rim and floor fractures.

PREVENTION[6]

Prevention of ocular injuries is as important as their management. The use of seatbelts, the avoidance of driving while intoxicated, and the use of safety helmets can help prevent much serious facial and ocular trauma. Other important factors involved in reducing the incidence of ocular injury include the determination of visual standards for particular athletic and occupational activities and the utilization of protective eyewear. Activities can be divided into those requiring better than average visual ability, average visual ability, and less than average visual ability. These categories are based on the amount of visual concentration and attention required, eye/hand coordination and skill, reflexes, and extent of required environmental awareness and interaction. At the highest level of visual ability, the necessary requirements are better than 20/30 vision in each eye, stereopsis, single binocular vision, the absence of any horizontal or vertical phorias, normal monocular and binoc-

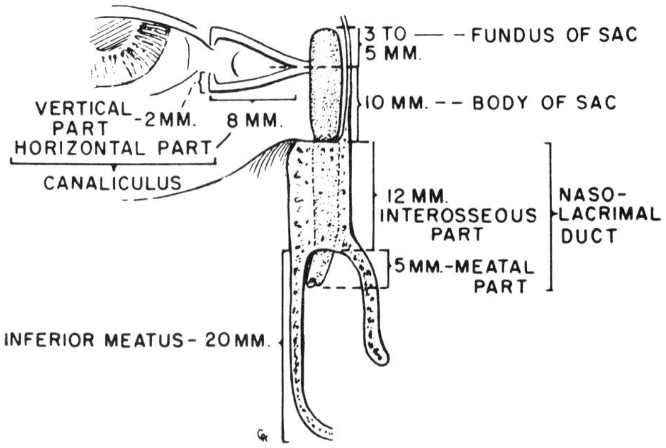

Figure 23–5. Lacrimal drainage system.

ular visual fields by confrontation, normal color vision, and the absence of any active eye disease. Average visual ability differs somewhat in not requiring stereopsis or the absence of phorias. Less than average visual ability requires 20/40 or better vision in each eye, average color discrimination, a complete monocular field by confrontation, the absence of active eye disease, and concurrence of an ophthalmologist.

Safety glasses are essential for athletic and occupational activities. Contact lenses alone do not provide adequate protection for environments involving projectile objects, chemicals, particulate matter, and intense heat or radiation energy. Ocular protection ranges from full face protection (wire mesh, polycarbonate, or both) attached to a helmet with a separate mouthguard for such sports as football and hockey to one-piece molded eye protectors with polycarbonate lenses backed by a posterior lip that is part of the molded front for use in racquet sports. Protective requirements for specific sports have been defined by the American Society of Testing Materials (ASTM), the American National Standards Institute (ANSI), the Canadian Standards Association (CSA), and the British Standards Institution (BSI).[6]

For occupational uses, a variety of ocular safety protectors are available, depending on the job requirements. The ANSI Z87.1-1979 Standard Practice for Occupational and Educational Eye and Face Protection defines three types of safety spectacles: style A has no side shields; style B has orbital-fitting cup-type side shields of wire mesh or perforated/nonperforated plastic; and style C has semi- or flat-fold plastic side shields. All have polycarbonate or CR-39 lenses. Style B glasses provide the best protection against hazardous material from the sides, above, below, in front, and behind. Additional protection is required for specific occupations involving radiation and light (welding goggles) or chemical splashes and dust (eye cups or rigid-cover goggles). Coverall polycarbonate goggles are very useful when a spectacle correction is required. These protectors fit over spectacles and are very convenient for use at home as well as on the job.[6]

When vision is 20/200 or less in one eye with the best spectacle correction, or when unilateral anophthalmos is present, a person is considered to have monocular sight. These individuals should not wear contact lenses for even recreational use, since no protection is afforded their only eye. It must be emphasized that in such cases polycarbonate lenses provide the best ocular protection and should be utilized at all times during both leisure and occupational activities. In addition, these individuals cannot be employed in occupations requiring stereopsis or binocular vision (e.g., airline pilots, police officers). They also may have restrictions on their driver's licenses, such as requiring bilateral outside mirrors or, for people in whom the better eye also has a visual deficit, being limited to daytime driving only. The motor vehicle administration of each state should be consulted for specific restrictions.

TRAUMA MANAGEMENT

When managing a trauma patient, it is essential to set priorities for the treatment of injuries. The ABCs of resuscitation must be adhered to; however, this course of events may have implications for the treatment of ocular trauma. Examination, diagnosis, and treatment of ocular trauma may need to be delayed until emergency and life-threatening injuries are treated and the patient has been adequately stabilized to allow further evaluation. The priorities established for treating each multitrauma patient require individualization based on the nature and severity of each injury. In accordance with the complexity of trauma patients, these patients may not be capable of assisting in an examination. The administration of paralytic agents, heavy sedation, intubation (compromising communication), confusion, disorientation or combativeness secondary to a head injury, coma, or cardiac instability are some of the variables inhibiting assistance by a patient. In such instances, it may be necessary to obtain an ocular history from other sources, when available, such as family, friends, or personal ophthalmologist. The evaluation of the severely injured comatose patient or the uncooperative and combative patient who needs sedation may be limited or incomplete. Such patients often require repeated examinations before a complete knowledge of any ocular pathology is possible.

Assessment[5–10]

The ocular trauma examination begins with an ocular history. Symptoms of visual loss or blurred vision that does not improve with blinking, double vision, sectoral visual loss (Fig. 23–6), and ocular pain are important findings and require immediate referral to an ophthalmologist. The time course of events and the inciting event must be determined as well as any treatment interventions that may have been provided. It is important to ascertain whether ocular disease or visual loss was present prior to the traumatic event and whether the patient is currently receiving any chronic ocular therapy that needs to be continued.

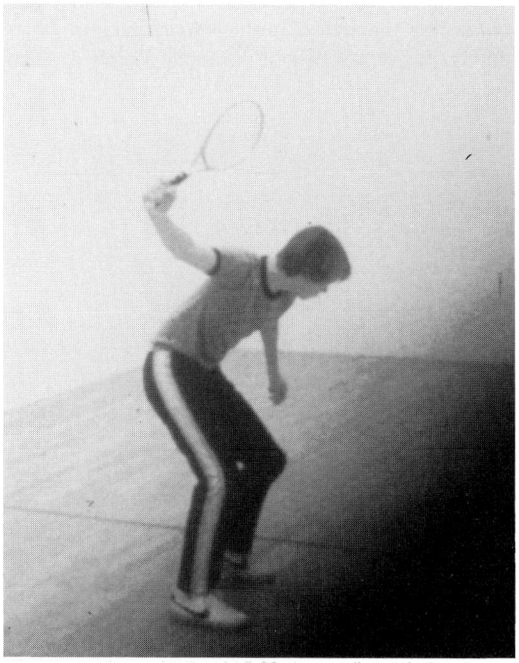

Figure 23–6. Sectoral vision. (Reprinted with permission from the Athlete's Eye. San Francisco, American Academy of Ophthalmology, 1984.)

To adequately examine the patient with ocular trauma, a few simple instruments are required. A near-vision chart, pinhole occluder, and loose +2.75 sphere spectacle lens (for the presbyopic patient) are useful in assessing visual acuity. A penlight with a cobalt blue filter, Schiøtz tonometer, Hertel exophthalmometer, and ophthalmoscope will help in the other parts of the examination. A slit-lamp biomicroscope, if accessible, will greatly aid in the evaluation of the conjunctiva, cornea, anterior chamber, iris, lens, and anterior vitreous cavity. Topical anesthetic agents such as tetracaine or proparacaine will help in examining patients who are unable to open their eyes because of corneal abrasions or erosions. A lid retractor or bent paperclip retractors (Fig. 23–7) may be required for patients with corneal injury or in evaluating infants. Sodium fluorescein test strips are needed to evaluate the extent of corneal epithelial loss. These are used with a cobalt blue filter covering a penlight. Short-acting dilating drops such as 2.5% or 10% phenylephrine HCl or 1% tropicamide, both of which have a duration of action lasting 3 to 6 hours, are essential for an adequate examination of the ocular fundus in patients with ocular trauma. However, these agents prevent evaluation of the pupils and must either be avoided or be used with great caution in any patient with intracranial trauma. Finally, it is important to have the name and phone number of an easily accessible and available ophthalmologist for emergency consultation and management.

Visual Acuity

The most essential aspect of the ocular examination is a determination of visual acuity. This is performed with the patient utilizing his spectacle correction for distance and near acuity. In a presbyopic patient who does not have a spectacle correction available, a loose +2.75 spherical lens can be used to aid near vision. If a standardized distance or near visual acuity chart is not available, a newspaper or some other printed material can be used. Visual acuity can then be recorded as the size of print (large, medium, or small) the patient sees at a specified distance, usually 14 inches. If the patient is a child or is unable to read, a picture chart such as an Allen chart or the "E" game (determination of which way the letter E points at specific distances) can be used. If the patient is unable to see any of these, the ability to count fingers or ascertain hand motions at a specific distance is determined. If these are inadequate, then the ability to perceive light with or without the ability to determine the direction from which the light is projecting must be ascertained. If no light perception is present, this is recorded as NLP. Vision is always measured for each eye separately, with the opposite eye covered. If a patient does not have his or her spectacle correction or if there is a question concerning the adequacy of a particular correction, a pinhole occluder will allow for the measurement of visual acuity to within one or two lines of the patient's expected best corrected vision. If the patient is comatose or otherwise unable to perform visual acuity testing, visual evoked response testing will help to determine the intactness of the visual system. In general, any patient with a best corrected visual acuity of 20/40 or worse needs to be evaluated by an ophthalmologist.

Pupils

The next aspect of the visual examination is an evaluation of the pupils. This is performed by having the patient look at a distant object (to prevent the pupillary constriction that occurs on viewing a near object) and shining a light first in one eye and then in the other. Initially, the pupils should be equal in size and then should constrict equally and briskly to the light stimulus. Unequal or nonreactive pupils can be seen in many conditions, including ocular trauma or surgery, acute glaucoma, topical drug instillation, Horner's syndrome, and lesions of the midbrain or third cranial nerve. The serious nature of these conditions makes it essential that any patient with unequal or nonreactive pupils receive immediate evaluation by an ophthalmologist.

The pupillary response to light also can be used to determine the presence of optic nerve damage. This pupillary response is called the *Marcus-Gunn pupil* or *afferent pupillary*

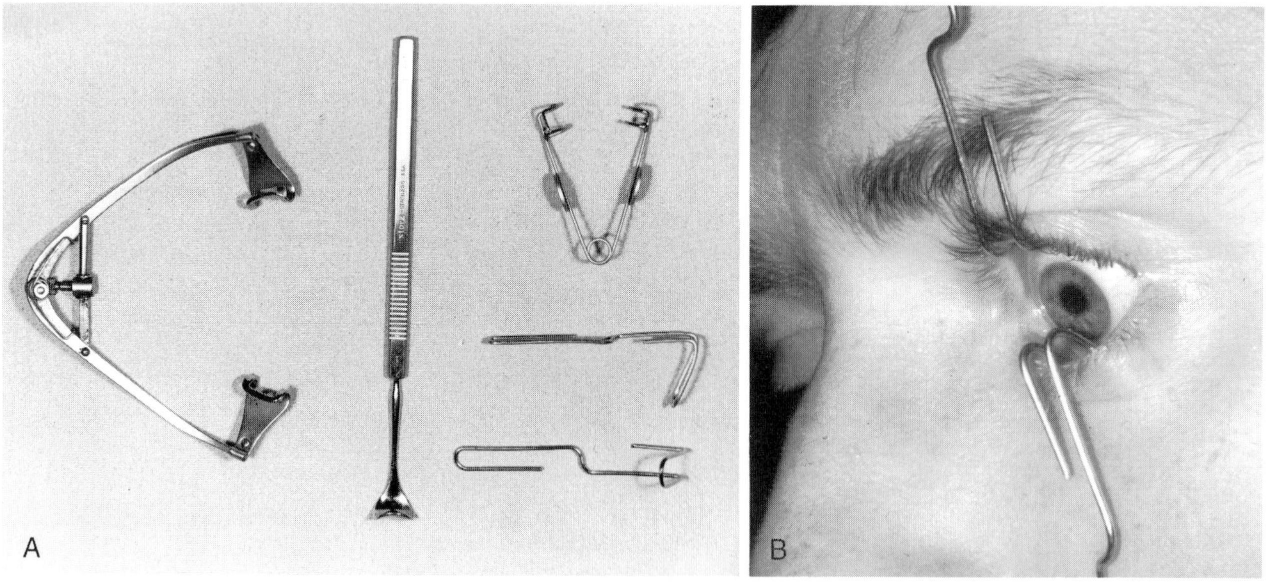

Figure 23–7. *A*, Eyelid retractors. *B*, Paperclip retractors.

defect. To understand this type of pupil, it must be remembered that normally the pupils are linked together in response to a light stimulus, each constricting an equal amount to the stimulus. If one optic nerve is normal and the opposite optic nerve is abnormal and a light stimulus is presented to the normal side, the pupils constrict equally on both sides. When the light stimulus is then presented to the abnormal side, the damaged optic nerve is only able to transmit a portion of the light stimulus. This causes it to falsely perceive that less light is present; therefore, both pupils will paradoxically dilate. This response only occurs in the presence of unilateral optic nerve damage and is an important examination technique to use when there is a question concerning optic nerve viability.

Ocular Motility

Evaluation of ocular motility is the next step in the examination process. The patient is asked to fixate on a penlight, which is moved to the right, left, up, and down. The eyes are linked in tandem and should move an equal amount in each gaze direction. In an uncooperative patient or in one with a depressed mental status, the "doll's head" maneuver (rapid passive head turning, with a normal response being movement of the eyes in the direction opposite to the head movement) or caloric testing (cold water stimulus to one ear, with a normal response being a slow deviation of the eyes toward the stimulus followed by a jerk movement of the eyes away from the stimulus) can be used to evaluate the ocular motor system. When there is a question regarding a restrictive component to an ocular motility abnormality, as in cases of orbital floor fractures, forced duction (Fig. 23–8) testing needs to be performed. This involves anesthetizing the eye with topical anesthesia, grasping the limbal conjunctiva and sclera with a toothed forceps, and rotating the globe up and down to test the vertical rectus muscles and right and left to test the horizontal rectus muscles while noting any restriction to free movement of the globe. Common causes of abnormal ocular movements include orbital edema, muscle entrapment, and cranial nerve damage. Any patient with a disturbance of ocular motility requires a thorough evaluation by an ophthalmologist.

Orbit

As part of the ophthalmic examination, it is important to assess the periorbital and orbital structures and the relationship of the globe to these structures. A determination of the position of the globe within the orbit and in comparison with the ocular structures on the opposite side is important for the diagnosis of such conditions as orbital fractures and foreign bodies, retrobulbar hemorrhage, and orbital cellulitis and abscess. Normally, a comparison of the two globes by Hertel exophthalmometry (Fig. 23–9) shows less than a 2-mm difference between opposite sides in the distance from the lateral orbital rim to the corneal apex. The normal measurement for this distance is approximately 18 to 20 mm. When the difference is 2 mm or higher and the globe is pushed out of the orbit or proptotic, orbital edema, a retained foreign body, retrobulbar hemorrhage, orbital abscess or cellulitis, dysthyroid ophthalmopathy, or orbital tumor should be considered. When the difference is 2 mm or higher and the globe is sunken back into the orbit or enophthalmic, orbital fractures must be considered. If a straight edge is held horizontally to bisect the pupil, the center of each pupil should be on the same horizontal plane. When one eye is lower than the other, an orbital floor fracture may be present (Fig. 23–10). The horizontal distance from the medial canthus to the middle of the nasal bones is approximately 16 mm. When this is widened or when there is inequality between opposite sides, telecanthus associated with a midfacial fracture may be present. The orbital rim should be smooth without any breaks or irregularities that might indicate an orbital rim fracture. Crepitus on palpation of the eyelids is another sign associated with fractures of the orbital bones. Periorbital edema and ecchymosis commonly accompany many types of orbital, head, and facial trauma and, while not specific signs, do indicate the possibility of severe ocular injury. In any case, where there is the possibility of orbital fracture, retrobulbar hemorrhage, or orbital infections or foreign bodies, an ophthalmologist should be consulted in order to fully evaluate and appropriately manage the patient.

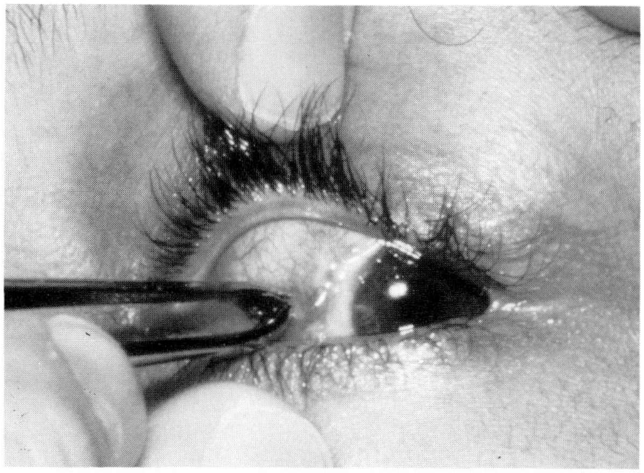

Figure 23–8. Forced duction.

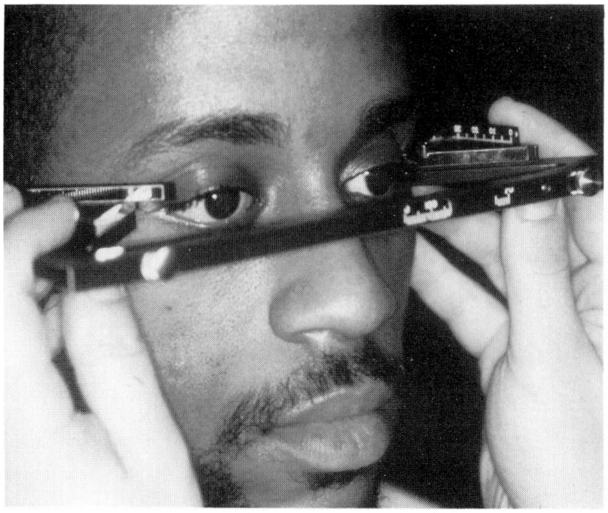

Figure 23–9. Hertel exophthalmometry.

Intraocular Pressure

Assessment of intraocular pressure is another important aspect of the examination following ocular trauma. This should not be performed when there is any question concerning the integrity of the globe, since any pressure on a

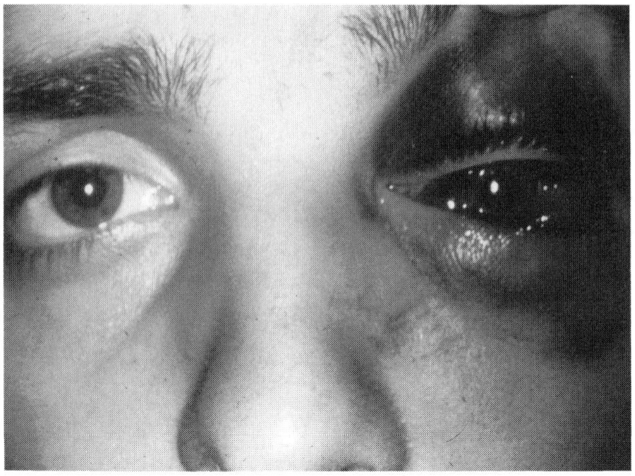

Figure 23–10. Acute orbital fracture with periorbital edema, ecchymosis, and hypophthalmos. (Reprinted with permission from the Athlete's Eye. San Francisco, American Academy of Ophthalmology, 1984.)

perforated eye will result in extrusion of the ocular contents and permanent loss of vision. To measure intraocular pressure, a topical anesthetic is instilled into the ocular cul-de-sacs. A Schiøtz tonometer (Fig. 23–11) with a 5.5 gm weight is used to measure the pressure. To do this, the patient's head is placed so that the face is toward the ceiling. The patient is asked to look straight up, and the footplate of the tonometer is placed on the central portion of the cornea. The scale value indicated by the tonometer needle is read and then translated into the appropriate intraocular pressure reading using a special table. Normal intraocular pressure is 20 mm Hg or less. Patients with dangerously high intraocular pressure (>30 mm Hg) may have angle closure glaucoma, pupillary block glaucoma, or a retrobulbar hemorrhage. Urgent treatment is needed to lower elevated pressure and prevent permanent loss of vision due to optic nerve damage. Patients with low intraocular pressure (<10 mm Hg) may have a perforated globe or severe intraocular trauma and may need immediate evaluation by an ophthalmologist.

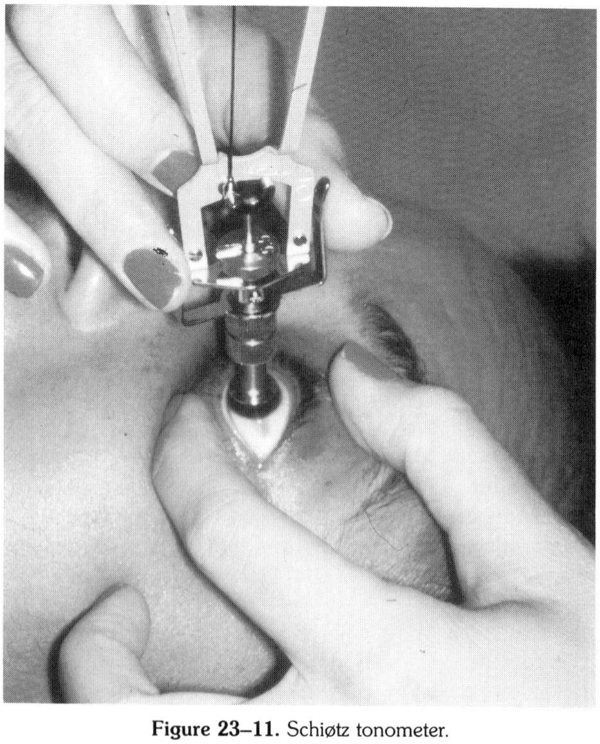

Figure 23–11. Schiøtz tonometer.

Eyelids

The eyelids protect the globe, remove excess tear secretions and debris, and facilitate complete and adequate corneal wetting. They are frequently involved in cases of trauma. Ptosis (Fig. 23–12) often accompanies periorbital edema and ecchymosis, but it also may be a result of direct damage to the levator complex or Müller's muscle or may be seen with enophthalmos associated with an orbital fracture. Inability to adequately close the eyelids is a more serious problem associated with damage to the seventh cranial nerve. It also may be seen with scarring following repair of eyelid lacerations. Decreased corneal sensation from damage to the fifth cranial nerve can result in a poor blink reflex and inadequate surfacing of the pericorneal tear film. Misdirected lashes can result in severe corneal damage. Conditions that result in damage to the cornea such as those due to an inability to close the eye, inadequate blinking, or poor corneal wetting need immediate referral to an ophthalmologist to prevent visual loss.

Lacerations involving the eyelids, while serious themselves, also can be associated with penetrating trauma to the globe (Fig. 23–13). Lacerations of this type are usually deep and may have concomitant prolapse or orbital fat. These injuries require a thorough ocular evaluation to eliminate the possibility of severe injury to the globe. When lacerations involve the eyelid margin or canalicular system or when they are deep or complicated, repair by an experienced ophthalmologist is essential to prevent permanent functional and cosmetic deficits.

Conjunctiva

Examination of the conjunctiva, tear film, cornea, anterior chamber, iris, lens, and anterior vitreous cavity is best performed with a slit-lamp biomicroscope. However, since this instrument is not usually available to nonophthalmologists, a penlight can be used. The eyelids must be everted (a cotton-tipped applicator facilitates this maneuver) to examine

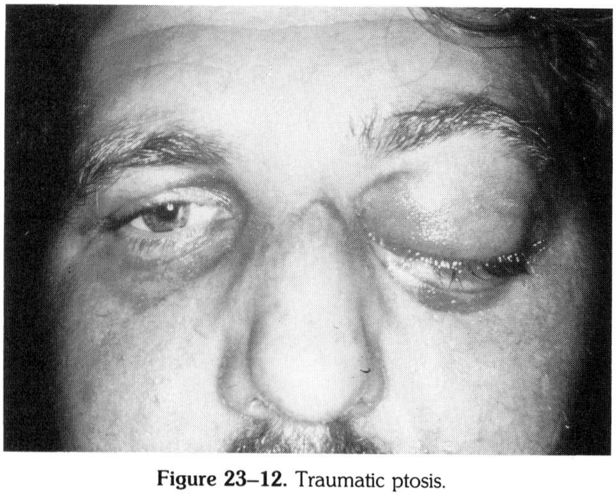

Figure 23–12. Traumatic ptosis.

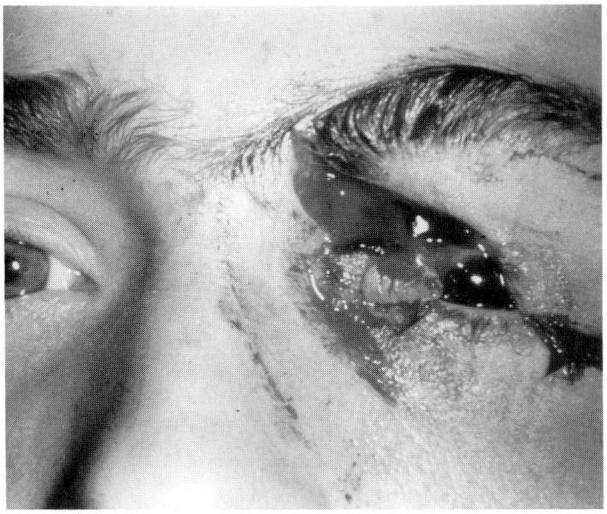

Figure 23–13. Severe eyelid laceration with associated penetrating trauma to globe. (Reprinted with permission from Eye Trauma and Emergencies. San Francisco, American Academy of Ophthalmology, 1985.)

their conjunctival surface thoroughly for foreign bodies or embedded material. It is also important to examine the anterior conjunctiva for injection, lacerations, foreign bodies, chemosis, or hemorrhage. The presence of any of these signs may indicate a perforated globe. In addition, conjunctival infection is often present posttraumatically owing to ocular inflammation and in cases of infectious and noninfectious conjunctivitis, corneal abrasions, acute glaucoma, and other types of ocular inflammation. Perilimbal (area where cornea and sclera blend together) dilated blood vessels often associated with proptosis can be a manifestation of a posttraumatic intracranial arteriovenous fistula. If there is any uncertainty regarding ocular integrity or the presence of severe ocular injury, an ophthalmologist should be consulted.

Cornea

Normally, the cornea is crystal clear and glistening. A penlight can easily demonstrate corneal lacerations, foreign bodies, abrasions, and irregularities. Instillation of sodium fluorescein, which stains areas denuded of epithelium, and utilization of a cobalt blue filter over a penlight will facilitate evaluation of the cornea. A cloudy cornea may indicate acute glaucoma, edema from trauma, a foreign body in the anterior chamber, or an infectious process. While many cases of conjunctivitis, corneal foreign bodies, and abrasion can be safely managed without an ophthalmologist, if there is any uncertainty about the seriousness of the disease process, an ophthalmologist should be consulted.

Anterior Chamber

On penlight examination, the anterior chamber should be clear and deep, with the iris well separated from the posterior corneal surface. When blood (hyphema) (Fig. 23–14) or white cells (hypopyon) are present, serious ocular injury has occurred, and immediate ophthalmologic consultation is required. Shallowing of the anterior chamber can be demonstrated by shining the beam from a penlight across the chamber from the temporal side of the globe. The beam should highlight the entire chamber without impediment. When the chamber is shallowed, the beam will fall on the iris, creating shadows, and will not illuminate the chamber. Acute angle closure glaucoma is a consideration in such cases, especially if there is an associated rise in intraocular pressure; clouding of the cornea; complaints of visual loss, halos around objects, or eye pain; nausea; or vomiting. Urgent ophthalmic consultation is needed if these symptoms and signs are present.

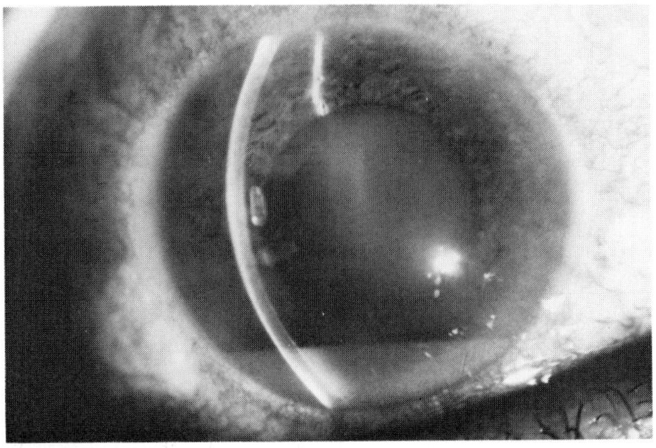

Figure 23–14. Hyphema involving 15 per cent of the inferior anterior chamber.

Iris

Examination of the iris in cases of ocular trauma may demonstrate tears and holes. These may cause pupillary irregularities (Fig. 23–15) or, more important, may be associated with hyphema (see Fig. 23–14) (from damage to iris blood vessels) or chronic glaucoma (from damage to the trabecular meshwork and aqueous drainage system). Iris tears and hyphemas can be associated with penetrating foreign bodies; when tears are seen, the globe must be considered perforated. This requires immediate evaluation by an ophthalmologist. Sometimes small foreign bodies will be embedded on the iris surface or may bounce off the iris and fall into the anterior chamber angle. Small colored foreign bodies may be confused with small pigmented nevi, which are normally present on the surface of the iris.

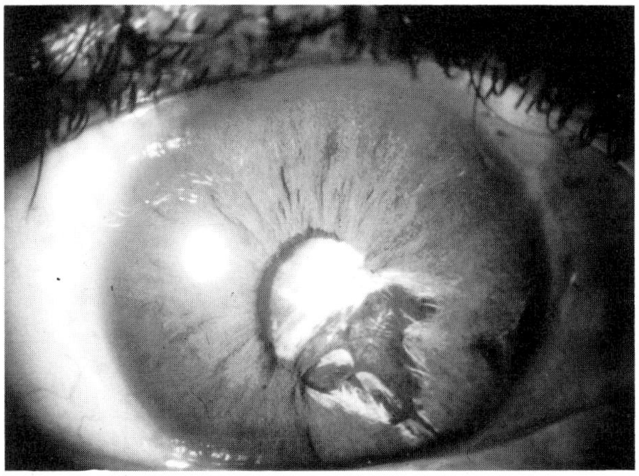

Figure 23–15. Traumatic pupillary irregularities with posterior synechiae and cataract formation.

Lens

The normal lens is a crystalline structure that is best examined by slit-lamp biomicroscopy. Following ocular trauma, it is not uncommon for the lens to develop opacities and become cataractous. These defects are often visible on penlight examination. If severe inflammation is associated with ocular injury, adhesions (posterior synechiae) (see Fig. 23–15) between the iris and the lens may develop. These may lead to an elevation of intraocular pressure and subsequent optic nerve damage. When a force of sufficient intensity is delivered to the globe, the lens can be torn from its moorings to the ciliary body. In such cases, it may be dislocated to float free in the vitreous or settle on the retina. More rarely, it may become positioned in the anterior chamber, blocking aqueous outflow and resulting in acute glaucoma. Proper evaluation and management of these serious conditions requires prompt ophthalmologic consultation.

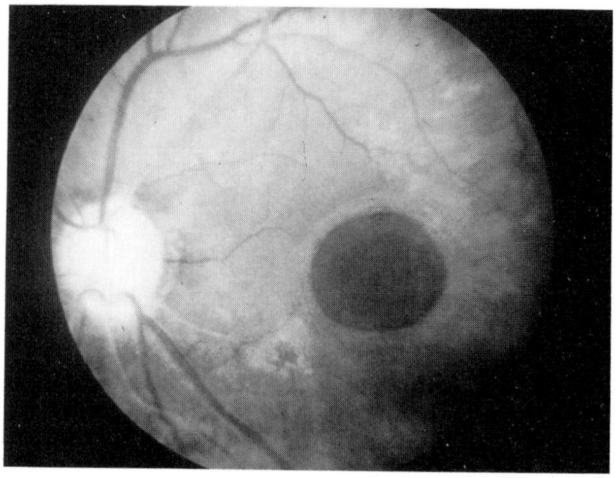

Figure 23–17. Macular hole.

Fundus

The fundus examination is the final aspect of the ocular evaluation. Normally, the vitreous is a clear structure that allows an unimpeded view of the retina. Hemorrhage (Fig. 23–16*A*) within the vitreous occasionally occurs in association with intracranial hemorrhage. It also may occur when a retinal vessel is torn and may indicate damage by a penetrating foreign body or a retinal detachment. The normal retina is thin, relatively clear, and colorless. The orange color imparted to it on fundus examination is due to the underlying retinal pigment epithelium and vascular choroid. Retinal edema (Berlin's edema, commotio retinae) is common after ocular trauma. In such cases, the retina appears milky-white and a pseudo-cherry red spot may be present. Although this condition usually subsides spontaneously, resulting in a return of vision, some patients go on to develop a macular hole (Fig. 23–17) and loss of central acuity. Traumatic hemorrhages (Fig. 23–16*B*) can occur on, within, or beneath the retina or choroid when the retinal or choroidal vessels are damaged. These may be associated with retinal tears and holes, retinal detachment, and choroidal layer ruptures. Hard exudates also may be associated with retinal trauma. Proliferation of glial tissue or neovascular fronds can occur following retinal trauma, resulting in retinal detachment or hemorrhage. Choroidal layer ruptures are another posttraumatic cause of visual loss and fibrovascular proliferation. All these pathological processes can cause severe and, in many cases, permanent visual loss and therefore necessitate careful ophthalmologic evaluation.

A

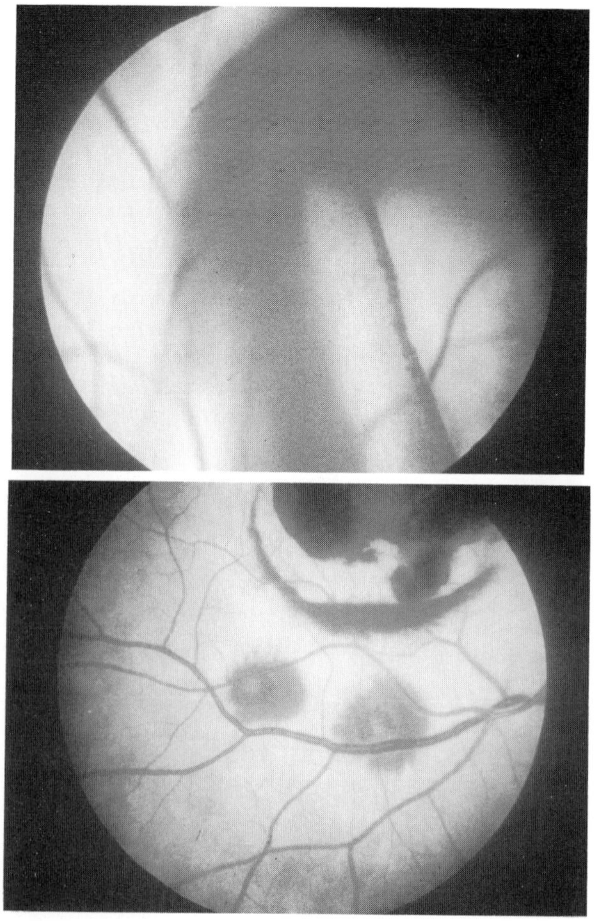

B

Figure 23–16. *A*, Vitreous hemorrhage. *B*, Traumatic intraretinal and periretinal hemorrhages.

Optic Nerve

The optic nerve head is usually somewhat yellow, with sharply defined margins. Its central cup constitutes approximately one-third of its substance and has a single branching central retinal artery and vein. Blurring of the disk margin due to edema of the nerve fibers is seen with an increase in intracranial pressure (papilledema) or pressure on the optic nerve (Fig. 23–18) (disk edema). Atrophy of the optic nerve following contusion or transection injuries results in a loss of disk substance and a whitening of the nerve head.

Diagnostic Studies

In addition to the ophthalmic examination, several other modalities can further aid in the evaluation of the eye and its adnexal structures following trauma. Computed tomographic (CT) scanning (Fig. 23–19) is essential to delineate completely the extent of orbital and optic canal fractures as well as intraocular and orbital foreign bodies. Coronal and anteroposterior cuts of 3 mm thickness overlapped by 2 mm

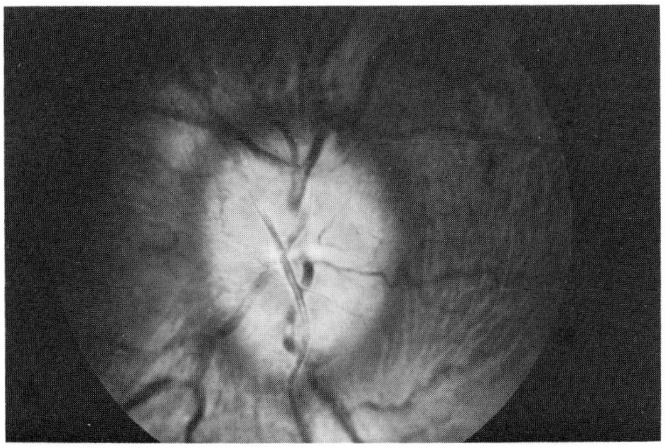

Figure 23–18. Edema of the optic nerve head (disk edema).

are required to obtain the most complete data concerning both the exact location of a foreign body and the extent of any orbital fractures. Thinner sections of 1.5 mm are needed to evaluate the optic canal and foreign bodies within the globe itself. Visual field examination with either a tangent screen or Goldmann perimeter is essential for delineating damage to the optic nerve, chiasm, and tract. This will provide additional important localizing information for intracranial pathology. Orbital and intraocular ultrasonography will greatly aid in the evaluation of retinal and choroidal detachments, intraocular and intraorbital foreign bodies, vitreous hemorrhage, dislocation of the lens, and lacerations of the globe. It can be performed at the bedside and is advantageous to use when an unstable patient cannot be moved or when the eye cannot be fully examined because of anterior segment opacities and disruption. A final modality for evaluating the patient with ocular trauma is the measurement of visual evoked responses. This test is helpful in the nonresponsive or uncooperative patient for determining whether the visual pathways are intact. Like ultrasonography, this too may be routinely performed at the bedside of a nonmobile patient.

Equipment for Management

After a patient with ocular trauma is thoroughly evaluated, any injuries need to be properly managed. Access to a variety of items is necessary for the successful treatment of ocular injury prior to ophthalmologic consultation. At least 2 liters of normal saline are needed for irrigation following chemical injuries. Intravenous acetazolamide (Diamox) and mannitol, 0.5% timolol maleate, 2% pilocarpine HCl, and either 50% oral glycerine or 45% isosorbide are needed for pressure reduction in cases of acute glaucoma. A short-acting mydriatic/cycloplegic, such as 1% tropicamide, 1% cyclopentolate HCl, or 5% homatropine HBr, and antibiotic eyedrops, such as gentamycin sulfate, tobramycin, sulfacetamide sodium, or chloramphenicol, are needed to treat corneal abrasions and bacterial conjunctivitis. A long-acting mydriatic and cycloplegic such as 0.25% scopolamine HCl or 1% atropine sulfate and the topical steroid drop 1% prednisolone acetate are needed to treat severe intraocular inflammations. Artificial teardrops and ointments are essential for managing patients with inadequate blinking or poor eyelid closure. Eye pads and tape (preferably Transpore by the 3M Company) are needed to treat corneal abrasions.

As part of a trauma patient's management, even in the absence of ocular trauma, it is important to determine whether contact lenses are being worn. Corneal abrasion can occur when contacts are worn for extended periods, especially during prolonged surgical procedures. Often it is necessary to examine the eye closely for contact lenses, since not all lenses are tinted. Clear ones are more difficult to see and locate. Following trauma, lenses frequently become dislodged from the cornea and can be found in the superior or inferior ocular cul-de-sacs. A bulb contact lens remover (Fig. 23–20*A*) uses suction to lift hard contact lenses from the cornea or sclera. Soft contact lenses can be removed by finger manipulation or by irrigating the eye with balanced salt solution or normal saline, which allows the lens to "float" off the globe (Fig. 23–20*B*). Once removed, lenses should be placed in the appropriate storage solution and stored in a contact lens case that delineates right from left lens.

Team Management—Resuscitation Cycle

Field Management

Field management of ocular trauma is very limited. The most important aspect is the protection of any injured eye, which is achieved by shielding the eye (Fig. 23–21). To decrease anxiety, it must be explained to the patient why this is being done. No ocular medicine should be given except in cases of chemical injury, where immediate "in the field" irrigation must be performed, or in severe facial burns, where the eyes must be vigorously lubricated with artifical tear ointments. It is best to keep the patient quiet and still. If any active bleeding is noted, a dressing can be applied; however, any pressure to the eye itself needs to be avoided.

The introduction of acidic or alkaline substances into the eye constitutes a medical emergency requiring immediate attention within minutes of injury. Accidents can occur at

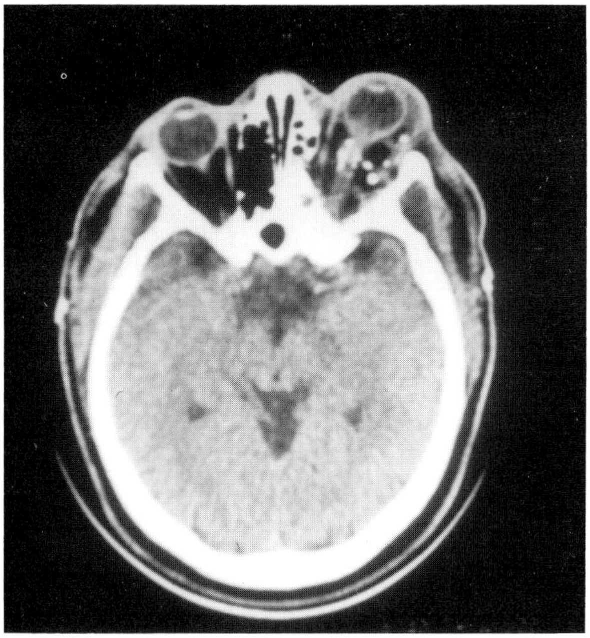

Figure 23–19. CT scan of bullet fragments in orbit and around optic nerve.

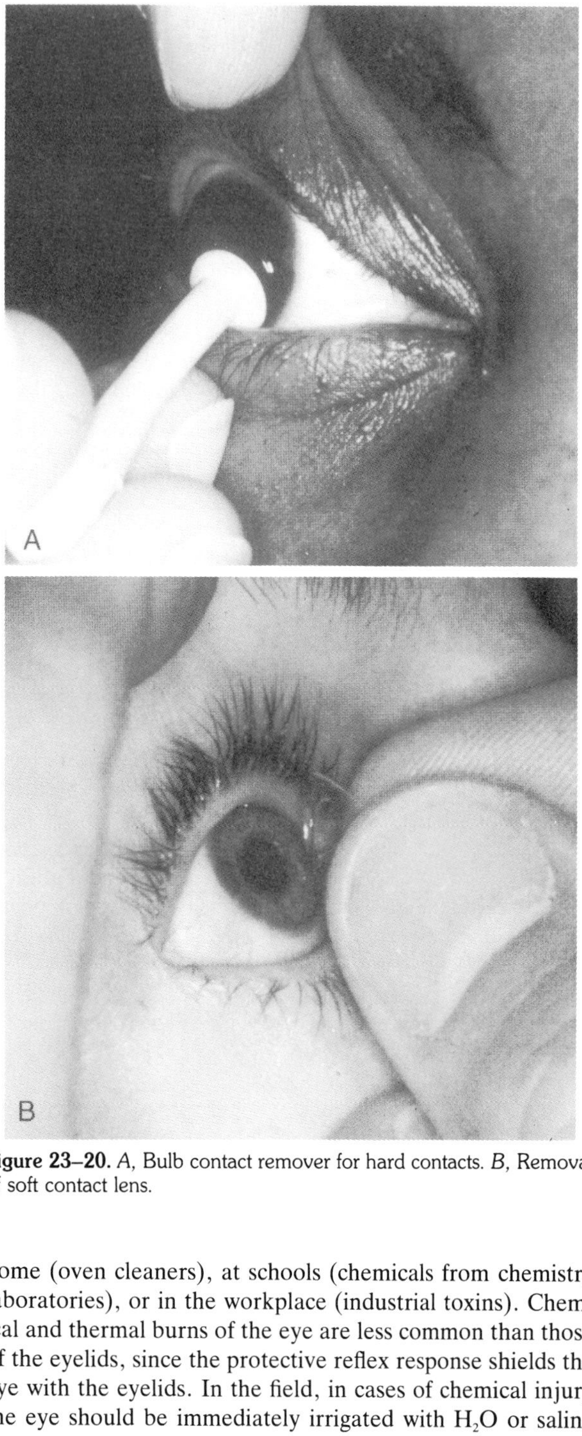

Figure 23–20. *A,* Bulb contact remover for hard contacts. *B,* Removal of soft contact lens.

home (oven cleaners), at schools (chemicals from chemistry laboratories), or in the workplace (industrial toxins). Chemical and thermal burns of the eye are less common than those of the eyelids, since the protective reflex response shields the eye with the eyelids. In the field, in cases of chemical injury the eye should be immediately irrigated with H_2O or saline for at least 15 to 20 minutes prior to transfer to an emergency facility. A loose, moist saline dressing can be applied until the patient arrives at a hospital.

In all cases, the period of acute management requires extensive emotional support and physical care. If there is any visual impairment (secondary to either patching or injury), the patient must be assured that the injury is being thoroughly assessed and appropriately and expertly treated. Explanation of what has happened and what is being done for the patient is essential to help alleviate fears of the unknown. When ocular trauma occurs in conjunction with other injuries, management needs to be prioritized. The treatment of an ocular injury may be delayed until more serious, life-threatening injuries are addressed and the patient stabilized. During this period a shield should be placed over any eye suspected of having sustained injury (see Fig. 23–21).

When managing a patient's nonocular injuries, it is essential to remember that if there is any suspicion that a globe may be perforated, the eyelids, ocular adnexa, orbit, and facial structures must not be manipulated in any way. In some cases it may be necessary to immobilize the head and administer pain medication and sedation while awaiting ophthalmologic consultation. In such cases, periorbital lacerations must not be sutured, and orbital fractures must not be palpated until the perforating ocular injuries are repaired. Generally, bleeding associated with eyelid lacerations and penetrating orbital trauma is minimal and will stop spontaneously. In any event, pressure should never be put on the eyelids, eyeball, or periorbita to stop bleeding if there is any suspicion that the globe is not intact. Any increased pressure on an open eye will result in loss of the intraocular contents and in irreparable damage to the eye (Fig. 23–22). Immediate ophthalmologic consultation should be obtained when any ocular injury is suspected.

Anesthetic ointments should never be used in cases of eye trauma because their prolonged effect may result in inadvertent self-mutilation. For a similar reason, anesthetic drops should not be used on a long-term basis or given to patients. Ocular ointments of any type should not be used when examination of the fundus is necessary (they obscure any view of the fundus) or when penetrating ocular trauma is present (they may enter the globe). In rare cases of eyelid

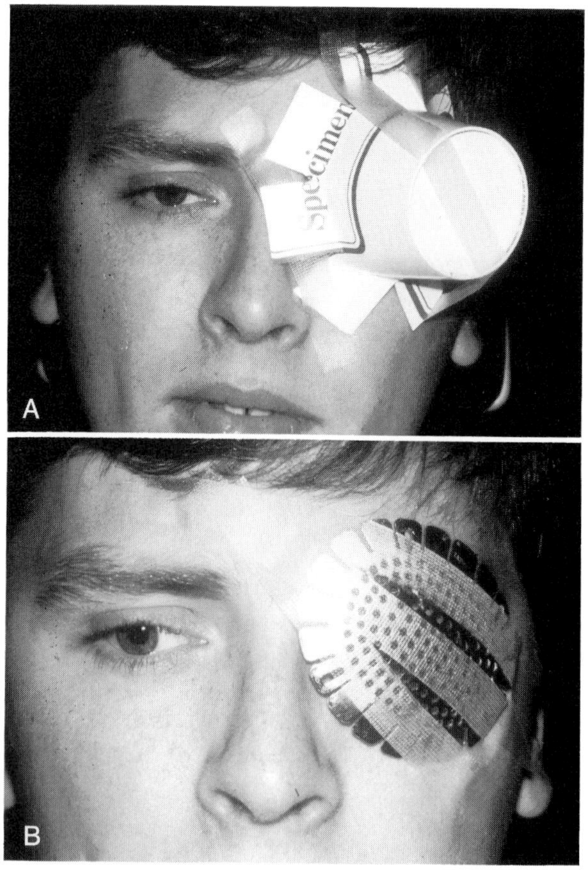

Figure 23–21. *A,* Cup shield. *B,* Metal shield.

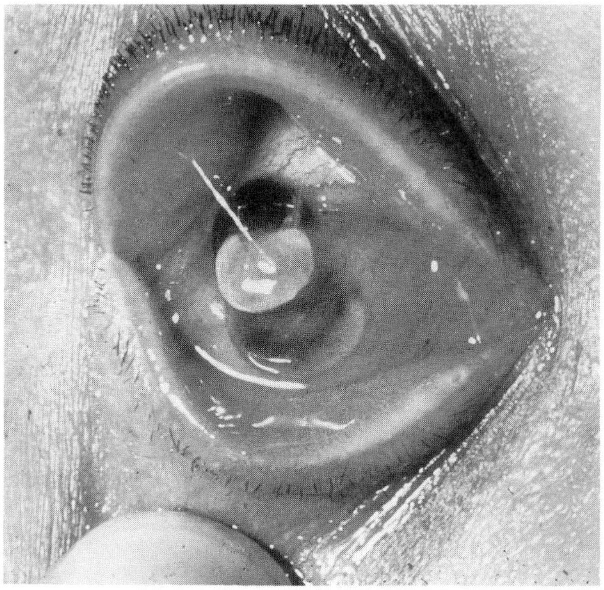

Figure 23–22. Extrusion of lens through corneal laceration.

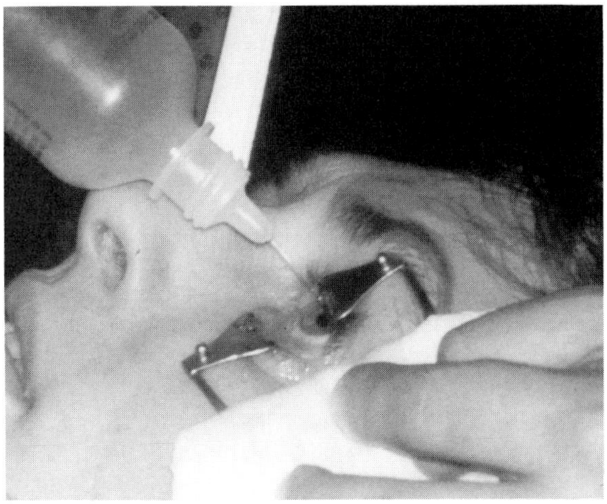

Figure 23–23. Ocular lavage.

avulsion or severe thermal injury, it may be necessary to apply artifical tear ointment to the cornea to protect it. Corticosteroid eyedrops should never be used if there are any diagnostic uncertainties or if infection with herpes simplex virus or any fungus is a possibility. Atropine eyedrops are not for routine use: Their effect is too long-lasting, and they can cause chemical and allergic reactions.

Ocular Emergencies—Management of Specific Injuries[5–10]

Chemical Injury

There are only two true ocular emergencies: chemical injuries and central retinal artery occlusion. Both require the institution of therapy within minutes of their occurrence to prevent permanent ocular damage. Chemical injuries are treated by immediate and copious irrigation of the eye with the most readily available source of water. The longer the period of time between injury and lavage, the worse is the prognosis. The lids must be held apart so that the injured globe can be copiously irrigated (Fig. 23–23). A cloth will help in holding the eyelids apart. Irrigation should be carried out for 15 to 20 minutes prior to transporting the patient to an emergency center. Lavage should be continued in the emergency center until 2 liters of normal saline have been irrigated over a 1-hour period. An IV infusion set for irrigation, eyelid retractors to hold the eyelids apart, and topical anesthetic drops to reduce the blepharospasm caused by corneal damage will all greatly help in carrying out adequate lavage. The eyelids need to be everted to ensure removal of any particulate matter clinging to the conjunctiva. After lavage, a cycloplegic/mydriatic such as 0.25% scopolamine HCl or 5% homatropine should be instilled to reduce pain from ciliary spasm and prevent synechiae (Table 23–1). Topical antibiotics also should be used as prophylaxis against infection. Increases in intraocular pressure frequently accompany serious alkali injuries; therefore, evaluation of intraocular pressure is very important. If the pressure is highly elevated, it should be treated with 500 mg intramuscular or intravenous acetazolamide, intravenous mannitol, and timolol maleate drops. Pain control with acetaminophen plus 60 mg codeine or another strong analgesic is also an important aspect of therapy. While this initial treatment is carried out, ophthalmologic consultation must be sought for further management. If an ophthalmologist is not immediately available, the eye should be pressure patched until one arrives.

Central Retinal Artery Occlusion

Central retinal artery occlusion is usually an embolic phenomenon characterized by sudden, painless, unilateral visual loss. Fundus examination reveals markedly narrowed arterioles, a milky edematous retina, and a cherry-red spot in the macula. While often unsuccessful, immediate treatment must be instituted nonetheless if there is to be any chance for recovery of visual acuity. Treatment includes digital massage of the affected eye and rebreathing into a paper bag or inhalation of a mixture of 95% O_2 and 5% CO_2. Intravenous acetazolamide and mannitol also may help to lower intraocular pressure and dislodge the embolus. An ophthalmologist should be sought for further management and, if necessary, to perform an anterior chamber paracentesis.

Elevated Intraocular Pressure—Glaucoma

An acute elevation in intraocular pressure requires vigorous treatment to prevent optic nerve damage. This is a true

TABLE 23–1. EYEDROP INSTILLATION PROCEDURE

1. Wash hands prior to instillation.
2. Check for correct medication and dosage instructions.
3. Consistently start with either right or left eye (prevents confusion if interrupted).
4. Have the patient look upward, tilting head backward.
5. Place either forefinger or thumb on bony rim of eye socket above cheek. Gently draw down lower eyelid, thus forming a small pocket between the lid and eye.
6. Instill ointment/drops into the pocket. Approximately 1/2 inch of ointment is sufficient.
7. Have the patient close the eye gently, allowing medication to evenly coat the eye.

emergency and always requires an immediate ophthalmological consult. Generally, pressure elevations between 30 and 40 mm Hg can be successfully lowered with a regimen of 2% pilocarpine HCl, one drop every 15 minutes for 1 hour, and then one drop every 6 hours, as well as 0.5% timolol maleate drops initially and every 12 hours. Apraclonidine 1% drops also may be helpful. If pressure fails to lower within 30 to 60 minutes or is higher than 40 mm Hg, then 500 mg intravenous or intramuscular acetazolamide is given as well as intravenous mannitol (1.0 to 2.0 gm/kg) and oral glycerol (1.0 to 1.5 gm/kg). Additional therapy is helpful in specific situations. If the lens is ruptured or is dislocated into the anterior chamber, surgical removal is necessary. If pupillary block or angle closure glaucoma is present, a surgical or YAG laser iridotomy is required. In alkali injuries, paracentesis of the anterior chamber with a phosphate buffer irrigation solution may be helpful. When hyphema is associated with acute intraocular pressure increases, pilocarpine drops are not used. Instead, a cycloplegic/mydriatic such as 5% homatropine or 0.25% scopolamine HCl is used with the other previously mentioned general measures. Paracentesis to irrigate blood from the anterior chamber may be necessary.

Hyphema

Hyphema (blood in the anterior chamber) often accompanies severe blunt and perforating ocular trauma. Until otherwise proven, the globe should be considered perforated in the presence of a hyphema and, therefore, should be protected with a plastic or metal shield or some other protection, e.g., a cardboard cup. An ophthalmologist should be consulted for further management. If the globe is intact, the involved eye should be dilated and kept dilated with a mydriatic/cycloplegic to prevent synechiae formation and to view the fundus. Both the visual acuity and the intraocular pressure should be evaluated. In general, all patients with hyphema need to be admitted to the hospital to facilitate daily examination of intraocular pressure and to decrease the incidence of rebleeding. However, adults with normal intraocular pressure and less than 15 per cent of the anterior chamber filled with blood can be managed at home. The usual hospital regimen consists of bed rest with bathroom privileges and patching of the involved eye for the prevention of rebleeding. Rebleeding has its maximum incidence 3 to 5 days after the initial trauma and can result in additional ocular pathology. Aminocaproic acid in a dose of 50 mg/kg orally every 4 hours (maximum dose 30 gm/24 hr) may be used to prevent rebleeding. Although this does not improve resorption of blood, it inhibits fibrinolysis of the clot at the site of the injured vessel.

There are several criteria for surgical intervention to prevent serious ocular complications associated with hyphema. Paracentesis and/or aspiration of the hyphema are the most common procedures to evacuate blood from the anterior chamber and to lower intraocular pressure. To prevent optic atrophy, surgery must be performed before the intraocular pressure has reached an average level of 50 mm Hg or higher for 5 days or 35 mm Hg or higher for 7 days. To prevent permanent opacification of the cornea from blood staining, surgery must be performed before the intraocular pressure has reached an average level of 25 mm Hg or higher for 6 days or if there is any indication of blood staining. To prevent the formation of anterior synechiae (adhesions of the iris to the trabecular meshwork, which can cause angle closure glaucoma), surgery must be performed before a total hyphema has persisted for 5 days or a diffuse hyphema for 9 days. The late incidence of glaucoma in patients with hyphema and damage to the aqueous drainage system (trabecular meshwork and anterior chamber angle) is significant. For this reason, it is necessary to carefully and routinely evaluate these patients for increases in intraocular pressure over many years after their traumatic episode.

Penetrating and Perforating Injuries

Penetrating and perforating injuries of the ocular structures are a major cause of traumatic visual loss. Such injuries may occur in isolation or in association with severe injuries including lacerations and fractures of facial structures or other areas of the body. Failure to aggressively manage lacerations of the cornea and sclera will almost assuredly result in visual loss.

When it is suspected that an injured patient has a ruptured globe, an eye shield or paper cup should be taped over the injured eye before any further manipulation of the patient is carried out. This prevents the application of any pressure on the periocular structures or the globe itself, which can result in the extrusion of the ocular contents with severe and irreparable ocular damage. Treatment of all non-life-threatening injuries of the face and head should be deferred until an ophthalmologist can evaluate the extent of the ocular injuries. In general, the surgical repair of penetrating or perforating ocular trauma can be delayed until all specialized ophthalmic surgical equipment, such as an ophthalmic operating microscope and vitrectomy instrumentation as well as skilled operating room staff, is available. In the interim, appropriate radiological evaluation, particularly thin-cut axial and coronal CT for the visualization of intraocular foreign bodies, laboratory tests, cultures, and administration of antibiotics and tetanus prophylaxis can be carried out.

Exploration/Repair of Globe

If there is any question concerning the presence of a penetrating ocular injury, the globe should be thoroughly explored while the patient is under general anesthesia. In general, every attempt should be made to salvage or to repair any lacerated globe. Such surgery is performed with the patient under general anesthesia. It is often complicated and can require several hours to perform. Few ruptured globes need to undergo primary enucleation due to the extent of the injuries they have sustained; if necessary, this procedure can be performed as late as 9 days after the initial attempt at repair.

Enucleation

The major indication for enucleation of a severely injured nonrepairable perforated globe or a globe following an initial repair attempt is the prevention of sympathetic ophthalmia. This is characterized by a severe, bilateral, granulomatous uveitis. It manifests as early as 9 days following penetrating ocular injury to as late as years later. It occurs in 3 to 5 per cent of eyes with such injuries. Although its exact etiology is unknown, it appears that the inflammation in the noninjured eye is an autoimmune response to the retinal S antigen from the injured eye. If untreated, the inflammatory response will result in bilateral loss of vision. Aggressive use of oral steroids is necessary to manage sympathetic ophthalmia, since enucleation will not improve this condition after the immune response has occurred. Therefore, in those cases in which enucleation is considered, such as a blind eye or one with severe irreparable damage, the procedure generally should be performed within 9 days following the initial injury to prevent any autoimmune response.

Orbital Fractures

Management of orbital fractures must be considered in the context of both functional and cosmetic deficits. Patients usually present with periorbital swelling (see Fig. 23–10), ecchymosis, crepitus, proptosis, chemosis, subconjunctival hemorrhage, ophthalmoplegia (decreased movement of the globe) (Fig. 23–24), infraorbital and buccal anesthesia, and palpable deficits in the bony orbital rims. Orbital fractures can be associated with optic nerve trauma as well as globe perforation. These must be managed as described elsewhere in this chapter. Radiological studies are essential for determining the extent of any orbital fractures. Immediate repair of these fractures is not necessary: The treatment of other injuries, especially those to the globe and optic nerve, may take precedence. As previously mentioned, if the globe is perforated, there should be no manipulation of the orbital bones or eyelids. Nose blowing should be discouraged because this may lead to the development of intraorbital and intraeyelid air, which can cause proptosis, pressure on the globe, and pressure on the optic nerve, with possible loss of vision. Since the extensive swelling associated with orbital injury may mask the true deficits that are present, waiting 7 to 10 days for this to subside can be very beneficial for determining further treatment. Both swelling and muscle entrapment can be causes of ophthalmoplegia. Forced duction testing (see Fig. 23–8) can help to determine whether either of these is present or whether there is nerve damage or muscle contusion. Indications for surgery include diplopia in primary gaze and downward gaze that shows no sign of spontaneous improvement, enophthalmos of 2 mm or more, and hypophthalmos (see Fig. 23–10) of 2 mm or more. Rim fractures with a 2-mm or greater displacement of the bony fragments and flattening of the malar eminence are indications for open reduction and wiring. Midfacial fractures and telecanthus and Le Fort fractures generally require repair.

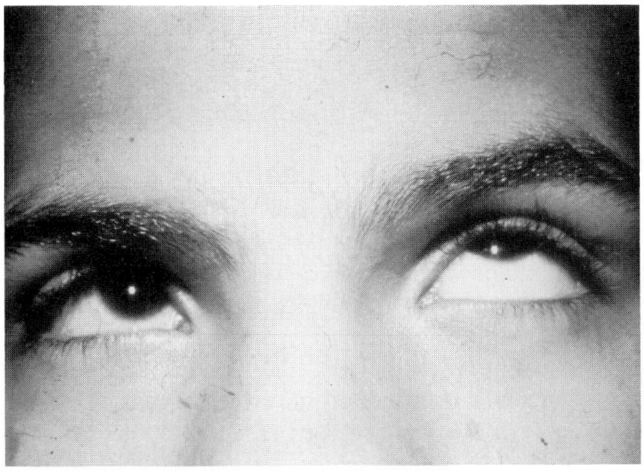

Figure 23–24. Orbital fracture with decreased upward mobility.

A

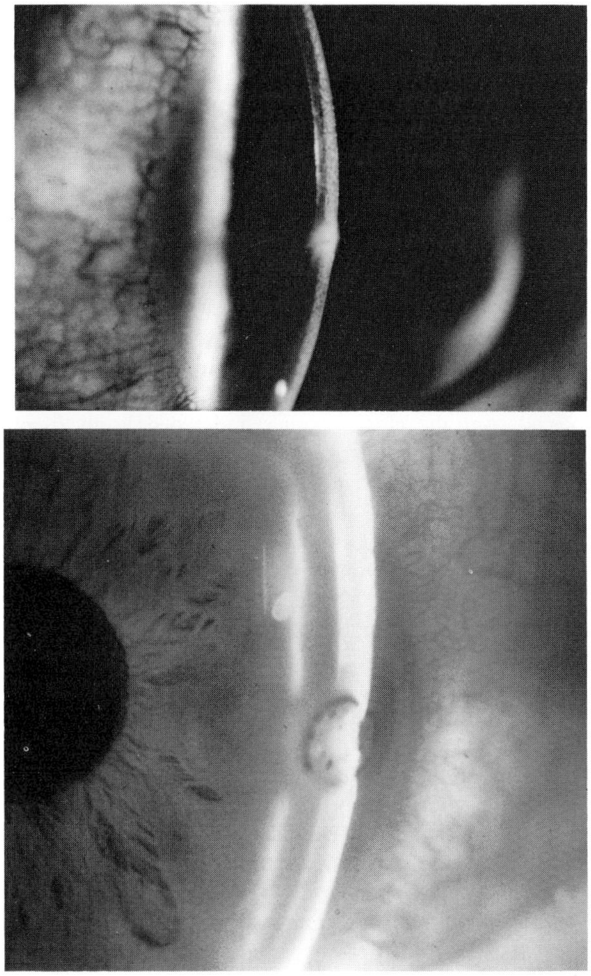

B

Figure 23–25. *A*, Foreign body (rose thorn) embedded in cornea. *B*, Rust ring after removal of foreign body.

Complications of orbital fracture repair include permanent loss of vision, persistent enophthalmos and diplopia, scarring and eyelid retraction, and implant extrusion. Some patients may feel that the cosmetic deficit does not justify surgery and its possible complications. Finally, fractures can easily be repaired 3 to 4 weeks after trauma, with only a slight increase in the difficulty over that of earlier repair.[8]

Corneal Foreign Bodies

The management of corneal foreign bodies (Fig. 23–25), corneal abrasions, and radiation injuries to the cornea (e.g., from welding arcs or sun lamps) is similar in certain aspects. Anesthetic drops and fluorescein staining to facilitate examination and short-acting cycloplegic drops, antibiotic drops, and firm pressure patching for 24 to 48 hours are the mainstays of management of these injuries. Topical anesthetic drops are essential for removing foreign bodies. If a foreign body is suspected or seen, it must be removed. Both the upper and lower eyelids need to be everted, and any clinging particulate matter must be removed. A cotton-tipped applicator can be used to remove superficial conjunctival foreign bodies. Some corneal foreign bodies also can be removed in this manner. More often, a 23- or 25-gauge needle on the end of a tuberculin syringe is needed to pry the foreign body from the cornea. To facilitate this maneuver and prevent perforation of the cornea, a slit lamp or high-powered loupe should be used. A small, hand-held, battery-driven burr can be used to remove rust rings associated with metallic foreign bodies. Deeply embedded foreign bodies should be removed by an ophthalmologist.[9] Contact lenses are another type of foreign body often requiring removal as part of trauma management. Hard lenses can be removed with a suction cup and soft lenses with fingertip manipulation (see Fig. 23–20). Lenses need to be placed in storage solution after removal and given to the patient. They may be reworn 2 or 3 days after a corneal abrasion has healed. An essential aspect of the management of corneal abrasions is pressure patching the eye for 24 to 48 hours. Two eyepads should be placed over the closed eyelids and taped firmly in place. Tape is positioned diagonally across the pads from the lower ear to the middle of the forehead. After patching for 24 hours, the cornea is reexamined for healing or persistent abrasion. Repatching for an additional 24 hours may be necessary. Certain abrasions, such as those caused by fingernails or paper, have a tendency to recur over a period of months or years after the initial incident. Often this necessitates the chronic use of sodium chloride drops or ointments at bedtime and upon awakening.[10]

Corneal Erosion

A corneal erosion can be caused by abnormal eyelid position, such as ectropion or lid retraction, abnormal eyelashes (trichiasis), poorly fitted contact lenses, abnormalities of the eyelid margin, an inadequate tear film, an inability to close the eyelids, poor closure of the eyelids during blinking, or infrequent blinking. Traumatic facial nerve damage is frequently associated with corneal abnormalities, as is eyelid and conjunctival scarring and injury. As with the opposite condition, traumatic ptosis, improvement in eyelid closure and blinking may occur spontaneously over 6 to 12 months. In the interim, vigorous use of artificial tears and ointments, as frequently as every hour, is essential. Pressure patching after taping the eyelids shut may be needed initially to allow the healing of large erosions. Surgical correction of eyelid abnormalities may be required in some cases. If drops and ointments are inadequate to prevent continued exposure keratopathy, taping the eyelids shut, various types of suture tarsorrhaphies, a cellophane vapor barrier, or various surgical tarsorrhaphies may be necessary. It is essential that patients with corneal pathology due to exposure be managed vigorously to prevent ocular discomfort and blepharospasm as well as permanent scarring, corneal ulcers, and corneal perforation.

Subconjunctival Hemorrhage

Subconjunctival hemorrhage and chemosis (see Fig. 23–24) frequently occur following trauma. Although these may herald serious intraocular and orbital trauma, they often occur as isolated signs. The management of these problems in the absence of more serious trauma involves waiting and watching. Generally, both subconjunctival hemorrhages and chemosis will resolve over a 1- to 3-week period. In extreme instances of conjunctival prolapse and drying, ocular ointments may be helpful in maintaining an intact conjunctiva.

A mild inflammatory reaction frequently occurs after blunt trauma. This is associated with photophobia, aching pain, perilimbal infection, minimally decreased vision, and either increased or decreased intraocular pressure. After serious ocular injury is eliminated by a thorough ocular examination, symptomatic relief can be achieved through the use of short-acting cycloplegic/mydriatic drops and topical steroid drops four times a day for 7 to 10 days.

Optic Nerve Injuries

Severe penetrating orbital injury can result in sudden visual loss. This type of injury is most frequently caused by a handgun, shotgun, or knife. Trauma to the optic nerve also can occur in association with blunt orbital trauma as well as orbital fractures. Loss of vision can be due to transection or avulsion of the optic nerve, optic nerve sheath hemorrhage, pressure on the optic nerve from bone fragments, orbital hemorrhage, direct contusion of the nerve, or disruption of the blood supply to the nerve and glove. Often, such injuries are irreversible. However, every effort must be made to try to restore vision. As an essential part of any evaluation of such injuries, a visual acuity must be obtained, if possible, and the pupils examined for an afferent defect. Thin-cut (1.5-mm) axial and coronal CT scans of the optic nerve and canal are important for evaluating the extent of optic nerve injury. Surgical intervention, such as unroofing the optic canal or opening the optic nerve sheath, may be required in those cases in which there is a nerve sheath hemorrhage or fracture of the optic canal. Intravenous high-dose steroids are essential for managing such injuries. The usual dosage in these cases is the same as for spinal cord injury: methylprednisolone, 30 mg/kg intravenously infused over a 20- to 30-minute period followed by an intravenous infusion of 5.4 mg/kg/hr for each of the next 23 hours. No further treatment is given after this 24 hours of infusion. An alternative to this regimen is an initial 30 mg/kg intravenous infusion followed by 15 mg/kg 2 hours later and at 6-hour intervals. Improvement in visual function has been seen even if therapy is begun several days following injury. However, initiation of treatment within the first 12 to 24 hours following injury gives the best chance for visual recovery.

Conjunctivitis

The management of conjunctivitis is based on the recognition of the etiological factors involved. Bacterial conjunctivitis (Fig. 23–26) is characterized by a copious purulent or mucopurulent discharge composed of polymorphonuclear leukocytes, bacterial organisms, and epithelial cells. The conjunctiva is usually markedly infected. Chemosis and subconjunctival hemorrhage may be present. After the discharge is cultured and Gram stained, treatment consists of broad-spectrum antibiotic drops or ointments every 3 to 4 hours for 7 to 10 days.

There are two exceptions to this treatment regimen. If a corneal ulcer is present, immediate ophthalmologic consultation should be sought, the patient should be admitted to the hospital, and vigorous topical therapy (every 30 minutes) should be started with fortified antibiotic drops such as gentamicin and bacitracin. If a fungal ulcer is present, appropriate antifungal therapy must be initiated. If gonococcal conjunctivitis is diagnosed, intravenous or intramuscular penicillin is necessary as well as topical erythromycin ophthalmic ointment.

Viral conjunctivitis is characterized by a minimal watery

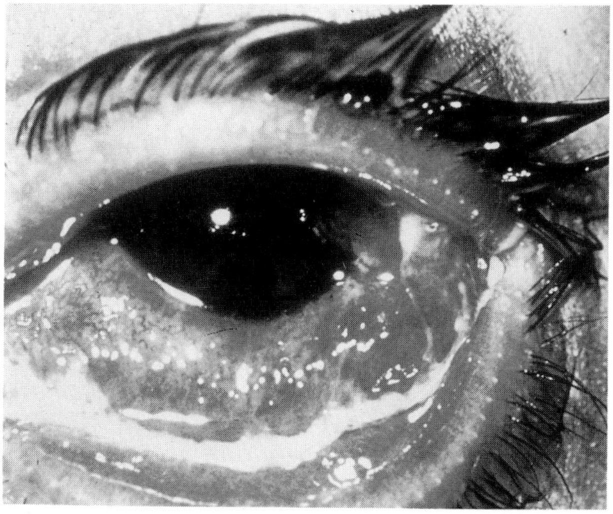

Figure 23–26. Bacterial conjunctivitis. (Reprinted with permission from Red Eye. San Francisco, American Academy of Ophthalmology, 1984.)

discharge, moderate conjunctival infection and hemorrhage, and palpable and sometimes painful preauricular nodes. Treatment is supportive and consists of topical tear supplements, ocular decongestants, and, in cases of herpes simplex virus, topical antiviral agents. Viral conjunctivitis is self-limited and generally lasts 10 to 14 days. Topical steroids should not be used in cases of viral conjunctivitis.

Allergic conjunctivitis is characterized by pruritus, mild to moderate conjunctival infection, and stringy discharge. Treatment involves avoidance of the responsible allergen, cold compresses, ocular antihistamines, ocular cromolyn sodium drops, and topical steroid drops.

Toxic conjunctivitis is related to a variety of ocular preparations, including antibiotics, antivirals, mydriatic/cycloplegics, and contact lens preparations. It is characterized by moderate infection, pain, and scant watery discharge. Treatment consists of identifying and discontinuing the offending agent and topical steroid preparations.

Other causes of ocular discharge are eyelid malpositions, exposure keratitis, and tear drainage abnormalities. The discharge in these situations ranges from watery to mucoid, with minimal to moderate conjunctival infection. Treatment is generally surgical and is related to the specific abnormality present.

Cellulitis

Preseptal or periorbital cellulitis (Fig. 23–27*A*) is commonly associated with breaks in the periorbital or eyelid skin occurring with both blunt and penetrating trauma. Several days may elapse between the time of injury and the occurrence of cellulitis. Commonly, there is marked eyelid edema and skin erythema. Usually, there is some degree of fluctuance in addition to skin tautness and inflammation. Edema may extend to the opposite lid and cheek and may be so severe as to prevent elevation of the eyelid in order to examine the globe. Associated with these suppurative changes are purulent drainage and superficial abscess formation (Fig. 23–27*A*). Despite the apparent severity of the adnexal signs, the globe is usually normal unless it is perforated. Proptosis, loss of vision, full ocular motility, and pain on eye motion are usually absent in contrast to orbital cellulitis. Usually, the patient does not appear ill. Staphylococci, streptococci, and hemophili are the most common pathogens. Treatment consists of oral antibiotics and incision and drainage of any suppurative area. In severe cases, intravenous antibiotics may be required.

Orbital cellulitis (Fig. 23–27*B*) is a serious disease and is associated with severe ocular, intracranial, and systemic morbidity, including loss of vision from optic nerve damage, glaucoma, corneal and retinal damage, brain abscess, cavernous sinus thrombosis, and sepsis. Patients appear ill and have a fever and leukocytosis. While the periorbital structures may appear normal, conjunctival hyperemia and chemosis, pain on eye movement, proptosis, resistance to globe retropulsion, increased intraocular pressure, and visual loss are signs of orbital cellulitis. There may be an associated orbital or subperiosteal abscess. The causes of this severe infective process may be exogenous (penetrating trauma or postoperative) or, more frequently, secondary to a paranasal sinusitis or oral infections. CT scan and orbital ultrasonography are important diagnostic modalities for determining the extent of the orbital disease process; CT scan is essential for assessing sinus and intracranial disease. It is important to obtain the aid of an otolaryngologist as well as an ophthalmologist to manage orbital cellulitis adequately. Intravenous antibiotics as well as sinus drainage are the mainstays of therapy. While cavernous sinus thrombosis may result from orbital cellulitis, it also may occur independently and be difficult to distinguish from orbital cellulitis. Patients with

A

B

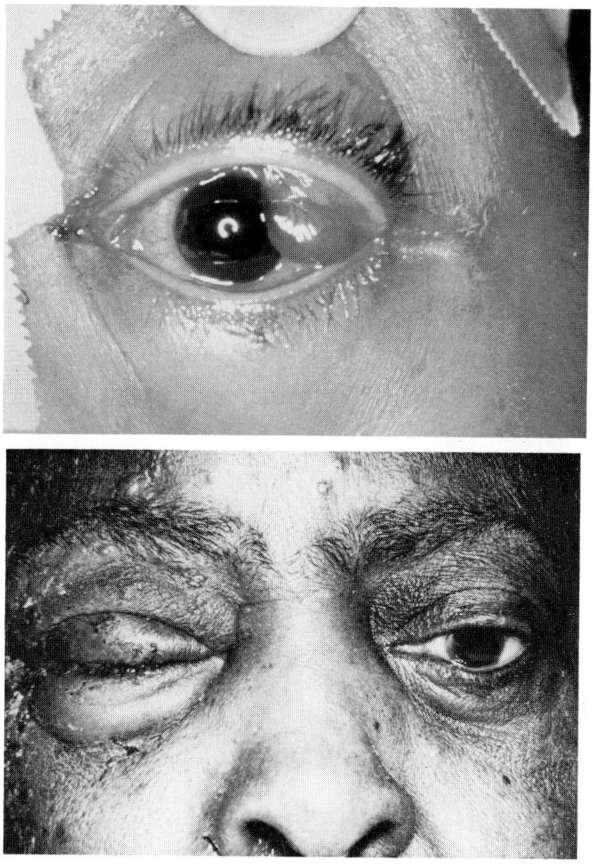

Figure 23–27. *A*, Periorbital cellulitis. *B*, Orbital cellulitis.

this process appear severely ill and have fever, nausea, vomiting, headache, and altered levels of consciousness in addition to some of the signs of orbital cellulitis. In addition, orbital pain is absent and cranial nerves III, IV, and VI are impaired owing to their compression within the cavernous sinus.

CRITICAL CARE/INTERMEDIATE CARE

Following the two initial phases (field management and initial resuscitation), the acute phase of nursing care will continue to place a high demand for physical care, patient and family education, and a significant emphasis on psychological and emotional support.

The major responsibility of the nurse during this cycle relates to the physical care of the patient with ocular injury. It is essential to closely monitor the patient for signs of infection, further visual loss, increasing pain, hemorrhage, or other complications. These changes must be promptly reported to the ophthalmologist so that proper therapy can be instituted and further visual loss prevented.

Pain Related to Ocular Injury

Pain evaluation is another important aspect of patient care. Although there is usually minimal or moderate pain following ocular surgery and trauma, pain medications and sedation may be helpful in many cases. Continuous ice compresses for the first 24 hours following eyelid surgery or orbital surgery will decrease swelling and its associated pain. Warm compresses over the next 48-hour period also may be helpful in reducing swelling. Keeping the head of the bed elevated to 30 degrees also may aid in promoting patient comfort. Increasing pain should be considered an indication for further ophthalmologic evaluation.

Potential for Disruption of Suture Site Related to Activity/Elevated Intraocular Pressure

Following surgical repair of many isolated traumatic ocular injuries, patients are often discharged to home within 1 to 2 days after the injury. Similarly, patients sustaining ocular injury requiring surgical intervention in conjunction with injuries to other body systems that are not of a critical nature may be ambulatory almost immediately. Patients in either of these situations are at risk for disruption of the surgical repair due to elevated intraocular pressure and accidental blunt trauma to the operative site. It is important that any eye which has undergone intraocular surgery be protected at all times with either a metal or plastic eye shield to prevent accidental trauma to the globe.

Elevated intraocular pressure may result from hemorrhage or edema following surgical repair. As previously stated, prolonged or sudden increases in intraocular pressure may lead to partial or total visual loss. Thus nursing measures must focus on the prevention of increased pressure and accurate assessment to detect its presence early. Activities that increase intraocular pressure include coughing, gagging, lying flat or in the Trendelenburg position, straining for bowel movements, bending over, and/or lifting heavy objects. In patients who have sustained ocular injury in conjunction with other system injuries, it is particularly challenging to institute effective nursing measures that will not potentially increase intraocular pressure. For instance, sedation and/or antiemetics may be necessary to prevent persistent coughing and/or vomiting.

Chest physiotherapy, which might normally be a routine intervention to prevent atelectasis and clear secretions, may be contraindicated for the patient who sustains thoracic injury in conjunction with an ocular injury.

Ambulatory patients must be cautioned not to lift heavy objects or to bend over to pick up objects. Stooping to retrieve objects is an acceptable alternative. Unnecessary coughing and/or sneezing should be avoided. Laxatives or stool softeners may be necessary to prevent straining for bowel elimination.

Fear Related to Lack of Education Regarding Ocular Injury

Teaching during the acute cycle should include information regarding the injury and its management, the symptoms the patient may expect, preoperative and postoperative management, and therapeutic interventions, especially regarding pressure patching, ocular medication, pain, and restrictions on mobility and activities.

Psychological Dysfunction Related to Potential or Actual Loss of Vision Secondary to Ocular Injury

Psychological and emotional support is essential for the temporarily or permanently, partially or totally visually impaired person.[11] Visual loss has been considered the "ultimate catastrophe" throughout the ages. Only death is feared more. For this reason, the person who has suffered a loss of vision requires increased support from medical personnel, friends, and family. The impact of blindness may be so severe as to require professional counseling to adjust to this unfamiliar situation. The emotional effects of shock, denial, and anger a patient experiences in order to adapt to a permanent visual loss are similar to the grieving process one experiences with the loss of a loved one (see Chapter 10).

The partially or totally blinded individual has lost the way he normally processed information from the environment. The major sense through which information is processed from the environment has now been eradicated. The individual is faced with learning new ways to retrieve and process this information. Activities of daily living and all social interactions are drastically altered. Pity and oversolicitousness on the part of the sighted are counterproductive in allowing a person to adapt to the new situation. Traditional agencies and/or schools for the blind may be helpful but also may emphasize the disability that is present and may further isolate an individual from the mainstream of society. Families of the newly blinded may encounter serious financial burdens if the wage earner has been disabled, and they must adjust their life-styles and activities of daily living to accommodate the patient with a visual disability within the home environment. Loss of sight for the adolescent, young people embarking on careers, or the elderly imposes additional psychological as well as financial adjustment.

The nurse, because of her continuous interaction with the patient, plays a significant role during the immediate period after a visual handicap is sustained. An understanding of her own fears, concerns, and anxieties is imperative to enable the nurse to individualize the care given to each patient.

To assist in alleviating fears of the unknown, frequent orientation to date, time, and place is necessary. Frequent orientation to the unfamiliar environment (including noises and smells) and introducing each person entering the patient's room are essential. The nurse or other health team members interacting with the patient should describe themselves (color of eyes, hair, height, weight), since the patient can now visualize people and the environment only through description. Ask the patient to "feel" your face if this will assist him. "Long distance" information is brought into the person through the sensory modality of vision. Size, dimension, color, shape, and density of objects are all normally quickly processed visually. With loss of vision, this input and assessment of the environment and people within it are lost. Only "short-distance" information receptors are available now to analyze the environment. The patient must now use other senses to bring in this information. This relearning takes time and requires thought, sensitivity, and above all patience from the care providers. Allow the patient to feel and smell objects. Describe them in color. Approach the patient with unilateral visual impairment from the sighted side. Explain procedures prior to carrying them out, and promote environmental stimulation through conversation, radio, television, or audio tapes.

The use of touch is also extremely important—a gentle hand on an arm or shoulder carries a message of concern and caring. Whether the visual loss is temporary or permanent, the absence of this vital and major sense is devastatingly frightening. Frequently, ocular trauma is not an isolated injury, especially if the patient has been involved in a motor vehicle or industrial accident. Multiple system trauma, combined with circumstances of the accident (if family or friends were involved), prognosis, pain, and potential morbidity, contributes to anxiety and fear, compounding the feelings of complete powerlessness felt by the patient. A gentle touch conveys many messages to a frightened patient—caring, concern, and a desire to help. It is reassuring and comforting to a patient to be able to identify a voice and gentle touch together. Anxiety, fear, and apprehension can be diminished, promoting a less terrifying experience for the patient and an easier recovery process.

In the acute phase of hospitalization, it may be difficult to promote the patient's sense of independence. Within the limitations imposed by other injuries and the patient's general condition, if the patient can assist with any small tasks, even as simple as washing his hands and arms, a sense of accomplishment is attained. As the patient faces needs requiring special considerations, so does the family.

Psychiatrists, psychologists, social workers, and spiritual leaders are important in helping the patient's family and the patient to adapt. Contact with rehabilitative services (occupational therapy, vocational rehabilitation, and community agencies providing services for the visually impaired) should be initiated and evaluated for future appropriateness of the available services for the particular and individualized needs of specific patients.

As the patient enters intermediate care, responsibility for physical care shifts from nurses (as in acute care) to the patient. Support measures outlined for the acute phase remain important throughout the hospitalization and are no less vital at this stage.

Potential for Self-Harm Related to Visual Impairment

The patient, depending on his general condition and injuries, should be encouraged to participate in personal care, which will promote a sense of independence. The patient's immediate environment will probably expand beyond the hospital bed to that of the hospital. The environment must be safe, stable, organized, and consistent for the person whose sight will not protect him from dangers. For a mobile patient this is crucial—the patient must be protected from sharp-edged furniture and equipment, small objects easily tripped over, objects that can be broken easily and cause injury, or objects hanging on walls or the ceilings. For this reason, environmental structure should be reorganized and the nurse should instruct the patient on the content and confines of the room. Since vision provides many clues relating to distance, simply explaining how far away something is may not be sufficient. Walking off the number of steps to the bathroom with the patient will be more meaningful. Activities of daily living (ADL) should be a part of the patient's therapy for recovery. Bathing and feeding oneself are usually the first tasks encouraged and accomplished. Consistency in the placement of objects in the room (e.g., phone on left side of bedstand, tissues on right, fork at left of plate) facilitates the patient's independence. Occupational therapists can greatly aid in helping a patient learn new ways to perform ADL. For a sense of security, a call bell or other means of attracting assistance when needed is important. The patient also may be taught how to perform simple tasks related to ocular therapy and management, e.g., the instillation of ocular medication or patching an eye.

As the trauma patient becomes less acutely ill, the patient and family members become more aware of the full impact that a permanent visual deficit will have on their lives. The family and patient must be allowed time and support to grieve and deal with this devastating injury. They should be encouraged to verbalize their feelings and concerns within an accepting atmosphere and should be assisted in finding resources to help with transitions. It must be acknowledged that the patient's self-image will be dramatically altered—a father and husband may no longer be the provider for the family, a mother no longer able to care for her children without assistance.

The nursing staff and other persons (social workers, clergy, rehabilitation services personnel) involved with the patient and family can direct the patient's and family's energy into dealing with these changes by finding alternatives and resolutions to the problems.

Providing quality nursing care for the temporarily or permanently visually impaired is challenging and yet rewarding. As with any injury, reactions to ocular injury and its sequelae will be individual, but an awareness of potential reactions by the health care team facilitates more effective care planning. Table 23–2 illustrates additional potential

TABLE 23–2. POTENTIAL NURSING DIAGNOSES FOR PATIENTS WITH OCULAR INJURY

	NURSING INTERVENTIONS		
NURSING DIAGNOSIS	**CRITICAL CARE**	**INTERMEDIATE CARE**	**REHABILITATION**
1. Potential for infection related to the loss of skin, structural integrity	Monitor for signs and symptoms of infection: elevated WBCs, wound discharge, erythema, tenderness, pain, inflammation. Wound/dressing care q ____°. Clean with half-strength H_2O_2 and NS. Apply thin layer of ophthalmic bacitracin. Apply dry sterile dressing or leave open to air if no drainage is present. Monitor visual acuity q____°. Instill medication as ordered.	Monitor for signs and symptoms of infection. Wound/dressing care q ____°. Instruct patient/family in wound care, medication instillation, monitoring for infection.	Instruction for home care by patient/family regarding: Obtaining necessary supplies/ equipment, medication. Monitoring for signs/symptoms of infection. Wound care. Instillation of medication. Prevention of injury. Posthospital follow-up care.
2. Potential for feelings of powerlessness related to visual impairment	Introduce all personnel involved with patient care. Explain all procedures and noises to patient. Give patient choices when appropriate. Encourage patient assistance with ADL and treatments. Orient frequently. Provide means of communicating (if patient is intubated). Consult OT/PT.	Promote mobility. Promote patient's responsibility for ADL. Encourage selection and use of diversional activities.	Expand environment. Obtain OT/PT consultation. Interventions to promote independence and patient's ability to perform ADL: mobility, personal hygiene, nutritional intake, safety precautions. Increase scope of diversional activities.
3. Potential for alterations in sensory perception related to visual impairment	Orient frequently to time, place, surroundings, and personnel. Promote sensory stimulation through media, conversation, and touch. Consult OT/PT. Institute safety precautions for patient with limited mobility. Monitor sensory assessment. Initiate referrals for discharge planning: vocational rehabilitation agencies/ organizations such as Society for the Blind, family, visiting nurses, support groups.	Orient frequently. Increase sensory stimulation through media, touch, and visitors. Consult OT/PT. Maintain stable environment: decrease unnecessary stimuli, promote continuity of environment. Institute safety precautions for patient with increasing mobility. Referrals for discharge planning: vocational rehabilitation, Society for the Blind, family, visiting nurses, support groups. Teaching: patient/family, home safety precautions, alternate functional activities.	Orient prn. Maintain normal sensory stimulation. Consult OT/PT. Maintain stable environment. Safety precautions for ambulatory patient. Confirmation of discharge plans/ referrals: restatement of discharge instructions, printed instruction sheets for family members. Patient/family teaching: safety precautions, alternate functional activities.
4. Potential for altered body image related to visual impairment	Monitor behavior responses: grieving process, confusion, coping mechanisms. Family involvement for support/ grieving process, assessment of coping mechanisms. Initiate consults: psychiatrist, support groups, spiritual leader. Encourage patient to assist with ADL, e.g., bath, treatments.	Monitor behavior responses. Family involvement. Surgical cosmetic correction of injury/scar. Cosmetic correction prn. Promote independence of ADL. Promote socialization.	Monitor behavior responses. Family involvement. Promote independence of mobility. Increase socialization.

nursing diagnoses and nursing interventions in the critical care, intermediate, and rehabilitative cycles following ocular injury.[12]

REHABILITATION AND COMMUNITY INTEGRATION

Rehabilitation efforts actually begin in the critical care phase, where some planning can be started, and takes special prominence in the intermediate phase and as the patient prepares for discharge. Decisions regarding care are determined by the individual requirements of each patient. Discharge placement will depend on the information and advice from the many persons involved: patient, family, nurse, physician, social worker, and therapist. Some visually impaired persons may have the capability of being discharged directly home, utilizing support services, while others may benefit best from admission to a rehabilitation facility. Another consideration is the type of services and/or facilities offered in the region where the patient resides. Programs will vary in the type of services offered: day programs, halfway house settings, or intensive overnight facilities.

The goal during this phase of recovery is to prepare the visually impaired person for a life of independence within the limitation of the disability. The patient must be encouraged and motivated to attain his maximum potential of independent functioning. Promotion of self-esteem, personal value, and self-confidence is essential for maximum recovery as well as learning to master living in a sightless world. Learning Braille and independent household management and increasing mobility (possibly using a seeing eye dog or cane) are examples of the priorities of this recovery phase. Rehabilitation is carried out closely in conjunction with community integration.

Community integration must be planned and initiated well before the patient is ready to go home, either from the hospital or rehabilitation facility. Housing arrangements and the availability of home care for the patient must be evaluated. Some patients may benefit from a visiting nurse to assess their progress. Some patients may need the temporary assistance of a delivered meal program. Each patient's needs require individualized evaluation for safe discharge planning. The nurse needs to utilize community resources fully for improved patient care at home. The patient, the family, and the involved health care providers should have a thorough understanding of the care required, including medications, activities, restrictions, signs and symptoms of complications, physician's follow-up appointments, and actions to take in an emergency situation.

Patients and families need to be educated concerning state and federal tax relief, Social Security and Medicare benefits, travel discounts (both local and national), and vocational rehabilitation. An ophthalmologist, as an essential resource for the patient with a visual disability, should be knowledgeable about community agencies and services available for the visually disabled. Visiting nurse agencies are appropriate for assisting the patient in utilizing available community and national organizations (Table 23–3). Introductions to other patients with visual disabilities who have adapted to disabilities and are functioning as productive members of society will greatly help the newly blinded. Social workers are also a great help in this area as well as in the area of financial, vocational, and social resources. The ophthalmologist needs to educate the family and the patient regarding the disease process, the visual prognosis, and possible therapeutic interventions. A sourcebook for additional information is the *Directory of Agencies Serving the Visually Handicapped in the U.S.* (20th ed. New York, American Foundation for the Blind, 1981).

TABLE 23–3. RESOURCE ORGANIZATIONS FOR THE VISUALLY IMPAIRED

1. American Foundation for the Blind, 15 W 16th St, New York, NY 10011
2. Independent Living Aids, Inc, 11 Commerical Ct, Plainview, NY 13137
3. National Braille Association, 85 Goodwin Ave, Midland Park, NJ 07432
4. Division for the Blind and Physically Handicapped of the Library of Congress, Washington, DC 20542
5. National Association for the Visually Handicapped, 205 E 24th St, 17-C, New York, NY 10010
6. National Federation of the Blind, Dupont Circle Building, Suite 212, 1346 Connecticut Ave, NW, Washington, DC 20036
7. National Association for Parents of the Visually Impaired, 2011 Hardy Circle, Austin, TX 78757
8. American Academy of Ophthalmology, 1833 Fillmore, PO Box 7424, San Francisco, CA 94120
9. Veterans Administration
10. Social Security Administration
11. U.S. Department of Health and Human Services
12. State Departments of Rehabilition

SUMMARY

Familiarity with ocular anatomy and function and the ocular examination form the basis for managing ocular trauma. The prevention of permanent damage from trauma depends on the utilization of appropriate management techniques. More important, ocular trauma may be avoided if proper safety measures are taken in the workplace, at home, and during recreational activities. If permanent visual disability occurs despite appropriate protective measures and trauma management, a variety of individuals and groups are available to aid in the adjustment of patients to a severe disability and their reintegration into the mainstream of society.

Although nursing management of patients with ocular injuries has advanced significantly, there are still many unknowns in this field. How do we identify the patient's priorities for rehabilitation? What are the most effective methods for promoting independence for the visually impaired? How do nursing measures affect intraocular pressure and ultimately healing of the eye? Research in this particular area of traumatic injury is relatively limited compared with other areas, which receive greater emphasis (e.g., shock, sepsis, pulmonary insufficiency). With further research in both medical and nursing management of ocular injury, it is hoped that patients will have less chance for the development of complications and greater chances for normal vision following ocular trauma.

REFERENCES

1. Leading work-related diseases and injuries—United States. MMWR 33:213–215, 1984.
2. Morris RE, Witherspoon CD, Helms HA Jr, et al: Eye Injury Registry of Alabama (preliminary report): Demographics and prognosis of severe eye injury. South Med J 80:810–816, 1987.
3. White MF Jr, Morris R, Feist RM, et al: Eye injury: Prevalence and prognosis by setting. South Med J 82:151–158, 1989.
4. Karlson JA, Klein BE: The incidence of acute hospital-treated eye injuries. Arch Ophthalmol 104:1473–1476, 1986.
5. Records RE: Primary care of ocular emergencies. Postgrad Med 65:157–160, 303–317, 1979.
6. Duane TD (ed): Clinical Ophthalmology, vol 5. Philadelphia, JB Lippincott, 1985.
7. Linberg JV (ed): Oculoplastic and Orbital Emergencies. Norwalk, CT, Appleton & Lange, 1990.
8. Shingleton BJ, Hersh PS, Kenyon KR (eds): Eye Trauma. St. Louis, Mosby–Year Book, 1991.
9. Spoor TC, Nesi FA (eds): Management of Ocular, Orbital, and Adnexal Trauma. New York, Raven Press, 1988.
10. Deutsch TA, Feller DB: Paton and Goldberg's Management of Ocular Injuries, 2nd ed. Philadelphia, WB Saunders Co, 1985.
11. Fenwick A, Wiley L: Traumatic blindness: A flexible approach for helping a blind adolescent. Nursing 79(9):36–41, 1979.
12. Baunner LS, Suddarth DS: The Lippincott Manual of Nursing Practice. 2nd ed. Philadelphia, JB Lippincott, 1978.

24

GENITOURINARY INJURIES AND RENAL MANAGEMENT

JOCELYN FARRAR, CHRISTINE COTTINGHAM, and MARY MURPHY RUTTER

Rapid diagnosis and treatment of genitourinary (GU) trauma can be very difficult. The trauma victim's most immediate requirement is restoration of cellular perfusion via establishment of a patent airway and an adequate circulating volume. Once these basic life support measures are implemented, immediate monitoring of their efficacy must be instituted. Assessment of the GU system often begins with the insertion of a Foley catheter to monitor urine output (as a reflection of fluid balance and/or shock state). This chapter will address the assessment, treatment, and care of the patient experiencing GU trauma. Attention also will be paid to the sequelae of acute renal failure and its impact on the recovering trauma patient.

GU trauma may be defined as any injury to the kidney, its collecting system, or the reproductive system. The kidneys are generally not susceptible to direct trauma because they are protected by the twelfth thoracic and fifth lumbar vertebrae. They are anchored in place by Gerota's fascia, surrounded by fat pads, and capped with adrenal glands. The left kidney is further protected by the spleen, chest wall, diaphragm, pancreatic tail, and descending colon. The right kidney is 1 to 2 cm lower than the left and is surrounded by the diaphragm, liver, and duodenum. The ureters are cushioned bilaterally by abdominal contents and surrounded by the pelvic bones. The urinary bladder is protected anteriorly and laterally by the pubic arch. The pelvic diaphragm supports the bladder inferiorly; the peritoneum covers the bladder superiorly and posteriorly. These anatomical guardians are consistent in both sexes.

The female urethra is protected by the symphysis pubis, as is the vagina. The uterus lies midpelvis, halfway between the sacrum and the symphysis pubis. It rests on the pelvic diaphragm, supported by six ligaments, and is cushioned by bowels and bladder. This same anatomical protection is afforded the ovaries and fallopian tubes on either side of the uterus.

The longer male urethra consists of two segments: the anterior segment, which is distal to the urogenital diaphragm, and the posterior segment, which passes through the urogenital diaphragm and includes the prostatic segment before attaching to the bladder. Comparatively minor anatomical protection is afforded the male urethra as well as the penis and scrotal sac. These anatomical considerations are important factors in the occurrence of distal GU trauma in men.

EPIDEMIOLOGY

Injuries to the GU tract account for 10 to 15 per cent of all abdominal trauma.[1] The most commonly injured organs are the kidneys (84 per cent) and the bladder and the urethra (8 per cent each).[2] Injury to the urethra is more common in men than in women.[2] Trauma to the ureters is rarely seen and most often has iatrogenic causes.[2] Occasionally, penetrating trauma, such as knife and gunshot wounds, induces ureteral injury.[2]

GU trauma is rarely an isolated injury.[3, 4] Approximately 60 to 80 per cent of patients with blunt renal trauma have associated major injuries to other organs.[5, 6] Injuries most often associated with GU trauma include fracture of the pelvis, lower rib fractures, gunshot wounds to the abdomen, and fracture of the transverse process of the lumbar spine.[7] Injury to the right kidney is most often seen in association with injury to the liver.[6] Injury to the left kidney is often associated with coexisting injury to the spleen.[6]

GU trauma can contribute to significant morbidity and mortality. Kreiger and associates[8] reported an overall mortality rate of 6 per cent in patients with renal trauma and associated multisystem injuries. Sagalowsky and associates[9] found a mortality rate of 12 per cent among their renal trauma patients.

MECHANISM OF INJURY

GU trauma may be induced by external violence or iatrogenic causes.[7] External violence may produce either blunt or penetrating trauma, with blunt trauma contributing to approximately 80 per cent of all GU trauma.[4, 5] Blunt GU trauma can result from many sources. These include motor vehicle accidents (MVAs), assaults, sports injuries, and occupational injuries.

The acceleration–deceleration, or contrecoup, injury is produced when a body in motion is halted abruptly. This situation can occur during a fall onto a rigid surface or in an MVA when the occupant makes contact with the dashboard or steering wheel of the vehicle. The kidney is then set in motion on its pedicle in relation to the more stationary body and aorta.[3, 10] This mobility may tear the intima of the renal artery, resulting in renal artery thrombosis. Other consequences of this type of blunt injury include disruption of the ureteropelvic junction[10] and contusion of the renal parenchyma (Fig. 24–1).

Causes of penetrating trauma include gunshots, stabbings, and impalement. MVAs account for a majority of GU injuries (42 per cent), followed by gunshots and stabbings (28 per cent), falls (16.5 per cent), and sports accidents (12 per cent).[12] The tremendous energy absorbed by internal organs during an MVA may account for the number of GU injuries seen. During an MVA, an unbelted victim slides forward, the femur is compacted into the pelvis, and the abdomen strikes the steering wheel (Fig. 24–2). The kinetic energy is then diffused into the internal organ structures, including the bladder, spleen, kidneys, and liver, resulting

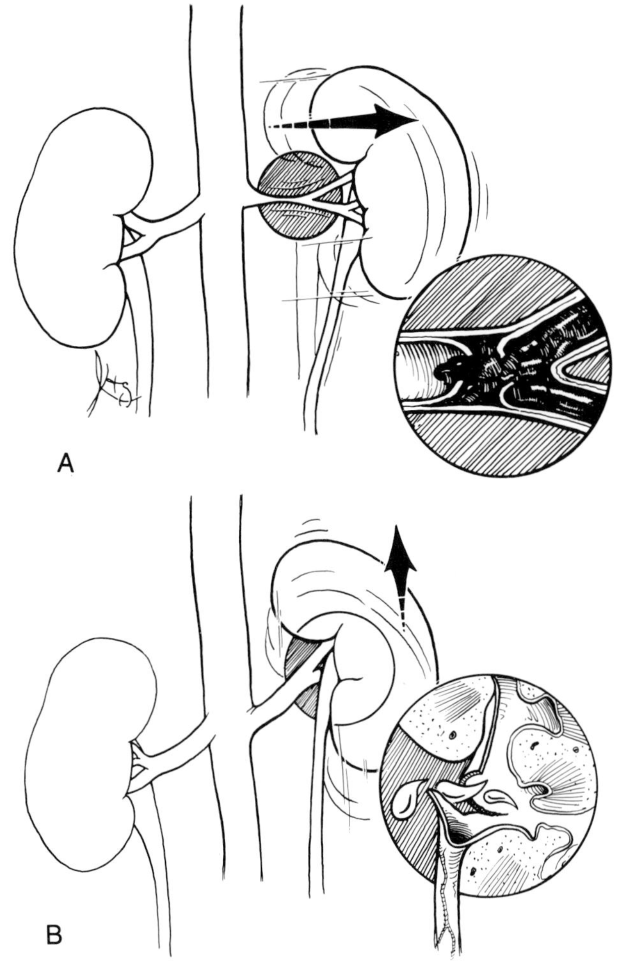

Figure 24–1. Acceleration–deceleration injury may produce disruption of renal artery *(A)*, and disruption of ureteropelvic junction *(B)*.

in traumatic injury. The use of seatbelts can decrease the incidence of organ injury by holding the occupant firmly against the seat and allowing the vehicle to absorb the impact of the collision.

Although the incidence of trauma to the ureters is rising with the increase in gunshot wounds, the most common cause of ureteral trauma remains accidental injury during surgery.[11] These iatrogenic injuries to the small ureters are most likely to occur during difficult pelvic procedures in which normal anatomical landmarks are obscured by obstruction, neoplasm, the effects of radiation, inflammation, congenital anomalies, or trauma displacement. Iatrogenic GU trauma also can result from radical surgery for malignancies, gynecological procedures, abdominal perineal resections, lumbar disk surgery, and laparoscopy.[7] A high index of suspicion must be established to detect and appropriately treat iatrogenic GU trauma.[7]

GENITOURINARY ASSESSMENT IN TRAUMA

The early detection of GU trauma is of paramount importance to optimal outcome in terms of organ salvage and patient survival. GU trauma may not present initially as a life-threatening situation, but delay in diagnosis and treatment can produce significant tissue loss from prolonged ischemia or from blood and urine extravasation.

Assessment of GU trauma is based on the results of multiple strategies. No one strategy is sufficient to diagnose GU trauma specifically. An accurate diagnosis is obtained through the interpretation of a multitude of diagnostic clues obtained from the history, physical examination, and radiologic and laboratory testing. In addition, the development of a high index of suspicion, based on knowledge of the mechanism of injury, assists in the detection of GU trauma when equivocal diagnostic results are obtained. GU trauma should be suspected in the following groups of patients: those with blunt mechanisms of injury associated with a fall or deceleration injury, MVA, or crushing incident; those with trauma to the abdomen, flank, lower chest, back, or pelvis[16]; anyone with a straddle injury; and those sustaining penetrating abdominal trauma.[10, 16, 17]

Accident Data Base

The initial step of the assessment is to obtain an accurate history of the events leading to injury.[14] Details about the mechanism of injury can provide valuable clues to the nature and extent of the GU trauma. For MVAs, it is important to determine the estimated speed of the vehicle when it crashed, the type of vehicle, and the use of seatbelts. What was the patient's position in the vehicle (driver, passenger)? Was the patient ejected from the vehicle?[14] When a patient sustains trauma from a fall, the height of the fall, objects struck during the fall, the patient's body position on landing, and the type of landing surface should be noted. Following penetrating trauma, information must be obtained regarding the type of weapon used (gun, knife, impaled object), the caliber of the gun, the size of the knife, and the occurrence of other events following the penetrating trauma (e.g., a fall).[14]

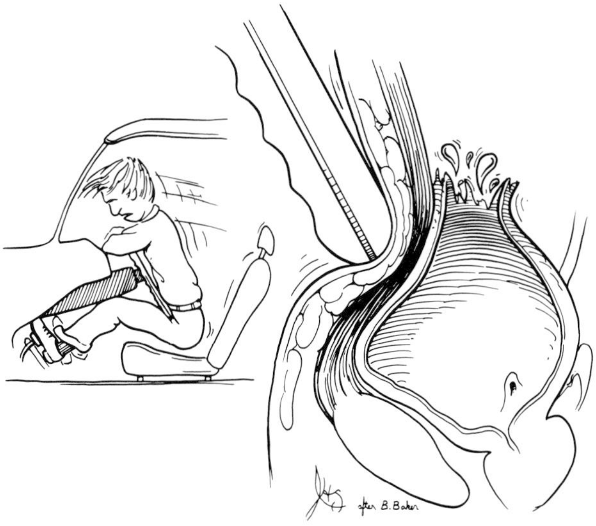

Figure 24–2. Compression injuries of abdomen that do not produce fracture may produce intraperitoneal bladder rupture. (From Guerriero WG, Devine CJ: Urologic Injuries. Norwalk, CT, Appleton-Century-Crofts, 1984, p 113.)

Various details about the condition of the patient at the scene of the trauma will affect clinical management decisions. Was the patient pinned in the vehicle, and what was the extrication time? Was there evidence of the use of drugs or alcohol? What care was provided in the field? Was there evidence of airway compromise or hemodynamic instability? Details such as these can be obtained from prehospital providers, witnesses, family, or police at the scene.[14]

Health History

A brief health history can provide valuable information that may help the nurse anticipate the patient's response to trauma. Essential information includes allergies, medications, previous diseases, last meal eaten, and the events leading to the trauma. Previous injuries, known anatomical abnormalities, and preexisting GU pathologies should be determined. The congenitally abnormal kidney is especially vulnerable to severe injury from minor trauma, so a history of tumors,[6] congenital hydronephrosis with cysts,[6] renal calculi,[6] polycystic disease,[6] and horseshoe or pelvic kidney[8] must be explored. Previous GU surgery may have contributed to the development of adhesions, strictures, or a predisposition to calculi formation or chronic GU infection, all of which can influence treatment modalities following GU trauma. Prior nephrectomy or previous GU disorders such as chronic renal failure, renal artery stenosis, or one of the glomerulopathies can influence profoundly both the initial treatment and long-term care of the trauma patient with GU injury.

Physical Examination

During the resuscitation phase, the assessment of life-threatening injuries to the cardiovascular, respiratory, and neurological systems takes priority.[1, 16] Until the patient is stabilized and the GU system can be assessed, a high index of suspicion should be maintained for GU trauma.

Inspection

The first phase of the physical examination is inspection. Abdominal and flank symmetry should be assessed[15]; evidence of torso or pelvic trauma may extend to evidence of GU trauma. The presence of a complex or open pelvic fracture,[16] the number of entrance/exit wounds due to penetrating trauma, or the position of impaled objects must be noted. Impaled objects should not be removed until the patient is in the operating room. Grey-Turner's sign, i.e., ecchymosis over the posterior aspect of the eleventh or twelfth rib or the flank, may indicate renal trauma or a retroperitoneal bleed.[15] Absence of this ecchymosis does not rule out renal trauma, since 24 per cent of patients with renal trauma do not have Grey-Turner's sign.[1, 15]

The urinary meatus must be inspected for signs of bleeding, which is a strong indicator of urethral injury.[10, 16] This assessment is of particular importance prior to passing a urinary catheter.[10] Attempting to pass a catheter past a urethral injury may convert a partial tear into a complete transection.[19] The perineal area should be assessed for evidence of trauma—lacerations, hematomas, swelling, or ecchymosis. A butterfly pattern of ecchymosis over the perineum is characteristic of urethral injury.[17] The scrotum may be edematous or contused because of extravasation of urine or blood in patients with urethral injury, pelvic fracture, or retroperitoneal hematoma.[17] Diffuse perineal bruising is a later sign of fracture of the symphysis pubis or pelvic rami.

The presence or absence of fractures must be noted.[4, 15] Fracture of the eleventh or twelfth rib or the lumbar transverse process may contribute to renal or ureteral injury.[17] Pelvic fractures may injure the urethra or bladder.[17]

A careful rectal examination should be performed. The presence of a palpable, boggy prostate or displacement of the prostate and bladder by an extravasated mass of blood and/or urine may indicate GU trauma.[16, 17] The flank must be inspected for signs of previous surgery. A patient who has had renal surgery for removal of a kidney is at greater risk if the remaining kidney has been injured.

Inability to void may indicate upper urinary tract injury, obstruction due to blood clots, bladder rupture with extravasation, or anuria.[17] Finally, the external genitalia should be inspected. In the male, lacerations and avulsion injuries to the penis and scrotum are readily apparent. Palpation of the scrotum establishes the presence and, to some extent, the condition of the testes. The female external genitalia are less easily examined. The external genitalia, mons, labia, and introitus may be visualized. The uterus and adnexa can be palpated using a bimanual abdominal and internal examination. In most blunt trauma patients, however, an internal examination is not necessary. For women with an altered level of consciousness, a brief internal examination should be performed to ascertain the presence of a tampon, diaphragm, or intrauterine device.

In blunt trauma patients with vaginal bleeding and/or pelvic fractures, the possibility of vaginal laceration should be considered. Evaluation for such injury is done under direct vision using a speculum or retractors. In the patient with a severe pelvic fracture, the examination usually must be done under anesthesia in an operating suite. Any patient with a penetrating wound that could have violated the vagina should have a speculum examination, particularly if there is vaginal bleeding. Such patients also should have an intravenous pyelogram and cystogram to evaluate for possible ureter and bladder injury. In both blunt and penetrating trauma with suspected or confirmed vaginal lacerations, rectal injury must be suspected. Such patients require a proctoscopic examination.

Auscultation

The presence and quality of bowel sounds must be assessed. Although the absence of bowel sounds is not specific to GU injury, a high index of suspicion must be maintained because trauma to other abdominal organ systems is frequently associated with GU trauma. Bowel sounds may be present or absent in patients with significant intra-abdominal injury.

Auscultation around the renal arteries is essential. A bruit in these areas may reflect turbulence at an intimal tear in the artery.[14]

Percussion

Percussion of the abdomen and flank allows assessment of abnormal areas of fluid or air collection.[15] Excessive dullness in the lower abdomen or flank may indicate the extravasation of blood or urine or the presence of a retroperitoneal hematoma.

Palpation

The flank, upper abdomen, lumbar vertebrae, and lower rib cage should be palpated for evidence of pain, mass, or crepitus—all potential indicators of GU trauma.[10, 15, 16] Renal colic or costovertebral angle pain may indicate renal trauma.[15] Renal colic may be the result of clots obstructing the renal collecting system.[15] Severe costovertebral angle pain may be caused by ischemia from a renal artery thrombosis.[10] Additional indicators of GU trauma include abdominal tenderness, with or without distention, a flank mass, or signs of a dislocated hip.[16]

The pelvic area should be palpated for evidence of tenderness or movable bony fragments, which may indicate pelvic fracture.[17] Palpation of the suprapubic area may reveal a distended bladder or a "doughy" swelling from extravasation of urine and/or blood.[17] Severe tenderness in the hypogastrium should raise the index of suspicion concerning bladder rupture.[4]

Diagnostic/Laboratory Tests

In addition to the history and physical examination, results from diagnostic and laboratory testing are essential to the assessment of the patient experiencing trauma to the GU tract.

On admission, blood work is drawn to establish baseline hematological, coagulation, ventilation–perfusion, electrolyte, and renal profiles. The results of these baseline studies give information regarding the status of the patient on admission and provide a basis for treatment decisions. These baseline tests may include the arterial blood gas, hemoglobin, hematocrit, white blood cell count, and platelet count.[16] Serum sodium, potassium, water content, osmolality, glucose, lactate, blood urea nitrogen (BUN), creatinine, and total solids are also assessed.[16] The urine is tested for electrolyte and creatinine levels.[16] A coagulation profile of prothrombin time (PT), partial thromboplastin time (PTT), and fibrinogen is also obtained.[16] Following admission, renal function is monitored by measurement of the urine output per hour. A urinary output of less than 30 ml/hr may reflect decreased renal blood flow, parenchymal dysfunction, or obstruction.[16] A creatinine clearance test is performed daily to monitor glomerular function.[16] Renal tubular function may be monitored via the results of free water clearance and urine sodium, specific gravity, and osmolality.[16] Trends in the BUN and creatinine levels are noted. A rise in BUN level may reflect renal insufficiency, catabolism, or hypermetabolism.[16] Urinalysis assists in the assessment of renal function, and a culture and sensitivity test helps to confirm the presence of urinary infection.[16]

The urine of any patient sustaining muscle damage, ischemia, or a transfusion reaction should be tested for the presence of hemoglobin or myoglobin.[16] Hemoglobinuria may be the result of a hemolytic transfusion reaction, while myoglobinuria is caused by muscle contusion or ischemia.[16]

Hematuria

The presence of hematuria may be a significant indication of GU trauma.[17] All patients who present with hematuria require additional evaluation with an intravenous pyelogram and cystogram.[7, 16]

The amount of hematuria does not correlate with the severity of the GU injury.[5, 7, 16, 19] Since urine obtained by catheterization contains 5 to 10 red blood cells per microscopic field,[20] it is optimal if the patient can be encouraged to void the initial specimen. This allows the differentiation between hematuria due to catheterization and hematuria due to GU injury. The absence of hematuria, however, should not lead the trauma team to falsely assume that there is no GU injury. In 2 to 20 per cent of all GU trauma, hematuria, even in microscopic amounts, is not present.[16, 17] Severe blunt and penetrating injury to the kidney may produce no hematuria. Gross hematuria may be present in only about 60 per cent of all patients with blunt renal trauma.[5] Similarly, an avulsed or lacerated ureter may not yield hematuria. Laceration of a major renal vessel may or may not be associated with hematuria. A normal urinalysis also can be obtained from a patient with blunt trauma to the ureters,[5] renal artery thrombosis,[5] renal pedicle injury,[7] and clots or an obstruction below the level of injury.[7]

Radiologic Techniques

Radiographic assessment of the patient with GU trauma may be the cornerstone of the diagnostic process.[5, 7]

Kidney-Ureter-Bladder (KUB) Radiography

The KUB, a radiograph of the kidneys, ureters, and bladder, is usually performed after the patient is stabilized. The purposes of the test are to visualize the position and size of the kidneys[5]; search for lower rib, pelvic, vertebral body, or transverse process fractures[7]; identify foreign bodies[7]; and evaluate diaphragmatic displacement.[5]

The psoas muscles may be obliterated or bulging, possibly the result of retroperitoneal hemorrhage or hematoma.[5] Overall, the KUB itself is not specific for GU trauma, so the lack of pathological findings on this examination does not rule out renal trauma.

Intravenous Pyelogram (IVP)

The IVP, also known as the *excretory urogram,* is a fundamental diagnostic procedure in the assessment of patients with renal trauma. The IVP evaluates both structural integrity and excretory function of the renal system. It also allows visualization of renal parenchyma, calices, and pelvis; assessment of perfusion to the injured kidney; evaluation of the status of both the injured and noninjured kidney; and assessment of the continuity of the collecting system.[7] Displacement or obstruction of the kidneys or collecting system also may be noted.[7]

With the patient in the supine position, an iodine-based dye is injected intravenously.[7, 10] Prior to the injection, the patient should be screened for allergy to the contrast medium. Patients who have experienced allergic reactions to shellfish or previous injections of contrast material should be given an initial test dose of the contrast dye and observed closely for hypotension with tachycardia or bradycardia, nausea, vomiting, or urticaria.[4]

One minute after the dye injection, a radiograph may be done, which allows visualization of the renal parenchyma. Additional films at 5-minute, 15-minute, and 30-minute intervals[10] allow visualization of the pelvocalyceal system, ureters, and bladder.[10] The IVP allows the evaluation of the presence and function of the contralateral uninjured kidney and the classification of injury to the traumatized kidney.

Abnormal findings on IVP include obliteration of the psoas muscle or shadow by extravasated blood or urine, decrease in excretion of contrast dye, extravasation of contrast material,[5, 10] scoliosis away from the injury due to ipsilateral spasm of the psoas muscle,[10] or nonvisualization of one or both kidneys.[5] The IVP is able to detect approximately 80 per cent of renal injuries.[10]

In addition to urological trauma, abnormalities such as polycystic kidneys, absent kidneys, renal calculi, hydronephrosis, and pyelonephritis may be assessed.

Urethrogram

The urethrogram is the diagnostic procedure of choice for a patient suspected of having an injury to the urethra.[21] To perform this test, a Foley catheter is attached to an irrigating syringe filled with contrast material. The catheter is gently inserted into the penile meatus until the catheter balloon is 2 to 3 cm proximal to the meatus.[21] The patient is then placed in a 25- to 30-degree oblique position, and radiographic studies are made as 25 to 30 ml of contrast material is injected.[21] Extravasation of the contrast material allows identification of urethral injury.[13]

In a male patient suspected of having urethral injury, a urethrogram must be done before any urethral catheterization to prevent extension of the existing injury.[13]

Cystogram

The cystogram is used to detect intraperitoneal or extraperitoneal bladder rupture. To perform the test, a urethral catheter is passed (after urethral injury is ruled out) and at least 250 to 400 ml[15, 22] of contrast medium is instilled by gravity.[23] An anteroposterior film is taken. The bladder is then emptied and washed out with saline, and another anteroposterior (wash-out) film is taken.[15] The wash-out film allows for visualization following removal of the contrast material. This film is important because the contrast material may adhere to the bladder mucosa and mimic extravasation.[17]

Radionuclide Imaging

Renal radionuclide scanning can provide valuable information regarding renal injury. This test is especially useful for patients who are allergic to contrast dyes.[17]

Abnormal results of this test may indicate renal hypoperfusion, fractures, urinary extravasation, and delayed excretion.[17] Renal blood flow can be assessed accurately, but parenchymal and collecting system injuries cannot be identified as accurately.[10] The urine of patients receiving radionuclide injections should be handled with gloves following the procedure.[5]

Ultrasound

Renal ultrasound is capable of detecting renal abnormalities with the use of high-frequency sound waves. The sound waves produce echoes which are amplified and converted via a transducer into electric impulses that are seen on an oscilloscope screen as anatomical pictures. This test is seldom used for early identification of injury because it is imprecise in differentiating among lacerations, urinary extravasation, and hematomas.[1, 10] Ultrasonography is most useful for the identification and serial evaluation of perinephric hematomas and urinomas.[10]

Renal Angiography

Renal angiography is indicated when there is incomplete or absent visualization of one or both kidneys on IVP, prolonged bleeding,[5] suspicion of renal pedicle trauma,[5] or clinical evidence of hemodynamic instability[5] and when renal viability is questioned.[10] Selective angiography allows more precise delineation of serious injury such as deep cortical lacerations and complete parenchymal fracture. It also gives information concerning the preservation of blood supply to the damaged renal parenchyma. Areas of devascularization must be identified, because necrosis or abscess formation may follow.[10]

Nonvisualization of the kidney on IVP is a potentially serious finding and may be caused by renal artery spasm, contusion, or intimal tear with thrombosis. Timely diagnosis of the lack of perfusion to the kidney can decrease the possibility of nephrectomy necessitated by massive parenchymal destruction.[10]

Renal arteriography involves cannulation of the femoral artery. Following the procedure, the site must be monitored closely for bleeding, and pulses distal to the site must be evaluated for presence and quality.[5]

Computed Tomography

Computed tomography (CT) provides the most precise delineation of GU trauma. The test is particularly sensitive in identifying the extent of renal lacerations, intrarenal and subcapsular hematomas, renal infarct, contrast extravasation, the size and extent of a retroperitoneal hematoma, and associated injuries to abdominal organs.[1, 5] Using contrast medium, arterial injury and lack of perfusion can be demonstrated.[1]

SPECIFIC ORGAN INJURY

Specific GU injuries vary widely in severity, the need for invasive therapy, and sequelae. In the following section, specific injuries, their diagnosis, and initial treatment are discussed.

Trauma to the Kidney

Approximately 3 per cent of all patients hospitalized for trauma have sustained trauma to the kidney.[6] Eight to ten per cent of all patients with abdominal trauma have coexisting renal injury.[6] Blunt trauma is responsible for 60 to 70 per cent of all kidney injuries.[6]

The kidneys lie in the retroperitoneal space between the twelfth thoracic and second lumbar vertebrae.[24] Each is surrounded by a layer of perirenal fat and Gerota's fascia, which, when intact, can tamponade a hemorrhage.[25] The kidney is well protected by major muscle groups, including the psoas and quadratus lumborum posteriorly, the latissimus dorsi and serratius posterior laterally, and the diaphragm superiorly.[26] The kidneys lie behind the liver and colon and are in close proximity to the spleen, stomach, jejunum, and pancreas.[26] Injury to these organs is often associated with renal injury.

The kidney is very mobile and is attached by a pedicle consisting of the renal artery, renal vein, and ureter. Its mobility can be detrimental in an acceleration–deceleration injury, whereby the organ is put into motion and contused by the ribs and abdominal viscera.[25]

Renal trauma is often classified according to mechanism of injury. Blunt renal trauma may be induced by a fall, MVA, assault, sports injury, or acceleration–deceleration injury. Penetrating renal trauma may be produced by knife or gunshot wounds or impalement injuries.[26]

Renal trauma also can be classified according to severity of injury. These classifications vary slightly among authors.[1, 4–6, 26] Sommers[5] uses the classification of minor, major, and critical renal trauma, as described below.

Minor Renal Trauma

Ninety per cent of blunt renal injuries are minor.[1] This degree of injury includes simple renal contusions,[4, 5] subcapsular hematomas,[4, 5] and superficial lacerations through the capsule into the parenchyma (Fig. 24–3). Minor injuries resulting from blunt trauma contuse the outer layers of functional renal tissue.[5] Thrombosis of small veins and arteries may occur. The renal parenchyma may swell because of small cortical tears and blood accumulation.[5] These injuries are associated with limited retroperitoneal bleeding[26] and usually do not involve associated organ injury.[5]

Patients with minor renal trauma will usually present with costovertebral angle pain upon palpation. A flank mass may indicate a tamponaded perirenal hematoma. Bruising may be evident over the eleventh and twelfth ribs.

Patients experiencing minor injury will typically have a normal IVP or will show a slight delay in function.[4] Microscopic or gross hematuria may be present.[1, 4] Patients with microscopic hematuria may be discharged home following evaluation or placed on partial bed rest with increased hydration.[17] Follow-up is provided until hematuria clears. A follow-up IVP or radionuclide study may be done at 6 weeks after injury to monitor healing.[17]

Patients with gross hematuria are admitted to the hospital and placed on strict bed rest.[1, 4] During this time, the nurse monitors trends in hemoglobin and hematocrit to assess the rate of bleeding, the need for transfusion therapy, and the potential need for surgery. Electrolytes, BUN, and serum creatinine levels are monitored. Changes from baseline may indicate renal dysfunction. Serial urinalyses are done to monitor the degree of hematuria, along with urine output, heart rate, blood pressure, respiratory rate, and temperature.[4, 5, 10] Gentle palpation of any flank mass by the same examiner over time allows assessment of expansion in size.[4, 17] Once gross hematuria has cleared, the patient is allowed to walk.[1, 4] If gross bleeding persists, CT or angiography may be indicated to identify the source of the bleeding.[1]

Definitive radiographic examinations include the KUB radiograph and IVP. Repeated CT scanning may be performed to monitor extravasation of blood and urine or expansion of a retroperitoneal hematoma.[1, 17]

Most patients with minor renal injury do well and rarely experience the complications of sepsis, loss of renal function, and hemorrhage.[5] However, approximately 5 per cent of patients require surgical exploration.[4] Indications for surgery include the development of sepsis, a falling hemoglobin and hematocrit despite blood replacement, an expanding perirenal mass, or the inability to maintain hemodynamic stability despite supportive care.[1]

Major Renal Trauma

Major renal trauma involves more severe injury to the kidney. These injuries include extensive lacerations through the cortex and deep into the medulla,[1, 5] lacerations involving the collecting ducts with extravasation of urine, and severe parenchymal injury with heavy bleeding from large renal vessels[1] (see Fig. 24–3). Renal function may be threatened because of damage to the nephrons.[5] Accumulation of free urine and blood in the collecting ducts and in the area surrounding the kidney may cause further renal damage.[5] Major renal injuries are produced by an impact of considerable force, which also may cause extensive injury to associated organs.[27]

On admission, patients with major renal trauma may present with grossly positive hematuria or shock and microscopic hematuria.[26] A palpable flank mass may be present.[26] These patients may complain of abdominal and flank tenderness, and ecchymosis may be evident over the flank and lower ribs. The eleventh and twelfth ribs may be fractured.[26] Life-threatening hemorrhage may occur from arterial and/or venous bleeding.

Radiologic studies must be done to assess the extent of damage. An IVP may demonstrate extravasation due to laceration.[2] There may be loss of the renal and psoas shadow due to blood and urine collected in the retroperitoneal space.[2] Arteriography is indicated when vascular injury is suspected.[2] Nephrotomography and CT also may be performed.[27]

Surgery is frequently necessary to treat not only the renal injury but also the associated injuries.[1] Extraperitoneal urinary extravasation should be drained to reduce the possibility of infection or fibrosis.[17] All expanding retroperitoneal hematomas should be explored.[16] Frentz and associates[17] describe seven principles of surgical management of renal trauma: (1) control of the vascular pedicle prior to opening Gerota's fascia, (2) delineation of injury, (3) debridement of damaged parenchyma, (4) meticulous hemostasis, (5) watertight closure of the collecting system, (6) reapproximation of parenchyma, and (7) extraperitoneal drainage. Timely exploration and repair of major renal trauma may save a greater amount of viable renal parenchyma and decrease the morbidity associated with complications of major renal injury.[4]

Despite appropriate intervention, large parts of the injured parenchyma may be lost. Extensive damage to the upper or lower pole of the kidney may result in a partial nephrectomy.[27] Damage to the midportion of the kidney may result in a renorrhaphy, in which the devitalized midportion of the renal parenchyma is removed and the parenchymal edges approximated.[27]

Nephrectomy is a possible consequence of major renal trauma. Prior to the nephrectomy, it is essential that the uninjured kidney be evaluated for function. If the noninjured kidney cannot be visualized by IVP and the patient's condition allows, an arteriogram should be considered prior to surgery.

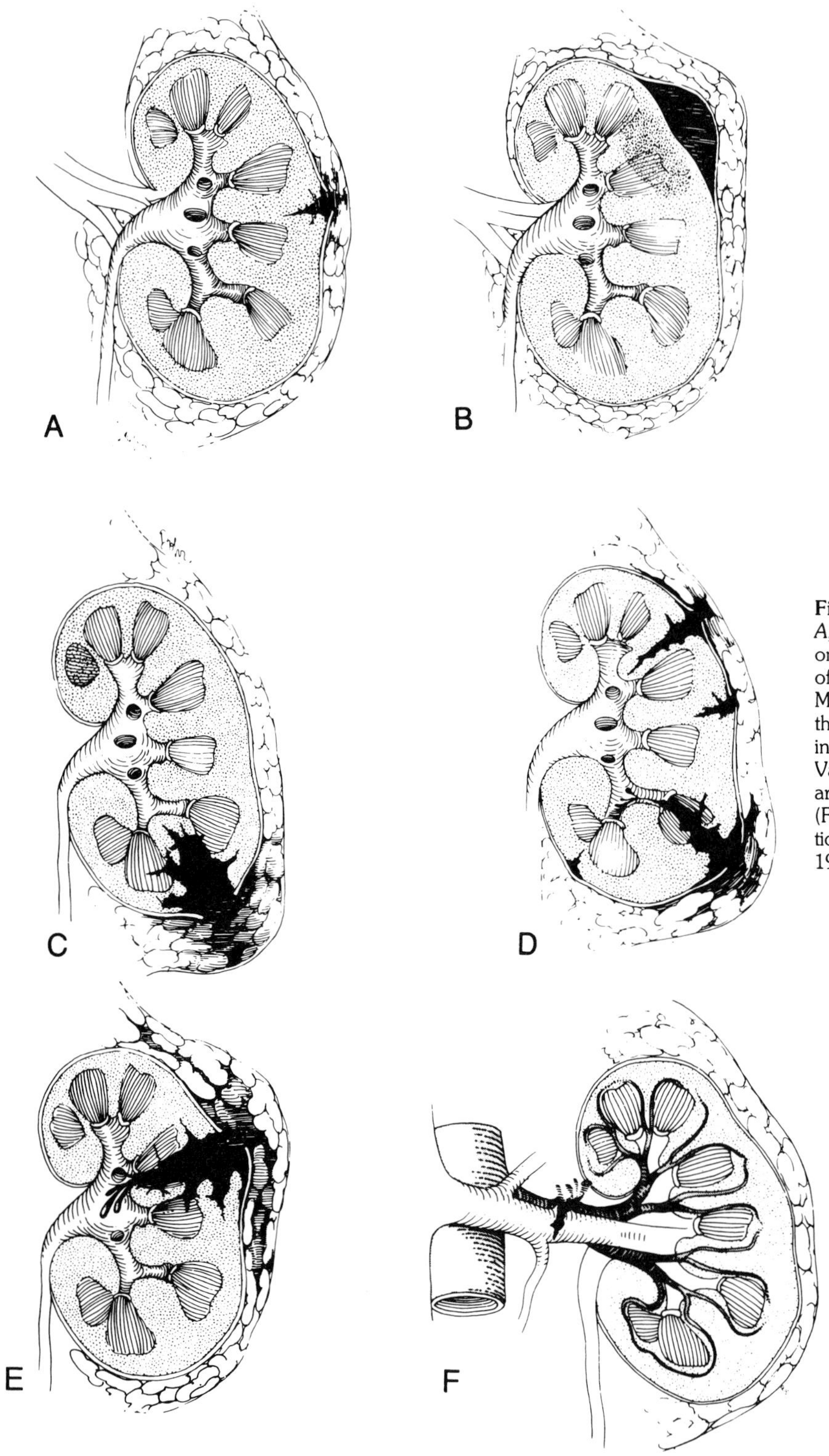

Figure 24–3. Classification of renal injuries. *A,* Minor parenchymal lacerations involving only renal cortex. *B,* Contusion has evidence of injury without parenchymal laceration. *C,* Major parenchymal lacerations extend through cortex and into renal medulla *(D)* and include lacerations of collecting system *(E)*. *F,* Vascular injuries include injuries to main renal artery or vein or their segmental branches. (From McAninch JW, et al: Renal reconstruction after injury. J Urol 1991; 145(5):993, 1991.)

Critical Renal Trauma

Critical renal trauma includes renovascular trauma as a result of a shattered kidney and injury to the renal pedicle (see Fig. 24–3). The renal pedicle may be injured in an acceleration–deceleration scenario, which may produce an intimal tear and thrombosis. The inelastic intima may rupture, producing hemorrhage and narrowing of the vessel lumen. A tear in the intima may produce a flap that causes a partial obstruction. A thrombosis may develop at the site and partially or completely occlude the artery. More severe trauma can lacerate or avulse the vessels.[28]

If the renal artery is lacerated or occluded, perfusion may be impeded to the renal parenchyma, producing an ischemic kidney.[5] The artery must be repaired within 8 hours to restore function to the kidney.[5] Consequently, timely diagnosis of a renal pedicle injury is essential. A shattered kidney is also at risk because major intrarenal arterial flow may be destroyed, which may contribute to ischemia, necrosis, or loss of function.

A patient with critical renal trauma may present with severe blood loss and shock. Gross or microscopic hematuria may be completely absent in the patient with renal pedicle injury.[29] An extensive renal hematoma may be present.[26] Diagnostic studies include an IVP, which may show extensive extravasation with renal fracture, or unilateral nonvisualization with renal pedicle injury.[26] A CT scan also may be performed, which can effectively identify renal pedicle injury.[26] Angiography may be indicated to identify the site of vascular injury.[26]

Critical renal trauma necessitates surgical intervention. Because of the extensive damage, the rate of nephrectomy is high.[28] Despite rapid diagnosis, most patients experiencing critical renal injury also have sustained life-threatening associated injuries and are not candidates for extensive vascular repair.[28] Even with vascular repair, normal renal function is not always restored.[28] Many patients may require a secondary nephrectomy 6 months to 10 years following the trauma because of the complication of refractory hypertension.[5, 28] Other complications of renal trauma include abscess formation, sepsis, fistula formation, and renal atrophy.[5]

Trauma to the Ureter

The ureter is a muscular tube with an adventitial sheath that acts as a conduit for urine from the kidney to the bladder.[30] The ureter is a mobile organ and has fixed points at the bladder and where the ureter crosses the pelvic brim.[30]

Ureteral injuries are typically the result of iatrogenic injury during surgery (see "Mechanism of Injury") or penetrating trauma.[30] Gunshot and stab wounds are common causes of penetrating ureteral injury and may produce a partial or complete transection.[1] The blast effect from high-velocity missiles may cause occult major damage that cannot be detected until ureteral necrosis produces urinary extravasation.[1]

Ureteral injury is rarely produced by blunt trauma but, when present, is usually in the form of disruption at the ureteropelvic junction.[1, 30] Blunt ureteral injury may be caused by the excessive force produced by a fall, ejection from a motor vehicle, or a major hyperextension of the lower thoracic or upper lumbar area.[1, 30] Other causes of ureteral injury include crush injuries, burns, devascularization, and rupture.[30]

Ureteral trauma can be described as a silent injury.[30] Often there are no presenting symptoms, or the findings are nonspecific.[1, 30] The patient may complain of pain only when the ureter is obstructed; transection produces no symptoms.[30] Hematuria, usually microscopic, is seen in 80 to 90 per cent of patients with penetrating injury but may be absent with iatrogenic injury.[30] Unilateral ureteral obstruction may produce a slight, transient increase in serum creatinine or BUN levels, but urine output typically does not change.[30] It is not unusual for a patient to lose complete kidney function secondary to unilateral ureteral injury and remain asymptomatic if the contralateral kidney is able to maintain renal function.[30] In patients with a solitary kidney, loss of function due to misdiagnosed ureteral injury can be life-threatening.[30] Bilateral ureteral injury is rare but may be induced iatrogenically.

Diagnosis of ureteral injury is based on a high index of suspicion. Any patient with a penetrating wound to the abdomen, flank, lumbar area, chest, or anywhere along the path of the ureter should be suspect.[1, 30] These patients should be assessed using an IVP, even if hematuria is absent. More than 90 per cent of ureteral trauma can be identified by this method.[30] If IVP results are inconclusive, a retrograde urethrogram may be obtained.[1]

Most patients with ureteral injury require surgical exploration for associated injuries, since 92 per cent of ureteral injuries are associated with injuries to other organ systems.[1, 30] It is not unusual for ureteral injury to be identified during this exploratory surgery.[1]

Laceration of the ureter must be repaired surgically immediately. Delay in repair may result in loss of a kidney.[30] The type of surgical repair used is dependent on the type of injury sustained by the patient. Trauma to the lower third of the ureter may be repaired by reimplantation into the bladder or ureteroureterostomy (the anastomosis of ureteral ends)[1] (Fig. 24–4). Injury to the upper and middle thirds of the ureter may be best managed by ureteroureterostomy.[22] Internal stenting silicone catheters may be placed to maintain alignment, ensure patency, prevent urinary extravasation, and provide support.[1] These stents remain in place for several weeks or months and are removed by cystoscopy.[1]

Loss of extensive segments of ureter may necessitate a transureteroureterostomy, the anastomosis of the injured ureter into the contralateral ureter[1, 30] (Fig. 24–5). If this procedure is not possible, the injured ureter may be replaced with ileum in an attempt to prevent loss of renal function.[1]

Following ureteral repair, the patient must be observed for signs of ureteral obstruction or seepage from the suture site. Fistulas may develop subsequent to stricture or obstruction. Persistent leakage of urine may follow. Correction of the underlying problem usually results in closure of the fistula.[1]

Stricture formation leading to hydronephrosis is another complication. This problem may develop slowly and may not be evident for months. To monitor the healing process and to observe for the development of stricture formation, an IVP is recommended at 6 weeks and again at 3 months following stent removal.[1]

Development of a retroperitoneal urinoma is a complication related to delay in diagnosis and prolonged extravasation

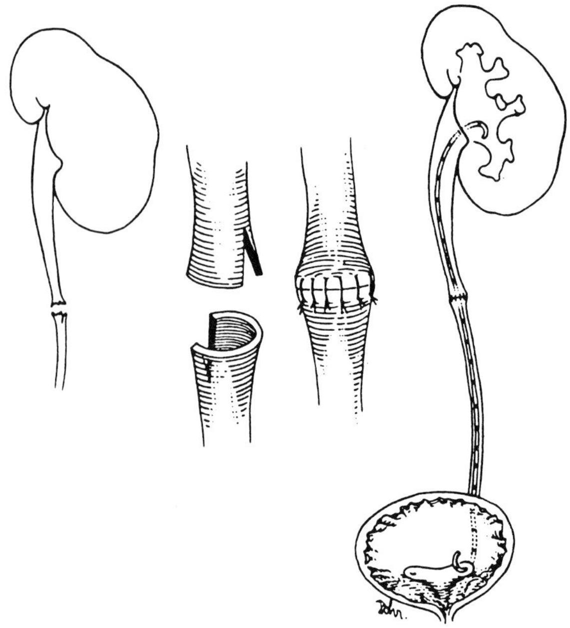

Figure 24–4. Spatulation of ureteral ends prior to ureteroureterosotomy over an internal ureteral stent. Watertight closure is accomplished. (From McAninch J: Injuries to the urinary system. In Blaisdell WF, Trunkey D (eds): Trauma Management, vol 1: Abdominal Trauma. New York, Thieme-Stratton, 1982; illustration by M. Dohrmann.)

at the repair site. This complication should be suspected in any patient experiencing penetrating ureteral trauma who has a low-grade fever, prolonged ileus, or flank pain.[1] Retroperitoneal drains may be placed until urine seepage ceases. These drains should be well protected from contamination and enclosed in a sterile bag.[1]

Infection is a threat to the patient experiencing ureteral trauma. Infection of the urine during the perioperative period may produce retroperitoneal scarring, abscess formation, or pyelonephritis.[1] The nurse must monitor the urine carefully for signs of infection, note urine culture results, and administer antibiotics as ordered.[1]

Trauma to the Bladder

The bladder is a hollow extraperitoneal organ located in the space of Retzius.[23] It is usually well protected from external trauma, especially if empty. It is normally attached laterally and at the base to the pelvic bones, with the pelvic ring offering additional protection.[23] When the pelvis is fractured or the bladder distended, the normal protective mechanisms are lost, and the bladder is at higher risk for injury.[13]

The most common cause of bladder injury is blunt trauma, as a result of MVAs, crush injuries, falls, or blows to the abdomen.[13] Deceleration injuries may damage the full bladder. In this case, the force of the trauma is exerted on the full bladder, which causes it to rupture. Examples of deceleration injuries include seatbelt injuries, situations in which the moving patient hits an unyielding object, and automobile–pedestrian accidents.[13, 22]

When the pelvis is fractured, the shearing force of the fracture may tear the bladder at its moorings.[23] Bone fragments can lacerate the bladder and produce injury.[13]

Penetrating injury to the bladder is often caused by gunshot and knife wounds.[13, 22] Bladder injury should be suspected in any patient with lower abdominal trauma, pelvic fracture, gross hematuria, the inability to void, or a history of a sudden violent deceleration injury.[22, 25] Patients who present with bladder rupture following minor trauma should be suspected of having preexisting bladder pathology, such as cancer, an infiltrative disease such as tuberculosis or amyloidosis, or previous radiation treatments.[22] On admission, patients with bladder trauma may present with nonspecific signs and symptoms. They may complain of abdominal pain or suprapubic tenderness.[2, 13] Pain in the shoulder area may indicate urine in the peritoneal cavity.[2] The patient may be unable to void.[13] A urine specimen will reveal hematuria, the hallmark of bladder rupture[13]—gross hematuria in 95 per cent of patients and microscopic hematuria in the remainder.[13] A suprapubic mass may be palpable.[2] The patient may be in shock and have multiple associated injuries.[2, 22] The most common coexisting injuries include bowel lacerations, a perforated hollow viscus, or laceration of major vessels, including the vena cava, mesentery, and renal or iliac arteries or veins.[22] Delay in diagnosis may produce symptoms similar to an acute abdomen.[25]

Definitive diagnosis is made by cystogram.[13] In the male, urethral injury must be ruled out prior to catheterizing the patient for cystogram.[13] Patterns of contrast extravasation assist in classification. Bladder injury may be classified as intraperitoneal or extraperitoneal rupture (Fig. 24–6). Intraperitoneal bladder rupture occurs as a result of a sudden increase in intravesicular pressure. This is most often due to a blow to the lower abdomen or pelvis.[13] This rise in pressure

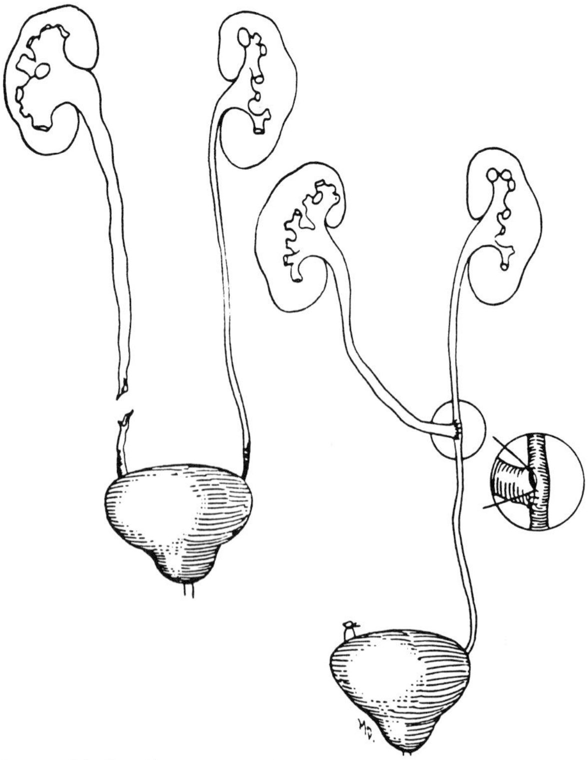

Figure 24–5. Technique of transureteroureterostomy. (From McAninch J: Injuries to the urinary system. In Blaisdell WF, Trunkey D (eds): Trauma Management, vol 1: Abdominal Trauma. New York, Thieme-Stratton, 1982; illustration by M. Dohrmann.)

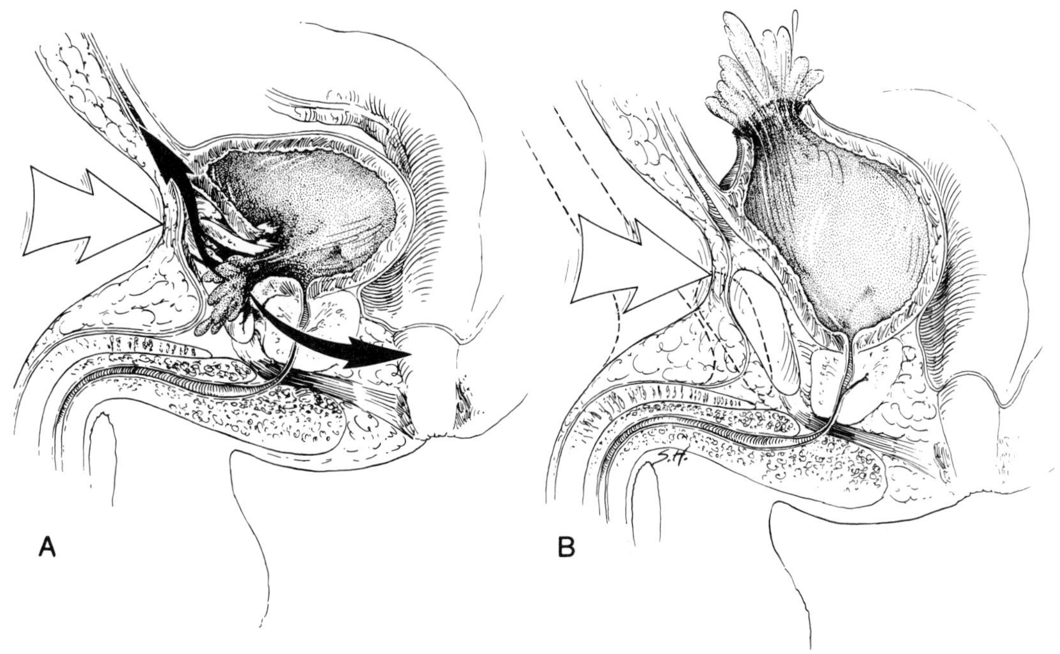

Figure 24–6. *A,* Mechanism of extraperitoneal urinary bladder rupture. The pubic rami are fractured, and the bladder is perforated by a bony fragment. *B,* Mechanism of intraperitoneal vesical rupture. A sharp blow is delivered to the lower abdomen of patient with distended urinary bladder. The distensive force is exerted on all surfaces of the bladder, and it ruptures at its weakest point, usually the dome. (From Peters P, Sagalowsky A: Genitourinary trauma. In Walsh P, Gittes R, Perlmutter A, Stamey T (eds): Campbell's Urology, 5th ed, vol 1. Philadelphia, WB Saunders Co, 1986.)

ruptures the bladder at its weakest and most mobile part, the dome. On cystogram, contrast material can be seen outlining bowel loops, filling the cul-de-sac, and extending into the paracolic gutters.[13] Urine and blood may collect in the peritoneal space.

An intraperitoneal bladder rupture must be surgically repaired, and extravasated urine and blood must be evacuated.[13] Nonviable bladder tissue is removed, the tear is sutured, and a suprapubic catheter tube is placed for urine drainage.[13]

Extraperitoneal bladder rupture is caused almost exclusively by pelvic fractures.[13] On cystogram, the simple rupture will become evident as contrast material extravasates in a classic flame-shaped pattern,[13] which is confined to the perivesicular area. A complex rupture may produce extravasation into the pelvis, scrotum, thigh, anterior abdomen, or retroperitoneal area as high as the kidneys.[23] The degree of extravasation is dependent not only on the extent of the injury but also on the amount of contrast material instilled. Therefore, the amount of extravasation does not correlate well with the severity of the injury.[1, 23]

Extraperitoneal bladder rupture is generally managed conservatively with catheter drainage. If the patient is to be explored surgically for associated injury, the bladder also may be repaired and a suprapubic tube inserted.[13]

A less severe form of bladder injury is bladder contusion. This injury to the bladder mucosa is caused by a more minor degree of trauma. The patient will present with hematuria,[25] and no extravasation of contrast material will be seen on cystogram.[13] Bladder contusion can be managed easily with urinary catheter drainage.[1]

Occasionally, the cystogram may reveal a bladder that is teardrop in shape. This change in shape is due to the presence of large lateral hematomas or urine extravasation. The pressure of these hematomas on the bladder creates the teardrop configuration.

The most serious complications of bladder rupture are a result of intraperitoneal rupture. Leakage of urine into the peritoneal space may produce peritonitis or uroacites with respiratory compromise.[3] Infected urine may contribute to septic complications.

Trauma to the Urethra

Injury to the female urethra is rarely seen.[13] When injury is present, however, it is usually associated with significant pelvic fracture or disruption and associated injury to the bladder neck and vagina.[13] This injury is seen more often in children than in adults. Immediate surgical repair is appropriate.[13] The female urethra also can be injured by obstetrical complications, foreign bodies, and vaginal operations.[2]

In the male, the urethra is divided into four segments: the prostatic urethra, the membranous urethra, the bulbous urethra, and the penile or pendulous urethra.[10] Injuries are classified according to their location. Urethral injuries below the urogenital diaphragm, involving the bulbous and penile urethrae, are classified as inferior or anterior urethral trauma.[4] Those above the urogenital diaphragm, upward toward the bladder neck and involving the prostatic and membranous urethrae, are classified as posterior or superior urethral trauma.[4]

Anterior Urethral Injury

Injuries to the anterior urethra, better known as *straddle injuries,* are most commonly caused by blunt trauma to the perineum.[13] The urethra is crushed against the symphysis pubis as the patient falls astride an object (such as a fence or bicycle) or takes a direct blow to the perineum.[4, 13]

Penetrating trauma to the anterior urethra may be produced by gunshot or stab wounds, self-inflicted instrumentation of the urethra with foreign bodies,[31] or iatrogenic trauma.[31] Power takeoff injury is another form of penetrating trauma and is sometimes seen in farm and industrial accidents.[31] In this case, the pants become caught in the power belt of a machine. The patient may sustain trauma involving the skin of the penis, the scrotum, and the urethra.[31]

The patient with anterior urethral injury will complain of local pain in the perineum.[25] Attempts to void will be painful and may cause perineal or penile swelling.[2] Blood will be present at the urethral meatus, a sequela of spasm of the bulbocavernosus muscle.[1] Extravasation may cause swelling of the scrotum, penis, and lower abdomen.[2] Areas of ecchymosis may be present. A patient with straddle injury will present with a characteristic butterfly-shaped ecchymotic area beneath the scrotum[4, 10] (Fig. 24–7).

Complications include infection of extravasated blood and urine and urethral stricture.[31]

The treatment of anterior urethral injury focuses on the following goals: prevention of extravasation of blood and urine, prevention of infection, prevention of further trauma to the urethra, and prevention of stricture formation.[19] Pierce[31] recommends suprapubic cystostomy drainage alone, allowing the urethra to heal for 10 to 14 days. At that time, contrast medium can be instilled into the bladder via a cystostomy tube. The patient is then encouraged to void. If extravasation is noted, the cystostomy tube is not removed.[31]

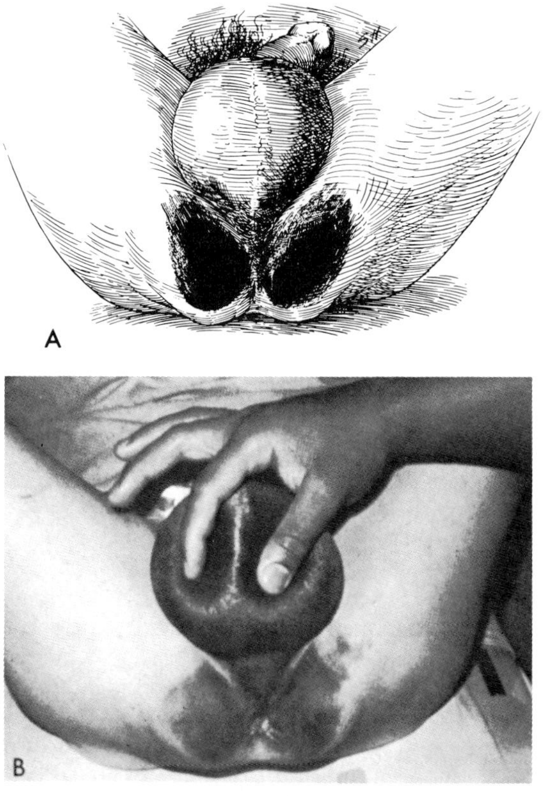

Figure 24–7. *A,* Diagram of a butterfly hematoma. *B,* Appearance of a patient with perineal butterfly hematoma. (From Peters P, Sagalowsky A: Genitourinary trauma. In Walsh P, Gittes R, Perlmutter A, Stamey T (eds): Campbell's Urology, 5th ed, vol 1. Philadelphia, WB Saunders Co, 1986.)

Posterior Urethral Injury

Posterior urethral injuries often occur in association with fracture of the bony pelvis[13] and are found in approximately 10 per cent of patients with pelvic fracture.[32] A vast majority of these injuries are caused by MVAs (90 per cent); the remaining result from falls, crush injuries, and sports accidents. Injury is most often induced by the shearing force produced by pelvic disruption, which pulls the prostate and puboprostatic ligaments in one direction and the membranous urethra attached to the urogenital diaphragm in another.[13]

Posterior urethral injury should be suspected in any patient with a pelvic fracture or separation of the symphysis pubis and in patients in whom a displaced prostate or soft boggy mass is found on rectal examination.[25] On admission, the patient will present with blood at the urethral meatus, the single best indicator of urethral trauma.[19] The meatus must be examined carefully to detect even the smallest amount of bleeding prior to urinary catheterization.[19] Passage of a catheter through a partially ruptured urethra can produce a catastrophic complete transection, with the development of infection or a retropubic hematoma.[19]

On rectal examination, the prostate may be found to be displaced superiorly by a hematoma.[19] The bladder may be distended, and the patient may be unable to void.[25]

Complications of posterior urethral injury can be devastating to the male, producing lifelong morbidity. The parasympathetic and sympathetic nerves that control erection and ejaculation surround the posterior urethra. The urogenital diaphragm contains the urinary sphincter and may be distorted as the prostate and bladder are displaced. Thus an injury to the posterior urethra may result in permanent impotence and/or incontinence.[2] Other complications of posterior urethral injury include extravasation with cellulitis[2] and sepsis. The long-term complication of urethral stricture may occur despite timely and appropriate treatment.[2]

Any patient with a suspected urethral tear must have a retrograde urethrogram prior to urethral catheterization. In complete transection, contrast material will not be visible proximal to the injury. With incomplete injury, some contrast material will be visible in the bladder.[19] Other diagnostic tests include abdominal and pelvic films to identify pelvic fracture, an IVP, or a cystogram.[2]

Management of urethral injury generally involves the placement of a suprapubic cystostomy to divert urine from the area of injury.[19] To avoid infection, the hematoma is usually not evacuated with drains.[19] The management of specific injuries varies according to the type of injury sustained and the preference of the surgeon.

Hanno and Wein,[2, 25] advocate a conservative approach to a contused or minimally torn urethra using urinary catheter drainage with or without suprapubic cystostomy. In the patient with a complete urethral rupture, Cass[2] advocates the use of an end-to-end urethral anastomosis with suprapubic cystostomy drainage and antibiotic coverage.

Penetrating injuries generally require surgical intervention. Debridement and cleansing are done along with reconstruction of the injury. A cystostomy tube is placed for urine drainage.[13, 25] Patients with posterior urethral trauma with minimal, partial injury may be treated with urethral catheter drainage for 14 to 21 days.[13] At that time, a voiding urethrogram is done to confirm healing.[13] A more severe partial tear or one that will not allow passage of a catheter can be managed with a suprapubic cystostomy tube.[13] Complete posterior urethral injury can be repaired surgically immediately after injury. This is often done for stable patients having pelvic exploration for associated injuries.[13] Delayed repair is also a consideration; it is most appropriate for a medically unstable patient who is not a good surgical candidate.[13] Suprapubic cystostomy can be performed in the interim to provide urinary drainage.[13]

Trauma to the Male Genitalia

Trauma to the genital organs, while often not life-threatening, can produce overwhelming loss and crisis for the patient and significant others. Genital trauma may be associated with injury to the perineum, bony pelvis, thighs, bladder, or rectum.[3] Blunt trauma; direct blows; thermal, electrical, or chemical burns; and industrial accidents all may produce genital trauma.[3] Fortunately, trauma to the genitals is not often seen, and surgical intervention can produce good results in both function and appearance.

Testis

The testis is usually spared from injury by its mobility, contraction of the cremaster muscle, and its tough capsular covering.[2, 3] However, injury can be produced by a direct blow that impinges the testis against the symphysis pubis, producing contusion or rupture. The tunica vaginalis sac may fill with blood (hematocele), and the patient may present with a large, tender, swollen scrotal mass.[2]

Immediate surgical intervention is the treatment of choice, with every attempt made to salvage the testis.[19] The tunica vaginalis is evacuated of blood clots, and the testicular rupture is repaired.[2] Delayed treatment may produce the possibility of infection of the hematocele or testis; testicular atrophy is also a potential consequence of pressure from the tense hematocele.[2] Orchiectomy is the least desired outcome of severe injury or complications of testicular trauma.[19]

Scrotum

Trauma to the scrotum may produce avulsion injuries, resulting in significant tissue loss.[2] When possible, the avulsed scrotum is reconstructed around the testis and usually regains normal size within a few months.[2, 19] If scrotal reconstruction is not possible, the testicles may be implanted in upper thigh pockets, where the temperature is similar to that of the scrotum.[2, 19]

Penis

Trauma to the penis may be a result of blunt trauma, strangulation injury, suction injury, amputation, or skin injury[2] (Fig. 24–8). Blunt trauma usually produces a penile fracture, with rupture of the tunica albuginea, hemorrhage, and hematoma formation.[2] Approximately one-third of these injuries result in injury to the urethra,[33] with possible urethral bleeding, hematuria, and urine extravasation.[2] The patient will present with pain, swelling, discoloration, and deviation away from the lesion.[2]

This injury may be treated either conservatively or via immediate surgical repair.[2] Conservative treatment includes urethral catheterization or suprapubic cystostomy, application of ice, elevation, and administration of anti-inflammatory drugs, sedatives, or analgesics.[2, 3] Potential complications of conservative treatment include infection of hematomas, painful lumps, inadequate erection, and permanent deformity.[2]

Surgical intervention is advocated as the treatment of choice by some practitioners.[2, 19, 33] Surgical evacuation of hematomas and repair of the injury may produce better long-term results and improved prognosis.[2, 3, 33]

Strangulation injuries may be produced by foreign objects or human hair constricting the penis.[2] The patient will present with pain and swelling distal to the constricting object. Urethral fistula formation and partial amputation may result from prolonged constriction.[2] The treatment of choice is immediate surgical intervention.[2]

Amputation of the penis may produce severe physical and psychological disability. A successful outcome requires cooperation of a urologist, plastic surgeon, and psychiatrist.[2] Surgical reattachment of the distal segment may be possible if ischemia time is 18 hours or less (this time may be longer if the segment is preserved in iced saline).[2] Microvascular repair may be advisable.[34] Immediate repair and local reshaping may be performed, with plastic surgical and cosmetic repair done at a later time.[34]

Trauma to the Female Genitalia

Trauma to the female genitalia is not well documented. Pelvic fractures account for the majority of female external genital trauma and most often injure the vagina and perineum.[35] Penetrating trauma also may injure the uterus and ovaries, which may require surgical repair, hysterectomy, or oophorectomy.

The most common clinical sign of vaginal trauma is vaginal bleeding, which may be hidden by spasm of the vagina.[35] Consequently, a speculum examination is essential in women who have sustained pelvic fracture.[35] Complications of vaginal tears include pelvic abscesses and septic consequences.[35]

NURSING THERAPEUTICS

Following GU trauma, nursing interventions address six significant nursing diagnoses. These diagnoses are potential for inadequate circulating volume, potential for infection, alteration in urinary elimination, potential for psychological dysfunction, alteration in comfort, and alteration in sexual and/or excretory bodily functions. Although these nursing diagnoses are applicable throughout the trauma cycles, some are more prevalent during specific phases of the injury. Therefore, each will be discussed in the cycle in which the diagnosis most commonly occurs.

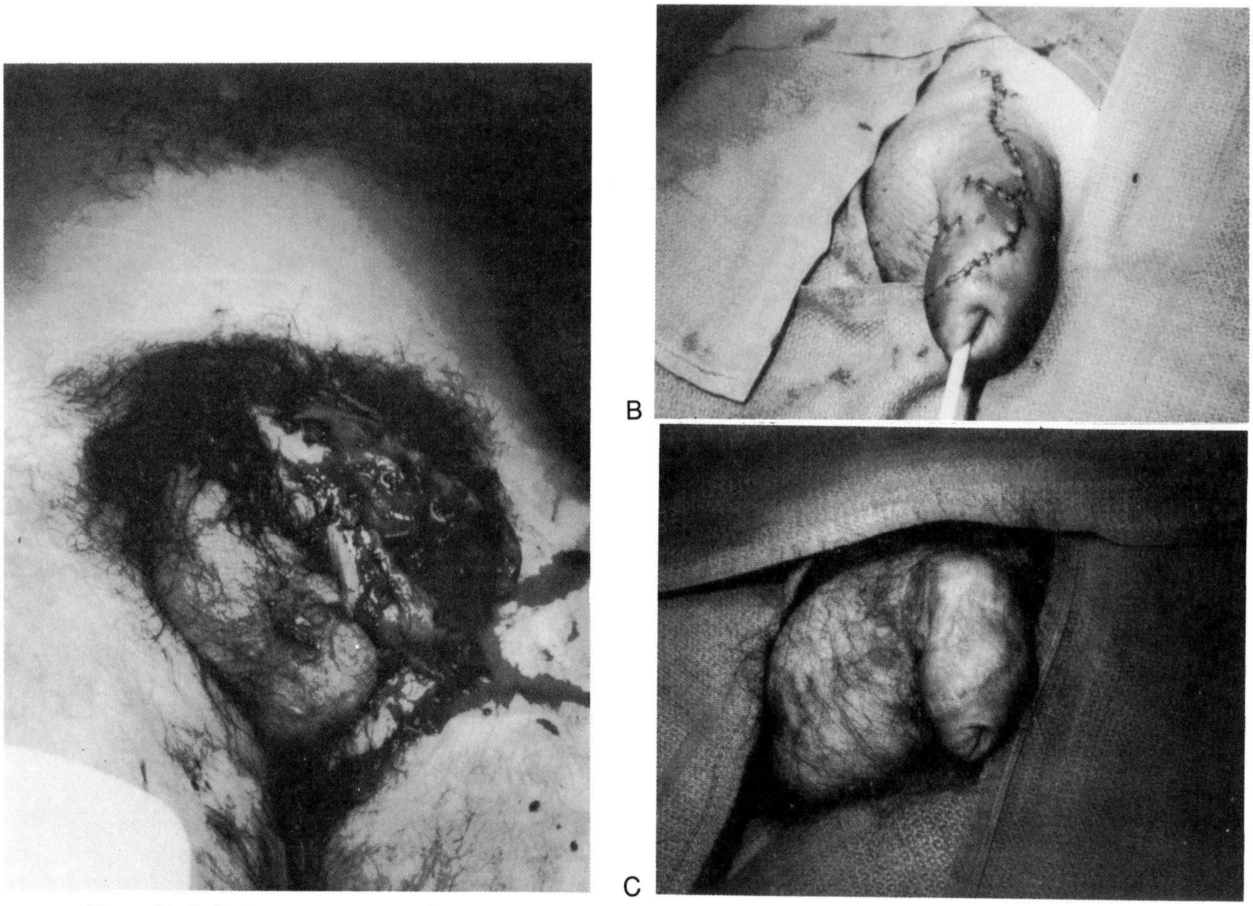

A B C

Figure 24–8. A, Power saw injury to the penis resulted in complete midline hemisection from symphysis through the glans penis, including the urethra. B, Appearance at the completion of reconstruction. A urethral stenting catheter was left in place. All tissue survived without additional debridement required. C, Genital appearance 6 months after injury. The patient had complete return of sensation, sexual function, and urethral voiding. (From McAninch JW, et al: Major traumatic and septic genital injuries. J Trauma 24:291–298, 1984.)

Critical Care Cycle

Potential Alteration in Circulating Volume Related to Bleeding and Hemorrhage

The potential for bleeding and subsequent hemorrhage is present following almost all GU trauma. During the resuscitation phase, maintenance of adequate circulating volume becomes a priority. Care is directed toward correcting blood loss and establishing an adequate circulating volume. The patient is rapidly assessed for evidence of hemorrhage. Multiple large-bore intravenous (IV) lines are placed for volume replacement with crystalloids, colloids, or blood.[5] Vital signs are obtained at frequent intervals. Blood samples are sent for type and cross-match and other appropriate cardiovascular and respiratory tests. If the patient does not stabilize hemodynamically, inotropic drips such as dopamine or dobutamine may be ordered.[5] The nurse must monitor trends in hemodynamic and respiratory parameters to assess improvement in circulatory volume[5] and oxygen delivery. During this phase, the nurse must be aware of the effects of inadequate circulating volumes and vasoactive drugs on renal function.

Following resuscitation, the patient must be monitored closely for signs of hemorrhagic shock, including tachycardia, hypotension, weakness, pallor, dyspnea, hypoxemia, oliguria, and downward trends in hemodynamic parameters.[5] Serial hemoglobin, hematocrit,[15] and coagulation studies will be ordered.[5] The patient must be observed closely for bleeding from surgical sites or drains, for evidence of hematuria formation,[15] and for expansion of an abdominal or flank mass. A pulmonary artery catheter may be utilized to allow the evaluation of circulating volume and the prevention of fluid overload.

It is essential to prevent hypotension or hypothermia, because both may contribute to oliguria, anuria, and loss of renal function.[15] Urinary output must be maintained; therefore, trends in intake and output must be monitored closely.[15] A rise in blood pressure during the critical care phase may indicate constriction of the renal parenchyma and potential deterioration in renal function.[15] Safeguarding the function of the renal parenchyma is essential to the patient experiencing unilateral nephrectomy.

In the critically ill patient, oxygen delivery to the kidney and all other organ systems is essential; therefore, ventilation–perfusion status must be assessed carefully and maintained.

Potential for Infection Related to Disruption of Skin Integrity Secondary to Surgical Procedures and Insertion of Monitoring and Drainage Devices

Following surgery, the critically ill patient with genitourinary injury will have a multitude of invasive monitoring and drainage devices. Consequently, this patient will be at high risk for infection. Strict aseptic technique must be maintained when caring for any drain, surgical site, or urinary drainage system. The urinary or suprapubic catheter must be secured to prevent accidental dislodgment. In females, the urinary catheter should be secured to the inner thigh by either adhesive tape or a Velcro strap. In males, the urinary drainage catheter should be secured to the abdomen. In this patient population, a dislodged urinary drainage catheter should not be replaced until a careful evaluation has been made by the physician.

Daily catheter care is essential in accordance with individual institution infection-control policies. The urinary drainage system must be kept closed to prevent the entrance of organisms.

The patency of all sumps and drains must be maintained.[5] A kinked or obstructed urinary catheter may allow the stagnation of urine and promote the growth of pathogens. An obstructed sump or drain may produce pooling of extravasated blood or urine, leading to abscess formation and sepsis.[15]

The patient must be observed for signs and symptoms of infection, including dysuria, frequency, low back pain, suprapubic pain, or foul, cloudy urine.[5] Infectious processes include perinephric abscess, renal abscess, and sepsis.[15] Trends in temperature and white blood cell counts should be monitored. Urine must be sent for culture and sensitivity and broad-spectrum antibiotics administered as ordered.[15]

Alteration in Elimination Related to Impaired Wound Healing or Renal Parenchymal Dysfunction

In the critical care phase, renal function must be monitored closely. The patient must be observed for signs of renal failure, including abnormal alterations in serum BUN, urine creatinine clearance, serum creatinine, and electrolytes. Other signs of renal dysfunction include edema, hypertension, confusion, nausea and vomiting, oliguria, and anuria.[5] Acute intrarenal failure may result from injury to the functional renal parenchyma. Postrenal failure may occur due to clots or obstruction.[5]

Infection or impaired wound healing may cause leakage of urine from repair sites. The patient must be observed closely for seepage of urine from surgical incisions. A flank or abdominal mass may develop as a result of urine leakage from the breakdown of an anastomosis or suture site.

Potential for Psychological Dysfunction Related to Fear of Altered Body Image, Loss of Control, Fear of Imminent Death

Severe genitourinary injury places the patient in crisis just as any other severe system injury can. Immediate psychological needs include reassurance and emotional support. As the level of crisis subsides, more in-depth information about the extent of the injury, operative repair, and potential complications should be provided.

Patients requiring nephrectomy and/or renal vascular repair may require extended care in a critical care unit.[9] Psychological needs of these patients are typical for any patient in an intensive care environment (see Chapter 10).

Alteration in Comfort Related to Pain Secondary to Massive Swelling, Contusion, and Surgical Repair

The patient experiencing GU trauma may experience severe pain due to edema from hemorrhage, tissue damage, and associated injuries. The patient on a ventilator will require IV narcotics for analgesia.[5] Less critically ill patients will require intramuscular or oral analgesics. The patient must be monitored closely for signs of abdominal pain, which may cause shallow breathing and reduce pulmonary excursion.[5] Ice packs placed on the scrotal area and/or penis also may be of benefit in reducing pain. Commercially available products may be utilized, or crushed ice may be placed in a surgical glove and secured with a rubber band to better cover the area. When ice packs are used, care must be taken to avoid cold burns, since the skin over these organs is thin and fragile. For severe scrotal swelling, a scrotal support may reduce pain aggravated by the additional weight of swollen tissue. Commercially available scrotal supports or handmade supports utilizing an Ace wrap or other material as a sling also may be effective.

Intermediate/Rehabilitation Cycle

Potential for Alteration in Circulating Volume Related to Delayed or Occult Bleeding

During the intermediate or rehabilitation phase, the nurse must continue to monitor the patient for signs of delayed or occult bleeding. The patient with minor renal injury or contusion will be placed on bed rest. Trends in vital signs and serial hemoglobin and hematocrit results must be monitored for evidence of hemorrhage.

Any flank or abdominal mass must be evaluated for increase in size. Gentle palpation allows more direct assessment of size but produces the risk of rupture of a tamponaded bleed. Changes in abdominal girth may allow more indirect but safer evaluation of the mass.

The patient with minor renal trauma will be allowed to ambulate once hematuria clears. After minor trauma, renal parenchyma typically heals in 4 to 6 weeks.[15]

Alteration in Urinary Elimination Related to Delayed Deterioration in Renal Function Secondary to Complications of Genitourinary Trauma

In the intermediate/rehabilitation phase, renal function must continue to be monitored. Changes in intake, output, serum BUN, creatinine, and electrolytes may indicate early deterioration in renal function.

The patient and family will require education about the care of any remaining drains or urethral or suprapubic catheters. Instruction should include information about potential delayed complications of GU trauma, including infection, sexual difficulties, incontinence, stricture formation, calculus formation, hypertension, hydronephritis, pyelonephritis, or chronic renal failure.

Alteration in Comfort Related to Pain Secondary to Surgical Intervention, Bladder Spasm, and/or Cystitis

Although postoperative pain is not as likely to be present once the patient reaches rehabilitation, bladder spasms may occur intermittently following bladder repair. Although antispasmodic medications are often effective in relieving bladder spasm, additional sedation may be required for effective pain relief. If cystitis does occur postoperatively, pain medication may be needed in conjunction with drugs, such as phenazopyridine hydrochloride (Pyridium), which produce an analgesic effect on the mucosa of the urinary tract, which in turn relieves burning, urgency, and frequency.

Potential for Infection Related to the Necessity for Indwelling Urinary Drainage Systems

The potential for infection remains a priority through the rehabilitation cycle. Some patients may require suprapubic and/or urinary catheterization for an extended time, depending on their injury. As long as urinary drainage systems are necessary, they constitute an avenue for bladder and/or kidney infection if handled improperly. Diligent catheter care and maintenance of a closed system must continue for as long as drainage is needed.

Fear Related to Concerns About Altered Sexual Functioning and/or Physical Disfigurement

Patients sustaining genitourinary injury may or may not have residual problems that can alter sexual functioning and/or bladder control. Such injuries may result in permanent sexual impairments that affect intercourse, masturbation, and fertility.[36] Certainly, those patients whose injuries are not likely to produce such sequelae should be reassured as soon as they are stable enough to comprehend such information.

Those patients whose injury will cause altered levels of normal bodily functions not only need intense psychological support but also may require professional counseling addressing sexual function. For instance, a male with urethral or external genital trauma is likely to be psychologically devastated once he understands the implications of this injury. He will need strong emotional support from family and nursing staff. A referral for counseling should be included in the patient's care plan. One can expect the usual phases of grief and loss (see Chapter 10).

Females who may have required a hysterectomy or oophorectomy also may experience significant psychological adjustment. Depending on her age and child-bearing status, a hysterectomy may cause severe emotional impact. The uterus is an important symbol of a woman's femininity. Its removal can have profound effects on how she perceives herself with respect to her reproductive role, sexuality, vitality, youth, and attractiveness. Each individual values these qualities differently.[37] Depression and/or mood swings can often occur as a result of these altered body image perceptions and/or normal hormonal changes.

It is not at all surprising that GU injuries that affect sexual functioning should precipitate such a crisis for the patient. One need only consider contemporary society's emphasis on physical characteristics as a component of one's "sexiness"—a preoccupation with the "whole body" or the "body beautiful." There is undoubtedly a chemistry in sexual relationships that is sparked by physical characteristics, and these dynamic features may pose exceptional difficulties for those with a disability.[38]

These problems are compounded by the fact that numerous myths and misconceptions abound concerning sexuality and disability.[39] Many people commonly believe, for example, that the disabled are asexual; only "normal" "able-bodied" people are sexual. A second common misconception is that orgasm is the goal of sex and is essential for sexual satisfaction. Closely aligned with this is the myth that sex equals intercourse.[40] To be a sexual man, one must be able to have an erection and ejaculation. To be a sexual woman, one must be capable of vaginal orgasm. Anything else is considered, by many, to be second rate.

Patients who have these misconceptions are understandably quite upset by an injury that affects their sexual functioning. Such misconceptions do not automatically vanish at the time of the traumatic incident. Instead, they persist and can generate tremendous turmoil unless they are adequately addressed. Patients may view themselves as unlovable and may begin to fear such things as rejection by loved ones and/or difficulty in meeting new people who will accept their altered body.

For these reasons, sexual concerns should not be ignored or postponed until the patient is in a rehabilitation unit. Patients may have concerns about sex even during the acute phase after injury. Such concerns may not override all others, yet they are significant and thus warrant attention by the nurse. The attainment of a rich and satisfying intimate relationship with a partner who loves and appreciates one's body should be a major goal in the patient's overall plan of care.

A first step toward meeting this goal is to recognize that patients may communicate their concerns about sexuality in a variety of ways, both verbally and nonverbally. Patients do not usually say, "Nurse, I have a question about sex." Concerns are communicated, instead, in a more cryptic way, such as through the use of subtle or symbolic language. For example, one patient remarked, "My pilot light is out." In this one simple statement, the patient summed up his feelings about his postinjury sexual impairment. Though the language was symbolic, the message was hard to miss.[41] Patients may also use terms peculiar to their own culture in their communication of sexual concerns. One patient asked if his "nature" would be affected by his injury. The nurse accurately guessed that he was referring to his ability to function sexually. This was an interesting choice of words, i.e., equating sexual function with one's very nature. It conveyed how vital the patient's sexuality was to him.

Sexual concerns also may be communicated through the patient's general behavior, such as patting or pinching the nurse, exposing oneself, or reading sexually explicit books and magazines. It is perhaps these types of behaviors that are most unsettling to the nurse. Yet the nurse must move beyond the anxiety that such situations invoke and attempt to address the sexual concerns that are often at the root of such behaviors.

Some patients may give no outward indication that they have concerns about sexuality. They may have falsely assumed that if their doctor or nurse did not discuss resumption of sexual activity, it must be beyond their capabilities and limits.[42] Doctors or nurses, on the other hand, may misinterpret the patient's reluctance to ask questions about sex as meaning the patient is not concerned about sex or believes he will return to normal levels of function.[43] Yet, for many patients, the inability to function sexually is an unspeakable loss, i.e., a loss so profound that they cannot begin to talk about it without help.

An excellent way to begin to assist the patient in dealing with his sexual concerns is to introduce the subject in a low-key fashion, letting the patient know that it is a legitimate topic for discussion whenever he is ready. One might say, "After an injury such as yours, many people have questions about their future capabilities." These questions often include concerns about sexual function. "I'd be happy to talk to you anytime about any questions you may have." Such an approach allows the patient to initiate the discussion and does not overwhelm someone who is still employing a significant amount of denial about his injury.[44] Also, discussing sexuality in the context of the variety of problems the patient faces does not make the subject uncomfortably conspicuous by segregating it for separate handling.[36]

Once the door for discussion of sexual concerns has been gently opened, take time to listen to the patient. Create an atmosphere wherein the patient feels free to talk about his injury and the meaning it has for him. Listening to a person describe his or her sexual concerns acknowledges that the person is indeed still seen as a sexual person. One should respond to these concerns with a balance of gentle reassurance and realism about the difficult adjustments that undoubtedly lie ahead. Simple acknowledgment that it is quite natural and understandable to feel anxious about one's sexuality can be tremendously reassuring.[45] While listening to patients, remember that the ties to a lost part or to a function that has been drastically altered are represented by hundreds of separate memories that must be sorted through. This is part of the work of mourning.[36] It helps to be able to talk about these memories to a receptive listener.

Offering the patient information about sexual function is another important intervention. Often, in the acute postinjury phase, many patients simply need reassurance that their sexual function is not totally lost. Actual details may not be important at a time when the patient must deal with many other concerns. Yet some patients may seek more detailed information, asking, "But what can I actually do?" Although genital intercourse is still possible for an overwhelming majority of disabled persons, it is crucial to remember that sexuality is more than genitalia or the sex act. Sexuality is reflected in all that a person is and all that one does. One must encourage a broader definition of sexuality when patients ask for detailed information on their capabilities.[47]

Specific answers to such questions might include information about foreplay of various types involving stimulation of secondary erogenous zones, alternate sexual techniques such as oral sex, use of vibrators, and massage. Masturbation also has been described as a very important option for disabled individuals for many reasons. It can be an alternate outlet if one is without a sexual partner. In addition, it helps one to relearn the potential of one's body, thus enabling the person to communicate to a partner what feels best. Finally, masturbation can become one really positive, pleasurable experience that makes the patient feel better about his body in general.[48] Patients should be encouraged to experiment, to try new positions and caresses. There is simply not enough information available to say what will or will not work. Instead, tell patients to try anything they can think of.[49] Realize, too, that a disabled person can enjoy real excitement and achieve feelings of adequacy through giving pleasure to another person. Such a realization may be of comfort to a newly disabled individual. One cautionary note is necessary when discussing all the above information. Before describing various sexual options, it is important to consider the patient's moral, religious, and cultural attitudes and those of his partner. One must work within the framework of these beliefs and not try to change them. Remember, too, that referring the patient to someone else is perfectly acceptable if the nurse is uncomfortable dealing with the patient's concerns or if he needs more detailed information than the nurse is capable of providing.

In the patient with genital trauma, specific counseling about the feasibility and safety of resuming sexual intercourse is necessary. Patients and their sexual partners need to know the details of the injury and how the surgical repair was performed. Prior sexual behaviors should be discussed so that the couple can be assured that resumption of these behaviors is safe. Information about how long to wait after injury before resuming intercourse is also necessary.

Patients whose genitourinary trauma involves total or partial scrotal avulsion warrant special mention. Loss of all or part of the scrotum can cause alterations in the male's self-image, necessitating sexual adjustment for both males and females. Since the scrotal sac is very sensitive to touch, damage or removal of the sac may result in a decrease or loss of pleasurable sensations derived from touching this area. Couples may find it helpful to know that sexual fulfillment can be achieved with patience and understanding and with exploration of other stimulating areas of each other's body.[50]

Allowing patients to have private time with their spouses or significant others is another important nursing measure. Such time can so easily be usurped by other concerns. Yet it is vital for people to be able to touch and to embrace each other without fear of interruption. In the case of the acutely ill, family members often need encouragement to touch, hug, and hold a person. They are afraid they will hurt the patient or disturb a tube or IV line. Yet the acutely ill are often "touch starved" and could benefit from the warm touch of another. One need only use a bit of ingenuity to create time and privacy for such interactions.

It is also of value for disabled individuals to experience consistency among their various care givers. This can promote the development of a trusting relationship between patient and staff. It is within the context of such a relationship that discussions about patient's sexual concerns will occur most easily.

Another intervention that may be helpful is to arrange for the newly disabled person to talk with someone who has made a successful adjustment to a similar disability. The opportunity to explore issues with someone in a similar circumstance may be just the outlet needed for one's concerns.

Offering positive comments about the disabled person's body also can be a comforting nursing measure. For example, women who were disabled reported that it is a tremendous value to hear a professional say things such as "this part of your body is in great shape. I just did a pelvic exam and the whole area looks just fine." Such comments work against the "body as enemy" stigma that a disabled person may harbor.[51]

One final intervention that may be useful is the technique of behavior rehearsal.[51] This is best described by an example. Suppose the nurse is working with a woman who is concerned about how a new partner will respond to the presence of her urinary catheter or to other features of her disability. In behavior rehearsal the nurse might say, "Pretend that I'm a new partner. You've been dating me awhile and we are on our way to the bedroom. How would you explain your catheter to me? What are you afraid of? What's the worst thing that can happen?" This technique helps a person to examine how she feels and how to prepare for new intimate experiences. Through this rehearsal, it is hoped, some of the anxiety surrounding such experiences will be diminished.

The measures described above are also appropriate for use with the patient's spouse or significant other. They too can have tremendous concerns about their future sexual relationship with the disabled individual. They are in danger of becoming the "forgotten other" if the nurse's concern is directed to the patient alone.

One final consideration of utmost importance to any discussion of patient's sexual concerns is the nurse's own comfort level regarding both sexuality *and* disability. Attitude is a critical determinant of one's effectiveness in this area. The intense issues surrounding sexuality and disability may be highly sensitive ones for the nurse for many reasons. Often patients are close in age to the nurse, who may be embarrassed to discuss sexuality in such a situation. Also, the nursing profession has until recently deemphasized sexual concerns, leaving many nurses feeling ill prepared to handle such discussions. A religious background that involves many prohibitions against sex also may be a discomforting factor for the nurse. Finally, patients with disabilities cannot but remind the nurse of his or her vulnerability to life's vicissitudes. This reminder can be anxiety provoking. Negative attitudes toward disability are reflected in statements or thoughts such as "If that happened to me, I'd kill myself" or "I'd give up completely." One may wonder secretly "Who would want to touch that person?" Yet that is not the nurse's question to answer but someone else's.[31]

It is crucial to take time for self-analysis regarding these issues, since nothing is communicated more surely to the patient than one's own attitudes. Negative attitudes can pose real barriers to the formation of rapport and openness, which is so vital in a caring relationship. It is so much better for the patient when the nurse conveys concern for his situation and respect for his beliefs and attempts to deal with them honestly, realistically, and compassionately. Patients typically are relieved when the nurse raises the one subject that perhaps had bothered them the most, i.e., their future as sexual, intimate beings.[52]

COMPLICATIONS OF GENITOURINARY TRAUMA

As with any traumatic injury, the potential for complications exists. In the acute phase of injury, these complications may include acute renal failure, renal infarction, urinoma, obstructive uropathy, and pyelonephritis. During the recovery phases, chronic renal failure, obstructive uropathy, renal calculi, urethral strictures, urinary retention, or urinary tract infections may develop. Complications that may arise during the rehabilitation phase of recovery include incontinence, impotence, sterility, and permanent physical disfigurement.

Acute renal failure is a potentially life-threatening, complication facing any trauma patient, with or without primary GU or renal injury. The following sections explore in detail the physiology, assessment, and treatment of this syndrome.

ACUTE RENAL FAILURE

Acute renal failure (ARF) is a syndrome characterized by an acute deterioration in renal function. ARF results in the inadequate excretion of various end products of cellular metabolism and an impaired ability to regulate fluid, electrolyte, and pH balance.

Normal Renal Function

Normal renal function begins with the formation of urine in the functional unit of the kidney, the nephron (Fig. 24–9). Hydrostatic pressure, created by the systemic blood pressure, forces water and electrolytes through a capillary membrane, the glomerulus, and then into the Bowman's capsule. In normal, healthy adults, this glomerular filtration rate (GFR) remains fairly constant at 125 ml/min.[53] The filtrate or urine flows from Bowman's capsule to the proximal convoluted tubule, where approximately 60 to 80 per cent of the water and salts are reabsorbed. From the proximal tubule, the urine enters the loop of Henle, where sodium ions are pumped from the tubule into the adjacent tissue. Using an osmotic gradient, water follows the sodium ions, resulting in a hypotonic urine solution. As the loop ascends, it becomes impermeable to water, while sodium and chloride are actively pumped back into the tubule. This so-called countercurrent exchanger is one mechanism for regulating urine concentration. As the urine enters the distal convoluted tubule and the collecting ducts, aldosterone and antidiuretic hormone (ADH) determine the final adjustments for water and electrolyte concentrations.

Acute renal failure results in a loss of this normal function and is subclassified by its etiology. *Prerenal failure* is a result of inadequate perfusion of the kidney without actual tissue damage. *Intrarenal failure* results from direct insult to the renal parenchyma by prolonged ischemia, injury to the nephron, or infectious/immunologic processes. *Postrenal failure* occurs as a result of an obstruction in the drainage system.[54]

Prerenal Failure

Trauma patients are at great risk for developing prerenal failure. Hypotension associated with hemorrhage, hypovolemia, and cardiac failure will lead to the same end point. Renal blood flow can remain relatively stable despite wide swings in the mean arterial pressure (MAP).[1] When the MAP falls below 50 mm Hg for any reason, these autoregulatory mechanisms fail, and the urine output falls.

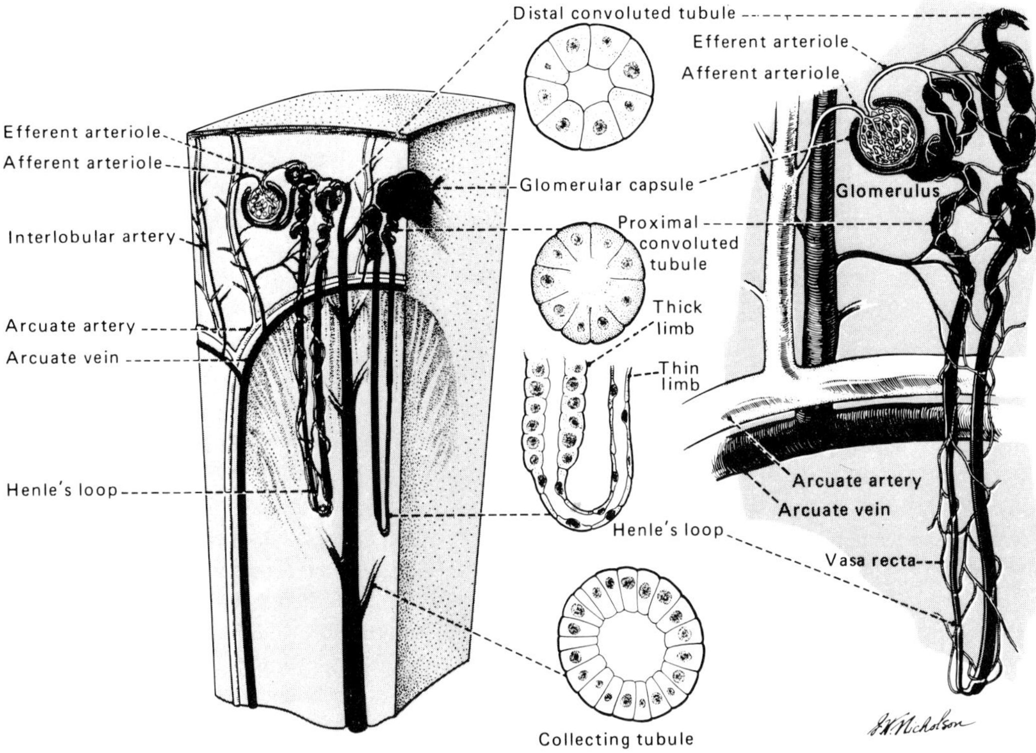

Figure 24–9. The nephron and its blood supply are shown at the sides of this figure. Sections of different portions of the tubule are shown in the center. (From Langley LL, Telford I, Christianson J: Dynamic Anatomy and Physiology. Figure 40–1, p 683. Copyright 1980 by McGraw-Hill, New York.)

Intrarenal Failure

The type of intrarenal failure is determined by the section of the kidney that is injured. The outer layer, or cortex, is the vascular portion containing the glomeruli and distal convoluted tubules. Damage occurs by vascular, infectious, or inflammatory processes which result in swelling at the capillary bed (Table 24–1).

The second type of intrarenal failure is caused by damage to the middle layer, or medulla. The medullary tissue is composed of the collecting tubules, ducts, and the long loops of Henle (Table 24–2). Nephrotoxic agents, particularly antibiotics or contrast media, release crystals that lodge in the tubules and obstruct the flow of filtrate. A source of ischemic injury frequently seen in trauma patients is rhabdomyolysis. Destruction of large muscles releases myoglobin into the circulation. These molecules are also too large to pass through the tubules and become lodged in the tubule system.

TABLE 24–1. INTRARENAL FAILURE: COMMON SOURCES OF CORTICAL DAMAGE

- Infectious
  - Acute glomerulonephritis
  - Acute pyelonephritis
- Immunologic
  - Goodpasture's syndrome
  - Systemic lupus erythematosus (SLE)
  - Severe hypercalcemia
  - Malignant hypertension

Postrenal Failure

Primary injury to any part of the urinary collection system, such as a ruptured bladder, interruption in ureteral or urethral integrity, or pressure from hematomas, may lead to postrenal failure. Other potential causes arise from sources of urinary retention, i.e., neurogenic bladder or a urinary tract infection (UTI).

Clinical Presentation

Acute tubular necrosis, an intrarenal failure, is the classic model for the clinical presentation of ARF. It consists of five

TABLE 24–2. INTRARENAL FAILURE: COMMON SOURCES OF MEDULLARY DAMAGE

- Nephrotoxic sources
  - Antibiotics
    - Aminoglycosides
    - Cephalosporins
    - Tetracyclines
  - X-ray contrast media
  - Heavy metals
    - Arsenic
    - Lead
  - Pesticides and fungicides
- Ischemic sources
  - Burns
  - Crush injuries
  - Massive hemorrhage
  - Prolonged hypotension
  - Sepsis
  - Transfusion reactions

stages: onset, oliguric phase, nonoliguric phase, diuresis, and recovery.[54, 55]

The onset or actual event initiates the pathology of renal failure. The kidney is still able to successfully compensate for changes in the renal blood flow or filtration pressures. The oliguric phase is reflected by a urine output of less than 25 to 30 ml/hr with the presence of electrolyte abnormalities. This phase generally lasts 10 to 20 days.

In the case of a less severe insult to the tubules, nonoliguric or high-output renal failure may develop. Electrolyte abnormalities occur, and the urine is poorly concentrated. Output is abnormally high, as much as 1 liter/hr; however, creatinine clearance remains low. The duration of this phase is shorter, approximately 5 to 8 days.

In comparison, the urine output in the diuretic phase is also elevated, to 125 to 150 ml/hr. However, as the kidneys begin to regain their function, the urine is more concentrated, and the electrolyte imbalances are corrected. The diuresis occurs because of an excess fluid volume and a hyperosmolar state created by the elevated urea level.

The final phase of renal failure is recovery, which can last between 3 and 12 months. It is characterized by gradual restoration of renal function. The degree of recovery is determined largely by the severity of the damage.

Assessment

Laboratory Data

The hallmark of ARF is a low urine output. This decrease in output reflects abnormalities in the GFR and regulation mechanisms. Laboratory analysis offers the clinician useful data in diagnosing and monitoring the progress of ARF. Pertinent values and their norms are summarized in Table 24–3.

Creatinine clearance is the gold standard for monitoring renal function. Creatinine, a normal by-product of tissue metabolism, is excreted via glomerular filtration into the urine. Since the rate of tissue metabolism is usually constant and clearance occurs solely at the nephron, renal function may be readily assessed by collecting urine over a fixed amount of time and measuring concurrent urine and serum creatinine levels. Once these values are known, the clearance is calculated by multiplying the urine creatinine (in mg/dl) by the urine volume (in ml/min) and dividing that figure by the serum creatinine (in mg/dl). As the GFR drops in renal failure, the amount of creatinine cleared by the kidney also drops, resulting in an elevation of serum creatinine levels.

Along with this increase in the serum creatinine, BUN levels also will rise. However, since the BUN level is affected by many other factors, i.e., hypovolemia, hypercatabolism, and gastrointestinal bleeding, it is an unreliable measure of the GFR when viewed in isolation of other values. A simultaneous rise in the BUN and serum creatinine levels with a ratio of greater that 10:1 is a better indicator of renal failure.

Other electrolyte values, serum and urine, will be affected as the ability of the nephron to regulate their movement becomes progressively more impaired. If the tubules are reabsorbing increasing amounts of sodium and free water, serum sodium levels will climb and urine values will fall. The failure of the collecting tubules to excrete potassium is responsible for elevated serum potassium levels.

Hemoglobin and hematocrit levels may be normal initially, but as the kidneys fail to produce erythropoietin, a chronic anemia may occur. White blood cell counts are valuable in monitoring the patient's infection status.

Urinalysis, specific gravities, and microbiology tests are also useful in determining and monitoring the progression of renal failure. Significant laboratory findings are summarized for each of the categories of renal failure in Table 24–4.

Physical Assessment

The physical assessment of a patient with ARF reveals changes in virtually every organ system. Neurologically, the patient's level of consciousness will vary because of azotemia and electrolyte abnormalities. The cardiovascular system will reflect the altered fluid volume, myocardial function, and stimulation of the renin–angiotensin system. Pulmonary function will be elevated in an attempt to correct acid–base imbalances. Gastric motility and appetite will be impaired. Table 24–5 outlines the primary signs and symptoms that are commonly seen with this population.

TABLE 24–3. IMPORTANT LABORATORY VALUES FOR ASSESSING RENAL FUNCTION

BLOOD CHEMISTRIES—ELECTROLYTES		URINE CHEMISTRIES	
Sodium	135–145 mEq/l	Urine should be yellow in color, clear with a mild ammonia odor.	
Potassium	3.5–5.0 mEq/l		
Chloride	96–109 mEq/l		
CO_2	24–30 mEq/l	Specific gravity	1.005–1.030
SUN	12–25 mg/dl	Osmolality	300–1200 mOsmol
Creatinine	0.4–1.5 mg/dl	pH	4.5–8
Glucose	70–115 mg/dl	Glucose	0
		Ketones	0
GENERAL CHEMISTRIES		Potassium	25–120 mEq
Magnesium	1.5–2.0 mEq/l	Sodium	40–220 mEq
Calcium	9.0–10.5 mg/dl	Calcium	50–150 mg
Phosphorus	3.0–4.5 mg/dl	Chloride	110–250 mEq
Total protein	6.0–8.5 gm/dl	Magnesium	100 mg
Albumin	3.2–5.3 gm/dl	Protein	<150 mg/24 hrs
pH	7.35–7.45	RBC	<3/HPF
		WBC	<4/HPF
HEMATOLOGY		Crystals	0
		Casts	0
WBC	4500–11000/mm^3	Creatinine clearance: 125 ml/min	
Hemoglobin	13.9–16.3 gm/dl		
PVC	41–53%		
Platelets	150,000–350,000/mm^3		
RBC	4.84 m/mm^3		

Treatment Goals

Treatment goals and nursing interventions for patients experiencing ARF focus on balancing or compensating for the deterioration in renal function.[56] This is particularly challenging when dealing with multiple trauma patients. Fluid, electrolyte, and pH balances may be exacerbated by postresuscitation fluid overload or fluid restrictions, such as those imposed with acute head injuries. Specific goals and interventions are summarized in Table 24–6.

Adequate nutrition, which assists in maintaining electrolyte balances, poses a special problem because of the high protein requirements experienced by trauma patients. Protein, vital for tissue healing, produces urea as a metabolic by-product. Elevations in BUN will contribute to the risk of developing significant azotemia. Thus early dialysis may be required to assist the patient in handling this increased protein load.[57]

TABLE 24–4. URINALYSIS IN RENAL FAILURE

	PRERENAL ETIOLOGY	INTRARENAL ETIOLOGY	POSTRENAL ETIOLOGY
Specific gravity	≥1.020	1.010	Normal
Myoglobin	May be positive	May be positive	Usually negative
Urine sodium	Low	High (>30 mEq/l)	Normal (<20 mEq/l)
Sediment	Normal	Renal tubular cells and cell casts Pigmented granular casts	Normal
Protein	<1 gm/24 hr	<1 gm/24 hr	<1 gm/24 hr
Red blood cells	Microscopic	Microscopic	Microscopic
White blood cells	Few	Few	Few

Hemodynamic stability is necessary for meeting the oxygen needs of all tissues, including the kidneys. Prolonged hypotension may exacerbate the existing renal failure, which could, in turn, diminish the amount of renal function recovered. Hypertension is a common result of renal failure. As the kidneys perceive a drop in the renal blood flow, the renin–angiotensin cascade is activated at the juxtaglomerular apparatus. Production of renal prostaglandins is also elevated. The resulting vasoconstriction and increases in the circulating plasma volume as a result of fluid overload, aldosterone production, and electrolyte imbalances will contribute to systemic hypertension.

In some cases, such as a prerenal pathology, patients in ARF will recover after treatment of the underlying cause with only careful management of fluids. Patients who experience actual damage to the nephrons will likely require some form of dialysis.

Treatment Options

All forms of dialysis strive to replicate normal kidney function, i.e., to regulate excess fluid and electrolytes and to remove metabolic wastes.[58] This is accomplished through the use of a porous membrane that, like the glomerular capillary bed, is only permeable to water and small molecules. This membrane essentially creates two compartments, one containing blood and the other a hypertonic solution called *dialysate* (Fig. 24–10).

Function of this system is governed by four principles. *Hydrostatic pressure* is the force that pushes the fluid through the system. In the kidney, this is created by the systemic blood pressure. *Osmosis* is the movement of fluid across the semipermeable membrane from an area of greater concentration to an area of lesser concentration. *Diffusion* is the movement of small molecules across the semipermeable membrane from an area of higher concentration to an area of lower concentration. Both processes will continue until equilibrium is reached. *Filtration* is the movement of fluid from an area of greater to lower pressure. Clinical applications of these principles are evident in all forms of dialysis.

Peritoneal Dialysis

Clinical use of peritoneal dialysis (PD) was reported as early as 1932.[59] Dialysis is accomplished by utilizing the mesenteric capillary bed as the semipermeable membrane. A hypertonic glucose solution is instilled into the abdominal cavity and left to dwell for 30 to 45 minutes. Water and solutes are pulled from the capillary bed to the dialysate. The greater the concentration of glucose, the more water and solutes are removed.[59, 60]

PD has the advantage of being relatively simple and inexpensive to perform. No special preparation is required for insertion of the abdominal trocar catheter, which may be done at the bedside. The procedure can be managed without use of costly equipment or specially trained personnel.

Physiologically, PD is a slow and gentle process, so no

TABLE 24–5. PHASES OF RENAL FAILURE

SYSTEM INVOLVED	SYMPTOMS		RECOVERY
	OLIGURIA	DIURESIS	
Neurological	Decreased level of consciousness, muscular twitches, fatigue, apathy, seizures, coma	Decreased level of consciousness, lessened potential for seizure activity, potential for fatigue, apathy, restlessness	Normal
Cardiovascular	Elevated blood pressure, pulse, cardiac output, potential for cardiac pump failure, anemia, cardiac arrhythmias, pitting edema	Low blood pressure, elevated pulse, elevated temperature, cardiac arrhythmias	Normal; may have residual blood pressure or arrhythmia problems
Pulmonary	Pulmonary edema, rales, Kussmaul's respiration	Tachypnea, Kussmaul's respiration	Normal
Metabolic	Hyperkalemia, hypermagnesemia, acidosis, hypernatremia	Hypokalemia, acidosis, hyponatremia	Normal
Gastrointestinal	Gastrointestinal bleeding, negative nitrogen balance, anorexia, nausea	Gastrointestinal bleeding, negative nitrogen balance, anorexia, nausea, thirst	Anorexia, nausea, thirst
Genitourinary	Decreased urine output	Increased urine output	Normal urine output, potential chronic renal failure, potential for impotence

TABLE 24–6. NURSING CARE PLAN FOR ACUTE RENAL FAILURE AND DIALYSIS

POTENTIAL FLUID AND ELECTROLYTE IMBALANCE RELATED TO IMPAIRED RENAL FUNCTION AND RENAL REPLACEMENT THERAPIES	
STG: Patient will remain euvolemic	Monitor for signs and symptoms of fluid volume deficit or excess *Deficit*—may be associated with nonoliguric or recovery phases of ARF and excessive fluid removal during dialysis Decrease in level of consciousness Decrease BP, PAP, CO Tachycardia or dysrhythmias Decrease in weight Poor skin turgor *Excess*—may be associated with oliguric or anuric phases of ARF Decrease in level of consciousness Increase BP, PAP, CO Dysrhythmias Congestive heart failure Increase in weight Edema Jugular vein distension
STG: Patient will remain free of electrolyte imbalances	Monitor patient's electrolytes, BUN, creatinine, creatinine clearance, pH and HCO_3 levels on a regular basis, before and after dialysis Assess for signs and symptoms of electrolyte abnormalities Treat imbalances as needed and as ordered
STG: Patient will maintain vascular stability during renal replacement therapies, e.g., dialysis	Monitor VS hourly during treatment Assess patient for signs and symptoms of hypotension during treatment Monitor thrill or bruit of AV fistula, if in place Treat hypotension with fluids or vasopressor agents as ordered
POTENTIAL FOR INFECTION RELATED TO ALTERED IMMUNE FUNCTION AND IMPAIRED SKIN INTEGRITY	
STG: Patient will remain free of infection	Monitor patient's temperature at regular intervals Monitor WBC and differential as needed Assess wounds, vascular access, and PD catheter for signs and symptoms of infection, i.e., erythema, induration, etc. Document condition of wounds and catheters every 24 hours Utilize strict sterile technique Assess for the development of skin breakdown associated with poor skin integrity, pruritus, etc. Monitor antibiotic levels and dosages carefully
POTENTIAL ALTERATION IN NUTRITION: LESS THAN BODY REQUIREMENTS RELATED TO INADEQUATE NUTRIENT INTAKE OR EXCESSIVE PROTEIN REQUIREMENTS	
STG: The patient will maintain adequate nutrient intake to facilitate wound healing	Assess for patient's appetite and diet (usual diet is restricted in protein, sodium, and potassium) Consider parenteral solutions, which are higher in protein, if needed Assess for hypercatabolic states, i.e., persistently elevated BUN, muscle wasting, etc. Monitor nitrogen balance and serum protein levels
KNOWLEDGE DEFICIT RELATED TO ARF AND RENAL REPLACEMENT THERAPIES	
STG: The patient/family will verbalize adequate understanding of pathology and treatments	Assess understanding of the following areas Etiology and pathology of ARF Parameters routinely monitored, including labs, VS, etc. Treatment equipment and routines Dietary and/or fluid restrictions Prognosis Periodically reevaluate learning because of potential decrease in level of consciousness associated with uremia and electrolyte abnormalities

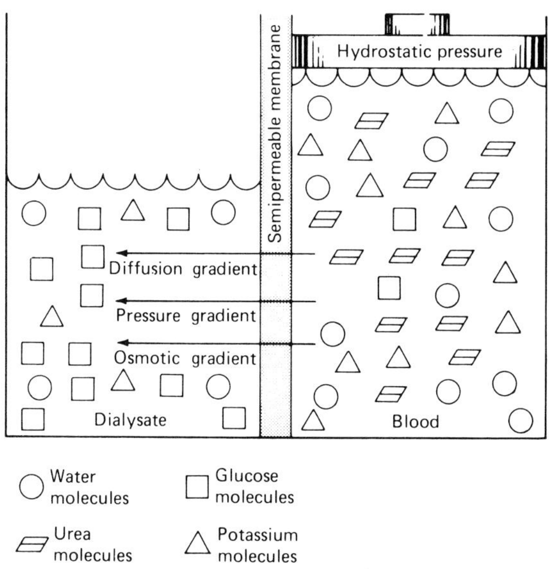

Figure 24–10. Osmosis, diffusion, and filtration in dialysis therapy. (From Baer CL: Dialysis therapy. In Kinney M, et al (eds): AACN's Clinical Reference for Critical Care Nursing, p 972. Copyright 1981 by McGraw-Hill, New York.)

rapid fluid or metabolic shifts are experienced by the patient. Because of this lack of rapid action, patients in acute uremic crisis, i.e., experiencing seizure activity, coma, or cardiac dysrhythmias, are not candidates for PD. Also, because of the pore size in the capillary bed, proteins are dialyzed. Patients can lose more than 5.0 gm/day.[60] Protein malnutrition is avoided by increasing the dietary intake.

In order for the procedure to work well, the peritoneum must be intact. In trauma victims, this is usually not the case. The use of PD in the presence of abdominal trauma, vascular anastomosis, or hematoma is at best controversial. This eliminates a large portion of the trauma population. Use of the hypertonic glucose solutions makes peritonitis the second major complication of PD. Another disadvantage is the effects of the increased intra-abdominal pressure during dwell times. This could lead to restriction of diaphragmatic motion and additional impairment of the patient's ventilatory status.

PD is an effective treatment for acute fluid overload and stable renal failure; however, these contraindications make it generally inappropriate for a multitrauma population.

Hemodialysis

Hemodialysis involves the extracorporeal circulation of blood through a hemofilter, which uses a synthetic semipermeable membrane between the blood and the dialysate.[61, 62] Figure 24–11 is a schematic representation of two commonly used filters. The blood is pumped through the extracorporeal circuit by a mechanical pump. Since management of the system requires specially trained personnel, the bedside nurse's primary function is monitoring the patient during the treatment.

Hemodialysis has two distinct advantages over any other form of dialysis. First, treatments are brief, usually between 4 and 6 hours. The process is also highly efficient in the removal of fluid, wastes, and electrolytes. These advantages are crucial to the survival of patients with life-threatening poisonings or those who are in uremic crisis.

The resulting rapid shift of fluid and electrolytes can lead to a disequilibrium syndrome. This manifests in a variety of ways: a decreased level of consciousness, dizziness, weakness, diaphoresis, vomiting, seizures, and hypotension. The neurological symptoms reflect the entry of water into the cerebrospinal fluid (CSF). This occurs because of a transient concentration gradient in which urea cannot be diffused rapidly enough from the CSF into the blood because of the blood–brain barrier. The cardiovascular signs are related to the rapid shifts of fluid, sodium, and potassium. These symptoms are most often evident when long-time abnormal blood chemistries are corrected too rapidly.

Another significant disadvantage is the risk of hemorrhage. Unlike PD, for hemodialysis patients must be anticoagulated. Many trauma victims are already coagulopathic due to such things as hepatic injuries, disseminated intravascular coagulopathies (DIC), thrombocytopenia, or multiple transfusions of banked blood.

Continuous Acute Renal Replacement Therapies

Continuous acute renal replacement therapies (CARRT) are a group of treatments that have been gaining popularity among critical care clinicians. Schematics of the various forms are presented in Figure 24–12.

Continuous arteriovenous hemofiltration (CAVH) was initially introduced in 1977.[63] In this arrangement, blood enters an extracorporeal circuit from an arterial access, passes through a hemofilter with a semipermeable membrane, and returns to the patient through a venous access. The hydrostatic pressure created by the patient's MAP forces plasma water and some small molecules across the membrane and into a collection system. Structurally, the hemofilter resembles that used in hemodialysis, but it is usually smaller in size.

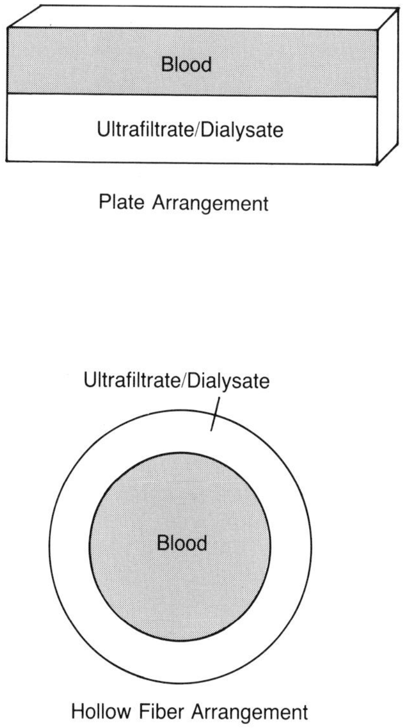

Figure 24–11. Schematic representation of two common hemofilters.

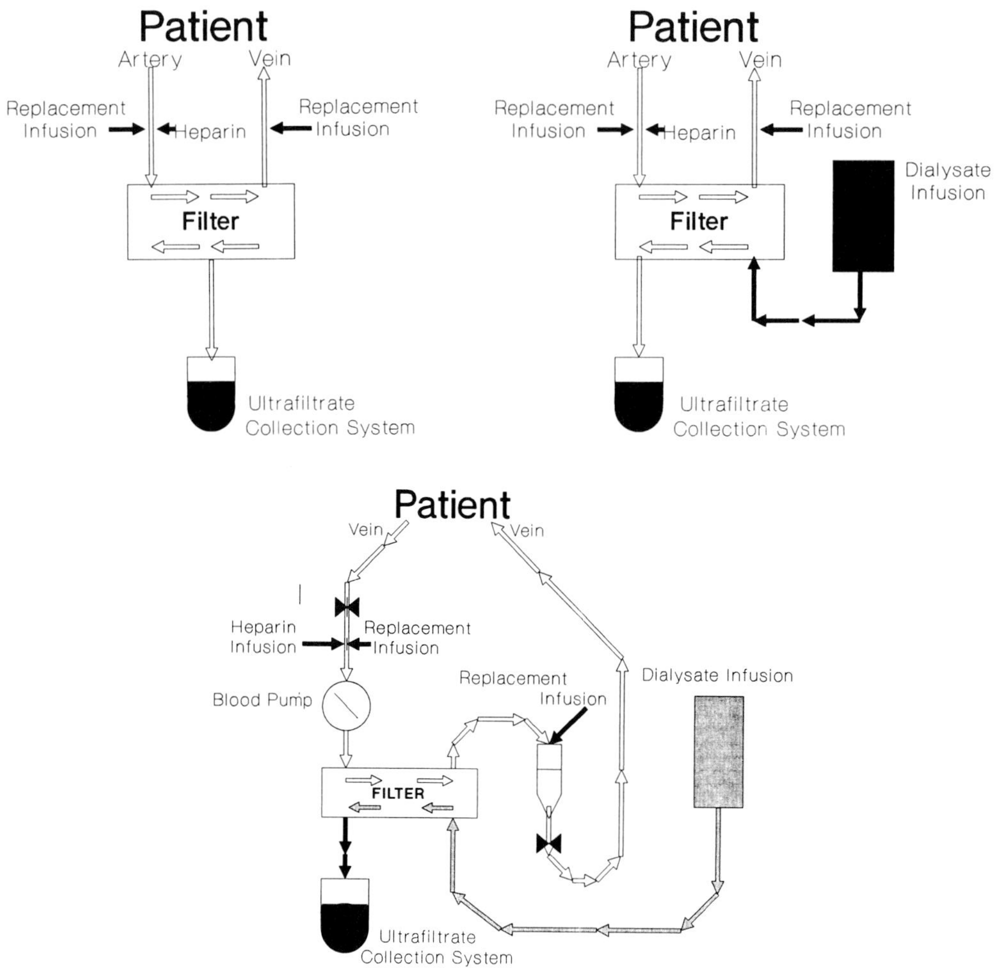

Figure 24–12. Schematic representations of various forms of continuous acute renal replacement therapies.

In 1983, the addition of a countercurrent dialysate infusion allowed for even greater removal of fluids and solutes because of the wider convective and diffusive gradients.[64] This new arrangement, continuous arteriovenous hemofiltration with dialysis (CAVH-D), has proven to be as effective as traditional hemodialysis in treating acute renal failure. This fact, coupled with the absence of a requisite specialized staff and capital investment for equipment, has caused it to gain great popularity among critical care clinicians.[65–69]

Both filter arrangements rely on the arteriovenous (AV) pressure gradient being greater than 60 mm Hg to create the hydrostatic pressure in the filter. The AV gradient (MAP − CVP) is a more reliable indicator than MAP alone because it incorporates the resistance the blood must overcome in returning to the systemic circulation.

Because the slow, continuous nature of both processes does not lead to rapid fluid or electrolyte shifts, they are generally well tolerated by patients. Like PD, this slow nature precludes the use of CAVH or CAVH-D for a life-threatening crisis.

Many trauma patients may have an inadequate AV gradient to support CAVH or CAVH-D. Inadequate MAP could be related to hypovolemia or septic shock. Significantly elevated venous pressures, such as with ARDS, may actually obstruct the blood in the filter from returning. When this pressure gradient narrows, flow through the filter slows and the blood clots. In such situations, a blood pump may be substituted between the arterial and venous access. In this case, a slower blood flow rate is maintained than that used in hemodialysis.[70, 71]

Arterial access may be undesirable or contradicted for some patients. In such patients, solely venous access can be utilized with a slow-running blood pump. This system, continuous venovenous hemofiltration with dialysis (CVVH-D), reveals several advantages.[72] Access can be established with one double-lumen catheter, minimizing the need for repeated central venous cannulation. Use of the pump enables clinicians to treat patients who would have been too hypotensive to support CAVH or CAVH-D.

Heparinization is also an issue in continuous hemofiltration. However, unlike hemodialysis, the goal is to localize the anticoagulation to the filter. This is accomplished using a low-dose heparin infusion located on the arterial side of the filter. Ideally, the heparin will be cleared by the filter prior to returning to the patient. The status is monitored via serial coagulation studies, partial prothrombin times (PTT), or activated clotting times (ACT).

Regardless of the dialysis therapy selected to treat the patient with ARF, optimal function will not return for up to 12 months. Renal function should be monitored at regular intervals. This should include serial laboratory tests in addition to detailed physical assessments. All treatment of these patients must be directed toward salvage and preservation of the kidney, unless this compromises more vital organs such as the brain, heart, and lungs. Failure to do so condemns the surviving patient to a life restricted by chronic dialysis or transplantation.

REFERENCES

1. McAninch J: Urologic injury: Kidney and ureter. In Moore EE (ed): Early Care of the Injured Patient. Philadelphia, BC Decker, 1990, pp 189–197.
2. Cass A: Genitourinary trauma. In Kreis D, Gomez G (eds): Trauma Management. Boston, Little, Brown, 1989, pp 263–280.
3. Althausen A: Injuries to the genitourinary tract. In Burke J, Boyd R, McCabe C (eds): Trauma Management: Early Management of Visceral Nervous System, and Musculoskeletal Injuries. Chicago, Year Book Medical Publishers, 1988, pp 126–139.
4. Peters P: Trauma to the genitourinary system. In Shires, T (ed): Principles of Trauma Care. New York, McGraw-Hill, 1985, pp 345–364.
5. Sommers MS: Blunt renal trauma. Crit Care Nurs 10(3):38–48, 1990.
6. Peterson N: Complications of renal trauma. In McAninch J (ed): Urologic Clinics of North America: Urogenital Trauma, vol 16. Philadelphia, WB Saunders Co, 1989, pp 221–236.
7. Taylor D, Fair W: Genitourinary trauma. In Zuidema M, Rutherford B, Ballinger W (eds): The Management of Trauma. Philadelphia, WB Saunders Co, 1985, pp 527–541.
8. Krieger JN, Algood CB, Mason JT, et al: Urological trauma in the Pacific Northwest: Etiology, distribution, management, and outcome. J Urol 132:70–73, 1984.
9. Sagalowsky AI, McConnell JS, Peters PC: Renal trauma requiring surgery: An analysis of 185 cases. J Trauma 23:131, 1983.
10. Peters PC, Sagalowsky AL: Genitourinary trauma. In Walsh PC, Gittes RF, Perlmutter AD, Stamey TA (eds): Campbell's Urology. Philadelphia, WB Saunders Co, 1986, pp 1192–1246.
11. Peters PC, Bright TC III: Trauma to the genitourinary system. In Shires GT (ed): Care of the Trauma Patient. New York, McGraw-Hill, 1979, p 360.
12. Cook LS: Genitourinary trauma. In Cardona V (ed): Trauma Nursing. Oradell, NJ, Medical Economics Books, 1985.
13. Corriere JN: Bladder and urethra. In Moore EE (ed): Early Care of the Injured Patient. Philadelphia, BC Decker, 1990, pp 198–203.
14. Weigelt JA, McCormack A: Mechanism of injury. In Cardona VD, Hurn PD, Mason PJ, et al (eds): Trauma Nursing: From Resuscitation through Rehabilitation. Philadelphia, WB Saunders Co, 1988, pp 105–126.
15. Cass AS: Diagnostic studies in bladder rupture: Indications and techniques. In McAninch JW (ed): Urological Clinics of North America: Urogenital Trauma, vol 16. Philadelphia, WB Saunders Co, 1989, pp 267–274.
16. Cowley RA, Dunham CM: Abdominal and pelvic injuries. In Shock Trauma/Critical Care Manual. Baltimore, University Park Press, 1982, pp 143–214.
17. Frentz GD, Lang EK: Trauma to the urinary tract. In McSwain NE, Kerstein MD (eds): Evaluation and Management of Trauma. New York, Appleton-Century-Crofts, 1987, pp 195–230.
18. Corriere JN, Sandler CM: Management of the ruptured bladder: Seven years experience with 111 cases. J Trauma 26:830–833, 1986.
19. McAninch JW: Genitourinary trauma. In Mattox EE, Moore EE, Feliciano DV (eds): Trauma. Norwalk, CT, Appleton & Lange, 1988, pp 537–552.
20. Guice K, Oldham K, Eide B, Johansen K: Hematuria after blunt trauma: When is pyelography useful? J Trauma 23:305–311, 1983.
21. Sandler CM, Corriere JN: Urethrography in the diagnosis of acute urethral injuries. In McAninch JW (ed): The Urologic Clinics of North America: Urogenital Trauma. Philadelphia, WB Saunders Co, 1989, pp 283–290.
22. Peters PC: Intraperitoneal rupture of the bladder. In McAninch JW (ed): The Urologic Clinics of North America: Urogenital Trauma, vol 16. Philadelphia, WB Saunders Co, 1989, pp 279–282.
23. Corriere JN, Sandler CM: Management of extraperitoneal bladder rupture. In McAninch JW (ed): The Urologic Clinics of North America: Urogenital Trauma, vol 16. Philadelphia, WB Saunders Co, 1989, pp 275–278.
24. McAninch JW: Injuries to the urinary system. In Blaisdell FW, Trunkey DD (eds): Trauma Management: Abdominal Trauma, vol 1. New York, Thieme-Stratton, 1982, pp 199–227.
25. Hanno PM, Wein AJ: Urologic trauma. In Cayten CG (ed): Emergency Medical Clinics of North America: Multiple Trauma, vol 2. Philadelphia, WB Saunders Co, 1984, pp 823–841.
26. Carroll PR, McAninch JW: Staging of renal trauma. In McAninch JW (ed): The Urologic Clinics of North America: Urogenital Trauma, vol 16. Philadelphia, WB Saunders Co, 1989, pp 193–202.
27. McAninch JW, Carroll PR: Renal exploration after trauma: Indications and reconstructive techniques. In McAninch JW (ed): The Urologic Clinics of North America: Urogenital Trauma, vol 16. Philadelphia, WB Saunders Co, 1989, pp 203–212.
28. Cass AS: Renovascular injuries from external trauma: Diagnosis, treatment, and outcome. In McAninch JW (ed): The Urologic Clinics of North America: Urogenital Trauma, vol 16. Philadelphia, WB Saunders Co, 1989, pp 213–220.
29. Mee SL, McAninch JW: Indications of radiographic assessment in suspected renal trauma. In McAninch JW (ed): The Urologic Clinics of North America: Urogenital Trauma, vol 16. Philadelphia, WB Saunders Co, 1989, pp 187–192.
30. Guerriero WG: Ureteral injury. In McAninch JW (ed): The Urologic Clinics of North America: Urogenital Trauma, vol 16. Philadelphia, WB Saunders Co, 1989, pp 237–248.
31. Pierce JM: Disruptions of the anterior urethra. In McAninch JW (ed): The Urologic Clinics of North America: Urogenital Trauma, vol 16. Philadelphia, WB Saunders Co, 1989, pp 329–334.
32. Webster GD, Ramon J: Repair of pelvic fracture posterior urethral defects using an elaborated perineal approach: Experience with 74 cases. J Urology 145(4):744–748, 1991.
33. Cumming J, Jenkins JD: Fracture of the corpora cavernosa and urethral rupture during sexual intercourse. Br J Urol 67:327, 1991.
34. Chen YT, Chen H: Penile reconstruction for a victim of electrical injury with bilateral below-elbow amputations. Plast Reconstr Surg 87(4):771–775, 1991.
35. Maull KI, Rozycki GS, Pedigo RE, Cruikshank SH: Injury to the female reproductive system. In Mattox EE, Moore EE, Feliciano DV (eds): Trauma. Norwalk, CT, Appleton & Lange, 1988, pp 553–560.
36. Cole T: Sexuality and the spinal cord injured. In Green R. (ed): Human Sexuality—A Health Practitioner's Text. Baltimore, Williams & Wilkins, 1979, p 155.
37. Drellich M, Bieber J: The psychological importance of a uterus and its functions; some psychoanalytic implications of a hysterectomy. J Nervous Mental Dis 126:322–336, 1958.
38. Hahn H: The social component of sexuality and disability—Some problems and proposals. Sexuality Disability Fall:224, 1981.
39. Latimer A: Accountability for the sexual awareness of the spinal cord-injured patient. Rehabil Nurs July-August:8, 1981.
40. Levitt R: Understanding sexuality and spinal cord injury. J Neurosurg Nurs 12:88, 1980.
41. Stewart T: Sex, spinal cord injury, and staff rapport. Rehabil Lit 42:347, 1981.
42. Otto H: The New Sex Education. Chicago, Follett Publishing Co, 1978, p 92.
43. Hott J: Sex and the heart patient: A nursing view. Top Clin Nurs 1:77, 1980.

44. Crigler L. Sexual concerns of the spinal cord-injured. Nurs Clin North Am 9:713, 1974.
45. Rodocker M, Bullard D: Basic issues in the sexual counseling of persons with physical disabilities. In Bullard D, Knight S (eds): Sexuality and Physical Disability: Personal Perspectives. St. Louis, CB Mosby, 1981, p 277.
46. Seller J: Psychological situation of the disabled with spinal cord injuries. Rehabil Lit 30:292, 1969.
47. Cole T, Glass D: Sexuality and physical disabilities. Arch Phys Med Rehabil 58:585, 1977.
48. Becker E: Sexuality and the spinal cord-injured woman. In Bullard D, Knight S (eds): Sexuality and Physical Disability: Personal Perspectives. St. Louis, CV Mosby, 1981, p 18.
49. Thornton CE: Sexuality counseling of women with spinal cord injuries. In Bullard D, Knight S (eds): Sexuality and Physical Disability: Personal Perspectives. St. Louis, CB Mosby, 1981, p 160.
50. Barnard M, Clancy B, Krantz K: Human Sexuality for Health Professionals. Philadelphia, WB Saunders Co, 1978, pp 238–239.
51. Bogle J, Shaul S: Body image and the woman with a disability. In Bullard D, Knight S (eds): Sexuality and Physical Disability: Personal Perspectives. St. Louis, CV Mosby, 1981, p 94.
52. Hanlon K: Maintaining sexuality after spinal cord injury. Nursing May:58, 1975.
53. Guyton AC: Textbook of Medical Physiology. Philadelphia, WB Saunders Co, 1991.
54. Stark JL: Acute renal failure. In Kinney MR, et al (eds): AACN's Clinical Reference for Critical Care Nursing, 2d ed. New York, McGraw-Hill, 1988.
55. Finn WF: Diagnosis and management of acute tubular necrosis. Med Clin North Am 74:873–890, 1990.
56. Solez K, Racusen LC (eds): Acute Renal Failure: Diagnosis, Treatment, and Prevention. New York, Marcel Dekker, 1991.
57. Weiss L, Danielson BG, Wikstrom B, et al: Continuous arteriovenous hemofiltration in the treatment of 100 critically ill patients with acute renal failure: Report on clinical outcome and nutritional aspects. Clin Nephrol 31:184–189, 1989.
58. Cogan MG, Garovoy MR: Introduction to Dialysis. New York, Churchill Livingstone, 1988.
59. Diaz-Buxo JA: Technology of peritoneal dialysis. In Jacobson HR, et al (eds): The Principles and Practice of Nephrology. Philadelphia, BC Decker, 1991.
60. Maher JF: Physiology of the peritoneum: implications for peritoneal dialysis. Med Clin North Am 74:985–996, 1990.
61. Jameson MD, Wieggmann EB: Principles, uses and complications of hemodialysis. Med Clin North Am 74:945–960, 1990.
62. Schulman G, Hakim RM: Complications of hemodialysis. In Jacobson HR, et al (eds): The Principles and Practice of Nephrology. Philadelphia, BC Decker, 1991.
63. Kramer P, Wigger W, Rieger J, et al: Arteriovenous haemofiltration: A new and simple method for treatment of overhydrated patients resistant to diuretics. Klin Wochenschr 55:1121–1122, 1977.
64. Geronemus R, Schneider W: Continuous arteriovenous hemodialysis: A new modality for the treatment of acute renal failure. Trans Am Soc Artif Intern Organs 30:822–826, 1984.
65. Gibney RT, Stollery DE, Lefebvre RE, et al: Continuous arteriovenous hemodialysis: An alternative therapy for acute renal failure associated with critical illness. Can Med Assoc J 139:861–866, 1988.
66. Golper TA: Continuous arteriovenous hemofiltration in acute renal failure. Am J Kidney Dis 4:373–386, 1985.
67. Lawyer LA, Velasco A: Continuous arteriovenous hemodialysis in the ICU. Crit Care Nurs 18:29–41, 1989.
68. Reynolds, HN, Borg U, Belzberg H, Wiles CE: Efficacy of continuous arteriovenous hemofiltration with dialysis in patients with renal failure. Crit Care Med 19:1387–1394, 1991.
69. Voerman HJ, Strack Von Schijndel RJ, Thijs, LG: Continuous arterial venous hemodiafiltration in critically ill patients. Crit Care Med 18:911–914, 1990.
70. Golper TA, Ronco C, Kaplan AA: Continuous arteriovenous hemofiltration: Improvements, modifications and future directions. Semin Dialysis 1:50–54, 1988.
71. Suddaby EC, Bell SB, Murphy KJ: Continuous hemofiltration in infants and children. Pediatr Nurs 16:79–83, 1990.
72. Canaud B, Garred LJ, Christol AS, et al: Pump assisted continuous venovenous hemofiltration for treating acute uremia. Kidney Int 33:S154–S155, 1988.

PART IV

Unique Patient Populations

25

THE PREGNANT TRAUMA PATIENT

LYNN GERBER-SMITH

Potential for Postpartum Hemorrhage
Potential for Postpartum Infection
Potential for Breast Engorgement
Alteration in Grieving Process Related to Maternal Injuries and Clinical Condition
Alteration in Maternal–Infant Bonding Related to Maternal Injuries and Clinical Condition
Alteration in the Family System and/or Potential for Family Stress Related to Maternal Hospitalization

INTERMEDIATE CARE/REHABILITATION CYCLE

Labor and Delivery Plans

Postpartum Care

Nursing Diagnosis and Therapeutics

Alteration in the Family System Secondary to Maternal Hospitalization and Clinical Needs
Potential Alteration in Breastfeeding Activities Related to Maternal Hospitalization

Fetal Death

COMMUNITY REINTEGRATION CYCLE

Perinatal Referrals

Home Health Care

The pregnant trauma patient presents a double challenge: two lives must be treated concurrently. When the trauma patient is pregnant, response to shock will be different, and unique injuries, life-threatening to both the mother and the fetus, can occur. While caring for the pregnant trauma patient from resuscitation through rehabilitation, the nurse must assess the patient, interpret the assessment findings, and make decisions pertinent to the patient's care. The nurse is the integral link between the many specialists consulting with the pregnant trauma patient. Therefore, it is essential for the nurse to develop a firm knowledge base and proficient assessment skills regarding the needs of this unique patient population so that sound decisions can be made to enhance the care of both mother and child.

EPIDEMIOLOGY

The national birth rate trended upward from 1975 to 1988, with a slight 1 per cent decline in 1983 and 1984.[1] With the increasing number of pregnant women in our society, it has been estimated that 7 per cent of pregnant women will suffer some type of accidental injury during their pregnancy.[2] The most common causes of traumatic injuries for the pregnant population include motor vehicle accidents, falls, firearm injuries, battering or spouse abuse, and burns. Actual statistics on the specific incidence of trauma during pregnancy are not known.[3] Several studies have identified the number of pregnant patients treated at specific trauma centers and emergency departments and their mechanisms of injury. In one such study at the Shock Trauma Center of the Maryland Institute for Emergency Medical Services Systems (MIEMSS), 79 injured patients admitted over a 9-year period were pregnant.[4] This total represents less than 1 per cent of total MIEMSS acute admissions, 1.7 per cent of all female admissions, and 2.6 per cent of the women of childbearing age (14 to 45 years of age).[4] Blunt mechanisms of injury in this study had been incurred by 96 per cent of the study population, and penetrating mechanisms had injured 4 per cent.

Timberlake and McSwain report that over a 10-year period at Charity Hospital of Louisiana at New Orleans, 28 patients were diagnosed as pregnant and incurred a traumatic injury.[5] Of the 25 patients studied, 68 per cent were found to have a blunt mechanism of injury and 32 per cent a penetrating mechanism of injury.[5]

During a 5-year study period at the Tampa General Hospital Regional Trauma Center, 318 pregnant women were identified as suffering traumatic injury. Twenty-five of these patients had injuries that warranted admission to the trauma service, and they represented 0.3 per cent of the general trauma admissions.[6] Of the subset of 25 pregnant women, 16 (64 per cent) sustained blunt trauma secondary to a motor vehicle accident, 4 (16 per cent) sustained burns, and 2 (8 per cent) were the victims of assault. One had an abdominal stab wound, one sustained a gunshot wound, and one had fallen.

Finally, in a multicenter study with a combined trauma registry base of 30,000 patients, 73 pregnant women were admitted to four level I trauma centers in Pennsylvania. The most common mechanism of injury was blunt trauma (76.7 per cent), followed by falls (15.1 per cent), penetrating trauma (6.8 per cent), and burns (1.4 per cent).[7]

Motor vehicle accidents are the leading cause of death for women ages 15 to 44,[8] which are generally considered the childbearing years.[8] There are nearly 10 times more fatalities from motor vehicle accidents than from any other mechanism of injury during the reproductive years.[9] In years past, pregnant women secluded themselves, traveling less often, but the pregnant woman of today continues to drive and ride in vehicles until the time of delivery.

For anatomical and physiological reasons, falls are more common during pregnancy. During the first trimester, the woman is more easily fatigued and prone to fainting. As the pregnancy progresses, the uterus extends beyond the pelvic confines and may alter the mother's gait and balance, thus increasing the potential for falls. Relaxation of the pelvic girdle ligaments causes pelvic tilt and increases lordosis, and hence a change in balance occurs. Falls can occur going down stairs, slipping on ice, and even doing simple tasks such as putting on boots.[10] During late pregnancy, the woman may desire to redecorate for the new baby (nesting syndrome) and is likely to climb on a ladder or a chair, further placing herself at risk.

Penetrating injuries secondary to ballistic trauma also can occur during pregnancy. Whereas there are no specific statistics concerning the incidence of these injuries during pregnancy, firearms are second only to motor vehicle accidents as a cause of fatal injury.[11] It has been suggested that penetrating trauma is more common in the urban environment; however, it is a problem faced in every emergency department.[12] The pregnant abdomen may be the target of penetrating trauma when angry behaviors are displayed or when attempts to abort the fetus are made. Domestic violence does not necessarily decrease during pregnancy; the pregnancy may actually be the precipitating factor for such action.[13]

Pregnant women also can receive burn and inhalation injuries, although these injuries occur less frequently than those previously mentioned. Traumatic injuries that result from the aforementioned sources account for the leading nonobstetrical causes of death in pregnant women.[14]

NURSING DATA BASE

Female trauma patients of childbearing age (15 to 40 years) should always be considered pregnant until proven otherwise. Sherer and Schenker[15] suggest that it is very difficult to determine the actual incidence of trauma during pregnancy because of lack of questioning and documentation. They cite two clinical examples in which this information may not be recorded: the very mild traumatic event that is poorly documented in the medical record and the life-threatening situation in which pregnancy may not be considered. Therefore, it is of utmost importance that an accurate data base and patient health history be obtained as soon as possible. This information not only helps to establish a pregnant condition but can often provide information that aids in both the diagnosis and management of traumatic injuries during pregnancy. An obstetrical history, starting with questions about pregnancy, should therefore be initiated immediately. If the patient is unconscious or the family is not available to answer questions, a pregnancy test should be obtained. A description of the events preceding an accident and, whenever possible, of the actual event itself is helpful in every traumatic injury, particularly when the trauma patient is pregnant. When a pregnant woman sustains a traumatic injury, obstetrical complications such as eclampsia must be ruled out as a precipitator. If loss of consciousness, headache, back pain, or abdominal pain precedes an accident, an underlying obstetrical problem that precipitated the event should be suspected. Information concerning the actual event can help the nurse to relate the mechanism of injury to possible injuries and must be included as part of the nursing data base.

Mechanism of Injury

Motor Vehicle Accidents

The information important to obtain following a pregnant woman's involvement in a road traffic accident includes whether she was a driver or passenger in the vehicle, whether she was wearing a seat belt and shoulder harness, and the severity of the crash. If the woman was the driver of the vehicle, then injury to the protuberant abdomen from the steering column may result, particularly if safety restraints were not utilized. Proper use of seat belts may decrease the severity of maternal injuries and increase maternal survival[16] (Fig. 25–1). Seat belts prevent ejection from the vehicle, decrease the likelihood of severe head injury, and, in general, lower mortality.[17, 18] Since the overall leading cause of fetal death is maternal death following motor vehicle accidents, seat belts increase the chance of fetal survival.[19]

When prehospital care providers have information about the events that precipitated the accident or the severity of the accident itself, this information should be conveyed to the health care providers at the receiving facility. One study examined the relationship between type of collision and resultant maternal injuries in 441 pregnant women who were involved in motor vehicle accidents.[20] It was reported that when there was minor damage to the vehicle, less than 1 per cent of the women were injured. When the damage to the vehicle was severe, more serious injuries were found, as expected. Seven per cent of those who were involved in severe accidents died, and 12.9 per cent suffered injury.

Falls

The enlarging uterus, loosened pelvic joints, and possible pain and neuromuscular dysfunction from pelvic pressure predispose pregnant women to falls.[2] An accurate history of the events preceding the fall and of the fall itself is helpful in determining an underlying pathological process that may have precipitated the fall and resultant injuries.

If possible, details of the actual fall event should be described, since the type and severity of injuries, which are related to the dissipation of mechanical energy, may be predicted.[11] The height a person falls in part determines velocity and may reflect injury severity. If a person is able to break the fall by grasping onto something, the velocity can be decreased. Impact forces also can affect injury severity. The energy-absorbing qualities of the structure one falls upon is an important factor to consider.

When a pregnant woman falls, she generally will land on her buttock or side, not the abdomen.[21] Injuries are therefore more likely to be sustained by the mother than by the fetus. Head and spinal cord injuries, as well as fractures of the

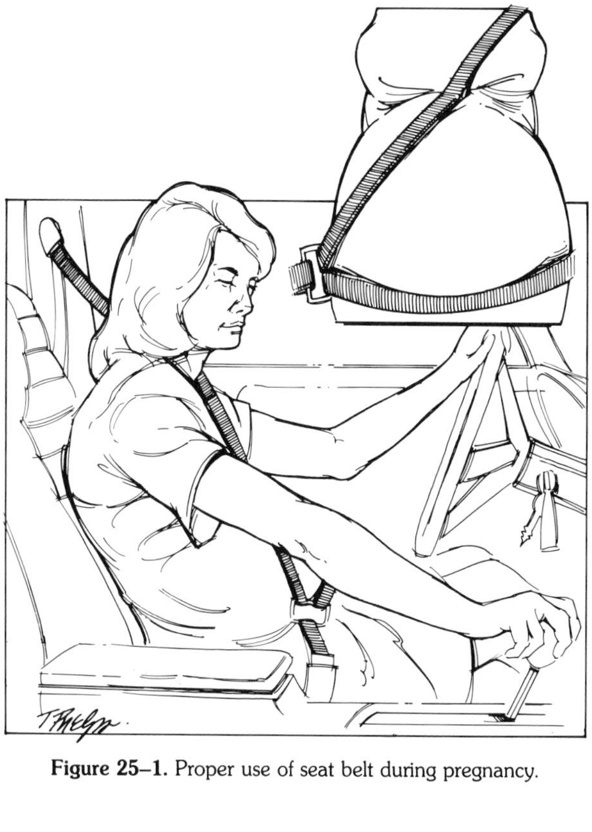

Figure 25–1. Proper use of seat belt during pregnancy.

pelvis and lower extremities, are common. But one must still be wary of obstetrical injuries such as an abruptio placentae.

Firearms and Other Weapons

Gunshot wounds are the most common type of penetrating trauma during pregnancy.[22] Other sources of penetrating trauma include stabbings with knives or other sharp objects. When the woman is pregnant, the enlarged abdomen is the most likely body part to be targeted, causing possible damage to the underlying uterus.[23]

Events surrounding a shooting are often vague, and witnesses or even the woman herself may claim the incident to be accidental. However, such violent crime may represent an attempt to damage or abort the fetus and must be suspected. The nurse must make every attempt to elicit this information from the patient, family members, or significant others. Information about the type of firearm involved and the distance between the individual and the weapon can aid in determining the severity of underlying injuries. Gunshot wounds usually require early surgical exploration and repair.

Stab wounds require that a description of the weapon be given to the emergency care personnel if the weapon does not accompany the patient. This information may need to be elicited from the victim or witnesses. The length and width of the object and how far it penetrated the abdomen or other body part are clues to possible underlying injury. Stab wounds may be explored locally to determine the extent of injury and the possible need for further surgical intervention.

Battering/Spouse Abuse

Battery, or intentional physical violence, is a major problem affecting the health and welfare of American women today.[24, 25] Up to one in three women has been battered by her male partner.[26] Numerous studies have indicated that battery or abuse occurs during pregnancy.[13, 27, 28]

In view of this strong epidemiological basis for violence during pregnancy, nurses should maintain a high index of suspicion and probe to ascertain information detailing the events leading to injury. Parker and McFarlane suggest that the routine prenatal assessment provides an excellent opportunity to obtain an abuse assessment screen.[29] An acute hospitalization for an unexplained traumatic event also should be a time to conduct such an assessment. As stated by Parker and McFarlane, a nonjudgmental, gentle approach is essential, but the questions must be direct.[29] An abuse assessment screen developed by the Nursing Research Consortium on Violence and Abuse is presented in Figure 25–2.

Investigators use a variety of terms that define or suggest the injury mechanism of battering (e.g., *beating, assault, biting*). Therefore, it is difficult to clearly ascertain the incidence of domestic violence as the cause of trauma during pregnancy when reviewing records. Several studies allow approximation: Three of the 25 pregnant trauma victims described by Timberlake and McSwain[5] had been beaten, and 1 had been bitten. Among the 73 pregnant women reviewed by Hoff[7] were 3 victims of assault. In Drost's study,[6] 2 (8 per cent) patients had been assaulted. However,

1. Have you ever been emotionally or physically abused by your partner or someone important to you?

YES ☐ NO ☐

2. Within the last year, have you been hit, slapped, kicked or otherwise physically hurt by someone?

YES ☐ NO ☐

If YES, by whom____________________________

Number of times____________________________

3. Since you've been pregnant, have you been hit, slapped, kicked, or otherwise physically hurt by someone?

YES ☐ NO ☐

If YES, by whom____________________________

Number of times____________________________

Mark the area of injury on body map.

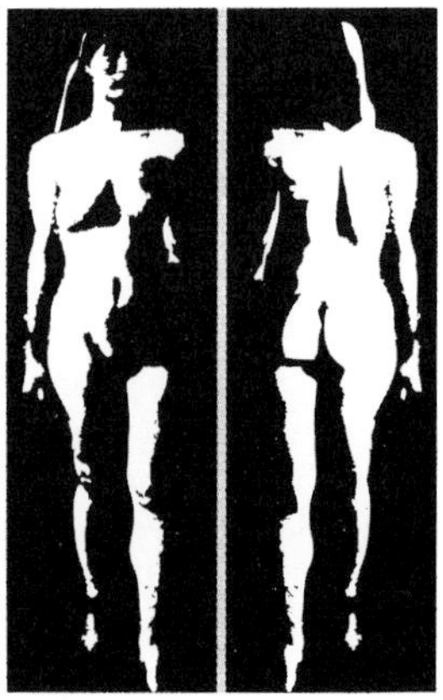

4. Within the last year, has anyone forced you to have sexual activities?

If YES, who____________________________

Number of times____________________________

5. Are you afraid of your partner or anyone you listed above?

YES ☐ NO ☐

**Developed by the Nursing Research Consortium on Violence and Abuse of which both authors are members. 1989. Readers are encouraged to reproduce and use this assessment tool.*

Figure 25–2. Abuse assessment screen. (Reprinted with permission from AJN Co, May/June 1991, Vol 16:3, Maternal Child Nursing, p 162.)

none of the 79 women described by Esposito was noted to be injured by battering, although one does not know if thorough questioning occurred.[30]

Burns and Inhalation Injury

When the burn patient is pregnant, fetal survival is primarily related to gestational age and maternal survival.[31] Initial management strategies include identification of the burn surface and rapid resuscitation efforts that focus on the provision of adequate oxygenation and restoration of circulating fluid volume[32] (refer to Chapter 28).

Carbon monoxide (CO) intoxication should always be suspected and carboxyhemoglobin levels measured, since carbon monoxide intoxication is the leading cause of all poisoning deaths, including fetal poisoning deaths, in the United States.[33] In addition to fires, automobile exhaust and faulty heating systems are major causes of CO poisoning.

The fetal effects of CO poisoning can be more severe than maternal effects, because the concentration of carboxyhemoglobin is 10 to 15 per cent higher in the fetus. Lethal fetal CO levels can exist in the face of nonlethal maternal levels.[34]

Fetal complications such as cerebral palsy may result, because the fetal partial arterial oxygen concentration (PaO_2) decreases in direct proportion to the increase in carboxyhemoglobin. CO poisoning impairs the release of oxygen from the mother to the fetus and from fetal hemoglobin to fetal tissue.[35, 36] Prompt diagnosis and appropriate management of inhalation injuries are therefore essential.

Obstetrical History

When pregnancy is suspected, an obstetrical history should be considered an important component of the patient's health history. The gestational age of the fetus and status of the pregnancy must be established, and a complete obstetrical history should be obtained as soon as possible. Suspicion of pregnancy increases if more than 41/2 weeks have lapsed since the last menstrual period (LMP).

To determine gestational age, a reliable historian can be most helpful. The LMP is the most accurate factor in determining the gestational age of the fetus and the expected date of confinement or due date.[37]

More thorough obstetrical history should include parity (Table 25–1), which will indicate any previous abortions or premature deliveries. Delivery history, including the number of hours of labor and types of birth (vaginal or cesarean), also should be obtained along with the maternal Rh factor. This information can alert medical personnel to potential problems, including premature labor and delivery as well as other fetal and maternal injuries. A spouse, family member, or significant other should be interviewed to obtain this information when possible.

TABLE 25–1. PARITY

In many institutions, obstetrical history is summarized by digits and dashes (e.g., 3–1–0–4).

First digit:	Number of term infants (≥ 38 weeks)
Second digit:	Number of premature infants (20–37 weeks)
Third digit:	Number of abortions (any loss prior to 20 weeks)
Fourth digit:	Number of children currently alive

In the example above (3–1–0–4), the woman had 3 term births and 1 premature infant and has 4 children alive.

Data from Pritchard J, MacDonald P, Gant NF: Williams Obstetrics, 17th ed. Norwalk, CT, Appleton-Century-Crofts, 1990, p 246.

TABLE 25–2. PRESUMPTIVE, PROBABLE, AND POSITIVE SIGNS OF PREGNANCY

Presumptive Signs
- Amenorrhea
- Breast changes
- Fatigue
- Frequent micturition
- Nausea and vomiting
- Quickening
- Skin changes
- Vaginal changes

Probable Signs
- Braxton Hicks contractions
- Fetal outline
- Laboratory pregnancy tests
- Uterine changes

Positive Signs
- Fetal heart movement recorded by sonogram
- Fetal heart sounds
- Fetal movement felt by examiner
- X-ray outline of fetal skeleton

Data from Pilliteri A: Maternal-Newborn Nursing Care of the Growing Family, 3rd ed. Boston, Little, Brown and Co, 1985, p 320.

RESUSCITATION CYCLE

Early recognition that the trauma patient is pregnant can lead the nurse through the dual on-going assessment of mother and fetus. Early signs of pregnancy may be easily overlooked. Therefore, the astute nurse must always be alert to even the most subtle changes that can occur during pregnancy (Table 25–2).

The general principles upon which trauma management is based must not be ignored when caring for a pregnant trauma patient. The implementation of a rapid primary survey followed by a secondary assessment is imperative, with the ABCs being acknowledged as first priorities.[30] Early recognition of pregnancy should trigger the nurse to be suspicious of unique injuries that can result and to be alert for the changes that occur during pregnancy that may alter assessment findings and mask signs of shock.

Clinical Management/Team Approach

The key to successful management of the pregnant trauma patient is the utilization of a team approach. Both emergency/trauma personnel and obstetrical personnel should be involved in the patient's care. Although obstetrical management is imperative, the ABCs of trauma resuscitation remain the first priority, since the best guarantee of fetal survival is prompt maternal care following traumatic injury.

In 1974, Crosby,[38] identified complications associated with the management of these patients:

> Among physicians who man emergency rooms, there is a lack of familiarity with the state of pregnancy and the physiological changes that accompany it . . . thus a state of therapeutic paralysis is often seen when the trauma victim is recognized as being pregnant. Attention is all too often directed away from the pregnancy, which may be unfamiliar, but potentially of major importance. . . . Lacerations are sutured, fractures are set, x-rays taken and abrasions cleaned while the fetus may die; a retroplacental clot may grow with shock-inducing speed during the time spent dealing with lesser problems.

The situation as Crosby describes it may not be as pervasive in the trauma setting today, but the concept of therapeutic paralysis does persist. The fact that aggressive maternal care is essential for the best fetal outcome must be emphasized.

Maternal Assessment

In order to render prompt and aggressive maternal care to the pregnant trauma patient, the nurse caring for the patient during the resuscitation phase must have knowledge not only about initial trauma management interventions but also about the normal anatomical and physiological changes that occur during pregnancy[38a] (Table 25–3). This knowledge must be applied during the initial assessment process and as resuscitation efforts continue. Care of the pregnant trauma patient becomes more complex when obstetrical complications are encountered in addition to traumatic injuries. These assessment considerations are not limited, however, to the resuscitation phase of care. These factors must be considered throughout all cycles of care.

Neurological Considerations

Neurologically, the pregnant woman has an increased risk of fainting and is more easily fatigued owing to the unpredictable physiological changes that occur during pregnancy.[2]

TABLE 25–3. NORMAL ANATOMICAL AND PHYSIOLOGICAL CHANGES DURING PREGNANCY

BODY SYSTEM	ALTERATION
Neurological	Increased risk of fainting
	Easily fatigued
Cardiovascular	Hypervolemic (increased volume of as much as 50 per cent above prepregnancy levels)
	Supine hypotension
	Physiological anemia
	Increased heart rate
	Hypercoagulability
Respiratory	Engorged upper respiratory passages
	Increased tidal volume
	Increased vital capacity
	Increased respiratory rate
	Elevated diaphragm
	Decreased functional residual capacity
Gastrointestinal	Physiological ileus
	Increased gastric acidity
	Compartmentalization of abdominal contents
Genitourinary	Increased urinary frequency
	Increased glomerular filtration rate
	Dilation of renal calyces, renal pelvis, and ureter
Musculoskeletal	Alterations in gait and balance
	Widened symphysis pubis
	Lordosis

TABLE 25–4. SIGNS AND SYMPTOMS OF PREECLAMPSIA

TRADITIONALLY DEFINED	CONSIDERED SEVERE IF ONE OR MORE OF THE FOLLOWING ARE PRESENT
Development of hypertension	BP ≥ 160/110
	Proteinuria (> 5 gm in 24 hr)
Proteinuria	HELLP* syndrome
Edema	Oliguria
With convulsions → Eclampsia	Epigastric pain
	Neurological effects

*Hemolysis, elevated liver enzymes, low platelets (thrombocytopenia).
Data from Berkowitz R: Critical Care of the Obstetric Patient. New York, Churchill Livingstone, 1983, p 299; and Chesley L: Hypertensive disorders in pregnancy. In Gleicher N (ed): Principles of Medical Therapy in Pregnancy. New York, Plenum, 1985, pp 751–752.

The pregnant woman also may experience changes in gait and balance, primarily during the third trimester. Changes in vision, history of headaches, or seizure activity is abnormal, and obstetrical complications such as preeclampsia and eclampsia should therefore be suspected (Table 25–4). Prompt identification of an obstetrical complication can guide care and prevent both maternal and fetal compromise.

Respiratory Considerations

The respiratory system is also altered during pregnancy. The upper respiratory passages become engorged by capillaries, making the pregnant patient more prone to nasopharyngeal bleeding and subsequent upper airway obstruction.

During pregnancy, there may be as much as a 40 per cent increase in tidal volume and a rise of 100 to 200 ml in vital capacity.[32] There also may be an increase in respiratory rate by 15 per cent,[39] or it may remain unchanged.[32] The combined effects of these respiratory changes place the pregnant woman in a chronic state of hyperventilation that results in arterial blood gas alterations. Pa_{CO_2} levels drop to approximately 25 to 30 mm Hg, and Pa_{O_2} increases to 101 to 104 mm Hg. A normal pH is maintained by the excretion of bicarbonate via the kidneys (Table 25–5).

As pregnancy progresses, the diaphragm becomes elevated, decreasing functional residual capacity by 20 per cent at times. This decreases the pregnant woman's oxygen reserve, predisposing her to hypoxia. Therefore, the airway and breathing of a pregnant trauma patient must be carefully monitored and supported as necessary to prevent maternal and subsequent fetal hypoxia.

Cardiovascular Considerations

Cardiovascular changes are perhaps the most profound physiological alterations that occur during pregnancy and the most critical to interpret when assessing the pregnant trauma patient. The pregnant woman is normally hypervolemic. Blood volume during pregnancy begins to increase by the 10th week of gestation; by the 34th week of gestation, a pregnant woman's circulatory volume can increase by as much as 50 per cent.[32] This increase can mask a 30 per cent gradual loss of maternal blood volume, or a 10 to 15 per cent acute blood loss. When this occurs, although the maternal vital signs may remain unchanged, the fetus can be at risk owing to a decrease in uterine perfusion; the woman's

TABLE 25–5. LABORATORY VALUE ADJUSTMENTS DURING PREGNANCY

VALUE	NONPREGNANT	PREGNANT
ELECTROLYTES AND ACID-BASE VALUES		
Sodium (mEq/l)	135–145	132–140
Potassium (mEq/l)	3.5–5.0	3.5–4.5
Chloride (mEq/l)	100–106	90–105
Bicarbonate (mEq/l)	24–30	17–22
P_{CO_2} (mm Hg)	35–50	25–30
P_{O_2} (mm Hg)	98–100	101–104
Base excess (mEq/l)	0.7	3–4
Arterial pH	7.38–7.44	7.40–7.45
BUN (mg/dl)	10–18	4–12
Creatinine (mg/dl)	0.6–1.2	0.4–0.9
Creatinine clearance (ml/min)	3.5–5.0	2.0–3.7
Osmolality (mOsmol/kg)	275–295	275–285
LIPIDS AND LIVER FUNCTION TESTS		
Total bilirubin (mg/dl)	1.0	1.0
Direct bilirubin (mg/dl)	0.4	0.4
Alkaline phosphatase (IU/ml)	13–35	25–80
SGOT (IU/ml)	10–40	10–40
Total protein (g/dl)	6.0–8.4	5.5–7.5
Albumin (g/dl)	3.5–5.0	3.0–4.5
Globulin (g/dl)	2.3–3.5	3.0–4.0
Total lipids (mg/dl)	460–1000	1040
Total cholesterol (mg/dl)	120–220	250
Triglycerides (mg/dl)	45–150	230
Free fatty acid (μg/l)	770	1226
Phospholipids (mg/dl)	256	350
HEMATOLOGICAL LABORATORY VALUES		
Complete blood count		
Hematocrit (%)	37–48	32–42
Hemoglobin (g/dl)	12–16	10–14
Leukocyte (count/mm³)	4300–10,800	5000–15,000
Polymorphonuclear cells (%)	54–62	60–85
Lymphocytes (%)	38–46	15–40
Fibrinogen	250–400	600
Platelets	150,000–350,000	Normal or slightly decreased
Serum iron (μg)	75–150	65–120
Iron binding capacity (μg)	250–410	300–500
Iron saturation (%)	30–40	15–30
Ferritin (ng/ml)	35	10–12
Erythrocyte sedimentation (mm/hr)	<20	30–90

Reprinted with permission from Elrad H, Gleicher N: Physiologic changes in normal pregnancy. In Gleicher N (ed): Principles of Medical Therapy in Pregnancy. New York, Plenum, 1985, pp 51–52.

risk is also increased, for these stable vital signs may change precipitously. Since the uterus cannot autoregulate, its flow is directly related to the pressure it receives from maternal circulation.

The electrical activity of the heart can be altered during pregnancy as well. As the uterus enlarges and elevates the diaphragm, the heart is pushed upward and rotated, causing a shift of the electrical axis by 15 degrees. This may precipitate changes such as T-wave flattening or inversion in lead III, Q waves in lead III, and augmented V lead (aVF), which are considered normal in pregnancy.[40]

Hematological Considerations

Although erythrocyte production increases during pregnancy, adequate levels cannot be maintained as plasma volume increases; therefore, the pregnant woman is physiologically anemic. A normal prepregnancy hematocrit of 40 to 41 per cent may drop to 31 to 34 per cent in late pregnancy.[32]

The coagulation profile of the pregnant woman is also altered, since fibrinogen and concentrations of factors VII, VIII, and IX are increased during pregnancy.[2] Bleeding time, clotting time, and prothrombin time should remain unchanged during pregnancy.[32] The increase in fibrinogen and other factors, coupled with a decrease in circulating plasminogen activator, can actually benefit the pregnant patient if hemorrhage occurs. These same changes, however, can pose a problem for the immobilized patient by increasing the risk of thromboembolic disease.[2]

The leukocyte count is normally elevated in pregnancy[32] to approximately 5000 to 15,000/mm³ and becomes even further elevated during labor and delivery. Except for an increase in phagocytes and a decrease in lymphocytes during pregnancy, the differential remains unchanged.[32] For other laboratory study adjustments that need to be made, refer to Table 25–5.

Hemodynamic Considerations

The most dramatic hemodynamic change that occurs during pregnancy is supine hypotension, also known as *vena cava syndrome.* In the supine position, the enlarging uterus compresses the vena cava and aorta, impeding venous return and decreasing cardiac output. Therefore, the pregnant trauma patient should never be placed in the supine position. During prehospital transport and until spinal injuries are ruled out, this position can be avoided by tipping the backboard 30 degrees, simulating the left lateral position[30, 41] (Fig. 25–3).

Hypotension therefore can occur normally in a pregnant woman who is in a supine position. When this occurs, the patient will become uncomfortable or nauseated until she is repositioned and blood pressure increases. Hypertension is never normal during pregnancy and suggests a possible obstetrical complication. During pregnancy, the heart rate will increase approximately 10 to 20 beats per minute above prepregnancy levels. Until recently, data on pregnant patients' central venous pressure and pulmonary artery wedge pressure were not established. Clark and associates[42] noted that most studies of hemodynamic assessment during pregnancy involved patients already compromised and critically ill. They assessed the central hemodynamic status of 10 normal pregnant patients who were screened carefully both in their third trimester and postpartum. In late pregnancy, the patients had a 43 per cent increase in cardiac output (4.3 to 6.2 l/min). Other significant findings included a 21 per cent decline in systemic vascular resistance, a 34 per cent decline in pulmonary vascular resistance, and a 28 per cent decline in the colloid oncotic pressure–pulmonary capillary wedge pressure gradient. There was no significant difference in mean arterial pressure, central venous pressure, or pulmonary capillary wedge pressure in late pregnancy and the nonpregnant state (Table 25–6).

The hemodynamic changes that occur normally during pregnancy cause confusion as the resuscitation team assesses the patient's condition. Tachycardia and hypotension that occur when the pregnant trauma patient is in a supine position may not be indicative of a shock state but may, instead, represent normal changes. Caution must be exercised, however, because the pregnant trauma patient, as previously stated, can mask a 15 to 30 per cent blood loss without evidence of shock while uterine perfusion decreases, risking fetal anoxia and dire maternal consequences. Laboratory values, including hematocrit and leukocyte count, further confuse the clinical picture.

Gastrointestinal Considerations

A physiological ileus or diminished emptying time of the bowel normally occurs during pregnancy. Also, the placental production of gastrin and progesterone increases the acidity of the stomach contents. Upon auscultation, bowel sounds may be absent, making interpretation difficult. It should always be assumed that the pregnant trauma patient has a full stomach and is at risk for vomiting, aspiration, and pulmonary complications.

Abdominal assessment by palpation is often unreliable in the pregnant patient. Typical indicators of abdominal injury, such as guarding, tenderness, and rigidity, can occur during

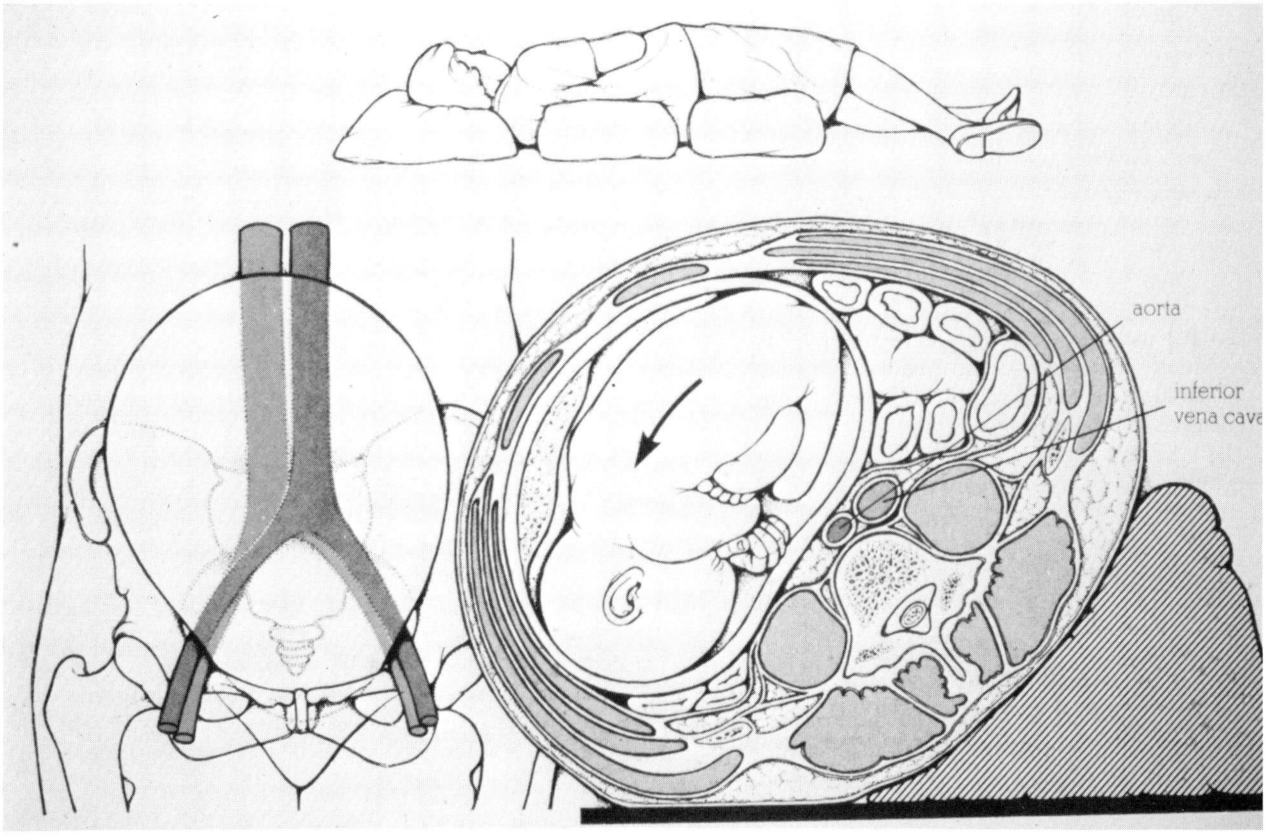

Figure 25–3. Left lateral positioning displaces the uterus and decreases compression of major abdominal vessels.

TABLE 25-6. CENTRAL HEMODYNAMIC CHANGES

	NONPREGNANT	PREGNANT
Cardiac output (l/min)	4.3 ± 0.9	6.2 ± 1.0
Heart rate (beats/min)	71 ± 10.0	83 ± 10.0
Systemic vascular resistance (dyne • cm • sec^{-5})	1530 ± 520	1210 ± 266
Pulmonary vascular resistance (dyne • cm • sec^{-5})	119 ± 47.0	78 ± 22
Colloid oncotic pressure (mm Hg)	20.8 ± 1.0	18.0 ± 1.5
Colloid oncotic pressure–pulmonary capillary wedge pressure (mm Hg)	14.5 ± 2.5	10.5 ± 2.7
Mean arterial pressure (mm Hg)	86.4 ± 7.5	90.3 ± 5.8
Pulmonary capillary wedge pressure (mm Hg)	6.3 ± 2.1	7.5 ± 1.8
Central venous pressure (mm Hg)	3.7 ± 2.6	3.6 ± 2.5
Left ventricular stroke	41 ± 8	48 ± 6

From Clark S, Cotton O, Lee W, et al: Central hemodynamic assessment of normal term pregnancy. Am J Obstet Gynecol 161:1439–1442, 1989.

pregnancy from the active and passive stretching of the abdominal wall as the enlarging uterus is accommodated.

Genitourinary Considerations

Genitourinary changes include an increase in urinary frequency throughout pregnancy. The increase in frequency during the first trimester is the result of an increase in glomerular filtration rate (GFR) by approximately 30.5 per cent of prepregnancy values.[43] During the third trimester, the further increased frequency is a result of the compression of the bladder by the enlarging uterus in addition to an increased GFR.

Following blunt trauma to the abdomen during late pregnancy, the bladder is more likely to spontaneously empty or rupture because the bladder may be elevated and out of the protection of the pelvic ring.[22] Assessment of the pregnant woman should include gentle palpation of the bladder above the symphysis pubis. If a stable condition allows, the patient should be encouraged to void. If unable to void spontaneously, the patient should be catheterized using strict aseptic technique. Urine testing revealing glucosuria is common during pregnancy, but the presence of frank or microscopic blood suggests genitourinary trauma. Diagnostic tests may be performed, including cystogram, intravenous pyelogram, and/or cystoscopy. Dilation of renal calyces, renal pelves, and ureter (particularly on the right side) may be evident. These conditions are present from about the 10th week of pregnancy until after delivery and are believed to be caused by ureteral obstruction from the ovarian vein plexuses and increased progesterone concentrations.[32] Normal changes that occur during pregnancy must be recognized so that interpretation of test results is enhanced.

Metabolic Considerations

As a normal change of pregnancy, the pituitary gland nearly doubles in weight. Shock and/or hypoxia in the pregnant patient can precipitate a sudden drop in pituitary blood flow, leading to necrosis.[44] Calcium, phosphate, and magnesium levels fall during pregnancy,[32] as well as creatinine and BUN. There is also an increased risk of glucose intolerance.

Obstetrical and Fetal Considerations

When the trauma patient is pregnant, primary and secondary assessment must focus on the fetus and possible obstetrical complications that can result following traumatic injury. The fetus may be compromised while the mother appears stable. As an initial response to shock, uterine perfusion decreases, causing stress to the fetus. Unique injuries to the uterus must be detected and treated immediately, or the lives of the fetus and mother are threatened.

Obstetrical Assessment

The obstetrical assessment must determine the viability of the fetus, establish the potential for impending delivery, and identify unique injuries.

Gestational Age. As previously mentioned, the LMP is the most accurate indicator of gestational age. However, in the emergency setting, it may not be possible to obtain this information. Other accurate physical assessment indicators of gestational age include measurement of the uterus at the umbilicus, the first auscultation of fetal heart tones, quickening, and fundal height.[37] In the emergency setting, if pregnancy history cannot be obtained, auscultation of fetal tones and determination of fundal height may be valuable.

The pregnant uterus is usually palpable at 12 to 14 weeks, and by 18 to 22 weeks it should be at the level of the umbilicus. Fundal height is reflected in centimeters and is determined by measuring the distance from the symphysis pubis to the top of the uterus. From 16 to 32 weeks from the LMP, this measurement approximates the weeks of gestation (Fig. 25–4). Although a multiple fetal pregnancy can alter the assessment of fundal height, as can uterine fibroids or polyhydramnios (increase in amniotic fluid), it is generally utilized as a guide in determining gestational age.

When immediately available, ultrasound has become extremely helpful in estimating gestational age. A mobile real-time unit that can be brought to the resuscitation area is the most appropriate method. It can be used to assess fetal well-being through fetal cardiac movement as well as to determine placental location.[45] If ultrasound is not readily available in an emergent situation, such as when a pregnant woman presents with vaginal bleeding and abdominal pain, clinical assessment and patient history must be relied on.

Determination of the gestational age of the fetus is also helpful in identifying possible injuries to both the mother and fetus. During the first 12 to 14 weeks (early pregnancy), the uterus is well protected in the pelvic confines. Cases of uterine and fetal injury in this stage have been documented, but they are rare.[2] During late pregnancy (greater than 12 to 14 weeks), the uterus becomes an abdominal organ and is no longer protected by the pelvis. The uterus and fetus may therefore absorb the impact of traumatic forces and consequently sustain unique injuries.

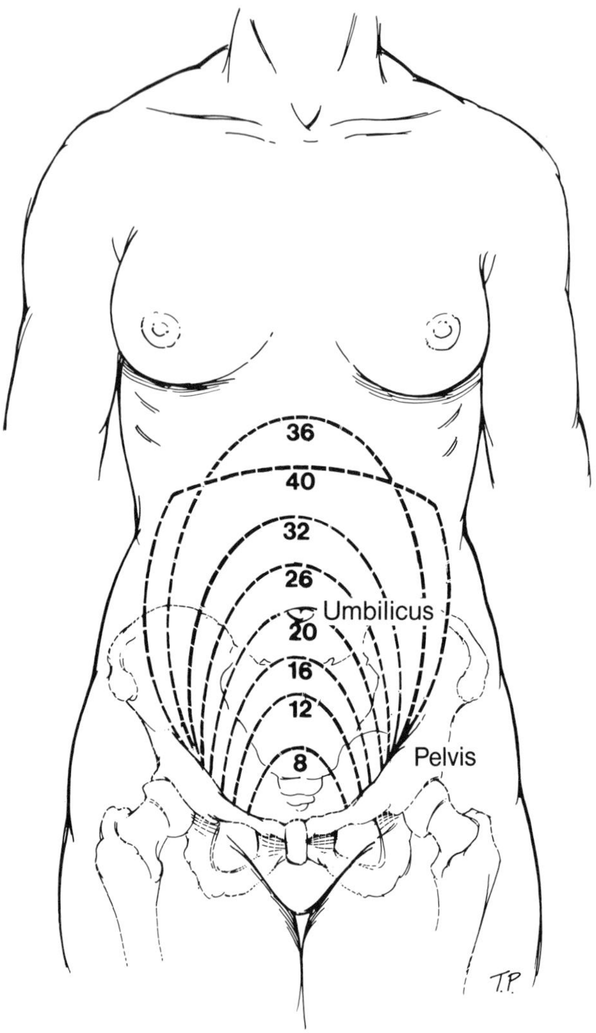

Figure 25–4. Uterine size and location reflecting gestational age.

Premature Rupture of Membranes (PROM). Following the estimation of gestational age and establishment of fetal well-being, the patient's amniotic membrane status (intact or ruptured) must be assessed. Indications of labor, if any, also must be noted. A history of a sudden gush of fluid following abdominal impact suggests a possible premature rupture of amniotic membranes but must be differentiated from a spontaneous bladder void. If a pool of vaginal fluid is present, it should be tested for pH. The normal pH of amniotic fluid is 7 to 7.5; that of urine is 4.8 to 6.0. The fluid also can be checked microscopically (place a drop on a slide and allow to dry) for the appearance of ferning, which is a more reliable sign of amniotic fluid presence.

Premature Labor. Determining if a patient is in labor is also a component of the obstetrical assessment. Labor consists of three stages: dilation of the cervix, expulsion of the baby via the birth canal, and the separation and expulsion of the placenta. The identification of the onset of labor is particularly important if the woman is not at term. Signs and symptoms of the onset of labor include bloody show, ruptured membranes, and contractions. Contractions can be difficult for the nonobstetrical staff to assess; therefore, obstetrical team expertise is most valuable. Contractions

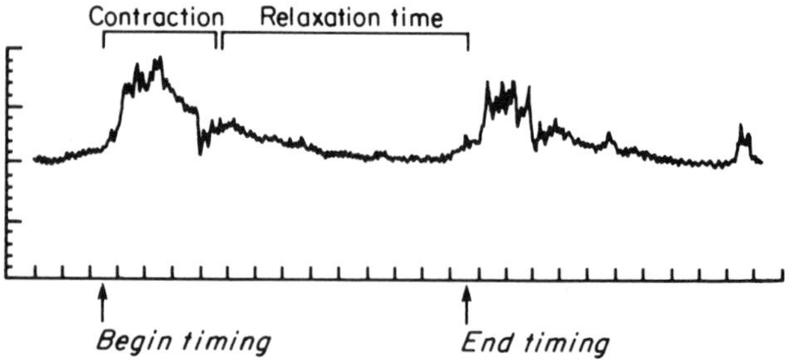

Figure 25–5. A uterine contraction consists of two periods, the contraction time and the relaxation time. The frequency of contractions is the interval of time from the beginning of one contraction period to the beginning of the next contraction period.

causing dilation of the cervix indicate that the patient is in labor. The duration and frequency of contractions must be assessed. The frequency of contractions is determined by noting the time from the beginning of one contraction to the beginning of the next contraction (Fig. 25–5). Premature labor following trauma may indicate fetal or uterine injury, which must be ruled out before measures are taken to inhibit the progression of labor.

Uterine Damage. As pregnancy progresses, the uterus becomes an abdominal organ and can be damaged following blunt or penetrating trauma. Uterine damage can consist of a laceration, a tear, or a partial or complete rupture. If uterine rupture has occurred, the uterus is usually, but not always, tender on palpation. The abdomen may be distended, and vaginal bleeding may occur (Table 25–7). When uterine rupture is severe, two distinct masses may be palpable in the abdomen: the uterus and fetus.[46] Milder forms of uterine damage are more common, although clinically less distinct.

Abruptio Placentae. Placental abruption, the premature separation of the placenta from the uterine wall, also can occur following trauma. It is the second leading cause of fetal death.[47] Abruption in mild forms can be difficult to diagnose. An abnormal fetal heart rate pattern (identified by obstetrical staff with expertise in this area) has been helpful in determining a placental abruption in women at greater than 20 weeks' gestation.[48, 49] The grave sign of a decrease or absence of fetal heart tones may indicate too late that there was injury to the placenta. Other signs and symptoms are listed in Table 25–8.[50] Placental abruption can occur more than 48 hours after the initial traumatic incident. The incidence of abruptio placentae following severe trauma ranges from 6.6 to 66 per cent.[51]

TABLE 25–7. SIGNS AND SYMPTOMS OF UTERINE DAMAGE

Mild uterine injuries (e.g., lacerations and contusions)
Varied and mild symptoms
Uterine rupture
Acute abdominal pain followed by no pain
Vaginal bleeding
Maternal shock
Loss of fetal heart tones
Uterine tenderness to palpation
Palpation of two abdominal masses (uterus and fetus)

Data from Whitney N: A Manual of Clinical Obstetrics. Philadelphia, JB Lippincott, 1985, pp 552–553.

TABLE 25–8. SIGNS AND SYMPTOMS OF ABRUPTIO PLACENTAE

Vaginal bleeding
Premature labor
Abdominal pain
Uterine tenderness to palpation
Uterine tetany or rigidity (uterine tone may be increased with small, frequent contractions superimposed)
Expanding or rising fundal height
Maternal shock
Fetal distress or absence of fetal heart tones
Abnormal fetal heart rate pattern

The signs and symptoms can often be vague, particularly in mild abruptions. Not all the symptoms may be present, particularly vaginal bleeding.

The mechanism causing the abruption is thought to be directly related to the trauma. Higgins and Garite describe the placenta in the uterus as a potato chip inside a tennis ball.[51] The uterus is elastic; the placenta is not. On impact, the placenta cannot reshape as the uterus does; instead, it separates or pulls away from the uterine wall, causing disruption of the maternal/fetal circulation and hemorrhage. Early detection of an abruption and appropriate action increase the chances of fetal survival.

Coagulation changes are rare following a mild abruption, but if the abruption is severe enough to cause fetal demise, as with any situation involving significant hemorrhage, the patient can develop a severe coagulopathy.

Fetomaternal Hemorrhage. Fetomaternal hemorrhage is the transplacental bleeding of fetal blood into the maternal circulation.[52] It occurs four to five times more often when the pregnant patient has incurred a traumatic injury.[48, 49] To detect fetomaternal hemorrhage, the Kleihauer–Betke acid-elution assay should be done on maternal blood. This test also can estimate fetal blood loss. It is especially significant for Rh-negative patients so that they can be administered Rh immune globulin to prevent development of isoimmunization.

Fetal Assessment

On-going fetal assessment is essential, since the mother can mask signs of shock and the fetus will be the first to show evidence of compromise.

The best indicator of fetal condition is the fetal heart rate. Normal fetal heart rate is 120 to 160 beats per minute and can be detected by an ultrasound device (Doppler) by 10 to 12 weeks of gestation.[53] If the fetus is viable, its heart rate should be monitored continuously. (Fetuses older than 24 weeks are considered viable if neonatal resources are available; infants born at 23 to 24 weeks have survived. In the absence of neonatal services, however, fetuses older than 27 weeks should be considered viable.) Only a Doppler designed for obstetrical evaluation should be utilized, since its frequency is adjusted to assess fetal heart tones. An adult Doppler of higher frequency may cause enough alteration that nothing is heard, even though the fetus is viable, thereby confusing the clinical picture. Fetal tachycardia followed by the more grave sign of fetal bradycardia suggests fetal anoxia and requires immediate action for fetal survival.

When the pregnant trauma patient is conscious, she is a resource for detecting an alteration in fetal activity, which is also an indicator of fetal well-being. Quickening, or the maternal perception of fetal movement, usually occurs about the 16th week of gestation in a second pregnancy and in the 20th week of the first. Although the fetus is not in constant motion, a prolonged period during which fetal movement is lacking can suggest fetal demise.

Additional diagnostic procedures that can aid in assessing the condition of the fetus include ultrasound and amniocentesis. Real-time ultrasound can identify fetal cardiac movement and detect fetal heart tones as well as fetal death.[54] Fetal biophysical assessment by ultrasound is a method used to determine if a fetus has been asphyxiated. Fetal biophysical profile scoring is based on five biophysical variables, four of which are monitored simultaneously by dynamic ultrasound imaging. The variables are fetal breathing movement, gross body movement, fetal tone, reactive fetal heart rate, and qualitative amniotic fluid volume.[55] Each is coded as normal or abnormal according to set criteria and given a rating of 2 (normal) or 0 (abnormal).

Based on the biophysical profile score, a management protocol is recommended. The biophysical profile looks for an alteration in the fetal central nervous system as an indication of fetal asphyxia. In the emergency setting, biophysical profile scoring may be helpful, but the test requires a 30-minute ultrasound observation period, which may not be appropriate during initial trauma resuscitation. The scoring and observation could be done postresuscitation while the patient undergoes acute monitoring.[41]

Amniocentesis can test for fetal maturity. Maturity of the fetal lungs is determined by the lecithin/sphingomyelin ratio and/or the presence of phosphatidyl glycerol.

Special Management Considerations

Other factors must be considered when caring for the pregnant trauma patient during intubation, radiographic examinations, medication administration, medical or pneumatic antishock garment (PASG) use, and invasive abdominal assessment procedures. The cardiac arrest situation is also unique for this patient population.

Intubation

Use of nasal airways or endotracheal tubes should be avoided to prevent nasal bleeding.[39] When intubation is required, a smaller (6.0 or 6.5 mm), well-lubricated endotracheal tube should be gently inserted.[56]

Radiographic Examinations

Radiographic examinations that are considered essential for diagnosing patient injuries following trauma should never be omitted during pregnancy. Exposure below 1 rad appears to carry little risk, and there is no correlation with childhood cancer at less than 2 rads. Exposures as high as 5 to 10 rads have not caused gross fetal abnormalities.[57, 58] Care must be taken, however, to protect the patient from unnecessary exposure. When possible, the uterus should be shielded with a lead apron prior to radiographic examination (Fig. 25–6). Duplication of radiographs should be avoided, and the purpose of each exposure should be validated as to its clinical implications. The patient should be assured that essential tests must be done to diagnose her injuries properly. If any questions arise after resuscitation, early consultation with a genetic counselor is appropriate.

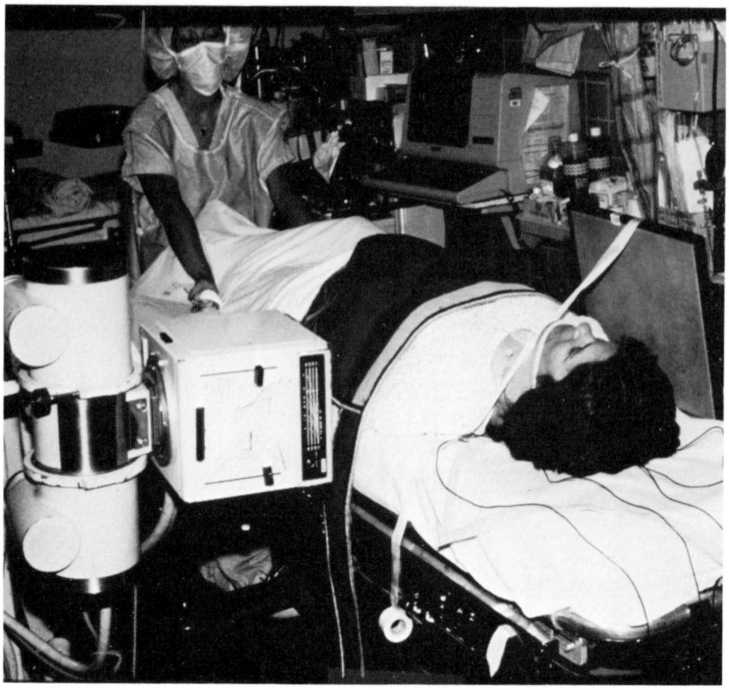

Figure 25–6. The pregnant patient's abdomen should be shielded by a lead apron from above the fundus to below the pelvic area.

Medications

All medications are, as a rule, contraindicated during pregnancy. Decisions concerning medication use during pregnancy must weigh the benefits to the mother against the risks to the fetus. The highest risk period for the fetus is during the period of organogenesis (days 15 to 56 after conception).[59] It is during this time that medications are most likely to have a teratogenic effect on the fetus (Table 25–9).

Tetanus prophylaxis with toxoid or human tetanus immune globulin, commonly given following trauma, should be given if the pregnant patient has not been immunized in the past 10 years.[60] If the patient requires anticoagulation therapy following trauma, heparin is the drug of choice, since coumadin crosses the placental membranes and is associated with fetal anomalies and an increased risk of stillbirth. The notion that the placenta is a barrier that keeps medications from the developing fetus has been disproved; a more appropriate analogy is that the placenta acts as a sieve.

Pneumatic Antishock Garment (PASG)

PASGs are commonly utilized in trauma resuscitation to augment circulatory support. Although once thought to autotransfuse blood from the lower extremities, new research suggests that the primary mechanism of action involves an increase in peripheral vascular resistance.[61] Regardless of the mechanism of action, the appropriateness of PASG use during pregnancy remains controversial. Generally, indications for PASG use include any patient in shock with a systolic blood pressure of less than 80 mm Hg. Clinical case studies have documented the use of PASGs during such obstetrical emergencies as abortion complications, ectopic pregnancies, hydatidiform mole bleeding, hypocoagulation states, postoperative hemorrhage, septic shock, and uterine atrophy.[62] In most of these obstetrical conditions, the uterus has been emptied of the fetus. The abdominal and leg portions can therefore be inflated, with the abdominal portion of the PASG controlling abdominal hemorrhage by tamponade.[63] During pregnancy, however, the effects of inflating the abdominal compartment over the uterus are not known; therefore, when PASG is utilized during pregnancy, it is suggested that only the leg compartments be inflated (Fig. 25–7) and that the patient's clinical status be monitored carefully.

Abdominal Assessment (Diagnostic Peritoneal Lavage, Computed Tomography, and Ultrasound)

Since abdominal assessment is usually unreliable for the pregnant trauma patient, an invasive or noninvasive procedure may be performed during the resuscitation phase to determine the presence of abdominal injury. Diagnostic peritoneal lavage (DPL), computed tomography (CT), and ultrasound are all useful for this patient population.

TABLE 25–9. SUMMARY OF THE EFFECTS OF DRUGS ON THE FETUS AND NEWBORN

All maternal drugs except those drugs with a large molecular weight cross the placenta and may affect the fetus
Effects may be immediate or delayed
Drug effect may be reflected in involvement of not one organ system, but many
Reported effects fall into 11 major categories:
- Fetal wastage
- Teratogenesis
- Carcinogenesis
- Impaired sexual reproductive capacity
- Abnormal prenatal growth
- Abnormal postnatal growth
- Abnormal adaptation to birth process
- Hematological changes
- Metabolic changes
- Mental retardation
- CNS sequelae

Adapted from Hill M, Stern L: Drugs in pregnancy: Effects on the fetus and newborn. Drugs 17:182–197, 1979.

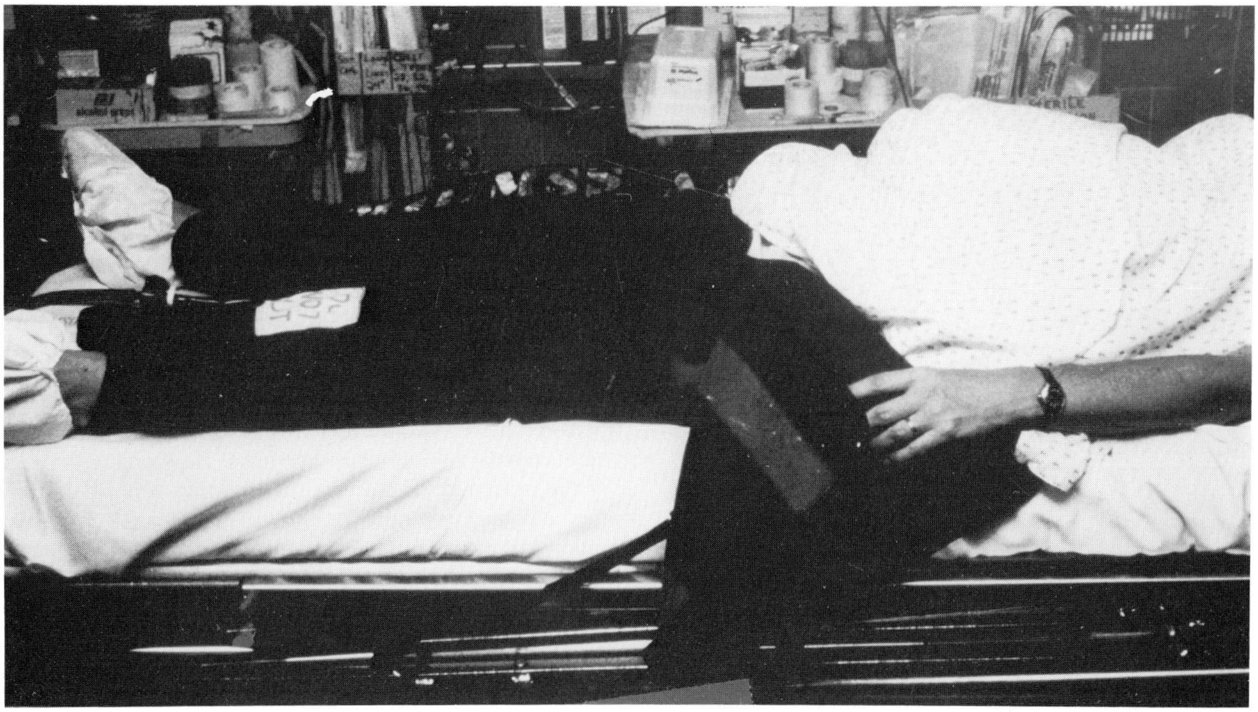

Figure 25–7. Pneumatic antishock garment with leg portion only to be inflated on pregnant trauma patients.

DPL is considered both safe and appropriate in pregnant trauma patients[32, 50, 54, 64, 65] (see Chapter 20). The stomach and bladder should be emptied prior to the procedure, and the uterus should be well defined. If clinical inspection following penetrating trauma suggests penetration of the abdominal wall, the lavage may be omitted in lieu of emergency laparotomy.

In general, CT has become a more popular modality for abdominal assessment in the trauma population.[66] It has the advantages of being noninvasive and providing information on the retroperitoneal and genitourinary tract. Some authors have recommended it for the gravid trauma patient.[67] Both fetal and uterine injuries can be identified and defined with an abdominal CT scan (Fig. 25–8). The amount of radiographic exposure to the fetus during abdominal CT depends on a number of factors, including patient age, type of machine, shielding of fetus, and fetal lie.[68]

Ultrasound is a relatively new modality in the evaluation of abdominal trauma in the United States. In the gravid trauma patient, ultrasound may have particular merit because it is noninvasive and does not expose the fetus to radiation. Ultrasound can be utilized to assess fetal well-being, gestational age, and placental and uterine injuries. A skilled radiologist also can employ ultrasound to evaluate abdominal viscera and pelvic fluid.[4]

Another diagnostic test that has been employed during pregnancy is culdocentesis. In selected patients, culdocentesis has been of clinical value,[32] but most traumatologists do not use this procedure because of its high false-positive rate.[30]

All these abdominal tests are frightening to the pregnant trauma patient, who may perceive the procedures as harmful to her baby. Reassurance and support as well as thorough explanations will be needed prior to and during the diagnostic testing.

Cardiac Arrest

When the pregnant trauma patient is in cardiac arrest, the principles of resuscitation are the same as those for nonpregnant patients. Standard cardiopulmonary resuscitation (CPR) procedures should be performed and advanced cardiac lifesaving (ACLS) measures instituted to ensure survival of both the mother and fetus. A team member should be assigned to manually displace the uterus to improve venous return. Defibrillation should be performed if necessary.[69] Drugs commonly administered during the cardiac arrest activities should be used during pregnancy as well.[70]

Postmortem Cesarean Section

When the patient is in cardiac arrest on admission, the decision to perform a postmortem cesarean section must be made. Obstetrical and neonatal personnel must be notified immediately. More than 150 cases of successful postmortem cesarean section have been documented.[71] The cesarean section should be performed while CPR is in progress and as soon after maternal death as possible. Two key factors that must be considered when making the decision to perform a postmortem cesarean section are gestational age of fetus and amount of time the patient has been in arrest. Neonatal resuscitation almost always will be necessary after delivery of the infant and should be managed by neonatal personnel, who must have emergency equipment immediately accessible (Table 25–10).

Nursing Diagnosis and Therapeutics

Blunt and Penetrating Trauma in Early Pregnancy

Potential for Maternal Hemorrhagic Shock Secondary to Traumatic Injury. The patient's vital signs

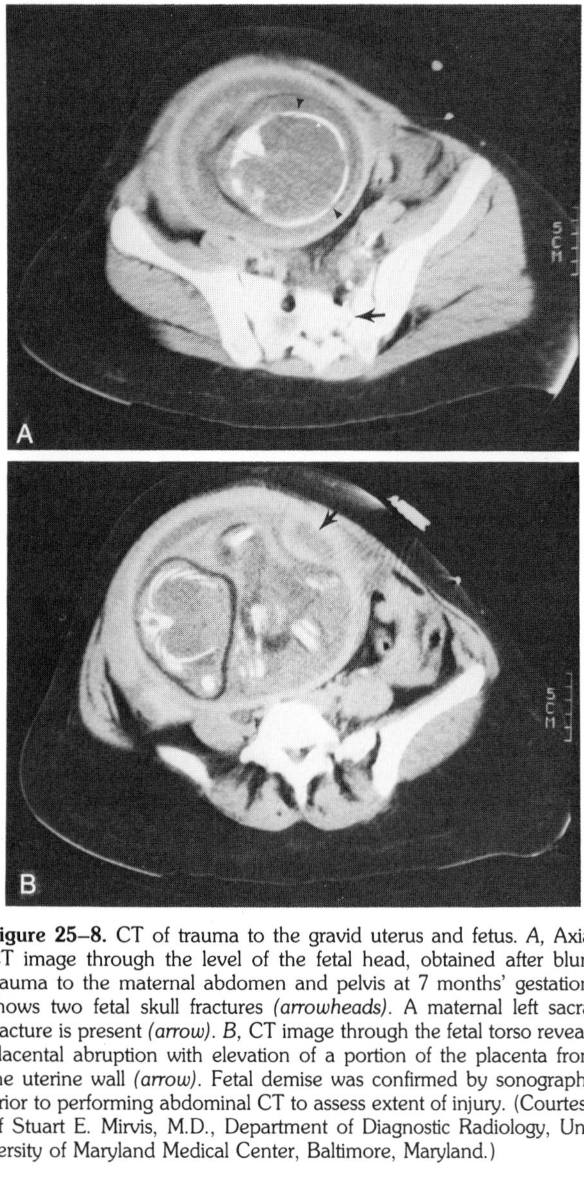

Figure 25–8. CT of trauma to the gravid uterus and fetus. *A,* Axial CT image through the level of the fetal head, obtained after blunt trauma to the maternal abdomen and pelvis at 7 months' gestation, shows two fetal skull fractures *(arrowheads).* A maternal left sacral fracture is present *(arrow). B,* CT image through the fetal torso reveals placental abruption with elevation of a portion of the placenta from the uterine wall *(arrow).* Fetal demise was confirmed by sonography prior to performing abdominal CT to assess extent of injury. (Courtesy of Stuart E. Mirvis, M.D., Department of Diagnostic Radiology, University of Maryland Medical Center, Baltimore, Maryland.)

should be monitored closely for signs and symptoms of shock throughout the resuscitation cycle so that aggressive volume replacement can be initiated as necessary. Hypotension can occur normally in a supine position during early pregnancy and may be subtle. Turning the pregnant patient to the left lateral position can produce a marked increase in cardiac output and should always be done as a resuscitative measure if possible (see Fig. 25–3). Care must be taken to stabilize the neck and maintain the spine in proper alignment when repositioning. When the patient is immobilized on a backboard, the board can be slightly elevated toward the left lateral position (Fig. 25–9). If the patient's injuries or resuscitation procedures prohibit this positional change, the uterus can be manually displaced. When audible, the fetal heart rate should be monitored continuously or auscultated with each check of maternal vital signs. The fetus may be the first to show evidence of shock. Laboratory value trends must be monitored closely as well and compared with normal pregnancy values (see Table 25–5).

As the initial assessment of the pregnant trauma patient progresses systematically, knowledge regarding the anatomical and physiological changes that occur during pregnancy must be integrated. Injuries of the liver and spleen are common during pregnancy. The patient's abdomen should be assessed carefully for pain, guarding, and rebound tenderness, considering the fact that results may be difficult to interpret in this patient population. Additional minutes should be spent in auscultating bowel sounds, since the diminished emptying time of the bowel can mimic a silent abdomen. A nasogastric or orogastric tube should be inserted early during the resuscitation phase of care.

The patient should be prepared for abdominal lavage or other diagnostic tests as indicated. The stomach and bladder should be emptied prior to the lavage. The patient may perceive the procedure as harmful to her baby and should be encouraged to verbalize her fears. Reinforcing the value of the procedure as a diagnostic tool that is not harmful to the baby may ease some of the mother's fears.[46, 64, 72] Preparation for surgical intervention may be indicated if abdominal exploration is deemed necessary.

Potential for Fetal Anoxia Secondary to Maternal Shock. Continuous fetal monitoring is ideal, since any change in maternal condition can be compared with fetal well-being. If continuous monitoring is not available, the fetal heart rate should be checked every 10 to 15 minutes and/or with each assessment of maternal vital signs. Since uterine perfusion decreases as an initial response to shock, the fetus may be the first to evidence shock. There is some question, though, over what, if any, action can be taken if

TABLE 25–10. RESUSCITATION OF THE NEONATE

. . . the goal of resuscitation and stabilization is to *gently* maintain an adequate stable flow of oxygenated blood to all parts of the body. . .

RESUSCITATION EQUIPMENT

Radiant heated bed
Aspiration equipment: No. 5, 8, and 10 French catheters
Oxygen source
Ventilation bag: nonrebreathing valve with pressure manometer, capable of delivering greater than 80% O_2
Face masks: newborn and premature sizes
Laryngoscope: blade sizes 0 and 1
Orotracheal tubes, straight: 2.5, 3.0, 3.5, 4.0 mm ID
Oral airways: sizes 000, 00, and 0
Stethoscope
Blood pressure apparatus (direct, Doppler, or oscillometry)
Umbilical catheter tray: No. 3.5 and 5.0 French catheters
Blood glucose reagent strip (Dextrostix or Chemstrip bG)
Portable x-ray unit available 24 hours
Blood gas equipment available 24 hours

EMERGENCY DRUGS FOR RESUSCITATION AND ACUTE STABILIZATION

DRUG	CONCENTRATION	DOSE/KG	
$NaHCO_3$	0.5 M (0.5 mEq/ml water)	2–3 mEq	= 4–6 ml
Glucose	10% (100 mg/ml)	200 mg	= 2 ml
Epinephrine	1:10,000 (0.1 mg/ml)	0.01 mg	= 0.1 ml
Calcium gluconate	10% (0.48 mEq Ca^{2+}/ml)	0.48 mEq	= 1 ml
or gluceptate	22% (0.9 mEq Ca^{2+}/ml)	0.45 mEq	= 0.5 ml
Atropine SO_4	0.1 mg/ml	0.03 mg	= 0.3 ml
Narcan	0.02 mg/ml	0.01 mg	= 0.5 ml
Plasma protein fraction (human) (Plasmanate)	5% protein	10–20 ml	
Dopamine	40 mg/ml (to be diluted)	2–5 μg/minute	
Tromethamine (Tham)	0.3 M (0.3 mEq/ml)	1–2 mEq	= 4–6 ml

From Edlich RF, Spyker DA: Current Emergency Therapy 2nd Edition. Rockville, Aspen Systems, 1986, p 1052.

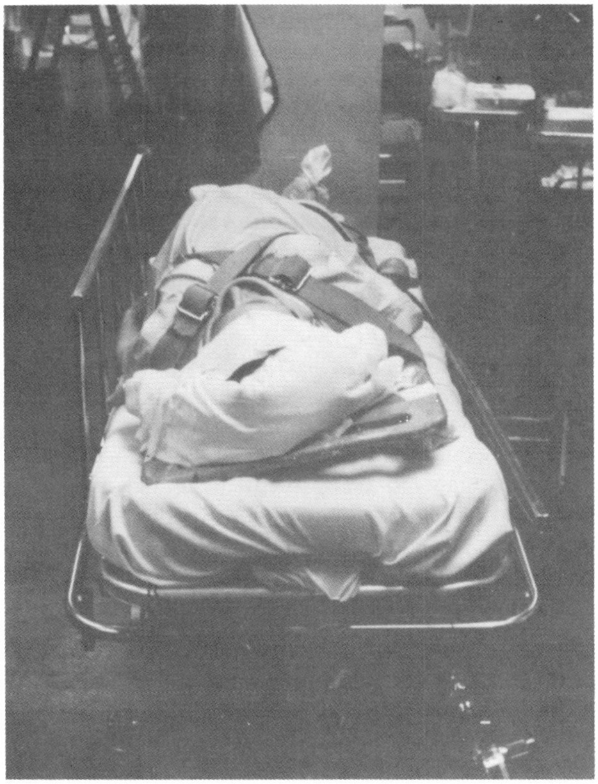

Figure 25–9. Placing a small roll under the right side of the backboard displaces the uterus to the left side.

the fetus is anoxic and not of viable age. A sudden change in fetal heart rate may prompt a change in maternal care but at the same time may be emotionally traumatic for the staff, who feel a sense of helplessness in facing the probability of fetal demise.

Blunt Trauma During Late Pregnancy

POTENTIAL FOR MATERNAL HEMORRHAGE AND SHOCK AND/OR FETAL ANOXIA SECONDARY TO UTERINE DAMAGE. When uterine damage is suspected, the patient's abdomen must be reassessed frequently (every 15 to 30 minutes), and fetal responses must be monitored closely (see Table 25–7). Fundal height should be measured and marked (on the patient's abdomen with indelible marker or with tape) on admission and every 30 minutes thereafter (Fig. 25–10). A rise in fundal height may indicate intrauterine hemorrhage.

Surgical intervention to repair the uterus is probable; disruption of the pregnancy will depend on the severity of the uterine injury and fetal assessment. Venous access is necessary in preparation for possible rapid transfusion.

POTENTIAL FOR MATERNAL HEMORRHAGE AND SHOCK AND/OR FETAL ANOXIA SECONDARY TO PLACENTAL ABRUPTION. The patient should be assessed every 15 minutes for signs and symptoms of abruptio placentae (see Table 25–8). Vaginal bleeding must be observed closely and accurate estimated blood loss records compiled.

Ultrasound procedures may be indicated, and clear explanations must be provided for the patient. If the fetus is alive, in distress, and of viable age, the patient should be prepared for an emergency cesarean section (refer to "Intraoperative Cycle"). The urgency of the patient's clinical condition may be alarming to the patient and family; therefore, they should be reassured that the best guarantee of both maternal and fetal well-being is the aggressive care that may be necessary. A nursing care plan for the patient with abruptio placentae is presented in Table 25–11.

The patient must be monitored for symptoms of disseminated intravascular coagulation (DIC) (Table 25–12). Coagulation studies should be obtained routinely, and arrangements for possible blood component therapy must be made.

POTENTIAL FOR PREMATURE RUPTURE OF MEMBRANES (PROM). The patient should be prepared for a sterile speculum examination with clear explanations provided. Ultrasound procedures may be indicated as well to determine gestational age and placental position.

POTENTIAL FOR PROLAPSED CORD SECONDARY TO PROM. Following a history of ruptured membranes, the perineum and vagina should be inspected for visualization of the umbilical cord. If the umbilical cord is present, immediate interventions are indicated (Table 25–13).

POTENTIAL FOR INFECTION RELATED TO PROM. The patient's core body temperature must be monitored closely, and white blood cell (WBC) counts should be obtained at regular intervals. If the patient develops signs of amnionitis (fetal tachycardia, WBC count > 22,000, maternal tachycardia, tender uterus, or temperature > 38°C [101°F]), she should be prepared for labor induction.

POTENTIAL FOR PREMATURE LABOR. The frequency and duration of contractions must be determined, and the patient must be continually assessed for signs of uterine and/or fetal distress, since premature labor may indicate fetal injuries. Strict bed rest (lateral position) is essential.

Since dehydration can precipitate premature labor, the patient must be kept well hydrated. Accurate intake and output records must be maintained. Tocolytic agents may be indicated (the current FDA-approved drug is ritodrine hydrochloride; however, most tertiary obstetrical centers use magnesium sulfate [$MgSO_4$]) and should be administered according to physician's order. The patient's labor activity and cardiovascular status should continue to be monitored. If measures to inhibit labor appear unsuccessful, the obstetrical and neonatal personnel must be notified of impending delivery.

POTENTIAL FOR DIRECT FETAL INJURY SECONDARY TO MATERNAL TRAUMA. The patient should be prepared for ultrasound to determine the existence of fetal injuries and to

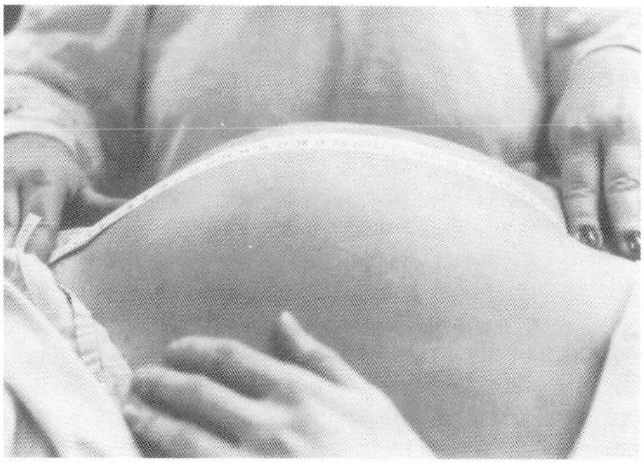

Figure 25–10. Measuring fundal height. The fundus is measured in centimeters from the symphysis pubis to the top of the fundus.

TABLE 25–11. ABRUPTIO PLACENTAE (OBSTETRICAL HEMORRHAGE) CARE PLAN

Nursing Diagnosis: Potential for maternal hemorrhage and shock and/or fetal anoxia secondary to placental abruption.

NURSING INTERVENTIONS	RATIONALE
1. Monitor maternal vital signs every 15 minutes and fetal heart rate continuously as appropriate. Note any trends or changes.	The abruption and subsequent hemorrhage can occur after the traumatic event. Maternal hypervolemia can mask signs of shock. Fetal distress may be the first indication of maternal hemorrhage.
2. Ensure placement of two large-bore intravenous catheters and maintain aggressive fluid resuscitation as ordered.	Maternal hypervolemia can mask a 15 to 30 per cent blood loss. Early aggressive fluid resuscitation is recommended to prevent maternal hypovolemia. Large volumes of fluid are necessary to maintain maternal hypervolemia.
3. Obtain and compare maternal laboratory values based on normal pregnancy values (include coagulation profile).	Laboratory values change acutely in pregnancy; an early, accurate baseline is essential for clinical observation. Coagulation profile is necessary because DIC is a possible complication.
4. Measure and mark fundal height on admission and every 30 minutes.	A rising fundal height may indicate intrauterine hemorrhage from abruptio placentae.
5. Monitor patient for clinical signs of abruptio placentae for 24 hours or longer. Vaginal bleeding Abdominal pain Uterine tenderness Uterine tetany or rigidity Rising fundal height Maternal shock/fetal distress	Symptoms can often be vague, and all do not necessarily occur. Abruption can occur 24 hours or more after injury.
6. Maintain continuous cardiotocographic monitoring in patients beyond 20 weeks' gestation.	Early, continuous monitoring has been shown to identify signs of abruption. Continuous monitoring can show fetal distress such as late decelerations and decreased beat-to-beat variability. Uterine contraction patterns should be noted because uterine irritability and preterm labor can indicate uterine hemorrhage.

From Smith LG: Assessment and resuscitation of the pregnant trauma patient. In Hoyt KS, Andrews J (eds): Contemporary Perspectives in Trauma Nursing. Berryville, VA, Forum Medicum, 1991.

approximate gestational age. The fetal heart rate should be assessed with each determination of maternal vital signs. If the fetus is of viable age and distressed, preparation should begin for emergency cesarean section. If fetal death has occurred, the fetus may be removed by cesarean section or allowed to remain in utero for a vaginal delivery. A dead fetus in a critically injured patient needs to be removed via a cesarean section if DIC is present or if a retroplacental clot is expanding; if a clot is stable, induction is indicated.

Potential for Maternal Hemorrhage and Shock Secondary to Bladder Rupture. The patient should void spontaneously or have a urinary catheter inserted. Urine samples should be obtained and checked for gross and microscopic blood. Additional diagnostic tests may be required, and the patient should be prepared accordingly.

Potential for Maternal and Family Anxiety Related to Sudden Hospitalization During Pregnancy. The patient must be reassured that prompt, aggressive care will offer the fetus the best chance for survival and should be kept informed of impending diagnostic tests and results. Allowing the patient to listen to the fetal heart beat and observe ultrasound images may help to lessen anxious feelings. The family needs to be kept informed of the status of the mother and baby. As appropriate, the family members should be permitted to be with the patient. In addition to fears concerning the baby, the patient and family may experience guilt feelings about the events leading to the accident. They should be encouraged to express their feelings and provided with nonjudgmental support.[73]

Case Study

A 34-year-old woman was admitted to a trauma center following a motorcycle accident. She was a passenger on the vehicle and was not wearing a helmet.

On initial nursing assessment, the patient had a compromised airway with blood in her nasopharynx and labored breathing with diminished breath sounds on the

TABLE 25–12. DISSEMINATED INTRAVASCULAR COAGULATION

Clinical Assessment

Uncontrolled bleeding at IV sites, from mucous membranes, and from traumatic wounds
Petechia, ecchymosis, and development of hematomas
Thrombosis of extremities evidenced by cyanosis and mottling
Organ dysfunction, including decreased urine production and impaired oxygenation

Laboratory Coagulation Value Alteration

Decreased platelet count
Prolonged prothrombin time (PT)
Prolonged partial thromboplastin time (PTT)
Decreased fibrinogen level
Normal clotting time

Goal of Therapeutics

Restore circulating blood volume
Provide adequate amount of red blood cells for oxygen transport
Replace hemostatic components

Nursing Therapeutics

Assist in identification and resolution of underlying cause
Continued assessment of bleeding sites for changes and blood estimation
On-going assessment of organ function, including oxygenation and urine production
Administration of blood products, including whole blood or packed red blood cells, fresh frozen plasma, and platelets per physician orders
Administration of fibrinogen, and cryoprecipitate per physician orders

Data from Mayberry L, Forte A: Pregnancy-related disseminated intravascular coagulation. Maternal Child Nursing: (MCN) 10:168–173, 1985; and Pilliteri A: Maternal-Newborn Nursing: Care of the Growing Family, 3rd ed. Boston, Little, Brown and Co, 1985, pp 905–907.

TABLE 25–13. IMMEDIATE TREATMENT FOR PROLAPSED CORD

Nursing Diagnosis: Potential for alteration in fetal cardiac and cerebral tissue perfusion secondary to cord compression.
Goal: Relieve cord compression and assure safe urgent fetal delivery.

NURSING INTERVENTION	RATIONALE
1. *Gently* insert a gloved hand into the patient's vagina, cradle the cord (level with the vagina), and elevate the fetal presenting part. Do not remove the examining hand until the fetus is delivered.	1. If the cord is being compressed by the presenting part, this will help relieve this compression.
2. *Extreme gentle* handling of the cord is essential; avoid manipulation, compressing, additional exposure of the cord to air.	2. Manipulation of the cord and its exposure to air can cause cord spasm, further compromising the fetus.
3. Position the mother in the knee-chest position and place the stretcher in Trendelenburg. (The Sim's lateral position may also be utilized.)	3. Positioning of the mother is aimed at helping to elevate the presenting part. If a long period of time occurs before delivery of the fetus, the Sim's lateral position may be less tiring for the mother.
4. Prepare the patient for emergency cesarean section.	4. Though sometimes these patients may have a vaginal delivery, a cesarean section is often clinically indicated and must be done in an emergent matter.
5. Monitor the fetal heart tones with an electronic monitor.	5. Determine fetal heart rate and note effectiveness of the emergency treatment.
6. Provide emotional support to mother and family during the procedures.	6. Answering patient and family questions and explaining the procedures may help decrease anxiety.

Make sure that the emergency department has a clinical plan in place for such obstetrical emergencies.

If obstetrical and neonatal personnel are available, they should be notified immediately to respond to the emergency department.

From Smith LG: Assessment and resuscitation of the pregnant trauma patient. In Hoyt KS, Andrews J (eds): Contemporary Perspectives in Trauma Nursing. Berryville, VA, Forum Medicum, June 1991.

left. The patient was tachycardic (rate 133 beats per *minute), hypotensive (88 systolic/56 diastolic), and decerebrate bilaterally.*

Nursing therapeutics focused on the ABCs of resuscitation. The nurses assisted in oral intubation and insertion of two large-bore IVs and a left chest tube. Vital signs were assessed every 5 minutes. Continued tachycardia and hypotension were noted.

Continued assessment identified a rigid abdomen, an open femur fracture, and left tibia fracture. With the airway maintained by intubation and fluid resuscitation with crystalloids and blood products, the patient was taken for a CT scan, then moved intraoperatively for repair of a liver laceration and fractured spleen. Patient history obtained from family at this time revealed that the patient was pregnant approximately 14 weeks.

The patient and fetus survived through the resuscitation and months of intensive care and rehabilitative care. A healthy full-term male, small for gestational age, was delivered via cesarean section near term.

COMMENT

During resuscitation of the pregnant trauma patient, the ABCs must remain the priority. The best guarantee of fetal survival is aggressive maternal care. At 14 weeks gestation, the fetus is not viable; therefore, continuous monitoring of the fetal heart at this time is of questionable value. Early knowledge or identification that the patient is pregnant would be useful in assessing for possible uterine injuries, although they are uncommon at this early gestation. Since all women of childbearing age should be considered pregnant until proven otherwise, shielding of the abdomen during radiographic procedures and left lateral positioning should be done. Once the patient is identified as pregnant, medication use may be altered (see Table 25–9).

Penetrating Trauma in Late Pregnancy

Potential for Maternal Hemorrhage and Shock and/or Fetal Injury Secondary to Penetrating Trauma. The patient should be monitored for signs and symptoms of uterine damage (see Table 25–7). In viable pregnancies, fetal heart rate must be monitored continuously, and fetal activity should be assessed in conjunction with maternal assessment. Local wound exploration may be necessary, and the patient should be prepared for emergency laparotomy if the wound extends into the abdominal cavity. The operating room personnel must be informed of the patient's pregnant condition (see "Intraoperative Cycle").

The obstetrical and neonatal personnel should be notified of impending surgery as well. The decision to empty the uterus intraoperatively will be based on gestational age, fetal distress, and control of hemorrhage around the uterus.

INTRAOPERATIVE CYCLE

When a pregnant trauma patient is admitted to a trauma center or emergency department, the operating room personnel should be notified of the possibility of an emergency cesarean section. A general surgery pack can be opened and additional surgical equipment added (Table 25–14), or an

TABLE 25–14. SURGICAL TOOLS TO BE ADDED TO GENERAL SURGERY PACK FOR CESAREAN SECTION

Bladder blade
Obstetrical forceps
Sponge sticks
deLee suction trap or bulb syringe
Suggested suture material
  1 chromic (uterine closure)
  00 or 000 chromic or vicryl on GI needle for bladder flap

obstetrical cesarean section pack can be opened. Other useful instruments are a small French suction catheter (no. 8 Fr) and several end clamps. The neonatal or pediatric personnel will need to be in the operating suite to manage the initial resuscitation and stabilization of the newborn.

Anesthesia

Anesthesia management of the pregnant trauma patient requires the expertise of anesthesia personnel familiar with both trauma and obstetrical anesthesia. If the pregnant trauma patient requires anesthesia, the care should be planned, recognizing that these patients are unique charges.[74] First, they have an increased metabolic demand secondary to pregnancy. Second, there are changes in hormonal activity. And finally, there are mechanical changes due to the enlarging uterus and breasts. The decision whether to administer regional or general anesthesia is one of many to be made prior to and during surgery.

When the pregnant trauma patient has multiple injuries and/or needs immediate surgery, general anesthesia may be the choice. The pregnant trauma patient given general anesthesia does have an increased risk of vomiting and aspiration, which is best controlled by first emptying the stomach with a gastric tube and administering 30 ml of a nonparticulate antacid (0.3 M sodium citrate), which increases gastric pH.[74] Cimetidine or ranitidine can be given to decrease acid production. Intubation using a cuffed endotracheal tube after rapid sequence induction with cricoid pressure and 5 minutes of preoxygenation should protect the airway and provide adequate oxygenation.[39]

Local or spinal anesthesia may be given during pregnancy. The location of injuries; length of procedure; cardiovascular, neurological, and psychological status of the patient; and risk of fetal distress are all determinants of the appropriateness of local or spinal anesthesia. For example, local anesthesia would be appropriate for repair of a facial laceration, whereas repair of extensive facial trauma would require general anesthesia. Lower extremity injuries resulting from trauma could be repaired with spinal or, preferably, epidural anesthesia, but general anesthesia may be more appropriate for other injuries. There is no difference in morbidity or mortality in pregnancy between regional or general anesthesia.[75] The circulating nurse must ensure that specialty drugs such as oxytocin (Pitocin) and methylergonovine maleate (Methergine) are available in the operating room suite for the anesthesia provider.

Surgical Procedures

Obstetrical Procedures

Exploratory laparotomy may be indicated to identify the type and severity of uterine injuries. Uterine lacerations, contusions, and tears are common following abdominal trauma and may need repair. Cesarean section for removal of the fetus is appropriate only if the fetus is in distress and of viable age (> 24 weeks' gestation) or, if necessary, to effect adequate uterine repair.

A cesarean section in a stable patient for a fetus that has died secondary to trauma is considered inappropriate in most instances, because it further burdens the mother with the probability of cesarean section as the method of delivery for future pregnancies.[40] A critically injured patient who is hemorrhaging could develop DIC, and in this instance a cesarean section may be necessary (although the fetus is dead) to prevent additional complications (i.e., DIC, sepsis). Cesarean section for an immature infant is also considered inappropriate, although here too a vaginal delivery is preferable.

When uterine rupture is identified in emergency surgery, the first task is to enlarge the tear and remove the fetus.[50] The fetus should be removed via a low transverse incision unless the tear is nearly large enough to remove the fetus. The fetus should be immediately handed to the neonatal personnel. When possible, the uterus is then repaired to preserve future childbearing capabilities. If there is uncontrollable hemorrhage, a hysterectomy or bilateral hypogastric ligation may need to be performed.[2]

Nonobstetrical Procedures

Abdominal laparotomy, multiple orthopedic procedures, and neurosurgery may be more common than obstetrical surgery during pregnancy.

When the fetus is of viable age, fetal heart rate should be monitored continuously during the surgical procedures to detect early signs of fetal distress.

To diminish surgical time and the anesthesia risk to the fetus, multiple surgical procedures should be done simultaneously, which may require that several scrub nurses assist with the operative procedures. The perioperative nurse preparing for this contingency must notify the charge nurse of the need for additional personnel. The procedures also might be done consecutively, which requires planning by the circulating nurse. When managing lower extremity orthopedic trauma during pregnancy, several factors must be considered. Although internal fixation of fractures exposes the patient to general anesthesia, it markedly reduces the pregnant patient's length of immobility. During pregnancy, a woman who must remain immobile faces the risk of developing phlebitis.

Nursing Diagnosis and Therapeutics

The nurse in the operating room is in a unique position to coordinate procedures and provide a therapeutic environment for the pregnant patient.

Potential for Patient and Family Fear and Anxiety Related to Pending Surgical Procedures and Possible Fetal Injury or Death. A calm preinduction environment must be maintained for the patient in the operating room, with discussions kept to a minimum. As time allows, the patient should be given the time to voice concerns and fears. The family should be kept informed of the surgical progress and fetal outcome.

Potential for Decreased Cardiac Output Related to Vena Cava Compression by the Enlarged Uterus. Patient positioning in the left lateral position is ideal but probably unrealistic during surgical intervention. An alternative is to displace the uterus using a towel roll or wedge under the hip and small of the back. A second alternative is to tilt the operating table laterally. Possible spinal damage may prohibit both these positions; manual displacement of the uterus by a team member may be required.

Potential for Emergency Delivery Secondary to Fetal Distress and/or Uterine or Placental Injuries. The surgical table should be prepared for possible cesarean section with the addition of several surgical instruments (Table 25–14). Neonatal personnel must be alerted, and space must be provided in the surgical suite or adjoining area for neonatal resuscitation at the time of delivery.

The circulating nurse must coordinate the intraoperative plan of care to include several disciplines (i.e., surgeons, labor and delivery nurses, neonatologists, and neonatal nurses). All these services must be ready within the operating room suite when the skin incision is made.

The time of birth and other birth-related details must be included with routine documentation procedures. The placenta must be obtained and prepared as a specimen for pathology test procedures.

Alteration in Maternal–Infant Bonding Related to Patient's Condition and Fetal Outcome. As the patient's and fetus's conditions allow, attempts should be made to provide an environment that will facilitate maternal–infant bonding. If the patient is awake and the fetus is alive and in no distress, the mother should be permitted to see and hold the infant.

If the infant is premature and/or in distress, the mother must be kept continually informed of the infant's progress and permitted to see the infant, even for a brief moment, if possible. Should the mother be under anesthesia, documentation of the birth can be shared with her later. The family or significant others should be permitted to see the baby when possible and kept informed of the baby's progress. Many intensive care nurseries (and labor/delivery suites) use a Polaroid camera to take a snapshot of the infant; the photograph provides the mother with what may be her only glimpse of the child for days.

Case Study

A 32-year-old woman at 38 weeks' gestation was admitted to a trauma center after being struck by an automobile. The patient was admitted directly to the operating room on a backboard with cervical collar in place for immediate intervention. The obstetrical and neonatal staff were on hand in the operating room when the patient arrived.

Immediate care included insertion of large-bore IVs, infusion of fluids, and anteroposterior and lateral C-spine films. Obstetrical and abdominal assessment was difficult. The patient's tachycardia made it impossible to differentiate fetal heart tones. The patient's abdomen was contused, bruised, and tender to palpation. While the patient was tipped in the left lateral position, an emergency cesarean section was performed by the obstetricians, and a female infant was delivered. The infant had 0/0 Apgar scores and was aggressively resuscitated and stabilized by the neonatal staff. After completion of the cesarean section by the obstetrical staff, the trauma surgical team performed a laparotomy with repair of liver lacerations, splenic hematoma, and mesenteric tears.

The patient was then placed in a pelvic Hoffman device, and open fractures were irrigated and debrided. The patient was then moved to the critical care unit.

CRITICAL CARE CYCLE

Following initial resuscitation, the pregnant trauma patient should be transferred to an appropriate critical care unit. The team approach, involving both the obstetrical and the trauma staff, will afford the patient the most comprehensive care. The bedside trauma nurse is the most likely person to detect subtle changes in the patient's status. It is therefore essential for the nurse to have a sound knowledge base in regard to the care of the pregnant trauma patient. The primary nurse assumes an important role in coordinating and integrating the care provided by the various services.

The general goal of care for the pregnant trauma patient following resuscitation is to provide aggressive maternal care while minimizing fetal stress. The patient should be kept well hydrated and provided with immediate nutritional support. Care should be focused on the immediate treatment of traumatic injuries and problems, while recognizing that the patient is pregnant.

The potential for delayed obstetrical complications, such as abruptio placentae and premature labor, should be considered. The critical care staff should be aware of the signs and symptoms of obstetrical emergencies and of the immediate action that must be taken, and obstetrical personnel must be notified (see Tables 25–7, 25–8, and 25–12). An emergency delivery plan should be established, as well as a neonatal resuscitation plan. Maintaining active communication with both the obstetrical and neonatal teams improves the quality of care.

Assessment for signs and symptoms of these obstetrical complications may be difficult in the critically injured patient for a number of reasons. Sedation or an unconscious state imposes limitations on the ability to communicate with the patient. Communicating with an intubated patient may be difficult as well. Following spinal cord injury, although the patient may be able to communicate, sensations that would otherwise indicate the onset of labor or signify the development of other problems may be lacking.

A communication link with the obstetrical staff should be prearranged. If an obstetrical complication is suspected or delivery appears imminent, the obstetrical staff should be notified immediately. If the patient cannot be moved from the critical care unit, obstetrical personnel should administer the appropriate treatment in the unit. Necessary emergency delivery equipment should be kept at the bedside. The potential need for neonatal personnel and emergency neonatal resuscitation equipment also should be addressed.

Collaboration with the obstetrical staff is essential. As the patient's hospitalization course continues, the obstetrical staff, as part of the critical care team, should monitor the status of the pregnancy and provide useful information for the staff caring for the patient. The frequency with which the obstetrical personnel have direct contact with the patient will depend in part upon the patient's unique needs and clinical condition.

Nursing Diagnosis and Therapeutics for the Antepartum Patient

Alteration in Nutritional Status Related to Metabolic Demands of Traumatic Injury and Pregnancy. Good nutrition is essential during pregnancy because of the metabolic demands of the fetus, placenta, and uterus in addition to the metabolic demands secondary to the normal physiological changes of pregnancy. When the pregnant patient is in critical condition following traumatic injury, meeting the metabolic demands of both the pregnancy and maternal healing becomes a challenge.

Dietary consultation should be initiated on admission to the critical care unit so that the patient's nutritional requirements can be determined. Tube feeding, parenteral nutrition, or a combination of the two may be necessary to meet metabolic demands. The goal is to prevent maternal protein–calorie malnutrition. In some cases, total parenteral nutrition (TPN) may be necessary. Although the use of TPN during pregnancy is considered relatively new, it has been utilized in selective cases.[76]

For patients who are able to tolerate oral feedings, food preferences should be acknowledged when possible. Smaller, more frequent meals are recommended for the pregnant patient to avoid unnecessary discomfort resulting from a full stomach. The nutritional status should be assessed continually so that adjustments can be made accordingly (refer to Chapter 14).

Potential for Alteration in Uterine/Fetal Perfusion Related to Cardiovascular Compromise Secondary to Maternal Positioning. The patient should be monitored closely. The frequency of vital sign recordings will depend on the patient's clinical condition. Trends in vital sign measurements for the pregnant patient should be acknowledged (see "Hemodynamic Considerations"). The pregnant trauma patient may require invasive monitoring for trend analysis of central venous pressure, pulmonary artery pressure, and cardiac output. Accurate intake and output records must be kept as well. Laboratory values should be monitored routinely and compared with normal pregnancy values (see Table 25–5). Decisions regarding intravenous fluid replacement therapy will be guided by the patient's hemodynamic status and cardiovascular response.

Positioning is an important aspect of nursing care for the pregnant trauma patient. Although the patient should be turned to the left side to prevent compression of the vena cava and aorta by the enlarging uterus, and thus improve cardiac output, this position cannot be maintained for long periods without pulmonary compromise. A turning schedule should be developed and followed to prevent the pregnant patient from remaining on her back for any length of time. The turning schedule should emphasize side-to-side turning with little, if any, time spent in the prone position. The patient's injuries may dictate the need to devise unique positioning strategies (i.e., musculoskeletal stabilization devices). Such requirements should be detailed in the patient's plan of care.

Potential for Venous Stasis and Pulmonary Emboli Related to Coagulation Alterations and Immobility. The normal physiological changes that occur during pregnancy place the pregnant woman at risk for venous stasis and phlebitis. Immobility during the critical care phase places the patient at further risk. It is therefore important for the pregnant patient to be mobilized as soon as possible to prevent such complications. Intermittent pneumatic compression of the calves is a safe and effective treatment modality that can be initiated. Also, minidose or prophylactic heparin therapy is indicated in this patient population.

A thorough respiratory assessment must be completed on every shift and as often as indicated. Vital signs, including pulse oximetry, must be monitored continually, and arterial blood gas trends must be examined routinely during the initial postresuscitation phase.

Potential for Fetal Damage Related to Pain-Control Methods. Special efforts are required to manage the pregnant patient's pain while minimizing fetal risks. Pain, if not managed effectively, can cause further stress for both the mother and fetus, further complicating the clinical course. The team approach is most useful in devising an effective pain-management plan. The critical care team should consult with both pharmacology and obstetrical experts in determining appropriate pain-management options that will minimize detrimental fetal effects while reducing maternal pain stress.

Nursing Diagnosis and Therapeutics for the Postpartum Patient

The trauma patient who has aborted or delivered during the resuscitation phase presents unique concerns during the critical care phase; therefore, appropriate priorities must be established. Immediately post partum, the patient must be monitored closely for hemorrhage and shock. The potential for postpartum infection also must be considered.

Telling the patient and family of a fetal loss, although a difficult task, also must be accomplished as soon as possible, and comfort measures should be provided as needed. Most obstetrical and neonatal units have a grief-management team. A group such as this can be invaluable not only to the patient and her family but also to the trauma team during what, even for them, can be a very difficult time. Important aspects of maternal–infant bonding must be a concern as well.

Potential for Postpartum Hemorrhage. The fundus should be assessed and massaged every 15 minutes for the first hour post partum and then every hour for at least 4 hours thereafter. A rise in fundal height, increased lochia, or a "boggy" uterus should be reported to the obstetrical staff. The amount of vaginal bleeding should be monitored closely. Pad counts are often helpful in assessing the extent of bleeding. An excessive amount of bleeding should be reported to the obstetrician immediately. The administration of oxytocin or Methergine is often necessary.

Potential for Postpartum Infection. The patient's temperature should be monitored routinely. A slight elevation can be expected after delivery. Persistent elevations, however, should be reported. The quantity and quality of vaginal drainage (lochia) should be monitored routinely for several days. The obstetrical team should be notified if a foul-smelling discharge is noted.

The perineum should be inspected routinely as well. Swelling is normal immediately following delivery but should decrease after several days. Ice should be applied directly to the perineal area to reduce swelling and to help alleviate local pain.

Potential for Breast Engorgement. If necessary, a breast binder should be obtained and applied for the patient who is planning to bottle feed or who has experienced a loss, provided that it does not restrict respiratory movement or interfere with necessary treatment activities. A snugly fitted bra may suffice.

Alteration in Grieving Process Related to Maternal Injuries and Clinical Condition. When the fetus is lost during resuscitation, the decision of when to tell the mother, the father, and other appropriate family members is difficult. The multidisciplinary team members should collaborate in making this decision. The mother's level of consciousness and clinical condition will be strong determining factors; once the mother can listen and comprehend, telling her should not be delayed. Input from family members is often helpful in determining the patient's ability to cope with such devastating news. Requests from family members should be respected and incorporated into the management plan if possible. Efforts should be made to allow family members to be present when the patient is told of the loss.

During the grieving process, the mother may request detailed information such as the time of birth, the baby's weight, or the color of the baby's hair. Pictures of the baby are often helpful. The grieving process will most likely extend beyond the critical care phase. A consistent approach will allow continued nursing support through all phases of care as grieving continues (refer to Chapter 11). Even though the mother may not request them at the time, many centers collect a lock of hair, a photograph, hand and foot prints, and baby's first cap and blanket and archive them, letting the mother know that the materials are hers whenever she wants them. Many mothers will request these keepsakes after their loss.

Alteration in Maternal–Infant Bonding Related to Maternal Injuries and Clinical Condition. The patient who has delivered a healthy or premature infant during the resuscitation phase of care presents an equal challenge to the critical care nurse. Every effort must be made to provide as much contact as possible between the mother and baby. The family should be encouraged to take frequent photographs of the baby to share with the mother. The mother will need to be assured that the baby is being properly cared for in the neonatal unit or at home. It might be suggested that the family keep a log of the baby's progress, which will be helpful to the mother as she becomes more stable. If the mother is not interested in the infant, however, her feelings should be accepted by the staff. The patient's injuries may be the focus of her attention during the critical care phase. During family visits, time also should be spent concentrating on the mother's injuries and concerns. Conversations should not always focus on the baby. Continued disinterest in the infant, however, may signal excessive guilt or denial. These feelings should be explored further with the patient.

Alteration in the Family System and/or Potential for Family Stress Related to Maternal Hospitalization. Following the delivery process, the disruption of the family unit will inevitably alter role functions. Family members should be encouraged to express their needs, concerns, and problems. Appropriate referrals should be made to social service personnel if necessary. The family will need assistance in developing a plan for maternal and infant care upon discharge from the hospital.

INTERMEDIATE CARE/REHABILITATION CYCLE

The pregnant trauma patient in the intermediate care/rehabilitation phase presents a challenging nursing situation. The patient and family have had to adapt to a sudden hospitalization and perhaps months of continuous care in the critical care setting. Depending on the patient's injuries and critical care course, the adaptation process may be more profound as the patient prepares for discharge.

Team members caring for the patient during this phase may include not only obstetrical personnel and trauma specialists but physical, occupational, and speech therapists as well.

During the critical phase of care, the primary goal was to provide aggressive maternal care with minimal fetal stress. As the pregnancy progresses and the patient's clinical condition shows continued improvement, the focus must be placed on the impending delivery. The family may begin to express fears about the fetal outcome. Changes in birthing plans must be made, and discharge planning should include delivery and home care requirements.

Concerns that existed during the critical care phase of care may carry over to the intermediate care/rehabilitation phase. The patient's nutritional status should continue to be a primary concern. Altered mobility and pain management concerns, although less intense, may continue to require consistent nursing intervention (refer to "Critical Care Cycle"). However, the patient's involvement in managing each of these concerns may become more active.

If the fetus was lost during the resuscitative or critical care phase, the patient and family must now deal with that loss as well as the effects of the trauma on the mother. The mother may feel guilt over the loss of the baby. Depending on the events leading to the accident, other family members may feel guilt about the accident. The adjustment process may be slow and tedious, and the family will need constant support. Pictures and a description of the baby may be appropriate to share with the mother for the first time. A Christian mother may need assurance that her baby was christened.

An assessment of how the mother and family are coping with the loss of the baby must be performed on a continual basis. Although the fetal death may have occurred weeks earlier, the rehabilitation phase may be the time when the family has the energy to focus on their grief and possible guilt. As the patient stabilizes, an obstetrical staff member may be asked to meet with the patient and family to review the fetal loss and discuss future pregnancies. In the grave event that the patient's injuries required a hysterectomy to be performed, the grieving process may be prolonged as the loss of future pregnancies is mourned. Many women equate loss of the uterus with a loss of femininity and desirability, a myth shared by some men as well. Therefore, the patient and family will need continued counseling. Appropriate referrals should be made as needed.

Labor and Delivery Plans

As the patient enters the third trimester, decisions should be made and plans established for the impending delivery. Initially, it must be decided where labor and delivery will take place. The decision should be a collaborative one, with both the obstetrical and rehabilitation staffs involved. Where the patient will receive optimal obstetrical care should be a strong consideration. Transfer from the rehabilitation setting to an acute care facility may be necessary. Transportation should be arranged for either an interunit or interhospital transfer at the time a decision is made concerning delivery plans. These transportation plans should be available 24 hours a day and be clearly stated in the patient's plan of care.

Signs and symptoms of labor should be assessed routinely. An organized plan of action should be included as part of the patient's care plan so that appropriate staff members are notified. All efforts should be made to ensure a smooth transfer when labor occurs.

The obstetrical staff should be educated by the rehabilitation clinical nurse specialist concerning the patient's current limitations. This may be accomplished during a meeting with the obstetrical staff, when a patient profile may be presented. The patient's neurological deficits and orthopedic limitations should be emphasized. If the patient has suffered a closed head injury and requires cognitive retraining, detailed information about the patient's current level of functioning should be presented to the obstetrical staff.

Orthopedic injuries that require special nursing interventions or that limit a patient's movement also should be explained. The obsetrical staff may not be familiar with musculoskeletal stabilization devices such as a Hoffman apparatus and will need detailed instructions.

Plans also should be made regarding alternative positions for vaginal delivery. The patient's primary nurse and the clinical nurse specialist may be able to help the obstetrical staff plan alternative positions. The obstetrical staff may need to be reminded of the advisability of the lateral Sims position. A birthing bed may be an alternative that will allow flexibility in patient positioning, as well as patient accessibility during delivery.

Childbirth classes should not be neglected and will need to be individualized according to the patient's special needs. For example, it may be appropriate for an obstetrical nurse to visit the pregnant patient regularly prior to the due date to discuss breathing techniques. The father or other support person should be included. This allows the obstetrical nurse to become familiar with the patient's special care needs while concurrently providing the opportunity for the patient and the father to ask questions and express concerns about the upcoming labor and delivery process. If the patient has suffered a head injury, it may be difficult for these instructions to be understood; therefore, alternative plans may need to be made.

The importance of planning ahead for the upcoming delivery must be emphasized. The establishment of a strong, supportive relationship between the trauma and obstetrical staff will foster effective communication patterns and facilitate a smooth delivery process.

Postpartum Care

Many trauma patients, owing to their injuries, are limited in their ability to care for themselves after delivery. This may be difficult for the postpartum nursing staff, who are not accustomed to caring for the trauma patient and therefore are unfamiliar with the special care needs. Postpartum staff members should be educated by either the rehabilitative clinical nurse specialist or the patient's primary nurse concerning the patient's ability to meet her own needs as well as those of the baby. Thorough attention will likely be focused on rehabilitation plans for discharge. There must be some consideration of family planning/contraception. The trauma/rehabilitation nurse should help the team remember this important aspect of postpartum care.

Nursing Diagnosis and Therapeutics

The situation is far from ideal when the newborn baby is in the nursery, the mother is in intermediate care or rehabilitation, and the family members are home. The nursing plan of care should include provisions to minimize family disruptions.

Alteration in the Family System Secondary to Maternal Hospitalization and Clinical Needs. When possible, the patient should be allowed to care for her infant. At times, it may be necessary for the nursing staff to offer alternative solutions if limitations imposed by the patient's injuries impede her caregiving abilities. For example, the patient may not be able to both hold and feed the baby, in which case the postpartum staff may assist the patient by holding the baby while allowing the patient to feed him or her. Early and frequent maternal–infant interaction is an important component of the bonding process; therefore, flexible visitation rights should be considered. The attachment or bonding that occurs between a mother and a newborn is a complex, unique emotional relationship.[77] Efforts should be made to allow the mother to hold the infant or to have the infant lie by her side. Physical communication between the newborn and mother allows the newborn to utilize sensual abilities (Table 25–15) and therefore is imperative.

When the patient's needs as a trauma patient are extensive, she may be transferred back to the rehabilitation or intermediate care unit after the immediate postpartum period (first 24 hours). This may be the most practical alternative for the patient's care but will produce maternal–infant separation. In this situation, every attempt should be made to arrange for regular and frequent maternal–infant interactions.

It also will be necessary for the family to identify who will provide infant care in the home after the baby's discharge. If infant care cannot be provided by family members or friends on a 24-hour basis, other alternatives must be explored. Reliable and competent contractual care providers may be identified by contacting an appropriate community agency.

Potential Alteration in Breastfeeding Activities Related to Maternal Hospitalization. If at all possible,

TABLE 25–15. PARENTAL-INFANT BONDING: NEWBORN SENSUAL RESPONSES OR ABILITIES UTILIZED IN BONDING

Touch
Eye to eye contact
Odor
Body warmth
Voice
Entertainment
Biorhythmicity

Data from Lowdermilk DL: Family dynamics after childbirth. In Bobak IM, Jensen MO (eds): Essentials of Maternity Nursing, 3rd ed. St. Louis, Mosby–Year Book, 1991, pp 560–577.

the mother's desire to breastfeed should be respected and accommodated. However, since the metabolic and emotional demands on the nursing mother will intensify, the status of the patient's clinical condition should be considered carefully by the rehabilitation team before a final decision regarding breastfeeding is made. An important aspect of this decision-making process will be any medications still required by the mother. Virtually all maternal medications appear in breast milk in a concentration similar to the serum concentration. The patient must be included in this decision-making process as well. If it is determined that breastfeeding is a viable option, the mother may need assistance while nursing the baby during visits.

It will be necessary for milk to be extracted from the breasts between visits; therefore, a breast pump must be made available to the patient, and instruction and assistance for use should be provided as needed. Plans for milk storage and a routine for delivery to the baby must be arranged in conjunction with the family.

Fetal Death

When a newborn dies or a pregnancy is lost, parents should be expected and encouraged to grieve. The death of an infant or a fetus is experienced as a deep loss to the mother, father, and other family members, and a variety of reactions and responses will be displayed by those who have invested emotional energy in the growth and development of the new life.[78] A supportive and accepting attitude by the nurse caring for the patient and family will be valuable as they address their feelings of grief (refer to Chapter 11). Consultation should be obtained from the perinatal grief-management service.

Home Health Care

The trend since the 1980s has been to plan for the patient's early discharge and to provide for continuation of care through home health services in order to decrease medical costs. Early discharge may be a possible alternative for the antepartum or postpartum trauma patient and will require special planning and educational preparation of home health providers.

Weeks before the patient is discharged, contacts should be made to the agency that will be providing care to the pregnant or postpartum trauma patient upon release from the hospital. Discharge planning conferences should be scheduled as needed and should include the patient, family, primary nurse, physician team members, social service team members, and members of the home health care team. This structured approach provides a forum for the patient's special care needs to be addressed and for the patient's and family's concerns to be expressed. These meetings also provide the opportunity for the patient and family members to begin to develop a trusting relationship with the home health care providers, thus fostering a smoother transition from hospital to home.

Family counseling sessions may be necessary. Physical or cognitive changes may alter the mother's ability to assume various role responsibilities. For example, the patient who returns home during the postpartum period with some cognitive dysfunction cannot assume full responsibility for the newborn baby. Another family member and/or a contractual infant care provider may be needed to assist with the care of the baby, while allowing the patient short and frequent interactions with the baby to encourage maternal–infant bonding.

COMMUNITY REINTEGRATION CYCLE

Preparation of the antepartum or postpartum trauma patient for discharge begins the day the patient is admitted. After weeks or possibly months of hospitalization, the patient must be prepared to return to home and to the community. The patient's obstetrical status is an important consideration when planning care during this cycle. If delivery occurred during the patient's hospitalization and the baby was discharged weeks before the mother, the priorities would be focused on maternal–infant interactions rather than delivery plans. For the patient who is pregnant during the discharge planning process, special attention must be placed on delivery plans, with careful consideration of injuries and restrictions imposed.

Perinatal Referrals

The antepartum trauma patient being discharged to home must continue to receive prenatal care. Referrals should be made to the patient's private obstetrician or to a high-risk maternity center if deemed necessary. The referral should include information about the patient's injuries and clinical course, current medications and treatment interventions, limitations that may affect the delivery process, and potential postpartum home care needs.

FUTURE TRENDS AND PREVENTION

Although future birth rates may be difficult to predict, it can be expected that pregnant women in modern society will remain active well into their third trimester of pregnancy. Presumably, modern women will continue to work outside the home and travel until the time of delivery. Driving or riding in automobiles is a reality for today's pregnant women. Trauma is often preventable, and public education that focuses on the proper use of safety belts during pregnancy may significantly decrease the number and severity of injuries resulting from vehicular accidents during pregnancy.

Safety belts should be worn during pregnancy, since they prevent ejection from the vehicle and impact against the steering wheel and dashboard. The seat belt should be worn low or under the fundus, across the pelvis.[79] The shoulder harness should be worn in the normal position, not against the neck, but between the breasts and off the shoulder (see Fig. 25–1). Padding the seat belt for comfort is discouraged, because the belt could shift upward on impact, causing injury to the thinner portion of the fundus.

Women are more likely to wear their seat belts than are men, but fewer women wear their seat belts when pregnant.[20, 80] The major myth concerning seat belt use during pregnancy is that the belt will hurt the unborn child. Lack of safety belt use by anyone increases the chances of ejection

TABLE 25–16. SAFETY PRECAUTIONS TO TAKE DURING PREGNANCY

AREA	PRECAUTION
Home	Do not stand on stepstools or stepladders, because it is difficult to maintain balance on a narrow base.
	Avoid throw rugs without a nonskid backing.
	Keep small items such as toys out of pathways, because it is difficult for a pregnant woman to see her feet.
	Use caution when stepping in and out of a bathtub, because the surface is slippery.
	Do not overload electrical circuits, because it is difficult for a pregnant woman to escape a fire because of poor mobility.
	Do not smoke (many fires are started by a person's falling asleep with a cigarette).
	Do not take medicine in the dark (an error may be made because of limited vision).
Work	Avoid handling toxic substances.
	Avoid working to a point of fatigue, which lowers judgment.
	Avoid long periods of standing, which can lead to orthostatic hypotension and fainting.
Automobile	Use a seat belt at all times.
	Refuse to ride with anyone who has been drinking alcohol or whose judgment might be impaired.

Adapted from Pilliteri A: Maternal–Newborn Nursing Care of the Growing Family, 3rd ed. Boston, Little, Brown and Co, 1985, p 954.

from the vehicle, which increases chances of death 20-fold.[81] This, in turn, of course, dramatically increases the risk of fetal death. Mandatory seat belt legislation and, more important, public education and enforcement may serve as major catalysts in increasing seat belt use during pregnancy and thus preventing injuries.

In addition to road traffic accidents, the number of accidental injuries during pregnancy can be decreased by preventive measures. Pregnant women should be educated concerning the normal changes that occur during pregnancy, which may place them at risk for accidental injuries. A pregnant woman should be encouraged to take short breaks from work or exercise. For example, if a teacher is pregnant, she should be encouraged to sit down and prop her feet up between classes. This may decrease her fatigue in early pregnancy. In late pregnancy, a pregnant woman's altered gait and balance should be of concern. Safety measures should be taken by pregnant women, including the avoidance of climbing on ladders or chairs (Table 25–16).

Legislative changes may affect the incidence of penetrating injuries. Stricter weapon control measures may decrease the total number of penetrating injuries sustained by the American public, including those experienced by pregnant women.

NURSING RESEARCH AND EDUCATION

The first step in research on the topic of trauma during pregnancy would be clarification of the scope of the problem. Baker estimates that 7 per cent of pregnant women will suffer trauma or accidental injury during pregnancy.[2] It is unclear how this figure was derived and whether it includes mild falls (which may not be recorded in hospital records) as well as severe trauma. Establishing a data base of pregnant trauma patients—their injuries and outcomes (both fetal and maternal)—would yield a wealth of information. In the absence of a national trauma registry, this would be most helpful. Several studies have been done to clarify the scope of the problem and address the issue of fetal outcome. Rothenberger and associates reviewed 103 cases of blunt maternal trauma and categorized the trauma as major, minor, and insignificant. In cases of minor or insignificant trauma, the incidence of fetal death or abortion was low.[50] However, a more recent study found a much higher incidence of fetal death following minor maternal trauma, suggesting that pregnant women in mild accidents should be hospitalized and monitored for at least 24 to 48 hours after injury.[82]

Another area open to nursing research is the use of PASGs during pregnancy. Advanced Trauma Life Support (ATLS) protocol states that only the leg portions should be inflated when the patient is obviously pregnant. However, some experts believe that in some situations, such as in the care of a ruptured uterus, inflation of the abdominal portion of the PASG can be useful. This remains a controversial issue.

Investigation of the adaptation of the antepartum or postpartum trauma patient after discharge home could affect future trends in discharge planning. Since current literature does not address this topic, it should be targeted in future nursing research endeavors.

REFERENCES

1. National Center for Health Statistics: The Advanced Report of Final Natality Statistics for 1988. Monthly Vital Statistics Report, vol 39, no 4, 1988.
2. Baker D: Trauma in the pregnant patient. Surg Clin North Am 62:275–289, 1982.
3. Stiffman L: The impact of injuries on the medical system. In Frey C (ed): Initial Management of the Trauma Patient. Philadelphia, Lea & Febiger, 1976, pp 3–8.
4. Esposito T, Gens R, Smith LG, et al: Trauma during pregnancy: A review of 79 cases. Arch Surg 126:1073–1078, 1991.
5. Timberlake G, McSwain N: Trauma in pregnancy: A 10-year perspective. Am Surg 55:151–153, 1989.
6. Drost TF, Rosemurgy AS, Sherman HF, et al: Major trauma in pregnant women: Maternal/fetal outcome. J Trauma 30:574–578, 1990.
7. Hoff WS, Amelio LF, Tinkoff GH, et al: Maternal predictors of fetal demise in trauma during pregnancy. Surg Gynecol Obstet 172:175–180, 1991.
8. Jackson F: Accidental injury; the problem and the initiatives. In Buschbaum HJ (ed): Trauma in Pregnancy. Philadelphia, WB Saunders Co, 1979, pp 1–21.
9. National Safety Council: Accident Facts. Chicago, 1975.
10. Lefton D: Expectant mothers and unexpected mishaps. Family Safety, winter 1980/81.
11. Baker S, O'Neill B, Karpf R: The Injury Fact Book. Lexington, MA, DC Heath, 1984.
12. Mauro LH, Cockrane SO, Cockrane P: Trauma and pregnancy in the urban environment. Trauma Q 6:69–82, 1990.
13. Hillard P: Physical abuse in pregnancy. Obstet Gynecol 66:185–190, 1985.
14. Buschbaum H: How serious is accidental injury during pregnancy? Medical Times 104:134–137, 1976.
15. Sherer DM, Schenker JG: Accidental injury during pregnancy. Obstet Gynecol Surv 44:330–338, 1989.
16. Pepperill R, Rubinstein E, MacIsaac I: Motor car accidents during pregnancy. Med J Aust 1:203–205, 1977.

17. Petrucelli E: Seat belt laws: The New York experience—Preliminary data and some observations. J Trauma 27:706–710, 1987.
18. Evans L: Fatality risk reduction from safety belt use. J Trauma 27:746–749, 1987.
19. Crosby W, King A, Stout L: Fetal survival following impact: Improvement with shoulder harness restraint. Am J Obstet Gynecol 112:April 1972.
20. Crosby W, Costiloe J: Safety of lap belt restraint for pregnant victims of automobile collisions. N Engl J Med 284(12):632–636, 1971.
21. Fort A, Harlin R: Pregnancy outcome after noncatastrophic maternal trauma during pregnancy. Obstet Gynecol 35:912–915, 1970.
22. Crosby W: Traumatic injuries during pregnancy. Clin Obstet Gynecol 26:902–912, 1983.
23. Morrovin V: Trauma in Pregnancy in OB/GYN Emergencies: The First 60 Minutes. Rockville, MD, Aspen 80, 1986.
24. Chez RA: Woman battering. Am J Obstet Gynecol 158:1–4, 1988.
25. McFarlane J, Parker B: Abstract: Intentional injury during pregnancy (research in progress).
26. Straus AM, Gelles RJ, Steinmetz SK: Behind Closed Doors: Violence in the American Family. New York, Anchor Books, 1980.
27. Helton AS, McFarlane J, Andersen ET: Battered and pregnant: A prevalence study. Am J Public Health 77:1337–1339, 1987.
28. Walker L: The Battered Woman Syndrome. New York, Springer, 1984.
29. Parker B, McFarlane J: Identifying and helping battered pregnant women. MCN 16:161–164, 1991.
30. Esposito T: Pitfalls in resuscitation and early management of the pregnant trauma patient. Trauma Q 5:1–22, 1988.
31. Deitch E, Rightmire D, Clothier J: Management of burns in pregnant women. Surg Gynecol Obstet 161:1–4, 1985.
32. Barrett S: Trauma during pregnancy. Prog Crit Care Med 1:248–272, 1984.
33. Winter PM, Miller JN: Carbon monoxide poisoning. JAMA 236:1502–1504, 1976.
34. Cramer CR: Fetal death due to accidental maternal carbon monoxide poisoning. Clin Toxicol 19:297–301, 1982.
35. Hollander D, Nagey O, Welch R, et al: Hyperbaric oxygen therapy in the treatment of acute carbon monoxide poisoning in pregnancy. J Reprod Med 32:615–617, 1987.
36. Myers RA: Hyperbaric oxygen therapy for gas gangrene and carbon monoxide poisoning. In Siegel J (ed): Trauma Emergency Surgery and Critical Care. New York, Churchill Livingstone, 1987, pp 1133–1169.
37. Anderson H, Johnson T, Barclay M, Flora J: Gestational age assessment. Am J Obstet Gynecol 139:173–177, 1981.
38. Crosby W: Trauma during pregnancy: Maternal and fetal injuries. Obstet Gynecol Surv 29:683–697, 1974.
38a. Maull KI, Rozycki GS, Pedigo RE, Cruikshank SH: Injury of the female reproductive system. In Moore EE, Feliciano D, Mattox KL (eds): Trauma. East Norwalk, CT, Appleton & Lange, 1987, pp 553–560.
39. Santos O: The obstetrical patient for nonobstetric surgery. Curr Rev Nurse Anesthetists 9:66–71, 1984.
40. Vander Veer J: Trauma during pregnancy. In Pieroz L, Deck K (eds): Topics in Emergency Medicine: Special Aspects of Trauma Care 1984, pp 72–77. Germantown, MD, Aspen Publishers, Vol 6 No 1, April 1984.
41. Smith LG: Assessment and resuscitation of the pregnant trauma patient. In Hoyt KS, Andrews J (eds): Contemporary Perspectives in Trauma Nursing. Berryville, VA, Forum Medicum, 1991.
42. Clark S, Cotton O, Lee W, et al: Central hemodynamic assessment of normal term pregnancy. Am J Obstet Gynecol 161:1439–1442, 1989.
43. Hytten F, Linda T: Diagnostic Indices in Pregnancy. Basel, Ciba-Geigy, 1973, pp 36–54.
44. Jacobs H: Hypothalamus and pituitary gland. In Hytten F, Chamberlain, G (eds): Clinical Physiology in Obstetrics. Oxford, Blackwell, 1980, pp 383–399.
45. Bang J, Holms HH: Ultrasonics in the demonstration of fetal heart movements. Am J Obstet Gynecol 102:956–960, 1986.
46. McCormick RD: Seatbelt injury: Case of complete transection of pregnant uterus. J Am Osteopath Assoc 67:1139–1141, 1968.
47. Foster C: The pregnant trauma patient. Nursing 84, November: 58–63, 1984.
48. Pearlman MD, Tintinalli JE, Lorenz RP: A prospective controlled study of outcome after trauma during pregnancy. Am J Obstet Gynecol 162:1502–1510, 1990.
49. Goodwin TM, Brun MT: Pregnancy outcome and fetomaternal hemorrhage after noncatastrophic trauma. Am J Obstet Gynecol 162:665–671, 1990.
50. Rothenberger D, Quattlebaum P, Zabel J, Fisher R: Blunt trauma: A review of 103 cases. J Trauma 18:173–177, 1978.
51. Higgins S, Garite T: Late abruptio placenta in trauma patients: Implications for monitoring. Obstet Gynecol 63[Suppl]:105–109, 1984.
52. Pearlman MD, Tentinolla JE, Lorenz RF: Blunt trauma during pregnancy. N Engl J Med 323:1609–1613, 1990.
53. Pilliteri A: Maternal-Newborn Nursing Care of the Growing Family, 3rd ed. Boston, Little, Brown, 1985.
54. Moylan J: Trauma and pregnancy. In Gleicher (ed): Principles of Medical Therapy in Pregnancy. New York, Plenum Medical Book Company 1985, pp 1136–1141.
55. Manning FA: Fetal biophysical assessment by ultrasound. In Creasy RK, Resnick R (eds): Maternal–Fetal Medicine: Principles and Practice, 2d ed. Philadelphia, WB Saunders Co, 1989.
56. Shnider S, Levinson G: Obstetric anesthesia. In Miller R (ed): Anesthesia, vol 3, no 47. New York, Churchill Livingstone, 1986, p 1683.
57. Wagner LK, Leslie RG, Saldona LR: Exposure of the Pregnant Patient to Diagnostic Radiations. Philadelphia, JB Lippincott, 1985, pp 1–34.
58. Mole RH: Radiation effects in prenatal development and their radiologic significance. Br J Radiol 52:89–91, 1979.
59. Howard F, Hill J: Drugs in pregnancy. Obstet Gynecol Surv 34:643–652, 1979.
60. Patterson R: Trauma in pregnancy. Clin Obstet Gynecol 27:32–39, 1984.
61. Kaback K, Sanders A, Merslin H: MAST suit update. JAMA 252:2598–2603, 1984.
62. Gunning J: For controlling intractable hemorrhage, the gravity suit. Contemp Obstet Gynecol 22:23–32, 1983.
63. Pearse C, Magrina J, Finley B: Use of MAST suit in obstetrics and gynecology. Obstet Gynecol Surv 37:416–422, 1984.
64. Dunham CM, Cowley RA: Shock Trauma/Critical Care Manual. Gaithersburg, MD, Aspen, 1991, pp 2–3, 54–62.
65. Esposito TJ, Gens DR, Gerber-Smith L, et al: Evaluation of blunt abdominal trauma occurring during pregnancy. J Trauma 29:1628–1632, 1989.
66. Kearney PA: Blunt trauma to the abdomen. Ann Emerg Med 18:1322–1325, 1989.
67. Alger LS, Crenshaw MC: Management of the obstetric patient after trauma. In Seigel JH (ed): Trauma: Emergency Surgery and Critical Care. New York, Churchill Livingstone, 1987, pp 1075–1098.
68. Maull KL, Rozychi GS, Pedya RE, et al: Injury to female reproductive system. In Mattox KL, Moore E, Feliciano DV (eds): Trauma. Norwalk CT, Appleton & Lange, 1988, pp 553–560.
69. Curry J, Quintana J: Myocardial infarction with ventricular fibrillation during pregnancy treated by direct current defibrillation with fetal survival. Chest 58:82, 1970.
70. Songster G, Clark S: Cardiac arrest in pregnancy: What to do. Contemp Obstet Gynecol 26:141–155, 1985.
71. DePace NL, Betesh JS, Kotler MN: Postmortem cesarean section with recovery of both mother and offspring. JAMA 248:971–973, 1982.
72. Auerbach P: Trauma in the pregnant patient. In Meislin H (ed): Priorities in Multiple Trauma. Germantown, MD, Aspen, 1980.
73. Smith LG: Abdominal trauma during pregnancy. In Strange J (ed): Shock Trauma Care Plans. Springhouse, PA, Springhouse Corp, 1987.

74. Mokriski BLK, Malinov AM: Anesthesia for the pregnant trauma patient. Probl Anesth 4(3):530–540, 1990.
75. Sendak M: Anesthesia in pregnancy. Emerg Med 18:111–131, 1986.
76. Berkowitz R: Critical Care of the Obstetric Patient. New York, Churchill Livingstone, 1983.
77. Bobak I, Jensen M: Essentials of Maternity Nursing. St. Louis, CV Mosby, 1984, pp 708–711.
78. Benfield DG, Nichols J: Living with newborn death. In Paul Almed (ed): Pregnancy, Childhood and Parenthood. New York, Elsevier, 1981.
79. Should I Wear a Seatbelt When I'm Pregnant? MIEMSS Brochure, 1984.
80. Automobile Passenger Restraints for Children and Pregnant Women, ACOG Technical Bulletin, no 74, Dec 1983, pp 1–3.
81. Tringa G: Medical aspects of seatbelt usage. J Traffic Med 8:37, 1980.
82. Agran P, Dunkle D, Winn D, Kent D: Fetal death in motor vehicle accidents. Ann Emerg Med 16:1355–1358, 1987.

26

PEDIATRIC TRAUMA

MARGARET WIDNER-KOLBERG and
PATRICIA MOLONEY-HARMON

Since the leading cause of death in children from 1 to 14 years of age is accidents, nurses must be able to recognize the patterns of pediatric injury and the appropriate treatment.

The purpose of this chapter is to explain the similarities and differences between critically ill children and adults and to bring the nurse up to date on the practical management of the pediatric trauma patient. The pathophysiological mechanism of traumatic injuries is basically the same for children and adults. In many respects, however, the management of trauma in children differs from that in adults. This chapter will describe in detail appropriate assessment and management strategies in caring for a critically injured pediatric patient through the resuscitation, critical care, and intermediate care/rehabilitation cycles of care. Special emphasis is placed on nursing management considerations as they pertain to the child rather than on specific injury types. The reader is referred to other sections of the book for injury-specific information.

Nurses often have the primary responsibility for recognizing and interpreting changes in the child's condition. The nurse must therefore understand how the child's normal circulating blood volume, cardiac output, thermoregulation, fluid and electrolyte requirements, and renal function are different from the adult's. Small variations may cause significant changes in the child's condition. These changes must be immediately recognized and acted on by the nurse. The intent of this chapter is to provide a systematic framework that allows nursing practitioners to relate to the pediatric trauma patient on the basis of the unique physiological and psychological dynamics inherent to this age group. Although various nursing diagnoses are implied throughout the text, they are not utilized as an organizational vehicle for chapter content (refer to Appendix 26–1).

EPIDEMIOLOGY/INCIDENCE

In the United States, children between the ages of 1 and 19 years are more at risk to die from injury than from all other diseases combined. Injury in this population is also the leading cause of disability. In 1986, more than 22,000 children in this age group died of injury.[1] The single largest cause of all trauma-related deaths is motor vehicle accidents. Other causes of traumatic injury in children include burns, drownings, poisonings, firearms, falls, and abuse, in order of decreasing frequency.

Two of three childhood accidents occur in males. The peak accidental age range is between 4 and 12 years, with the highest incidence at 8 years. This is easy to understand because children in this age group are starting school, and parents generally are allowing them to experience some independence. Accidental injury is not the leading cause of death in children under 1 year of age, but it does account for 30 per cent of infant deaths.

PATTERNS OF INJURY

The most common injuries seen in children are blunt as opposed to penetrating injuries. At least 80 per cent of life-threatening injuries in children occur from blunt trauma.[1] Blunt injuries are associated with rapid deceleration, which can occur in automobile accidents or from direct blows resulting from child abuse or from contact sports activities. Blunt injuries can complicate the management of the child because they are commonly associated with multiple injuries, including head injuries.[2] Evaluation of the semicomatose child is a problem if language skills are not yet fully developed. Feedback from the child is therefore limited. This often makes it difficult to complete a systems assessment as well, especially the abdominal component. In addition, few signs of injury may be visibly apparent following blunt trauma, but life-threatening internal damage may result. Nurses need to exercise a high index of suspicion when caring for children with blunt trauma.

Penetrating injuries represent approximately 20 per cent of abdominal trauma. These are not as difficult as blunt injuries to evaluate and manage in children because the injury is obvious, and therefore, appropriate intervention may be determined and initiated earlier. After the child has been totally evaluated and has relatively stable vital signs, preparation for surgical exploration usually begins.

The anatomical make-up of children renders them especially vulnerable to traumatic injury. The head of the child is proportionately larger in relation to the body mass as compared with these proportions in an adult. It is not surprising, then, that the head is especially vulnerable to injury in the child. Head injury occurs in up to 79 per cent of pediatric trauma patients and accounts for the highest mortality rate; the incidence is reported to be between 6 and 17 per cent.[3,4] The frequencies for other general types of injuries seen in pediatric trauma are extremities (29 per cent), abdominal (14 per cent), and thoracic (9 per cent).

In pedestrian trauma, injuries to the left side of the patient are predominant, perhaps owing to the fact that vehicles are driven on the right side of the road in the United States. Skeletal injuries usually involve long bones, especially of the lower limbs.[5] Chest injuries generally occur as a result of blunt trauma. Because of differences in the child's compliant chest wall, rib fractures and flail chest are less common than in adults, but pulmonary contusions are more frequent.[5] Injuries to the liver and spleen are the most common blunt abdominal injuries seen in children; other injury sites include the bowel and pancreas. Because the kidneys in children are less protected and are more mobile than in an adult, genitourinary system injuries often involve the kidneys, less frequently the bladder and urethra.[6]

TRAUMA AND CHILD ABUSE

Child abuse and neglect are the cause of approximately 4000 deaths a year in the United States. It is estimated that an overwhelming 1.4 per cent of all children in our population experience some form of child abuse and neglect.[7] Child abuse and neglect are broadly defined as the maltreatment of children and adolescents by their parents, guardians, or other caretakers. The nurse has two main responsibilities in such cases: detection and reporting. The laws on child abuse reporting are straightforward. In all states it is mandatory for nurses to report suspected cases of child abuse and neglect to the local protective service agency. The law protects health professionals from liability suits if suspicion proves to be wrong. It is important to remember that reluctance to report such information can lead to a recurrence of injury. The opportunity to help these children lies in the ability of the emergency department staff not only to appropriately treat the child but also to recognize the chronic and recurring nature of the underlying problem.

An important facet of the evaluation of pediatric trauma should be a careful examination of the child for other signs that might suggest the possibility of nonaccidental or inflicted injury. Inconsistencies between the accident history and the injuries sustained should alert the nurse to a potential child abuse situation. Orbital ecchymosis in the absence of a clear causative factor may be a significant indicator. This is a serious concern because of the high incidence of subdural hematoma formation associated with vigorous shaking or jarring of an infant's head. Skull fractures, particularly if out of magnitude with the history, should always alert one to the possibility of inflicted injury. The general appearance and nutritional state of the child also may suggest nonaccidental injury. Other diagnostic signs may include cigarette burns; unusual bruising, especially over the back or soft tissue areas of the body; and any situation whereby the circumstances are not clearly defined as causative in the injury. Old fracture sites revealed on radiographic examination also should raise suspicion. Careful examination of the genitalia and anal areas should always be part of the evaluation of the injured child. Any injury in these areas should raise suspicion of sexual abuse.

The nurse's role also should be to give the child the necessary emergency treatment and protection and to help alleviate the parents' distress at the same time. It is important to tell the parents the need for the child's treatment and protection and to verbalize interest in helping the parents through the crisis. This is a difficult task for nurses who are experiencing feelings of anger toward the parents; therefore, it is imperative for nurses to explore and come to terms with their own feelings regarding child abuse before therapeutic intervention can be expected. A helping relationship needs to be established early with the family to lay the groundwork for future intervention. If nonaccidental injury is raised as a legitimate consideration in the causation of the child's injury, the child protection team must be alerted so they can help clarify the circumstances surrounding the injury.

PREVENTION STRATEGIES

With the recognition that nonintentional injury and death are major public health problems, nurses should play a major role in injury prevention. Based on clinical experiences and the identification of patterns and trends related to pediatric trauma, nurses' contributions are paramount in all multidisciplinary efforts to determine sound trauma prevention strategies.[8]

Most children who are killed or injured in automobile-related mishaps are passengers. These casualties occur when an automobile collides with another vehicle or fixed object.[9] The use of safety belts decreases fatalities from motor vehicle accident injuries by 40 to 50 per cent, injury severity by 51 to 60 per cent, and hospital admissions by 64 per cent.[10] By communicating these facts, health professionals involved in the care of pediatric patients have been instrumental in promoting the passage of safety restraint laws in all states. Nurses also can have an impact on these legislative changes by teaching parents how to protect their children and how to use these devices correctly.

With the tremendous increase in the popularity of pedal cycling, pedal cycle injuries are now the most common cause of injuries severe enough to require treatment in an emergency department. Epidemiological studies indicate that 76 per cent of deaths resulting from bicycle crashes involving either motorized or nonmotorized vehicles were due to severe head injuries. The single most effective way to make bicycle riding safer is to insist that riders wear helmets. Improved bicycle design also would contribute to the reduction of injury and injury severity.

Drowning, the fourth leading cause of death in children, is most common in children under 4 years of age and in adolescent males 15 to 19 years of age.[11] Prevention strategies to decrease the incidence of drowning include teaching parents never to leave an infant or young child alone during a bath, providing supervised swimming instruction for children, and installing safety fences around pools. Cardiopulmonary resuscitation (CPR) also would help to decrease the number of deaths if initiated early and executed effectively; therefore, CPR education is paramount. Adult supervision, however, is by far the most effective defense strategy, although difficult to teach and impossible to legislate.

Fire-related deaths among children can be reduced in several ways. Since many fires are started by ignited cigarettes, the incidence of fires could be decreased by manufacturing cigarettes that self-extinguish. Parents also should be taught never to leave small children home alone, even for brief periods, and matches and lighters should be kept out of the reach of children. Smoke detectors in the home can provide early warning of fires and are, therefore, considered valuable devices in preventing asphyxiation and burns. Nurses could be instrumental here by teaching parents the necessity of having smoke detectors in the home as well as the importance of checking the battery routinely. Home fire drills involving all family members are important to establish so that safe practices are reinforced.

Falls by children are not uncommon, and even though many are minor, they account for a large number of injuries and deaths each year. Deaths are often due to falls from second-story windows by wandering toddlers. A preventive program was developed in New York City using a light-weight inexpensive bar that could be installed easily in second-story windows.[12] Reportedly, deaths were reduced by 47 per cent in children less than 16 years of age by this program. Nurses need to educate parents about the importance of constant adult supervision in and around the home, the installation of safety gates at the tops and bottoms of stairwells, and diligent use of window locks. Playground safety is also an area requiring community education and awareness. Playground design should be in accordance with available safety standards.

RESUSCITATION CYCLE

The assessment of the pediatric trauma patient during the resuscitation phase of care must take into account a broad spectrum of factors that will affect the priorities established for management. Immediate interventions will depend on the severity of injuries and the critical nature of the patient's responses. The primary and secondary survey provides a structured and systematic approach to the physical assessment of the patient. Other factors that must be taken into consideration are the growth and development patterns of the child. In addition, the child's family must be cared for as they face the traumatic experience with their child. Pertinent nursing diagnoses will be implied throughout various portions of this section. They have been generalized for the pediatric patient population and are not injury-specific. Specific injury-related nursing diagnoses can be found in the respective chapters. A more detailed summary of the nursing diagnoses that are appropriate for this cycle are presented in Appendix 26–1 in the Sample Care Plan for the Pediatric Trauma Patient.

Assessment Considerations

The Trauma Pediatric History

A thorough history should be obtained during the early evaluation of a child who has sustained multiple injury and included as part of the nursing data base. The purpose of the history is to learn and record the nature, location, and time of injury. The history of the injury may be crucial to the child's treatment and should first be taken at the scene of the accident. Paramedics or emergency medical technicians can often give valuable information regarding the child's level of consciousness at the scene of the injury and whether it has changed since that time. Documentation of any neurological changes, especially deterioration, is of the utmost importance. The history should include events leading to the accident, mechanism and time of injury, clinical course following the injury, contamination of wound sites, previous history of chronic illness or injury, allergies, medications, and time of the last meal eaten before injury. The American College of Surgeons recommends taking an AMPLE history:[13]

A = allergies
M = medications
P = past medical history
L = last meal
E = events leading to the accident

An allergy history must be obtained in children, as with all patients. The parents should be asked if the child is allergic to any medicine, adhesive tape, or environmental substances.

The nurse should establish if the parents have given the child any medications recently. It also should be determined if the child takes medication routinely for diabetes, seizures, lung disease, heart disease, or other disease entities.

In gathering the medical history, the nurse should establish if the child is under medical care for reasons other than routine well-child health care. Does the child have any chronic illness, such as diabetes, seizures, lung disease, or heart disease? Has the child been hospitalized previously? If so, for what? Are the child's immunizations up to date?

Also, try to establish when the child's last meal was eaten. This information is important if the child needs to be intubated and/or needs surgery.

Finally, whatever the presenting problem, specific questions can give more insight into the problem. What were the events leading to the accident? What were the mechanisms and time of injury?

Because of limitations in verbal and communication skills, neither the infant nor the very young child can give a complete history, but it is useful to obtain whatever information is possible from the child. Younger children are likely to remember recent events. Events somewhat farther back in time may be better remembered by a parent or caretaker even though their accuracy may be clouded by their emotional state following the injury. In general, once a child reaches school age, taking a history becomes considerably easier.

The nurse will begin to establish a relationship with the family and the child during this information-gathering session. It is important for nurses to remember as they are gathering this information that this crisis has disrupted the entire family unit and that fear and anxiety prevail. The family will need as much feedback information from the medical/nursing professionals as is possible on an on-going basis. Establishing a supportive rapport with the family during this initial phase will help to foster a closer working relationship among the child, the parents, and the health care team members throughout the child's hospitalization. Early interactions with family members and information presented should be documented in the nurse's notes. An assessment of the family's initial reactions, responses, concerns, and coping abilities should be included, serving as a baseline for other nurses who will continue the care for the patient and family.

Physical Examination

Nurses caring for children must be familiar with the normal physiological parameters for children at different ages. A small child responds differently to major injuries than an older child or adult. Special considerations that can compromise management in children include less respiratory reserve, abdominal distention, fluid–electrolyte and caloric imbalances, differences in blood volume, and heat loss.

Vital Signs. Pulses are obtained at the radial, brachial, carotid, or femoral arteries and should be counted for a full minute because there are often irregularities in an anxious or injured child. The child under normal circumstances has a faster heart rate and respiratory rate and a lower blood pressure than the adult. Tachycardia is usually found in such conditions as fever, shock, and the initial response to stress. Bradycardia can result from increased intracranial pressure, hypoxia, hypothermia, and hypoglycemia.

The respiratory rate also should be counted for a full minute for the same reason mentioned previously. Tachypnea is a normal initial response to stress in children. If a stressed child does not hyperventilate, head injury, spinal cord injury, or other reasons such as a distended abdomen should be considered.

Blood pressures should be obtained using a cuff size that is no less than one-half and no more than two-thirds the length of the upper arm. If pediatric cuffs are not available, an adult cuff can be used on the child's thigh. In the field a palpable systolic blood pressure is adequate; precious time should not be wasted to obtain a diastolic reading. The normal systolic blood pressure for individuals from 1 to 20 years of age is 80 plus two times the age in years. The diastolic pressure should be approximately two-thirds the normal systolic pressure. An example for a 5-year-old is

$$\text{Systolic: } 80 + (5 \times 2) = 90 \text{ mm Hg}$$
$$\text{Diastolic: } \tfrac{2}{3} \times 90 = 60 \text{ mm Hg}$$

Fear and distress can increase the child's heart rate and respiratory rate. The nurse may have to differentiate between emotional stress and hypoxia or shock. It is also important for the nurse to refer back to the medical history. A pediatric trauma patient may have a congenital heart problem and be tachypneic normally; if that child has a normal respiratory rate, ventilatory assistance may be required.

Normal heart rates, respiratory rates, and blood pressures for children, including upper limits of normal, are shown in Tables 26–1 through 26–3. The nurse can couple these ranges

TABLE 26–1. NORMAL HEART RATES IN CHILDREN

AGE	BEATS/ MINUTE
Infants	120–160
Toddlers	90–140
Preschoolers	80–110
School-age children	75–100
Adolescents	60–90

TABLE 26–2. NORMAL RESPIRATORY RATES IN CHILDREN

AGE	BREATHS/ MINUTE
Infants	30–60
Toddlers	24–40
Preschoolers	22–34
School-age children	18–30
Adolescents	12–16

TABLE 26–4. CALCULATION OF MAINTENANCE FLUIDS (PER 24 HOURS) IN CHILDREN

WEIGHT (kg)	KILOGRAM BODY WEIGHT FORMULA
0–10	100–120 ml/kg
11–20	1000 ml for the first 10 kg and 50 ml/kg for each kg over 10 kg
21–30	1500 ml for the first 20 kg and 25 ml/kg for each kg over 20 kg

with knowledge of the child's condition to determine the appropriate vital signs for the child.

Respiratory Reserve. The infant has less respiratory reserve than the adult for several reasons: (1) the infant's vital capacity is smaller, (2) the chest wall is soft because the ribs and sternum are cartilage, and (3) the ribs are horizontal with poorly developed intercostal muscles.

An infant whose lung capacity is decreased will compensate for it by increasing the respiratory rate and will easily start to retract. Retractions are an early sign of respiratory difficulty and will compromise the infant's tidal volume. Most of the child's normal respiratory activity is affected by abdominal movement until age 6 or 7 years; there is very little intercostal motion. A child who develops a paralytic ileus following blunt abdominal trauma may go into respiratory distress because abdominal distention may elevate the diaphragm and interfere with pulmonary function. As a result, children in respiratory distress who are spontaneously breathing should be treated in a semi-Fowler position when spinal injury has been ruled out.

Fluid and Electrolyte Balance. The daily fluid requirement of the child is larger per kilogram of body weight than that of an adult because the child has greater insensible water losses per unit of body weight. This is due to the fact that the child has a larger surface area and a higher metabolic rate than the adult. Even with these factors, the absolute amount of fluid required by a child is small. Nurses must be alert to the fluid volume administered to the child to avoid overhydration. The calculation of maintenance fluid requirements is shown in Table 26–4.

If the child's fluid intake is adequate, the urine volume should average 0.5 to 1.0 ml/kg/hr. The nurse should be attentive and keep accurate records of all possible sources of fluid loss, including blood drawing samples, blood loss from any source, gastric drainage, vomitus, or diarrhea.

Because the child's metabolic rate is higher than that of an adult, he or she will require more calories per kilogram of body weight. The critically ill child, even if immobile, will still require most of the normal maintenance calories. This is discussed in more detail in the critical care phase.

TABLE 26–3. NORMAL PEDIATRIC BLOOD PRESSURE RANGES

AGE	SYSTOLIC (mm Hg)	DIASTOLIC (mm Hg)
Infants	74–100	50–70
Toddlers	80–112	50–80
Preschoolers	82–110	50–78
School-age children	84–120	54–80
Adolescents	94–140	62–88

Some forms of electrolyte imbalance are more likely to occur in children than in adults, leading to complications. Serum glucose, calcium, and potassium are three electrolytes that should be monitored closely in the child. Infants have high glucose needs because of high metabolic rates and low glycogen stores; therefore, the infant can become hypoglycemic quickly during periods of stress. A $D_{25}W$ bolus (0.5–1.0 gm/kg) will help correct this. Changes in serum potassium concentration can occur with changes in acid–base status and diuretic administration. The critically ill child does not seem to be as sensitive to hypokalemia as the adult, so cardiac dysrhythmias from hypokalemia are not often seen in pediatric patients until the serum potassium is less than 3 mEq/liter.[14] Ventricular fibrillation is rarely seen in pediatric patients but may result from severe hypokalemia or hyperkalemia.

The administration of citrate phosphate dextran (CPD) blood will produce precipitation of serum ionized calcium.[15] An infant who requires frequent transfusions is at risk for developing hypocalcemia, a condition which can interrupt normal cardiovascular function. The calcium concentration should therefore be monitored closely so that calcium supplements can be administered as needed.

The child's circulating blood volume (80 ml/kg) is larger per unit of body weight than the adult's. The loss of a small amount of blood in a child, however, is proportionately more significant than in an adult because of the child's miniature total blood volume, potentially leading to hypovolemic shock. A closed fracture of the femur, for example, in a 10-year-old may result in a loss of 300 or 400 ml of blood. The same amount of blood loss in an adult may not cause a significant problem, whereas in the child, this may represent 15 to 25 per cent of the total circulatory blood volume. The child's total circulating blood volume should be calculated on admission, and all blood lost due to hemorrhage or drawn for laboratory tests should be accurately tabulated and recorded.

Body Temperature. Major heat losses can occur in a young child who is unclothed for even a short time. Infants and young children have a large surface area and therefore lose more heat to the environment through radiation, conduction, convection, and evaporation. During resuscitation, children are often exposed, losing much of their body heat and therefore dropping their core body temperature. Hypothermia will interfere with the resuscitation attempt, causing apnea, progressive metabolic acidosis, decreased cardiac output, and ventricular dysrhythmias. The nurse can minimize this stress by monitoring the child's temperature rectally, keeping the child covered as much as possible, using heat lamps if indicated, and warming all fluids prior to infusion.

Growth and Development

Physical Development. The initial encounter with the child should include an assessment of the child's growth and physical development. This information will help identify existing alterations that will determine the approach used during the examination. Owing to the critical nature of the child's injury, this assessment must be done quickly. An accurate estimate of the size and weight (Table 26–5) must be made as soon as possible so that therapy can be initiated. When time allows, however, an exact weight should be obtained because medical treatment that involves drug and fluid therapy, calculated on a per-kilogram basis, must be accurately determined.

Psychosocial Factors. The multisystem injuries and hospitalization of a critically ill child are devastating for the child and the family. Nurses have the responsibility to do everything possible to minimize the psychological trauma that will accompany the hospital visit. Since stressful medical situations can become the foci of fears and the source of new symptoms for the child, pediatric emergency care must include not only physical management but also consideration of the child's psychological reactions to the illness. By relying on some basic age-appropriate developmental characteristics, nurses can be astute to the general psychological responses expected of the child. Table 26–6 summarizes the essential issues in this assessment process based on the age of children; their state of language, motor, and social development; and related fears. Appropriate nursing implications are also outlined.

General Principles. Several general principles should be applied when working with a pediatric patient, regardless of the age or developmental level of the child. For most children, security in the world comes from their parents. Wanting his parents with him may be the child's first priority, even above that of having the nurse help or relieve pain. When taking care of a child, the nurse should observe the following guidelines:

- Let the child know someone will call his or her parents, and tell the child when they arrive.
- If the child brought a toy with him or her, let him or her hold it.
- When speaking to the patient, get down to the child's eye level and let him or her see your face. Speak clearly and slowly so the child can hear you.
- Never assume the child has understood you. Find out by questioning the child.
- Do not let children witness treatment given to a seriously ill adult. Take the time to segregate the child to avoid additional emotional trauma.
- Never lie to the child. Be honest that there might be pain during the physical examination. If the child asks about being sick or hurt, tell the truth, but give reassurance by telling him or her you are there to help. It is important to smile at the child. If you appear calm and in control, it will be more reassuring to the child.
- Touch the child and hold his or her hand. Acceptance of you by the child will show in the reaction to your touch. Talking with the child and smiling can provide comfort.
- Always explain to the child what you are going to do during the primary and secondary survey.
- Do not try to explain the entire procedure at once. Explain one step, do the procedure, then explain the next step.
- Children of all ages should be respected for feelings of bashfulness and modesty. In particular, school-age children and adolescents are modest about exposing their bodies to strangers. Keep all children covered with a hospital gown, allowing exposure of only different body parts during the physical examination.

Children are a unique patient population because they are in a dynamic state of growth and development. By practicing these few general principles while considering appropriate developmental tendencies, the nurse can lessen the trauma that the child experiences.

TABLE 26–5. APPROXIMATE WEIGHTS FOR CHILDREN

AGE	WEIGHT (kg)
Newborn	1
6 months	6
1 yr	10
3 yr	15
5 yr	20
8 yr	25
10 yr	30
16 yr	50

Assessment in Head Trauma

Head injuries are common in children. Each year approximately 100,000 to 250,000 acute brain-injured children are admitted to hospitals in the United States.[16, 17] In children, the brain tissues are thinner, softer, and more flexible; the head size is greater in proportion to the body surface area; and a relatively larger proportion of the total blood volume is in the child's head. Thus the child's response to head injury differs significantly from that of an adult. Mass lesions following head injuries are less common, and intracranial hypertension and cerebral hypoxia are more common, rendering the child more susceptible to secondary brain injury. Secondary brain injury is, in part, considered to be more treatable than primary brain injury. This contributes to a significantly better outcome in the pediatric patient. Mortality in children with severe head injuries is 6 to 10 per cent, as opposed to 30 to 50 per cent in the adult with severe head injuries.[18] Expandable fontanelles and opening sutures allow more room for swelling, providing an advantage for the head-injured infant. The primary disadvantage in the evaluation of the head-injured child is the developmentally imposed limitation in verbal expression, which can complicate assessment endeavors.

Neurological Assessment. A thorough neurological assessment should be done as soon as possible after the primary survey is complete and initial stabilization interventions (airway, breathing, circulation—ABC's) are under way. The neurological examination should consist of the deter-

TABLE 26–6. DEVELOPMENTAL APPROACH TO PEDIATRIC EMERGENCY CARE PATIENTS

AGE (yr)	IMPORTANT DEVELOPMENT ISSUES	FEARS	USEFUL TECHNIQUES
Infancy (0–1)	Minimal language Feel an extension of parents Sensitive to physical environment	Stranger anxiety	Keep parents in sight Avoid hunger Use warm hands Keep room warm
Toddler (1–3)	Receptive language more advanced than expressive See themselves as individuals Assertive will	Brief separation Pain	Maintain verbal communication Examine in parent's lap when possible Allow some choices when possible
Preschool (3–5)	Excellent expressive skill for thoughts and feelings Rich fantasy life Magical thinking Strong concept of self	Long separation Pain Disfigurement	Allow expression Encourage fantasy and play Encourage participation in care
School age (5–10)	Fully developed language Understanding of body structure and function Able to reason and compromise Experience with self-control Incomplete understanding of death	Disfigurement Loss of function Death	Explain procedures Explain pathophysiology and treatment Project positive outcome Stress child's ability to master situation Respect physical modesty
Adolescence (10–19)	Self-determination Decision making Peer group important Realistic view of death	Loss of autonomy Loss of peer acceptance Death	Allow choices and control Stress acceptance by peers Respect autonomy

From Fleisher GR, Ludwig S: Textbook of Pediatric Emergency Medicine. © 1983, Williams & Wilkins, Co, Baltimore.

mination of level of consciousness, pupillary response, and motor response.

Evaluation of the level of consciousness after a head injury is probably the single most important aspect of the neurological assessment but often the most difficult to perform in an infant or young child. Since "level of consciousness" means different things to different people, a uniform system like AVPU or the Glasgow Coma Scale should be used. The AVPU method is described below:

A Patient is *alert.*
V Patient responds to *vocal* stimuli. (This unfortunately is of little value in a very young child.)
P Patient responds to *painful* stimuli.
U Patient is *unresponsive.*

The Glasgow Coma Scale (GCS) is used worldwide as a neurological assessment tool. Developed in 1974 as a prognostic tool, the GCS also helps to grade the depth of coma by standardizing assessments.[19] The scale consists of three sections, each of which measures a separate function of the person's level of consciousness: the patient's eye opening response, verbal response, and motor response. The total score ranges from 3 to 15, with the higher scores indicating more favorable neurological function. However, since it is difficult to use this tool to evaluate verbal response in infants and preverbal children, many clinicians use a modified GCS (Table 26–7).[20]

TABLE 26–7. GLASGOW COMA SCALE

RESPONSE	ADULTS AND CHILDREN	INFANTS	POINTS
Eye opening	No response	No response	1
	To pain	To pain	2
	To voice	To voice	3
	Spontaneous	Spontaneous	4
Verbal	No response	No response	1
	Incomprehensible	Moans to pain	2
	Inappropriate words	Cries to pain	3
	Disoriented conversation	Irritable	4
	Oriented and appropriate	Coos, babbles	5
Motor	No response	No response	1
	Decerebrate posturing	Decerebrate posturing	2
	Decorticate posturing	Decorticate posturing	3
	Withdraws to pain	Withdraws to pain	4
	Localizes pain	Withdraws to touch	5
	Obeys commands	Normal spontaneous movement	6
Total score			3–15

From Nichols D, Yaster M, Lappy D, Buck JR: In Golden Hour: The Handbook of Advanced Pediatric Life Support. St. Louis, Mosby–Year Book, 1991, p 180.

With children, as with adults, pupil reactivity, size, shape, and symmetry are responses used to assess brainstem function. Size can be described as pinpoint, midpoint, or dilated, but measuring in millimeters is more accurate. Reaction to light is checked by shining a bright light into each eye separately. When increased intracranial pressure develops, the oculomotor nerve is compressed by general expansion of the brain, an intracranial lesion, or herniation of the brain; the pupil dilates but does not constrict in response to light. Eye movements also should be noted. Abnormal eye movements include deviation of one or both eyes from midline or back and forth movements.

Any difficulty in movement of the extremities should be described and the nature of the movement indicated as spontaneous or in response to pain. The extremity in which the response is elicited also should be recorded. The child with increased intracranial pressure will have a decrease in motor function as well as abnormal posturing or reflexes. Babinski reflex is positive when the toes fan out and the great toe moves dorsally. The reflex is assessed by scratching the sole of the foot with an object such as the blunt tip of a tongue depressor. A positive reflex is normal in a child under 18 months but abnormal in any child who is walking and may indicate the presence of increased intracranial pressure.

Continuous monitoring is essential. After the initial neurological examination, serial neurological checks must be repeated as often as every 15 minutes in the acutely ill child. Any changes should be reported to the physician immediately and documented in the nurse's notes or flow record.

Vital Signs. In addition to the importance of the vital signs in the assessment of the general status of the pediatric trauma patient, the vital signs may be an observable manifestation of what is going on inside the patient's cranial vault.

An increase in the child's core body temperature may cause increased cerebral blood flow, increased intracranial volume, and therefore, increased intracranial pressure. Since children are very sensitive to environmental temperatures and their body temperature can drop quickly, care should be taken to keep the child in a neutral thermal environment.

Bradycardia in the presence of increasing blood pressure (Cushing phenomenon) may indicate increasing intracranial pressure. A rapid pulse rate is a grave and late sign in a head-injured patient unless it is due to some other cause. In children, shock will be associated with tachycardia even if intracranial pressure is increased. Cushing phenomenon, often not seen in infants, is a late sign and should not be relied on as an early sign of deterioration.

An elevated blood pressure also can indicate a rise in intracranial pressure, although hypertension in a multiply injured child should never be assumed to be the direct result of a head injury. Hypertension may be precipitated by anxiety or pain or may be present as a result of preexisting illness. Careful assessment therefore is imperative. Generally, increased intracranial pressure is accompanied by an increase in systolic arterial blood pressure, producing a widening of the pulse pressure. This compensatory mechanism occurs as the body attempts to maintain adequate cerebral perfusion pressure by initiating a rise in blood pressure.

The child with a head injury may have several types of abnormal respiratory patterns. When intracranial pressure rises and signs of the Cushing phenomenon are evident, the child will typically develop apnea. Development of the Cheyne-Stokes pattern of breathing (alternating hyperpnea and bradypnea) following the presence of a normal respiratory pattern should alert the nurse to suspect neurological deterioration. Hyperventilation usually indicates injury to the brainstem at the level of the pons.[21]

Head and Neck Examination. All pediatric trauma patients must be suspected of having a cervical spine injury, especially those who have sustained facial or head trauma or who complain of pain in the neck or back. Anteroposterior, lateral, and open-mouth radiographic views of the cervical spine are necessary diagnostic studies.[21] Although spinal cord injury occurs infrequently in children, anytime the C-spine x-rays appear normal but the child is symptomatic, it is imperative that a neurosurgical consultation be obtained.

After the initial parameters for head and neck injury have been obtained (vital signs and cervical spine films), the child's head and neck are examined rapidly to look for obvious injury, including depressed or open skull fractures, lacerations, or leakage of cerebrospinal fluid (CSF). The nurse should look in the child's ears for blood or otorrhea and behind the child's ears for obvious ecchymosis (Battle sign), indicating the presence of a basilar skull fracture. CSF drainage from the nose may indicate the presence of a fractured cribriform plate. Finally, the face and oral cavity should be examined closely for lacerations or possible fracture sites.

Further neurodiagnostic evaluation is indicated in children with head injuries to identify the type and extent of injury. The need for skull radiographs in the management of severely head-injured patients has been under debate in recent years. For patients who require computed tomographic (CT) scan for possible intracranial lesions, skull radiographs add nothing to the diagnosis. Skull radiographs, however, can complement CT scan results in diagnosing depressed fractures and in identifying the location of foreign bodies and are indicated in cases of suspected child abuse.[22]

In patients with a head injury less than 72 hours old, CT scanning remains the procedure of choice for several reasons, including the limited potential for magnetic resonance imaging (MRI) to diagnose acute subarachnoid hemorrhage or acute parenchymal hemorrhage, the ease of monitoring unstable patients during the CT scan procedure, and the short time frame required to complete this procedure.[23] MRI is a technique used for imaging intracranial structures and is superior in imaging the posterior fossa, spinal cord structure, small vascular lesions, and most brain tumors.[24] Lengthy procedure time, difficulty in monitoring critically ill patients during the procedure, cost, and the inability to visualize bone directly are among the drawbacks of this procedure.

Assessment of Thoracic Trauma

Although chest trauma in children is not as common as it is in adults, it can cause a number of problems in diagnosis and management. Due to major advances in the transport and treatment of the injured child, the mortality rate associated with thoracic trauma has decreased. The absence of preexisting disease states in children also contributes to the low morbidity rate associated with thoracic trauma.

One of the unique features of the child who has sustained thoracic trauma is the amazingly compliant thorax resulting from the flexibility of the bony and cartilaginous structures. It is not unusual, therefore, for the child to have major internal injury from compression of the chest without fracture of the bony thorax. A child's mediastinum is freely mobile and capable of wide anatomical shifts, causing the potential for life-threatening situations with dislocation of the heart, angulation of the great vessels, compression of the lung, and angulation of the trachea. Children with any type of traumatic injury experience aerophagia (swallowing of air), which results in gastric dilation that limits diaphragmatic excursion and leads to reflex ileus. In a small child, this also can compromise the breathing pattern.

Cardiopulmonary Examination. Many injuries to the thorax can cause severe cardiorespiratory problems soon after injury; the result is fatal if prompt and accurate diagnosis and treatment are not initiated. This requires a rapid but thorough assessment. Continual reassessment of the child's condition after the initiation of therapy is of utmost importance.

Abnormalities in the child's breathing pattern, e.g., flaring nostrils, chest wall retractions, and prominent use of accessory muscles, suggest ventilatory impairment. If the child is inadequately oxygenated, cyanosis of the fingers, toes, and lips will be seen. When the airway is obstructed, cyanosis becomes prominent on both the face and trunk. A flail chest is usually apparent on visual inspection. The child will be moving air poorly; movement of the thorax is asymmetrical and uncoordinated. A child with tension pneumothorax and massive hemothorax will show poor respiratory exchange, unilateral chest wall movement, or decreased unilateral chest wall movement. The presence of a tension pneumothorax will result in distended neck veins and a tracheal and mediastinal shift to the opposite side. A child with cardiac tamponade also will present with distended neck veins; however, with a massive hemothorax, the neck veins are often flat due to decreased cardiac output. Any penetrating wounds to the thorax should be noted and treated immediately. When an entrance wound is found, an exit wound also should be sought. In the traumatized child, all aspects of the thorax, neck, and upper abdomen should be examined for abrasions, lacerations, and contusions.

Palpation should be performed gently and in a nonthreatening manner using warm hands. The area of injury should be palpated last during the examination. Talking softly may have a calming effect on the child and may lessen the pain experienced as injured portions of the chest are assessed.

The nurse should palpate the neck, clavicles, sternum, and thorax. Any signs of tenderness, swelling, or crepitus should be noted. Subcutaneous emphysema is a finding of significant concern. Subcutaneous air can be palpated near penetrating chest wounds. If it is found in the neck area, a proximal tear or avulsion of the tracheobronchial tree or an esophageal perforation is suggested.

During examination of the thorax, any instability should be noted. Unilateral tenderness in the upper abdomen may indicate a chest injury such as a fractured rib.

The small size of the chest in infants and children makes it difficult to use auscultation and percussion to determine the exact location of injury. Despite this limitation, however, these procedures are considered to be valuable in assessing thoracic injury. The presence of a pneumothorax is partially diagnosed through auscultation of breath sounds; since the chest wall of the young child is so thin, breath sounds are easily transmitted from other areas of the lung. Decreased breath sounds may not be heard over the involved lung; however, the nurse may note a difference in the quality or pitch of the breath sounds between the right and left sides. Auscultation also can be used to identify a shift in the heart sounds corresponding to a tracheal shift caused by a tension pneumothorax on one side of the chest. Cardiac tamponade is associated with muffled heart tones. In massive hemothorax, dullness to percussion is present, although the limited thoracic surface area in an infant makes this assessment technique difficult.

In examining the thorax, the nurse also should assess for the presence of any specific sounds, such as inspiratory stridor or expiratory wheezes, that might result from bronchial injury.

Radiographic and Laboratory Studies. To optimally evaluate a child with a thoracic emergency, a quality thoracic roentgenogram is needed. Roentgenograms of the chest should include posteroanterior (PA) and lateral views done in an upright position, *after* cervical spine injury has been ruled out. With an upright chest radiograph, the clinician can better visualize the degree of mediastinal shift. It is easier to diagnose abnormalities in the lung, pleural cavity, and diaphragm with this view as well.

Standard blood studies for any pediatric trauma patient should include an arterial blood gas determination. Other more involved studies such as pulmonary function tests, tomograms, barium contrast studies, sonograms, and CT scans may be indicated depending on other clinical findings.

Assessment of Abdominal Trauma

Intra-abdominal injuries account for only a small percentage of total pediatric trauma deaths, but failure to diagnose and successfully manage these injuries promptly accounts for the majority of preventable deaths following multiple trauma.[25] Serious abdominal injury tends to be quite subtle compared to injuries of the head, chest, or limbs. Isolated abdominal injuries are relatively easy to treat and manage; however, confusion in establishment of priorities is common when evaluating a child with multiple trauma and possible abdominal injury.

Physical Examination. The physical examination of an acute abdomen in children is similar to the procedure for adults, but objective findings are often masked or misinterpreted. This assessment may be difficult because the child, if conscious, is often apprehensive and may be unwilling to cooperate. In the unconscious child, many of the voluntary responses are gone; therefore, few clinical signs will be available to facilitate diagnosis. The key to making an accurate diagnosis of serious abdominal injury is careful examination with constant reassessment and the initiation of several diagnostic studies.

The abdomen and lower chest should be examined for contusions, abrasions, and lacerations that may indicate compression injury. It should be noted whether the abdomen is scaphoid or distended. If a conscious child is pulling up the lower extremities, it may be in an attempt to relieve tension on the abdominal wall, thereby reducing pain.

Penetrating wounds must be checked for involvement of intra-abdominal organs. The back should be examined for signs of surface injury, bony instability, or pain.

Since children up to about 6 years of age breathe primarily with their diaphragms, peritoneal irritation from blood or intestinal contents may result in an alteration of the child's breathing pattern. This child may now breathe shallowly with the chest muscles to avoid pain. A distended abdomen may indicate significant injury and be caused by the accumulation of gas or liquid, such as blood, bile, pancreatic juice, urine, or intestinal contents. To examine the abdomen adequately, a nasal or orogastric tube should be inserted. The drainage from the nasogastric tube should be examined for blood, which might indicate upper abdominal injury.

The abdomen should be auscultated, although absence of bowel sounds may be normal or indicate an ileus. An intra-abdominal hemorrhage or bowel perforation may initially give hypoactive or hyperactive bowel sounds. A quiet abdomen can be suggestive of an acute intraperitoneal injury.

Palpation. Frightened children are often uncooperative, making palpation of the abdomen a difficult part of the examination. The nurse must be gentle and creative in the approach to this portion of the assessment. Palpation should involve separate evaluation of the anterior and posterior abdominal wall and intra-abdominal contents. Gentle pressure may bring about a voluntary response or guarding by the child, which may be localized to the abdominal wall or intra-abdominal organs. Any physical signs of trauma should be compared with this response to help identify injuries. With deeper palpation, an involuntary response of muscle spasm may be present. In the pediatric trauma patient, this peritoneal irritation is usually a sign of intra-abdominal bleeding. Rebound tenderness may be difficult to interpret because it causes pain and therefore crying and voluntary guarding. The best way to elicit rebound tenderness in a child is by gentle percussion, shaking of the child, or asking the child to cough rather than by rapidly releasing manual pressure over portions of the abdomen. This part of the examination will help determine if peritoneal irritation is present.

Pelvic and Genitourinary Assessment. The last part of the abdominal examination is evaluation of the pelvis and genitourinary system. A pelvic fracture is suspected if pain is present upon compression of the wings of the ilium or symphysis pubis or with abduction of the legs. Rupture of the bladder frequently accompanies pelvic fractures, although a full bladder may rupture without a pelvic fracture. This injury should be suspected when the child has lower abdominal pain, hematuria, and an inability to void. Urethral injuries should be suspected when the child presents with perineal swelling, blood at the meatus, a floating prostate, a distended bladder, and an inability to void. Use of a urethral catheter is contraindicated, since it may change an incomplete urethral tear into a complete urethral disruption. A rectal examination is necessary to evaluate the tone of the anal sphincter, position of the prostate, and integrity of the bony pelvis and bowel wall. The presence of blood strongly indicates perforation of the colon or rectum.

Injury to the kidney is common in pediatric trauma patients. Parenchymal contusion is the most common injury seen and most often results from blunt trauma.[26] An indication of this injury may be hematuria, although up to 40 per cent of children with renal injury caused by blunt trauma may have no hematuria.[27] Flank pain and tenderness also may be present. Further radiological studies may be indicated, including contrast-enhanced CT scan, an intravenous pyelogram, and a renal scan.[26]

Diagnostic Studies. CT scan is a definitive method of evaluation for the child with blunt abdominal trauma. The CT scan provides superior detail of anatomy and allows for clear imagery of multiple abdominal organs simultaneously. An enhanced scan allows for the assessment of organ perfusion and evaluation of intraperitoneal bleeding, clearly defining the nature and extent of the injury.[28]

Penetrating abdominal trauma is rare in the child and is often the result of a rib fracture.[29] Owing to the unpredictable nature of penetrating injuries, surgical exploration is usually indicated.[30]

Peritoneal lavage is not performed as frequently in children as in adults because it interferes with serial abdominal examination and because an isolated posttraumatic intra-abdominal bleed is not necessarily an indication for surgery in pediatric patients.[31] Peritoneal lavage irritates the peritoneum for 24 to 48 hours, so it is not performed early in the clinical setting. In children with isolated abdominal trauma, the main determinations for surgical intervention are physical findings, deteriorating vital signs, and falling hematocrit. In a child with multitrauma, especially a head injury, clinical findings may not be as accurate in reflecting intra-abdominal bleeding. Peritoneal lavage may be an appropriate diagnostic tool in the following circumstances:[32]

1. Altered pain responses
   a. Head injury
   b. Alcohol or drug ingestion
   c. Fractures of ribs, pelvis, lumbar spine
   d. Chest wall injury
2. Equivocal abdominal findings
3. Hemodynamic instability
4. General anesthesia
5. Stab wound with no peritonitis

Initially the abdominal examination may be negative, but continual reassessment is needed to rule out the development of a significant problem. It may take 12 to 24 hours for intra-abdominal findings to become obvious in a child with suspected abdominal injury.

Following the physical examination, appropriate laboratory studies are obtained. These include a complete blood count, type, and cross-match; blood gas analysis; prothrombin time; partial thromboplastin time; platelet count; and serum amylase determination.

Assessment of Musculoskeletal Trauma

Injuries to the extremities are usually obvious or readily identified with radiographic examination. Except for cervical and displaced pelvic fractures, orthopedic trauma is rarely life-threatening. However, the importance of extremity injuries should never be underestimated because mismanagement could result in serious sequelae, such as infection, growth disturbance, or paralysis.

The high incidence of fractures in children can be explained by the combination of their relatively slender bone structure and their high activity level. Some of these injuries, e.g., buckle and greenstick fractures, are not serious compared with intra-articular and epiphyseal plate fractures, which can impair normal bone growth if they are not treated properly.

TABLE 26-8. CLASSES OF HEMORRHAGE FOR CHILDREN

CLASS	BLOOD LOSS	SIGNS	TREATMENT
Class I	15% or less 40-kg child = 500 ml blood	Pulse: Slight ↑ BP: normal Respiration: normal Capillary refill: normal Tilt test*: normal	Crystalloids
Class II	20–30% 40-kg child = 800 ml blood	Tachycardia > 150 BP: ↓ systolic; ↓ pulse pressure Tachypnea > 35–40 Delayed capillary refill Positive tilt test Urine output normal (1 ml/kg/hr)	Crystalloids
Class III	30–35% 40-kg child = 1200 ml blood *Major Bleed*	Blood pressure drop Narrow pulse pressure Urine output affected	Crystalloids Packed red cells
Class IV	40–50% 40-kg child = 1600 ml blood	Nonpalpable blood pressure and pulse No response to verbal or painful stimuli	Crystalloids Packed red cells

BP, blood pressure.
*A tilt test is done by sitting the child upright. The test is normal if the child can stay up more than 90 seconds and maintain blood pressure.

Examination of the Extremities. During the secondary survey, the nurse should palpate all extremities to detect pain, swelling, bruising, lacerations, and deformities. The neurovascular status of each limb should be noted and documented. The presence of a distal extremity pulse does not exclude an associated proximal artery tear. Soft tissue injuries should be thoroughly inspected for the presence of foreign bodies or dead tissue.

Temperature of the extremities should be noted, with special care being given to determine whether the temperature is equal on both sides. Differences in temperature are usually due to neurological or vascular abnormalities. Extremities may be cold and pale following sympathetic nervous system stimulation. This condition also can be a sign of venous or arterial thrombosis or embolism.

Radiological studies are used to confirm the diagnosis. Roentgenograms should always include the joint above and below the fracture to avoid missing an associated dislocation. Roentgenograms taken in two projections (i.e., PA and lateral) will help to avoid overlooking a fracture with deformity in only one location. Fractures in children often do not present a clear-cut picture; diagnosis may require additional effort. It is possible to overlook a severe injury such as an epiphyseal separation with only a small degree of displacement or a fracture involving unossified epiphyses. Radiological examination of both limbs, allowing for comparison of the injured and uninjured extremities, will assist in avoiding this error.

Shock in Children

In essence, shock is a generalized failure of adequate tissue perfusion resulting in impaired cellular and subcellular respiration. The basic cellular responses and general pathophysiological mechanisms of the disease appear to be identical among different age groups. However, because of the differences between children and adults previously mentioned (e.g., vital sign parameters, thermoregulation, and response to head injury), shock is quite different in pediatric patients than in the adult population. The pediatric trauma patient is in shock most often because of hypoxia and blood loss. Children rarely suffer from diseases that predispose them to the development of other kinds of shock. In addition, there is a thin margin of error in the recognition and treatment of pediatric patients with multisystem injury.

In infants and younger children, 70 per cent of the total body weight is water and 50 per cent of the total body water is located in the child's extracellular space. Therefore, hypovolemia will occur more rapidly in the child than in the adult, whose extracellular space contains only 23 per cent of total body water.

Children have the ability to vasoconstrict effectively and can compensate for up to 25 per cent of their blood loss. Therefore, when hypotension does occur in the pediatric shock patient, it usually indicates a significant degree of blood loss. A traumatized child who is tachycardic; has cold, mottled extremities; and is hypotensive should be considered to be in shock.

Clinical Presentation. In assessing the child in shock, several clinical signs will become apparent. Tachycardia and tachypnea will be present. Due to the peripheral vasoconstriction, the extremities will be cold, clammy, and mottled and the pulses will be weak or nonpalpable. The child's level of consciousness will be altered owing to decreased cerebral perfusion. Urinary output will be decreased or absent. The decrease in the systolic blood pressure is a late indicator; a narrowing of the pulse pressure is usually seen first. Table 26–8 differentiates the four classes of hemorrhage and lists the clinical signs and treatment for each.

Infants in shock may present differently from children or adults in shock. They may develop erratic hemodynamic parameters, mottling, hyperventilation or hypoventilation, glucose intolerance, and metabolic instability.[33] The process is often insidious and requires accurate assessment.

The key elements involved in the successful management of hemorrhagic shock in the pediatric population are early recognition of hemodynamic instability, replacement of circulating blood volume, and arrest of further bleeding. Nurses should be aware of the pathophysiological processes of shock as well as the signs and symptoms that these processes produce. If inadequate tissue perfusion is allowed to continue, a potentially correctable problem may well lead to a fatal outcome.

Clinical Management

In order to provide efficient and effective care to pediatric trauma patients, it is imperative that appropriate equipment and supplies be readily available. A general emergency department where both adults and children are seen must have equipment specifically for children. A separate pediatric trauma cart should be available, and pediatric resuscitation drug dosages should be posted in the area to make them readily accessible. A list of essential equipment that can be used as a guide in planning a pediatric resuscitation area can be found in Appendix 26–3.

In managing the critically ill child who has sustained multiple injuries, a systematic approach must be used. This approach must be practiced frequently so that it becomes automatic and can be applied even in a disorganized setting.

Children are assessed and treatment priorities are established on the basis of existing and potential life-threatening problems as well as the stability of the child's vital signs. The primary survey involves assessing the airway (while protecting the cervical spine), breathing, and circulation, with attention given to the diagnosis and treatment of shock. When indicated, appropriate resuscitative measures must be instituted concurrently with the primary survey. Time is of the essence.

Primary Survey

AIRWAY/BREATHING. The first priority in the sequential evaluation and management of the traumatized child is assessment of the airway. Airway patency must be ensured. There exists a great variation in the anatomy of the upper airway depending on the age of the child. In infants, the oral cavity is small and the tongue is relatively large. The infant's larynx is more cephalad than the adult's. The glottis is higher than in adults; it is located at the level of the third cervical vertebra at birth and descends about one to two vertebrae with maturity. The vocal cords slant upward and backward behind a narrow U-shaped epiglottis. However, for all ages the best method for initial assessment of the airway is to apply the chin lift or jaw thrust.

As with an adult, in-line cervical traction should always be applied in the traumatized child to maintain stability of the neck until a cervical fracture has been ruled out. Although cervical injury is rare in children (frequency of 1 per 100,000 in children under age 14), they should be treated as if such injury has occurred until it is ruled out by roentgenogram. In addition to positioning for airway patency, foreign matter should be quickly removed with a finger or gentle suction. This should be done carefully, especially if a facial injury or basilar skull fracture is suspected. Close, continuous observation is essential, since the child's ineffective efforts to clear the airway may quickly result in an obstructed airway once again.

The Conscious Child. In a conscious child who is breathing spontaneously but whose airway is obstructed despite the foregoing measures, a nasopharyngeal airway device is useful. The length of the nasopharyngeal airway is estimated by measuring the distance from the nares to the tragus of the ear. Nasopharyngeal airway sizes that should be available in the airway equipment kit for pediatric resuscitation are French sizes 12, 16, 20, 24, and 28. The tube should be lubricated, advanced gently along the floor of the nasal cavity, and rotated if resistance is met. If unsuccessful, the procedure should be repeated on the opposite side. Epistaxis, avulsion of adenoid tissue, or damage to conchae can occur if a gentle technique and lubrication are not utilized during insertion. This method is contraindicated if rhinorrhea is present.

The Unconscious Child. In an unconscious child, an oropharyngeal airway can be used. The selection of an appropriately sized airway is of paramount importance and can be facilitated by placing the airway alongside the child's face so that the flange is at the level of the central incisors and the bite block portion is approximately at the angle of the mandible. An airway device too small or too large can obstruct the airway (Fig. 26–1).

The airway is inserted by opening the child's mouth and lifting the tongue with a tongue depressor. The airway is slid into position with care to avoid pushing the tongue backward and thus obstructing the airway. The practice of inserting the airway in an inverted position and rotating it 180 degrees is not recommended in pediatric patients because trauma to the teeth or soft tissue may occur. In the conscious child, gagging may occur with an oral airway, and it is generally tolerated poorly.

When a clear and stable airway has been established, the child should be reassessed continually. The nurse should look, listen, and feel for evidence of air exchange. In infants, adequacy of ventilation is assessed by observing for expansion at the lower chest and upper abdomen. This differs from the reassessment of older children and adolescents, in whom adequate ventilation and expansion are checked at the upper chest. Air exchange should be assessed through auscultation, listening first over the trachea to establish that air exchange is occurring through the central airway and then listening for breath sounds bilaterally to assess for peripheral air exchange. Observing for symmetrical lung expansion is also essential.

Once the airway has been established and the child is spontaneously breathing, supplemental oxygen (50 to 100 per cent saturation) should be provided. Children, being quite resistant to the effects of hypercarbic and respiratory acidosis, do not tolerate even short periods of oxygen deprivation.

The Apneic Child. In the apneic child, ventilation is immediately accomplished by either a mouth-to-mouth, mouth-to-nose, or bag-and-mask technique. Using the mouth-to-mouth or mouth-to-nose technique, the nurse should establish an airtight seal and deliver two gentle breaths in slow succession. These two slow breaths serve as a means of checking for airway obstruction as well as for opening the small air sacs in the lungs. The lungs of a child, especially in an infant, are smaller than those of an adult and have a correspondingly smaller volume. Ventilation should be limited to the amount of air needed to cause the chest to rise. However, it should not be forgotten that the smaller air passages provide a greater resistance to airflow, and the rescuer's blowing pressure will probably have to be greater than imagined.

In the past, greater emphasis has been placed on not blowing too hard for fear of causing rupture of the air sacs. This is indeed an on-going concern, but more often than not, most infants and children are being underventilated rather

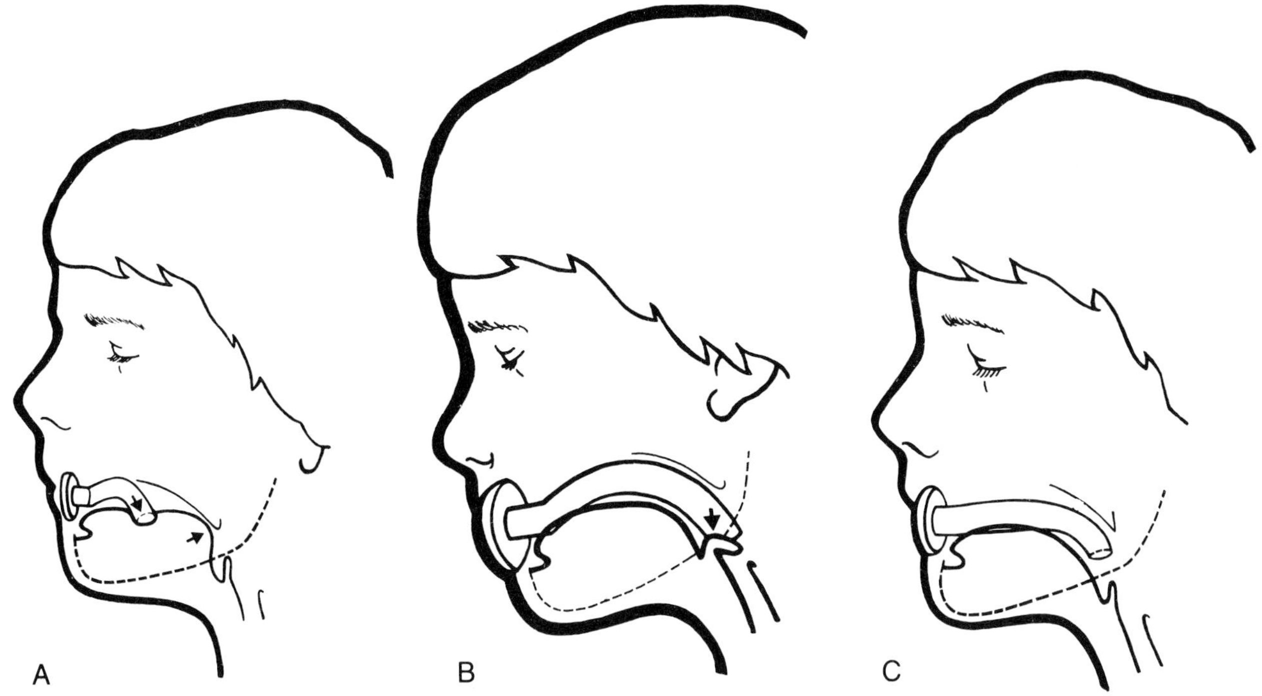

Figure 26–1. Choosing the appropriate size airway. *A*, Airway too small. *B*, Airway too large. *C*, Airway correct size.

than overventilated. The key is to watch for a rise in the chest; if it does not occur, airway patency must be reassessed followed by a gradual increase in breathing pressure.

Bag-Valve Mask Ventilation. The bag-valve mask provides a method that the nurse can use to ventilate the patient. Hand-squeezed, self-inflating resuscitators are most commonly used for infants and children because they are easy for the inexperienced operator to manage. Many of the self-inflating bags are equipped with a pressure-limiting pop-off valve to prevent delivery of high pressures. Resuscitator bags that are capable of delivering 100 per cent oxygen should be used. In most cases this involves use of an oxygen reservoir adaptation to the unit. Units without oxygen reservoir adaptations often deliver low concentrations of supplemental oxygen and therefore should be avoided.

The mask should be selected to fit the size of the patient. A tight fit is critical. The advantage of a mask that is transparent is that vomitus can be easily visualized. Resuscitators, masks, and endotracheal tubes should be standardized so that any resuscitator can connect with any mask or endotracheal tube. When using a bag-valve mask to ventilate, the fingers should be kept on the lower jaw to avoid compressing the soft tissue under the infant's chin. Placing the fingers on the soft tissue forces the tongue back into the posterior pharynx and then obstructs the airway (Fig. 26–2).

Endotracheal Ventilation. Indications for endotracheal intubation are the inability to ventilate the child adequately by the mouth-to-mouth or bag-and-mask method and the need for prolonged control of the airway, including prevention of aspiration.

The oral route for endotracheal intubation is preferred for the child in the emergent phase. A nasotracheal tube is generally more stable in the pediatric patient, but nasal intubation usually takes longer and is not recommended in patients who are not breathing or who have cranial, maxillary, or facial injuries. Children are also likely to have hypertrophied lymphoid tissue (adenoids and tonsils), which can cause problems with the passage of a nasotracheal tube. The higher location of the larynx in the pediatric patient creates a more acute angle from the nasopharynx, making successful nasal intubation less likely. When cervical injury is suspected, oral intubation must be done with in-line traction applied and without extension of the neck, as in the adult population.

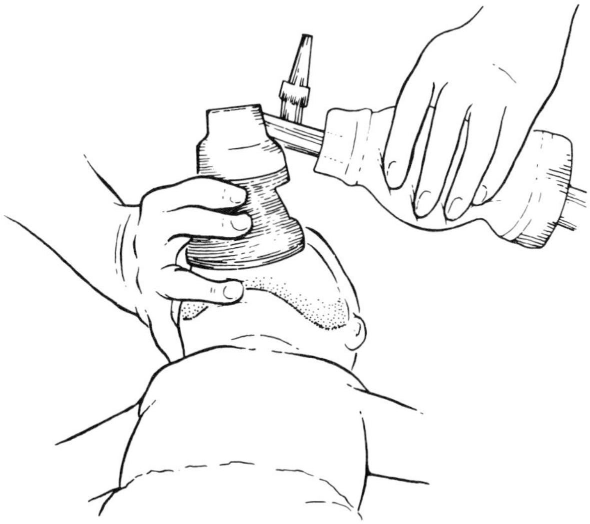

Figure 26–2. Proper placement of hand and fingers on lower jaw when using a bag-valve mask. (From Eichelberger MR, et al.: Brady Pediatric Emergencies. © 1992, p. 49. Adapted by permission of Prentice Hall, Englewood Cliffs, NJ.)

Uncuffed endotracheal tubes (ETTs) are used in pediatric patients up to 7 years of age to avoid subglottic edema and stenosis. The appropriate interior diameter (ID) of the ETT for a particular child can be estimated by using the following formula:

$$\frac{16 + \text{age in years}}{4} = \text{ID of ETT}$$

For example, for a 2-year-old child, the following calculation applies:

$$\frac{16 + 2}{4} = 4.5$$

This is an approximate rule, so it is recommended that tubes of the next higher and lower sizes also be readily available. Another approximate measure often used to determine ETT diameter is the size of the internal naris. If the tube will fit into one naris, it will probably fit comfortably down the trachea.

A rapid-sequence intubation is indicated in the child with a full stomach or in the child with a potential for increased intracranial pressure. All pediatric trauma patients are assumed to have a full stomach, and a rapid-sequence intubation will minimize the possibility of regurgitation.[34] This technique also will blunt the response of increased intracranial pressure that can be stimulated by intubation. Intubation should always be preceded by ventilation with 100 per cent oxygen. The medications commonly administered in a rapid-sequence intubation are atropine, a sedative, and a muscle relaxant.

The technique of cricoid pressure (Sellick's maneuver) is used during a rapid-sequence intubation to prevent passive regurgitation of stomach contents into the pharynx. In this technique, the upper esophagus is compressed against the cervical vertebral column by applying anteroposterior pressure on the cricoid cartilage.[35] Cricoid pressure must be maintained until correct placement of the endotracheal tube has been confirmed.

Successful intubation also requires proper positioning of the head and neck, opening the mouth widely, proper insertion of the laryngoscope with clear visualization of the vocal cords, and proper placement of the endotracheal tube.

If an ETT cannot be placed within 30 seconds, ventilation should be resumed for several minutes prior to a second attempt. After the tube has been placed, to ensure proper placement of the tube in the trachea, the nurse should auscultate both lung fields and observe for symmetrical chest expansion. As in adults, it is extremely easy for the endotracheal tube to slide into the child's right mainstem bronchus, causing atelectasis and further decreasing ventilation. After the nurse's assessment by auscultation and observation of chest expansion, the tube should be secured to the upper lip with tincture of benzoin and adhesive tape until proper tube position is verified by chest roentgenogram. An effective method for taping the ETT is described in Figure 26–3. Securing the endotracheal tube carefully and restraining the child's hands are necessary interventions because dislodgment can occur easily due to the short length of the child's trachea.

Surgical Intervention. If the airway obstruction persists following implementation of the preceding methods, direct injury to the larynx or trachea or uncontrollable hemorrhage should be suspected. Although cricothyroid puncture may be a lifesaving procedure, it is virtually never the first choice for establishing an airway and adequate ventilation. Almost all children can be adequately ventilated and oxygenated without surgical intervention. When necessary, the preferred surgical method in children is needle cricothyroidotomy, which can provide up to 30 minutes of airway control when used with jet ventilation. Great care should be taken to ensure that the catheter remains patent. Arterial blood gases should be drawn to assess the adequacy of oxygenation and ventilation endeavors.

If inadequate ventilation is due to chest injury, e.g., tension pneumothorax, open pneumothorax, or large flail segment, these alterations must be addressed immediately. A tension pneumothorax may be relieved by needle insertion or chest tube placement, an open pneumothorax must be covered with a sterile petrolatum gauze dressing, and a flail segment must be supported and, if necessary, positive-pressure controlled ventilation should be instituted. Adequate ventilation does not ensure adequate tissue oxygenation; the potential for impaired gas exchange remains a concern throughout the emergent and critical phases of care. An attempt should be made to maintain arterial Po_2 in the 80 to 100 mm Hg range.

Circulation. During the primary survey, the adequacy of circulation is first assessed by noting the quality, rate, and regularity of central and peripheral pulses. Peripheral perfusion is also assessed initially by looking at capillary refill. Capillary refill is easily tested by applying pressure to the nail beds and observing the time required for return of skin color. Under normal circumstances, the color should return within 2 seconds. If the child has been in a cold environment, refill in the extremities may be prolonged, in which case it should be assessed on mucous membranes.

If circulatory support is needed during the primary survey, it may be achieved by the following:

1. External cardiac massage
2. Control of active hemorrhage
3. Intravenous fluid and crystalloid/blood replacement
4. Drug therapy
5. Defibrillation
6. Application of pediatric pneumatic antishock garment (PASG)

External Cardiac Massage

Checking the Pulse. Once the airway has been opened and two breaths have been delivered, it must be determined whether only breathing has stopped or whether a cardiac arrest also has occurred. Cardiac arrest is recognized by absence of a pulse in the large arteries in an unconscious patient who is not breathing. The pulse in a child can be felt over the carotid artery in a manner similar to that for the adult. Feeling a pulse in an infant is more of a challenge. Unfortunately, the very short and, at times, fat neck of an infant makes the carotid pulse difficult to palpate. Use of the apical pulse is not recommended because precordial activity can represent an impulse rather than a pulse and therefore is not reliable. Some infants with adequate cardiac activity may have a quiet precordium, leading to the erro-

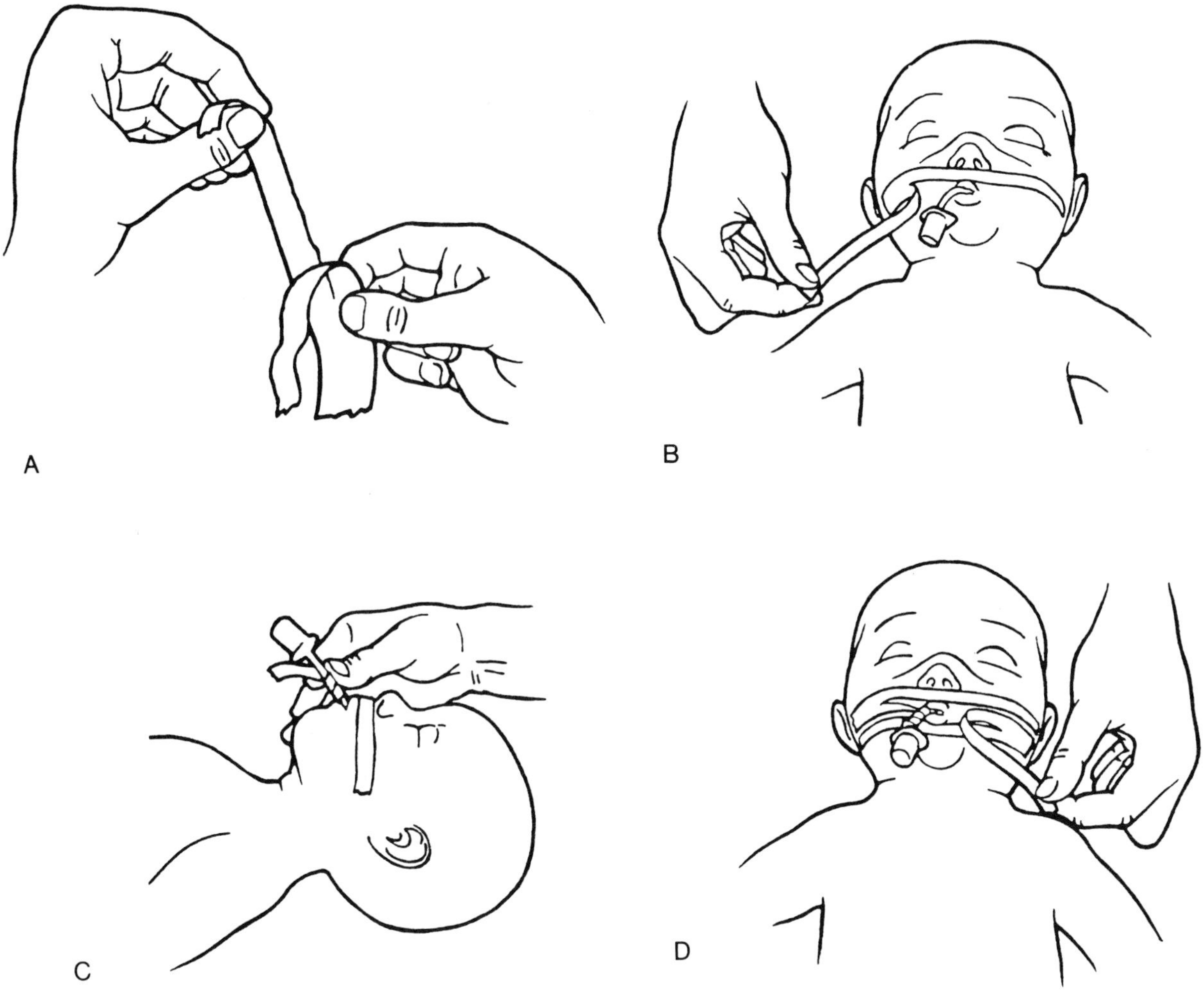

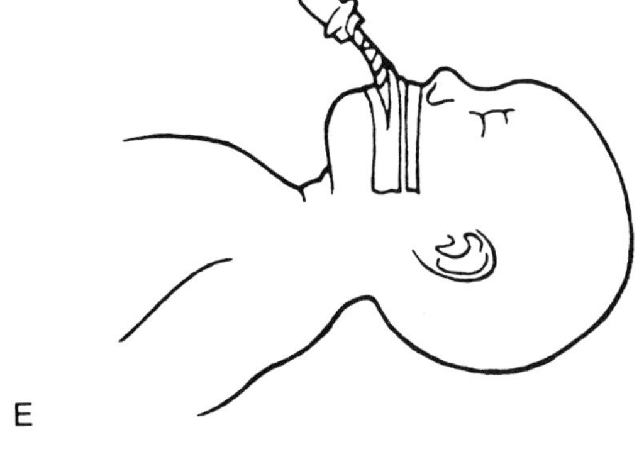

Figure 26–3. Securing the airway. *A*, Step one. Tear a 1-inch piece of tape in half. *B*, Step two. Place one-half the tape across the child's upper lip. *C*, Step three. Wrap the other half of the tape around the endotracheal tube. *D*, Step four. Tear a second piece of tape in half and bring one-half of it around the child's lower lip. *E*, Step five. Take the other half of that piece of tape and wrap it around the endotracheal tube in the opposite direction from the first piece of tape. (From Moloney-Harmon P: Managing Pediatric Emergencies: Cardiopulmonary Arrest. Baltimore, Resource Applications, Inc, 1984, pp 22–24.)

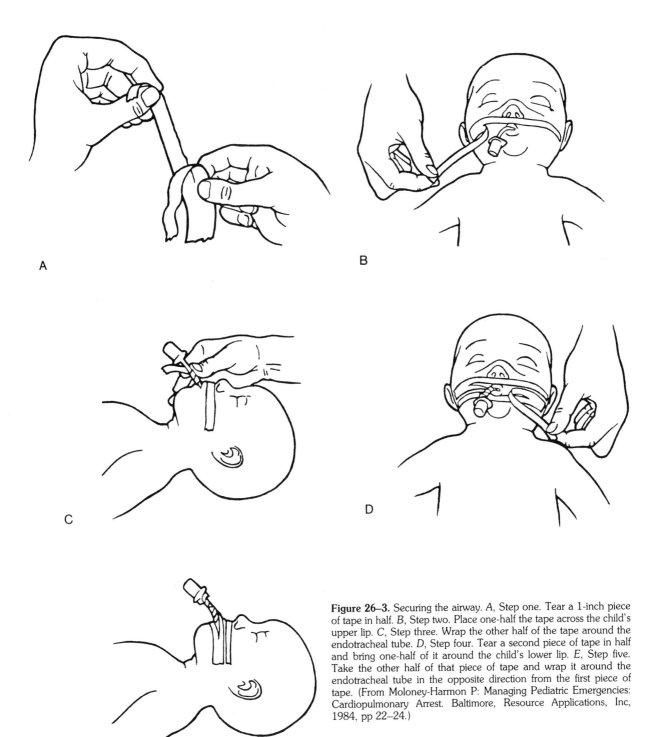

neous impression that chest compression is indicated. Because of this difficulty, it is recommended that the brachial pulse be palpated in infants. With practice, this can be as easily mastered as palpating a carotid pulse.

External Chest Compression. If the child's pulse is not palpable, a combination of rescue breathing and chest compression is indicated to circulate blood through the body and provide oxygenation and ventilation. Rescue breathing alone is indicated when breathing has stopped but a pulse is still palpable. In the technique of external chest compression, differences among infants, children, and adults become most apparent.

The differences are related to the position of the heart within the chest, the size of the chest, and the faster heart rate of the infant and child compared with that of the adult. The proper area of compression in the infant is midsternum. If an imaginary line is drawn between the nipples, the index finger of the hand farthest from the infant's head is placed under the intermammary line. The area of compression is one finger's width below this intersection, at the location of the middle and ring fingers (Fig. 26–4). A child's heart is lower than an infant's but not as low as an adult's. Using the technique as described for the adult, the notch where the ribs join in the center of the chest is located with the middle finger. The area just above the index finger is the appropriate area of compression in the child (Fig. 26–5).

The infant or child should be on a hard surface before compressions are begun. In an infant, compressions are performed with two to three fingers. In a child, more force will have to be exerted so the heel of one hand should be used, keeping the fingers off the chest. The rate and depth of the compressions are

Infant:	At least 100 comp/min	½ to 1 inch
Child:	80–100 comp/min	1 to 1½ inches

External chest compression and rescue breathing must be coordinated. In the infant and the child, the ratio of compressions to respiration is 5:1 for both one- and two-rescuer resuscitation. In infants and small children, positioning of the head creates a dead space. A firm support beneath the back is therefore required for external chest compression and can be provided by the rescuer's slipping one hand beneath the child's back while using the other hand to compress the chest. A folded blanket or other adjunct also can be used beneath the back to provide support (Fig. 26–6). This helps to maintain head positioning to facilitate the establishment of a patent airway. At the end of every fifth compression, a pause should be allowed for ventilation (1.0 to 1.5 seconds per breath).

Control of Active Hemorrhage. Active bleeding should be controlled immediately with a direct pressure dressing. If the bleeding is from an open extremity fracture or from a presumed pelvic fracture, the PASG serves a dual purpose: it applies direct pressure to the site of injury and shunts blood to vital organs of the body.

Intravenous Lines and Fluid Therapy. Intravenous access

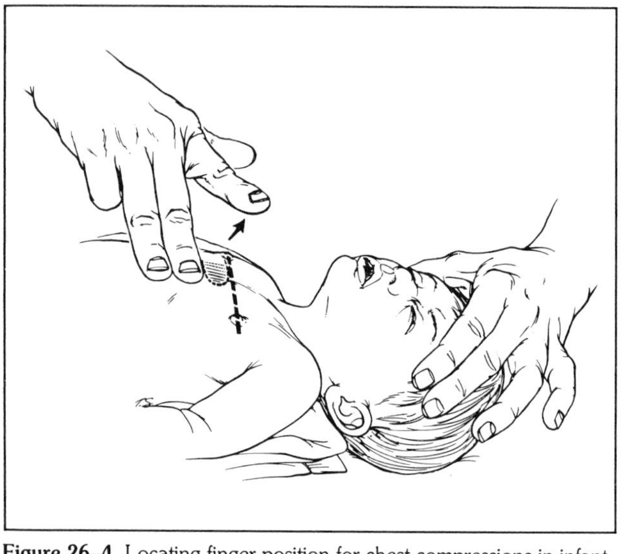

Figure 26–4. Locating finger position for chest compressions in infant. (From Standards and guidelines for cardiopulmonary resuscitation [CPR] and emergency cardiac care [ECC]. JAMA 255:2958, 1986. Copyright 1986, American Medical Association.)

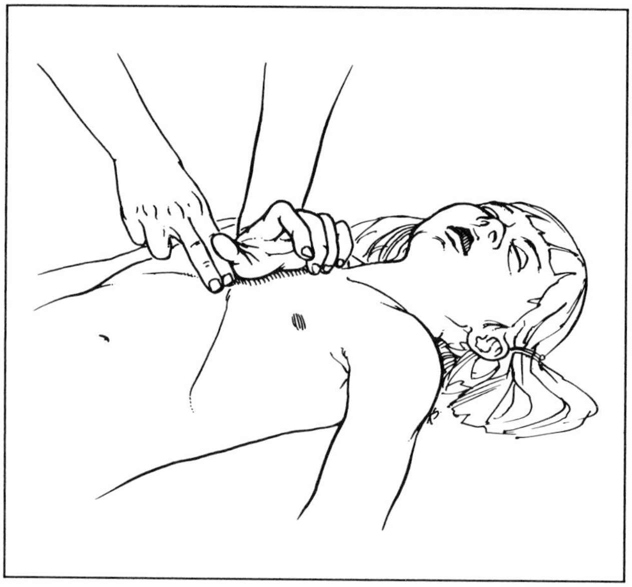

Figure 26–5. Locating hand position for chest compressions in child. (From Standards and guidelines for cardiopulmonary resuscitation [CPR] and emergency cardiac care [ECC]. JAMA 255:2958, 1986. Copyright 1986, American Medical Association.)

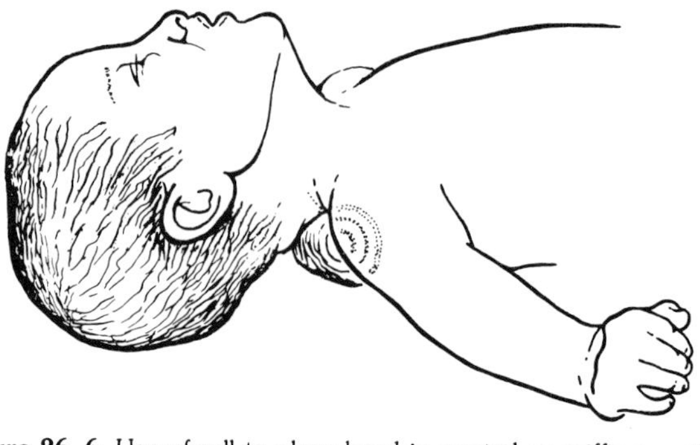

Figure 26–6. Use of roll to place head in neutral or sniffing position. (From Eichelberger MR, et al.: Brady Pediatric Emergencies. © 1992, p. 59. Adapted by permission of Prentice Hall, Englewood Cliffs, NJ.)

is critical in infants and children in severe shock or cardiac arrest. However, it is in this clinical situation that venous access may be most difficult and time-consuming because of the smaller vessel size in children and the fact that veins often collapse when a child is in shock. Intravenous access should be attempted either by percutaneous catheter placement or by peripheral cutdown. Recommended areas for catheter placement are

1. Saphenous vein (distal)
2. Upper extremity vessels
3. Femoral vein (cutdown with 20- to 18-gauge needle and plastic cannulae)
4. Subclavian vein (last resort)

Cannulation in small children can be made easier by following some simple rules. First, the extremity should be firmly secured to an armboard or footboard to prevent movement and subsequent dislodgment of the catheter during or after placement. Second, a tourniquet should be placed proximal to the site, and when possible, warm compresses should be placed over the vein to cause dilation. Third, the catheter should be flushed with normal saline with 1 unit of heparin per milliliter, which will cause more rapid return of blood and possibly prevent through-and-through puncture of the vessel. Fourth, transillumination with a high-intensity light will help to locate the veins. Fifth, application of the pediatric PASG may increase the filling of upper extremity veins, allowing easier cannulation. Finally, the bevel of the needle should face upward during insertion and then be rotated 180 degrees to allow more room for the advancement of the catheter once venous access is confirmed.[36]

If percutaneous peripheral vein cannulation cannot be performed easily and rapidly, alternative methods must be pursued. Two safe and rapid alternative methods for venous access are peripheral venous cutdown and intraosseous infusion. Most clinicians prefer to use the saphenous or brachial vein for peripheral cutdown; the external jugular vein is used less commonly. Cutdown procedures, however, require experienced clinicians and, in some cases, take a considerable amount of time.

Intraosseous Infusion. Intraosseous infusion is a technique used to establish venous access that was described over 60 years ago. For intraosseous infusion, a bone marrow needle is inserted into the medial flat surface of the anterior tibia, approximately 2 fingerbreadths below the tibial tuberosity. The needle is inserted perpendicular to the bone or at a 45 degree angle away from the growth plate to avoid injury to this structure. This is considered an effective route for the administration of sodium bicarbonate, calcium, bretylium, and glucose, none of which can be given via the endotracheal route. In addition, infusions of crystalloids, colloid, blood, dopamine, epinephrine, and dobutamine can be given while attempts at intravenous cannulation are under way. The main advantages of intraosseous infusion are that it is a readily available route, requires little skill, and has a low rate of complications. The most common complications attributed to this procedure are the subcutaneous infiltration of fluid (although minimal) and leakage from the puncture site following the removal of the needle. Osteomyelitis and subcutaneous infections have been noted, but they occurred only after the intraosseous infusion was maintained for extended periods of time or when hypertonic fluids were infused via this route.[37]

Volume Replacement. Volume replacement with a crystalloid solution of Ringer's lactated solution (20 ml/kg) is given to raise blood pressure and improve circulation. If vital signs do not stabilize with the administration of one bolus, a second bolus of 20 ml/kg should be given rapidly, keeping in mind that half of the child's blood volume has been replaced. If the blood pressure returns to normal, the intravenous line is maintained at 5 ml/kg/hr. If the child remains hypotensive, the replacement of whole blood is needed. In children with exsanguinating hemorrhage, either type-specific or type O blood should be immediately infused.

Fluid therapy is guided by special attention to preinfusion and postinfusion parameters, since these will indicate whether a child has continued fluid losses. In the past, platelets and clotting factors were routinely administered when patients received large amounts of blood products. At present, it is recommended that platelets and fresh frozen plasma be given only when the patient's clinical status and laboratory studies indicate that they are necessary.[38]

Drug Therapy. The essential drugs utilized for advanced life support are oxygen, sodium bicarbonate, epinephrine, calcium chloride, atropine, lidocaine, dopamine, and isoproterenol. Each agent has specific actions, indications, and dosages. The recommended drug doses are based on kilograms of body weight. Refer to Table 26–9 for guidance in determining drug dosages for children.

For use in emergency situations, when the exact weight of the child is not known, nurses should have on hand completed emergency drug cards for various weights (e.g., 2 kg, 5 kg, 10 kg, 15 kg). The approximate weight card can be pulled out and used during the emergency situation. (Approximate weights for children are discussed earlier in the chapter.) The key to successful resuscitation efforts is being prepared with predetermined charts for drug dosages before the arrest takes place. Nurses should be knowledgeable about the

TABLE 26–9. EMERGENCY MEDICATIONS FOR CARDIAC ARREST IN CHILDREN

DRUG	DOSE	INDICATIONS
Epinephrine (1:10,000)	0.01 mg/kg	Asystole Ventricular fibrillation
Sodium bicarbonate	0.05 mEq/kg	Asystole Ventricular fibrillation Prolonged arrest
Calcium chloride (10%)	10 mg/kg (dilute to 1%)	Asystole Electromechanical dissociation
Atropine	0.02 mg/kg	Asystole Bradycardia with hypotension
Lidocaine	1.0 mg/kg (bolus) 10 μg/kg/min (infusion)	Ventricular fibrillation Ventricular tachycardia
Dopamine	10–20 μg/kg/min	Asystole Low cardiac output
Isoproterenol	0.05–1.0 μg/kg/min	Asystole Low cardiac output

actions, indications, and adverse effects of the standard drugs used in resuscitation.

Defibrillation. Since ventricular fibrillation is an uncommon occurrence in pediatric cardiopulmonary arrest, defibrillation is a relatively uncommon intervention. Prior to any attempt to defibrillate, the rhythm should be confirmed; unmonitored defibrillation is not recommended. When fibrillation is monitored, defibrillation should be attempted only after the child has been prepared. Acidosis and hypoxemia should first be corrected. If the child's arrest was unobserved or if a long interval of poor perfusion has occurred, 100 per cent oxygen and sodium bicarbonate should be administered. Coarse fibrillation may be more easily treated than fine fibrillation. Fine fibrillation may be converted to coarse fibrillation with the administration of epinephrine or calcium.

Pediatric paddles are smaller in diameter than those used for an adult and are available with most defibrillators. The electrodes should be prepared with electrode paste or saline-soaked pads. The paste or pads should be placed carefully. Any electrical bridging will result in ineffective defibrillation and possible burning of the skin surface. Both electrodes may be placed on the anterior chest wall, one at the right of the sternum below the clavicle and the other at the level of the xyphoid along the left midclavicular line. Anteroposterior placement of the electrodes is also acceptable; however, this is sometimes difficult to achieve during resuscitation. Using either placement, firm pressure should hold the paddles in contact with the skin. All personnel should be instructed to be clear from the child and the bed.

An acceptable dose of current for the initial shock is 2 watt-sec/kg. Having this dosage taped to your machine ensures that the information is quickly available during resuscitative efforts. If the first defibrillation effort is unsuccessful, cardiopulmonary resuscitation should be continued for 3 to 5 minutes before the dose is doubled to 4 watt-sec/kg for a second attempt. If a third defibrillation is needed, the dose is again doubled to 8 watt-sec/kg.

Pediatric Pneumatic Antishock Garment (PASG). An additional means for increasing the circulatory volume is use of the pediatric PASG. The pediatric PASG is identical in design and operation to the adult PASG. The pediatric PASG is specifically designed to fit children ranging in height from 46 to 58 inches and who weigh between 40 and 100 pounds (usually indicated for children 4 years of age and older). The prime indication for the pediatric PASG is hypovolemic shock, including traumatic and nontraumatic cases. An absolute indication for the use of this garment is for a child with a systolic blood pressure below 60 mm Hg. When deciding whether the pediatric PASG should be used in pediatric patients with systolic blood pressures above 60 mm Hg, other signs of shock such as tachycardia, delayed capillary refill, and cool and clammy skin should be considered. The child's normal blood pressure for age is also a factor that should be determined and used as a baseline indicator (see Table 26–3). Children with leg or pelvic fractures and those with major abdominal or lower extremity bleeding also may benefit from use of the trousers. The only absolute contraindication to the use of the pediatric PASG is the presence of pulmonary edema.

The PASG should be deflated slowly, since sudden removal may produce profound hypotension. Deflation should begin only after adequate fluid replacement has brought the vital signs toward normal limits. Deflation should be gradual, one segment at a time, beginning with the abdominal compartment. After the blood pressure drops 5 mm Hg, the deflation process should be stopped and intravenous fluid replacement should be increased until blood pressure stabilizes again. At this point, deflation may be carefully resumed.

Secondary Survey

Following the primary survey, initial stabilization of the cardiopulmonary system, and aggressive treatment of shock, each child should undergo a secondary survey. As in adults, this secondary survey consists of a timely, systematic, and directed evaluation of each body region to assess for injury. Specific injuries more common to the pediatric population are discussed earlier in the chapter. The assessment process should progress with these factors in mind.

While performing the systematic head-to-toe survey in children, several principles should be applied. First, any child with one injury should be assumed to have additional injuries until proven otherwise. Second, isolated head injuries rarely cause shock; therefore, a child with a head injury who is in shock must be evaluated thoroughly. Third, verbal reassurance should be offered to the child who is conscious, and the treatment plan should be explained in terms that are easily understandable. Finally, appropriate physiological parameters and laboratory studies should be obtained and recorded frequently, and the child should be monitored closely and reassessed continually. Laboratory study trends should be analyzed consistently as well. To aid in laboratory data interpretation, normal laboratory values for the pediatric patient population are included in Appendix 26–2.

The Family of the Child

An important aspect of the care of the pediatric trauma patient is care of the family. The family experiences the circumstances surrounding trauma as a crisis situation. Since trauma is unexpected, the parents do not have time to adjust to the possible death or disability of their child. Parents initially may experience shock and disbelief. Normal reactions include confusion, disorganized behavior, and an increase in tension and anxiety.[39, 40] They may also have difficulty in accepting the situation as real. The normal coping mechanisms they have always used to deal with previous crises may no longer be effective. Decision-making abilities may be impaired.[41] The parents often experience feelings of guilt that may be indicated by feelings of anger at themselves, each other, the child, or the health care team. These feelings of anger may occur immediately or later as the family passes through the shock and disbelief phase to the developing awareness phase.[42]

These families require compassionate support through their adjustment to this crisis in their lives and need to be informed about what is happening to their child. Too often parents are whisked away to a waiting area and left to wonder about what is happening. Someone from the health care team should talk to the parents as soon as possible, since the parents are often imagining the worst; they wonder if the child is still alive. Parents should therefore be allowed to see their child as soon as possible. As the child stabilizes, other concerns that the family members may have must be addressed.

Family Assessment

An assessment of the family network should be accomplished as soon as possible. Information should be gathered about the family's knowledge of the situation. Does the family have any kind of support system, e.g., friends, relatives, or clergy? Where will they stay while their child is in the hospital? Does the family have other children? From this assessment, some inferences can be made about the family's perception of the situation and their ability to cope.[43] Information about the family's medical insurance coverage should be obtained as well. Many families express early concerns about hospitalization and health care costs and may require the services of a financial counselor. Referrals should be made accordingly.

Providing Information

Parents should be given information about their child in a simple, straightforward manner, since it is often difficult for them to synthesize a lot of information at this time. Any misconceptions that the family may have about the situation and/or their child's injuries and treatment plan should be addressed. In preparing the family to see the child, they should be told about the change in their child's appearance and about the equipment and personnel that will be at the bedside. Parents should be asked how the child appears to them, and explanations can then be based on their perceptions.

Response to the Death of a Child

Some children may not survive resuscitation efforts; following emergent efforts to save the child, care will shift to the family. These parents will need support from the nursing staff when the news about the death of the child is shared. The immediate reactions of the family will be shock, numbness, and disbelief—a period of time when parents often feel out of touch with reality. They are often immobilized and unable to make decisions.[44] Guilt also is a feeling that parents often experience when a child dies, especially if it is an accident-related death.

Following the initial shock of a child's death, the phase of intense grief begins. This may begin immediately or may be delayed for weeks. During this phase, parents may experience loneliness and an intense yearning for their child. They may feel extremely helpless, which often leads to feelings of anger and despair. At this time, they are at risk for the development of physical symptoms also, such as loss of appetite, and may experience sleep disturbances as well.[44]

The phase of reorganization follows. Parents report that they never recover completely from a child's death, but most are able to regain their previous level of functioning with support and care from others. This is evidenced by a return to normal daily activities, more happy memories of the child, and a decrease in feelings associated with intense grief.

Nursing Interventions. For nurses working in an emergency department setting, telling the family of a child's death is a very difficult task. Initial interactions with the family will usually occur as they experience the shock and numbness of their loss. At this time, it is important to let parents know that all extraordinary measures were taken to save the child. The family is often comforted, too, to know that the child did not suffer. Further conversation should be guided by the family's expressed need for more information. Quiet time is often needed and appreciated. The nurse's physical presence while the family begins to experience their loss is often helpful. Many families are comforted to know of the care and concern that can be expressed more effectively in silence.

Some parents may feel a need to express their great pain and sorrow. Guilt feelings also may surface as the family begins to grieve. Such feelings should not be negated, since they are a significant part of the process through which the family must progress in order to come to terms with their loss.

Anger and rage also may be experienced at this time and are often directed toward hospital personnel. Such feelings often pass, once expressed, and the family members may become extremely confused by the various emotions that have overcome them. The most appropriate intervention at this time is for the nurse to listen, reinforce the positive aspects of their parenting role, and explain the normalcy of their feelings.

Parents may need assistance with problem solving as they face the many decisions that must be made during this time of great stress. Many families will benefit from the support offered through social service programs. Appropriate referrals should be made at this time. Clergy members and social workers may assist the family by providing guidance in making funeral arrangements and by offering emotional and spiritual support.

It is also helpful if the nurse who cared for the child makes contact with the family shortly after the child's death. This conveys to the family that they have been remembered and provides them the opportunity to ask questions and express feelings that have surfaced since the child's death. Many parents need reassurance and continued support as they experience various aspects of their personal grief (refer to Chapter 11).

CRITICAL CARE CYCLE

Once resuscitation and stabilization measures have been taken, the child is prepared for the definitive treatment regimen. Although not always the case, surgical intervention may be necessary at this time. The patient then progresses through a critical period that requires close observation and intensive interventions. Identified in this text as the critical care cycle, it is during this phase of care that complications resulting from earlier resuscitation efforts may become evident. It is imperative that the pediatric critical care nurse develop and refine the necessary skills for detecting signs of impending danger. Early recognition of even the most subtle changes and rapid and efficient intervention may positively affect the outcome of care.

Appropriate nursing diagnoses for the pediatric trauma patient and family in the critical care phase of care have been integrated into various portions of this section. The nursing diagnoses included have been generalized for the pediatric trauma population and are not injury-specific, since these are found in other chapters of the text. The Sample Care Plan for the Pediatric Trauma Patient is included in Appendix 26–1 and summarizes the nursing diagnoses and interventions that are appropriate for each cycle of care.

Total Systems Assessment

As in the resuscitation phase of care, the pediatric trauma patient requires a systems assessment that will help to identify priorities for critical care management. The assessment during the critical care cycle focuses more broadly on the integrated function of the child's body systems, psychological status, and response to resuscitative and operative therapies. For example, the neurological status must be monitored closely. The child's level of consciousness, pupillary response, movement, and reflexes should be assessed continually. In assessing body movement, it should be noted if the child's movements are spontaneous or in response to pain. The type of movement should be documented as well. Does the child withdraw or posture? Is the child able to grasp? Grasp activity should be evaluated for strength, equality, and the ability to release upon command. The Glasgow Coma Scale (see Table 26–7) is a useful assessment tool and should be utilized during the critical care phase as well as during the resuscitation phase of care (refer to Chapter 17).

The child's cardiovascular status, including heart rate and rhythm, blood pressure, quality of pulses, and perfusion, must be assessed routinely. Clinical examination findings as well as hemodynamic parameters are part of the assessment data. The child should continue to be assessed for the presence of shock, either septic or hypovolemic. Hypovolemic shock may be present if the child continues to bleed as a result of the traumatic injuries.

Infection is a risk in any posttrauma patient, including the pediatric patient. When disruption of the body's normal defense mechanisms takes place, septic shock may occur following exposure to infectious agents. Infants, because of their immature immune systems, are more prone to infection. Vital signs (including core body temperature), white blood cell (WBC) count, and the condition of all wounds, surgical sites, and vascular sites should be monitored closely.

Intravenous infusion sites should be examined, and an estimate of fluid intake and output should be documented. Signs of infection such as redness, swelling, and purulent drainage must be noted.

The potential for impaired gas exchange, ineffective airway clearance, and altered breathing patterns necessitates a thorough respiratory assessment. Assessment parameters include respiratory rate, pattern and effectiveness of respirations, and quality of breath sounds. If the child is intubated, the presence or absence and quality of the child's own respirations should be assessed. For infants, an increase in respiratory rate is the mechanism of compensation for respiratory dysfunction, since they cannot increase the tidal volume because of the shape of the ribs.

The ventilator delivering rate should be checked routinely and respiratory patterns must be monitored closely to ensure that the child's breathing is synchronized with the ventilator. Note the amount of oxygen being delivered, the positive end-expiratory pressure, and the peak inspiratory pressure. An increase in peak inspiratory pressures often indicates difficulty in delivering volume, which may be the result of progressive atelectasis or the development of a pneumothorax (refer to Chapter 19).

Serial arterial blood gases should be obtained to determine the adequacy of oxygenation and ventilation. Pulse oximetry is useful for continuously monitoring O_2 saturation, and if appropriate, end-tidal CO_2 monitoring also should take place. Thoracic roentgenograms should be monitored for the development of a pathological respiratory process, such as atelectasis or pneumothorax. If the child has chest or mediastinal tubes in place, the color and amount of drainage should be noted.

Abdominal assessment includes monitoring the abdominal girth and the presence or absence and quality of bowel sounds. The amount and quality of nasogastric drainage should be noted and recorded. The child should be monitored for bleeding by noting the hematocrit, abdominal girth and tension, and bleeding through the nasogastric tube. If the child has had surgical repair of the abdomen, a postoperative ileus will probably be present due to surgical manipulation and the body's response to trauma. The nasogastric tube should be irrigated every 2 hours with saline. There may be signs of hypovolemia and shock if the child starts to bleed intra-abdominally. The nasogastric fluid should be tested for the presence of occult blood as well as obvious bleeding. A stress ulcer can occur in the child not receiving food or antacids. The pH of the nasogastric drainage should be monitored every 2 hours, and antacids should be administered to keep the pH greater than 4.0 to prevent the development of a stress ulcer (refer to Chapter 20).

Renal assessment includes monitoring the amount and characteristics of urine output, the presence of hematuria, specific gravity, serum blood urea nitrogen and creatinine, urine electrolyte levels, and creatinine clearance.

Hematuria may be associated with the trauma of inserting a urinary catheter or may be due to genitourinary trauma related to the child's injury. Monitoring the renal parameters is important in assessing for the development of acute tubular necrosis. Acute tubular necrosis is a postresuscitation complication that may be seen in children who have experienced a profound decrease in circulating blood volume.[45] It also can result from hypoxemia or septicemia. A significant decrease in circulating fluid volume leads to hypotension, causing a decrease in renal perfusion. This reduces the glomerular filtration rate and renal cortical blood flow, stimulating renin and aldosterone secretion and producing sodium and water retention as well as diminished urine output (refer to Chapter 24).

The condition of the child's skin should be assessed, noting any lacerations or abrasions that may have been overlooked during the resuscitation phase. The condition of dressings, casts, traction, and pin sites should be noted. Fracture reduction, necessitated as a result of musculoskeletal trauma, may be accomplished in a number of ways: closed reduction with immediate casting, continuous traction using Buck's or skeletal traction, external fixation devices such as a Hoffmann device, or open reduction and internal fixation. The child in any traction device should be assessed for skin breakdown related to immobility resulting from cast pressure sites. The child also should be assessed for signs of infection at pin sites and under the cast. The potential for circulatory compromise in the injured extremity exists and should be assessed by checking pulses, color, temperature, capillary refill, and sensation (refer to Chapter 21).

Body temperature remains an important parameter to monitor in the child. Hypothermia may produce dysrhythmias during the critical care phase as well as during the resuscitation phase. A temperature of less than 30°C (86°F) can produce a life-threatening dysrhythmia with a resultant decrease in cardiac output. Elevated temperatures may signal the development of an infection. Early detection and intervention may prevent the development of serious complications that increase the morbidity and/or mortality associated with the initial injury.

Clinical Management

The clinical management of the pediatric trauma patient in the critical care unit requires the team approach that was necessary during the resuscitation cycle. There is a need for coordination of disciplines to provide the best care for the child. The purpose of placing the child in the critical care unit is to provide continued monitoring and treatment.

The first step of clinical management is preparation. A report should be given to the receiving unit from the emergency department/resuscitation area, operating room, or radiology department to facilitate continuity of care. The report should include the child's injuries and interventions, the level of consciousness, fluids received, expected blood loss, airway and ventilatory support, intravenous lines and location, and any special equipment that is needed or that will be accompanying the child. It is the nurse's responsibility to ensure that all necessary equipment and supplies are in the receiving area and functioning properly.

Monitoring Hemodynamic Stability

On-going management will depend on the injuries and resultant problems. One of the main objectives of clinical management in the postresuscitation period is to restore hemodynamic stability and adequate perfusion to ensure viability of all organs and to prevent complications related to decreased perfusion, such as renal failure and hypoxic encephalopathy. This objective is accomplished by close, astute monitoring. Vital signs (including blood pressure, pulse, and respirations) should be checked every 15 minutes until the child stabilizes.

Central venous lines, often inserted during the resuscitation phase of care, allow for trend analysis during the critical care phase. Pulmonary arterial pressure catheters may be inserted in the critical care unit for the following indications: (1) poor peripheral perfusion despite maximal fluid therapy, (2) pulmonary edema, or (3) a need for measurement of cardiac output or pulmonary venous oxygen levels.[46] Central venous and pulmonary artery pressure trends provide information regarding fluid volume status and cardiac function, thus serving as a guide for fluid and pharmacological therapy. Normal values are shown in Table 26–10. Decreased central venous pressure readings indicate fluid deficit; elevated readings indicate fluid overload, congestive heart failure, or cardiac tamponade. The readings also may be elevated as a result of positive-pressure ventilation.

Intake and output should be monitored and recorded accurately. If possible, the child should be weighed daily so that appropriate fluid and nutritional calculations can be determined. Serum electrolytes should be measured daily or more often if appropriate. Depending on the goals of the treatment regimen, the child may be receiving maintenance or less than maintenance fluids.

TABLE 26–10. NORMAL PRESSURE VALUES FOR CHILDREN

Central venous pressure	4–12 mm Hg
Systolic pulmonary artery pressure	20–30 mm Hg
Diastolic pulmonary artery pressure	<10 mm Hg
Mean pulmonary artery pressure	<20 mm Hg
Pulmonary capillary wedge pressure	4–12 mm Hg

Monitoring Neurological Status

The child with neurological impairment due to head injury requires close monitoring and prompt intervention if evidence of increased intracranial pressure exists. The management of the pediatric patient with head injury is similar to that of an adult. A more detailed discussion of neurological management is presented in Chapter 17.

Intracranial pressure monitoring devices are used in managing pediatric head trauma. If an intracranial pressure monitoring device is in place, the child's intracranial pressures should be monitored closely and recorded accurately. If it is necessary to remove excess CSF or to drain blood, a ventricular drain is inserted, and physician orders should include the frequency and amount of fluid to be drained. Meticulous care of the catheter and insertion site is imperative to prevent infection. Specific instructions for intraventricular catheter site care and dressing changes should be included in the child's plan of care. Methods of caring for these catheters are standardized in many institutions.

Ventilatory therapies are also used in children to reduce intracranial pressure. The child should be hyperventilated in an effort to maintain the $Paco_2$ between 25 and 30 mm Hg to decrease blood flow to the brain. The child's head is kept in a midline position and, if not contraindicated, elevated to 30 degrees to facilitate venous drainage from the brain.

If the child is not in hypovolemic shock, fluids should be restricted to one-half to two-thirds of maintenance levels. Nonosmotic diuretics such as furosemide (Lasix) are administered to promote excretion of free water in an attempt to decrease intracranial pressure. Lasix not only promotes excretion of body water but also reduces production of CSF. The recommended dose of Lasix for children is 0.5 to 1.0 mg/kg every 4 to 6 hours. Osmotic diuretics such as mannitol (0.25 gm/kg) may be given to children with increased intracranial pressure who are not responsive to other forms of therapy; however, these agents are used with caution. Following head trauma, children are at risk for the development of *malignant brain edema*—a significant cerebral hyperemia; as many as 50 per cent of head-injured children may develop this condition.[47] Since mannitol can increase cerebral blood flow dramatically because of the shift of fluid from the cellular to the vascular space, the use of loop diuretics for the first few days following pediatric head injury is viewed as a more favorable approach.[48] When the administration of mannitol is necessary, serum osmolality should be monitored every 6 hours and should not exceed 320 mOsm.

Posttraumatic seizures, which can occur in the child as a result of a severe head injury (GCS 3–8); diffuse cerebral edema; or an acute subdural hematoma must be pharmacologically controlled.[49] Diazepam (0.1–0.3 mg/kg) or phenobarbital (20–30 mg/kg) may be given in the acute situation, with phenytoin (5 mg/kg/day) used for long-term control. Posttraumatic seizures may occur for up to 1 to 2 years after injury.

Steroids may be used because of their ability to reduce cerebral edema, although their efficacy with cerebral edema related to head trauma has not been proven. Dexamethasone, 0.25 to 1.0 mg/kg every 6 hours, or methylprednisolone, 10 to 15 mg/kg every 6 hours, may be administered.[50]

If all measures to control increased intracranial pressure have failed, barbiturate coma may be the therapy of choice. High-dose barbiturates reduce cerebral blood flow and decrease cerebral metabolic demand.[51] The barbiturate of choice is pentobarbital given in an initial dose of 3 to 5 mg/kg. This is followed by a continuous infusion of 2 to 3.5 mg/kg/hr (to maintain serum levels between 25 and 40 μg/ml). High-dose barbiturates have a significant effect on the circulatory system in that they reduce systemic vascular resistance, which may produce profound hypotension. Fluid therapy and vasopressors may be required. These patients require close supervision with continuous blood pressure, cardiac output, and pulmonary capillary wedge pressure monitoring.

Spinal cord injury is an infrequent occurrence in children, yet the implications for rehabilitation are far-reaching. Some of the complications that may develop in the spinal cord–injured patient are systemic hypertension or hypotension, cutaneous vasomotor instability, constipation, neurogenic bladder, urinary tract infections, stress ulcers, pneumonia, pulmonary embolism, decubiti, and deformities such as scoliosis. Nursing interventions such as frequent turning, effective pulmonary toilet, range-of-motion exercises, monitoring of bowel movements, and initiation of a bladder training program may help prevent complications (refer to Chapter 18).

Reorientation of the child to the surroundings is important as the child awakens. Family members, in conjunction with the nursing staff, can play an important role in stimulating the child's memory and assisting with mobility and activities of daily living.

Respiratory Support

Respiratory support is usually provided via an endotracheal tube, and mechanical ventilation may be required for a prolonged period. Emergent intubation of the child is usually done with an oral tube, although some physicians prefer initial use of a nasal tube for long-term placement. An oral tube may be changed to a nasal tube after the child has stabilized. This would not be appropriate, however, for a child with hemodynamic instability, uncontrollable increased intracranial pressure, or a basilar skull fracture. If the child needs to be intubated for a prolonged time, a tracheostomy may be performed. Special creative methods for communicating with the intubated child should be implemented.

Determination of ventilator settings will be based on the child's ability to breathe spontaneously and on arterial blood gas trends, with consideration of the presence of pulmonary disorder. The child may need to be pharmacologically paralyzed to receive the full benefit of ventilatory support. Pancuronium bromide (Pavulon) (0.1 mg/kg) may be used and should be administered with appropriate analgesia or sedation. Morphine sulfate (0.1 mg/kg) or fentanyl (1–2 μg/kg) may be used in conjunction with Pavulon. If the child has sustained a flail chest injury, mechanical ventilation with positive pressure will be necessary for internal stabilization. The child should be observed closely for the development of posttraumatic respiratory insufficiency. Early signs include increased respiratory rate, nasal flaring and retractions, and cyanosis on room air. Auscultation may reveal sparse rales. The nurse should monitor the patient for hypoxemia that does not respond to increased levels of inspired oxygen, decreased lung compliance, and diffuse infiltrates that may progress to consolidation. If the child does develop posttraumatic respiratory insufficiency, massive respiratory and hemodynamic support will be necessary (refer to Chapter 19).

Chest physiotherapy should be provided for the intubated child to promote adequate ventilation and clearing of secretions. The frequency of physiotherapy is individualized and depends on the respiratory disorder and the child's condition.

Extubation. Once the child has passed through the critical phase and is able to oxygenate and ventilate adequately as well as clear secretions, extubation will be the next step. If the child is to be extubated, vital capacity and negative inspiratory force should be assessed to ensure that the child can sustain spontaneous respirations. The vital capacity should range from 15 to 30 ml/kg; the negative inspiratory force should be greater than -20 cm H_2O. If the child cannot be extubated due to a continuing need for assisted ventilation, a tracheostomy will be required. Once the child with a tracheostomy no longer requires mechanical ventilation, oxygen or humidified air can be provided via a tracheostomy collar. The child will require rigorous pulmonary toilet and suctioning to maintain a patent airway. Frequent turning and repositioning and, when possible, getting the child up in a chair facilitate secretion removal.

Complications of Abdominal Injuries

Many children who experience liver or splenic trauma are managed nonoperatively and therefore require close observation for the possible development of complications. Indications for intraoperative management include hemodynamic instability, signs of increasing peritoneal irritation, and the requirement of a transfusion of more than 30 to 50 per cent of the child's total estimated blood volume (20–40 ml/kg).[52]

Complications of Immobility

The child is at risk for developing complications resulting from immobility. As soon as the child's condition has stabilized, a referral should be made to a physical or occupational therapist so that appropriate range-of-motion exercises can be incorporated into the plan of care. Splints also should be utilized as soon as possible to prevent contractures. Collaboration between the nurses caring for the child and the occupational and/or physical therapist will enhance the benefits of the treatment regimen. When appropriate, the child and parents or significant others should be included in the treatment plan as well.

Skin care should be meticulous. The child should be placed on an eggshell or air mattress. Mouth care should be provided by lubricating the mouth and cleansing the teeth at least once a shift. Eye care should be provided by the use of an ophthalmic ointment if the child's blink reflex is absent.

Nutritional Support

Adequate nutrition is essential for the pediatric trauma patient. Table 26–11 gives the estimated caloric and protein needs of the child. Children are more at risk than are adults for developing protein–calorie malnutrition in the critical care unit. They have increased energy requirements, small nutritional reserves, and greater obligate energy needs than do adults. Protein–calorie malnutrition can develop in 5 to 7 days in critically ill children who were previously healthy.[53] Nutritional support should be started as soon as possible after resuscitation is complete. Wound healing and immunocompetence depend on the provision of adequate nutrition.

Enteral feedings are preferable because they are more physiologically normal and more efficient. Individual caloric requirements and the child's general tolerance of a particular formula are among the factors that must be considered when choosing from a variety of available enteral formulas. Excess protein is not beneficial because it is not utilized efficiently by the body.[54] For children who have been NPO (nothing by os) for an extended period of time, a lactose-free formula is necessary, since, after a period of no gastrointestinal intake, the gut will not produce lactase, which is essential for the breakdown of lactose.

If the child is unable to tolerate enteral formulas, total parenteral nutrition (TPN) should be initiated via a central venous catheter. The choice of TPN formulas greatly depends on the child's individual calorie needs. Once the child is receiving TPN, response to the therapy must be monitored. Metabolic complications may result from electrolyte, glucose, and fat imbalances. Therefore, serum levels should be monitored routinely. Weight gain and progressive wound healing will indicate the child's positive response to nutritional support.

Close observation for complications resulting from TPN therapy is indicated as well. Infection is the most frequent complication and is most often due to poor aseptic technique during catheter placement, during the solution preparation process, or while performing routine catheter care. Care also must be taken to avoid dislodgment of the catheter upon insertion or during routine maintenance activities. Such mechanical complications may result in the development of a pneumothorax or air embolism. Close, continuous observation and meticulous catheter care will serve as the best preventive methods.

TABLE 26–11. ESTIMATED NUTRIENT NEEDS PER KILOGRAM FOR CHILDREN

AGE (yr)	CALORIES/ kg	PROTEIN/ kg
0–0.5	115	2.2
0.5–1	105	2.0
1–3	100	1.8
4–6	85	1.5
7–10	85	1.2
Male		
11–14	60	1.0
15–18	42	0.85
Female		
11–14	48	1.0
15–18	38	0.85

Adapted from Walker W, Hendricks K: Manual of Pediatric Nutrition. Philadelphia, WB Saunders Co, 1985.

Pain Management

Pain is a part of every child's experience in the critical care unit. The nurse caring for the child must develop an individualized plan for helping the child cope with alterations in comfort levels. The child's developmental level is the most influential factor in the child's pain response. The ability to understand the reason for pain and to develop ways to cope with it is dependent on the child's level of psychological maturity.[55]

Serving as adjuncts to analgesic therapy, nursing interventions that may assist the child to deal with pain include the use of touch therapy, relaxation or distraction techniques, and the provision of verbal explanations and support. The presence of parents and other family members often helps to lessen the burden of pain as well.

With infants, touching and holding—especially when they are rhythmic—may be effective, since these may stimulate some cutaneous receptor sites that decrease the perception of pain by inhibiting painful impulses.[56] Toddlers will often seek out parents for comfort as well as use self-regulating behaviors such as sucking and rocking. Toddlers are often comforted by parents' talking to them because it serves as a distraction. Also utilized as a distraction technique, a discussion about siblings or family pets is often a useful method to initiate conversation with preschool children. School-age children can be taught methods for relaxation such as deep-breathing exercises, which often work as a distraction technique as well as a tension release modality. Touch therapy in the form of massage can also reduce a child's perception of pain.[57]

Prior to painful procedures, verbal explanations should be given in simple terms, geared specifically to the child's level of understanding. To help prepare for the procedure, the nurse can allow the child to think through how he or she might deal with the pain and to verbalize fears and concerns.

Adolescents may respond favorably to many of the same techniques as younger children, such as distraction and relaxation. They also use verbalization as a method of pain relief. Preparation via verbal explanations is as important for this age group as it is for the younger patient population.

Despite these efforts, however, there are situations when the administration of pain medication is the intervention of choice. Analgesics are useful for all age groups to decrease painful impulses and may enhance the effectiveness of other nursing interventions as well. Pain medication should never be withheld from the child if it seems to be the only effective means of pain relief.

The stimulating atmosphere and fast-paced routines of the critical care unit can contribute to the development of altered sleep patterns. The child's normal sleep patterns should be accommodated if at all possible. Special efforts should be made to reduce activity at the bedside and to create a quiet environment to promote quality sleep time.

INTERMEDIATE CARE/ REHABILITATION CYCLE

Many of the associated nursing diagnoses and clinical management strategies that were addressed in the critical care cycle may be appropriate during the intermediate care/ rehabilitation cycle as well. To avoid unnecessary repetition, the reader is asked to refer to the discussion of these issues in previous sections. The discussions in this section focus primarily on general rehabilitation issues as they pertain to the pediatric trauma patient.

Many children, resilient by nature, tend to recover quickly. They often progress rapidly from the critical care phase to the rehabilitation phase of care, breezing quickly through or skipping entirely a clearly identifiable intermediate care stage.

Rehabilitation issues should actually be addressed at the time of admission. Even during the resuscitation cycle, the nurse should be astute to the measures that can be taken to lessen or prevent conditions that may otherwise result in short- or long-term disability. All efforts must be taken to assist the child and parent in adapting to the life changes that the trauma experience has elicited. Early recognition of available or lack of available support systems for the pediatric patient and family can facilitate the process of rehabilitation planning as assistance is offered from appropriate resource programs (e.g., social services and financial assistance services). Information elicited for further development of the nursing data base should include details that greatly potentiate the creation of a comprehensive rehabilitation plan of care. (Refer to Chapter 16 for more detailed information.)

Trauma, in addition to being the leading cause of death in children, is also a major cause of long-term disability. It is estimated that more than 30,000 children suffer permanent disabilities resulting from injury every year.[58] The goal of rehabilitation is to provide a better quality of life for the child and to return the child to maximum potential within the family/social unit.[59]

Assessment of Adjustment/Adaptation to Injury

It is important to first understand how the child adjusts to illness based on the individual cognitive/affective developmental level.[60] This will affect how the child perceives the situation as well as what range of responses are available to the child (see Table 26–6).

Toddlers

The first 2 years of life pose a difficult time for the child because of a smaller repertoire of coping skills.[61] The child does not understand the reasons for the illness or treatments, and neither parents nor the health care team can explain them. The child's coping ability is greatly influenced by the parent's presence.

Preschool-Age Child

Preschoolers (3 to 6 years) have acquired some inner resources for coping with stress and thus have more coping abilities than the younger child.[62] The parents remain the major source of coping strength; however, children tolerate short periods of separation from their parents. The child at this age fears bodily intrusion and injury because of an inability to perceive long-term effects. Fantasy and guilt can distort the child's perception about the injury.

School-Age Child

The school-age child (7 to 12 years) has developmentally made enough progress to enhance coping abilities. This child has usually developed a peer group by this time and can tolerate longer periods of separation from the parents. The child, because of increasing cognitive abilities, is able to understand more cause-and-effect relationships and can think about the future.[61] However, the child still fears bodily injury and loss of control of bodily function.

Adolescent

The adolescent (13 to 18 years) has developed skills that enhance the ability to cope.[61] The adolescent is working to establish identity and does not rely as heavily upon parents for coping strength. The adolescent is able to think abstractly and can apply general principles to specifics. Some of the biggest fears of the adolescent, however, are bodily disfigurement and loss of control. This becomes a critical issue with an adolescent trauma patient who has suffered an amputation, a spinal cord injury, or some other disfiguring injury. Part of the challenge of rehabilitation with this age group involves helping the adolescent adjust to an altered body image and a level of dependency during a developmental period when independence is being sought.[63]

Clinical Management

Interdisciplinary conferences that include the parents and, if appropriate, the patient should be held on a regular basis. Mutual goal setting is imperative; goals that have been established by the health team without the involvement of the family and adolescent can actually hinder progress.[64]

The child and family will need much support during the rehabilitation phase. Families need to be involved in the child's care as well as long-range plans. They need honest, accurate information from the health care team. Many times these families are feeling guilt, frustration, and anger. These feelings need to be recognized and channeled appropriately. The nurses working with the families may help them assess their own support systems.[64] The family may identify other family members, friends, a minister, or other people they know as support systems. It is helpful that they know it is beneficial for them to maintain relationships during this time. Other support systems, such as community and government agencies that provide assistance with financial problems or child care, should be discussed.

Planning for Discharge

As the child continues to improve, plans for discharge are discussed by the team, again including the parents. Some children may require total care and have little or no rehabilitation potential due to a persistent vegetative state. Other children may make progress toward higher levels of consciousness and rehabilitation with proper stimulation. Children with spinal cord injury will require an extended rehabilitation program to help them become as functional as possible relative to their injury. Because of the restorative and regenerative powers of the child and the potential for a long and productive life, every attempt should be made to locate a rehabilitation program that will provide what the child needs to become a functional member of the family/social unit.

Some parents may choose to take their child home. For some families this is a viable alternative, but one that requires a tremendous amount of preparation. Families that are considering this option need to take into consideration the impact this child will have on the family unit. Does the child require special equipment, such as a ventilator and monitors? Will the child need home care nurses? How does the family feel about having a stranger in the home? How will bringing this child home affect the parents' relationship with each other and with their other children?

Once these considerations have been addressed and the decision is made to take the child home, preparations are begun. The family must be taught new skills such as skin care, catheter care, tracheostomy care, or suctioning procedures so that care of the child continues in the home environment. Education and instruction about bowel and bladder regimens and range-of-motion exercises also must be accomplished. Electrical safety in the home environment is an issue that must be addressed if special equipment will accompany the child. Family members also must learn to operate and maintain the equipment, such as ventilators and monitors. The tremendous advantage is that children do benefit from the stimulation they receive from their home environment. These families should be encouraged to make contact with rehabilitation centers and appropriate community or government agencies as soon as possible for continued support, guidance, and direction as needed. A nursing assessment tool (Table 26–12) and sample teaching checklist (Table 26–13) will assist in the discharge planning process.

Community Reintegration

As the child progresses through the rehabilitation phase, discharge planning should continue. Discharge planning, although it can be exciting for the child and family, also may be an extremely frightening time. They are losing the protective environment of the health care facility.

A comprehensive discharge plan will adequately prepare the family and child to go home and will help make the transition back into the community easier. The discharge plan should have begun as the child began rehabilitation, because the success or failure the family experiences after leaving the hospital will depend on how the staff has assessed and worked with the family during the hospital stay.[65] The family should be involved from the very beginning of the discharge planning process.

The discharge planning process should include a thorough assessment of the family dynamics and their outside support systems, as well as their ability to cope with stress. This is often assessed by observing the family with the child in the hospital as well as by asking pointed questions. These details need to be incorporated into the discharge plan, and appropriate referrals to community agencies must be initiated.

It is often helpful for the child to go home for a day or weekend before the actual discharge date. This gives the family an idea of unforeseen difficulties and helps them gain insight into living again with their child. It also helps the family gain a level of confidence as they realize that they can cope outside of the hospital environment.

Another alternative is to have the family spend the weekend at the hospital caring for the child. This approach is especially useful for families of ventilator-dependent children who are going home. Children with spinal cord injuries are included in this population. These families can gain experience with special equipment such as ventilators and feeding pumps. This will help them capture a more realistic view of what it will be like to live with the child and gain a higher level of confidence while receiving the support of the nursing staff.

The development of the discharge plan requires a team effort, often coordinated by the primary nurse. The family should be included in the plan, since they will be implementing the care measures at home. (An example of a discharge plan is shown in Appendix 26–4.)

TABLE 26–12. NURSING ASSESSMENT: GUIDELINES FOR HOME CARE

Will patient have tracheostomy and/or ventilator indefinitely?

Options
- Remain in hospital.
- Place patient in nursing home.
- Place patient in rehabilitation center.
- Send patient home with 24 hr/day or some nursing care.
- Send patient home with family care.

Explore family's feeling about patient's status.

Have a meeting including patient's physicians, primary nurse, appropriate family members, and social worker to discuss above options and what each would mean to them.

If family does want to care for patient at home,
- Determine whether the patient's physician is willing to be responsible for this patient once sent home.
- If patient does not have physician, a hospital physician will be needed to help the family choose one.
- If patient has problems and needs to be rehospitalized, will he or she be taken to the nearest hospital or must the patient return to this hospital? Discuss this with family members and patient's physician.
- Determine how much and what kind of resources will be required.

Resources
- Who will supply equipment?
- Who will service equipment and how often?
- Who will provide nursing care (e.g., family, visiting nurse association, public health, nursing agencies)?
- Who will pay for supplies, nurses, and other needs?

Responsibilities of the hospital (e.g., physician, nursing, social work)
- Make home assessment: Is home environment (physical and mental) appropriate for this patient?
- Teach and train all people who will be caring for this patient at home.
- Make appropriate referrals (e.g., supply company, nursing agencies).
- Make sure all equipment is set up at home and working at time of discharge.
- Make sure family has appropriate phone numbers. Be available for phone consultation.
- May want to visit family one or two times after discharge or at least make a few follow-up phone calls.

From Lawrence PA: Home care for ventilator-dependent children: Providing a chance to live a normal life. Dimens Crit Care Nurs 3:1, 1984.

TABLE 26–13. SAMPLE TEACHING CHECKLIST

	Explanation	*Observation*	*Demonstration*	*Return Demonstration*	*Independent Function*
Tracheostomy care					
Tracheostomy site care					
Tracheostomy dressing change					
Tracheostomy ties change					
Tracheostomy tube change					
Suctioning					
Hyperinflate and hyperoxygenate before, during, and after					
Insert suction catheter and withdraw while applying suction					
Instill 2–3 ml normal saline solution prn to loosen secretions					
Chest physiotherapy					
Ventilator					
Circuit change					
Clean and disinfect equipment					
Check and change rate					
Check and change tidal volume					
Check inspiratory pressure					
Trouble shoot problems					
Check alarms are on					
Tracheostomy collar					
Humidified RA/oxygen					
Sterile water change					
Tubing and collar change					
Cardiac monitor					
Lead placement					
Setting alarm limits					
Intervention for bradycardia or tachycardia					
Nasogastric tube					
NG tube insertion					
Placement verification					
Gavage feeding					
NG tube removal					
Cardiopulmonary resuscitation					
Medications					
Name					
Dose and frequency					
Actions					
Side effects					

From Lawrence PA: Home health care for ventilator-dependent children: Providing a chance to live a normal life. Dimens Crit Care Nurs 3:1, 1984.

Topics that need to be considered along with the discharge plan include finances, equipment, and supplies. Decisions must also be made about the child's care givers. It is not uncommon for one or two family members to inadvertently be singled out by other family members as the primary caregiver(s). This will inevitably happen if a plan for shared responsibilities is not arranged and agreed upon by all involved family members prior to the child's homecoming. The most effective plan will be one that takes into consideration the needs of the caregiver(s) and provides periodic relief. This will lessen the stress experienced by all involved.

Anyone who will be caring for the child at home also must master skills such as suctioning, tracheostomy care, and CPR, which are necessary to safely care for that child. Family members must be taught to problem solve for any emergencies that may arise, such as power outages and equipment failure. They also need to be made aware of the resources that are available in the hospital and in the community. The family should be encouraged to contact the local emergency response agency prior to the child's discharge to home to inform them of the situation. This helps to ensure that the response team arrives at the home with appropriate equipment and supplies and is adequately prepared to care for the child if called on for an emergency at a later date. It often helps for the family to be linked with a support group as well. This provides the opportunity for them to be in touch with others who can relate to what they are experiencing and with whom they can exchange information.

Family involvement in the discharge plan and reintegration into the community is imperative. A comprehensive plan that prepares the child and family and takes into account all aspects of their physical, emotional, intellectual, and spiritual well-being has a favorable chance for success. Families can provide a strong motivation for the child to work toward recovery by being prepared to take the child home and support him or her through the reintegration process.

SUMMARY AND CONCLUSIONS

Trauma is the primary killer of children between the ages of 1 and 14 years. One of every two children who die during these years will do so because of an unexpected injury. Trauma is also a major cause of disabling injuries in children. This has serious implications for the expenditure of resources and personnel at a time when more constraints are occurring in the health care system. The resulting need for rehabilitation also has tremendous implications when one considers the termination of work potential, the length of rehabilitation, and the adjustments affecting the growth and development of the child.

Further research endeavors may include activities that attempt to answer the following questions. Is the use of touch effective in reducing the child's intracranial pressure? What is the relationship between the nutritional status of the child and long-term outcomes? What are the effects of an accidental injury on the growth and the development of the child? What are the effects on the family when the child with special needs is returned to the home? What coping mechanisms do the child and/or family typically use? What are the long-term psychological effects that the head-injured child experiences? What nursing interventions are most effective in supporting the child in the adjustment to an altered body image? Many of the studies undertaken in the area of adult trauma should be redesigned to study the pediatric trauma population as well.

Efforts are needed to improve the pediatric emergency medical systems. Such efforts must be focused on regional centers that can develop a systematic approach to the care of pediatric trauma patients.[66] The health care team caring for the pediatric trauma patient must be well trained in the area of pediatric trauma. The facility also must be equipped to handle an injured child.

Legislators and other community leaders must be aware of the devastating sequelae of traumatic injury. Pediatric trauma can be considered to be at epidemic proportions in our society today. Mandatory car seat and seat belt laws, where they do not already exist, could result in the saving of many young lives. Motorcycle and bicycle helmet laws could do the same. More attention needs to be focused on safety issues that affect the child. Nurses can do this by writing letters to senators, congressional representatives, and editors and by testifying at legislative hearings that are concerned with pediatric trauma and safety issues.

Nurses, by virtue of their expert knowledge and skills, can provide educational leadership in a variety of ways. Nurses should expand the scope of practice by speaking to local agencies, parent groups, and children themselves about child safety issues and by teaching other colleagues about caring for the pediatric trauma patient. Legislators should be kept informed of all issues that currently affect the pediatric trauma population. Funding that supports extensive public awareness programs must be sought. Training and instruction must be provided by knowledgeable professionals, and more stringent safety laws must be pursued with diligence. The nurse's role in supporting all aspects of preventive care is paramount. Prevention will remain the most effective treatment regimen for preserving the precious young lives in our society.

REFERENCES

1. Fingerhut L, Kleinman J: Trends and current status in childhood mortality, United States, 1900–1985. Vital Health Stat 326:1, 1989.
2. King DR: Trauma in infancy and childhood: Initial evaluation and management. Pediatr Clin North Am 32:1299, 1985.
3. Walker ML, Mayer TA, Storrs BB, et al: Pediatric head injury: Factors which influence outcomes. Concept Pediatr Neurosurg 6:84, 1985.
4. Mayer T, Walker ML, Johnson DG, et al: Causes of morbidity and mortality in severe pediatric trauma. JAMA 245:719, 1981.
5. Snyder CL, Jain VN, Saltzman DA, et al: Blunt trauma in adults and children: A comparative analysis. J Trauma 30:1239–1245, 1990.
6. Klauber G: Genitourinary trauma in children. Emerg Care Q 3:51–56, 1987.
7. Wodorski JS, Kurtz PD, Gardin JM, Howing PT: Maltreatment and the school age child: Major academic socio-emotional and adaptive outcome. Social Work 35:506, 1990.
8. Widner-Kolberg MR: The nurse's role in pediatric injury prevention. Crit Care Nurs Clin North Am 3:3, 1991.
9. National Committee for Injury Prevention and Control: Injury Prevention: Meeting the Challenge. Oxford, Oxford University Press, 1989, p 27.
10. Newman K, Bowman L, Eichelburger M, et al: The lap belt complex: Intestinal and lumbar spine injury in children. J Trauma 30:1133–1139, 1990.
11. Centers for Disease Control: Childhood injuries in the United States. Am J Dis Child 144:627–646, 1990.
12. Rivara FB: Epidemiology of childhood injuries. In Bergman AB (ed): Preventing Childhood Injuries (Report of the 12th Ross Roundtable on Initial Approaches to Common Pediatric Problems). Columbus, OH, Ross Laboratories, 1982, pp 13–18.
13. Subcommittee on Advanced Trauma Life Support of the American College of Surgeons Committee on Trauma: Initial Assessment and Management, 1984, p 11.
14. Hazinski MF, Weinberg M Jr: Care of the surgical pediatric cardiac patient. In Neville WE (ed): Intensive Care of the Surgical Cardiopulmonary Patient, 2nd ed. Chicago, Year Book, 1983.
15. Management of infants undergoing cardiac surgery. In Behrendt DM, Austen WG (eds): Patient Care in Cardiac Surgery, 3rd ed. Boston, Little, Brown, 1982.
16. Kraus JF, Black MA, Hessul N, et al: The incidence of acute brain injury and serious impairment in a defined population. Am J Epidemiol 119:186, 1984.
17. Mayer T, Walker ML, Matlak ME, Johnson DG: Causes of morbidity and mortality in severe pediatric trauma. JAMA 245:719, 1981.
18. Walker M, Storrs B, Mayer T: Head injuries. In Mayer T (ed): Emergency Management of Pediatric Trauma. Philadelphia, WB Saunders Co, 1985, p 273.
19. Raphaely RC, Swedlow DB, Downes JJ, et al: Management of severe pediatric head trauma. Pediatr Clin North Am 27:715, 1980.
20. Raimondi AJ, Hirschauer J: Head injury in the infant and toddler: Coma scoring and outcome scale. Child's Brain 11:12, 1984.
21. Kling TF: Spine injury in the multiply injured child. In Marcus RE (ed): Trauma in Children. Rockville, MD, Aspen, 1986, p 182.
22. Vernon Levett P: Head injuries in children. Crit Care Nurs Clin North Am 3:3, 1991.
23. Snow RB, Zimmerman RD, Gandy SE, et al: Comparison of magnetic resonance imaging and computed tomography in the evaluation of head injury. Neurosurgery 18:45, 1986.
24. Marshall SB, Marshall LF, Vas HR, et al: Head injury and the treatment of increased intracranial pressure. In Neuroscience Critical Care. Philadelphia, WB Saunders Co, 1990, p 169.
25. Eichelberger MR, Mangibat EA, Sacco WJ, et al: Outcome analysis of blunt injury in children. J Trauma 28:1109, 1988.
26. Hensle TW, Dillon P: Renal injuries. In Touloukian RJ (ed): Pediatric Trauma, 2nd ed. Philadelphia, Mosby–Year Book, 1990, p 358.
27. Guerriero WG: Trauma to the kidneys, ureters, bladder, and urethra. Surg Clin North Am 62:1047, 1982.
28. Amparo EG, Hayden CK, Schwartz MZ, et al: Computerized tomography and ultrasonography in evaluating blunt abdominal trauma in children. In Brooks BF (ed): The Injured Child. Austin, University of Texas Press, 1985, p 61.
29. Lebit RM: Abdominal and genitourinary trauma in children. Crit Care Nurs Clin North Am 3:3, 1991.
30. Yaster M, Haller JA: Multiple trauma. In Rogers MC (ed): Textbook of Pediatric Intensive Care. Baltimore, Williams & Wilkins, 1987, p 1295.
31. McAnena OJ, Moore EE, Marx JA: Initial evaluation of the patient with blunt abdominal trauma. Surg Clin North Am 70:495, 1990.
32. Matlack ME: Abdominal injuries. In Mayer TA (ed): Emergency Management of Pediatric Trauma. Philadelphia, WB Saunders Co, 1985.
33. Crone R: Acute circulatory failure in children. Pediatr Clin North Am 27:525, 1980.
34. Moloney-Harmon PA: Initial assessment and stabilization of the critically ill child. Crit Care Nurs North Am 3:3, 1991.
35. The Johns Hopkins University School of Medicine and the Johns Hopkins Pediatric Trauma Center: An Advanced Pediatric Life Support Course. Baltimore, Johns Hopkins University Press, 1990, p 37.
36. Mayer TA: Initial evaluation and management of the injured child. In Mayer T (ed): Emergency Management of Pediatric Trauma. Philadelphia, WB Saunders Co, 1985, pp 1–38.
37. Fiser DH: Intraosseous infusion. N Engl J Med 322:1579, 1990.
38. Committee on Trauma, American College of Surgeons: Early Care of the Injured Patient. Philadelphia, WB Saunders Co, 1982.
39. Lindenmann E: Symptomatology and management of acute grief. Am J Psychol 101:141–148, 1944.

40. Aquelera D, Messick J: Crisis Intervention: Theory and Methodology. St. Louis, CV Mosby, 1982.
41. Lust B: The patient in the ICU: A family experience. Crit Care Q 6:49–57, 1984.
42. Miles M, Perry K: Parental responses to the sudden accidental death of a child. Crit Care Q 8:73–82, 1985.
43. Miles M, Demi A: Sources of guilt in bereaved parents: Toward the development of a theory of bereavement guilt. Omega 14:299–314, 1983.
44. Schultz C: The dynamics of grief. J Emerg Nurs 5:25–30, 1979.
45. Czerwinski S: Complications of pediatric trauma. Crit Care Nurs Clin North Am 3:479, 1991.
46. Smith J, Giblin M, Koehler J: The cardiovascular system. In Smith J (ed): Pediatric Critical Care. New York, Wiley, 1983.
47. Bruce DA, Alavi A, Bilaniuk L, et al: Diffuse cerebral swelling following head injuries in children: The syndrome of "malignant brain edema." J Neurosurg 54:170, 1981.
48. Bruce DA, Raphaely RC, Goldberg AI, et al: Pathophysiology, treatment, and outcome following severe head injury in children. Childs Brain 5:174, 1979.
49. Hahn YS, Fuchs S, Flannery AM, et al: Factors influencing post-traumatic seizures in children. Neurosurgery 22:864, 1988.
50. Davis RJ, Dean JM, Goldberg AL, et al: Head and spinal cord injury. In Rogers MC (ed): Textbook of Pediatric Intensive Care. Baltimore, Williams & Wilkins, 1987, p 649.
51. Vernon-Levett P: Head injuries in children. Crit Care Nurs Clin North Am 3:411, 1991.
52. Lebet RM: Abdominal and genitourinary trauma in children. Crit Care Nurs Clin North Am 3:433, 1991.
53. Seashore J: Nutritional support of children in the intensive care unit. Yale Biol Med 57:111–134, 1984.
54. Walker W, Hendricks K: Manual of Pediatric Nutrition. Philadelphia, WB Saunders Co, 1985.
55. Broome M: The child in pain: A model for assessment and intervention. Crit Care Q 8:47–55, 1985.
56. Melzack R, Wall P: Pain: Theory, research, and nursing practice. Adv Nurs Sci 2:43–59, 1980.
57. Zeltzer LK, Jay SM, Fisher DM: The management of pain associated with pediatric procedures. Pediatr Clin North Am 36:941, 1989.
58. Division of Injury Control, Center for Environmental Health and Injury Control, Centers for Disease Control: Childhood injuries in the United States. Am J Dis Child 144:627, 1990.
59. Symington D: The goals of rehabilitation. Arch Phys Med Rehabil 65:38, 1984.
60. Smith J: Nursing process in pediatric critical care. In Smith J (ed): Pediatric Critical Care. New York, Wiley, 1983, pp 1–19.
61. Ferguson C: Childhood coping: Adaptive behavior during intensive care hospitalization. Crit Care Q 6:81–93, 1984.
62. Granger R: The psychologic aspects of physical trauma. In Touloukian R (ed): Pediatric Trauma, 2nd ed. St Louis, Mosby–Year Book, 1991, p 93.
63. King R, Ducas S: Rehabilitation of the patient with a spinal cord injury. Nurs Clin North Am 15:225–242, 1980.
64. Kelly T: Emotional support of the injured child and family. In Joy C (ed): Pediatric Trauma Nursing. Rockville, MD, Aspen, 1989, p 239.
65. Jacus C: Working with families in a rehabilitation setting. Rehabil Nurs 14:10–14, 1981.
66. Haller J: Organization of a regional pediatric trauma and emergency center. In Mayer T (ed): Emergency Management of Pediatric Trauma. Philadelphia, WB Saunders Co. 1985, p 502.

27

TRAUMA IN THE ELDERLY

JUDITH K. BOBB

Projections by the U.S. Bureau of the Census[1] for the 21st century indicate that approximately one-fifth of the population of the United States will be age 65 years or older. This represents a significant change in the national character, which has a major impact on the delivery of health care.

Normal aging is a gradual process. From the moment of conception, a person undergoes progressive change: Youth and immaturity give way to adulthood and maturation. The summation of all the unique experiences of an individual is known as *aging*.

Research on the effects of aging on human function has provided greater understanding of the process but has also generated many new questions. To date no universal agreement exists as to when a person becomes "old." The chronological age of 65 years is most often cited, although many authors now differentiate between the "young old" and the "old old" as suggested by Neugarten and Havighurst.[2] A better description appears to be one that differentiates between the "healthy" old and the "infirm" old. These distinctions indicate that age alone is not adequate to explain the term *elderly*. That definition must await some future time when methods have been developed to assess biological rather than chronological age.

Within the natural human life span, the individual's experience is like no other. Illness and injury may contribute to shortened life expectancy, or the biological clock that regulates function may begin to slow. Differences among individuals are expressed as differences in the capacity to function. Because of the wide variability among individuals, it becomes more and more difficult to estimate when an individual becomes "old." That is, any two 40-year-old persons are more alike than they are different; any two 70-year-old persons are more different than they are alike. Although chronological age is inadequate, for purposes of this chapter *elderly* will be defined as an individual of chronological age 60 years or greater.

The lack of distinction concerning a definition of aging creates problems for the nurse who is trying to anticipate potential problems related to trauma, for it is unlikely that protocols developed for a younger population base will be as effective for older persons. However, present data bases do not provide sufficient information to indicate where changes should be made. Health care literature lacks sufficient data describing the responses of the elderly to injury.

This chapter will attempt to provide the nurse with a summary of what is presently known of age-related changes in mind, body, and spiritual functions; how these changes relate to the elderly trauma patient; and suggestions for modifications to nursing care plans for the elderly.

EPIDEMIOLOGY

Three statistical statements help to define the differences in the elderly trauma population compared with the "typical" younger group: (1) the older segment of the population, as a group, tends to be injured less frequently than people under age 50, (2) older individuals who are injured are much more likely to experience a fatal outcome from their injuries, and (3) injury of relatively low severity is more likely to result in death in an older person.[3, 4]

Since the previous edition, the proportion of licensed drivers aged 65 years and older has increased from 6.1 to 7.2 per cent, yielding approximately 16.5 million drivers.[4, 5] As Table 27–1 illustrates, both the automobile accident rate and the rate of fatal accidents involving the elderly have increased since 1980. During the same period, the rates have fallen slightly for younger drivers. However, drivers between the ages of 25 and 34 years continue to have the highest rates for accidents and for fatalities. Falls remain the most common cause of elderly death (33 per cent), followed by motor vehicle accidents (26 per cent) and fire and burns (5 per cent).

TABLE 27–1. ACCIDENT INVOLVEMENT OF THE ELDERLY: COMPARATIVE FIGURES

	1980*	1988†	CHANGE
Accident Rate‡			
>65 years	6.1	7.2	+ 1.1
20–24	19.8	16.9	− 2.9
<44	76.8	76.5	− 0.3
Fatal Accident Rate‡			
>65 years	6.3	8.9	+ 2.6
20–24	20.8	17.5	− 3.3
<44	76.9	74.4	− 2.5
Death Rates‡	**1978**	**1986**	**CHANGE**
15–24 years	64	51.2	−12.8
65–74	61	49	−12
75+	166	141.9	−24.1

*Data from National Safety Council: Accident Facts. Chicago, National Safety Council, 1981.

†Data from National Safety Council: Accident Facts. Chicago, National Safety Council, 1989.

‡Per 100,000 population

In contrast to the accident rate, the death rate for all accidents remains highest for the elderly despite a drop in rates for all age groups (Table 27–1). Death from accident is most likely to occur in those over the age of 75 years, even when the injuries sustained are relatively moderate.

Baker and associates[6] developed an Injury Severity Score in 1974 which permits comparison of anatomical injuries among injured individuals. The results obtained from a study of 2128 patients hospitalized as a result of motor vehicle injury show that Injury Severity Scores above 20 to 29 are associated with close to 50 per cent mortality in those over age 70, while the mortality for similar injury severity in the 50- to 69-year group is approximately 25 per cent and is 10 per cent for those younger than 50 years of age. This finding of low injury severity and high mortality in the elderly has been confirmed in additional reports by Oreskovich and associates[7] and others.[8–11]

CAUSES OF DEATH

Comparative data from the National Safety Council[4, 5] continue to indicate that 65 per cent of deaths in the older trauma population are due to three causes: falls, thermal injury, and motor vehicle accidents. Falls are the leading cause of death for both elderly men and women, accounting for approximately 33 per cent of all fatalities. The most common injuries associated with falls are fractures of the hip, femur, and proximal humerus; Colles' fracture of the wrist; and head injury.[12]

Motor vehicles are responsible for approximately 26 per cent of deaths in those over age 65 years.[5] The number of deaths and injuries can be expected to increase as the number of drivers over age 65 increases in coming years. In 1988, 10 per cent of all licensed drivers were over age 65.[5] Despite the fact that the number of miles driven annually decreases after age 50, the elderly have a higher incidence of collisions than any group except those under 25 years of age.[8]

Death as a result of thermal injury accounts for approximately 6 per cent of all accidental deaths in those 65 years of age and older.[5] Thermal injuries include burns and inhalation injury, contacts with sources of heat, and electrical injury. Scalds, flame burns, and contact with hot objects are the types of thermal injuries most commonly reported in the literature.[8]

INJURY THRESHOLD

Increased Personal Risk

The aging process produces unique changes in an individual's functional status, which contribute to increased susceptibility to injury and to increased mortality. Body systems most often cited as showing evidence of age-impaired function include the cardiovascular, respiratory, renal, musculoskeletal, and endocrine systems. Neurological function is generally considered intact, with one notable exception: a deterioration in special senses. The elderly also tend to accumulate the effects of chronic disease, which may add further limitations to those imposed by aging alone.

Age-related deterioration in function and chronic disease have been implicated as causative factors in accidental injury. Tripping over furniture, stairs, scatter rugs, and other obstacles is often cited as the immediate precursor to a fall. Among the factors leading to falls are decreasing function of the special senses, such as loss of peripheral vision, syncope, postural instability, transient impairment of cerebrovascular perfusion, alcohol ingestion, and medication use.[13–16] The elderly also seem more susceptible to falls when exposed to a new environment. Tinker[17] noted that the highest incidence of falls in nursing home residents occurred during the first week after admission.

Alterations in perception and delayed response to stressors also may contribute to injury. Diminished or impaired proprioception reduces awareness of an impending fall. The onset of corrective measures may then be too late to avoid falling. Loss of visual acuity limits the elderly person's ability to see traffic hazards and to avoid them. When the sensation of temperature is diminished, a hot object remains in contact with the body longer, resulting in a more severe degree of injury.

The role of chronic disease has been implicated as a contributing factor in injury but primarily in an anecdotal fashion. Chronic conditions that are associated with loss of consciousness, such as epilepsy, certain cardiac dysrhythmias, and cerebrovascular disease, have been documented as leading to injury.[16, 18] However, no control study has been done to examine a comparably impaired group without accident history. Additionally, the implication that chronic disease may be the cause of increased mortality in the older trauma patient has been recently questioned. Studies since 1984[19–25] have repeatedly attempted to demonstrate a relationship between chronic disease, as measured by medical diagnosis, and mortality in the elderly. Use of medical diagnoses existing prior to injury has proven unsuccessful. The Acute Physiology Score,[19] in so far as it reflects preexisting function, appears to be a better descriptor of the role of chronic disease.

Use of medications by the elderly has not been clearly related to increased injury rates, but it can be expected to contribute in some cases. Often an individual is under the care of more than one physician for more than one condition that requires medication. Drug interactions among prescribed medications (in addition to over-the-counter self-medication practiced by some persons) are likely causes of impaired perception and/or response. Reidenberg[26] noted that the number of adverse reactions to polypharmacy increased as the number of drugs taken and as the complexity of the drug regimen increased. The concept of drug interactions also should include the use of alcohol.

Increased Societal Risk

We live in a society that has been dominated for four decades by the fantasy of everlasting youth and health. Communicable diseases have all but been eradicated, lifespans have increased, and we are indeed enjoying healthier lives. However, such permutation of youthful social values increases the degree of hazard for the elderly. For example, the average traffic signal in the United States assumes that a pedestrian walks at 4 ft/sec, a rate that is too fast for many persons over 60 years of age.[27]

Environmental hazards abound. Road traffic areas were designed 40 to 50 years ago, when the standard automobile was larger and heavier and the average age of drivers was younger. Increases in the number of distractions present on modern streets and highways may overload the information-processing capabilities of anyone, but especially elderly drivers and pedestrians.

In the home, design and furnishings favor the decorating tastes of younger persons. Scatter rugs, tables with sharp corners, open flames on stoves, cabinets located above eye level, stairs without railings, tap water heated to greater than 130°F, and inadequate lighting increase the risk of accidental injury for the elderly.

As we look toward a future with greater numbers of elderly citizens, it becomes apparent that not enough is known about the special needs of our aging citizens. Hogue[13] points out the need for better reporting of injury events so that injury control procedures can be designed and implemented. Nurses must become aware of the risks faced by the elderly. They are in a position to support the efforts of epidemiologists to engineer reduced environmental hazards as well as to promote modification of social attitudes and values.

RESUSCITATION CYCLE

Those who attempt to plan for resuscitation of the elderly trauma patient are faced with two immediate problems. First is the wide variability in prior function that exists in this patient population. Generalizations concerning injuries and response to injury, which are possible with younger patients, are difficult, if not impossible, in the elderly. Second is the lack of adequate documentation concerning the initial response of these patients to injury.

As a result, much is assumed about the elderly trauma patient, but little is known. Widespread beliefs that the elderly have significantly impaired cardiovascular function sometimes lead to inadequate fluid replacement and persistence of hypovolemia. Conversely, the elderly may be treated without due consideration for potential cardiovascular impairment, and fluid overload may result.

Beliefs that the elderly as a group have significantly impaired function are easily acquired from the literature. For example, DelGuercio and Cohn[28] have noted that a significant percent of elderly people admitted for elective surgery present with some impairment in function. They documented impairment in oxygenation (decreased oxygen tension, increased alveolar to arterial oxygen differences) and impairment in cardiovascular function (abnormal pulmonary vascular pressures, decreased myocardial contractility). They also reported that nearly 60 per cent of the 148 patients they studied exhibited mild to moderate abnormality. Only 13 per cent of the sample was considered normal for their age. Reports such as this are typical of the health care literature that tends to document only disease and disability.

In contrast, data[29] from 122 elderly patients admitted to the Maryland Institute for Emergency Medical Services Systems (MIEMSS) Shock Trauma Center showed an approximately even distribution of hypotension, normotension, and hypertension in the sample. The mean arterial oxygen tension was 80 mm Hg, with a mean respiratory rate of 20. Thirty per cent of the sample reported a history negative for chronic disease and showed no evident clinical impairment at the time of admission.

The difference between these two studies raises the question of different health subsets among the elderly population. It may be postulated that some elderly are healthy at any age, in which case chronological age is a poor criterion for decisions about patient management. At present there is insufficient data to explain differences found in the studies.

TABLE 27–2. FREQUENCY OF INJURY* BY BODY REGION AND NUMBER OF SUBJECTS FOR TWO AGE GROUPS

SAMPLE	TOTAL (PER CENT)	AGE GROUPS (NUMBER OF SUBJECTS)	
		55 TO 70	71 TO 101
Head and neck	60.6	45	29
Face	18.9	16	7
Chest	42.6	32	20
Abdomen and pelvic contents	10.7	9	4
Extremities and pelvis	49.2	34	26
External	60.6	49	25

*More than one body region may be injured.

Data from Bobb JK: A descriptive study of the impact of injury sustained by persons age 55 years and older in road traffic accidents. Master's thesis, University of Maryland, 1986.

Patterns of Injury

Falls are the most frequent cause of injury to the elderly. As noted previously, the most common injuries associated with falls are fractures of the hip, femur, and proximal humerus; Colles' fracture of the wrist; and head injury.[7] The reports from the literature suggest that some alteration in health status immediately precedes a fall. These changes frequently are related to the level of consciousness or the musculoskeletal system[16–18] and may involve the use of alcohol as well.

Scalds, especially from tap water in the home, are frequent causes of thermal injury in the elderly. This has been related to diminished thermal perception. Flame burns result from use of matches and cigarette lighters and ignition of clothing.[13] Thermal injuries in the elderly are also associated with higher mortality when compared with similar injuries in the young. Data from the National Burn Information Exchange[30] indicate that victims aged 60 to 74 have a survival potential one-half that of a person aged 35 to 49 with a similar injury. For persons over 74 years of age, the projected survival from a 40 per cent burn is only 6 per cent, compared to 78 per cent survival for someone aged 35 to 49 years.

The data from studies of the biomechanics of motor vehicle crashes indicate that crashes involving the elderly should be expected to result in injury patterns similar to those seen in younger patients. Comparisons between the young and the elderly are difficult because of variation in the manner of documenting injury in published reports and the fact that the elderly are seldom analyzed separately from the young. However, examination of the medical records of 122 patients over age 55 admitted directly to the MIEMSS Shock Trauma Center following motor vehicle injury shows differences in the expected distribution of injuries across body areas.[29] Injuries to the head and neck and injuries classified as external (abrasions, lacerations) were seen most frequently, followed by injuries to the extremities, the chest, the face, and the abdomen and pelvic contents. As shown in Table 27–2, the incidence of injury to the abdominal and pelvic contents region in the older age group is remarkably low. In published reports,[31, 32] the incidence of injuries to the abdomen varies from 15 to 39 per cent. The mortality from abdominal injuries has been shown to be 4.7 times greater for the elderly.[10] Despite a growing interest in this population, the question of distribution of injuries remains unanswered.

Assessment

Resuscitation of the trauma patient is characterized by a need for speed and efficiency. To determine the magnitude of injury, the individual's response, and the potential for complications, the nurse relies on knowledge and experience to direct patient assessment. Experience is limited in resuscitation of elderly patients. Assessment is crucial in all emergencies; it is more difficult to perform in elderly patients because previous assumptions may not be valid, yet there are little data available from which to form new generalizations. Assessment itself is complicated when an older person presents with the accumulated effects of prior disease and injury.

Gerontological literature offers some preliminary guidance for how the elderly may differ from the young; this is shown in Table 27–3.

An increase in the degree of monitoring is indicated because the elderly are noted for high mortality rates even when apparent injury is of low severity. In younger populations, increases in Injury Severity Score parallel increases in mortality. For the older population, however, death often results from injuries that would be survived by younger persons. In 1985, Baker and associates[6] reported Injury Severity Scores for the age groups under age 50 years, between 50 and 69 years, and 70 years and older. For mild injury (Injury Severity Score of 20 or less), the mortality increased from 1 per cent in those under 50 years to 14 per cent in those 70 years and older. Moderate injury (Injury Severity Score of 20 to 29) produced mortality rates of 10 per cent in those under age 50, 26 per cent in those between 50 and 69 years, and 45 per cent in persons aged 70 years and older. With Injury Severity Scores between 30 and 50 (moderate to severe), the mortality rate ranged from 62 to 85 per cent in the elderly compared with 39 per cent in subjects under age 50.

TABLE 27–3. CHANGES IN FUNCTIONAL STATUS ASSOCIATED WITH AGING

Perfusion	Thickening heart valves
	Thickening of blood vessels
	Diminished cardiac output
	Delayed response to stress
Ventilation	Limited rib cage expansion
	Atrophy of respiratory muscles
	Decreased arterial oxygen tension
	Decreased vital capacity
	Diminished cough
Perception	Loss of visual acuity
	Diminished hearing
	Decreased sense of taste
	Lower sensitivity to touch
	Decreased proprioception
Elimination	Decreased peristalsis
	Decreased intestinal enzymes
	Diminished glomerular filtration
	Decreased bladder capacity
Mobility	Muscle atrophy
	Decreased bone mass
	Loss of skin subcutaneous fat
	Decreased flexibility
Consciousness	Short-term memory loss
	Slower thought processing
	Decreased pain threshold

Cardiovascular Considerations

The general decline in cardiovascular function noted in the aged implies a diminished ability to respond to traumatic stresses. This change may be characterized by a delay in activation of responses, diminished magnitude of compensatory responses, a failure to sustain life following injuries usually survived by younger persons, or a combination of all these factors.

As is true for all trauma patients, initial measurements of blood pressure are likely to be misleading because of compensation or because of prior dysfunction. In the elderly, for example, the literature notes an increased incidence of hypertension.[33] Thus an initial normal blood pressure may mask hypotension. The report of Oreskovich and associates,[7] however, noted that the elderly conformed to standard clinical parameters regarding the presence of shock. In a study of 100 patients over 70 years of age admitted with severe injuries (67 per cent falls), they diagnosed shock based on a systolic pressure less than 90 mm Hg for 15 minutes. They found a mortality of 100 per cent in those patients who presented in shock.

A different result was found in data from the MIEMSS Shock Trauma Center.[29] Thirty of 122 elderly patients admitted following motor vehicle injury presented with initial blood pressures less than 70 mm Hg. Eleven died, resulting in a mortality of 37 per cent.

Frequent monitoring should be instituted rapidly in elderly patients in order to assess trends and patterns of response. Invasive monitoring should be considered, despite the additional risk, since it provides more reliable assessment of cardiovascular performance and guidance of replacement fluid therapy. Scalea and associates[25] have suggested that the elderly may appear hemodynamically stable while experiencing inadequate perfusion. Their experience further showed that delays in recognition and treatment of underperfusion were associated with increasing mortality. Although the sample was small, they showed that invasive monitoring can help identify those elderly who have cardiovascular impairment and help reduce the risk of iatrogenic complications and death.

Although many elderly have chronic dysrhythmias,[34] the presence of initial cardiac dysrhythmias should be evaluated for causes related to the trauma, such as hypoxemia or myocardial contusion, before assuming they are due to cardiac disease. Myocardial infarction is often hypothesized as a cause of accident, but there is little evidence to support this assumption. However, acute infarction may be found by the time the patient is admitted. Therefore, the patient should be assessed to rule out an acute process. A 12-lead electrocardiogram should be obtained initially to provide baseline data. When clinical and/or electrocardiographic evidence supports a diagnosis of myocardial infarction, serial EKGs and serial cardiac enzymes should be obtained, with special reference to the cardiac isoenzyme creatinine phosphokinase.

Pulmonary Considerations

Aging reduces lung mass and elasticity, limits the expansion of the rib cage, decreases vital capacity, and reduces the ability to cough. These aging-related changes should not be mistaken for chronic lung disease. Common clinical findings in the elderly are a lowered arterial oxygen tension, a decrease in lung mechanics, and a marked tendency to develop pneumonia when hospitalized.[19, 28, 35] Arterial blood gas measurements typically show a moderately reduced oxygen tension (e.g., Pa_{O_2} of 80 mm Hg), while other values are within normal limits. Changes in values other than the Pa_{O_2} should be interpreted in the context of the injury. Measurements across time remain essential for determining trends.

Neurological Considerations

Initial neurological assessment should include a brief examination of the patient for impairments of the special senses, especially vision and hearing, since alterations in these functions may cloud further assessment. Cognitive function can be superficially tested if the patient is capable of verbal response. Assessment of cognitive function may also be complicated by loss of short-term memory, the presence of senile dementia, or slow responses due to an overload of sensory input.

Careful assessment should be made for evidence of intracerebral bleeding, particularly in trauma associated with falls. While the younger trauma victim tends to sustain closed head injuries with cerebral edema, the older victim is more prone to bleeding incidents. A retrospective examination of the medical records of 94 patients aged 65 and older admitted to the MIEMSS Shock Trauma Center[29] in 1985 was done to determine the frequency and type of head injuries sustained. There were 30 injured in falls, 41 injured in road traffic accidents, and 23 injured from other causes. Forty-three patients sustained head injuries secondary to falls or motor vehicle accidents. Of the 43, 20 were associated with intracranial bleeding (including hematomas). The overall mortality rate in this group was 30 per cent (29 of 94). However, when head injury was involved, the mortality rate was

41 per cent (18 of 43); when intracranial bleeding was present, the mortality rate rose to 60 per cent (12 of 20).

Musculoskeletal Considerations

Musculoskeletal assessment should be performed with consideration of age-related changes: limitations in mobility and joint flexibility, muscle atrophy, loss of subcutaneous fat, preexisting deformity, and increased pain threshold. Hielema[12] reviewed epidemiological data on hip fractures. He noted that hip fractures are often associated with additional musculoskeletal injury, such as other fractures or head injury. These data suggest that the nurse should be alert to the potential for Colles' fractures of the wrist, fractures of the upper humerus, and skull fractures, in addition to the hip or femur fracture in patients admitted following falls.

Osteoarthritis is a common finding in the elderly[36] that may result in deformity and/or limitation in joint mobility. When the cervical spine is involved, difficulty may be encountered in interpretation of initial assessment of the neck.

Capillary fragility often leads to large ecchymoses that can be associated with minor injury. The elderly also have a tendency to develop large hematomas that migrate to dependent locations.

While conventional assessment techniques are presumed effective, some fractures may be missed if the patient has impaired perception of pain. Absence of pain should not be relied on to rule out the possible fracture. Where a question exists, radiological confirmation is indicated.

Renal Considerations

Papper[37] summarized the effects of age on renal function as decreased renal blood flow (reduced glomerular filtration rate), impaired water reabsorption, decreased bladder capacity, decreased diluting ability, and delayed accommodation to stresses. These changes may manifest through inappropriately high urinary output in the face of hypovolemia. Insertion of a retention urinary catheter carries a greater risk of infection in older persons but is justified for its monitoring value. Modest elevations in the BUN (22 mg/dl) and serum creatinine (1.2 mg/dl) are reflective of age.[20, 37]

Metabolic Considerations

No evidence exists that there is a decline in endocrine functions essential to the stress response, such as epinephrine or norepinephrine secretion.[38, 39] Adaptive responses in the elderly seem to be intact, but greater time is required for adaptation to occur.[40–42] Some endocrine secretions, most notably estrogen, do diminish with age. The most frequent endocrine disorders found in the elderly are diabetes mellitus and hypothyroidism.[41]

Psychosocial Considerations

The unique personal and health history of the individual should be obtained as soon as possible. If the patient is a reliable historian, immediate information concerning relevant past medical history, including use of medications, can be obtained. If this is not possible, family members or friends often can provide valuable information. Contacting the patient's personal physician may provide insight into the prior health of the patient. (Remember that the elderly tend to utilize several physicians.) In addition to data helpful during initial assessment and treatment, questions concerning the individual's daily activity and degree of independence will prove helpful during later assessment and in formulating long-term plans.

Management Considerations

Although initial assessment and treatment priorities of elderly patients do not differ from those of the young, specific procedures may have to be modified. Should the elderly person require intubation, potential difficulty should be anticipated with positioning if the patient has cervical osteoarthritis. The procedure should be attempted under the best possible conditions in order to minimize incidental damage to the larynx or friable mucous membranes. Asepsis is essential because of the great risk of pulmonary infection in the elderly. Mechanical ventilation should be instituted rapidly, if indicated, since the elderly have limited ventilatory reserve. Allen and Schwab[19] investigated elderly patients with blunt chest trauma. They found that nearly 90 per cent of the subjects who required mechanical ventilation sustained injury in motor vehicle accidents. The mechanically ventilated group had a higher morbidity than nonventilated. They suggest that it may be possible to avoid mechanical ventilation when the trauma is not secondary to motor vehicle accident. Further, they reported successful ventilatory management of elderly patients with blunt chest trauma when local anesthesia was used to control pain.

Fluid resuscitation must be monitored closely to ensure adequate, rapid replacement without excess administration of fluids. The general belief that rapid rates of administration tend to produce fluid overload in the elderly has not been substantiated through research. Conservative treatment based on this belief may prolong periods of hypovolemia, when placement of central lines and close monitoring can provide the means for determining if replacement therapy is adequate. Scalea and associates[25] have emphasized the possibility of prolonged periods of low flow which may contribute to increased mortality. Because of the greater incidence of preexisting cardiac disease among the elderly, the suggestion of DelGuercio and Cohn[28] to monitor intravascular pressures should be considered early. For the same reason, early consideration should be given to the use of inotropic support when the patient fails to respond adequately to fluid replacement.

Nursing Management Considerations

The same principles and concepts that underlie nursing management in young trauma victims apply to care of the elderly. A notable exception concerns the special senses.

Initially, it seems advantageous to presume significant deterioration in vision, hearing, touch, and thermoregulation until assessment indicates otherwise. Nursing care should emphasize communication with the patient through combined mediums, including vision, touch, and hearing. Although it is difficult to accomplish during resuscitation, the nurse should seek eye contact in a direct line of vision and should speak slowly and clearly and in low tones when talking to the patient. Phrase questions simply, with little reliance on medical terms. Verbal communication should be reinforced by purposeful touch that is gentle yet firm. Restraints, while often necessary for patient protection and for facilitation of resuscitation efforts, should be released periodically to allow the patient to explore the new extensions of his or her physical space.

Older people experience poor tolerance for cold, partly due to peripheral vascular changes and partly due to diminished thermoregulatory ability. Faulty thermoregulation also has been related to undernutrition and to falls.[43] Injury responses as well as exposure to ambient temperatures may produce significant heat loss, indicating a need for close monitoring of core body temperatures. Keeping the skin covered during resuscitation when the body is uncovered for assessment and routine procedures is difficult, but it helps to reduce losses. In some cases, passive rewarming (e.g., warmed intravenous fluids, heated humidification) may be necessary.

Health care providers, like others in our society, are undergoing a revision of attitudes toward the elderly. However, there still exists a tendency to limit aggressive therapy at some point merely because of the individual's age. The health care team should recognize that survival to age 75 earns the individual a potential life expectancy of 9.1 additional years.[5] Age alone is no criterion for limitation of resuscitation efforts.

PERIOPERATIVE CYCLE

Perioperative management of the elderly should adhere to the same general principles that are applied to the young. Some age-related adaptation may be necessary for certain individuals.

In nonemergency situations, additional time should be allowed for obtaining operative consent. The elderly individual may have difficulty understanding the choices offered or arriving at a decision. Additional visits by the health care team may be indicated, as may be consultation with family or other support persons. Care must be exercised so that the patient understands the consequences of consent and also those of refusal to consent.

Because of the higher mortality associated with surgery in the elderly compared with the young, every possible step should be taken to reduce the risk for these patients. This includes consideration of prophylactic antibiotics to reduce infection risk and reduced amounts of premedication in those persons who have minimal anxiety. If time permits, correction of underlying physiological deficits is known to be effective.[28]

Potential problems with airway management should be anticipated. Loss of orofacial structures make mask ventilation difficult. Endotracheal intubation provides airway protection but may be difficult to accomplish because of deformity and/or rigidity of the cervical spine. Vigorous manipulation of the head and neck should be avoided because of the risk of impairing vertebral circulation.

Positioning in the operating room should be done with consideration for fragile bones and stiff joints. The incidence of osteoporosis is nearly the same for men and women after age 70. Iatrogenic fractures can occur if the patient is not protected.

Diminished function of the thermoregulatory mechanisms in the elderly make them more vulnerable to loss of body heat. Core body temperature should be monitored frequently. The nurse should be alert to the potential need to warm inspired gases or to administer warm fluids during the procedure.

Anesthesia has the potential for disruption of regulatory systems for perfusion, whether it is general or regional. General anesthesia is recommended for upper abdominal, thoracic, and intracranial procedures, while regional anesthesia is indicated for lower extremity procedures. Regional anesthesia can be used when preexisting respiratory disorders would be adversely affected by anesthetics; general anesthesia is recommended if airway control is essential.[38]

CRITICAL CARE CYCLE

Two considerations, over and above those for trauma alone, govern nursing care planning for the elderly in critical care units. First is to anticipate complications that are related to aging rather than to trauma. Second is modification and negotiation of rehabilitation goals.

Anticipating Complications

As noted earlier, the cardiovascular, respiratory, and neurological systems are most critical for assessment and management during the resuscitation cycle. They continue to play a major role during the critical care cycle, along with renal, endocrine, and integumentary systems.

The older person, by virtue of living to "a ripe old age," has a greater propensity for chronic disease that may impair cardiac contractility or systemic perfusion. The individual may function quite adequately during usual activities but may decompensate under the stresses of trauma. The health care team must be diligent in assessing the actual impact of chronic health care problems rather than assuming they play a major role.

Assessment

Cardiovascular Considerations

Cardiac and vascular system changes do not necessarily increase the risk of death to the elderly unless there is significant underlying heart disease. Mohr[44] noted that reduction in surgical mortality during the past 25 years resulted primarily from correction of underlying defects during the preoperative and postoperative phases of care. Trauma provides little opportunity for preoperative intervention. Therefore, much of the corrective therapy must be attempted in the critical care setting.

Continuous monitoring of intravascular pressures is indicated until the patient is stable. Inotropic support may be needed during the acute phase, along with close attention to fluid balance. The elderly also should be monitored for water-handling capabilities. Because of potential renal dysfunction, monitoring should include frequent electrolyte measurements, with attention given to the development of hypo-osmolality–hyponatremia. This finding could indicate potential water overload, even when intravascular pressures are within acceptable limits.

The prevalence of peripheral vascular stiffening that accompanies aging increases the likelihood that perfusion may be compromised at some time despite adequate volumes and contractility. Extremities should be inspected frequently for temperature and/or color changes. Keeping the patient warm, which includes the use of special covering for the hands and feet, is of benefit in warding off some effects of vasoconstriction and in adding to the patient's comfort. For those who are critically ill, monitoring of systemic vascular resistance will help detect indications for institution of vasodilators.

The incidence of cardiac dysrhythmias, particularly atrial in origin, increases with age.[34] In many cases they are secondary to previous myocardial infarction. Each dysrhythmia should be evaluated for its impact on perfusion before therapy is instituted. Arrhythmias need to be examined for origin, since they may indicate a hypoxic problem, electrolyte imbalance, or decrease in perfusion, or they may reflect a prior problem. Continuous electrocardiographic monitoring is essential.

With no prior knowledge of the individual's tolerance to fluid administration, each patient has the potential for pulmonary edema. Early fluid therapy should be carefully monitored, but rates of administration need not be slow just because of the person's age. Patient responses, including pulmonary artery pressures, should provide individual guidelines. It may be of benefit to plot ventricular function curves and/or to administer a fluid challenge to assess the impact of fluid volume and type.

Respiratory Considerations

Seymour and Pringle[45] found a 40 per cent incidence of respiratory complications in a study of 158 postoperative elderly surgical patients. They noted that the overall rate of complications for emergency patients was higher than that for elective patients and that respiratory complications were related to the surgical site. As with young patients, surgery involving the abdomen produced greater potential for respiratory compromise in the elderly. DelGuercio and Cohn[28] found preoperative oxygen tension deficits (44 per cent) and abnormal pulmonary artery pressures (45.5 per cent) in their study of elderly patients. The literature also reflects an elderly propensity to develop respiratory infections. DeMaria and associates,[22] Osler and associates,[9] and Finelli and associates[10] confirm that the pulmonary system is the leading site of posttraumatic complications, that the elderly have a higher rate of complications, and that these complications are related to mortality. The data from Allen and Schwab[19] suggest that respiratory complications are related to impaired ventilation secondary to pain and to the use of mechanical ventilation. They also noted that patients requiring mechanical ventilation were usually injured in motor vehicle accidents.

Despite the risk of infection, this is a patient group that also frequently requires airway and ventilatory support. They are less able to defend the airway because of decreased sensitivity of the gag reflex and diminished strength of the respiratory muscles. The elderly person who requires endotracheal intubation will often need tracheostomy for long-term protection. Expect the early institution of mechanical ventilation to be followed by a long period of ventilatory support. Just as the older person may be slow to respond to stresses initially, the recovery of function will take longer. Weaning from ventilatory support may take as much as twice the time needed for a younger person with similar injuries. Intermittent mandatory ventilation appears to be the method of choice for weaning, as it allows respiratory muscle strength to be regained. Weaning should be closely monitored and it should not be started before the patient has had sufficient time to recover from the injuries.

Cognitive Considerations

Seymour and Pringle[45] also noted acute confusion postoperatively in approximately 10 per cent of elderly surgical patients. This is consistent with the 10 to 15 per cent noted in the literature for hospitalized elderly.[14, 41] Much of this can be attributed to information and sensory overload, short-term memory losses, and delays in information processing. Additional causes of confusion in the elderly include medications, pain, stress, metabolic imbalance, alterations in thermoregulation, and brain disorders. The need for comprehensive differential diagnosis is readily apparent.

Estimates place the level of mental health disorders in the elderly as high as 25 per cent. Primary causes of dementia include Alzheimer's disease and multiinfarct disease (e.g., diabetes, atherosclerosis). These conditions also have been associated with a higher mortality from trauma.[14, 39, 41]

Psychosocial Considerations

Psychosocial factors also may contribute to deterioration in neurological functions. The best outcomes noted for the hospitalized elderly occur in those persons who were relatively independent at the time of injury and who did not live alone.[14] Family dynamics also appear to play a significant role, increasing the chances for good outcomes when the older person feels needed and wanted.[14, 16] Conversely, factors such as social isolation, loneliness, residence in a nursing home, and infirmity seem to contribute to increased levels of dependence postinjury.

Nickens[14] poses several questions concerning the relationship of psychosocial factors to occurrence of and outcome from hip fractures. He questions the role of depression or recent loss, hopelessness, diminished self-image, or perceived family rejection as causal factors. Most of these questions also could be raised in regard to the trauma population in general.

Renal Considerations

Major derangements in renal function will be evident from laboratory assessment. Less evident may be the decreased ability of the kidney to concentrate and to excrete waste products. The potential for water intoxication exists, as does a possible need to alter drug dosage. In some cases the kidneys may respond to trauma with development of acute renal failure. Anecdotally, this condition most often presents as polyuric failure. Routine examination of renal function studies is indicated for each patient.

Musculoskeletal Considerations

Musculoskeletal system injury, particularly hip fracture, has been documented extensively in the literature. Recall that hip fracture is also frequently associated with other injury and is associated with a poor outcome when return to preinjury state is used as a criterion.[12] Recovery from musculoskeletal injury is related to age, sex, intellectual functioning, and social factors.

Isolated hip fracture occurs most often in women and in those with evidence of osteoporosis. The incidence also increases with advancing age and where there is evidence of decreased intellectual capability.[13] Beyond age 70, the incidence of hip fracture is similar for men and women.[13] Those persons who are active before injury, independent in the activities of daily living, and relatively free of social services appear to have the best opportunity for recovery of preinjury function.[12]

The major musculoskeletal complication to be anticipated is loss of mobility. Older bones and muscles tend to develop stiffness and loss of motion more quickly, and they also tend to recover function more slowly. Recovery may be complicated by arthritic changes. Nursing care should be directed to maintaining mobility early in the critical care cycle. Passive and active range-of-motion exercises are indicated while bed rest is maintained. At the earliest opportunity, the patient should be out of bed, even if this entails taking the ventilator with the patient.

The benefits of early mobilization cannot be stressed enough. It helps reorient the older person, improves cardiac and pulmonary performance, maintains musculoskeletal integrity, minimizes damage to the integument from prolonged bed rest, promotes healing, provides evidence of progress for the patient, and generates a sense of hope.

Immune System Considerations

There is some evidence to show that aging reduces immune competence. This, combined with the reduction in immune competence noted for major trauma, puts the older patient at increased risk for both wound infections and bacteremia. Seymour and Pringle[45] found a 16.4 per cent incidence of wound complications in elderly surgical patients, although they did not specify the nature of the complications. Delays in wound healing have been noted,[42] leading to additional problems such as dehiscence and infection. Wound complications are also more likely when diabetes is present.

Chronic Disease Considerations

Since the first edition, several additional authors have contributed to the geriatric trauma data base. Many have attempted to correlate preexisting chronic disease with mortality. Using a history of recent physician care or the medical diagnosis as evidence of chronic disease, these attempts have been uniformly unsuccessful. It is clear that prior diagnosis does not give sufficient information about the patient's physiological reserve to draw conclusions or make predictions of mortality. Yet it seems both reasonable and logical that some chronic diseases could lessen the physiological reserve to the point where survival is in jeopardy. Finelli and associates[10] provided support for this hypothesis through autopsy results of a sample of geriatric nonsurvivors. They found a high incidence of coronary artery and cerebrovascular disease, along with left ventricular hypertrophy and renal and hepatic pathology. These findings, along with those of DelGuercio and Cohn[28] and Scalea and associates,[25] imply that preexisting disease does make a difference in survival. What is lacking is an acceptable measure of the impact of such disease on the individual's ability to survive.

Management Considerations

In any discussion of management of trauma in the elderly it is important to recognize that age alone does not dictate changes in therapeutic approach. The elderly should not be treated more or less conservatively than younger patients merely because they are 65 years of age or older. What age does point out is the need for more intensive monitoring and assessment in order to determine which patients do require modification of care plans for age-related changes.

All members of the team should contribute to the on-going assessment of prior health status and the level of activity the individual enjoyed. The latter, according to Seymour and Pringle,[45] may be the best single predictive parameter. Planning for long-term care must begin at this point, and the team should not lose sight of the ultimate goal of treatment—return to the best possible functional state—even if unusual modifications to therapy prove necessary.

Assessment and treatment priorities should parallel those indicated by the nature and extent of the injuries. Cardiovascular and respiratory function take priority, as usual. Intensive monitoring of both systems is indicated, since aging does increase the probability that chronic disease will be present and may influence the outcome.

Respiratory Considerations

The need for pulmonary artery measurements should be indicated by the patient's status. However, placement of a Swan-Ganz catheter increases the probability that dysfunction will be noted rapidly, and it may provide some protection against fluid excesses. It also offers the opportunity for cardiac output measurements and plotting of ventricular function curves. Because the elderly may be slow to respond to stresses, the use of inotropic support of cardiovascular function may be considered early in the patient's course. Scalea and associates[25] suggest that invasive monitoring is of greatest benefit in patients who have no obvious serious injury. They also suggest that optimizing oxygen delivery and oxygen consumption may indicate an avenue to lowered mortality.

Respiratory support, in the form of endotracheal intubation and mechanical ventilation, is a two-edged sword. Once such devices are in place, they increase the risk of pulmonary infection in a population noted for pneumonia. Oreskovich and associates[7] studied 100 patients aged 70 or greater with severe trauma. They found pulmonary sepsis to be the cause of death in 80 per cent of the nonsurvivors ($n = 15$). Survivors differed from nonsurvivors in that the former spent an average of 2 days in intensive care compared with 16 days for the latter. Horst and associates[8] reported pneumonia in 10 of 39 patients, the most common septic complication in their population. Pneumonia also was reported as the leading complication in the study of Finelli and associates.[10] These studies confirm the increased risk of pulmonary sepsis in the elderly.

In contrast, Allen and Schwab[19] studied 48 elderly patients with blunt chest trauma. They found multiple fractured ribs to be the most common injury following both falls and motor vehicle injury. When adequate pain relief was achieved, they were able to avoid mechanical ventilation in 41 of the patients. The authors also found the duration of ventilation to range from 2 to 31 days, with a mean of 14.3 days. Complications included three cases of pneumonia and one case of pulmonary embolus. They suggest that indications for institution of mechanical ventilation include a high Injury Severity Score (25 or over), flail chest, and preexisting disease.

Indications from respiratory and medical intensive care units are that the elderly, once placed on mechanical support, will require such intervention for a longer period than younger patients and that weaning time also will be extended. McLean and associates[46] studied 1018 patients admitted to a respiratory intensive care unit. There were 267 patients 65 years of age and older. The average length of stay in the respiratory intensive care unit was 6.8 days for the 65- to 74-year-old group (n = 213) and 7 days for those over 75 years of age (n = 54). The longest duration for mechanical ventilation (13.8 days) was in the subgroup admitted from postoperative emergency noncardiac surgery. Overall mortality for the elderly in the respiratory intensive care unit was 11.2 per cent. These authors also calculated the Acute Physiology Score,[19] noting that the overall Acute Physiology Score of 18.8 in the elderly "suggests a higher mortality rate adjusted for severity of illness than for comparable groups of younger patients."

When the patient requires ventilatory support, the full range of nursing care measures should be instituted rapidly. Special attention should be placed on pulmonary asepsis to minimize pulmonary infection. Measures to facilitate removal of secretions, such as turning and humidification of inspired gases, should be intensified in light of the elderly's diminished pulmonary clearance capability. Strategies should be formulated to maximize coughing effectiveness, such as planned cough exercises in the upright position.

Renal Considerations

Close attention to renal function through laboratory measurements is indicated. Even brief periods of hypovolemia and hypotension may compromise the kidneys. Evidence of rising serum creatinine level or decreased creatinine clearance will alert the health care team to modify drug dosage, if indicated, and to determine free-water clearance. Constant monitoring of fluid balance and serum electrolytes will be necessary to avoid water intoxication. Renal failure may respond favorably to conservative management and protection of the patient from iatrogenic complications. Alternatively, the patient may require hemofiltration or dialysis just as the younger individual.

Musculoskeletal Considerations

Priorities for musculoskeletal management include decisions about operative procedures. The full range of options should be explored in order to achieve early mobilization and provide the best possible outcome for the individual. It is conceivable that some procedures may be delayed in order to correct underlying functional deficits. All possible steps should be taken to keep bed rest to a minimum.

Cognitive Considerations

Several alternatives exist for the nurse to deal with confusion. Short-term memory loss means frequent repetitions of the same information, such as orientation to time and place. The physical and personal environment should be maintained as constantly as possible. Increased levels of lighting help adjust for loss of visual acuity and disorientation. The addition of familiar objects to the hospital setting may be of benefit when this is possible. Family members and significant others can contribute to recovery of orientation by providing familiar relationships and a sense of comfort and security.

Nursing Management

In addition to participation in formulation of team management goals, nursing has special responsibilities in the areas of monitoring, communication, nutrition, and protection from further injury.

Monitoring needs have been previously outlined. The systems most vulnerable during the critical care phase are the cardiovascular, respiratory, and renal systems. Communication with older patients is likely to be much more difficult than usual. In addition to potential problems associated with artificial airways, the older person may have a communication impediment as a result of diminished hearing and vision. This, along with sensory overload, loss of short-term memory, and delays in information processing, calls for special attention to communication strategies.

Communication Strategies

The first rule for communication is gain the individual's attention. Verbal communication begins with facing the individual. Language should be kept in simple terms, spoken slowly in lower tones, and repeated frequently. If a hearing deficit is determined, speaking into the better ear may be helpful. Speech should be clearly enunciated in a volume loud enough to be audible. Beware of shouting, since this tends to garble spoken words. The nurse should identify herself clearly and often. Nurses should verify that the patient heard what was spoken, since hearing losses may cause spoken words to sound garbled to the patient. Verify the content of spoken messages. Communication techniques should be included in the written care plan to foster consistency in methods of approach and to provide a data base from which potential changes in approach can be determined.

Use touch as a form of communication. It reinforces verbal communication and can convey caring and worth as well as comfort. Older persons are often deprived of this form of communication, since their perception of touch may be decreased, and there exists a tendency to avoid touching the older person.

Visual communication may consist of written materials, but it is often more subtle, such as facial expressions. Visual communication extends into the physical environment as well, including, perhaps, family pictures and other objects within the visual field. Maintaining constancy in the physical environment helps convey a sense of respect for the individual and helps improve orientation. While this may be difficult for the staff, it is beneficial for the patient. Bright lighting helps compensate for losses of visual acuity and may help reduce nighttime disorientation.

Nutritional Strategies

Providing for the nutritional needs of critically ill trauma patients can be vexing at best. If age, infirmity, and poverty combine to produce prior undernutrition, significant modifications in care plans are indicated. Present needs must be met, and prior deficits must be corrected.

Initially, intravenous feedings are indicated if the gastrointestinal system recovers function slowly. Decreases in gastric secretions and intestinal motility are features of aging that predispose the individual to intolerance of enteral feedings. Enteral feedings can be attempted once the patient recovers bowel sounds and movement. Caution should be used to ensure the airway is protected. Diminished sensitivity of the gag reflex increases aspiration potential, particularly if the level of consciousness is impaired. Resumption of diet will be addressed in the next section.

Infection Considerations

In addition to preventing cardiovascular and respiratory complications, the elderly patient has increased need for protection from infection. This includes monitoring vascular access sites and indwelling devices, such as urinary catheters and endotracheal tubes. Removal of such devices should be planned at the earliest opportunity. Older persons are very susceptible to pneumonia, as mentioned earlier, and to urinary tract infections secondary to placement of catheters and loss of mobility. They also exhibit increased incidence of wound infections.

Integumentary Considerations

Early mobilization of the older patient helps reduce the potential for integumentary injury. Aging reduces the elasticity of the skin, decreases the subcutaneous fat layer, and may reduce perfusion. The skin becomes vulnerable to pressure and abrasion, but breakdown can be prevented in most cases. Normal care of the aged skin includes minimal bathing, avoiding harsh soaps, use of lubricating lotions, and avoidance of abrasive and irritating materials. The patient's skin should be kept free from prolonged wetness (urinary incontinence) or prolonged contact with irritating secretions (fecal incontinence). To this should be added frequent changes in position in order to minimize pressure areas. Excessive reliance should not be placed on devices (e.g., foam pads or rings) to minimize pressure. If the patient is not capable of moving independently, nursing care plans should be modified to assist in position changes.

Modification of Goals

Advancing age has been called a time when the major goal in life is learning to live with losses. It is also a time when attitudes, goals, and values undergo significant revision. Nurses in critical care units also must revise their values for patient outcomes and modify goals of patient care accordingly.

It is of particular importance that the patient and family be directly involved in the care planning process. Since the goals usually set for younger people may not be achievable in the aged, more effort must be placed on determining the goals of individual patients. Following a hip fracture, for example, an older person may expect to walk with a cane and be satisfied with this achievement. On the other hand, the patient may know friends who have been placed in nursing homes after fractures and may perceive death as a better goal. Talking with the patient and with the family helps elucidate attitudes and values that underlie the direction for care planning.

The foundation for rehabilitation of the patient is developed during the critical care phase. Assessment of the potential for return of function is shared with the patient and family in a realistic manner. Advising them of available health care support services allows them time to investigate and to begin necessary arrangements. For the patient and family, this is a time to concentrate on short-term goals. Both may be discouraged when anticipating a long recovery period.

Primary attention should be placed on maintaining function as near to the preinjury state as possible. Emphasis on prevention of complications and early mobility is needed. When the stress of critical care is eased, more specific objectives can be defined.

Unfortunately many of the elderly do not recover from injuries. Epidemiologists have shown that nonsurvivors tend to die in the critical care unit after a prolonged stay. Oreskovich and associates[7] found that the average stay before death was 16.3 days. When the prognosis and outlook are poor, the attitudes and values toward death need to be determined. For some, "death with dignity" is paramount; for others, it is a need to feel that everything possible was done. Often the patient cannot be consulted, so the family is the main source of information. However, the family should be encouraged to consider the expressed wishes of the individual as well as their own desires. It behooves the health care team to respect these wishes when they no longer can offer a reasonable chance of recovery. At the same time, the team must resist the temptation to develop a negative outlook based primarily on the age of the patient. Recall that the average life expectancy of a 75-year-old is an additional 9.1 years.

INTERMEDIATE CARE AND REHABILITATION

Once the patient is removed from the critical care environment, plans for return to the community and/or rehabilitation become more specific. Assessment of the potential for return to the preinjury functional state should be completed. Correction of underlying problems secondary to chronic disease or nutritional deficits should be accomplished and support services mobilized.

The key to assessment at this stage is determination of the degree of change in function from the preinjury state. This assessment should include the patient's attitude, participation in the activities of daily living, mobility, social activities, and the type of support systems available. Comparison of preinjury function with the limitations imposed by the type and nature of present injuries permits the formulation of initial rehabilitation goals. When formulating these goals, it is best to recall that many of the aged cannot return to their prior functional state. This is most true for those who have sustained fractures in the lower extremities. The best prognostic indicator at this time seems to be activity and independence of the person before injury, along with the patient's outlook toward life.[14] The active aged have the best chance of returning to an independent state. However, Oreskovich and associates[7] found that only 8 per cent of those over 70 years of age regained independence following severe injuries. Seventy-two per cent of the patients in this study required full nursing care 1 year postinjury.

Steffl[47] has tabulated a list of feelings and behaviors that are useful in psychosocial assessment (Table 27–4). These are listed as positive behaviors that correlate with an improved mental and emotional outlook and behavioral disabilities. Using this framework as a tool, nursing is in a position to document those factors which contribute to or hinder the return of the elderly to a functional state.

Correction of underlying problems associated with chronic disease helps prepare the patient for discharge. Some of the aged have not been under regular physician care before injury. This can mean the discovery of health deficits that were previously unknown. When indicated, initial therapy can be started. Alternative discharge plans should include referral to the appropriate health care providers. The team should be alert to conditions such as diabetes, hypothyroidism, and carcinoma, which may be discovered in this manner.

Nutritional evaluation should not be limited to the hospital course. Estimation of prior status can give clues to preexisting problems, whether of a financial or a social nature. In this case, nutritional management must attempt to correct past as well as present deficits.

Cadigan[48] lists potential obstacles to adequate nutrition in the elderly, including physiological changes, psychosocial factors, and sensory alterations. Inadequate nutrition may be related to limited income, decreased function of the special senses (especially taste), social isolation, medication use, and/or depression and loneliness. Dietary patterns are also governed by social and cultural values that tend to be fixed in the older person. When assessment reveals an underlying problem, this must be included in the nutritional plan for the individual.

In general, baseline nutritional requirements should be age adjusted to the reduced needs of the older person.[48] To this baseline should be added increased nutritional requirements imposed by recovery from acute injury (see Chapter 14).

TABLE 27–4. PSYCHOSOCIAL ASSESSMENT CONSIDERATIONS

BEHAVIORAL DISABILITIES TO LOOK FOR AND RECORD	POSITIVE BEHAVIORS TO LOOK FOR AND RECORD
Forgetful	Communicates easily
Communicates with difficulty	Seems satisfied with self
Periods of agitation	Finds things to keep busy
Periods of depression	Wants to do for others
Wanders off	Likes to reminisce about good things of the past
Nuisance to neighbors	Talks about self and family
Drinking problem (social setting upset)	Curious—wants to know what is going on
Panics readily	Sometimes critical of younger generation
Loses personal belongings (money, glasses)	Well groomed
Fire and burn hazard	Has a routine
Severe and specific fears	Enjoys eating
Hallucinations and delusions	Makes plans for the future
Spends time in bed	Creative
Signs of deterioration in personal habits:	Strives to maintain leadership/ responsibility
1. Incontinence of bladder	Interested, active—a doer
2. Incontinence of bowels	Friendly—outgoing
3. Perspiration odor	Smiles a lot
4. Clothing soiled	Jokes with workers
5. Hair uncombed	Responds to friendly approach
6. Fingernails long and dirty	Shares freely
Short tempered and irritable	Reads the paper
Withdrawn from surroundings—passive	Interested in mail
Dependent—repeatedly asks for help	Writes letters and cards
Submissive—excessive capitulation to suggestion	Sometimes sings and/or whistles
Hostile, challenging	Good appetite—enjoys eating
Nervous, tense, "jumpy," anxious	Reaches out for touch and has warm personal touch
Ashamed of, and tries to hide, disability	Concerned about governmental affairs
Indecisive, uncertain, hesitant	Copes with limitations
Demanding—constantly seeks attention	
Overly affectionate	
Domineering, dogmatic	
Nagging dissenter; objects, complains	
Unrealistic, immature	
Lonely	
Negative, rejecting	
Suspicious, distrustful of others	

Adapted from Steffl BM: Handbook of Gerontological Nursing, New York, Van Nostrand Reinhold, 1984, p 46.

Nursing Management

The patient's needs for communication become, if anything, more important at this time. It is likely that verbal methods will be used more often at this stage. Continuing care should be taken to verify that the patient understands what is said. Lighting should be sufficiently bright so that the patient can see who is talking. This will also help the patient remain oriented to the physical environment.

Loss of short-term memory will continue to require frequent repetition of instructions and communication that orients the patient. Plans for moving the patient should be communicated early to allow the patient time to adjust. Constancy of the physical environment is more important as the patient becomes increasingly aware. Tables, chairs, and other items become part of the patient's personal space and contribute to orientation as well as a sense of security. They should remain in the same location or be returned if they must be moved.

Once the dietary requirements are determined, attention to the particular likes and dislikes of the individual can help ensure adequate intake. Frequent small feedings may be better tolerated than traditional meals. When indicated, the family can contribute foods prepared at home. Meals should provide a variety of tastes, textures, and colors but be limited in the amount of salt and sugar. Meals also should be enjoyed in the company of others whenever possible.

Loneliness, fear, and depression often accompany the hospitalization of the older person. The availability of support systems for the patient should be determined. These might include family, local church or civic groups, or friends and neighbors. Visitors can help alleviate some of the sense of isolation the patient may feel.

Rehabilitation goals for the patient are continued through the intermediate cycle of care. The goals for older persons are often not the same as those for younger patients. Restoration of "normal" function is often not possible, so emphasis should be placed on achieving the maximum function possible. Age should not be a cause to deny the patient maximum benefit to be achieved from rehabilitation.

Achievement of rehabilitation goals must include the family and/or other support systems throughout the planning stages. Assessment of the family's ability to assist in care needed by the patient is crucial to the eventual placement of the patient. Consider the following questions. Will the patient require support in mobility, such as a walking device? Can the nutritional needs of the patient be met? Will there be assistance in complying with complicated medication regimens? The home environment is another consideration. Are modifications necessary? Can an elderly person manage such modifications financially?

Community Reintegration

The outlook for return of some elderly people to the community is not good. Oreskovich and associates[7] found that only 8 per cent of the elderly trauma victims returned to an independent life-style 1 year following severe injury. The majority (72 per cent) required full nursing care. Contrast this to the experience at the MIEMSS Shock Trauma Center,[29] where elderly trauma victims are often admitted with minimal injury and return home within 2 to 3 days.

The probable outcome for a given individual should be assessed early in the hospital course so that plans can be developed for alternative care if that proves necessary. For some, return to a home environment is likely. For others, it may be possible to provide limited assistance in the form of home health care as an alternative to placement in a long-term care facility.

Support systems that have been identified previously can be mobilized just prior to discharge. Health care teaching needs for professionals and nonprofessionals alike should be implemented early enough to allow time for assessment of learning. Written reinforcement of teaching should accompany the patient.

Part of the health care teaching should include measures that can be taken to prevent future injury. Assessment of the home environment by interview or by home health visits can help correct identified hazards. When financial considerations limit preventive strategies, social services may offer access to additional financial support.

NURSING RESEARCH IMPLICATIONS

Throughout this chapter the inadequacies of the data base for trauma in the elderly have been noted. With the possible exception of hip fractures, too little is known of how the elderly respond to injury to make possible more than theoretical or anecdotal recommendations for nursing care. As the number of elderly people increases, there is an even greater need for guidance in the care of these patients. Epidemiologists have described the problem in terms of incidence and expense, but they offer little clinical data. If trauma is today's neglected disease, then trauma to the elderly is yet to be recognized as a problem. The need for systematic research of a descriptive nature is widespread. The scope of research potential in this population can be best addressed by considering unanswered questions.

Still undefined in the realm of epidemiology are those questions dealing with the mechanism of injury. We know that falls are the most common mechanism, but less clear are the circumstances surrounding them. How many falls (or other injuries) are related to age alone? Are injuries often or seldom preceded by transient losses of consciousness? What is the relationship between injury and psychosocial factors? Do falls precede admission to nursing homes? Are they causally related to nutritional status, thermoregulation, or osteoporosis? What environmental factors are associated with injury? How does the preinjury functional status compare with that of those who are not injured?

With regard to injury severity, what role does chronic disease play? How shall chronic disease be measured? Are there differences in injury severity or response to injury between those who fall and those injured in motor vehicle accidents? Are the disabled more prone to injury than the active? Do the elderly actually succumb to injuries of low severity, as it appears, and if so, why? What factors contribute to the apparent poor return to the preinjury functional level? Is there a time in health care when the wisest action is no action at all? Should a goal of health care include attention to the quality of life to which the patient returns?

These questions and many more need to be answered before looking to the possibilities for therapy. Currently, the need for descriptive data is paramount. It is not possible to consider alternative therapy for the elderly until we have a better grasp on how they differ from younger trauma patients.

Once the data base is large enough, attention can be turned to modifications of therapy. For now it is not possible to do more than hypothesize changes that appear to be indicated by aging changes in function.

PREVENTION

Data available from studies of accidental injury show that the elderly have a high risk of death from three major causes: falls, motor vehicle injuries, and thermal injuries.[13] Accidental injury is the fifth leading cause of death in the elderly population.[6] Evidence is also present that the cost of treatment is higher for the elderly than for the young but that the outcome may be less satisfactory.[7] Since most "accidents" are not accidents at all, prevention of injury should be a priority for health care professionals.

Public health history indicates that individual change is the prevention strategy least likely to succeed.[27] A more successful approach includes environmental modification and modification of support systems. Nurses can participate in public decisions through professional organizations and legislative action.

Despite the fact that modification of the individual has the least potential for success, there are situations when this is the only available approach. The foundation of patient teaching rests on the professional's ability to persuade an individual to change. Education and training of the elderly individual are complicated by health, financial limitations, values, and attitudes that make change difficult to accomplish.

Prevention of Falls

Factors that increase the probability of falls in the elderly include deterioration in health, physical changes associated with aging (e.g., loss of visual acuity), use of prosthetic devices (e.g., canes, walkers), and environmental hazards (e.g., slippery surfaces, stairs, poor lighting, unexpected objects in walkways).

Physical changes and deterioration in health increase the vulnerability of the elderly person to falling and to injury as a result of a fall. Correction of underlying deficits can lessen the chance of a fall when there is a medical condition predisposing the individual. For example, placement of a pacemaker can eliminate syncope from some cardiac dysrhythmias. Better information on the benefits of diet and exercise also may be useful in reducing the frequency of falls. When walking devices are necessary, the patient should receive instruction on proper use and be advised as to how tripping can occur.

Home and public environments are not designed with the elderly in mind. To lessen the chances of falls, floor surfaces should be covered with nonslip materials and handgrips provided on both sides of walkways. Handgrips are especially helpful in bathrooms. Floors and stairs can be covered with resilient materials that lessen the chance of injury if a fall occurs. Improved lighting in hallways and on stairs helps the elderly avoid tripping. Lighting should be concentrated on landings, where falls are most likely to occur. Lighting should provide uniform levels so that the elderly do not have to make rapid visual adjustments to variable light intensity.

Prevention of Motor Vehicle Accidents

The most effective reduction in morbidity and mortality associated with motor vehicle injury comes from engineering of the vehicle and the environment. Recommendations for changes have been documented elsewhere.[27] Driver and pedestrian modifications are less effective in producing change in the population, but nurses can have an impact on individuals.

Most elderly pedestrians are injured at intersections and most often by vehicles turning right rather than left.[27] Education of elderly pedestrians, and drivers in general, can increase their awareness of the potential problems. The elderly should be alerted to driver behaviors, such as turning right on red without looking for pedestrians, that increase the risk of collisions. The pedestrian walking at night also should wear light-colored clothing or reflective material to increase his visibility to drivers.

Elderly drivers tend to voluntarily restrict their driving to familiar conditions and daytime hours. This behavior can be encouraged in the individual. Training in defensive driving skills also may be of benefit to the older driver. As important, perhaps, is education of younger drivers to the behaviors of elderly drivers. Emphasis should be placed on use of seatbelts or other safety devices to reduce mortality and injury.

Prevention of Burns

A frequent cause of burns in the elderly is hot liquid. Many of these injuries are caused by tap water whose temperature exceeds 130°F. This temperature is enough to produce a full-thickness burn in 30 seconds.[27] The simple reduction in hot water heater temperatures to 120°F or less can reduce the frequency and/or severity of scalds. Hot liquids from cooking are another source of potential burn wounds. Use of special aprons and specially designed containers while cooking has been recommended as a prevention strategy.[27]

Causes of flame injuries include smoking, open flames (gas stoves), and house fires. The elderly are overrepresented in the burn fatalities from house fires,[13] possibly because they are less able to remove themselves once fire starts. Smoke detectors should be required in all elderly housing, along with use of flame retardant materials in construction and furnishings. The elderly homeowner should be cautioned against household storage of flammable materials, such as old newspapers and gasoline. Lastly, smoking in bed should be eliminated.

SUMMARY

In a health care environment in which initial care is based on rapid institution of protocols, the elderly trauma patient presents a unique challenge to the nurse. Not only are usual protocols in question for this patient population, but variability among individuals is greater with advancing age. The challenge is to provide essential care while drawing on a limited data base.

The elderly offer the nurse a true opportunity to individualize nursing care plans. They present with a great potential for altered responses to trauma. This may be only as a result of normal aging, or it may reflect the impact of chronic disease on the response to stress. Because little guidance is available from experience or from the literature, the nurse must institute an intense degree of monitoring to detect those deviations from the expected norms that characterize the elderly individual. The nurse also must be prepared to modify care plans based on the findings of assessment and the responses of the individual patient.

This patient population also offers nearly unlimited potential for the nurse researcher. Few descriptions of the elderly individual's response to trauma are available. Differences between the young and the old must be documented before changes in therapy can be explored. Methods for determining the impact of chronic disease need to be explored. Once the descriptive data base is adequate, the most effective methods for treating the elderly trauma patient can be tested. Until that time, the nurse must depend on the gerontologist to supplement knowledge regarding the effects of trauma.

REFERENCES

1. United States Bureau of the Census: Current population reports (Series P-70, Household Economic Studies). Washington, DC, U.S. Government Printing Office, 1984.
2. Neugarten BL, Havighurst RJ: Aging and the future. In Neugarten BL, Havighurst RJ (eds): Social Policy, Social Ethics, and the Aging Society. Washington, DC, U.S. Government Printing Office, 1976, pp 3–7.
3. Baker SP, O'Neill B, Karph RS: The Injury Fact Book. Lexington, MA, Lexington Books, 1985.
4. National Safety Council: Accident Facts. Chicago, National Safety Council, 1981.
5. National Safety Council: Accident Facts. Chicago, National Safety Council, 1989.
6. Baker SP, O'Neill B, Haddon W, et al: The Injury Severity Score: A method for describing patients with multiple injuries and evaluating emergency care. J Trauma 14:187–196, 1974.
7. Oreskovich MR, Howard JD, Copass MK, et al: Geriatric trauma: Injury patterns and outcome. J Trauma 24:565–572, 1984.
8. Horst HM, Obeid FN, Sorensen VJ: Factors influencing survival of elderly trauma patients. Crit Care Med 14:681–684, 1986.
9. Osler T, Hales K, Baack B, et al: Trauma in the elderly. Am J Surg 156:537–543, 1988.
10. Finelli FC, Jonsson J, Champion HC, et al: A case control study for major trauma in geriatric patients. J Trauma 29:541–548, 1989.
11. Smith DP, Enderson BL, Maull KL: Trauma in the elderly: Determinants of outcome. South Med J 83:171–177, 1990.
12. Hielema FJ: Epidemiology of hip fracture. Phys Ther 59:1221–1225, 1979.
13. Hogue CC: Injury in late life: Epidemiology. J Am Geriatr Soc 30:183–190, 1982.
14. Nickens HW: A review of factors affecting the occurrence and outcome of hip fracture, with special reference to psychosocial issues. J Am Geriatr Soc 31:166–170, 1983.
15. Prudham D, Evans JG: Factors associated with falls in the elderly: A community study. Age Aging 10:141–146, 1981.
16. Waller JA: Injury in aged. NY State J Med 74:2200–2208, 1974.
17. Tinker GM: Accidents in a geriatric assessment department. Age Aging 7:196–198, 1978.
18. Sheldon JH: On the natural history of falls in old age. Br Med J 2:1685–1690, 1960.
19. Allen JE, Schwab CW: Blunt chest trauma in the elderly. Am Surg 51:697–700, 1985.
20. Bobb JK: A descriptive study of the impact of injury sustained by persons age 55 years and older in road traffic accidents. Unpublished Master's thesis, University of Maryland, 1986.
21. Degutis LC, Baker CC: Trauma in the elderly: A statewide perspective. Conn Med 51:161–164, 1987.
22. DeMaria EJ, Kenny PR, Merriam MA, et al: Aggressive trauma care benefits the elderly. J Trauma 27:1200–1206, 1987.
23. DeMaria EJ, Kenny PR, Merriam MA, et al: Survival after trauma in geriatric patients. Ann Surg 206:738–743, 1987.
24. Martin RE, Teberian G: Multiple trauma and the elderly patient. Emerg Med Clin North Am 8:411–420, 1990.
25. Scalea TM, Simon HM, Duncan AO, et al: Geriatric blunt multiple trauma: Improved survival with early invasive monitoring. J Trauma 30:129–136, 1990.
26. Reidenberg MM: Drug interactions and the elderly. J Am Geriatr Soc 30:S67–S70, 1982.
27. Waller PF: Preventing injuries to the elderly. In Phillips HT, Gaylord SA (eds): Aging and Public Health. New York, Springer, 1985.
28. DelGuercio LR, Cohn JD: Monitoring operative risk in the elderly. JAMA 243:1350–1355, 1980.
29. Bobb JK: Trauma in the elderly. J Gerontol Nurs 13:8–31, 1987.
30. Praiss IL, Feller I, James MM: The planning and organization of a regionalized burn care system. Med Care 18:202–210, 1980.
31. Gill W, Long WB: Shock Trauma Manual. Baltimore, Williams & Wilkins, 1979.
32. Cox EF: Blunt abdominal trauma. Ann Surg 199:467–474, 1979.
33. Kannel WB, Brand F, McGee D: Hypertension in the elderly. In Cape RDT, Coe RM, Rossman I (eds): Fundamentals of Geriatric Medicine. New York, Raven Press, 1983, pp 275–285.
34. Moser M: The management of cardiovascular disease in the elderly. J Am Geriatr Soc 30:S20–S29, 1982.
35. Astrand I, Astrand PO, Hallback I, et al: Reduction in maximal oxygen uptake with age. J Appl Physiol 35:649–654, 1973.
36. Seimon LP: Complaints related to the spine. In Cape RDT, Coe RM, Rossman I (eds): Fundamentals of Geriatric Medicine. New York, Raven Press, 1983, pp 163–170.
37. Papper S: The effects of age in reducing renal function. Geriatrics 28:83–86, 1973.
38. Avakian EV, Horvath SM: Influence of aging and thyroxine hydroxylase inhibition on tissue levels of norepinephrine during stress. J Gerontol 37:257–261, 1982.
39. Elahi D, Miller DC, Tzankoff SP, et al: Effect of age and obesity on fasting levels of glucose, insulin, glucagon, and growth hormone in man. J Gerontol 37:385–389, 1982.
40. Green MF: The endocrine system. In Pathy MSJ (ed): Principles and Practice of Geriatric Medicine. New York, Wiley, 1985, pp 909–973.
41. Goldman R: Aging changes in structure and function. In Carnevale D, Patrick M (eds): Nursing Management for the Elderly. Philadelphia, JB Lippincott, 1986, pp 73–101.
42. Shock NW: Aging of regulatory mechanisms. In Cape RDT, Coe RM, Rossman I (eds): Fundamentals of Geriatric Medicine, New York, Raven Press, 1983.
43. Bastow MD, Rawlings J, Allison SP: Undernutrition, hypothermia, and injury in elderly women with fractured femur: An injury response to altered metabolism? Lancet 1:143–144, 1983.
44. Mohr DN: Estimation of surgical risk in the elderly. J Am Geriatr Soc 31:99–102, 1983.
45. Seymour DG, Pringle R: Postoperative complications in the elderly surgical patient. Gerontology 29:262–270, 1983.
46. McLean RF, McIntosh JD, Kung GY, et al: Outcome of respiratory intensive care for the elderly. Crit Care Med 13:625–629, 1985.
47. Steffl BM: Handbook of Gerontological Nursing. New York, Van Nostrand Reinhold, 1984.
48. Cadigan M: Nutrition and the elderly. In Steffl BM (ed): Handbook of Gerontological Nursing. New York, Van Nostrand Reinhold, 1984.

28

THERMAL INJURIES

JANET MARVIN

CARE OF THE BURN-INJURED PATIENT

Advances in the care of the burn-injured patient have improved survival significantly in the last 30 years. In the early 1960s, a patient with a 50 per cent total body surface area (TBSA) burn had only a 30 to 40 per cent chance of survival. In the 1990s, a patient with a 50 per cent TBSA burn has at least a 70 to 80 per cent chance of survival. In specialized centers, older children and young adults with greater than 80 per cent TBSA burns routinely survive. The advances that have led to this improved survival are legion. Some of the more significant ones are improved methods of resuscitation, infection control, surgical management, nutritional support, pulmonary support, and the development of biologic and synthetic wound covers. Along with these are more global advances, such as improved critical care techniques, safe blood supply, and increased knowledge of the mechanisms of wound healing.

PATHOPHYSIOLOGY OF BURN INJURY

Tissue Injury

Tissue injury in burns is related to the coagulation of cellular protein as a result of heat produced by thermal, chemical, electrical, or radiation energy. The coagulation associated with thermal injury is related to the temperature of the wounding agent and the length of exposure to a given temperature. This is demonstrated in Figure 28–1.[1] The coagulation associated with chemical injuries is related to the type, strength, concentration, duration of contact, and mechanism of action. The chemical agents may be divided into several groups depending on the mechanism by which they coagulate protein.[2] Table 28–1 shows the chemicals within the various groups and the mechanism by which these chemicals cause coagulation.

Electrical injury is produced by the conversion of electrical energy into heat and from the direct physicochemical effects of electric current on tissue. Two laws govern the relationship

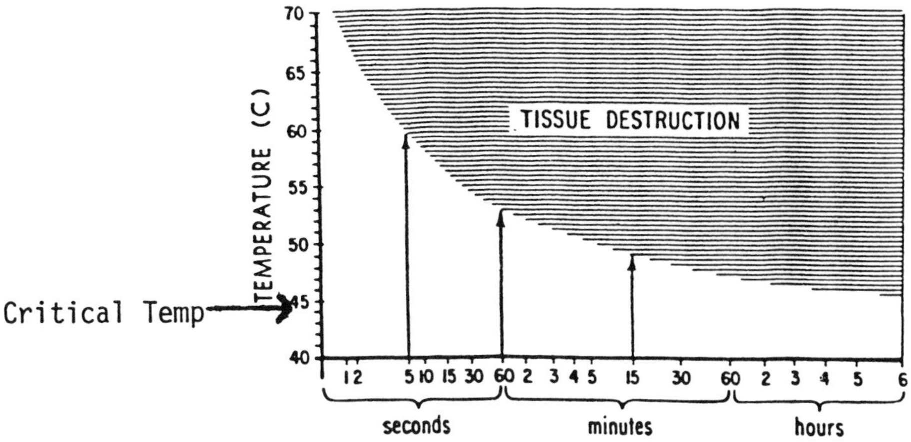

Figure 28–1. Temperature duration curve. Tissue destruction proceeds logarithmically with increasing temperatures as a function of time exposure. (From Robson MC, Kucan JO: The burn wound. *In* Wachtel TL, Kahn V, Frank HA (eds): Current Topics in Burn Care. Rockville, MD, Aspen Publications, 1983, p. 56.)

between electric current and injury. Ohm's law describes the relationship between current flow (amperage), potential difference (voltage), and resistance (current = voltage/resistance). Thus the amount of current flowing in a circuit is directly proportional to voltage and inversely proportional to resistance. Joule's law states that the quantity of heat produced by an electric current is directly proportional to the square of the current, the resistance of the conductor, and the duration of contact. Each type of tissue within the body absorbs the heat energy according to its own electrical resistance. Studies of tissue injury from heat show that neural derangement and irreversible coagulation occur at a temperature around 45°C.[3] High-voltage current can produce tissue temperatures in excess of 80°C. In addition to the heat injury, electric current can produce tissue injury by causing movement of intercellular and extracellular ions and polarization of large, electrically charged molecules.[4]

Tissue coagulation is the irreversible effect of tissue injury and results in full-thickness injury. Jackson's description of the zonal concept shows that not all heat injury results in coagulation.[5] As seen in Figure 28–2, the burn wound is conceptualized in three zones. The center-most zone is the *zone of coagulation* and would represent an area of the burn where the tissue temperature reached at least 45°C. The adjacent area is considered the *zone of stasis*. This zone may not show areas of coagulation initially but may proceed to a zone of coagulation over the initial 24 hours. Although providing adequate fluid resuscitation and maintaining normal tissue oxygenation may limit this progression in some injuries, the complex interaction of the prostaglandins, thromboxanes, and other active tissue agents may participate in this progressive coagulation despite adequate resuscitative measures. The outer zone is called the *zone of hyperemia* and has sustained minimal injury. This zone will usually heal very rapidly.

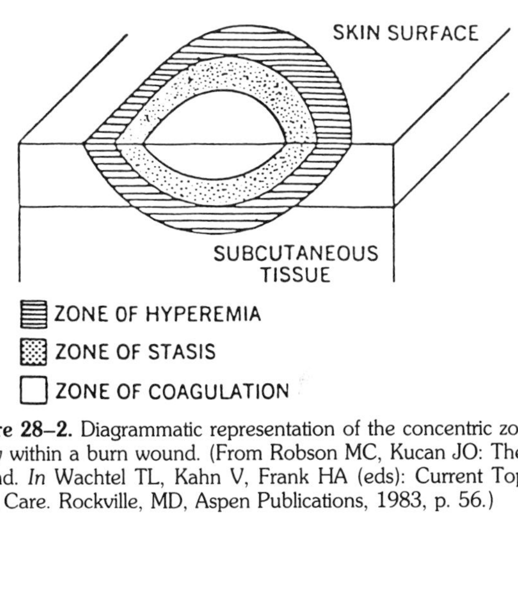

Figure 28–2. Diagrammatic representation of the concentric zones of injury within a burn wound. (From Robson MC, Kucan JO: The burn wound. *In* Wachtel TL, Kahn V, Frank HA (eds): Current Topics in Burn Care. Rockville, MD, Aspen Publications, 1983, p. 56.)

TABLE 28–1. CLASSIFICATION OF CHEMICAL AGENTS AND THE RESULTANT CAUSE OF INJURY

CHEMICAL AGENTS	REACTION RESULTING IN COAGULATION
Oxidizing agents	Oxidization
Chromic acid	
Sodium hypochlorite	
Potassium permanganate	
Corrosives	Denaturization
Phenol	
White phosphorus	
Dichromate salts	
Lye	
Desiccants	Severe cellular dehydration
Sulfuric acid	
Muriatic acid	
Vesicants	Produce blisters and release tissue amines, producing local anoxic tissue damage
Cantharides	
Dimethyl sulfoxide (DMSO)	
Poisonous gases (warfare chemicals)	
Protoplasmic poison	Produce coagulation by forming salts or binding cations, thus impairing cellular function
Formic acid	
Acetic acid	
Cresylic acid	
Trichloroacetic acid	
Tannic acid	
Sulfosalicylic acid	
Tungstic acid	
Oxalic acid	
Hydrofluoric acid	
Hydrochloric acid	

Extent and Depth of Injury

Two important concepts in the clinical diagnosis and management of burn injuries are the extent and depth of thermal injury. The *extent of burn* refers to the total surface area of injured tissue. This is usually calculated as percentage of TBSA using either the Berkow,[6] Lund and Browder,[7] or rule of nines[8] formula. The rule of nines is an easy-to-remember, rapid, gross estimate of the extent of burn. The body is divided into seven areas which represent 9 per cent or multiples of 9 per cent of the body surface area, with the remaining area, the genitalia, representing 1 per cent TBSA (Fig. 28–3). Both the Berkow and the Lund and Browder charts divide the body into multiple areas and take into consideration the changes in the contribution of the head and lower extremities over the age range from infancy to adulthood (Fig. 28–4). The extent of body surface area injured is important both as a predictor of morbidity/survival and also as a predictor of the physiological response in relation to fluid shifts initially and, later, to the metabolic and immunological responses.

Also, the concept of depth of injury is an important predictor of survival as well as overall morbidity, including surgical management, functional outcome, and cosmesis. Descriptions of the depth of burn are often confusing because a variety of nomenclature is used (Table 28–2). In general, the more shallow the wound depth, the more rapidly the wound heals, which results in less scarring. In addition, the more superficial the wound, the more likely the patient with a very extensive burn will survive.

Tissue Injury and the Immunological Response

In the last decade, much knowledge has been generated about the relationship of tissue injury and immunological function. Recent work in the histochemical response to tissue injury has further elucidated the mechanisms of inflammation, infection, sepsis, sepsis syndrome, and multiorgan system (MOS) failure. The tissue injury related to burns not only refers to the local response of the coagulation produced by heat but also to the systemic responses that lead to inflammation, fluid shifts, and ultimately to multiorgan system failure without proper treatment. Early work in burn research led to an understanding of how local inflammatory processes resulted in fluid shifts and burn shock if untreated. Figure 28–5 is a simplistic diagramatic representation of the local and systemic factors that result in burn shock. Although this initial cardiovascular response to the burn injury may be corrected with fluid resuscitation, the local inflammatory effects of the wound continue to interact with the body's host defense response. The beneficial aspects of this reaction prevent local and systemic sepsis.

However, not all the effects of the inflammatory response are beneficial. Pathophysiological effects related to thermal injury of the skin may be both local and systemic. Ward and Till have elucidated some of the local pathophysiological responses in rats.[9] As has been shown previously, the progressive vascular permeability is associated with complement activation and histamine release (Fig. 28–6). Ward and Till have further described the interaction of histamine with xanthine oxidase to enhance the release of the toxic oxygen products of xanthine oxidase. This causes the release of superoxides (O_2^-), H_2O_2, and its conversion products, the hydroxyl radical (HO), with resultant microvascular injury to endothelial cells and edema formation. In the future, as this response is better understood in humans, the local pathophysiological effects of histamine release, complement activation, and xanthine oxidase conversion may be prevented by the administration of inhibitors of xanthine oxidase such as allopurinol and lodoxamide or hydroxyl radical scavengers such as DMSO (dimethyl sulfoxide), DMTU (dimethylthiaurea), cimitadine, or similar agents.

Ward and Till have described similar systemic pathophysiological events associated with thermal injury of the skin. These systemic events are depicted in Figure 28–7 and are related to complement activation, especially C5a, which leads to activation of intravascular neutrophils. Neutrophil activation causes a respiratory burst and results in the generation of O_2^-, H_2O_2, and HO. The release of the oxygen radicals is thought to be the genesis of red blood cell lysis and pulmonary vascular endothelial cell injury, resulting in intravascular hemolysis, pulmonary interstitial edema, and intra-alveolar hemorrhage. As with the local pathophysiological effects, in the future, specific therapies to block complement activation or the effects of oxygen radicals may reduce or prevent the systemic immunological effects of tissue injury.

In addition to the complement-derived factors described by Ward and Till, nutritional factors and gut-derived factors also have been suggested by Alexander to exert a profound effect on the immune system.[10] The primary nutritional factor that negatively alters the immune response in burn patients

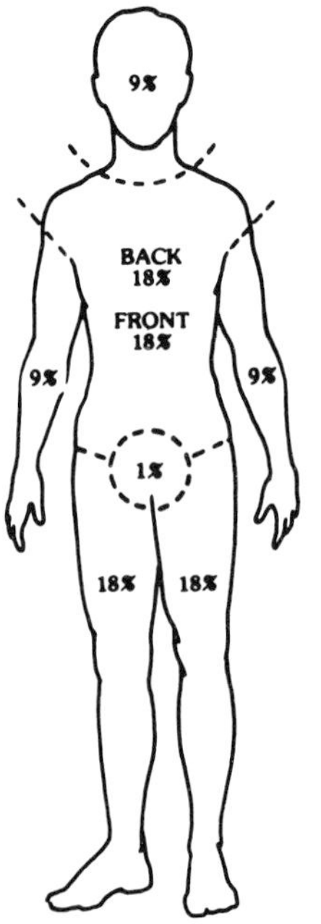

Figure 28–3. An estimate of the percentage of total body surface area (% TBSA) burned can be obtained using the "rule of nines," whereby TBSA is divided into nine per cent segments of total. Second- and third-degree burn is added and presented as a percentage of total skin. (From Boswick JA (ed): The Art and Science of Burn Care. Aspen Publications, Rockville, MD, 1987, p. 193.)

Area	Birth 1 yr.	1-4 yr.	5-9 yr.	10-14 yr.	15 yr.	Adult	2°	3°	Total	Donor Areas
Head	19	17	13	11	9	7				
Neck	2	2	2	2	2	2				
Ant. Trunk	13	13	13	13	13	13				
Post. Trunk	13	13	13	13	13	13				
R. Buttock	2½	2½	2½	2½	2½	2½				
L. Buttock	2½	2½	2½	2½	2½	2½				
Genitalia	1	1	1	1	1	1				
R. U. Arm	4	4	4	4	4	4				
L. U. Arm	4	4	4	4	4	4				
R. L. Arm	3	3	3	3	3	3				
L. L. Arm	3	3	3	3	3	3				
R. Hand	2½	2½	2½	2½	2½	2½				
L. Hand	2½	2½	2½	2½	2½	2½				
R. Thigh	5½	6½	8	8½	9	9½				
L. Thigh	5½	6½	8	8½	9	9½				
R. Leg	5	5	5½	6	6½	7				
L. Leg	5	5	5½	6	6½	7				
R. Foot	3½	3½	3½	3½	3½	3½				
L. Foot	3½	3½	3½	3½	3½	3½				
						TOTAL				

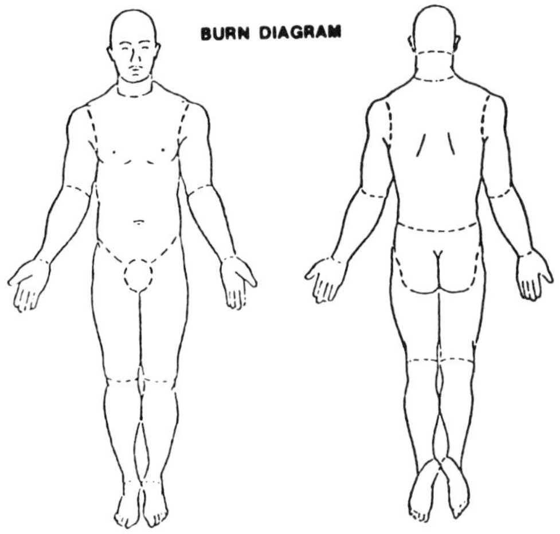

Figure 28–4. Lund and Browder method of calculating burn size. (Modified from Robson MC and Kucan JO: The burn wound. In Wachtel TL, Kahn V, Frank HA (eds): Current Topics in Burn Care. Rockville, MD, Aspen Publications, 1983, p. 56.)

TABLE 28–2. CLASSIFICATION OF BURN INJURY

BY DEPTH	FIRST DEGREE	SECOND DEGREE		THIRD DEGREE
By skin thickness	Superficial partial thickness	Moderate partial thickness	Deep partial thickness	Full thickness
By anatomic description	Epidermal	Superficial dermal	Deep dermal	Subdermal (fat, muscle, bone)
Appearance/diagnosis of depth	Pink to red; no blisters; skin remains intact when rubbed gently; may appear slightly edematous	Red or mottled red and pink; contains blisters; skin easily rubbed off; moist weeping, edematous; if pulled, hair remains intact; blanches with pressure	Pink to pale ivory; can see a reticulated pattern; wound may appear somewhat dry; contains blisters and bullae; hair removes easily; does not blanch with pressure or return of color is slow	White, cherry red, brown, or black; may or may not contain blisters; may contain thrombosed vessels; appears dry, hard, leathery; and may be depressed
Cause	Radiation (sunburn), flash from low-intensity explosion	Brief contact with hot liquids, steam, or hot objects; high-intensity flash	Longer contact with hot liquids or hot objects; chemicals; and brief contact with flames	Prolonged contact with hot liquids or objects; flames; chemicals; electrical
Pain response	Uncomfortable to touch	Very painful	Pain response variable; hyper- and hypoalgesia	Painless to pinprick; pain is aching in nature
Time to heal	3–5 days	<3 weeks	>3 weeks	Requires grafting

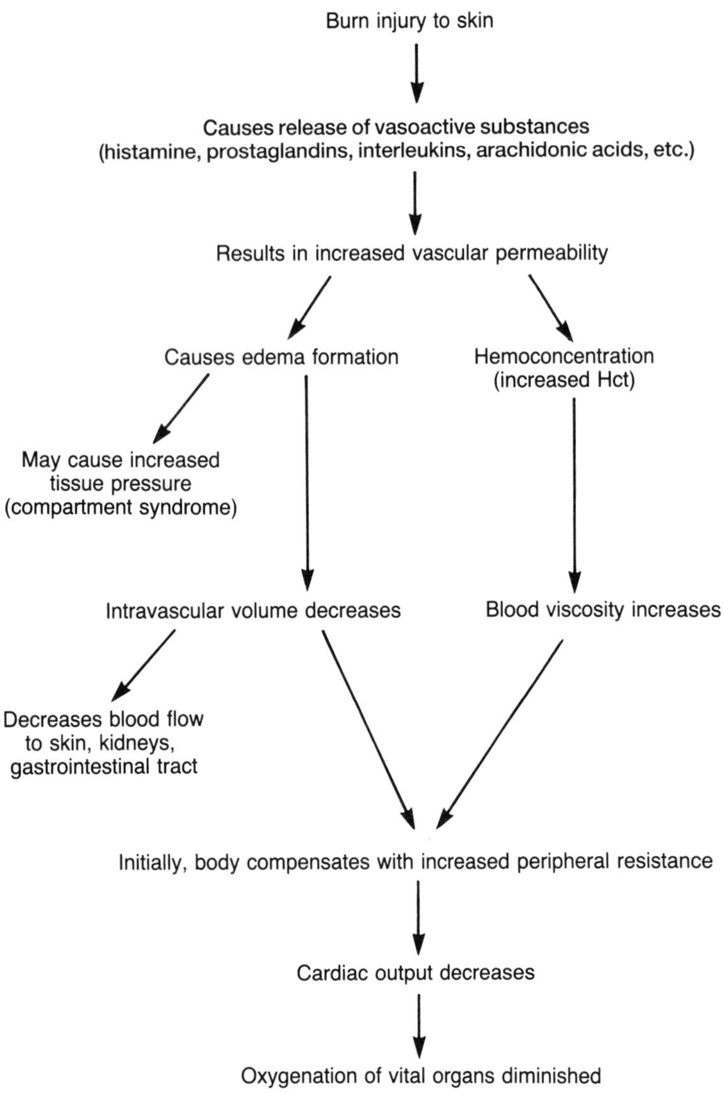

Figure 28–5. Physiological response to burned skin.

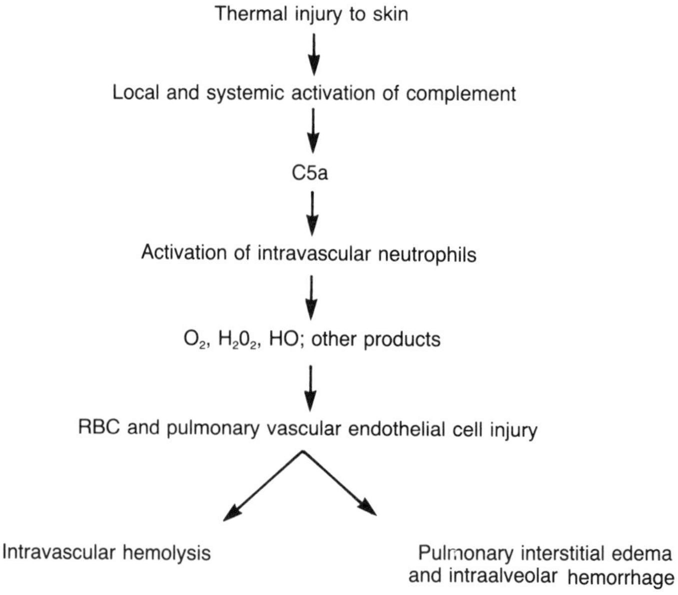

Figure 28–6. Remote pathologic events associated with thermal injury of skin. (From Ward PA, Till GO: Pathophysiological events related to thermal injury of the skin. J Trauma 30(12): 77, 1990. Copyright 1990 by the Williams & Wilkins Co., Baltimore, MD.)

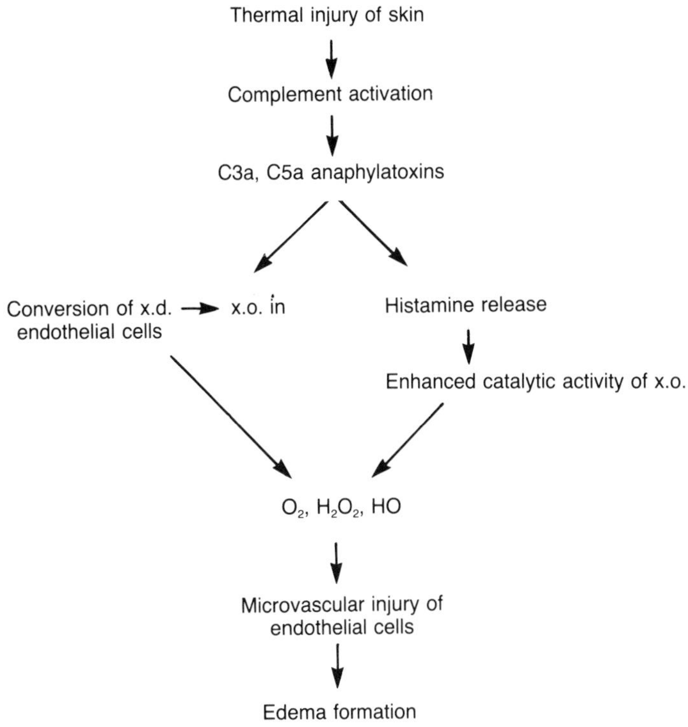

Figure 28–7. Local events associated with thermal injury of skin. (From Ward PA, Till GO: Pathophysiological events related to thermal injury of the skin. J Trauma 30(12):78, 1990. Copyright 1990 by the Williams & Wilkins Co., Baltimore, MD.)

is lipids of the omega-6 fatty acid series, such as linoleic acid. The omega-6 fatty acids have been shown to inhibit many immune functions related to delayed hypersensitivity responses and opsonic index. On the other hand, omega-3 fatty acids (fish oil) have been shown to improve immunological functions. Another nutritional factor that improves immune function, releases growth hormone, and stimulates wound healing is arginine. When these nutritional concepts were incorporated into a new enteral feeding formula and compared with Osmolite (Ross Laboratories), Promix (Corpak), and Traumacal (Mead Johnson), the occurrence of wound infection and the average length of stay, as expressed in days of hospitalization per per cent burn, were significantly decreased using the new formula.[11] This new diet incorporated 2 per cent of energy from arginine, 20 per cent of energy from whey protein, and 12 per cent of energy from lipids, comprised equally of safflower oil (rich in omega-6 fatty acid) and fish oil (rich in omega-3 fatty acids). It contained the same amount of protein as the other formulas with which it was compared; thus the difference could be attributed to arginine and the lipid mixture.

Translocation of gut microbes and endotoxin has been shown to occur rapidly after burn injury and lead to activation of macrophages, neutrophils, the arachidonic acid pathway, the complement cascade, the production of cytokines, the generation of proteases, and stimulation of the metabolic response, all of which adversely affect the immune response.[10] Recent work by Moore and associates has shown that enteral feeding is superior to intravenous feeding in patients with abdominal trauma in reducing sepsis.[12] Inoue and associates demonstrated that a single enteral feeding results in prevention of yeast translocation in animals with burn injury.[13] Thus early enteral feedings are currently recommended in burn patients. As noted in this brief review, a variety of immunological abnormalities can be attributed to the nutritional intake of adequate calories and specific nutrients and route of administration.

Metabolic Response to Tissue Injury

The metabolic response to burn injury has been studied extensively over the past three decades. As early as 1930, Cuthbertson described the metabolic response to injury.[14] He noted that there were increased urinary nitrogen losses as well as losses of other intracellular substances such as potassium and phosphorus. Over the years, the study of the catabolic response to injury has been fascinating. Numerous studies have documented increased oxygen consumption, negative nitrogen balance, and excessive muscle wasting and weight loss in these patients. Early work ruled out hyperthyroidism as the reason for increased oxygen consumption and related the response to increased activity of the sympathetic nervous system.[15, 16] Caldwell and associates[17] and Barr and associates[18] explored the question of whether the elevated heat production was related to the thermoregulatory response to the increased evaporative heat losses from the wound surface. Although increasing the environmental temperatures to thermoneutral levels and decreasing the ambient humidity showed a substantial reduction in basal metabolic rates with increased evaporation of water from the burn surface, subsequent studies by Zawacki and associates[19] and Wilmore and associates[20] suggest that evaporative cooling from the burn wound is not the major factor in the hypermetabolic response to thermal injury. This led Wilmore to deduce that "although there may be thermal regulatory influences on burn hypermetabolism, the increased rate of heat production is primarily determined by metabolic factors: that is, *burn hypermetabolism is temperature-sensitive, but not tempera-*

TABLE 28–3. FORMULAS FOR ESTIMATING NUTRITIONAL REQUIREMENTS

AUTHOR(S)	DATE	AGE RANGE	TBSA BURNED	NUTRITIONAL CALORIES	PROTEIN REQUIREMENT
Davies and Liljedahl[25]	1971	Child	Any %	60 kcal/kg/day + 35 kcal/%TBSA/day	3 gm/kg/day + 1 g/%TBSA/day
		Adult	Any %	20 kcal/kg/day + 70 kcal/%TBSA/day	1 gm/kg/day + 3 g/%TBSA/day
Wilmore[26]	1972	Child	<40%	1350–1450/m²/day	
			>40%	1950–2050/m²/day	
		Adolescent	<40%	1200–1300/m²/day	
			>40%	1675–1850/m²/day	
		Adult	<40%	1100–1150/m²/day	
			>40%	1550–1625/m²/day	
Wilmore[27]	1974	Adult	>40%	2000–2200/m²/day	94 gm/m²/day
Curreri et al.[28]	1974	Adult	Any %	25 (body weight kg) + 40 (%TBSA burned)	
Muir and Barclay[29]	1974	Adult	<20%	35 kcal/kg/day	1.5 gm/kg/day
			20–30%	40 kcal/kg/day	2 gm/kg/day
			30–40%	50 kcal/kg/day	3 gm/kg/day
			40–50%	60 kcal/kg/day	5 gm/kg/day
Wachtel et al.[30]	1980	Any age	Any %	1.4 kcal (BMR × m² × 24 hr) + wt (growth + 0.6 BSAB)	wt × (RDA + 0.05 BSAB)
Bell et al.[31]	1982	Child	<20 kg	BEE × 1.75	3 gm/kg/day
		Adult	>20 kg	BEE × 2.0	1.5–2.5 gm/kg/day

From Wachtel TL: Nutritional support of the burn patient. In Boswick JA Jr (ed): The Art and Science of Burn Care. Rockville, MD, Aspen, 1987.

ture-dependent."[21] More recently, investigation related to the role of the stress hormones (cortisol, glucagon, and epinephrine) has been carried out. Bessey and associates[22] have shown that infusion of the three stress hormones into normal individuals produces the same alterations as seen in burn-injured patients. These responses are significant hypermetabolism, negative nitrogen and potassium balances, glucose intolerance, hyperinsulinemia, insulin resistance, sodium retention, and peripheral leukocytosis. In addition to the role that the sympathetic nervous system plays in mediating this catabolic response, a role for inflammatory mediators in this response also has been posed. Watters and associates[23] gave normal volunteers the pyrogen etrocholanolone, with and without infusions of the stress hormones. Although the infusion of etrocholanolone alone resulted in fever, local inflammation, increased white blood cell count, increased C-reactive protein, and a fall in serum iron, the subjects remained in nitrogen equilibrium and their carbohydrate metabolism was normal. Administration of the pyrogen and stress hormone produced a catabolic response similar to the stress hormone response alone. Yet the simultaneous administration of both the inflammatory and endocrine mediators was necessary to demonstrate a response more similar to the complete manifestation of the response to thermal injury. Thus the question as to what mediates the metabolic response is still not known in its entirety.

More recently, with the advent of early excision and removal of the major portion of the burn wound with immediate coverage, the question has surfaced: Will excisional therapy reduce this hypermetabolic response? Wolfe compared excised and nonexcised burn patients matched for burn size and showed that even with excision and complete wound coverage the burn patients continued to have metabolic rates 30 to 50 per cent higher than normal.[24]

Since the sympathetic response seems to be the major determinant of the metabolic response to burn injury, and since the sympathetic nervous system can be stimulated by a variety of responses, including lower than normal environmental temperatures, pain, psychological responses, and the body's response to inflammatory mediators, it would seem that the use of nutritional replacement formulas based on the size of the burn injury would no longer be appropriate. Thus current recommendations, on which to base nutritional replacement therapy in the burn patient, should be based on frequent measurements of oxygen consumption. With the advent of the metabolic cart, these measurements can be made easily at the bedside. The measurements should be made daily or several times each day at specific times over several days to obtain meaningful data on which to base adjustment in nutritional therapy. Unfortunately, metabolic carts are very expensive and may not be available in all burn care facilities. When measurement of oxygen consumption is not possible, caloric and protein needs may be based on one of several formulas (Table 28–3). Nutritional formulas vary as much as resuscitation formulas, and there is little consensus as to which is most appropriate. In part this lack of consensus has to do with the great variability in nutritional needs from patient to patient and for the same patient over time. This is why actual measurement of oxygen consumption allows for more accurate nutritional repletion.

MANAGEMENT OF THE PATIENT WITH BURN INJURY

Physiological Response—Changes in Hemodynamics

As noted in Figure 28–5, the initial host defense response leads to a shift in fluids from the vascular tree into the interstitial and intracellular spaces. When the burn involves large areas of skin (i.e., > 20 per cent TBSA), this response may become an overall systemic response, with fluids shifting into interstitial spaces throughout the body. This massive fluid shift may lead to shock. To prevent shock, large volumes of salt-containing solutions must be given. A number of formulas have been suggested for optimal replacement of this fluid. Some of the early formulas, such as the Evans[32] formula and the original Brooke[33] formula, recommended a mixture of sodium-containing fluids and plasma, since both sodium-rich fluids and plasma proteins are lost as a result of this fluid shift. Baxter and Shires demonstrated that plasma given in the first 24 hours was no more effective than Ringer's lactate alone in maintaining normal plasma volume.[34] Thus newer formulas have primarily concentrated on the replacement of sodium and water. Baxter and Shires estimated that the sodium deficit from the extracellular space was 0.5 to 0.6 mEq per per cent TBSA per kilogram of body weight. Thus, to maintain urine output at about 0.5 ml/kg body weight per hour, the Baxter or Parkland formula suggests that a patient will need approximately 3 to 4 ml per per cent TBSA per kilogram of body weight.[35] Other formulas containing sodium also have been promulgated. These include the modified Brooke formula,[36] the hypertonic sodium formula of Monafo,[37] and the New Mexico formula (another hypertonic sodium formula).[38] More recently, Demling and his group have revived an interest in early protein replacement.[39]

The results of the 1979 National Institutes of Health consensus conference would suggest that the burn patient may be adequately resuscitated by a variety of formulas and that, to date, no one formula is preferred over the others.[40] Thus the recommendation in the Advanced Trauma Life Support Course[41] and the Advanced Burn Life Support Course[42] is to use a simple formula that is readily available in any hospital. The recommended resuscitation is to use either the Baxter or modified Brooke formula (Table 28–4).

The controversy over which resuscitation formula to use is similar to the controversy over what parameters to follow to assess the adequacy of resuscitation. Adequacy of organ perfusion is usually assessed by measurement of the normal function or output of the individual organ system. The function of the central nervous system is measured by noting the level of consciousness. The normal function of the gastrointestinal system is inferred by the return of normal bowel sounds and absence of ileus. The function of the kidneys is monitored by measurement of urine output, urine specific gravity, urine glucose level, and urine electrolyte content. Urine volume is a frequent parameter cited, yet the appropriate hourly rate recommended ranges from 0.4 to 1.0 ml/kg body weight. Urine output may be affected by glucosuria as a result of the stress response or in response to administration of hypertonic saline or dextran as part of resuscitation. Haynes suggests that the hematocrit should be followed frequently to detect hemoconcentration or excessive volume expansion.[43]

Because of the early release of catecholamines, the blood pressure may be artificially elevated in relation to the degree of hypovolemia. Thus trends obtained from the frequent monitoring of blood pressure may not reflect the status of resuscitation. Frequent monitoring of heart rate trends may be more useful in monitoring the cardiovascular response to resuscitation. In the well-resuscitated patient, the heart rate should be in the upper limits of normal for age. For the elderly patient or the patient with preexisting cardiac disease, the heart rate may not increase as the patient becomes hypovolemic; thus the heart rate is a less reliable resuscitation parameter in these patients.

Other cardiovascular parameters that may be monitored include central venous pressure, pulmonary artery wedge pressure, and cardiac output. Filling pressures are frequently very low for the first 24 hours after a burn, and if one tries to improve filling pressures during this period, overresuscitation may be the outcome. As long as other signs of adequate tissue perfusion are within normal ranges, the temptation to improve filling pressures should be avoided. Likewise, cardiac outputs are often very low in the first 24 hours and then trend upward over the second and third 24 hours until they are 1½ to 2 times normal. This is thought to be the result of the hypermetabolic response observed in patients with larger burns. Thus the use of invasive monitoring devices such as Swan-Ganz catheters for measurement of wedge pressure and cardiac output may add little to the ability to monitor resuscitation and may increase long-term morbidity because of the increased risk of infectious complications. Only in the elderly patient, the cardiac patient, or the patient with severe smoke inhalation is it truly necessary to monitor filling pressures. In these patients, the goal is to monitor and prevent increased filling pressures as a result of overresuscitation.

Thus, for most burn patients, frequent monitoring of urine output, urine glucose level, pulse rate, bowel sounds, and sensorium will allow for assessment of the adequacy of resuscitation. These parameters, when monitored together, allow one to evaluate tissue perfusion, and only in very extreme cases, as noted above, are invasive monitoring techniques required to assess the adequacy of resuscitation.

TABLE 28–4. FLUID RESUSCITATION FORMULAS

Baxter (Parkland formula)
1st 24 hours, *administer*
4 ml Ringer's lactated/%TBSA/kg body weight
1/2 volume in first 8 hours
1/4 volume in second 8 hours
1/4 volume in third 8 hours
2nd 24 hours, *administer*
Dextrose in water plus potassium in quantities sufficient to maintain normal electrolyte balance.
Plasma or albumin in boluses to maintain hemodynamic stability.*
Modified Brooke formula
1st 24 hours, same as Baxter *except*
2 ml Ringer's lactated/%TBSA/kg body weight
2nd 24 hours,
Same as above

*Plasma or albumin may be given as early as 12 hours if needed to maintain hemodynamic stability.

Nutritional Management

The nutritional needs can best be met in most burn patients with a mixture of glucose, as a source for nonprotein calories, and essential amino acids, as a source of protein. The ratio of calories to nitrogen is also a source of controversy. The suggested ratios range from 150:1 to 100:1.[44] Fat also may be used as a source of carbohydrates and in moderate-sized burns has been shown to have similar protein-sparing effects.[45, 46] Long and associates have suggested that the protein-sparing effect of fat is not as effective as carbohydrates in equal caloric doses in larger burns.[47]

In addition to the major nutrients, vitamins appear to be important, even though their requirements remain poorly defined in the burn patients. Of primary importance is the replacement of water-soluble vitamins (B complex and C), since these are not stored in the body and may not be supplied in sufficient quantities in enteral or parenteral nutritional products. The fat-soluble vitamins (A, D, E, and K) are stored in fatty tissue and are released slowly, so repletion of these is necessary only with prolonged use of parenteral nutrition. Most enteral nutrition formulas contain adequate amounts of fat and fat-soluable vitamins. Therefore, the guidelines for daily vitamin replacement of the National Advisory Group of the American Medical Association are adequate unless deficiencies occur.[48] The one exception to this is vitamin C, which plays a major role in wound healing. Thus, in the case of vitamin C, repletion with twice the recommended amount is usually recommended.[49]

In most severely burned patients, electrolyte imbalances are a common occurrence. Frequent measurement of serum sodium, potassium, chloride, phosphorus, calcium, and magnesium levels is necessary to prevent major electrolyte derangements. In addition, deficiencies in trace metals may occur in the burned patient; thus it is recommended that zinc, copper, manganese, and chromium levels be measured periodically and repleted if found deficient. Zinc is an important cofactor in wound healing and has been shown to be deficient after burn injury.

Nutritional support for the burned patient should utilize the normal route of alimentation whenever possible. Most patients with minor to moderate burn injuries can take in the required calories with a normal diet that is high in protein and carbohydrate supplements. If for some reason the patient cannot maintain adequate intake, enteral support with high-protein, high-calorie formulas via tube feeding may be used. Only in the very sickest burn patient is it necessary to utilize parenteral nutrition. Parenteral nutrition in the burned patient carries with it a much higher rate of septic complications and is used only when absolutely necessary.

Recently, studies in burned patients suggest beginning enteral feeding within the first 12 to 24 hours after injury. Early feeding can be accomplished by feeding the patient in the duodenum. As a matter of fact, duodenal feedings may help resolve the early ileus seen in these patients. Alexander has reported that early feeding may reduce the septic complications in burn patients by decreasing bacterial translocation across the gut membrane.[10] As cited previously, this early bacterial translocation is thought to contribute significantly to sepsis or multiorgan system failure, even without clinical documentation of bacteremia.

Management of Pulmonary Injury

For the burned patient, pulmonary injury may be the result of inhalation of the by-products of smoke or may be the result of a systemic process related to sepsis syndrome or multiorgan failure (MOF). Inhalation injury may or may not produce direct tissue injury to the lung. One component of inhalation injury is carbon monoxide (CO) intoxication. CO does not affect the lining of the lung but produces its effect on the body by competing with oxygen (O_2) for uptake by hemoglobin. Since hemoglobin has 200 times more affinity for CO than for O_2, CO replaces O_2, thus reducing the delivery of O_2 to tissues. This may lead to severe anoxia and related brain injury. In addition, CO combines with myoglobin in muscle cells and the cytochrome oxidase system of the brain, producing muscle weakness and coma, respectively. The initial effects of muscle weakness and confusion from decreased O_2 uptake occur within approximately 5 minutes of exposure and may contribute to the inability of the person to escape from the fire. The long-term neurological effects occasionally associated with smoke inhalation are most likely related to both prolonged anoxia and inhibition of the cytochrome oxidase system of the brain. Levels of CO necessary to produce significant neurological effects are usually predicted to be above 40 per cent COHbg (carboxyhemaglobin) at the time of exposure. CO has a half-life of 4 hours if the patient breathes room air and 1 hour if the patient is breathing 100 per cent oxygen. COHbg levels measured in the emergency room must be interpreted in relation to the time after exposure and the concentration of oxygen administered to the patient since the exposure. Thus a level of 25 per cent COHbg 1 hour after exposure in a patient on 100 per cent O_2 would be predicted to have been about 50 per cent COHbg at the time of exposure.

Other components of inhalation injury are upper airway injury and chemical injury to the lung parenchyma. Upper airway injury is the result of inhalation of superheated air and may cause blisters and edema in the subglottic area around the vocal cords. This may cause upper airway occlusion and is best treated by early endotracheal intubation. Chemical injury to the lung is caused by the inhalation of a variety of oxides of sulfur and nitrogen, aldehydes, and acrolein which are given off as the by-products of combustion. Although the exact mechanics of injury may differ with each of these by-products, the end result of each of these is loss of ciliary action, decreased surfactant production, hemorrhagic tracheobronchitis, increased interstitial edema, and decreased macrophage function. This results in a typical adult respiratory distress syndrome (ARDS) response, usually evident about 12 to 24 hours after injury. The typical presentation is one of decreasing lung volume, evidence of obstructive disease with reduction in flow rates, an increase in dead space, a rapid decrease in compliance, and a decreased ability to maintain adequate oxygenation.[50]

The treatment of chemical injury to the lung secondary to smoke inhalation is primarily one of supportive care. Of early primary concern is the need for increased volume of fluid resuscitation.[51] Although patients with smoke inhalation require additional fluid resuscitation to maintain organ perfusion, excessive fluid resuscitation may lead to fluid overload and further compromise pulmonary function. For the patient with minimal injury, the administration of warm, humidified oxygen and incentive spirometry may result in adequate oxygenation. In patients with mild injury, maintenance of ventilation and prevention of atelectasis are of prime importance. Administration of oxygen, incentive spirometry, and removal of secretions may be adequate. For the individual with more severe disease, endotracheal intubation and mechanical ventilation may be necessary. Cioffi and associates

TABLE 28–5. COMPARISON OF ADVANTAGES AND SIDE EFFECTS OF CURRENTLY USED ANTIMICROBIAL AGENTS IN BURNED PATIENTS

ANTIMICROBIAL AGENT	ADVANTAGES	SIDE EFFECTS
Silver nitrate solution	Effective against most gram-positive and some gram-negative organisms	Hyponatremia, hypokalemia, and hypochloremia Decreased penetration of eschar—not effective against established infection Requires large bulky dressings which limit mobility
Mafenide acetate cream	Effective against wide range of gram-positive and gram-negative organisms Rapidly diffuses through eschar (improved effectiveness in established infections) Permits open treatment of wound, thus increasing mobility	Painful on application May cause hypersensitivity reaction in 5–7% of all patients Associated with acid-base derangements
Silver sulfadiazine cream	Effective against a wide range of gram-positive and gram-negative organisms Soothing on application Softens the eschar and increases joint mobility Absorbed slowly, reducing the chance of nephrotoxicity	May cause a hypersensitivity reaction in 5–7% of all patients Associated with an initial decrease in leukocytes

From Patrick ML, Woods SL, Craven RF, Rokosky JS: Comparison—Burn injuries and skin trauma. In Medical-Surgical Nursing: Pathophysiologic Concepts. Philadelphia, J. B. Lippincott, 1991.

have shown that the prophylactic use of interrupted-flow, high-frequency positive-pressure ventilation may improve the morbidity and mortality of patients with severe smoke inhalation.[52] Some patients with smoke inhalation also experience bronchospasms, which may be treated with administration of aerosolized isoproterenol, albuterol, or systemic aminophylline. Steroids have been shown to be contraindicated in treating the burned patient with smoke inhalation because of the increased incidence of infection and mortality.[53, 54]

In addition to lung injury caused by smoke inhalation, the burned patient also may exhibit lung injury associated with MOF. This process is the result of vascular and perivascular inflammation which causes a diffuse microvascular leak. There is an increasing body of literature that suggests that the tissue injury of MOF is caused by circulating inflammatory cells induced by a massive inflammatory response. Neutrophils and platelets have both been implicated in the genesis of this response.[55–57] Neutrophils have the ability to produce reactive oxygen metabolites such as superoxides, which, in turn, produce extensive tissue injury. Anderson and Harkin suggest that this response is not caused by a single factor but rather by a constellation of events that lead to cellular priming and activation; in the future this may be prevented by the administration of a platelet-activation factor antagonist.[58] At this time, the primary treatment of lung injury related to MOF is supportive care and correction of the underlying cause of the induced inflammatory response, i.e., sepsis or hypovolemia.

Wound Management—Prevention of Infection

In the not too distant past, the goal of wound care was to find an antimicrobial cream or solution that would prevent infection and allow the wound to heal or granulate so that the wound could be grafted. During this time, a number of the wound care products used today were developed. These products include mafenide acetate cream, silver sulfadiazine cream, and silver nitrate. The advantages and side effects of these agents are listed in Table 28–5.

More recently, the emphasis in wound care has been on early removal of eschar or devitalized tissue of deep dermal and full-thickness burns and use of a variety of biological and synthetic dressings. See Table 28–6 for a comparison of some of the currently available dressings. This change in the focus of wound care has had a dramatic effect on burn care. The length of hospital stay has decreased by 50 to 70 per cent, and patients have less frequent septic episodes.[59] The emphasis has changed from survival at all cost to concerns for survival with the most acceptable functional and cosmetic results possible. This has improved not only survival but also rehabilitation of the burned patient. The surgical and plastic surgical literature abounds with studies of early facial excision and grafting,[60] the use of microvascular free flaps and composite grafts to close large deep defects,[61, 62] especially in the electrical burn, and the use of tissue expansion in reconstructive procedures.[63]

In all areas of wound management, the maintenance of a clean, well-nourished wound through meticulous nursing care is imperative. Careful cleansing of the wound several times a day may be necessary to remove wound exudate. Healing wounds require adequate circulation, so care must be taken to apply a snug dressing that will remain on the wound but will not cause restriction to blood flow. Similarly, the patient's position must be changed frequently to reduce pressure and maintain blood flow to dependent areas. Adequate nutrition is also imperative to prevent infection and maximize wound healing.

With modern wound-management practices, the use of systemic antibiotics in burn care has been significantly reduced in all but those with extensive injuries (>70 per cent), since most of the devitalized tissue is removed early and the wound is closed with a autograft or other biological or synthetic dressing. Often systemic antibiotics are used in the perioperative period as prophylaxis against infection. In this case, it is important to administer the antibiotic so that its peak period of effectiveness will be during the surgical

TABLE 28–6. SPECIALIZED BURN WOUND DRESSINGS AND SYNTHETIC SKIN SUBSTITUTES

TYPE OF DRESSING	PROPERTIES OF DRESSINGS	UTILIZATION
Biological dressings Allografts Living related donor Cadaver grafts Fresh Frozen Amniotic membrane Xenografts (pigskin) Fresh Frozen Lyophilized	Decrease bacterial proliferation Decrease desiccation of wound Decrease evaporative water loss Prevent further contamination Prevent physical damage to underlying skin structures Prepare granulation tissue for autografting	Allografts are commonly used to cover excised wounds when autografts are not available or to cover widely expanded mesh. Xenografts may be used to cover clean partial-thickness wounds, to cover donor sites, or to temporarily cover excised or granulating wounds.
Cultured epithelial cells	Cells grown in tissue culture to form sheets of epidermal tissue. The benefit to the patient is that this is an autologous graft grown from the patient's own cells; thus the rejection factor is avoided and small biopsies of tissue can be used to grow large sheets of skin. Disadvantages: requires 3 weeks to grow skin and resultant skin is thin, with no skin appendages and is easily rubbed off, even months after grafting.	Used on patients with extensive injury when autografts are very limited (i.e., >90%TBSA). Applied to excised wounds or over allografted dermal tissue.
Synthetic gels Omniderm (Omikron Scientific) Geliperm (Geistlich) Duoderm (Convatec, Squibb)	The structure of these gel-like dressings allows them to absorb large quantities of aqueous materials without deterioration of the dressing.	Superficial partial-thickness wounds and donor sites. Dressing may be left in place until wound heals or may be changed if excessive drainage occurs.
Synthetic laminates Biobrane (Dow B. Hickham) Epigard (Parke Davis)	These materials contain two or more layers of biological or synthetic materials, designed to replicate the two layers of skin. Outer layer is water vapor permeable. The inner layer is usually a porous adherent material and allows migration of fibroblast.	May be used over partial-thickness wounds or donor sites. May also be used as a temporary cover of excised wounds until autografts are available.
Synthetic films OpSite (Smith & Nephew, Ltd.) Bioclusive (Johnson & Johnson) Tegaderm (3M Company)	Homogeneous thin plastic-like membranes with variable permeability to water. Secretion may pool beneath dressing and require the removal of the dressing.	Initial dressing for more superficial partial-thickness wounds and donor sites.

procedure. This may vary with the prescribed antibiotic. When systemic antibiotics are used to treat bacteremias or sepsis, it is imperative to follow blood levels to ensure maximal effectiveness without toxicity and untoward effects. The burned patient is known to handle a variety of drugs differently than other patients.[64, 65] These changes in drug pharmacokinetics must be considered when administering drugs to the burned patient. For example, Zaske and associates found that some burned patients required two to three times the amount of gentamicin normally prescribed for severe gram-negative sepsis.[66]

The future of wound healing and management for the burned patient appears to lie in a better understanding of the role of growth hormone and growth factors on wound healing. Growth hormone is normally secreted by the hypothalamus and is important to normal growth and development. Recent work by Herndon and associates has shown more rapid reepithelialization of wounds of patients treated with growth hormone.[67] Early experiments with growth factors in animals suggest that in the future a variety of these factors may be used to improve wound healing.[68–72]

NURSING MANAGEMENT OF THE BURNED PATIENT

Management of the burned patient can be divided into several cycles. These cycles lend themselves well to a discussion of nursing management. The initial cycle is resuscitation and usually extends over the first 72 hours. The second cycle is the reparative cycle, which spans the time from resuscitation until complete wound closure occurs. The time varies depending on the depth and extent of burn, the method of wound management employed, and the variety of complications that may extend this phase, such as smoke inhalation, sepsis, multiorgan failure, etc. The third cycle involves rehabilitation and reconstruction and may extend over years. Nursing management during each of these cycles depends on accurate assessment and diagnosis and the development of a nursing plan based on data-based problem solving. Table 28–7 lists a number of nursing diagnoses relevant to the various cycles of care. This is not intended to be an exhaustive list of relevant diagnoses but only an example of the more common ones that may be appropriate to the individual burned patient. The nursing management will be discussed using the three cycles and elaborating on some of the more common or more critical problems associated with each.

Resuscitative Cycle

Nursing management during this cycle is centered around maintenance of homeostasis, treatment of life-threatening complications, prevention of infection, management of pain, and management of anxiety and fear. As noted in Table 28–7, a number of nursing diagnoses may be applied to the

TABLE 28–7. NURSING DIAGNOSES APPROPRIATE THROUGHOUT THE CYCLES OF BURN PATIENT MANAGEMENT

	CYCLE OF BURN CARE		
NURSING DIAGNOSIS	RESUSCITATION	REPARATIVE	REHABILITATIVE AND RECONSTRUCTIVE
Alteration in skin integrity	+	+ +	+
Fluid volume deficit	+ +	+	
Potential for fluid volume excess	+	+	
Potential for fluid and electrolyte imbalances	+	+	
Potential for impaired gas exchange	+	+	
Potential for infection	+ +	+ +	+
Potential for altered tissue perfusion	+	+	
Altered nutrition, less than body requirements	+ +	+ +	+
Pain	+ +	+ +	+
Decreased physical mobility	+	+ +	+ +
Alterations in sensory perception	+	+	
Alterations in sleep patterns	+	+	+
Potential self-care deficits	+ +	+ +	+
Fear, anxiety, and spiritual distress	+ +	+ +	+
Anticipatory grieving and social isolation		+	+ +
Alterations in self-concept		+	+ +
Activity intolerance			+ +
Potential noncompliance		+	+ +
Potential sexual dysfunction			+ +

Note: +, May be a problem during this cycle; + +, most likely to occur during this cycle.

patient during this cycle. The obvious ones are alteration in skin integrity and fluid volume deficit or potential for fluid volume deficit depending on the extent of the burn injury. Also high on the list of nursing diagnoses in this cycle are altered nutrition less than body requirements, potential for infection, and impaired gas exchange in the patient with smoke inhalation.

Altered Skin Integrity

The management of this problem is a collaborative one, and the major therapies have been discussed previously. The assessment of wound healing, though, is a major nursing issue. Initially, the extent and depth of injury must be accurately assessed. An accurate assessment of the extent of the wound should be made by an experienced health care professional. Research has shown that the more experienced health care professional, nurse, or physician is the one most likely to make the most accurate determination.[73, 74] One technique that may increase accuracy is to calculate the burned area using either the Berkow or Lund and Browder formula and then to calculate the unburned area using the same formula. When these two calculations are then compared, the total percentage of body surface area may be more or less than 100 per cent. Once the calculations of burned and unburned areas are compared, a more accurate calculation can be made in areas of discrepancies, thus providing an accurate assessment of the extent of injury. The tendency is to overcalculate burns in adults and undercalculate burns in children.

Depth of injury requires even more judgment. Table 28–2 may be helpful in the assessment of depth. The very superficial first-degree burn and the truly deep third-degree burn are fairly obvious. The difficulty comes in distinguishing the different depths of second-degree or dermal injuries. Again, experience is helpful, but even the most experienced observer may be wrong as much as 50 per cent of the time, especially during the first 24 hours.[75] As noted previously, the wound is dynamic, and the depth may change over time if edema, pressure, and low-flow states decrease the circulation to the wound. Careful documentation of wound appearance over time as the nurse provides wound care is useful in the assessment of depth or in the early recognition of wound infection. Increased erythema around the wound, increased tenderness or pain around wound, exudate that becomes more yellow or green, and discoloration within the wound, such as black or purple areas, are all signs of wound infection. The appearance of wound changes should be documented and followed carefully. An easy way to monitor increasing erythema is to use a marker to delineate the edges of the reddened area, noting the date and time. If the redness extends past these margins over the next few hours, this may indicate the need for a change in wound therapy or administration of systemic antibiotics to control wound infection.

Evaluation. The outcome criteria for this problem are an accurate initial assessment of the depth and extent of burn and daily wound assessments that indicate the lack of wound changes associated with infection and sepsis.

Alteration in Skin Integrity (Nonburn)

Although in the burned patient alteration of skin integrity usually is considered in relation to the burn injury, the potential for other alterations in skin integrity exist. These patients often have their mobility restricted by invasive line placement, management of respiratory problems, sedation and narcotic administration, and positioning necessary to prevent graft loss after excision and grafting. Any or all of these may contribute to prolonged bed rest, decreased ability to move in bed, and the development of pressure sores. The management of these patients on specialized beds to reduce pressure problems is useful. Even though the patient is managed on a bed that supposedly reduces pressure, it is still possible for the patient to develop pressure sores, so frequent position changes continue to be necessary. With each bath and dressing change, the dependent areas of the body should be inspected carefully for evidence of increased pressure. Common areas for the development of pressure sores for burn patients treated on specialized beds are the heels and the occiput. Burn injuries to these areas often mask the beginning of pressure problems.

Fluid Volume Deficit

The burned patient is prone to fluid and electrolyte disorders until the burn wound is healed or covered with a permanent or semipermanent wound cover. Initially, fluid volume deficit is a major concern. As fluid shifts occur in relation to the initial injury, the circulating volume decreases rapidly. Without rapid infusion of sodium-containing fluids, the patient develops hypovolemia and shock. Burn fluid resuscitation has been discussed previously. Monitoring the patient frequently to assess response to fluid therapy is a major nursing concern in the first 24 to 48 hours. The well-resuscitated patient should have a normal urine output for age, urine that is free of glucose, a pulse rate that is in the upper limits of normal for age, a clear sensorium, a hematocrit that is below 50 per cent and be free of ileus. Urine output can be a very sensitive measure of adequate organ and tissue perfusion, but a variety of things should be considered when monitoring urine output. First, there is a normal variation in urine output from hour to hour and most especially at night when cortisol levels normally diminish. Therefore, when using urine output as a parameter to monitor resuscitation efforts, an average of 3 or 4 hours of urine should be assessed before changes in flow rates of intravenous fluids are made unless other signs of hypovolemia are present. Urine flow rates usually decrease over time in response to hypovolemia rather than dropping abruptly. An abrupt decrease or absence of urine flow usually is related to a mechanical problem, i.e., a kink in the catheter or drainage system or a clot or plug in the catheter. Manipulation or irrigation of the catheter may correct this problem immediately. Glycosuria is a common response to stress and may cause the urine output to be falsely elevated. If the patient has other signs of hypovolemia and a high urine output, this is often the cause. The use of dextran or mannitol also may cause the urine output to increase in the face of hypovolemia. Thus, although urine output can be a sensitive measure of organ perfusion, each of these issues should be considered when monitoring urine output.

In patients with electrical injuries, the urine may contain hemochromogens, i.e., hemoglobin or myoglobin. The treatment for myoglobin in the urine is to flush the kidney to prevent permanent injury. In this case, fluids are given to increase hourly urine output to twice or three times normal. Also, osmotic diuretics are given to increase urine output. Thus normal parameters of urine output are no longer appropriate for monitoring.

Pulse rate also varies for a variety of reasons. Age is a common source of variation; i.e., infants and young children have significantly higher pulse rates. Elderly patients tend to have lower pulse rates and may not be able to increase their rate in response to hypovolemia because of preexisting heart disease. Young athletes often have a normal pulse rate of 50 or 60 beats per minute. When stressed by hypovolemia, their rate may increase only to 80 or 90 beats per minute and may seem a little low for the normal response to hypovolemia. Pain may cause an increased pulse rate and may be associated with agitation, both of which may mimic some of the signs of hypovolemia.

Unless the burned patient also has experienced head trauma, the sensorium should be clear; i.e., the patient should be oriented to time, place, and person. Often patients may appear to be somnolent and confused because they have been given narcotics or sedatives for pain management. For the most part though, patients who are somnolent or confused from medication are oriented to time, place, and person when aroused.

A hematocrit that is greater than 50 per cent is usually a clear indication of hypovolemia and hemoconcentration. It is the rare patient with a normal hematocrit above 50 percent. Ileus is another indication of decreased organ perfusion. This is common in the early hours of burn management, but once fluid replacement is well under way, it should no longer remain a problem.

As noted above, each of these parameters has its limitations. It is only when all the parameters are considered in combination that a true picture of the patient's volume status can be assessed. When more than one of these parameters indicate that a fluid volume deficit has occurred, then the volume of administered fluid should be adjusted. This may be done by administering boluses of fluid or by increasing the flow rate for a specified period of time. It is important to monitor the patient's response to this fluid challenge continuously to note whether the monitored parameters return to normal or not. If the parameters continue to be abnormal, other causes of hypovolemia should be considered.

Evaluation. The outcome criteria for this problem should be that the assessment parameters are maintained within normal limits. The assessment parameters monitored in all burn patients should include mental acuity, pulse rate, urine output, urine glucose level, hematocrit, and bowel sounds to assess bowel function. In patients with extensive burns (> 70 per cent TBSA), patients with smoke inhalation, or patients with preexisting cardiac disease, monitoring also should include measurement of central venous pressure, pulmonary artery pressure, and cardiac output.

Other Fluid and Electrolyte Problems

Although fluid volume deficit is the most common fluid and electrolyte problem in burned patients, one must be alert to a variety of other fluid and electrolyte issues. *Fluid volume excess* may become an issue with overresuscitation. This is a rare problem except in infants, patients with preexisting cardiac conditions, patients with severe smoke inhalation, patients with preexisting renal disease, or patients who have had delayed resuscitation intervention and have sustained a renal insult. The parameters that indicate that this is a problem are: CVP > 12 cm H_2O, PCWP > 18 mm Hg, confusion, dyspnea, rales, inadequate oxygenation, low cardiac output, normal or increased urine output, decreased urine specific gravity, normal or decreased heart rate, peripheral edema unrelated to burn site, decreased serum sodium level, and decreased serum and urine osmolality. Therapy may include more judicious administration of fluids, administration of diuretics, administration of oxygen if dyspnea is present, and evaluation and treatment of any underlying problems.

Hyponatremia, hypernatremia, hypokalemia, or *hyperkalemia* also may occur with some frequency during the resuscitation cycle. Frequent monitoring of electrolytes and adjustments in fluid replacement regimens may be necessary to prevent complications associated with electrolyte imbalances.

Evaluation. Outcome criteria related to fluid and electrolyte problems in burned patients are to maintain assessment parameters within normal limits or limits appropriate to the therapy instituted; i.e., if hypertonic saline is used for resuscitation, the expectation would be for the serum sodium level to be slightly elevated. Likewise, if a diuretic has been given, the expectation would be that the urine output would increase for several hours. Other outcome criteria may include ensuring that monitoring equipment functions properly, that patients receive the necessary volume of fluid over the appropriate period of time, that intravenous lines remain in place and patent, and that indications of fluid or electrolyte imbalances are recognized promptly and treated appropriately.

Potential for Impaired Gas Exchange

Impaired gas exchange is second only to fluid volume deficit as a life-threatening problem encountered in the resuscitation cycle. This problem may occur as a result of smoke inhalation, fluid overload, inadequate expansion of the chest wall related to full-thickness circumferential third-degree burns, or ARDS related to impaired immune function and multiorgan failure. The nursing goals for this problem are that the problem will be recognized early and that in collaboration with the physician the problem will be treated expeditiously. The parameters to be monitored are rate and character of respiration, signs of increasing hoarseness, increased pulmonary secretions, decreased chest wall expansion, chest wall retractions in children, and changes in mentation. If patients exhibit some or all of these parameters, blood gases should be analyzed. A P_{O_2} of less than 120 mm Hg on an F_{IO_2} of 40 per cent indicates significant hypoxia. A P_{CO_2} greater than 45 mm Hg indicates hypercarbia. Actual changes in P_{O_2} and P_{CO_2} are usually late signs of impending problems and occur when the patient is no longer able to compensate. The treatment for impaired gas exchange is intubation and ventilatory support as needed. Endotracheal intubation in the burned patient may be difficult if the upper airway is swollen and may be difficult to maintain especially if the patient's face is burned. The antibacterial creams and ointments used on burn wounds tend to make securing the endotracheal tube exceptionally difficult. Although a tracheostomy may be easier to maintain, it is particularly difficult to perform in the often edematous neck of the burned patient, resulting in inappropriate placement and long-term complications. If tracheostomy tubes are placed early before edema formation has reached its maximum, the tissue swelling may cause the tube to be pulled out of the tracheal opening, thus losing access to the airway. In either case, the patient with an endotracheal tube or tracheostomy should be observed frequently for tube placement, and the straps securing the tubes should be tightened or loosened accordingly, to account for increases and decreases in edema formation over time. Also, care should be taken when securing the nasally placed endotracheal tube not to put pressure on the nares or the burn-injured face, ears, or scalp. Pressure on the nares may lead to necrosis and loss of the normal contour of the nose. Pressure on the injured tissue of the face, ears, and scalp may cause further loss of tissue and result in a poorer cosmetic result. Intubation may increase the burned patient's already altered sensory perception. Patients who have facial burns often have eyes that are swollen shut so that they cannot see, and if they can no longer talk, they are likely to become even more agitated. This may make it more difficult for them to cooperate with mechanical ventilation. Frequent explanation, reassurance, and sedatives are necessary to ensure their cooperation.

Since these patients often have increased pulmonary secretions, frequent suctioning may be necessary. The utmost care should be taken to maintain sterility when suctioning the immunocompromised patient. Pneumonia is a major cause of morbidity and mortality in the intubated burn patient.

Evaluation. Outcome criteria include prompt recognition of impaired gas exchange; prompt referral to the physician when an impending problem is recognized; respiratory parameters should be maintained within normal limits once treatment is initiated; intubation tubes should be maintained in place and patent; further tissue injury should be prevented; anxiety should be relieved; compliance should be maintained; pulmonary secretions should be removed as needed; and pulmonary infections should be avoided.

Potential for Infection

The burned patient is an immunocompromised vessel with open wounds waiting for the invasion of microorganisms. The nursing management to prevent infection focuses on four areas of concern: (1) vigilant monitoring for signs of impending wound infection and systemic sepsis, (2) maintenance of the external and personal hygienic environment to reduce the reservoir of microorganisms, (3) use of aseptic technique for wound care and all invasive procedures, and (4) timely administration of antibiotics and appropriate use of topical antibacterial agents. Since the assessment of wounds for infection was discussed previously, this discussion will be limited to signs of systemic infection. The diagnosis of sepsis in the burned patient is complicated by the hypermetabolic response, as well as by pain and anxiety, which may account for abnormalities in a variety of parameters monitored. Thus the diagnosis of sepsis depends on the presence of several abnormal parameters. The parameters to be monitored include mental acuity; changes in body temperature, heart rate, respiratory rate, blood pressure, urine output, and gastrointestinal function; and changes in laboratory values such as urine glucose level, blood pH, white blood cell count, and platelet count. A patient is considered to be septic if three or more of the following signs and symptoms exist: disorientation, hypo- or hyperthermia, tachypnea, tachycardia, ileus, glycosuria, unexplained acidosis, hypotension, anuria, white blood cell count > 5000 cells/mm^3, and decreased platelet count. Thus frequent, accurate monitoring of these parameters will lead to timely diagnosis and treatment.

The second concern for infection prevention is to provide an external environment that will limit the access of microorganisms to the wounds of the burned patient. This includes the environment that is external to the patient: the patient's room; other areas of the hospital to which the patient is exposed, i.e., the operating room, treatment rooms, hydrotherapy rooms, etc.; as well as the staff who care for the patient. The most important aspect of providing a protective environment is to place a protective barrier between the patient and the environmental hazards. This may sound complicated but, in fact, can be quite simple. As to the inanimate objects within the environment, as long as these areas are cleansed with standard hospital disinfectants and are dried, they should present little, if any, risk to the patient. The major concern in the environment is porous materials that cannot be cleaned, such as chairs with cloth covers, mattresses without intact plastic covers, and similar hard-to-clean items. The biggest problem in maintaining a protective environment is the personnel. Most transfer of microorganisms in the hospital environment is via the hands and apron area of the staff.[76, 77] Meticulous handwashing, wearing of gloves, and covering the apron area of the health care workers' clothing during direct patient care will eliminate the major sources of microorganisms from the patient's immediate environment.[78] During wound care and invasive procedures, wearing surgical mask and hair covers may increase the protection. These simple precautions can produce an acceptable external environment.

The other environment that is of concern is the patient's own body. Providing meticulous hygienic measures is important to reduce infection. Especially of concern is hygiene of hair-bearing areas and skin folds in the groin, axilla, under nail beds, etc. Oral care is also important, especially in the intubated patient. Johnson and associates have demonstrated an association between respiratory tract infections and increased adherence of gram-negative bacilli to epithelial cells of the oral cavity.[79, 80] This increased adherence is especially prominent in the critically ill patient who is intubated; thus frequent oral care may reduce the bacterial count and lessen the threat of pulmonary infection.

Wound care should be managed aseptically. Careful attention to the removal of exudate and devitalized tissue several times a day will reduce the bacterial load and maximize the use of antibacterial creams or solutions to control bacterial proliferation. The choice of antibacterial agents should be based on knowledge of the usual bacterial flora prevalent within the burn care facility; routine, periodic cultures of the patient's wounds; and the antibacterial spectrum of the particular antibacterial agents. The advantages and side effects of some of the more commonly used antibacterial agents are listed in Table 28–5.

Invasive procedures in burned patients carry increased risk for infection. Often, intravenous or arterial lines must be placed through burned areas, thus increasing the risk of infection. Meticulous care should be taken to keep the area around venous and arterial access lines as clean as possible. Usually, the topical antibacterial agent used on the surrounding burn wound is used at the insertion site to decrease the risk of infection. Suturing lines in place will keep them from being easily displaced or slipping within the vein, which may increase the chance of infection. Intravenous catheters should be changed frequently to reduce the risk of bacteremia and systemic sepsis.[81]

As mentioned previously, burned patients often exhibit altered pharmacokinetics in relation to the administration of certain drugs. For this reason, it is important when administering antibiotics to draw frequent peak and trough levels so that the dose and frequency of administration can be adjusted to obtain appropriate drug levels.

Evaluation. The outcome criterion is that the patient will not exhibit signs of local or systemic infection and that if systemic antibiotics are required, the dose and frequency of administration will be adapted to provide adequate blood levels.

Reparative Cycle

The second cycle is the reparative cycle. Here, the major focus is to support the body's natural healing properties and to provide psychosocial support to allow both physical and psychological repair. The major new nursing concerns during this cycle include provision of adequate nutritional support to enhance healing, pain management, prevention of contracture formation, self-care deficit management, management of alterations in sensory perception and disturbances in sleep, management of anticipatory grieving and social isolation, and management of fear, anxiety, and spiritual distress. Many of these nursing issues are common to all critically ill or injured patients; thus only those with specific concern to the burn-injured patient will be discussed. These will include nutrition, pain, and prevention of contracture formation. Each of these is a shared concern with other health care disciplines, but nursing continues to have a major management role in each of these areas.

Altered Nutrition, Less than Body Requirements

As discussed previously in this chapter, the burned patient has greatly increased metabolic needs. The increased metabolic demands actually begin during the resuscitation cycle and continue for some time after wound closure occurs, as evidenced by increased oxygen consumption for several months after complete wound closure.[82] The goal of the health care team is to continually assess the nutritional requirements and to assist the patient in meeting these needs. The nutritionist and respiratory therapist may be helpful in actually measuring and calculating the patient's nutritional needs. The nutritionist is also usually responsible for estimating the total calorie and protein requirements for the individual patient. To determine if the nutritional needs of the patient are being met, measurement of weights, intake and output, serum proteins (albumin, prealbumin, transferrin), and nitrogen balance are usually considered. Accurate measurements of weights and intake and output and urine collection for nitrogen balance determinations are extremely important. Indications of inadequate nutrition include weight loss of greater than 10 per cent of preinjury weight, serum albumin levels of less than 3.5 gm/dl, serum prealbumin levels of less than 19 mg/dl, transferrin levels less than 200 mg/100 ml, and a negative nitrogen balance.

The delivery of appropriate nutrition is a major nursing consideration. Since most burned patients experience lack of appetite or may not be able to cooperate with attempts to get them to eat the large amounts of food required, alternative methods of alimentation may be necessary.

Tube Feeding. Tube feeding is the most common way to meet the burned patient's nutritional needs during the early cycles of care. This approach allows for a prescribed amount of calories and protein to be administered without requiring the patient to comply with a level of therapy that may be virtually impossible to achieve. Providing nutrients by this method is safer than intravenous hyperalimentation and takes advantage of the normal route of alimentation. As discussed previously, early alimentation by the nasogastric route may decrease bacterial translocation and reduce the risk of sepsis and multiorgan failure.

Concerns to be considered, when tube feedings are administered, include hyperosmolar diarrhea, hyperglycemia, ileus, aspiration, and fluid and electrolyte imbalance. Hyperosmolar diarrhea may occur if the osmolarity of the enteral feeding product is high or if the tube feeding is infused too rapidly. Careful monitoring of flow rates and feeding of a progressively concentrated solution will usually eliminate this problem. Some patients will experience hyperglycemia related to the high carbohydrate content of tube feeding. This can be controlled by a change in the components of the feeding solution or administration of insulin. Symptoms of hyperglycemia will include osmotic diuresis, glycosuria, and an increased serum glucose level. Ileus related to fluid and electrolyte imbalances and sepsis is a common problem in the burned patient and may complicate the administration of tube feedings. To guard against complications related to ileus, if the feeding is administered gastrically, gastric residuals should be monitored hourly. If the level of gastric residuals is greater than the amount fed over the previous 2 hours, the feedings should be discontinued and the physician notified. Often duodenal feedings are used to bypass the stomach and reduce the risk of aspiration associated with gastric feedings. The debate as to whether to use gastric or duodenal feeding routinely centers around two factors: Duodenal feedings are less likely to be related to vomiting and aspiration but leave the lining of the stomach unprotected, which may lead to gastric ulceration. Tube feedings administered into the stomach protect the gastric mucosa but may be more prone to the complication of aspiration. To prevent ulceration when duodenal feedings are used, antacids or histamine blockers are prescribed routinely. To reduce the risk of aspiration, it is also recommended that the head of the patient be maintained at 30 degrees of elevation. There is little evidence that elevation of the patient's head reduces the incidence or severity of aspiration, but it is a generally held opinion that it may be beneficial.

While tube feedings may be the primary means of nutritional support during the early cycles of care, frequent consideration should be given to beginning oral feedings. Offering small amounts of food that the patient likes or is craving may begin to stimulate the patient's appetite and improve his overall morale. In some patients, to make the transition from tube feedings to oral alimentation, it may be necessary to use tube feedings at night to make up the calories not taken during the day. All too often health care workers use the threat of tube feeding to encourage the patient to eat. This rarely accomplishes an increase in oral intake and often leads to feelings of failure for the patient who just cannot eat enough. If it is apparent that the patient cannot eat enough, tube feedings should be presented as an adjunct or alternative rather than as a threat.

Intravenous Alimentation. Intravenous alimentation in the burned patient represents both lifesaving technology and a major threat to life because of the increased risk of sepsis. For the burned patient in whom enteral feedings are contraindicated, i.e., the septic patient, the patient with a prolonged ileus, or the patient with injury to the gastrointestinal system, the only method of adequate alimentation may be with intravenous solutions high in calories and protein. Intravenous alimentation should be carefully managed and monitored to prevent complications. The major complications are hyper- or hypoglycemia, sepsis, and iatrogenic injury related to venous access such as pneumothorax or hydrothorax. The rapid administration of glucose in this already maximally stressed patient may lead to stress-related diabetes and eventually hyperosmolar coma. Careful control of fluid administration rates and frequent monitoring of urine and blood sugar levels can detect periods of hyperglycemia early. The treatment of hyperglycemia is usually the administration of insulin either by subcutaneous injection, intravenous bolus, or continuous drip. Hypoglycemia may occur if the administration is abruptly discontinued. This is especially true if insulin is being administered concomitantly. If the administration of these concentrated glucose solutions must be interrupted, a solution of 10% dextrose should be administered via a peripheral intravenous infusion to reduce the risk of hypoglycemia. The major symptom of hypoglycemia in the burned patient is mental confusion which may rapidly progress to coma.

Catheter-related sepsis is another common complication of intravenous alimentation. Meticulous attention to aseptic technique during placement and care of the catheter and frequent catheter changes can reduce the incidence of catheter-related sepsis. Symptoms of catheter-related sepsis include all the signs and symptoms of sepsis previously discussed and may include local signs of infection around the catheter insertion site. Any burned patient receiving intravenous alimentation who exhibits signs of sepsis should be considered to have catheter sepsis until proven otherwise. The only way to diagnose catheter-related sepsis is to remove the catheter and see if the patient's condition improves.

Iatrogenic complications such as pneumothorax or hydrothorax are related to difficulties encountered in placement of central venous lines. Routine chest x-ray immediately after catheter insertion will lead to rapid diagnosis and treatment of this problem. To reduce the complications of a hydrothorax, the rate of fluid administration should be reduced until the result of the chest x-ray is known.

Oral Feedings. For patients with smaller burns or patients in the later cycles of burn care, the oral administration of a high-calorie, high-protein diet is appropriate. Yet, even with these patients, a reduced appetite, nausea related to pain or pain relief medication, and psychological problems may interfere with their ability to take in an adequate diet. To encourage eating, the meal time should be as pleasant as possible. The food should be served in an attractive, unhurried manner. The timing of meals, painful procedures, and administration of pain and antiemetic medications should be carefully scheduled to achieve the utmost symptom relief at meal times. Although self-feeding should be encouraged to promote active exercise and maximal independence, if self-feeding causes excessive pain, assistance with feeding should be provided. Pain is a powerful appetite depressant and may interfere with the necessary caloric intake.

When oral feeding is the sole means of nutritional support,

frequent, small feedings and high-calorie, high-protein supplements are useful in increasing calorie and protein intake. The intake of fluids low in calories and protein such as coffee, tea, diet sodas, etc. should be discouraged or offered as positive reinforcers when adequate oral intake has been achieved.

Evaluation. Outcome criteria include a weight that returns to normal or does not decrease more than 10 per cent of baseline, serum protein levels that return to normal, and a positive nitrogen balance.

Pain

Pain is a major problem for the burned patient. Although the character and intensity may vary throughout all cycles, it is no less a problem. Pain is related to tissue injury and the healing process and is complicated by fear, anxiety, depression, and the chronicity of the healing process. The goal of pain control throughout burn care should be to provide maximal comfort given the nature of the injury and the treatments required for recovery.

Establishing a partnership with the patient as to how to manage pain relief early in the course of care may prevent problems and disappointments in the management of the patient's pain. One of the first goals in pain management is to establish an objective system by which the patient can measure and communicate the intensity of pain. Simple adjective scales using three to five descriptors (i.e., none, mild, medium, moderate, severe) may be used with patients from early school age to the elderly. Scales using numbers should be tailored to the cognitive state of the patient. Rating pain on a scale of 0 to 5 may be used with children of 4 or 5 years (if they know their numbers and have a concept of which is greater). This scale also can be used with young school age children (6 to 9 years) and in patients who seem to have limited cognitive abilities, especially those in the later years of life (i.e., > 70 years). Older school age children, adolescents, and adults who can adequately discriminate between a larger group on the numbers may use 0 to 10 scales or even 0 to 100 scales. In addition to asking patients to rate their pain, health care workers can observe the frequency or intensity of certain physiological responses or behaviors that are indicative of pain. These include increased pulse rate, diaphoresis, increased agitation, grimacing, and rhythmical movements or no movement at all. Observation of these symptoms or behaviors can be especially helpful in diagnosing pain in preverbal children, confused patients, or patients who are intubated and cannot communicate verbally.

As important as the measurement or diagnosis of pain is an assessment of the effectiveness of various pain relief measures. The absence of symptoms or pain behaviors or verbal reports of relief using adjective or numerical scales are necessary to tailor pain management therapies.

The burned patient may experience two types of pain. *Background pain* is the pain related to tissue injury and the inflammatory response, which may be exacerbated by movement, breathing, or pressure. *Procedural pain* is pain brought on by manipulation of the wound, as in dressing changes, debridement, or intensive exercise to prevent skin contractures and improve immobility.

The mainstay of pain management in the acutely injured burn patient is opioids. Morphine may be used during the initial cycle of care to manage both background and procedural pain. Initially, it should be administered in small, frequent doses intravenously or by intravenous drip. Over the first 48 to 72 hours, an adequate level of medication to relieve background pain can be established, and the background medication needs can be converted to oral morphine equivalents. When the patient's condition permits, a long-acting oral opioid can be used to manage background pain. Slow-release oral morphine preparations or methadone can be used for background pain control. The most important aspect of background pain control is to realize that this pain is always present to some degree and is best relieved by administering pain medication on a non-pain-contingent schedule. Background pain control in patients with high anxiety levels may be supplemented with an anxiolytic such as a benzodiazepine. Patient-controlled analgesia (PCA) is another method that may be used to control background pain. This technique works especially well in young male adults who want and need to have some control over their care.

Procedural pain is intermittent and of high intensity. It is also best managed by an opioid. During the initial cycle of care, intravenous morphine or fentanyl may be used. An intravenous morphine bolus should be given 15 to 20 minutes prior to the procedure, and smaller boluses may be given during the procedure, if necessary. Allowing the patient to deliver small doses every 5 minutes using a PCA pump is often very effective during wound care. Fentanyl has a much shorter half-life than morphine and can be used when a short-acting drug is needed. Fentanyl is also useful for the patient with decreased cardiac reserve, exhibited by a labile blood pressure and periods of hypotension when given morphine. Once the patient's condition improves, oral opioids can be used for procedural pain. Immediate-release morphine, hydromorphone, oxycodone, and other opioids or synthetic opioids can be used. Unlike patients with cancer pain, in whom the objective is to begin with the weaker opioid and work up, the objective in burned patients is to begin with potent opioids for the severe pain associated with the fresh open wound and use opioids of decreasing strength as the wounds heal and the pain is less intense. Anxiety and fear, especially fear of the unknown, is a major component of procedural pain. Many patients report that the use of anxiolytics in conjunction with pain medication is very helpful. In this case, the benzodiazepines are useful. When opioids and benzodiazepines are both administered for pain management, the time of peak effectiveness may be different and may necessitate giving them at different times before procedures to obtain maximal effectiveness.

Once the wounds are essentially healed, the need for opioids should diminish. At this point, most of the patient's pain can be managed with regularly scheduled doses of nonsteroidal anti-inflammatory agents. During the later cycles of care, antidepressants may be useful in some patients and may act as an adjunct to pain management.

Nonpharmacological therapies may be useful throughout the various cycles of burn care as an adjunct to other pain-management regimens. The goal of this type of therapy is to assist the patient to relax and to control the perception of pain. The type of nonpharmocological therapy is dependent on individual coping styles and the age of the patient.

Techniques that may be used include distraction, imagery, breathing techniques, hypnosis, and biofeedback. A variety of distraction techniques may be used, such as music, cartoons (especially in children), or talking to the patient about hobbies, etc. Imagery, breathing techniques, and hypnosis are similar and require that the patient actively concentrate on an activity (i.e., breathing) or a mental image that allows the patient to perceive something other than the pain and thus relax. Biofeedback, like imagery, breathing techniques, or hypnosis, requires the patient to concentrate on something other than the pain. In biofeedback, a bodily function such as lowering the heart rate is used to assist the patient with the intense concentration and gives a specific measurement as to when relaxation is maximized. Distraction techniques are external to patient control and require less energy and less cognitive effort on the part of the patient. Imagery, breathing techniques, hypnosis, and biofeedback all require intense patient participation and are energy consuming. When these techniques are used, the patient will often complain of being tired and energyless and may have increased pain complaints after the procedure. Administering less potent pain medications at the end of the procedure may prevent the let-down feeling and decrease pain complaints when nonpharmocological therapies are used.

Evaluation. Outcome criteria should include patient reports of decreased pain and anxiety, increased cooperation with treatments, cooperation with nonpharmocological therapies used as adjuncts to pain management, and satisfaction with the overall pain-management plan.

Prevention of Wound Contractures

Contracture prevention begins immediately and continues until the scar has matured and the patient has completed the rehabilitation cycle. Physical and occupational therapists play a major role in this aspect of care in that they provide a variety of splints and positioning devices and explicit exercise programs aimed at reducing contracture formation. The nurse must provide consistent and frequent monitoring of the patient's position, use of splints, and adherence to an exercise regimen. The nurse must understand the importance of positioning the patient in an anticontracture position and to integrate the use of these positions in the overall management of the patient. Often the use of special antipressure beds or mattresses to prevent tissue breakdown may require an adjustment in the preferred position or the use of a special splint. Understanding the importance of each aspect of care will allow the nurse to work with the therapist to maximize care, reduce tissue breakdown, and prevent contractures at the same time. Likewise, elevation of the patient's head to prevent aspiration or to improve respiratory effort may be contrary to the usual positioning techniques to reduce neck contractures; continued assessment and adjustment in patient positioning may allow all objectives to be accomplished over time. Another area that may pose problems is the need for intravenous access in extremities, which may limit or require alteration of the usual splints used to prevent contractures of extremities. Likewise, a thorough understanding of the goals and priority of all aspects of the burned patient's care allows the nurse to optimize patient care.

Evaluation. Outcome criteria are that contractures will be reduced or prevented while all aspects of patient care are coordinated and optimized.

Rehabilitative and Reconstructive Cycle

As noted in Table 28–7, a variety of nursing issues must be considered for the burned patient during this cycle of care. Of prime concern are potential for impaired skin integrity after healing, activity intolerance, alteration in self-concept, and potential noncompliance secondary to pain, cognitive impairment, lack of motivation, or depression.

Potential Impaired Skin Integrity after Healing

Burn wounds may break down after primary healing for a variety of reasons, such as thinner than normal epithelial cover, excessive dryness with itching, trauma to scar tissue, exposure to sun or extremes of temperatures, and pressure from pressure garments and splinting devices. Burn wounds are especially prone to blistering and tissue breakdown for several months after healing. Without proper cleansing and application of therapies to encourage reepithelialization and prevent infection, these small wounds may become infected and cause additional tissue loss. If treated with gentle cleansing and small adherent pieces of fine-mesh gauze when wounds are smaller than nickel size, these wounds will usually heal in 5 to 7 days. In addition, if the wounds are caused by excessive pressure or active exercise, then adjustment to splints, pressure garments, and exercise routines should be made immediately. It is imperative that discharge teaching cover this type of preventative care so that infection and large open wounds can be minimized. Discharge instructions should be accompanied by a booklet of simple instructions about the aftercare of burns and the telephone number of a nurse or therapist who can answer questions and guide adjustments in the patient's care as necessary.

Evaluation. The outcome criteria are that the burned patient will have no areas of breakdown in healed wounds and if areas of breakdown occur, the patient will be able to manage these wounds without infection and further tissue loss.

Activity Intolerance

Activity intolerance is prevalent in all cycles of burn care but becomes a special concern during this cycle when the patient is striving to regain independence in the activities of daily living and returning to work or school. The problem is related to the prolonged metabolic consequences of the burn injury and decreased range of motion caused by scar maturation and contraction. The goal is for the patient to increase activity tolerance gradually as the scars mature, range of motion improves, and physical stamina increases. Indications of activity intolerance include concern about not being able to complete desired activities, need for frequent rest periods, and exercise intolerance as evidenced by shortness of breath, need for more sleep at night, and a general complaint of malaise. Often the diagnosis of activity intolerance is confused with depression, either or both of which may be prevalent during this cycle of burn care. Usually over time, if the problem is activity intolerance, a planned program of increasing activity with planned periods of rest will result in improvement. This type of plan should be a part of discharge planning. If the patient and patient's family recognize that this is a normal part of rehabilitation, they will be able to plan for this and cope with it. It is often helpful as the patient prepares to return to work or school that the nurse contact the supervisor or teacher and explain the issues related to activity intolerance. Usually allowances can be made for a part-time or limited work schedule that includes additional rest periods. It is also important to explain the patient's need to get back into a normal social environment as soon as possible, since remaining off work or out of school until the patient is completely physically recovered may be detrimental to his psychosocial recovery.

Evaluation. Outcome criteria include decreasing complaints of fatigue and shortness of breath, less need for frequent rest periods, and return to preinjury sleep patterns.

Alterations in Self-Concept

During the resuscitative and reparative cycles, the patient is usually in a state of denial as to what the final outcome of the physical injury will be. Even during the early stages of rehabilitation, the patient may have feelings that with scar maturation and reconstructive surgery, the physical deformities will be corrected and their appearance will return to the preinjury state. This early denial may actually be therapeutic in that the patient is motivated to do what is necessary to return to normal. Sometime during rehabilitation, though, the patient will begin to deal with the alterations in his physical appearance. As incorporation of the new physical appearance occurs, the self-image must change as well. The patient may go through the various stages of grief as the process proceeds. Eventually, the patient will develop a revised self-image. How the patient copes with this revised self-image will depend on the patient, the patient's support system, and the patient's preinjury emotional or psychological status. Interestingly, the final physical appearance may have little correlation with how the patient copes with this revised self-image.[83–85]

Evaluation. Because the alteration in self-image is a lifelong process and may take months to years to evolve after a major insult such as a changed physical appearance, the actual measurement of this outcome is difficult. How patients approach reconstructive procedures, whether they have unrealistic expectations after such procedures, and whether they continue to be motivated to work for even small gains in their rehabilitation plan may suggest how well such patients are adjusting to a revised self-image.

Potential Noncompliance with Treatment Measures

Noncompliance occurs when patients do not follow a treatment regimen or do not behave in the manner expected by the health care team. The reasons for noncompliance are legion, but for the most part, they are the result of lack of communication between patients and members of the health care team. This lack of communication on the part of the health care team usually occurs because we are unclear in our instructions, have expectations that are unachievable by patients, or do not listen to what patients are trying to tell us. Lack of communication on the part of patients occurs because they do not understand the instructions, they lack the cognitive ability to understand, they do not have the social or environmental support to comply with the regimen or expectations, or they lack understanding of the consequences of noncompliance. Symptoms of noncompliance may include wound breakdown, decreased range of motion, increased contracture formation, splints that are not worn because they no longer fit properly, increased complaints, and apparent lack of motivation. Noncompliance is a frustrating problem for both patients and members of the health care team and because of its negative connotation does not foster solutions to the problem. When the problem is considered one of communication breakdown, it can be more readily addressed and corrected. When symptoms of noncompliance appear, the responsibility for the problem lies with the health care worker not the patient. This approach allows the health care worker to diagnose the problem and deal with it. The first question to ask is: Are our plans and expectations realistic? Second, we must diagnose the patient issues. The keystone to diagnosing the patient problem is to listen intently to what patients say or do not say concerning the issues. If patients demonstrate the cognitive ability to understand and perform the recommended care, then other avenues of miscommunication should be explored. What in the environment or in the patient's social relationships impinges on the problem? Does the patient have increased pain related to an undiagnosed physical problem such as heterotopic bone formation? Is the patient showing signs of depression?[86] Usually the cause for the communication problem can be found and corrected, and the symptoms of noncompliance should resolve.

Evaluation. The cause for noncompliance will be explored, and communication problems will be corrected. The outcome criterion is that the symptoms of noncompliance exhibited by the patient will be resolved.

RESEARCH PRIORITIES IN NURSING MANAGEMENT OF THE BURNED PATIENT

A Delphi study to ascertain the research priorities in the care of the burned patient was undertaken in 1990.[87] The goal of this study was to delineate those areas in which nursing practice-based research could improve burn care. The research method used, the Delphi technique, consisted of a series of four questionnaires to reach consensus on the priorities. The final questionnaire contained 101 questions distilled from a total of 548 questions submitted in the initial round of the study. Table 28–8 lists the top 20 priorities for research.

The 2 questions to receive the highest priorities dealt with the management of pain.[88] In addition, 3 other questions in the top 20 were related to pain management. Thus pain-management questions occupied 25 per cent of the top 20 priorities. These questions dealt with nursing interventions to reduce anxiety and pain, the choice and administration of pharmacological modalities, the relief of unpleasant side effects of pharmacological modalities, and the measurement of pain. Research to improve the nursing therapies and to manage the pharmacological therapies related to pain relief was seen as a major area in which scientific inquiry could lead to improved patient management. Questions related to infection control and wound management were the most frequent issues addressed and accounted for 7 of the 20

TABLE 28–8. PRIORITIES: IMPACT ON PATIENT WELFARE

RANK	SCORE	QUESTION
1	6.40	What nursing interventions reduce anxiety and pain during dressing changes and other painful procedures?
2	6.33	What is the role of anesthetic agents used in subanesthetic doses for pain control during painful procedures in burned adults and children?
3	6.25	What modalities are effective in controlling postburn itching? Are some of these more effective than others?
4	6.17	What nursing interventions are most effective in the prevention or minimization of contractures (both short and long term)?
4	6.17	What stategies can nurses employ to optimize intake of prescribed nutritional requirements for pediatric and/or adult patients with burns?
6	6.15	What nursing interventions are most effective in stress reduction in the patient with burns (physiological and psychologic)?
7	6.13	What is the best method to measure the pain of the patient with burns?
8	6.09	What community-based follow-up would best meet the physical and emotional needs of the patient with burns?
9	6.05	What nursing interventions promote healing of donor sites and skin grafts?
10	6.04	What methods are effective in helping patients with burns (children, adolescents, adults) deal with social reentry?
10	6.04	What is the relationship between type of donor-site dressing, patient pain, mobility, and infection?
12	6.03	What is the relationship between the frequency of performing range-of-motion exercises and maintenance of function?
13	6.02	What nursing interventions are most effective in preventing diarrhea from contaminating the burn wound?
14	5.98	What is the relationship between onset of activity and graft take?
14	5.98	What are the most effective routes and methods of narcotic administration in the adult patient with burns at various times after injury?
16	5.97	What is the most effective wound closing protocol for the patient with burns (timing, method, temperature regulations, etc.)?
16	5.97	What is the effect of early use of elastic wraps or pressure garments on healing of the burn wound?

highest priorities.[89] Four questions in the top 20 priorities were related to issues of rehabilitation and discharge planning or aftercare of the burn wound. Three of the top 20 questions were related to psychosocial adjustment of the burn patient.[90] Each of these questions appeared in the 11 questions of highest priority, thus highlighting the importance of this area in future research. Of interest, only 1 question regarding physiological issues was rated among the top 20 priorities; this question was related to nutritional support and was ranked fourth.[91]

An in-depth discussion of these and other research priorities in the nursing management of burn care can be found in a series of articles in the *Journal of Burn Care and Rehabilitation* 1991 through 1992.[87–92]

SUMMARY

The care of the burned patient is complex. Nursing management over the three cycles of care requires the nurse to explore many areas of nursing, continually evaluating signs and symptoms of physical dysfunction as well as addressing psychosocial impairment associated with the injury. Continued research is needed to improve many aspects of patient care and to ensure optimal rehabilitation.

REFERENCES

1. Robson MC, Kucan JO: The burn wound. In Wachtel TL, Kahn V, Frank HA (eds): Current Topics in Burn Care. Rockville, MD, Aspen Publications, 1983, p 56.
2. Luterman A, Curreri PW: Chemical burn injury. In Boswick JA (ed): The Art and Science of Burn Care. Rockville, MD, Aspen Publications, 1987, p 234.
3. Sances A, Myklebust JB, Sanford JD, et al: Experimental electrical injury studies. J Trauma 21:589–597, 1981.
4. Rudowski W, Nasilowski W, Zietkiewicz W, Zietkiewicz K: Burn Therapy and Research. Baltimore, John Hopkins University Press, 1976, pp 262–271.
5. Jackson DM: The diagnosis of the depth of burning. Br J Surg 40:588, 1953.
6. Berkow SG: A method for estimating the extensiveness of lesions (burns and scalds) based on surface area proportions. Arch Surg 8:138, 1924.
7. Lund CC, Browder NC: Estimation of areas of burns. Surg Gynecol Obstet 79:352, 1944.
8. Artz CP, Moncrief JA, Pruitt BA: Burns: A Team Approach. Philadelphia, WB Saunders Co, 1979, p 153.
9. Ward PA, Till GO: Pathophysiological events related to thermal injury of skin. J Trauma 30(suppl):S75–S85, 1990.
10. Alexander JW: Mechanism of immunologic suppression in burn injury. J Trauma 30(suppl):S70–S75, 1990.
11. Gottschlich MM, Jenkins M, Warden, G, et al: Differential effects of three enteral dietary regimens on selected outcome variables in burn patients. JEPN 30:453–456, 1990.
12. Moore FA, Jones TN, McCroskey BC, et al: TEN versus TPN following major abdominal trauma: Reduced septic morbidity. J Trauma 29:916–923, 1989.
13. Inoue S, Epstein MD, Alexander JW, et al: Prevention of yeast translocation across the gut by a single enteral feeding after burn injury. JPEN 13:565–571, 1989.
14. Cuthbertson DP: The disturbance of metabolism produced by bone and nonbony injury with notes on certain abnormal conditions of bone. Biochem J 24:1244–1263, 1930.
15. Wilmore DW, Long JA, Mason AD Jr: Catacholamines: Mediator of the hypermetabolic response to thermal injury. Ann Surg 180:653–668, 1974.
16. Aulick LH, Hander EH, Wilmore DW, et al: The relative significance of thermal and metabolic demands on burn hypermetabolism. J Trauma 19:559–566, 1979.
17. Caldwell FT Jr, Osterholm JL, Sower ND, et al: Metabolic response to thermal trauma of normal and thyroprivic rats at three environmental temperatures. Ann Surg 150:976–988, 1959.
18. Barr PO, Birke G, Liljedahl SO, et al: Oxygen consumption and water loss during treatment of burns with warm, dry air. Lancet 1:164–168, 1968.
19. Zawacki BE, Spitzer KW, Mason AD Jr, et al: Does increased evaporative water loss cause hypermetabolism in burned patients? Ann Surg 171:236–240, 1970.

20. Wilmore DW, Mason AD Jr, Johnson DW, et al: Effect of ambient temperature on heat production and heat loss in burn patients. J Appl Physiol 38:593–597, 1975.
21. Wilmore DW: Metabolic changes after thermal injury. In Boswick JA (ed): The Art and Science of Burn Care. Rockville, MD, Aspen Publications, 1987, p 138.
22. Bessey PQ, Watters JM, Aoki TT, et al: Combined hormonal infusion simulates the metabolic response to injury. Ann Surg 200:264–280, 1984.
23. Watters JM, Bessey PQ, Dinarello CA, et al: Both inflammatory and endocrine mediators are necessary to simulate host response to sepsis. Ann Surg 121:179–190, 1986.
24. Wolfe RR: Caloric requirements of the burned patient. J Trauma 21:712–714, 1981.
25. Davies JWL, Liljedahl SO: Metabolic consequences of an extensive burn. In Polk HC, Stone HH (eds): Contemporary Burn Management. Boston, Little, Brown & Company, 1971, pp 151–169.
26. Wilmore DW: Energy requirements of seriously burned patients and the influence of caloric intake on their metabolic rate. In Cowan GSM Jr, Sheetz W (eds): Intravenous Hyperalimentation. Philadelphia, Lea & Febiger, 1972, pp 96–108.
27. Wilmore DW: Nutrition and metabolism following thermal injury. Clin Plast Surg 1:603–619, 1974.
28. Curreri PW, Luterman A: Nutritional support of the burned patient. Surg Clin North Am 58:1151–1156, 1978.
29. Muir IFK, Barclay TL: Burns and Their Treatment, 2nd ed. Chicago, Year Book Medical Publishers, 1974, pp 113–114.
30. Wachtel TL, Yen M, Fortune JB, et al: Nutritional support for burned patients. In Wachtel TL, Kahn V, Frank HA (eds): Current Topics in Burn Care. Rockville, MD, Aspen Publications, 1983, pp 107–123.
31. Bell SS, Molnar JA, Mangino JE, et al: Manual of Nutritional Support of Adult and Pediatric Burn Patients. Boston, Massachusetts General Hospital and Shriners Burns Institute, 1982.
32. Evans EL, Purnell OJ, Robinett PW, et al: Fluid and electrolyte requirements in severe burns. Ann Surg 135:804, 1952.
33. Reiss E, Stirman JA, Artz CP, et al: Fluids and electrolyte balance in burns. JAMA 152:1309, 1953.
34. Baxter CR, Shires T: Physiologic response to crystalloid resuscitation of severe burns. Ann NY Acad Sci 150:874, 1968.
35. Baxter CR: Fluid and electrolyte changes in the early post burn period. Clin Plast Surg 1:693–709, 1974.
36. Pruitt BA Jr: Fluid and electrolyte replacement in the burned patient. Surg Clin North Am 58:1291–1312, 1978.
37. Monafo WW, Chuntrasakal C, Alvasian V: Hypertonic sodium solution in the treatment of burn shock. Am J Surg 126:778–783, 1973.
38. Wachtel TL, Fortune JB: Fluid resuscitation for burn shock. In Wachtel TL, Kahn V, Frank HA (eds): Current Topics in Burn Care. Rockville, MD, Aspen Publications, 1983, p 47.
39. Harms BA, Kramer GC, Bodai B, Demling RH: Effect of hypoproteinemia on pulmonary and soft tissue edema formation. Crit Care Med 9:503–508, 1981.
40. National Institutes of Health: Consensus Conference. J Trauma 19(11)S89, 1979.
41. Advanced Trauma Life Support Committee on Trauma Instructors Manual. Chicago, American College of Surgeons, 1988.
42. Advanced Burn Life Support. Lincoln, Nebraska, National Burn Institute, 1987.
43. Haynes BW Jr: Early fluid treatment of severe burns: Hemodynamic alterations and the use of dextran and blood. Ann NY Acad Sci 150:907–911, 1968.
44. Dominioni L, Trocki O, Fan CH, et al: Nitrogen balance and liver changes in burned guinea pigs undergoing prolonged high-protein enteral feedings. Surg Forum 34:99, 1983.
45. Gassaniga AB, Barlett RH, Shode JB: Nitrogen balance in patients receiving either fats or carbohydrates for total intravenous nutrition. Ann Surg 182:163, 1975.
46. Jeejeebhoy KN, Anderson GH, Nakhooda AF, et al: Metabolic studies in total parenteral nutrition with lipid in man. J Clin Invest 57:125, 1976.
47. Long JM, Wilmore DW, Mason AD Jr, et al: Effect of carbohydrate and fat intake on nitrogen excretion during total intravenous feeding. Ann Surg 185:417, 1977.
48. Gottschlich MM, Warden GD: Vitamin supplementation in the patient with burns. J Burn Care Rehabil 11(3):275–279, 1990.
49. Lund CC, Levenson SM, Green RW, et al: Ascorbic acid, thiamine, riboflavin and nicotinic acid in relation to acute burns in man. Arch Surg 55:557–583, 1947.
50. Petroff TA, Hander EW, Clayton WH: Pulmonary function studies after smoke inhalation. Am Surg 132:246–351, 1976.
51. Herndon DN, Barrows RE, Linares HA: Inhalation injury in burned patients: Effects and treatments. Burns 14:349–356, 1988.
52. Cioffi WG, Graves TS, McManus WF: High-frequency percussive ventilation in patients with inhalation injury. J Trauma 29:350–354, 1989.
53. Moylan JA, Chan CK: Inhalation injury: An increasing problem. Am Surg 188:34–37, 1978.
54. Robinson NB, Hudson LD, Reiml M, et al: Steroid therapy following isolated smoke inhalation injury. J Trauma 22:876–879, 1982.
55. Pomashefski JF, Davies P, Boggis C, et al: The pulmonary vascular lesions of the adult respiratory distress syndrome. Am J Pathol 112:112–126, 1983.
56. Wedmore CV, Williams TJ: Control of vascular permeability by polymorphonuclear leukocytes in inflammation. Nature 289:646–650, 1981.
57. Weiss SJ: Tissue destruction by neutrophils. N Engl J Med 320:(6)365–376, 1989.
58. Anderson BO, Harkin AH: Multiorgan failure: Inflammatory priming and activation sequences promote autologous tissue injury. J Trauma 30(12):544–549, 1990.
59. Gray DT, Pine RW, Harner TS, et al: Early surgical excision versus conventional therapy in patients with 20–40 percent burns: A comparative study. Am J Surg 144:76–79, 1982.
60. Engrav LH: Acute care and reconstruction of head and neck burns. In Boswick JA (ed): The Art and Science of Burn Care. Rockville, MD, Aspen Publishers, 1987, pp 331–338.
61. Ohmori S: Correction of burn deformities using free flap transfer. J Trauma 22:104, 1982.
62. Niam Yang Zeng, Hao-Man Shih, Laing Chao, et al: Free transplantation of subaxillary lateral thoracodorsal flap in burns. Surg Burns 10:164, 1984.
63. Kenny JG, DiMercurio S, Angel M: Tissue-expanded radial forearm free flap in neck burn contracture. J Burn Care Rehabil 11(5):443–445, 1990.
64. Perry S, Inturrisi CE: Analgesia and morphine deposition in burn patients. J Burn Care Rehabil 4:276–279, 1983.
65. Bloedaw DC, Goodfellow LA, Marvin JA, Heimbach DM: Meperidine deposition in burn patients. Res Commun Chem Pathol Pharmacol 54:87–89, 1986.
66. Zaske DE, Sawchuk RJ, Gerding DS, Strate RG: Increased dosage requirements of gentamycin in burn patients. J Trauma 16:824, 1976.
67. Herndon DN, Barrow RE, Kunkel KR, et al: Effect of recombinant human growth hormone on donor site healing in severely burned children. Ann Surg 212:424–429, 1990.
68. Brown GL, Curtsinger L, Brightwell JR, et al: Enhancement of epidermal regeneration by biosynthetic epidermal growth factor. J Exp Med 163:1319–1324, 1986.
69. Lynch SE, Nixon JC, Colvin RB, et al: Role of platelet-derived growth factor in wound healing: Synergistic effects with other growth factors. Proc Natl Acad Sci USA 84: 7697–7700, 1987.
70. Schultz GS, White N, Mitchell R, et al: Epidermal wound healing enhanced by transforming growth factor alpha and vaccine growth factor. Science 235:350–352, 1987.
71. Lynch JB: Enhancement of wound healing by topical treatment with epidermal growth factor. N Engl J Med 321:76, 1989.
72. Hunt TK: Basic principles of wound healing. J Trauma 30(suppl 12):S122–S128, 1990.
73. Miller SF, Finley RK, Waltman M, Lincks J: Burn size estimation reliability: A study. J Burn Care Rehabil 12:546–559, 1991.
74. Berry CC, Wachtel T, Frank HA: Differences in burn size estimates between prehospital reports and burn center evaluation. J Burn Care Rehabil 3:176–177, 1983.
75. Heimbach DM, Afromowitz MA, Engrav LH, et al: Burn depth estimation: Man or machine? J Trauma 24(5):373–378, 1984.

76. Lynch P, Jackson MM, Cummings MJ, Stamm WE: Rethinking the role of isolation practices in the prevention of nosocomial infection. Ann Intern Med 107:243–246, 1987.
77. Ransjo U: Attempts to control clothes-borne infection in a burn unit: 3. An open-rooted plastic isolator or plastic aprons to prevent contact transfer of bacteria. J Hgy (Camb) 82:369–384, 1979.
78. Lee JJ, Marvin JA, Heimbach DM, et al: Infection control in a burn center. J Burn Care Rehabil 11:575–589, 1990.
79. Johnson WG, Pierce AK, Sanford JP: Changing pharyngeal bacterial flora of hospitalized patients: Emergence of gram-negative bacilli. N Engl J Med 281:1137–1139, 1969.
80. Johnson WG, Woods DE, Chaudhuri T: Association of respiration tract colonization with adherence of gram-negative bacilli to epithelial cells. J Infect Dis. 139:667–669, 1979.
81. Harris GJ, Kealey GP, Massanari MD, Pfaller MA: Comparison of two techniques of central vein catheterization in burn patients. In Proceedings of American Burn Association New Orleans, Louisiana, March 29–April 1, 1989.
82. de Lature BJ: Increased O_2 consumption. Personal communication, 1992.
83. Questad KA, Patterson DR, Boltwood MD, et al: Relating mental health and physical function at discharge to rehabilitation status at three months postburn. J Burn Care Rehabil 9(1):87–89, 1988.
84. Willis-Helmich JJ: Reclaiming body image: The hidden burn. J Burn Care Rehabil 13(1):64–67, 1992.
85. Cobb N, Maxwell G, Silverstein P: Patient perception of quality of life after burn injury: Results of an eleven year survey. J Burn Care Rehabil 11:330–333, 1990.
86. Stoddard FJ, Stroud L, Murphy JM: Depression in children after recovery from severe burns. J Burn Care Rehabil 13(3):340–347, 1992.
87. Marvin JA, Carrougher G, Bayley B, et al: Burn nursing Delphi study: Setting research priorities. J Burn Care Rehabil 12:190–197, 1991.
88. Marvin JA, Carrougher GJ, Bayley EW, et al: Research priorities in burn nursing: Pain assessment and management. J Burn Care Rehabil (in press).
89. Carrougher GJ, Marvin JA, Bayley EW, et al: Research priorities for burn nursing: Report of the wound care and infection control group. J Burn Care Rehabil 12:272–277, 1991.
90. Knighton J, Carrougher GJ, Marvin JA, et al: Research priorities for burn nursing: Report of the psychosocial issues group. J Burn Care Rehabil 13:97–104, 1992.
91. Rutan RL, Carrougher GJ, Marvin JA, et al: Research priorities for burn nursing: Report on physiologic issues. J Burn Care Rehabil 13:373–377, 1992.
92. Bayley EW, Carrougher GJ, Marvin JA, et al: Research priorities for burn nursing: Patient, nurse and burn prevention education. J Burn Care Rehabil 12:377–383, 1991.

29

THE TRAUMA PATIENT WITH A PREEXISTING PSYCHIATRIC DISORDER

NEIL WARRES and PAUL McCLELLAND

Trauma patients with psychiatric disorders pose many problems from the time of admission through their return to the community. The recognition, assessment, and diagnosis of these disorders may include contributions from ambulance staff, surgeons, and psychiatrists, but the role of the nurse in all these efforts is crucial. Considerable knowledge and skill in history taking and interviewing are essential to this role. Among the most common psychiatric disorders in the general population,[1,2] schizophrenia, depression, personality disorders, and alcohol abuse are of special importance in the trauma unit. The nurse needs to know the principal symptoms and signs, natural history, and techniques of management applicable in the intensive care setting. In addition, the nurse should be familiar with commonly used psychotropic medications and the assessment of both therapeutic efficacy and side effects. Equally important is an appreciation of the behavioral and psychological changes that result from head injuries, sepsis, medications, and other factors that mimic or exacerbate the disorders listed above. The nurse needs to be able to identify when a disorder is acute or dangerous and requires immediate, aggressive intervention; when a disorder is not immediately treatable or changeable but requires special management techniques; and when the most appropriate intervention is simply good discharge referral for definitive treatment in another setting. Discharge planning requires an understanding of the strengths and limitations of community mental health centers and other typical community resources. A very important, related issue is when and how to use the psychiatric consultant to assist in the assessment, treatment, and referral of patients. Finally, a task of unsurpassed importance is the recognition and management of the feelings of anger, fear, and rejection that such patients often evoke in nurses and other care providers, as well as in their own families.

This chapter begins with a discussion and case presentation

of each of the disorders mentioned above. With this foundation, the remaining issues are discussed.

SCHIZOPHRENIA

Although great strides have been made in the control of certain symptoms of schizophrenia, it remains a devastating, often progressive disease of unknown etiology. This accounts for some of the feelings of hopelessness and helplessness frequently experienced by medical staff members when they encounter schizophrenics. Most of its victims will suffer chronic or intermittent disruptions of several functions, including the ability to discriminate between fantasy and reality. This inability is synonymous with psychosis; its symptoms, often bizarre hallucinations and delusions, are largely responsible for the difficulties in empathizing with and relating to the schizophrenic. Medical personnel must overcome these difficulties if they are to establish the effective communication necessary to perform adequate medical assessment and ensure satisfactory compliance with medical treatments. Listening to, speaking with, understanding, and making oneself understood all hinge on a rudimentary insight into the disorder of thinking that underlies the many symptoms of these patients. This insight advances communication in a number of ways, perhaps most importantly by making such patients appear more human and less bizarre.

There are different types of schizophrenia with somewhat different symptoms, prognoses, and etiologies. Nevertheless, all schizophrenic patients share certain features that are known as *cardinal,* or *core, symptoms* and signs. By way of analogy, pneumonia can present with bizarre behavior, agitation, confusion, and many other symptoms or signs, but most patients have fever, cough, and tachypnea, the cardinal signs for this syndrome of many etiologies.

Supervised work with schizophrenics is the most effective way to learn how to recognize this disorder and to overcome the many hurdles to taking care of these patients. This can occur in the trauma unit with supervision provided by the unit's psychiatric liaison nurse and/or psychiatrist. As preparation for this type of training, reading the next section will provide an awareness of the more common presenting symptoms as well as a rudimentary understanding of their origins and meanings.

Case History

Mr. Wright is a 34-year-old single man who was admitted to a trauma center after jumping from a highway bridge and sustaining multiple fractures of both legs. In the resuscitation area he was fully alert. A neurological examination revealed no deficits. There was no spontaneous speech, but his responses to questions were coherent and goal-directed. The patient appeared hypervigilant, but there was no suggestion of paranoia. He did not volunteer any information about hallucinations or delusions, and he was not questioned about these symptoms. After surgery and a brief stay in the intensive care unit, both of which were uneventful, he was transferred to the step-down unit. In this setting, he initiated no interactions with any of the staff and remained hypervigilant. Several staff members remarked that they felt distinctly uncomfortable around him and said they wondered if he was suspicious about something. One physician raised the question of possible drug abuse. A review of the toxicology screen obtained at admission revealed a positive assay for phenothiazines but was otherwise negative. A psychiatric consultation was requested because of the suicide attempt and because the patient's silence suggested withdrawal due to depression. The psychiatrist elicited a history of five hospitalizations in mental institutions over the prior 7 years. Since the most recent hospitalization Mr. Wright had been taking trifluoperazine hydrochloride (Stelazine) in an attempt to treat several symptoms, including "hearing voices" that told him to kill himself. A week before the accident, for no apparent reason, the voices had become more intensely insistent that he kill himself. He abruptly made the decision to follow their command and thus made the suicide attempt that resulted in his admission. At the time of the evaluation, he was alert and very paranoid, and the voices were still present. He was placed on suicide precautions and Stelazine, 20 mg PO b.i.d. The next day he reported considerable reduction in his paranoia despite the fact that the voices remained. After 5 days, the suicide precautions were removed and he was transferred to a rehabilitation hospital, where he was maintained on Stelazine and followed by the hospital psychiatrist.

This patient demonstrates many of the typical features of schizophrenia, which will be discussed in the following section. It is noteworthy that several of the staff members sensed that Mr. Wright had some type of mental disorder, but they were not sure whether this was depression, drug abuse, or something else. Many schizophrenics evoke similar feelings in staff. It is important to trust these feelings and request a psychiatric evaluation in such cases.

Common Symptoms

Irrational Statements

Trauma patients often make irrational statements such as "You doctors are trying to kill me!" "This is not a hospital—you're not a nurse!" or "You're trying to hurt me." The most common explanation for such behavior is that the patient is delirious—perhaps from shock, from alcohol intoxication or withdrawal, as a side effect of administered medications, from head injury or infection. Since delirium is so common and since it often spontaneously disappears as the patients' medical problems are successfully treated, this type of behavior is often overlooked and not investigated. It is important to note that virtually all cases of delirium also include clouding of consciousness (the absence of a continual state of alertness). Delirious patients also typically have memory deficits and are disoriented to time and often place. Sometimes they cannot identify their own name. Thus irrational statements particularly raise the possibility of schizophrenia when there is no clouding of consciousness (the cardinal symptom of delirium)—and even more so when there is no accompanying memory impairment or disorientation and there is no obvious reason for delirium to be present. This was the case for Mr. Wright when he was evaluated by the psychiatrist.

Certain types of statements are strongly suggestive of schizophrenia. Reports of having one's thoughts or actions controlled by machines or people and complaints that others can hear one's own thoughts are two examples. Descriptions of thoughts having been inserted into the patient's mind or of thoughts having been removed from his head are additional examples. Finally, complaints of any bizarre physical experiences, such as snakes or other animals crawling within the patient's abdomen or of "rays" being directed at the patient and causing a headache or other symptoms, are unusual and raise the possibility of schizophrenia. Although delirious patients occasionally report such experiences, these patients deserve psychiatric evaluation. This is especially true when these complaints persist for several days or when there is a history of schizophrenia in the patient or his family.

Psychiatric consultation may be helpful even when a patient who makes irrational statements is suspected to be delirious rather than schizophrenic. For example, if the irrational statements contain suicidal thought content, risk of suicide may need to be evaluated. If the patient is agitated, the psychiatrist can often help the treatment team choose appropriate medication, assess the risk of violence, and clarify any need for physical restraints.

Hallucinations

Reports of unusual sensations are common in the trauma unit because of severe pain, spinal cord injuries, medication toxicity, alcohol withdrawal, and many other factors. Some patients may mislabel shadows as animals or people. These mislabelings or misidentifications can involve sounds, smells, or other sensory modalities and are usually short-lived and rarely significant. *Hallucinations* refer to situations in which the patient reports sounds, sights, or smells that others cannot perceive. Although still commonplace in trauma patients, such symptoms should be recorded as evidence that the patient is psychotic. A psychiatric evaluation is indicated because even though the majority of cases will have a physical basis such as intoxication or sepsis, treatment with an antipsychotic medication may be required to diminish or avoid agitation. Furthermore, some of these patients will be found to have schizophrenia.

The schizophrenic patient may describe hearing two or more voices conversing ("He is no good." "He is too!") or one voice commenting about his behavior or thoughts. The voices are usually described as being outside the patient's head and may have been present for months or years. This symptom is rarely seen in patients other than schizophrenics and should always prompt evaluation by a psychiatrist.

Bizarre Behavior and Inappropriate Affect

The preceding phenomena often strike the observer as bizarre, an experience that the nurse can learn to use as a cue that psychosis such as schizophrenia may be present. Other schizophrenic patients may present in different but equally bizarre ways. Abnormal body posture itself or the patient's explanation that he assumes this position "to atone for my sins" may hint at the presence of schizophrenia.

Many schizophrenic patients have a noticeably strange affect. That is, their facial expressions seem either oddly blank, bizarre, or in some other way inappropriate to the situation. "Flat" or "inappropriate" affect is considered to be a hallmark of schizophrenia, and whenever this is noted, schizophrenia should be a major part of the differential diagnosis. This is also true whenever a patient appears very strangely aloof or socially withdrawn.

Myriad examples of strange behavior by schizophrenics could be discussed, but there are two essential points to be made. First, bizarre behaviors or experiences should not be ignored. Second, the nurse's investigation of these phenomena should include careful questioning of the patient to elicit his explanations for their occurrence. In addition to providing information about the patient's speech (a focal neurological function), the patient's explanation may reveal the presence of psychosis.

Underlying Psychopathology

The preceding examples suggest something of the range of possible presentations or chief complaints and raise the question of how all these cases can be given one diagnosis. The answer is that psychiatric evaluation of these patients will reveal a few underlying characteristics. Although an understanding of these characteristics is not essential to the nurse's or nonpsychiatric physician's primary roles of seeing that these patients receive psychiatric evaluations, such understanding can be invaluable in continuing to work and communicate with the schizophrenic and his family. A rudimentary knowledge of the basis or meaning of otherwise bizarre and meaningless symptoms will make these patients seem more human and normal. This information is useful in understanding the family's experience with such a patient. The following section provides some basis for such understanding.

Disturbance in Thinking

One of the cardinal signs of schizophrenia is a serious and often profound difficulty with thinking. Irrational statements are the result of illogical and disorganized thought processes; therefore, schizophrenia is regarded as a "thought disorder" and not a "mood disorder" (such as depression). Machines do not put thoughts into the schizophrenic's mind, but the patient and the interviewer may have no better explanation for the way the patient connects two thoughts.

A schizophrenic with abdominal pain might first think of his intestines as a source or location of the pain. If the thought of his intestines makes him think of snakes (because of the similarity in shape or for some other reason), he may then illogically conclude that snakes within his abdomen are the cause of his pain.

Sometimes bizarre comments by schizophrenics can be understood as if they were metaphorical statements. For example, a schizophrenic's statement, "I am possessed by demons!" might be understood to mean: "I feel like I'm possessed by demons; I feel like I'm a bad person."

Although many of the bizarre statements and behaviors can be explained as the result of disordered thinking, auditory hallucinations require a different type of explanation, which illustrates another way of understanding schizophrenic symptoms. One of the monumental problems resulting from the thought disorder is misunderstandings in relationships. As a result, many people with schizophrenia are socially isolated and profoundly lonely. For some schizophrenics, the voices soften this painful state by providing the illusion of companionship. Since relationships are often so confusing and painful, the voices also can shield the patient from pain by keeping other people at a distance. (The typical response to the hallucinating patient is to avoid him.)

Etiology

If disordered thinking is the core deficit in schizophrenia, what is its etiology? Currently, the answer to this question remains obscure. There is an increasing body of evidence that indicates that schizophrenics have metabolic, chemical, and perhaps structural brain abnormalities and that some of these abnormalities are inherited. However, not everyone with an inherited vulnerability to schizophrenia seems to get the disease itself. Some theories suggest that schizophrenia develops when there is a combination of genetic predisposition along with pathological early development. (That is, personality traits learned in childhood predispose the individual to psychotic responses to a variety of stressful circumstances such as living independently, working, or forming relationships.) Although further discussion of this issue is beyond the scope of this chapter, it is important to note that genetic, biological, personality, and social factors are all presumed to interact in combination in producing schizophrenic symptoms. This has important implications for treatment, both within the trauma center and elsewhere. In particular, as discussed below, medication, individual and family therapy, and hospitalization all play a role in treatment.

Disease Course and General Treatment Goals

Schizophrenia is usually diagnosed for the first time during early adulthood. Typically, the process starts insidiously and gradually. The patient becomes withdrawn, unmotivated, and begins behaving oddly. He suffers a progressive deterioration in function at school or work and begins to have increasingly disordered and peculiar thought processes. He may exhibit poor personal hygiene, and the withdrawal from the people and events in his environment may become profound. Eventually, the typical patient develops more flagrant psychotic symptoms. He begins to experience delusions (false beliefs) such as that he is possessed. His thoughts may become grossly disjointed and incoherent. He may begin experiencing hallucinations similar to the auditory hallucinations described previously. The typical schizophrenic patient stops being grossly psychotic after a period of several weeks to several months but may never return to his premorbid level of functioning even though he is no longer overtly psychotic. Instead, his overall functional capacity may remain decreased. Most schizophrenic patients experience multiple recurrences of psychotic episodes. Treatment is very effective in decreasing the duration and severity of these episodes but is less effective in improving patients' chronically decreased level of functioning during the quiescent intervals in between.

This discussion described the typical schizophrenic patient, but there is considerable variability. Some patients gradually deteriorate over time; their baseline level of functioning between psychotic episodes worsens throughout the course of their lives. Other patients return to a fully normal or near-normal functional state whenever their psychosis abates. Some never recover from their first psychosis. Others recover fully and never have any relapses. This latter group is not considered to have true schizophrenia but instead is diagnosed as having a "schizophreniform disorder."

The goals of treatment are limited and difficult to achieve. One is to reduce the number and duration of psychotic episodes. Another is to maximize recovery after each episode. Additionally, one wants to help the patient avoid hospitalization and maintain employment and functional independence. An important but easily overlooked goal is preventing suicide and other self-destructive behaviors during and between psychotic episodes.

Antipsychotic medications are often effective in controlling agitation, lowering anxiety, decreasing social withdrawal, and reducing or eliminating the hallucinations and delusions that appear during acute episodes. Individual psychotherapy can help the patient develop a more reality-based assessment of day-to-day events, identify sources of stress in the environment as well as appropriate coping methods, provide respite from loneliness, enable the monitoring of effects of antipsychotic medications, combat noncompliance with medications which so often defeats treatment programs that rely solely on medications, and generally support the patient. Family therapy is used to teach the family how to support the patient without unduly compromising his independence, provide support for family members, and identify any other family members needing individual attention. Psychiatric hospitalization may be required to protect the acutely suicidal patient, safeguard the extremely agitated or combative patient, eliminate environmental stresses, evaluate the effects of medications, initiate individual and/or family therapy, and, less desirably, provide safe shelter.

All these treatments are available to most patients. Many need a mental health worker who is skillful at coordinating these and other services. The psychiatric consultant is usually the best source of information about community services of this type.

Screening and Management Through the Trauma Cycles

Resuscitation and Critical Care

The preceding discussion included most of the information necessary to screen patients for schizophrenia, a task that sometimes can be performed during the resuscitation and critical care cycles of treatment. Of course, life-threatening and potentially debilitating injuries must receive first priority for care. A psychiatric history should be obtained for any patient suspected of having this disorder, although identification of the symptoms and signs described above already constitutes sufficient grounds for requesting psychiatric consultation. Examples of particularly relevant historical questions for the patient and family members are these: (1) Has the patient ever been hospitalized in a psychiatric unit (including admission for detoxification from alcohol or other drugs)? (2) Has the patient ever taken antipsychotic or other psychotropic medicine? (3) Has the patient ever been seen by a psychiatrist or other mental health worker? (4) Has the patient ever attempted suicide or been violent? (5) Has the patient ever experienced hallucinations? (6) Is the answer to any of these questions "yes" for any of the patient's relatives?

The patient also might be asked if he is currently "hearing voices others don't hear" or having any type of hallucination, and whether he is having any thoughts of hurting himself or anyone else. If the patient answers "yes" to either of these questions, or if the patient seems very agitated or distraught, psychiatric evaluation should be requested on an emergency basis.

When a psychiatrist confirms that a patient has schizophrenia, a number of management strategies should be instituted. All these are best understood as strategies for dealing with the aforementioned disorder of thinking which characterizes schizophrenia. Most important is providing careful explanations of the rationale and meaning of tests, physical examinations, medications, and other treatments so that the patient is less likely to develop irrational and paranoid explanations of his own. Similarly, the patient should be questioned daily about pain and other symptoms so that these experiences can be discussed and explained. This is especially important with respect to any experienced hallucinations or other misperceptions or misinterpretations, since schizophrenic patients have so much difficulty maintaining an accurate sense of reality.

It is important to monitor the patient for suicide or other violent impulses. Although the psychiatrist will be attuned to this potential, the nursing staff will have much greater opportunity to observe suspicious behaviors such as hiding scissors or other potential weapons. It is essential to ask the patient about thoughts or plans of violence. The nurse might say, "Many of our patients get very upset while they're here. Some think about giving up or hurting themselves. Others find themselves afraid of losing control and hitting the staff or other people. Have you had thoughts like this?" If the patient acknowledges having these thoughts or feelings, this should be treated as a dangerous situation, and the psychiatrist should be called immediately. This is especially true for thoughts of this type that are described as intrusive or beyond the patient's control. Hearing voices that tell the patient to kill himself or someone else would be an extreme example of this.

Many schizophrenic patients are characterized as "loners." They typically find interpersonal relationships stressful and threatening and prefer relative solitude. Staff caring for these patients should bear this in mind and not increase these patients' anxiety by mistakenly pushing them to socialize.

Intermediate Care and Rehabilitation

Treatment for an exacerbation of schizophrenia may begin in the resuscitation area, critical care unit, or intensive care unit, but this will usually be restricted to antipsychotic medication and supportive individual psychotherapy. When the patient is no longer critically ill and has been transferred to an extended care or rehabilitation unit, treatment may become more aggressive, including higher doses of antipsychotics [doses of 50 to 80 mg per day of haloperidol (Haldol) or equivalent doses of other agents would not be unusually high] and involvement of the family. Alternatively, especially if the patient fails to respond to these treatments, transfer to a psychiatric unit may be necessary at this time.

The goals of treatment are to end the psychotic episode quickly, avoid psychiatric hospitalization if possible, involve the family in the patient's treatment, and motivate the patient and his family to continue with appropriate psychiatric treatment after discharge. It is important to note that the current psychotic episode may be the patient's first or the first for which he received treatment. In either case, successful intervention may have a significant effect on the patient's prognosis by showing the patient and family the desirable consequences of early and thorough treatment. Moreover, since the trauma nurses and surgeons often have saved the patient's life, their belief in and support of psychiatric treatment may be invaluable in getting the patient and family to remain compliant after discharge to the community.

When these patients are treated in the trauma or rehabilitation units, the nurse can play a major role by monitoring and recording the treatment response of "target symptoms." Often the treating psychiatrist will specify which of the patient's symptoms should be monitored. Early in treatment, the target symptom will usually be agitation. Subsequently, withdrawal from the environment and, later still, hallucinations and delusions may become the focus of treatment.

While monitoring treatment response, the staff should be alert for potential side effects of antipsychotic medication. By far the most common are acute dystonia, akathisia, and pseudoparkinsonian states. Acute dystonia is a sudden episode of dramatically increased muscle tension or spasm, which often presents as torticollis but which may involve any muscle group, including those of the larynx. With the exception of the latter (laryngeal stridor, a potentially fatal complication with death resulting from asphyxiation), this is not life-threatening. However, the fear and pain that often accompany this condition frequently produce considerable agitation. Fortunately, this state is easily reversed with 1 to 2 mg benztropine mesylate (Cogentin) or biperiden (Akineton), both of which can be given orally or parenterally. Another common treatment is 50 mg diphenhydramine (Benadryl) given orally or parenterally, but this can cause problems with sedation or respiratory depression. Acute dystonia usually occurs during the first few days of treatment. Usually it is treated for days to weeks with daily doses of benztropine mesylate.

Akathisia usually presents after a few weeks of treatment but can begin as early as 5 days after an antipsychotic agent is started. This adverse effect consists of a poorly defined sense of motor restlessness, usually in the calf muscles. Although less dramatic than the dystonic reaction, this condition is unpleasant and may result in refusal to take the antipsychotic or noncompliance with other medical or psychiatric treatments. Reduction of the dose of the antipsychotic agent may be beneficial. The medications listed for treatment of acute dystonia are often ineffective. Propranolol (Inderal), 20 to 80 mg a day, is probably the most effective drug. Sometimes benzodiazepines such as diazepam (Valium) are helpful.

The signs of the pseudoparkinsonian syndrome are those of the idiopathic Parkinson's disease, including mask-like facies, increased muscle tone and rigidity, pill-rolling tremor, difficulty initiating and terminating movement, and sometimes drooling. This condition typically develops 5 to 30 days after initiation of treatment with antipsychotic medication. It responds to the same medications as acute dystonia. (A typical treatment might be Cogentin, 1 to 2 mg PO b.i.d.) This drug side effect is often mistaken for depression.

The key to discovering any of these side effects is observation, plus asking the patient about each set of symptoms.

DEPRESSION

For psychiatrists, *depression* refers to a syndrome of psychological and physical signs and symptoms that, like schizophrenia, has multiple etiologies. Many depressive illnesses are also chronic, with numerous relapses. Unlike schizophrenia, however, many of the etiologies and their specific remedies are known. A variety of effective treatments exists even for those cases in which the cause is unknown. The natural history of this disorder also differs in that its victims do not generally demonstrate the deteriorating course often seen in the schizophrenic. Because of these differences, and because the symptoms and signs are less bizarre than those of schizophrenia, nurses, doctors, and family members generally do not have the same degree of difficulty in empathizing with these patients. Similarly, since the core symptoms and signs of depression center around a disturbance of mood or feeling state rather than a disturbance of thinking, communication with the depressed patient is not as great a challenge. Diagnosis and choice of treatment, however, can be very difficult with trauma patients. Very severe depressions can be disguised by physical symptoms so that they appear minor. Medical considerations can make pharmacological treatment difficult. However, effective identification and treatment are essential. Depression can last for months and result in virtually total incapacitation. Depressed patients are at significant risk for suicide and alcohol and drug abuse. It is imperative that trauma staff ensure that depressed patients and those suspected of being depressed are referred for psychiatric evaluation. The following section will focus on this task.

Case History

Mr. Wilson is a 38-year-old married man who was admitted after being struck by an automobile while crossing a street. In the resuscitation area he was found to have a hemopneumothorax, multiple rib fractures, a positive minilaparotomy, and hematuria. Following surgery and a stormy postoperative course marked by two septic episodes, he was transferred to the intensive care unit. His recovery was uneventful from this point on, and he felt ready for discharge after a total stay of 26 days. Five days prior to discharge, his wife asked the staff to obtain a psychiatric evaluation because she was concerned about a personality change she had observed in him over the prior 2 or 3 months. The patient did not want to see the psychiatrist but was convinced by the primary nurse that such evaluations were routine in the trauma unit. Mr. Wilson denied feeling depressed and denied that his personality had changed. He acknowledged several stressful events during the previous 6 months, including a financial setback that had threatened his plans to send his daughter to a private secondary school. When asked about his "strengths," he first denied that he had any and then mentioned a former interest in woodworking, which the wife described as a skill of professional quality. He had not entered his woodworking shop or attempted to play his piano (another activity that his wife and friends described as one that he used to perform with great talent and enthusiasm) for several months. Mr. Wilson attributed this to lack of time but finally acknowledged that the thought of engaging in either activity no longer gave him any pleasure. He slept poorly and ate little for several weeks prior to his accident; both of these were attributed by him to his recent excessive consumption of alcohol. He denied any thoughts of suicide. He was preoccupied with thoughts about his own death and blamed this experience on his near death over the previous few weeks. Later he admitted that he had been troubled by these thoughts for several months and that he thought that all responsible people had similar experiences during middle age. His mother and her brother had both been treated for depression. A detailed investigation of his accident failed to reveal any evidence that it was a suicide attempt. He agreed to return as an outpatient to see the psychiatrist.

This patient denied that he had many of the symptoms of depression and specifically denied that he was depressed. Furthermore, he did not want to see the psychiatrist. This resistance was easily countered, and psychiatric evaluation confirmed the presence of depression. Subsequent treatment with an antidepressant led to a dramatic reversal of his condition over a 3-week period. All this is very typical. Also common was the wife's concern about his condition and her labeling of his problem as a personality change. All family concerns about a trauma patient's premorbid emotional status and their requests for a psychiatric consultation should be taken seriously. The most common presenting symptoms and signs are discussed in more detail in the following section.

Common Presentations

Depression is more than a sad or gloomy mood and more than a feeling of unhappiness related to adverse circumstances. It is a serious psychological disorder with a constellation of symptoms and signs. Characteristically, a mood disturbance is present, but additional abnormalities involve somatic function, thought, and motivation.

Depressed or Irritable Mood

"Sad," "lonely," "down," "gloomy," "empty," or "depressed" might be the words used by six different individuals to describe essentially the same mood. It is easy to overlook the possible significance of this symptom because it represents a common and, most would agree, normal experience. In fact, the mood of the depressed patient differs only in the intensity and duration of these feelings. Any patient who reports a depressed mood and describes it as new, deeper, more intense than usual or unduly persistent should be evaluated further. With respect to duration, most moods last several hours to a day or two at most. The depressed patient, by comparison, may report this mood as a predominant experience for weeks to months. As the severity of the depression increases, the patient becomes progressively less responsive to the usual daily experiences that provoke nondepressed moods in most of us. Inspiring music, humorous movies, invigorating activities, and interesting or stimulating people all lose their impact when one becomes depressed.

Disorders of Sleep, Appetite, or Other Somatic Functions

An alteration in the sleep–wake cycle, especially the pattern of waking 2 to 4 hours earlier than normal, is well known as a classic symptom of depression, but some patients experience difficulty falling asleep or begin sleeping excessively. Many patients' appetites worsen and they lose weight, but some eat excessively and gain weight. Physical and mental fatigue, profound slowing of all motor activity, loss of libido, and decreased ability to concentrate are additional, generally accepted features of this disorder. Less familiar findings include constipation, agitation, and a striking daily fluctuation in the severity of all symptoms, with morning hours dreaded as the worst of the day.

Depressive Thoughts

Just as the mood disturbance in depression is best understood as a deepening and prolongation of normal feelings, the disturbance in thinking represents a preoccupation with commonplace and essentially normal thoughts. Most people will admit to at least occasional thoughts about their shortcomings, the inevitability of physical deterioration and death, feelings of hopelessness about whether certain problems in their life will go away, a sense of helplessness or inability to effect changes in their job or in other areas of their life, and some degree of guilt about past activities. For the depressed patient, one and often several of these themes becomes incorporated into intense, persistent, and intrusive thought patterns. The patient's preoccupation with them precludes other more "normal" thought processes. The patient may begin dwelling on how helpless and hopeless things seem, or how guilty he feels, and thus may stop thinking about eating, or working, or playing, or loving, or being with others. An excessive focus on physical symptoms is a common finding in depressed patients. Normal aches and pains are less likely to be overlooked. Physical symptoms of depression may be interpreted as having much more serious portent. Thus a patient's experience of weight loss, fatigue, and loss of appetite may lead to hypochondriacal or, in the extreme, delusional concerns about having cancer or some other serious disorder. This characteristic presents serious problems and will be discussed below.

Impaired Motivation

Perhaps the most distressing symptom of severe depression is the loss of interest in other people, work, hobbies, food, and ultimately, virtually everything. Hours seem like days, days like weeks, and nothing breaks the monotony and emptiness. As with the mood changes and the abnormalities of thought, this symptom occurs in nondepressed people, but for much shorter periods and with much less intensity. Survivors of suicide attempts that have occurred during a serious depression frequently describe this experience as the most troubling and least tolerable of all that they endured.

Etiology

There are many causes of the depressive syndrome. A partial list of medical causes includes increased or decreased thyroid or adrenal function, vitamin B_{12} deficiency, hypercalcemia, a variety of other metabolic abnormalities, viral illnesses, abdominal neoplasms, stroke, and Parkinson's disease. The physical stigmata of each of these conditions and the absence of a personal or family history for depression suggest the diagnosis.

Several drugs and medications are notorious for causing depression. Alcohol, cocaine, and other sedatives and stimulants can cause severe depressions. Antihypertensive medications, especially alpha-methyldopa, reserpine, and clonidine, are also important causes. Other agents associated with depression include birth control pills, corticosteroids, and benzodiazepines (Valium, Librium). An onset of symptoms within days to weeks after the initiation of therapy is the usual clue. It is noteworthy that people with a history of depression are more susceptible to this complication, so a history of depression does not make the diagnosis of drug-induced depression less likely.

Although many depressions will have identifiable etiologies, the majority of serious depressions are best understood with psychological theories. For example, many of these depressions appear to develop when the patient is forced to accept a real or threatened loss. The loss may involve a person, job, home, self-respect, or anything else greatly valued. It may be, though, that many of those patients who are prone to depression have an inherited vulnerability. That is, these patients may respond to loss by becoming depressed in a way which is analogous to how the schizophrenic patient responds to stress by becoming psychotic. Depression, like schizophrenia, seems to have a genetic component involving inherited vulnerability to the disease. As with schizophrenia, the mechanism whereby genetic or biological factors are expressed is unknown.

Treatment Through the Trauma Cycles

Resuscitation and Critical Care

Depression is not generally likely to interfere with medical treatment in these settings. However, one important exception is the acutely suicidal patient. Nursing staff should always be alert to the possibility that a patient may be depressed and potentially suicidal—especially if he was admitted with a self-inflicted wound, has a history of depression, or is being treated with antidepressant medication. When a recent suicide attempt or current suicidal intent is suspected, the patient should be questioned about his mood, about any wishes to die, and about any thoughts of hurting himself. The patient's family and friends also should be questioned about whether they have noticed any change in mood or behavior or have become aware of physical symptoms suggestive of depression or suicidal ideation. If there is even minimal continued suspicion that a patient might intend to harm himself, prudence dictates that staff watch him closely and that all potentially harmful objects and substances be removed from the bedside. A psychiatric evaluation should be requested immediately to determine the need for continued suicide precautions and to begin instituting appropriate psychiatric treatment. It is important to note that the risk for suicide is increased considerably whenever a depressed patient has a coexistent organic brain syndrome (head injury, delirium, dementia). These patients' poor judgment and increased impulsiveness impair their ability to exercise restraint if they begin thinking about killing themselves.

Often, if a patient was taking antidepressant medication prior to admission, the medication will temporarily be stopped because of the effects of these agents on blood pressure and cardiac function and because of the interactions with other medications. Excessive sedation may result from the combination of antidepressants and analgesics, for example. Symptoms from antidepressant withdrawal are not dramatic. If they occur, they consist of cholinergic rebound (from the very potent anticholinergic effects of these medications), which resembles an upper respiratory illness.

Occasionally, patients are admitted who were taking a kind of antidepressant called an *MAO inhibitor*. Examples of medications in this class are phenelzine (Nardil) and tranylcypromine (Parnate). It is important to be aware of this because serious adverse drug interactions can occur when a patient who took an MAO inhibitor is given meperidine (Demerol) or pressor agents or other catecholamines. Also, there are serious adverse effects from many foods, and dietary restriction is necessary. Special precautions are necessary for 2 weeks after discontinuation of the drug.

The definitive evaluation and treatment of depression are usually deferred until the patient is stabilized and moved to a less acute care setting. It is crucial that any information about possible depression which was obtained from the patient or his family at the time of admission be communicated to intermediate care and rehabilitation staff so that the patient can be evaluated and appropriately treated in those settings.

Intermediate Care and Rehabilitation

A serious depression can interfere significantly with recovery by impeding the patient's ability to engage in rehabilitative therapies. The risk of suicide both before and after hospital discharge supports the need for aggressive treatment with medication and/or psychotherapy during these cycles of treatment. A response to treatment may require several days or weeks. During this time, the nurse bears the burden of observing the patient for activities suggesting suicidal ideation. Fortunately, most suicidal patients will address this issue with the nursing staff. Many will initiate this by complaining of hopelessness or by exhibiting other symptoms of depression. Such patients should be asked directly and repeatedly if they are bothered by thoughts of hurting themselves or "ending it all." They also should be evaluated by the unit's psychiatrist. For those patients started on antidepressants, it is crucial that the nurse monitor the patient for side effects and therapeutic response. Unpleasant side effects often occur, and unless the patient is encouraged and told that these symptoms are usually short-lived and not dangerous, they may refuse to continue therapy. The typical side effects of antidepressant medication include feelings of drowsiness, dizziness when rising suddenly (due to orthostatic hypotension), dry mouth, constipation, blurred vision, and possible urinary retention. Many of the tricyclic antidepressants are given as a bedtime dose to minimize these side effects. On the other hand, Fluoxetine (Prozac) and amphetamines such as methylphenidate (Ritalin) are typically given in the morning because these drugs interfere with sleep. The selection of the drug is dependent on the patient's medication history (response to a particular medication or a family history of response to one drug) and the clinical utility of particular side effects such as sedation or stimulation.

The desired effects of the medication should be clear to the patient and nurse so that decisions can be made about modifying the dosage. Patients usually begin to sleep better before experiencing more energy and a lifting of their mood. The depressive thinking and lack of motivation are usually the last symptoms to disappear. Targeted on these four symptoms, nursing observations play an essential role in the treatment of depression. Therapeutic response to traditional antidepressant agents usually takes a minimum of 2 weeks.

PERSONALITY DISORDER

Demanding, dissatisfied, and generally intolerable patients frequently are labeled as having personality disorders requiring strict limit setting. This management approach rarely works well. One problem stems from the difficulty differentiating in the trauma unit between a personality disorder and the temporary use of primitive or otherwise pathological behavior as a response to extreme stress. (Fear, panic, and physical suffering often "bring out the worst" in a person.) Another problem is that the understandably negative response of members of the medical team often results in the "lumping together" of patients with differing types of personality disorders so that similar approaches are used for these patients when, in reality, they have very different needs and demands. Better techniques can be employed in place of, or in addition to, limit setting. It is important to realize that limit setting in the trauma unit will not change or cure any personality disorder. Definitive treatment of personality disorders usually requires years of intensive psychotherapy. However, accurate diagnosis and the utilization of more effective strategies can lead to successful management of trauma patients with personality disorders and facilitate appropriate referral for treatment.

It is important to understand personality disorders in the context of trauma. Certain personality disorders are associated with impulsive, risk-taking, and otherwise dangerous behaviors, as well as with alcohol and drug abuse. Identification and subsequent treatment of these problems may lead to prevention of future admissions. In addition, major psychiatric disorders can be initially misidentified as personality disorders, and thus without psychiatric evaluation, covert depressions, delirium, subtle psychoses, or schizophrenia might remain undiagnosed and untreated. However, the definitive diagnosis of personality disorders remains significantly more difficult than is true for schizophrenia or depression, even in the rehabilitation unit, where the patient is less stressed and where there is more time for comprehensive psychiatric evaluation. Referral for further outpatient evaluation and treatment is often necessary.

This section will start with a description of the nature, etiology, and treatment of personality disorders. This background will be used to discuss the management of demanding patients (regardless of their diagnosis) in the trauma unit, the evaluation of patients with apparent personality disorders, and the referral of such patients to psychiatrists.

Case History

Mr. Jones is a 23-year-old man who was admitted to the trauma unit 6 days after sustaining multiple fractures and a ruptured spleen in an automobile accident. Since being transferred to the intensive care unit from the critical care unit, he was noted by the nursing staff to be demanding, depressed, and easily agitated. His demands included more frequent and larger doses of pain medication, faster response to his shouted summonses, and fewer dressing changes. Attempts to set modest limits on these demands led to crying episodes as well as temper tantrums, during which he insisted on being discharged against medical advice. His vital signs were stable, and there was no evidence of delirium. The family spokesperson stated that the patient is unmarried, has many friends, and works as a sheet metal worker. Because his blood alcohol level on admission was 221 mg%, he was evaluated by the alcohol counselor. This revealed that Mr. Jones worked for seven different employers in the past 2 years and that temper tantrums, not alcohol use, played a major role in each move. Although he apparently did not drink before or during work, he did consume in excess of 12 drinks each Friday and Saturday night. The patient noted that on a given night he could consume far more than his drinking companions without becoming more intoxicated. The counselor also noted that despite the family's description of many friends, the only visitor since his admission had been his mother. A psychiatric consultation was requested to evaluate his depression and to recommend management. After several visits, the consultant found that although he was friendly and seemingly interested in the opinions of others, Mr. Jones actually only related to other people in a very superficial manner. Expecting to be used by others, he evaluated other people in terms of their usefulness to him. Although he described feelings of loneliness and emptiness, he did not describe any close friends or family members whom he missed. His history was notable for a general inability to tolerate strong feelings or to delay gratification of any of his desires (e.g., food, possessions, sexual release). He experienced these desires or needs as overwhelming and felt that he was entitled to their gratification even when this brought him into conflict with other people. Shoplifting, casual sexual encounters, and similar examples involving abuse of other people were described without remorse, although he did remember being afraid that his victim of the moment might discover his intent. As for the present, he felt terrified that his needs for pain relievers, food, a television, and numerous other items would be ignored or get low priority and then become overwhelming to him. Doctors and nurses were seen solely in terms of their ability and willingness to meet his needs. Accordingly, staff members were seen as important or unimportant, good or bad, respectively. Other patients and their needs were of no interest. There was no evidence of depression or schizophrenia.

The psychiatric consultant recommended that several changes be made in the management of Mr. Jones. For the next 2 days, his dosage of meperidine hydrochloride (Demerol) would be increased to 100 mg every 3 hours unless the patient refused it. Family members would be asked to make arrangements for a television (he was no longer in the ICU) and to bring in special foods and other requests. In general, the staff was encouraged to focus on gratifying his demands or getting his family to do so. The psychiatrist would see Mr. Jones for 10 to 15 minutes several days each week for supportive therapy. No additional medications were ordered. Over the next few days in the trauma unit and during his several-week stay on an orthopedic service, these interventions resulted in a modest reduction in Mr. Jones' demands and marked reduction in the number of temper tantrums.

Mr. Jones displayed many of the features of an antisocial personality disorder. The diagnosis is based on a thorough evaluation of the patient's relationships with other people and the exclusion of a diagnosis of depression or schizophrenia. Patients with other types of personality disorders may be impulsive, demanding, or manipulative, but they will not exhibit the same degree of disturbance in their sense of obligation to other people and to society. The patient with schizophrenia might resemble Mr. Jones in many respects, but this patient did not have the key symptoms and signs of schizophrenia. Brain-damaged individuals and delirious patients often demonstrate impulsive and demanding behaviors, but a review of their history or the current medical picture should reveal these causes. The differential diagnosis also includes maladaptive coping in the normal individual exposed to overwhelming stressors. Here, too, the history is vital.

This type of evaluation is often too time-consuming to be completed in the trauma unit. Fortunately, antisocial patients as well as the much larger group of demanding patients (composed of both normal individuals and patients with other types of personality disorders) all respond to certain similar management approaches. The psychiatric intervention described above is aimed at smoothing the hospital stay of such patients by reducing their fears, addressing their needs, and providing staff with an organizing principle for their interaction with the patient. Understanding the rationale for this approach and appreciating the reasons for the medical staff's initial aversion to its use follow from a discussion of the natural history and presumed etiology of all personality disorders.

In general terms, the individual with a personality disorder has a relatively permanent disturbance in relationships with other people, and he perceives this disturbance as something outside his control or responsibility. In fact, the problem is most often seen by the patient as stemming from the behavior or attitudes of the other person. This blindness to his own behavior and the blaming of others for these difficulties are often as annoying as the behaviors themselves. There are several classifications of personality disorders, but the following is a conventional one often utilized in descriptions of medical–surgical patients.

Patients with a dependent personality disorder perceive themselves as incapable of meeting their own basic needs (e.g., food, shelter, clothing, acceptance). Such individuals seek out companions and friends who will take responsibility for providing these things, but they often fear that these people will abandon them. Relationships with family members, employers, nurses, and other care providers usually take the same form. Their demands to be cared for and constantly reassured that they will not be abandoned often seem primitive to the point of being purely manipulative. The understandable response of the staff is a categorical refusal to meet such demands.

Compulsive patients are usually struggling over issues involving control. The possibility of emotional loss of composure can be very frightening, and any perceived lack of control in interpersonal relationships can seem very threatening. Examples include internal and external struggles over being compliant or disobedient of rules, regulations, or even the requests of other people. Such individuals often complain about tardiness or sloppiness in others. More generally, these patients seem to expect or demand perfection. The staff's natural or intuitive response to such behavior in the hospitalized patient is again to refuse to meet such demands. In addition, there is a tendency for power struggles to develop between the patient and staff, which prompts staff to feel particularly strongly about setting limits and establishing authority.

Histrionic patients may best be understood as demanding attention from others. They wish to be seen as interesting and desirable and need reassurance that staff and others continue to view them in that way despite their illness, disability, or disfigurement. Their attention-seeking behavior often takes on a demanding quality in the hospital and results in a general avoidance by the staff. In many ways the mirror image of the obsessive, these individuals give flamboyant, colorful descriptions of their experiences but tend to be unconcerned with details. This indifference makes their stories seem implausible and perhaps manufactured.

Patients with a paranoid personality disorder are usually seen as suspicious, distant, and dissatisfied. When tests or procedures are needed, legitimate requests for explanations about their rationale or about results are often presented as hostile demands. Attempts at reassurance—"Everything is OK," "We're taking care of you"—may result in more demands and more suspicions. At times, their general sense that others are intent on taking advantage of them may result in paranoid delusions of the type seen in some schizophrenics. The deterioration over time and other features of schizophrenia will be absent, however. Staff members understandably often react negatively to what they experience as an insulting atmosphere of distrust.

Schizoid patients demand to be left alone. This demand may suggest the withdrawal of a depressed, schizophrenic, or psychotic patient and therefore often leads to requests for psychiatric evaluation. Such patients will prove to have had a long-standing inability to tolerate close ties to other people. Often appearing odd or idiosyncratic, they lead very isolated lives. The usual and fully appropriate response of staff is to request a psychiatric evaluation for depression or schizophrenia. Sometimes, however, these patients are seen to be demanding special treatment and in need of strict limit setting.

The masochistic patient presents a very difficult management problem because his demands are rarely understood. The prototype for this situation is the patient with chronic pain who has undergone multiple treatments, often exhausting the armamentarium of the medical staff. Each consultant or new member on the team is seen as having the ultimate solution, and each is destined to fail. If such patients are understood to be merely demanding a cure for their pain, then failure is inevitable. These individuals place great value on persevering despite great suffering. Relief of pain—their explicit demand—threatens that position. Implicit or explicit guarantees of successful treatment are likewise threatening, although they represent the natural response to staff members. It is more useful and more accurate to perceive such patients as demanding acknowledgment of their suffering rather than reassurance or immediate relief.

The patient with a narcissistic personality disorder is particularly difficult to deal with. This individual often insists on very special treatment with specific demands, varying from special visiting hours to direct service by the unit's head surgeon. It is useful to know that the patient's underlying fear and source of insecurity are that people might believe he is inconsequential, and the basic demand that underlies his behavior is that the patient's personal power and prestige be acknowledged. As with many of the other personality styles, the characteristic response of the staff is a blanket refusal to honor all demands.

Patients with borderline personality disorders are also very problematical. They are very impulsive, unhappy, anxious, self-destructive people who are unable to maintain stable relationships and who often abuse alcohol or drugs. Their behavior is perplexing and inconsistent. Their comments and opinions change from moment to moment and are typically mutually contradictory. They are provocative and notorious for sowing staff dissention—for causing "staff splitting." They idealize some staff and vilify others. They give distorted, often inflammatory versions of events or conversations. They play individuals off against one another, promoting intense staff discord. Much of this activity seems purposefully manipulative but often results from unconscious behavior patterns. These patients create chaos and strife, but what they need and behaviorally demand is that staff members restore and maintain an ordered hospital environment imbued with consistency and structure.

Regardless of type, and most individuals will have mixtures, the prognosis for patients with personality disorders is poor. Although few deteriorate over time, relatively little change can be expected in these behavior patterns. Personality disorders are generally believed to develop in conjunction with the formation of character in the first few years of life. During this period, individuals develop their characteristic characterologic patterns of coping and dealing with anxiety and adversity. Their early interactions with parents or other primary care providers shape all future relationships. Modification of these styles of coping, containing anxiety, and relating to others will occur throughout life, but the most basic features tend to be very resistant to change.

The types of personality disorders described above also represent extremes of normal behavior. With varying degrees of accuracy, the personalities of normal individuals can be seen as mixtures of these habitual styles of coping and relating. At times of great stress, and this is a crucial point, otherwise normal individuals may rely more heavily on these types of behaviors. Similarly, the patient with a true, preexisting personality disorder is likely to appear much more severely impaired when hospitalized and under great stress. One way to understand this process is to regard such behaviors as defenses against anxiety and other potentially overwhelming feelings. When reasoning or other more mature defenses fail to contain such feelings, more primitive defenses are used. It follows that attempts to set limits on such defensive behaviors run the risk of provoking still more primitive behavior. A more rational approach to management is to help the patient find other coping mechanisms to reduce anxiety.

Attempts to modify personality disorders through psychiatric treatment face very significant hurdles. The first is the patients' characteristic failure to see their personality as the cause of their difficulties with other people. There is little likelihood of patients being motivated for treatment unless or until they perceive their habitual styles of relating to other people as being problematical. Even then, individual psychotherapy can be very difficult. This form of treatment relies on a trusting relationship in which the patient's demands and wishes are often not gratified and in which fantasies, wishes, ideas, and impulses are talked about instead of acted out. Group psychotherapy is sometimes preferable because the other patients can take over the role of pointing out the patient's inadequacies, leaving the therapist to support the patient and to suggest alternative behaviors.

Although no psychotropic medications directly treat personality disorders, anxiolytics, antidepressants, and occasionally, antipsychotics are sometimes used as an adjunct to individual or group treatment. The use of such agents may help to keep these patients in treatment by partially satisfying their needs for relief from anxiety and other painful feelings and by giving them a "longer fuse" when their demands go unsatisfied.

Management of Demanding Behavior

The key to the initial management of demanding patients, including those with personality disorders, is to first determine the exact nature of their demands. The next step is to either gratify the demands or find substitutes that seem feasible and which are acceptable to the patient. Excessive demands usually indicate that a person is overwhelmed by fear or anxiety or other painful feelings. Meeting the demands reduces the likelihood of the patient's use of even more primitive behaviors. More important, since the nature of a given patient's demands often reflects his underlying fears, satisfying the demand addresses these unconscious issues, thereby reducing the motivation for future demands. For example, the obsessive patient's demands for control reflect his fears of loss of control, which are addressed and reduced by granting him more control. Even when the patient is in the critical care unit this can be accomplished by allowing the patient to make decisions such as when he will have a bath, when he takes p.r.n. medications, and who is allowed to visit and for how long. A dependent patient often demands and requires reassurance that he or she will be cared for and not abandoned. Staff can gratify the demands and provide reassurance by encouraging family and friends to stay with the patient and by making frequent, brief patient contacts part of the care plan.

Again, the crucial step is determining the nature of the patient's demands. Table 29–1 summarizes characteristic demands of patients with personality disorders. (Borderline personality disorder was omitted because of its complexity.) A therapeutic response consists of giving the patient what he wishes whenever possible. However, appreciating that seemingly similar demands may actually reflect very different needs and fears is important so that the nature of a patient's requirements can be accurately and precisely identified. For example, the dependent patient and the paranoid patient may both demand information about the treatment regimen, but the former is seeking reassurance that he will continue to be taken care of, while the latter wants evidence that no one is plotting to harm him. Although their questions should be answered in both cases, reassurance ("We're taking care of everything. . . .there's no need to worry") is appropriate for the dependent patient but irrelevant and perhaps even terrifying for the paranoid patient ("Why shouldn't I worry? Are you trying to hide something?").

TABLE 29–1. COMMON PERSONALITY STYLES

LABEL	DEMAND
Dependent	Reassurance
Compulsive	Control
Histrionic	Attention
Paranoid	Explanation
Schizoid	Isolation from others
Masochistic	Acknowledgment of suffering
Narcissistic	Acknowledgment of power and superiority

In most cases, the nature of the patient's needs, fears, and demands will be clear, but the staff will be very uncertain about the advisability or feasibility of gratifying them. One reason for this is the concern that gratifying these demands will reinforce them and lead to more in the future. This is plausible, but clinical experience suggests that it is wrong. In most cases, this approach will lead to a decrease rather than an increase in subsequent demands. As suggested above, this is presumably because the patient's anxiety has been reduced. Another reason staff might resist following this approach is the fear that it might somehow exacerbate the patient's personality disorder—that it might make him worse or "teach" him undesirable behavior patterns. This is an intuitive, unspoken, and often unconscious staff concern that is not plausible. All our understanding of personality disorders strongly indicates that personality traits cannot be altered—for better or for worse—by any intervention lasting only a few weeks. Still another concern regarding this approach stems from the fear that special treatment of one patient will lead to similar demands by other patients and their families. Certainly this is possible, especially when adolescent patients are involved. Usually, however, this does not happen. Most patients realize that each patient's treatment is individualized.

Sometimes patients' behaviors seem so hateful or obnoxious that staff members feel emotionally unwilling to gratify the demands because they feel so angry and frustrated. In other cases, the treatment team's own need to feel in charge may be threatened by patients' demands for special treatment. In both these instances, the best way to deal with these feelings is for staff to acknowledge them and talk about them.

When dealing with patients with borderline personality disorders who "split" staff, staff members again need to be able to engage in honest and frank discussion among themselves. They need to be able to discuss the conflicts these patients cause or exploit, and they need to be able to resolve differences so that they can be unified and extremely consistent in their approach to the patient. A more detailed discussion of borderline personality disorder is beyond the scope of this chapter. It is an extremely severe personality disorder that is complex and difficult to manage. Early psychiatric intervention should be requested for any patient suspected of having this disorder or any other severe personality disorder.

One challenge already mentioned is that of finding ways to gratify patients' demands when they seem excessive or unreasonable. It is unrealistic to demand that a staff member provide reassurance numerous times each day, but suitably prepared family members can meet this demand. Narcissistic demands for very special treatment can be dealt with by substituting other indications that the patient's special position in life is recognized. For many such patients, merely showing an interest in that position will suffice ("Your job sounds like it would be enough for two people. . . . How did you go so far at such a young age?").

The major challenge, however, is overcoming the causes of staff resistance described above. Once this has been done, the actual interventions are often very straightforward.

Referral for Psychiatric Consultation

If a patient's suspected personality disorder seems severe, or if the approach outlined above does not work, psychiatric consultation should be requested. It also should be considered before discharge and prior to the formulation of rehabilitation plans for any patient thought to have this type of problem. Although specific treatment for these disturbances is very difficult, interventions targeted at preventing future trauma admissions must be considered. Many patients may benefit from appropriate outpatient referral for treatment. Alcohol abuse and other treatable conditions often associated with personality disorders may be identified and then addressed. Finally, quite different approaches to management during the rehabilitation cycle may be suggested by the psychiatrist. The dependent patient, for example, must be encouraged to adopt a more independent posture during the rehabilitation cycle. Otherwise, a successful transition from rehabilitation back to the community may be delayed or blocked.

ALCOHOL ABUSE

Compulsive use of alcohol may be the most important of the treatable behavior disorders that lead to trauma admissions. It is a major risk factor for trauma. In studies of trauma patients, blood alcohol levels have been positive in at least a third of admissions.[3, 4] Furthermore, a recent study showed that a quarter of the patients admitted were legally intoxicated.[4] These numbers, plus the importance of knowing whether a confused and potentially brain-damaged patient is inebriated, justify the inclusion of blood alcohol levels as a part of the routine evaluation of all trauma patients. Of even greater importance is the key role played by these test results in the screening of trauma admissions for alcohol abuse. Despite the fact that diagnosis is often straightforward and treatment is usually available, there are several hurdles that may interfere with both diagnosis and referral. Screening, diagnosis, referral, and, more generally, the approach to the alcohol-abusing trauma patient are illustrated in the following case.

Case History

Ms. Williams is a 27-year-old divorced woman who was admitted to the trauma unit with a closed head injury and a fractured femur sustained in an automobile accident. Her blood alcohol level on admission was 240 mg%. Initially comatose, she regained consciousness after 48 hours and remained drowsy and intermittently stuporous until the seventh day, when she became alert. Between days 2 and 7, she was agitated on several occasions, and the possibility of alcohol withdrawal was considered. On day 12, prior to being transferred to the orthopedic service, Ms. Williams was evaluated by the alcohol counselor. Evaluation was incomplete because she continued to exhibit poor recent memory and other deficits, presumably due to the head injury. Contact with the family revealed the following: Ms. Williams graduated from college and held several secretarial positions during the prior 4 years. Alcohol was involved in one previous accident and in two traffic violations. Family members disagreed over the extent and causes of her drinking. Some felt that she drank socially, while others felt that she might be an alcoholic. One thought that she drank when she got depressed; the others were not sure that there was any pattern. On day 28 she was reevaluated by the counselor and found to be largely recovered from her head injury. Evaluation at this time revealed that she had a reputation for being able to tolerate significantly larger quantities of alcohol than her friends. It was not unusual for her to consume 20 drinks before driving home. She insisted that she was not addicted to alcohol, but she acknowledged that she often needed a few drinks "to feel normal." She admitted that her drinking concerned her and that she had unsuccessfully tried to cut down her alcohol intake. There had been at least two episodes when she was unable to recall the events of the previous evening when she was drinking. She denied any episodes of delirium tremens or seizures but admitted occasionally experiencing "morning shakes" and downing a drink to stop them. A psychiatric consultation was recommended to evaluate her depressive episodes. The psychiatrist found no evidence for a thought disorder and felt that her depression was probably secondary to her abuse of alcohol. The patient agreed to attend an Alcoholics Anonymous meeting in her community.

This patient demonstrates many of the features of alcoholism. Many alcoholic patients will admit they consumed alcohol prior to admission but deny that their habitual pattern of alcohol use is problematical. Increased tolerance, as suggested by this patient's ability to handle larger quantities of alcohol than her peers and by her ability to operate an automobile after 20 or more drinks, is an important warning sign. If there had not been a head injury, then a relatively alert state on admission despite a blood alcohol level of 240 mg% would have confirmed that she had tolerance. The involvement of alcohol in at least two accidents and at least two traffic violations also supports this diagnosis. The same is true for the family's concern over her drinking. Another fruitful area to explore with Ms. Williams would be her frequent job changes. Although these may not be related to alcohol, it may be that she has had a poor attendance record with frequent Monday absences, a common finding in heavy drinkers. Similarly, her use of alcohol to "feel normal" should be investigated. Questions in this area may get to the root of her abuse of alcohol. One possibility is that she has any of a number of psychiatric symptoms that make her feel abnormal and that she is trying to ameliorate with alcohol. Anxiety, depression, guilt, and other painful feelings may be temporarily relieved by alcohol. Although less likely, persecutory voices and other symptoms of schizophrenia also might lead to alcohol abuse. In such cases, the patient usually reports that the voices remain but are of less concern when the patient is intoxicated.

A medical history in a relatively young person who abuses alcohol may be negative, but many alcoholics will report blackouts (amnesia for the previous evening's drinking bout), occasional morning shakes (tremulousness) and the need for a morning drink, and gastric distress. A few may have already experienced withdrawal seizures or delirium tremens.

It is difficult to describe a typical history for alcohol abusers. Some will have a family history; some will not. Many, but not all, will have started abusing alcohol by the time they were in high school; a few will have started at an earlier age. Most will have tried to reduce, stop, or otherwise regulate their drinking, with varying degrees of success. One of the most alarming discoveries many will make is that they are prone to loss of control over the amount of alcohol consumed in a given setting. Similarly, the craving for and preoccupation with alcohol become distressing over time. Many will be surprisingly productive despite their consumption of alcohol. Many will enter treatment through Alcoholics Anonymous, other group therapy, or individual therapy, and the majority will ultimately achieve progressively longer periods of sobriety. The minority of such patients who also have a major psychiatric disorder will usually require treatment for both disorders.

The etiology of alcohol abuse is best considered from the same "systems" standpoint used in the discussions of the etiology of schizophrenia and depression. Some individuals may have a genetic predisposition expressed as an increased tolerance for alcohol. The physical effects of the alcohol also must be considered because the withdrawal symptoms can be powerful incentives to drink. Potent environmental factors are virtually always found. An alcoholic parent will usually play a major role in determining an individual's attitudes about drinking. Current living partners may conceivably encourage continued abuse of alcohol in several ways. An alcoholic's partner may know from personal experience all the most effective ways to sabotage efforts to stop drinking, or a nondrinking spouse may overtly complain about the patient's drinking while covertly (unconsciously) facilitating its continuation by encouraging ties with alcoholic friends. Psychological factors cover the entire spectrum of psychopathology and lie beyond the scope of this chapter. Suffice it to say that there is no convincing evidence for a prealcoholic personality or neurosis.

Understanding the etiology of a particular individual's abuse of alcohol is a very complicated and involved process that is made more difficult by the various stereotypes of alcoholics as weak or pleasure-seeking individuals. Clarification of etiology is not crucial in the trauma unit. What is crucial, however, is that alcohol abusers be identified, dealt with compassionately, and appropriately referred for treatment.

Treatment is usually directed toward abstinence, with an intermediate goal of progressively longer periods of sobriety. Much has been written about the success of Alcoholics Anonymous, which takes a self-help approach predicated on the need to acknowledge publicly that one is an alcoholic. Although many patients complain initially about the style of Alcoholics Anonymous meetings, the clinical success and cost-effectiveness of this form of treatment cannot be denied. Some patients respond better to group therapy of the type often provided for patients with personality disorders. Others benefit from individual therapy, especially if there is coexisting depression. Many benefit from a mixture of treatment modalities, including the use of disulfiram (Antabuse), a medication that produces a severe headache and other noxious effects when combined with alcohol. All these treatments have in common the need for the patient to acknowledge the abuse of alcohol, a step that can be greatly facilitated by interaction with members of the trauma team.

Management Through the Trauma Cycles

Resuscitation

The high prevalence of alcohol abuse in trauma patients requires that alcohol intoxication be considered in every admission, especially in those patients with a depressed level of consciousness. Although not definitive, a high blood alcohol level helps in the differentiation between a head injury and intoxication. The administration of sedatives, especially long-acting agents like diazepam, is best done with caution because of the synergistic sedative effects of alcohol and these agents. The greatest value of testing blood alcohol levels on admission, as discussed below, is the process of screening for alcohol abuse. When blood toxicology results are not immediately available, the presence of elevated blood alcohol levels can be suspected when patients have unexplained elevations of serum osmolality (especially if also their breath smells of alcohol). A serum osmolality of 306 mOsmol roughly corresponds to a blood alcohol level of 70 mg%, and a serum osmolality of 315 mOsmol roughly correlates with a blood alcohol level of 100 mg%.[5]

Critical Care

Alcohol withdrawal seizures are often suspected during the first 24 to 48 hours after a trauma admission, but the wide range of other possible etiologies makes this diagnosis difficult. Treatment is usually with anticonvulsants if the seizures recur. Other alcohol withdrawal symptoms include tremor, sweating, increased blood pressure and heart rate, decreased appetite, insomnia, and nightmares. These symptoms usually begin within 12 hours of admission but can last for several days. Alcohol withdrawal is often treated successfully with either an alcohol drip or with a benzodiazepine such as chlordiazepoxide (Librium) or diazepam (Valium). If untreated, these withdrawal symptoms can become more severe and progress to frank delirium tremens, which unfortunately is far from uncommon in trauma patients. Delirium tremens usually presents during the first 5 days of hospitalization but sometimes can occur more than twice as long after admission.[6, 7] Untreated, this condition is usually described in nontrauma patients as having a mortality rate of 15 per cent. In other settings its presence is usually suggested by agitation, clouding of consciousness, fever, autonomic hyperactivity, and visual hallucinations. Because these findings occur commonly in the trauma patient, it is important to keep a high index of suspicion that delirium tremens is at least part of the etiology. Treatment usually consists of aggressive doses of intravenous chlordiazepoxide (Librium) or diazepam (Valium) or an alcohol drip. Sometimes antipsychotic agents are also utilized.

Intermediate Care and Rehabilitation

The trauma team can play a crucial role in the treatment of alcohol abuse by screening for alcohol abuse, by providing referral information to patients and their families, and by encouraging identified or likely patients to seek treatment. It is reasonable to assume that these efforts also will reduce the rate of readmissions, perhaps more so than ensuring the passage of mandatory motorcycle helmet laws or any other activity open to the trauma team.

Determination of the blood alcohol level is the first step in screening. The trauma unit can establish a policy of offering or requiring evaluations by an alcohol counselor for all patients with positive values or with values above the level of impairment as legislated by the state. Few patients will refuse evaluations, even when these are not mandatory.

The nurse can supplement this process by eliciting positive histories of the type previously described. This is especially critical for identifying alcoholic patients who otherwise would remain unsuspected because of a negative toxicology. Any family concerns about a trauma patient's use of alcohol should be thoroughly evaluated.

The trauma team's attitude about alcohol evaluations and referrals for treatment can have an enormous effect on a patient's compliance with both processes. Successfully treated patients often describe interactions with medical staff that had a crucial effect on their decision to pursue treatment.

SUMMARY AND CONCLUSIONS

Nurses play a central role in the recognition and management of psychiatric disorders in the trauma unit. As the most consistent providers of bedside care, they are able to observe behavior changes, elicit symptoms, record treatment responses, and deal appropriately with the demands of patients with major mental disorders. Superior management can speed recovery from physical injuries, reduce suffering, and prevent psychiatric admissions. These goals can be achieved if care is both coordinated and consistent. A thorough written plan of care is absolutely essential because of the large number of care providers and diverse treatment settings encountered by patients as they cycle back to the community. Because arrangement of outpatient or inpatient psychiatric treatment is often time-consuming, discharge planning should begin soon after admission.

Prevention of repeat trauma admissions is an important but neglected area. Effective treatment of alcoholism and other psychiatric disorders could be expected to lower rates of suicide, drunk driving, and other causes of repeat injuries in former trauma patients, an area that may be targeted with future research endeavors.

REFERENCES

1. Robin LN, Helzer JE, Weissman MW, et al: Lifetime prevalence of specific psychiatric disorders in three sites. Arch Gen Psychiatry 41:949–958, 1984.
2. Regier DA, Boyd JH, Burke JD, et al: One month prevalence of mental disorders in the United States. Arch Gen Psychiatry 45:977–986, 1988.
3. Champion HR, Baker SP, Benner C, et al: Alcohol intoxication and serum osmolality. Lancet 1:1402, 1975.
4. Soderstrom CA, Trifillis AL, Shankar BS, et al: Marijuana and alcohol use among 1023 trauma patients. Arch Surg 123:733–737, 1988.
5. Redetzki HM, Koerner TA, et al: Osmometry in the evaluation of alcohol intoxication. Clin Toxicol 5(3):343–363, 1979.
6. Behnke RH: Recognition and management of alcohol withdrawal syndrome. Hosp Pract November:79–84, 1976.
7. McNichol RW, Hoshino AY: Therapy for deliria. Curr Psychiatr Ther 15:181–193, 1975.

BIBLIOGRAPHY

Andreasen NC, Black DB: Introductory Textbook of Psychiatry. Washington, DC, American Psychiatric Press, 1991.

American Psychiatric Association: Diagnostic and Statistical Manual of Mental Disorders, 3rd ed. Washington, DC, American Psychiatric Association, 1987.

Appleton WS: Practical Clinical Psychopharmacology, 3rd ed. Baltimore, Williams & Wilkins, 1988.

Cassem NH: Massachusetts General Hospital Handbook of General Hospital Psychiatry, 3rd ed. St Louis, Mosby–Year Book, 1991.

Gelenberg AJ, Bassuk EL, Schoonover SC: The Practitioner's Guide to Psychoactive Drugs, 3rd ed. New York, Plenum Medical Books, 1991.

Jellinek EM: The Disease Concept of Alcoholism. New Haven, CT, Hillhouse Press, 1960.

Kahana RF, Bibring GL: Personality types in medical management. In Zinberg NE (ed): Psychiatry and Medical Practice in a General Hospital. New York, International Universities Press, 1964, pp 108–123.

MacKinnon RA, Michels R: The Psychiatric Interview in Clinical Practice. Philadelphia, WB Saunders Co, 1971.

Schuckit MA: Drug and Alcohol Abuse: A Clinical Guide to Diagnosis and Treatment. New York, Plenum Medical Books, 1989.

Strauss JS, Carpenter WT: Schizophrenia. New York, Plenum Press, 1981.

30

THE TRAUMA PATIENT WITH A HISTORY OF SUBSTANCE ABUSE

PATRICIA E. McCABE and ERKAN HASSAN

The number of Americans who use drugs either habitually or intermittently is poorly approximated. A recent government report reveals that approximately 10 per cent of the adult population in the United States has alcohol misuse problems.[1] Other sources have reported that 20 per cent of adults who are seen in medical consultation have an alcohol misuse problem at some time during their lives.[2–6] Results from the 1987 National Behavioral Risk Factor Surveillance System indicate that among individuals older than 18 years of age, an estimated 15.3 per cent participated in "binge drinking" on at least one occasion in the month prior to survey and 5.6 per cent consumed 60 or more drinks per month.[7] The economic burden associated with alcohol abuse and/or dependence, projected to be at $117 billion in 1993, is likely to increase to $150 billion by the year 1995.[1]

Gross estimates show that almost 28 million Americans used illicit drugs at some point in time during 1988, with a direct purchase price of over $79 billion.[8] Marijuana is the most commonly used illicit substance in the United States, with an estimated 65 million lifetime users and 21 million recent new users.[8] Other studies suggest that nearly 50 per cent of high school seniors admit to having used marijuana, 7 per cent of whom employed the drug on a daily basis.[9]

In addition to alcohol and marijuana, the cocaine epidemic has created an unprecedented health care crisis. It is believed that 30 million Americans have used cocaine, and each day another 5000 people will try it for the first time.[10] At least 10 million Americans are cocaine-dependent, according to the National Institute on Drug Abuse. Cocaine-related hospital admissions in 10 major cities climbed from 8831 in 1984 to 46,020 in 1988—an increase of over 421 per cent.[11]

Substance abuse reaches across all socioeconomic and educational boundaries, as documented by a study of medical students who self-reported that approximately 27 per cent were users of alcohol, marijuana, cocaine, and/or tranquilizers.[12] In addition, there is a growing body of evidence that links drug use to violent behaviors, traumatic events, and fatalities. Ethanol, marijuana, and cocaine represent the largest proportion of drugs associated with these events.

INCIDENT AND ACCIDENT DATA

Trauma and Alcohol

Alcohol use has been linked to all types of injury,[2, 7, 13–20] particularly injury sustained in vehicular crashes.[21, 22] During the years 1982 through 1988, by conservative estimate, 314,187 individuals were killed in vehicular crashes, alcohol being a factor in 53 per cent of them.[21] In 1987, alcohol-related crashes accounted for 57 per cent of the years of potential life lost due to roadway trauma.[23] A positive correlation also has been demonstrated between the temporal use of alcohol and the occurrence of vehicular crashes.[24] Further, a correlation has been demonstrated relative to the probability of causing both fatal and nonfatal vehicular crashes and driving with increasingly elevated blood alcohol concentrations.[24]

In addition to vehicular trauma, alcohol is a significant factor in fatal falls, drownings, suicides, and occupational injuries.[7, 13, 14] Alcoholic and heavy-drinking men have been shown to have a two to eight times greater risk of dying as the result of injury compared with other individuals.[25, 26] In 1987, the leading cause of alcohol-related deaths was trauma, which accounted for 45.5 per cent of deaths. These figures are probably too low, since there are indications that alcohol-related deaths due to injury are most likely underreported.[27] A factor that has hampered the accumulation of such knowledge is the reluctance of clinicians to procure admitting blood alcohol specimens,[28] a basic screening test for blood alcohol levels.[7, 29]

Trauma and Marijuana

One trauma center study conducted between 1985 and 1986 was the first to prospectively document alcohol and marijuana use among a large number of patients admitted to a major trauma center.[15] This study found that 35 per cent of the 1023 patients admitted showed evidence of having used marijuana prior to the time of injury and 33 per cent had used alcohol. The study is the only one in which a radioimmunoassay (RIA) test for serum delta-9-tetrahydrocannabinol activity has been used among a large number of hospitalized trauma patients. RIA measurements enable the determination of *Cannabis* use proximal to the time of injury. A recent funded follow-up project will address crash characteristics, including crash culpability and alcohol, marijuana, and other drug use among injured drivers. Smart found that a group of marijuana-using students had twice the frequency of traffic mishaps in the 6 to 12 months before their marijuana convictions when compared with a control group of students.[30] Other research concludes that deleterious effects of varying degrees have been shown to influence those abilities necessary to operate a vehicle and some elements of driving performance in experimental situations using marijuana.[31]

Trauma and Cocaine

Marzuk and associates noted an 18.2 per cent rate of cocaine use in motor vehicle accident fatalities.[32] In a study of 169 trauma cases, Lindenbaum and colleagues noted that 74.5 per cent of the patients tested positive for the presence of illicit or prescription drugs—more than half of which involved the use of cocaine.[33] In a similar study of urban trauma patients, positive rates for cocaine and marijuana use were found to be 37 and 34 per cent, respectively.[34]

ETIOLOGY

The absence of consistent scientific evidence concerning the etiology and basic characteristics of alcoholism and other addictions has created some ambiguity and uncertainty among professionals in the addiction field. No single theory or perspective has yet proved sufficiently broad or flexible to explain the addiction phenomenon. However, most fall within four broad categories: biological, psychological, sociological, and behavioral.

Medical/Disease Perspective

Proponents of the medical or disease perspective agree that alcoholism and drug addiction occur in persons whose body chemistry makes them susceptible to addiction. The most impressive evidence for genetic transmission comes from studies of children reared apart from their alcoholic biological parents. Since the 1950s, studies have repeatedly shown that the likelihood of a person developing alcoholism increases with the number of alcoholic relatives and the degree of genetic closeness to the alcoholic relative.[35, 36] On the basis of stringent criteria for diagnosis of alcoholism, Goodwin and associates found that adopted sons whose biological fathers were alcoholic were more than three times as likely to become alcoholic as the adopted sons of nonalcoholics.[36, 37]

Fewer studies have been conducted supporting the influence of genetic factors; thus evidence of hereditary predisposition for these forms of addiction is less convincing. Limited data do exist showing a correlation between drug use in groups of young men and drug problems among their parents.[38] Most of the research concentrating on possible biochemical influences on drug addiction has focused on neurotransmitters and receptor sites. Benzodiazepine and opiate receptors have been identified in the central nervous system. In addition, the discovery of endorphins, endogenous chemical substances that look and behave like opiates, led to the hypothesis that people who become addicted (particularly to narcotics) may have inborn abnormalities in their opiate receptor–endorphin systems.

Addictive Behaviors Perspective

Theories of cause and consequence have often tended to emphasize a particular biological, psychological, or sociocultural perspective. It has become increasingly apparent, however, that behavioral disorders are determined by more complex factors. Over the past two decades there has been a trend to view addiction from a multidimensional learning-based perspective.[39] Such a perspective emphasizes a behavioral learning model with careful attention to social and environmental influences on learning.

Marlatt[40] has combined the principles of social-learning theory, cognitive psychology, and experimental social psychology to formulate the addictive behaviors model. Rather than viewing the recipient as a victim, as guilty, or as lacking willpower, proponents of this perspective view the alcoholic or drug abuser as a person who has developed or "overlearned" maladaptive ways of coping. Conceptualized as the "maladaptive habit pattern" rather than distinct or dichotomous entities such as abstinence and loss of control, addictive behaviors are thought to exist along the entire continuum of use or practice.

Substance Abuse Terms and Definitions

Understanding substance abuse behaviors is a complex task, and the relatively new field of addiction research is not limited to one scientific data base: Epidemiology, chemistry, medicine, psychology, nursing, and, most important, pharmacology have all made significant contributions to the total understanding of the patient who is a substance abuser. The interpretation of such data, however, depends on the comprehension of a number of related terms (Table 30–1).

The American Medical Association, integrating a broad spectrum of concepts, defines drug abuse as

> The ingestion of a psychoactive substance in an amount and at a frequency likely to result in overt intoxication or to lead to physical or psychological problems.[41]

Drug abuse occurs with the deliberate nontherapeutic continued use of a psychoactive substance resulting in detrimental physical or psychological effects.

TABLE 30–1. SUBSTANCE ABUSE TERMS AND DEFINITIONS

Alcoholism: A chronic behavioral disorder manifested by repeated drinking of alcoholic beverages in excess of dietary and social uses of the community and to an extent that interferes with the drinker's health or social or economic function.
Alcohol Dependence: The use of alcohol to the point of impairment of social or occupational functioning, but with the presence of tolerance or withdrawal symptoms.
Psychological Dependence: Variable degrees of obsessive preoccupation with drugs, preference for the intoxicated state, and chronic or recurrent abuse.
Physical Dependence: An altered physiological state produced by repeated drug use and requiring continued drug use to prevent the emergence of withdrawal symptoms.
Withdrawal: Physical signs or symptoms associated with discontinuation of drug use after the development of tolerance.
Tolerance: A diminished response to a constant dose of a drug reflecting changes in pharmacodynamic and cellular mechanisms.
Addiction: A person's pattern of drug use that is characterized by compulsive drug use, overwhelming involvement in the use and procurement of its supply, and relapse into use after a period of abstinence.

Adapted from Research Issues 26, U.S. Department of Health and Human Services.

PHARMACOLOGICAL EFFECTS OF PSYCHOACTIVE DRUGS

Drug abuse usually stems from the use of psychoactive substances, which are classified under three broad categories: depressants, stimulants, and psychogenic agents (hallucinogens) (Table 30–2).

When a drug is used therapeutically, the initial effect observed in the individual is most often due to the drug itself. However, this is not always the case with psychoactive substances. These agents are typically used socially and in small doses. Therefore, the final effect observed will be influenced by other factors, specifically set and setting. The *set* refers to the frame of mind the individual is in at the time of drug use; the drug's effect for the individual who is in a good, pleasant mood will be different from its effect for an individual who is upset or depressed. The *setting* refers to the environment that exists at the time of drug use. The final effect from the drug may differ, for example, if it is used at a private party with close friends versus in a bathroom in a public facility. In addition, the set and/or setting may change from minute to minute; for example, an adolescent is having a marijuana party for his friends while his parents are out of town when, suddenly, the parents come home early and unexpectedly or a policeman appears at the door to investigate the source of loud noise. As this occurs, the effect obtained from the drug also may change. The set and setting are as important as the pharmacological properties of the drug itself on the final behavioral effects observed in an individual patient.

Alcohol Pharmacology

Ethanol will serve as the prototype central nervous system (CNS) depressant. Although differences exist between agents for such factors as potency, onset, elimination, and toxicity, the drugs in this category produce similar pharmacological effects.

Pharmacokinetics

Absorption. Although a small amount of ethanol can be absorbed systemically from the stomach, the upper portion of the small intestine represents the principal site of absorption. Absorption is generally rapid (30 to 60 minutes) and virtually complete. The critical determinant of the rate of absorption is gastric emptying time. A number of other variables also may affect ethanol absorption and are listed in Table 30–3.

Distribution. Ethanol is distributed throughout the total body water. The rate at which ethanol enters tissues is dependent on the blood supply to the tissue. Since the CNS is highly vascularized, systemic and CNS concentrations of ethanol quickly equilibrate.

Elimination. Ethanol is primarily (90 per cent) metabolized to acetaldehyde in the liver by the enzyme alcohol dehydrogenase. The metabolism is the rate-limiting step in ethanol elimination.[42] The metabolic pathway becomes saturated at ethanol concentrations between 13 and 30 mg/dl. Therefore, a 70-kg man can metabolize 7 to 10 gm of ethanol per hour, which is approximately one drink per hour regardless of the form (i.e., one 12-ounce beer = one 4-ounce wine = 1 ounce whiskey). Acetaldehyde is then further metabolized to acetate, which is broken down to acetylcoenzyme A, which ultimately enters the Krebs cycle.

Only a small percentage of ingested ethanol (5 to 10 per cent) is excreted unchanged in the lungs, sweat, and kidneys. The concentration of ethanol in alveolar air is approximately 0.05 per cent that of blood. The amount of ethanol in 2100 ml of expired air approximates the amount of ethanol in 1 ml of blood, serving as the basis for the Breathalyzer test.

The liver is the site of many drug–alcohol interactions. Acute alcohol ingestion may inhibit the liver oxidative enzyme system responsible for the metabolism of many drugs. Acutely intoxicated patients will have impaired metabolism of benzodiazepines, barbiturates, chloral hydrate, meprobamate, tolbutamide, and warfarin.[43] Administration of these agents may result in an enhanced or prolonged pharmacological effect.

Chronic ethanol use may have an opposite effect by inducing hepatic microsomal enzymes, resulting in increased drug metabolism. This interaction has been reported with barbiturates, meprobamate, phenytoin, tolbutamide, and warfarin[44] and may result in the patient's requiring a larger dose of these agents to achieve the desired effect.[43]

Mechanism of Action

As a CNS depressant, ethanol depresses neuronal excitability, conduction of impulses, and neurotransmitter releases, although the exact molecular mechanisms resulting in alcohol intoxication remain unknown.[44] The effects of ethanol on the brain are concentration-dependent. At low blood ethanol concentrations (20 to 80 mg/dl), the highly integrated functions of the cerebral cortex are affected; therefore, thought processes are impaired. Although ethanol may occasionally be considered a stimulant drug, this is not true. Individuals who have ingested ethanol may appear to be stimulated and exhibit extroverted behavior, but this activity is due to

Table 30–2. CATEGORIZATION OF PSYCHOACTIVE DRUGS OF ABUSE

		PSYCHOGENICS	
DEPRESSANTS	STIMULANTS	MINOR	MAJOR
Sedative-hypnotics	Amphetamine (Dexedrine)	Marijuana	LSD (lysergic-acid diethylamide)
Alcohol	Methamphetamine	Hashish	Mescaline
Barbiturates	Nonamphetamines*		Psilocybin
Short-acting	Ritalin		STP (DOM) (dimethoxymethylamphetamine)
Thiopental	Preludin		DMT (dimethyltryptamine)
Intermediate-acting	Ionamin		THC (tetrahydrocannabinol)
Seconal	Others		Hash oil
Nembutal	Caffeine (coffee)		
Tuinal	Nicotine (tobacco)		
Amytal	Cocaine (coca)		
Long-acting	Freon (propellants and refrigerants)		
Phenobarbital			
Barbital			
Nonbarbiturates†			
Methaqualone (Quaalude)			
Doriden			
Chloral hydrate (Noctec)			
Placidyl			
Meprobamate			
Minor Tranquilizers			
Valium			
Librium			
Serax			
Dalmane			
Narcotics			
Natural			
Morphine			
Codeine			
Synthetic			
Methadone			
Propoxyphene (Darvon)			
Dilaudid			
Demerol			
Percodan			
Semisynthetic			
Heroin			
Major Tranquilizers			
Thorazine			
Mellaril			
Others (phenothiazines)			
Volatile Solvents			
Anesthetics			
Phencyclidine (PCP)			
Nitrous oxide			
Ether			

*Many drugs used as anorexiants are also stimulants, although they are chemically different from amphetamines.
†Many drugs used as hypnotics are unrelated chemically to the barbiturates, although they produce similar effects.
Modified with permission from Student Committee on Drug Abuse Education, University of Maryland School of Pharmacy.

ethanol's ability to depress the control one exerts on inhibitions.

As the concentration of ethanol increases, motor function, sensory function, and memory become more impaired. Legal intoxication in most states occurs at a blood ethanol concentration of 100 mg/dl. As this concentration is approached, individuals will manifest impaired judgment, increased reaction time, and decreased motor control. At concentrations above 150 mg/dl, gross intoxication will be evident in most individuals. Individuals with concentrations in the 200 to 300 mg/dl range may manifest ataxia and diplopia. Due to effects on the chemoreceptor trigger zone, vomiting also may occur. This may be a physiological defense mechanism utilized in an attempt to inhibit further ethanol absorption from the gastrointestinal tract.

At concentrations in the 300 to 400 mg/dl range, a patient may be stuporous, hypothermic, and amnesic. Death, commonly due to respiratory arrest, occurs when blood ethanol concentrations exceed 400 to 500 mg/dl.[45]

In addition to alcohol and water, alcoholic beverages contain varying amounts of coloring agents, flavoring additives, and other substances such as lead, iron, cobalt, histamines, tannins, and phenols. These contents are called *cogeners* and contribute to the toxic effects of alcohol. Chronic alcohol abuse can cause an accumulation of cogeners that may potentiate pathological changes in the CNS. These

TABLE 30–3. FACTORS AFFECTING BLOOD ALCOHOL CONCENTRATIONS

The primary factor affecting blood alcohol concentrations is the amount of alcohol consumed. Other important factors are time, body weight and build, and food consumption.

Body Weight and Build	Fat absorbs only 20% of the alcohol from the blood stream in contrast to muscle. A small person consuming the same amount of alcohol as a large person will have a higher blood alcohol level than the larger person because there is less body water to dilute the alcohol. Women's bodies generally are smaller in frame and contain a higher portion of fatty tissue; consequently, more alcohol will remain in the system. The average man weighing 70 kg (154 lb) metabolizes ⅔ of one standard drink per hour.
Time	**Constant Rate of ¾ Ounce of Pure Alcohol per Hour:** This rate of metabolism is ⅔ of one standard drink per hour. A standard drink is 1.5 oz of 80 proof distilled spirits, 3 oz of fortified wine such as sherry, 5 oz of table wine, or 12 oz of beer.
Food Consumption	Food in the stomach, especially food high in fat and protein, delays absorption. The closer to eating, the better.

cogeners are associated with headaches, nausea, shaking, and dizziness during the "hangover" period. Each type of alcoholic beverage has its own amount and types of cogener, although darker-colored alcoholic beverages tend to contain higher concentrations than lighter-colored beverages.

Potentiation

The comcomitant use of alcohol and other CNS depressants (e.g., barbiturates, opiates, sedative–hypnotics) may result in a potentiation of each drug's effect. Therefore, the combination of CNS depressant drugs may result not in additive effects but rather in synergistic effects.[46] The clinical importance of this finding on morbidity and mortality is not completely known. Rangno and associates[47] found that the presence of ethanol did not correlate with coma, altered vital signs, or mortality in 196 overdose patients.

Dependence and Tolerance

Chronic use of ethanol will result in the development of psychological and physical dependence as well as tolerance. The psychological dependence that develops is very difficult to interrupt. This is evidenced by the high rate of relapse occurring in alcoholics after they have gone through the alcohol withdrawal syndrome.

The clinical manifestations of withdrawal indicate that a patient is physically dependent on ethanol. A report as early as 1939 demonstrated that withdrawal from ethanol is of significant concern. Isbell and associates[48] studied the withdrawal effects of 95 per cent ethanol in 10 healthy former narcotic addicts. The authors confirmed the relationship between ethanol and the withdrawal syndrome and therefore the occurrence of physical dependence. In addition, the severity of the withdrawal syndrome following the discontinuation of ethanol ingestion was related to the dose and duration of ethanol ingestion.

Tolerance is a state that occurs with chronic drug use in which a larger dose of the drug is required in order to achieve the same effect. Tolerance develops to psychoactive drugs and is reversible with time and abstinence.

There are several types of tolerance. *Tissue tolerance* refers to the biological adaptation that occurs at the cellular level in response to prolonged exposure to a drug. *Metabolic tolerance* is characterized by an enhanced rate of inactivation of a drug.[48] Metabolic tolerance to ethanol may occur from the induction of a number of factors, including alcohol dehydrogenase, NAD, or acetylcoenzyme A. The degree of tolerance a given patient will manifest is unpredictable. Since tolerance to ethanol exists intrinsically in some individuals, the degree of tolerance that occurs in the population is characterized by wide interindividual variability.[49] The development of tolerance in these individuals probably stems from the development of tissue tolerance, metabolic tolerance, or both.

Clinicians caring for the ethanol-tolerant patient also must be aware that these patients develop cross-tolerance to other CNS depressants.[50] For the ethanol trauma patient, this implies that the patient also will be tolerant to the analgesic effects of narcotics as well as the sedating effects of commonly used tranquilizers. These agents should be used with caution in the tolerant patient who continues to consume alcohol.

A major difference between ethanol and narcotics revolves around the issue of tolerance. Patients will develop tolerance to the pharmacological effects of both drugs. Tolerance does not develop to the toxic effects of ethanol. However, tolerance does develop to the toxic effects (respiratory depression) of narcotics. Tolerance to narcotic-induced respiratory depression develops in an almost parallel fashion to the pharmacological effects (Fig. 30–1). This does not mean a patient cannot overdose from narcotics. If the blood concentration with any degree of tolerance exceeds the toxic level threshold, toxic effects will occur.

Other Pharmacological Effects

Cardiovascular System. Ethanol's cardiovascular effects center on its direct myocardial depressant and vasodilating effects. Following acute ethanol ingestion in individuals without cardiac disease, these two pharmacological properties counteract each other, so the net effect is minimal.[51] Similar findings are reported in alcoholic patients without cardiac disease.

Studies in nonalcoholic and alcoholic patients with cardiac disease demonstrate that myocardial function is quite sensitive to ethanol's depressant effects. Patients with various cardiac disorders who were given 2 to 6 ounces of whiskey demonstrated a fall in cardiac output, stroke work, blood pressure, and left ventricular end-diastolic pressure. Patients with severe congestive heart failure may have a decrease in preload and afterload following ethanol ingestion. This is most likely due to ethanol's peripheral vasodilating effects. In addition, administration of ethanol in the patient with cardiac disease may produce both atrial and ventricular dysrhythmias.[52–54]

Chronic ethanol intake may ultimately result in congestive

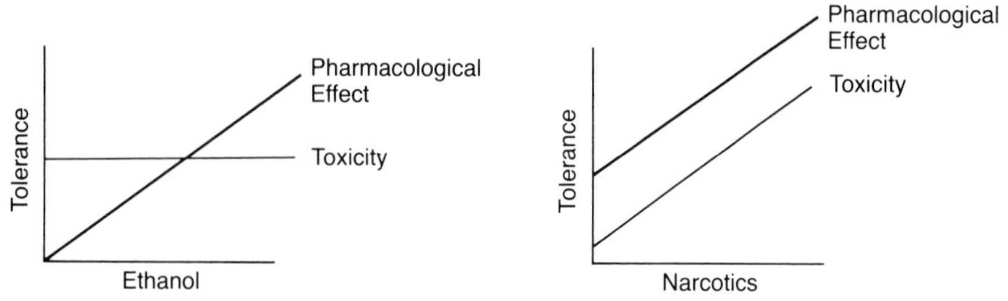

Figure 30–1. Tolerance (*A*) does not develop to the toxic effects of ethanol and (*B*) does develop to the toxic effects of narcotics.

cardiomyopathy, although the exact amount of ethanol and the duration of consumption required to produce this condition are not known and vary among individuals.[51] Typically, for this condition to develop, a large quantity of ethanol ingested over a 10- to 15-year period is required. Alcoholic cardiomyopathy should be suspected in any patient with a congestive cardiomyopathy who provides a history of chronic ethanol use. The clinical findings in these patients are consistent with the diffuse cardiac hypertrophy present and are the same as for other causes of congestive heart failure. Abstinence or a significant decrease in ethanol consumption may help improve the patient's status.

Gastrointestinal System. The ability of ethanol to induce injury to the gastric mucosa has been known since the early 19th century. In animal models, ethanol has been shown to stimulate gastric acid secretion.[55] Although the exact mechanism of action of this effect is unknown, it may involve gastric or histamine stimulation. The relevance of these findings to human patients is not clear. Data that demonstrate a clinically significant effect from ethanol ingestion on gastric acid secretion in humans are lacking.

Esophagus. Reflux esophagitis occurs as a result of local irritation to the esophageal mucosa by alcohol and hydrochloric acid following vomiting or regurgitation.[56] The alcoholic is also predisposed to epidermoid carcinoma of the esophagus, and esophageal varices can occur in conjunction with liver disease.[57]

Stomach. Ethanol has a concentration-dependent effect on the gastric mucosal barrier.[58] Ethanol concentrations between 8.2 and 14 per cent are associated with mucosal damage. If the gastric mucosal barrier is disrupted, acute gastritis may occur. This condition may occur after an acute ethanol binge and is reversible with abstinence. The presence of a severe gastritis decreases the mucosal barrier and allows gastric acid to further irritate the mucosa. When ethanol is used in conjunction with other mucosal irritants, a potentiation of gastric mucosa irritation may occur, resulting in gastrointestinal hemorrhage. Gastric acid reduction or neutralization is therefore an important therapeutic modality in this patient population.

Small Intestine. Abnormalities occurring in the small intestine include malabsorption of fat, xylose, folic acid, and vitamin B_{12}.[58] Altered nutrient absorption arises as a result of poor dietary habits, liver disease leading to decreased storage of folic acid, a decrease in pancreatic enzyme, and direct inhibition of tissue utilization of folate.

Pancreas. Acute pancreatitis syndrome resulting from alcohol intake is clinically manifested by upper abdominal pain, nausea, vomiting, hypotension, and elevated serum amylase and lipase concentrations. It is speculated that alcohol causes an increase in pancreatic spasm of the sphincter of Oddi, resulting in an increase in pancreatic intraductal pressure. Relaxation of the sphincter allows duodenal contents to enter the pancreatic duct. A change in the chemistry of the pancreatic juices leads to calculus formation.

Chronic pancreatitis may result from the cumulative effects of the above or perhaps the direct toxic effects of alcohol on the pancreas.[59] The development of chronic pancreatitis is insidious, although patients may complain of chronic pain, which may lead to analgesic or narcotic abuse. The signs of exocrine insufficiencies include weight loss, malnutrition, and foul bulky stools, often with diarrhea.

Liver. Alcohol, as well as many other drugs, can cause severe liver damage. The three common liver diseases that are attributed to alcohol use and abuse include alcoholic fatty liver, alcoholic hepatitis, and alcoholic cirrhosis.[60]

Alcoholic fatty liver occurs secondary to free fatty acid accumulation in liver cells, forming fat deposits. It is rarely symptomatic and can be present with moderate quantities of ethanol ingestion. Alcoholic hepatitis may result in fatty liver if continued ethanol ingestion occurs; however, frank jaundice is unusual. Alcoholic fatty liver is usually a benign disease and will resolve in 4 to 6 weeks with abstinence.

Alcoholic hepatitis is secondary to inflammatory necrosis of liver cells producing cell death and fibrosis. Alcoholic hepatitis consists of a spectrum of illnesses ranging from a totally asymptomatic condition to full-blown life-threatening acute liver failure. The clinical presentation usually includes hepatomegaly, jaundice, hepatic pain, fever, elevated liver function tests, marked leukocytosis, and ascites. Many of these patients will proceed to develop cirrhosis.

Alcoholic cirrhosis is characterized by advanced cell necrosis with scarring, nodule formation, and an altered hepatic structure. It is essentially an irreversible condition. Clinical evaluation usually reveals the presence of portal hypertension, ascites, edema, and, in some cases, an enlarged spleen. Abnormal serum chemistries, such as hyperbilirubinemia and hypoprothrombinemia, may also result from prolonged abuse of alcohol. Late-stage conditions related to cirrhotic liver disease include esophageal varices, deteriorating mental alertness, elevated temperature, anorexia, increased jaundice, and ascites.

Central Nervous System. Alcohol ingestion produces both acute and chronic neuropathy due to thiamine deficiency; the acute phase is referred to as *Wernicke encephalopathy,* and the chronic phase as *Korsakoff syndrome.*[61] Thiamine deficiency in alcoholics is due to a number of contributing factors, including inadequate dietary intake and altered absorption, storage, and use.[62]

Wernicke encephalopathy is characterized by an abrupt

onset and a triad of symptoms: oculomotor disturbances, ataxia, and mental confusion. Oculomotor disturbances range from nystagmus and various gaze palsies to total ophthalmoplegia. Ataxia results from cerebellar involvement, which causes instability of the lower extremities and trunk and an impaired gait. Mental confusion ranges from drowsiness to disorientation and coma.[63, 64] Mortality associated with Wernicke encephalopathy is approximately 17 per cent.[65]

Korsakoff psychosis represents the chronic phase of neuropathological changes and is characterized by short-term (few years) memory loss; long-term memory remains intact. The exact cause of this psychosis is not known. Recovery may occur, but it is incomplete in over 50 per cent of cases.[64] The use of clonidine, 0.3 mg twice a day, has been reported to be beneficial.[66] Other CNS problems associated with chronic ethanol ingestion are outlined in Table 30–4.[64]

Respiratory System. Decreased diaphragmatic excursion may be seen in alcoholics related to diminished respiratory drive or long-term effects of a phosphate-depletion syndrome, which affect the respiratory muscles.[67] In addition, ethanol may alter the level of consciousness and has been shown to impair glottal reflexes and ciliary motility. These processes will inhibit bacterial clearance mechanisms.[68, 69] Aspiration pneumonia in an alcoholic patient is likely to be due to gram-negative aerobic bacilli.[70] Its higher incidence is due to ethanol's direct depressant effects on respiratory clearance.[71]

Alcoholic cirrhosis also may impair lung function. The mass effect of severe ascites can restrict lung volumes.[72] Vascular shunts in the lung parenchyma of unknown cause may decrease arterial oxygen saturation and may, therefore, result in hypoxemia.[73, 74] Alcoholics with cirrhosis and hypoproteinemia may accumulate lung fluid, which causes impaired oxygen diffusion from alveoli to capillary blood.[75] Finally, cirrhotic patients may present with hyperventilation and a respiratory alkalosis. The cause of the hyperventilation is unknown but may be related to blood ammonia concentrations.

Activated pancreatic enzymes released during acute alcoholic pancreatitis may produce pulmonary endothelial damage.[76] The resulting consequences include pulmonary vasospasm, adult respiratory distress syndrome, and elevated pulmonary vascular and hydrostatic pressures.[77] Hyperlipidemia associated with acute pancreatitis also may contribute to hypoxemia by impairing oxygen uptake.[78]

Hematological System. Ethanol may exert a direct toxic effect or interfere with normal physiological processes, disrupting erythrocyte, leukocyte, and hemostatic mechanisms.[79, 80] Megaloblastic anemia due to folate deficiency is the most common anemia reported in alcoholic patients. Decreased dietary intake, malabsorption, direct "antifolate" effects, and inhibition of folic acid enterohepatic circulation are all possible effects.[81, 82]

Iron deficiency anemia is the second most common type of anemia seen in alcoholic patients. The depletion of iron stores and the inability to use iron result in sideroblastic anemia. The more severe cases are seen in malnourished patients.[83]

Ethanol also can affect the morphological features, production, and function of leukocytes.[84] Enlarged WBCs with multiple nuclear lobes may occur with folic acid deficiency. Phagocytic function of macrophages is also impaired. Lymphocyte activity and lymphocyte transformation to T lymphocytes are impaired in alcoholic patients as well. These processes tend to persist for 1 to 2 weeks after ethanol ingestion is halted.

Patients with acute or chronic ethanol ingestion may experience a prolonged bleeding time.[79] A 25 to 50 per cent decrease in the life-span of circulating platelets is associated with ethanol ingestion.[85] Platelet function also may be impaired by ethanol. Enlarged platelets result in a sluggish response and small, loose platelet aggregation.[86] In addition, defective collagen in vessel walls secondary to vitamin C deficiency in the malnourished alcoholic patient may affect platelet function. Ethanol-induced liver disease also may prevent the formation of vitamin K–dependent clotting factors.[85]

TABLE 30–4. OTHER ALCOHOL-RELATED CNS DISEASES

NAME	SYMPTOMS	TREATMENT
Alcoholic polyneuropathy	Variable pain, glove-stocking type of paresthesias, weakness starting in legs A slow, insidious process	Vitamin B complex, abstinence, improved nutrition Recovery often slow and incomplete
Alcoholic cerebellar degeneration	Wide-based stance, ataxia of various degrees Lower extremities > upper; men > women	Abstinence and improved nutrition may improve symptoms Etiology unknown, may involve Na and H_2O abnormalities
Central positive myelinolysis	Progressive quadriparesis Difficulty with speech and swallowing Partial or complete paralysis of eye movements Usually fatal in 2–3 weeks Progresses to extensive brainstem dysfunction	No treatment available Etiology unknown May involve Na abnormality; slowly correct hyponatremia
Marchiafava-Bignami disease	Demyelinating disease Diverse and nonspecific symptoms Dysarthria, aphasia, impaired gait, mental status changes Increased muscle tone, urinary incontinence	Etiology unknown May be associated with excessive red wine consumption
Alcoholic dementia	Diffuse cognitive defects caused by cortical atrophy	Exact mechanism controversial May be associated with thiamine deficiency; administer thiamine

Cocaine Pharmacology

Cocaine, a major alkaloid found in the *Erythroxylon coca* plant, is an agent with potent CNS stimulant properties and will serve as the prototype for this discussion. Coca leaves were chewed as early as the 16th century by the Incas. By the mid-1880s, coca was added to many medicinal tonics and was an active ingredient in Coca-Cola. With the 1914 Harrison Narcotic Act, cocaine was classified as a narcotic. Legally, the possession and/or sale of cocaine is subject to the same legal penalties as those for morphine and heroin.

Since the early 1970s, the use of cocaine has increased substantially. With this increase in use, there has been a concomitant increase in morbidity and mortality. From the mid-1970s to 1981 there was a sixfold increase in cocaine-related admissions to drug treatment programs, a threefold increase in cocaine-related deaths, and a threefold increase in cocaine-related emergencies.[87] Smoking and intravenous use of the drug also increased during the same time. Data collected between 1981 and 1983 also reveal a continued upward trend.

Pharmacokinetics

Cocaine is absorbed from all sites of application. The effects of the administration of cocaine are thought to be limited owing to inactivation within the gastrointestinal tract. Although Wilkinson and associates[88] demonstrated that similar plasma concentrations existed following oral and intranasal administration of a 2 mg/kg dose of cocaine, it was not reported whether similar pharmacological effects occurred from the two routes of administration.

Intranasal cocaine administration (snorting) produces local vasoconstriction, which may limit further systemic absorption. When an intranasal dose is repeated at intervals more frequent than the rate of elimination, drug accumulation may occur. Intranasal cocaine administration produces a subjective "high" in 15 to 20 minutes, which dissipates in 60 to 90 minutes.[89] Serum concentrations parallel both the "high" and heart rate changes. In contrast, intravenous cocaine produces an onset within 3 to 5 minutes, and the effects dissipate in 30 to 40 minutes. Intravenous administration produces higher serum concentrations as well as a greater increase in heart rate.

Cocaine in hydrochloride salt form has a combustion point of 197°C; the combustion point for the freebase form is 98°C.[90] Due to the lower combustion point, the freebase is the more suitable form for smoking. With similar doses, Perez-Reyes and associates[91] compared the intravenous use of the salt form with the inhalation of the freebase and found that there was no significant difference between the two routes of administration in heart rate, blood pressure, or the subjective "high" achieved. The results indicate that the physiological and psychological effects of smoking cocaine freebase must be considered equivalent to intravenous cocaine hydrochloride administration.

In the mid-1980s, "crack" cocaine became a popular form of cocaine use. Crack is produced by mixing cocaine with water and an alkali (baking soda or sodium bicarbonate). Once the water has been evaporated by boiling, chunks of waxy "crack" cocaine remain.[92] Due to its small particle size, crack is rapidly absorbed when smoked, producing a peak effect in 6 to 8 minutes.

Following systemic absorption, cocaine is eliminated by liver metabolism, with only a small fraction excreted in the urine. The liver can detoxify one minimum lethal dose of cocaine per hour.

Pharmacology

The only medical use of cocaine is as a local anesthetic. The stimulation properties of cocaine affect the CNS by stimulating the cortex and the lower portions of the cerebrospinal axis. Eventually, it causes medullar depression and respiratory failure.[90] Peripherally, cocaine inhibits catecholamine reuptake, the major mechanism by which the effects of catecholamines are reversed; therefore, a picture of sympathetic stimulation or the "fight-or-flight" response is reflected. Expected effects include increases in heart rate and blood pressure, vasoconstriction, dilated pupils, tremors, excitability, restlessness, and decreased gastrointestinal motility.

With chronic (≥2 years) cocaine administration of up to 7 gm/day, the most common physical symptoms reported in 32 patients were blurred vision (34.3 per cent), black sputum (34.3 per cent), muscle pain (34.3 per cent), tremors (28.1 per cent), and weight loss (25 per cent).[93] Blurred vision was secondary to chronic mydriasis; black sputum was secondary to residues from lighters, matches, or contaminated smoke; and back and shoulder muscular pain was associated with bending over pipes during extended smoking sessions.

Psychological Effects

As with other psychoactive substances, the final effects one experiences with cocaine are largely influenced by the environment where drug use occurs (setting) and the frame of mind of the individual at time of use (set). Immediately after inhalation, a period of marked euphoria, pleasure, hyperalertness, hyperactivity, anorexia, and insomnia develops. After approximately 20 minutes, the state of arousal is replaced by irritability as the drug effects dissipate. This phase also may be accompanied by dysphoria and may lead to repeated use to recapture the initial rush.

Depending on the set, setting, dosage, and chronicity of cocaine use, individuals are predisposed to two further stages of psychological effects. The first stage is of paranoia characterized by suspiciousness, insomnia, and possibly delusions. The second stage is of psychosis marked by delusions with possible hallucinations, disorientation, and loss of impulse control.[93] Paranoia has been reported to be the most common (62.5 per cent) psychological effect associated with chronic cocaine use in 32 patients admitted to a drug treatment program. Visual "hallucinations" can occur with the eyes open (objects) or closed (flash of light) and may include pulsating or vibrating geometric patterns. Tactile "hallucinations" have been reported with binge cocaine use and may consist of itching, feelings of foreign particles moving under the skin ("cocaine bugs"), and sensations of people brushing against the body. Although these experiences are called "hallucinations," true hallucinations whereby the subject believes the perceptions are real rarely occur.

Tolerance and Dependence

Animal and human data indicate that tolerance develops to cocaine use. Reverse tolerance to some of cocaine's effects (less drug is required to produce the desired effect) has been described in animal models.

There is no clear evidence that true physical dependence to cocaine develops. Twenty-four to 48 hours after abrupt discontinuation of continued cocaine use (>4 days), a patient may manifest a depressed mood, fatigue, and sleep disturbances. These findings, however, are more a reflection of the strong psychological dependence produced by cocaine rather than a true physical dependence.[90] Cocaine is capable of producing the psychological dependence seen with psychoactive substances. Intense drug-seeking behavior to cocaine has been demonstrated in animal studies.[94, 95]

Toxicity

The fatal dose of cocaine varies but is approximately 1.5 gm orally and 800 mg parenterally or by inhalation. The purity of street cocaine averages approximately 50 to 55 per cent.[90] The amount of cocaine administered intranasally is, therefore, approximately 14.5 mg but has been reported to be as high as 200 mg. Most subjects who were given various intravenous doses of cocaine and asked to subjectively rate the effect experienced stated that 16 mg produced the stimulant effect they were accustomed to by self-administering illicitly acquired drugs.[96]

As little as 25 mg of cocaine absorbed systemically will produce a noticeable rise in pulse and blood pressure (30 to 50 per cent and 15 to 20 per cent rise above baseline, respectively).[97] Following a large dose of cocaine, a vagally mediated effect may produce a slowing of the pulse. This effect is short-lived and is followed by a sinus tachycardia. Since norepinephrine reuptake is inhibited, myocardial effects manifest as ventricular dysrhythmias. With a severe exposure, ventricular fibrillation and death may occur. Hypotension due to loss of sympathetic tone also may occur.

Respirations may be rapid and shallow. Cheyne-Stokes respirations also may be observed; central respiratory collapse may be a cause of death.

The major neurological complications associated with cocaine use are seizures and cerebral hemorrhages.[98] Seizures typically occur following significant use of cocaine; however, they also have been reported with first-time use. Wetti and Wright reported that terminal seizures occurred in 6 of 14 (43 per cent) patients whose death was caused by acute cocaine use. The seizures occurred without warning, and the onset was between 36 and 60 minutes after oral ingestion and between a few minutes and 60 minutes after snorting cocaine. Once seizures began, death occurred within a few minutes up to 60 minutes later in those patients receiving medical attention.[99] Mental status changes ranging from anxiety to acute psychosis also may occur. The role that other drugs contribute to these side effects is difficult to evaluate in cases of polydrug abuse. The clinician should be cognizant of this difficulty and attempt to obtain a full drug history.

Marijuana Pharmacology

Marijuana, the psychogenic prototype used in this discussion, comes from the *Cannabis sativa* plant, which contains at least 420 different alkaloids called *cannabinoids*. There are four major cannabinoids: delta-9-tetrahydrocannabinol (delta-9-THC), delta-8-THC, cannabidiol, and cannabinol. Delta-9-THC is the major psychoactive component of *Cannabis*.

Delta-9-THC is available in various forms and concentrations. Marijuana is made of the leaf with or without the stem of the *Cannabis* plant and has a THC concentration of approximately 5 per cent. Hash or hashish is a resin produced by the plant and contains up to 10 per cent THC. When extracted and concentrated, the resin forms hash oil, which may be up to 40 per cent THC.

Pharmacokinetics

After smoking, marijuana has an onset of action of a few minutes, a peak effect in 10 to 30 minutes, and a duration of approximately 1 hour and seldom greater than 3 to 4 hours.[100] When ingested, the onset of action is delayed up to 1 hour; the peak effect occurs in 2 to 3 hours, with a duration of action up to 5 hours.

Following oral absorption in the animal model, THC is found in the brain, heart, lungs, and liver 3 hours postingestion. By 12 hours, concentrations are not detectable in the brain or heart but are present in the fat pads and lungs. This demonstrates THC's affinity for fat tissues; THC easily enters fat tissue but does not rapidly exit.

Delta-9-THC is rapidly metabolized to 11-hydroxy-THC, a pharmacologically active form that is further converted to 8, 11-dehydroxy-THC. This is subsequently eliminated in the urine and feces.

Physiological Effects

The most common and prominent effect of THC is tachycardia and occasionally an increase in blood pressure. Tachycardia-induced increases in myocardial oxygen consumption may be a cause for concern in patients with underlying cardiovascular disease.[101]

Ocular effects of THC include conjunctival injections (red eyes), an increase in the amount of time needed to recover from light-induced glare, and a decrease of up to 40 per cent in intraocular pressure.[102] THC does not have a prolonged (>5 minutes) effect on pupil size.

Psychomotor coordination also may be impaired.[101] Therefore, driving and activities requiring mental alertness may be affected. Marijuana smoke also may produce a dry mouth and throat irritation. Acute inhalation generally produces a bronchodilatory response, whereas chronic and excessive use may contribute to obstructive airway disease.[103, 104]

Delta-9-THC has been reported to produce a small, reversible decrease in the number and motility of human sperm, although there is no conclusive evidence that marijuana affects male fertility.[101] There also exist no convincing data of THC's detrimental effect on female hormonal function. Gynecomastia with marijuana use has been reported in a very small number of patients. The small number of case reports makes it unlikely that a significant correlation exists.[90]

Psychological Effects

Similar to other psychoactive drugs, the set and setting are important determinants of the final effect observed with the use of marijuana. Therefore, the same person may react differently to the same dose on two different occasions if the set or setting is varied. With small doses of marijuana, one experiences euphoria, heightened perception, time and space distortion, and sedation. Lapses of attention and short-term memory loss also may occur without gross brain abnormalities.[101]

Marked sensory disturbances may occur with large doses of marijuana. These changes include decreases in color discrimination, auditory effects, and visual detection of small moving objects. Impairment in thought process and disturbed muscle coordination also may occur.

The most common adverse reaction to *Cannabis* use is the acute panic anxiety reaction.[90] The patient may be hysterical because he feels he is going crazy. Acute panic reactions are most common in novice users with substance containing high THC concentrations. In addition, these reactions generally occur with an adverse set and/or setting. Although not conclusively documented, patients with an underlying psychiatric disorder may be more prone to this type of reaction.[105]

Tolerance and Dependence

There is strong evidence that tolerance can develop to many of the psychological and physical effects of marijuana. A true physical dependence and, therefore, withdrawal syndrome as seen with narcotics has not been observed following moderate amounts of marijuana intake containing 1 to 2 per cent THC. Large doses (up to 10 joints per day of 2 per cent THC for 7 to 64 days) may produce symptoms consistent with a type of withdrawal.[106, 107] Symptoms include a sense of inner unrest, irritability, insomnia, anorexia, and nausea.

Reverse tolerance may occur with marijuana use. The proposed mechanisms for this reverse tolerance include (1) an enhanced metabolic rate of delta-9-THC to the more active component; (2) with cumulative doses, the fat stores become saturated, therefore requiring less drug to produce CNS effects; (3) increased receptor sensitivity; and (4) with continued use, it becomes easier to recognize the THC-induced "high" state.

Other Considerations

Marijuana users who are given atropine have been reported to manifest a prolonged tachycardia postoperatively.[90] Chronic marijuana smokers also have been shown to have a higher rate of theophylline clearance than nonsmokers.[108] Marijuana users may therefore require larger than usual doses of theophylline to achieve plasma concentrations in the 10 to 20 μg/ml range.

A number of investigations have examined the potential role of THC as a therapeutic agent.[109] Although some studies do indicate a beneficial effect, the available data are currently incomplete. The potential uses include THC as an agent in the treatment of glaucoma, chemotherapy-induced nausea and vomiting, asthma, hypertension, and seizures and for analgesia. In addition, THC has been investigated as an antispasmodic, antitussive, antidepressant, and sedative–hypnotic agent.

Chronic Effects of Marijuana Use

Experienced marijuana smokers inhale smoke longer, inhale a larger volume of smoke, and hold the smoke in their lungs for a longer period of time when compared with naive marijuana smokers or tobacco smokers.[110] Chronic marijuana use by experienced users may predispose them to a number of complications.

Marijuana smoke contains a higher amount of polynuclear aromatic hydrocarbons (PAH) than does tobacco smoke; PAH is the content thought to contribute to the carcinogenic activity of smoke condensate.[111] In addition, marijuana smoke has a higher amount of tar than tobacco cigarettes.[112] This combination of higher amount of tar and PAH may result in carcinogenic effects of long-term marijuana use. In the animal model, applications of *Cannabis* residue to the skin resulted in tumor formation.[113] However, extrapolation to humans cannot be made at this time. Although a correlation between marijuana smoking and lung cancer may exist, years of epidemiological research are needed before this can be documented.

Another concern that exists for the long-term marijuana smoker is altered pulmonary function. Clinical reports in this area are conflicting.[103, 104] Respiratory tract symptoms from *Cannabis* smoking include pharyngitis, rhinitis, bronchitis, and asthma.[114] Long-term marijuana smokers in Jamaica and India have been reported to have a high incidence of chronic bronchitis.[115, 116] Other studies in Jamaica and Costa Rica, however, did not find this correlation.[117, 118] Interpretation of these results is difficult owing to study design flaws.

Tashkin and associates[103] examined the effects of chronic marijuana use (>2 years) in 74 regular users. When compared with controls, the marijuana users demonstrated a mild but significant decrease in specific airway conductance. Their results indicate that chronic marijuana smoking may produce a functional impairment of the large airways. The full implications of these studies are not known, although it seems prudent to advise patients with pulmonary disease not to smoke marijuana. However, the nonconclusive nature of the existing studies mandates further evaluation on this topic.

Clinical Application

Drug and alcohol abusers suffer from a complex disorder that has physiological, psychological, and sociological dimensions and are also subjected to an increased risk of both acute and chronic medical problems (Fig. 30–2). The nurse caring for the trauma patient with a substance abuse history is faced with a variety of complex clinical challenges and therefore must acquire knowledge and skills pertaining to alcoholism and drug abuse, including prevention strategies, diagnosis, and management of associated problems, to deliver the highly specialized care required by this patient population.

The clinical application discussion that follows is organized in accordance with the cycles of trauma care format. The resuscitation cycle will detail assessment considerations, including identifying the substance abuser, psychosocial factors associated with substance abuse, and laboratory findings. Medical management priorities are identified first, followed by nursing management considerations for each cycle.

Because of the dramatic increase of cocaine-related deaths and traumatic events, a case-flow summary highlighting the systemic effects of acute intoxication from initial ingestion of "crack" cocaine is presented (Fig. 30–3). Trauma nurses need an expanded knowledge base pertaining not only to the physiological effects of cocaine intoxication but also to the

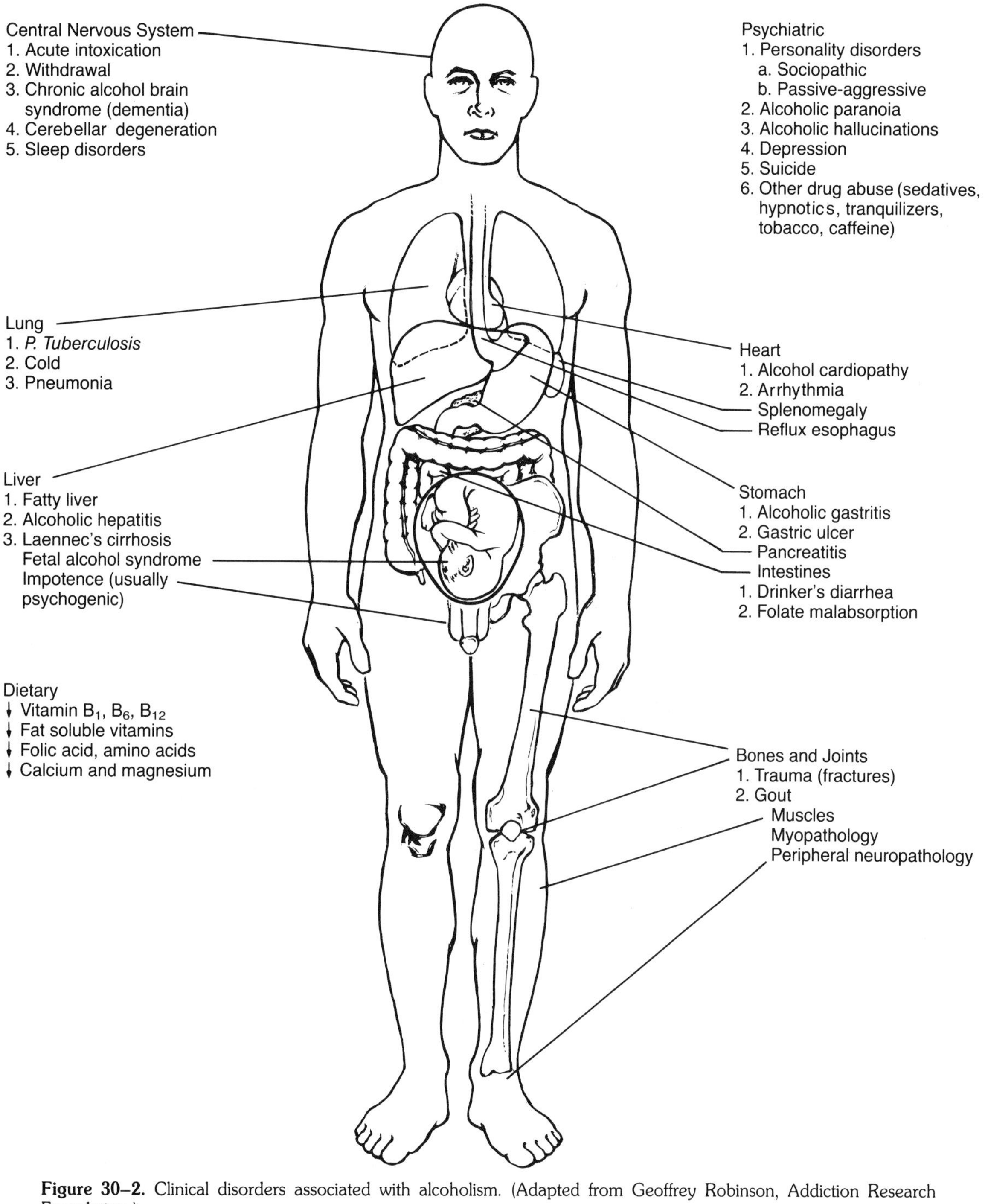

Figure 30–2. Clinical disorders associated with alcoholism. (Adapted from Geoffrey Robinson, Addiction Research Foundation.)

Acute "Crack" Intoxication
Bilateral Tibia-Fibula Fractures

Resuscitation Cycle
Glasgow Coma Scale 3 Profound Hypotension
↓
Fluid Resuscitation Vasopressors Dopamine
PASG Pulmonary Artery Catheter
↓
Improved Level of Consciousness
Prepare for OR
↓
Perioperative Cycle
Intubation Fluid Resuscitation Surgical Phase Unremarkable
Extubation Stable Postop Phase
↓
Critical Care Cycle
Systems Stable for 18 Hours
Then
Decreased Level of Consciousness Noted
SVT (190–200 beats/min) Cardiac Arrest
↓
ACLS Measures Initiated Intubation Vasopressors
Successful Resuscitation
EEG Reveals Alpha Pattern Coma
↓
Stable ABGs Ventilator Assistance Maintained
No Changes for 48 Hours Extubation
↓
Progressive Hypotension Dopamine Vasopressors
Cardiogenic Shock Possible Myocarditis
Intra-aortic Balloon Pump (IABP)
↓
48 Hours Later Stable Weaned Off Dopamine
Response to Verbal Commands Noted
↓
IABP Discontinued Repeat Two-Dimensional ECHO
Revealed Improved Ejection Fraction
Increased Responsiveness Left-sided Weakness Noted
↓
Intermediate Care/Rehabilitation Cycle
Systems Stable with Cardiac Reserve Limitation
Resting Ejection Fraction of 40%
Awake and Oriented
Inconsistent Ability to Assist With ADLs

Figure 30–3. Acute "crack" intoxication case-flow summary—system response through trauma cycles.

wide range of therapeutic modalities involved in caring for a patient with multisystem involvement.

RESUSCITATION CYCLE

During the resuscitation cycle, the primary goals of care for the trauma patient who is a substance abuser, as for any trauma patient, are directed toward (1) stabilization of the cardiovascular, respiratory, and neurological systems, (2) prevention of circulatory–respiratory collapse, and (3) monitoring of the patient's response to detect detrimental and beneficial physiological changes in condition. Since detailed assessment and management priorities of the multiple trauma patient are discussed elsewhere in this text, this information will not be repeated. Rather, clinical care issues that are peculiar to the trauma patient with a substance abuse history are the focus of subsequent discussions.

Assessment Considerations

The assessment of the trauma patient who is a substance abuser is complicated by several factors. In a majority of cases, the patient's history is unknown, thereby increasing the possibility that significant clinical findings related to substance abuse go unrecognized. In addition, differentiating clinical findings that occur secondary to traumatic injury from those which are related to ethanol or drug ingestion can be difficult. Therefore, it is essential that the assessment of the patient be complete and progress rapidly and systematically. Findings that correlate with substance abuse patterns (refer to "Pharmacological Effects") should be incorporated as specific injury-related data are accumulated. (Refer to injury-specific assessment considerations detailed in other chapters.)

Identifying the Substance Abuser

Accident Data Base. The collection of information about the accident is vital. Repeated automobile accidents, falls, and injuries are clues to a possible substance abuse history. Accidents or falls resulting from carelessness, loss of coordination, risk-taking, and impaired judgment should trigger suspicion of a possible substance abuse history and be further explored. Reports that the patient exhibited bizarre behavior before or after the occurrence of trauma, particularly if the individual has a history of drug abuse, strongly suggest the presence of psychogenic agents.

Substance Abuse History. Information regarding the substance abuse history, if provided by the patient, should not be considered a reliable predictor because substance abusers often deny their habits or provide inaccurate information. It is important, therefore, to minimize the development of denial behavior by the patient and to build some degree of trust during the admission process by demonstrating sensitivity and discretion when questioning the patient and family.

Ethanol History. An attempt to elicit an ethanol history from the patient or family member should be initiated as soon as possible. Brief questioning, focusing on validating drug use patterns, is appropriate at this time; the completion of a thorough health history may need to be delayed until a later phase of care.

The type and amount of ethanol that the patient usually drinks should be determined. A description of one's drinking habits such as "social drinking" is not acceptable, since this term has many possible interpretations. Specific information regarding the following issues should be collected: (1) type of alcoholic beverage consumed, (2) largest volume patient usually drinks at one sitting, (3) duration of drinking habit, and (4) frequency of drinking activities (e.g., every day, twice a week). To identify symptoms characteristic of alcohol withdrawal syndrome (AWS), the patient or family should be asked the following questions:

What was the date and time of the last drink?
Have any of the following symptoms been experienced after drinking or following a drinking episode: shakes, sweats, restlessness, sleeping problems, decrease in appetite, hallucinations, convulsions or seizures, or delirium tremens (DTs)?

Drug History. A drug history also must be obtained. Questions that elicit information about the severity of the substance abuse problem are posed. Sample questions include:

Do you take any medication by prescription from a physician?
Have you ever used drugs that were not prescribed by a physician?
What are the types of drugs used?
How often? What is the usual amount?
In what way have you used these drugs: oral, smoking, inhalation, intravenous, intramuscular?

In addition, drug withdrawal information can be obtained by asking the following questions:

Have you had any drug-free periods during your drug use?
What do you experience when you stop taking drugs?

Combination abuse is common. This occurs when one or more substances in addition to ethanol are abused; thus the magnitude of the problem is intensified. Barbiturates and ethanol or ethanol and other drugs, when ingested, could prove to be lethal combinations.

Psychosocial Assessment

Information pertaining to the patient's psychological and emotional well-being should be obtained as well. The use of ethanol and drugs may be an attempt to self-medicate a depression or schizophrenic psychosis. As continued ethanol and drug use cause deterioration and disintegration of vital social relationships and support systems, deeper levels of emotional and psychological despair are experienced. Excessive use of ethanol or drugs may ultimately result in overdose, the most common means of suicide attempt.[119] Specific questions that relate to social relationships, communication patterns, coping abilities, and general life-style patterns are posed. The following issues should be considered when assessing drinking and drug use behaviors:[120]

1. Marital discord
2. History of four or more intoxications in the previous year
3. History of driving-related arrests

4. History of injuries while intoxicated
5. Legal profile related to drinking/drug use history
6. History of "drinking on the job" or reported intoxications at the workplace
7. Family history of alcoholism/drug use

A direct but sensitive approach by the nurse will often engender the patient's trust; however, denial and hostility are factors that frequently deter the data-collection process. Family members and significant others may be helpful in corroborating information in these situations. Nevertheless, despite all efforts made to obtain accurate information, it is often necessary for the nurse to rely on astute observation skills to assist in the recognition of subtle cues.

Laboratory Assessment

Toxicology Screening. The initial diagnostic workup of a trauma patient with a possible substance abuse history should include a toxicology screen of both urine and serum. Whenever samples are sent for toxicology analysis, be aware of the laboratory capabilities. Toxicology screens are most reliable when the laboratory technician knows what drugs are suspected. Many drugs are not found on a routine toxicology screen (Table 30–5); therefore, it may be necessary to request a specific drug screen for the suspected drug. Most of the psychogenic drugs are not included in a typical screen.

Serum Osmolarity and Blood Alcohol Levels. A close correlation exists between serum osmolarity and blood alcohol concentration (BAC) in trauma patients.[121] Estimating the blood alcohol level from serum osmolarity is often beneficial, since blood alcohol determinations are not always readily available (Table 30–6). Serum osmolarity provides a rapid and convenient means of detecting intoxication with dangerously high blood ethanol levels and ethanol-complicated drug overdoses. It is not a substitute for direct determination of blood ethanol levels in medicolegal cases, however, since it slightly overestimates the amount of ethanol present.[122]

Serum osmolarity is indicative of the blood alcohol level at the time of measurement, not at the time of injury; therefore, the BAC level should be determined as soon as possible after admission, since a delay can cause difficulty with interpretation of the results. Intravenous infusions and metabolism of alcohol will lower the serum osmolarity levels. Other factors, such as renal disease, diabetes, vomiting, dehydration, hyperproteinemia, hyperlipidemia, and ingestion of methanol or ethylene glycol (antifreeze), can increase the serum osmolarity.

The blood alcohol level is expressed as the number of milligrams of alcohol per 100 ml (or per deciliter [dl]) of blood. Therefore, 50 mg of alcohol per 100 ml (1 dl) of blood would be expressed as 0.05 mg%. The relationship between blood alcohol concentration and clinical symptomatology is characterized in Table 30–7. The common legal blood alcohol concentration is 0.10 mg%. At concentrations above 0.30 mg%, patients may be unconscious and close to respiratory and/or cardiovascular compromise. A linear relationship between blood alcohol concentration and incidence of motor vehicle accidents has not been clearly established. However, an increased risk of involvement in a motor vehicle mishap has been associated with blood alcohol concentrations as low as 0.047 mg%.[123]

Other Laboratory Indicators. Several other tests are helpful in confirming suspicion of alcoholism. Liver enzymes are commonly examined, but caution must be exercised because changes in liver enzymes are insensitive and indicate a higher level of alcohol consumption for a long time. Aspartate aminotransferase (AST, SGOT) and alanine aminotransferase (ALT, SGPT) are nonspecific (elevated in fatty liver, cirrhosis, alcoholic hepatitis, as well as nonalcoholic liver disease). The AST may well be higher than ALT because alcohol may selectively inhibit ALT synthesis. Gamma-glutamyl transferase (GGPT, GGT) changes are sensitive for alcoholic intake, although they do not signify liver damage. GGPT changes are induced over several weeks and return to normal weeks to months after abstinence.[124]

An elevated or high-normal high-density lipoprotein (greater than 60 HDL) and elevated mean corpuscular volume (MCV) are also commonly found with high alcohol intake levels. The MCV changes may be a combined result of vitamin deficiency and direct alcoholic toxicity on the bone marrow.[125]

Medical Management Priorities

Drug Overdose in the Trauma Patient

Management priorities for the trauma patient with a drug overdose are the same as for the multiple-system injured trauma patient. Initial resuscitation efforts must focus on stabilization of cardiopulmonary function, and intervention must be timely, since a shock state can result. A patent airway must be secured, adequate ventilation must be provided, and adequate circulation must be supported and maintained.

Naloxone Administration. Naloxone is frequently administered to unconscious patients in an attempt to rule out narcotic exposure.[122] The initial intravenous dose recommendation for naloxone is 0.2 mg in children and 2 mg in adults. If no effect is observed, the dose may be repeated. The dose commonly administered to an adult, however, is 0.8 mg (2 ampules); this dose is frequently inadequate. If a response is not observed following the administration of up to 10 mg, narcotic exposure may not have occurred.[124]

If the patient has narcotic substances in the bloodstream, naloxone will improve the respiratory pattern as well as the mental status of the patient. Naloxone also has been reported to produce beneficial results in reversing the effects of benzodiazepines, alcohol, nitrous oxide and halothane, pentobarbitone–oxymorphone combination, and valproic acid.

Naloxone must be administered with caution. Overaggressive administration may not only awaken the patient but also may produce narcotic withdrawal symptoms. Therefore, naloxone should be administered gradually until a level of awakeness occurs, thus preventing respiratory depression and coma.

Patients who have overdosed from long-acting narcotics (e.g., methadone) will respond favorably to naloxone initially. However, since naloxone has a duration of action of 1 to 4 hours, with time the beneficial effects of naloxone will dissipate while the quantity of narcotic substances in the blood remains substantial. In this situation, the patient may

TABLE 30–5. TYPICAL TOXICOLOGY SCREEN REPORT

Collection Date ________ Rec'd Date ________
Time ________ Time ________
Blood ________ Urine ________ Other ________

TEST	SCREEN RESULTS: Tested In	SCREEN RESULTS: Neg	SCREEN RESULTS: Pos	CONFIRMATION/QUANTITATION: Fluid Tested	CONFIRMATION/QUANTITATION: Results
Ethanol	Blood				
Methanol	Blood				
Acetaminophen	Blood				
Amphetamine	Urine				
	Blood				
Barbiturates	Urine				
	Urine				
Benzodiazepines	Blood				
Cocaine	Urine				
Ethchlorvynol (Placidyl)	Blood				
	Blood				
Glutethimide (Doriden)	Urine				
Meperidine (Demerol)	Urine				
Methadone	Urine				
Opiates	Urine				
Phencyclidine (PCP)	Urine				
Phenothiazines	Urine				
	Blood				
Phenytoin (Dilantin)	Urine				
Propoxyphene (Darvon)	Urine				
Quinine	Urine				
	Blood				
Salicylates	Urine				
Tricyclic Antidepressants	Blood				

relapse into a comatose state with severe respiratory depression following an initial period of improvement.

Flumazenil Administration. Flumazenil is a competitive antagonist at the benzodiazepine receptor site. Similar to naloxone, flumazenil has no pharmacological effects of its own.[126] Clinically, it rapidly reverses the effects of benzodiazepine within 10 minutes.[127] Flumazenil has been reported to effectively reverse coma and excessive sedation induced by benzodiazepine overdose and mixed overdoses with benzodiazepine and ethanol.[128] The duration of flumazenil's reversal of benzodiazepine effects is dose-dependent and ranges from 15 to 180 minutes.

TABLE 30–6. ESTIMATING THE BLOOD ALCOHOL LEVEL FROM SERUM OSMOLARITY

To determine the blood alcohol level, subtract the low, normal value of 280 milliosmols/liter (mOsmol/l) from the patient's serum osmolarity. Then, divide that number by 25 to approximate the blood alcohol level.

For example: Given a serum osmolarity of 350 mOsmol/l

1. 350 − 280 = 70
2. 70 ÷ 25 = 2.8
3. 2.8 = Approximate blood alcohol level

In an acute benzodiazepine overdose, a patient may present with depressed CNS function, and respiratory depression may occur if the benzodiazepine has been mixed with other CNS depressant agents. Although the administration of flumazenil will awaken the benzodiazepine overdose patient and have some effect on patients who have ingested ethanol, if the duration of action of the benzodiazepine taken is longer than that of flumazenil, the patient may once again lapse into a state of depressed CNS function once the effects of flumazenil have dissipated. Therefore, care must be taken to closely monitor these patients.

One of the greatest concerns with the use of flumazenil is in the patient with a history of chronic benzodiazepine use. In this situation, administration of flumazenil may precipitate

TABLE 30–7. ALCOHOL INGESTION AND ALCOHOL BLOOD LEVELS

PERCENT OF ALCOHOL IN BLOOD	SYMPTOMS
0.05%	Not under the influence, appears normal
0.10% (common legal limit for operation of motor vehicle)	Beginnings of outward physical symptoms: • Emotional lability (boastfulness, exhilaration, talkativeness, remorse, belligerence) • Slight muscular incoordination, such as slowed reaction time, ataxia • Decreased inhibitions
0.15%	"Under the influence": • Sensory disturbances (decreased pain sense, diplopia, vertigo, slurred speech) • Confusion • Staggering gait • Rapid pulse • Diaphoresis
0.20%	"Acutely intoxicated": • Marked decrease in response to stimuli • Muscular incoordination approaching paralysis • Nausea and vomiting • Drowsiness and/or stupor • Symptoms listed for 0.15%
0.30–0.40%	• Complete unconsciousness • Impaired or absent tendon reflexes • Peripheral vascular collapse (hypotension; tachycardia; cold pale skin; hypothermia; slow, stertorous respiration) • Seizures (if present may also indicate hypoglycemia)
0.50%	• Death due to cardiac or respiratory arrest or aspiration pneumonitis

Adapted from Anspaugh P: Emergency management of intoxicated patients with head injuries. J Emerg Nurs 3(3):9–13, 1977.

benzodiazepine withdrawal and seizures. In addition, patients who have overdosed on both benzodiazepines and tricyclic antidepressants receiving flumazenil also may manifest seizures.[129]

For patients with a benzodiazepine overdose, flumazenil is administered in 0.2- to 0.5-mg dosage increments intravenously over 30 seconds in 1-minute intervals. Cumulative doses beyond 3 mg do not reliably produce additional beneficial effects. In rare cases, patients with a partial response at 3 mg may require additional doses up to a total cumulative dose of 5 mg. If 5 mg of flumazenil has been administered without a response in a suspected drug overdose patient, the sedation is not likely to be due to benzodiazepine administration, and additional doses are not likely to have an effect. Alternative drugs and/or causes of altered mental status should be investigated.

Neurological Management Issues

Intoxication and drug use should never be assumed to be the sole cause of abnormal neurological findings. The dangers of delayed diagnosis and misdiagnosis in patients with traumatic intracranial hematomas have been emphasized.[125] The most common reason for failing to recognize an intracranial hematoma is that a depressed level of consciousness is incorrectly attributed to a cerebrovascular accident or excessive ethanol intake.

Clinical assessment trends play a key role in the differential diagnosis of neurological impairment and must therefore be closely monitored (see Chapter 17). If clear evidence of clinical deterioration exists or focal neurological signs become evident, the presence of a traumatic hematoma must be excluded before the clinical presentation is attributed to ethanol intake or drug use. Other causes of CNS depression that are associated with the trauma population include hypoxia, shock, and hypothermia.

Cardiac Disturbances

Acute and prolonged ingestion of ethanol has a direct deleterious effect on left ventricular function.[130] In addition, vasodilation of the peripheral blood vessels occurs with vasoconstriction of the larger vessels producing resistance to blood flow, thus increasing the work load of the heart. Alcoholic cardiomyopathy is characterized by a slow or sudden onset of left- and right-sided congestive heart failure, cardiomegaly, elevated diastolic blood pressure, and peripheral edema. Congestive failure associated with early alcoholic disease responds readily to diuretic and digitalis therapy early in the progression of failure.

Fatal dysrhythmias, conduction disturbances, pathological Q waves, or left ventricular hypertrophy with abnormal T waves also can occur. Differential diagnosis and management of cardiac disturbances are complicated by the fact that EKG abnormalities also can occur secondary to blunt thoracic trauma, although this is more likely to occur during the critical care phase.[131] Decisions regarding the treatment of cardiac disturbances are based on clinical symptoms. All measures should be taken to ensure optimal cardiopulmonary function.

Respiratory Management Issues

Acute respiratory failure is often precipitated in patients with chronic obstructive pulmonary disease (COPD) by the sedative effects of drugs such as ethanol, barbiturates, tranquilizers, and narcotics. Intubation and mechanical ventilation are measures that are frequently necessary to maintain pulmonary parenchymal expansion, and an extended period of ventilatory support may be required.

Hemostatic and Hematological Mechanisms

Ethanol exerts a direct toxic effect on normal physiological processes, disrupting erythrocyte, leukocyte, and hemostatic mechanisms.[86] Bleeding tendencies and a poor response to hemorrhagic episodes result from ethanol-induced thrombocytopenia, poor platelet response, ineffective platelet plugs, depletion of plasma coagulation factors, and altered fibrinolytic response.[79] These alterations contribute significantly to the complexities of clinical management, since these patients are at risk for problems associated with oxygen transport, infection, and hemorrhage.

Clinical management decisions are based on the degree to which hemostasis is affected. Blood component therapy in conjunction with vitamin K administration may be indicated.

Fluid/Electrolyte Imbalances

Numerous fluid and electrolyte dysfunctions are commonly found in alcoholic patients. Abnormal findings may include hypomagnesemia, hypocalcemia, hypophosphatemia, sodium and water imbalance, and hypokalemia.

Electrolyte and IV fluid volume replacement must be accomplished. An indwelling urinary catheter is inserted; strict recording of intake and output is vital. Laboratory values should be monitored closely as well.

Hypomagnesemia. Poor nutritional intake, malabsorption, and the direct effects of ethanol can cause magnesium deficiency.[132] As a result, the CNS is greatly stimulated, causing irritability, delusions, or aggressive behavior.[133] Hypoactive reflexes, facial twitching, jerking, and convulsions also can occur. Cardiovascular functioning may be affected as well, resulting in hypotension and tachycardia.

In addition, since magnesium is a necessary cofactor for thiamine-dependent cofactors, hypomagnesemia may cause an altered response to thiamine administration in the alcoholic patient. Thiamine resistance is overcome, however, with the administration of magnesium.[61]

Hypocalcemia. Hypocalcemia occurs in alcoholism secondary to low protein and calcium intake. Consequently, neuromuscular functioning and blood coagulation processes are impaired. Painful tonic muscle spasms, facial spasms, laryngospasm, and fatigue often occur as a result of hypocalcemia.[133, 134]

Hypophosphatemia. Low phosphate levels in the alcoholic patient may be due to poor intake or to diarrhea. Phosphate depletion is often severe and is characterized by dysfunction of leukocytes and erythrocytes, defective platelets, and myocardial failure.

Sodium and Water Imbalance. Alcohol ingestion causes a rapid but limited water diuresis, followed by an antidiuretic phase during alcohol withdrawal. Sodium imbalances occur in conjunction with altered fluid balances.

Hypokalemia. Hypokalemia can occur in the alcoholic as a consequence of inadequate intake, diarrhea, vomiting, or hyperaldosteronism. Adequate potassium levels are required for skeletal and muscle tissue functions and for regulation of intracellular osmolarity.[135] Cardiac dysrhythmias can occur secondary to potassium imbalances.

Nursing Management Considerations

Potential for Hypoxia, Decreased Vital Capacity, and Reduced Lung Expansion Related to Respiratory Center Depression Secondary to Substance Abuse

The breathing pattern of the intoxicated patient may be slow and shallow owing to CNS depression. The patient with altered sensorium may lose consciousness and be prone to aspiration or airway obstruction.

Establishing and maintaining a patent airway is a first priority during the resuscitation phase of care. Although airway management is usually the responsibility of the anesthesiology staff, the nurse's role includes frequent respiratory assessment, including inspection of chest wall, palpation, and auscultation of breath sounds. Arterial blood gas trends should be monitored as well. If the patient is being artificially ventilated, airway pressures should be monitored closely. Scrupulous pulmonary toilet must be accomplished. All clinical assessment findings must be correlated with injury-specific criteria for accurate identification of underlying pathological processes (see Chapter 19).

If drug overdose is suspected and respiratory inadequacies are apparent, the medical treatment may include the administration of the narcotic antagonist naloxone (Narcan) (refer to earlier discussion). An improvement in respiratory rate and depth should be observed within ½ to 2 minutes if narcotic intoxication has occurred. Recovery is often dramatic, but precautionary measures should be taken to protect the patient as well as team members because the patient may emerge from a narcotic-induced coma in an agitated state.

Potential for Alterations in Cardiac Function Related to:

- Fluid volume deficit secondary to impaired hemostatic mechanisms
- Cardiac dysrhythmias secondary to substance abuse
- Hypothermia secondary to ethanol intake
- Altered erythropoietic mechanisms

Early detection of cardiovascular disturbances is facilitated by close observation and continuous monitoring of EKG, blood pressure, central venous pressure, cardiac output, urine output, skin color, core body temperature, and peripheral circulation throughout the resuscitation phase of care. Knowledge regarding the common dysrhythmias and cardiopulmonary symptoms that often develop with ethanol abuse should be applied during the assessment process. This information coupled with other findings related to ethanol abuse will assist in determining the origin of specific patient problems (refer to earlier discussions). Laboratory study results must also be considered. Trends in hemoglobin, hematocrit, osmolarity, electrolytes, isoenzymes, and coagulation values must be observed. These values will assist with the assessment of the trauma patient's response to injury or to therapeutic interventions. All data must be correlated with the history and physical assessment findings.

Administration of intravenous fluid therapy is based on clinical findings and hemodynamic stability. Efforts should be taken to maintain normal core body temperature.

Potential for Self-Harm or Harm to Others Related to Combativeness or Uncooperative Behavior Secondary to Drug Abuse

If a patient presents a danger to himself or others on admission, care provisions become complex. The use of restraints is indicated if the patient is combative, restless, or attempting to interfere with resuscitative care activities. A reasonable amount of force may be necessary to protect the patient or health team members until restraints can be applied. The health care facility's policies and procedures regarding use of restraints should be followed. In some cases, sedation becomes the only alternative to calm the patient, but it should be avoided if at all possible until a thorough neurological assessment has been completed.

The nurse should be alert to the effect that set and setting can have on the patient's response to treatment. Attempts should be made to orient the patient to the surroundings. Simple, honest explanations regarding resuscitation activities should be offered. A calm, nonthreatening approach is often helpful in gaining the patient's trust and eliciting cooperation.

Stress levels intensify among the trauma team members when the patient's behavior interferes with the delivery of care. A calm approach on the part of the nurse often has a positive effect on team functioning as well.

Alterations in Neurological Status Related to Dulled Consciousness and Neuropathy Secondary to Substance Abuse

Sudden changes in the patient's neurological status can occur quickly; therefore, close observation is essential. A thorough neurological assessment should be completed immediately on admission and every 15 to 30 minutes thereafter (refer to Chapter 17). Interpretation of neurological abnormalities in a critically injured trauma patient with a substance abuse history can be difficult, and the process can extend beyond the resuscitation cycle. Data collection continues through the perioperative and critical care cycles. Continuity of expert nursing care is dependent on efficient communication and accurate documentation.

PERIOPERATIVE CYCLE

The drug-dependent trauma patient presents unique problems during the perioperative cycle of care. Difficult clinical decisions must be made that involve the choice of an appropriate anesthetic agent, the management of hematological alterations, and the prevention of detoxification.

Medical Management

Anesthesia Considerations

An understanding of anesthetic pharmacology is important to prevent a variety of drug interactions that may occur in the traumatized substance abuse patient. Drugs will alter the amount of inhalant anesthetic needed to achieve the desired pharmacological end point. Several agents (e.g., diazepam, opiates, pentazocine, meperidine, morphine) have been shown to increase the potency of anesthetic vapors.[136, 137]

When used alone, nitrous oxide has apparent sympathomimetic activity that is due to elevated catecholamine concentrations.[138] The major mechanism of action for most CNS stimulants is to block the reuptake of catecholamines from the synapse, thereby inducing a sympathomimetic effect. The effects of drug combinations (i.e., a cocaine abuser who receives nitrous oxide) may potentially be addictive or synergistic. Although not documented conclusively, this combination may lead to increases in cardiac output, mean arterial pressure, and mean pulmonary artery pressure. Conversely, nitrous oxide used in the presence of narcotics may produce a decrease in cardiac output and an increase in systemic vascular resistance.[139]

The halogenated anesthetics (halothane, enflurane, isoflurane) have been reported to decrease systemic vascular resistance.[140] The pulse increases following enflurane and isoflurane use but tends to remain constant or decrease with halothane.[141] The final cardiovascular response observed is determined by the patient's preoperative autonomic tone. Patients with an increased sympathetic baseline (i.e., CNS stimulant users) may manifest the largest decrease in blood pressure and cardiac output.

Hematological Considerations

The altered hematological system may leave the patient at risk for tissue hypoxia, thromboembolism, and cardiac failure.[86] Care of the patient is dependent on the degree to which hemostasis is affected. Potential complications must be recognized early so that appropriate measures can be taken (refer to earlier discussion).

During the perioperative cycle, the physician may elect to administer vitamin K or to transfuse platelets, fibrinogen, or fresh frozen plasma in addition to transfusing blood.

Preventing Detoxification

During long intraoperative procedures, the potential for drug withdrawal exists. This is especially true for the drug-dependent trauma patient who abuses short-acting agents such as heroin. Abstinence syndromes are delayed with some agents, such as ethanol. Identification and treatment of withdrawal syndromes must be accomplished as soon as possible. (Refer to more in-depth discussion in "Critical Care Cycle.")

CRITICAL CARE CYCLE

The team approach during this part of the trauma patient's recovery centers on continued stabilization of body systems and management of the complications that may arise as a result of ethanol or drug abuse. Respiratory or cardiovascular disturbances remain a constant threat. Because of the special problems associated with withdrawal, efforts are directed toward prevention, differentiation, and treatment of any withdrawal syndrome.

Withdrawal Syndromes

A key component in critical care assessment is the recognition of a previous ethanol or drug abuse problem. It is

TABLE 30–8. SYSTEMATIC APPROACH FOR THE DIFFERENTIAL DIAGNOSIS OF WITHDRAWAL IN TRAUMA PATIENTS

Validate drug history with patient or family
Rule out hypoxia and pulmonary emboli
Rule out intracranial pathological processes
Rule out electrolyte imbalances
Rule out sepsis
Rule out medication/blood interactions
Rule out sleep deprivation
Rule out ICU psychosis or acute schizophrenia

possible for the trauma patient to progress through resuscitation and initial management without being diagnosed as a substance abuser. Previous data, i.e., the health history and toxicology screen reports, are reviewed and validated with the patient and/or family members. Subtle clues such as unusual coping patterns, altered pain tolerance, and frequency of narcotic or sedative requests may suggest a substance abuse history. In some cases, however, a valid diagnosis may not be made until the patient actively presents symptoms that are consistent with a withdrawal syndrome.

Differential Diagnosis

A systematic approach facilitates the diagnosis process and is summarized in Table 30–8. The patient who exhibits signs of agitation, restlessness, tachycardia, and confusion is carefully assessed for potential withdrawal. However, the diagnosis is complicated by the many potential problems in the trauma population that can mimic a withdrawal syndrome. Hypoxia, pulmonary emboli, primary intracranial or psychiatric disorder, sepsis, medication or blood transfusion reactions, and sleep deprivation must all be considered and excluded. Fluid and electrolyte imbalances, particularly hypokalemia and magnesium depletion, can cause symptoms that mimic a withdrawal syndrome. Close evaluation of laboratory trends is essential.

Assessment of Alcohol Withdrawal Syndrome (AWS)

Although the symptoms and time frame for development of AWS display individual variation, there is considerable consistency and a progressive order to the clinical picture of ethanol withdrawal. The severity of the syndrome is directly proportional to the length and extent of the trauma patient's drinking pattern, but the development of symptoms is not necessarily dependent on cessation of alcohol intake.[142] Sudden withdrawal even after fewer than 30 days of regular ethanol use can result in anxiety, agitation, tremors, seizures, and hallucinations. Cessation from any alcoholic beverage, including beer and wine, can cause the syndrome. Many times, an event beyond the patient's control, such as a traumatic accident, precipitates the syndrome.[143]

The sequence of AWS development is described in stages (Table 30–9). The patient in stage 1 is anxious and has mild tremors. This patient may be hyperreflexic as well. In stage 2, some patients exhibit mild disorders of perception, whereas others have frank hallucinations. The patient is usually very difficult to control and may require physical restraints. These patients may be diaphoretic and incontinent.

TABLE 30–9. STAGES OF THE ALCOHOL WITHDRAWAL SYNDROME

STAGE	ONSET	CLINICAL MANIFESTATIONS
1	Approximately 8 hours after cessation or reduction in drinking (e.g., overnight abstinence)	Mild tremulousness, nervousness, nausea, tachycardia, hypertension
2	Approximately 24 hours; occasionally up to 8 days	Marked tremors, hyperactivity, insomnia; some patients have nightmares, illusions, or hallucinations
3	From 12–48 hours	Same as stage 2, only more marked; distinguishing feature: grand mal seizures, often multiple
4	Usually 3–5 days, sometimes up to 12 days	Delirium tremens includes severe autonomic hyperactivity, global confusion, hypertension, increased temperature, and diaphoresis

Adapted from Behnke RH: Recognition and management of alcohol withdrawal syndrome. Hosp Pract November:79–84, 1979.

The autonomic hyperactivity of stage 1 continues through stage 3 and becomes more pronounced. Classic grand mal seizures, the hallmark symptom, can occur. If untreated, 30 to 40 per cent of these patients go on to develop delirium tremens (DTs).

Delirium tremens is the most dramatic and serious manifestation of the alcohol withdrawal syndrome. The clinical picture is impressive with its profound disorientation and perception disorders. The patient has gross motor tremors and suffers from extreme restlessness. A 15 per cent mortality rate exists for patients who develop DTs,[144] and although lower mortality rates have been reported, these may reflect milder forms of withdrawal. In most fatalities associated with delirium tremens, there is an associated infection or injury. However, other deaths are related to hyperthermia or peripheral circulatory collapse.

The cause of AWS remains controversial. The signs and symptoms of AWS appear over a wide and variable time course, suggesting that several pathophysiological mechanisms underlie their development[145] (Table 30–10). Neural hyperexcitability is a predominant symptom, particularly in early withdrawal.

Two consistent biochemical changes occur with ethanol withdrawal: fluctuations in the respiratory center sensitivity to CO_2 and marked depression of serum magnesium levels.

TABLE 30–10. PROPOSED PATHOPHYSIOLOGICAL MECHANISMS OF ALCOHOL WITHDRAWAL

Unopposed compensatory mechanisms
Respiratory alkalosis and hypomagnesemia
Hypokalemia
Prostaglandin E (PGE_1)/zinc deficiency

Adapted from Brown CG: The alcohol withdrawal syndrome. Ann Emerg Med 11:276–280, 1982.

The patient may hyperventilate early in the phases of withdrawal, leading to a respiratory alkalosis and a propensity for generalized seizures. Exactly how hypomagnesemia occurs in AWS is unknown. The alkalosis and hypomagnesemia are usually resolved spontaneously within 18 to 48 hours.

Treatment. Treatment modes and therapies for AWS vary. Early treatment of patients with drugs that are cross-tolerant with ethanol decreases the frequency of both seizures and the DTs. The two most common pharmacological interventions are benzodiazepines and ethanol. Both intravenous and oral ethanol can be used in prophylaxis or in treatment of withdrawal. Appendices 30–1 and 30–2 provide suggested guidelines for nursing administration of ethanol.

Bias against the therapeutic use of ethanol does exist, however, and arises primarily from earlier misconceptions of its role in metabolism. Its use in the treatment of patients with alcoholism, therefore, is not always supported because of concern for possible toxic effects. Gower and Kersten[146] indicate that the need of the alcoholic addict cannot be satisfied by sedative drugs. Readaptation of the patient's metabolism during abstinence from ethanol is variable but is usually completed within 10 days. Withdrawal symptoms can be prevented by providing small amounts of ethanol at a rate that is insufficient to cause measurable blood alcohol levels.[147]

If ethanol administration is considered appropriate, it is ordered either orally or intravenously for a 10-day period. Ethanol should be used cautiously in patients with potential gastroduodenitis, pancreatitis, or known end-stage liver disease.

If ethanol prophylaxis is contraindicated, the use of benzodiazepines is suggested (Table 30–11). The effects of benzodiazepines for the prevention of AWS are considered superior to those obtained from other agents. Benzodiazepines tend to be more effective than phenothiazines in preventing seizure activity. They also cause less drowsiness than barbiturates and are less toxic. In addition, benzodiazepines do not induce hepatic microsomal enzymes or produce substantial changes in coagulation parameters. There is also a marked reduction in anxiety, tremors, and agitation without significant respiratory depression or stupor. Phenothiazines, on the other hand, adversely affect thermoregulation and thus may potentiate hyperthermia. Use of these agents also can result in profound hypotension.

More important than the choice of a particular therapeutic agent is its early initiation to prevent the occurrence or progression of detrimental withdrawal effects. Since alcohol may interfere with the absorption of water and a number of nutrients, including folic acid, amino acids, vitamins (B_{12}, thiamine), potassium, phosphorus, magnesium, and glucose, supportive therapy also must include adequate hydration, vitamin supplements, potassium and magnesium replacement, and other nutrient support.[148]

Assessment of Opiate Withdrawal

Opiate withdrawal is seldom life-threatening in a normal, healthy individual. However, the traumatized patient may be unable to tolerate the additional stress of opiate withdrawal. Therefore, it is recommended that patients who are physically dependent on opiates be maintained on the drug until the acute illness is over.

Symptoms of withdrawal from various types of opiates are similar. The time frame and intensity of withdrawal symp-

TABLE 30–11. BENZODIAZEPINES

DRUG	FACTORS INFLUENCING DRUG USE
Diazepam	Active metabolite Incompletely and slowly absorbed from IM injections; should be given PO or IV The *total body clearance* is *inversely proportional* to the *age* and directly proportional to liver function. The half-life of diazepam in hours is approximately equal to the *patient's* age.
Chlordiazepoxide	Long-acting drug with active metabolites The smallest effective dose should be used to avoid oversedation in geriatric or debilitated patients. Usual dose is 5–10 mg 3 or 4 times daily. Manufacturers state that in acute alcohol withdrawal, dosage should not exceed 300 mg daily.
Lorazepam	Short-acting agent Half-life of 5 to 20 hours; peaks more slowly, 2–4 hours No active metabolites Less dependent on hepatic function, only glucuronidation
Oxazepam	No active metabolite Only oral route For severe agitation, 15–30 mg given 3–4 times daily Dosage should be individualized, especially in geriatric patients and those with low serum albumin.
Flurazepam	Administered at bedtime Usual dose is 15–30 mg
Clorazepate	Active metabolite Peaks quickly 30 mg may be necessary initially, followed by an additional 30–60 mg in divided doses on day 1; the maximum daily recommended dose is 40 mg; on day 2, 45–90 mg of clorazepate is given in divided doses; 22–45 mg in divided doses on day 3; 15–30 mg in divided doses on day 4; thereafter, daily doses are periodically reduced to 7.5–15 mg.
Temazepam	Administered orally at bedtime No active metabolites Usual dose 15–30 mg in the elderly

toms are related to the duration of drug action.[90] Short-acting agents (morphine, heroin, meperidine) have a brief, more intense abstinence syndrome, whereas long-acting agents (methadone) have a prolonged, milder withdrawal syndrome. The first signs of withdrawal begin 4 to 6 hours after the last dose of short-acting opiates. Patients appear anxious and express a craving for the drug. Six to 12 hours after the last dose, rhinorrhea, lacrimation, diaphoresis, and yawning may be present. Twelve to 14 hours after the last dose, these symptoms intensify. Shaking chills, restlessness, irritability, anorexia, dilated pupils, and pilomotor erection (goose flesh) may occur. The syndrome of opiate withdrawal peaks in 48 to 72 hours after the last dose. At this time, symptoms increase and the patient may develop nausea, vomiting, diarrhea, central nervous system hyperactivity, muscle spasms with kicking movements, pain, tachycardia, and an elevated blood pressure. Cardiovascular collapse is a major concern during this phase of withdrawal.

Treatment. Opiate withdrawal is abated at any time during the course of withdrawal by the administration of a narcotic agent. Methadone is frequently recommended but should not be administered until the first signs of withdrawal are present.[149] The patient is monitored closely, since the onset of oral methadone action may be delayed up to 2 to 4 hours. If the symptoms have not improved following methadone administration, a short-acting agent (e.g., morphine) also may be given to treat withdrawal until the methadone effects begin. Methadone dosage can be prescribed using a graded opiate withdrawal scale. Fultz and Senay grade withdrawal on a scale of 1 (lacrimation, rhinorrhea, diaphoresis, yawning, restlessness, insomnia) to 4 (diarrhea, vomiting, dehydration, hyperglycemia, hypotension, curled-up position).[149] Grade 1 requires 5 mg of methadone as an initial dose, whereas grade 4 requires 20 mg (Table 30–12).

Pain-Management Considerations. Traumatized opiate abusers frequently require analgesia. These individuals fall into two groups: patients currently receiving methadone maintenance and opiate abusers not on methadone maintenance. Within 12 hours of hospitalization, it is readily apparent which patients in the latter group will require methadone therapy. The pain-management techniques for both groups of patients are similar.[149] Initially, the patient's pain should be treated with normal doses of a short-acting narcotic agent (e.g., hydromorphone, morphine). Those patients on methadone should continue to receive their normal daily dose of methadone in addition to the pain medication. Because of the tolerance present in patients who have previously received methadone, the duration of analgesic effect is short. Therefore, more frequent dosing may be necessary in these patients. Narcotic agonist–antagonists (e.g., pentazocine, butorphanol, nalbuphine, nalorphine, levallorphan) are not used in analgesic therapy, since such agents may potentiate withdrawal symptoms.

TABLE 30–12. RELATIONSHIP BETWEEN SIGNS AND SYMPTOMS OF OPIATE WITHDRAWAL AND INITIAL METHADONE DOSE

	SIGNS AND SYMPTOMS	INITIAL METHADONE DOSE
Grade 1	Lacrimation, rhinorrhea, diaphoresis, yawning, restlessness, and insomnia	5 mg
Grade 2	Dilated pupils, piloerection, muscle twitching, myalgia, arthralgia, and abdominal pain	10 mg
Grade 3	Tachycardia, hypertension, tachypnea, fever, anorexia, nausea, and extreme restlessness	15 mg
Grade 4	Diarrhea, vomiting, dehydration, hyperglycemia, hypotension, and curled-up position	20 mg

From Guidelines for the management of hospitalized narcotic addicts. Ann Intern Med 18:816, 1975.

Assessment of Sedative–Hypnotic Withdrawal

Abstinence symptoms generally begin within 24 hours after the last dose of a sedative–hypnotic agent.[90] The patient experiences insomnia, anxiety, twitching, tremors, weakness, and orthostatic hypotension. Major symptoms generally appear on days 2 or 3 and may last 3 to 14 days. Central nervous system manifestations consist of a wide spectrum of findings ranging from agitation and disorientation to hallucinations, tonic–clonic seizures, or status epilepticus. Death may occur from sedative–hypnotic withdrawal.

Treatment. Treatment of sedative–hypnotic withdrawal centers on the administration of another sedative–hypnotic agent to minimize or prevent the withdrawal symptoms. Regardless of the agent being abused (i.e., chloral hydrate, meprobamate, ethchlorvynol), it is generally recommended that the withdrawal syndrome be treated with a barbiturate. There are several possible methods for patient stabilization and drug tapering. Wikler recommends administration of pentobarbital (200 to 400 mg every 4 to 6 hours) to eliminate withdrawal signs and symptoms.[150] After 48 to 72 hours of a stable dose, the pentobarbital is slowly tapered. Smith and Wesson[151] recommend using phenobarbital at a dose related to the amount of drug previously consumed by the patient. Thirty milligrams of phenobarbital are given for each of the following: 100 mg of secobarbital or pentobarbital, 400 mg of meprobamate, 250 mg of chloral hydrate, 200 mg of ethchlorvynol, or 125 mg of glutethimide. Care should be taken in the use of this conversion method, since the history provided by drug abuse patients is frequently inaccurate.

Regardless of the method used, the barbiturate should be administered until the signs and symptoms of withdrawal dissipate, while the patient is constantly monitored for undesirable oversedation. As with narcotics, the patient should be maintained on the barbiturate until the acute injuries have resolved. Once the patient has been stabilized, the barbiturate should be gradually tapered (i.e., decreased by 10 per cent per day over a 10-day period). As the dose is being tapered, the patient should be monitored for signs of withdrawal indicating that the tapering process has been too rapid. In these circumstances, the dose of barbiturate is increased and later decreased at a slower rate.

Assessment of CNS Stimulant Withdrawal

Although CNS stimulants do not induce physical dependence to a degree comparable to narcotics and sedatives, withdrawal is not symptom-free. Hypersomnia occurs for the first few days. Depression, fatigue, and apathy are typical and may persist for weeks or months, depending in part on the extent of drug abuse preceding withdrawal. These symptoms may reflect the unmasking of an underlying exhaustion resulting from chronic overstimulation. Relief is often sought through renewed use of stimulants.

Discontinuation of prolonged episodic heavy cocaine use, referred to as "binges," results in a clinical syndrome called the *postcocaine crash*. The postcocaine crash is separated into three phases[152] (Fig. 30–4). Phase 1 begins within a few minutes of the last dose and is characterized by depression, agitation, and insomnia. These early symptoms, coupled with the high degree of craving for more cocaine, perpetuate the binge as long as cocaine supplies are available. Phase 1 may last from 9 hours to 4 days, with the latter stage of phase 1 characterized by exhaustion, hypersomnolence, and hyperphagia.

Phase 2 is the acute withdrawal phase, which may last 1 to 10 weeks. Although initially manifesting normal affective function, anxiety, dysphoria, and a high degree of cocaine craving rapidly ensue over a period of 1 to 5 days. Once again, the patient is prone to relapse and may begin a new binge cycle.[153]

Phase 3 is characterized by certain conditioned cues triggering intense cocaine cravings with the risk of relapse. Cues vary among individuals but may consist of environmental cues (places associated with using or buying cocaine) or emotional cues (seeing cocaine-using friends). If the patient is able to avoid the use of cocaine with each craving, the possibility of long-lasting abstinence improves.[153]

TREATMENT. Treatment of stimulant withdrawal generally focuses on symptoms, since the major acute syndrome tends to dissipate on its own within 1 to 3 days. Senay and Lewis[154] observed that many cases of stimulant withdrawal are resolved after a deep sleep period, which may be 24 to 48 hours. If symptoms of depression, sleep disturbances, suspiciousness, or hostility appear, the treatment is designed to restore biological health. Sedatives that do not produce dependence may be prescribed for nighttime use until a normal sleep cycle is restored. Vitamin-fortified diets are recommended. Major tranquilizers should be used only if a psychosis persists. Similarly, antidepressants should be used cautiously during the first weeks of treatment, since residual blood levels of stimulants cause an undesirable interaction between the two classes of drugs.

Cannabis *Withdrawal*

Withdrawal phenomena are not seen after discontinuation of psychogenic drug use. Interruption of regular use of *Cannabis* can lead to irritability, sleeping difficulties, and nausea.[106, 107] These symptoms are generally mild and subside rapidly without treatment. Psychological support with drug abuse education is suggested.

Nursing Management Considerations

The focus of nursing care is on identification of the withdrawal syndrome and initiation of appropriate treatment. Vital signs, neurological status, autonomic responses, and psychological stability are constantly monitored. If symptoms appear or if the patient has a known substance abuse history, the physician is consulted for medication orders.

The patient may need continual reassurance about his condition and reorientation to the environment. All sources of unnecessary stimuli at the bedside are avoided, and

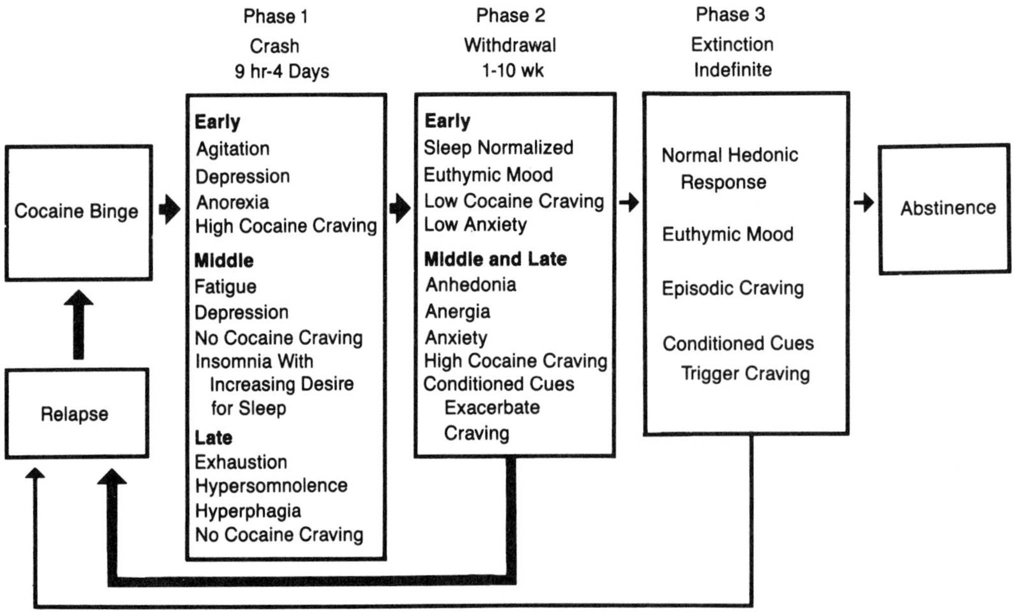

Figure 30–4. Duration and intensity of symptoms vary based on binge characteristics and diagnosis. Binges range from under 4 hours duration to 6 or more days. High cocaine craving early in phase 1 continues for up to 20 hours, but usually lasts less than 6, and is followed by period of noncraving with similar duration in next subphase (middle-phase 1). Substantial craving then returns only after lag of up to 5 or more days, during phase 2. (From Gawin F, Kleber H: Abstinence symptomatology and psychiatric diagnosis in cocaine abusers: Clinical observations. Arch Gen Psychiatry 43:110, 1986.)

patient/staff interactions should be calm, quiet, and controlled. The patient may need protection from self-harm and require physical restraints. Seizure precautions, such as padded side rails and immediately available suction and airway equipment, are instituted as needed.

The patient who presents with withdrawal symptoms requires intravenous access and an indwelling Foley catheter. Accurate intake and output records are essential because many of these patients have potential fluid and electrolyte alterations. Overhydration or dehydration from ethanol-related fluid losses must be identified and corrected.

Alterations in Nutritional Status Related to Dietary Deficiencies Secondary to Ethanol or Drug Abuse

Alterations in nutritional status are common in trauma patients with substance abuse problems. Nutritional management in these patients may be complicated by the extent of preexisting nutritional deficiencies and hepatic dysfunction. Support may include total or partial parenteral nutrition, enteral alimentation, or a combination of these therapies. The reader is referred to Chapter 14 for a detailed discussion of nutritional assessment and management. Electrolyte imbalances and vitamin deficiencies should be corrected to prevent poor wound healing and to improve hemopoietic processes.

Potential for Infection

Respiratory and wound infections are of special concern in this patient population. The patient should be monitored closely for signs of inflammation and infection. Respiratory care is particularly a priority and should include chest physiotherapy, daily chest radiographs, and periodic cultures of tracheal aspirate or sputum. Wounds are carefully examined to assess the healing process. Strict aseptic technique is always required for invasive procedures and dressing changes.

Role of the Alcohol and Drug Counselor

As the patient is stabilized and becomes increasingly awake and alert, support from the alcohol/drug counselor should be requested. Education about substance abuse and its relationship to the traumatic injury and recovery must be initiated early in the patient's hospital course. Although policy varies from institution to institution, any patient with an elevated blood alcohol concentration (i.e., greater than 80 mg/dl) or positive toxicology screen should be interviewed and evaluated by the substance abuse counselor. Recommendations are then incorporated into the nursing plan of care.

The role of the counselor as part of the clinical management for these patients is vital. Even patients who are intubated or receiving mechanical ventilation can be interviewed and the teaching process begun. The counselor may choose to coordinate a conference with the patient, the primary nurse, and the family. Possible interventions include (1) confronting the patient about the admission toxicology results, (2) explaining the consequences of ethanol or drug abuse, (3) offering educational support, (4) initiating follow-up visits, and (5) planning for therapy in a residential treatment center on discharge.

INTERMEDIATE CARE/ REHABILITATION CYCLE

Nursing care during this phase of the trauma patient's hospitalization continues to focus on the assessment of resolving system alterations in relationship to the substance abuse history and the prevention of complications. The effectiveness of current therapeutic interventions must be evaluated and modified as needed. In addition, independent functioning and compliance with the treatment regimen are assessed in conjunction with patient and family coping abilities as plans for discharge are developed.

Patient/Family Conferences

During this phase of the patient's recovery, the patient and family members should become actively involved in the discharge planning process, which is facilitated through scheduled patient/family conferences. These conferences provide a forum for the trauma team to share information regarding the patient's injuries, rehabilitation potentials, and the status of the substance abuse habit as it relates to the patient's current well-being. It also provides the opportunity for the patient and family to ask questions, to express concerns, and to tap the resources that are available for trauma rehabilitation as well as for drug rehabilitation.

As the patient and family adapt to the aftermath of traumatic injury, they need to become knowledgeable about the physical, psychological, emotional, and social ramifications of the substance abuse behavior. The continued involvement of an alcohol/drug counselor is essential as the patient and family come face-to-face with the reality of the substance abuse problem and are encouraged to make decisions that will lead toward a more healthful outcome for all involved.

As mentioned previously, the patient and family are told as soon as possible of the blood alcohol level or positive toxicology screen results from the day of admission. If the patient's critical condition prevented this from occurring earlier, this information should now be shared to assist the patient in understanding the significance of his drinking or drug use as it relates to the traumatic injury.

If the trauma patient had an elevated blood alcohol level on admission, it is helpful to correlate the blood alcohol level with the approximate amount of alcohol consumed. The patient can thereby better relate to the laboratory results. This correlation should initially be done with the patient in private. The patient is often unwilling to discuss the issue openly at this time. During subsequent conferences, however, the primary nurse and alcohol/drug counselor may succeed in encouraging the patient to participate in conversations pertaining to the substance abuse topic. A referral for psychiatric consultation may be appropriate for patients who are unwilling to participate in these discussions or who display behaviors that are characteristic of personality disorders (refer to Chapter 29).

The patient/family teaching that occurs should include information about the physiological effects of the ethanol or drug use and resultant complications that occurred during the patient's clinical course. The patient and family should be informed of the medical treatments incorporated to prevent or to treat withdrawal. Information about the patient's nutritional status also should be shared. Liver function deficits and respiratory, cardiovascular, and gastrointestinal disorders should be explained as well as how such conditions relate to the substance abuse habit.

Nursing Management Considerations

Potential for Continued Nutritional Deficit Related to Poor Dietary Habits and Loss of Appetite Secondary to Ethanol/Drug Abuse

The nurse continues to assess eating habits and determine caloric intake as postdischarge dietary considerations are addressed. The nutritional management of each substance abuse patient should be individualized. Careful attention must be given to food preferences and dislikes, since basic changes in lifelong eating habits rarely occur. The patient should understand the basis for the dietary regimen as it relates to the substance abuse history and gain an appreciation for the role of good dietary habits in expediting healing processes and in improving overall health. Support from a dietary counselor is often helpful in developing creative alternatives for patients who experience a loss of appetite secondary to substance abuse.

Potential for Anxiety and Guilt Secondary to Consequences of Ethanol or Drug Abuse

A supportive, therapeutic environment must be maintained for the patient to stimulate expression of feelings. During scheduled conferences, constructive guidance should be offered so that the patient can identify effective and ineffective personal coping patterns. The patient should be encouraged to redirect the feelings of anxiety and guilt into a positive energy that can better be utilized for rehabilitative activities and planning for discharge. Referrals should be made to psychiatric consultants, alcohol/drug counselors, and social services as needed.

Diminished Self-Esteem Related to Alcoholism or Drug Abuse

The nurse should acknowledge the patient's value as an individual by providing choices and permitting involvement in decision making regarding care needs. An atmosphere of acceptance should be created by listening to the patient's concerns. It is important to build on strengths and resources that the patient can utilize in recovering from alcoholism. Pride can be fostered by identifying the patient's courageous efforts in recuperating from the traumatic injuries. Daily progress should be acknowledged, and possibilities for long-term recovery should be emphasized.

The nurse should always be alert for teaching opportunities. Emotional appeals to halt drinking or drug use habits should be avoided, however. Patients will rarely respond positively to this approach. Rather, the nurse who displays a nonjudgmental attitude regarding the patient's substance abuse habits while appearing knowledgeable about alcohol/drug-related issues may gain the patient's trust. Helping the patient to identify the negative physiological, psychological, emotional, and social consequences of his substance abuse behavior is often the most effective approach in stimulating the initiation of subsequent behavior modifications. A more positive self-image may, therefore, begin to emerge.

Providing written information about Alcoholics Anonymous (AA) and other substance abuse programs may stimulate motivational efforts on the part of the patient to prepare for discharge. An awareness of such programs provides the patient with supportive alternatives and perhaps a more hopeful attitude. The patient should be encouraged to speak with the alcohol/drug counselor or psychiatric consultant for detailed information as needed.

COMMUNITY REINTEGRATION

Trauma patients with a history of substance abuse present a particularly unique challenge to the health care professionals with whom they will interact during the community reintegration process. The issues that must be faced by the patient during this cycle include those that relate to the physical limitations that are imposed as well as the psychological and emotional adjustments that take place following traumatic injury (refer to Chapter 10). In addition, the trauma patient's preexisting substance abuse habits and the intricate social networks and relationship patterns that precipitated and fostered the substance abuse behavior must be acknowledged and addressed. The role that ethanol and drugs play in the development and maintenance of family, social, and work relationships is paramount and presents an additional dimension to the complexities of therapeutic endeavors. The patient's reintegration into the community becomes a difficult task not only for the patient but for the family as well.

Substance Abuse and the Family

Alcoholism and drug abuse are conceptualized as a symptom of family or social unit dysfunction.[155] Forming the basis for this thinking is the assumption that significant people within the family structure contribute to the way that individual family members function in relation to each other and, therefore, to the way that the symptom emerges (refer to Chapter 11). Excessive drinking or drug use by an individual tends to occur when family or social group anxiety is high, which can, in turn, cause even higher anxiety levels among group members. The process of drinking or abusing drugs that is stimulated by spiraling anxiety levels can lead to a functional collapse of primary relationships or to the development of a chronic pattern.

A majority of substance abusers remain closely tied to their families, and their behavior remains functionally related to the emotional processes that occur within the family structure. There is, for example, a tendency for an adult substance abuser to continue to live with parents.[156] The family is viewed as a central component in the development and maintenance of a drug abuse problem owing primarily to a strong emotional interconnectedness. Viewed within the context of the family structure, the substance abuser plays an integral part in the malfunctioning of the family system.

Noone[156] suggests that

1. The abuse of ethanol and other drugs by an individual is directly related to the emotional processes of that individual's family.

2. Change in substance abuse behavior is generally indicative of changes in the family emotional process.
3. Substance abuse serves as an adaptive mechanism for the individual and family.
4. The presenting problem of substance abuse is generally indicative of the family's protective process.
5. Substance abuse generally serves as a distancing mechanism in response to the anxiety generated by increased fusion (as in marriage).
6. Substance abuse is generally seen in highly cohesive families, which have traditionally utilized intrapsychic distancing mechanisms.
7. A decrease in chronic substance abuse behavior by an individual will be disruptive to a family's equilibrium and result in increased anxiety within the family.

The chronic substance abuser often maintains a stabilizing function in one or more important family triangles (with mother–father or mother–grandmother, for example). The decision to halt the use of drugs is a threat to the functional structure, and the anxiety experienced will be related to the degree to which the drug abuse serves as a stabilizing factor.[157] If the abuse of drugs or ethanol has been temporary and in response to an acute upset in a family's equilibrium, the cessation of drug use will not be met with resistance and may even be accompanied by relief on the part of the family. However, a move toward the cessation of chemical dependence on the part of an individual who has been abusing drugs for a lengthy period will be met with some resistance from family members, who may view this process as a mechanism to facilitate increased autonomy.

Observing a family's response to an individual's cessation of chronic drug use provides the nurse with a clearer understanding of the importance of behavioral adaptive mechanisms that are employed by the patient and family members.

Community Support Systems

Proper management of the detoxified patient who expresses some motivation for continued treatment is extremely important to the overall community reintegration process. Motivation can wane and the patient's attitude toward further substance abuse treatment may become more ambivalent if active therapeutic interventions are not maintained. The continued involvement of the alcohol/drug counselor is, therefore, essential. In addition to providing psychosocial support, the counselor can provide the link between the patient/family and available community substance abuse services.

Numerous therapeutic communities and inpatient residential substance abuse treatment centers exist.[158] Therapeutic aftercare programs, including quarterway houses and halfway houses, aim to provide residential supervision and structure. Such an atmosphere allows the patient to initiate behavioral and cognitive changes by practicing assertiveness and problem-solving skills. In-house programs vary in length (from 30 days to 1 year) and may provide follow-up outpatient services after discharge.

Other support systems exist for the substance abuser, family member, and/or significant others, such as Alcoholics Anonymous, Narcotics Anonymous, and Al-Anon.[159, 160] These programs help participants to develop confrontational skills while providing a supportive environment that facilitates the resocialization process. Individual and group counseling are other therapeutic options that can be explored by the substance abuser and/or family members.

Nursing Management Considerations

Potential for Continued Lack of Control Over One's Life Related to Unresolved Dependence on Drugs or Ethanol

Helping the substance abuser to recognize and accept the problem becomes a challenging task. It involves measures that will prepare the individual to make a commitment to change—a change that involves the abandonment of a powerful reinforcer.

If the patient continues to deny the substance abuse problem, an assertive and persistent communication style is essential, yet the integrity of the patient's self-esteem must be supported. The patient may need time to cope with the fear of rehabilitation from drugs or ethanol. Appropriate referral services should be utilized as needed; alcohol or drug counseling should be offered routinely. Realistic goal-directed encouragement must be offered by the nurse, who serves as a source of continuing positive reinforcement.

FUTURE TRENDS IN SUBSTANCE USE AND ABUSE AND THE IMPACT ON TRAUMA

An attempt to predict future trends in drug or ethanol abuse based on the incomplete data that are available is merely speculative. Although current trends can provide some insight, future trends will depend on a number of factors, including public awareness, values clarification, and legislative action. In addition, the outcome of clinical research endeavors will continue to affect future treatment modalities.

Prevention

An ever-increasing number of people are reacting strongly to the consequences of drunk driving. Citizen action groups, such as Mothers Against Drunk Driving (MADD), Remove Intoxicated Drivers (RID), and Students Against Driving Drunk (SADD), have increased the public's awareness and have prompted legislative action on the local, state, and federal levels. The widespread social and health problems created by substance abuse are the focus of a number of governmental initiatives.[161] Relying heavily on integrated and cooperative efforts of federal, state, and local governments, as well as the close involvement of the private sector, the Federal Strategy for the Prevention of Drug Abuse and Trafficking sets the tone for the government's overall efforts to reduce drug abuse.[162]

Minimum drinking age laws and driving while intoxicated (DWI) laws are examples of prevention strategies targeted at the state level. In addition, trauma-prevention programs, educational programs that bring adolescents face-to-face with the risks and consequences of drinking and driving, have been developed.[163]

Future Research Endeavors

Individuals who are involved in ethanol- and/or drug-related accidents represent a unique study group from which valuable data can be derived. More thorough retrospective investigations need to be conducted[164] and may provide the answers to such questions as what types of individuals are at highest risk for accidental injury, and what predictor factors exist. Other potential research endeavors may arise from the field of behavioral genetics. Further studies that examine the relationship between heredity and substance abuse are necessary. The effects of various substances on aggressiveness and risk-taking behaviors is another area worthy of attention.

Information is also needed that will elucidate the reaction of various injured organ systems to ethanol. The role of psychoactive substances, either alone or in combination, on injury severity score results also requires further delineation.

More clinical research focusing on the treatment of withdrawal in hospitalized ethanol abusers following trauma is warranted as well. The use of ethanol (oral or IV) needs to be further evaluated. No study has clearly demonstrated the relationship of infusion rates to toxicity and blood levels of alcohol. In addition, the amount of alcohol necessary to prevent withdrawal is not known and may, in fact, be less than the amount routinely prescribed.

Additional clinical management issues pertaining to the trauma patient with a history of substance abuse have been identified. How should pain be measured in a substance abuse patient? Are nursing interventions perceived as supportive by the patients and/or family? How does the team management plan affect long-term recovery outcomes? The effects of having an alcohol/drug counselor available in a trauma center and the nurse's collaborative efforts with the counselors to educate the trauma patient have been described.[165] This area warrants more research to identify and define beneficial results.

CONCLUSION

Health problems associated with alcoholism and drug abuse are of epidemic proportions in our society, and the nurse's contact with this unique patient population has increased. Nurses are challenged to develop creative and comprehensive management plans for the trauma patient with a history of substance abuse. This chapter has emphasized the need to develop specific nursing interventions that pertain not only to the care of the trauma patient but to the special care needs of the substance abuser as well.

REFERENCES

1. Secretary of Health and Human Services: Seventh Special Report to the U.S. Congress on Alcohol and Health. Rockville, MD, US Department of Health and Human Services, DHHS no 90-1656, January 1990.
2. National Research Council: Injury in America: A Continuing Public Health Problem. Washington, DC, National Academy Press, 1985.
3. Rice DP, MacKenzie EJ, Jones AS, et al: Cost of Injury in the United States: A Report to Congress. San Francisco, Institute for Health and Aging, University of California and Injury Prevention Center, Johns Hopkins University, 1989.
4. Centers for Disease Control: Estimated years of potential life lost before age 65 and cause-specific mortality, by cause of death: U.S., 1985. MMWR 36:447, 1987.
5. Centers for Disease Control: Alcohol-related mortality and years of potential life lost: United States, 1987. MMWR 39:173–178, 1990.
6. Whitfield RA, Zador P, Fife D: Projected mortality from injuries. Accid Anal Prev 17:367–371, 1985.
7. Secretary of Health and Human Services: Seventh Special Report to the US Congress on Alcohol and Health. Rockville, MD, US Department of Health and Human Services, DHHS no 90-1656, January 1990.
8. National Institute of Drug Abuse: National Household Survey on Drug Abuse: Population Estimates, 1988. Rockville, MD, NIDA, 1989.
9. Blum R: Contemporary threats to adolescent health in the United States. JAMA 257:3390, 1987.
10. Cregler LL, Mark H: Special report: Medical complications of cocaine abuse. N Engl J Med 315:1495–1500, 1986.
11. US Drug Enforcement Administration Yearly Reports. Jacksonville, FL, USDEA, 1988–1989.
12. Kamerow DB, Pincas HA, MacDonald DI: Alcohol abuse, other abuse, and mental disorders in medical practice. JAMA 255:2054, 1986.
13. National Committee for Injury Prevention and Control: Injury Prevention Meeting the Challenge. New York, Oxford University Press, 1989.
14. Smith GS, Kraus JF: Alcohol and residential, recreational, and occupational injuries: A review of the epidemiologic evidence. Annu Rev Public Health 9:99–121, 1988.
15. Soderstrom CA, Trifillis AL, Shankar BS, et al: Marijuana and alcohol use among 1023 trauma patients: A prospective study. Arch Surg 123:733–737, 1988.
16. Lindenbaum GA, Carroll SF, Daskal H, Kapusnick BS: Patterns of alcohol and drug abuse in an urban trauma center: The increasing role of cocaine abuse. J Trauma 29:1654–1657, 1989.
17. Rivara FP, Mueller BA, Fligner CL, et al: Drug use in trauma victims. J Trauma 29:462–470, 1989.
18. Sloan EP, Zalenski RJ, Smith RF, et al: Toxicology screening in urban trauma patients: Drug prevalence and its relationship to trauma severity and management. J Trauma 29:1647–1653, 1989.
19. Thal ER, Bost RO, Anderson RJ: Effects of alcohol and other drugs on traumatized patients. Arch Surg 120:708–712, 1985.
20. Ward RE, Flynn TC, Miller PW, Blaisdell WF: Effects of ethanol ingestion on the severity and outcome of trauma. Am J Surg 144:153–157, 1982.
21. National Highway Traffic Safety Administration: Fatal Accident Reporting System 1988: A Review of Information on Fatal Traffic Crashes in the United States in 1988. Washington, DC, US Department of Transportation, DOT HS 807 507, December 1989.
22. Council on Scientific Affairs, American Medical Association: Alcohol and the driver. JAMA 255:522–527, 1986.
23. Centers for Disease Control: Premature mortality due to alcohol-related motor vehicle traffic fatalities—United States, 1987. MMWR 37:753–755, 1988.
24. Arfken CL: Temporal pattern of alcohol consumption in the United States. Alcohol Clin Exp Res 12:137–142, 1988.
25. Anda RF, Williamson DF, Remington PL: Alcohol and fatal injuries among US adults: Findings from the NHANES I epidemiologic follow-up study. JAMA 260:2529–2532, 1988.
26. Popham RE, Schmidt W, Israelstam S: Heavy alcohol consumption and physical health problems: A review of epidemiologic evidence. In Smart RG, et al (eds): Research Advances in Alcohol and Drug Problems, vol 8. New York, Plenum Press, 1984, pp 149–182.

27. Centers for Disease Control: Underreporting of alcohol-related mortality on death certificates of young US Army veterans. MMWR 36:437–440, 1987.
28. Simel DL, Feussner JR: Blood alcohol measurements in the emergency: Who needs them? Am J Public Health 78:1478–1479, 1988.
29. Popkin CL, Kannenberg CH, Lacey JH, Waller PF: Assessment of Classification Instruments Designed to Detect Alcohol Abuse. Washington, DC, National Highway Traffic Safety Administration, Department of Transportation, DOT HS 807 475, December 1988.
30. Smart RG: Marijuana and driving risk among college students. J Safety Res 6:155, 1979.
31. Klonoff H: Marijuana and driving in real-life situations. Science 186:317–324, 1974.
32. Marzuk PM, Tordeff K, Leon AC, et al: Prevalence of recent cocaine use among motor-vehicle fatalities in New York City. JAMA 263:250, 1990.
33. Lindenbaum GA, Carrol SF, Daskal I, et al: Patterns of alcohol and drug abuse in an urban trauma center: The increasing role of cocaine use. J Trauma 29:1654, 1989.
34. Sloan EP, Zalenski RJ, Smith RJ, et al: Toxicology screening in urban trauma patient: Drug prevalence and its relationship to trauma severity and management. J Trauma 29:1647, 1989.
35. Goodwin DW: Is Alcoholism Hereditary? New York, Oxford University Press, 1976.
36. Goodwin DW: Drinking problems in adopted and nonadopted sons of alcoholics. Arch Gen Psychiatry 31:164, 1974.
37. Goodwin DW, Schulsinger F, Hermansen L, et al: Alcohol problems in adoptees raised apart from alcoholic biological parents. Arch Gen Psychiatry 28:238–243, 1973.
38. Annes HM: Patterns of intra-familial drug use. Br J Addict 69:361–369, 1974.
39. Brownell KD, Marlatt GA, Lechtenstein E, Wilson GT: Understanding and preventing relapse. Am Psychol 41:765–782, 1986.
40. Marlatt GA: Relapse prevention: Theoretical, rationale, and overview of the model. In Marlatt GA, Gordon JR (eds): Relapse Prevention: Maintenance Strategies in the Treatment of Addictive Behaviors. New York, Gilford Press, 1985.
41. Wilford BB: Drug Abuse: A Guide for the Primary Care Physician. Chicago, American Medical Association, 1981.
42. Von Wartburg JP: The metabolism of alcohol in normals and alcoholics: Enzymes. In Kissin B, Begleiter H (eds): The Biology of Alcoholism, vol 1: Biochemistry. New York, Plenum Press, 1971.
43. Hansten PD (ed): Drug Interactions, 4th ed. Philadelphia, Lea & Febiger, 1979.
44. Ritchie JM: The aliphatic alcohols. In Goodman LS, Gilman A (eds): The Pharmacological Basis of Therapeutics. New York, Macmillan, 1980.
45. Johnston RE, Reier CE: Acute respiratory effects of ethanol in man. Clin Pharmacol Ther 14:501–508, 1973.
46. Morland J, Setekleiv J, Haffner JFW, et al: Combined effects of diazepam and ethanol on mental and psychomotor functions. Acta Pharmacol Toxicol 34:5–8, 1974.
47. Rangno RE, Dumont CH, Sitar DS: Effect of ethanol ingestion on outcome of drug overdose. Crit Care Med 10:180–185, 1982.
48. Isbell H, Fraser HF, Wikler A, et al: An experimental study of the etiology of "rum fits" and delirium tremens. Q J Stud Alcohol 16:1–33, 1955.
49. Lindblad B, Olsson R: Unusually high levels of alcohol? JAMA 236:1600–1602, 1976.
50. Thompson WL: Management of alcohol withdrawal syndromes. Arch Intern Med 138:278–283, 1978.
51. Segel LD, Klausner SC, Gnadt JTH, et al: Alcohol and the heart. Med Clin North Am 68:147–161, 1984.
52. Gould L, Zahir M, DeMartino A, et al: Cardiac effects of a cocktail. JAMA 218:1799–1802, 1971.
53. Greenberg BH, Schutz R, Grunkemeir GL, et al: Acute effects of alcohol in patients with congestive heart failure. Ann Intern Med 97:171–175, 1982.
54. Ettinger PO, Wu CF, DeLacruz C, et al: Arrhythmias and the "holiday heart": Alcohol-associated cardiac rhythm disorders. Am Heart J 95:555–562, 1978.
55. Davenport HW: Ethanol damage to canine oxyntic glandular mucosa. Proc Exp Biol Med 126:657–662, 1967.
56. Kaufman SE, Kaye MD: Induction of gastroesophageal reflux by alcohol. Gut 19:336–338, 1978.
57. Tuyas AJ: Epidemiology of alcohol and cancer. Cancer Res 39:2840–2843, 1979.
58. Burbige EJ, Lewis R, Halsted CH: Alcohol and the gastrointestinal tract. Med Clin North Am 68:77–89, 1984.
59. Geokas MC, Lieber CS, French S, et al: Ethanol, the liver, and the gastrointestinal tract. Ann Intern Med 95:198–211, 1981.
60. Witt LG, Witt LD: Alcohol abuse. In Katcher BS, Young LY, Koda-Kimble MA (eds): Applied Therapeutics: The Clinical Use of Drugs, 3rd ed. Spokane, WA, Applied Therapeutics, 1983.
61. Traviesa DC: Magnesium deficiency: A possible cause of thiamine refractoriness in Wernicke-Korsakoff encephalopathy. J Neurol Neurosurg Psychiatry 37:959–962, 1974.
62. Thomson AD, Ryle PR, Shaw GK: Ethanol, thiamine, and brain damage. Alcohol 18:27–43, 1983.
63. Torvik A, Lindboe CF, Rogde S: Brain lesions in alcoholics. J Neurol Sci 56:233–248, 1982.
64. Nakada T, Knight RT: Alcohol and the central nervous system. Med Clin North Am 68:121–131, 1984.
65. Victor M: The Wernicke-Korsakoff syndrome. In Vinken PJ, Bruyn GW (eds): Handbook of Clinical Neurology. Amsterdam, Elsevier–North Holland Press, 1976.
66. McEntee WJ, Mair RG: Memory enhancement in Korsakoff's psychosis by clonidine: Further evidence for a nonadrenergic defect. Ann Neurol 7:466–470, 1980.
67. Burkhalter PK: Nursing Care of the Alcoholic and Drug Abuser. New York, McGraw-Hill, 1975.
68. Laurenzi G, Guarneri J: Study of the mechanics of resistance to infection: The relationship of bacterial clearance to ciliary and alveolar macrophage functions. Am Rev Respir Dis 93(suppl):134–141, 1965.
69. Greenhouse BS, Hook R, Hehre FW: Aspiration pneumonia following intravenous administration of alcohol during labor. JAMA 210:2393–2395, 1959.
70. Cameron L, Mitchell WH, Zuidema GD: Aspirational pneumonia: Clinical outcome following documented aspiration. Arch Surg 106:49–52, 1973.
71. Green G, Kass E: Factors influencing the clearance of bacteria by the lung. J Clin Invest 43:769–776, 1964.
72. Snell AM: Effects of chronic disease of liver on composition and physiochemical properties of blood: Changes in serum proteins; reduction in oxygen saturation of arterial blood. Ann Intern Med 9:690–711, 1935.
73. Tunahoski A, Kutty A, Prater S: Hypoxemia and cirrhosis of the liver. Thorax 31:303, 1976.
74. Ruff F, Hughes JMB, Stanley N, et al: Regional lung function in patients with hepatic cirrhosis. J Clin Invest 50:2403, 1971.
75. Arndt H, Buchta T, Schameras H: Analysis of factors determining resistance to diffusion in patients with liver cirrhosis. Respiration 32:21–31, 1975.
76. Hayes MF Jr, Rosenbaum RW, Zebelman M: Adult respiratory distress syndrome in association with acute pancreatitis. Am J Surg 127:314, 1974.
77. Interiana B, Stuard ID, Hyde RW: Acute respiratory distress syndrome in pancreatitis. Ann Intern Med 77:923, 1972.
78. Warshaw AL, Lesser PB, Rie M, et al: The pathogenesis of pulmonary edema in acute pancreatitis. Ann Surg 182:505, 1975.
79. Haut MJ, Cowan DH: The effect of ethanol on hemostatic properties of human blood platelets. Am J Med 56:22–33, 1974.
80. Hornbaker AE: Hematological disorders in the critically ill alcoholic. Crit Care Q 8:29–39, 1986.
81. Estes NJ, Heinemann ME: Alcoholism: Development, Consequences, Interventions, 2nd ed. St. Louis, CV Mosby, 1982.
82. Lindenbaum J: Tolate and vitamin B_{12} deficiency in alcoholism. Semin Hematol 17:119–125, 1980.

83. Lindenbaum J: Alcohol and the hematologic system. In Lieber CS (ed): Medical Disorders of Alcoholism: Pathogenesis and Treatment. Philadelphia, WB Saunders Co, 1982.
84. Coleman N, Herbert V: Hematologic complications of alcoholism: Overview. Semin Hematol 17:164–175, 1980.
85. Cowan DH: Thrombokinetic studies in alcohol-related thrombocytopenia. J Lab Clin Med 81:64, 1973.
86. Davis JW, Phillips PE: The effect of ethanol on human platelet aggregation in vitro. Atherosclerosis 11:473, 1970.
87. National surveillance of cocaine use and related health consequences. MMWR 31:265–273, 1982.
88. Wilkinson P, Van Dyke C, Jatlow P, et al: Intranasal and oral cocaine kinetics. Clin Pharmacol Ther 27:386–394, 1980.
89. Javaid JI, Fischman MW, Schuster CR, et al: Cocaine plasma concentration: Relation to physiological and subjective effects in humans. Science 202:227–228, 1978.
90. Inaba DS, Dunphy TW: Drug abuse. In Katcher BS, Young LY, Koda-Kimble MA (eds): Applied Therapeutics: The Clinical Use of Drugs, 3rd ed. Spokane, WA, Applied Therapeutics, 1983.
91. Perez-Reyes M, Di Guiseppi S, Ondrusek G, et al: Free base cocaine smoking. Clin Pharmacol Ther 32:459–465, 1982.
92. Washton AM, Gold MS, Pottash AC, et al: "Crack:" Early report on a new drug epidemic. Postgrad Med 80:52–58, 1986.
93. Seigal RK: Cocaine smoking. J Psychoactive Drugs 14:277–341, 1982.
94. Johanson CE, Balster RL, Bonese K: Self-administration of psychomotor stimulant drugs: The effects of unlimited access. Pharmacol Biochem Behav 4:45–51, 1976.
95. Yanagita T: An experimental framework for evaluation of dependence liability in various types of drugs in monkeys. Bull Narc 25:57–64, 1973.
96. Fischmann MW, Schuster CR, Resnekov L, et al: Cardiovascular and subjective effects of intravenous cocaine administration in humans. Arch Gen Psychiatry 33:983–989, 1976.
97. Gay GR: Clinical management of acute and chronic cocaine poisoning. Ann Emerg Med 11:562–572, 1982.
98. Smart RG: Crack cocaine use: A review of prevalence and adverse effects. Am J Drug Alcohol Abuse 17:13–26, 1991.
99. Wetti CV, Wright RK: Death caused by recreational cocaine use. JAMA 241:2519–2522, 1979.
100. Ohlsson A, Lindgren JE, Wahlen A, et al: Plasma delta-9-tetrahydrocannabinol concentrations and clinical effects after oral and intravenous administration and smoking. Clin Pharmacol Ther 28:409–416, 1980.
101. Relman AS: Marijuana and health. N Engl J Med 306:603–605, 1982.
102. Hepler RS, Frank IM, Underleider JT: Pupillary constriction after marijuana smoking. Am J Ophthalmol 74:1185–1190, 1972.
103. Tashkin DP, Shapiro BJ, Frank IM: Acute pulmonary physiologic effects of smoked marijuana and oral delta-9-tetrahydrocannabinol in healthy young men. N Engl J Med 289:336–341, 1973.
104. Tashkin DP, Calvarese BM, Simmons MS, et al: Respiratory states of seventy-four habitual marijuana smokers. Chest 78:699–706, 1980.
105. Ablon SL, Goodwin FK: High frequency of dysphoric reactions to tetrahydrocannabinol among depressed patients. Am J Psychiatry 131:448–453, 1974.
106. Jones RT: THC and the marijuana-induced social "high" or the effects of the mind on marijuana. Ann NY Acad Sci 191:155–163, 1971.
107. Nowlan MA, Cohen S: Tolerance to marijuana: Heart rate and subjective "high." Clin Pharmacol Ther 22:550–556, 1977.
108. Juskows J, Gardner MJ, Mangione A, et al: Factors affecting the phylline clearances: Age, tobacco, marijuana, cirrhosis, congestive heart failure, obesity, oral contraceptives, benzodiazepines, barbiturates, and ethanol. J Pharm Sci 68:1358–1366, 1979.
109. Hollister LE: Cannabis: Finally a therapeutic agent? Drug Alcohol Depend 11:135–145, 1983.
110. Rosenkrantz H, Fleishman RW: Effects of cannabis on the lungs. In Nahas CG, Puton WDM (eds): Marijuana: Biological Effects. Elmsford, NY, Pergamon Press, 1979.
111. Lee L, Novotny M, Bartle KD: Gas chromatography/mass spectrometric and nuclear magnetic resonance spectrometric studies on carcinogenic polynuclear aromatic hydrocarbons in tobacco and marijuana smoke condensate. Anal Chem 48:405–416, 1976.
112. National Institute on Drug Abuse: Marijuana Research Findings: Research Monograph Series No. 31. Rockville, MD, NIDA, 1980.
113. Hoffman D, Brunneman KD, Gori GB, et al: On the carcinogenicity of marijuana smoke. Res Adv Phytochem 9:63–81, 1975.
114. Henderson RL, Tennant FS, Guerny R: Respiratory manifestations of hashish smoking. Arch Otolaryngol 95:245–251, 1972.
115. Rubin V, Comitas L: Respiratory Function and Hematology in Ganja in Jamaica: A Medical Anthropological Study of Chronic Marijuana Use. The Hague, Mouton, 1975, pp 87–102.
116. Chopra IC, Chopra RN: The use of cannabis drugs in India. Bull Narc 9:4–29, 1975.
117. Hernandez BJ, Swenson EW, Coggins WJ: Presentation of pulmonary function in regular, heavy, long-term marijuana smokers (abstract). Am Rev Respir Dis 113:100, 1976.
118. Hall JAS: Testimony in marijuana-hashish epidemic hearings of the committee on the judiciary. United States Senate, Washington, DC, U.S. Government Printing Office, 1975, pp 147–154.
119. Miller M: Suicide Interventions by Nurses. New York, Springer, 1982.
120. Redetzki HM, Koerner TA, Hughes JR, et al: Osmometry in the evaluation of alcohol intoxication. Clin Toxicol 5:343–363, 1972.
121. Glasser L, Sternglanz PD, Combie ZJ, et al: Serum osmolarity and its applicability to drug overdose. Am J Clin Pharmacol 60:695–699, 1973.
122. Haddad LM, Winchester JF: Clinical Management of Poisoning and Drug Overdose. Philadelphia, WB Saunders Co, 1983.
123. Zylman R: Accidents, alcohol and single-cause explanations: Lessons from the Grand Rapids Study. Q J Stud Alcohol (suppl 14):212–233, 1968.
124. Goldfrank L: Opiates. Poisondex Micromedic, vol 53, May 1987.
125. Galbraith S: Misdiagnosis and delayed diagnosis in traumatic intracranial haematoma. Br Med J 12:1438–1439, 1976.
126. Brogden RN, Goa KL: Flumazenil: A preliminary review of its benzodiazepine antagonist properties, intrinsic activity and therapeutic use. Drugs 35:448–467, 1988.
127. Tefakis Karavokiros KA, Tsipis GB: Flumazenil: A benzodiazepine antagonist. DICP Ann Pharmacother 24:976–981, 1990.
128. O'Sullivan GF, Wade DN, Phil D: Flumazenil in the management of acute drug overdosage with benzodiazepines and other agents. Clin Pharmacol Ther 42:254–259, 1987.
129. Burr W, Sandham P, Judd A, et al: Death after flumazenil. Br Med J 298:1713, 1989.
130. Spondick DH, Pigott VM, Chirife R: Preclinical cardiac malfunction in chronic alcoholism. N Engl J Med 287:677–680, 1972.
131. Cowley RA, Dunham CM: Shock Trauma/Critical Care Manual. Baltimore, University Park Press, 1982.
132. Kalbfleisch JM, Lindeman RD, Ginn HE: Effects of ethanol administration on urinary excretion of magnesium and other electrolytes in alcoholics and normal subjects. J Clin Invest 43:1471–1475, 1963.
133. Johnson D: Fluid and electrolyte dysfunction in alcoholism. Crit Care Q 8:53–62, 1986.
134. Luckmann J, Sorensen KC: Fluid and electrolyte imbalances. In Medical-Surgical Nursing: A Psychophysiologic Approach. Philadelphia, WB Saunders Co, 1980.
135. Groer MW: Potassium imbalances. In Physiology and Pathophysiology of the Body Fluids. St. Louis, CV Mosby, 1981.
136. Hoffman JL, DiFazio CA: The anesthetic sparing effect of pentazocine, meperidine, and morphine. Arch Int Pharmacodyn 186:261, 1970.
137. Tsunoda Y, Hattori Y, Tokatsuka E, et al: Effects of hydroxy-

zine, diazepam, and pentazocine on halothane minimum alveolar concentration. Anesth Analg 52:390, 1973.
138. Lunn JK, Lui WS, Stanley TH: Peripheral and cardiac effects of nitrous oxide in the bovine. Can Anaesth Soc J 24:571, 1977.
139. Stanley TH: Nitrous oxide: New concepts about an old agent. Anesthetist Update Series, no 16, 1978.
140. Coyle JP, Cullen DJ: Anesthetic management of the critically ill. In Chernow B, Lake R (eds): The Pharmacologic Approach to the Critically Ill Patient. Baltimore, Williams & Wilkins, 1983.
141. Duke PC, Fownes D, Wade JG: Halothane depresses baroreflex control of heart rate in man. Anesthesiology 46:184, 1977.
142. Behnke RH: Recognition and management of alcohol withdrawal syndrome. Hosp Pract 11:79–84, 1976.
143. Koch-Weser J: Alcohol intoxication and withdrawal. N Engl J Med 294:757–762, 1976.
144. Victor M: Treatment of alcoholic intoxication and the withdrawal syndrome. Psychosom Med 27:636–646, 1966.
145. Brown CG: The alcohol withdrawal syndrome. Ann Emerg Med 2:276–280, 1982.
146. Gower WE, Kersten H: Prevention of alcohol withdrawal symptoms in surgical patients. Surg Gynecol Obstet 151:382–384, 1980.
147. Hansbrough JF, Zapata-Sirvent RL, Carroll WJ, et al: Administration of intravenous alcohol for prevention of withdrawal in alcoholic burn patients. Am J Surg 148:266–269, 1984.
148. Burbige EJ, Lewis DR Jr, Halsted CA, et al: Alcohol and the gastrointestinal tract. Med Clin North Am 68:77, 1984.
149. Fultz JM, Senay EC: Guidelines for the management of hospitalized narcotic addicts. Ann Intern Med 82:815–818, 1975.
150. Wikler A: Diagnosis of treatment of drug dependence of the barbiturate type. Am J Psychiatry 125:758–761, 1968.
151. Smith DE, Wesson A: A new method for treatment of barbiturate dependence. JAMA 213:294–295, 1970.
152. Gawin FH, Kleber HD: Abstinence symptomology and psychiatric diagnosis in cocaine abusers: Clinical observations. Arch Gen Psychiatry 43:107–113, 1986.
153. Hall WC, Talbert RL, Ereshefsky L: Cocaine abuse and its treatment. Pharmacotherapy 10:47–65, 1990.
154. Senay CC, Lewis DC: The Primary Physician's Guide to Drug and Alcohol Abuse Treatment. Medical Monograph Series, vol 1. Rockville, MD, National Institute on Drug Abuse, 1980.
155. Bowen M: The use of family theory in clinical practice. Compr Psychiatry 7:345–374, 1966.
156. Noone R: Observations on drug abuse and the family. Family 9:46–52, 1981.
157. Steinglass P: Experimenting with family treatment approaches to alcoholism, 1950–1975: A review. Fam Process 97–123, 1976.
158. National Directory of Drug Abuse and Alcoholism Treatment Programs. National Institute on Drug Abuse Clearinghouse, 5600 Fishers Lane, Rockville, MD, 20857.
159. Twelve Steps and Twelve Traditions. Alcoholics Anonymous. New York, World Services, 1953.
160. Peyrot M: Narcotics Anonymous: Its history, structure, and approach. Int J Addict 20:1509–1522, 1985.
161. National Commission Against Drunk Driving: A Progress Report on the Implementation of Recommendations by the Presidential Commission on Drunk Driving, December 1985. Washington, DC, U.S. Department of Transportation, National Highway Traffic Safety Administration, 1985.
162. Federal Strategy for Prevention of Drug Abuse and Drug Trafficking 1982. Washington, DC, U.S. Department of Agriculture, 1982.
163. Dearing-Stuck B: Trauma prevention. In Cardona G (ed): Trauma Nursing. Oradell, NJ, Medical Economics, 1985.
164. Walsh JM: Polydrug and alcohol use. Alcohol, Drugs and Driving, Abstracts and Reviews 1:115–119, 1985.
165. Soderstrom CA, Cowley RA: A national alcohol and trauma center survey: Missed opportunities, failures of responsibility. Arch Surg 122:1067–1071, 1987.

31

THE ORGAN DONOR

PAMELA PHILLIPS GAUL and
MARGARETA K. CUCCIA

In recent decades, research and extraordinary developments in technology have given biomedicine an array of possibilities once unimaginable. Today, organ transplants are almost commonplace, yet the future of transplantation may quite possibly be as dramatic as its inception. Surgical techniques have been refined, techniques for preserving organs are becoming more sophisticated, and research continues to produce more effective immunosuppressive drugs so vital to the postoperative success of transplants. However, all these advances will be of little consequence without an enlarging pool of potential organ donors. The public has responded to this growing need: The dramatic rise in the number of transplantations attests to this support. Yet it cannot only be the responsibility of an increasingly better informed public. The future of organ transplant programs nationwide, even worldwide, must be a responsibility shared by a knowledgeable and enthusiastic physician/nursing community that can transform the potential of this life-giving process into a workable, efficient reality.

Organ transplantation is an accepted mode of therapy for those with end-stage organ disease. Since the first kidney transplant was performed in 1954, many changes have occurred in both surgical technique and immunosuppressive therapy. To date, there are 25 solid organs and tissues that can be transplanted. Throughout the United States, there are at any given time over 26,000 men, women, and children waiting for transplants. Approximately every one-half hour, one new person is added to the list. Those who are on the waiting list for a heart, lung, or liver may not live long enough to gain a second chance at life.

One of the reasons for the current success of transplantation is the development of a more specific immunosuppressive agent, cyclosporine. Cyclosporine is a polypeptide derived from a fungus. It may be given intramuscularly, intravenously, or orally. The precise mode of action is not completely understood except that it inhibits the action of the T helper cells and is therefore one of the most useful drugs in fighting rejection without suppressing the body's entire immune system. This drug is used by almost all patients who receive organ transplants. Side effects include dose-related liver and renal toxic effects, hirsutism, and tremor, which are commonly reversible if the dosage is decreased. Cyclosporine also may be used in combination with conventional drugs such as Solu-Medrol, azathioprine, antihymocyte globulin, and prednisone to prevent rejection. All organ recipients remain on immunosuppressive therapy for the rest of their lives. Immunosuppression decreases recipients' vulnerability to systemic infections, which has increased the overall survival rate of recipients over the past 5 years.[1] Statistics show a 1-year graft (the transplanted organ) survival rate of 60 per cent when azathioprine is used as the drug of choice versus an 80 per cent graft survival rate when cyclosporine is used.[2] Additional immunosuppressive drugs are now being investigated at various transplant institutions, specifically FK506 and Rapamycin. These new drugs are proving to have fewer side effects than cyclosporine, allow the use of lower dosages of steroids, and demonstrate comparable success rates.

Advances in the field of transplantation have given rise to many issues that were not confronted before its widespread success. The shortage of donor organs remains the largest issue. Ideas about how to increase the supply to meet the demand are currently being considered by legislators and task force members throughout the country. One proposal is *presumed consent*. This is based on the idea that all persons would be considered organ donors unless an objection was registered before their death. This would mean, contrary to the current practice of carrying an organ donor card, that one would have to carry a *non*organ donor card. This procedure is practiced in many European countries. Another proposal that has found favor in the United States is *required request*.[3] The required request law was federally instituted in 1986 and has since been adopted in most states. This law makes it mandatory at the time of one's death that the next of kin be approached by hospital personnel about organ donation. The purpose is to allow each family to have an opportunity to consider organ donation as an option.

The purpose of the signed organ donor card is to allow individuals to make their own decisions *before* their death. The problem with this system is that often those who meet the criteria are unidentified at the time of admission; therefore, donor information is not known. The responsibility then falls on health care professionals to raise the question or on family members to make their wishes known. There are differing attitudes among nurses and physicians in their perception of organ donation and brain death.[4] Consequently, organ donation may be forgotten or ignored. Over the past decade, media coverage of successful transplants has increased family awareness and willingness to initiate the process. Parents of children who have suffered fatal head injuries often are quick to ask about donation even before they are approached.

In designated trauma centers where the most severely injured patients are treated, brain death is more common than in other medical facilities, and fewer problems are associated with the concept of organ donation. For example, over 50 per cent of all organ donors in Maryland come from these institutions. Most patients admitted to trauma centers are between the ages of 15 and 40 years and were healthy prior to their trauma.[5] Thus many of them meet the criteria for potential organ donors. So it is the trauma nursing personnel and physicians who must *first* identify the patient as a potential organ donor.

The ability of trauma care providers to recognize and understand donor criteria creates a vital link in the chain of the donation process. Each organ has both unique and shared criteria that determine its selection for transplantation.

DONOR REFERRAL AND IDENTIFICATION

Every death, with the exception of those who are confirmed HIV-positive, has the potential for some type of donation. For the purposes of this chapter, we will focus on those patients who are declared brain dead and have the potential for organ donation. No patient should be ruled out before the organ procurement agency is contacted.

Once a patient is recognized as a potential donor, the next step is referral. The referral call is made by a physician or nurse to the certified organ procurement agency. If the nurse refers the potential donor, she should inform the attending physician of the action. This allows the nurse, physician, and procurement personnel to work together in ensuring the best possible course of action for both patient and family.

One criterion that is common to all organ donors is brain death. No organs may be taken from someone who does not meet this basic criterion. Many times referrals are received *before* the declaration of brain death. This provides the time needed for an initial evaluation to screen for medical suitability. It presents no conflict, since the family should not be approached about organ donation before being told that brain death is imminent or has occurred. When a referral call is made, it is the beginning of the process of organ donation. The care of the patient is not changed until brain death is declared.

DONOR PROFILE

A 17-year-old white male is admitted to the emergency room after being involved in a motor vehicle accident. The only injury sustained by the patient is a severe closed head injury. The patient is transported for a computed tomography scan for evaluation of his injury, which reveals diffuse cerebral swelling. The patient's prognosis at this time is guarded to poor. (This would be an appropriate time for the physician or nurse to make a referral call.) The physician's plan is to insert an intraventricular catheter and admit the patient to the intensive care unit for observation.

Later that evening, despite all efforts to control his intracranial pressure, the patient exhibits signs of herniation. Blood flow studies show no evidence of cerebral perfusion. The clinical bedside testing for brain death was performed by a physician, and the patient was established as brain dead.

TABLE 31–1. GENERAL CRITERIA AND SPECIFIC EVALUATION TESTS FOR ORGAN DONORS

ORGAN	CONTRAINDICATIONS	UNIQUE EVALUATION
Heart	Prolonged cardiac massage (>20 min) Intracardiac injections Cardiomyopathy Extracranial malignancy	EKG Chest x-ray Echocardiogram Accurate weight in kilograms Cardiac isoenzymes Cardiac catheterization*
Lung	Tracheostomy† Same as heart Pulmonary edema, contusion, or infection Extracranial malignancy	Same as heart Normal ABGs Sputum cultures O_2 challenge Accurate weight and height for size match Normal tidal volume and lung compliance
Kidney	Chronic renal disease History of hypertension (uncontrolled) Diabetes mellitus, insulin-dependent Extracranial malignancy	Serum BUN, creatinine, and creatinine clearance Microscopic urinalysis Urine culture
Pancreas	History of diabetes mellitus Pancreatitis Extracranial malignancy	Serum amylase and glucose
Liver	Abdominal trauma, penetrating History of hepatitis, drug abuse, or severe alcoholism Extracranial malignancy	Liver function tests: AST, ALT, CPK, LDH Direct and indirect bilirubin PTT and PT, platelets Patient's weight in kilograms
Tissue		
Cornea	Local injuries, conjunctivitis	
Skin	Local wounds or malignancy	
Bone	Open injuries	
Heart valves	Open cardiac massage	

*Requested only in specific elderly donors.
†The area of the donor tracheostomy is too close to the anastomosis site in the recipient and therefore is considered contaminated.
EKG, electrocardiogram; ABGs, arterial blood gases; BUN, blood urea nitrogen; AST, aspartate aminotransferase; ALT, alanine aminotransferase; CPK, creatine phosphokinase; LDH, lactate dehydrogenase; PTT, partial thromboplastin time; PT, prothrombin time.

EVALUATION OF THE POTENTIAL DONOR

After the hospital personnel have made a referral call, an evaluation must be made by an organ procurement coordinator, who will visit the unit to review the chart. Table 31–1 lists criteria that serve as general guidelines in evaluating a potential donor. Each case is evaluated on an individual basis. Hospital personnel should never rule out a potential donor. The organ procurement coordinator should always make the final determination for medical suitability. A toxicology screen may be ordered in some cases to determine if the donor has taken any toxic drugs or narcotics. To facilitate these tests, the attending physician is requested by procurement personnel to order them. The specific tests outlined in Table 31–1 are performed only after consent is obtained from the family for the specific organs to be donated.

The tests listed in Table 31–2 are routinely ordered for any potential organ donor. Concerns about communicable diseases have made it necessary to test for the HTLV I, HIV, and hepatitis C viruses, as well as other infectious processes.

The nurse taking care of the donor should understand the importance of having this blood work drawn and sent to the laboratory in an expeditious manner. The results will determine the suitability of the organs for transplantation.

General Contraindications

Some general contraindications to organ donations are

1. Chronic disease in the organ
2. Diabetes mellitus, insulin-dependent
3. Communicable diseases
4. Malignancy, except primary brain tumor and skin cancer
5. Untreated sepsis
6. Documented IV drug abuse or high-risk behavior

TABLE 31–2. ROUTINE TESTS FOR POTENTIAL ORGAN DONORS

TEST	RATIONALE
VDRL	Venereal disease
Hepatitis B surface antigen	Hepatitis, active or latent
Blood and urine culture	Current infections
ABO	Determines the blood type of the donor
Electrolytes	Metabolic status of the donor
HTLV III* (HIV)†	Presence of the HIV antibodies
Hepatitis C	Non A, non B
HTLV I and II	Presence of antibodies
Toxoplasmosis	
CMV	

*Human T-cell lymphotropic virus type III
†Human immunodeficiency virus

TISSUE DONATION

Although this chapter deals primarily with organ donation, it would not be complete without mentioning the advances and discoveries made in the field of tissue donation. If a patient has been declared "cardiac" dead, it is appropriate for the nurse to mention the possibility of tissue donation to the physicians involved. This process, as in organ donation, requires a referral call to be placed to the tissue bank in accordance with the federal law.[3]

Corneas have been successfully transplanted for a number of years. The overall graft survival rate is 90 per cent in the first year.[6] The practice of cryopreserving or "banking" of other tissues such as skin, bone, and heart valves has benefited many patients suffering from burns, degloving injuries, vascular deficiencies, and trauma.[7] Tissue transplant recipients do not need immunosuppressive therapy like organ recipients. The quality of their lives is vastly improved. Most areas now have established tissue banks that procure all these tissues for the purpose of transplantation and/or research. The criteria for tissue donation are broader than those for organ donation. The donor does not need to be maintained on ventilatory support, and the procurement can take place up to 24 hours after death. Almost any person who dies who is not confirmed as HIV-positive can donate at least one form of tissue, such as corneas/eyes.

BRAIN DEATH

As stated earlier, all patients considered for organ donation must meet the criteria for the declaration of brain death. Nurses caring for the organ donor should be familiar with the law governing brain death declaration in their state and the associated hospital policies.

Most laws state that there must be no spontaneous brain or brainstem function. Death is to be pronounced before any mechanical life-support systems are terminated or any vital organ is removed for transplantation.[8] The attending physician or neurosurgeon determines this diagnosis in accordance with the standards of medical practice. Hypothermia, barbiturate poisoning, metabolic imbalances, and shock must be ruled out as the cause of central nervous system depression before clinical testing is performed. Criteria for the determination of brain death are as follows:[9]

1. No spontaneous movement
2. No response to painful stimuli
3. No spontaneous respiration after 100 per cent O_2 for 10 minutes, then tested for a period of 4–6 minutes with a P_{CO_2} reaching 60 mm Hg. Oxygen therapy should not be removed. If available, an oxygen saturation monitor can be used to monitor oxygenation during the test.
4. Absence of brainstem reflexes:
   a. Fixed and dilated pupils
   b. No corneal reflexes
   c. Absent doll's eyes
   d. Absent cough and gag reflex
   e. Absent vestibular response to caloric stimulation

Ancillary tests include:

1. Demonstration of a "no flow" state to the brain using arteriography or nucleotide scan.
2. A flat EEG repeated in a 6- to 12-hour period.
3. Rudimentary spinal reflexes, when present, should not influence the determination of brain death.

Some states require that two brain death notes be entered on the patient's chart and signed by the attending physician and neurosurgeon or neurologist. The time of brain death declaration is the time of death documented in the chart and death certificate.

OBTAINING CONSENT

The Nurse's Role

The nurse's role in the consent process may vary. In most states, it is the responsibility of the organ procurement coordinator to approach the family for consent. The nurse should be involved with the physician in the discussion of brain death with the family. The concept of brain death is difficult for many families and should be explained clearly. Often, the nurse is asked questions after the physician has left to reconfirm the explanation. The scenario for requesting organ donation should, ideally, be set up by the physician, nurse, and procurement coordinator. There are advantages and disadvantages to this approach.

There are advantages and disadvantages for the nurse to approach the family for donation. Although the nurse is aware of the patient's history and present status, some families may be unable to accept the role change of the nurse from providing care to requesting organs for transplant. Procurement personnel are not directly involved with the care of the patient and therefore present no possible conflict of interest. Although the nurse may have established a rapport with the family of the patient and feels comfortable broaching the topic of organ donation, she may not know how to answer the family's questions about the organ donation process. When approaching a family, it is helpful to know which organs to request. Nurses do not have this information readily accessible to them. The nurse's role here is an important, albeit a passive, one. When the physician and/or the organ procurement coordinator discusses the organ donation question with the family, the nurse's presence provides the family with some sense of comfort, since the nurse had cared for the patient with whose death the family is now trying to come to terms. In most cases, it is the nurse whom the family has come to trust and to rely upon for information, the one who has offered them consistent support. The nurse has been the caregiver, so it may be unreasonable to expect her to be the one to seek the family's consent for organ donation. However, it is the nurse's sympathetic presence that helps create a less stressful atmosphere in which the family can reach a decision.

In those situations in which the nurse is called on to seek consent for organ donation, there are certain family dynamics she may find helpful to understand in making the initial approach to the family. When confronted by the sudden death of a loved one, family members often feel lost. They have had no time to resolve their feelings about the deceased relative. The nurse cannot remove their grief but can offer the option of organ donation as a positive action. Faced with a decision, relatives have something tangible to deal with and something that offers another human being a chance at life or an improved quality of life.

Suggested Locations for Obtaining Consent

A quiet area may be available in the emergency room or intensive care unit. If not, then an empty nurses' lounge will suffice. It is not uncommon in this setting to have to inform a family of a death or impending death. A quiet area is of the utmost importance, since families must have a place to respond to such news privately. The simple request for a family to move to an area away from other waiting families helps prepare them for the worst.

In the intensive or intermediate care facility, family privacy remains important. Because family members have had time to work through some of the grieving process, they may realize that death is a distinct possibility. This response usually is based on the consistent information communicated to them over a period of time by the nursing staff and physicians.

Who May Give Consent

When approaching a family for organ donation, consent must be obtained from the next of kin as defined by law. The accepted legal order is as follows:

1. Spouse: If a couple is separated but not divorced, the spouse remains the legal next of kin.
2. Adult son or daughter: In the event of a parent's death and there is no spouse, the children of that parent over the age of 18 are considered the legal next of kin.
3. Parents: Legal next of kin for any unmarried child.
4. Siblings: In the event that both parents are deceased and the donor is unmarried or divorced without adult children, the siblings would be considered legal next of kin.
5. Legal guardian: An adult or agency who has been awarded legal custody of the potential donor by a court of law, e.g., a foster child or an elderly person.[8]

Consent may be obtained by phone conversation if witnessed by one other person in person or by fax. The nurse can help in this situation by asking any family member or friend present at the time of admission the identity of the legal next of kin. Health care professionals are protected in obtaining consent by the "good faith" law. This means that the family members actually are who they represent themselves to be and that the professional accepts this in good faith.

If the next of kin cannot be found, the police department conducts a "reasonable search." This search is performed in cases of homicide and suspicious deaths. If the police cannot locate the next of kin, then consent may be granted by the medical examiner's office. The nurse has no responsibility in initiating this procedure.

Medical Examiner's Cases

A common misconception is that patients falling under the medical examiner's or coroner's jurisdiction cannot be organ donors. The medical examiner's law accepts under its jurisdiction anyone who has died as a "result of violence or by suicide, or by casualty or suddenly when in apparent good health or when unattended by a physician or in any suspicious or unusual manner."[10] Based on the criteria given earlier, it is true that most organ donors *are* medical examiner cases. The final consent for organ donation is given by the medical examiner's office after it is contacted by the procurement personnel. Nursing has no responsibility in obtaining this consent. It is the medical examiner's responsibility to determine the exact cause of death; therefore, an investigation by the medical examiner's office *must* be conducted. In most cases, when given sufficient information to determine the cause of death, the medical examiner will give consent for organ donation. The medical examiner's consent must be documented in the chart.

Approaching the Donor's Family

Studies show that the organ recovery coordinator is the most trained individual who could speak to the family. It is not recommended for an R.N. or M.D. to approach the family unless they feel comfortable doing so. Some *very* general guidelines are discussed here, but remember that if the nurse does approach the family, it is helpful to have a recovery coordinator nearby to be available to answer any specific questions the family may have. Consider this scenario: The parents of a 16-year-old girl have just been told that their daughter is brain dead. They are stunned and helpless. Time should *always* be given to the family to understand that their loved one is dead and to begin their grieving process before the subject of donation is approached. Many different indicators could be given by the family to direct the health care team as to that moment; Questions such as "What do we do now?" or using the deceased's name in the past tense, and so on. The approach should not occur until that family can reiterate in these or other ways that they realize their loved one is dead. Many families will seize an opportunity to turn their own tragedy into something perceived as meaningful.

A fair approach under these circumstances is to ask the parents what they think their daughter would have wanted. In this case, the parents respond by saying how "loving and giving" their daughter was. "Yes, she would have wanted to do this," they conclude.

This is a common family response when the deceased is young. The family can take comfort that, in a sense, their loved one lives on. Organ donation is an option and should be presented as such without pressure. No matter what the family's decision is, it should be made clear there is no *wrong* decision.

If the patient has signed a donor card or has such a designation on his or her driver's license, it is still customary to obtain consent from the next of kin. In these circumstances, consent is rarely denied.

If the family response to organ donation is uncertainty or reluctance, then the relatives should be allowed time to consider the option in privacy. They may need help from other family members or clergy members, or they may have conflicting views. It is important, however, to set a time limit. If a decision is not reached within an hour, then clearly the organ donation issue may be provoking unreasonable stress. In this case, the person making the request may suggest that it is better for the family to abandon the idea of organ donation than to exacerbate an already stressful situation. Once again, the family should be reassured that even the indecision is perfectly appropriate.

After Consent

An accurate and detailed medical/social history must be obtained from the family after consent is given. The person who obtains the consent (nurse, physician, or organ procurement coordinator) should also explain to the family how the donation process works: The donor will be maintained on mechanical support until taken to the operating room, and once the organs are recovered, the body will go to the morgue. The purpose of the explanation is to account for the time lapse between brain death declaration and termination of ventilatory support. The family should be assured that there will be no visible signs of disfigurement as a result of the organ donation procedure. Families frequently have questions:

Q: Who will get the organs?
A: The identity of the recipients is not immediately known because there are so many people in urgent need of a transplant. (Procurement agencies usually send a follow-up letter to families to tell them the ages and progress of the recipients.)
Q: How much time is involved in the procedure?
A: Generally, organ recovery will be completed within a 4- to 8-hour period depending on the availability of an operating room.
Q: What do we do now?
A: The family should be instructed to go home and make funeral arrangements. The funeral home and the morgue will coordinate the release of the body.

DONOR MANAGEMENT

Maintaining brain dead patients for the purpose of organ donation is a challenge. The focus of care shifts from treating a brain injury to that of preserving the organs. Hormonal changes occur as well as the failure of the sympathetic nervous system. Therefore, the cardiovascular and respiratory systems are particularly taxed, leading to fundamental problems, such as metabolic and electrolyte disturbances, hypotension, hypovolemia, and poor oxygenation. Prevention of infection and the treatment of hypothermia are also concerns for management. Nursing care priorities involve establishing a homeostatic environment with aggressive monitoring and therapies.[11]

The nurse, physician, and organ procurement personnel work as a team while managing the donor. The recovery coordinator directs and establishes the priorities of care depending on which organs are being procured for transplant. Optimal care of donor organs is imperative for successful outcomes of transplanted organs.

It is possible that, despite optimal care, the potential organ donor will arrest. This event usually presents as ventricular fibrillation or asystole.[12] If the family has given consent for donation, cardiopulmonary resuscitation should be instituted in an attempt to maintain perfusable organs. Kidneys, in particular, can often still be successfully retrieved and transplanted. For example, an unstable donor may arrest en route to the operating room. If CPR is initiated, the surgical teams can work quickly to remove the organs. In these situations, the efforts of the family, medical, nursing, and procurement teams to enhance and save the lives of the future recipients are carried out to the maximum potential. However, if it appears that attempts at cardiopulmonary resuscitation are not being successful, then the efforts should be discontinued and the donor case brought to a close.

Nursing Management Guidelines for the Organ Donor

Hydration and Hypotension

One of the principal objectives of donor management is to keep the donor normotensive. Hypotension is caused by a variety of factors, such as hypovolemia, endocrine changes, and a decrease in the systemic vascular resistance. Acceptable blood pressure ranges between 90 and 150 mm Hg systolic, with a diastolic range of 40 to 100 mm Hg. The mean arterial pressure should be kept above 70 mm Hg to ensure adequate organ perfusion.

Assessment includes accurate monitoring of the donor's intake and output of fluids. No longer having to consider the donor's intracranial pressure allows the nurse the freedom of replacing the output on a milliliter for milliliter basis with IV fluids. If the donor is hypotensive as a result of hypovolemia, a fluid challenge of 500 ml of lactated Ringer's solution may be given over a 30-minute period. If the blood pressure rises, subsequent fluid challenges may be given until the donor is adequately hydrated. Colloids, such as Hespan and albumin, are excellent volume expanders and may be utilized as well. The type of fluid given should be guided by hemoglobin and hematocrit levels and serum electrolytes. Large amounts of fluids containing dextrose or high Na^+ concentrations should be avoided if diabetes insipidus is a problem. Although a central venous pressure (CVP) line is not mandatory, it may be useful in helping the nurse differentiate between a labile blood pressure secondary to hypovolemia and one that is secondary to loss of vasomotor tone. If a CVP line is available, the central venous pressure should be maintained between 8 and 12 mm Hg. Frequently, if the heart or lungs are to be donated, a Swan-Ganz line may be inserted for more specific and accurate readings. If so, the pulmonary artery wedge pressure should be maintained between 8 and 12 mm Hg. The more monitoring devices that are used, the easier it is to determine volume status and the effects of pressors given.

Inotropic Support

When adequate intravascular volume is replaced and hypotension persists, the nurse should consider inotropic agents for support of the blood pressure. The drugs most commonly preferred by transplant surgeons include dopamine, dobutamine, and Neo-Synephrine. Drugs such as norepinephrine bitartrate (Levophed), epinephrine, and isoproterenol (Isuprel) are not contraindicated but may decrease organ perfusion. However, dobutamine may give false indicators of contractility and cardiac output, which could pose a problem if the heart is to be donated. The main objective in the use of inotropics is to support the blood pressure of the donor without decreasing organ perfusion. This may be accomplished by using a concentration of either dopamine, <10 to 15 μg/kg/min, or dobutamine, not exceeding 10 to 15 μg/kg/min.

If, as a result of hypotension, the urine output is decreased and the donor has received adequate volume replacement and inotropic support, the nurse may give furosemide (Lasix), 40 mg IV. Mannitol should not be given because it may exacerbate pulmonary edema. Many times in the resuscitation phase of both head-injured patients and organ donors there can be an initial 1- to 2-hour period of anuria. This is usually secondary to hypotension and does not preclude kidney donation. In the majority of cases, once the patient has been hydrated and a mean blood pressure of 60 to 70 mm Hg is established, the organs will function normally. Close monitoring of the serum electrolytes, especially the blood urea nitrogen (BUN) and creatinine levels, is important. The recipe for inotropic support will change depending on which organs are going to be procured and the transplant physician's preference. The organ procurement personnel will control the communication with the teams and discuss the best possible solutions.

Electrolyte Disturbances

Serum electrolytes should be monitored closely in the potential organ donor to ensure organ viability and cardiovascular stability. The most common electrolyte disturbances are hypokalemia, hypernatremia, hypocalcemia, hyperglycemia, and hypophosphatemia. The causes of these imbalances can be multifactoral; therefore, donor medical histories should be obtained as well as an accurate review of the hospital course. The electrolyte changes also may present from diabetes insipidus. Treatment includes potassium and Ca^{2+} supplements, Na^{+} restriction, and close monitoring of serum electrolyte levels.

Diabetes Insipidus

Most patients suffering massive head injuries will exhibit signs of diabetes insipidus. The frequency of diabetes insipidus in brain dead patients ranges from 85 to 87 per cent.[13] This poses a problem in the management of both hypotension and hydration. Diabetes insipidus presents as polyuria (300 to 1000 ml of urine per hour). The urine osmolality is usually less than 150 mOsmol/kg, with associated serum hypernatremia. For the patient whose intake of fluids was restricted from the time of admission while being treated as a survivor, this type of urine output is enough to cause severe hypotension when the volume is not replaced or the polyuria is uncontrolled.

The management of diabetes insipidus in the organ donor may include replacing the urine output volume plus 50 to 100 ml with intravenous 0.25 normal saline. If the urine output is excessive and there is risk of volume overload and pulmonary edema, it is recommended that a vasopressin (Pitressin) drip be started. The Pitressin drip should begin at 0.08 unit/ml/hr; urine output must be monitored hourly. Adequate urine output for kidney donors ranges between 100 and 200 ml/hr. If urine output falls below 50 ml/hr, the Pitressin is weaned and the urine output should increase immediately. When using this therapy, the preference for IV versus SC or IM Pitressin is based on the fact that patients are more easily regulated on IV Pitressin because of improved and predictable absorption. Pitressin is a potent vasoconstrictor; its use should be limited to the lowest possible effective dose.

Hypertension

Although not always exhibited, hypertension can present a problem in the organ donor. Whether to treat this hypertension depends on the cause. If it is due to hypervolemia, then the treatment would include diuretics and/or fluid restriction. Hypovolemia also may cause hypertension secondary to a catecholamine response. In this case, the treatment would be volume expansion, not vasodilators. If necessary, sodium nitroprusside (Nipride) may be used to control hypertension and is easy to regulate by IV drip to gain the desired effect. Hypothermia also may contribute to hypertension, and the steps mentioned in the preceding section should be taken.

Oxygenation

Monitoring oxygenation in a potential donor is important to maintain organ viability. The patient's oxygen should be optimally maintained between 70 and 100 mm Hg at the lowest possible FIO_2. Pulmonary edema is a frequent complication in brain dead patients caused by a sympathetic response and capillary leakage.[14] Treatment includes ventilation with positive end-expiratory pressure, infrequent suctioning, possible fluid restriction, and diuretics. Continuous monitoring of arterial oxygen saturation and/or mixed venous saturation is very useful and helps keep the number of arterial blood gas levels needed to a minimum.

Coagulopathy

In cases in which the donor has sustained an open skull fracture, severe scalp lacerations, or lower extremity fractures, a significant amount of blood may have been lost. The hematocrit and hemoglobin should be maintained within normal limits by replacing lost blood volume with packed red cells. This will help to ensure adequate oxygenation of the organs and increase perfusion by replacing the blood volume. Arterial blood gases also should be monitored and maintained within normal limits to ensure adequate oxygenation of the tissues. Another complication due to the mechanism of injury is the release of large amounts of tissue fibrolytic agents from the injured brain that initiates a coagulopathy. These patients with a coagulopathy or disseminated intravascular coagulation (DIC) are very difficult to maintain. Treatment is palliative with transfusion of packed red blood cells, fresh frozen plasma, and platelets. The patient should be brought to the operating room as soon as possible to prevent further complications.

Temperature Regulation

Patients must be normothermic before brain death can be pronounced. A core body temperature of 95°F (35°C) is considered sufficient both for declaration of brain death and for organ recovery. Objectives for organ donation are to decrease vasoconstriction and to prevent a decrease in perfusion, which may be due to the hypothermia commonly seen in these patients. Hypothermia also may cause myocardial depression with subsequent bradycardia, hypotension, and decreased cardiac output. The cause of hypothermia in the resuscitation phase is commonly a patient's exposure to the elements prior to admission. In the ICU or IMCU, the cause of a low temperature may be the irreversible brain swelling and consequent damage to the hypothalamus.

Prevention and treatment for hypothermia consist of using warming blankets above and below the patient. The use of heated humidity also works well when applied to the ventilator. Other therapies include irrigating the nasogastric tubes with warmed fluids and administering IV fluids for central warming, as well as wrapping the top of the head with warm towels. By raising the temperature to 95°F (35°C), vasoconstriction due to hypothermia can be decreased, thus increasing perfusion to the organs.

Infection Control

Across all cycles of care from admission through maintenance and eventually organ recovery, the nurse's role in monitoring strict aseptic technique cannot be overemphasized. Even though a patient has made the transition from viable patient to organ donor, his care cannot be compromised. Recipients of transplanted organs will be on immunosuppressive therapy for the rest of their lives; with this knowledge comes the responsibility for nurses caring for the donor organs to be diligent in using aseptic technique during routine procedures. The sources of nosocomial infections do not differ for survivors and organ donors: The most common are dressing changes, invasive procedures, suctioning, blood drawing, and Foley catheters. Nurses either perform these functions or oversee their implementation by physicians or other members of the health care team. The nurse serves as the monitor of infection control and therefore has a primary responsibility to see that all protocols for the prevention of infection are followed. In doing this, the nurse fulfills the responsibility of providing quality care for the organs that are being preserved for transplantation into someone who will be susceptible to infection. Urine, sputum, and blood cultures are taken in the ICU, and additional cultures are taken during operative procedures. Complete blood counts (CBC) with differentials should be followed closely.

Antibiotic Therapy

The decision to use prophylactic antibiotics to prevent infection in the organ donor depends on the protocols of the recovery team. When questions arise, the nurse or physician should consult organ procurement personnel or the policy concerning what, if any, antibiotics are to be used. The use of aminoglycosides is not contraindicated, but blood levels should be monitored because of their nephrotoxic effect.

The nurse's role in caring for the organ donor, whether single or multiple, is diverse. In management, it is the nurse who monitors all parameters of organ function.

Organ-Specific Considerations

The decision as to which organs will be procured is initially made by the family. Each individual donor situation is different. The mechanism and extent of injuries to the potential donor, the age and medical history, and the hospital course will determine which, if any, organs meet the criteria for transplantation.

Whatever organs are to be procured, the goal is to establish a homeostatic environment as best one can. The objectives for care remain the same: monitoring for electrolyte and metabolic disturbances, managing hypotension and hypovolemia, and maintaining oxygenation, normothermia, and an infection-free environment.

Each organ-specific transplant team will request particular management goals. It is the responsibility of the organ procurement personnel to coordinate communication and direct the donor care.

OPERATING ROOM

Time and Personnel Requirements

It is important that the operating room staff be adequately prepared for the procedure of single or multiple organ retrieval. The circulating nurse should ask the organ recovery personnel what procedures will be done, what the time requirements and special instrumentation needs are, and how many physicians will be present. By having this information beforehand, the nurse can decide which operating room will be most suitable and can make the proper arrangements. Most recovery teams will have written information on the specific needs of the surgeons. Any special instruments will be provided by the recovery teams as well.

Multiple organ recoveries are performed in stages. The hosting operating room provides a single scrub nurse, circulator, and an anesthesiologist. The length of the procedure will vary for single-organ versus multiorgan procurement (Table 31–3). Equipment needs for the various surgeries are shown in Table 31–4.

If the operating room personnel have been adequately prepared for the organ retrieval procedure by the recovery personnel, all sequences of the surgery should flow smoothly and quickly. Most recovery teams procuring extrarenal organs are familiar with the multiorgan retrieval process, and the responsibility for communicating the sequence of dissection, perfusion, and ultimately removal of the organs rests with them.

Surgical Requirements for Organ Removal

Under ideal circumstances, the organ donor is scheduled for organ removal as an emergency surgical procedure after completion of all medical, legal, and administrative requirements. In general, one circulating nurse, one scrub nurse, and an anesthesiologist are needed for the procedure. The teams will bring an extra scrub nurse, if desired. The number of people in a recovery team may necessitate a large room. The teams bring the specific medications, sterile ice, and

TABLE 31–3. TIMES REQUIRED FOR ORGAN PROCUREMENT

PROCEDURE	TIME (hr)	OPERATING ROOM PERSONNEL	SEQUENCE OF SURGERIES
Cardiectomy	0.5–1	1 scrub nurse* 1 circulator	Dissected and taken first
Hepatectomy	2	1 scrub nurse 1 circulator	Dissected and taken second if done with cardiectomy
Nephrectomy	1.5	1 scrub nurse 1 circulator	Dissected and taken with pancreas, last if done with cardiectomy and hepatectomy
Pancreatectomy	2	1 scrub nurse 1 circulator	Dissected and may be taken with nephrectomy
Lung	1–2	1 scrub nurse 1 circulator	Dissected and taken first

*Some recovery teams bring an extra scrub nurse to assist them.

packaging materials needed, as well as specialized instruments.

Premedication

In the operating room, it is often confusing as to why the skills of an anesthesiologist are needed in an organ recovery because the donor is dead and needs no anesthesia. Anesthesia personnel monitor the fluid management and vital signs of the donor. It is requested by procurement personnel that the anesthesiologist give a series of drugs at a time designated by the transplant team. Diuretic agents are also given for renal cortical vasodilation and to protect donor renal integrity during the ischemic period. Heparin is given intravenously to prevent blood clotting during circulatory arrest. Examples of required drugs include Lasix, 40 mg IV; mannitol, 25 to 50 gm IV; and sodium heparin, 10,000 to 30,000 units IV. The suggested doses are based on adult donors. The recovery coordinator will provide these medications to the anesthesiologist, if necessary.

The nurse may be asked by procurement personnel to have these drugs available so that the anesthesiologist may give them when so instructed by the procurement surgeons.

Operative Procedure for Single-Organ Procurement

Nephrectomy

Many centers use the en bloc technique. The best strategy is to have a well-prepared diuresing donor, use the technique with which the surgical team is most proficient, preserve the anatomical integrity of the kidneys, and minimize the warm ischemia period. Exposure should be through the abdomen using either a long midline or a cruciate incision (Fig. 31–1).

En bloc nephrectomy (Fig. 31–2) is quite different from individual nephrectomy and requires detailed orientation and prior experience to be performed satisfactorily.[12] This method ensures the removal of the renal arteries in continuity with a large aortic cuff, thus facilitating later transplantation. The aorta is cleared of anterior branches, and the inferior mesenteric, superior mesenteric, and celiac axis roots are ligated and divided. (At this point, the kidneys may be perfused with a cold flush solution through the aorta if cardiac arrest occurs. This is done by ligating the aorta above and below the renal artery level and injecting the cold perfusate through a large cannula until the kidneys become blanched and cold. At this time, the en bloc nephrectomy can be completed.) Both kidneys and ureters should be carefully and gently mobilized and the ureters divided just above the bladder. The aorta and vena cava are ligated and divided distally, and the posterior lumbar branches are serially ligated with hemoclips. The proximal suprarenal aorta and vena cava are transected, and the kidneys are removed to a back table set up for trimming and separating the kidneys[12] (Fig. 31–3). When kidneys are taken from a donor, lymph nodes and spleen also should be taken for use in tissue typing and crossmatching. The kidneys are preserved in two ways. One method is to place them in a cold electrolyte solution known as Belzer's solution (Viaspan or UW solution). They are packaged individually and sterilely and placed on ice until transplanted (Fig. 31–4). The "life" of a kidney begins with the cross-clamping of the aorta. It is placed in ice and must be transplanted within a 40- to 48-hour period of cold ischemic time. On rare occasions, kidneys also may be preserved on a perfusion machine, which pumps cold oxygenated perfusate through the renal artery. Kidneys on the pump have a maximum "cold life" of 72 hours before transplantation (Table 31–5).

Cardiectomy

Cardiectomy (Fig. 31–5) is often performed with nephrectomy and hepatectomy. In these cases, it is imperative to understand the sequence of events to facilitate effective procurement of all organ recovery.

A standard median sternotomy incision is used.[12] The pericardium is opened vertically with a T inferiorly and suspended with suture laterally. The heart is inspected at this time for any evidence of damage or congenital anomaly. Once the surgeon is satisfied with the condition of the heart, the procedure continues. The ascending aorta is cleared

TABLE 31–4. SPECIAL EQUIPMENT NEEDED FOR ORGAN RECOVERY

HEART/LUNG	LIVER	KIDNEY	PANCREAS
10 liters cold saline Sternal saw Large chest retractors Sterile large basin Large vascular clamps	10 liters cold saline Sternal saw Large Balfour retractor Sterile large basin	Large Balfour retractor Vascular clamps Large Deaver retractor Sterile large basin	Large Balfour retractor Vascular clamps Deep retractors Sterile basin
2 large basins of ice, sterile Nonsterile ice	2 large basins of sterile ice Nonsterile ice	1 large basin of sterile ice Nonsterile ice	1 large basin of sterile ice Nonsterile ice

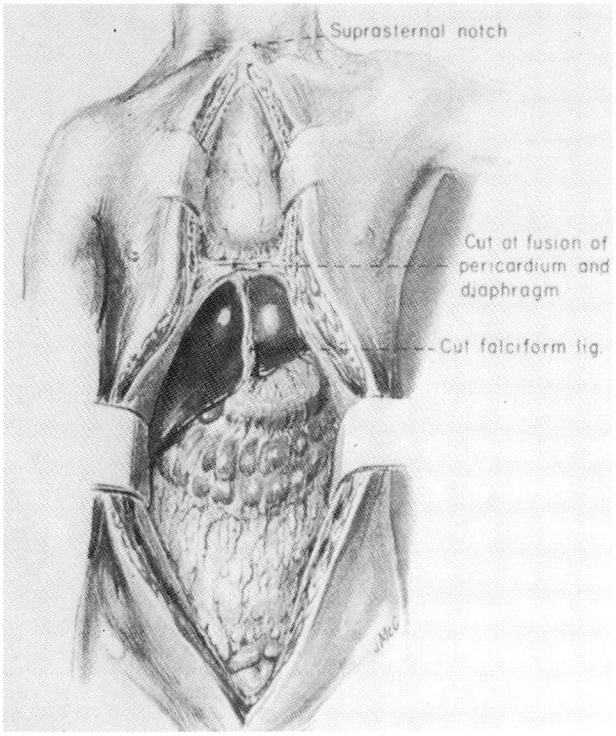

Figure 31–1. Incision used for multiple organ recovery. (From Starzl TE et al: A flexible procedure for multiple cadaveric organ procurement. Surg Gynecol Obstet 158:224, 1984.)

circumferentially and looped with an umbilical tape. The superior vena cava is then cleared circumferentially approximately 2.5 cm below the azygos vein. An umbilical loop is placed superiorly, and a suture loop is placed inferiorly. The inferior vena cava is cleared in the same manner from the pericardial reflection. Thirty thousand units of heparin are given in the superior vena cava, and the cardioplegia or flush solution is prepared. The flush is placed in a pressure bag with an extension tube to the patient. A 14-gauge short catheter is placed into the anterior surface of the ascending aorta. If a central line is in place, it will be removed at this time. Downward traction is now applied to the suture ligament of the superior vena cava while upward traction is applied to the intravenous catheter as it is clamped. The heart is allowed to empty partially, and the cold cardioplegia solution is infused. The distal ascending aorta is cross-clamped also. The pulmonary veins and the inferior vena cava are divided. The heart is then rinsed in situ with several liters of cold sterile saline as the cardioplegia solution is infusing. Once the solution has infused, the cardioplegia line is removed. The aorta is transected distally, and the superior vena cava and inferior vena cava are also completely transected. After the posterior pulmonary veins as well as the right and left pulmonary arteries are transected, the heart is ready to be removed.[12] It is placed in a basin of sterile iced saline and totally immersed. After a second rinsing, it is packaged in several intestinal bags with cold saline between each one and placed in a hard plastic container. It is then put in ice until it reaches its destination. Once the aorta is cross-clamped, the "life" of the heart begins (Table 31–5).

TABLE 31–5. PRESERVATION TIMES BETWEEN RETRIEVAL AND TRANSPLANT

ORGAN	TIME ALLOWED FOR COLD ISCHEMIA	STORAGE METHOD
Heart	<4 hours	On ice
Lung	<4 hours	On ice
Kidney	<48 hours	On ice
	<72 hours	On perfusion
Pancreas	<24 hours	On ice
Liver	<36 hours	On ice

Hepatectomy

To remove the liver, a standard midline incision is used (Fig. 31–6) in an approach similar to that in nephrectomy.[12] After the abdomen is open, the liver is inspected for color and texture and any sign of injury or anomaly. Provided the anatomy is normal, the left gastric and splenic arteries are ligated and divided, and a dissection of the celiac axis is

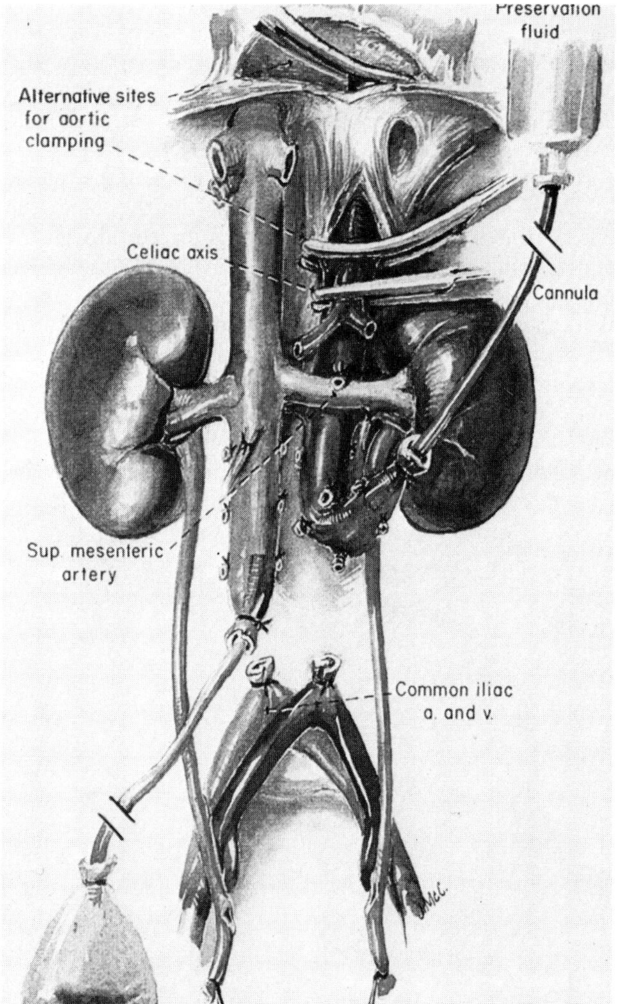

Figure 31–2. En bloc nephrectomy. (From Starzl TE et al: A flexible procedure for multiple cadaveric organ procurement. Surg Gynecol Obstet 158:225, 1984.)

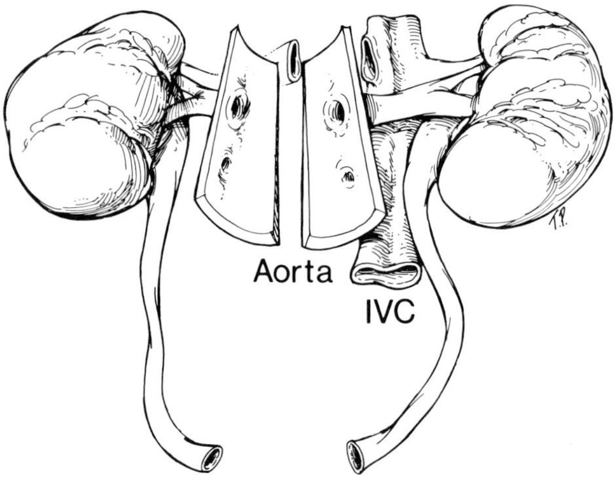

Figure 31–3. Kidneys are divided by splitting the aorta and vena cava.

done toward the aorta. A loop is placed around the aorta above the celiac axis. The gastroduodenal and, when present, the right gastric artery are ligated and divided. The portal vein is found beneath the gastroduodenal artery. The common bile duct is mobilized to as low a level as possible, and then it is transected. Simultaneously, an incision is made in the gallbladder, and care is taken to wash out all bile to prevent autolysis of the mucosa of the biliary tract. The portal vein is cleaned inferiorly to the junction of the splenic vein and the superior mesenteric vein. At this time, the splenic vein is ligated, and a catheter is placed through the central end. Belzer's solution at 4°C (39.2°F) is started through this catheter. The superior mesenteric vein is encircled, and the pancreas should be divided, if necessary, for exposure. The abdominal aorta (distal) and inferior vena cava are now freed and ligated. After systemic heparinization, cannulas are placed in the aorta and vena cava. The encircled superior mesenteric artery is tied, and this should be followed by ligature of the superior mesenteric vein. Donor circulation remains intact as the liver is cooling. Portal

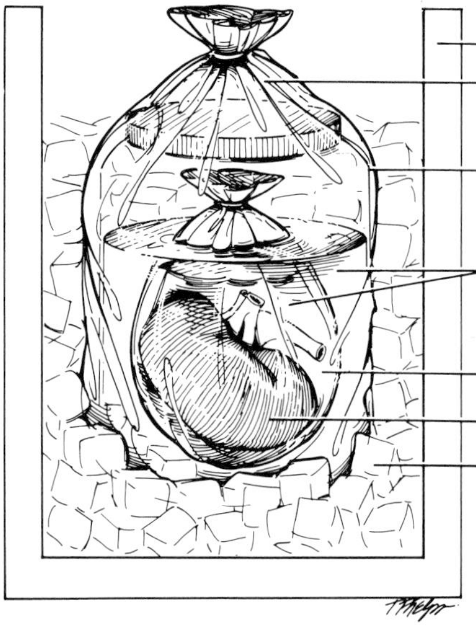

Figure 31–4. Organ transport box.

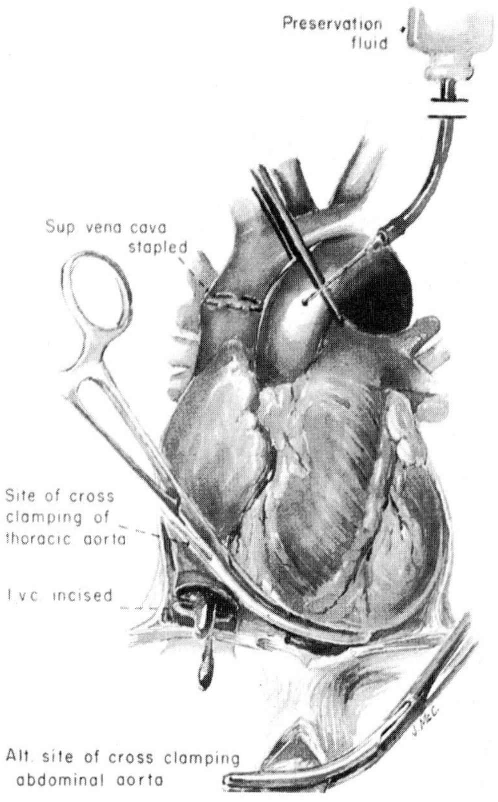

Figure 31–5. In situ flush of the heart. (From Starzl TE et al: A flexible procedure for multiple cadaveric organ procurement. Surg Gynecol Obstet 158:229, 1984.)

infusion with the Belzer's solution is stopped after 1 to 2 liters have been infused, and the aorta is cross-clamped. The kidneys, as well as the liver, are cleared of blood and are core cooled. The celiac axis is detached from the aorta with an aortic patch.

The suprahepatic vena cava is dissected along with the surrounding cuff of diaphragm. Now the liver is removed inferiorly, and the posterior structures are cut, including the right adrenal veins. Once removed, the liver is again flushed, and it is packaged in Belzer's solution and packed in ice until transported.[15] The cold ischemic time allowed for the liver is about 24 hours before it must be implanted.

Multiple organ donors are more frequent today than ever. Recent techniques allow procurement with optimal function of multiple grafts. There are many combinations of multiple organ recovery; the most common sequence is heart, liver, pancreas, and kidneys. With proper dissection and cannulation of these structures, it is possible to remove all, in that order, with minimal, if any, warm time for each individual graft.

ORGAN SHARING

The transplant coordinator notifies the surgeon once all the evaluations are finished and laboratory results are available to determine the suitability of the donor candidate.

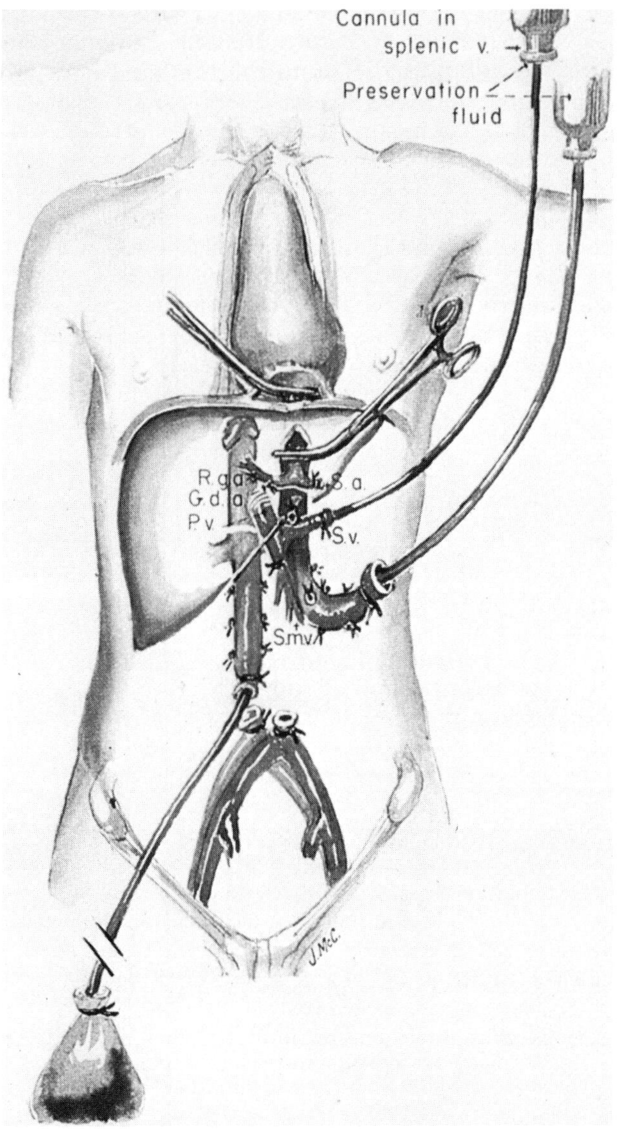

Figure 31–6. In situ flush of the liver. (From Starzl TE et al: A flexible procedure for multiple cadaveric organ procurement. Surg Gynecol Obstet 158:229, 1984.)

After evaluations are complete and the recipients have been located, the surgical team performs the procurement.

Multiple organ donor information, including age, weight, and blood type, is entered into a 24-hour computerized network, the United Network for Organ Sharing (UNOS) in Richmond, Virginia. A list of potential recipients is generated by a prioritized point system that determines those individuals best suited for the available organ. This enables procurement coordinators to know where the needs for specific organs are, as well as whom to contact. It is not unusual to have a heart and liver retrieval team arrive from two separate geographical areas. The lifetime of each organ (Table 31–5) is always considered when calling a retrieval team; there must be enough "cold ischemic time" to get the organ back and transplanted within that critical time frame. Much of the coordinator's time is allocated to scheduling the procurement teams and then placing the organs.

Although the nurse is not directly responsible for coordinating the transportation of these teams to and from their destination, she can expedite the departure of the procurement team by understanding the need for a well-planned organ recovery.

Choosing Recipients in Kidney Donation

The nationwide computer network, UNOS, is used for the matching process. Kidney matching is more complicated than for other organs and is therefore explained here in some detail.

Leukocyte Cross-Matching

Each potential kidney recipient has serum samples at the tissue typing laboratory that are individually mixed with the donor leukocytes. This is a cross-match. Its result ultimately determines whether the donor kidney is transplanted into the recipient. Each tissue typing laboratory is supplied with cross-match trays containing a high-antibody serum from highly sensitized patients at regional transplant centers. Any serum giving a positive cross-match indicates that the potential recipient has preformed antibodies against the specific donor and is therefore excluded from receiving a kidney from that donor.

The cross-matches on extrarenal recipients are usually done after the transplant if the recipient has not required multiple transfusions and thus has no preformed antibodies.

Human Leukocyte Antigen Testing

The other type of testing done to match a donor kidney with a recipient is human leukocyte antigen (HLA) testing.[13] This process is used to detect inherited antigenic determinants that are present on all surfaces of nucleated cells throughout the body and that participate in cellular recognition and rejection. The sources of cells used for the test are the lymph nodes, blood, and spleen. To identify the inherited tissue antigens, the lymphocytes are incubated with a panel of known antisera. The three main series of antigens (A, B, and DR) have over 30 such specifications. Since the lymphocytes of one individual usually have two A and two B series antigens, the matching between two persons can range from all four antigens in common to no antigens in common. The best match is when all six antigens are shared.

HLA-matching is one of the few predictors of long-term graft survival. The better the match, the better is the long-term outcome. Kidneys are frequently transplanted from one family member to another. This is known as *living related transplants*.

The time involved in the actual tissue typing process varies. Blood type O kidneys usually take 8 hours, whereas blood types A, B, and AB generally require 4 to 5 hours. After the antigens are identified from the donor, the information is entered into a computer. The computer will integrate this information and print out a list of compatible recipients. The recipients are sorted by blood group, degree of match, degree of presensitization, and location.

Extrarenal Organ Placement

As mentioned earlier, when a patient is referred, the procurement personnel contact the referral center and make an initial evaluation, including the donor's age, blood type, sex, and weight. UNOS matches extrarenal donors with recipients who are waiting. Recipients on the list are classified by the severity of their illness as determined by the transplant surgeons who have evaluated the recipient's medical condition. The heart, lung, and liver are not HLA-sensitive, unlike kidneys. Therefore, these former organs can be placed first. Pancreata are transplanted with a kidney for ease of surgical technique and highest rate of success.

These classifications apply to all extrarenal organ recipients and enable the coordinator to know which recipient is in urgent need of the donor organ. In addition to the recipient status, the transplant center's name and phone number are provided. Such information allows the coordinators on both ends to work out the logistics of the donation and transplant.

Organ Sharing

Organ sharing is essential in the field of transplantation. In the United States, tens of thousands of people are waiting for a transplant. With the help of organizations such as UNOS, organ procurement centers are able to find the best matches for organs in patients across the country. The computerized network for sharing has saved the lives of many who otherwise would have died waiting. The list of recipients grows daily, and with the limited number of donor organs available, there must be a mechanism by which the most seriously ill will be served first. The number of transplant centers in the United States continues to increase; in recent years, it has more than doubled. Almost every state has at least one transplant center. The number of active heart transplant centers has increased dramatically over the past few years. Heart, lung, liver, and pancreas transplants also are on the rise, with many centers now performing them.

When kidneys cannot be used in the United States, they are shared with other countries such as England, Canada, and Japan. Kidneys are only shared after the list for recipient matches has been exhausted in the United States. Centers in Canada also have shared extrarenal donors with the United States programs.

CONCLUSION

Clearly, there are difficulties, both physical and emotional, that confront the trauma nurse in the role she undertakes in the organ procurement process. One may well be confronted by feelings of helplessness and frustration from the stark fact that the patient for whom she has cared so attentively is dead. Her patient "didn't make it." And now she is being asked to exert possibly even more effort to maintain and monitor her dead patient so that the patient can "make it" in another, seemingly less tangible way. These very organs may be effectively preserved long enough to be transplanted in another unknown patient who desperately needs them to live or continue life more fully. From an altruistic point of view, such a transition may seem reasonable and worthwhile, but it may well take a conscious effort on the part of the trauma nurse to make such a rapid adjustment without any slippage of her professional attitude of vigilant caring. Such an adjustment can be made more easily if the nurse is confident of her knowledge and skills in the proper maintenance of organ donors. In effect, rather than "losing" a patient, she is now confronted with another professional and, in a sense, just as humanitarian a challenge: allowing a living patient the chance to "win." It is also valuable for the nurse to realize that donor families gain a sense of comfort by salvaging something positive from the tragedy.

The federal law governing required request, requires hospitals participating in Medicare and Medicaid to develop protocols to identify potential organ donors that

- Ensure that families of potential donors are made aware of the option of organ donation
- Encourage sensitivity with respect to the views and beliefs of the family
- Require that a certified procurement agency be notified of potential donors.

This law became effective in November 1987.[3] As of April 1988, hospitals must work with a certified procurement agency in order to receive their Medicare/Medicaid reimbursement for procurement costs.

Routine inquiry or required request ensures that families of all donor candidates are provided with the opportunity to make their own decision about donation rather than have the decision "made" for them because of a lack of information about their options. Donation also can provide families with a source of solace during their grief. Routine inquiry can increase the number of organs recovered while supporting the tradition of informed consent.

Things to look for in the future of organ and tissue transplantation may include

- Closer monitoring by JCAHO of which hospitals comply with the federal law for reimbursement purposes.
- The idea of incentives to donor families has been discussed and remains possible in the future.
- The improvement of public and professional education on a national level.
- A change in attitudes with regard to organ and tissue donation as more people are directly affected by their use.

As more medical centers across the country seek the necessary licensing to perform transplants, the pressure to find suitable donors will intensify. Thus the care given any potential organ donor in the trauma setting will become even more important. While the demand for transplantable organs will increase dramatically, the organ pool is not likely to expand nearly as rapidly. The organ procurement agencies are stepping up their efforts to create hospital development programs. These programs promote education and awareness of organ and tissue donation. Public education is increasingly altering family attitudes about donation. Families may now approach the health care team.

It is in the long run not so much the system, the physician, the organ procurement coordinator, or sometimes even the family that makes the difference between the possibility and the reality of a successful organ transplant. The trauma nurse is the consistent and most effective force in the care of the patient, in the support of the family, and in the successful maintenance of the donor. It is, then, the trauma nurse who fully can assure that the gift of life is not wasted.

The authors gratefully acknowledge Arthur C. Kurz, B.S., for his review and contributions to this chapter.

REFERENCES

1. McKenzie N: Cardiac transplantation. Transplantation Today 1:20–24, 1984.
2. Dossetor JB: Kidney transplantation: A medical perspective. Transplantation Today 1:28–30, 1984.
3. Required request legislation. 52 *FR* 147; 28666–77, July 31, 1987; and 53 *FR* 40; 6526–6551, March 1, 1988.
4. Stark JL, Reiley P, Osiecki A, et al: Attitudes affecting organ donation in the intensive care unit. Heart Lung 13:400–404, 1984.
5. Lewis JC, Miskosky PD: Organ procurement. JEMS 2:32–33, 1985.
6. Dixson WS: Corneal transplant. Transplantation Today 1:47–49, 1984.
7. Spence RJ: The banking and clinical use of human skin allograft in trauma patients: History. Maryland Med J 35:50–52, 1986.
8. Annotated Code of Maryland: Anatomical Gift Act, Article 43, Annapolis, 1974, p. 91.
9. Black PM, Zervas NT: Declaration of brain death in neurosurgical and neurological practice. Neurosurgery 15:170–174, 1984.
10. Maryland Post Mortem Examiners Commission: Maryland State Post Mortem Examiners Law and Regulations Governing Medical Examiner Cases. Annapolis, State of Maryland Department of Post Mortem Examiners, 1981, p 6.
11. Minkosky PD: Introduction to the Johns Hopkins Heart and Lung Donor Protocol. Unpublished manuscript, 1984.
12. Starzl TE, Hakala TR, Shaw BW, et al: A flexible procedure for multiple cadaveric organ procurement. Surg Gynecol Obstet 158:223–230, 1984.
13. Dausset J: The role of human leukocyte antigen (HLA) in transplantation. In Slavin S (ed): Bone Marrow and Organ Transplantation. New York, Elsevier, 1984, pp 1–12.
14. So SK, Simmons RL, Fryd DS, et al: Improved results of multiple renal transplantation in children. Surgery 98:729–738, 1985.
15. Task Force on Organ Transplantation: Organ Transplantation, Issues and Recommendations. U.S. Department of Health and Human Services, 1986, pp 2–7.

BIBLIOGRAPHY

Bartucci MR: Organ donation: A study of the donor family perspective. J Neurosci Nurs 10:305–309, 1987.

Batten HL, Prottas JH: Kind strangers: The families of organ donors. Health Affairs: 35–47, 1987.

Baumgartner WA, Reitz BA, Achuff SC: Heart and Heart-Lung Transplantation. Philadelphia, WB Saunders Co, 1990.

Bernat JL: Ethical and legal aspects of the emergency management of brain death and organ retrieval. Emerg Med Clin North Am 5:661–676, 1987.

Bidigow SA, Oermann MH: Attitudes and knowledge of nurses regarding organ procurement. Heart Lung 20:20–24, 1991.

Cate FH, Laudicina SS: Transplantation white paper. Prepared for the Annenberg Washington Program and the United Network for Organ Sharing, 1991.

Coolican MB: Healing by giving. Dialysis Transplant 19:239–240, 1990.

Covner AL, Shinn JA: Cardiopulmonary transplantation: Initial experience. Heart Lung 12:131–134, 1983.

Cowley RA, Dunham CM: Shock Trauma/Critical Care Manual. Baltimore, University Park Press, 1991.

Darby JM, Stein K, Grenvik A, Stuart S: Approach to management of the heartbeating "brain dead" organ donor. JAMA 261:2222–2228, 1989.

Definition of irreversible coma: Report of the Ad Hoc Committee of the Harvard Medical School to examine the definition of brain death. JAMA 205:85–88, 1968.

Evans RW: Organ donation: Facts and figures. Dialysis Transplant 19:234–237, 1990.

Evans RW, Orians CE, Ascher NL: The potential supply of organ donors: An assessment of the efficiency of organ procurement efforts in the United States. JAMA 267:239–246, 1992.

Fisher JC: Skin—The ultimate solution for the burn wound. N Engl J Med 311:466–467, 1984.

Garrison RN, Bentley FR, Rague GH, et al: There is an answer to the shortage of organ donors. Surgery Gynecol Obstet 173:391–396, 1991.

Gideon MD, Taylor PB: Kidney donation: Care of the cadaver donor's family. J Neurosurg Nurs 13:248–251, 1981.

Harwood CH, Cook CV: Cyclosporine in transplantation. Heart Lung 14:529–540, 1985.

Howard S: "How do I ask?" Requesting tissue or organ donations from bereaved families. Nursing: 70–73, 1989.

How other countries handle consent. Hastings Cent Rep 13:30, 1983.

Levey AS, Hou S, Bush HL: Kidney transplantation from unrelated living donors (editorial). N Engl J Med 314:914–916, 1986.

Machersic RC, Bronstiher OL, Shackford SR: Organ procurement in patients with fatal head injuries: The fate of the potential donor. Ann Surg 213:143–150, 1991.

Mair J, Artner-Dworzak E, Dienstl F, et al: Routine inquiry about organ donation: An alternative to presumed consent. N Engl J Med 325:1246–1250, 1991.

Movitsky D, Cooper C, Reichart B: Hemodynamic and metabolic responses to hormonal therapy in brain-dead potential organ donors. Transplant 43:852–854, 1987.

Nube MJ, Persijn GG, Kalff MW: Kidney transplantation, presensitization, and transplant survival. Dialysis Transplant 9:543–547, 1980.

Painvin GA, Frazier OH, Chandler LB, et al: Cardiac transplantation: Indications, procurement, operation and management. Heart Lung 14:484–489, 1985.

Pallis C: Brain stem death: The evolution of a concept. In Kidney Transplantation: Principles and Practice, 2nd ed. New York, Grune & Stratton, 1984, pp 101–127.

Peele A, Salvatierra O: Is routine inquiry the answer to solving the organ donor shortage? Contemp Dialysis Transplant 7(2):5–43, 1986.

Phillips M: Organ Procurement, Preservation and Distribution in Transplantation. Washington, DC, William Byrd Press, Inc, 1991.

Potter P: Making required request work. Nurs Management 19:50–58, 1988.

Prottas J, Batten HL: Health professionals and hospital administrators in organ procurement: Attitudes, reservations, and their resolutions. Am J Public Health 78:642–645, 1988.

Prottas JM, Batten HL: Neurosurgeons and the supply of human organs. Health Affairs: 120–130, 1989.

Roberts AJ: Organ transplantation. Surg Clin North Am 66:425–657, 1986.

Ropper AH: Unusual spontaneous movements in brain dead patients. Neurology 34:1089–1092, 1984.

Ropper AH, Kennedy SK, Russel L: Apnea testing in the diagnosis of brain death. J Neurosurg 55:942–946, 1981.

Slamenda MB: Brain death determination and management in children. Crit Care Nurs 3:63–66, 1983.

Spital A: The shortage of organs for transplantation: Where do we go from here? N Engl J Med 325:1243–1246, 1991.

Stuart FP, McKearn TJ, Fitch FW: Immunological enhancement of renal allografts by antireceptor antibody. Surgery 80:130–135, 1976.

Swerdlow JL: Matching Needs, Saving Lives. Prepared for the Anneberg Washington Program, 1989.

Toledo-Pereyra LH: Complications of Organ Transplantation. New York, Marcel Dekker, 1987.
Tolle SW, Bennett WM, Hickam DH, et al: Responsibilities of primary physicians in organ donation. Ann Intern Med 106:740–744, 1987.
Weber P: The human connection: The role of the nurse in organ donation. J Neurosci Nurs 17(2):119–122, 1985.
Youngrer SJ, Landefield S, Counton CJ, et al: Brain death and organ retrieval: A cross-sectional survey of knowledge and concepts among health professionals. JAMA 261:2205–2210, 1989.

Appendix 1–1. Hospital Criteria for Trauma Center Designation

The following table shows levels of categorization and their essential (E) or desirable (D) characteristics.

	LEVELS I	LEVELS II	LEVELS III
A. HOSPITAL ORGANIZATION			
1. Trauma Service	E	E	D
2. Surgery Departments/Divisions/Services/Sections			
Cardiothoracic Surgery	E	D	—
General Surgery	E	E	E
Neurologic Surgery	E	E	—
Ophthalmic Surgery	E	D	—
Oral Surgery—Dental	E	D	—
Orthopaedic Surgery	E	E	—
Otorhinolaryngologic Surgery	E	D	—
Plastic and Maxillofacial Surgery	E	D	—
Urologic Surgery	E	D	—
3. Emergency Department/Division/Service/Section[1]	E	E	E
4. Surgical Specialties Availability			
General Surgery	E[2]	E[2]	—
Neurologic Surgery	E[3]	E[3]	—
Orthopaedic Surgery	E[4]	E[4]	—
On call and promptly available from inside or outside the hospital:[5]			
Cardiac Surgery	E	D	—
General Surgery	—	—	E[6]
Neurologic Surgery	—	—	D
Microsurgery Capabilities	E	D	—
Hand Surgery	E	D	—
Obstetric/Gynecologic Surgery	E	D	—
Ophthalmic Surgery	E	E	D
Oral Surgery (dental)	E	D	—
Orthopaedic Surgery	—	—	D
Otorhinolaryngologic Surgery	E	E	D
Pediatric Surgery	E	D	—
Thoracic Surgery	E	E	D
Urologic Surgery	E	E	D
5. Nonsurgical Specialties Availability			
In-house 24 hours a day:			
Emergency Medicine	E[7]	E[7]	E[10]
Anesthesiology	E[8]	E[8, 9]	—
On call and promptly available from inside or outside the hospital:			
Anesthesiology	—	—	E
Cardiology	E	E	D
Chest Medicine	E	D	—
Family Medicine	D[11]	D[11]	D[11]
Gastroenterology	E	D	—
Hematology	E	E	D
Infectious Diseases	E	D	—
Internal Medicine	E[11]	E[11]	E[11]
Nephrology	E	E	D
Pathology	E	E	D
Pediatrics	E[11, 12]	E[11, 12]	E[11, 12]
Psychiatry	E	D	—
Radiology	E	E	D
B. SPECIAL FACILITIES/RESOURCES/CAPABILITIES			
1. Emergency Department (ED)			
a. Personnel			
1. Designated physician director	E	E	E
2. Physician who has special competence in care of critically injured and who is a designated member of the trauma team and is physically present in the ED 24 hours a day	E	E	E
3. A sufficient number of RNs, LPNs, and nurses aides to handle caseload	E	E	E
b. Equipment for resuscitation and to provide life support for the critically or seriously injured shall include but not be limited to:			
1. Airway control and ventilation equipment including laryngoscopes and endotracheal tubes of all sizes, bag-mask resuscitator, pocket masks, oxygen, and mechanical ventilator	E	E	E
2. Suction devices	E	E	E
3. Electrocardiograph-oscilloscope-defibrillator	E	E	E
4. Apparatus to establish central venous pressure monitoring	E	E	E
5. All standard intravenous fluids and administration devices, including intravenous catheters	E	E	E
6. Sterile surgical sets for procedures standard for ED, for example, thoracostomy, venesection, lavage	E	E	E
7. Gastric lavage equipment	E	E	E

Appendix 1–1. Hospital Criteria for Trauma Center Designation *Continued*

	LEVELS I	II	III
B. SPECIAL FACILITIES/RESOURCES/CAPABILITIES *Continued*			
8. Drugs and supplies necessary for emergency care	E	E	E
9. X-ray capability, 24-hour coverage by in-house technician	E	E	D
10. Two-way radio linked with vehicles of emergency transport system	E	E	E
11. Skeletal traction device for cervical injuries	E	E	E
12. Swan-Ganz catheters	E	D	D
13. Arterial catheters	E	D	D
14. Thermal control equipment			
a. for patient	E	E	E
b. for blood and fluids	E	E	E
2. Operating suite			
a. Personnel			
Operating room adequately staffed in house and immediately available 24 hours a day	E	E	D
b. Equipment: special requirements shall include but not be limited to:			
1. Cardiopulmonary bypass capability	E	D	—
2. Operating microscope	E	D	—
3. Thermal control equipment:			
a. for patient	E	E	E
b. for blood and fluids	E	E	E
4. X-ray capability including c-arm image intensifier with technologist available 24 hours a day	E	E	D
5. Endoscopes, all varieties	E	E	E
6. Craniotome	E	E	D
7. Monitoring equipment	E	E	E
3. Postanesthetic recovery room (surgical intensive care unit is acceptable)			
a. Registered nurses and other essential personnel 24 hours a day	E	E	E
b. Appropriate monitoring and resuscitation equipment	E	E	E
4. Intensive care units (ICUs) for trauma patients			
a. Personnel			
1. Designated surgical director	E	E	E
2. Surgeon, credentialed in critical care by the trauma director, on duty in ICU 24 hours a day or immediately available in hospital	E	E	D
3. Minimum nurse-patient ratio of 1:2 on each shift	E	E	E
b. Equipment			
Appropriate monitoring and resuscitation equipment	E	E	E
c. Support services			
Immediate access to clinical diagnostic services	E[13]	E[13]	E
5. Acute hemodyalysis capability	E	D	D
6. Organized burn care	E	E	E
a. Physician-directed burn center staffed by nursing personnel trained in burn care and equipped properly for care of the extensively burned patient OR			
b. Transfer agreement with nearby burn center or hospital with a burn unit			
7. Acute spinal cord/head injury management capability	E	E	E
a. In circumstances in which a designated spinal cord injury rehabilitation center exists in the region, early transfer should be considered; transfer agreements should be in effect			
b. In circumstances in which a head injury center exists in the region, transfer should be considered in selected patients; transfer agreements should be in effect			
8. Radiological special capabilities			
a. Angiography of all types	E	E	D
b. Sonography	E	D	D
c. Nuclear scanning	E	D	D
d. Computed tomography	E	E	D
e. In-house CT technician 24 hours	E	D	D
f. Neuroradiology	E	D	—
9. Rehabilitation medicine			
a. Physician-directed rehabilitation and service staffed by personnel trained in rehabilitation care and equipped properly for care of the critically injured patient, OR	E	—	—
b. Transfer agreement when medically feasible to a nearby rehabilitation service	—	E	E
10. Clinical laboratory service (available 24 hours a day)			
a. Standard analyses of blood, urine, and other body fluids	E	E	E
b. Blood typing and cross-matching	E	E	E
c. Coagulation studies	E	E	E
d. Comprehensive blood bank or access to a community central blood bank and adequate hospital storage facilities	E	E	E
e. Blood gas levels and pH determinations	E	E	E
f. Serum and urine osmolality	E	E	D
g. Microbiology	E	E	E
h. Drug and alcohol screening	E	E	D[14]

Appendix 1–1. Hospital Criteria for Trauma Center Designation *Continued*

	LEVELS I	II	III
C. QUALITY ASSURANCE			
1. Organized quality assurance programs	E	E	E
2. Special audit for all trauma deaths and other specified cases	E	E	E
3. Morbidity and mortality review	E	E	E
4. Trauma conference, multidisciplinary	E[15]	E[15]	D[15]
5. Medical nursing audit, utilization review, tissue review	E	E	E
6. Trauma registry	E[16]	E[16]	E[16]
7. Review of prehospital and regional systems of trauma care	E	D	D
8. Published on-call schedule must be maintained for surgeons, neurosurgeons, orthopaedic surgeons, and other major specialists	E	E	E
9. Times of and reasons for bypass must be documented and reviewed by quality assurance program	E	E	E
10. Quality assurance personnel—dedicated to and specific for the trauma program	E	E	D
D. OUTREACH PROGRAM			
Telephone and on-site consultations with physicians of the community and outlying areas	E	D	—
E. PUBLIC EDUCATION			
Injury prevention in the home and industry and on the highways and athletic fields; standard first-aid; problems confronting the public, medical profession, and hospitals regarding optimal care for the injured	E	E	D
F. TRAUMA RESEARCH PROGRAM	E	D	D
G. TRAINING PROGRAM			
1. Formal programs in continuing education provided by hospital for:			
a. Staff physicians	E	E	D
b. Nurses	E	E	E
c. Allied health personnel	E	E	E
d. Community physicians	E	E	D
H. TRAUMA SERVICE SUPPORT PERSONNEL			
Trauma coordinator	E	E	D

[1]The emergency department staff should ensure immediate and appropriate care for the trauma patient. The emergency department physician should function as a designated member of the trauma team. The relationship between emergency department physicians and other participants of the trauma team must be established on an individual hospital basis, consistent with resources but adhering to established standards that ensure optimal care.

[2]Evaluation and treatment may be started by a team of surgeons that will include, at minimum, a PGY 4 or senior general surgical resident who is a member of that hospital's surgical residency program. The trauma attending surgeon's participation in major therapeutic decisions and presence at operative procedures are mandatory and must be monitored by the hospital's trauma quality assurance program.

[3]An attending neurosurgeon must be promptly available and dedicated to that hospital's trauma service. The in-house requirement may be fulfilled by an in-house neurosurgeon or surgeon who has special competence, as judged by the chief of neurosurgery, in the care of patients with neural trauma, and who is capable of initiating measures directed toward stabilizing the patient as well as initiating diagnostic procedures.

[4]An attending orthopaedic surgeon must be promptly available and dedicated to that hospital's trauma service. The in-house requirement may be fulfilled by an in-house orthopaedic surgeon or a surgeon who has special competence, as judged by the chief of orthopaedic surgery, in the care of patients with orthopaedic trauma, and who is capable of initiating measures directed toward stabilizing the patient as well as initiating diagnostic procedures.

[5]The staff specialists on call will be immediately advised and will be promptly available. This capability will be continuously monitored by the trauma quality assurance program.

[6]Communication should be such that the general surgeon will be present in the emergency department at the time of arrival of the trauma patient.

[7]In Level I and Level II institutions, requirements may be fulfilled by emergency medicine chief residents capable of assessing emergency situations in trauma patients and providing any indicated treatment. When chief residents are used to fulfill availability requirements, the staff specialist on call will be advised and be promptly available.

[8]Requirements may be fulfilled by anesthesiology chief residents who are capable of assessing emergent situations in trauma patients and of providing any indicated treatment, including initiation of surgical anesthesia. When anesthesiology chief residents are used to fulfill availability requirements, the staff anesthesiologist on call will be advised and be promptly available.

[9]Requirements may be fulfilled when local conditions assure that the staff anesthesiologist will be in the hospital at the time of or shortly after the patient's arrival. During the interim period, prior to the arrival of the staff anesthesiologist, a certified nurse anesthetist (CRNA) capable of assessing emergent situations in trauma patients and of initiating and providing any indicated treatment will be available.

[10]This requirement may be fulfilled by a physician who is credentialed by the hospital to provide emergency medical services.

[11]The patient's primary care physician should be notified at an appropriate time.

[12]The pediatrician is not required in a system that has a designated pediatric trauma center to which all patients are taken.

[13]Blood gas measurements, hematocrit level, and chest x-ray studies should be available within 30 minutes of request. This capability will be continuously monitored by the quality assurance program.

[14]Toxicology screens need not be immediately available but are desirable. If available, results should be included in all quality assurance reviews.

[15]Regular and periodic multidisciplinary trauma conferences that include all members of the trauma team should be held. These conferences will be for the purpose of quality assurance through critiques of individual cases.

[16]Documentation will be made of severity of injury (by trauma score, age, ISS) and outcome (survival, length of stay, ICU length of stay), with monthly review of statistics.

From Committee on Trauma, American College of Surgeons: Resources for Optimal Care of the Injured Patient. Chicago, American College of Surgeons, 1990.

Appendix 6–1. Master Care Plan for Spinal Cord Injury (SCI)

DATE STARTED	NURSING DIAGNOSIS/GOALS	DATE RESOLVED	NURSING INTERVENTIONS	DATE DISCON-TINUED	EVALUATION
	Potential for changes in sensory and motor function related to disruptions in skeletal integrity and spinal cord edema secondary to SCI. STG: Patient will maintain or improve present neurological status as evidenced by spinal cord sensory/motor assessment ______.		Baseline sensory/motor levels (per neurosurgery). Monitor NSDOs q ______. Maintain adequate cervical/body alignment. Head of bed flat at all times (per order) Reverse Trendelenburg position for head of bed elevation (per order). Log roll only. Philadelphia collar at all times (per order). Cervical traction: check bolts/pins q4° ______. *Monitor weights: Number of lbs. Maintain head in neutral position along axis with cervical alignment. Weights to be hanging freely *at all times.* Traction knot should be 1 to 2 inches from pulley at all times in order to maintain adequate traction. Stryker frame (turn q2°) unless otherwise ordered: Monitor body alignment on frames. To pull patient down on frame, he must be supine only. Three people needed (one person to place one hand on rope to weights, the other hand on stabilization device) in order to guide weights and maintain traction. Pull down patient with one fluid motion. *Never* pull patient up on a Stryker frame. Turn slowly to avoid orthostatic hypotensive episodes (rapid drop in heart rate). Avoid hyperflexion/extension by using padded chin/forehead straps at all times. Specific measures (per order neurosurgery) for flexion/extension: Immobilization device Check bolts q4°. Wrench attached at all times.		
	Potential for decreased cardiac output, retained secretions, venous stasis, contractures, skin breakdown, impaction, urinary retention related to immobility, and sympathetic disruption secondary to SCI. STG: Patient will maintain cardiac output > 4 liters as evidenced by ______ cardiac output readings ______.		Monitor for vasovagal responses: Report sudden episodes of bradycardia especially when associated with hypotension (e.g., spinal shock). Follow trends in hemodynamic parameters (e.g., CO, CVP, PAW, SVR). Note: Sympathetic paralysis often leads to fluid overload.		

Appendix 6–1. Master Care Plan for Spinal Cord Injury (SCI) *Continued*

DATE STARTED	NURSING DIAGNOSIS/GOALS	DATE RESOLVED	NURSING INTERVENTIONS	DATE DISCON-TINUED	EVALUATION
	STG: Patient will maintain heart rate > 50 as evidenced by monitored pulse rate ____.		Keep IV atropine at bedside.		
			Record activity at time of decreased heart rate.		
			Hyperoxygenate prior to suctioning.		
			Monitor closely during suctioning (15 to 30 seconds only) for signs and symptoms of vagal response.		
	STG: Patient will be free of retained secretions as evidenced by clear CXR, $Pa_{O_2} > 70$, $Pa_{CO_2} < 50$ ____________.		CPT q ____________.		
			Trendelenburg position (when placing patient be sure weights hang freely).		
			Monitor type of breathing (abdominal or diaphragmatic).		
			Abdominal binder.		
			Avoid abdominal distention.		
			Monitor respiratory parameters (CXR, ABGs, breath sounds).		
			Maintain normothermia.		
			Incentive spirometer.		
			Cough and deep breath (may need assistive coughing with impaired diaphragmatic excursion).		
	STG: Patient will be free of venous stasis as shown by unchanging calf/thigh measurements, absence of unusual warmth, redness or induration of extremities, and absence of calf pain ____________.		Calf/thigh measurements q ________.		
			Teds/Ace wraps: Remove q ________ with skin assessment.		
			Avoid prolonged pressure/rubbing of extremities.		
			Circulation checks q ____________		
	STG: Patient will remain free of skin breakdown ____________.		Skin care (per routine) q ________.		
			Philadelphia collar: (may use alcohol to clean).		
			Monitor chin, earlobes, occipital area for redness, and signs and symptoms of breakdown.		
			To remove collar:		
			Patient flat in bed (supine).		
			Remove front of collar (immobilizing head/neck).		
			Replace front of collar.		
			Remove back of collar (two people). One person stabilizes head/neck by placing one hand on front of collar and the other hand and arm along the patient's neck to back.		

Appendix 6–1. Master Care Plan for Spinal Cord Injury (SCI) *Continued*

DATE STARTED	NURSING DIAGNOSIS/GOALS	DATE RESOLVED	NURSING INTERVENTIONS	DATE DISCON-TINUED	EVALUATION
	STG: Patient will retain full range of motion of all extremities ____________.		Range of motion q ____________		
			Activity: OOB (order by physician) .		
			Type of chair: ____________.		
			Tolerance time OOB: ____________		
			Shift weight q15 minutes.		
			Method of transfer: ____________		
			Sitting program in conjunction with physical therapy: ____________.		
			Teds/Ace wraps.		
			Abdominal binder.		
			Gradual head elevation.		
			Monitor blood pressure (signs and symptoms of hypotension).		
	STG: Patient will have bowel movement QOD ____________.		Check for impaction qd ____________.		
			Initiate bowel regimen.		
	STG: Patient will remain free of impaction qd. ____________.				
	STG: Patient will remain free of urinary retention ____________.		Strict input and output records.		
	STG: Patient will remain free of urinary tract infection ____________.		Fluid restriction (per order).		
			Intermittent catheterization program: (if urinary output > 500 ml when patient is catheterized, notify physician).		
			Catheterize q ____________.		
			Monitor urine cultures, urinalysis, appearance of urine.		
			Chart erections in males.		
	Potential for prolonged frustration and feeling of powerlessness related to dependency and lack of control of environment secondary to SCI.		Activities of daily living.		
			Assisted:		
			Unassisted:		
	STG: Patient will participate in activities of daily living as appropriate for patient's neurological deficit level as documented in nurse's notes ____________.		Consults:		
	STG: Patient will communicate feelings of control and decreasing frustration as evidenced by written or verbal statements ____________, participation in treatment regimen ____________, and increasing tolerance of obstacles to activities of daily living ____________		*Daily schedule (asterisk means patient may choose time sequence of activity).		
			Encourage patient to assist to fullest potential.		
			Remember independence through rehabilitation is ultimate goal.		
			Remember to answer all questions honestly with patient.		
			Specific psychological interventions:		

Reference Books
1. Goldberg, S: Clinical Neuro Anatomy Made Ridiculously Simple. Miami, Medmaster, Inc, 1979.
2. Hanak M, Scott A: Spinal Cord Injury, An Illustrated Guide for Health Care Professionals. New York, Springer Publishing Co, 1983.
3. Mason D: Neurologic Critical Care. New York, Litton Education Publ Inc, 1979.
4. Nikas DL: The Critically Ill Neurosurgical Patient. New York, Churchill Livingstone, 1982.

Appendix 6–2. Critical Pathway for Acute Cervical Spinal Cord Injury

Admission
↓

NURSING DIAGNOSIS: Alteration in neurological function
DESIRED OUTCOME: No further loss in neurological function.
Steroids ⟶
SCI assessment every 8 hours and prn ⟶ till stable ⟶ every 24 hours
Maintain osmolarity at or > normal ⟶
Maintain _____ lb traction on _____/ Surgical fixation Date: _____ Surg _____ ⟶ fit for braces ⟶ OT consult
_____/ Somatosensory evoked potential
Bedrest ⟶ ↑ HOB 30° _____ 60° _____ 90° _____ ⟶ OOB to chair; Mtn brace

NURSING DIAGNOSIS: Alteration in tissue perfusion.
DESIRED OUTCOME: Will monitor systemic BP to enable adequate tissue perfusion.
VS every 1 hour ⟶ VS every 2 hours ⟶ VS every 4 hours
Hemodynamic push MABP ≥ 75 mm Hg ⟶
Atropine kept at bedside ⟶
Avoid rapid position changes ⟶
/Spinal Shock resolved ⟶ Observe for autonomic dysreflexia →
Provide patient/family teaching
/ace wraps; √ abdominal binder to maintain BP when OOB

Admission
↓

NURSING DIAGNOSIS: Impaired gas exchange.
DESIRED OUTCOME: Maintain adequate gas exchange.
Maintain on ventilator support _____/wean from vent ⟶
CPT every _____ hours _____/_____ Incentive spirometer every _____ hour(s); quad cough
Initiation PT consult

NURSING DIAGNOSIS: Alteration in bowel and urinary elimination.
DESIRED OUTCOME: Patient will have adequate bowel/bladder elimination.
Initiate bowel regimen: _____
Foley to straight drainage _____/able to PO restrict _____ cc/day
every _____ hour(s) intermittent cath

NURSING DIAGNOSIS: Self-care deficit.
DESIRED OUTCOME: Patient discharged to Rehab Center.
Instruct family on patient injuries _____/family conference to plan rehabilitation ⟶ (transfer to SA-PN report to SA nurse)
⟶ continue to discuss rehabilitation with patient & family ⟶ medically cleared
⟶ transfer to _____
Initiate family service consult

Admission
↓

NURSING DIAGNOSIS: Ineffective coping: Individual/Family.
DESIRED OUTCOME: Patient will cope appropriately with injury.
Inform patient of actions ⟶ formulate a schedule with patient
limit setting: _____ ⟶
Speech consult for alternative communication ⟶ Instruct patient/family at SCI hotline and other resources available.
Neuropsych Evaluation Consult

NURSING DIAGNOSIS: Impaired physical mobility.
DESIRED OUTCOME: Skin will remain intact.
Turn every 2 hours ⟶
/OOB every _____ hours for _____ minutes ⟶
√ chair cushion _____
/Transfer technique _____
Type of mattress
DESIRED OUTCOME: Deep vein thrombosis will be prevented.
Venodynes ⟶
DESIRED OUTCOME: Patient will not develop contractures.
ROM every _____ hour(s)
Splints to _____
Remove splints _____

Appendix 6–2. Critical Pathway for Acute Cervical Spinal Cord Injury *Continued*

Cervical Spinal Cord Injury (Nursing Documentation Component)

DIAGNOSIS	OUTCOME GOALS	PROJECTED DATE OR DAYS	TREATMENT PLAN		DATE D/C	EVALUATION/ REVISION
Alteration, neurological function	Maintain or improve neurological function	Day 1	Steroid start	_____		
			D/C	_____		
		Day 1	SCI assessment:			
			q 4 × 24 till stable	_____		
			then q 8	_____		
			q 24	_____		
			q week	_____		
		Day 1	Cervical stability:			
			traction _____ lbs			
			device _____			
			Halo _____			
			tongs _____			
		Day 1	Type of Bed:			
			Stryker	_____		
			Rotorest	_____		
			TxBoard	_____		
			Regular Bed	_____		
		Day 1	Initiate OT/PT/ Speech consult			
			Brace	_____		
			type			
			Collar	_____		
			Halo vest	_____		
		Day 1–7	Surgically fixated	_____		
			Bed rest	_____		
			HOB ↑ 30	_____		
			60	_____		
			90	_____		
			OOB	_____		
		Day 1–3	Initiate/evoke potentials			
		Day 1–D/C	*Diagnostic studies*			
			MRI	_____		
			CT myelogram	_____		
			Tomogram	_____		
			Flexion/extension	_____		
Alteration in tissue perfusion	Monitor systemic BP to enable adequate tissue perfusion	Day 1–5	VS q 1°	_____		
			VS q 2°	_____		
			VS q 4°	_____		
			VS q 8°	_____		
		Day 1–5	Hemodynamic push			
			start _____ D/C'd _____			
			MAP > _____			
			Atropine at bedside			
			Avoid sudden increase in position changes			
		Day 1–D/C	Maintain normovolemia			
		Day 1	Monitor sign/sym.			
			Spinal shock			
			Labs unstable	_____		
			stable	_____		
			other	_____		
			Monitor signs/sym.	_____		
			for vasovagal response			
		Day 5–D/C	Observe for autonomic dysreflexia			
			Pt/family teaching			
		Day 1	Measure calf/thighs			
			q 8° × 72° then q day	_____		
		Day 1	Venodynes _____			

Appendix 6–2. Critical Pathway for Acute Cervical Spinal Cord Injury *Continued*

Cervical Spinal Cord Injury (Nursing Documentation Component) *Continued*

DIAGNOSIS	OUTCOME GOALS	PROJECTED DATE OR DAYS	TREATMENT PLAN	DATE D/C	EVALUATION/ REVISION
Impaired gas exchange	Maintain adequate gas exchange	Day 1	Airway management: natural ______ endotracheal tube ______ tracheostomy ______ O_2 therapy: ventilator ______ mask/cannula ______ room air ______ other ______		
		Day 1	Weaning program CPT q 2 ______ q 4 ______ IS q 2 ______ q 4 ______ quadcough ______		
Alteration in bowel/ bladder elimination	Maintain adequate bowel/bladder elimination	Day 1	Check impaction q day ______		
		Day 1	Bowel regimen ______ Check abdominal distention ______		
		Day 5	Foley ______ Fluid restriction 2400 ml/day ______ ___ cath. q 4 hr ______ q 6 hr ______		
Impaired physical mobility		Day 1	Initiate antacid regimen		
	Skin will remain intact	Day 1	Skin intact yes ______ no ______ Monitor sacrum and bony prominences for breakdown		
		Day 5–D/C	Sitting program in conjunction with PT transfer method ______ chair ______ cushion ______ tolerance time ______		
	Maintain full ROM of extremities		Teds/leg wraps ______ Abdominal binder ______ OT splints ______		
Ineffective Pt/family coping	Pt/family will experience ______ feelings of dependency, frustration, powerlessness	Day 1	Explain procedures ______ Develop schedule with patient ______ Family participation in care ______		
		Day 1	Initiate Family Services consult ______		

Appendix 6–3. Trauma Outcome Guide: Critical Care

	PROBLEMS/ NEEDS	OUTCOMES	INITIAL ASSESSMENT	ADMISSION DAY 1	DAY 2
Respiratory	Airway	1. Patent airway 2. Airway maintained independently or by tracheostomy 3. Suctioning/airway clearance measures <q2h	Nonintubated	Assess for: airway obstruction resp failure ↑ workload of breathing/ fatigue Acute change: ______ Chest assessment RR effort q ___ BS Assess ability to clear secretions	⟶ Acute change: ______ Chest assessment q ___ (↑ freq w/resp distr) ⟶
			Intubated	Appropriate tube size Assess tube security Pre/post hyperinflation w/suctioning	Extubation plan ___ (Assess extubation criteria daily) ⟶ ⟶ ⟶
			NT ___ R ___ L ___ Size	Assess nasal drainage for signs of infection and/or pressure necrosis q4h	NT removal plan ______
			OT ___ cm lip ___ size	Assess: ET position (BS, cm lip) -tube security -lip/mucosal necrosis Change tube to opposite side q24h (if not contraindicated)	⟶ ⟶ ⟶ ⟶

Appendix 6–3. Trauma Outcome Guide: Critical Care *Continued*

Day 3	Day 4	Day 5	Day 6	Day 7
⟶ Acute change ______ Chest assessment q ______ ⟶	⟶ Acute change ______ Chest assessment q ______ ⟶	⟶ Acute change ______ Chest assessment q ______ ⟶	⟶ Acute change ______ Chest assessment q ______ ⟶	⟶ Acute change ______ Chest assessment q ______ ⟶
Extubation plan ______ ⟶ ⟶ ⟶	Extubation plan ______ ⟶ ⟶ ⟶	Extubation plan ______ ⟶ ⟶ ⟶	Extubation plan ______ ⟶ ⟶ ⟶	Consider trach if nonneuro, vent supported pt unable to initiate weaning or fails weaning attempts ⟶ ⟶ ⟶
Consider elective reintubation to OT or trach: ______				
⟶ ⟶ ⟶ ⟶ Consider trach if GCS<8	⟶ ⟶ ⟶ ⟶ Trach plan ______	⟶ ⟶ ⟶ ⟶ Trach plan ______	⟶ ⟶ ⟶ ⟶ Trach plan ______	⟶ ⟶ ⟶ ⟶ Trach plan ______

KEY:

⟶ = Same outcome as previous column

Appendix 6–3. Trauma Outcome Guide: Critical Care *Continued*

	PROBLEMS/ NEEDS	OUTCOMES	INITIAL ASSESSMENT	ADMISSION DAY 1	DAY 2
Respiratory	Breathing	1. Oxygenation & ventilation needs met by effective breathing pattern w/ or w/o supplemental O_2 *$SpO_2 \geq 91\%$ of $FIO_2 \leq 0.6$ *Respiratory status stable for 12 hr w/o mechanical ventilation or CPAP *Stabilization of ABGs for 12 hr prior to transfer *Clinical or radiological evidence of improvement –clearing lungs –improving breath sounds –improving vital capacity		Continuous SpO_2 (transport w/ oximetry if intubated) Titrate FIO_2 to achieve $SpO_2 > 0.91$ HOB 30° if not contraindicated ABG at 6 AM q AM	Reassess need q shift ⟶ ⟶ Reassess need daily Chest x-ray 6 AM "R/O Atelectasis" (Daily if intubated)
			Nonintubated	IS q1h while awake & w/VS at night. Volume & attempts recorded	IS: Avg volume ___ Avg # attempts ___
			Intubated	<u>Initial Vent Orders:</u> mode: SIMV f: 12 (unless head inj) TV: 15 cc/kg PEEP: 5 cm PS: 5 FIO_2: 1.0 Lowest flow rate to support work of breathing Avoid RR >14 if possible	<u>Daily Vent Mgt Plan:</u> mode: ___ f: ___ TV: ___ wt: ___ PEEP: ___ PS: ___ FIO_2: ___ desired pCO_2: ___ Flow rate: ___ Sens: ___ Peak pressure: ___ Wean by: ___
				Initial ABG in 30 min, repeat ABG for any change in TV or rate Oximeter to monitor FIO_2 changes	⟶ ⟶
				<u>Vent Adjustments:</u> $FIO_2 > 0.50$: ↑ PEEP 2.5–5.0 cm q30m Desired pCO_2: adjust rate to achieve (target rate = present pCO_2/ desired pCO_2 × present rate) ↑ resp distress and/or ↑ WOB: ↑ flow rate or sensitivity Change to CMV/AC Change to PB7200 ↑ PS to 20 cm (PB7200) ? sedation/ paralysis at higher rate if all above fails	Review Vent needs q4h or w/ clinical changes Sedation: ___ NMB: ___ (Assess pt response & need for dosage change)

Appendix 6–3. Trauma Outcome Guide: Critical Care *Continued*

Day 3	Day 4	Day 5	Day 6	Day 7
→	→	→	→	→
→	→	→	→	→
→	→	→	→	→
→	→	→	→	→
Reassess daily need	→	→	→	→
IS: Avg volume ______ Avg # attempts ______	IS: Avg volume ______ Avg # attempts ______	IS: Avg volume ______ Avg # attempts ______	IS: Avg volume ______ Avg # attempts ______	IS: Avg volume ______ Avg # attempts ______
Daily Vent Mgt Plan: mode: ______ f: ______ TV: ______ PEEP: ______ PS: ______ FIO_2: ______ desired pCO_2: ______ Flow rate: ______ Sens: ______ Peak pressure: ______ Wean By: ______	Daily Vent Mgt Plan: mode: ______ f: ______ TV: ______ PEEP: ______ PS: ______ FIO_2: ______ desired pCO_2: ______ Flow rate: ______ Sens: ______ Peak pressure: ______ Wean By: ______	Daily Vent Mgt Plan: mode: ______ f: ______ TV: ______ PEEP: ______ PS: ______ FIO_2: ______ desired pCO_2: ______ Flow rate: ______ Sens: ______ Peak pressure: ______ Wean By: ______	Daily Vent Mgt Plan: mode: ______ f: ______ TV: ______ PEEP: ______ PS: ______ FIO_2: ______ desired pCO_2: ______ Flow rate: ______ Sens: ______ Peak pressure: ______ Wean By: ______	Daily Vent Mgt Plan: mode: ______ f: ______ TV: ______ PEEP: ______ PS: ______ FIO_2: ______ desired pCO_2: ______ Flow rate: ______ Sens: ______ Peak pressure: ______ Wean By: ______
→	→	→	→	→
→	→	→	→	→
Sedation: ______ NMB: ______	Sedation: ______ NMB: ______	Sedation: ______ NMB: ______	Sedation: ______ NMB: ______	Sedation: ______ NMB: ______

Appendix 6–3. Trauma Outcome Guide: Critical Care *Continued*

	PROBLEMS/ NEEDS	OUTCOMES	INITIAL ASSESSMENT	ADMISSION DAY 1	DAY 2
Respiratory (cont)	Breathing (cont)		Intubated (cont)	Atelectasis on CXR TV 15 m/kg ↑ PEEP to 10 cm Chest PT q4h, if not contraindicated by injury Aerosol q4h for thick secretions *0.5 cc albuterol/2 cc *10% Mucomyst	Chest PT q ____ Aerosol Rx: ____ Secretions: ____
				Patient Position: Turn q2h or more frequently Position for optimal oxygenation/ventilation and drainage Consider therapeutic bed for rotational therapy	Turn q ____ Position: ____ Bed: ____
			Chest tube(s) R__ #__ size__ L__ #__ size__	Assess: breath sounds air leak subQ air tension pneumo hemo/pneumo	 ⟶ ⟶ ⟶ ⟶ ⟶
				Suction: ____	Suction: ____
				Drainage (24h total)	Drainage: ____
				Dressing q ____	Dressing q ____

Appendix 6–3. Trauma Outcome Guide: Critical Care *Continued*

DAY 3	DAY 4	DAY 5	DAY 6	DAY 7
Chest PT q ______ or d/c	Chest PT q ______ or d/c	Chest PT q ______ or d/c	Chest PT q ______ or d/c	Chest PT q ______ or d/c
Aerosol Rx: ______ Secretions: ______	Aerosol Rx: ______ Secretions: ______	Aerosol Rx: ______ Secretions: ______	Aerosol Rx: ______ Secretions: ______	Aerosol Rx: ______ Secretions: ______
Turn q ______ Position: ______	Turn q ______ Position: ______	Turn q ______ Position: ______	Turn q ______ Position: ______	Turn q ______ Position: ______
Bed: ______	Bed: ______	Bed: ______	Bed: ______	Bed: ______
→ → → → →	→ → → → →	→ → → → →	→ → → → →	→ → → → →
Suction: ______	Suction: ______	Suction: ______	Suction: ______	Suction: ______
Drainage: ______	Drainage: ______	Drainage: ______	Drainage: ______	Drainage: ______
Dressing q ______	Dressing q ______	Dressing q ______	Dressing q ______	Dressing q ______

Appendix 6–3. Trauma Outcome Guide: Critical Care *Continued*

	PROBLEMS/ NEEDS	OUTCOMES	INITIAL ASSESSMENT	ADMISSION DAY 1	DAY 2
Cardiovascular	Circulation *Hemodynamic stability *Drip titration *Assess sites *Thermoregulation	1. Normovolemic (unless on dialysis) 2. BP >100 mm Hg (adult) 3. BP w/o variation>300 mm Hg for 12 hr w/o vasoactive agents prior to transfer 4. Strong palpable pulse 5. External hemorrhage controlled 6. Absence of active bleeding for 24 hr prior to transfer 7. Skin & mucous membranes normal in color & temperature 8. Capillary refill<3 sec	Art line site: ____ size: ____ PA site: ____ type: ____	EKG monitor VS: q ____ CIRC √: q ____ Acute change: ____ DX test: ____ Appropriate call orders (assess daily) Maintain BP/PAP within call orders Assess for A Line/PA complications Hemo profile 6AM daily & PRN w/hemodynamic instability/therapy changes Assess adequacy of resuscitation DO_2>600 ml/kg/m_2 ____ VO_2>150 ml/kg/m_2 ____ Lactate decreases or WNL ____ PCWP 16–18 w/PEEP ≤15 cm HgB 10–13 Dobutamine to ↑ SV and/ or achieve DO_2/VO_2 goals Avoid vasodilators Drip Status: Dobutamine: ____ Dopamine: ____ Levophed: ____ ____ ____ Trend I & O	→ VS: q ____ CIRC √: q ____ Acute change: ____ DX test: ____ → → → D/C PA≤36h (if not reassess need daily) → → DO_2 ____ VO_2 ____ Lactate ____ PCWP ____ HgB ____ Drip Status: Dobutamine: ____ Dopamine: ____ Levophed: ____ ____ ____ →
		9. IV sites patent & noninfected	PIV site: ____ size: ____ ____ ____ ____ ____	Change field lines PIV: ____ change/DC ____ change/DC	Assess sites q4h PIV: __ change/DC __ change/DC
			TL site: ____ size: ____ 8.5 Fr Introducer site: ____	TL: ____ change/DC 8.5 Fr ____ change/DC	TL: ____ change/DC 8.5 Fr __ change/DC
		10. Normothermia (97.5–100°F)	Hypothermia (<96°F) ____ °F Hyperthermia (>101°F) ____ °F	Temperature sensing Foley T q ____ Temp control measures: ____ ____	→ T q ____ Temp cont: ____ ____

Appendix 6–3. Trauma Outcome Guide: Critical Care *Continued*

Day 3	Day 4	Day 5	Day 6	Day 7
→ VS: q ____ CIRC $\surd$: q ____ Acute change: ____ DX test: ____ → → → PA: ____ change/DC A-line: ____ change/DC → → DO_2 ____ VO_2 ____ Lactate ____ PCWP ____ HgB ____ Drip Status: Dobutamine: ____ Dopamine: ____ Levophed: ____ ________ ________ →	→ VS: q ____ CIRC $\surd$: q ____ Acute change: ____ DX test: ____ → → → PA: ____ change/DC A-line: ____ change/DC → → DO_2 ____ VO_2 ____ Lactate ____ PCWP ____ HgB ____ Drip Status: Dobutamine: ____ Dopamine: ____ Levophed: ____ ________ ________ →	→ VS: q ____ CIRC $\surd$: q ____ Acute change: ____ DX test: ____ → → → PA: ____ change/DC A-line: ____ change/DC → → DO_2 ____ VO_2 ____ Lactate ____ PCWP ____ HgB ____ Drip Status: Dobutamine: ____ Dopamine: ____ Levophed: ____ ________ ________ →	→ VS: q ____ CIRC $\surd$: q ____ Acute change: ____ DX test: ____ → → → PA: ____ change/DC A-line: ____ change/DC → → DO_2 ____ VO_2 ____ Lactate ____ PCWP ____ HgB ____ Drip Status: Dobutamine: ____ Dopamine: ____ Levophed: ____ ________ ________ →	→ VS: q ____ CIRC $\surd$: q ____ Acute change: ____ DX test: ____ → → → PA: ____ change/DC A-line: ____ change/DC → → DO_2 ____ VO_2 ____ Lactate ____ PCWP ____ HgB ____ Drip Status: Dobutamine: ____ Dopamine: ____ Levophed: ____ ________ ________ →
→ PIV: ____ change/DC ____ change/DC	→ PIV: ____ change/DC ____ change/DC	→ PIV: ____ change/DC ____ change/DC	→ PIV: ____ change/DC ____ change/DC	→ PIV: ____ change/DC ____ change/DC
TL: ____ change/DC 8.5 Fr ____ change/DC	TL: ____ change/DC 8.5 Fr ____ change/DC	TL: ____ change/DC 8.5 Fr ____ change/DC	TL: ____ change/DC 8.5 Fr ____ change/DC	TL: ____ change/DC 8.5 Fr ____ change/DC
→ T q ____ Temp cont: ____ ________	→ T q ____ Temp cont: ____ ________	→ T q ____ Temp cont: ____ ________	→ T q ____ Temp cont: ____ ________	→ T q ____ Temp cont: ____ ________

Appendix 6–4. Trauma Resuscitation Cubicle Supplies

CABINET A–1 **LEFT SIDE**

	Philadelphia collars 2 Each of Small Medium Large	
A-line catheters–Femoral and radial Tongue blades Applicators Lubricant Band-Aids	Penrose drains Alcohol pads Betadine ointment Lidocaine with Epi. 5:1 connectors	Trach tape Lidocaine ABD pads
IV catheters ABG syringes NSS for lavage	12 cc syringes 6 cc syringes T.B. syringes Insulin syringes	
Single 4 × 4–1 box Tape–various widths Suture removal kits Xeroform dressing Tegaderm Vaseline dressing	Single 2 × 2–1 box Telfa pads	
Unsterile ABD pads Blue pads		

CABINET A–2 **RIGHT SIDE**

Heparin saline	NSS 500 cc–2 NSS 1000 cc–2 D5.45 NSS 500 cc–4	
Plasmanate–6	RL 500 cc–10	D5RL 500 cc–4 NSS 500 cc–2
4 × 4–10 Packs	Pump tubing–2 Kerlix–10 Stopcocks–12	Y tubing–12 Solution sets–4 Extension sets–10 Cath guards–12 Luer Locks–10
Four NSS Pour H_2O	H_2O_2 Pour ETOH	Benzoin spray
Restraints–2 Denture cups Contact lens cases Medication labels	2-Liter urine bottles Sputum trays Urine cups Bedpan Urinals	

Appendix 6–4. Trauma Resuscitation Cubicle Supplies *Continued*

COMBO & DPL TRAY CART

Combo Trays

Suture Material
Scalpel Blades
1 Box Each Size

DPL Tray

DPL
Catheters

G-W Tongs

Plastics Tray

T & A Add On Tray

Trach Tray

Scalpel Blades
#10–#11–#15–#20

Suture Material

4.0 Nylon PC-1
5.0 Nylon PC-1
6.0 Nylon PC-1
3.0 Nylon PS-1
2 Nylon Retention
0 Silk Ties
3.0 Silk Ties
2.0 Vicryl SH
3.0 Vicryl SH
3.0 Vicryl PC-5
4.0 Vicryl PC-5
5.0 Vicryl PC-5
3.0 Nylon KS

CABINET B

Thoradrain	Disploxes	Cordis kits
Thoradrain refills	Sterile gowns	Triple lumens
Green tubing	3/4 sheets	Double lumens
Clear tubing	PA catheters	Pressure tubing
NG tubes	Foley insertion sets	
Irrigation sets	DPL catheters	
Sterile drapes	Guidewires	
Urine meters	Chest tubes–#36 & #40	
	Foley catheters	

Needle box

Suction outlets

Suction canisters

CABINET C

Anesthesia equipment
ETT tubes
Anesthesia drugs

Trachs
Sizes 6–7–8

Computer terminal

IV pump located behind computer

Gloves 6½	Gloves 7
Gloves 7½	Gloves 8

Appendix 6–4. Trauma Resuscitation Cubicle Supplies *Continued*

CUBICLE CART

Top Basket

Cordis kit
Double lumen
Femoral A-lines
Arrow A-lines

Alcohol
Benzoin
Betadine
Pour NSS
Pour H_2O

Bottom Basket

Nonsterile gloves
Gloves–sizes 6–8

4 × 4–10 packs
Kerlix
Box of single 4 × 4
Box of single 2 × 2

Lubricant   NSS lavage
Betadine ointment
ABG syringe caps

Blood tubes
Syringes   Needles

ABD pads
Blue pads

Suction setups with tubing

IV pole on side
Heparin saline
Pressure tubing
Plasmanate–500 cc
RL–500 cc

Front Tray

IV catheters
EKG pads   Alcohol pad
NG tube
Irrigation set
Tape   Lidocaine
ABG syringes
Suture material

Bottom Basket

Yankauer & tracheal suction catheters

1) O_2 nebulizer setup attached to flow meter located on front of cubicle cart
2) Guidewires and pressure extension tubing located on left side of cubicle cart

Appendix 6–5. Trauma Resuscitation Unit Admission Nursing Protocol*

PREPARATION FOR AN ADMISSION
Turn on cubicle lights
Open sterile trays
Flush intravenous lines
Prepare monitor
Turn on suction

ADMITTING A PATIENT
Respond to heliport/ambulance entrance
Gather history from conscious patients
Perform primary, rapid secondary survey
Receive report from medic
Transport patient to admitting area
Report initial assessment and information from medic to team
Take position on right side of patient (circulating nurse is positioned on patient's left when appropriate)
Help undress patient
Obtain blood pressure, heart rate, and respiratory rate and announce to team
Obtain core temperature
Document vital signs, assessment findings
Assist with right side intravenous insertions
Insert Foley catheter
Collect urine specimen, test with Chemstrip, document results
Monitor and document fluid administration
Obtain 12 lead EKG
Protect chain of evidence (suspected criminal case)
Assist with emergent procedures, e.g.:
- ICP/IVC insertion
- Gardner-Wells tongs insertion
- Intubation/tracheostomy/cricothyroidotomy
- Chest tube insertion
- Defibrillation/cardioversion
- Diagnostic peritoneal lavage
- Thoracotomy

Initiate autotransfusion if indicated
Review initial and subsequent laboratory results
Draw blood for follow-up laboratory tests
Monitor sterile technique of team members
Monitor and document backboard time
Transport patient for diagnostic studies
Communicate with family
Communicate with police
Collect and document valuables (place in safe) and clothing
Obtain needed equipment not in cubicle

*These are the major responsibilities of the admitting primary nurse, not a comprehensive description of the role of the admitting nurse. The designated primary nurse should be assisted by a circulating nurse who has delegated responsibilities, e.g., obtain supplies, assist with procedures, collect valuables.

Appendix 6–6. Patient Assessment Form

PATIENT ASSESSMENT

UNIVERSITY OF MARYLAND MEDICAL SYSTEM

MARYLAND INSTITUTE FOR
EMERGENCY MEDICAL SERVICES SYSTEMS

DATE	TIME	ALLERGIES	WEIGHT

NEUROLOGICAL

LOC

PUPILS

SENSORY & MOTOR FUNCTION

OTORRHEA RHINORRHEA

NUCHAL RIGIDITY

ICP

SEDATION

MODE OF STABILIZATION

RESPIRATORY

AIRWAY PATENCY AND TYPE

VENTILATOR SETTINGS

RESPIRATIONS

BREATH SOUNDS

CHEST TUBE DRAINAGE

SECRETIONS

OTHER

CARDIOVASCULAR

SKIN COLOR   TEMP

PULSES CRT'S

EDEMA

HEART SOUNDS

MONITORING LINES	CVP	PA	PCWP

OTHER

METABOLIC

HAS

GASTROINTESTINAL

ABD

BOWEL SOUNDS

STOOL/ FLATUS

DRAINS DRAINAGE

* SEE NURSES NOTES

50032 (3/91)

GASTROINTESTINAL (continued)

DIET

INCISIONS

OTHER

GENITOURINARY

URINE OUTPUT

METHOD OF VOIDING   TEXAS   FOLEY   VOIDING

INFECTION

TEMP / WBC

WOUND DRAINAGE

SKIN / EXTREMITIES

DISCOLORATION

PRESSURE AREAS

INCISIONS/ ABRASIONS

CASTS

TRACTION

CIRCULATION

ROM   ACTIVE   PASSISVE

PSYCH - SOCIAL

1. SENSORIUM

   A. ORIENTATION

   B. MEMORY

   C. INTELLECTUAL FUNCTION

   D. JUDGEMENT

II. PERCEPTION

III. THOUGHT PROCESSES

   A. FLOW

   B. FORM

   C. CONTENT

IV. MOOD & AFFECT

SIGNATURE

Appendix 6–6. Patient Assessment Form *Continued*

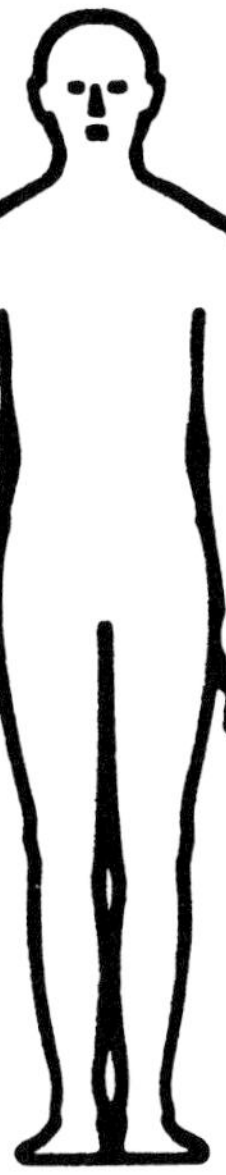

FRONT

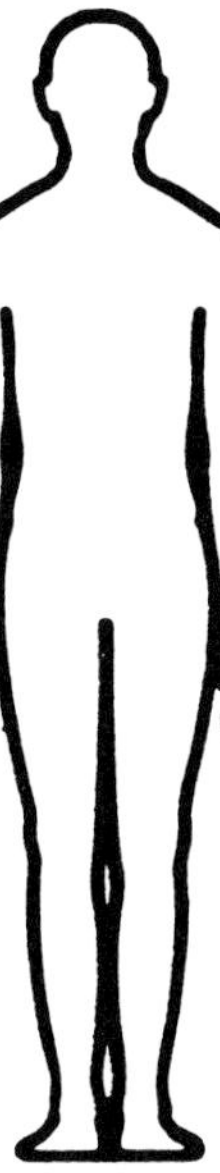

BACK

EKG

A-LINE

PA/CVP

ICP

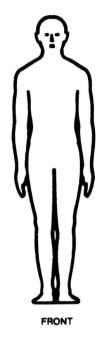

Appendix 6–7. Major Complications in Trauma

COMPLICATION	ASSOCIATED CONDITIONS	LOOK FOR	NURSING INTERVENTIONS
Hypovolemia	Internal hemorrhage Multiple systems injuries Fractures of major bones Coagulopathies	Decreased blood pressure Tachycardia, tachypnea Cool, clammy skin Pallor Decreased urine output Frank hemorrhage Anxiety Obtunded sensorium	Notify physician immediately Type and cross-match patient's blood Check amount of blood on hand in blood bank Administer transfusion as ordered Elevate patient's legs while patient is supine, with head elevated as necessary to facilitate respiration Administer medications as ordered Monitor vital signs q 15 minutes
Sepsis	Systemic infection Peritonitis	Increased WBCs Increased or decreased temperature Tachycardia Sudden hypotension Increased serum glucose Decreased platelets Decreased Pa_{O_2} Confusion/disorientation Diaphoresis/flushed face	Monitor ABGs Notify physician Monitor VS q 15 minutes Administer fluid replacement and medications as ordered Monitor arterial blood gases (ABGs), electrolytes, and CBC Maintain normothermia
Neurogenic shock	Spinal cord injury	Hypotension Hypothermia with absence of sweating below injury level Flaccid paralysis below injury level Bradycardia	Notify physician Administer medications and IV fluids as ordered Monitor VS q 15 minutes Insert Foley catheter and nasogastric tube as ordered
Pulmonary embolism	Immobility Fracture of the long bones, pelvis, or ribs Improper handling of fractures before and during admission	Chest pain Shortness of breath Sudden disorientation Petechiae over axillae and chest (fat) Decreased Pa_{O_2} Tachycardia	Notify physician Assist with transport to lung SCAN Monitor EKG Administer O_2 Draw ABGs STAT and serially Assist ventilation as ordered
Adult Respiratory Distress Syndrome (ARDS)	Chest trauma Sepsis Multiple transfusions Brain injuries Multiple systems injuries	Decreased Pa_{CO_2} Decreased Pa_{O_2} Decreased lung compliance Decreased tidal volume Increased airway pressures Increased WBC	Assess chest Draw serial ABGs Administer O_2 or ventilator therapy as ordered Suction PRN Administer medications as ordered Monitor EKG Monitor lung volumes and compliance
Pneumonia	Blunt chest trauma Immobility Atelectasis Endotracheal intubation	Increased temperature Increased WBC Decreased breath sounds Rales, some bronchi on auscultation Radiologic changes Positive sputum cultures	Assess chest Use sterile suction technique and chest physiotherapy for pulmonary hygiene PRN Supplemental O_2 PRN Serial chest x-rays as ordered
Wound dehiscence	Abdominal surgery Wound infection Poor nutritional status	Pink serous wound exudate Poor wound edge approximation	Notify physician Have sterile saline and dressings on hand Prevent/correct abdominal distention
Gastrointestinal fistula	Penetrating abdominal trauma Sepsis	Bile, fecal, or pancreatic drainage from wounds or drain sites	Monitor amount, odor, and color of drainage Meticulous skin care around drainage sites Perform dressing changes as necessary
Stress ulcers	Multiple system trauma Patient kept NPO for prolonged periods Head injury Sepsis Continuous mechanical ventilation Prolonged ICU	NG aspirate hemopositive Decreased pH of NG aspirate Stools hemopositive Decreased hematocrit Melena	Administer medications as ordered Chilled saline lavage until clear Administer transfusions, medications, and fluid replacement as ordered
Pneumothorax (simple)	Mechanical ventilation	Decreased or absent breath sounds Radiologic evidence Decreased Pa_{O_2} Cyanosis Unequal chest expansion Hyper-resonance over affected area	Notify physician Administer supplemental O_2 Assist with chest tube insertion or thoracentesis

Appendix 6–7. Major Complications in Trauma *Continued*

COMPLICATION	ASSOCIATED CONDITIONS	LOOK FOR	NURSING INTERVENTIONS
Pneumothorax (tension)	PEEP Improper CVP line placement	Decreased Pa_{O_2} Decreased tidal volume Decreased lung compliance Breath sounds absent Tracheal deviation Increased airway pressures Restlessness Cyanosis Unequal chest expansion Hyper-resonance over affected area Hemodynamic instability	Notify physician STAT Insert 18-gauge needle into 2nd intercostal space laterally if certified Assist with chest tube insertion If chest tubes in place, check for patency and suction Monitor Vs q15 minutes
Renal failure	Prolonged hypotension Sepsis Ruptured aorta Toxic drug reaction ARDS	Increased serum BUN and creatinine Decreased specific gravity Decreased urine output Increased serum potassium Increased confusion Uremic frost	Record hourly intake and output Foley catheter care daily Monitor lab values Administer hemodialysis or peritoneal dialysis as ordered Daily weights
Bronchoesophageal fistula	Prolonged tracheostomy Overinflation of cuff balloon Prolonged need for NG tube	Gastric contents suctioned through tracheostomy Radiologic confirmation Respiratory distress	Maintain NPO Maintain proper positioning of endotracheal tube to maintain ventilation Administer feedings as ordered via gastrostomy or jejunostomy Deflate cuff to check pressure twice per shift
Diabetes insipidus	Brain injuries	Increased urine output Decreased urine specific gravity Decreased urine osmolality Severe thirst	Record hourly intake and output Maintain fluid balance Replace urine output as ordered Administer Pitressin as ordered Check urine specific gravity q4h
Ruptured innominate artery	Tracheostomy Tracheal tube too long Inadvertent traction on tracheal tube when moving patient Prolonged overinflation of tracheal tube cuff	Visible pulsation of trachea Frank bleeding from trachea	Elevate tracheal flange with 4 × 4's if arterial pulsations present If rupture occurs, slide finger down outside of outer cannula and attempt to tamponade innominate against clavicle
Atelectasis	Immobility Prolonged anesthesia Blunt chest trauma Pain Endotracheal intubation	Radiologic changes Decreased Pa_{O_2} Inability to cough Decreased breath sounds	Provide pulmonary hygiene and chest physiotherapy Turn and position q1–2h Kinetic therapy Encourage coughing and deep-breathing Draw serial ABGs Administer O_2 PRN Incentive spirometer
Empyema	Blunt chest trauma Pneumonia Prolonged atelectasis Pleural effusion Open chest wound	Purulent chest drainage Increased temperature Increased WBC Generalized malaise Radiologic confirmation Sepsis	Monitor amount and consistency of chest tube drainage as ordered Culture chest tube drainage as ordered Maintain chest tube patency Provide pulmonary hygiene and chest physiotherapy
Aspiration	Unconscious patients Spinal cord injury Sudden vomiting Malfunctioning NG tube Decreased gag reflex Prolonged endotracheal intubation	Suctioning of gastric contents from tracheal tube or ET tube Radiologic confirmation Increased temperature and WBCs Decreased Pa_{O_2}	Notify physician immediately Take chest x-ray STAT Turn patient to side or suction if he vomits Elevate head of bed when giving tube feedings
Meningitis	Brain injury Skull fracture Maxillofacial trauma Intraventricular catheter placement	Increased temperature Increased WBC Positive spinal fluid cultures Changes in neurological status	Administer medications as ordered Monitor VS q1h Do neurological checks q1h Assist with spinal tap Draw serial WBCs
Sensory deprivation/ICU psychosis	Prolonged stay in ICU Sleep deprivation	Confusion Disorientation Hallucinations Restlessness Combativeness	Arrange for psychiatric consult if necessary Provide quiet environment Plan nursing care in blocks of time to promote sleep Administer medications as ordered Use consistent nursing approach to orient to reality

Appendix 6–8. Critical Care Daily Record

UNIT / BED NUMBER ____________

Date ______/ ________/ ________

Diagnosis ______________________

____

Fluid Limit: ________________ cc/24°

24° Urine: __________ to __________

Maryland Institute For Emergency Medical Services Systems
CRITICAL CARE DAILY RECORD

7906 - 015 REV 7/86

WEIGHT

TODAY ___ kg

Net ± ___ kg

PREDIALYSIS ___ kg

Net ±

POST DIALYSIS ___ kg

Net ±

Abdominal Girths/Calf & Thigh Measurements

07-15: ________ cm ________ cm

15-23: ________ cm ________ cm

23-07: ________ cm ________ cm

BSA ________ Hgt. ______

TRACTION ____________________ lbs.

FEVER PACK ____________________

LAB CATEGORY: (Unstable) ____________ (Stable) ____________

Allergies: ____________________

____

Pt: Addressograph

Diet ____________________

____

Mobility: ____________________

VITAL SIGNS		07	08	09	10	11	12	13	14		15	16	17	18	19	20	21	22		23	24	01	02	03	04	05	06	
TEMPERATURE	40.0									104									40.0									104
VITAL SIGN CODE	39.4									103									39.4									103
R	38.9									102									38.9									102
• Rectal	38.3									101									38.3									101
0	37.8									100									37.8									100
• Oral	37.2									99									37.2									99
A	36.7									98									36.7									98
• Axillary	36.1									97									36.1									97
Hypothermia	35.6									96									35.6									96
BLOOD PRESSURE	200									200									200									200
PULSE	190									190									190									190
RESPIRATION	180									180									180									180
	170									170									170									170
B.P. M	160									160									160									160
X Monitor	150									150									150									150
C	140									140									140									140
X Cuff	130									130									130									130
	120									120									120									120
• Apical	110									110									110									110
	100									100									100									100
H.R. O Radial	90									90									90									90
	80									80									80									80
Resp. R ⊗	70									70									70									70
	60									60									60									60
	50									50									50									50
OHP, PAC [ ]	40									40									40									40
	30									30									30									30
	20									20									20									20
	10									10									10									10
	0									0									0									0

Appendix 6–8. Critical Care Daily Record *Continued*

MBP																												
PAP M																												
S/D																												
PCWP																												
CVP (RAP)																												
ICP/CPP																												
CARDIAC OUTPUT																												
INTAKE	07	08	09	10	11	12	13	14	8 HR. TOTAL	15	16	17	18	19	20	21	22	8 HR. TOTAL	23	24	01	02	03	04	05	06	8 HR. TOTAL	24 HR. TOTALS
A.																												
B.																												
C.																												
D.																												
E.																												
F.																												
G.																												
H.																												
I.																												
J.																												
K.																												
L.																												
M.																												
N.																												
O.																												
P.																												
Q.																												
INTAKE TOTALS Yesterday 24 Hr. Total						8' COL./BLOOD		8'							8' COL./BLOOD		8'		16'					8' COL./BLOOD		8'		I
OUTPUT	07	08	09	10	11	12	13	14	8 HR. TOTAL	15	16	17	18	19	20	21	22	8 HR. TOTAL	23	24	01	02	03	04	05	06		COL./BLOOD
Routine																												
Specific Gravity																												
Sugar/Acetone																												
Ph Urine/NG																												
Hematest																												
S. N-G Tube																												
T. Chest Tube Drainage																												
U.																												
V.																												
W.																												
X.																												
Y. Stool																												
OUTPUT TOTALS Yesterday 24 Hr. Total			8'					8'									8'		16'							8'		O
I & O BALANCE: Yesterday		+ or – NET	8'					8'									8'		16'						8'			

Appendix 6–8. Critical Care Daily Record *Continued*

RESPIRATORY TIME	07	08	09	10	11	12	13	14	15	16	17	18	19	20	21	22	23	24	01	02	03	04	05	06
Ventilator-O_2 Apparatus																								
FIO_2 (%)																								
Liters-Air O_2 /Mode																								
Tidal Volume (mix/ EXP																								
Rate / minute machine patient																								
P.E.E.P./C.P.A.P. (cm H_2O)																								
PIP (cm H_2O) Plateau																								
Respiratory Pressure + -																								
SaO_2																								

MED.-AMT.-ROUTE-FREQ.

MEDICATIONS

START	RENEW	TIME	07	08	09	10	11	12	13	14	15	16	17	18	19	20	21	22	23	24	01	02	03	04	05	06

		STAT / PRN MEDS	07	08	09	10	11	12	13	14	15	16	17	18	19	20	21	22	23	24	01	02	03	04	05	06

50036 (REV. 3/92)

Nurse's Signature: 07-15 ____________ 15-23 ____________ 23-07 ____________

RECOPIED BY: ____________

Appendix 6–8. Critical Care Daily Record *Continued*

NURSING OBSERVATIONS

TIME	07	08	09	10	11	12	13	14	15	16	17	18	19	20	21	22	23	24	01	02	03	04	05	06
Cardiac Rhythm																								
Respiration																								
Breath Sounds																								
Sputum Character																								
Skin																								
Pulses: (R/L)																								
(R/L)																								
(R/L)																								
Medications																								
Stimulus																								
Eye Opening																								
Verbal Response																								
Orientation																								
Pupil Equality																								
Pupil Reaction (R/L)																								
Corneals (R/L)																								
Facial Grimace (R/L)																								
Best Motor Response																								
*Strength Arms (R/L)																								
*Strength Legs (R/L)																								
* Record Strength if																								
Motor Response 4 or greater																								
Nurses Initials																								

PUPIL SIZE: DILATED 8 | LARGE 7, 6 | MEDIUM 5, 4 | SMALL 3, 2 | PINPOINT 1

PUPIL EQUALITY (R/L)
= ; L>R; R>L

CODE FOR NURSING OBSERVATIONS

Cardiac Rhythm: NS – Normal Sinus, ST – Sinus Tachycardia, SB – Sinus Bradycardia, PAC'S – Premature Atrial Contractions, AF – Atrial Fibrillation, PVC'S – Premature Ventricular Contractions, VT – Ventricular Tachycardia, VF – Ventricular Fibrillation, B – Bigem, · HB – · Heartblock, CA – Cardiac Arrest

Respiration: N – Normal, L – Labored, HP – Hypernea, CS – Cheyne-Stokes, A – Apnea, PV – Paralyzed on Ventilator, V – Ventilator

Breath Sounds: N – Normal, W – Wheezing, R – Rales, RH – Rhonchi, D – Distant, A – Absent (Note R/L below line) C – Coarse

R – Right, RU – Right Upper, RM – Right Middle, RL – Right Lower, LU – Left Upper, LL – Left Lower B – Bilateral

Sputum: N – None, S – Small, M – Moderate, C – Copious, T – Thin, Th – Thick, F – Foul, BT – Blood-tinged

Skin: W – Warm, D – Dry, M – Moist, R – Rubor, C – Cyanosis, P – Pallor, M – Mottling, J – Jaundice

Pulses: (Scale 0 to 4 +, where 3 + is normal e.g. R-3, L-2)

Medications:

Sedation	S
Paralytic	PL
Tranquilizer	T
Pain	P

Stimulus

Voice	4
Shake or shout	3
Peripheral pain	2
Deep pain	1

Eye Opening:

Spontaneously	4
To speech	3
To pain	2
None	1
Untestable	U

Verbal Response

Orientated	5
Confused	4
Inappropriate (words)	3
Incomprehensible (sounds)	2
None	1
Untestable	U

Orientation:

Time, place person	3
2 of the 3	2
1 of the 3	1
None Untestable	U

Best Motor Response

Obeys	6
Localizes	5
Withdraws	4
Flexes	3
Extends	2
None	1
Untestable	U

Pupil, Reaction, Corneal Reflex and Facial Frimace

Normal	3
Decreased or abnormal	2
Absent	1
Untestable	U

Strength (R/L)

Strong	5
Mild weakness	4
Moderate weakness	3
Severe weakness	2
Trace	1
None	0
Untestable	U

Appendix 6–8. Critical Care Daily Record *Continued*

ROUTINE TREATMENTS

TIME	07	08	09	10	11	12	13	14	15	16	17	18	19	20	21	22	23	24	01	02	03	04	05	06
TURN (direction)																								
SKIN CARE (area)																								
NG IRRIGS.																								
MOUTH CARE & EYE CARE																								
TRACH CARE																								
FOLEY & PERI. CARE																								
NSDO'S q ______																								
IV TUBINGS (which) & DRESSING																								
BATH & SHAMPOO																								
SUCTION & CHEST PT. q ______																								
CULTURES (which)																								
LAB. STUDIES (which done)																								
X-RAY (Type)																								
TIME	**07**	**08**	**09**	**10**	**11**	**12**	**13**	**14**	**15**	**16**	**17**	**18**	**19**	**20**	**21**	**22**	**23**	**24**	**01**	**02**	**03**	**04**	**05**	**06**
TED STOCKINGS OFF 1 hr.																								
✓ IMPACTION q ______																								
CARDIAC OUTPUT																								
ROM (PCP)																								
WEIGH q ______																								
NEURO-VASC CHECKS q ______																								
MILK CT q ______																								
✓ PATIENT CARE PLAN																								
#1 q ______																								
#2 q ______																								
#3 q ______																								
PCS																								
FAMILY CALLS																								

CULTURE REPORTS:

	ORGANISM/SENSITIVITY	DATE CULTURE TAKEN:
Blood:		
Urine:		
Sputum:		
Wound:		
Other:		

PROCEDURES	TIME	COMMENTS
Daily Chest X-Ray		
Angio		
Ultrasound		
CT-Head		
CT-Body		
Scans-Lung		
Liver/Spleen		
Echo		
Doppler		
EEG		
Dialysis - On/Off		

OPERATIVE DATA

Procedure: ______ OR Time ______

Anesthesiologist: ______

Type of Anesthesia

General: ______

Regional: ______ Local: ______

Reversal: ______

Appendix 6–8. Critical Care Daily Record *Continued*

NURSING INTERVENTIONS

7A - 3^{30}_{P}	3P - 11^{30}_{P}	11P - 7^{30}_{A}

Nurse's Signature 07-15 ______ 15-23 ______ 23-07 ______

Appendix 9–1. Pneumatic Antishock Garment (PASG)

Indications for Use

1. Hypotension secondary to (a) hypovolemic or traumatic shock or (b) relative hypovolemia due to neurogenic shock, drug overdose, septic shock, or anaphylaxis. Hypotension is defined as a systolic blood pressure less than 80 mm Hg or a systolic blood pressure less than 100 mm Hg accompanied by symptoms of shock.
2. Stabilization of lower extremity or pelvic fracture.
3. Control of hemorrhage within confines of garment.
4. Maintenance of upper torso perfusion when intravenous fluids cannot be initiated.
5. Circulatory support during volume replacement.

Equipment

1. Pneumatic antishock garment (PASG).
2. Foot pump.
3. Blood pressure cuff.
4. Stethoscope.
5. Long spine board.

Application

NURSING ACTION	RATIONALE
1. Assess the patient's vital signs (pulse, blood pressure, respirations), level of consciousness, skin, and possible sites of hemorrhage.	The patient should be assessed to establish baseline data, from which changes in the patient's condition can be evaluated. Once the trousers are applied, the area beneath the trousers will be difficult to assess.
2. Explain procedure to patient.	
3. Remove lower body clothing.	Wrinkled clothing beneath PASG may increase risk of skin breakdown.
4. Unfold the PASG and lay flat on long spine board.	
5. Carefully log roll the patient, *always maintaining spinal alignment,* and place the suit under the patient.	The patient's spinal alignment should always be maintained until spinal injury has been ruled out.
6. Position the top of the PASG just below the patient's lowest rib.	Be sure that the abdominal section of the PASG does *not* encase the thoracic cavity and inhibit chest expansion.
7. Search for and remove sharp objects that get between the patient and the suit.	Removal of sharp objects prevents patient injury or suit rupture during inflation.
8. Fold the trousers around the left leg first and fasten.	
9. Fold the trousers around the right leg and fasten.	
10. Fold the trousers around the abdominal section and fasten.	
11. Attach the air tubes and foot pumps to the connections on the PASG. Be sure all stopcocks are open.	

Inflation and Maintenance

NURSING ACTION	RATIONALE
1. Reassess the patient's vital signs.	Establish a vital sign baseline prior to inflation.
2. *Always* inflate the leg compartments first by closing the stopcock to the abdominal section and pumping the foot pump.	Inflation should increase systemic vascular resistance to raise blood pressure and improve perfusion to tissues above the diaphragm.
3. If the foot pumps are inoperable, inflation can be done by mouth.	
4. Monitor the blood pressure frequently and stop inflation when it is maintained within acceptable limits (90 to 100 mm Hg systolic).	The amount of inflation necessary is determined by the patient's perfusion status.
5. *Do not* inflate the trousers on the basis of the intrasuit pressures.	
6. If the patient's perfusion status and vital signs remain unimproved with leg compartment inflation, the abdominal section should be inflated. Close the leg valves and open the abdominal stopcock to allow for abdominal compartment inflation.	Tamponade of intra-abdominal hemorrhage may be achieved with abdominal compartment inflation.
7. Monitor the patient's blood pressure and respiratory status frequently as the abdominal compartment is inflated. Stop inflation when blood pressure is adequate or when respiratory embarrassment is noted. Onset of respiratory distress signals the need to immediately deflate the abdominal compartment.	The patient's perfusion guides inflation. Respiratory embarrassment may signal the presence of diaphragm rupture and abdominal viscera herniation.
8. When optimal blood pressure levels are obtained, turn the stopcocks to the hold position.	Turning the stopcock to the hold position prevents escape of intrasuit air and maintains the desired inflation pressures.

Appendix 9–1. Pneumatic Antishock Garment (PASG) *Continued*

9. Insert an IV and infuse fluid volume as ordered to maintain blood pressure.	The PASG is *not* a substitute for fluid-volume replacement.
10. Monitor the patient's blood pressure and add pressure to the suit as needed, to maintain optimal blood pressure levels.	
11. If the trousers are inflated to the point of pop-off valve activation and there is or has been no hemodynamic response in 30 minutes, the inflation pressure should be reduced as resuscitation continues.	As a safety mechanism, release valves are activated when intrasuit pressures exceed just over 100 mm Hg to prevent lower extremity ischemia.
12. Protect the patient from sudden removal of the PASG.	Sudden removal of the PASG may cause lethal hypotension.
13. To assess intrasuit pressure, when no gauge is present, attach a T-connector to a mercury manometer and place the manometer between the foot pump and the garment.	The intrasuit pressure may be assessed to determine the amount of pressure exerted on the tissues beneath the garment. This value does not determine the need for inflation or deflation of the trousers.
14. Monitor and document how long the PASG is inflated. Assess feet for evidence of ischemia.	Avoid prolonged inflation to prevent lower extremity tissue ischemia, compartment syndrome, and/or skin breakdown.

Deflation

NURSING ACTION	RATIONALE
1. Prepare the patient for PASG deflation: a. Insert at least two large bore IVs and reestablish blood volume. b. Monitor EKG and vital signs. c. Assemble qualified personnel and a surgical team.	Ensure intravascular volume is being restored and shock has been adequately managed prior to PASG deflation.
d. Have additional fluids and sodium bicarbonate on hand.	As the trousers are deflated, additional intravascular volume repletion may be necessary. Acids that have accumulated in the tissues beneath the trousers will be washed out as deflation occurs so that bicarbonate therapy may be necessary.
e. Have pump readily available.	Pump should be available in case reinflation is necessary.
2. Deflate the PASG *slowly* by opening the stopcock while monitoring the patient's blood pressure. a. *Always* start with deflation of the abdominal compartment first. b. *Stop* deflation when the patient's systolic blood pressure drops by 5 mm Hg and hold at that point until additional fluids are given to return and maintain the patient's blood pressure. c. Continue deflation slowly, while monitoring the vital signs and infusing IV fluids to maintain the blood pressure.	The patient's systolic blood pressure serves as a guide throughout the deflation process.
d. Once the abdominal compartment is completely deflated and vital signs remain stable, deflate the right or left leg compartment slowly. e. Continue to assess vital signs, and if the patient remains stable, deflate the other leg compartment. f. Should the patient's blood pressure fall suddenly, the PASG should be reinflated until more fluid can be given and/or hemorrhage can be surgically controlled. g. After the shock state has been adequately managed and vital signs are stable the PASG may be removed.	Compartments are deflated sequentially to allow for a gradual return of blood flow from the central circulation back into the extremities to prevent a sudden drop in circulating blood volume.

Adapted from Committee on Trauma, American College of Surgeons: Advanced Trauma Life Support Program: Instructor Manual, 1989, pp 87–88; MIEMSS Medical Antishock Trouser Procedure. MIEMSS Advanced Trauma Life Support Management for Nurses, Code #300. Baltimore, MD, 1986; Cowley RA, Dunham CM: Shock Trauma/Critical Care Manual. Rockville, MD, Aspen, 1991).

Appendix 10–1. The Mental Status Examination: An Assessment Tool for the Trauma Patient

- I. Initial general impressions
  - A. Dress
    1. Neat and groomed
    2. Meticulous
    3. Disheveled or unkempt
    4. Inappropriate or bizarre (specify)
  - B. Posture
    1. Erect and comfortable
    2. Slouched or slumped
    3. Tense or rigid
    4. Unusual or bizarre
  - C. Facial expression (suggests)
    1. Sadness
    2. Anger
    3. Suspicion
    4. Anxiety
  - D. Behavior toward examiner
    1. Cooperative
    2. Uncooperative
    3. Inaccessible (coma, negativistic)
    4. Apathetic or detached
    5. Suspicious or mistrustful
    6. Aggressive, antagonistic, or defiant
    7. Attention seeking or exaggerated behavior
  - E. Observed abnormal behaviors
    1. Tics
    2. Repetitive behaviors—mannerisms, compulsions
    3. Posturing
- II. Specific observations
  - A. Sensorium
    1. Orientation
       - a. Time
       - b. Place
       - c. Person
       - d. Situation
    2. Memory
       - a. Recent
       - b. Remote
       - c. Immediate retention and recall
    3. Intellectual functioning
       - a. Counting
       - b. Calculation
       - c. Ability to abstract
       - d. General fund of knowledge
       - e. Vocabulary
       - f. Ability to read and write
    4. Judgment
  - B. Perception: Process of organizing and interpreting sensory data by combining them with previous experience
    1. Illusions: Perceptual misinterpretation of a real, external sensory experience
       - a. Auditory
       - b. Visual
       - c. Tactile
    2. Hallucinations: Apparent perception of an external object when no correspondingly real object exists
       - a. Auditory
       - b. Visual
       - c. Olfactory
       - d. Taste
       - e. Tactile
       - f. Kinesthetic
       - g. Hypnogogic: occur when falling asleep and suddenly awakened
       - h. Hypnopompic: occur when waking from sleep
    3. Depersonalization
       - a. Distorted perception of body image or part
       - b. Feelings of unreality
  - C. Thought processes
    1. Flow: rate of speech
       - a. Normal, spontaneous
       - b. Retarded
       - c. Speeded
       - d. Blocking present
    2. Form: manner in which thought segments are related to each other
       - a. Logical sentences and speech sequences
       - b. Association disorder
         - 1) Tangential—circumstantial
         - 2) Looseness
         - 3) Incoherencies (total disorganization)
       - c. Flight of ideas
    3. Content
       - a. Delusions: false ideas that cannot be corrected by reasoning
         - 1) Grandiose
         - 2) Persecutory
         - 3) Depressive
         - 4) Of being influenced—referential
       - b. Obsessive ideas
       - c. Bizarre or unusual ideation
       - d. Intellectualization—overworking "rational" excuses and reasons
       - e. Other: phobias
  - D. Mood and affect
    1. Behavior
       - a. Facial expression
         - 1) Warm and friendly
         - 2) Fixed—grim
         - 3) Perplexed
         - 4) Depressed
         - 5) Apprehensive
         - 6) Suspicious
         - 7) Elated
         - 8) Other
       - b. Motor Activity
         - 1) Slow or retarded movement
         - 2) Fast or hyperactive movement
         - 3) Restless movement
         - 4) Agitated movement
       - c. Vocal tone
         - 1) Expressive range
         - 2) Monotone
         - 3) Affected (dramatic)
    2. Verbal content (statements indicating)
       - a. Sadness
       - b. Fear or anxiety
       - c. Persecution
       - d. Rambling, elation
       - e. Anger
       - f. Self-condemnation
       - g. Impoverished ability to experience
       - h. Preoccupation (recurrent themes)
    3. Physiological signs
       - a. Flush
       - b. Pallor
       - c. Perspiration
       - d. Tears
    4. Affective status (for thought content)
       - a. Normal and appropriate
       - b. Inappropriate
       - c. Flat or blunted
       - d. Labile (rapidly changing emotions)
    5. Mood (prevailing affect)
       - a. Depression
       - b. Anxiety
       - c. Elation
       - d. Resentment, anger
       - e. Other (apathetic, detached)
       - f. Normal (none dominant)

Appendix 14–1. Nutritional/Metabolic Laboratory Assessment Strategies

LABORATORY TEST	ABNORMALITY	SIGNIFICANCE	NORMAL VALUE
BUN/Cr	Increased > 20	Impending or actual renal failure	10
Glucose	Increased Decreased	Diabetes mellitus, sepsis, hypermetabolism, steroids, rapid discontinuance of hypertonic glucose, hyperinsulinemia	70 to 110 mg/dl
Calcium	Increased Decreased	Dehydration, renal damage, lethargy, coma, tetany, seizures, Vitamin D deficiency, pancreatitis, Mg^+ deficiency	8.8 to 10.5 mg/dl
Phosphorus	Increased Decreased	Hyperthyroidism, ↑ GH secretion, hypervitaminosis D, hypoparathyroidism, refeeding, hyperglycemia, excess PO_4 binding antacids	3.0 to 4.5 mg/dl
Chloride	Increased Decreased	Metabolic acidosis Metabolic alkalosis	95 to 109 mEq/l
Uric acid	Increased	Gout, chronic renal failure, diuretics	2.0 to 7.8 mg/dl
Cholesterol	Increased Decreased	Biliary obstruction, pancreatectomy, pancreatic dysfunction, malnutrition, extensive liver disease	150 to 250 mg/dl
Magnesium (mg^+) (serum)	Increased Decreased	Chronic renal failure Malabsorption, TPN, ETOH abuse, NG suction	1.5 to 2.5 mEq/l
Zinc (serum)	Decreased	Impaired wound healing, TPN, diarrhea, loss of taste, dermatitis, hair loss, smell acuity	55 to 150 gm/dl
Copper (serum)	Decreased	Anemia, hypoproteinemia, leukopenia	85 to 140 gm/dl
Manganese	Decreased	Weight loss, nausea, vomiting, dermatitis	2 to 3 gm/dl
Selenium	Decreased	Long-term TPN	0.1 to 0.34 gm/ml
Molybdenum	Decreased	Increased dental caries, decreased growth	0.4 to 0.6 ng/ml
Triglyceride	Increased	Hyperlipidemia, sepsis, coronary artery disease	10 to 190 mg/dl
Transferrin	Increased Decreased	Increased visceral proteins, dehydration, malnutrition with decreased visceral proteins	200 to 400 gm/dl
Chromium	Decreased	Weight loss, glucose intolerance, diabetic neuropathy	< 0.05 ng/ml

Appendix 14–2. Nutritional Assessment Parameters—Use in Trauma/Critically Ill Patient

ASSESSMENT PARAMETER	PURPOSE (DESCRIPTION)	PROS	CONS	APPLICATION
Medical and dietary history	Determine patients at risk 1. Change in eating habits 2. Recent weight loss or gain 3. GI disorders 4. Past diet history—special diet, types of foods eaten 5. Chronic illness.	Detection of potential patients at risk prior to trauma—identification of preexisting dietary or disease processes that would further complicate recovery.	Difficult to obtain accurate information since patient critically ill. Family sources not necessarily reliable.	
History of trauma	Determine estimate of energy expenditure related to injury-tissue damage and potential infection.	Gives clue to general energy demands. Nomograms available (Wilmore, Rainey-MacDonald).	Does not allow for individual metabolic variation.	
Physical examination	Detection of physical signs of nutritional deficits.	Detection of overt body wasting. May detect vitamin and mineral deficiencies not routinely tested. Good for ongoing general analysis of nutritional status. Inexpensive.	Needs quantification. Limited due to overt mechanical disruption in total body integrity. More accurate through other assessment parameters.	
Weight/height	Gross body composition.	Indicator of nutritional risk when compared with patient's usual weight, desirable weight, or both. Recommend use of usual body weight. Preweight/height ratios provide baseline index. Use in patients who are hemodynamically stable, with adequate serum osmolarity to note trends.	Incorrectly detects malnourishment in normally ectomorphic patient. Overlooks depletion in obese patient. Avoid use of Metropolitan Life Insurance tables. Use in patients with fluid overload, edema—patients with rapid weight loss and gain in response to differing colloid osmotic pressures. Falsely elevates weight and difficult to use in patients with body casts.	
Anthropometric measures 1. Tricep skin fold (fat reserves) 2. Midarm circumference (skeletal muscle protein) 3. Arm muscle area (skeletal muscle protein)	Evaluation of somatic stores—fat, protein. Depressed values indicate protein calorie malnutrition (PCM). Marasmus type malnutrition—balanced deficit diets, low calories, adequate protein.	Inexpensive, noninvasive, losses easily measured. May help to note trends in trauma patients due to severe catabolic processes, thus useful in patients with intact arm muscles to note trends in nutritional interventions.	Accuracy of measurements requires standardization of site, body position (preferable standing position), and use of appropriate equipment. Utilization may be impossible in patients with orthopedic, neurological, burn, and other injuries who are unable to sit or stand upright because of limitations imposed by traction, mental status, or massive injury. Presence of edema or subcutaneous emphysema will falsely elevate. IV administration may change pliability of skin. Magnitude of "malnutrition" ill-defined. Table of normal values must be available for age, sex, and fat pad—such tables remain to be fully developed.	
Biochemical measures Creatinine/height index (CHI)	Estimate of skeletal mass. Urinary creatinine levels are dependent primarily upon extent of skeletal muscle catabolism especially during protein depletion. 24-hour urine creatinine.	Protein depletion can be detected over time.	Dependent upon normal renal function. Multiple medications may affect creatinine excretion; therefore, drug history must be obtained before interpretation. Effective collection of urine. To ensure reliability, three consecutive 24-hour urine collections must be obtained.	

Appendix 14–2. Nutritional Assessment Parameters—Use in Trauma/Critically Ill Patient *Continued*

ASSESSMENT PARAMETER	PURPOSE (DESCRIPTION)	PROS	CONS	APPLICATION
Serum proteins	Note: Plasma concentrations depend on rate of synthesis and utilization, intravascular transfer, catabolism, excretion, and hydration. Help to estimate the degree of visceral protein depletion (kwashiorkor type malnutrition). Visceral protein—all other proteins (not stored somatically), including such vital functions as enzymes, antibodies, plasma proteins, and involvement in function of visceral organs and immune system.			
1. Albumin		Valuable screening indicator. Repeated studies have correlated hypopalbuminemia with increased morbidity and mortality, especially < 3.0 gm/dl.	During protein deprivation, may require days or weeks to decrease because of large extravascular stores and relatively long serum half-life (20 days). Liver damage may cause depression; however, must be severe, i.e., 10 to 25 per cent of hepatic cells are required for normal serum albumin levels. Corticosteroids result in shift from extravascular albumin to intravascular space.	
2. Transferrin		Accurately reflects rapid changes in nutritional status based on shorter half-life and smaller body pool. Documentation of depressed transferrin concentrations in severe PCM is conclusive.	Interpretation is limited in the presence of iron deficiency anemia (elevations would be seen). Calculations vary in different clinical settings, i.e., direct or indirect with use of total iron binding capacity. Indirect may carry significant error. Arbitrary cut-off points.	
3. Prealbumin- and retinol-binding capacity		Sensitive indicator of early changes in protein status. Short half-life.	Controversy still exists over its practical application in clinical settings. High level sensitivity with even minor stress.	

Appendix 14–2. Nutritional Assessment Parameters—Use in Trauma/Critically Ill Patient *Continued*

ASSESSMENT PARAMETER	PURPOSE (DESCRIPTION)	PROS	CONS	APPLICATION
Nitrogen balance	Index of protein nutritional status. Nitrogen primary component that differentiates protein from other basic nutrients. In stresses such as severe trauma and sepsis, balance between anabolism and catabolism in terms of protein is altered. Estimated via 24-hour urine collection (nitrogen excreted), nitrogen intake, and correction for occult losses. Nitrogen balance reflects homeostasis if it is approximately zero.	Negative nitrogen balance reflects greater degree of protein catabolism and therefore serves as an indication of the magnitude of injury. Allows for serial evaluation of nutriment adequacy.	Nitrogen depletion cannot be prevented during peak catabolic response. Accurate 24-hour urine collection. Need meticulous evaluation of all nitrogen intake (oral, enteral, parenteral) and all nitrogen excretion (urinary, fecal, dermal). Renal disease and specific medications must be examined before interpretation. Must consider occult losses in trauma patient through burns, diarrhea, vomiting, fistula drainage.	
Immunological parameters	Identification of protein losses—WMB, antibody response to antigens.	Protein-calorie malnutrition (PCM) is generally recognized as the most common cause of immune dysfunction. Close association exists between increased susceptibility to infection and PCM, although the exact relationship between nutrition and host defense mechanisms remain unclear. It has been found that preoperative lymphocytopenia was associated with depressed albumin levels, and if both were depressed, an increased rate of postoperative sepsis was observed. Also note trends in relation to clinical picture.		
1. Total Lymphocyte Count (TLC)	TLC particularly reflects humoral immunity as well as cell mediated immunity.			
2. Skin antigen testing	Inability to respond (anergy) is related to visceral protein depletion.	Serial testing can serve as a sensitive guide to prognosis and adequacy of clinical management. Anergic states have identified postoperative and posttrauma patients who are at an increased risk for sepsis and mortality and have presaged those complications in patients studied preoperatively. Use in patients with questionable nutritional status.	No universal standards for interpretation exist. Most subjects tested repeatedly exhibit accelerated response. Should not be applied immediately following an operation or thermal injury, since stress can obliterate the response.	

Appendix 14–2. Nutritional Assessment Parameters—Use in Trauma/Critically Ill Patient *Continued*

ASSESSMENT PARAMETER	PURPOSE (DESCRIPTION)	PROS	CONS	APPLICATION
Energy expenditure metabolic rate	Estimate of energy needs.			
1. Harris and Benedict equation (HBE)	Based on age, sex, height, and weight—estimate of basal energy expenditure (the BEE is the metabolic rate after a 12-hour fast and after lying completely still for at least 30 minutes).	Simple equation, most commonly used, inexpensive. Reported reliability—difference between actual and predicted findings only 4.6 per cent.	Found that stress factor adjustment to HBE for trauma significantly overestimates the energy needs when compared with true energy needs as measured by indirect calorimetry. Overestimates caloric need in obese patients.	
2. Nomograms used to estimate energy requirements	Scale analysis. Usually based on age, height, weight, and surface area. Corrections that account for percentage increase due to injury, trauma, sepsis.	Simple method for supplying an estimate of energy needs.	Individual variations or extreme cases are generalized. Cookbook approach.	
3. Indirect calorimetry (Beckman metabolic cart, mass spectrometry)	Gas analysis—measure of gas exchange. $\dot{V}_{O2}$ and CO_2 production are related to the release of energy from the body.	Very reliable and accurate technique.	Expensive technical equipment. Accuracy depends on trained technician and properly functioning equipment. Must use average, not one-time measure. Instrument not available in all hospitals.	
Respiratory quotient (RQ) range (0.7 + 1.0)	RQ is the ratio of volume of carbon dioxide produced divided by the volume of oxygen consumed during the same period of time. It varies with substrate oxidation.	Identification of nutritionally depleted patients in whom large glucose loads result in excess glucose being utilized for lipogenesis, i.e., CO_2 produced in excess of O_2 consumed (carbohydrate exceeds needs). RQ = > 1.0. Identification or prolonged fasting with almost complete fat oxidation—0.70 RQ. Excess carbohydrate may precipitate respiratory failure and is of particular interest in patients being weaned from mechanical ventilation. RQ of < 0.70 has been associated with oxidation of keytones or synthesis of carbohydrate from fat.	RQ in septic hypermetabolic patients may remain below 1.0 even with excessive glucose loads because endogenous fat (RQ = 0.70) is preferentially used and glucose is stored as glycogen. Hyperventilation increases the RQ often > 1.0 and reflects an inaccurate test situation. Values of < 0.70 may reflect methodological error—regard with skepticism. To use RQ in determining protein utilization, must use formula that incorporates urinary nitrogen excretion.	

Prepared by GL Stiver Stanek, RN, MS, Clinical Specialist, Maryland Institute for Emergency Medical Services Systems, Baltimore, MD, 1986.

Appendix 14–3. Dietary Department, University of Maryland Medical Systems, Nutrition Flow Sheet

NUTRITION GOALS: _____ kCAL _____ gm protein usual body wt. _____ kg IBW _____ kg MGU _____ gm CHO

DATE

NUTRITION RX

Tot. kCAL in														
Tot. Protein/N_2 in														
Kcal:N_2														
PO Protein/kCal														
TPN ml 24 hr														
TPN—carbohydrate														
TPN—protein														
Lipids kCAL														
Other IV														
TF ml 24 hr														
TF—carbohydrate														
TF—protein														
TF—fat														
I/O net ±														
UUN/N_2 balance														
Measured RE—mean														
Measured kCAL—mean														
V_{CO2}/V_{O2}														
Weight (kg)														
Residuals (ml)														
Temperature maximum														
Stool frequency														

MGU = maximum glucose utilization; TF = tube feeding; RE = respiratory exchange.

Appendix 15–1. Trauma Pain Data Base and History Guidelines

This information should be obtained from the patient. Family, police, medics, or other witnesses are secondary sources. Some questions may only be answered many hours or days after the accident.

1. Describe the accident (include type of vehicle, where the accident occurred, whether it was work-related).
2. Describe the injury.
3. What is the relationship of others involved in the accident to the patient (specify injuries)?
4. Were there any deaths in the accident (specify relationship of the deceased to the patient)?
5. Did the patient lose consciousness? If so, for how long?
6. Is the toxicology screen positive for alcohol or drugs? If so, what are the actions of the drug(s) and when might withdrawal occur if used regularly.
7. Describe rescue events (time between accident and rescue and any further injury related to rescue).
8. Describe other consequences of the accident: driver at fault, legal charges against patient, damage to patient's vehicle.

Appendix 15–2. Pain Assessment Factors in the Critical, Intermediate, and Rehabilitation Cycles of Trauma

1. Patient report of pain
   a. Rating on 0 to 10 scale
   b. Description (continuous, intermittent, percentage of time in pain, sharp, dull, burning, aching)
2. Blood pressure, pulse and respiratory rates
3. Mobility (sit, stand, lift, bend)
4. Food and fluid intake
5. Elimination
6. Sleep and rest
7. Location of injury
8. Type of injury (fractures, ruptured viscera, head, nerves, burns, infection, loss of body part)
9. Affect (anxious, worried, oblivious, happy, sad, fearful, angry)
10. Behavior (crying, lethargic, restless, motionless)
11. Energy level (patient's report)
12. Past experience with pain
13. Meaning of pain (to patient and family)
14. Oriented to person, place, date, situation
15. Memory functioning
16. Ability to follow instructions
17. Knowledge of injuries
18. Past health history
    a. Chronic pain history (in spouse, family of origin)
    b. Physical illnesses
    c. Emotional illnesses
    d. Medications (name, dose, frequency, last taken)
19. Social functioning
    a. Education, occupation
    b. Family history (siblings' and parents' functioning)
    c. Behavioral problems
    d. Drug use (name, amount, length of time used, last used, treatment, withdrawal reactions).

Appendix 15–3. Tools for the Measurement of Pain

Visual Analogue Scale

|————————————|

The reliability and validity of the visual analogue scale (VAS) has been well established. Typically, a VAS is a 10-cm line with right-angle stops at either end of the line. The stops are critical to contain marks made by the patient. Descriptive anchors should be placed at either end of the line beyond the stops. The use of numbers or words placed on or below the line tends to produce non-uniform scores. Both the vertical and the horizontal orientations have been used. Researchers report conflicting results with the vertical scale. One researcher[1] noted that scores tended to be skewed compared with the horizontal orientation, whereas Gift[2] noted that asthmatic patients had greater difficulty scoring the horizontal scale. Gift noted higher scores with the vertical VAS.

The advantages of the VAS include ease in administration and scoring and usefulness for subjective phenomena. Because the VAS does not force subjects into a limited number of categories for the expression of pain, it is considered more sensitive.[1]

A disadvantage of the VAS is that specific instructions are necessary for the subject to properly rate pain. Even with instructions, some researchers report that some patients have difficulty translating the subjective nature of pain to an abstract line. Another disadvantage is that the VAS measures only the intensity of pain.

McGill Pain Questionnaire

The McGill Pain Questionnaire (MPQ) was developed by Melzack and Torgerson[3] by dividing words descriptive of pain into classes and subclasses that represent the sensory, affective, and evaluative dimensions of pain. The MPQ is a multidimensional tool that provides quantitative data about pain. Strong evidence for the reliability and validity of the MPQ has been published.[4–6]

Criticisms of the MPQ center on the time required to complete the tool. Melzack stated that initially the tool takes 15 to 20 minutes to complete and with increased experience, only 5 to 10 minutes. Researchers state it takes about 20 to 30 minutes to complete.[7] A shorter version of the MPQ (sf-MPQ), developed by Melzack,[8] is reported to take 2 to 5 minutes to administer.

The MPQ is useful for the assessment of the multiple dimensions of pain. The drawing on the tool is useful to document whether and where the location of pain changes

BEHAVIORAL DEFINITION AND SCORING OF THE CHEOPS

ITEM	BEHAVIOR		DEFINITION
Cry	No cry	1	Child is not crying.
	Moaning	2	Child is moaning or quietly vocalizing silent cry.
	Crying	2	Child is crying, but the cry is gentle or whimpering.
	Scream	3	Child is in a full-lunged cry; sobbing; may be scored with complaint or without complaint.
Facial	Composed	1	Neutral facial expression.
	Grimace	2	Score only if definite negative facial expression.
	Smiling	0	Score ony if definite positive facial expression.
Child verbal	None	1	Child not talking.
	Other complaints	1	Child complains, but not about pain, e.g., "I want to see Mommy" or "I am thirsty."
	Pain complaints	2	Child complains about pain.
	Both complaints	2	Child complains about pain and about other things, e.g., "It hurts; I want Mommy."
	Positive	0	Child makes any positive statement or talks about other things without complaint.
Torso	Neutral	1	Body (not limbs) is at rest; torso is inactive.
	Shifting	2	Body is in motion in a shifting or serpentine fashion.
	Tense	2	Body is arched or rigid.
	Shivering	2	Body is shuddering or shaking involuntarily.
	Upright	2	Child is in a vertical or upright position.
	Restrained	2	Body is restrained.
Touch	Not touching	1	Child is not touching or grabbing at wound.
	Reach	2	Child is reaching for but not touching wound.
	Touch	2	Child is gently touching wound or wound area.
	Grab	2	Child is grabbing vigorously at wound.
	Restrained	2	Child's arms are restrained.
Legs	Neutral	1	Legs may be in any position but are relaxed; includes gentle swimming or serpentine-like movements.
	Squirming/kicking	2	Definitive uneasy or restless movements in the legs and/or striking out with foot or feet.
	Drawn up/tensed	2	Legs tensed and/or pulled up tightly to body and kept there.
	Standing	2	Standing, crouching, or kneeling.
	Restrained	2	Child's legs are being held down.

From McGrath P, Johnson G, Goodman JT, et al: CHEOPS: A behavioral scale for rating post-operative pain in children. In Advances in Pain Research and Therapy, Vol 9. New York, Raven Press, 1985, p 398; with permission.

Appendix 15–3. Tools for the Measurement of Pain *Continued*

McGill-Melzack
PAIN QUESTIONNAIRE

Patient's name ______________ Age __________

File No. ______________ Date __________

Clinical category (e.g., cardiac, neurologic)

Diagnosis: ____________

____

____

Analgesic (if already administered):

1. Type ______________________
2. Dosage ______________________
3. Time given in relation to this test ______

Patient's intelligence: circle number that represents best estimate.

1 (low) 2 3 4 5 (high)

****

This questionnaire has been designed to tell us more about your pain. Four major questions we ask are

1. Where is your pain?
2. What does it feel like?
3. How does it change with time?
4. How strong is it?

It is important that you tell us how your pain feels now. Please follow the instructions at the beginning of each part.

Part 1. Where Is Your Pain?

Please mark, on the drawings below, the areas where you feel pain. Put E if external, or I if internal, near the areas you mark. Put EI if both external and internal.

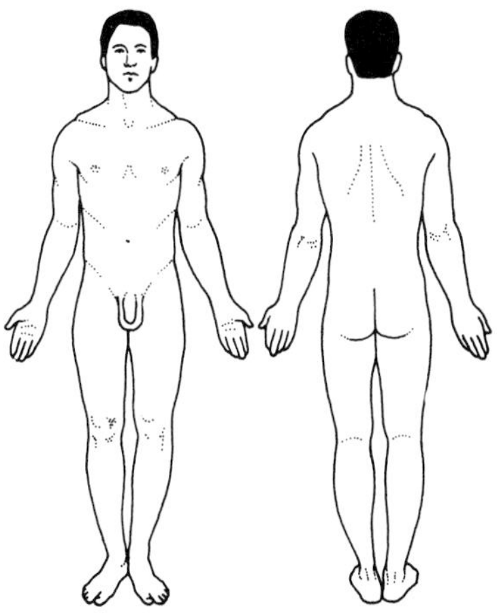

Part 2. What Does Your Pain Feel Like?

Some of the words below describe your *present* pain. Circle *ONLY* those words that best describe it. Leave out any category that is not suitable. Use only a single word in each appropriate category—the one that applies best.

1: Flickering, Quivering, Pulsing, Throbbing, Beating, Pounding

2: Jumping, Flashing, Shooting

3: Pricking, Boring, Drilling, Stabbing, Lancinating

4: Sharp, Cutting, Lacerating

5: Pinching, Pressing, Gnawing, Cramping, Crushing

6: Tugging, Pulling, Wrenching

7: Hot, Burning, Scalding, Searing

8: Tingling, Itchy, Smarting, Stinging

9: Dull, Sore, Hurting, Aching, Heavy

10: Tender, Taut, Rasping, Splitting

11: Tiring, Exhausting

12: Sickening, Suffocat-ing

13: Fearful, Frightful, Terrifying

14: Punishing, Grueling, Cruel, Vicious, Killing

15: Wretched, Blinding

16: Annoying, Troublesome, Miserable, Intense, Unbearable

17: Spreading, Radiating, Penetrating, Piercing

18: Tight, Numb, Drawing, Squeezing, Tearing

19: Cool, Cold, Freezing

20: Nagging, Nauseating, Agonizing, Dreadful, Torturing

Part 3. How Does Your Pain Change With Time?

1. Which word or words would you use to describe the *pattern* of your pain?

1	2	3
Continuous	Rhythmic	Brief
Steady	Periodic	Momentary
Constant	Intermittent	Transient

2. What kind of things *relieve* your pain?
3. What kind of things *increase* your pain?

Part 4. How Strong Is Your Pain?

People agree that the following 5 words represent pain of increasing intensity. They are:

1	2	3	4	5
Mild	Discomforting	Distressing	Horrible	Excruciating

To answer each question below, write the number of the most appropriate word in the space beside the question.

1. Which word describes your pain right now? ____
2. Which word describes it at its worst? ____
3. Which word describes it when it is least? ____
4. Which word describes the worst toothache you ever had? ____
5. Which word describes the worst headache you ever had? ____
6. Which word describes the worst stomach ache you ever had? ____

Appendix 15–3. Tools for the Measurement of Pain *Continued*

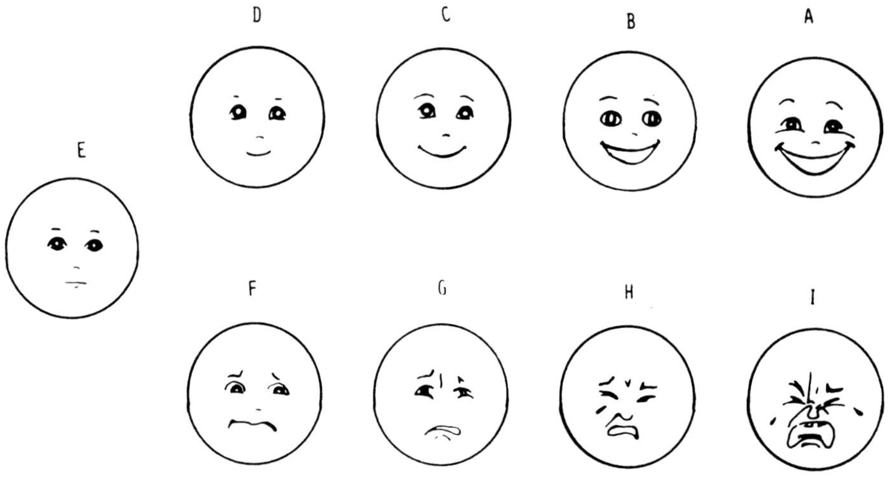

Nine-face interval scale developed in a pilot study as a measure for pain affect. Faces A–D represent varying magnitudes of positive affect; faces F–I represent varying magnitudes of negative affect. Face E was initially assumed to represent a neutral face. From McGrath PA, deVeber LL, Hearn MT: Multidimensional pain assessment in children. In Advances in Pain Research and Therapy. New York, Raven Press, 1985, p. 390.

over time. The questionnaire has been used successfully for both acute and chronic pain. The reader is referred to Melzack[5] for administration and scoring instructions.

Children's Hospital of Eastern Ontario Pain Scale

The Children's Hospital of Eastern Ontario Pain Scale (CHEOPS), developed specifically for children, involves observing a child for behaviors indicative of pain. These behaviors are then tallied to form an overall score.

Reliability and validity for this tool were established in the postanesthesia care unit by the authors.[10] To use the tool, the nurse looks at each item and assigns the score that corresponds to the observed behavior. The scores correspond to 0 = behavior that is the antithesis of pain; 1 = behavior that is not indicative of pain and is not the antithesis of pain; 2 = behavior that indicates mild or moderate pain; and 3 = behavior that indicates severe pain. Definitions of each behavior are helpful for consistent use of the tool.

Faces Pain Scale

McGrath and colleagues[9] tested the reliability of the faces pain scale using brightness matching and visual analogue scales (VAS). Children were asked to make a light "as bright as the container is heavy" and to make the VAS line as long "as the container is heavy." The researchers then compared the brightness and line lengths assigned by the children to the representative pain intensity of each face.

The results of the study showed that the intervals between the positive faces (A through E) were about equal, whereas the intervals for the negative faces (F through I) were not. Face E was intended but not interpreted by the children as neutral. Because the intervals were not equal, the authors recommend the following scale for scoring the approximate magnitude of a child's pain: A = .8; B = .22; C = .34; D = .47; E = .60; F = .78; G = .82; H = .90; and I = .97.

The authors used the faces pain scale with normal children who experienced everyday falls and scrapes and with children who have cancer and undergo frequent painful interventions. The VAS and faces pain scale can be used for patients aged 5 and above.

REFERENCES

1. Sriwanatakul K, Kelvie W, Lasgna L, et al: Studies with different types of visual analogue scales for the measurement of pain. Clin Pharmacol Ther 34:234–239, 1983.
2. Gift AG: Validation of a vertical visual analog scale as a measure of clinical dyspnea. Rehab Nurs 14:323–325, 1989.
3. Melzack R, Torgerson WS: On the language of pain. Anesthesiology 34:50–59, 1975.
4. Kremer E, Atkinson JJ, Ignelzi RJ: Measurement of pain: Patient preference does not confound pain measurement. Pain 10:241–248, 1981.
5. Melzack R: The McGill Pain Questionnaire; major properties and scoring methods. Pain 1:277, 1975.
6. Prieto EJ, Hopson L, Bradley LA, et al: The language of low back pain: Factor structure of the McGill Pain Questionnaire. Pain 8:45–56, 1980.
7. Slack JF: Personal communication, October 10, 1990.
8. Melzack R: The short-form McGill Pain Questionnaire. Pain 30:191–197, 1987.
9. McGrath PA, deVeber LL, Hearn MT: Multidimensional pain assessment in children. Advances in Pain Research and Therapy 9:387–393, 1985.
10. McGrath PJ, Johnson G, Goodman JT, et al: CHEOPS: A behavioral scale for rating postoperative pain in children. Advances in Pain Research and Therapy 9:395–402, 1985.

Appendix 17–1. Rancho los Amigos Scale

Levels of Cognitive Functioning

I. No Response

Patient appears to be in a deep sleep and is completely unresponsive to any stimuli presented to him.

II. Generalized Response

Patient reacts inconsistently and nonpurposefully to stimuli in a nonspecific manner. Responses are limited in nature and are often the same regardless of the stimulus presented. Responses may be physiological changes, gross body movements, and/or vocalization. Often the earliest response is to deep pain. Responses are likely to be delayed.

III. Localized Response

Patient reacts specifically but inconsistently to stimuli. Responses are directly related to the type of stimulus presented, as in turning the head toward a sound or focusing on an object presented. The patient may withdraw an extremity and/or vocalize when presented with a painful stimulus. He may follow simple commands in an inconsistent, delayed manner, such as closing his eyes or squeezing or extending an extremity. Once the external stimulus is removed, he may lie quietly. He may also show a vague awareness of self and body by responding to discomfort by pulling at the nasogastric tube or catheter or by resisting restraints. He may show a bias by responding to some persons (especially family, friends) but not to others.

IV. Confused-Agitated

Patient is in a heightened state of activity with severely decreased ability to process information. He is detached from the present and responds primarily to his own internal confusion. Behavior is frequently bizarre and nonpurposeful relative to his immediate environment. He may cry out or scream out of proportion to stimuli even after removal, may show aggressive behavior, attempt to remove restraints or tubes, or crawl out of bed in a purposeful manner. He does not, however, discriminate among persons or objects and is unable to cooperate directly with treatment efforts. Verbalization is frequently incoherent and/or inappropriate to the environment. Confabulation may be present; he may be euphoric or hostile. Thus, gross attention to environment is very short, and selective attention is often nonexistent. Being unaware of present events, patient lacks short-term recall and may be reacting to past events. He is unable to perform self-care (feeding, dressing) without maximum assistance. If not disabled physically, he may perform motor activities such as sitting, reaching, and ambulating. He does these as part of his agitated state and not as a purposeful act or on request, necessarily.

V. Confused, Inappropriate, Nonagitated

Patient appears alert and is able to respond to simple commands fairly consistently. However, with increased complexity of commands or lack of any external structure, responses are nonpurposeful, random, or at best fragmented toward any desired goal. He may show agitated behavior, not on an internal basis as in level IV, but rather as a result of external stimuli and usually out of proportion to the stimulus. He has gross attention to the environment but is highly distractable and lacks ability to focus attention on a specific task without frequent redirection to it. With structure, he may be able to converse on a social, automatic level for short periods of time. Verbalization is often inappropriate; confabulation may be triggered by present events. His memory is severely impaired, with confusion of past and present in his reaction to on-going activity. Patient lacks initiation of functional tasks and often shows inappropriate use of objects without external direction. He may be able to perform previously learned tasks when structured for him, but is unable to learn new information. He responds best to self, body, comfort, and often family members. The patient can usually perform self-care activities with assistance and may accomplish feeding with maximum supervision. Management on the ward is often a problem if the patient is physically mobile, as he may wander off either randomly or with vague intention of "going home."

VI. Confused-Appropriate

Patient shows goal-directed behavior but is dependent on external input for direction. Response to discomfort is appropriate, and he is able to tolerate unpleasant stimuli (such as nasogastric tube) when need is explained. He follows simple directions consistently and shows carryover for tasks he has relearned (such as self-care). He is at least supervised with old learning; he is unable to maximally assist for new learning with little or no carryover. Responses may be incorrect because of memory problems, but they are appropriate to the situation. They may be delayed to immediate stimuli, and he shows decreased ability to process information with little or no anticipation or prediction of events. Past memories show more depth and detail than recent memory. The patient may show beginning immediate awareness of his situation by realizing he does not know an answer. He no longer wanders and is inconsistently oriented to time and place. Selective attention to tasks may be impaired, especially with difficult tasks and in unstructured settings, but he is now functional for common daily activities (30 minutes with structure). He shows at least vague recognition of some staff, has increased awareness of self, family, and basic needs (such as food), again in an appropriate manner, which is in contrast to level V.

VII. Automatic-Appropriate

Patient appears appropriate and oriented within hospital and home settings, goes through daily routine automatically although frequently robotlike, with minimal to absent confusion, but has shallow recall of what he has been doing. He shows increased awareness of self, body, family, foods, people, and interaction in the environment. He has superficial awareness of, but lacks insight into, his condition, demonstrates decreased judgment and problem-solving ability, and lacks realistic planning for his future. He shows carryover for new learning but at a decreased rate. He requires at least minimal supervision for learning and for safety purposes. He is independent in self-care activities and supervised in home and community skills for safety. With structure he is able to initiate tasks as social or recreational

Appendix 17–1. Rancho los Amigos Scale *Continued*

activities in which he now has interest. His judgment remains impaired, such that he is unable to drive a car. Prevocational or avocational evaluation and counseling may be indicated.

VIII. Purposeful and Appropriate

Patient is alert and oriented, is able to recall and integrate past and recent events, and is aware of and responsive to his culture. He shows carryover for new learning acceptable to him and his life role, and needs no supervision once activities are learned. Within his physical capabilities, he is independent in home and community skills, including driving. Vocational rehabilitation, to determine ability to return as a contributor to the community (perhaps in a new capacity), is indicated. He may continue to show a decreased ability, relative to premorbid abilities, in reasoning, tolerance for stress, and judgment in emergencies or unusual circumstances. His social, emotional, and intellectual capacities may continue to be at a decreased level for him but are functional for operating in society.

Reprinted with permission from Hagen C, Malkmus D, Durham P: Communication Disorders Service, Rancho Los Amigos Hospital, Downey, CA, 1972. Revised 1974 by Malkmus D, Stenderup K.

Appendix 19–1. Trauma Airways Procedures

PURPOSE: Maintain an open airway for ventilation (spontaneous or mechanical ventilation).

Oropharyngeal Airway

EQUIPMENT
1. Oral airway (sizes 000 to 10 mm)
2. Tongue blade
3. Adherent tape

Nursing Action	Rationale
1. Clear the mouth of potential obstructing agents.	
2. Insert the airway between the patient's teeth with the curved portion toward the patient's feet.	Avoid pushing the tongue back and obstructing the airway.
3. As the airway passes the tongue, rotate it so that the curved portion follows the natural curve of the pharynx.	
4. Alternative: Use a tongue blade to depress the tongue while passing the airway into the pharynx.	
5. Secure in place with adherent tape if required.	To secure the airway and prevent dislodging.

Nasopharyngeal Airway

EQUIPMENT
1. Nasal airway
2. Water soluble lubricant

Nursing Action	Rationale
1. Select the desired size, determined by the largest size that will fit comfortably into the patient's nostril. Examine both nostrils for internal injuries or obstruction and select the clearest opening.	Avoid nasal trauma and patient discomfort.
2. Lubricate the airway.	
3. Pass the airway gently with the bevel facing the nasal septum along the floor of the nose.	The floor of the nose lies parallel to the oral cavity. Proper insertion reduces trauma and bleeding.

Esophageal Obturator Airway (EOA)

Note: Insertion and removal of the EOA as a nursing responsibility varies with the nurse's training and certification and institutional policy.

EQUIPMENT
1. EOA and mask (15 inches long, open at the top and blind at the bottom. Holes are located near the upper end to allow for air flow into the pharynx.)
2. 50 ml syringe
3. Water soluble lubricant
4. Suction equipment
5. Oxygen source
6. Ambu bag

Appendix 19–1. Trauma Airways Procedures *Continued*

NURSING ACTION	RATIONALE
1. Check the cuff and connect the esophageal tube to the face mask.	
2. Set the syringe at 35 ml.	Avoid overinflation and esophageal trauma. Avoid underinflation and risk of aspiration.
3. Lubricate the tube.	
4. Ventilate and oxygenate the patient. Position the patient's head in a neutral position. Do *not* hyperextend.	
5. Grasp the lower jaw and tongue; lift the jaw straight up.	The neutral position allows the tube to pass most readily into the esophagus.
6. Insert the tube while the patient's head is maintained in a neutral position. Advance the tube until the mask is properly seated on the face.	
7. Ventilate and auscultate both lung fields.	To ensure that the EOA is not positioned in the trachea.
8. Inflate the cuff with 35 ml of air.	
9. With the cuff inflated, check again for breath sounds.	To ensure proper position and ventilation.
10. Remove only when (a) the patient is breathing spontaneously and adequately awake so as to protect his own airway and (b) an endotracheal tube is in place.	
11. To remove, turn the head to side. Have suction immediately available.	Vomiting is **expected**.
12. Deflate the cuff and remove.	

Endotracheal Intubation

EQUIPMENT

1. Laryngoscope with MacIntosh and straight blades
2. Endotracheal tube
3. Stylet (optional)
4. Water soluble lubricant
5. Syringe
6. Stopcock
7. McGill forceps
8. Tracheal suction with sterile catheters
9. Oropharyngeal suction
10. Oral airway
11. Tongue blade
12. Adherent tape
13. Benzoin solution or spray (optional)
14. Ventilator
15. Oxygen supply and tubing
16. Ambu bag with mask

NURSING ACTION	RATIONALE
1. Explain the procedure to the patient.	To decrease apprehension and gain the patient's cooperation.
2. Test oxygen supply and ventilator.	
3. Assist with anesthesia and muscle relaxant administration, as appropriate.	
4. Apply cricoid pressure as directed by anesthesia provider.	Trauma patients are assumed to have a full stomach. This will decrease the possibility of aspiration.
5. Stay with the patient throughout the procedure.	To monitor the patient's response to the procedure, to record baseline measurements upon establishing airway and ventilation, and to provide reassurance for the patient.
6. Secure the tube to the patient's maxilla with benzoin and tape.	
7. Auscultate bilateral breath sounds and chest excursion. A postintubation chest film must be obtained.	To ensure that the patient is being properly ventilated, to definitively determine tube position, and to identify any complications of the procedure.
8. Note and document time and type of intubation, any complications, and the patient's response to the procedure.	

Appendix 19–2. Autotransfusion

PURPOSE: To collect and reinfuse a patient's own blood for intravascular volume replacement.

DEFINITIONS

Autotransfusion: reinfusion of patient's own blood.
Autologous blood: the patient's own blood.
Homologous blood: bank blood donated by another individual.

TYPES OF AUTOTRANSFUSION

Preoperative: patient donates own blood preoperatively, which is stored and used later during elective surgery (days or weeks later).
Perioperative: immediately before surgery, blood is drawn off (may or may not be diluted with plasma) and infused during surgery.
Intraoperative: blood collected (in trauma center or emergency room) from chest/abdomen and reinfused.
Postoperative: usually after cardiac surgery, shed blood is collected from mediastinum and reinfused.

EQUIPMENT

1. Collection device with detachable reservoir
2. Suction tubing/apparatus
3. Sterile water for creating underwater seal
4. Minidrip Buretrol infusion set
5. Citrate anticoagulant
6. Filter tubing for reinfusion

The responsibility of the nursing and physician staff in managing the autotransfusion system during collection and reinfusion is dependent on institutional policy.

PREPARATION

1. Suspect need for use of autotransfusion equipment on any patient with acute intrathoracic or intra-abdominal bleeding.
2. Gather necessary equipment.
3. If patient is conscious, inform of the procedure and offer support.

NURSING ACTION	RATIONALE
1. Fill suction chamber with sterile H_2O to 20 cm suction	Sterile H_2O should be used instead of tap H_2O.
2. Fill underwater seal chamber with sterile H_2O to level indicated by product specifications.	To create underwater seal
3. Attach suction tubing to collection device and turn on suction source.	
4. Attach collection device tubing to patient's intrathoracic or intra-abdominal catheter.	
5. Upon collection of the shed blood in the reservoir, instill citrate anticoagulant via minidrip Buretrol at a ratio of 1:10 (1 part anticoagulant to 10 parts shed blood).	To prevent clotting
6. Clamp catheter and remove reservoir and attach patient tubing to underwater seal device (suction). Unclamp catheter.	To restore suction and underwater seal
7. Force air out of reservoir prior to attaching filtered reinfusion tubing.	To prevent the otherwise likely chance of air embolism
8. Invert reservoir and reinfuse shed blood via intravenous access.	
9. Monitor patient's physiological response to transfusion.	Watch for signs and symptoms of transfusion reaction, air embolism, and coagulopathies
10. Document volume of blood shed and reinfused.	

Appendix 19–3. Pericardial Tap

Purpose: To remove fluid from the pericardial sac and thereby relieve cardiac tamponade. Cardiac tamponade is the compression of the heart by blood, effusion, or a foreign body in the pericardial sac that restricts normal heart action.

EQUIPMENT

1. Instrument tray
2. Povidone-iodine (Betadine) scrub
3. Povidone-iodine (Betadine) solution
4. 1 per cent lidocaine
5. Sterile gloves
6. 18 gauge arterial needle
7. Have available EKG monitor, thoracoabdominal tray, defibrillator, and emergency drugs, i.e., atropine, lidocaine

PROCEDURE

NURSING ACTION	RATIONALE
1. Premedicate patient.	To reduce patient's apprehension and discomfort
2. Place EKG leads on patient.	To monitor patient's cardiac performance during procedure
3. Place patient supine.	This position makes it easier to insert needle into pericardial sac.
4. Have defibrillator and pacemaker available in room.	In case of cardiac complications
5. Using aseptic technique, open tray and prepare setup.	
6. While the procedure is in progress, monitor patient's EKG and blood pressure continuously.	There is a danger of laceration of myocardium and coronary artery and cardiac arrhythmias. ST segment will rise with contact of needle to ventricle. PR segment will elevate when needle contacts atrium. Large, erratic QRS complexes will indicate penetration of myocardium.
7. Observe for presence and rapid accumulation of bloody fluid. Thoracotomy may be indicated.	Bloody pericardial fluid may be due to trauma. Bloody pericardial effusion fluid does not clot; blood obtained from inadvertent puncture of heart chambers does clot.
8. Following procedure, apply sterile dressing.	
9. Complete data sheets.	To document times, surgeons, and place of surgery for medicolegal reasons

FOLLOW-UP

NURSING ACTION	RATIONALE
1. Following pericardial tap, careful monitoring of EKG and blood pressure is necessary to indicate possible recurrence of tamponade.	
2. Be aware of complications resulting in unsuccessful pericardial tap, including inadvertent puncture of heart chamber; arrhythmias; puncture of lung, stomach, or liver; and laceration of coronary artery or myocardium.	These would result in need for emergency surgical intervention.

Adapted from the Nursing Procedure Manual, Maryland Institute for Emergency Medical Services Systems, Baltimore, MD, 1987.

Appendix 19–4. Summary of Chest Physiotherapy Treatment

Frequency of Treatment

As Indicated (PRN)

1. Ideal frequency for patient's status.
2. Therapist must be well trained in clinical evaluation.
3. Close communication with the physician is essential.
4. Works well with experienced therapists assigned to a specific unit.

Every Four Hours

1. Usual frequency that is necessary for critically ill patients.
2. Treatment is continued throughout a 24-hour period for mechanically ventilated patients.
3. Spontaneously breathing patients in no acute distress usually benefit from sleep at night; cooperation is then improved with daytime treatments.

More Frequently Than Every Four Hours

1. Patients with copious secretions that are not removed by four hourly chest physiotherapy treatments, turning, and suctioning or coughing.
2. Patients with closed head injuries and secretion retention who are limited in the amount of time they may remain in the head-down position.
3. The need for treatment more frequently than q4h should be reevaluated after 12 to 24 hours of treatment.
4. Increased frequency of treatment often makes optimal treatments impossible because of multiple other therapeutic interventions.

Less Frequently Than Every Four Hours

1. Mobilized patients.
2. Patients who clear their secretions spontaneously with deep breathing and coughing.
3. Patients with minimal secretions with or without radiological evidence of atelectasis or pneumonia.
4. Acute lobar collapse usually responds to one to two vigorous chest physiotherapy treatments, which may then be replaced by patient mobilization.

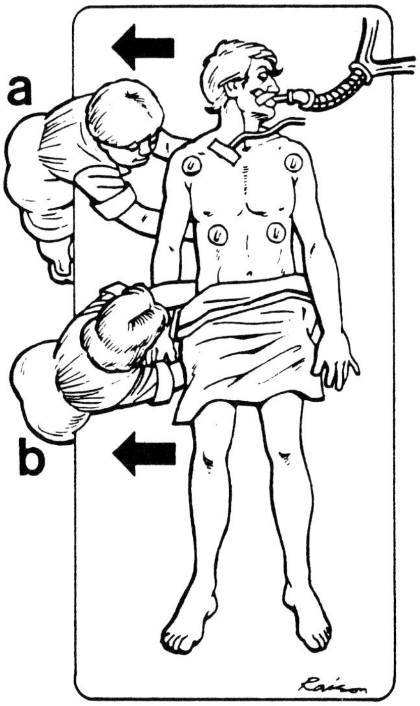

Both hands are placed under the trunk *(a)* while a second person places both hands under the hips *(b)*. The patient is lifted to the side of the bed.

Appendix 19–4. Summary of Chest Physiotherapy Treatment *Continued*

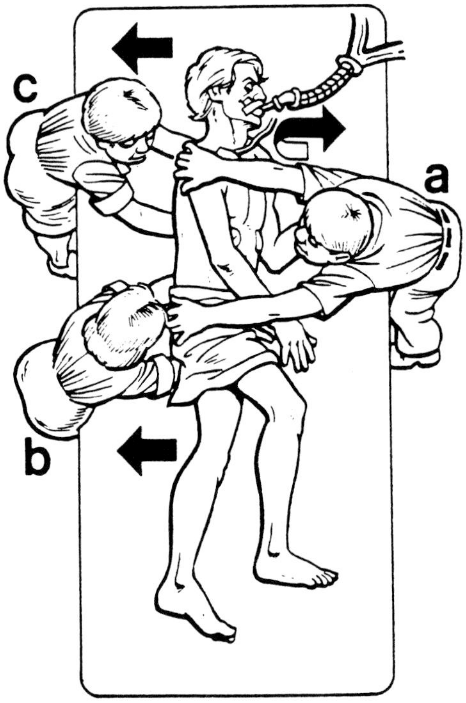

a. With one hand over the uppermost shoulder and the other over the uppermost hip, the patient is pulled onto the side. (Crossing the patient's legs prior to turning facilitates rolling the patient.) *b*. A second person lifts the hips back. *c*. For obese or difficult patients, a third person may simultaneously lift the shoulders back.

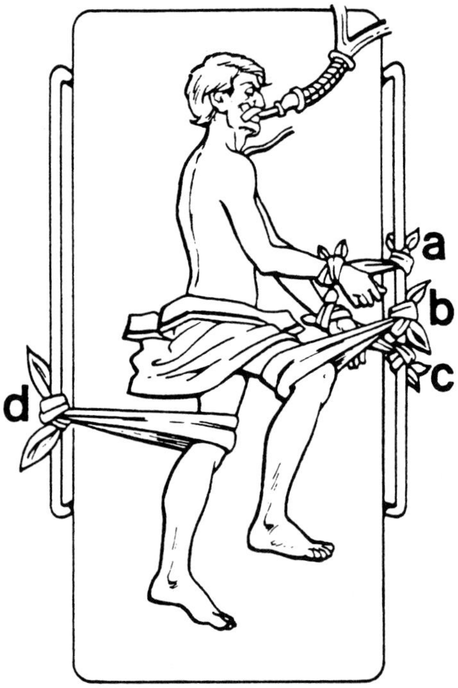

To keep an agitated patient sidelying, the wrists are restrained (*a* and *c*), and sheets are tied around the thighs to the bed rail. The upper hip is flexed *(b)* and the lower hip is extended *(d)*.

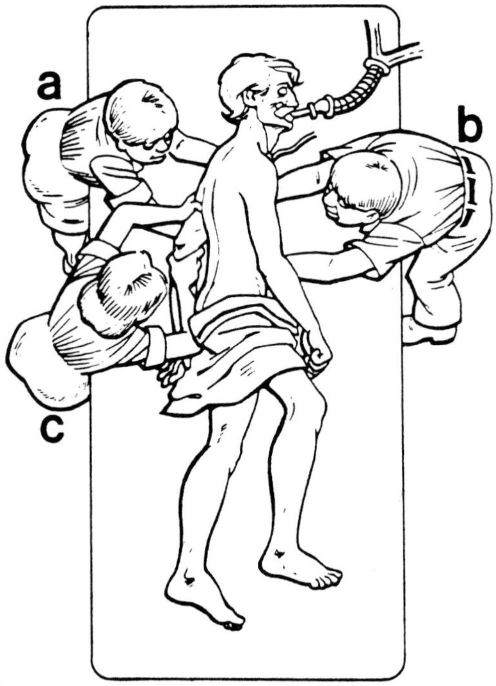

To turn the patient from the side to prone position, two people (*a* and *b*) lift the trunk while a third person *(c)* pulls the dependent arm under the patient.

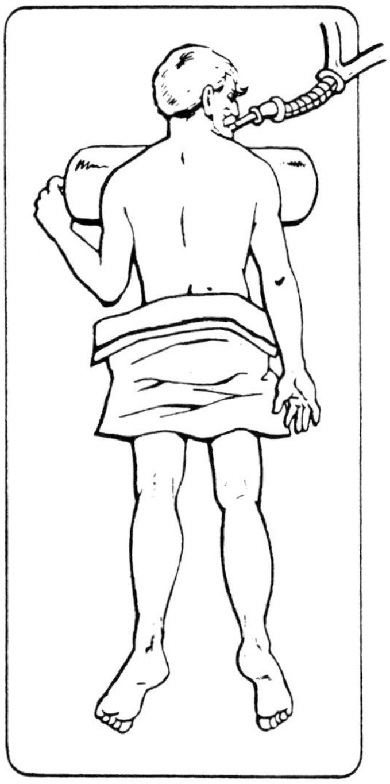

If a tracheal tube is present, while two people hold up the patient's trunk, the third places a roll under the upper thorax. The patient remains positioned as shown.

Appendix 19–4. Summary of Chest Physiotherapy Treatment *Continued*

ESSENTIALS OF CHEST PHYSIOTHERAPY TREATMENT

TREATMENT COMPONENTS	PURPOSE	HOW TO PERFORM	WHEN TO USE	THINGS TO AVOID	IMPORTANT DETAILS TO REMEMBER
Postural drainage	Mobilize retained secretions through assistance of gravity.	Patient positioned so that involved segmental bronchus is uppermost.	When coughing or suctioning, breathing exercises, and patient mobilization are not adequate to clear retained secretions.	Avoid significant changes in patient's vital signs, increase in intracranial pressure, and stress to intravascular lines and indwelling tubes.	Patient must be properly positioned for bronchial drainage of lung segment involved; this can be attained despite the presence of multiple injuries, monitoring equipment, and lines.
Percussion	As an adjunct to postural drainage for mobilization of secretions.	Rhythmical clapping of cupped hands over bare skin or thin material covering area of lung involvement; performed during inspiration and expiration.	Same as above.	Avoid redness or petechiae of skin (indicates improper hand positioning by therapist, or patient coagulopathy).	May be performed in the presence of rib fractures, chest tubes, and subcutaneous emphysema; should produce a hollow sound; should not cause undue pain, does not need to be forceful to be effective if performed properly.
Vibration	As an adjunct to postural drainage for mobilization of secretions.	Intermittent chest wall compression over area of lung involvement; performed during expiration only.	Same as above.	Avoid pinching or shearing of soft tissue and digging of fingers into soft tissue.	Should not be performed over rib fractures or unstable thoracic spine injuries; be sure to vibrate chest wall, not just shake soft tissue; forcefulness should vary according to patient's needs and tolerance.
Breathing exercises	Assistance in removal of secretions, relaxation, and to increase thoracic cage mobility and tidal volume.	Patient taught to produce a full inspiration followed by a controlled expiration; use hand placement for sensory feedback; for diaphragmatic, costal excursion, and lateral costal excursion techniques.	For use with spontaneously breathing patients.	Avoid use of accessory muscles of respiration.	May be used independently or in conjunction with other chest physiotherapy techniques; with practice, breathing exercises lead to increased chest expansion; breathing exercises should promote relaxation, not increase the work of breathing.
Coughing	Removal of secretions from the larger airways.	Steps: 1. Inspiratory gasp. 2. Closing of the glottis. 3. Contraction of expiratory muscles. 4. Opening of the glottis.	For use with spontaneously breathing patients.	Avoid bronchospasm induced by repetitive coughing.	Coughing is less effective in tracheally intubated patients; coughing ability can be improved by manual support of the patient's incision; stomas, following tracheal tube removal, should be covered with an airtight dressing to improve cough efficiency; an effective cough must be preceded by a large inspiration; methods of cough stimulation, including "huffing," vibration, summed breathing, external tracheal compression, and oral pharyngeal stimulation, are used.

Appendix 19–4. Summary of Chest Physiotherapy Treatment *Continued*

ESSENTIALS OF CHEST PHYSIOTHERAPY TREATMENT *Continued*

Treatment Components	Purpose	How to Perform	When to Use	Things to Avoid	Important Details to Remember
Suctioning	Removal of secretions from the larger airways.	Use aseptic technique. Steps: 1. Provide supplemental oxygen. 2. Insert suction catheter without applying suction, as fully as possible; be gentle. 3. Apply suction while withdrawing catheter. 4. Reexpand lung with mechanical ventilator or manual inflation by resuscitator bag attached to tracheal tube.	Tracheal suctioning for use only with patients who have an artificial airway in place.	Avoid hypoxemia (cyanosis and significant changes in vital signs) and cardiac arrhythmias, mechanical trauma and bacterial contamination of tracheobronchial tree, and increase in intracranial pressure.	In intubated patients, suctioning is performed routinely and is an integral part of chest physiotherapy; frequency of suctioning is determined by the quantity of secretions; the suctioning procedure should be limited to a total of 15 seconds; the suction catheter can reach only to the level of the main stem bronchus; it is more difficult to cannulate the left main stem bronchus than the right; nasotracheal suctioning should be avoided.
Bagging	Provide artificial ventilation, restore oxygen, and reexpand the lungs after suctioning.	Coordinate with patient's breathing pattern Steps: 1. Attach manual resuscitator bag to oxygen source. 2. Connect manual resuscitator bag to tracheal tube. 3. Squeeze bag rhythmically to deliver volume of air to patient. 4. Patient expires passively.	Before and after suctioning patients who are not mechanically ventilated and who cannot be mechanically sighed.	Avoid barotrauma	Bagging can be used in conjunction with vibration when treating patients not breathing deeply; hyperinflation can produce alterations in cardiac output.
Patient mobilization	To prevent the detrimental sequelae of bedrest and immobilization; to decrease rehabilitation time.	Turning and passively positioning the patient; appropriate splint usage; passive and active range of motion; active and resistive exercises; sitting, standing, and ambulating the patient.	Used to some degree with every patient according to patient's diagnosis and tolerance.	Avoid stress to intravascular lines and indwelling tubes, orthostatic hypotension, significant changes in vital signs, and dyspnea.	Mobilization is possible to some degree for every patient; minimal supplies are needed for mobilization; emphasis should be placed on functional activities; proper positioning may decrease spasticity in patients with head injuries; EKG leads and arterial and central venous pressure lines should be temporarily disconnected from the recording module during ambulation; at the physician's discretion, chest tubes and abdominal sumps may be disconnected from wall suction to allow ambulation.

Appendix 20–1. Peritoneal Lavage

PURPOSE: To detect free blood in the peritoneal cavity.

INDICATIONS

Immediate

History of trauma with the following:

1. Altered state of consciousness.
   a. Head injury.
   b. Intoxication—alcohol or drugs.
2. Spinal cord injury.
3. Multiple trauma.
4. Unstable vital signs—especially blood pressure.
5. Prolonged anesthesia for nonabdominal procedures.
6. Penetrating chest trauma.

Latent

7. Decreasing hemoglobin and hematocrit.
8. Change in abdominal status—loss of bowel sounds, increase in distention.
9. Unexplained fall in blood pressure.

Note: This is not a nursing procedure. It is the nurse's responsibility to assemble the equipment, to offer patient support, and to assist the physician as needed.

EQUIPMENT:

1. Foley catheter (#16 or size determined) with 5 ml balloon
2. Catheter insertion set

   } Only needed if patient does not have one previously inserted. (items 1–2)
3. Drainage bag
4. Naso- or oral gastric tube
5. Gastric suction

   } Only needed if patient does not have one previously inserted. (items 4–5)
6. Irrigation set
7. Razor
8. IV pole
9. 1000 ml normal saline solution in glass bottle (peritoneal lavage solution).
10. Solution administration set
11. Abdominal tap tray
12. Peritoneal dialysis catheter
13. Sutures: One 3–0 nylon on P_3 needle, one 2–0 nylon on reel, one 2–0 chromic on taper needle, or any other suture the physician requires
14. Bottle of 1 per cent lidocaine with epinephrine
15. Alcohol swab
16. Povidone-iodine (Betadine) scrub and prep
17. 10 packs of 4 × 4 gauze sponges
18. Surgical attire
19. 2 sterile barriers
20. Laboratory slip for peritoneal lavage
21. Laboratory slip for chemistry/special fluids
22. Two red top tubes, 30 ml syringe, and 18 gauge needle
23. Dressing supplies

Appendix 20–1. Peritoneal Lavage *Continued*

Preparation

NURSING ACTION	RATIONALE
1. Inform patient of the procedures and provide privacy.	
2. Insert Foley catheter and connect to drainage bag.	To reduce the risk of accidental puncture of the urinary bladder during insertion of dialysis catheter.
3. Insert nasogastric tube and attach to gastric suction.	To decompress the stomach, which prevents vomiting and possible aspiration and minimizes risk of bowel perforation during insertion of dialysis catheter.
4. Shave the patient's abdomen, umbilicus to pubic areas.	To decrease risk of infection.
5. Place liter bottle of normal saline solution on IV pole and flush line.	
6. Prepare abdominal tap tray in aseptic manner. a. Add povidone-iodine scrub and solution. b. Add suture material. c. Add dialysis catheter. d. With alcohol swab, clean rubber stopper on vial of 1 per cent lidocaine with epinephrine and hold vial so physician can withdraw the anesthetic. e. May need to add 10 pack of 4 × 4 gauze sponges.	To decrease risk of infection of the peritoneum, which could lead to peritonitis. Correct assembly of tray and equipment ensures proper function of all components and decreases delay in performing procedure.
7. Inform patient of procedure and reinforce as needed. It may be necessary to restrain patient's hands lightly.	To remind patient not to put hands in sterile field.
It may be necessary to stay at head of bed to help patient relax and to encourage cooperation during procedure.	To decrease risk of complications.
8. Assist surgeon with procedure as needed.	

Procedure

NURSING ACTION	RATIONALE
1. The physician prepares the skin using sterile technique. a. The skin of the abdomen is cleansed.	
b. The area is draped with sterile towels.	To create a sterile field.
c. Local anesthetic is injected into desired site.	Used on *all* patients for anesthesia and to maintain hemostasis.
d. An incision is made (usually midline), dissecting down to peritoneum.	Hemostasis must be maintained in order not to create a false-positive result.
e. The peritoneal catheter is inserted into the peritoneal cavity using either the open or closed method. Fluid is aspirated and examined: if positive, exploratory laparotomy is indicated. If negative, 1 l of normal saline solution is infused. Note: Physician will hold sterile peritoneal catheter. Nurse plugs sterile tip of IV tubing into catheter. Do *not* position unsterile tubing over sterile field. Run it up to sterile field and physician can make a pocket with the sterile drape.	
f. While fluid is infusing, cover sterile fields (tray and abdomen) with sterile barriers.	To decrease risk of contamination.
g. After fluid has infused, perform the following: 1. Clamp tubing. (Physician may wish to rock patient side to side, position patient in Trendelenburg and/or reverse Trendelenburg position.) 2. Place normal saline solution bottle below the level of the patient's body. 3. Remove tubing from infusion port and place into vent port. 4. Unclamp tubing.	To distribute fluid throughout peritoneum unless contraindicated (e.g., spinal cord injury). To allow fluid to return by gravity and to vent bottle (such venting is unnecessary with plastic bags).
h. After fluid has returned and sample is requested, ask physician which tests are needed: 1. Culture and Sensitivity 2. RBC and WBC	
i. Rotate bottle vigorously. Use syringe to withdraw fluids and fill appropriate containers: 1. 5 ml specimen container 2. 10 ml red top tube 3. 10 ml red top tube	To thoroughly mix fluid.
j. Label specimens and send to appropriate laboratories.	

Appendix 20–1. Peritoneal Lavage *Continued*

Follow-Up

NURSING ACTION	RATIONALE
Note: Positive test results: WBC > 500/mm^3; RBC > 100,000/mm^3	
1. If necessary, prepare patient for surgery and for transport to operating room.	
2. If the peritoneal lavage is negative, physician removes catheter and sutures the incision.	
3. Place sterile dressing over suture line.	
4. Discard disposable equipment.	
5. Return all equipment to proper area for cleaning and resterilization.	To ensure that equipment is not inadvertently thrown away in linen.
6. Document: quantity of fluid infused and returned, specimens obtained, patient's tolerance, and complications noted.	To maintain concise, thorough medical record.

Special Considerations

COMPLICATIONS

Iatrogenic injuries: Perforated bladder
Perforated mesenteric vessels
Perforated small bowel } may cause peritonitis
Perforated omental injury }

False-positive results: Related to insufficient hemostasis
Puncture of a retroperitoneal hematoma
Production of intraperitoneal hemorrhage by an injury of an adjacent normal structure during the insertion of the catheter

False-negative results: Capsular injury
Catheter not in peritoneum (usually fluid will not flow in or out)

Respiratory compromise: Especially in patients already experiencing respiratory distress, instillation of fluid may cause additional stress precipitating respiratory arrest.

Reprinted with permission from Nursing Procedure Manual, Maryland Institute for Emergency Medical Services Systems, Baltimore, MD, July, 1983.

Appendix 21–1. Nursing Care Plan for the Patient With Crush Injury

Hypovolemia

Nursing Diagnosis	Assessment/Intervention	Expected Outcome
Fluid volume deficit related to third spacing into affected extremity	1. Monitor BP, CVP, and EKG. If patient has Swan-Ganz, evaluate data from hemodynamic parameters, PAP, PCWP, CO for deviation from the norm. 2. Administer IV fluids via infusion pump. 3. Observe for fluid overload during fluid resuscitation (hypertension, congestive heart failure, pulmonary edema). a. Auscultate lungs q 4 hrs or more frequently if pulmonary edema develops. b. Monitor intake and output every hour. 4. Monitor pulses of all extremities, q 1 hr, use Doppler flow detector if necessary.	Fluid volume will be stabilized at patient's norm. Patient will exhibit no signs of fluid deficit/overload.
Knowledge deficit related to invasive procedures and complexity of information	1. Teach patient and family about angiography, preparation, post procedure, dressings. 2. Prepare patient and family for insertion of CVP and Foley catheter. 3. Prepare patient and family for fasciotomy, appearance of wound, potential for plastic closure. 4. Listen to patient, offer emotional support. Physical touch is reassuring. 5. Keep the family apprised of patient's condition and prognosis. 6. Contact Pastoral Care to help provide additional support.	Patient and family will verbalize accurate knowledge.

Increased Compartment Pressure

Nursing Diagnosis	Assessment/Intervention	Expected Outcome
Altered tissue perfusion: peripheral	1. Instruct patient of the symptoms that necessitate prompt action; increasing pain, paresthesia, paralysis. 2. Assess for increased pain with passive movement q 1–2 hrs, evaluate response to pain medications. 3. Monitor pulses of injured extremity at least q 2 hrs. 4. Observe for sluggish capillary (>3 sec), increasing limb edema, consult physician if deficits noted. 5. Monitor compartment pressure serially or q 8 hours.	Patient has adequate perfusion to tissue as noted by brisk (<3 sec) capillary refill, peripheral pulses >1+ on a 4+ scale, normal compartment pressure (<8 mm Hg)

Fasciotomy

Nursing Diagnosis	Assessment/Intervention	Expected Outcome
Impaired skin integrity with potential for infection	1. Monitor vital signs, especially temperature q 4 hrs. 2. Inspect wounds for odor, swelling, drainage, obtain culture of draining wound. 3. Aseptic technique with dressing and tubing changes. 4. Dressing changes to fasciotomy wounds at least q 8 hrs to assess wounds. Place sterile towels under limb. 5. Maintain sterility of all lines (IV, Swan-Ganz, arterial). 6. Monitor lab values for increased WBC, sed rate. 7. Administer antibiotics. Review renal function indices and consult physician to adjust antibiotic dosage.	Patient will remain infection free as noted by presence of normal temperature, WBC, sedimentation rate. Wounds will be free of drainage, odor, inflammation. Wound will be vascularized with healthy tissue.

Appendix 21–1. Nursing Care Plan for the Patient With Crush Injury *Continued*

Rhabdomyolysis

NURSING DIAGNOSIS	ASSESSMENT/INTERVENTION	EXPECTED OUTCOME
Alteration in tissue perfusion: renal	1. Administer alkaline crystalloid solution at 500 ml/hour. 2. Monitor urine to maintain pH >6.5 (normal range 4.5–7.5) q 1 hr. 3. Maintain accurate intake and output. The patient may maintain normal urine output for the first 24–36 hours only to develop progressive oliguria over the next 2–3 days. 4. Observe for signs of pulmonary edema, congestive heart failure, hypertension. 5. Administer diuretics and observe for urine output of 300 ml/hr in response to forced diuresis. 6. Monitor muscle enzymes, potassium, and serum pH.	Patient's urine will remain free of precipitates. Patient will respond with diuresis of 300 ml/hr. Urine pH will be >6.5. Serum potassium, pH, enzymes will remain within normal range.

Chemical Imbalance

NURSING DIAGNOSIS	ASSESSMENT/INTERVENTION	EXPECTED OUTCOME
Acid base imbalance, metabolic acidosis related to muscle ischemia and anaerobic metabolism	1. Obtain daily serum pH via arterial blood gases. 2. Administer alkaline crystalloid solutions. 3. Monitor respiratory pattern and maintain adequate ventilation, obtain blood gas if distress occurs. 4. Monitor EKG pattern continuously; consult physician if dysrhythmia or pattern change occurs.	Patient serum pH will remain between 7.35 and 7.45.
Intracellular electrolyte excess/calcium deficit	1. Monitor EKG for high peaked T waves, S-T segment depression, absence of U wave, and QRS duration and P-R interval increase. 2. Monitor daily lab values for deviation from the norms. 3. Treat elevated potassium levels (potassium >6.0) a. Administer IV calcium to stabilize the myocardium or sodium bicarbonate to buffer acidosis and drive potassium into the cell. b. Administer Kayexalate in divided doses orally or as enemas. Mixed with sorbitol it removes potassium from the body in exchange for sodium. c. Administer 5–10 units insulin and 50 ml of 50% glucose IV to temporarily move potassium into the cell. 4. Observe for prolonged Q-T interval consistent with hypocalcemia, administer calcium as ordered.	Patient's serum potassium will remain between 3.5 and 5.5 mEq/l; phosphorus will remain between 1.7 and 2.6; calcium will remain between 4.8 and 5.2.

Reprinted with permission from Peck SA: Crush syndrome: Pathophysiology and management. Orthopaedic Nursing National Association of Orthopaedic Nurses May/June 9(3):36, 1990.

Appendix 21–2. Pin Care Procedure for Steinmann Pins, Kirschner Wires, and Hoffmann Pins

PURPOSE: To maintain aseptic conditions surrounding pin insertion sites.

EQUIPMENT

1. Normal saline
2. Hydrogen peroxide
3. Alcohol
4. 4 x 4 gauze sponges
5. 2 x 2 gauze sponges
6. Sterile applicators
7. Needle and syringe (for draining wounds at pin sites)
8. 0.01 per cent neomycin solution

For Nondraining Pin Sites

Nursing Action	Rationale
1. Leave original dressing on for 24 hours.	To protect open wounds until hemostatic plugs and early granulation form; to decrease skin flora entrance into pin sites.
2. Remove dressing and observe for signs of infection and/or hemorrhage and report to physician.	
3. If the skin around the pin sites is under tension, report this to the physician.	
4. Using sterile applicators, cleanse with alcohol around each pin site. Do not remove scabs or push skin away from pins. If patient cannot tolerate alcohol, use half-strength hydrogen peroxide and saline.	Scabs are a normal healing process. Skin adhering to the pin keeps skin flora from entering the bone. Alcohol is the preferred solution because it will remove blood and residue and will help decrease the bacterial count.
5. Do *not* use any antibiotic ointment at the pin sites.	The antibiotic ointment will occlude drainage from around the pin site.
6. The orthopedic surgeon will write orders leaving the *specific* solution to be used with the *specific* type of dressing (dsg) change to be done, e.g., a. Leave pin sites open without dsg. b. Apply dry sterile dsg. c. Apply dsg. wet with 0.01 per cent neomycin or povidone-iodine solution and/or saline and then cover with dry dsg.	Any dressing instruction starting "soak with," "wet with," or "moistened with" means the 2 × 2 or 4 × 4 is wet with the appropriate solution and then wrung out so that the solution does not go through the next outer layer of dry 2 × 2 or 4 × 4.
7. Do this pin care procedure tid (once per shift) unless otherwise ordered by the orthopedic surgeon.	

For Draining Pin Sites

Nursing Action	Rationale
1. Remove exudate and crusts with half-strength peroxide and saline or sterile applicator from around the pins.	
2. On open draining wounds at pin sites, using a needle on a syringe, irrigate thoroughly into the wound with half-strength peroxide and saline.	This will free up any exudate and cleanse the wound.
3. Clean into the open wound thoroughly with applicators soaked in half-strength peroxide and saline.	This will help remove any encrusted materials and cleanse the wound to allow healing.
4. Pack the open wound with 2 × 2s moistened in (a) saline, (b) 0.01 per cent neomycin, or (c) povidone-iodine solution.	The 2 × 2s will act as a drain to prevent accumulation of infected fluid and/or material.
5. Apply dry 2 × 2s or 4 × 4s as a top layer of dressing.	This will help prevent bacteria from entering the wound via wet 2 × 2s or 4 × 4s and will collect any infected fluid that may drain from the wound.
6. Do this pin care procedure q4h unless otherwise ordered by the orthopedic surgeon.	This will help decrease bacteria in the wound, which will promote wound healing; will also prevent further bacterial growth on dirty dressing if left on for long periods.

Appendix 21–2. Pin Care Procedure for Steinmann Pins, Kirschner Wires, and Hoffmann Pins *Continued*

Other Important Points to Remember

Nursing Action	Rationale
1. The various articulations and rods of the Hoffmann apparatus or traction should be kept clean by wiping them with peroxide or alcohol.	This will prevent bacteria formation and growth; if the patient requires surgery, this will make the preparation of the apparatus for traction easier.
2. The entire Hoffmann apparatus should be checked for integrity. If a joint or rod feels loose, call the orthopedic surgeon immediately.	This will prevent loss of acceptable bone alignment; any loose piece of equipment can be easily adjusted at the bedside by the orthopedic physician with the proper equipment from the operating room.
3. The affected limb may be safely moved by moving the extremity using the Hoffmann apparatus, not the limb itself.	This will prevent possible malalignment of the affected fractured bones.
4. The affected limb may be safely suspended by tying traction rope around the Hoffmann frame.	This will prevent the development of pressure sores.

Reprinted with permission from the Nursing Procedure Manual, Maryland Institute for Emergency Medical Services Systems, Baltimore, MD, 1992.

Appendix 21–3. External Fixator Care

PURPOSE: To maintain alignment of the fracture, to maintain the integrity of the Hoffmann device, and to decrease incidence of infection.

Note: Each Hoffmann apparatus is individually designed to maintain alignment of fracture fragments. The orthopedic physician may have special orders for each (e.g., turning instructions, elevation).

NURSING ACTION	RATIONALE
1. Inspect entire Hoffmann apparatus every 8 hours for integrity. If a joint or rod feels loose, notify the orthopedic physician immediately.	Prevents loss of bone alignment.
2. Wipe articulations and rods of the Hoffmann apparatus with alcohol every 24 hours.	Decreases the potential for bacterial growth.
3. Move the affected limb using the Hoffmann apparatus, not the limb itself.	Prevents possible malalignment of the affected fractured bones.
Note: If the patient has a pelvic Hoffmann apparatus applied, he may turn side to side to the limitation of the apparatus or as per the orthopedic physician's order. *Never* use the pelvic Hoffmann apparatus itself to turn or position the patient because pelvic fracture fragments do not have the stability of an extremity fracture.	
4. Suspend the affected limb by tying a traction rope around the Hoffmann frame and attaching it to the overhead traction bar. When suspending the leg, always do so with the knee bent.	This will decrease edema and prevent development of pressure areas. If the knee remains straight while suspended, it will be very painful for the patient.
5. Cover exposed sharp ends of Hoffmann pins with rubber caps.	Prevents harm to the patient and staff members.
6. If pillows are utilized to support a suspended extremity or elevate an extremity during transport, arrange pillows so that they are supporting the Hoffmann frame, and *not* the leg itself.	Sustained pressure on muscle groups may cause increased damage and possible compartment syndrome.

Appendix 21–4. Continuous Passive Motion Machine

The continuous passive motion machine is a device that provides continuous passive exercise to a patient's joint through automatic flexion and extension movements. Two models of this device that are both for exercising the lower extremities will be discussed.

Which Patients Benefit from CPMM?

1. Patients with soft tissue injury
2. Patient with (most frequent use)
   a. Tibial plateau fractures
   b. Supracondylar fractures
   c. Patella fractures
   d. Acetabular fractures.

How Does CPMM Benefit Patients?

The leg exerciser provides continuous passive exercise to the leg of a patient who has undergone reparative or reconstructive joint surgery. It moves the joint passively through its range of motion (ROM). Clinical evidence indicates that passive motion restores or increases flexion and extension and inhibits formation of adhesions and contractures.

1. Continuous motion with a CPMM causes early closure of the subcondylar bone plate, which prevents the ingrowth of capillaries, which creates low O_2 tension—the stimulus for the formation of cartilage.
2. Cartilage forms in the joint instead of the formation of degenerative bone changes, which would ultimately lead to arthritis.
3. A secondary effect from the CPMM is increased patient comfort. The motion causes decreased swelling, thereby decreasing pain, and allowing increased ROM.
4. The motion also stimulates increased production of synovial fluid, which lubricates and provides nutrition to the articular surface.
5. To achieve maximum benefit, the CPMM should be applied within the first postoperative week.

Nursing Implications

1. The CPMM may or may not be used with traction. If it is utilized with traction, the traction bar overhead is usually turned out so that the weights do not catch on the bed while the machine is in operation.
2. If the patient utilizing the CPMM also needs a Clinitron bed, the old "square" model must be ordered. The new oval-shaped Clinitron is not large enough for the machine to sit on the bed.
3. With the Richards-Kinetec model (see diagram, below, right) the acrylic protective guard must be in place. This prevents the patient's opposite limb from inadvertently getting caught and being compressed by the machinery during the flexion cycle.
4. Routine skin and neurovascular checks should be done even when machine is in motion.
5. The CPMM should be removed only if:
   a. The patient is unable to provide his own pressure relief, i.e., lift up with a trapeze or push himself up in bed.
   b. The patient gets out of bed.
   c. The patient needs to be turned for chest physiotherapy.
6. The orthopedic surgeon must write the order for the CPMM and designate the settings for the amount of flexion and extension. The settings will be increased by the physical therapist or orthopedic surgeon according to the patient's tolerance.

The leg exerciser's range of motion is established by the settings of the extension angle and the flexion angle control knobs. The range of motion will automatically adjust to the flexion/extension settings regardless of the adjustments made to the leg support frame.

Reprinted with permission from the Nursing Education Department, Maryland Institute of Emergency Medical Services Systems, Baltimore, MD, 1986.

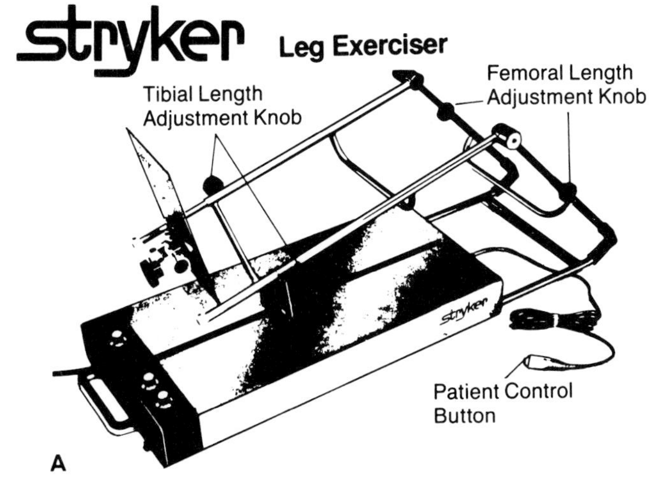

A

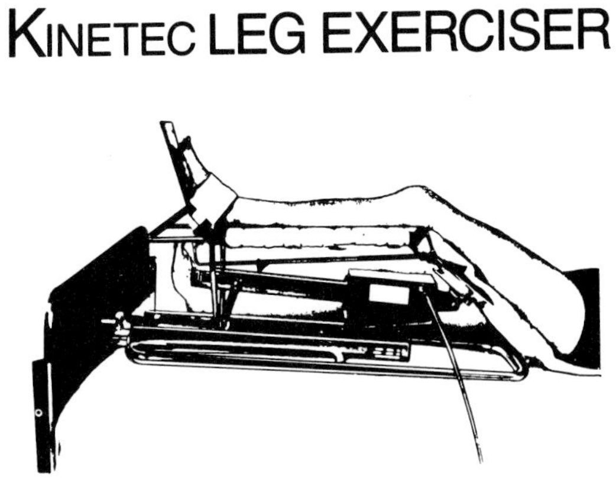

B

Appendix 24–1. Continuous Arteriovenous Hemofiltration (CAVH)

Attachment Procedure

Nursing Action	Rationale
1. Baseline vital signs, weight, and laboratory work (including activated clotting time) must be documented on the flow sheet and/or the computer.	
2. Obtain appropriate loading dose and maintenance drip of heparin as well as replacement fluid mixture (from pharmacy). Attach heparin drip tubing to the arterial ports nearest the filter. Attach the replacement fluids to the venous infusion port.	If patient is on CAVH therapy for volume overload, replacement fluid may not be ordered. Loading dose of heparin may be omitted if coagulation studies so indicate.
3. Perform shunt care per institution protocol. Be sure shunt connectors are available as adapters to the filter tubing.	The filter tubing has bevelled edges and may stretch the shunt tubing if connectors are not used.
4. Administer loading dose of heparin as ordered (usually 20 units/kg). Wait a minimum of 3 minutes before connecting hemofilter to shunt.	The time interval allows for systemic anticoagulation.
5. Attach hemofilter tubing to shunt connectors, making sure that arterial and venous accesses and ports match. Securely tape all connections.	
6. Begin the heparin infusion.	
7. Release clamps on both the arterial and venous blood tubings. After 5 minutes, release the clamp on the ultrafiltrate tubing and push the "reset" switch on the Vitalmetric monitor.	The time interval allows the blood to establish a flow pattern through the filter.
8. Begin infusing replacement fluid as ordered.	
9. Apply sterile dressing to shunt per institution protocol. Attach bulldog clamps to exterior edge of dressing.	Clamps must be on the dressing in case of accidental disconnection to prevent exsanguination.

Filter Maintenance

Nursing Action	Rationale
1. Monitor the ultrafiltration rate (UFR) every hour as digitally displayed on the Vitalmetric unit. Notify physician if UFR is < 200 ml/hr.	The UFR is a reflection of the patency and efficacy of the filter.
2. Monitor ACT every 2 hours for 8 hours then every 8 hours. Notify physician if ACT > 300 seconds.	
3. Monitor electrolytes every 4 hours for 8 hours, then every 8 hours for 24 hours, then every 12 hours.	
4. Monitor vital signs closely (within CCRU protocols). Clamp ultrafiltrate tubing for severe hypotension but leave blood tubing open.	Clamping ultrafiltrate tubing will prevent free water loss; leaving blood tubing open will increase possibility of continued filter patency.
5. Monitor shunt patency every hour per institution protocols.	
6. Monitor ultrafiltrate for signs of visible blood. Clamp *all* tubings if blood is noticed and notify physician.	A rupture in the filter risks contamination and possible blood loss.
7. Monitor position of ultrafiltrate tubing to maximize the distance between the filter and the ultrafiltrate collector. The bed may need to be elevated to its highest position.	The greater the distance between the filter and the collector, the greater the flow rate through the filter (prevents clotting of the filter).

Adapted from Continuous Arterio-Venous Hemofiltration Clinical Protocol, Department of Surgery, University of Michigan. Reprinted with permission from Nursing Procedure Manual for Maryland Institute for Emergency Medical Services Systems, Baltimore, MD, 1992.

Appendix 26–1. Sample Care Plan for the Pediatric Trauma Patient

As the child progresses through the cycles from resuscitation to home, it is imperative that the plan of care be consistent and continuous. The plan of care for each phase should provide for appropriate interventions in the next phase. All aspects of the child's care—physical, psychosocial, emotional—and care of the family must be considered.

NURSING DIAGNOSIS	EXPECTED OUTCOME	NURSING INTERVENTIONS
Alteration in cardiac output: decreased.	Adequate cardiac output, blood volume.	*Resuscitation Cycle*: Monitor and document changes in vital signs, heart and lung sounds, and fluid balance. Monitor EKG for rate and rhythm. If arrhythmias occur, document, notify appropriate physician, and treat per protocol. Administer fluids and medications per physician orders. Provide O_2 as ordered. Use emergency procedures as necessary. *Critical Care Cycle*: Monitor and document: heart rate and rhythm, blood pressure, central venous pressure, pulmonary artery pressures, peripheral pulses, capillary refill, color, temperature of skin, urine output, respiratory rate, core body temperature, laboratory data, hemodynamic profile. Administer medications and fluids as ordered. Prepare for emergency measures as necessary.
Alteration in tissue perfusion: cerebral, cardiopulmonary, renal, gastrointestinal, peripheral.	Absence or resolution of increased intracranial pressure. Adequate cardiac output and blood volume. Absence or resolution of respiratory distress. Respiratory sufficiency. ABGs within normal limits for patient. Kidney function within normal limits. Urine output at least 1 ml/kg/hr. Absence or resolution of gastrointestinal bleeding. Adequate tissue perfusion.	*Resuscitation Cycle*: Monitor and document changes in vital signs and heart and lung sounds. Provide O_2 as ordered. Administer medications and fluids per physician orders. Monitor and document changes in child's level of consciousness, pupil reactions, spontaneous movements, and reflexes. Monitor and document presence of seizures. Correctly position patient to decrease cerebral edema (head of bed elevated). Insert Foley catheter per physician orders. Note color and characteristics of urine. Monitor and document changes in child's urine output. Monitor and document changes in abdominal size and bowel sounds. Insert nasogastric tube. Note characteristics of gastric contents. Monitor and document changes in color and warmth of skin and extremities. *Critical Care Cycle*: Cerebral: Monitor and document intracranial pressure, pupillary reactions, level of consciousness, reflexes, motor response, seizures, abnormal respiratory pattern, widening pulse pressure, bradycardia, and intake and output. Keep head of bed elevated to 30 degrees and head in a midline position. If changes do occur, administer medications and treatments as ordered, noting patient's response. Prepare patient for tests as ordered, such as CT scan. Provide nursing care, especially care that stimulates the child, in such a way as to provide rest periods.

Appendix 26–1. Sample Care Plan for the Pediatric Trauma Patient *Continued*

NURSING DIAGNOSIS	EXPECTED OUTCOME	NURSING INTERVENTIONS
Alteration in tissue perfusion: cerebral, cardiopulmonary, renal, gastrointestinal, peripheral. *Continued*		Cardiopulmonary: Monitor and document vital signs, ABGs, hemodynamic parameters, temperature, and ventilator settings. Provide O_2 as ordered, noting child's response. Provide medications as ordered, noting child's response. Renal: Monitor and document fluid intake and output, serum and urine electrolytes, serum BUN, creatinine, and weight. Administer therapy aimed at providing adequate renal blood flow. Gastrointestinal: Monitor and document abdominal girth, bowel sounds, characteristics of NG drainage, pain, tenderness or rigidity, and decrease in hematocrit. Observe for signs and symptoms of hypovolemic shock. Provide antacids as ordered. Peripheral: Monitor and document core temperature, pulses, especially those distal to injury, capillary refill, temperature of skin, color of skin, diameter of extremities for development of compartment syndrome, and condition of cast if applicable. Position correctly to maintain adequate perfusion to extremities. Administer medications and fluids as ordered, noting child's response. Monitor appropriate laboratory values. Monitor core body temperature.
Impaired gas exchange.	Pa_{O_2}, Pa_{CO_2}, arterial saturations within normal limits.	*Resuscitation Cycle*: Monitor and document patency of airway, amount of secretions, respiratory rate and pattern, breath sounds, color, agitation and restlessness, ABGs, presence of pneumothorax or hemothorax, and response to airway support measures. Maintain correct position for open airway. Deliver O_2 as per nursing judgment or physician orders. Provide emergency measures as necessary. Prepare child for and assist with intubation or chest tube insertion. *Critical Care Cycle*: Monitor and document respiratory rate, presence or absence of respiratory distress, adequacy of ventilation, chest movements, ABGs, respiratory profile, presence and quality of breath sounds, chest radiograph, ventilator settings, and changes in vital signs. Provide chest physiotherapy as ordered, noting the child's response. Suction as necessary. Turn patient every 2 hours to allow for full lung expansion.

Appendix 26–1. Sample Care Plan for the Pediatric Trauma Patient *Continued*

NURSING DIAGNOSIS	EXPECTED OUTCOME	NURSING INTERVENTIONS
Ineffective airway clearance.	Adequate oxygenation and ventilation. Absence of respiratory distress. Clear lungs as evidenced by chest radiograph.	*Resuscitation Cycle*: Monitor and document absence of respirations, amount of secretions, ABGs, presence of respiratory distress, and chest movements. Suction as necessary to clear airway. Prepare child for intubation as necessary. *Critical Care Cycle*: Monitor and document presence or absence of respiratory distress, adequacy of ventilation, ABGs, presence and quality of breath sounds, chest radiograph, ventilator settings, and quantity and characteristics of secretions. Provide chest physiotherapy as ordered, noting child's response. Suction as necessary.
Alteration in fluid volume: excess or fluid volume deficit—actual or potential.	Adequate blood volume. Hemodynamic parameters within normal limits for patient. Urine output 1 ml/kg/hr. Clear lungs as evidenced by radiograph. Absence of pulmonary or systemic edema.	*Resuscitation Cycle*: Monitor and document vital signs, presence of signs and symptoms of shock (marked hypotension, tachycardia, weak or absent pulses, peripheral vasoconstriction), pallor, restlessness, decreased urine output, external blood loss, results of hematocrit and hemoglobin, and child's response to fluids. Administer fluids, blood, and blood products as ordered. Maintain PASG as appropriate. Assist with insertion of CVP and PAP lines. Monitor CVP and PAP pressures every 15 minutes during resuscitation. *Critical Care Cycle*: Monitor and document fluid intake and output, body weights, presence of edema, presence of dehydration, vital signs (including CVP and PAP), chest radiograph, signs of congestive heart failure or hypovolemic shock, hematocrit and hemoglobin, presence or absence of pulses, and peripheral vasoconstriction. Administer fluids carefully, noting correct fluid requirements for the child. Administer medications as ordered, noting child's response. Administer blood and blood products as ordered.
Impaired physical mobility.	Absence of problems associated with immobility: contractures, decubiti, venous stasis, and renal calculi.	*Critical Care Cycle*: Provide active and passive range-of-motion exercises. Turn child every 2 hours and maintain proper body alignment. Maintain extremities in position of function. Assist child in getting out of bed and in chair as soon as possible.

Appendix 26–1. Sample Care Plan for the Pediatric Trauma Patient *Continued*

NURSING DIAGNOSIS	EXPECTED OUTCOME	NURSING INTERVENTIONS
Potential for infection.	Absence or resolution of infection. Temperature within normal limits. Normal wound healing.	*Critical Care Cycle*: Monitor and document vital signs (especially temperature, redness, inflammation), purulent drainage from vascular catheter sites or wounds, restlessness or confusion, changes in WBC count, cloudy or bloody urine, culture results, and response to antibiotics. Meticulous handwashing by all personnel caring for or touching patient. Aseptic care of all invasive lines and tubes. Aseptic care of all wounds. Meticulous patient hygiene. Send appropriate cultures.
Alteration in nutrition: less than body requirements.	Positive nitrogen balance. Absence of weight loss. Appropriate weight gain. Nutritional parameters within normal limits.	*Critical Care Cycle*: Monitor and document child's weight, appropriate laboratory data (serum albumin, transferrin, lymphocyte count, electrolytes, total protein, and intradermal skin test results), anthropometric data, type of nutritional support, and complications of nutritional support. Provide appropriate nutritional support, noting child's response. Follow established protocol for central line maintenance.
Alteration in comfort: pain.	Absence or resolution of pain.	*Critical Care Cycle*: Monitor and document heart rate, blood pressure, irritability, diaphoresis, response to painful stimuli, and response to pain medications. Administer analgesics, noting child's response. Provide supportive measures such as distraction techniques, massage or rhythmic rubbing of the painful area, relaxation techniques such as deep breathing, teaching various pain relief methods child and/or parent may try, maintain ongoing assessment of child's pain, and prepare child for all painful procedures.
Fear and anxiety Disturbance in self-concept: body image, self-esteem, role performance, personal identity.	Reduction in child's fears and anxieties.	*Resuscitation Cycle*: Provide explanations of procedures when and where appropriate. Provide comfort measures and emotional support. *Critical Care Cycle*: Infancy—the major fear is separation from parents. Take time to get acquainted with infant while parents are there. Encourage parents to spend as much time as possible with child. Explain child's behavior to parents. Attempt to minimize parent's stress. Allow as much motor activity as possible; if infant must be restrained, allow as much movement as safe. Provide age-appropriate toys. Toddlers—fears are separation from parents and loss of control at a time when attempting to attain autonomy. Encourage parents to spend as much time as possible with child.

Appendix 26–1. Sample Care Plan for the Pediatric Trauma Patient *Continued*

NURSING DIAGNOSIS	EXPECTED OUTCOME	NURSING INTERVENTIONS
Fear and anxiety Disturbance in self-concept: body image, self-esteem, role performance, personal identity. *Continued*		Minimize caretakers for toddlers. Allow toddlers as much freedom of movement as safe. Provide as much of a routine as possible for the child. Provide activities for child to channel anger. Provide activities that allow for play and provide sensory stimulation different from that of the ICU. These include age-appropriate toys, brightly colored pictures, tape recordings from child's family, soft music, cartoons, or favorite TV show. Preschool—the child has difficulty separating fantasy from reality and has fear of the unknown, the dark, being left alone, and of bodily injury and mutilation. Provide clear, concise explanations to the child. Anticipate concerns about wounds and scars. Provide explanation. Offer realistic choices when possible. Let child know someone will be there. Provide activities that allow for large muscle movement when possible. Provide play activities that allow child to act out fears and stressful situations. School-age—fears are loss of control at a time they are attempting to achieve independence and possible mutilation and injury. The child is also establishing relationships with a peer group. Allow privacy for the child. Provide clear explanations of all procedures. Provide realistic choices in scheduling activities. Allow child to receive letters, telephone messages, and visits from peers and siblings. Help parents understand child's behavior if the child does not wish parents there during procedure. Encourage child to communicate feelings. Provide appropriate play objects such as books, collections, or competitive games. Adolescent—major fears are altered body image, loss of control and identity, and separation from peer group. Allow adolescent to be an active participant in plan of care when appropriate. Provide assistance to adolescent in coming to terms with the illness and any real or imagined alterations in body image. Provide privacy for adolescent. Facilitate peer group contact as much as possible. Provide information about the illness and procedures. Provide for play activities appropriate for the adolescent such as watching TV, listening to music, reading, or playing cards or games. Allow for daydreaming.

Appendix 26–1. Sample Care Plan for the Pediatric Trauma Patient *Continued*

NURSING DIAGNOSIS	EXPECTED OUTCOME	NURSING INTERVENTIONS
Sleep pattern disturbance.	Normal sleep patterns. Absence or resolution of signs and symptoms of ICU psychosis.	*Critical Care Cycle*: Provide a sense of day-night as much as possible. Plan care to allow for undisturbed rest periods. As child stabilizes, delete some treatments at night when possible. Attempt to minimize noise level as much as possible during the night.
Family coping: potential for growth.	Reduction in family's anxiety. Verbalization of fears and grief. Family exhibits appropriate coping behavior. Family is able to make realistic goals for and/or with child. Family is able to seek out appropriate resources.	*Resuscitation Cycle*: Allow family to express fears and anxieties. Provide family with clear, simple, honest explanations. Allow family to see child as soon as possible. *Critical Care Cycle*: Encourage parents to communicate their feelings. Prepare parents as much as possible for the unit and how their child will appear to them. Provide help for parents to adapt to changes in their parenting role and their child's behaviors and emotions. Provide help for parents to cope with their child's pain. Provide parents with honest communication. Limit the number of people who interact with them. Give parents clear explanations of what is happening, realizing they may need to be repeated. Encourage parents to be involved in child's care. Provide encouragement to parents as they touch, talk to, and care for their child. Encourage bringing in toys and items familiar to child from home. Listen to concerns and information parents offer about their child. If possible, incorporate them into the plan of care. *Intermediate/Rehabilitation Cycle*: Include family in realistic goal-setting for themselves and the child. Allow them to be part of the team. Allow family to explore discharge alternatives for the child. Encourage family to participate in plan of care. Allow family to go through grieving process. Help family to channel feelings of anger and frustration. Make appropriate referrals to family counselor, social services, minister, or other appropriate community agencies. Make appropriate referrals, if family desires, to support groups. Allow family and child to experience hope and a sense of future; however, assist family in dealing with unrealistic hopes.

Appendix 26–1. Sample Care Plan for the Pediatric Trauma Patient *Continued*

NURSING DIAGNOSIS	EXPECTED OUTCOME	NURSING INTERVENTIONS
Impaired home maintenance and management (related to lack of support systems and insufficient use of community resources).	Family verbalizes knowledge of discharge information. Family verbalizes knowledge of appropriate support systems and community resources.	*Intermediate/Rehabilitation Cycle*: Assist family in setting realistic goals for child. Help family assess and identify support systems. Suggest strategies for utilization of appropriate support systems. Assist family in identification of and recognition of need for community resources. Assist family in identification of learning needs to prepare for discharge.
Knowledge deficit (related to child's injury).	Family verbalizes knowledge of child's injury and appropriate treatments. Family is able to describe plan for rehabilitation.	*Intermediate/Rehabilitation Cycle*: Assess family's knowledge of child's injury. Instruct parents about child's injury and any treatments, especially those that may involve the parents. Prepare specific discharge plan for child with parent's input. Assist family and child in relearning activities of daily living. Provide consistency in teaching approach for family. Allow families to tour therapy areas, providing explanations for equipment and activities. Teach families skills in memory stimulation and activities of daily living.
Alteration in bowel elimination: constipation and diarrhea.	Normal bowel elimination patterns.	*Intermediate/Rehabilitation Cycle*: Assess child and family's current level of knowledge as well as child's previous pattern of defecation. Administer appropriate stool softener and/or stimulant. Establish time of day and frequency for bowel control program. Teach child, if appropriate, and family bowel control program. Assess child for development of impaction; if the child does become impacted, initiate appropriate measures.
Alterations in pattern of urinary elimination.	Normal urinary elimination patterns.	*Intermediate/Rehabilitation Cycle*: Assess child for signs of urinary tract infections and for bladder overdistention. Catheterize child as ordered. Assess child for appropriateness for catheterization program. Assess fluid intake and output. Teach child, if appropriate, and/or parents proper technique for catheterization. Teach aseptic performance of procedure. Teach importance of avoidance of bladder distention. Teach correct catheter care.

Appendix 26–1. Sample Care Plan for the Pediatric Trauma Patient *Continued*

NURSING DIAGNOSIS	EXPECTED OUTCOME	NURSING INTERVENTIONS
Impairment of skin integrity: actual or potential.	Absence or resolution of skin integrity.	*Intermediate/Rehabilitation Cycle*: Assess child for development of pressure sores. Turn child every 2 hours. Provide mattresses that distribute pressure more evenly, such as an egg crate mattress. Use supportive devices as appropriate. Teach child, if appropriate, and family proper techniques for assessing skin and providing skin care. Educate staff in aspects of prevention of skin care problems.
Disturbance in self-concept: body image.	Child/family exhibits behaviors that demonstrate acceptance of new body image.	*Intermediate/Rehabilitation Cycle*: Allow child to express fears and concerns about altered body image. Allow child to vent anger and frustration and know he is still accepted. Support the child through the grieving process of adjusting to a new body image. Support the family in adjusting to the differences in their previously healthy child. Teach the child and family new ways of self-care if child has experienced loss of function. Allow child to experience realistic challenges. Success will help restore child's sense of self-worth.
Sensory-perceptual alteration: visual, auditory, kinesthetic, gustatory, tactile, olfactory.	Behavior that exhibits orientation to time, person, place.	*Critical Care Cycle and Intermediate/Rehabilitation Cycle*: Keep child oriented to time, place, and person. Explain all procedures to child. Provide for sense of day and night: turn lights down at night, try to keep noise level lower at night. Encourage parents to bring familiar items from home to the child, e.g., toys, pictures, posters. Encourage parents to bring in tape recordings of familiar voices and music. Encourage parents to spend time with child, talking to and touching child. Assist, if appropriate, in activities that help child regain sense of balance and reorient child to environment.

Appendix 26–2. Normal Laboratory Values for the Pediatric Patient

Sodium	135 to 145 mEq/l	Serum glutamic oxaloacetic	
Potassium	3.5 to 5.5 mEq/l	transaminase (SGOT)	5 to 20 IU/l
Chloride	96 to 106 mEq/l	Serum glutamic pyruvic	
Glucose		transaminase (SGPT)	4 to 25 IU/l
Newborn	20 to 110 mg/dl	Amylase	25 to 125 IU/l
Child	60 to 105 mg/dl	Lactate	
Adult	70 to 115 mg/dl	Venous	5 to 18 mg/dl
Blood urea nitrogen (BUN)	5 to 25 mg/dl	Arterial	3 to 7 mg/dl
Creatinine	0.5 to 1.3 mg/dl	Hematology	
Calcium	9 to 11 mg/dl	Hematocrit (Hct)	
Bilirubin (total)	0.25 to 1.5 mg/dl	Birth	44 to 68 %
Magnesium	1.2 to 1.8 mEq/l	3 mo to 1 yr	30 to 40 %
Phosphorus		4 to 15 yr	31 to 43 %
Newborn	4.2 to 9.0 mg/dl	Hemoglobin (Hb)	
1 yr	3.8 to 6.2 mg/dl	Birth	14 to 24 gm/dl
2 to 5 yr	3.5 to 6.8 mg/dl	1 mo	11 to 17 gm/dl
Adult	3.0 to 4.5 mg/dl	1 yr	11 to 15 gm/dl
Osmolality	285 to 295 mOsm/kg	4 to 15 yr	13 to 15.5 gm/dl
Protein (total)		Prothrombin time (PT)	11 to 14 sec
1 to 3 mo	4.7 to 7.4 gm/dl	Partial thromboplastin time	
3 to 12 mo	5.0 to 7.5 gm/dl	(PTT)	25 to 35 sec
1 to 15 yr	6.5 to 8.6 gm/dl	Platelet count	150,000 to 400,000/liter
Ammonia		Fibrinogen	150 to 450 mg/dl
Newborn	90 to 150 gm/dl	White blood cell (WBC) per $mm^3 \times 100$	
Child	45 to 80 gm/dl	Newborn	7 to 35
Adult	18 to 48 gm/dl	3 mo to 1 yr	6 to 17
Alkaline phosphatase		2 to 10 yr	7 to 13
Newborn	122 to 231 IU/l	11 to 15 yr	5 to 12
1 mo to 1 yr	109 to 265 IU/l	Urine volume	
1 to 6 yr	95 to 218 IU/l	Infant	>0.5 mg/kg/hr
6 to 12 yr	122 to 323 IU/l	Child	>1.0 mg/kg/hr
12 to 19 yr	55 to 367 IU/l (male)	Osmolality	50 to 1200 mOsm/kg urine
	27 to 221 IU/l (female)		water
> 19 yr	37 to 108 IU/l	Specific gravity	1.002 to 1.030
Creatine phosphokinase	0 to 70 IU/l	Pulmonary	
(CPK)		Pa_{O_2}	60 to 80 mm Hg (newborn)
Lactate dehydrogenase			80 to 100 mm HG (child)
(LDH)		Pa_{CO_2}	35 to 45 mm Hg
Newborn	290 to 501 IU/l	pH	7.35 to 7.45
1 day	185 to 404 IU/l	Bicarbonate	22 to 26 mEq/l
1 mo to 2 yr	110 to 244 IU/l	Base excess	−2 to +2
3 to 17 yr	80 to 165 IU/l		

Appendix 26–3. Essential Equipment for Pediatric Resuscitation

Electrocardiograph with pediatric and adult leads
Defibrillator with infant, pediatric, and adult paddles; include pediatric and adult internal paddles
Blood pressure cuffs: 5, 7.5, 9 mm sizes
Doppler ultrasound flowmeter
Pediatric PASG
Laryngoscope handles: large and small
Extra bulbs for laryngoscope: large and small
Laryngoscope blades
  Miller 0, 1, 2, 3
  McIntosh 2, 3, 4
Oral airways: sizes 000 to 3
Masks: infant, child, adult
Endotracheal tubes
  Uncuffed, 2.5 to 7.5
  Cuffed, 5.5 to 9.0
Stylets: child and adult
Pediatric Magill forceps
Resuscitation bags: pediatric and adult
Suction catheters: sizes 6 to 16 French
Tonsil suction
Nasogastric tubes: sizes 5 to 14 French
Needles
  25 gauge, ⅝ inch
  21 gauge, 1 inch
  20 gauge, 1 inch
  18 gauge, 1½ inch
Butterflies: 19, 21, 23, 25 gauge
Angiocaths: 20, 22, 24 gauge
Cutdown trays: pediatric and adult
Micro-drip Buretrols
Tape
Pediatric arm and foot boards
Intravenous infusion pump
Cardiac board
Pediatric rigid cervical collars
Foley catheters: sizes 5 to 12 French
Chest tubes: sizes 8 to 16 French
17-gauge, 3-inch needles for thoracentesis
Syringes: 1, 3, 5, 10, 20, 50 ml

Appendix 26–4. Michael's Care Plan

The following is a sample discharge care plan for a child who sustained a closed head injury as a result of a motor vehicle accident.

PROBLEMS AND GOALS	INTERVENTION
Potential respiratory distress or failure secondary to vasomotor abnormality. Goal: Maintain adequate respiratory status.	1. No. 2 Shiley tracheostomy tube to maintain patent, accessible airway. 2. Home oxygen therapy. a. Humidified RA/O_2 via tracheostomy collar: Use as much as possible when Michael is off ventilator and at home. Change sterile water q day. Change tubing every 3 days. Allow long enough tubing for mobility. b. RA/O_2 via ventilator: Use during nap times, bedtime, and as needed for respiratory distress unrelieved with oxygen via tracheostomy collar. Check rate, inspiratory pressure, and tidal volume every time before placing Michael on ventilator. Ensure that alarms are on. Change circuit daily. Change sterile water every day.
Increased potential for respiratory infection and atelectasis secondary to tracheostomy. Goal: Prevent respiratory infection.	1. Daily tracheostomy care. a. Clean tracheostomy site with one-half strength hydrogen peroxide twice daily and as needed. b. Change tracheostomy dressing bid and as needed. c. Change tracheostomy ties as needed. d. Change tracheostomy tube every week: Clean thoroughly and rinse with sterile water. Reuse tube three times and then discard. 2. Pulmonary toilet. a. Suction every 3 to 4 hours as needed, before meals, and before bedtime. b. Instill normal saline solution as needed to loosen secretions. c. Perform chest physiotherapy as needed. d. Note any change in sputum color, amount, and consistency. Obtain culture and send to clinic as needed. e. Encourage patient to cough.

Appendix 26–4. Michael's Care Plan *Continued*

PROBLEMS AND GOALS	INTERVENTION
Potential seizure activity. Goal 1: Control seizures. Goal 2: Protect from harm during seizure activity.	1. Give anticonvulsive medications as ordered. a. Phenobarbital. b. Phenytoin sodium. 2. Record time, duration, focal onset, apnea, and any loss of consciousness during seizure. 3. Protect from injury during seizure. a. Clear area. b. Loosen clothing. c. Use Ambu bag if apneic. d. Use suction as needed. e. Notify pulmonary intensive care unit and transport if seizure activity is sustained.
Growth retardation and weight loss. Goal 1: Increase weight gain. Goal 2: Increase muscle strength.	1. Weigh daily and record. 2. Encourage oral intake. 3. Offer small, frequent, high caloric meals and snacks. 4. Supplement oral intake. a. Insert nasogastric tube before bedtime. b. Gavage-feed Isocal (Mead Johnson) 6 to 8 oz every 4 hr while sleeping. c. Check for aspirate before each feeding. d. Remove nasogastric tube in morning.
Potential parental fatigue, isolation, anxiety, and lack of privacy. Goal 1: Time away from Michael to pursue own interests. Goal 2: Time alone. Goal 3: Private time with each other.	1. Private duty nurses. a. Every night (10 p.m. to 7 a.m.) to allow parents to get a good night's sleep. b. Several hours during the day per week: Allow parent(s) to do errands outside the house. Transport Michael to weekly clinic appointments. Provide emotional/medical support during times of crisis. Help take Michael on outings (e.g., for haircuts, ice cream cones). c. Evening hours as needed to allow parents a night out together. 2. Social worker. a. Weekly visits. b. Assess for problems, family interactions, adequate supplies. 3. Physician. a. Weekly telephone call to assess any problems and/or concerns.

Adapted from Lawrence PA: Home health care for ventilator-dependent children: Providing a chance to live a normal life. Dimens Crit Care Nurs 3:1, 1984.

Appendix 30–1. Procedure for Administration of Oral Ethanol

PURPOSE: To prevent or treat the alcohol withdrawal syndrome.
EQUIPMENT
1. 80 proof ethanol from pharmacy
2. Beer or ethanol (patient's brand from home)

Oral Ethanol Dosage Guidelines

Oral Ethanol Dose	Actual Ethanol Delivered
15 ml (½ oz) 80 proof whiskey	6 ml
30 ml (1 oz) 80 proof whiskey	12 ml
1 can beer (12 oz)	12 to 13 ml
6 cans beer	Approx. 75 ml

Nursing Action	Rationale
Prepare oral ethanol dose for administration.	
1. Validate physician's order.	As per department of nursing policy.
2. Obtain oral 80 proof ethanol from pharmacy, or when necessary, obtain the patient's favorite brand of whiskey or beer from home.	Some patients prefer a specific beer or whiskey and will not drink the brand carried by the pharmacy.
Prepare the patient for administration of oral ethanol.	
1. Assess and document baseline vital signs and record neurological assessment on flow sheet before beginning administration. Note level of awareness, orientation, and level of arousal. Document any signs of alcohol withdrawal.	Ethanol is a central nervous system depressant, and each patient possesses varying capacities for metabolizing this drug.
2. Assess the need for a nasogastric tube.	The patient with a decreased level of consciousness or swallowing disorder is prone to aspiration. An uncooperative patient may need a nasogastric tube to ensure that the proper dose is delivered.
3. Obtain orders for antacids.	Ethanol is known to stimulate gastroduodenitis.
Administer oral ethanol as ordered.	
1. Dosing ranges may vary but usually begin with 15 to 30 ml of 80 proof whiskey every 1 to 4 hours. The dosage guidelines summarize the actual amount of ethanol in various doses.	Obtaining a significant blood-alcohol level is not necessary to prevent the withdrawal syndrome. The goal is to meet the *minimum* metabolic requirements for ethanol in patients long accustomed to regular daily consumption.
2. Continue to assess and document the neurological assessment every 2 hours while ethanol is being administered. Note any signs of euphoria, analgesia, inebriation, or oversedation.	Manageability of the patient is the key physiological end point. Do not induce stupor with excess ethanol administration.
Wean or discontinue the dose of ethanol as ordered.	Oral doses of ethanol may be necessary for the entire readjustment period, which could vary from a few hours to 9 to 10 days.

Appendix 30–2. Procedure for Administration of Intravenous Ethanol

PURPOSE: To prevent or treat the alcohol withdrawal syndrome with IV ethanol.

EQUIPMENT

1. Administration rate–controlling device (IV pump)
2. IV solution of 5 per cent ethanol in D_5W
   or
3. IV solution of 10 per cent ethanol in D_5W

Dosage Guidelines for Intravenous Ethanol

5 PER CENT ETHANOL IN D_5W

Rate Per Hour (ml)	Actual Ethanol Delivered (ml)
50	2.5
75	3.7
100	5
125	6.25
150	7.5
200	10

10 PER CENT ETHANOL IN D_5W

Rate Per Hour (ml)	Actual Ethanol Delivered (ml)
25	2.5
37	3.7
50	5
62	6.25
75	7.5
100	10

NURSING ACTION	RATIONALE
Prepare ethanol infusion or oral doses for administration. 1. Validate physician order.	As per department of nursing policy.
2. Obtain 5 per cent ethanol or 10 per cent ethanol from pharmacy.	
3. Check physician's order for ml of ethanol per hour. Orders must be written in *ml* or *cc* of *ethanol to be delivered.* Do not accept an order stating only the rate of the infusion. Clarify that the physician is aware that 5 and 10 per cent solutions are available.	If the patient presents with a diagnosis in which fluids should be limited, e.g., head injury, fluid electrolyte imbalances, the 10 per cent solution should be utilized.
4. Calculate the rate of solution and validate the rate with another nurse. a. Physician's order must state: (1) type of ethanol preparation, (2) solution (fluid) rate (ml/hr), and (3) ethanol rate (ml/hr). b. Example: 5 per cent ethanol: 5 per cent dextrose Solution: (fluid) rate: 100 ml/hr Ethanol rate: 5 ml/hr	Calculating the rate: In a 5 per cent solution 200 ml of the solution is equal to 10 ml of ethanol. Therefore: 200 ml: 10 ml = x ml: 5 ml (10 ml) (x ml) = (200 ml) (5 ml) 10x = 1000 x = 100 ml/hour In a 10 per cent solution 100 ml of the solution is equal to 10 ml of ethanol. Therefore: 100 ml: 10 ml = x ml: 5 ml (10 ml) (x ml) = (100 ml) (5 ml) 10x = 500 x = 50 ml/hour

Appendix 30–2. Procedure for Administration of Intravenous Ethanol *Continued*

Dosage Guidelines for Intravenous Ethanol *Continued*

NURSING ACTION	RATIONALE
5. Prime solution set according to procedure for controlling device utilized.	Ethanol infusions must be administered by IV pumps to avoid overdose.
Maintenance of ethanol infusion	
1. Assess and document baseline vital signs. Note level of awareness, orientation, and level of arousal. Document any signs of withdrawal.	
2. Assess and document manageability of the patient, e.g., patient cooperates with chest physiotherapy. The patient is monitored hourly for signs of euphoria, analgesia, inebriation, or oversedation.	
3. Assess patency of IV line. 4. Flag IV controller with a bright sticker labeled ETHANOL. 5. Set controlling device for: a. rate to be delivered (ml/hr) as ordered by physician. b. volume limit to deliver no more than 4 hours of the dose.	Remember that if the patient has a known history of alcohol dependency, he is capable of metabolizing ethanol at a rate of approximately 25 ml of ethanol/hour. It is not necesary to obtain that same rate! Doses should range from 2.5 ml ethanol to 10 ml of ethanol/hour. The rate the solution should be infused depends on whether a 10 or 5 per cent solution is used.
6. Assess and document in progress notes or flow sheet vital signs and any signs or symptoms of ethanol withdrawal. Also continue to document facts indicating patient manageability. Utilize the neuro assessment section of flow sheet and document neuro assessment every 2 hours.	
7. Document IV volume infused hourly on intake and output sheet.	
8. Verify IV solution and dose rate at each change of shift with on-going and off-going RNs.	Institution nursing policy.
9. Change solution and IV tubing according to department of nursing policy.	
10. Weaning patient from ethanol infusion.	Continuous infusions may be necessary for the entire readjustment period, which could vary from a few hours to 9 or 10 days. As soon as possible the patient should be changed from IV to oral ethanol.

Reprinted with permission from Nursing Procedure Manual, Maryland Institute for Emergency Medical Services Systems, Baltimore, MD, 1987.

Index

Note: Page numbers in *italics* refer to illustrations; page numbers followed by t refer to tables.

ISBN 0-7216-4333-7
90038
9 780721 643335